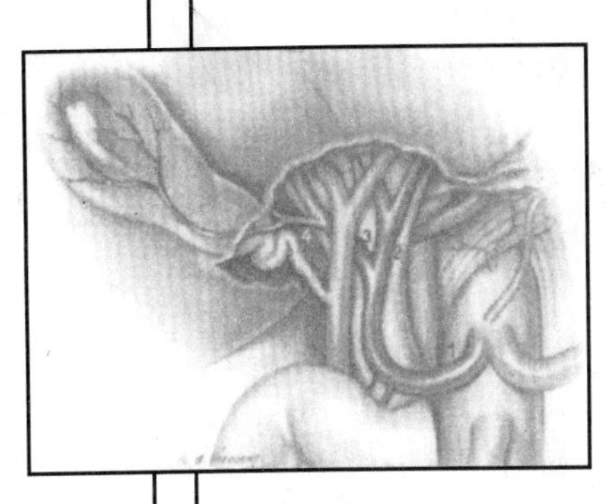

Atlas of Gastrointestinal Surgery

胃肠道外科手术图谱

（上卷）

Volume Ⅰ

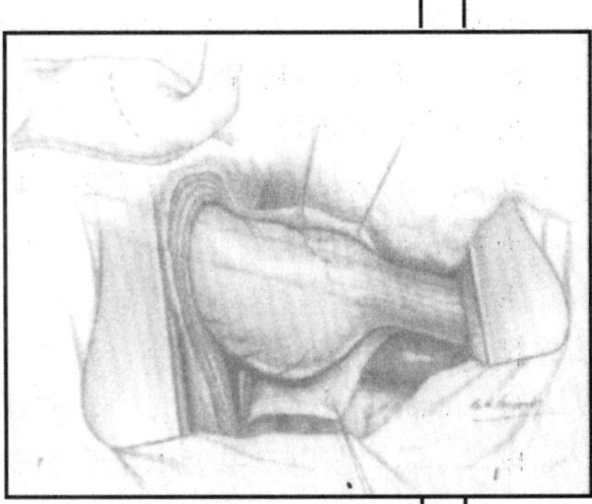

Emilio Etala

Lippincott Williams & Wilkins Inc. 授权
天津科技翻译出版公司出版

著作权合同登记号:图字:02-2002-6

图书在版编目(CIP)数据

胃肠道外科手术图谱/(美)埃泰赖(Etala,E.)编著.—影印版.—天津:天津科技翻译出版公司,2002.6
ISBN 7-5433-1499-1
书名原文:Atlas of Gastrointestinal Surgery

Ⅰ.胃...　Ⅱ.埃...　Ⅲ.胃肠病-外科手术-图谱　Ⅳ.R656-64

中国版本图书馆 CIP 数据核字(2002)第 010729 号

Copyright © 1997 by Lippincott Williams & Wilkins Inc.

All right reserved. This book is protected by copyright. No part of this book may be reproduced in any form or by any means, including photocopying, or utilized by any information storage and retrieval system without written permission from the copyright owner.

Reprint authorized by Lippincott Williams & Wilkins Inc. Reprint is authorized for sale in the People's Republic of China only.

授权单位:Lippincott Williams & Wilkins Inc.
出　　版:天津科技翻译出版公司
出 版 人:邢淑琴
地　　址:天津市南开区白堤路 244 号
邮政编码:300192
电　　话:022-87893561
传　　真:022-87892476
E - mail:tsttbc@public.tpt.tj.cn
印　　刷:天津市蓟县宏图印务有限公司印刷
发　　行:全国新华书店
版本记录:880×1230　16 开本　157.5 印张　3700 千字
2002 年 6 月第 1 版　2002 年 6 月第 1 次印刷
定价:430.00 元(上、下卷)

(如发现印装问题,可与出版社调换)

Atlas of Gastrointestinal Surgery

Volume I

Edited by

Dr. Emilio Etala
Buenos Aires, Argentina

Translated by

Dr. Alfred L. Axtmayer
Guaynabo, Puerto Rico

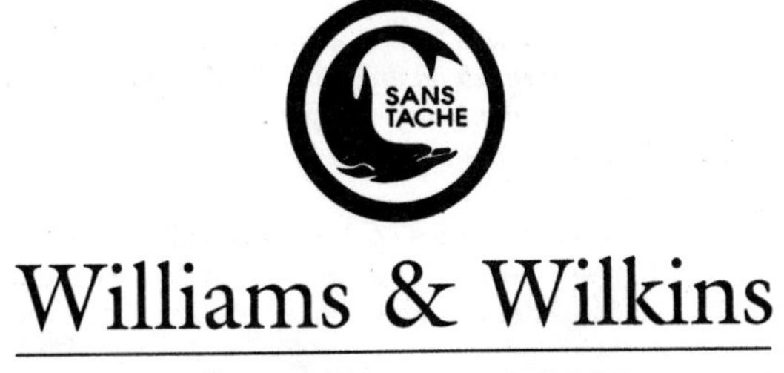

A WAVERLY COMPANY

BALTIMORE • PHILADELPHIA • LONDON • PARIS • BANGKOK
HONG KONG • MUNICH • SYDNEY • TOKYO • WROCLAW

Editor: Carroll C. Cann
Managing Editor: Susan Hunsberger
Production Coordinator: Peter J. Carley
Copy Editor: Robert Magee
Designer: Nancy Hagan Abbott
Illustration Planner: Danielle Hagan
Cover Designer: Nancy Hagan Abbott
Typesetter: Graphic World, Inc.
Printer: RR Donnelley & Sons Company
Digitized Illustrations: Graphic World, Inc.
Binder: RR Donnelley & Sons Company

Copyright © 1997 Williams & Wilkins

351 West Camden Street
Baltimore, Maryland 21201-2436 USA

Rose Tree Corporate Center
1400 North Providence Road
Building II, Suite 5025
Media, Pennsylvania 19063-2043 USA

All rights reserved. This book is protected by copyright. No part of this book may be reproduced in any form or by any means, including photocopying, or utilized by any information storage and retrieval system without written permission from the copyright owner.

Accurate indications, adverse reactions and dosage schedules for drugs are provided in this book, but it is possible that they may change. The reader is urged to review the package information data of the manufacturers of the medications mentioned.

First Edition.

Library of Congress Cataloging-in-Publication Data

Atlas of gastrointestinal surgery / edited by Emilio Etala : translated by Alfred Axtmayer.
p. cm.
Includes index.
ISBN 0-683-02837-5
1. Gastrointestinal system—Surgery—Atlases. I. Etala, Emilio, M.D.
[DNLM: 1. Gastrointestinal System—surgery—atlases.
2. Gastrointestinal Diseases—surgery—atlases. WI 17 A8793 1996]
RD540.A845 1996
617.4'3—dc20
DNLM/DLC
for Library of Congress

96-21197
CIP

The publishers have made every effort to trace the copyright holders for borrowed material. If they have inadvertently overlooked any, they will be pleased to make the necessary arrangements at the first opportunity.

To purchase additional copies of this book, call our customer service department at **(800) 638-0672** or fax orders to **(800) 447-8438.** For other book services, including chapter reprints and large quantity sales, ask for the Special Sales department.

Canadian customers should call **(800) 268-4178,** or fax **(905) 470-6780.** For all other calls originating outside of the United States, please call **(410) 528-4223** or fax us at **(410) 528-8550.**

Visit Williams & Wilkins on the Internet: **http://www.wwilkins.com** or contact our customer service department at **custserv@wwilkins.com.** Williams & Wilkins customer service representatives are available from 8:30 am to 6:00 pm. EST. Monday through Friday, for telephone access.

97 98 99
2 3 4 5 6 7 8 9 10

To my wife Celia
To the memory of my parents

Foreword

I first met Dr. Emilio Etala in Ireland at the meeting of the International Society of Surgery in 1961. A true friendship having been established there, it remains to this day.

Dr. Etala has garnered many honors as a surgeon, among them: membership in the Societe Internationale de Chirurgie (1956) and election to the Honorary Fellowship in the American College of Surgeons (1971). It was my honor as Presenter to him of that election to the ACS.

Without reservation, this is an important work, destined to become an integral part of every general surgeon's library. Unique in its single authorship, *Atlas of Surgery of the Gastrointestinal Tract* provides detailed explanations of all techniques performed on all organs of the gastrointestinal tract and a wealth of exquisitely detailed clinical observations not readily available in the existing surgical literature. This can only serve to improve the safety of each operation and to prevent complications. All of these qualities are evident throughout the book, but none are more evident than in the chapters on *Choledochal Cysts* and *Portal Hypertension,* which mandate reading from anyone who is preparing to perform any of these procedures.

Illustrations are critical to the explanation of any surgical procedure and I give this presentation here the highest possible praise. The outstanding art throughout this volume is the work of a single artist who worked closely with Dr. Etala throughout the performance of every operation depicted. Each illustration rendered is from the surgeon's perspective, which provides the reader with a highly accurate view of the operative field and the related surgical anatomy at each step of each operation.

I am pleased to see this wonderful book come to fruition. Dr. Etala is a surgeon *non pareil.* His work here is destined to become a world classic. Shakespeare may best describe Dr. Etala and his work:

I dare do all that becomes a man, who dares do more is none.

John L. Madden, MD

Preface

The completion of the Atlas of Gastrointestinal Surgery would have filled Master Professor of Surgery Pablo L. Mirizzi, whose name is inseparable from operative cholangiography and biliary tract surgery, with satisfaction.

This book describes the surgical procedures used to treat diseases of the gastrointestinal tract. However, the author has always had the conviction that an atlas of surgery should not be limited to a description of surgical techniques, because this means an incomplete vision of reality. So, in addition to the description of the surgical anatomy, the clinical picture, the preoperative and intraoperative diagnosis, and the surgical indications are also presented. It has been proven that the success of an operation does not depend exclusively on surgical technique but is influenced by other factors, such as the stage of the illness, the opportunity of the operation, and the selection of the procedure to be used. All these factors should be carefully contemplated by the surgeon, since they may be decisive in diminishing the number of complications.

For more than 30 years, the author has conducted courses in gastrointestinal surgery for graduate students with surgical sessions transmitted directly. This has allowed the author to understand the most common difficulties that affect graduates with a desire to learn.

The surgical procedures described in this atlas are those that are practiced by the author, and they have produced good results. Alternative techniques are described in separate chapters for when the usual procedures are inappropriate or contraindicated.

Care has been taken to avoid publishing an encyclopedia which could lead to confusion or uncertainty. Afflictions have been detailed that, though rare, can be mortal if not treated adequately and promptly. These illnesses are not usually included in an atlas of surgery. Examples of these illnesses are complicated diverticuli of the second or third portion of the duodenum, gastric ulcers of the cardia, pancreaticocutaneous fistulas, and duodenal fistulas.

The descriptions of surgical techniques have been written to include both manual suturing and staplers. The most accepted laparoscopic procedures have also been described.

This atlas has been written by a single author. This is not the usual present day practice. However, a book written by a single experienced author offers great uniformity and, at times, is a necessity.

The illustrations are the work of the excellent artist Carlos A. Vescovo. The author and the artist have collaborated very closely to present the most representative and, at the same time, didactic illustrations. The illustrations were made directly in the operating room and later modified to make them more representative and explicit for teaching purposes.

This atlas can be useful for both general surgeons and gastrointestinal surgeons. Colonic surgeons and anorectal surgeons will also find it useful, as well as senior surgeons who may need a concise update of infrequently performed procedures.

The atlas was translated into English by Dr. Alfred L. Axtmayer of Puerto Rico, who has realized the difficult task of interpreting the author's concepts with fidelity. The author would like to express his deepest gratitude.

The author has also been privileged by Dr. John L. Madden of New York, who has written the Foreword. Dr. Madden is one of the world's masters of surgery and the author of an Atlas of Surgery that has spread to all the countries of the world. The author is grateful for Dr. Madden's constant encouragement.

Williams and Wilkins has not limited its efforts in producing an excellent book, for which the author expresses deep gratitude.

Mr. Carroll C. Cann, Executive Editor, has been a great proponent of the book, and the author is grateful for the continuous and extraordinary enthusiasm shown by him in overcoming all difficulties

The author is also grateful to Ms. Susan Hunsberger for her excellent work in organizing and coordinating the atlas.

To Mr. Peter Carley, Production Coordinator, whose work was a decisive factor in publishing the Atlas, as well as to Mr. Andrew Potter for his brilliant task in correcting manuscripts, the author gives his sincere gratitude.

Emilio Etala, M.D.
Buenos Aires

CONTENTS 目　录

Volume Ⅱ 第Ⅱ卷

PART I

Surgery of the Hepatobiliary Tract and Pancreas

Section A

Surgery of the Biliary Tract

CHAPTER 1

Surgical Anatomy of the Extrahepatic Biliary Tree

Guy de Chauliac (1300–1368), a famous surgeon from Avignon, France, stated that "good surgery cannot be performed without knowing anatomy." This knowledge of anatomy is fundamentally important in surgery of bile ducts. The biliary tract surgeon confronts a situation of innumerable anatomic variations, which may present at the hepatic hilum and extrahepatic bile structures. The surgeon must be thoroughly familiar with the normal anatomy and with the more frequent variations that occur. Before ligating or dividing a structure it must be precisely identified to avoid dire consequences.

GALL BLADDER AND CYSTIC DUCT

The gall bladder is located on the inferior surface of the liver and held to its bed by peritoneum. The dividing line between the right and left lobes of the liver passes through the bed of the gall bladder. The gall bladder is a pear-shaped sac 8 to 12 cm in length and 4 to 5 cm in maximal diameter, with a capacity of 30 to 50 mL. When distended, however, it may reach a capacity of some 200 mL. The gall bladder serves the function of receiving the bile and concentrating it. It is normally bluish in color, a combination of its translucent walls and the contained bile. This translucence is lost when the walls are opacified by inflammation.

The gall bladder is described as divided in three segments, which are, however, without precise demarcation: the fundus, the body, and the infundibulum.

1. The fundus of the gall bladder is that part which projects beyond the anterior border of the liver and is completely covered with peritoneum. The fundus is the segment of the gall bladder that becomes palpable when the gall bladder is distended. The fundus projects onto the anterior abdominal wall at the in-

tersection of the ninth costal cartilage with the lateral border of the right rectus muscle, although numerous variations occur.

2. The body of the gall bladder follows the fundus, and its diameter diminishes progressively more distally. The body is not totally covered with peritoneum; the peritoneum binds it to the inferior surface of the liver. Thus the inferior surface of the gall bladder is covered by peritoneum while the superior surface is in contact with the inferior surface of the liver, from which it is separated by a layer of areolar connective tissue through which blood vessels, lymphatics, nerve fibrils and, occasionally, accessory hepatic ducts traverse. At cholecystectomy, the surgeon should enter and exploit this areolar cleavage plane. This will permit bloodless surgery. When the cleavage plane has been obliterated by disease, the hepatic parenchyma is frequently traumatized and bleeding results.
3. The infundibulum, the third portion of the gall bladder, follows the body with diminishing diameter and is covered by peritoneum. It is within the hepatoduodenal ligament and usually protrudes anteriorly. The infundibulum is referred to as Hartmann's pouch, but we believe that Hartmann's pouch is the result of a pathologic process consequent to impaction of a calculus at the inferior infundibulum or in the neck of the gall bladder. This in turn produces dilation of the infundibulum and this dilation results in the formation of the pouch. The pouch, in turn, hinders the cholecystectomy owing to the adhesions it provokes to the cystic or the common duct. Hartmann's pouch is to be considered a pathologic alteration insofar as the normal infundibulum does not have the form of a pouch.

The gall bladder consists of a layer of tall epithelial cylindrical cells and a thin fibromuscular layer consisting of longitudinal, circular, and oblique muscle fibers plus fibrous tissue covering the mucosa. The gall bladder has no submucosa nor muscularis mucosa. It has no mucous glands and occasionally may present scant mucous glands, which may be more numerous in cases of inflammation. The mucous glands are located almost exclusively in the neck. The fibromuscular layer is covered by a layer of areolar connective tissue through which blood and lymphatic vessels and nerves traverse. This is the plane to be sought to perform a subserosal cholecystectomy. This areolar plane is in continuity with that which separates the gall bladder from the liver at the hepatic bed. The infundibulum is in continuity with the neck whose length is 15 to 20 mm and angles acutely upward with the angle opening superiorly.

CYSTIC DUCT

The cystic duct joins the gall bladder and the hepatic duct to form the choledochus. It is 4 to 6 mm long, although it may measure up to 10 to 12 cm. It may be short or even nonexistent. The proximal diameter of the cystic duct is usually 2 to 2.5 mm, somewhat smaller than the distal diameter, which is some 3 mm. Viewed from the outside it appears irregular and convoluted specially in its proximal half or two-thirds owing to the presence of Heister's valves. Viewed from the inside, it presents Heister's valves, which are semilunar and present in alternate sequence giving the impression of a continuous spiral. This is inexact, however, since the valves are individually separate from each other. Heister's valves regulate the flow of bile between the gall bladder and the biliary passages. The cystic duct usually joins the hepatic duct in the superior half of the hepatoduodenal ligament, usually at the right border of the hepatic duct and usually at an acute angle, thus forming the cystohepatic angle. The cystic duct may enter the common duct perpendicularly. The cystic duct may also join the hepatic duct after coursing parallel to the hepatic duct joining it behind the first portion of the duodenum, in the pancreatic area, and even near to or at the papilla forming a parallel junction. It may join the hepatic duct in front or behind the hepatic duct, entering it, not on the right side of the hepatic duct, but on its left border or its anterior wall. This rotation about the hepatic duct would be described as a spiral union. Mirizzi has called this variant a banding cystic duct. This may give rise to the hepatic syndrome of Mirizzi (27, 29). Rarely the cystic duct enters the right or left hepatic duct.

HEPATIC DUCT

The biliary ducts originate within the liver as bile canaliculi that receive the bile excreted by the hepatic cells and join among themselves, forming larger and larger ducts, giving rise to the right and left hepatic ducts from the right and left lobes of the liver respectively. The right and left hepatic ducts join to form the common hepatic duct, usually extrahepatically. The right hepatic duct is generally more intrahepatic than the left. The length of the common hepatic duct is very variable and depends on the level at which the left and right hepatic ducts join. The length of the common hepatic duct also depends on the level of its union with the cystic duct to form the choledochus. The common hepatic duct is usually 2 to 4 cm long, although a length of 8 cm is not infrequent. The diameter of the common hepatic and the common bile duct is usually 6 to 8 mm. The normal diameter may be up to 12 mm. However, ducts of normal diameter may harbor calculi as seen in recent cases

(27, 30). There is obviously an overlap of normal and pathologic common ducts as to their size and diameter. Previously cholecystectomized patients may increase the diameter of their choledochus and so may the elderly. The hepatic duct is covered with high cylindrical epithelium over a lamina propria that contains mucous glands. A fibroelastic tissue layer covers the mucosa and contains some muscular fibers. Mirizzi described a sphincter at the distal portion of the hepatic duct. Because no muscle cells were found, he labeled it a functional sphincter of the common hepatic duct (27, 28, 29, 32). Lang (23), Geneser (39), Guy Albot (39), Chikiar (10, 11), and Hollinshead and others (19), have demonstrated muscle fibers in the hepatic duct. To demonstrate these muscle fibers, it is essential to proceed immediately to fixation of the tissue upon obtaining the sample, since autolysis rapidly supervenes both in biliary and in pancreatic ducts. With these precautions in mind, we have confirmed with Dr. Zuckerberg the presence of muscle fibers in the hepatic duct.

CHOLEDOCHUS

The choledochus is 5 to 15 cm in length (usually 8 to 10 cm). It is situated, like the common hepatic duct, at the free border of the hepatoduodenal ligament. To its left and in the same anterior plane is the hepatic artery. The portal vein is in a posterior plane and closer to the hepatic artery than to the choledochus. The cystic duct joins the hepatic duct generally superior to the first portion of the duodenum. The choledochus passes behind the first portion of the duodenum, continues downward and to the right along a groove or tunnel provided by the head of the pancreas, and enters the second portion of the duodenum along the internal (lesser curvature) portion of the duodenum and at an angle of 45 degrees. The choledochus enters the wall of the duodenum and joins the pancreatic duct, forming a common channel that empties through the duodenal papilla.

The common duct may be described in four segments:

1. Supraduodenal, usually 20 mm long. This is the segment more readily accessible at surgery and with the lower hepatic duct provides access for choledochotomy and biliary tract exploration (39).
2. Retroduodenal segment, 15 to 20 mm in length.
3. Infraduodenal extrapancreatic segment, 20 to 30 mm in length, which courses along the head of the pancreas in a groove or tunnel to reach the duodenum at its second portion.

   A cleavage plane between the choledochus and the pancreas can usually be found because the pancreas and choledochus do not adhere to each other except in cases of chronic pancreatitis in the area of the head of the pancreas. In these cases it is quite impossible to separate the choledochus and the pancreas, and the choledochus may even be obstructed by the pancreatic thickening and fibrous tissue infiltration. If the situation of choledochal-pancreatic fusion does not exist, retropancreatic choledochotomy may be performed to remove an impacted calculus that has not been removable from above nor by transduodenal sphincterotomy.
4. Intraduodenal or intramural segment. As the choledochus traverses the wall of the duodenum its caliber diminishes considerably and its walls get thicker. This is to be borne in mind when interpreting cholangiography. Furthermore, at operative cholangiography the dye that has passed into the duodenum can give rise to superimposition of shadows, hindering a clear view of the intramural segment of the choledochus. In these cases films should be repeated and a clear view of the terminal choledochus obtained. The length of the intramural choledochus is very variable but always more than the thickness of the duodenal wall. This is explained by the oblique trajectory of the choledochus as it traverses the duodenal wall. The length of the transduodenal choledochus is 14 to 16 mm (39). During its intramural path the choledochus and the pancreatic duct join in various forms. These may be described as occurring in three principal manners (18, 21, 22, 48), as follows:
   - I. The choledochus and the pancreatic duct join shortly after penetrating the wall of the duodenum sharing a short common tract. This is the more frequent occurrence.
   - II. Both ducts course in parallel fashion, in contact but not joined, emptying separately into the duodenal papilla. Occasionally the pancreatic duct may empty 5 to 15 mm below the papilla.
   - III. The pancreatic duct and the choledochus join at a higher level before entering the duodenal wall forming a common channel longer than usual. Only in few occasions does the union of Type I or Type III present a dilation giving rise to being designated as an "ampulla" (10, 11, 16, 18, 48, 50).

HISTORICAL REVIEW OF PAPILLA OF VATER AND AMPULLA OF VATER

Abraham Vater, in 1720 (49), gave a lecture at the University of Wittenberg, Germany, titled "Novus bilis diverticulum," in which he described a diverticulum localized at the distal end of the choledochus. Vater thus described a diverticulum of the choledochus, a most rare instance of choledochocele (10, 50). Vater searched for another such case, but was not successful in finding one (10, 50). Vater never made reference to the papilla, nor did he describe the ampulla that bears his name. However, in the medical literature both the papilla and the ampulla bear his name. What is called the ampulla of Vater is the duct formed by the union of the choledochus and the pancreatic duct as these pass through the wall of the second portion of the duodenum to empty at the papilla. This generally short but occasionally longer joined segment has the configuration of a duct and not of an ampulla. This duct can dilate when the papilla is obstructed by inflammation or by an impacted stone. It is probable that the duct may acquire a larger diameter "post mortis" owing to autolysis of the choledochus and pancreatic duct (10) without obstruction. We believe, as other authors do, that the term "ampulla" should not be used because what is observed is a duct and not an ampulla. The eponym "Vater" should also not be used, since he never referred to it (10). Some authors believe that the error in naming it ampulla of Vater arose from Claude Bernard (1, 10, 11, 50), who, in writing his book in 1856, quoted Vater as saying "ampoule commune nommé ampoule de Water," and spelling Vater with a "W" instead of with a "V."

Vater never referred to the papilla that bears his name. The papilla was first described by Sir Francis Glisson in England in 1654 (15) in the first edition of his book *Anatomie Hepatis,* the second edition of which was published in 1681 (3–5, 15). Some authors (48) attribute the first description of the papilla to Gottfried Bidloo of the Hague in 1685 (2). Other authors attribute it to Giovanni Domenico Santorini (42) in 1724, that being the reason why in some texts the duct is called the papilla of Santorini. Santorini did make an excellent description of the papilla in the dog, sheep, and ox, but he was not the first to describe it. Santorini did not add a drawing to his description.

The sphincter of Oddi was also first described by Sir Francis Glisson in 1654, when he described the papilla (3, 4, 5, 15). In his description Glisson describes the annular muscle fibers of the terminal choledochus, affirming that these muscular fibers served to close off the choledochus to avoid reflux of duodenal content. In 1887 (36), Ruggiero Oddi also described the terminal sphincter of the choledochus and related it to biliary physiology. Thus we find that the papilla described by Glisson has been named after Oddi. The ampulla named Vater has not been described by anyone and there are serious doubts that it exists under normal, nonpathologic circumstances, but it is still called the ampulla of Vater.

Hendrickson (17) studied the sphincter at the end of the choledochus in 1898, in the United States. He added details unknown at that time. In 1937, Schwegler and Boyden (46) studied the sphincter of Oddi, and Boyden later added much to our knowledge of the sphincter of Oddi (3, 4, 5).

To avoid confusion in nomenclature we believe that the following should be considered as synonyms: papilla of Vater, papilla of Santorini, papilla of Bedloo, duodenal papilla, major duodenal papilla, and major duodenal caruncle.

PAPILLA OF VATER

This is ovoid in shape and projects into the lumen of the duodenum at its posteromedial wall somewhat beyond the midportion of the second portion of the duodenum. At times the papilla may be more distally located, close to the third portion of the duodenum (19, 21, 22, 39). The usual distance from the pylorus to the duodenal papilla is 10 cm. It may be closer to the pylorus, with the choledochus emptying into the proximal half of the second portion of the duodenum, or more rarely because it empties into the first portion of the duodenum. In patients with duodenal ulcer or postbulbar ulcer with pancreatic penetration and fibrous retraction of the duodenum, the papilla may come to be dangerously close to the pylorus and should be kept in mind during gastrectomy.

The papilla is covered by duodenal mucosa, but its lumen is lined by choledochal mucosa. The two mucosas meet at the orifice of the papilla (10). At its superior border, the papilla is usually partially covered by a transverse fold that gives the impression of a eave (39, 48). Less frequently a vertical duodenal fold is located under the papilla and with the previously mentioned transverse fold forms a "T"(19, 48).

At the end point at the papilla the choledochus occupies the superior portion of the papilla and the terminal end of the pancreatic duct is situated interiorly corresponding to the 4, 5, or 6 o'clock positions.

The papilla is easily recognized in more than 60% of cases because of its size when it is increased, owing to its prominence into the duodenal lumen, because it is erect or because of the folds disposed as a "T" indicate its presence. Because of its fibrous and muscular fiber its consistency is palpably enhanced (22, 48). But the papilla may be difficult to detect in the absence of these factors (48) or owing to its being completely covered by duodenal folds (48).

To locate the papilla, a longitudinal incision is made at the second portion of the duodenum starting at about its midpoint and continuing distally where it is usually to be found (22). Palpation should complement visual exploration passing the finger posteromedially along the second portion of the duodenum. It is often possible to palpate a small ovoid mound of consistency greater than the duodenal folds (22). During the exploration, excessive traction of the duodenum is to be avoided as this maneuver distorts and irons out the duodenal folds (48). The transverse fold present in some cases and that forms as it were a shed over the papilla can completely cover and hide it. If the papilla has not been identified and the gall bladder is present, this may be gently squeezed to provoke visual exit of bile through the papilla thereby revealing it. If the gall bladder has been previously removed another recourse is to introduce a physiologic solution or a catheter or dilator through the cystic duct or through a supraduodenal choledochotomy. A jutapapillar duodenal diverticulum may add to the difficulty in identifying the papilla (22, 48). The papilla is easily identified by endoscopy and an experienced endoscopist may expeditiously catheterize the ampulla and perform papillotomy (22).

SPHINCTER OF ODDI

Boyden's description of the sphincter of Oddi, which he studied extensively, is today the most accepted (2–5). Boyden describes four groups of muscle fibers:

1. Superior sphincter of the choledochus
2. Inferior sphincter of the choledochus
3. Sphincter of the pancreatic duct
4. Sphincter of the papilla

The fibers of the superior sphincter are not constantly found, and the fibers of the inferior sphincter are not all annular. Muscles fibers of the pancreatic sphincter are not constant, being present in only 20% of cases, and are rarely annular. Boyden affirms that the sphincter of Oddi is embryologically and functionally distinct from the muscular fibers of the duodenum (5). Several authors hold that there exists an interconnection leading to functional interplay between the muscular fibers of the sphincter of Oddi and those of the duodenum. The structure of this sphincter complex varies according to the manner of union of the choledochus with the pancreatic duct. There are also bundles of longitudinal fibers that connect both ducts which in turn connect with muscular fibers of the duodenum. There are other fibers, designated as reinforcing fibers, which go from the muscular fibers of the duodenum proper to the longitudinal fibers.

Cinecholangiographic, manometric, and electromyographic studies confirm that the muscular fibers of the sphincter of Oddi and the muscular fibers of the duodenum act synchronously (7, 8, 20, 22, 33, 34, 38, 44, 45, 51). Relaxation of the sphincter of Oddi and relaxation of the adjacent duodenal musculature occur synchronously; contraction of both also occurs at the same time. It has been established that the sphincter of Oddi opens from above downward and closes from below upward (22). These cycles of contraction–relaxation–contraction can be initiated by the presence of food in the duodenum, by the injection of cholecystokinin, or by a duodenal peristaltic wave passing through the sphincter zone. This sequence is known as duodenosphincteric synergy (22).

HEPATIC ARTERY, CYSTIC ARTERY, AND VENOUS CIRCULATION IN THE EXTRAHEPATIC BILIARY TREE

Hepatic Artery

After giving off the gastroduodenal artery, the hepatic artery courses vertically upward within the hepatoduodenal ligament in an anterior plane to the left of the choledochus, which occupies the free border of the hepatoduodenal ligament. The portal vein courses behind the hepatic artery. Proximal to the hepatic hilus the hepatic artery divides into right and left hepatic arteries. The right hepatic artery passes behind the common hepatic duct and enters the triangle of Calot. In some cases the right hepatic artery, as will be seen later, passes in front of the common hepatic duct.

Cystic Artery

In the majority of cases, the cystic artery takes its origin from the right hepatic artery within the triangle of Calot to the right of the hepatic duct. Hence it approaches the cystic duct and the neck o. the gall bladder, usually passing above and in a rather posterior plane. On arriving at the gall bladder it divides into two branches, one anterior, which travels in the subperitoneal surface of the gall bladder, the other posterior, which travels in the bed between the gall bladder and the liver. The cystic artery may present numerous variations. It may arise from the right hepatic but course behind the common hepatic duct instead of anterior to it. It may also originate from the left hepatic artery and course in front of the common hepatic duct. The cystic artery may arise from the common hepatic artery, the gastroduodenal artery, the left gastric artery, the right gastric artery, or the superior mesenteric artery. In 20% of cases there may be two cystic arteries, one anterior and one posterior (19, 21, 26, 48).

Triangle of Calot

In 1891, Jean François Calot described a triangle that is of crucial importance to gall bladder surgery. This triangle is formed by the cystic duct and neck of the gall bladder on the right and the common hepatic duct on the left (this is the hepatocystic angle), with the inferior base of the liver forming the triangle. It is in this triangle that the hepatic and the cystic arteries are identified.

Arterial Supply to the Hepatocholedochus

The arterial supply to the hepatocholedochus is very variable. Multiple small-caliber arteries arise from the superior and posterior pancreaticoduodenal artery, the supraduodenal artery, the cystic artery, the common hepatic artery, the right hepatic artery, and so on. Trauma to these vessels at reoperations could well result in hepatocholedochal strictures (19). It has been shown that repair of this hepatocholedochus is effected more easily transversely than longitudinally, which could be an aggravating factor in longitudinal strictures of the hepatocholedochus.

Venous Drainage of the Extrahepatic Biliary Ducts

Venous return from the gall bladder is by way of multiple veins of small caliber that go from the gall bladder to the hepatic parenchyma. These veins arise from all aspects of the gall bladder, both from the bed and the subperitoneal areas. Rarely a cystic vein that enters the portal vein or its right branch is found (19, 22, 26).

The venous return from the hepatocholedochus is by way of a plexus that covers the anterior wall of the choledochus. This is used to identify the choledochus. The plexus may give rise to troublesome bleeding during surgery in this area.

LYMPHATICS OF THE GALL BLADDER AND BILIARY DUCTS

The lymphatics of the gall bladder go to the hepatic parenchyma, to the nodes of the hepatocholedochus, and to the suprapancreatic and celiac nodes.

Above and next to neck of the gall bladder there is usually a lymph node known as the cystic node or node of Mascagni. This is useful as an anatomic point of reference.

Behind the inferior portion of the choledochus a commonly present lymph node known as the choledochal node is often used to help identify the common duct.

Surgery of the Biliary Tract

Surgery of the Biliary Tract

FIGURE 1.1

Semischematic drawing of the extrahepatic biliary ducts and their relationship to the duodenum:

1. Fundus of the gall bladder totally covered by peritoneum;
2. Body of the gall bladder bound to the hepatic bed by peritoneum;
3. Infundibulum of the gall bladder completely covered by peritoneum;
4. Neck of the gall bladder;
5. Cystic duct (pars spiralis);
6. Cystic duct (pars glabra);
7. Lymph node of the cystic duct or node of Mascagni (first anatomist to have described it);
8. Hepatic duct;
9. Choledochus, with its four choledochal segments: supraduodenal, retroduodenal, transpancreatic, and transmural or introduodenal;
10. Papilla of Vater;
11. Major pancreatic duct.

FIGURE 1.2

This depicts the relation of the structures at the hepatic hilus considered as normal, although found in less than 40% of cases:

1. Common hepatic artery arising from the celiac axis and following a horizontal course to the right, reaching the hepatoduodenal ligament and ascending to the hepatic hilum. After giving off the gastroduodenal artery the hepatic artery becomes the hepatic artery proper. As it approaches the hepatic hilum the hepatic artery divides in two, the left hepatic artery
2. to the left lobe of the liver and the right hepatic artery
3. going to the right lobe of the liver.

The right hepatic artery passes behind the common duct and enters the triangle of Calot, where it gives off the cystic artery. The cystic artery, upon approaching the neck of the gall bladder, divides into two branches, an anterior one that goes subperitoneally on the gall bladder and a posterior or deep branch that courses between the gall bladder and its hepatic bed.

The drawing shows the triangle of Calot formed on the left by the common hepatic duct, on its right side by the cystic duct and neck of the gall bladder, and at its base by the inferior surface of the liver. It is in this triangle that the right hepatic artery and the cystic artery should be identified.

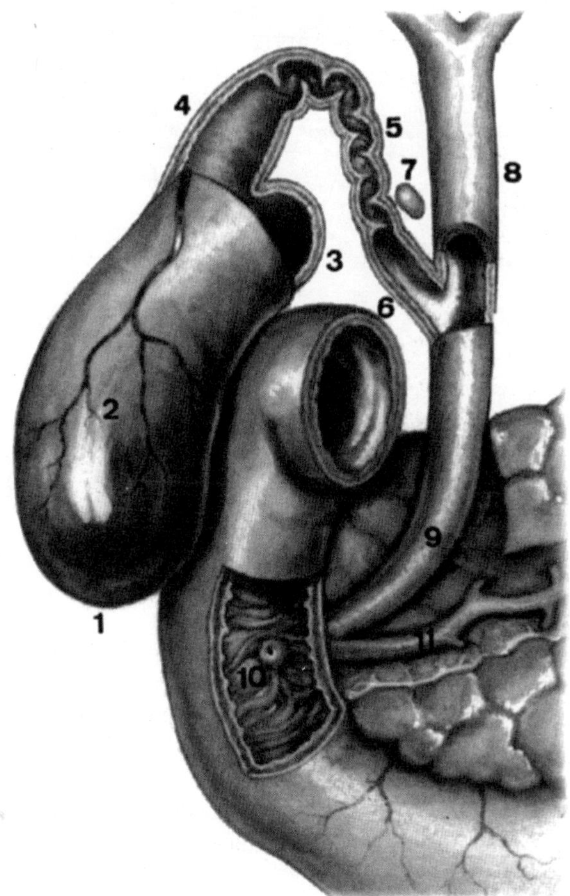

FIGURE 1.1

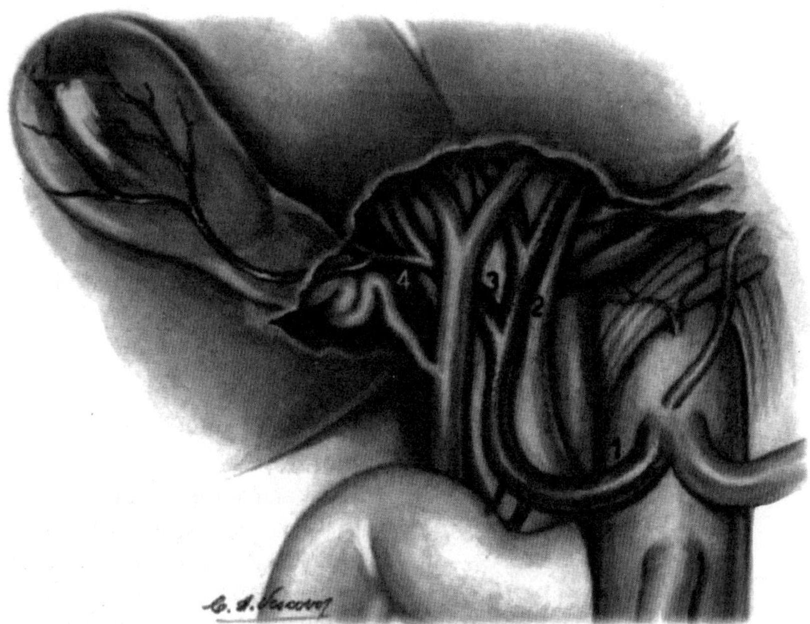

FIGURE 1.2

FIGURE 1.3
This drawing is very similar to the previous one but please note that here the left hepatic artery (which gives rise to the middle hepatic) courses in front of the left hepatic duct. This arrangement can be a very serious obstacle if one has to anastomose the left hepatic duct to the jejunum in a Roux-en-Y fashion in cases with high biliary tract lesions requiring difficult techniques of Hepp-Couinaud or similar.

Surgery of the Biliary Tract

FIGURE 1.4
The right and left hepatic ducts may join variously in the hepatic hilum or pedicle; high, midlevel or very low. Here depicted is a very low joining of the left and right hepatic ducts as seen at cholangiography after cholecystectomy: The joining is so near to the ampulla of Vater that there is no common hepatic duct and no choledochus to speak of.

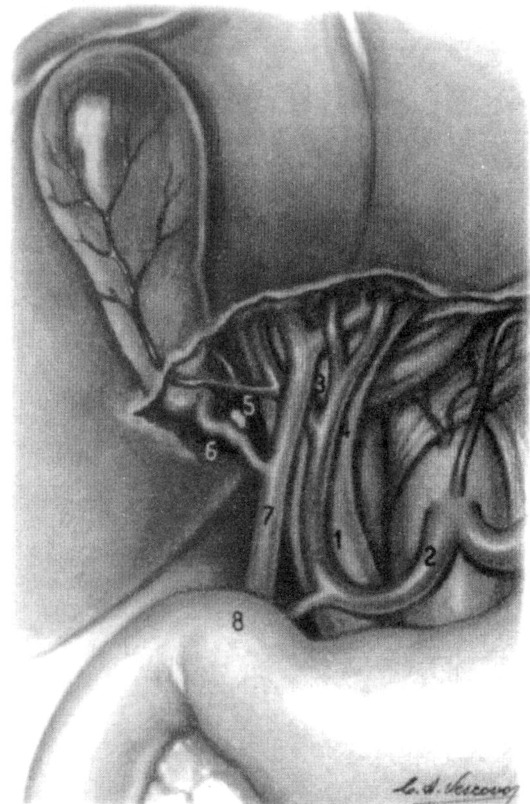

FIGURE 1.3

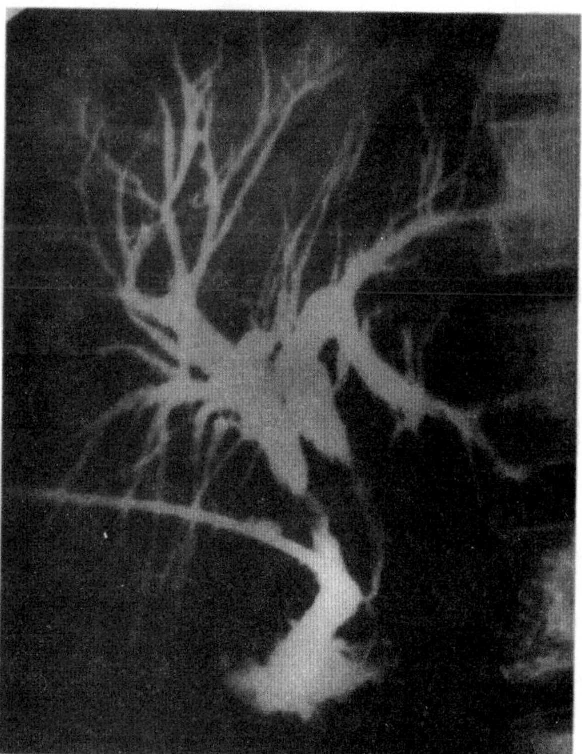

FIGURE 1.4

FIGURE 1.5
A. Aberrant right hepatic duct emptying into the cystic duct. If the cystic duct were ligated distal to its entrance into the aberrant hepatic duct, serious consequences would ensue. Operative cholangiography clarifies the presence of the aberrant hepatic duct. **B.** In the lower drawing we see a hepatic duct entering the common hepatic duct. The anomalous duct can be confused with the cystic duct during cholecystectomy. Operative cholangiography contributes to identifying the anomaly (see Figure 1.7). Aberrant ducts may enter the choledochus though rarely. Aberrant bile ducts of small caliber at the hepatic bed (retro–gall bladder aberrant ducts) may give rise to significant bile drainage after cholecystectomy (14, 19, 30, 40, 52).

Surgery of the Biliary Tract

FIGURE 1.6
Operative cholangiography showing aberrant right hepatic duct entering the cystic duct.

FIGURE 1.7
Operative cholangiography showing aberrant right hepatic duct draining into the common hepatic duct.

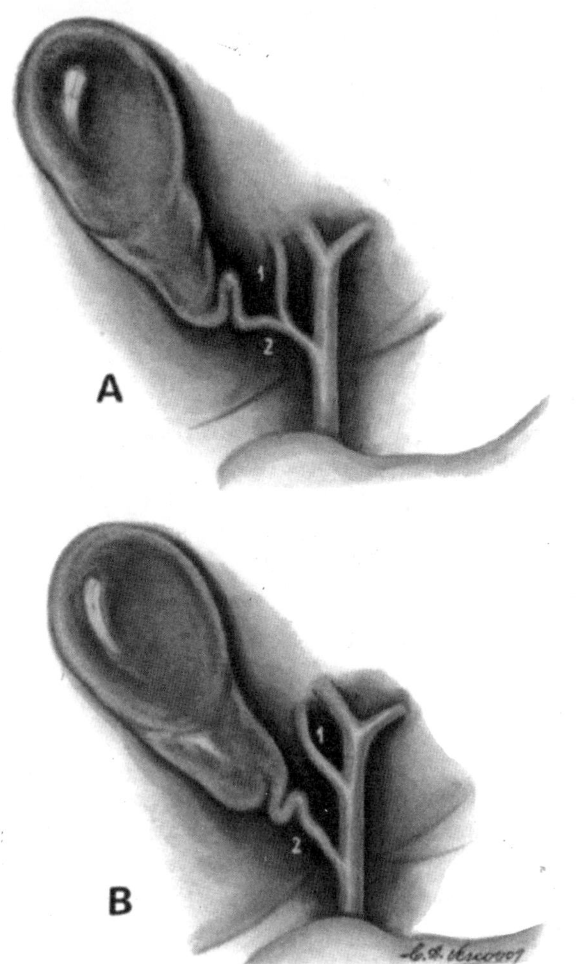

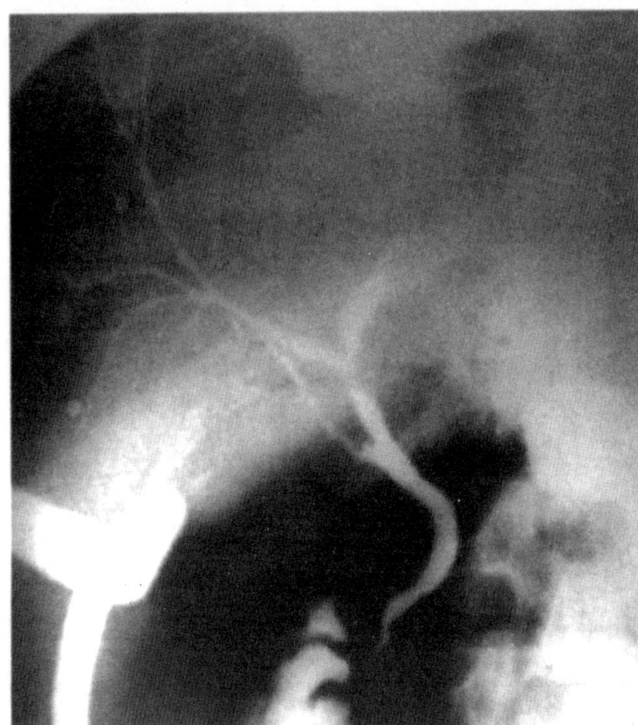

FIGURE 1.5

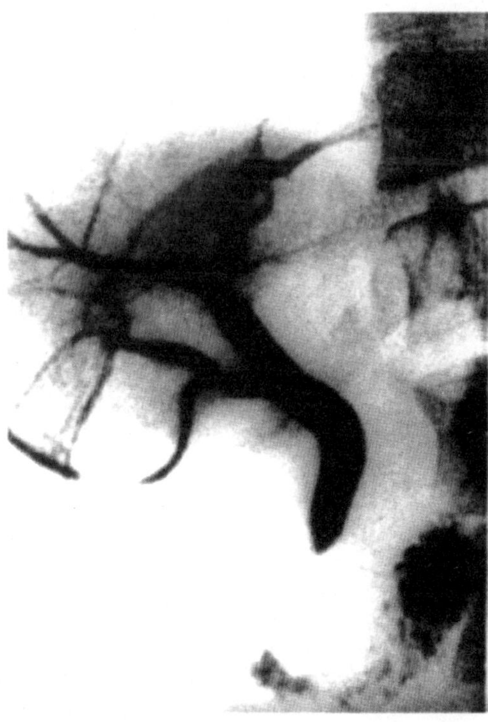

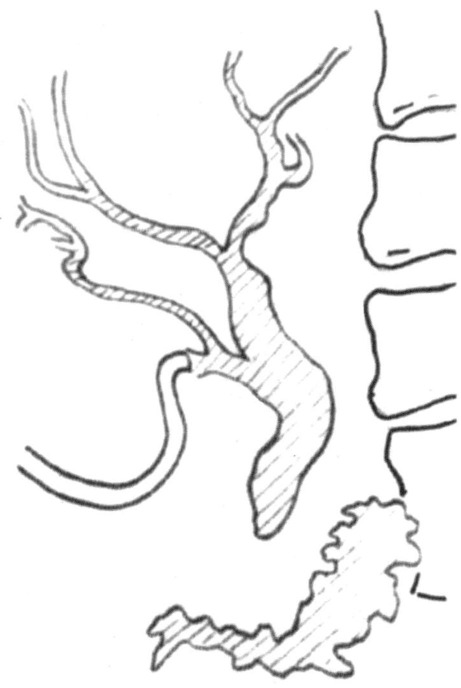

FIGURE 1.7

FIGURE 1.8
Choledochus joining the pancreatic duct shortly after entering the wall of the duodenum. Thus a short common channel is formed usually called the ampulla of Vater. This is the more common finding.

Surgery of the Biliary Tract

FIGURE 1.9
The choledochus and the pancreatic ducts never join to form a common duct as in Figure 1.8. They stay in contact, run in parallel fashion and empty independently at the duodenal papilla. Occasionally the pancreatic duct does not enter the duodenum at the papilla but does so 5 to 15 mm distally.

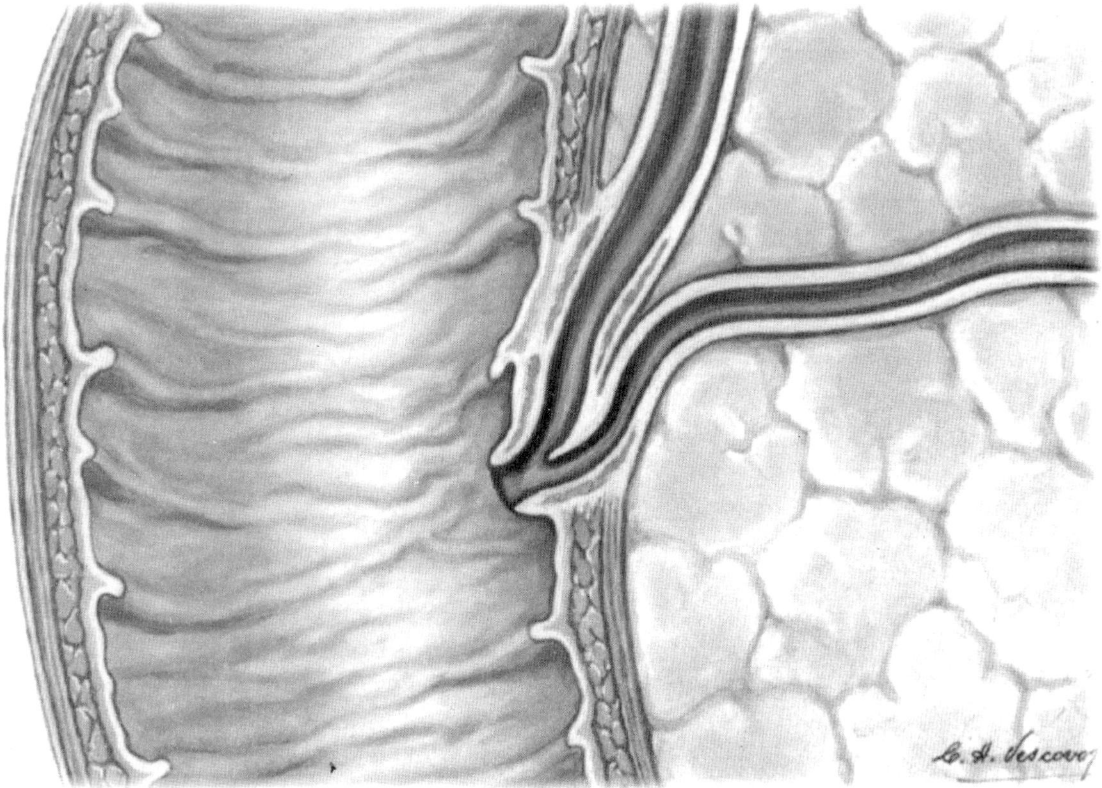

FIGURE 1.8

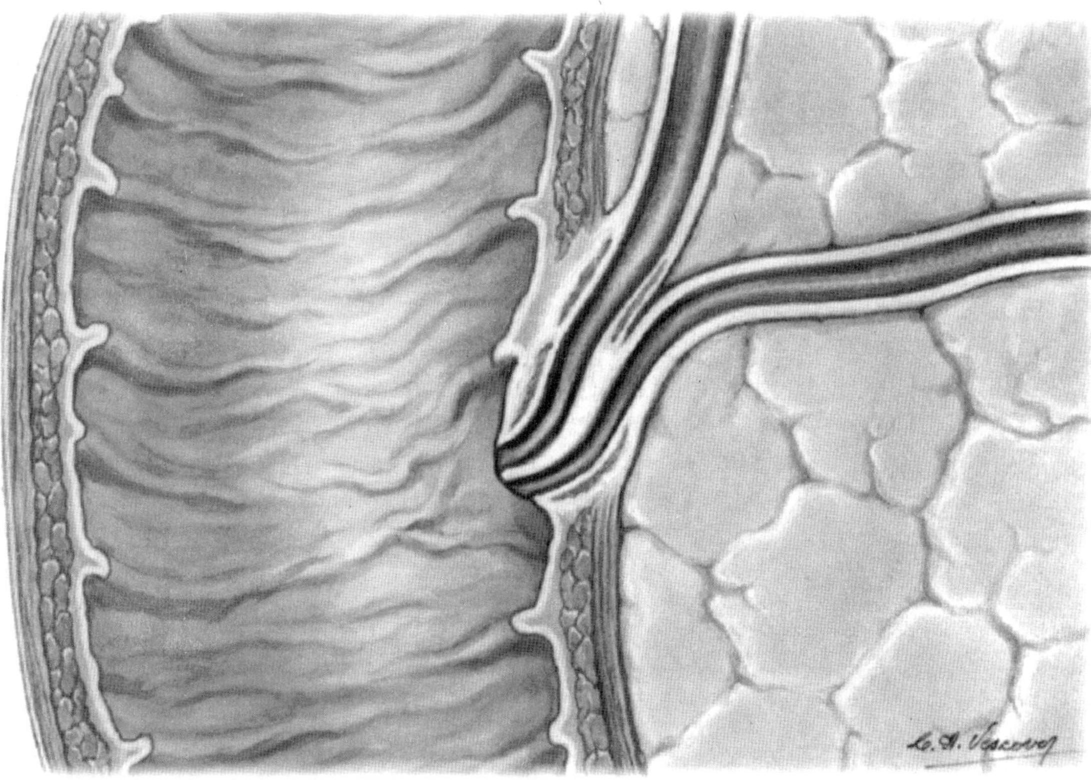

FIGURE 1.9

FIGURE 1.10
The pancreatic duct and choledochus may join prior to entering the wall of the duodenum. A longer common channel is thus formed.

Surgery of the Biliary Tract

FIGURE 1.11
The choledochus and pancreatic ducts end at the papilla after forming a common channel or may do so independently through separate paths, as previously seen..

The papilla is usually to be found in the distal half of the second portion of the duodenum (B). However, variations occur: It may be located in the inferior bend of the duodenum (distal part two) (C) or in the third portion of the duodenum (D). Less frequently it may be found in the proximal half of the second portion (A) and even more rarely at the first portion of the duodenum. The papilla is usually 10 cm from the pylorus but this distance can be very shortened in ulceration of the duodenum. If the ulcer is penetrating the resultant retraction of tissue enhances the danger during gastric surgery.

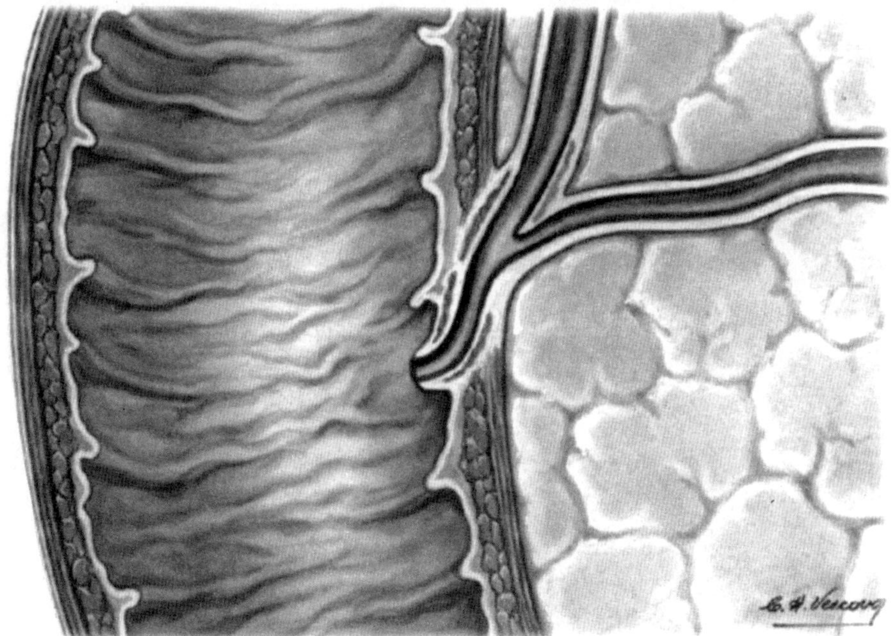

FIGURE 1.10

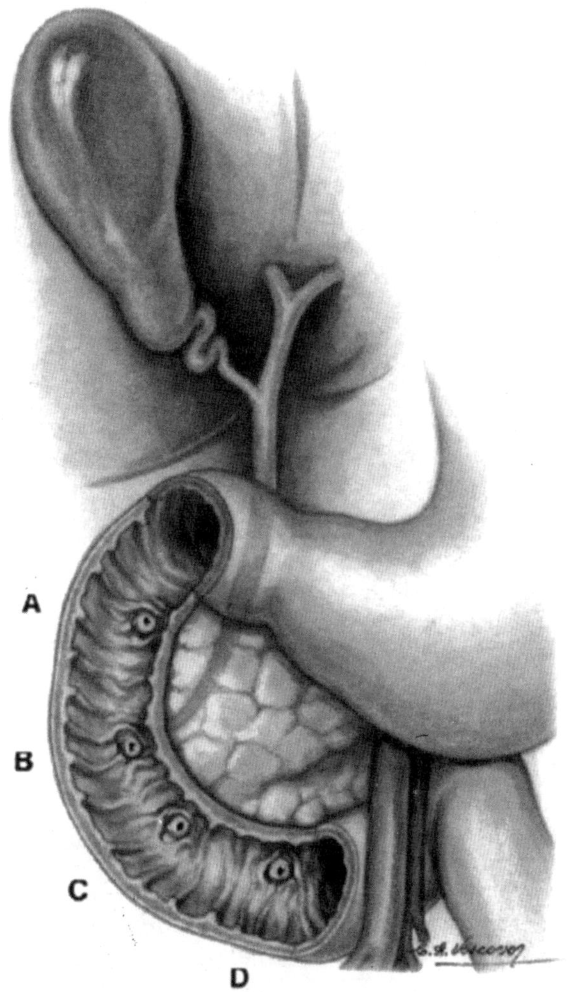

FIGURE 1.11

FIGURE 1.12
This drawing depicts the sphincter of Oddi complex as described by Boyden and his predecessors. According to Boyden the sphincter of Oddi consists of:

1. The sphincter proper of the choledochus consisting of annular muscle fibers about the terminal choledochus. Boyden postulates two such sphincters, one superior and the other inferior.
2. The sphincter of the pancreatic duct; this is not constant and is found only in 20% of cases. Its fibers are usually not annular.
3. The sphincter of the papilla is made up of annular, longitudinal and oblique fibers. Boyden affirms that the sphincter of Oddi is embryologically and functionally independent of the muscular fibers of the duodenum. However, there is proof that interconnections and functional synergy exist between the fibers of the papilla and of the duodenum.

Surgery of the Biliary Tract

FIGURE 1.13
This is the usual union between the cystic and common hepatic ducts. In 70% of cases this takes place at an acute angle, to form the choledochus at the right border of the hepatic duct. This is known as the angular union.

FIGURE 1.14
The cystic duct courses parallel to the common hepatic and joins it at the inferior border of the posterior wall of the first portion of the duodenum. This is known as the parallel union.

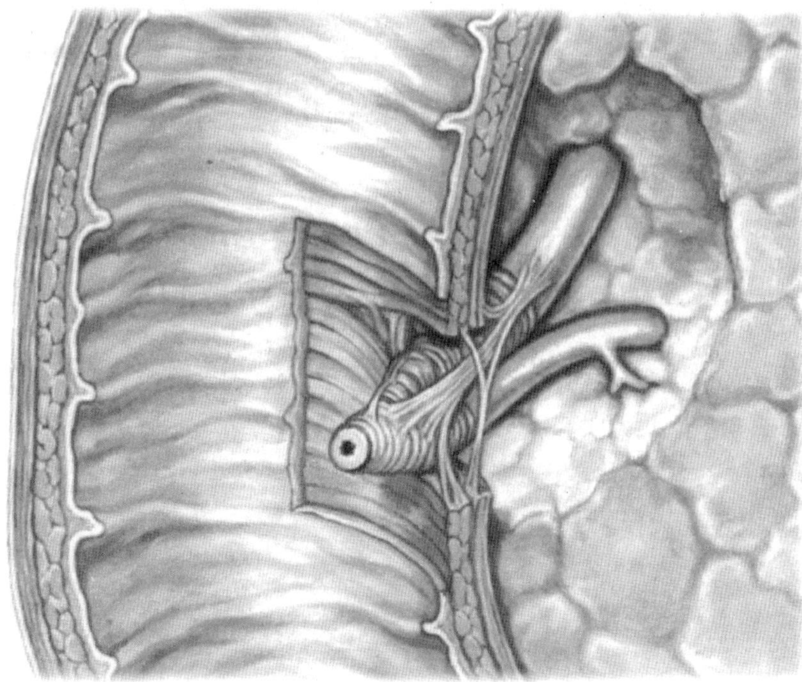

FIGURE 1.12

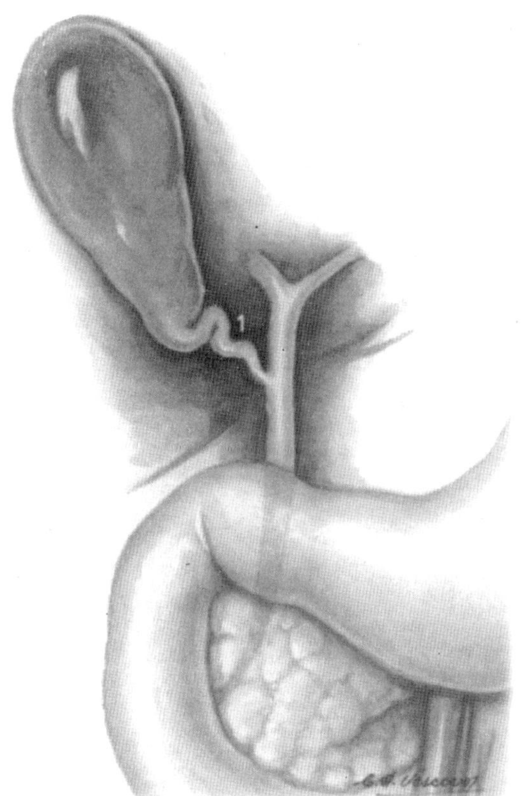

FIGURE 1.13

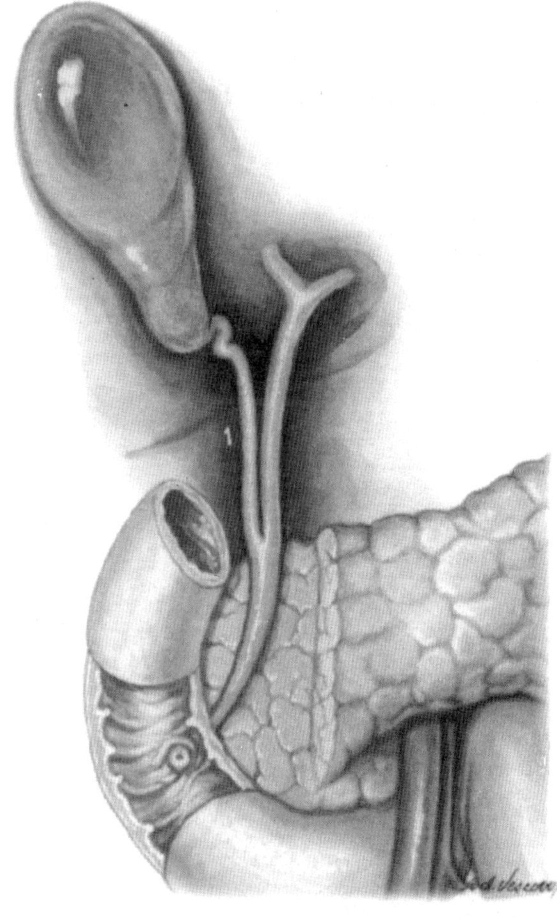

FIGURE 1.14

FIGURE 1.15
The cystic duct, 1, runs parallel to the common hepatic and joins it close to the papilla. This is another variation of parallel union.

FIGURE 1.16
Operative cholangiography showing a long parallel course of the cystic duct joining the bile duct at the papilla.

Surgery of the Biliary Tract

FIGURE 1.17
The cystic duct, 1, courses behind the hepatic duct in a spiral fashion entering the hepatic duct at its left border. This is designated the "spiral posterior union." Mirizzi called this "cystic in posterior band" because the cystic crossed the hepatic duct in band form.

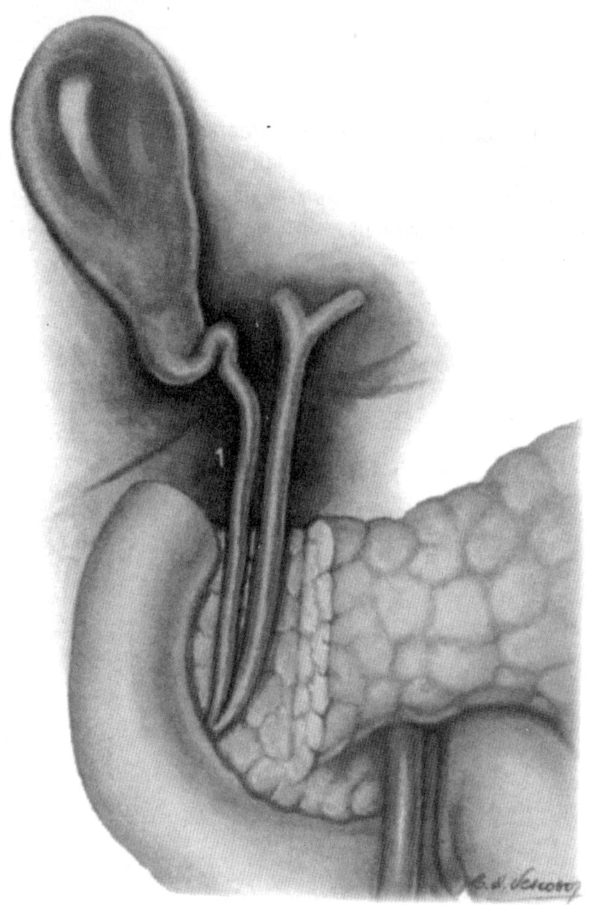

FIGURE 1.15

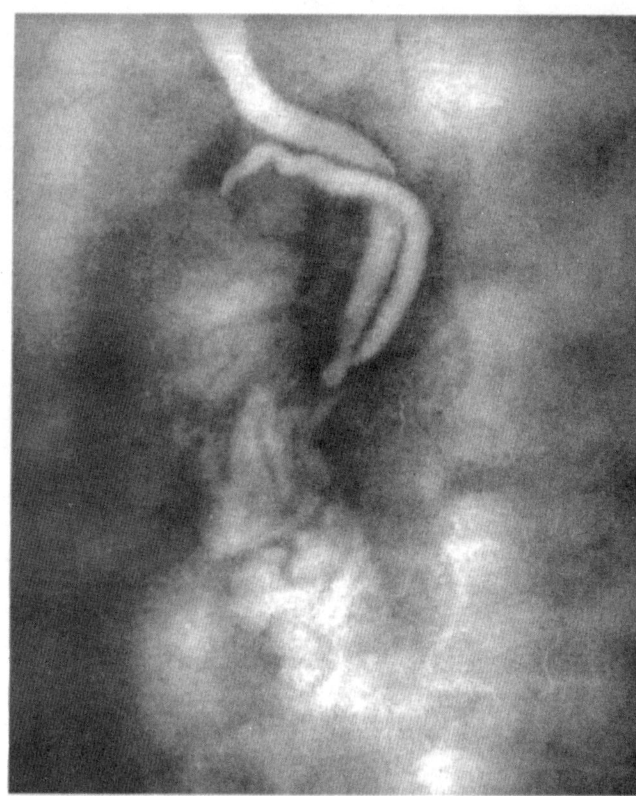

FIGURE 1.16

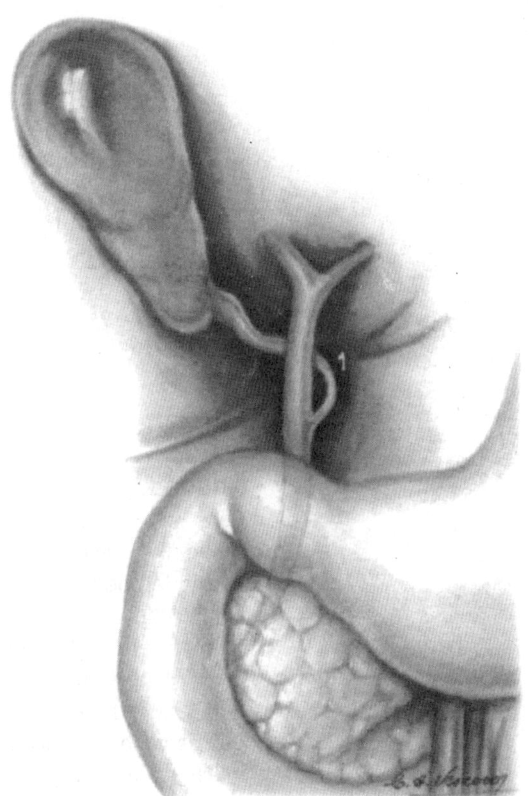

FIGURE 1.17

FIGURE 1.18
The cystic duct runs in front of the hepatic duct forming a spiral and enters the hepatic at its left border. This is designated "union in anterior spiral"; Mirizzi called this "cystic in anterior band." This arrangement could well give rise to the Mirizzi hepatic duct syndrome.

FIGURE 1.19
Cystic duct entering the right hepatic duct. Rarely the cystic duct enters the left hepatic duct.

Surgery of the Biliary Tract

FIGURE 1.20
Here we see the common hepatic artery, 1, rising from the celiac axis, which after a short trajectory divides into a right, 2, and left hepatic, 3, artery. The right hepatic artery passes behind the common hepatic duct and enters the triangle of Calot, where it gives rise to the cystic artery. The left hepatic artery courses upward to the left lobe of the liver. In some elderly and arteriosclerotic patients and in younger ones also, the right hepatic artery may bend markedly to the right so much so that it comes into contact with the neck and infundibulum of the gall bladder constituting a real danger during cholecystectomy.

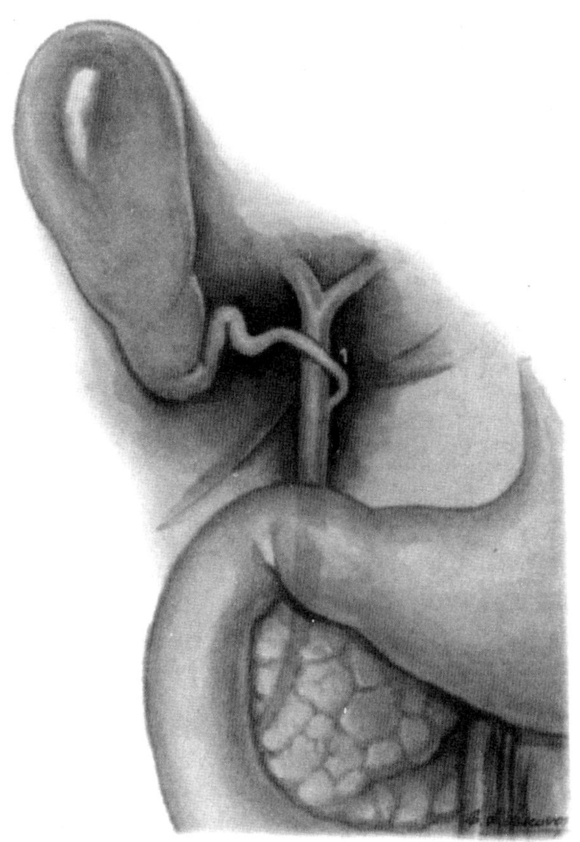

FIGURE 1.18

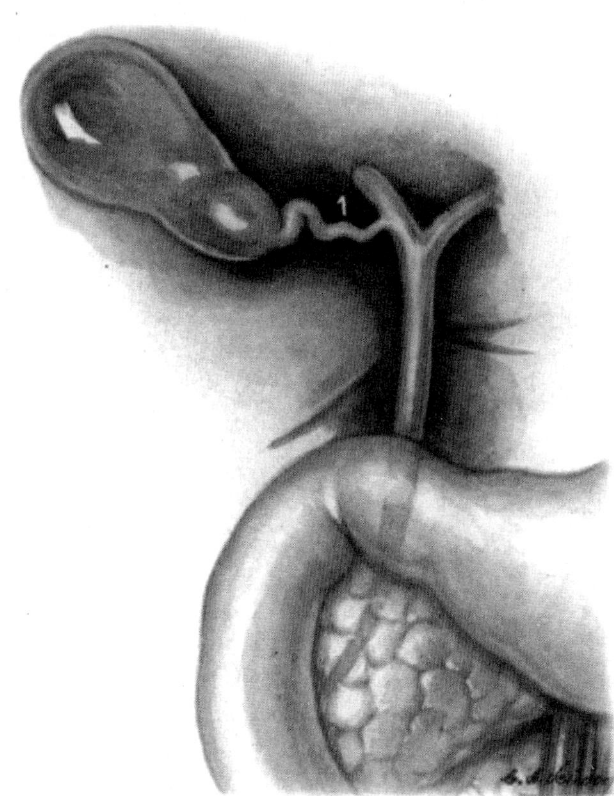

FIGURE 1.19

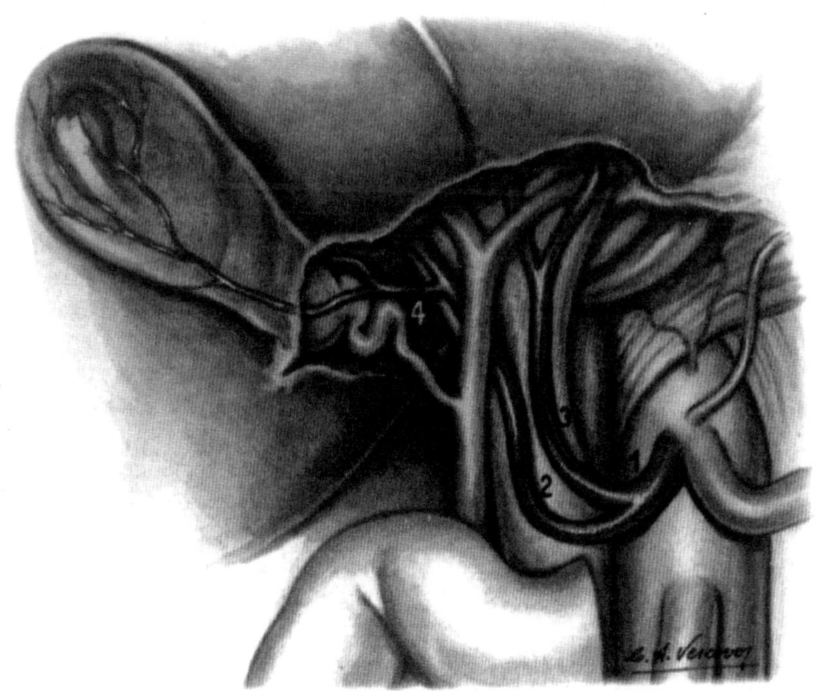

FIGURE 1.20

FIGURE 1.21
The right and left hepatic arteries have separate origins. The left hepatic artery, 1, arises from the celiac trunk and after running upward, goes directly to the left lobe of the liver. The right hepatic artery, 2, arises from the superior mesenteric artery, travels behind the head of the pancreas and enters the hepatoduodenal ligament, passes in front of the common hepatic duct and gives origin to the cystic artery, 3.

Surgery of the Biliary Tract

FIGURE 1.22
The left hepatic artery, 1, rises from the left gastric (coronary) artery and courses upward to the left lobe of the liver as its only arterial supply. The right hepatic artery, 2, originates from the celiac axis, passes behind the common hepatic duct, and enters the triangle of Calot, where it gives off the cystic artery, 3. In this situation the left hepatic artery is the only arterial supply to the left lobe and is definitely not an accessory artery. Ligation of this left hepatic artery would produce fatal necrosis of the left lobe. In the insert the left hepatic also arises from the left side from the coronary (gastric) artery, but in this case it is definitely an accessory artery. This is so because here the common hepatic artery originates in the celiac trunk, travels its usual path, and divides near the hepatic hilum to yield the right and left hepatic arteries to their respective lobes of the liver. Ligation of the hepatic artery rising from the gastric artery would not have the dire consequences indicated above because the left lobe is well supplied by the artery from the celiac axis. In this situation the left hepatic artery rising from the coronary (left gastric) artery is truly an accessory artery. Differentiation between these two is essential prior to ligation.

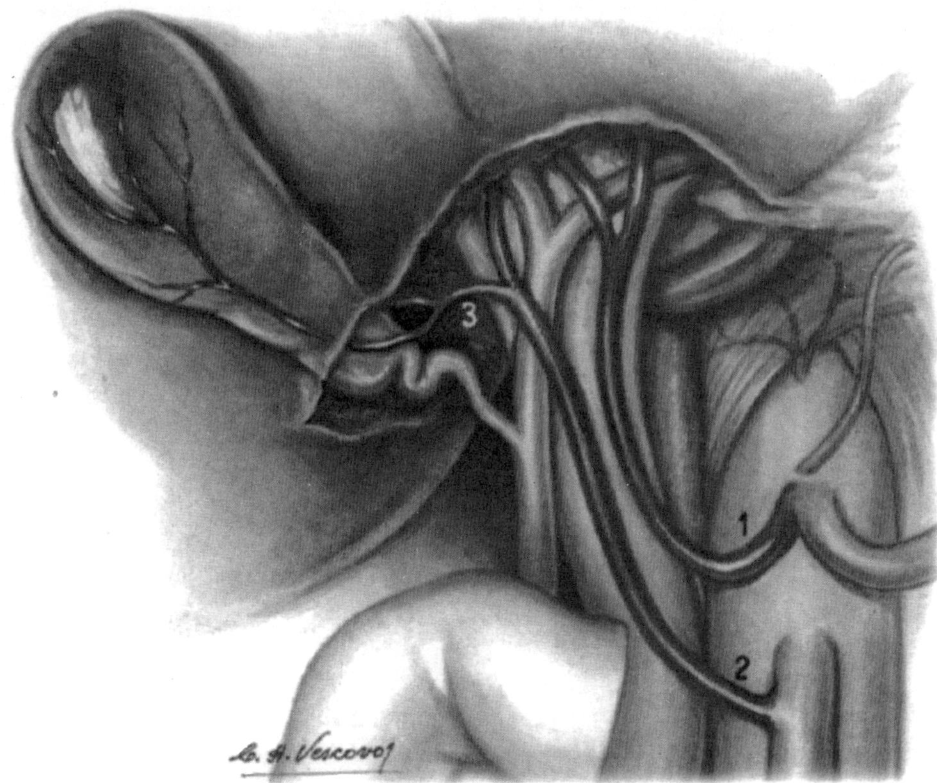

FIGURE 1.21

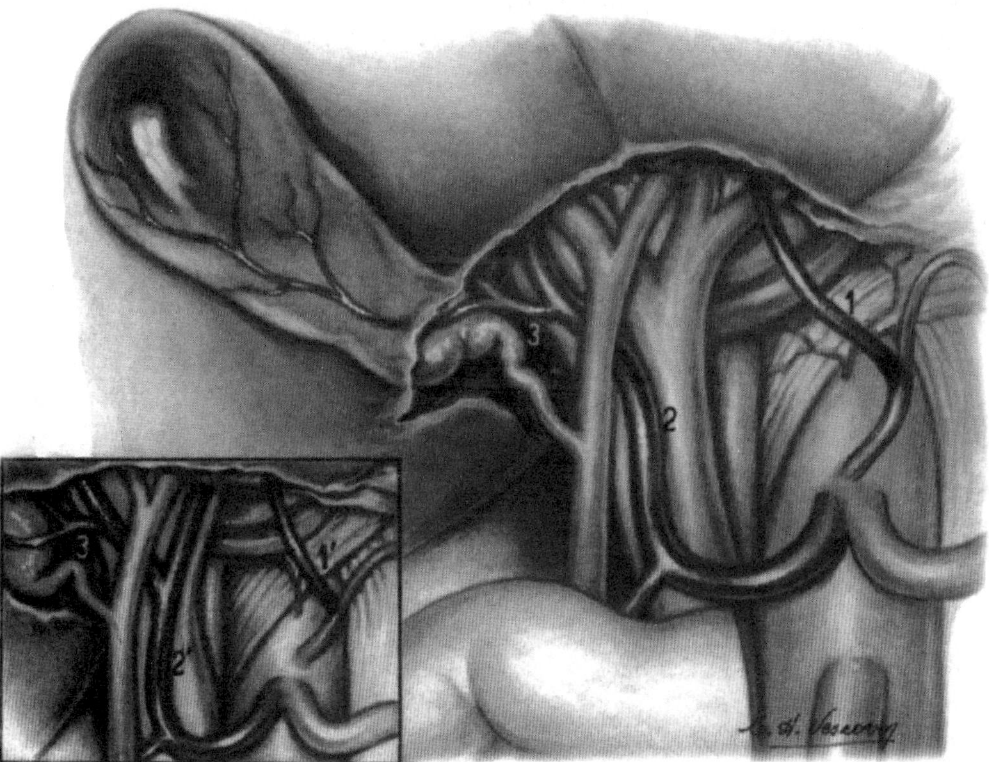

FIGURE 1.22

FIGURE 1.23
Cystic artery arises from the right hepatic in the triangle of Calot, the more common situation among numerous variations.

FIGURE 1.24
The cystic artery arises from the right hepatic artery outside the triangle of Calot and passes anterior to the common hepatic duct rather than posterior to it.

Surgery of the Biliary Tract

FIGURE 1.25
The cystic artery, 1, arises from the left hepatic instead of the right and courses to the neck of the gall bladder passing in front, anterior to the common hepatic duct.

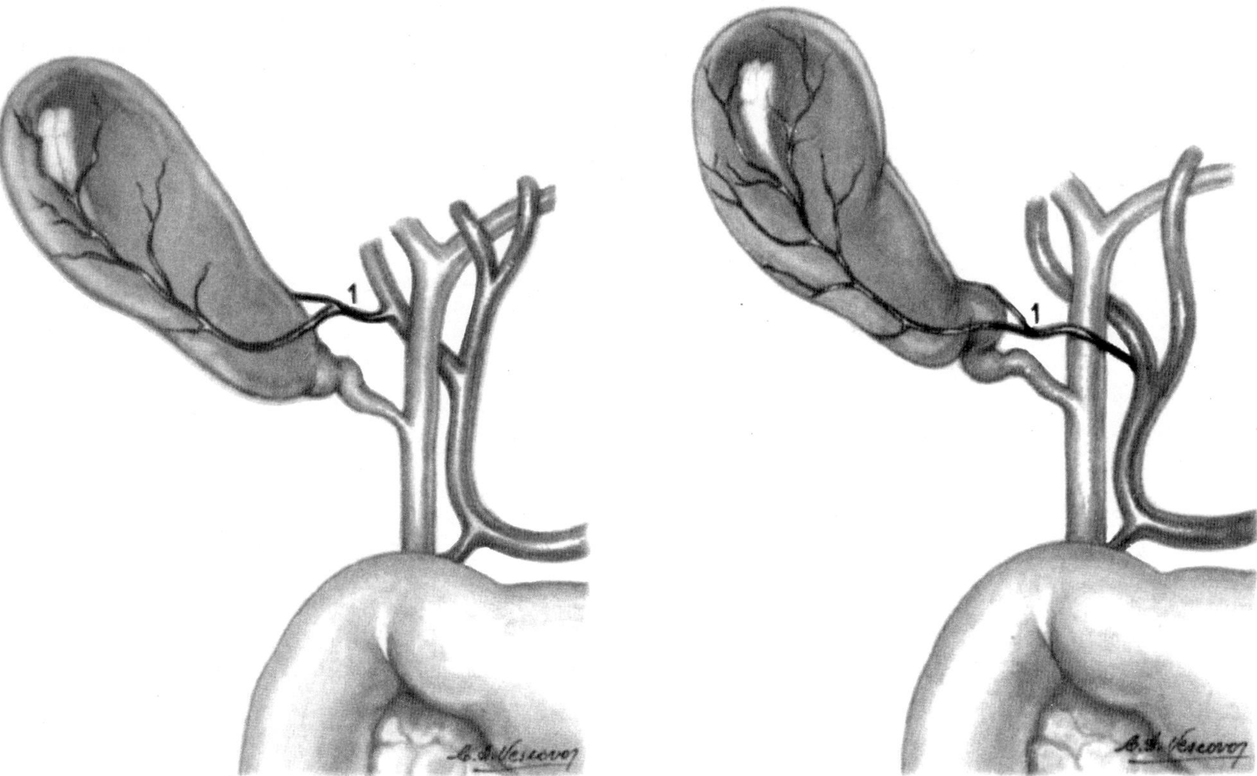

FIGURE 1.23

FIGURE 1.24

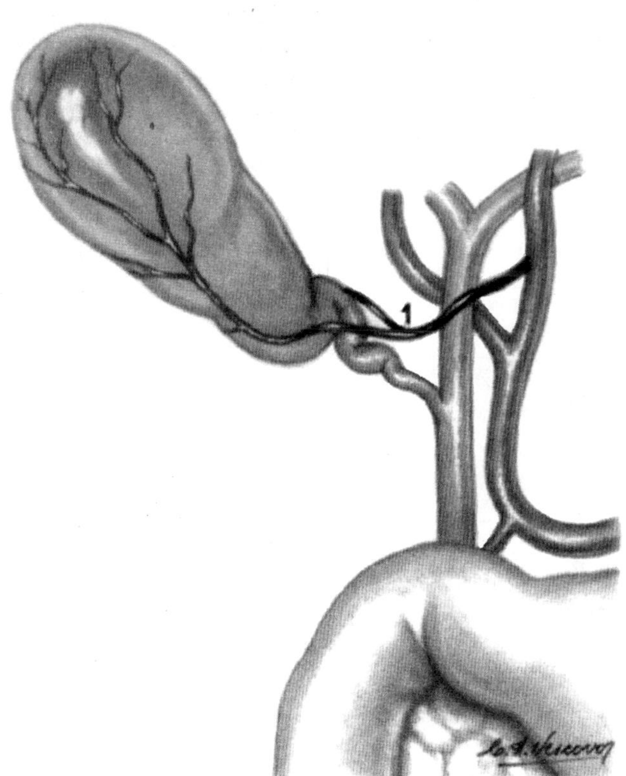

FIGURE 1.25

Surgery of the Biliary Tract

FIGURE 1.26

The cystic artery, 1, presents numerable variations in its origin and its courses: from the celiac axis, from the gastroduodenal, superior mesenteric, and so on. In this illustration it arises from the common hepatic artery and courses in front of the common hepatic duct.

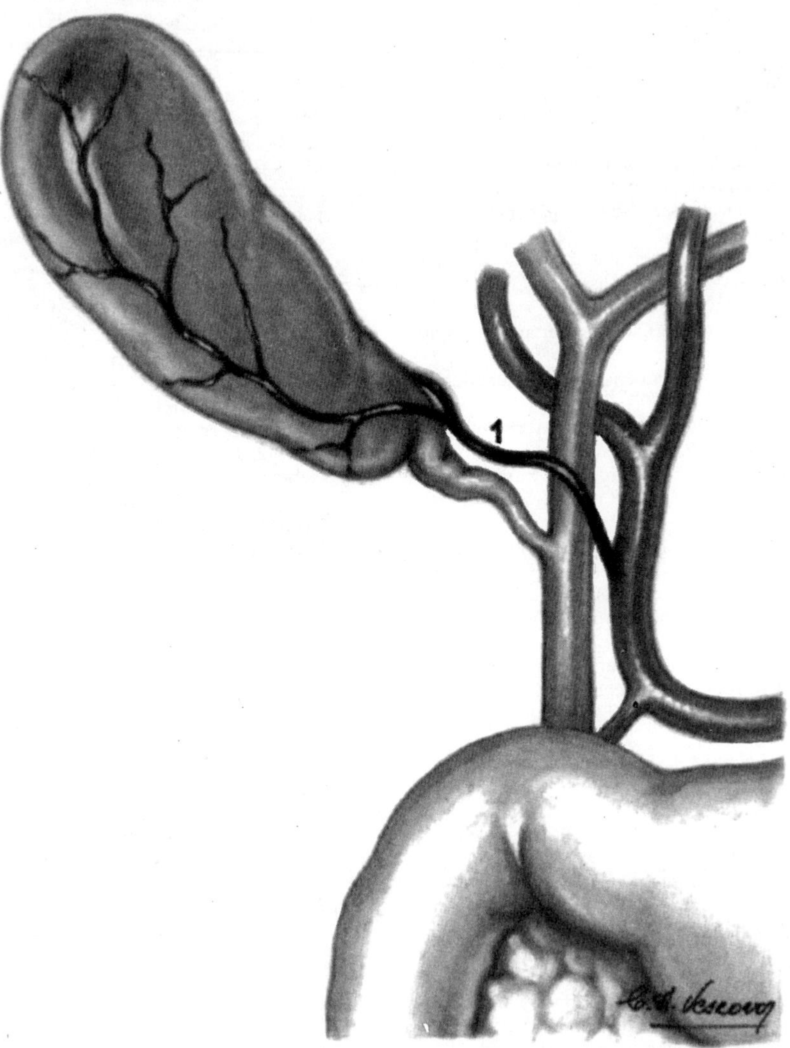

FIGURE 1.26

References

1. Bernard, C. Mémoire sur le pancréas et sur le rôle du suc pancréatique dans les phénomènes digestifs, particulièrement dans la digestion des matières grasses neutres. Baillières, Paris, 1856.
2. Bidloo, G. Quoted in Skandalakis, J.E., Gray, S.W., Skandalakis, L.J. Surgical anatomy of the pancreas. In Howard, J.M., Jordan, G.L., Jr., Reber, H.A. (Ed.) Surgical diseases of the pancreas. Lea & Febiger, Philadelphia, 1987.
3. Boyden, E.A. The pars intestinalis of the common bile duct, as viewed by the older anatomists (Vesalius, Glisson, Bianchi, Vater, Haller, Santorini, etc.). Anat. Rec. 66:27, 1936.
4. Boyden, E.A. The sphincter of Oddi in man and certain representative mammals. Surgery 1:25, 1937.
5. Boyden, E.A. The anatomy of the choledochoduodenal junction in man. Surg. Gynecol. Obstet. 104:641, 1957.
6. Brittain, R.S., Marchioro, T.L., Hermann, G. et al. Accidental hepatic artery ligation. Am. J. Surg. 107:822, 1964.
7. Caroli, J., Porcher, P., Pequignot, G., Delattre, M. Contribution of cineradiography to study the function of human biliary tract. Am. J. Digest. Dis. 5:677, 1960.
8. Caroli, J., Plessier, J., Plessier, B. Endogenous cholecystokinin and its inhibitor method of assessment in humans; its role in normal and pathologic physiology. Am. J. Digest. Dis. 6:646, 1961.
9. Chassin, J.L. Operative strategy in general surgery. Vol. II, p. 59. Springer-Verlag. New York, 1984.
10. Chikiar, A., Eguía, O., Ghinelli, C. Estructura fibromuscular del colédoco. XIII Congreso Pan Amer. Gastroenterología, 1973.
11. Chikiar, A., Szurman, N., Cederbaum, E. El colédoco. Enfoques Terapéuticos 2:15, 1981.
12. Del Valle, D., Dónovan, R. Colédoco-Odditis esclerorretráctil. Concepto clíníco y quirúrgico. Arch. Argent. Enfer. Ap. Digest. 1:1, 1926.
13. Ferris, D.O., Vibert, J.C. The common bile duct: Significance of its diameter. Ann. Surg. 149:249, 1959.
14. Foster, J.H., Wayson, E.E. Surgical significance of aberrant bile duct. Am. J. Surg. 104:14, 1962.
15. Glisson, F. Anatomia hepatis. Ed. 2. London, Hagae, 1681.
16. Hand, B.H. Anatomy and function of the extrahepatic biliary system. Clin. Gastroenterol. 2:3, 1973.
17. Hendrickson, W.F. A study of the entire extrahepatic biliary system including that of the duodenal portion of the common bile duct and the sphincter. Bull. Johns Hopkins Hospital 1:221, 1898.
18. Hermann, R.E. Manual of surgery of the gallbladder, bile ducts, and exocrine pancreas. p. 3. Springer-Verlag, New York, 1979.
19. Hollinshead, W.H. Anatomy for surgeons. Vol. 2, p. 345. Hoeber Harper, New York, 1956.
20. Jacobsson, B., Lanner, L.O., Radberg, C. The dynamic variability of the choledocho-pancreatico-duodenal junction. Acta Radiol. 52: 269, 1959.
21. Kune, G.A. Surgical anatomy of common bile duct. Arch. Surg. 89:995, 1964.
22. Kune, G.A., Sali, A. The practice of biliary surgery. Ed. 2, p. 1. Blackwell Scientific Publications, Oxford, 1980.
23. Lang, F.J. Die arterielle blutversogung der tiefen galenwage. Chirurgie 18:67, 1946.
24. Livingston, E.M. A clinical study of the abdominal cavity and peritoneum. Paul B. Hoeber, New York, 1932.
25. Longmire, W.P., Jr., Tompkins, R.K. Lesions of the segmental and lobar hepatic ducts. Ann. Surg. 182:478, 1975.
26. Michels, N.A. The hepatic, cystic and retroduodenal arteries and their relations to the biliary ducts with samples of the entire celiacal blood supply. Ann. Surg. 133:563, 1951.
27. Mirizzi, P.L. Fisiopatología del hepatocolédoco. Colangiografea operatoria. El Ateneo, Buenos Aires, 1939.
28. Mirizzi, P.L. Physiologic sphincter of hepatic bile duct. Arch. Surg. 41:1325, 1940.
29. Mirizzi, P.L. Functional disturbances of the choledochus and hepatic bile ducts. Surg. Gynecol. Obstet. 74:304, 1942.
30. Mirizzi, P.L. La colangiografía operatoria. Ejemplos que fundamentan sus ventajas y justifican su práctica sistemática. Bol. Acad. Argent. Cir. 26:917, 1942.
31. Mirizzi, P.L. La peristalsis del colédoco. Pren. Méd. Argent. 33:1009, 1946.
32. Mirizzi, P.L. Chirurgie du système du canal hépatique. Masson et Cie., Paris, 1962.
33. Myers, R.V., Haupt, G.J., Birkhead, N.C., Deaver, J.M. Cinefluorographic observations of common bile duct physiology. Ann. Surg. 156:442, 1962.
34. Nebesar, R.A., Pollard, J.J., Potsaid, J.J. Cine-cholangiography: Some physiologic observations. Radiology 86:475, 1966.
35. Norman, O. Study on the hepatic ducts in cholangiography. Acta Radiol. (Suppl 84) 1951.
36. Oddi, R. Una disposizione a sphincter espeziale della oberture del canale choledoco. Arch. Ital. Biol. 8:317, 1887.
37. Parke, W.P., Michels, N.A., Ghosh, G.M. Blood supply of the common bile duct. Surg. Gynecol. Obstet. 117:47, 1963.
38. Plessier, J. The use of cholecystokinin in the roentgenological examination. Clinical aspects. Handb. Exp. Pharm. 34:311, 1973.
39. Pi-Figueras, J. Práctica quirúrgica. Ed. 2, Vol. II, p. 563.
40. Prinz, R.A., Howell, H.S., Pickleman, J.R. Surgical significance of extrahepatic biliary tree anomalies. Am. J. Surg. 131:755, 1976.
41. Saint, J.H. The epicholedochal venous plexus and its importance as a means of identifying the common bile duct during operations on the extrahepatic biliary tract. Brit. J. Surg. 48:489, 1961
42. Santorini, G.D. Observationes anatomicae. Venezia, Recurti, 1724.
43. Santorini, J.D. Anatomici summi septemdecim tabulae quas nunc primum edit atque eplicat parmae ex regis typographia, 1775.
44. Sarles, J.C., Bidart, J.M., Devaux, M.A. et al. Action of cholecystokinin and caerulein on the rabbit sphincter of Oddi. Digestion 14:415, 1976.
45. Schein, C.J., Beneventano, T.C. Choledochal dynamics in man. Surg. Gynecol. Obstet. 126:591, 1968.
46. Schwegler, R.A., Jr., Boyden, E.A. The development of the common bile duct in the human fetus with special reference to the origin of the ampulla of Vater and the sphincter of Oddi. Surg. Gynecol. Obstet. 68:17, 1937.
47. Shapiro, A.L., Robillard, L. The arterial blood supply of the common and hepatic bile ducts with reference to the problems of common duct injury and repair. Surgery 28:1, 1948.
48. Skandalakis, J.E., Gray, S.W., Skandalakis, L.J. Surgical anatomy of the pancreas. In Howard, J.M., Jordan, G.L., Reber, H.A. (Eds.) Surgical diseases of the pancreas, p. 11. Lea & Febiger, Philadelphia, 1987.
49. Vater, A. Dissertatio anatomica. IV. Novum bilis diverticulum circa orificium ductus coledochia. Wittenberg, Paulo Gotlop Berger. 1720.
50. Velasco Suárez, C. La mal llamada ampolla de Vater. Estudio de revisión histórica. Pren. Méd. Argent. 62:139, 1975.
51. Watts, J., Dunphy, J.E. The role of the common bile duct in biliary dynamics. Surg. Gynecol. Obstet. 122:1207, 1966.
52. Williams, C., Williams, A.M. Abnormalities of the bile ducts. Ann. Surg. 141:498, 1955.

Section A

Surgery of the Biliary Tract

CHAPTER 2

Cholecystectomy

Cholecystectomy is indicated in gallbladder lithiasis and most cases of acalculous acute cholecystitis. It may be indicated in chronic acalculous cholecystitis, but poor selection in this group of patients leads to an increase in the number of patients with postcholecystectomy syndrome.

Nobody doubts that cholecystectomy means resection of the gallbladder. However, the surgeon who performs a cholecystectomy should always perform an act of significant importance—exploration of the bile ducts. Cholecystectomy should be considered an incomplete operation if exploration of the biliary tract and treatment of the pathologic alterations that may be present are not carried out at the same time.

In relation to cholecystectomy, several questions are a subject of discussion among surgeons. Some of these are

1. Is cholecystectomy indicated in asymptomatic biliary lithiasis?
2. Should operative cholangiography be used systematically, selectively, or not at all?
3. Should cholecystectomy be performed from the cystic duct to the fundus or from the fundus to the cystic duct?
4. Should the hepatic bed be peritonealized?
5. Should drainage be routine after cholecystectomy?

ASYMPTOMATIC BILIARY LITHIASIS

The great majority of surgeons (7, 9, 10, 12, 14, 21, 29, 30, 32, 34, 35, 40, 42, 44, 46, 48, 51) recommend surgery in patients with asymptomatic biliary lithiasis. Many studies (5, 10, 12, 21, 23, 44) have demonstrated that asymptomatic lithiasis may become symptomatic at any moment, leading to serious complications with increased morbidity and even death (46, 53, 54, 56). Elderly patients and particularly diabetics frequently develop acute cholecystitis, with perforation and/or gangrene and acute cholangitis owing to increased frequency of choledocholithiasis (53, 54, 56). Some asymptomatic patients may continue to be asymptomatic even while developing complications such as: biliobiliary or bilio–intestinal fistulas, chronic cholecystitis with an enlarging Hartmann's pouch, chronic cholecystitis simulating tumors, and so on, all of which complicate cholecystectomy and increase morbidity (21). The pathologic process may progress asymptomatically, giving rise to the above complications (25, 32, 46, 53, 55, 56).

It has been shown that cancer of the gallbladder usually develops in the presence of stones, and 1 to 2% of gallbladders removed for lithiasis present carcinoma of the gallbladder (6, 13, 14, 30, 32, 43, 45, 55). The longer the stones have been present and the older the patient, the higher the incidence of malignancy (13, 14). Elective cholecystectomy has a mortality of 0.1 to 0.5%. The mortality in cholecystectomy for acute cholecystitis is much higher (32, 35).

The author believes that, given the low mortality of cholecystectomy, it is the best prophylaxis of the complications and of cancer of the gallbladder. Years ago, when surgery carried a high mortality and morbidity, advising elective cholecystectomy may not have been prudent, but not at present.

Cholecystectomy is not recommended in asymptomatic lithiasis if the patient is more than 70 years of age or has significant cardiac, respiratory, or renal disease.

Some authors do not believe that patients with asymptomatic biliary lithiasis should be operated on because they believe that the incidence of complications and development of cancer in these cases have been exaggerated (4, 24). Other authors believe that the following are indications for surgery:

1. Small calculi which may give rise to acute pancreatitis.
2. Large calculus, more than 2 cm in diameter, because of the chance of acute cholecystitis or of biliary fistula or gall stone ileus.
3. Diabetic patients because acute complications are more frequent and more severe in them.
4. Calcified gallbladder walls (porcelain gallbladder) because of its association with cancer.
5. Patients who live far from adequate surgical facilities.
6. Patients who must travel a lot.

SHOULD OPERATIVE CHOLANGIOGRAPHY BE PERFORMED?

Operative cholangiography, proposed by Mirizzi in 1931, is the most effective, objective, and innocuous manner in which to explore the biliary tract (8, 9, 17, 18, 22, 25, 38, 39, 41, 47) and should be employed in all cases. By means of cholangiography the surgeon is offered a complete view of the biliary tree before invading it. We can see the caliber, anatomic variations, pathologic alterations, the presence of calculi, and their number, size, and location. Cholangiography will permit considerable assurance that all calculi have been successfully removed. It will also afford evaluation of the sphincter of Oddi. To perform operative cholangiography only selectively enhances the possibility of errors in diagnosis and treatment.

With a good set–up the time consumed by cholangiography should be no more than 5 or 6 minutes. The surgeon should be well versed in the interpretation of the operative cholangiogram without requiring the attendance of a radiologist. Practice simplifies implementation. If image amplifiers with televised fluoroscopy are available one can observe filling, flow, and function of the duct as well as passage of dye into the duodenum. Films are nevertheless essential for a permanent record and details not well seen in fluoroscopy.

CHOLECYSTECTOMY FROM THE CYSTIC DUCT TO THE FUNDUS OR VICE VERSA?

The experienced surgeon can use either technique with equally good results. The important consideration is that the anatomy be completely and correctly identified before any ligation or section is performed.

Although many surgeons (4, 7, 10, 21, 26, 29, 34, 52) affirm that cholecystectomy should be done from the cystic duct to the fundus, many recommend changing the technique to fundus to cystic duct if needed in order to identify the cystic artery, the right hepatic and/or common hepatic artery, and the common duct. This attitude evidences that the latter method is safer (4, 22, 26, 29) and the author prefers to use it in teaching (20, 40). Entering the correct cleavage plane with this technique allows practically a bloodless resection even though ligature of the cystic artery is delayed until all the gallbladder has been separated from its bed. If inflammatory reaction is so intense that it is not possible to find the cleavage plane, the Pribram technique, modified by Mirizzi, may be used, as described further ahead. Cholecystectomy through the hepatic parenchyma results in very troublesome bleeding and should not be attempted.

SHOULD THE HEPATIC BED BE PERITONEALIZED?

At present many surgeons object to this, claiming that it is unnecessary and may trap blood draining from the bed. The author prefers peritonealization, which is usually feasible, for the following reasons:

1. To avoid adhesion of small bowel and even intestinal obstruction, which we have seen.

2. Peritonealization facilitates better hemostasis of the hepatic bed.
3. Aberrant bile ducts, which may have been sectioned inadvertently, are better sealed off.
4. Peritonealization has not produced any complication in more than 2,000 cholecystectomies performed by the author.

SHOULD DRAINAGE BE USED AFTER CHOLECYSTECTOMY?

The great majority of surgeons drain the abdomen after cholecystectomy using either a Penrose drain or a suction drainage tube. Other surgeons believe that draining is unnecessary and may be harmful and may lead to infection. The author favors leaving a suction drainage tube for 48 hours, not to drain blood but to detect bile in case a biliary duct has been traumatized inadvertently. This will allow early recognition so appropriate measures can be taken. If there were no drain, the bile would remain intraperitoneallv and diagnosis would be delayed. Some surgeons place the drain at Morison's pouch or in the foramen of Winslow. The important thing is to drain the undersurface of the liver. This gave rise to the term "subhepatic drain" coined by Mirizzi.

INCISIONS

Alternative incisions are many: subcostal and variations thereof, right paramedian, Mayo-Robson, hockey stick, Mallet-Guy, midline xipho– umbilical, and so on.

We employ only two of these incisions: the subcostal and the Mirizzi incision. The Mirizzi incision, to be described later, offers the advantages of the subcostal and the vertical incisions and gives excellent exposure.

Mirizzi Incision

This incision affords an excellent operative access in biliary or gastric surgery and for the repair of hiatus hernia, truncal or selective vagotomy, and so on. Drainage and T-tube extrusion may be made through the incision without debilitating the abdominal wall. Mirizzi, in 4,000 cholecystectomies observed no eviscerations. The author shares this experience in more than 2,000 cases.

Incisions

FIGURE 2.1 SUBCOSTAL INCISION

This is the most commonly used incision for cholecystectomy. It is placed 3 to 4 cm below and parallel to the costal margin. The incision may be extended upward and to the left, and may extend beyond the midline. It may also be extended beyond the lateral border of the anterior rectus muscle. The skin and subcutaneous tissue are incised and the incision continued with division of the anterior fascial sheath of the right rectus and the external oblique muscle. Incision of the rectus and of the internal oblique follow. The peritoneum is divided with the posterior fascia of the rectus muscle and with division of the transversus and its aponeurosis.

At closure the posterior rectus fascia and transversus muscle and aponeurosis are closed together with the peritoneum. The internal oblique aponeurosis and the anterior sheath of the rectus abdominus are sutured followed by closure of the anterior oblique, the subcutaneous tissue and skin. All sutures are interrupted and synthetic material of slow reabsorption is used.

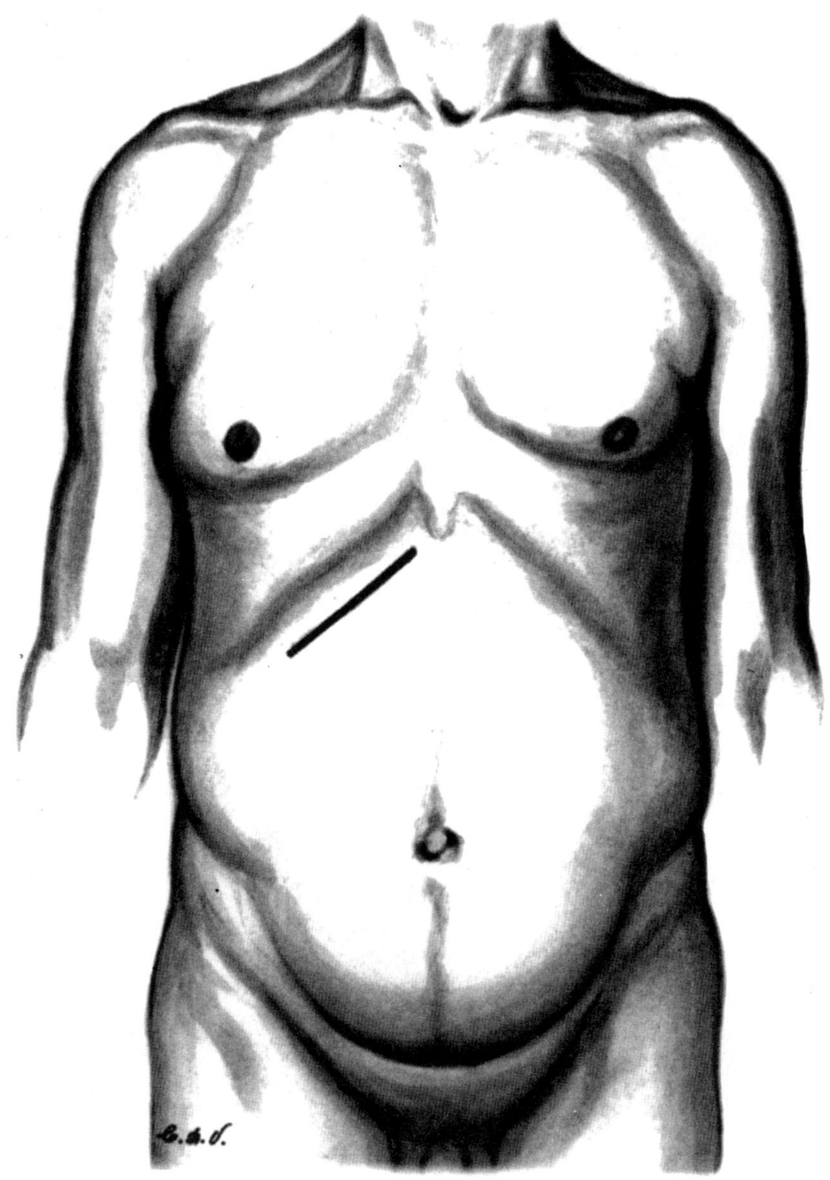

FIGURE 2.1 SUBCOSTAL INCISION

Mirizzi Incision

FIGURE 2.2
The Mirizzi incision consists of two parts: a vertical incision that divides the superficial planes and a subcostal incision that divides the deep layers. The vertical incision is transrectal, starting at the costal border extending downward 3 to 4 cm from the umbilical line. The incision should pass along a line between the medial third and the lateral two-thirds of the right rectus muscle.

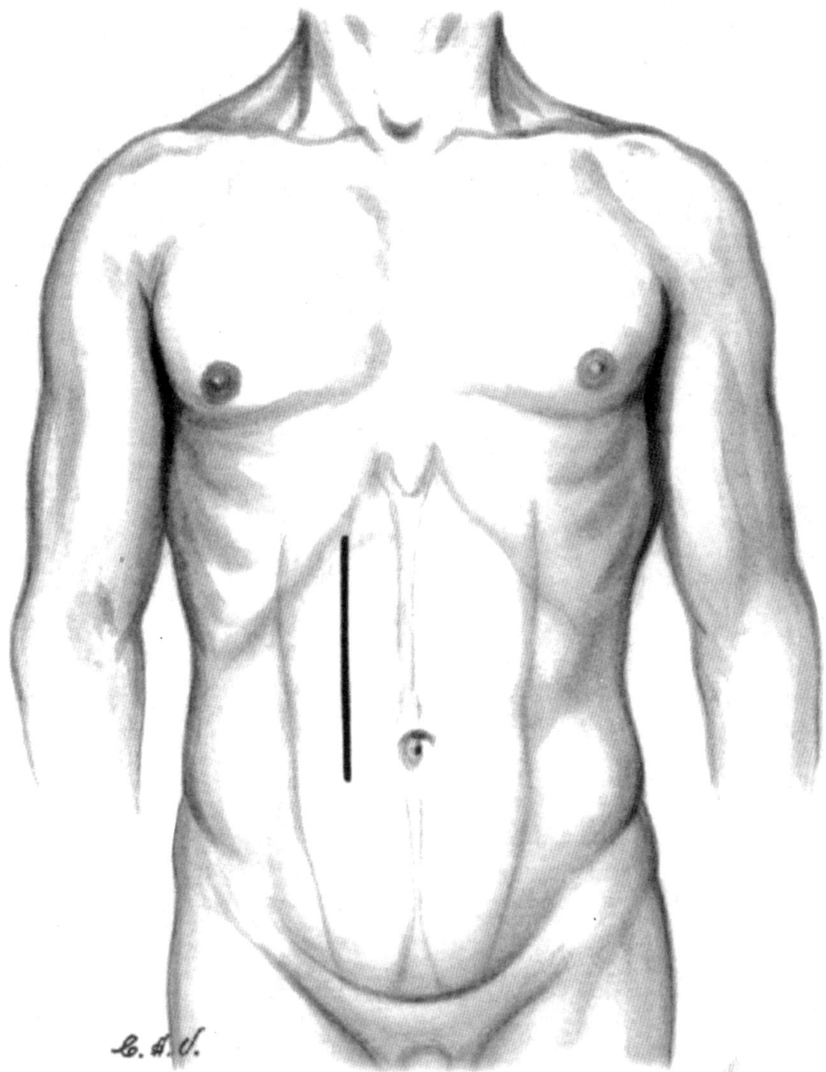

FIGURE 2.2

Mirizzi Incision

FIGURE 2.3
After opening the skin and superficial tissue and the rectus, the anterior rectus sheath is opened and the rectus fibers separated, exposing the deep layer made up by the transversus abdominis muscle and its aponeurosis, the transversus fascia and the peritoneum, as shown in the drawing.

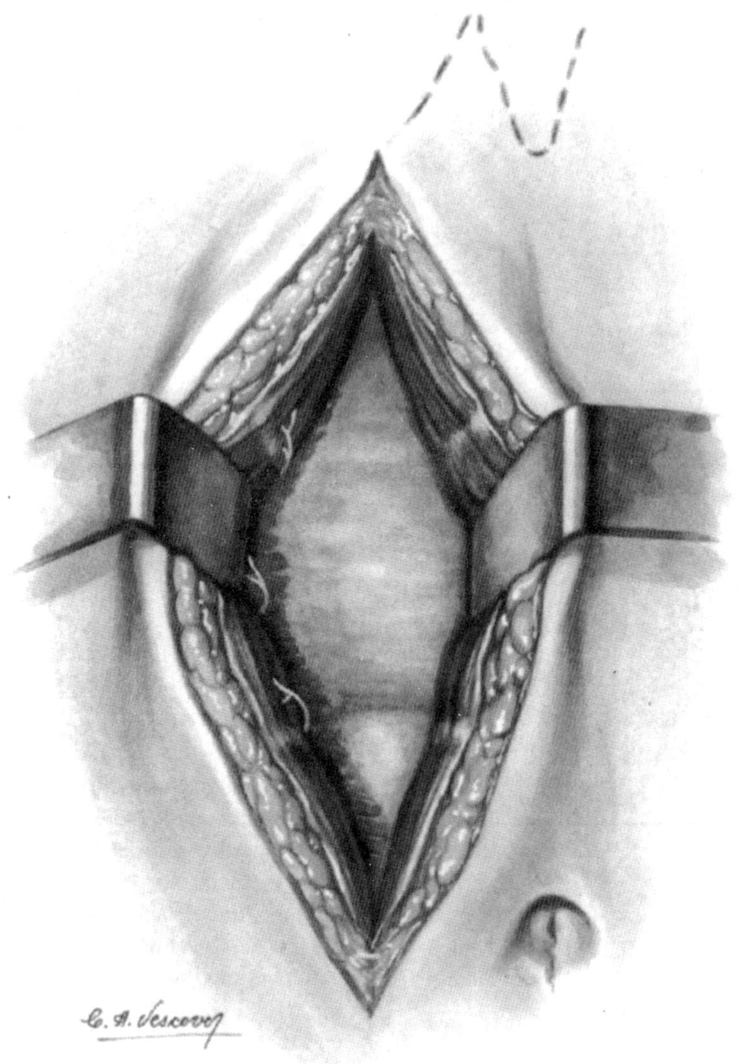

FIGURE 2.3

FIGURE 2.4

The borders of the rectus muscle are separated using retractors on either side. More traction is applied on the lateral side, permitting exposure of the costal border and the entrance of the intercostal nerves that enter the anterior rectus muscle from this deep plane. Though rarely necessary, the intercostal nerves and vessels may be dissected and displaced toward the costal border for 1 to 2 cm. The aponeurosis of the transversus is grasped with an Allis clamp and retracted downward and to the left. If the muscle is very developed, it, and not the aponeurosis, is grasped with the Allis clamp. The first assistant continues to exert traction, and this permits a subcostal incision 3 to 4 cm from this costal border as shown by the line in the drawing. This in turn permits division of the transversus, its aponeurosis, the transversalis fascia, and the peritoneum.

Mirizzi Incision

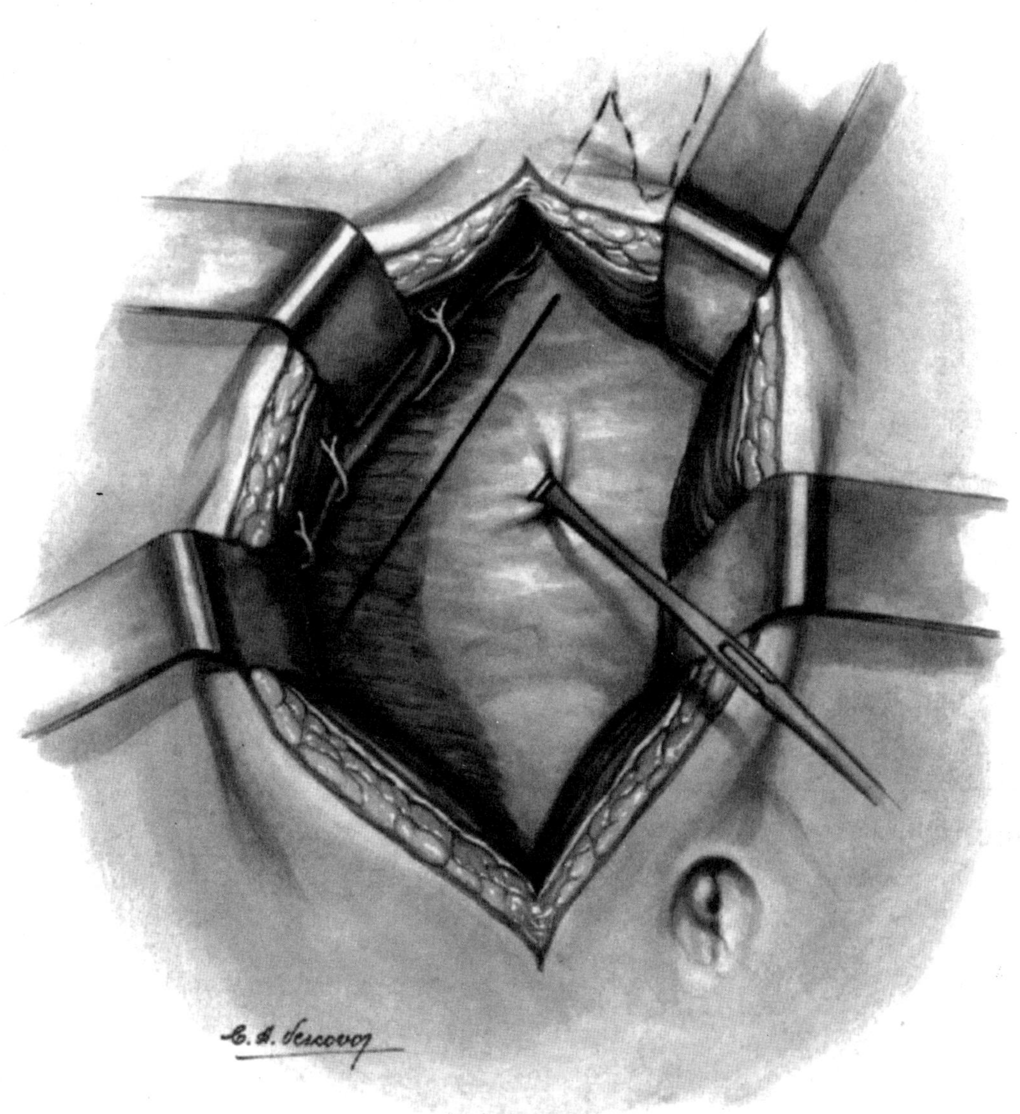

FIGURE 2.4

Mirizzi Incision

FIGURE 2.5
The drawing shows the deeper part of the Mirizzi incision. Allis clamps hold up the borders applying moderate traction. The superior portion of the incision is made with scissors. Extension of the incision beyond the linea alba may be made, even excising the xiphoid process, if need be.

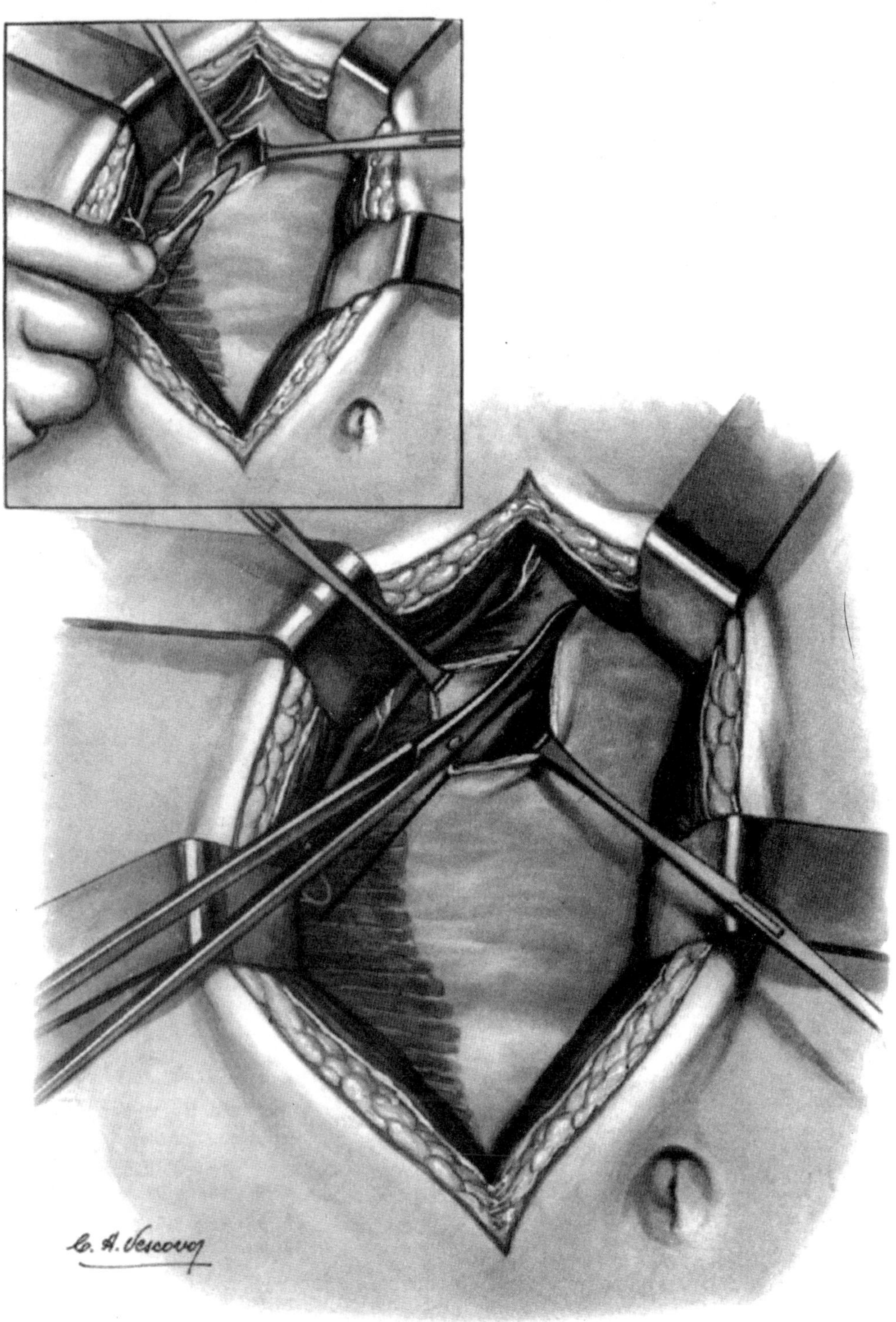

FIGURE 2.5

Mirizzi Incision

FIGURE 2.6
The inferior portion of the deep plane is made with a scalpel. The surgeon retracts with two fingers of the left hand in the abdominal cavity to permit incision with the scalpel. The intercostal nerves are visible, and the surgeon may thus decide to section the ninth intercostal nerve or not. In the subcostal incision the ninth intercostal nerve is always divided.

The need to section the ninth intercostal nerve depends on the need for extension of the incision. The division of the rectus muscle seldom makes it necessary to extend the deeper part of the incision.

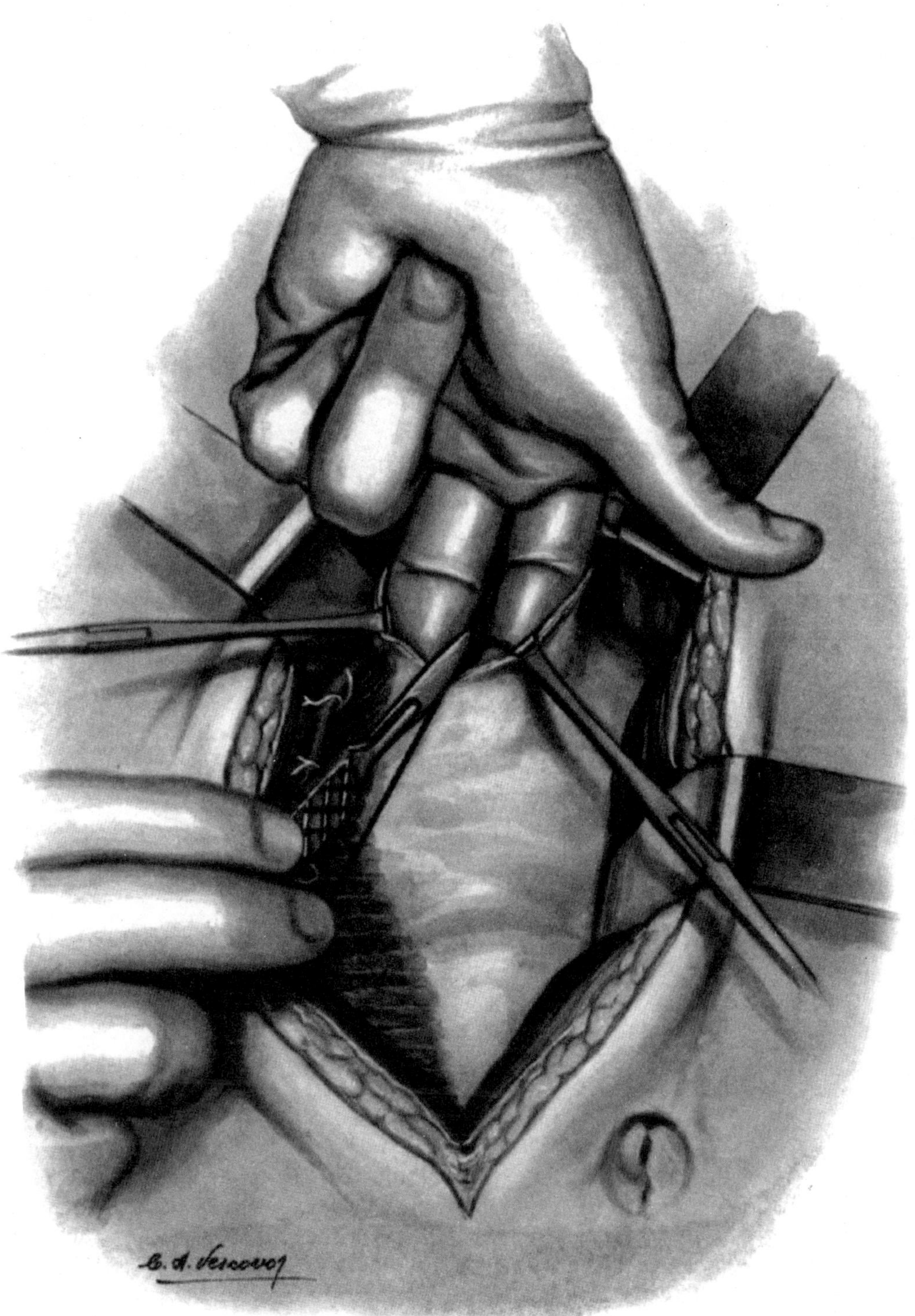

FIGURE 2.6

Mirizzi Incision

FIGURE 2.7
Mirizzi's self-retaining retractor is inserted once the abdominal cavity has been opened, amplifying the operative field. The deeper blade retracts the lateral portion of the incision and the smaller one retracts the medial portion.

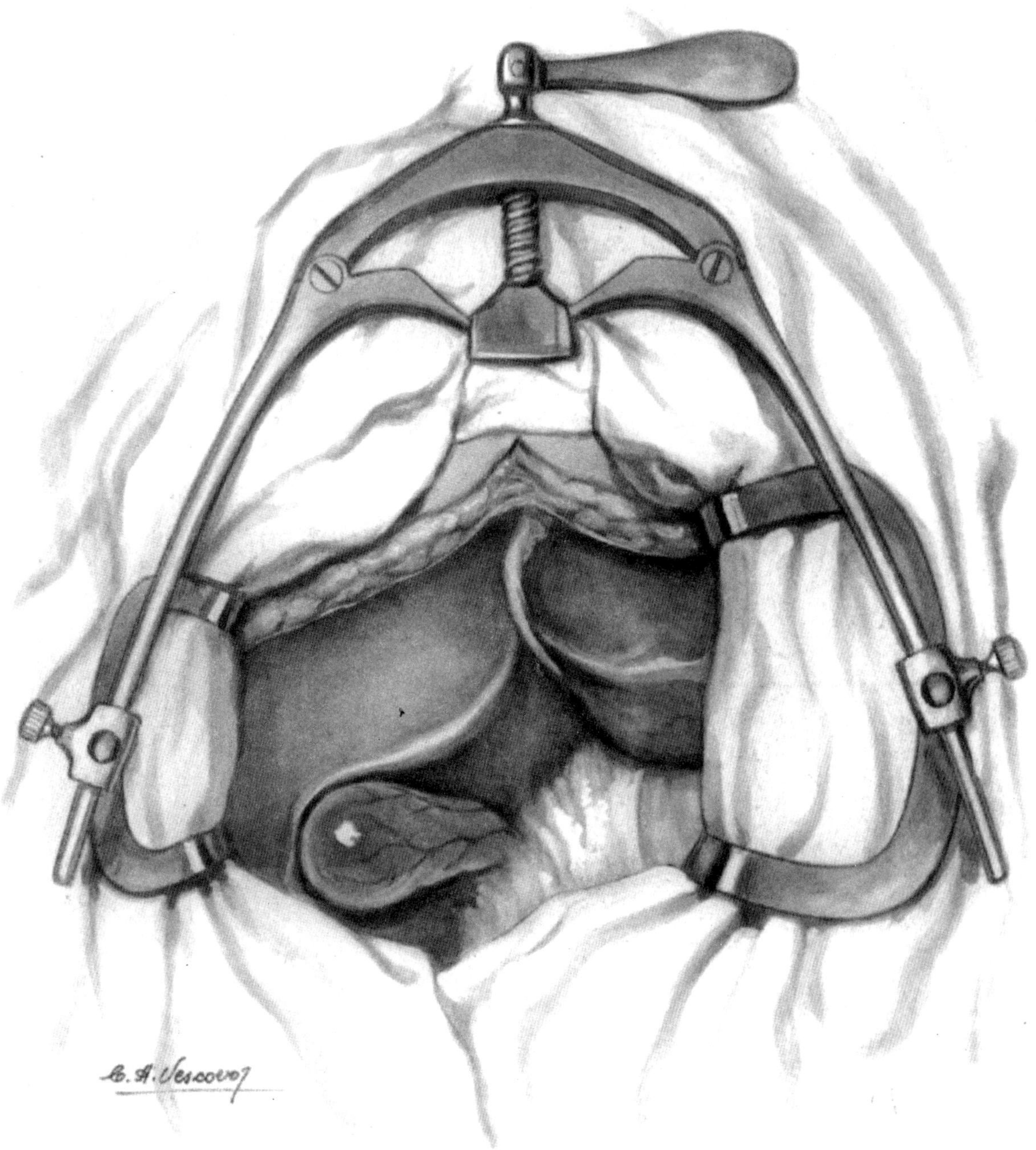

FIGURE 2.7

Mirizzi Incision

FIGURE 2.8
Mirizzi's incision is closed starting with the deeper incision at its inferior angle and using interrupted sutures of synthetic material of slow absorption. This plane is very strong because it consists of the aponeurosis of the transversus muscle plus fascia transversalis and peritoneum. Care must be taken to avoid including the neighboring intercostal nerves in the suture.

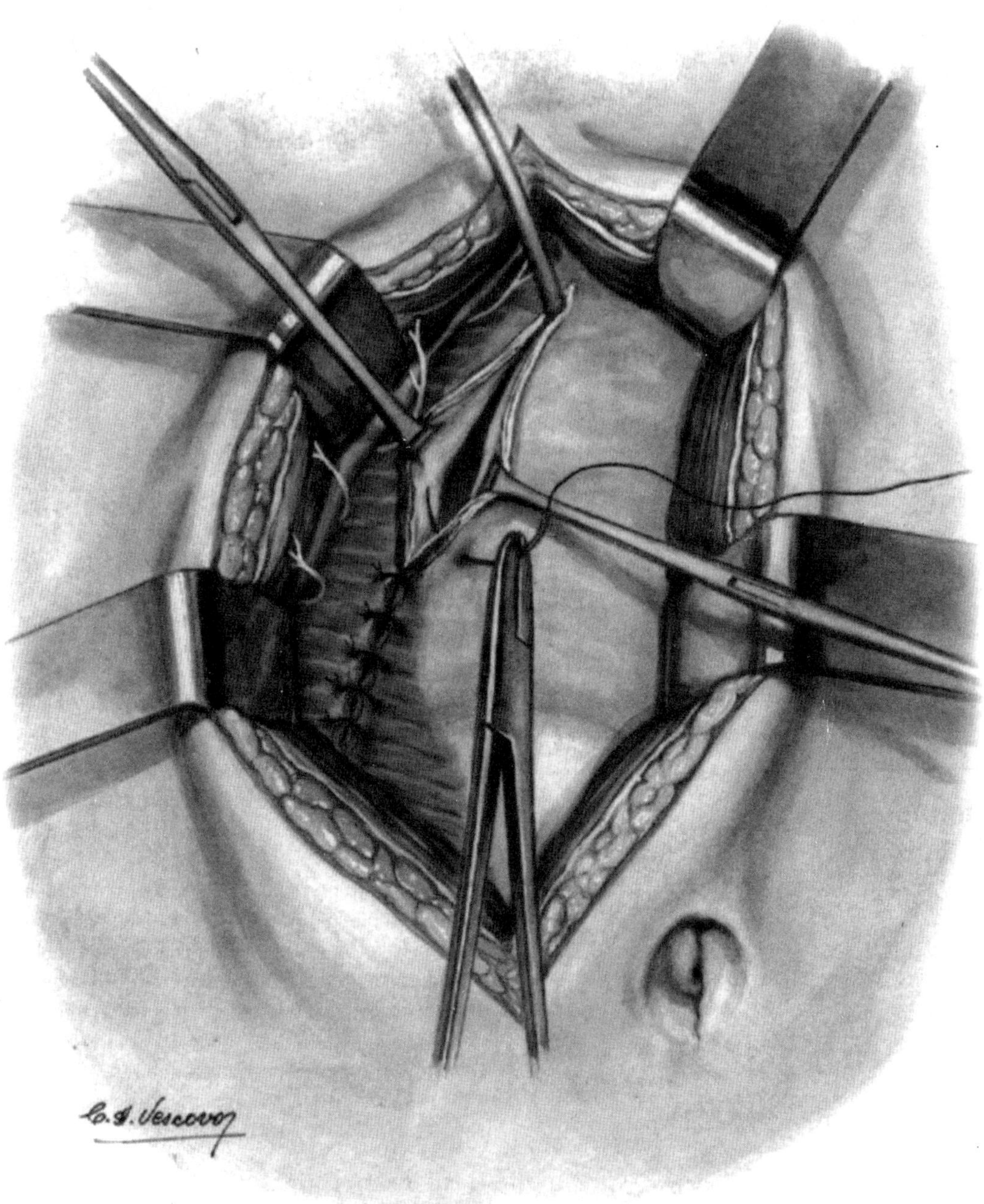

FIGURE 2.8

Mirizzi Incision

FIGURE 2.9
The drainage tube to the subhepatic area is placed as desired before completing closure. We usually place this at the superior angle of the incision to drain the subhepatic space. A T-tube would be similarly placed. The T-tube should exit as directly as possible in case manipulation becomes necessary (36, 37). Closure of the anterior fascia of the rectus muscle follows with similar interrupted sutures. Please note that the layers of closure are not superimposed on each other. Drains and the T-tube are fixed with sutures to the skin.

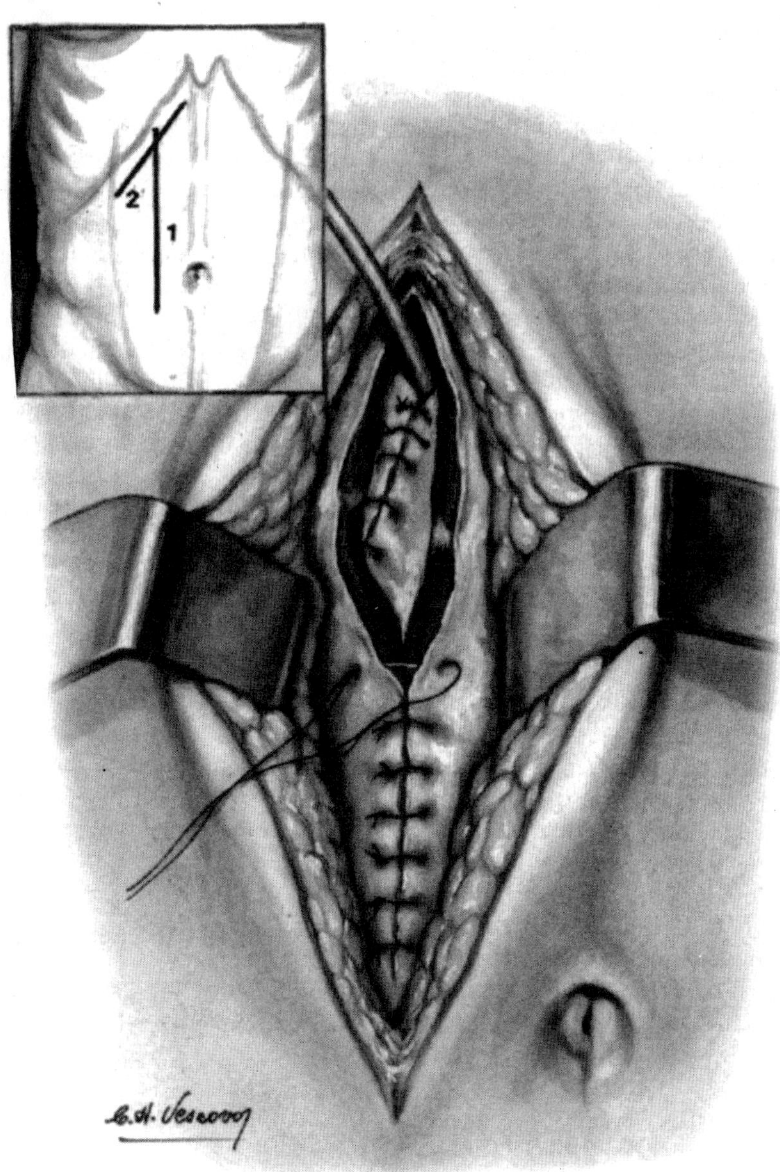

FIGURE 2.9

CHOLECYSTECTOMY BY MINILAPARATOMY

Cholecystectomv by minilaparatomy is being proposed and preferred in increasing numbers. Experienced surgeons know well that some gallbladders are easy to remove whereas others tax the ingenuity of the most experienced surgeon. We prefer an adequate incision to obtain a good operative field, good illumination, and good anesthetic relaxation. All of these precautions minimize serious problems and errors that could be fatal. A mini-incision becomes a funnel and results in more errors. Adequate exposure is one of the most important factors in any surgical procedure.

CHOLECYSTECTOMY FROM FUNDUS TO CYSTIC DUCT

Once the abdomen is open, a complete exploration is carried out in search of other lesions. Attention is then directed to the gallbladder, hepatocholedochus, duodenum, papilla of Vater, and pancreas. At this time the existence of calculi is confirmed. If the gallbladder presents normal or inflammatory adhesions to adjacent organs, duodenum, colon or greater omentum, these should be carefully divided. This should be done near the gallbladder, since at this level there is less hemorrhage. Besides, entering the gallbladder is less serious than entering the duodenum or the colon. The gallbladder is isolated and traction is applied on the fundus with a Duval clamp held in the surgeon's right hand while the left hand is introduced between the liver and diaphragm and the liver rotated forward and to the right. Exposure of the biliary structures is thus enhanced. It may be necessary to aspirate a tense gallbladder to facilitate this maneuver. In some cases the gallbladder is tense not owing to fluid but because it is full of calculi. Several seromuscular sutures on the gallbladder may be used to apply traction with a clamp. Before proceeding with the cholecystectomy, the surgeon should confirm the presence of calculi. This is usually easily done by palpation, but in some cases the gallbladder is tense and does not allow the palpation of small calculi, even though they may be numerous. In these cases the infundibulum, the neck of the gallbladder, or the cystic duct should be palpated, since it is easier to feel calculi in these areas. If calculi are still not felt, the gallbladder can be punctured and aspirated, removing part of its liquid contents, allowing caluli to be felt. The gallbladder should always be palpated gently, especially with small calculi, since too much pressure on palpation may force calculi into the bile ducts, where they may be hard to find, especially if they have migrated to the hepatic duct or its branches. In some cases the gallbladder has the same appearance as in cases of cholelithiasis but does not contain calculi because these have migrated to the ducts or further on. In these cases the gallbladder should be removed. Exploration of the bile ducts will show if they contain calculi or if they have been eliminated.

Preparation of the Operative Field

Methodical and orderly surgery is facilitated by preparation of the operative field.

Cholecystectomy From Fundus To Cystic Duct

Cholecystectomy From Fundus To Cystic Duct

FIGURE 2.10

The Mirizzi incision has been made and the Mirizzi self-retaining retractor is in place, giving excellent exposure. The gallbladder has been freed of adhesions, and an atraumatic triangular Duval clamp applied for traction upward and forward. The liver has been rotated and a gauze pack placed to displace and hold the transverse colon and its mesentery downward, held in place with a wide Deaver retractor. The stomach and duodenum are held to the left under a gauze pack and another Deaver. Visualization of biliary structures is very adequate. The broken line indicates where the peritoneum over the gallbladder is to be sectioned, 2 cm from the liver.

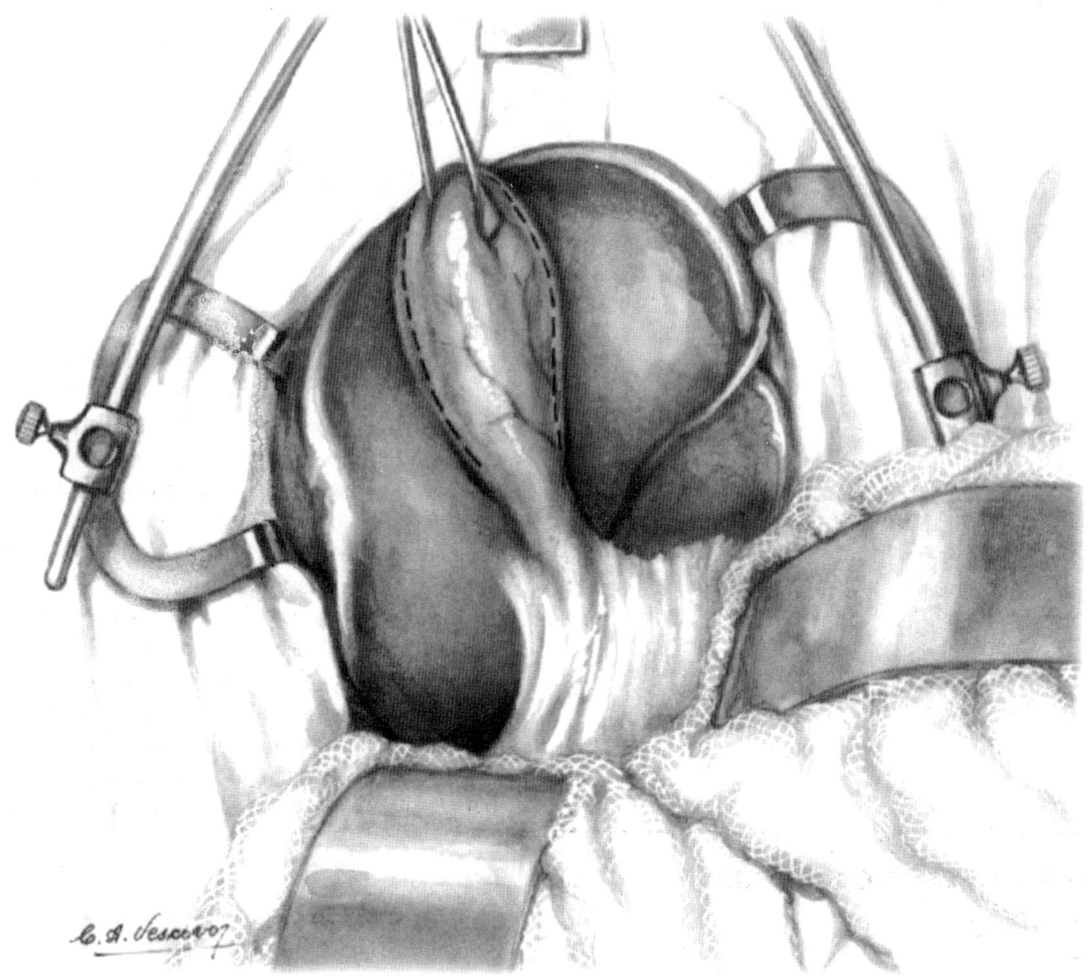

FIGURE 2.10

FIGURE 2.11
The serosa over the fundus of the gallbladder has been incised with a scalpel, and the cut edges are held with two hemostatic clamps. Once this is done we proceed with the important step of finding the correct cleavage plane, which will allow the resection of the gallbladder in bloodless fashion without having to previously ligate the cystic artery. To do this the surgeon places traction with his or her left hand on the clamps that hold the peritoneum, upward and backward, while with the right hand he or she places traction on the triangular clamp, holding the gallbladder in the opposite direction. This simple maneuver allows the finding of the cleavage plane between the fibromuscular layer of the gallbladder and the areolar layer that separates the gallbladder from the liver bed. The rest of the dissection should remain in this plane. The dotted line shows the rest of the peritoneal incision over the gallbladder.

Cholecystectomy from Fundus to Cystic Duct

FIGURE 2.12
The drawing shows the dissection of the body of the gallbladder in the correct cleavage plane. Traction on the peritoneum is applied by the second assistant holding the hemostats while traction on the gallbladder is applied by the first assistant. The surgeon continues the dissection of the gallbladder using scissors in the correct plane.

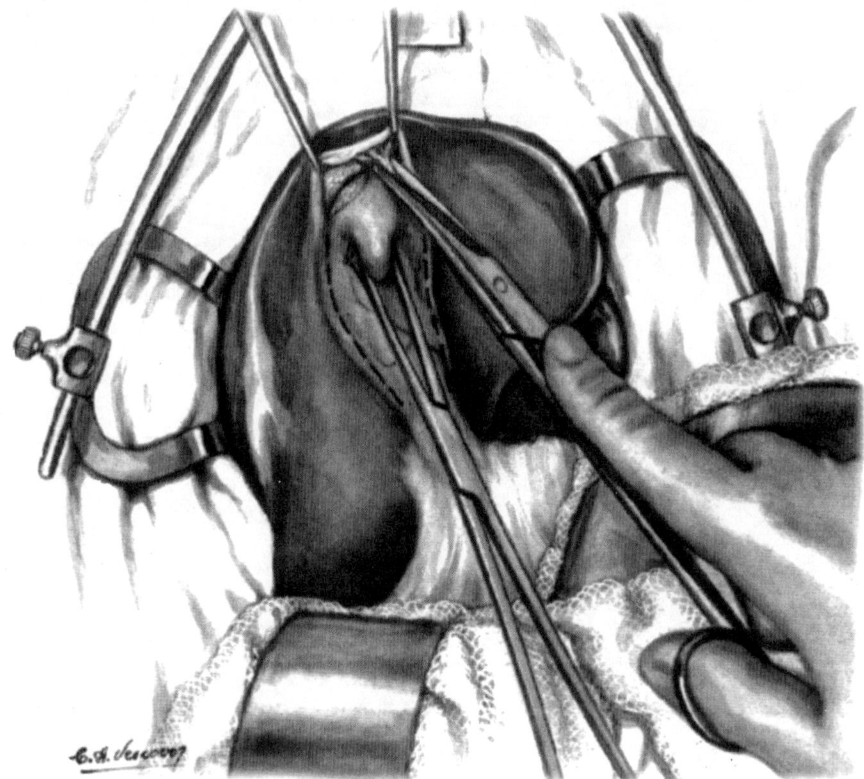

FIGURE 2.11

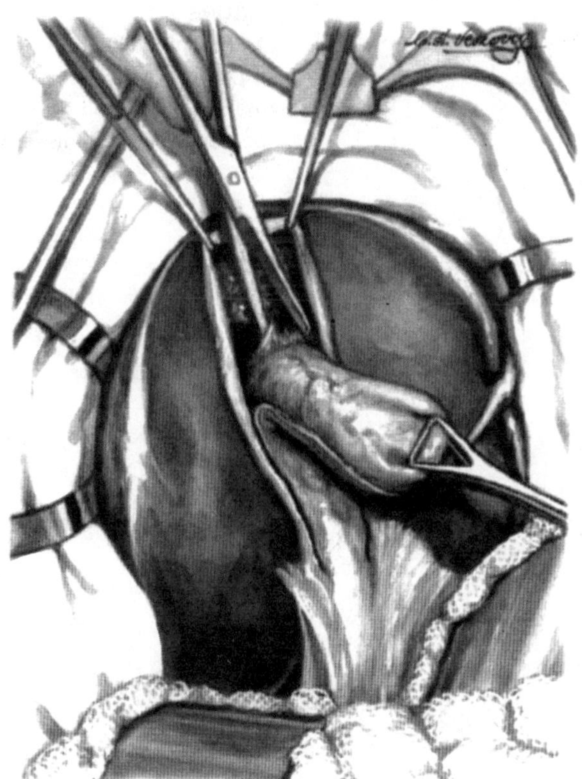

FIGURE 2.12

Cholecystectomy from Fundus to Cystic Duct

FIGURE 2.13
As the infundibulum is reached the clamps are withdrawn and a Doyen retractor is used to displace the liver bed backward making dissection of the gallbladder easier. This may at times be done by digital dissection.

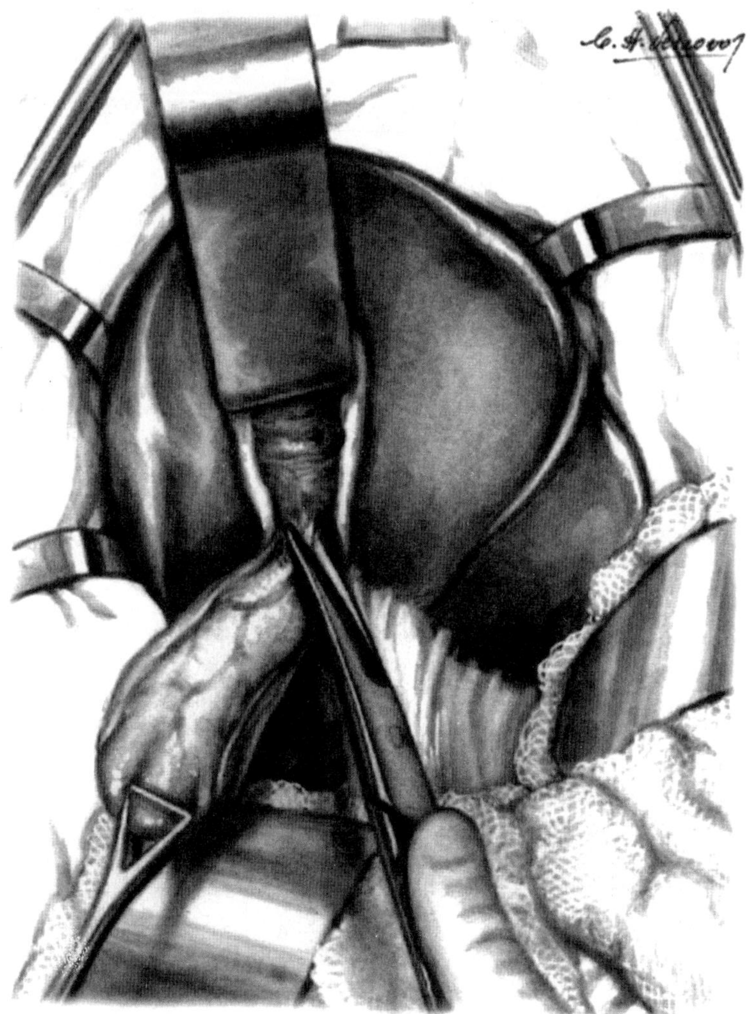

FIGURE 2.13

FIGURE 2.14

The dissection proceeds to the neck of the gallbladder. The cystic artery is identified at the neck, where it usually courses above and behind the gallbladder. The whole course of the cystic artery from its origin to its entering the gallbladder, where it divides in two branches, an anterior and a posterior branch, should be followed. The cystic artery usually arises from the right hepatic artery within the triangle of Calot constituted by the neck and cystic duct to the outside and the common hepatic duct to the inside. The cystic artery is not divided or ligated until its origin and termination have been established without doubt. The right hepatic and even the common hepatic artery may present as the cystic artery, leading to many accidents in biliary surgery. The right hepatic artery may even curve markedly and abut into the vestibule of the gallbladder. This is frequently associated with a very short cystic artery, making it easy to confuse with the right hepatic artery. Once the cystic artery is identified and dissected, two ligatures are applied to it, well apart from each other, one at the junction with the gallbladder and the other toward its origin. The cystic artery is then divided between the ligatures (see insert). During all this procedure the common anatomic variations of the cystic artery must be kept in mind.

Cholecystectomy from Fundus to Cystic Duct

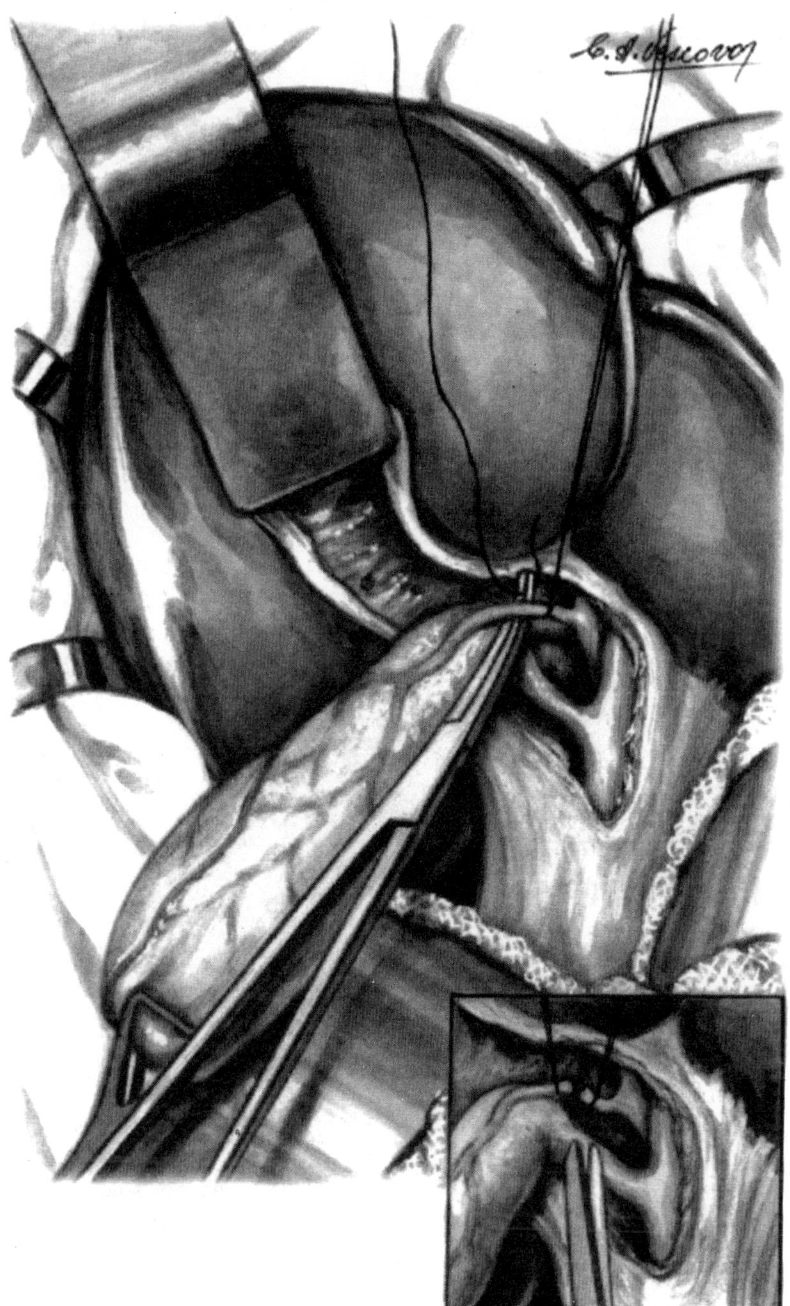

FIGURE 2.14

Cholecystectomy from Fundus to Cystic Duct

FIGURE 2.15

Ligature of the cystic artery makes it easier to straighten out the cystic duct. The duct should be freed to its junction with the hepatic duct. Stones in the cystic duct or infundibulum should be squeezed up toward the gallbladder. A clamp is then placed across the neck to prevent spillage of bile when the cystic duct is transected. As this is done, two guide sutures are placed on the distal cystic duct to avoid retraction on sectioning it. The insert shows the gallbladder being removed. The gallbladder must be opened and carefully examined by the surgeon before it is sent to the pathologist.

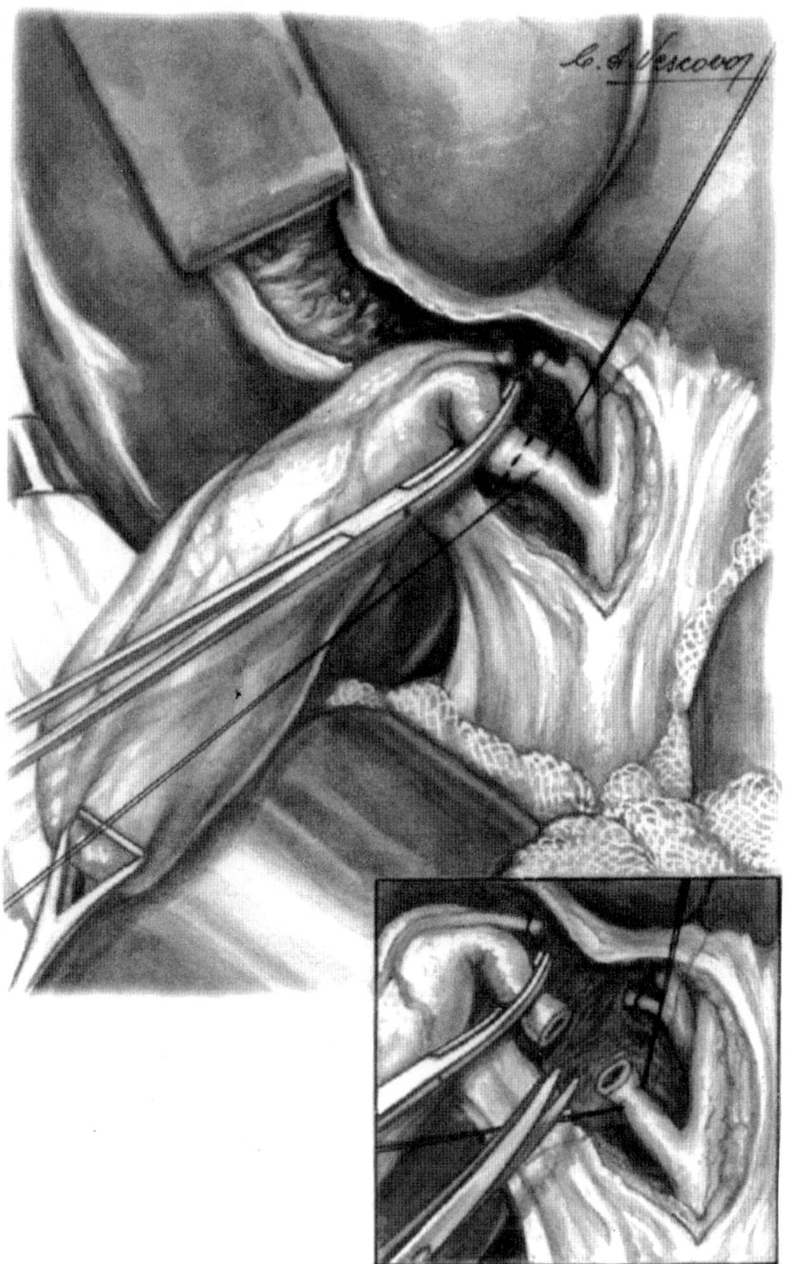

FIGURE 2.15

FIGURE 2.16
The two guide sutures on the cystic duct, placed there to prevent its retraction, have been removed. Four sutures have been placed on the border of the cystic duct to enlarge its lumen. Heister's valves constitute an inconvenience in the introduction of the polyethylene catheter used in the cholangiography. They are ironed out by introducing a thin hemostat within the duct and gently opening and closing it within the duct so as to stretch the duct and facilitate insertion of the cholangiogram tubing. This facilitates passing the cholangiogram tube into the choledochus. The tube, filled with a radiopaque solution diluted to 25 to 30% and weaned of air bubbles, is introduced gently into the common duct. Injection of fluid should be gentle to avoid displacing calculi upward. Five mL are injected and a film taken to study the distal common duct and to obtain an image clear of superimposition with the dye passing into the duodenum. Now 10 mL are injected to study the hepatocholedochus. If the duct is dilated, 10 mL or more are injected, according to the degree of dilation of the common duct. An image amplifier and televised fluoroscopy afford a dynamic study of the biliary tree.

Cholecystectomy from Fundus to Cystic Duct

FIGURE 2.17
If the cholangiography is normal the cystic duct is ligated next to the choledochus and the cystic duct resected up to the ligature. The hepatic bed is closed with interrupted suture, beginning either proximally or distally.

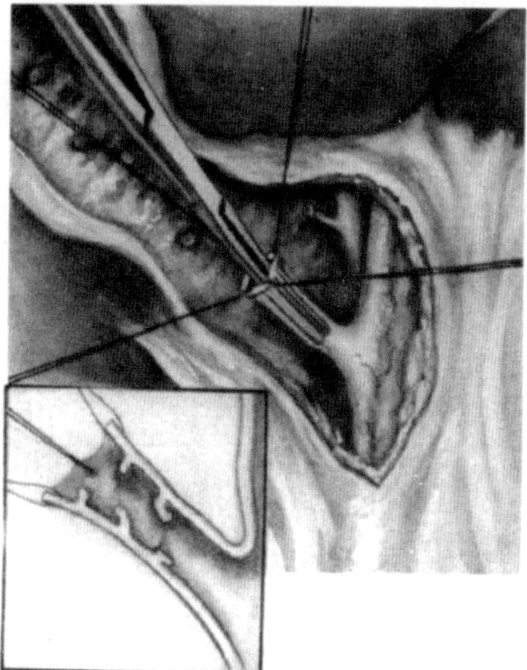

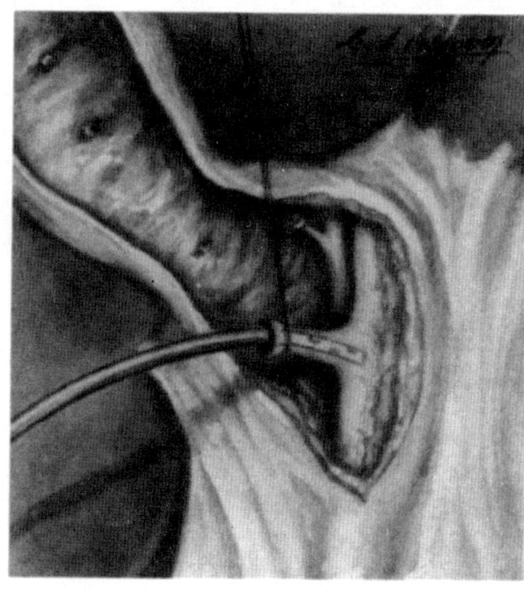

FIGURE 2.16

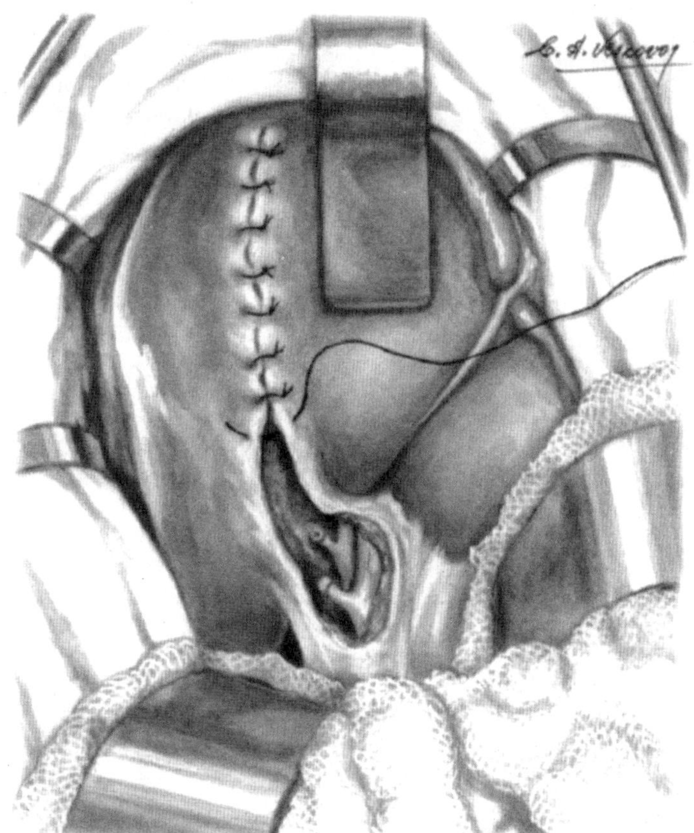

FIGURE 2.17

Cholecystectomy from Fundus to Cystic Duct

FIGURE 2.18
Peritonealization has been completed, including the gallbladder bed, choledochus, cystic duct, and cystic artery stumps. The drawing shows a drainage tube exiting from the foramen of Winslow. This tube is usually left in place for about 48 hours.

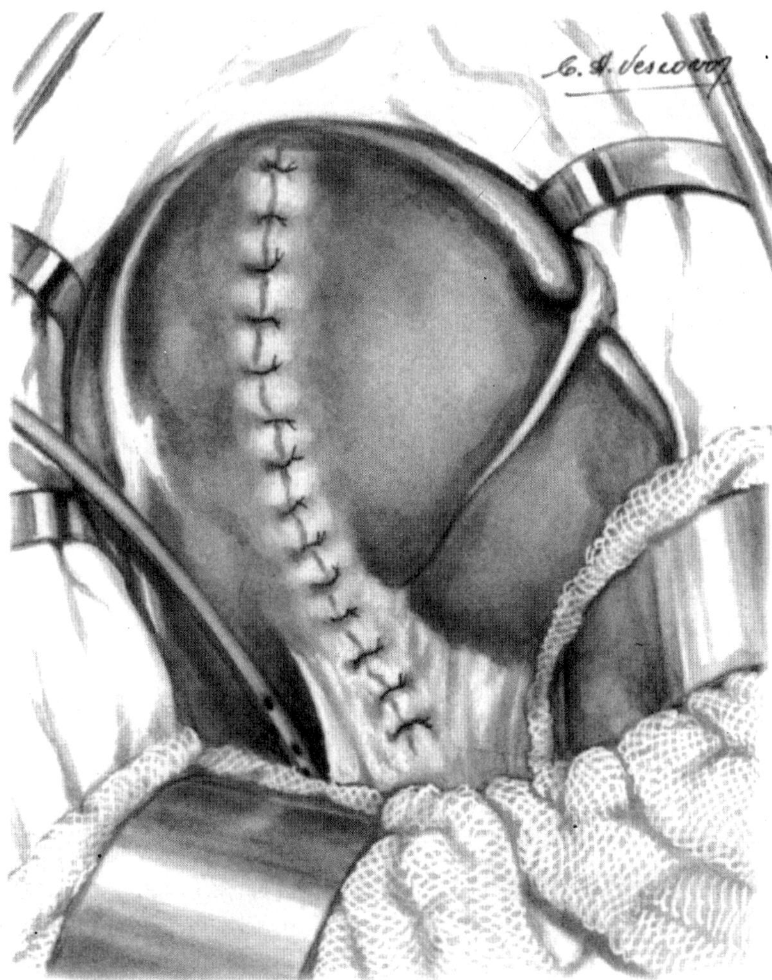

FIGURE 2.18

Cholecystectomy from Cystic Duct to Fundus

FIGURE 2.19

After the same exposure previously described, the fundus of the gallbladder is grasped with an atraumatic triangular Duval clamp and retracted gently upward and backward. The next step is designed to identify the cystic artery and duct. The peritoneal border of the hepatoduodenal ligament is incised, grasping the anterior edge of the incision with forceps and continuing this incision parallel to the choledochus. We use a scissors for this step, which allows us to identify the cystic artery and the cystic duct.

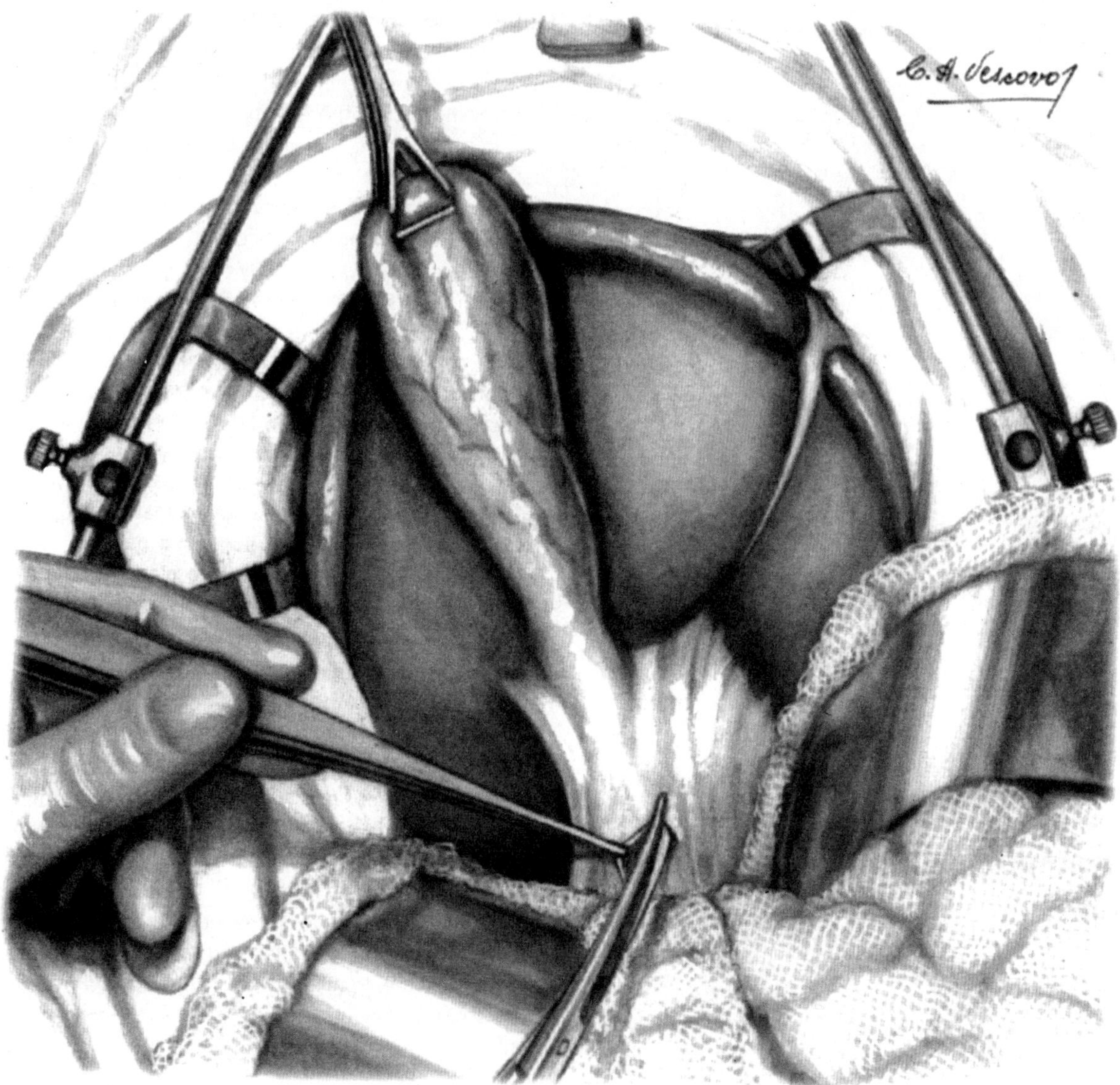

FIGURE 2.19

FIGURE 2.20

The peritoneum is cut with scissors and then separated with scissors or a gauze dissector in order to identify the junction of the cystic duct to the hepatic duct where it forms the cystohepatic angle of the triangle of Calot in which we can then investigate the cystic artery.

To be sure that it is the cystic artery that has been identified, it must be followed throughout its entire extent, from its origin in the right hepatic artery to its penetration into the gallbladder. The cystic artery may present many anatomic variations, in its origin as in its course. Therefore, the other structures in the hepatic pedicle must be identified before ligating the cystic artery. This artery can be confused with the right hepatic or even with the common hepatic artery. The cystic artery should be ligated close to the gallbladder, as shown in the drawing. The cystic artery can at times be lacerated if it is surrounded by an inflammatory reaction, leading to an intense hemorrhage that may test the surgeon's patience. In these circumstances one should not rush to place hemostatic clamps without clearly seeing the bleeding vessel, which generally retracts toward the hepatic artery. Blind clamping may cause damage to the right hepatic or common hepatic arteries or the common bile duct, with dire consequences. It is fundamental that the surgeon remain calm and transmit this calm to the team by actions and not by words. The blood should be rapidly suctioned, and the Pringle maneuver performed. This consists of compression of the hepatic artery in the hepatic pedicle between fingers to stop the bleeding. The blood should again be aspirated and, with a clean field, the pressure on the artery partially and intermittently released to clearly see the bleeding cystic artery so it can be clamped and tied with great care. In some cases the Pringle maneuver using the surgeon's left hand is not sufficient because it immobilizes one of the surgeon's hands at a decisive moment—particularly if the assistants are not experienced. In these cases temporary hemostasis can be attained using an atraumatic vascular clamp such as a bulldog clamp. See Figures 2.21 and 2.22 for these explanations.

Cholecystectomy from Cystic Duct to Fundus

FIGURE 2.21 PRINGLE MANEUVER

This maneuver consists of compression of the hepatoduodenal ligament between the index finger of the left hand posteriorly and the thumb anteriorly to compress the hepatic artery and obtain temporary hemostasis in order to better visualize the bleeding vessel and proceed with its ligation without injuring other structures.

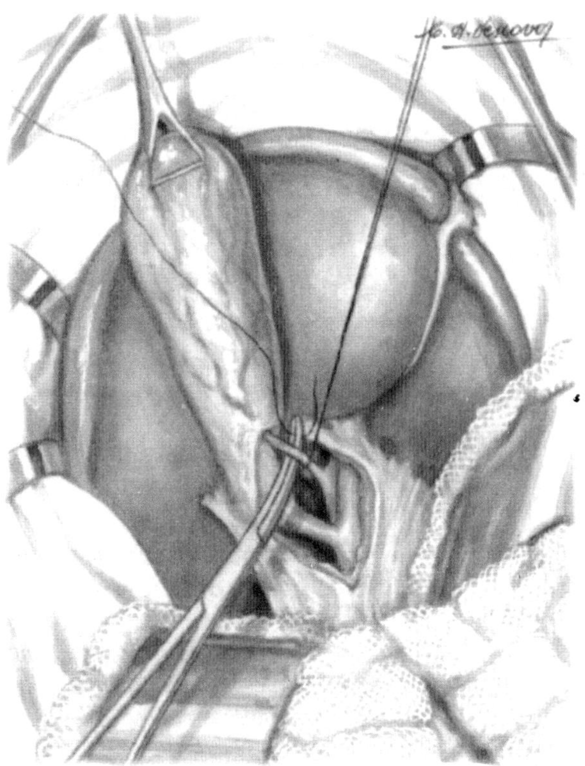

FIGURE 2.20

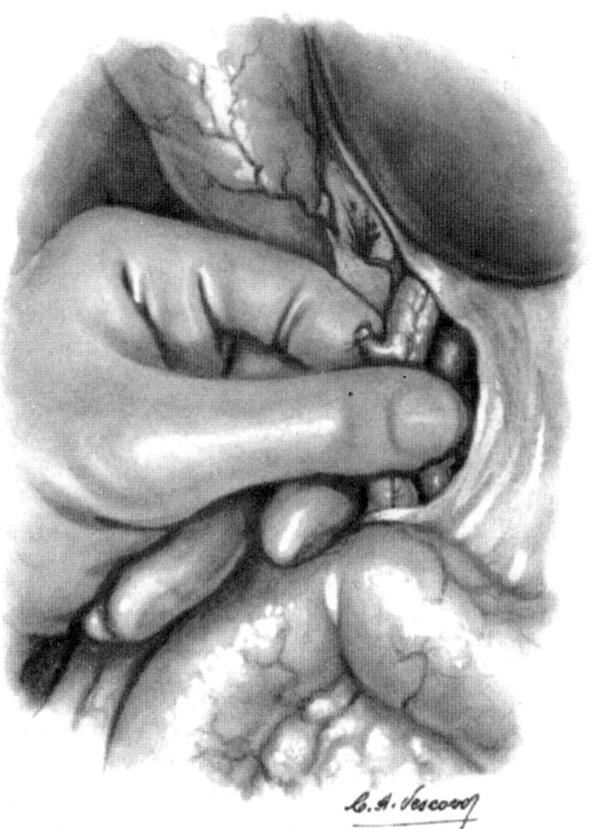

FIGURE 2.21 PRINGLE MANEUVER

FIGURE 2.22 HEPATIC ARTERY COMPRESSION WITH BULLDOG CLAMP

This modality frees a hand of the surgeon using a vascular clamp, giving the surgeon and the team more mobility. It is advisable not to clamp the hepatic artery for more than 20 minutes at a time.

Cholecystectomy from Cystic Duct to Fundus

FIGURE 2.23

The cystic artery has been tied and divided near the gallbladder. A clamp has been applied at the neck of the gallbladder to avoid spillage of bile. Two guide sutures placed in the cystic duct distally are evident. The insert indicates the site of division of the cystic duct in broken lines.

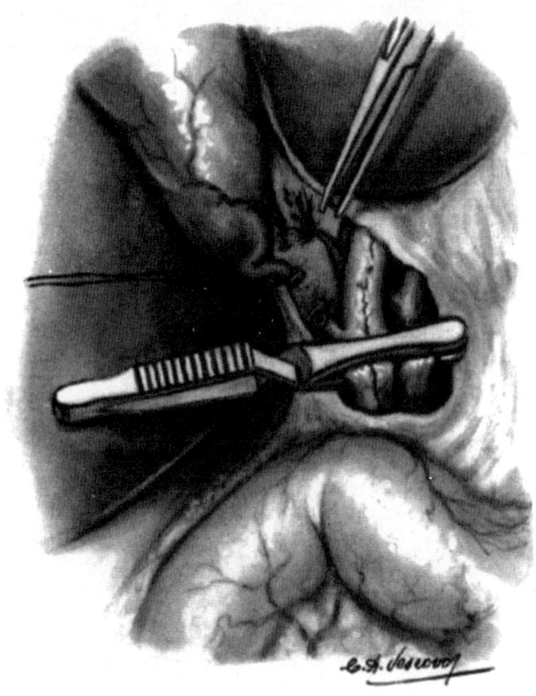

FIGURE 2.22 HEPATIC ARTERY COMPRESSION WITH BULLDOG CLAMP

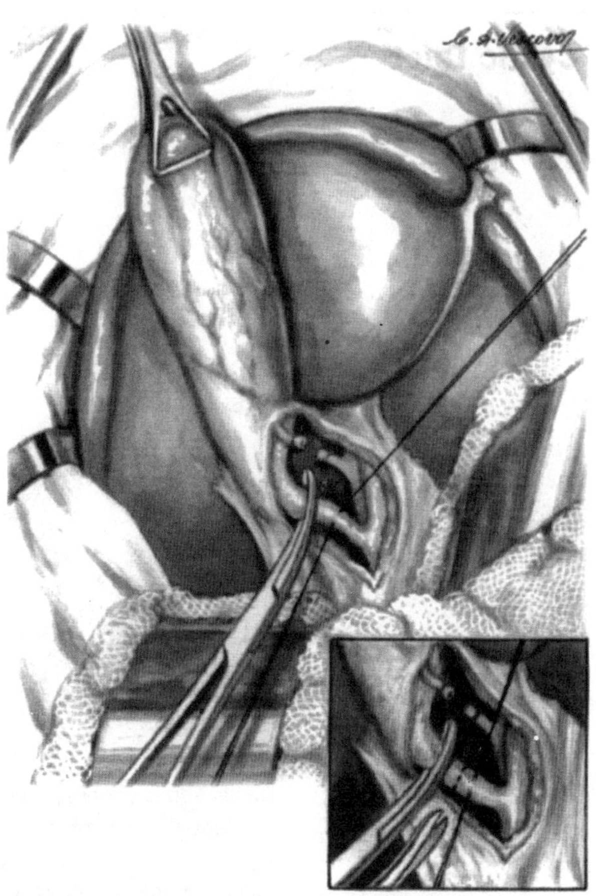

FIGURE 2.23

FIGURE 2.24
After dividing the cystic duct, upward traction on the clamp at the neck of the gallbladder permits resection of the gallbladder within the correct cleavage plane, avoiding entering the liver substance which may lead to troublesome bleeding.

Cholecystectomy from Cystic Duct to Fundus

FIGURE 2.25
Dissection proceeds, sharply or bluntly in the cleavage plane. Incidentally appearing small bleeders are electrocoagulated. Aberrant bile ducts are suture ligated to prevent postoperative bile drainage. Peritonealization may proceed during or after gallbladder resection.

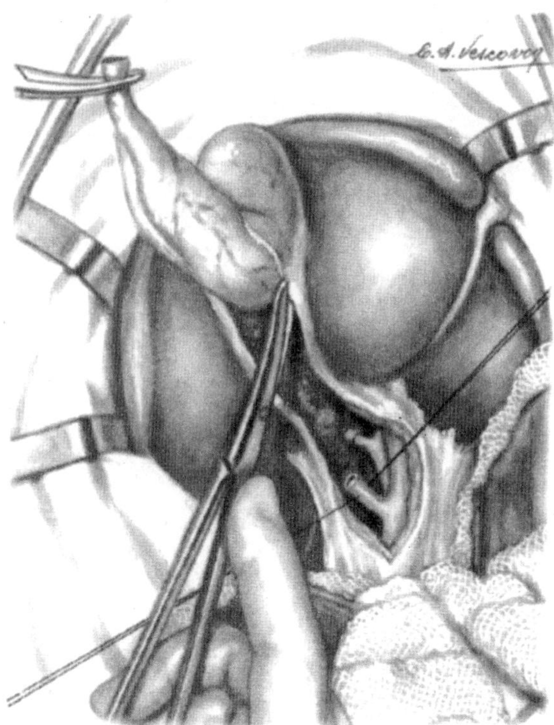

FIGURE 2.24

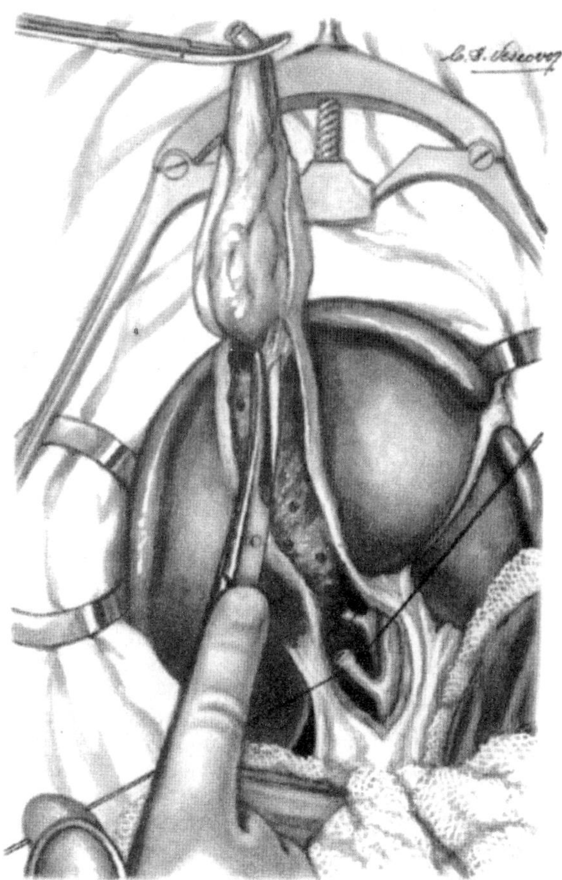

FIGURE 2.25

FIGURE 2.26
A cholangiography tube has been placed within the cystic duct and ligated in place. If the study is normal, the cystic duct is ligated next to the common hepatic duct and the redundant cystic duct is removed. Peritonealization can then be completed.

Cholecystectomy from Cystic Duct to Fundus

FIGURE 2.27
Peritonealization proceeds with interrupted sutures. The author prefers peritonealization of the hepatic bed for the following reasons:

1. To eliminate raw surfaces and attendant adhesions of small bowel with possible postoperative bowel obstruction.
2. For better hemostasis.
3. To avoid bile drainage from aberrant ducts in the gallbladder bed.
4. The author has never had a complication caused by having peritonealized the liver bed.

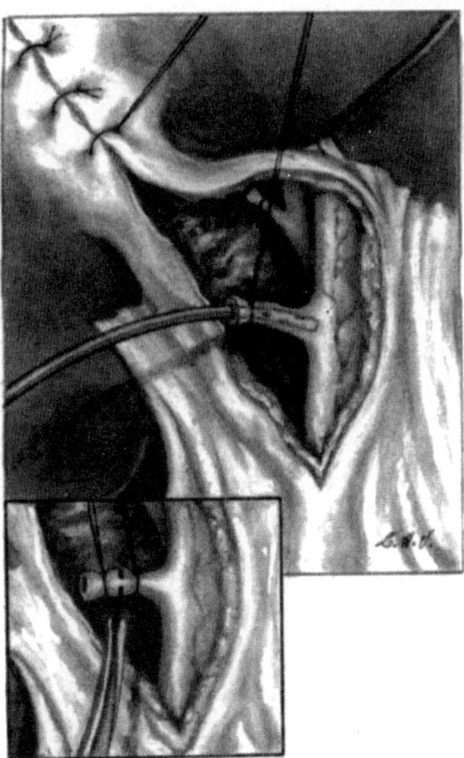

FIGURE 2.26

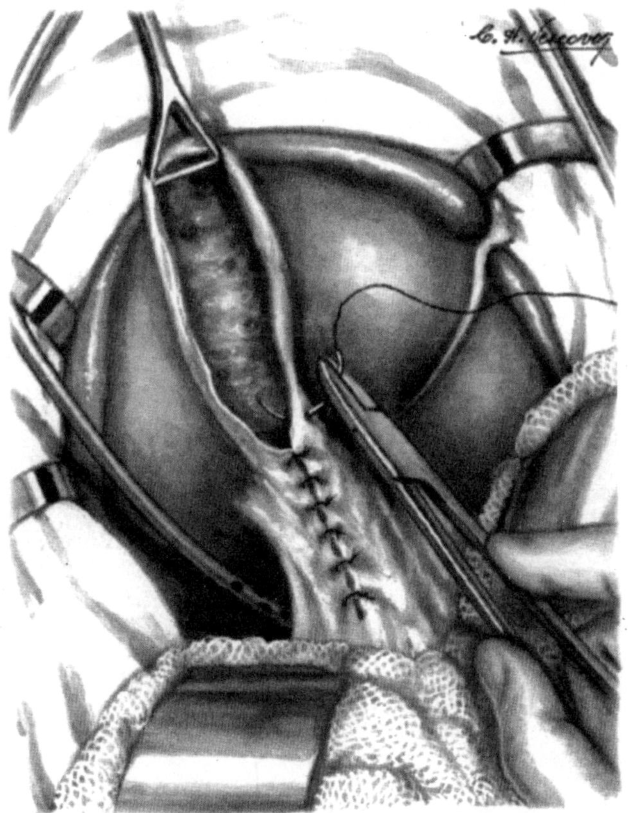

FIGURE 2.27

CHOLECYSTECTOMY BY THE PRIBRAM TECHNIQUE

Pribram's technique was described in 1928 and later modified by the same author and by Mirizzi and Olmedo (40, 43) in Argentina. It is indicated in severe inflammatory processes, acute or chronic, where the anatomy has been altered and no cleavage plane, as previously described, exists between the gallbladder and the hepatic bed.

Cholecystectomy performed by the modified Pribram technique converts a difficult cholecystectomy to an easy one. A well-performed modified Pribram technique gives good results. Torek (50) also used a modification of the Pribram technique, which will not be described since we do not consider it practical.

Cholecystectomy by the Pribram Technique

FIGURE 2.28
The preparation of the operative field is the same as previously described plus the addition of gauze pads around the gallbladder to protect the peritoneal cavity from spillage of bile and calculi. The fundus is grasped with a Duval clamp and, with the suction nearby, the fundus is incised, using scalpel or electrocautery. (See drawing)

Cholecystectomy by the Pribram Technique

FIGURE 2.29
Once the fundus of the gallbladder is open, its contents are suctioned and all the calculi removed with a Desjardins clamp. If necessary, the gallbladder can be squeezed from the cystic duct toward the fundus to remove impacted distal calculi.

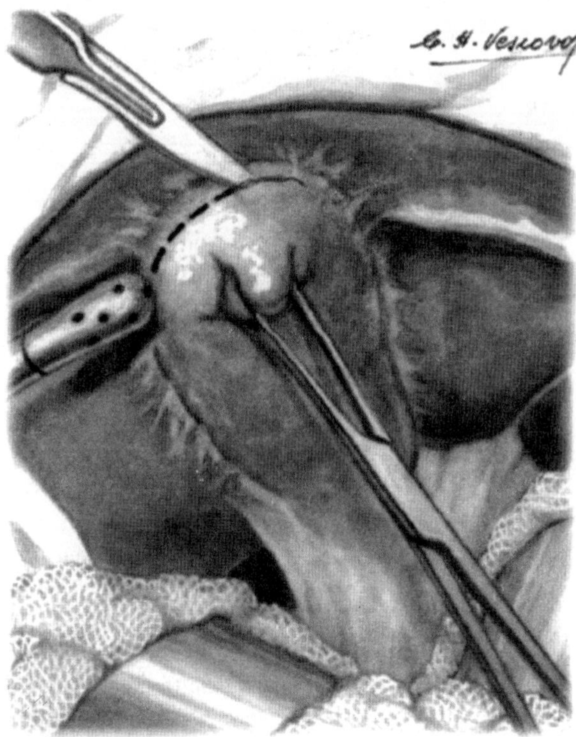

FIGURE 2.28

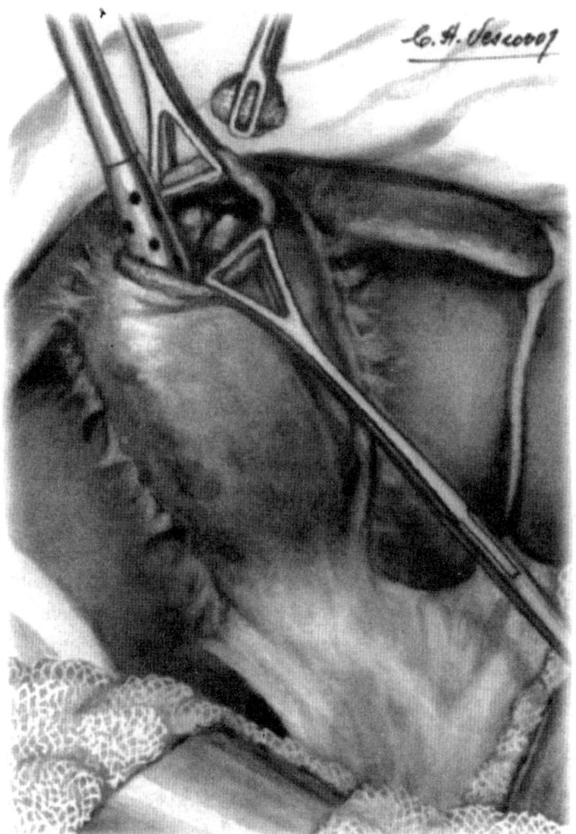

FIGURE 2.29

FIGURE 2.30
Once the gallbladder is empty, it is cut with scissors or electrocautery along a line 2 cm from the liver. As it is sectioned the remaining gallbladder wall is grasped with curved clamps. The clamps should include generous portions of the gallbladder wall to obtain adequate hemostasis of the numerous vessels, which tend to bleed profusely. Hemostasis is attained with electrocautery. The dotted line shows where the gallbladder is cut.

Cholecystectomy by the Pribram Technique

FIGURE 2.31
The fundus and body of the gallbladder have been cut in two halves. One remains adherent to the liver bed and its mucosa is electrocauterized, and the other half is resected. The gallbladder is cut down to the infundibulum. The gallbladder is not incised further down. The mucosa is sectioned at its limit between the body and the infundibulum, as shown in the drawing. This stage of the procedure is known as separation of the mucosa of the body and infundibulum. This point is easily recognizable because the infundibulum is completely covered with peritoneum and not held against the liver bed as is the body. Sectioning the mucosa at the level of the infundibulum will separate this segment of the gallbladder together with the neck and cystic duct from the portion that remains adherent to the liver bed, the mucosa of which will be electrofulgurated. The wall of the infundibulum is held with a traction suture.

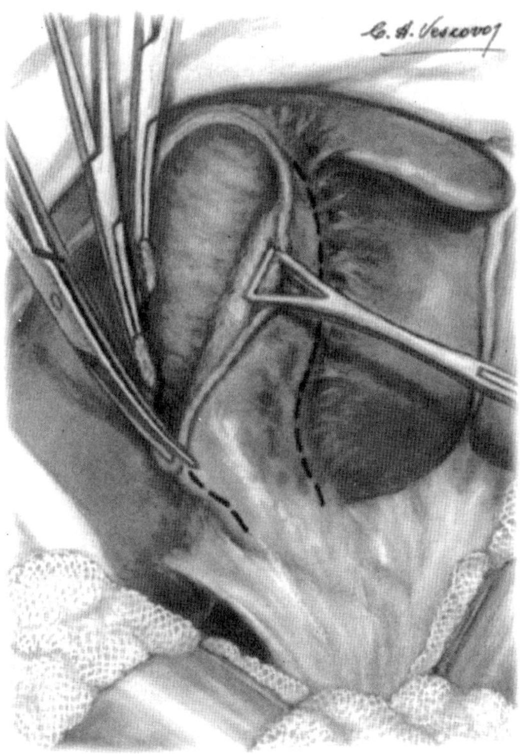

FIGURE 2.30

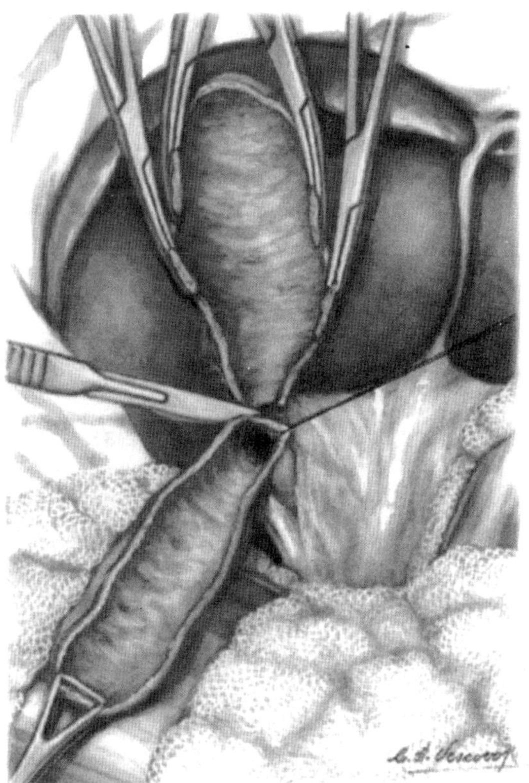

FIGURE 2.31

Cholecystectomy by the Pribram Technique

FIGURE 2.32
The infundibulum is held with two traction sutures and the seg ment to be removed is cut along the dotted line.

FIGURE 2.33
The infundibulum, neck, and cystic duct have been separated from the rest of the gallbladder and will be handled in the same manner as in the classical cholecystectomy. This means that the cystic artery should be identified in the triangle of Calot together with the right hepatic artery and the cystic artery tied near its entrance into the neck of the gallbladder. The mucosa of the remnant in the liver bed is totally destroyed by electrocautery, and the vessels in the hemostatic clamps are also electrocoagulated (see drawing). The destroyed mucosa is removed with a curette. If all the mucosa has not been destroyed, the bed is again electrocoagulated and curetted, as shown in the insert.

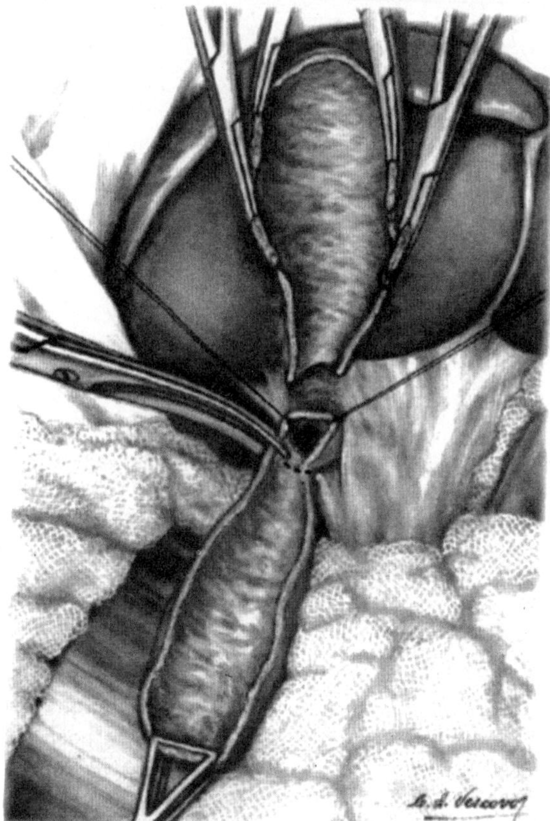

FIGURE 2.32

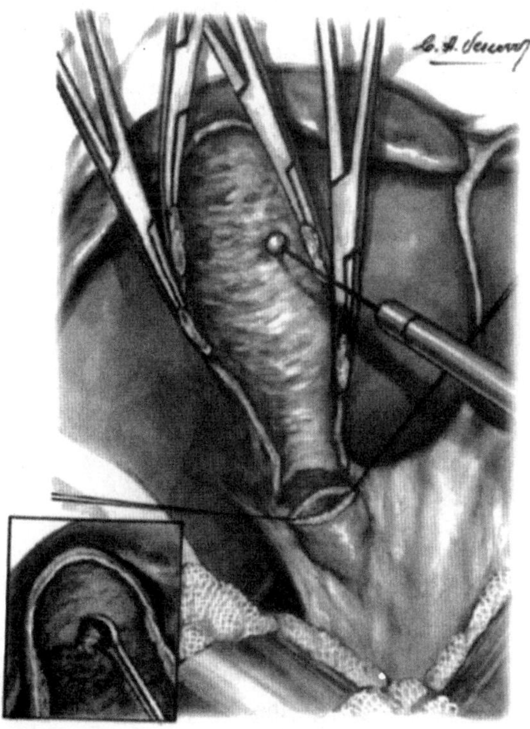

FIGURE 2.33

FIGURE 2.34
This drawing shows the gallbladder bed completely electrofulgurated and curetted, leaving no mucosal remnants. The cystic artery has been identified and tied, the operative cholangiogram has been obtained, confirming that the common bile duct is normal, and radiopaque substance passes into the duodenum. The cystic duct has been ligated near the common duct.

Cholecystectomy by the Pribram Technique

FIGURE 2.35
The drawing shows the peritonealization of the liver bed as in the classical cholecystectomy, using interrupted sutures. A drainage tube is left in the vicinity of the foramen of Winslow, to be removed 48 hours postoperatively.

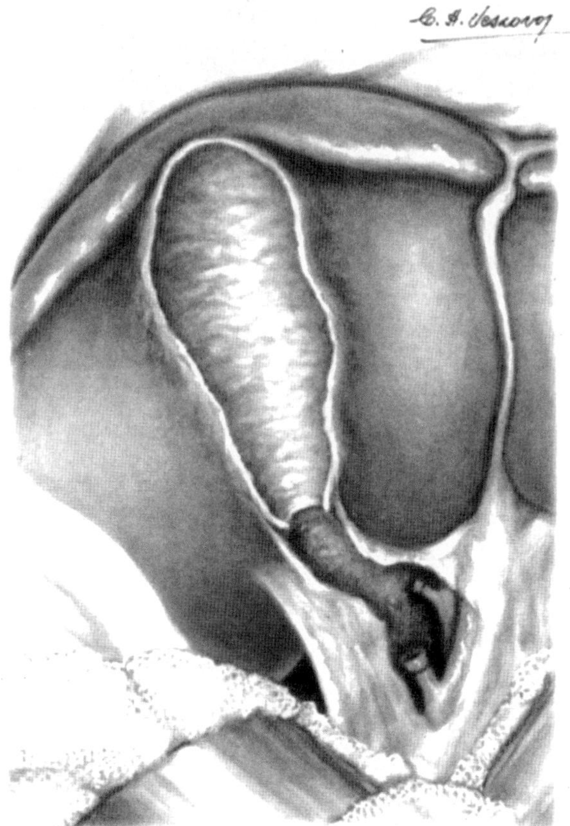

FIGURE 2.34

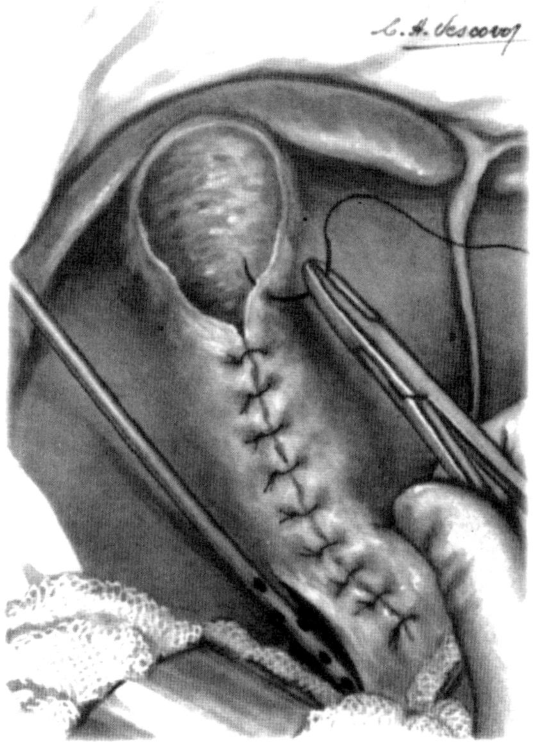

FIGURE 2.35

CHOLECYSTECTOMY WITH VERY LARGE HARTMANN'S POUCH ADHERENT TO THE BILIARY TRACT

Hartmann's pouch is used as a synonym of infundibulum of the gallbladder. Normally, the infundibulum is not shaped like a bag, but may acquire this shape when it is enlarged by the impaction of a calculus in its neck or in the infundibulum itself. In these cases the infundibulum increases in size, at times considerably, showing a great protrusion in the silhouette of the gallbladder. This pouch generally becomes adherent to the hepatic or common bile ducts, making cholecystectomy difficult. This alteration is the one that should be designated as Hartmann's pouch, meaning that Hartmann's pouch should be considered a pathologic process and not a normal anatomic variation.

A Hartmann's pouch, even though greatly developed, will not make cholecystectomy more difficult technically if it is not adherent to the hepatocholedochus. When firm adhesions are present, they can make cholecystectomy complicated due to the danger of injuring structures in the hepatic pedicle. In these cases it is usually necessary to vary the operative technique to avoid these injuries to arteries or bile ducts.

Cholecystectomy with Very Large Hartmann's Pouch Adherent to the Biliary Tract

FIGURE 2.36
The drawing shows an acute cholecystitis with a large Hartmann's pouch and firm adhesions to the common and hepatic bile ducts. The insert shows a section of the gallbladder with Hartmann's pouch and a large calculus in it. Adhesions to the hepatic and common ducts can be seen. In this situation it is difficult and dangerous to perform cholecystectomy from cystic duct to fundus as well as from fundus to cystic duct. In these cases it is preferable to resect the fundus and body of the gallbladder transecting it at the upper edge of the Hartmann's pouch, leaving the pouch to be dissected separately, as will be shown later.

Cholecystectomy with Very Large Hartmann's Pouch Adherent to the Biliary Tract

FIGURE 2.37
The fundus and body of the gallbladder have been resected, the gallbladder having been transected at the upper edge of the Hartmann's pouch. The pouch is then cut along the dotted line seen in the drawing.

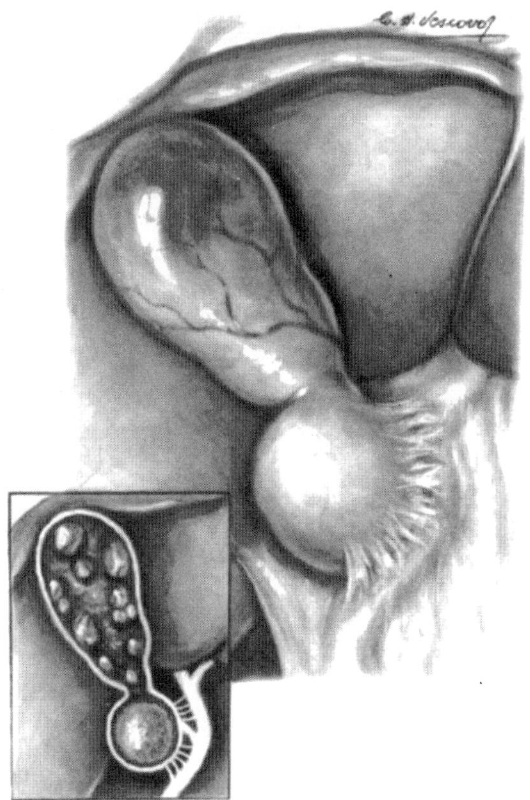

FIGURE 2.36

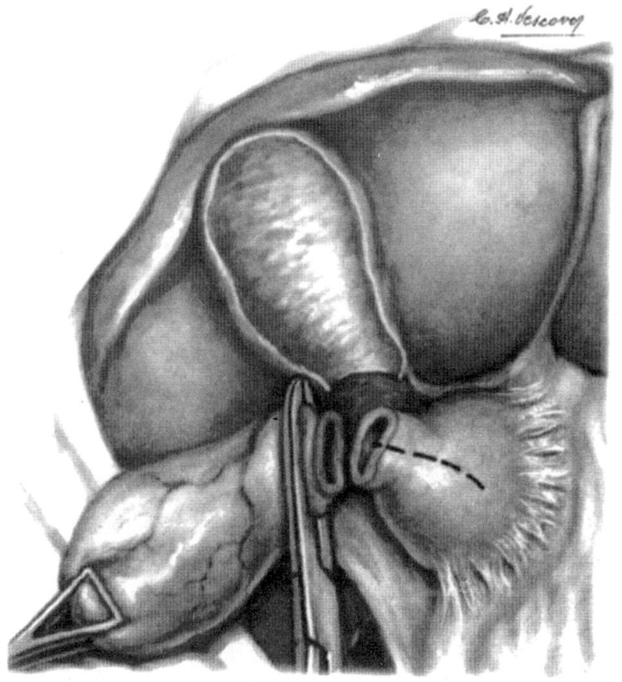

FIGURE 2.37

FIGURE 2.38
The large calculus in Hartmann's pouch is removed using a Desjardins clamp.

Cholecystectomy with Very Large Hartmann's Pouch Adherent to the Biliary Tract

FIGURE 2.39
Once Hartmann's pouch is empty, the left index finger is introduced in it and its wall is grasped between this finger and the thumb, exerting gentle traction and proceeding to carefully and delicately divide the adhesions between the pouch and the common bile duct. Adhesions between the pouch and the hepatic duct are then divided. This dissection may reveal the presence of a fistula between the pouch and the hepatocholedochus (biliobiliary fistula), making the procedure more complex.

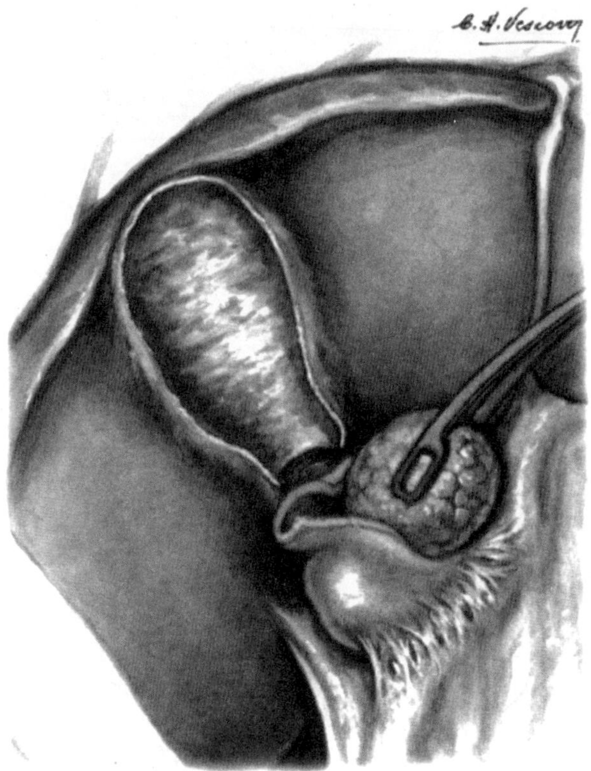

FIGURE 2.38

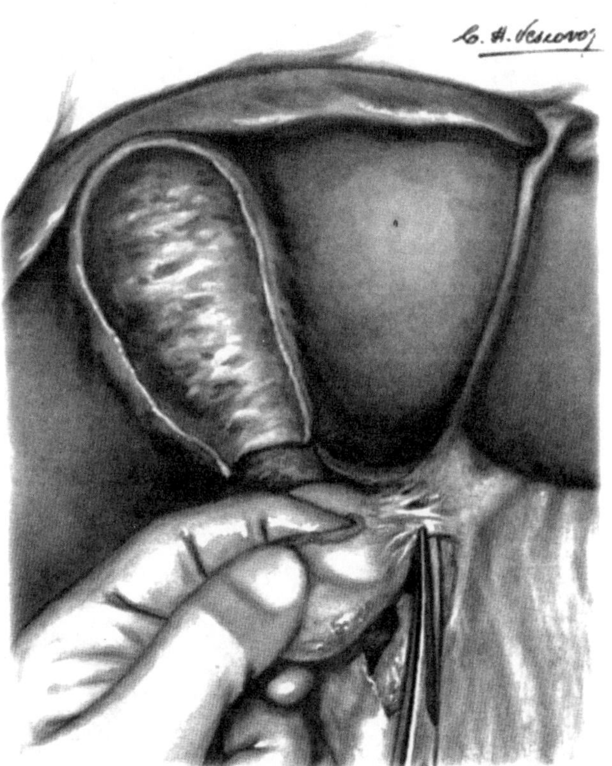

FIGURE 2.39

Cholecystectomy with Very Large Hartmann's Pouch Adherent to the Biliary Tract

FIGURE 2.40

Once Hartmann's pouch has been freed, and the cystic artery identified and ligated, the pouch is resected to the level of the cystic duct. This duct is then grasped with traction sutures to allow the polyethylene catheter to be introduced to perform the operative cholangiogram. If the common duct is normal, the cystic duct is ligated and the gallbladder is peritonealized, leaving a drainage tube for continuous suction near the foramen of Winslow.

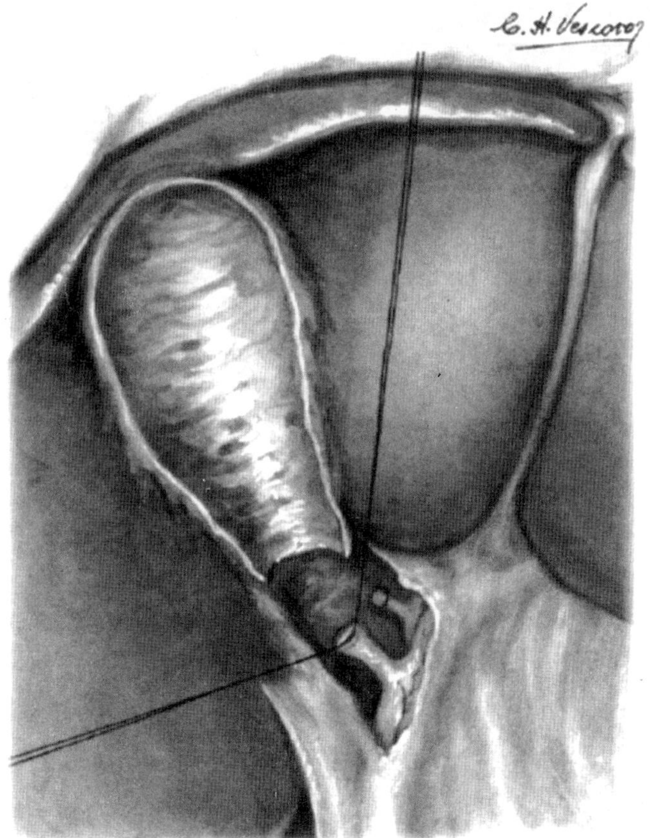

FIGURE 2.40

CHOLECYSTECTOMY IN PATIENTS WITH VERY DEVELOPED AND TRANSPOSED HARTMANN'S POUCH (41)

In some cases Hartmann's pouch can rotate and, instead of being located in its normal position, come to lie on the superior border of the gallbladder. The causative factors for this rotation are not clear, but they may be unusual mobility of the gallbladder or strong retraction exerted by the fibrosis caused by pericholecystitis. A transposed Hartmann's pouch may make cholecystectomy more technically difficult.

Cholecystectomy in Patients with Very Developed and Transposed Hartmann's Pouch

Cholecystectomy in Patients with Very Developed and Transposed Hartmann's Pouch

FIGURE 2.41
The drawing shows a Hartmann's pouch lying on the superior border of the gallbladder with intense cholecystitis and pericholecystitis. The procedure in this case is very similar to that described when Hartmann's pouch is located in its more common position. In this patient cholecystectomy from fundus to cystic duct could not be performed using the classical technique due to the absence of an adequate cleavage plane, for which reason resection of the fundus and body of the gallbladder had to be done using the Pribram technique.

FIGURE 2.42
Once the fundus and body of the gallbladder have been resected, using the Pribram technique, the gallbladder is transected at the superior border of Hartmann's pouch. The pouch is then incised and the impacted calculus removed with a Desjardins clamp.

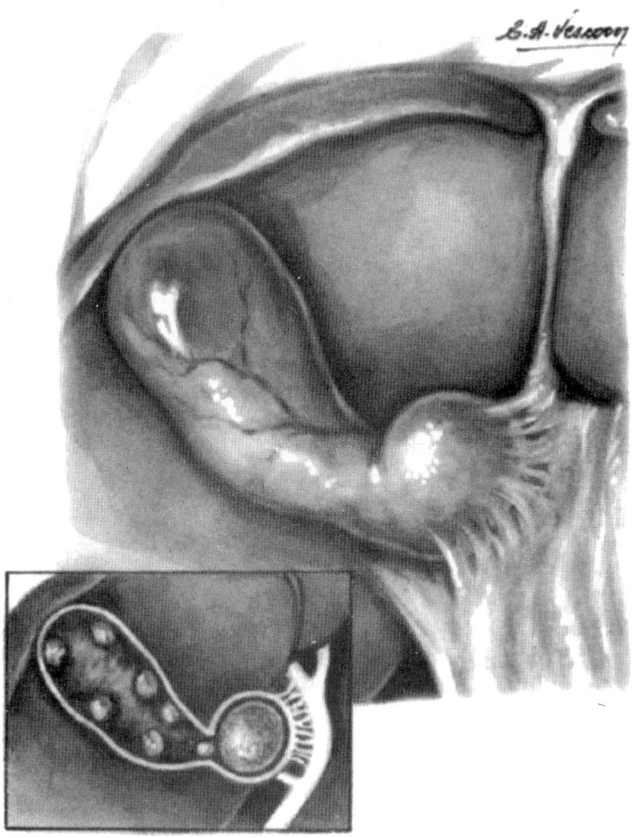

FIGURE 2.41

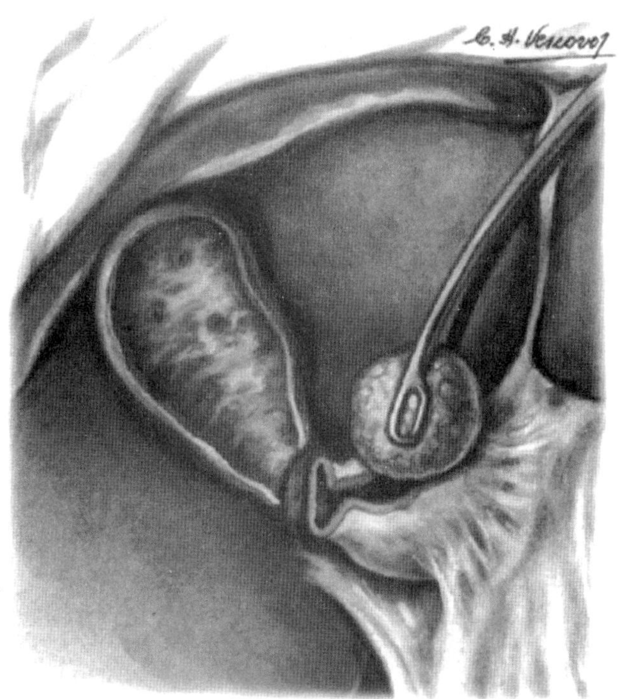

FIGURE 2.42

FIGURE 2.43
The left index finger is introduced into the empty pouch and the lateral wall of the pouch grasped with a Duval clamp to apply moderate traction and cut, with scissors, the fibrous adhesions between the pouch and the common and hepatic ducts, as observed in the drawing.

Cholecystectomy in Patients with Very Developed and Transposed Hartmann's Pouch

FIGURE 2.44
Once Hartmann's pouch has been freed, the cystic artery identified and ligated, the cystic duct identified, and Hartmann's pouch resected, operative cholangiography is performed. If the hepatocholedochus is normal, the cystic duct is ligated near to it. Then the mucosa of the body and fundus of the gallbladder is electrocoagulated by the Pribram method and the abdomen closed in layers, leaving a continuous suction drainage tube near the foramen of Winslow.

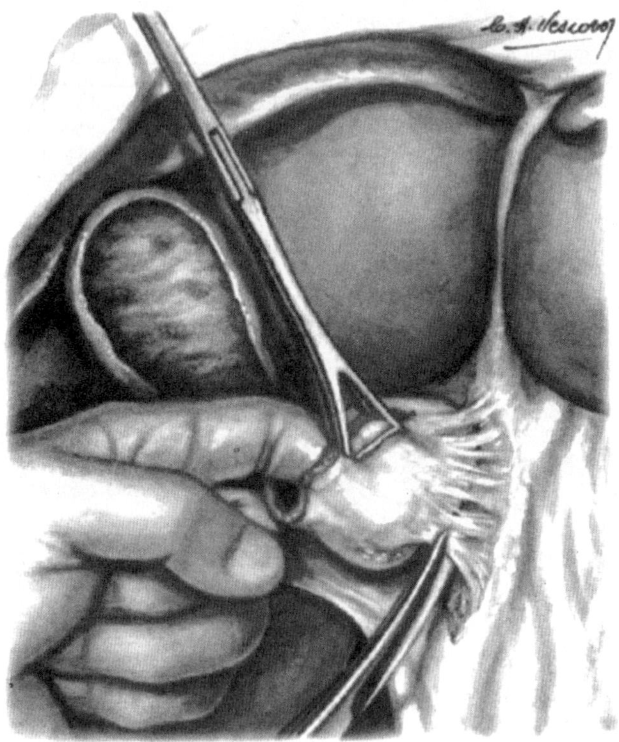

FIGURE 2.43

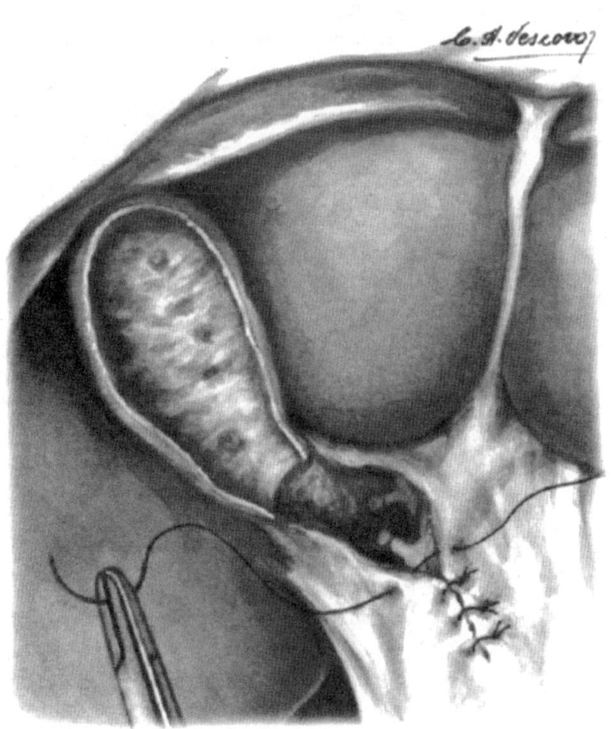

FIGURE 2.44

References

1. Acosta, J.M., Ledesma, C.L. Gallstone migration as a cause of acute pancreatitis. N. Engl. J. Med. 290:484, 1974.
2. Berci, G. Intraoperative biliary diagnosis modalities: present and future. Ital. J. Surg. Sci. 17:67, 1987.
3. Berci, G., Hamlin, J.A. Operative Biliary Radiology, p. 63. Williams & Wilkins, Baltimore, 1981.
4. Cameron, J.L. Atlas of surgery. Vol. I p. 2. B.C. Decker, Toronto, Philadelphia, 1990.
5. Comfort, M.W., Gray, H.K., Wilson, J.M. The silent gallstone: A 10–20 year follow-up study of 112 cases. Ann. Surg. 128:931, 1948.
6. Cooke, L., Jones, F.A., Keech, M.K. Carcinoma of the gallbladder. A statistical study. Lancet 2:585, 1953.
7. Coppe, D. Gallbladder and calculous biliary tract diseases. In Fromm, D. (Ed.) Gastrointestinal surgery. Vol. 2, p. 717. Churchill Livingstone, New York, 1985.
8. Corlette, M.R., Schatzki, S., Ackroyd, F. Operative cholangiography and overlooked stones. Arch. Surg. 113:729, 1978.
9. Champeau, M., Pineau, P. Chirurgie des voies biliaires de l'adulte et du nourrisson. p. 97. Masson et Cie., Paris, 1952.
10. Chassin, J.L. Operative strategy in general surgery. Vol. II p. 59. Springer-Verlag, New York, 1984.
11. Chatterjee, D.K., Jones, W.M. Value of operative cholangiography. Br. J. Surg. 32:105, 1978.
12. Editorial. Br. Med. J. Danger of silent gallstones. 41:415, 1975.
13. Etala, E. Tumores benignos de la vesícula biliar. Su significación clínico-patológica. Soc. Cir. Buenos Aires. Bol. Trab. 49:250, 1955.
14. Etala, E. Tratamiento del cáncer de la vesícula biliar. Soc. Int. Chir. XVII Congrès, México, p. 550. Imprimerie Médical et Scientifique, Bruxelles. 1957.
15. Etala, E. Tumores de la vesícula biliar. Arch. Ital. Malattie Apar. Digerente 26:5, 1957.
16. Etala, E. Litiasis incipiente del colédoco. Importancia de la colangiografía operatoria. Pren. Méd. Argent. 48:2128, 1961.
17. Etala, E. Valor de la colangiografía operatoria para el diagnóstico del cáncer de la cabeza del páncreas y de la ampolla de Vater. Soc. Inter. Chir. XX Congrès, Rome, p. 1198. Imprimerie Médical et Scientifique, Bruxelles, 1963.
18. Etala, E., Russo, R. Operative cholangiography in the diagnosis of tumoral obstruction of the distal end of the common duct. In Recent advances in gastroenterology. Vol. IV, p. 537. 3rd World Congress of Gastroenterology, Tokyo, 1966.
19. Farha, G.J., Pearson, R.N. Transcystic duct operative cholangiography. Am. J. Surg. 131:228, 1975.
20. Finochietto, R. Cirugía Básica. p. 288. López Libreros, Buenos Aires, 1962.
21. Glenn, F., Hays, D.M. The age factor in the mortality rate of patients undergoing surgery of the biliary tract. Surg. Gynecol. Obstet, 100:11, 1955.
22. Glenn, F. Surgical techniques illustrated. Vol. 1/1. Cholecystectomy and cholangiography. p. 17. Little, Brown & Co., Boston, 1977.
23. Glenn, F. Silent gallstones. Ann. Surg. 193:251, 1981.
24. Gracie, W.A., Ranschoff, D.F. The natural history of silent gallstone: The innocent gallstone is not a myth. N. Engl. J. Med. 307:798, 1982.
25. Hacker, K.A., Schultz, C.A., Helling, T.S. Choledochotomy for calculous disease in the elderly. Arch. Surg. 160:610, 1990.
26. Hermann, R.E. Manual of surgery of the gallbladder, bile ducts and exocrine pancreas. p. 116. Springer-Verlag, New York, 1979.
27. Hermann, R.E., Hoerr, S.O. The value of the routine use of operative cholangiography. Surg. Gynecol. Obstet. 121:1015, 1965.
28. Kelley, T.R. Gallstone pancreatitis. Pathophysiol. Surg. 88:345, 1976.
29. Kune, G.A., Sali, A. The practice of biliary surgery. Ed. 2, p. 137. Blackwell, Oxford, 1980.
30. Lund, J. Surgical indications in cholelithiasis. Prophylactic cholecystectomy elucidated on the basis of long-term followup on 526 non operated cases. Ann. Surg. 151:153, 1960.
31. McCormick, J.S., Bremner, D.N., Thomson, J.W.W. et al. The operative cholangiogram: Its interpretation, accuracy and value in association with cholecystectomy. Ann. Surg. 180:902, 1974.
32. McSherry, C.K., Glenn, F. The incidence and causes of death following surgery for non malignant biliary tract diseases. Ann. Surg. 191:271, 1980.
33. Madden, J.L. Atlas of technics in surgery. Ed. 2, Vol. I, p. 474. Appleton-Century-Crofts, New York, 1964.
34. Maingot, R. Abdominal operations. Ed. 7, Vol. 1, p. 1033. Appleton-Century-Crofts, New York, 1980.
35. Martin, J.K., Jr., van Herden, J.A. Surgery of the liver, biliary tract and pancreas. Mayo Clin. Proc. 55:333, 1980.
36. Mazzariello, R. Review of 220 cases of residual biliary tract calculi treated without re-operation. An eight year study. Surgery 73:299, 1973.
37. Mazzariello, R. Comunicación personal. Buenos Aires, 1989.
38. Mirizzi, P.L. La colangiografía durante las operaciones de las vías biliares. Bol. Soc. Cir. Buenos Aires 16:1133, 1932.
39. Mirizzi, P.L. Fisiología del hepatocolédoco. Colangiografía operatoria. El Ateneo, Buenos Aires, 1939.
40. Mirizzi, P.L. Cirugía de la litiasis biliar. p. 93. Imprenta Universidad de Córdoba, Córdoba, Argentina, 1948.
41. Mirizzi, P.L. Lithiase de la voie biliaire principale. p. 21. Masson et Cie., Paris, 1957.
42. Moosman, D.A., Coller, F.A. Prevention of traumatic injuries to the bile ducts. Am. J. Surg. 82:132, 1952.
43. Olmedo, F.A. Electrocoagulación en la cirugía de las vías biliares en Mirizzi, P.L. Cirugía de la litiasis biliar. p. 291. Imprenta de la Universidad de Córdoba, Córdoba. Argentina. 1948.
44. Peskin, G.W. The treatment of silent gallstones. Surg. Clin. North Am. 53:1063, 1973.
45. Prehler, J.M., Crichlow, R.W. Primary carcinoma of the gallbladder. Surg. Gynecol. Obstet. 147:929, 1978.
46. Pi-Figueras, J. Práctica quirúrgica. Ed. 2, Vol. II, p. 612. Salvat, Barcelona, Madrid. 1986.
47. Roux, M., Debray, Ch., Le Canuet, R., Laumonier, R. Pathologie chirurgicale des voies biliaires extra-hépatiques. p. 159. Masson et Cie., Paris, 1961.
48. Seltzer, M.H., Steiger, E., Rosateo, F.E. Mortality following cholecystectomy. Surg. Gynecol. Obstet. 130:64, 1970.
49. Schwartz, S.I. Gallbladder and Extrahepatic Biliary System. In Schwartz, S.I. (Ed.). Principles of Surgery, Ed. 3 Vol. 2 p. 1317: McGraw-Hill, New York, 1979.
50. Torek, M. Modern Surgical Technic. Ed. 2 Vol. 3 p. 2376. Lippincott, Philadelphia, 1953.
51. Thorbjarnarson, B. Surgery of the Biliary Tract. Ed. 2. W. B. Saunders, Philadelphia, 1982.
52. Valdoni, P. Abdominal Surgery. An Atlas of Operative Techniques. p. 80. W.B. Saunders, Philadelphia, 1976.
53. Walsh, D.B., Eckhauser, F.E., Ramsbeirgh, S.R. et al. Risk associated with diabetes mellitus in patients undergoing gallbladder surgery. Surgery 91:254, 1982.
54. Wangensteen, O.H. Personal communication, 1971.
55. Wenckert, A., Robertson, B. The natural course of gallstone disease: Eleven-year review of 781 non-operated cases. Gastroenterology 50:376, 1966.
56. Wright, H.K., Holden, W.D. The risks of emergency surgery for acute cholecystitis. Arch. Surg. 81:34, 1960.

Section A

Surgery of the Biliary Tract

CHAPTER 3

Cholecystostomy

Cholecystostomy is a surgical procedure that is rarely performed at present. Out of every 100 cases of acute cholecystitis, only one or two cholecystostomies are done. About the end of the 19th century and the early years of the 20th century the procedure was performed frequently, but because of recurrent lithiasis and cholecystitis in 50% of patients and because of persistent postoperative fistulas, cholecystostomy was gradually abandoned until at present it is done only by necessity, to save a patient's life and allow the performance of a definitive operation later (1–13, 18).

Cholecystectomy has replaced cholecystostomy because of its unquestionable advantages (15):

1. Cholecystectomy removes the organ where calculi develop.
2. It eliminates a site where infection may persist.
3. Cholecystectomy is generally a definitive operation, whereas cholecystostomy generally is not.
4. Resection of the gallbladder logically prevents recurrence of lithiasis, whereas in cholecystostomy recurrence of biliary lithiasis occurs in 50% of patients (13).
5. Cholecystectomy prevents the development of a biliary or mucous fistula, which cannot always be avoided with cholecystostomy.
6. Cholecystectomy eliminates the dangers of developing malignancy of the gallbladder.

Cholecystostomy is usually indicated in three situations:

1. In patients with gallstones who are a high surgical risk because of coexisting severe cardiac, pulmonary, renal, or neurologic problems in whom it is more prudent to perform an operation less risky than cholecystectomy (1, 2, 4). In these patients a cholecystostomy can be done through a small incision under local anesthesia. The operation in these patients should be strictly limited to the removal of easily accessible calculi, forgetting calculi that are impacted in the infundibulum or neck of the gallbladder or in the cystic duct. A tube should be left in place to drain the gallbladder.

2. Cholecystostomy may be indicated in some patients with septic acute cholecystitis and severe pathologic changes, such as multiple adhesions, that make surgery very difficult or make it impossible to identify the hepatic hilar structures, thereby converting cholecystectomy into a very risky procedure because of the possibility of injury of the common bile duct or the hepatic artery (5, 6, 8, 14).
3. It is better that, under special circumstances, surgeons with limited experience in biliary surgery who are forced to operate on a case of severe acute cholecystitis should lean toward cholecystostomy, since it is a simpler and less risky procedure.

Cholecystostomy, even though it is a simple procedure, may present technical difficulties in obese patients with the fundus of the gallbladder far from the anterior abdominal wall. On the other hand it is very difficult to perform a cholecystostomy under local anesthesia in very obese patients.

CHOLECYSTOSTOMY UNDER LOCAL ANESTHESIA THROUGH A SMALL INCISION

Cholecystostomy through a small incision under local anesthesia may be indicated in very high-risk patients in whom only minimal surgery should be done to save their lives. It is important to localize the fundus of the gallbladder previously, either by palpation or ultrasonography, to perform the incision in the exact position of the abdominal wall. Once the incision is made, an ample purse-string suture is placed on the gallbladder fundus and its contents are aspirated. A 2 to 2.5 cm incision is then made and the easily removable calculi are extracted with a Desjardins clamp. A Pezzer tube is placed in the gallbladder and the purse string suture tied. A second purse string suture is then placed around the first one to prevent leakage as much as possible. Under local anesthesia and through a small incision palpation and extraction of impacted calculi cannot be done.

Besides, with local anesthesia and a small incision a patch of gangrene away from the fundus may be missed. In the same way, common duct calculi as well as obstruction or cholangitis may be overlooked.

CHOLECYSTOSTOMY UNDER GENERAL ANESTHESIA WITH A CONVENTIONAL CHOLECYSTECTOMY INCISION

If the general condition of the patient will allow it, cholecystostomy should be performed under general anesthesia with a long enough incision to allow both cholecystostomy and adequate exploration of the gallbladder with removal of free and impacted calculi as well as the exploration of the common bile duct and pancreas (2).

The operative field is prepared as for a cholecystectomy. After the gallbladder and biliary tract have been explored visually and by palpation, the entire field is covered, leaving only the fundus of the gallbladder exposed. This protection of the operative field has the object of preventing spillage of gallbladder liquid contents, biliary mud, and calculi into the peritoneal cavity when the fundus of the gallbladder is opened. Using chromic catgut a 3 cm purse-string suture is applied to the gallbladder fundus without trying it. The fundus is punctured with needle and syringe to remove fluid for bacteriologic culture and sensitivity. A trochar is then introduced at the puncture site to remove the rest of the liquid as well as the mud and small calculi in the gallbladder.

Once the trochar is removed, a 2 to 2.5 cm incision is made in the fundus within the limits of the purse-string. A Desjardins or Randall clamp is then used to remove all the calculi. To be sure that all calculi have been removed, the left index finger is introduced into the gallbladder. Direct palpation is the surest method for recognizing calculi. Another useful maneuver is introducing the left index finger into the gallbladder and using the thumb on the outside for the same purpose. To confirm the pressure of residual impacted calculi in the cystic duct or in the neck of the gallbladder, the cystic duct is grasped between the right index finger and thumb, trying to mobilize calculi upward. In some cases it is useful to grasp the infundibulum between the left thumb and index fingers to free calculi in this location. Once mobilized, the calculi are removed with the appropriate clamp. In patients with severe inflammatory processes of the gallbladder wall, these maneuvers may lead to rupture of the cystic duct or the neck or infundibulum of the gallbladder. In these cases a cholecystectomy, which we were trying to avoid, will have to be done. For this reason, when calculi are too impacted it is advisable not to insist on their removal. It is preferable to remove them postoperatively through the cholecystostomy without morbidity (9). When the inflammation and edema of the gallbladder wall subside, calculi usually become free and can be easily removed (9). Through the cholecystostomy calculi can be removed from the common bile duct after dilation of the cystic duct (9). After the calculi are removed a Malecot, Pezzer, or Foley catheter, 16 to 18 F, is then left in place. These catheters should be introduced some 5 cm into the gallbladder. The purse string suture is then tied and adjusted so that the closure is as snug as possible. Another purse-string suture is then placed and adjusted around the first one.

In some patients the gallbladder wall is very thick, and it is extremely difficult to close the fundus by means of a purse string suture. In these cases it is advisable to close the fundus around the tube using interrupted sutures through the entire gallbladder wall. Before closing the abdominal wall a cholecystocholangiogram through the Pezzer tube should be done to confirm permeability of the cystic and common bile duct. The cholecystostomy tube is brought out through the incision or through a small counterincision. If possible, the fundus of the gallbladder around the Pezzer tube is fixed to the abdominal wall with several sutures to prevent leakage. If the fundus cannot be fixed to the parietal peritoneum, the entire gallbladder is wrapped with the greater omentum, allowing only the drainage tube to exit through it. The tube should be carefully fixed to the abdominal wall to prevent its displacement postoperatively. A subhepatic suction drainage tube should be left in place. It can be brought through the incision or through a stab wound. This tube can be removed in 3 to 4 days. The cholecystostomy tube should drain by gravity in a closed system. It should not be removed for 15 days postoperatively. It is advisable that the cholecystostomy tube be irrigated with a physiologic solution daily to prevent it from being blocked by biliary mud. Before removing the cholecystostomy tube, a cholecystocholangiogram should be obtained to confirm that the cystic and common ducts are open. If these are patent, removal of the tube will not result in a biliary or mucous fistula. If calculi are shown in the gallbladder or in the cystic or common ducts, they should be removed through the cholecystostomy (9).

Some patients with septic acute cholecystitis may present a gangrenous plaque in the fundus of the gallbladder. In these cases the necrotic area should be resected and the drainage tube placed in the opening, which is then closed with interrupted chromic catgut sutures. If, besides the gangrenous patch in the fundus, there is another gangrenous patch in the body of the gallbladder, the surgeon must weigh the convenience of doing a partial cholecystectomy with a drainage tube or performing a complete cholecystectomy.

The most frequent complications of cholecystostomy are subphrenic abscess and biliary and mucous fistulas.

PERCUTANEOUS CHOLECYSTOSTOMY

At present cholecystostomy can be done percutaneously in patients with very precise indications (10, 11). However, this technique needs 2 to 3 weeks for the establishment of the percutaneous tract and the extraction of calculi from the gallbladder. This indispensable waiting period makes this technique inadequate in cases of septic acute cholecystitis who need urgent surgery. Percutaneous cholecystostomy has its most precise indication in high-risk patients who do not need urgent surgery.

LAPAROSCOPIC CHOLECYSTOSTOMY

Cholecystostomy can also be done by laparoscopic means. This procedure, which has generated great enthusiasm among young surgeons, necessarily involves pneumoperitoneum and general anesthesia, which may not be advisable in high risk patients.

Cholecystostomy

FIGURE 3.1
Acute cholecystitis with very distended gallbladder. An ample purse-string suture using chromic catgut has been performed. The center has been aspirated with syringe and needle, removing fluid for culture and sensitivity. A trochar is introduced at the same site as the aspiration needle to remove all the liquid content as well as biliary mud and small calculi from the gallbladder.

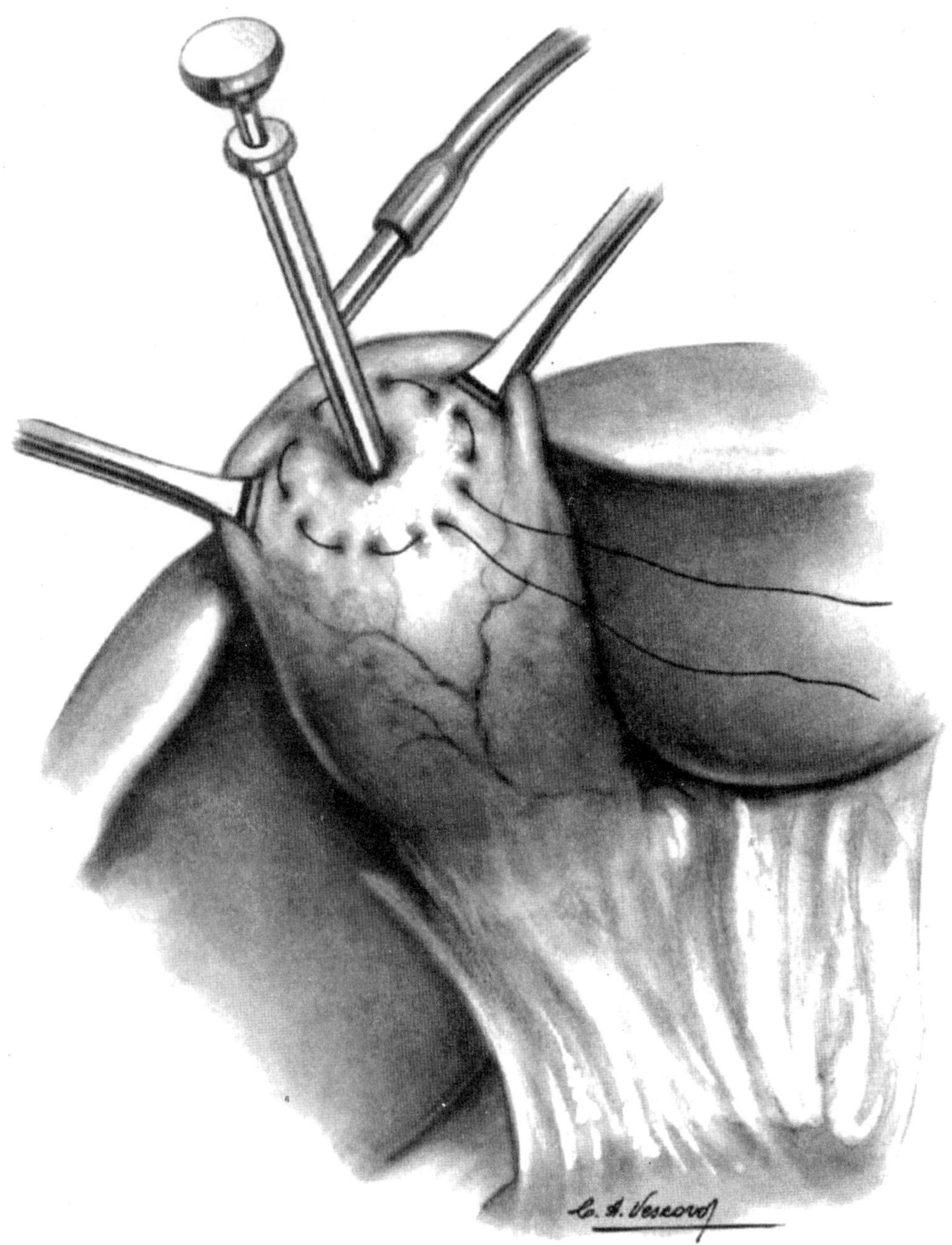

FIGURE 3.1

Cholecystostomy

FIGURE 3.2
An incision is made with a scalpel, in the gallbladder fundus, 2 to 2.5 cm long, within the purse string suture to allow for the removal of the calculi using a Desjardins clamp, as shown in the drawing.

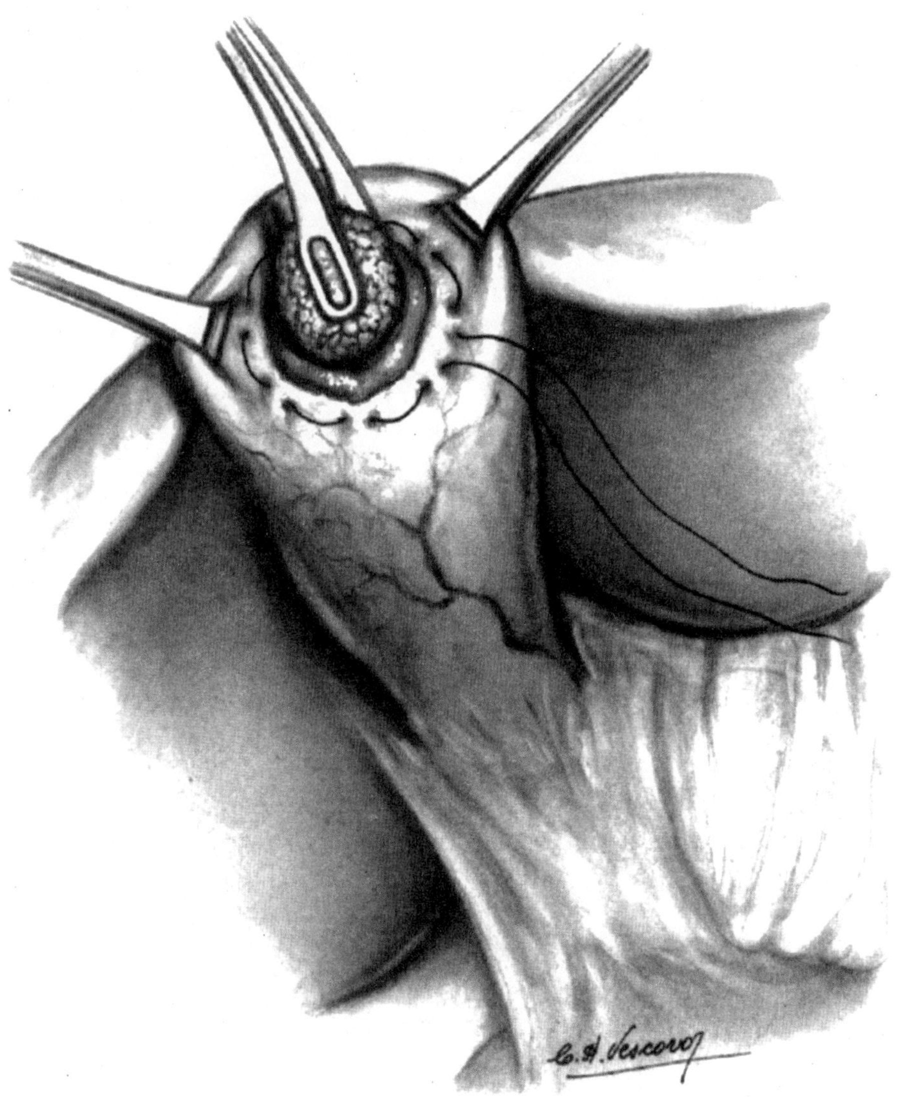

FIGURE 3.2

Cholecystostomy

FIGURE 3.3

If there are impacted calculi in the distal part of the gallbladder or in the cystic duct, one should proceed to mobilize them using digital maneuvers. One of these is that shown in the drawing, in which the cystic duct, the gallbladder neck, and the infundibulum are compressed by grasping them between the left thumb and index finger. Another maneuver that may be successful in mobilizing impacted calculi is performed by grasping the cystic duct and gallbladder neck between the right index and thumb, compressing them to place the calculi within reach of the Desjardins clamp. These maneuvers can only be done if the patient is under general anesthesia. It is practically impossible to do these maneuvers under local anesthesia. On the other hand, these maneuvers must be performed gently so as not to traumatize the wall of the gallbladder or cystic duct, which would make it necessary to perform a cholecystectomy instead of a cholecystostomy.

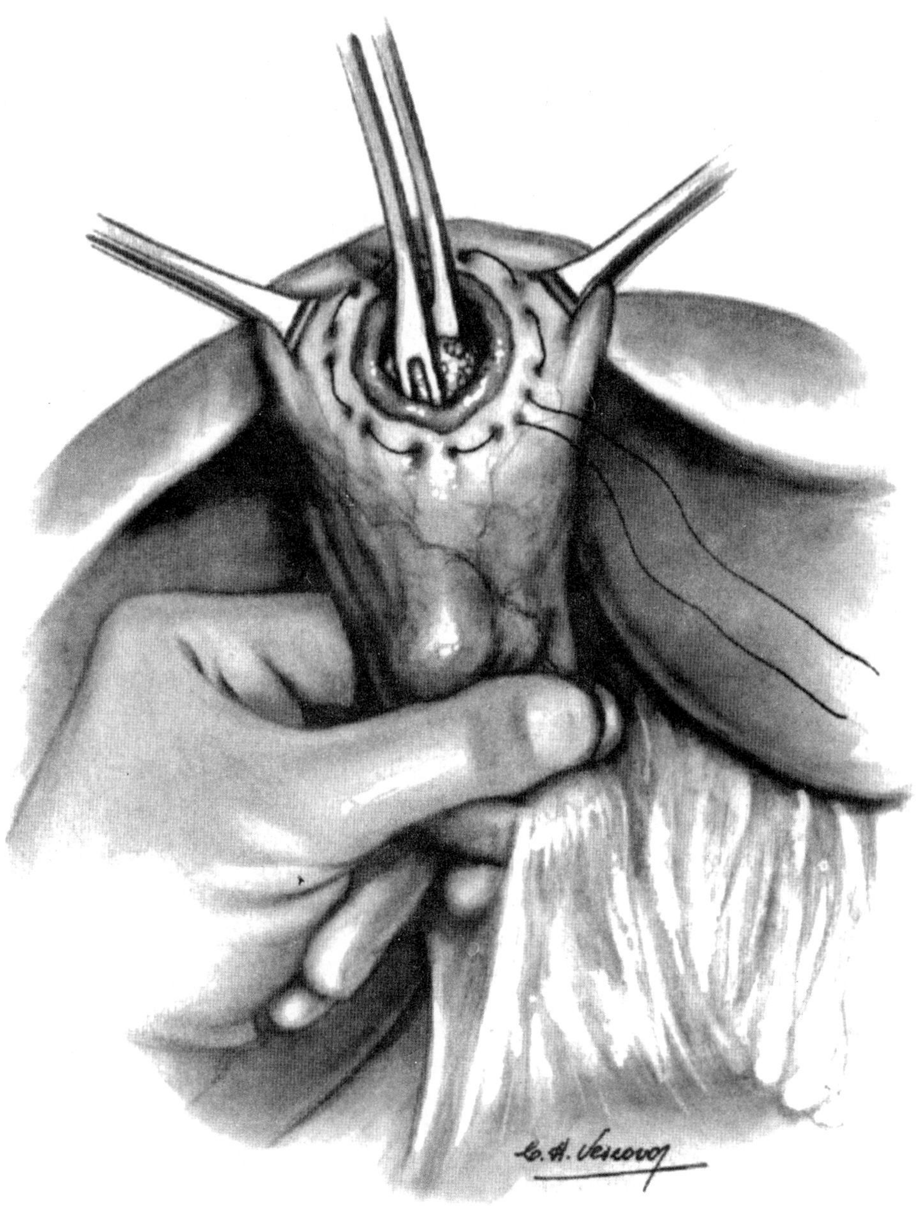

FIGURE 3.3

Cholecystostomy

FIGURE 3.4
After removing all the calculi a tube is placed in the gallbladder. This can be a Pezzer tube, a Malecot tube or a 16 to 18 F Foley catheter. The drawing shows a Pezzer tube being placed in the gallbladder. The tube has had part of its head cut off, leaving two lateral openings to keep it from becoming obstructed. The tube is introduced some 5 cm into the gallbladder and the purse string suture adjusted. Another purse-string suture is then placed to assure a more hermetic closure. The Pezzer tube is brought out through a stab wound or the incision itself. If possible, some sutures are placed between the gallbladder and the parietal peritoneum, around the cholecystostomy tube. Before final closure a continuous aspiration drainage tube should be left near the foramen of Winslow. The Pezzer tube is carefully fixed to the abdominal wall to avoid its displacement, especially in the immediate postoperative period.

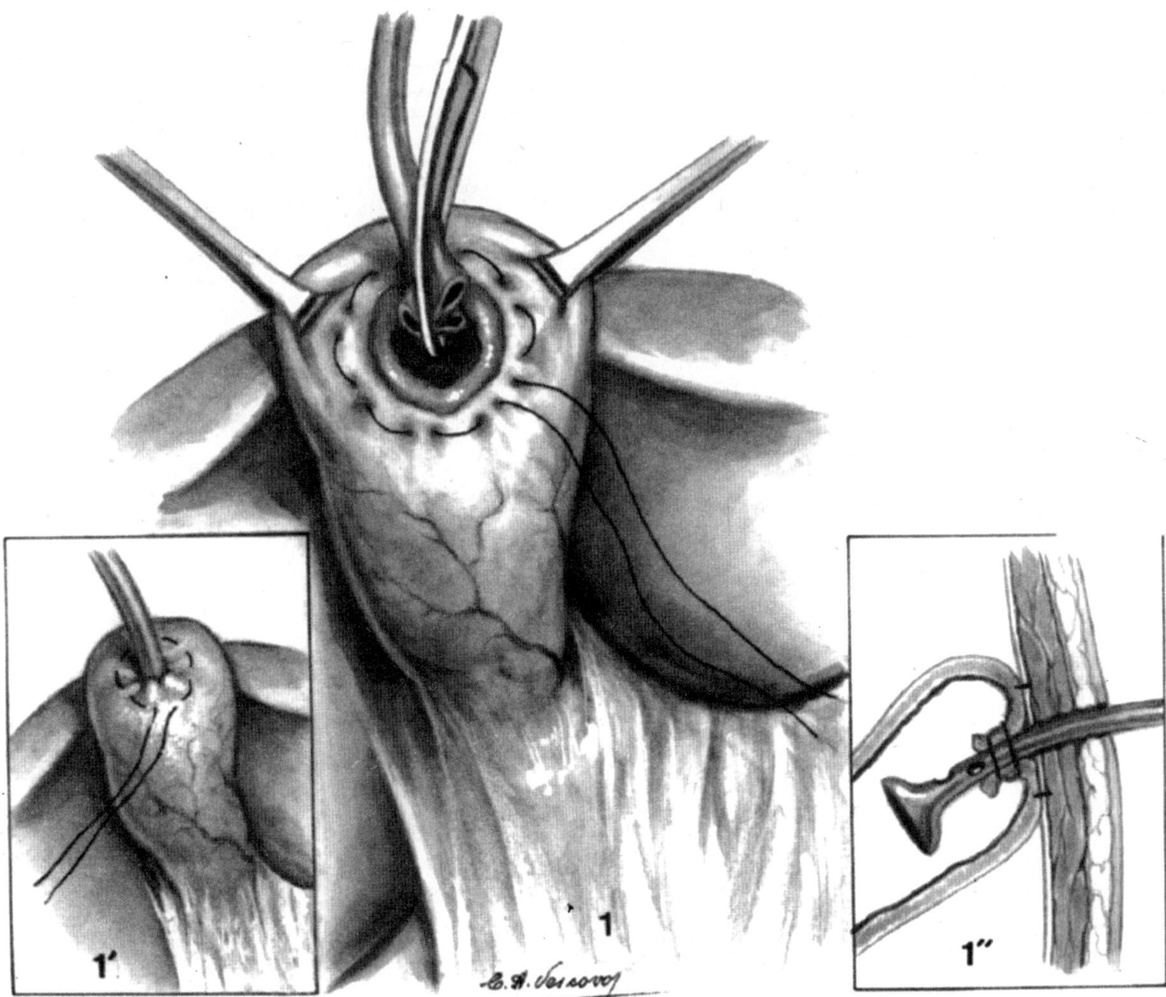

FIGURE 3.4

References

1. Coppe, D. Gallbladder and calculous biliary tract diseases. In Fromm, D. (Ed.) Gastrointestinal surgery. Vol. 2, p. 717. Churchill Livingstone, New York, 1985.
2. Chassin, J.L. Operative strategy. In General surgery, an expositive atlas. Vol. II, p 79. Springer-Verlag, New York, 1984.
3. Gagic, N., Frey, C.F. The results of cholecystostomy for the treatment of acute cholecystitis. Surg. Gynecol. Obstet. 140:868, 795.
4. Glenn, F., Thorbjarnarson, B. In Cooper, P. (Ed.) The craft of surgery. Vol. 2, p. 953. Little, Brown & Co., 1964.
5. Glenn, F. Cholecystostomy in the high risk patient with biliary tract disease. Ann. Surg. 185:185, 1976.
6. Hermann, R.E. Manual of surgery of the gallbladder, bile ducts and exocrine pancreas. p. 123. Springer-Verlag, New York, 1979.
7. Kune, G.A., Sali, A. The practice of biliary surgery. Ed. 2, p. 137. Blackwell Scientific Publications, Oxford, 1980.
8. Maingot, R. Abdominal operations. Ed. 7, Vol. I, p. 1,033. Appleton-Century-Crofts, New York, 1980.
9. Mazzariello, R. Extraccion transcolecistica de los calculos biliares residuales coledocianos. Bol. Soc. Argent. Cir. 34:558, 1974.
10. Mazzariello, R. Extraccion de grandes calculos por via transparietohepatica. Rev. Argent. Cir. 56:241, 1988.
11. Mazzariello, R., Novas, O., Perrone. R., Barbella, J.C. Colecistolitotomia percutanea. Pren. Méd. Argent. 78:20, 1991.
12. Nora, P.F. Operative surgery. Ed. 2, p. 552. Lea and Febiger, Philadelphia, 1980.
13. Pi-Figueras, J. Practica Quirúrgia. Ed. 2, Vol. II, p. 690. Salvat, Barcelona, 1986.
14. Puestow, C.B. Surgery of the biliary tract, pancreas and spleen. Ed. 3, p. 158, Year Book, Chicago, 1964.
15. Rintoul, R.F. Farquharson's textbook of operative surgery. Ed. 6, p. 591. Churchill Livingstone, Edinburgh, London, 1978.
16. Sparkman, R.S. Planned cholecystostomy. Am. Surg. 149:746, 1959.
17. Thorbjarnarson, B. Surgery of the biliary tract. p. 46. W.B. Saunders, Philadelphia, 1975.
18. Warren, K.W., Jenkins, R.L., Steele, G.D., Jr. Atlas of surgery of the liver, pancreas and biliary tract. p. 6. Appleton-Lange, East Norwalk, CT, 1991.
19. Welch, J.P., White, C.E. Outcome of cholecystectomy. Surg. Gynecol. Obstet. 135:717, 1972.

Section A

Surgery of the Biliary Tract

CHAPTER 4

Exploration of the Common Bile Duct

Exploration of the common bile duct should be performed in all patients subjected to cholecystectomy for biliary lithiasis (21, 28, 31, 33, 34, 40, 56, 57). A cholecystectomy for biliary lithiasis should not be considered complete without the complement of this exploration (59, 60, 70, 71, 81). Among the various procedures that are at present used to explore the biliary tract, operative cholangiography is the most efficacious because of its diagnostic accuracy, objectivity, and simplicity. To these advantages one must add that it is not necessary to open the common bile duct, which allows the surgeon to plan beforehand the therapeutic procedure to be followed. If operative cholangiography shows a common bile duct of normal caliber without images of calculi within it and passage of the radiopaque dye freely into the duodenum, revealing no suspicious images, the operation is complete. If, on the contrary, operative cholangiography reveals calculi in the common bile duct or difficulty in the passage of the radiopaque substance into the duodenum, opening the common bile duct will be necessary to remove the calculi and explore the duct with instruments designed for that purpose.

METHODOLOGY OF EXPLORATION OF THE COMMON BILE DUCT

The common bile duct can be explored in several ways, be it with the common duct closed or the common duct open.

Exploratory Methods Without Choledochotomy

The common bile duct can be explored without performing a choledochotomy visually, by palpation, by operative ultrasonography, by transcystic choledochoscopy, and by operative cholangiography. To all these procedures, fluoroscopy with a magnifying image has been added.

Exploratory Methods with Choledochotomy

To perform this exploration the common duct is opened by means of a supraduodenal choledochotomy through which instrumental exploration of the common bile duct is carried out, calculi are removed if they were present, and the papilla explored. This instrumental exploration can be complemented by means of choledochoscopy with choledochoscopes that are rigid or flexible, of different calibers, which permit the interior of the duct to be visualized and calculi to be removed. Choledochoscopy can be complemented with video-choledochoscopy.

Different methods of exploring the common bile duct will be described in the following.

Visual and palpatory examination of the common bile duct

Upon opening the abdominal cavity the surgeon generally performs an exploration of the entire abdomen and then concentrates on exploration of the gallbladder, the biliary ducts, the head of the pancreas, the duodenum, and the papilla of Vater. This is an incomplete exploration because in order to perform an adequate visual and palpatory examination it is an indispensable requirement to perform the Vautrin-Kocher maneuver. This maneuver, however, should not be overused. It should be used only when necessary. For this reason the maneuver should be postponed until an operative cholangiogram is obtained. If the operative cholangiogram reveals the presence of calculi or some other pathologic changes, the Vautrin-Kocher maneuver should be performed to complete the visual and palpatory examination, which will be a step to be performed prior to choledochotomy and instrumental exploration. If the cholangiogram reveals that the common bile duct is normal and radiopaque substance passes readily into the duodenum, it is not necessary to perform the Vautrin-Kocher maneuver nor the choledochotomy to do the instrumental exploration.

Operative ultrasonography

Operative ultrasonography is used to determine if there are calculi within the common bile duct (14, 78). Some authors (77) have been able to show the presence of small calculi that had not been noticed in other exploratory maneuvers. However, up to the present time, exploration of the common bile duct by operative ultrasonography has not become very popular.

Exploratory choledochoscopy performed through the cystic duct

In patients with a wide cystic duct it is possible to introduce a fiberoptic choledochoscope to look inside the common bile duct (63, 83). In cystic ducts of normal diameter that can be dilated it is also possible to introduce a fine flexible choledochoscope (63). Exploration of the common bile duct by endoscopy through the cystic duct has, up to the present time, not become very popular.

Operative cholangiography

This method of exploration of the common bile duct was originally proposed in 1931 by Mirizzi of Argentina (56). This exploratory procedure extended throughout the world and it is now unusual for a surgical center not to perform cholangiography. Operative cholangiography is optimal when it is performed in every patient with biliary lithiasis. Systematic practice of operative cholangiography leads to better technique, better quality x-rays, shortening of the time for the procedure, and a better interpretation of the films. It is rare in operating rooms organized for the performance of operative cholangiography that the procedure takes more than 7 minutes. In operating rooms not prepared for this examination, the radiographic technique is generally of inferior quality and takes longer, leading to a greater number of errors of interpretation (1). Cholangiography of poor quality should be discarded, since it has many more disadvantages than benefits. Actually, most operating rooms are equipped with fluoroscopic cholangiographic apparatus including image amplifiers, which are very helpful in the dynamic study of the biliary tract and particularly the sphincter of Oddi. In spite of the presence of televised fluoroscopy, one should not neglect obtaining x-rays because the neatness of the images and the radiographic details are superior to those in televised fluoroscopy and the x-ray has a documentary value.

The presence of a radiologist in the operating room is not indispensable. One only needs the presence of an assistant or radiologic technician who can obtain the x-rays. The x-rays should be interpreted by the surgeon, who acquires experience in this with daily practice.

Some patients, particularly those with jaundice, come to the operating room with a previously performed transparietohepatic cholangiogram or an endoscopic retrograde cholangiogram. If the x-rays are of good quality and the diagnosis clear, it is not necessary to perform transcystic operative cholangiography. However, if it becomes necessary to perform a choledochotomy with removal of calculi, a cholangiogram should be obtained through the T-tube to be sure that the common bile duct is free of calculi and that radiopaque substance passes readily into the duodenum.

It is useful to point out that both transparieto-hepatic cholangiography and endoscopic retrograde cholangiopancreatography are not completely innocuous, since they do carry some morbidity and mortality and should therefore be limited in their use.

The principal indication for operative cholangiography is in the diagnosis of calculi in the common bile duct. However, there is no doubt that cholangiography is very important in the diagnosis of other afflictions of the common bile duct or other problems that are related to the common bile duct (22, 25, 26, 39).

It is a proven fact that when surgery for biliary lithiasis does not include an operative cholangiogram, there is an increase in the number of unnecessary instrumental explorations of the common bile duct with the possibility that in some cases calculi of the common bile duct may be overlooked and patients not be explored whose bile ducts contain calculi, even though they are normal in caliber and have had no preoperative symptoms of calculi in the common bile duct. There is no doubt that operative cholangiography can diagnose cases of intrahepatic calculi, small calculi in a dilated common bile duct, calculi in the papilla (particularly when they are small and soft in consistency), calculi lodged in a diverticular cavity of the terminal common bile duct, and so on. On the other hand, cholangiography through the previously placed T-tube will allow us to verify if the common bile duct is free of calculi and if the radiopaque dye passes normally into the duodenum.

Operative cholangiogram, besides demonstrating the presence of calculi in the common bile duct, is very useful in making other diagnoses among which the following can be pointed out:

1. The existence of anatomic anomalies, whose frequency is 8 to 10% of cases, making it possible to avoid trauma to the biliary tract.
2. Operative cholangiography is useful in differentiating between organic and functional alterations of the sphincter of Oddi (24, 39).
3. In the diagnosis of surgical strictures of the common bile duct.
4. It is of importance in the diagnosis of the hepatic duct syndrome of Mirizzi (19, 58, 61).
5. To diagnose patients in whom the common bile duct and the pancreatic duct empty into a diverticulum in the second portion of the duodenum.
6. To demonstrate the presence of a peripapillary diverticulum.
7. Operative cholangiography may contribute to the diagnosis of hemobilia by showing the presence of a cavity in the hepatic parenchyma communicating with intrahepatic biliary ducts (39).
8. To diagnose the presence of hydatid cysts communicating with the intrahepatic biliary tract and to show the presence of daughter cysts in the common bile duct.
9. Operative cholangiography is of great importance in the diagnosis of jaundice due to calculi in the common bile duct, carcinoma of the head of the pancreas, carcinoma of the papilla, carcinoma in a segment of the common bile duct, and chronic pancreatitis with partial obstruction of the retropancreatic common bile duct (22, 25, 26).
10. Operative cholangiography is useful in the diagnosis and to determine the extent of sclerosing cholangitis.
11. Operative cholangiography contributes to the diagnosis of cystic dilations of the intrahepatic ducts or Caroli's disease (39).

Some surgeons (42) maintain that operative cholangiography unnecessarily increases the operative expenses of cholecystectomy. However, one should remember that this expense is minimal if compared to the expense and time that is lost if residual calculi are left in place. Six to eight weeks postoperatively patients have to undergo instrumental extraction of calculi through the fistulous tract left in place by the T-tube or removal of calculi through an endoscopic sphincterotomy. If both of these alternative methods fail, the patient has to be submitted to a reoperation.

Medical literature frequently mentions the term "unsuspected lithiasis" when operative cholangiogram reveals the presence of calculi in the common bile duct of patients who never had symptoms or in common bile ducts of normal size with thin cystic ducts, and so on. The surgeon who operates on a case of biliary lithiasis should always suspect that stones may be present in the common bile duct even though the patient has not had any symptoms and the caliber of the common bile duct is normal.

Interpretation of operative cholangiography is based on the following:

1. Caliber of the common bile duct.
2. Appearance and function of the narrow distal end of the common bile duct.
3. Passage of the radiopaque substance into the duodenum: easy, slow, or absent.
4. The presence of calculi in the common bile duct, their number, and their location.
5. The presence of anatomic anomalies.
6. The presence of other pathologic changes: strictures, diverticula, and so on.

If any doubts arise in the interpretation of the cholangiography, repetition of the x-rays will in many cases contribute to dissipate these doubts.

TECHNIQUE OF OPERATIVE CHOLANGIOGRAPHY

The patient should be correctly positioned on the operating table so that the hepatobiliary region rests on the radiologic Bucky cassette. At the moment of obtaining the x-rays the operating table should be tilted 10 to 15° to the right so that the shadow of the common bile duct would not be superimposed on the vertebral column.

Once cholecystectomy is performed the cystic duct is prepared in order to facilitate the introduction of a polyethylene catheter into it of an adequate caliber according to the diameter of the cystic duct to perform the injection of the radiopaque substance. To facilitate the introduction of the polyethylene catheter, it is convenient to place four sutures on the edges of the stump of the cystic duct to exert gentle traction, making the lumen of the cystic duct more accessible. If the diameter of the cystic duct is ample, the catheter can be easily introduced. If, on the contrary, the lumen of the cystic duct is narrow or the valves of Heister are an obstruction to the introduction of the catheter, it is very useful to rupture the valves of Heister and dilate the cystic duct. This is obtained by introducing the closed lower end of a fine hemostat into the lumen of the cystic duct and breaking the valves of Hister with gentle opening and closing movements of the clamp, thereby obtaining dilation of the cystic duct to be able to introduce the catheter more easily. Before the catheter is introduced the cystic duct should be flushed with physiologic solution to avoid the introduction of air bubbles into the system. The catheter should not be introduced more than 2 cm into the common bile duct. Excessive introduction of the catheter into the common bile duct makes the radiopaque substance run downward and pass into the duodenum without filling the common hepatic or the intrahepatic ducts. A ligature is placed around the cystic duct to hold the catheter in place. Some authors, instead of using a ligature, use a clip.

Many authors perform operative cholangiography through the cystic duct before removing the gallbladder. To introduce the polyethylene catheter, they make a small incision in the anterior wall of the cystic duct. This technique has no advantages over the one previously described. Operative cholangiography through the cystic duct before removal of the gallbladder has the inconvenience that the gallbladder occupies space in the operative field, which may interfere with the surgical maneuvers. On the other hand, if the cystic duct is narrow and it is necessary to rupture the valves of Heister to increase the lumen of the cystic duct, the maneuver is more difficult.

Once the x-ray apparatus is adequately focused, the perfusion of the radiopaque substance is performed using gentle pressure. It is not convenient to use excessive pressure, since this can lead to displacement of small calculi within the common bile duct into the common hepatic duct or the intrahepatic ducts. It can also lead to spasm of the sphincter of Oddi. One should also avoid injecting excessive amount of radiopaque substance, since this can lead to an artificial dilation of the common hepatic duct, affecting the interpretation of the cholangiogram.

If the common bile duct is normal in caliber or moderately dilated some 5 mL of radiopaque substance are infused and two x-rays taken. This first infusion of 5 mL of radiopaque substance has the object of clearly demonstrating the distal narrow end of the common bile duct before the radiopaque substance passes into the duodenum and becomes superimposed on the cholangiographic image of the distal end of the common bile duct. An additional 5 mL of radiopaque substance are then injected to see the rest of the common bile duct. If the common bile duct is dilated, one should inject a greater amount of radiopaque substance. The radiopaque substance should be infused after diluting it to 35% because greater concentration may impede the vision of small calculi. While the radiographs are being developed, the surgeon can continue with the peritonealization of the gallbladder bed.

If fluoroscopic equipment is available with an amplifying screen it is possible to observe the dynamic functioning of the common bile duct and the sphincter of Oddi. Normally the sphincter of Oddi contracts and relaxes synchronous with the contraction of the muscular layer of the duodenum. When the sphincter of Oddi is relaxed, bile and radiopaque substance pass into the duodenum. At the moment of contraction, the bile or radiopaque substance ceases to pass into the duodenum. Normally the sphincter of Oddi opens from above downward and closes from below upward. An x-ray may be taken at the moment of contraction of the sphincter of Oddi, which will prevent the surgeon from observing the narrowed zone at the end of the common bile duct. This may lead the surgeon to believe that there is spasm of the sphincter, stenosis, or an impacted calculus. A second x-ray may clear up the diagnosis. For this reason it is important to obtain two x-rays when the first injection of radiopaque substance is performed. Fluoroscopic examination with image amplifier is very useful to study the functional status of the sphincter of Oddi. If there is a permanent spasm of the sphincter, an injection of glucagon or cholecystokinin will lead to relaxation of the sphincter. Amyl nitrate or trinitrin will have a similar action. Spasm of the sphincter of Oddi is not usually associated with dilation of the common bile duct, whereas there is always dilation in cases of fibrosis of the sphincter of Oddi.

OPERATIVE CHOLANGIOGRAPHY IN CHOLECYSTECTOMIZED PATIENTS

If the patient has been previously cholecystectomized, operative cholangiography should be performed by puncture of the common duct. The puncture should be carried out close to the site where the choledochotomy is to be performed, using a 21 gauge needle with a 10 mL syringe filled with 35% radiopaque solution. It is important to carry out the puncture from below upward and at an acute angle to the common duct. If the puncture is carried out at an obtuse angle or in a vertical direction, the posterior wall of the common duct can be perforated, without aspirating bile and with perforation of the vena cava, with consequent confusion owing to aspiration of blood. The puncture should not be carried out parallel to the duct to avoid perforation of one of the veins of the venous plexus, which covers the duct and is frequently very well developed. Once the puncture has been carried out and a few mL of bile have been aspirated to be sure that the needle is in the duct, the radiopaque solution is injected very slowly. The amount of solution injected is related to the diameter of the duct, rarely more than 10 to 15 mL. If the cholangiogram does not reveal a need for a choledochotomy and instrumental exploration of the common duct, the puncture should be closed with a 5-0 synthetic reabsorbable suture to close the puncture site. Collections of bile in the peritoneal cavity have been known to complicate the procedure even though bile has not been seen at the time of the operation.

OPERATIVE CHOLANGIOGRAPHY IN PATIENTS WITH TUMORAL OBSTRUCTIONS OF THE COMMON BILE DUCT

In patients who present an obstructed common bile duct caused by carcinoma of the head of the pancreas, carcinoma of the papilla, or carcinoma of the distal common bile duct, as well as in strictures of the retropancreatic common bile duct caused by chronic pancreatitis, injection of the radiopaque substance should be made into the gallbladder. Prior to injection of the radiopaque substance a purse-string suture is placed in the fundus of the gall bladder and its contents aspirated. These contents are usually thick and gelatinous. Some 50 to 80 mL of radiopaque substance are then injected and the purse-string suture around the puncture site closed, leaving the ends of the suture long to apply traction to the gallbladder upward and to the right so that the image of the gallbladder will not be superimposed on that of the common bile duct. The amount of radiopaque substance to be injected in these cases is greater because it is injected into the gallbladder and because the entire biliary tract is generally dilated (22, 25, 26, 39).

CHOLEDOCHOTOMY AND INSTRUMENTAL EXPLORATION OF THE COMMON BILE DUCT

Instrumental exploration of the open common bile duct is performed when an operative cholangiogram reveals the presence of shadows that suggest calculi associated or not with other pathologic changes. If operative cholangiography is not performed systematically on every patient, opening and exploring the common duct with instruments should be based on a series of indications. Some of these had already been pointed out by Kehr in 1913, by Hartmann in 1923, and by Walzel in 1928 (30, 39, 56, 57, 60, 70, 71). These indications are the following:

1. Palpable calculi in the common bile duct.
2. Presence or history of jaundice.
3. History of biliary colic with fever and chills.
4. History of nonalcoholic acute pancreatitis.
5. Chronic pancreatitis.
6. Elevated alkaline phosphatase.
7. Multiple small calculi in the gallbladder.
8. Dilated thick-walled common bile duct.
9. Sclerotic or atrophic cholecystitis.
10. Cystic duct increased in diameter.
11. Drainage of cloudy bile from the cystic duct.

At present, one can add to these classical indications the information obtained from preoperative ultrasonography when the biliary tract is dilated; and in some 50 to 60% of cases when ultrasonography shows calculi, especially those in the common hepatic duct and less frequently calculi in the distal common bile duct. Computed tomography may also reveal the presence of dilation of the biliary tree.

In spite of these classical indications to open the common bile duct there are some cases in which the common bile duct is normal in caliber, there is no history of clinical symptoms of calculi, and the patient can still have calculi in the common bile duct. There can be cases in which the gallbladder contains one large calculus and has a thin cystic duct with a common bile duct of normal caliber but can still contain calculi in the common bile duct. There are some patients with a history of obstructive jaundice or frequent biliary colics with fever and chills who may or may not have calculi at the moment of surgery.

Instrumental exploration of the common bile duct no matter how carefully it is performed cannot recognize the presence of intrahepatic calculi or small or midsize calculi in a dilated common bile duct, calculi in the papilla, and so on. Kehr maintained in 1913 (60) that more than 50% of patients operated upon for biliary calculi should be subjected to an instrumental exploration of the common bile duct. Zollinger (87) maintained that, when operative cholangiography is not performed, more than 40% of patients operated upon for biliary calculi should undergo an instrumental exploration of the common bile duct.

The frequency of calculi in the common bile duct varies considerably according to race, country, age of the patient, duration of preexisting calculi, presence of acute cholecystitis, and so on. In the United States, the frequency of calculi in the common bile duct is estimated to be between 12 to 15% (84). According to Mirizzi, in Argentina, it is some 20% (60). In the Far East, the frequency of common bile duct calculi is much greater. In a recent study performed in Chinese patients immigrating into the United States (16), the frequency of common duct calculi was found to be 37.2% while in immigrants that were not Chinese the frequency of common duct calculi was only 11.8%. The greater age of the patient, the greater duration of calculi, and the complication of acute cholecystitis increases the frequency of common duct calculi.

TECHNIQUE OF INSTRUMENTAL EXPLORATION OF THE COMMON BILE DUCT

To perform an exploration of the common bile duct by means of palpation and instrumentation it is indispensable to perform the Vautrin-Kocher maneuver. To perform this maneuver the transverse colon and its mesocolon is displaced downward, exposing the distal half of the second portion of the duodenum and the lateral segment of the third portion. The peritoneum of the external border of the second portion of the duodenum is then incised, and the duodenum is mobilized with the pancreas toward the midline. Identification of the common bile duct is usually easy. However, if simple traction is placed on the cystic stump it stretches the common bile duct, facilitating its recognition. In cases of intense fibrosis it may be necessary to puncture the common bile duct to identify it. To perform this puncture a No. 21 caliber needle is attached to a 10 mL syringe. The puncture should be performed directing the needle from below upward, following an acute angle in relation to the hepatoduodenal ligament to avoid perforation of the posterior wall of the common bile duct, which may lead the surgeon to believe that it was a negative puncture.

CHOLEDOCHOTOMY

Choledochotomy is usually performed in the supraduodenal portion of the common bile duct because this is the most accessible segment of the duct. It is important to verify the exact location of the junction of the cystic duct with the common bile duct before opening the duct. This is because there are cases in which the cystic duct runs parallel to the common bile duct and at times even shares one of its walls. The surgeon may believe that he or she has opened the common bile duct when in fact the cystic duct has been opened. In some cases this inconvenience occurs more when the cystic duct runs a spiral course over the anterior wall of the common bile duct entering its medial border. In other cases incision of the common bile duct may fall too close to the entrance of the cystic duct tending to form a real spur, leading to confusion.

In some patients, owing to pathologic or anatomic reasons, it is more convenient to perform an incision in the common hepatic duct than into the common bile duct. The author favors making a transverse choledochotomy in the anterior wall of the common bile duct, below the entrance of the cystic duct, for the following reasons:

1. Exploration of the common bile duct and the papilla, as well as extraction of any size calculi, are performed with the same certainty as with the vertical incision of the common bile duct.
2. In common bile ducts of normal caliber with thin walls, the opening and closure of a transverse in cision does not lead to strictures, while closure of a vertical incision in these cases may lead to stenosis.
3. If the diameter of the common bile duct is ample, more than 20 mm, a transverse incision may serve to perform a choledochoduodenostomy (21, 26, 60). It is not necessary to divide the entire extent of the anterior wall of the common bile duct. Prior to incising the common bile duct the peritoneum that covers it should be incised if this has not previously been done. In some cases the venous plexus covering part of the anterior wall of the common bile duct is very well developed and when the choledochotomy is performed rather bothersome bleeding may occur. To prevent this it is advisable to place some hemostatic sutures so that the choledochotomy will not bleed. To open the common bile duct two sutures are placed one below and the other above the line where the transverse incision will pass. These sutures should be 3 to 4 mm apart from each other. The incision is then made transversely, using a scalpel, while gentle traction is applied to the previously placed sutures. Once the common bile duct is open, the two edges of the incision and the two angles of the incision are grasped with sutures to apply gentle traction giving greater amplitude to the opening. A vertical incision of the common bile duct is preferred by the great majority of surgeons because it can be extended upward and

downward, an extension that is hardly ever practiced. If one desires to make the incision vertically, two traction sutures are placed to the right and left of the anterior wall of the common bile duct and the common bile duct incised for about 15 mm. The edges of the incision are grasped with sutures and gentle traction applied to amplify the opening in the common bile duct.

If the operative cholangiogram has shown the presence of one or two calculi in the common hepatic duct, malleable spoons of adequate size are used to remove the calculi. If the patient shows numerous calculi, nearer to the choledochotomy, they have a tendency to show through the opening in the common bile duct. These calculi can be grasped with a Desjardins or Randall clamp. Calculi that are further away from the incision but palpable may be pushed between the index and thumb, leading them toward the orifice of the choledochotomy to be grasped with the stone forceps. This maneuver can be repeated with calculi in the common hepatic duct or in the common bile duct, in its retropancreatic segment. To remove calculi that are farther away from the common bile duct, a malleable spoon of adequate size according to the calculi is introduced into the common bile duct and the calculi are removed by the most practical technique, which is as follows: The spoon is introduced with the left hand, and the index and thumb of the right hand are used to introduce the stone into the cavity of the spoon. While the spoon is being removed, the fingers of the right hand maintain the calculus in the cavity of the spoon so that it will not fall off into the lumen of the common bile duct. This maneuver is repeated as many times as necessary to remove all the calculi from the common bile duct. Using the same spoon, some calculi that are impacted in the papilla of Vater can be removed. In spite of what is stated in many surgical textbooks, it is rarely possible to introduce a Desjardins or Randall clamp into the common bile duct to remove calculi except when the common bile duct is very dilated and the calculi are well formed. Calculi in the papilla of Vater that cannot be removed easily with the malleable spoon should be removed through a transduodenal sphincterotomy. In some cases it is necessary to remove calculi from the common bile duct using a Fogarty or Dormia catheter. Calculi that are lodged in a diverticular cavity of the distal common bile duct should not be removed through the supraduodenal choledochotomy and should be removed through a transduodenal sphincterotomy. In some exceptional cases one or two large calculi may become impacted in the retropancreatic common bile duct, making it impossible or very traumatizing to remove them through the supraduodenal choledochotomy. These calculi should be removed through the retropancreatic approach.

If the operative cholangiogram reveals that there are calculi in the intrahepatic ducts, these can be removed by means of malleable spoons, Dormia catheters of different sizes, or modified Fogarty catheters (to remove calculi from the biliary ducts). At times it is necessary to resort to irrigation with physiologic solutions or suction to remove small calculi and biliary mud.

EXPLORATION OF THE PAPILLA

The best way to explore the papilla of Vater is operative cholangiography. If the operative cholangiogram reveals adequate passage of radiopaque substance into the duodenum and through the narrow segment of the distal common bile duct, which can be clearly seen, it is not necessary to perform instrumental exploration of the papilla. If the cholangiography has in addition been performed with fluoroscopy using a magnifying screen, the sphincter of Oddi and its functional state can be better evaluated. However, if it has been necessary to perform a choledochotomy to remove calculi in the common bile duct, an instrumental exploration of the papilla is commonly performed in spite of the normal anatomy and function shown by the operative cholangiogram. If examination of the papilla by means of cholangiogram reveals an anatomic or functional abnormality of the sphincter of Oddi or the presence of an impacted calculus, instrumental exploration of the papilla is mandatory.

To perform an exploration of the papilla it is safest to use explorers with tapering olive shaped explorers made of rubber, plastic, or silk. These plastic and silk tissue explorers are considered semirigid in relation to those made of rubber, which are soft, and metallic ones, which are rigid. Metallic explorers should be used only occasionally, since they may traumatize the common bile duct and the papilla. If metallic Bakes dilators are used (in spite of their name. since they were originally designed to dilate the papilla), they should not be used for this purpose and only should be used as explorers. It is sufficient that the Bakes 3 mm dilator pass through the papilla to consider that the papilla is not strictured. It is completely unnecessary to dilate the papilla, since recurrence in a short period of time is the rule and because of the possibility that trauma of the papilla produces spasm, edema, hematomas, and even lacerations of the same. On the other hand, attempts to dilate the papilla, at times forced, may lead to dangerous false tracts. It is also not advisable that the explorer that has passed easily into the duodenum be passed several times unnecessarily through the papilla with the object of reconfirming the papilla's permeability. This is enough to traumatize the papilla, giving rise to spasm, edema, and congestion of the same.

At the moment of instrumental exploration of the papilla it is necessary to establish if the exploring instrument passed through the lumen of the papilla or if the papilla was pushed by the exploring instrument. To perform this distinction these elements of judgment are involved:

1. If the explorer has passed through the lumen of the papilla, it makes the duodenal wall opposite the papilla prominent, giving the impression that it is about to perforate it. If the explorer used is metallic, it produces a shiny metallic color which is characteristic and was described by Walzel in the year 1919. Walzel's sign will not appear if the explorer is pushing the papilla forward.
2. If the explorer passes through the papilla, its end moves freely in the duodenal lumen, something that does not occur if it pushes the papilla.
3. If the explorer passes through the papilla it generally descends 4 to 5 cm below the level at which the papilla is found.
4. Palpation of the explorer reveals that it is not surrounded by tissue but lies free in the duodenum.

When exploration of the papilla is performed, one must keep in mind that in certain patients the lumen of the distal common bile duct does not coincide with the lumen of the narrowed segment of the common bile duct (39) (intraparietal segment), so that the lumen of the narrowed segment has an eccentric or lateral position with respect to the segment of the common bile duct located above it and wider in diameter. As a consequence, when the explorer, which passes easily through the distal common bile duct, reaches the narrowed segment, it bumps into the wall that separates both instead of entering directly into the lumen of this segment, which is placed laterally, and makes one believe that there is a narrowing of the papilla, which is not exactly true.

CHOLEDOCHOSCOPY

After having removed the calculi in the common bile duct a choledochoscopic examination can be performed contributing efficiently to verify if any calculi have remained in the lumen of the common bile duct before proceeding to place the T-tube and performing final control operative cholangiography. Choledochoscopic examination was performed in the year 1953 (86). Choledochoscopy not only permits visualization of the inside of the common bile duct and its calculi, but also facilitates their removal.

Choledochoscopes have been perfected in recent years. Accessories have been added to choledochoscopes for the removal of calculi and for the performance of biopsies. There are basically two principal models of choledochoscopes: a rigid model and a flexible model. The rigid model is composed of a longitudinal stem and another horizontal stem connected at right angle. The horizontal portion may be 4 to 6 cm long. This instrument is easy to manipulate and gives excellent visualization. The flexible model is more complex and somewhat more difficult to manipulate, but it has the advantage that it can be introduced into the common hepatic duct and its principal branches. This instrument can also be introduced into the common bile duct through the papilla. To be able to visualize the inside of the common bile duct it is indispensable to dilate it with a flow of physiologic saline during the examination (1, 5, 27, 65, 66).

The best application for choledochoscopy is in patients with intrahepatic lithiasis and patients with multiple stones. Some surgeons have replaced control operative cholangiography at the end of the procedure, through the T-tube, with choledochoscopy (13, 15). Some of the reasons given by these surgeons are these:

1. A control cholangiogram with the T-tube in place is difficult to interpret due to the frequent presence of air bubbles in the common bile duct.
2. Control cholangiography performed after the removal of calculi and exploration of the papilla frequently reveals spasm of the sphincter of Oddi, which makes interpretation difficult.

The first objection, the presence of air bubbles, is a technical fault that is easy to avoid if habitual care is taken. In relation to the second objection, spasm of the sphincter of Oddi, it is not produced if the papilla is explored very carefully. Spasm of the papilla occurs if forced dilations of the papilla are carried out or if exploring instruments are passed several times through the papilla, traumatizing the papilla, or when false tracts have been produced. Exploration of the papilla should be performed with plastic or woven silk explorers with conical ends. The papilla should never be dilated. If a 3 mm explorer passes through the papilla it is enough to show that the papilla is permeable. Choledochoscopy should be employed to perform a more complete exploration of the common bile duct but should not replace the control operative cholangiogram, which should be performed every time the common duct has been opened and explored (83).

In recent years video choledochoscopy has been added to the methods of exploration of the common bile duct. This exploratory method permits the vision of the interior of the common bile duct by all the members of the surgical team through the television screen, greatly facilitating complementation of the maneuvers between the surgeon and his or her assistants for the removal of calculi.

COMPLICATIONS OF INSTRUMENTAL EXPLORATION OF THE COMMON BILE DUCT

Exploration of the common bile duct may produce lesions, some of them serious, if the instruments used are not managed with extreme care, particularly if they are metallic. Exploration of the intrahepatic duct may produce lesions of the hepatic parenchyma when metallic spoons or explorers are used to remove calculi. The hepatic parenchyma may also be traumatized by Fogarty catheters or with Dormia baskets.

The most serious lesions, however, are usually produced when the papilla is explored. The most frequent cause of trauma to the papilla are attempts to dilate the papilla, which may lead to false tracts. The false tract may occur over the duodenum or over the pancreas. The surgeon who is attempting to pass the papilla with the dilator perforates the common bile duct entering the duodenal lumen believing he or she has done so through the papilla and then continues to pass dilators of progressively greater diameter, believing the papilla is being dilated when in fact it is the false tract produced by the surgeon (81). A more serious and at times mortal false tract occurs when the explorer perforates the inferior common bile duct into the pancreatic parenchyma. The appearance of bile on the surface of the pancreas is indicative of this complication and should be confirmed with an operative cholangiogram (15). It is very important that the surgeon realize that he or she has produced a false tract in order to try to correct it during the surgical procedure, since not doing so may lead to loss of the patient's life. If the surgeon realizes that he or she has produced a false tract into the pancreas, he or she should immediately proceed to transect the common bile duct, closing the distal end and anastomosing the proximal end of the common bile duct or preferably the hepatic duct to a jejunal loop in Roux-en-Y fashion (15). Before the abdomen is closed, a suction drainage tube should be placed under the liver for 5 to 6 days. A false tract into the lumen of the duodenum carries less serious complication and in many cases is not recognized although it occurs more frequently than a false tract into the pancreas.

INTRODUCTION OF THE T-TUBE INTO THE COMMON BILE DUCT

Final Control Cholangiogram

Once the calculi have been removed from the common bile duct and the instrumental exploration and choledochoscopy have been performed, a T-tube is placed in the common bile duct. The final operative control cholangiogram is performed with the T-tube in place, with the object of verifying that all the calculi have been removed and the radiopaque substance passes readily into the duodenum. If the cholangiogram reveals that the common bile duct is free of calculi and the radiopaque substance passes normally into the duodenum, the surgical procedure is terminated, leaving a closed suction drainage tube in the foramen of Winslow and closing the abdominal wall. If, on the contrary, the control cholangiogram reveals that there are residual calculi, the T-tube is removed and the calculi seen in the cholangiogram are removed. The T-tube is again replaced in the common bile duct and a new cholangiogram obtained to be sure that all calculi have been removed. The surgeon should never leave a stone behind if at all possible, except in cases in which the patient's condition does not permit continuation of the operation or the calculi are located in a duct from which they cannot be removed (usually intrahepatic). It is not advisable to leave calculi that can be removed in the operation to be removed postoperatively, be they by instrumental removal or endoscopic sphincterotomy.

Conditions To Be Met by the T-tube

One of the basic conditions that a T-tube must meet is that it be made of good quality rubber and that the long limb be solidly united to the short limb. Before placing the T-tube in the common bile duct, traction should be applied to the short and the long limbs to verify that they are well joined. One should never use a T-tube made of Silastic because this material does not produce a fibrous reaction in the tissues and there is danger of leakage of bile into the peritoneum when the tube is removed. In addition the tract produced by the long limb of the Silastic tube does not develop tissue reaction sufficient to develop a tract that will permit removal of retained calculi postoperatively. On the other hand, a T-tube should never be smaller than 14 to 16 F to facilitate instrumental removal of calculi that may have been retained. The greater the diameter of the long limb of the T-tube, the easier it is to introduce instruments to remove retained calculi. For this reason T-tubes are now made of rubber whose long limb is of greater caliber than the short limb. The greater caliber of the long limb is to facilitate removal of retained calculi postoperatively. The short limb should only allow the passage of bile and therefore its diameter can be much smaller.

The T-tube should be prepared before it is placed in the common bile duct. To facilitate its postoperative removal, the posterior side of the short limb should be removed, that is, the T-tube should be converted so that its short limb is a canal and not a tube. In addition the short limb that is to be placed in the common bile duct should not be too long or too short. It should not be too long to make drainage of bile more difficult nor too short to be easily extruded postoperatively. An incorrect placement of the short limb in the common bile duct may lead to a series of complications, as we will demonstrate later.

Placement of the short limb of the T-tube in the common bile duct is a simple task. The short limb is grasped with a toothed clamp and placed deeply into the hepatic duct so that the entire short limb is in the hepatic duct. It is later placed in such a way that part of the short limb is in the common hepatic duct and part in the common bile duct so that the long limb of the T-tube will come to the outside through the choledochotomy. Once the T-tube is correctly placed, the opening in the common bile duct is closed with 3-0 chromic catgut or with absorbable synthetic material using interrupted sutures. Once the wall of the common bile duct is closed, the peritoneum over the common bile duct is sutured so that a watertight closure is obtained. This should also be done using 3-0 chromic catgut or reabsorbable synthetic suture material.

There are surgeons who do not leave T-tubes in patients in whom they establish that the common bile duct is free of calculi and that the radiopaque substance passes normally into the duodenum. Most surgeons, however, leave a T-tube in place when the common bile duct has been opened (32, 39, 40, 59, 85). The reasons for this are these:

1. The T-tube partially drains bile to the outside, which does not represent a significant loss.
2. The T-tube acts as a security valve so that if there is postoperative spasm or edema of the sphincter of Oddi and the pressure in the common bile duct increases, an incident may occur that could lead to the leakage of bile through the closure of the common bile duct, into the peritoneal cavity.
3. With the T-tube in place it will be possible to perform postoperative cholangiography to verify that no calculi have remained in the common duct.
4. Through the T-tube tract it may be possible to remove calculi retained in the common bile duct.

The T-tube should be brought out of the abdomen in the most direct direction possible without curves or turns to facilitate the removal of residual calculi. if this should be necessary.

The author prefers to bring the T-tube out through the same incision as the surgery without ever having had a complication caused by this. Other surgeons bring the T-tube out through a small counter incision. In either way the T-tube should be fixed by suturing it to the skin and then taped to the abdominal wall using wide tape to avoid displacement of the T-tube during the transportation of the patient from the operating room or caused by some act by the patient himself in the first postoperative hours.

Bile drained through the T-tube by gravity is collected in a plastic sterile bag located at the side of the bed. After a cholecystectomy with or without exploration of the common bile duct, a closed subhepatic suction drainage tube is left in place and brought out through the same operative wound or through a small counter incision. This drainage tube is left in place about 48 to 72 hours. If there is considerable bile drainage, the drainage tube is left in place as long as it is considered necessary.

MULTIPLE CALCULI IN THE COMMON BILE DUCT

When patients have many calculi in the common bile duct one should always attempt to remove all of the calculi in the same operative procedure. Once the calculi have been removed, choledochoscopy is useful in cases in which there are many calculi. Once the endoscopy has been completed, a T-tube is placed in the common bile duct and the control cholangiogram obtained. If calculi are still present the T-tube is removed and the retained calculi extracted. This maneuver can be repeated as many times as necessary until choledochoscopy and operative cholangiogram reveal that there are no further calculi in the common bile duct. If in spite of all these measures a calculus is found in the cholangiogram performed postoperatively, this calculus can be removed through the fistulous tract formed by the long limb of the T-tube (9, 11, 48, 51). This is the procedure of choice for the great majority of surgeons when treating multiple stones in the common bile duct. However, when calculi are very numerous, some surgeons, after removing calculi in a systematic form, do a choledochoduodenostomy or a sphincteroplasty as a method of treatment in case a calculus has been retained or calculi reform in the common bile duct (36, 44, 46, 56, 72, 73). The author believes, as other surgeons (15, 32, 33, 39, 40, 60), that these prophylactic measures increase the mortality and morbidity rates even in experienced hands. It is logical to think that these figures will be even higher in less experienced hands (15). The author believes that bypass procedures between the biliary and digestive tract or sphincteroplasty should be indicated in cases of stricture of the sphincter of Oddi, in stricture of the retropancreatic duct, or in those patients in whom the surgeon is sure he or she has left calculi in the common bile duct because he or she could not remove them. This possibility can occur in some cases of intrahepatic calculi, to which we will refer later.

Calculi in the common bile duct, according to the great majority of authors, have migrated from the gallbladder (15, 18, 28, 31, 33, 39, 40, 60, 83, 87). However, some authors maintain that these calculi may form in the common duct itself, designating them as primary calculi. These calculi have very typical morphologic characteristics (44, 45, 73). According to some authors, primary calculi develop when there is biliary stasis, particularly in common bile ducts that are dilated. Other authors admit that calculi can develop without there being any biliary stasis. Some surgeons maintain that primary calculi of the common bile duct are frequent in occurrence (44–46) and therefore advise that a choledochoduodenostomy or a sphincteroplasty be performed in these cases to prevent the frequent recurrences of primary common duct lithiasis. Other surgeons, however, believe that choledochoduodenostomy and sphincteroplasty should only be used in patients with primary lithiasis who have fibrosis of the sphincter of Oddi or stenosis of the retropancreatic common bile duct.

The choice between a choledochoduodenal anastomosis and a sphincteroplasty depends on several factors:

1. Caliber of the common bile duct.
2. Age of the patient.
3. General condition of the patient.
4. Stricture limited to the sphincter of Oddi.
5. Stricture extending proximal to the sphincter of Oddi.
6. Stenosis of the retropancreatic common bile duct.

Choledochoduodenal anastomosis is performed when the common bile duct is greater than 20 mm in diameter, in patients of advanced age or poor general condition, or in patients with stenosis of the retropancreatic duct. Sphincteroplasty is indicated in patients with only slight dilation of the duct, in younger patients, and in patients in good health in whom the stricture is limited to the sphincter of Oddi.

MEGACHOLEDOCHUS

There are patients who have a very dilated common bile duct without calculi or stricture in their distal segment. This condition is commonly known as megacholedochus. Some surgeons routinely perform a choledochoduodenostomy or a sphincteroplasty in these patients. It is the author's opinion that these very dilated common bile ducts without a stricture in their distal segment proven by operative cholangiography, instrumental exploration, or choledochoscopy do not need to have either a bypass between the bile tract and the digestive tract or sphincteroplasty. In these patients, as in all patients in whom an instrumental exploration of the common bile duct is performed, a T-tube is left in place, which will allow us to confirm that there are no residual calculi and dye passes readily into the duodenum.

INTRAHEPATIC LITHIASIS

Intrahepatic calculi that are not impacted or lodged in a diverticular sac or behind a stricture of the ducts can be removed by means of the diverse instruments used to remove calculi from the common bile duct. These are malleable spoons of different sizes, modified Fogarty catheters, Dormia basket catheters of different sizes, Desjardins or Randall calculi forceps, catheters that can be managed through the supraduodenal choledochotomy, dilating plastic catheters, irrigations of physiologic solutions, suction, and so on.

The flexible choledochoscope contributes efficiently to the extraction of intrahepatic calculi. Fluoroscopy with an image amplifier is also very useful, since it assists in performing the maneuvers to extract the calculi. It is more frequent to find calculi in the left branch of the common hepatic duct because its diameter is greater and its direction more horizontal than the right branch. In addition, there may be a stricture at the site of junction of the left hepatic duct with the common hepatic duct, which would contribute to calculi remaining in the left hepatic duct.

In patients that have intrahepatic calculi above a stricture of the ducts or lodged in a sacciform dilation of a segment of the left hepatic duct their extraction may be very difficult and sometimes impossible during the surgical procedure. Removal of these calculi is usually performed postoperatively through the tract formed by the T-tube. This removal should be performed by expert surgeons, in several sessions, following progressive dilation of the narrowed segments (51).

When the surgeon is certain that he or she has left calculi intrahepatically due to not having been able to remove them, it is advisable to terminate the procedure with a choledochoduodenostomy, if the caliber of the common bile duct allows this, or if not by means of a sphincteroplasty, foreseeing that some of the calculi may spontaneously pass postoperatively through the common bile duct into the duodenum. Before proceeding to remove intrahepatic calculi instrumentally, it is better to wait at least 4 months, since during this period calculi can spontaneously pass into the common bile duct.

In some patients a large calculus may be retained in the left branch of the hepatic ducts. Removal of this calculus during the operative procedure can at times be attained by incising the left common hepatic duct where the calculus is present and removing it, as we will show later.

Intrahepatic calculi are not frequently seen in Western countries but are common in the Far East, especially in Chinese, Korean, or Japanese patients. In these countries cholangitis is common and adds a very serious factor to the process, in some cases making it necessary to remove a segment of the liver or a hepatic lobe.

IMPACTED STONES IN THE PAPILLA

In the majority of cases, calculi in the common bile duct are localized above the intramural or narrowed portion of the distal common bile duct. In some cases, however, calculi can become localized within the narrowed zone of the distal common bile duct and in the papilla. Generally, calculi of the papilla that are not impacted can be removed relatively easily by means of malleable spoons, and in some cases even impacted calculi can also be removed. When a calculus that is impacted in the papilla presents some difficulty in its removal, the surgeon should not insist but should recur to removal of the calculus by means of a transduodenal sphincterotomy. Insistence on removal of the impacted calculi by means of the supraduodenal choledochotomy can traumatize the papilla, leading to edema, hematoma, laceration of the papilla, or a false tract. When a calculus becomes impacted in the papilla, at first it leads to spasm and edema of the papilla but later fibrosis develops, which traps the calculus. Sometimes it is not only one calculus that is impacted but several small calculi, which join when they are soft in consistency, forming a sort of paste-like obstruction. In these cases, even though this paste-like material is removed, one is never sure that the papilla is free of calculi. The technique for the removal of calculi that are impacted in the papilla will be described later.

CALCULI LODGED IN A DIVERTICULUM-LIKE FORMATION OF THE DISTAL COMMON BILE DUCT

The localization of calculi in a sort of diverticular sac at the lower end of the common bile duct is not frequently seen but when present leads to difficulty in their diagnosis and removal. Exploring instruments do not find any difficulty in passing through the common bile duct and the papilla. Sometimes these calculi can be felt, but since the explorers pass without difficulty to the duodenum it is believed that they are chronic pancreatitis nodules. A sure and objective diagnosis of this localization can only be obtained by means of operative cholangiography, which will show the presence of one or more calculi lodged in the diverticular sac. At times these calculi are very adherent to the wall of the diverticulum making their mobilization difficult. Attempts at removal of these calculi through the supraduodenal choledochotomy is usually a very difficult and dangerous task owing to the lesions that can be provoked. In spite of the fact that these diverticular sacs usually develop above the narrow zone of the distal common bile duct, with the passage of time the dilation usually extends into the narrowed zone. The most appropriate technique to remove calculi in these diverticula is through a transduodenal sphincterotomy, as will be seen later.

CALCULI IMPACTED IN THE RETROPANCREATIC COMMON BILE DUCT

In the great majority of cases calculi of the retropancreatic common bile duct including those that are impacted can be removed through the supraduodenal choledochotomy. There are, however, some rare cases in which one or more retropancreatic calculi are so firmly adherent to the wall of the common bile duct that removal is difficult and risky. Under these circumstances it is advisable to recur to the retroduodenal pancreatic approach through the pancreatic groove or the posterior surface of the pancreas, making an incision in the common bile duct at the same site where the calculus is impacted. These calculi are generally large. The technical details of their removal will be given later.

EXTRACTION OF CALCULI FROM THE COMMON BILE DUCT THROUGH THE CYSTIC DUCT

In patients with common bile ducts of normal caliber with one or two calculi within them, it is possible to attempt their extraction through the cystic duct to avoid having to perform a choledochotomy in a narrow common bile duct.

To perform this technique it is necessary that the cystic duct be dilated or dilatable. In addition, the common bile duct should contain one or two calculi that are perfectly well localized by means of operative cholangiography. This technique cannot be performed when the cystic duct joins the common bile duct in a very acute angle or when it runs parallel to the common bile duct. It will also be impossible to perform the removal of these calculi when the cystic duct joins the common bile duct on its inner border or on its anterior or posterior wall such as in cases where the cystic duct has a spiral tract. It is not advisable to use this technique if the common bile duct contains more than two calculi. This technique should also not be attempted for the removal of calculi in the common hepatic duct or the intrahepatic ducts. The calculi in the common bile duct are removed by means of a fine malleable spoon. It is also possible to explore the papilla by this method. Once the calculus is removed, a control operative cholangiogram is obtained through the cystic duct to prove that the common bile duct is free of calculi and that the passage of radiopaque substance into the duodenum is normal. If that is the case, the operation is finished by tying off the cystic duct, leaving a subhepatic drainage, and closing the abdominal wall. It is, however, advisable to leave a thin tube in the common bile duct through the cystic duct to partially drain bile to the outside in the immediate postoperative period in case hypertension in the common bile duct caused by edema or spasm of the sphincter of Oddi should occur. The details of this technique will be given later.

Extraction of calculi from the common bile duct by the transcystic approach is an interesting option. It is easy to perform and gives good results when the indication is precise and the technique correct and delicately performed. If the calculi cannot be removed through the cystic duct, a supraduodenal choledochotomy will be performed. The author always uses a horizontal (transverse) choledochotomy, which prevents stenosis in a common bile duct of small diameter. Some authors perform the removal of calculi from common bile ducts of normal caliber through a transduodenal sphincterotomy (13).

POSTOPERATIVE CONTROL CHOLANGIOGRAPHY

In patients in whom a T-tube has been placed in their common bile duct, a control postoperative cholangiogram is obtained 8 to 10 days following surgery. If the common bile duct appears normal without images of calculi and the radiopaque substance passes normally into the duodenum, the T-tube can be removed 2 to 3 days later. If the cholangiogram reveals images of calculi, instrumental removal of these calculi through the T-tube tract is indicated. Removal of these calculi should not be performed until 6 weeks following surgery. Allowing this time as necessary for the development of a fibrous tract, which will permit the introduction of specially designed instruments to perform removal of the calculi without producing false tracts or traumatizing neighboring organs.

INSTRUMENTAL REMOVAL OF RESIDUAL CALCULI FROM THE COMMON BILE DUCT THROUGH A FISTULOUS TRACT OF A T-TUBE

Removal of calculi from a common bile duct through the fistulous tract of a T-tube is a method that was first proposed and used in Argentina by the surgeon Dr. Rodolfo Mazzariello in 1964. Additionally, Dr. Mazzariello has designed and perfected numerous instruments with the object of facilitating removal of residual calculi from the common bile duct with the help of fluoroscopy and an image amplifier (48–51). At present calculi of any size and number can be removed from any localization. Large calculi can be fragmented in order to remove them, and some small calculi can be pushed into the duodenum. An important contribution to this procedure was made by Burhenne, a radiologist from Vancouver, Canada since 1973 (9–11). A precursor of this procedure was, without doubt, Dr. A. Mondet, a surgeon from Argentina (62). The removal of calculi should be performed 6 weeks after the operation, when the fibrous tract has already formed. This is performed using special clamps of different lengths and of different diameters and flexibility, by catheters with baskets at their ends of different sizes, and so on.

To facilitate the removal of calculi by this method it is necessary to leave T-tubes in the common bile duct that are no less than 14 to 16 F. These tubes should be brought to the outside in a direct line, without lateralizations or angulations. At present, T-tubes are made whose long limb is of greater caliber than the short limb to facilitate removal of calculi and in order not to leave very thick tubes within the common bile duct.

Residual calculi that are most difficult to remove are those that are intrahepatic and those that are impacted in the papilla. When intrahepatic calculi cannot be removed owing to the presence of zones of narrowing in the ducts, one should dilate the narrowed segments until adequate instruments can be introduced for the removal of the calculi.

When residual intrahepatic calculi are present, it is convenient not to attempt their removal until 4 months following surgery, since it is possible that in that period of time some of the calculi may descend into the common bile duct.

Patients who were subjected to cholecystostomy because of their serious condition but who have calculi in their common bile duct, can have these removed through the cholecystostomy by previously dilating the cystic duct. Calculi of the common bile duct can also be removed by a transcutaneous hepatic route in patients whose general condition is very precarious (52–54).

REMOVAL OF COMMON BILE DUCT CALCULI BY THE TRANSCUTANEOHEPATIC ROUTE

Calculi in the common bile duct, the common hepatic duct, and the intrahepatic ducts can be removed by the transcutaneo-hepatic approach (54). Mazzariello (54), in 34 high risk patients with large calculi in the common bile duct or intrahepatic ducts and zones of narrowing below these, was able to remove all the calculi without mortality and with minimal morbidity. The large calculi were fragmented with clamps and catheters with baskets designed to break up the calculi (54). The procedure is performed with local anesthesia, and patients do not need to be hospitalized except those that may be seriously ill. Indications for this procedure are very precise and care must be extreme. It is possible to carry out this procedure in patients with a high surgical risk and in those in whom attempts to remove the calculi through T-tube tracts or endoscopically may have failed (54).

REMOVAL OF CALCULI FROM THE COMMON BILE DUCT BY ENDOSCOPIC SPHINCTEROTOMY

Endoscopic sphincterotomy was first practiced in 1973 by Classen and Demling, in Germany (17). At present there is a large body of experience acquired by means of this procedure. If the patient does not have a T-tube in place, this is the procedure of choice. If the patient has a T-tube in place, the indicated procedure is that of removal of the calculi through the T-tube tract. Sometimes sphincterotomy is enough for the calculi to be spontaneously eliminated. In other cases, it is necessary to remove them by catheters with a basket at their end. Removal of calculi by means of endoscopic sphincterotomy is effective in more than 90% of cases. This procedure should be performed by an experienced endoscopist trained in this therapeutic method. The indications for this procedure should be very exact, and the procedure should not be abused, since it is not exempt of serious or even mortal complications. It has been shown that the complications and mortality of this procedure are considerably higher than those published, probably because patients who become complicated are taken care of by emergency services and are not brought to the attention of the endoscopist who performed the procedure.

Complications that can occur due to endoscopic sphincterotomy include hemorrhage, retroperitoneal perforation, simultaneous hemorrhage and perforation, acute cholangitis, and acute pancreatitis. The patient should be informed of the possibility of these complications and of the possibility that some patients may have to be operated on an emergency basis following endoscopic sphincterotomy. Endoscopic sphincterotomy should not be performed in patients with altered blood clotting, patients with calculi larger than 20 mm in diameter or in patients with stricture of the sphincter of Oddi extending beyond the duodenal wall. Sphincterotomy should not be performed in patients with peripapillary duodenal diverticula. In patients in whom the gallbladder has not been removed, sphincterotomy may lead to functional complications of the gallbladder and, at times, cholecystitis.

Exploration of the Common Bile Duct

Exploratory Methods Without Choledochotomy

FIGURE 4.1 TRANSCYSTIC CHOLANGIOGRAM

Operative cholangiography is a valuable procedure to explore the common bile duct. To carry out this procedure it is not necessary to perform the Vautrin-Kocher maneuver nor is it necessary to open the common bile duct. These procedures will be performed if the operative cholangiogram reveals findings that make them necessary. Operative cholangiography is performed after the gallbladder is removed. Many surgeons, however, practice cholangiography with the gallbladder in situ. The cystic duct is held by four sutures and its edges, facilitating the introduction of the polyethylene catheter, which should have been previously flushed with a physiologic solution to eliminate the possibility of air bubbles entering the common bile duct. The catheter is introduced some 2 or 3 cm. It is not advisable to introduce it more than 3 cm. (Figure 4.1B). The catheter is fixed in the cystic duct with half a knot and perfused with 5 mL of hydrosoluble radiopaque solution diluted to 35%. This original 5 mL perfusion is with the purpose of opacifying the distal common bile duct and observing the function of the sphincter of Oddi. If an image amplifier is available, the dynamic changes in the sphincter of Oddi can be observed more clearly. Another 5 mL are then infused to observe the rest of the common bile duct. If the common bile duct is dilated an additional amount of radiopaque substance should be infused according to the diameter of the common bile duct. It should be pointed out, however, that it is not advisable to inject an excessive amount of radiopaque substance and this substance should not be infused under pressure. If the cystic duct is narrow, and the valves of Heister present an obstruction to the introduction of the polyethylene catheter, it may be necessary to break the valves of Heister and dilate the cystic duct as shown in Figure 4.1A and in the insert.

FIGURE 4.2

This patient has had a cholecystectomy for biliary lithiasis. Operative cholangiography reveals a common bile duct of normal caliber without any symptoms of obstruction. One can, however, observe a calculus that is impacted in the distal common bile duct.

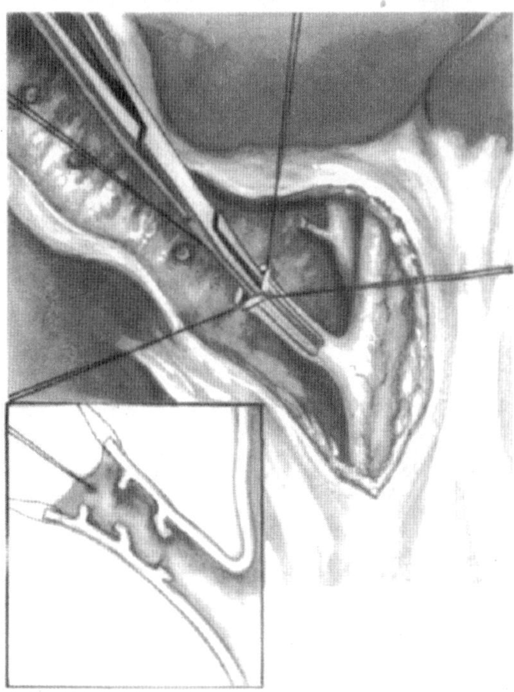

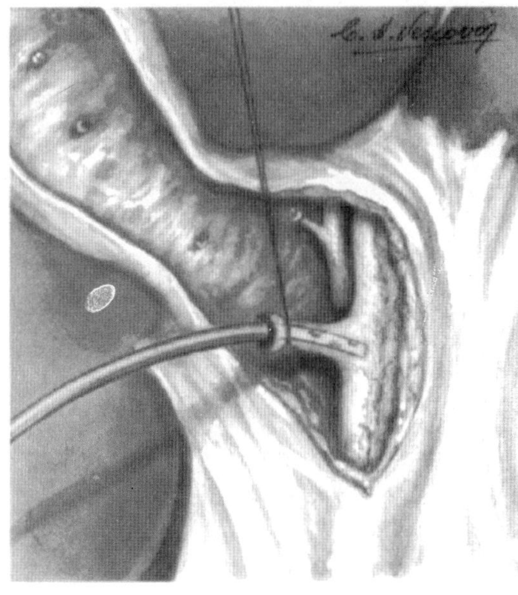

FIGURE 4.1 TRANSCYSTIC CHOLANGIOGRAM

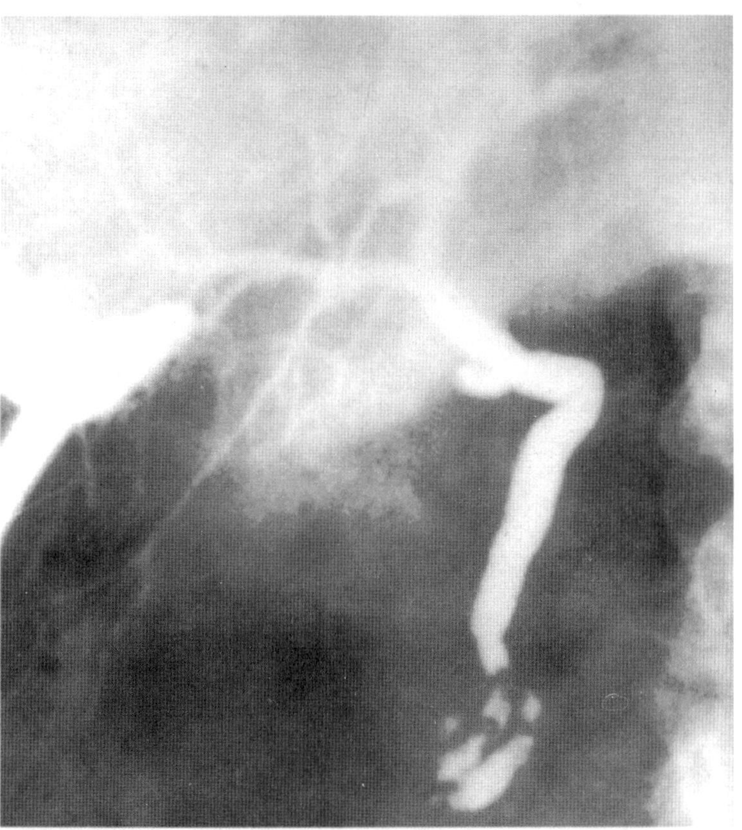

FIGURE 4.2

FIGURE 4.3
This patient presented a single large calculus in the gallbladder with a dilated cystic duct. Operative cholangiography, however, revealed a common bile duct of normal diameter with an image typical of a calculus in its distal end. The patient had presented symptoms that did not suggest obstruction of the common bile duct.

FIGURE 4.4
A patient with previous cholecystectomy for biliary lithiasis. Operative cholangiogram shows that the common bile duct is of normal caliber, without calculi in its interior but revealing an aberrant hepatic duct emptying into the cystic duct. Lack of knowledge of the existence of this anomaly may lead to serious consequences.

Exploratory Methods Without Choledochotomy

FIGURE 4.5
A patient with previous cholecystectomy for biliary lithiasis. The surgeon did not perform an operative cholangiogram. Instrumental exploration did not reveal the presence of calculi in the common bile duct. In the immediate postoperative period the patient developed significant hemobilia and had to be operated on the fourth postoperative day, revealing a lesion of the hepatic parenchyma communicating with the intrahepatic biliary tract caused by instrumental exploration performed in the first operation. The operative cholangiogram reveals the existing communication between the hepatic parenchyma and the intrahepatic ducts.

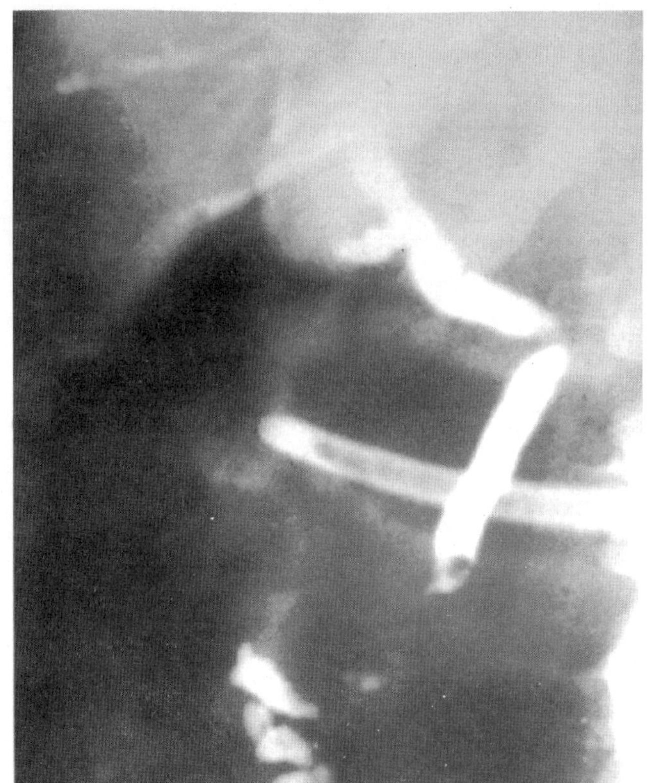
FIGURE 4.3

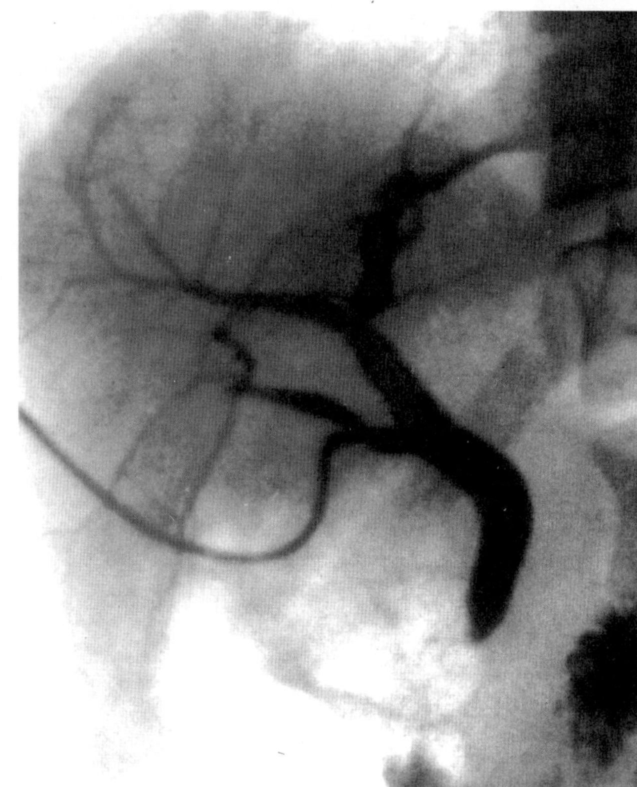
FIGURE 4.4

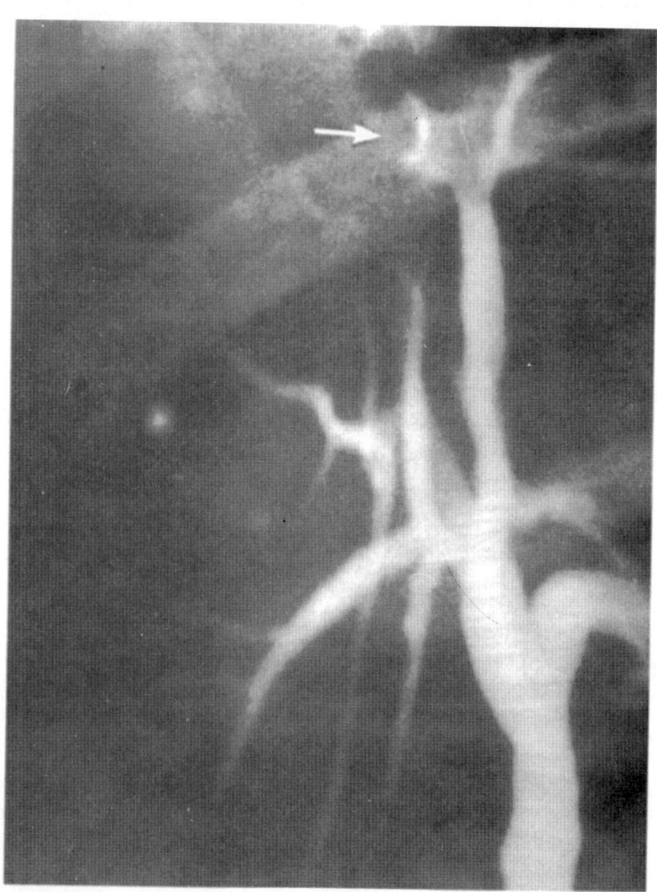
FIGURE 4.5

FIGURE 4.6
Control operative cholangiogram through the T-tube. The surgeon was convinced that he had removed all the calculi in this patient with multiple calculi of the common bile duct. An operative control cholangiogram, however, revealed, as shown in the illustration, that there are several residual calculi in the left hepatic bile duct and in the common hepatic bile duct, as well as a small calculus adherent to the left wall of the common bile duct and a calculus impacted in the papilla. The radiopaque substance scarcely passes in a sufficient amount into the duodenum.

Exploratory Methods Without Choledochotomy

FIGURE 4.7
Operative cholangiogram in a patient with a dilated common bile duct and two large rounded calculi in the common bile duct as well as a calculus impacted in the papilla. One can clearly observe the filling defect between the extra and intramural common bile duct. The rounded image with calcified walls corresponds to a hydatid cyst of the liver with no relation to the biliary tract.

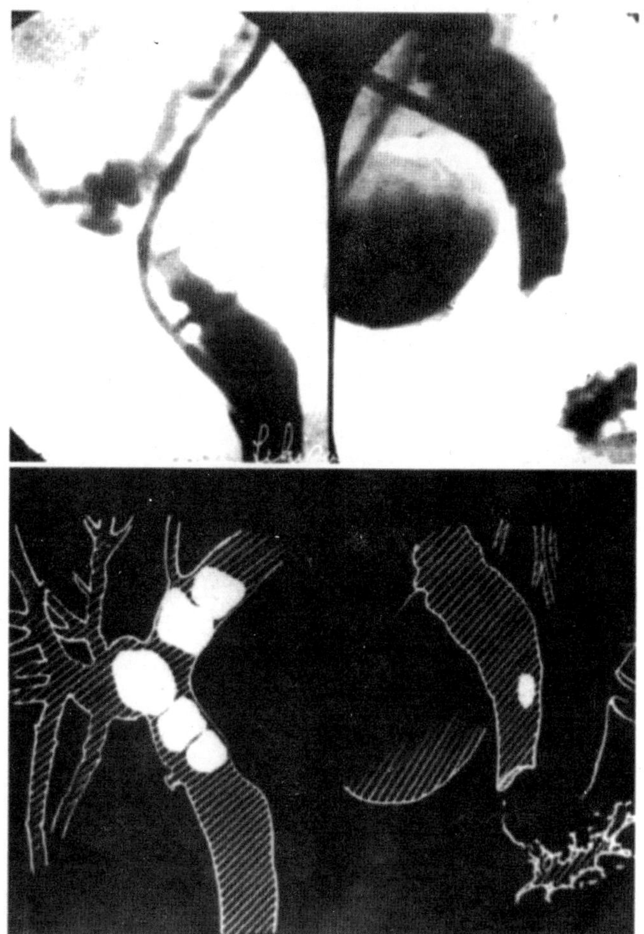

FIGURE 4.6

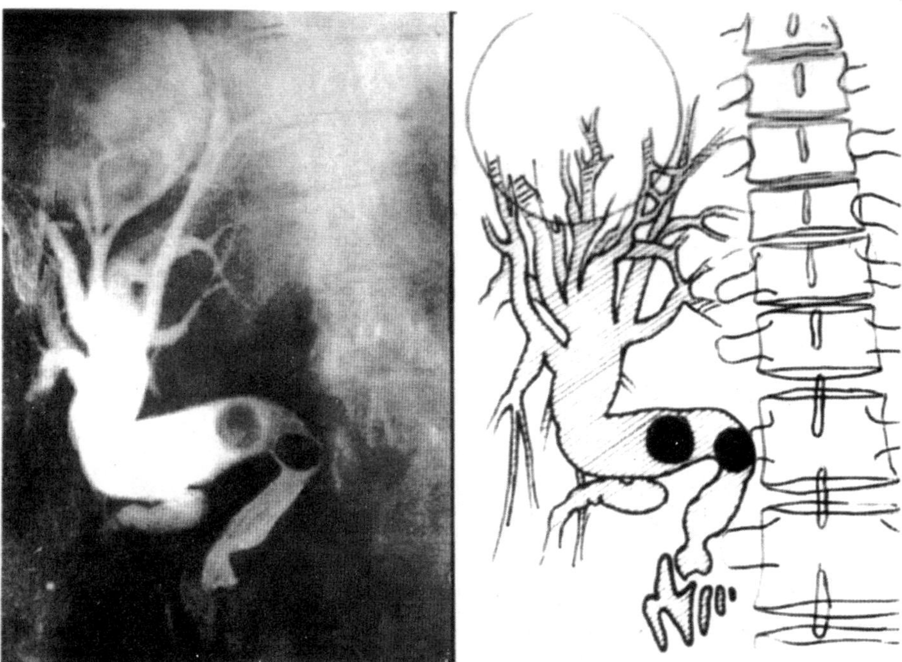

FIGURE 4.7

Exploratory Methods Without Choledochotomy

FIGURE 4.8
Operative cholangiogram in a patient cholecystectomized because of multiple biliary calculi. The common bile duct is moderately dilated with no calculi within it and emptying into a diverticulum of the second portion of the duodenum. The pancreatic duct also empties into the same diverticulum.

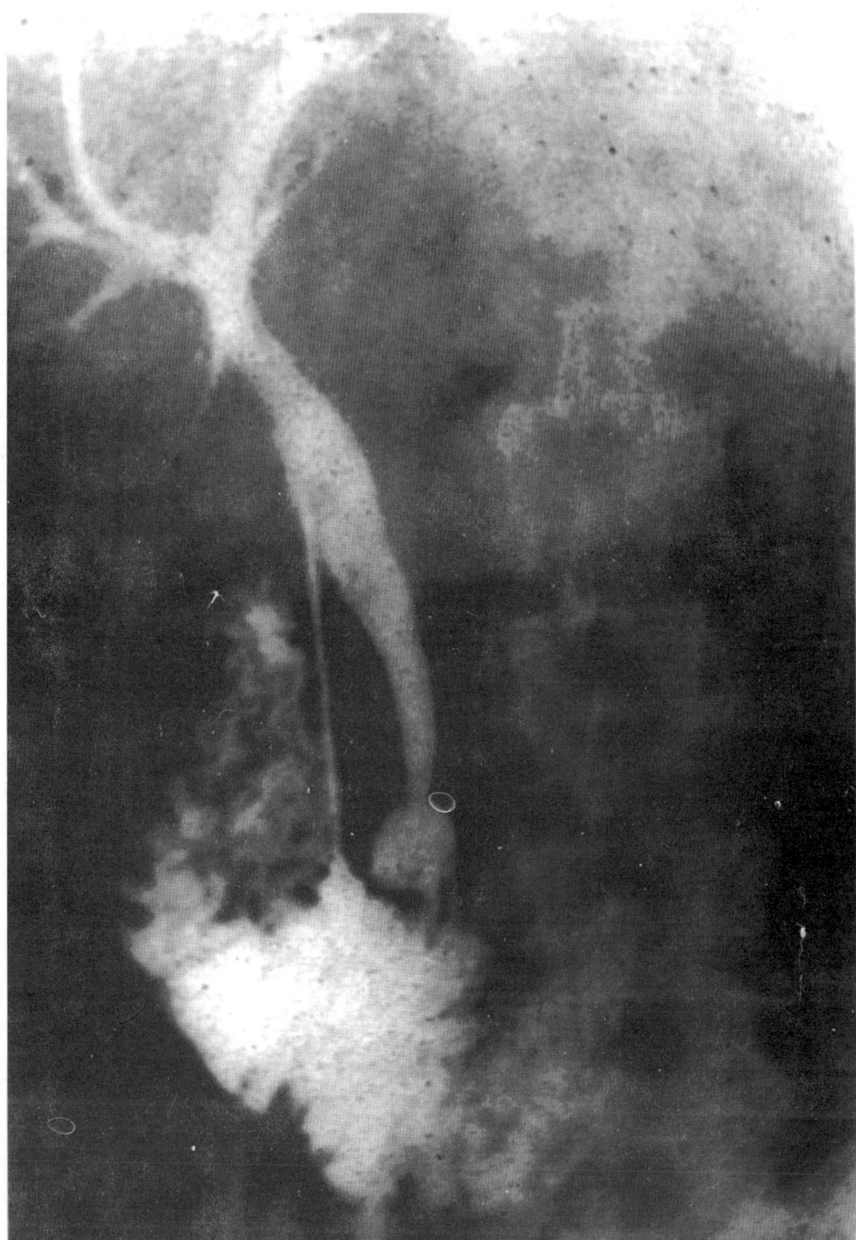

FIGURE 4.8

Exploratory Methods Without Choledochotomy

FIGURE 4.9
Cholecystectomized patient for biliary lithiasis. The control operative cholangiogram through the T-tube reveals that there are still calculi in the common bile duct and that this duct empties into a diverticulum of the second portion of the duodenum.

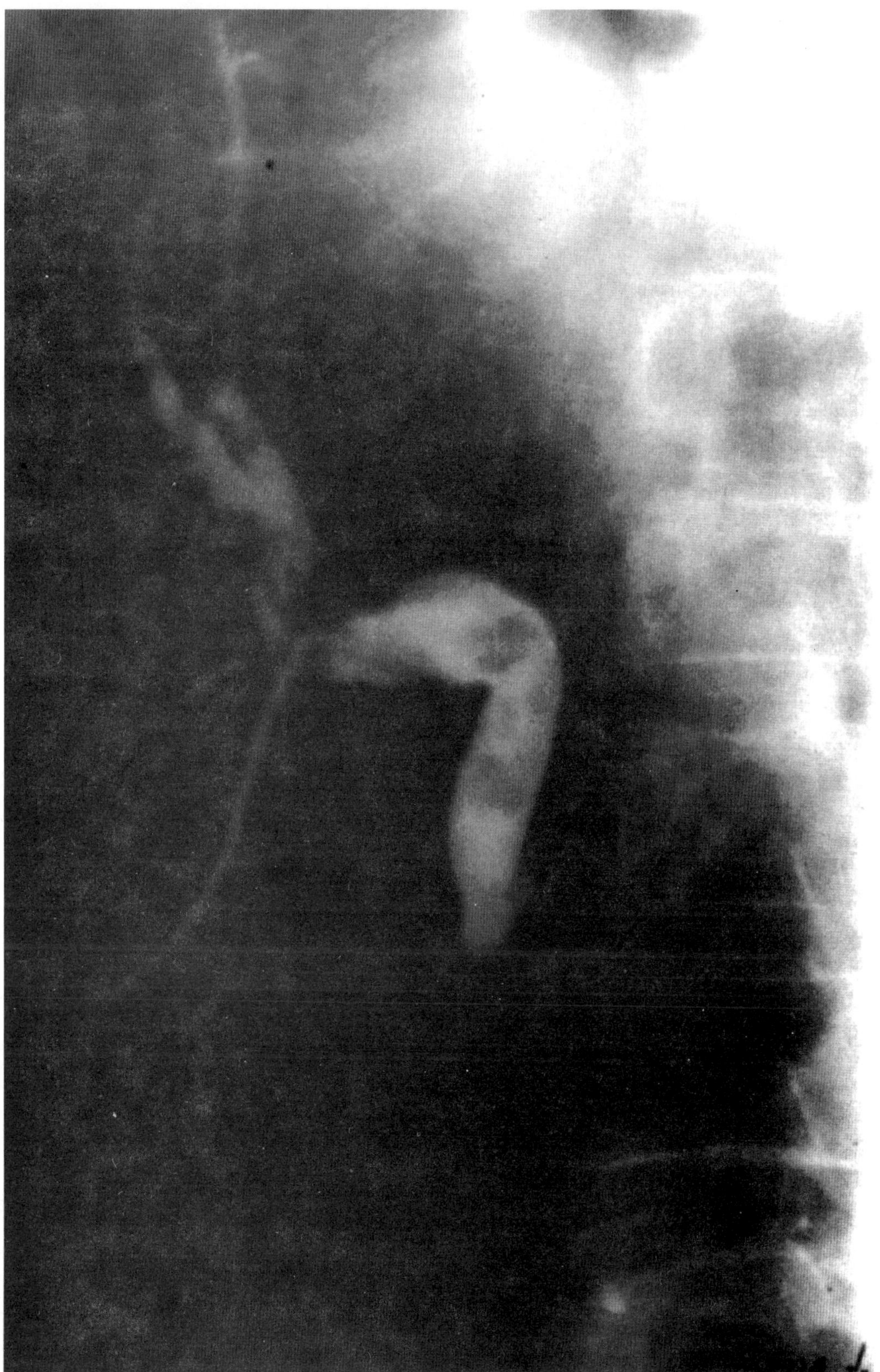

FIGURE 4.9

FIGURE 4.10
Cholecystectomized patient for multiple biliary calculi. A calculus in the common bile duct had been removed. Operative control cholangiogram reveals that there is a peripapillary duodenal diverticulum.

Exploratory Methods Without Choledochotomy

FIGURE 4.11
In patients who have been previously cholecystectomized and have to be reoperated, an operative cholangiogram should be performed by puncture of the common bile duct. It is very easy to identify the common bile duct when it is dilated. On the contrary, if the common bile duct is normal in caliber or only slightly dilated and covered by thick and fibrous tissue due to the previous surgery, its identification may be more difficult and performance of the operative cholangiogram also difficult. To puncture the common bile duct one usually uses a No. 23 needle adapted to a 10 mL syringe. The needle should not have a long bevel. The needle should be directed from below upward as shown in the drawing, following an acute angle in relation to the hepatoduodenal ligament with the object of preventing the needle from passing through the posterior wall of the common bile duct or entering the portal vein. Either possibility may lead to confusion. The puncture should be made in the area of the suprapancreatic portion of the common bile duct where choledochotomies are usually performed. Puncture into the lumen of the common bile duct generally reveals bile. Using the same needle 10 mL of a radiopaque substance diluted to 35% is slowly injected and two x-rays obtained.

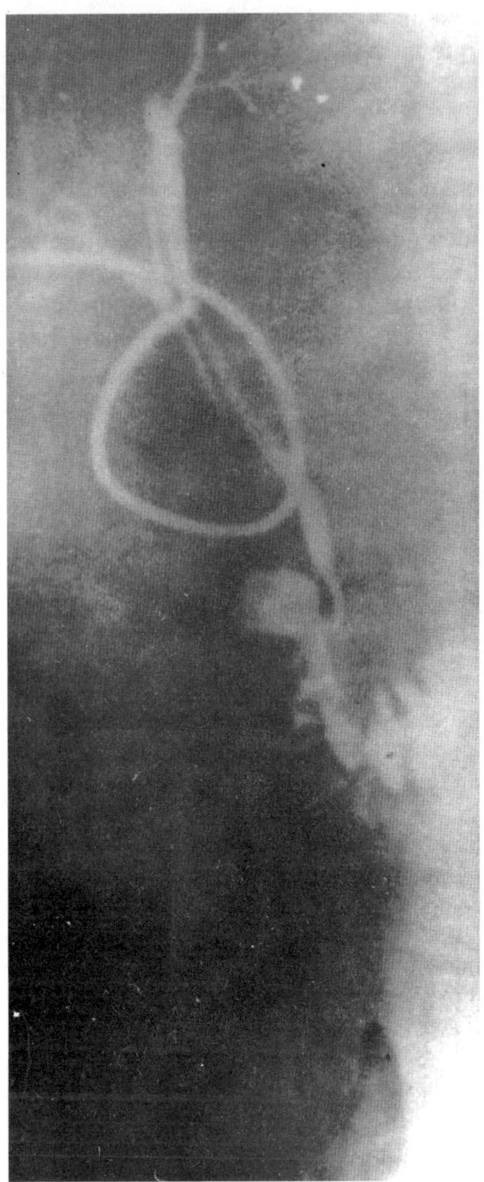

FIGURE 4.10

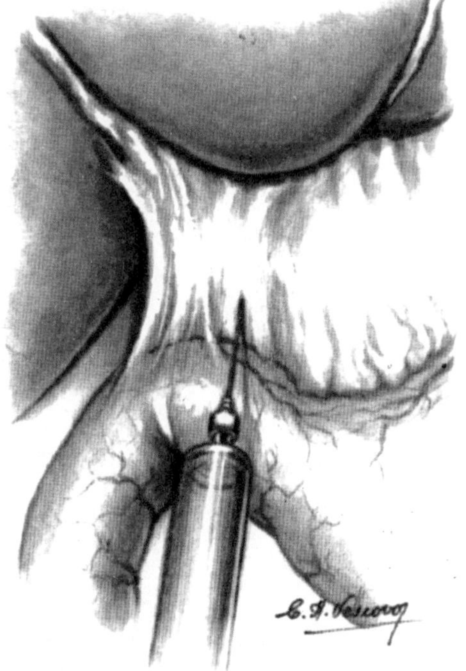

FIGURE 4.11

Operative Cholangiography in Patients with Neoplastic Obstructions of the Common Bile Duct

The most common neoplastic obstructions of the common bile duct are those caused by carcinoma of the head of the pancreas, carcinoma of the papilla, carcinoma of the distal end of the common bile duct, or chronic pancreatitis with compression of the retropancreatic common bile duct. The gallbladder and the common bile duct above the narrowed segment are generally very dilated, making it necessary to inject a large amount of radiopaque material. A purse-string suture is placed on the fundus of the gallbladder in the center of which the gallbladder is punctured with a Trocar and the thick gelatinous contents removed by electric suction. Some 60 to 80 mL of radiopaque substance are then injected through the puncture site. The purse-string suture is tied, leaving the ends long to apply traction to the fundus of the gallbladder upward and to the right so that the shadow of the gallbladder will not become superimposed on the shadow of the common bile duct.

Operative Cholangiography in Patients with Neoplastic Obstructions of the Common Bile Duct

FIGURE 4.12
Operative cholangiogram in a patient with carcinoma of the head of the pancreas. The gallbladder and the biliary tract are very dilated. The obstruction of the common bile duct is complete, blunt shaped, and proximal to the papilla, giving the impression that the common bile duct has been amputated. One can observe the horizontal direction of the common bile duct. The cystic duct empties near the tumor.

Operative Cholangiography in Patients with Neoplastic Obstructions of the Common Bile Duct

FIGURE 4.13
Operative cholangiogram in a previously cholecystectomized patient for biliary lithiasis. One can observe the dilation of the common bile duct and the ribbon-like narrowing of the retropancreatic portion of the common bile duct produced by chronic pancreatitis, predominantly cephalic, obstructing the retropancreatic duct. Obstruction of the common bile duct can be produced by hypertrophy of the pancreas, by pseudocyst of the head of the pancreas, or by peripancreatic fibrosis. Above the stricture one can observe a very dilated common bile duct and a big rounded stone located at the beginning of the stricture.

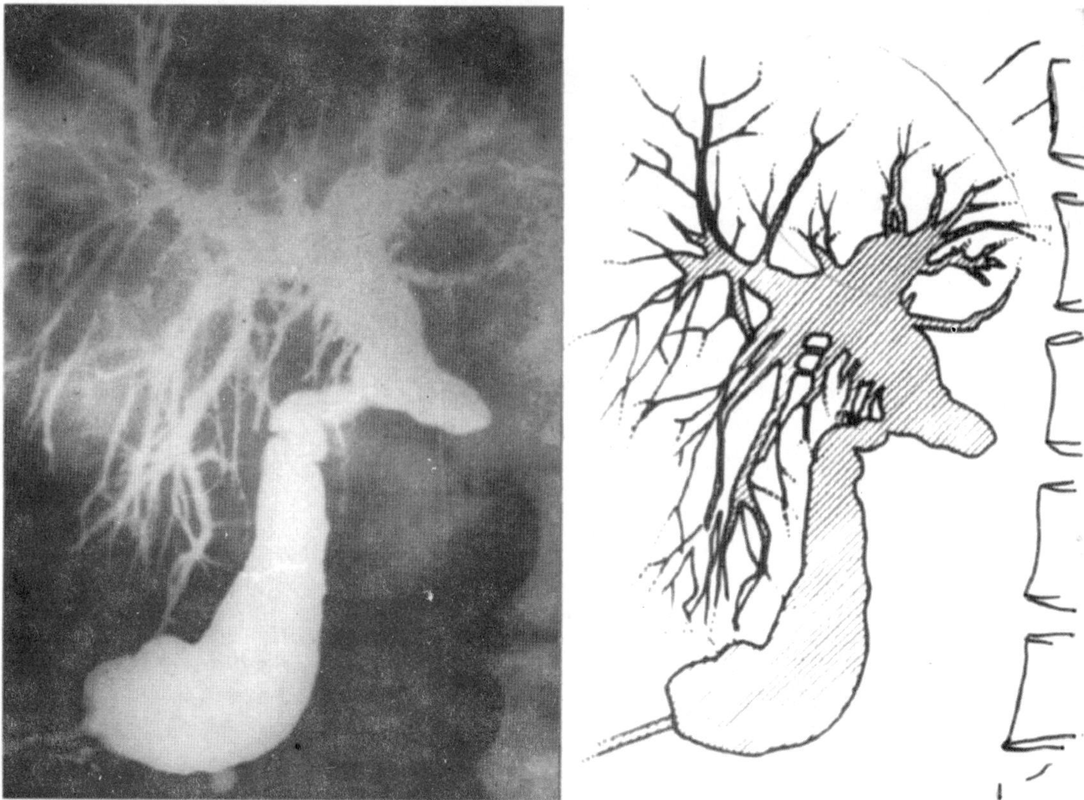

FIGURE 4.12

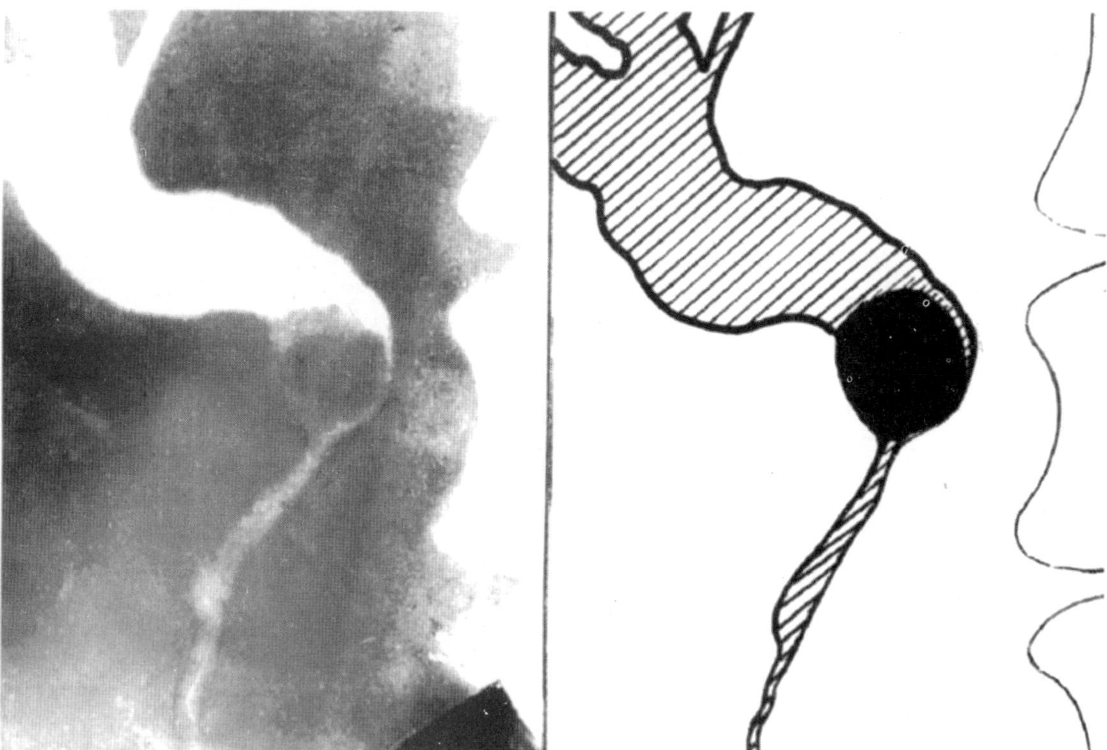

FIGURE 4.13

FIGURE 4.14
Operative cholangiogram in a patient with carcinoma of the papilla. The gallbladder and the biliary tract are very dilated. There is a complete obstruction of the common bile duct at the level of the papilla. The irregularity in the area of the obstruction is produced by the neoplasm protruding and growing into the lumen of the common bile duct. This cystic duct empties in the common bile duct, far from the tumor.

Operative Cholangiography in Patients with Neoplastic Obstructions of the Common Bile Duct

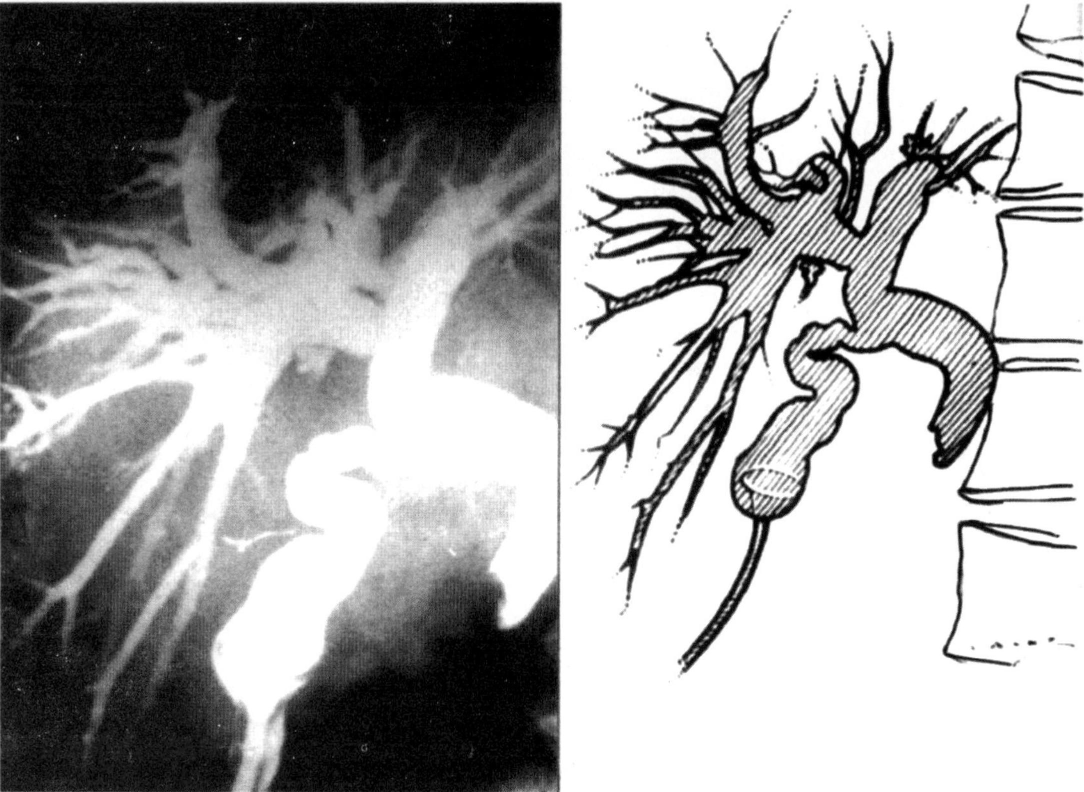

FIGURE 4.14

Exploration of the Common Bile Duct by Palpation

A superficial palpation of the common bile duct is usually performed when the abdomen is open in a procedure for biliary lithiasis. To perform an adequate palpation of the common bile duct and neighboring organs such as the pancreas and duodenum, it is necessary to perform a Vautrin-Kocher maneuver. This maneuver should be performed if the operative cholangiogram shows the presence of any pathology. On the contrary, if the cholangiogram reveals that the common bile duct is normal in caliber without abnormal images of calculi and the dye passes readily into the duodenum, it is not necessary to perform the Vautrin-Kocher maneuver.

Technique of the Vautrin-Kocher Maneuver

Technique of the Vautrin-Kocher Maneuver

FIGURE 4.15
The Vautrin-Kocher maneuver is begun by bringing the transverse colon and its meso-colon downward exposing the entire second portion of the duodenum and the lateral segment of the third portion of the duodenum.

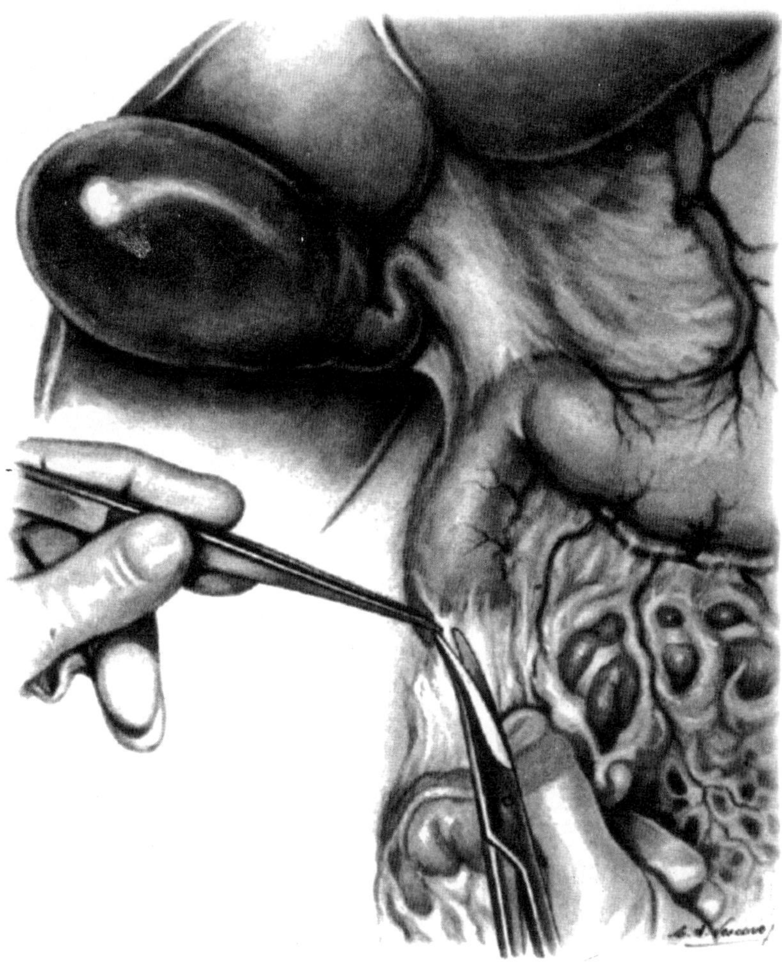

FIGURE 4.15

Technique of the Vautrin-Kocher Maneuver

FIGURE 4.16
The transverse colon and its meso-colon are held downward by means of a gauze compress held in place by a Deaver retractor.

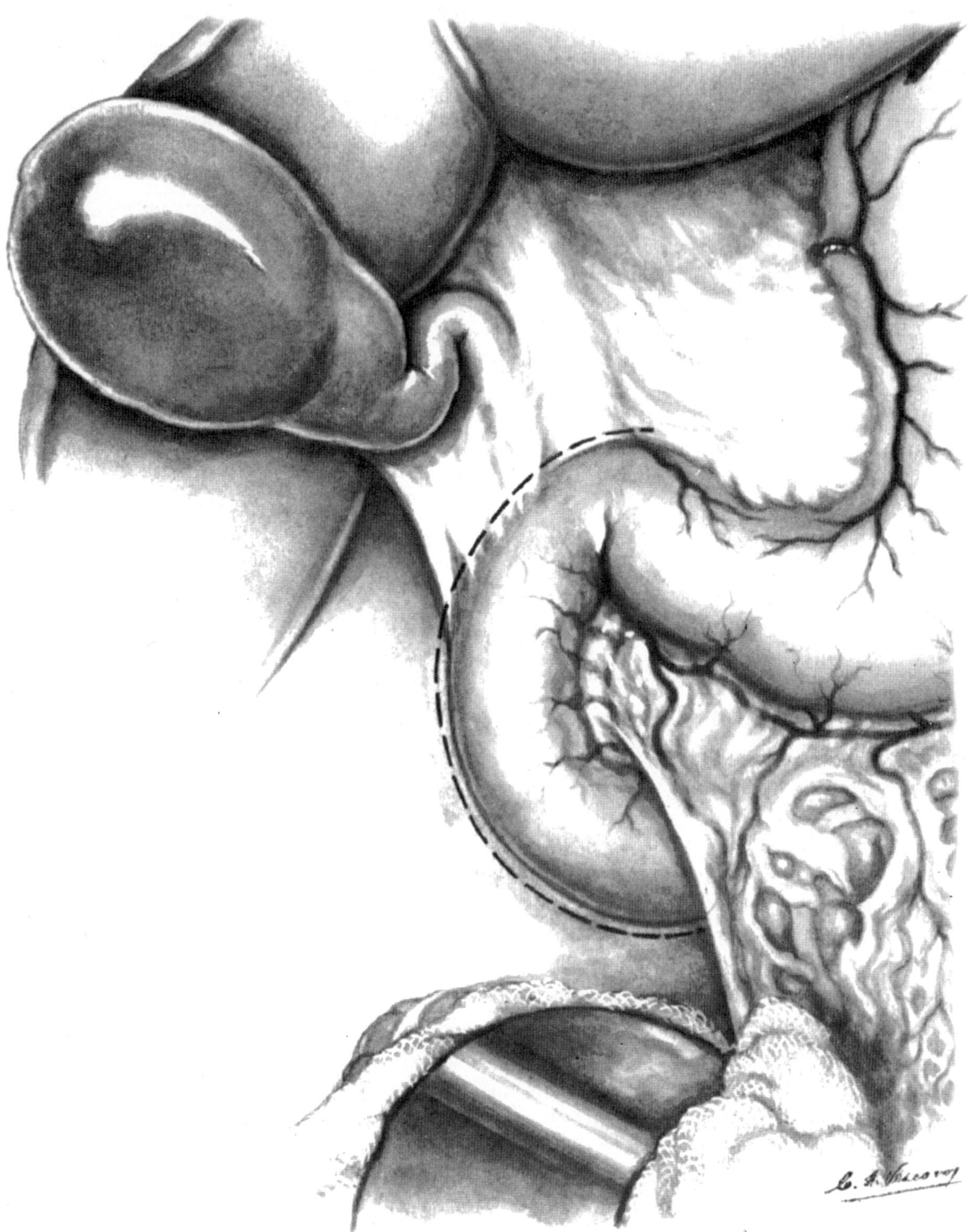

FIGURE 4.16

FIGURE 4.17

The peritoneum along the external border of the second portion of the duodenum is incised. To perform this maneuver the first assistant grasps the second portion of the duodenum with both hands and applies traction to it gently toward the left while the surgeon, using scissors, transects the peritoneum near the lateral border of the second portion of the duodenum, as can be seen in the drawing.

Technique of the Vautrin-Kocher Maneuver

FIGURE 4.18

The peritoneum of the external border of the second portion of the duodenum and the lateral segment of the third portion of the duodenum have been incised as well as the anterior leaf of the peritoneum of the hepatoduodenal ligament.

FIGURE 4.19

The duodenum and the head of the pancreas have been mobilized and retracted to the left of the patient being held in place by the first assistant's hands or by two Babcock or Foerster clamps applying gentle traction so that the duodenal wall will not be torn.

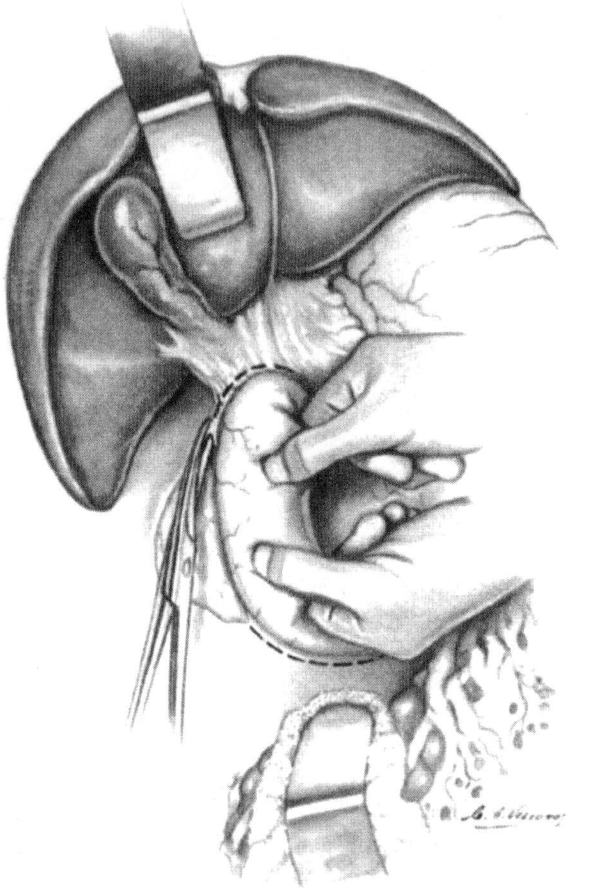

FIGURE 4.17

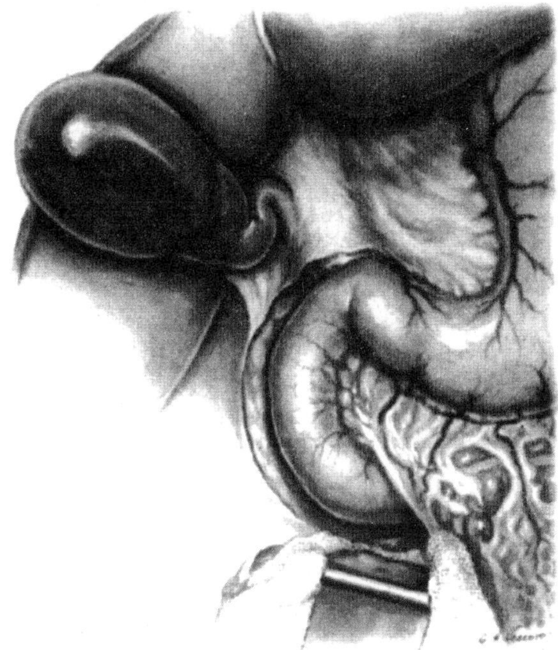

FIGURE 4.18

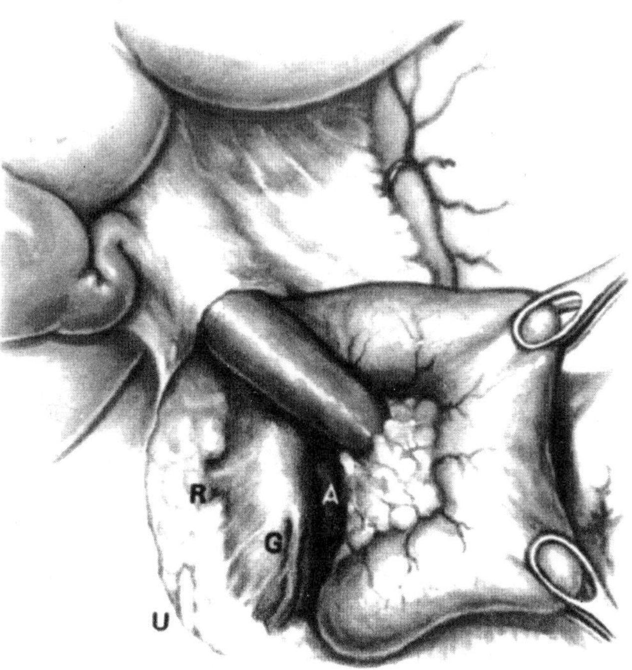

FIGURE 4.19

FIGURE 4.20
With the left index and middle fingers placed behind and the thumb in front of the duodenum and pancreas, the common bile duct is palpated, as can be seen on the drawing. With the same hand the duodenum, head of the pancreas, and papilla can be palpated.

Palpation of the Common Bile Duct

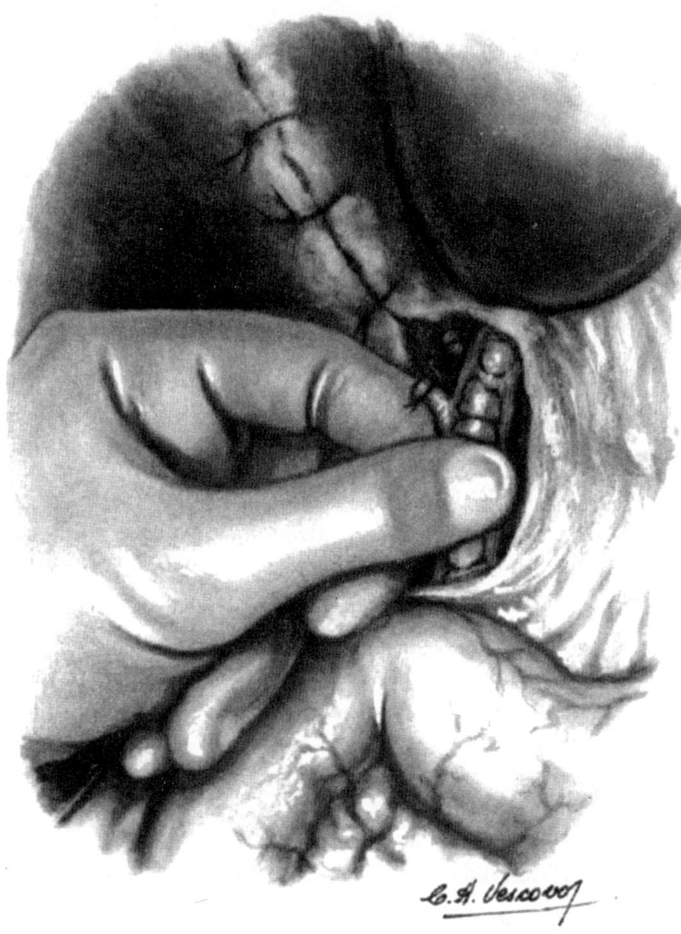

FIGURE 4.20

FIGURE 4.21

To perform an instrumental exploration of the common bile duct it is necessary to perform a choledochotomy. This choledochotomy is made in the supraduodenal segment of the common bile duct. The majority of surgeons perform a longitudinal choledochotomy as shown in the figure to the right. The author, like Mirizzi, prefers to perform a transverse choledochotomy, below the opening of the cystic duct, as shown in the figure to the left.

Choledochotomy and Instrumental Exploration of the Common Bile Duct

FIGURE 4.22

The transverse choledochotomy is performed by grasping the common bile duct with two sutures using fine cotton on an atraumatic needle, one above the other and separated by some 3 mm. The surgeon applies gentle traction to the ends of the sutures to raise the anterior wall of the common bile duct. Part of the anterior wall of the common bile duct is incised between the previously placed sutures. The extent of the transverse incision will be directly related to the diameter of the common bile duct and the size of the calculi to be removed. In the great majority of cases it is not necessary to incise the entire anterior wall of the common bile duct. Once the anterior wall of the common bile duct has been incised, the edges of this incision and the angles are grasped with traction sutures that significantly amplify the opening of the common bile duct.

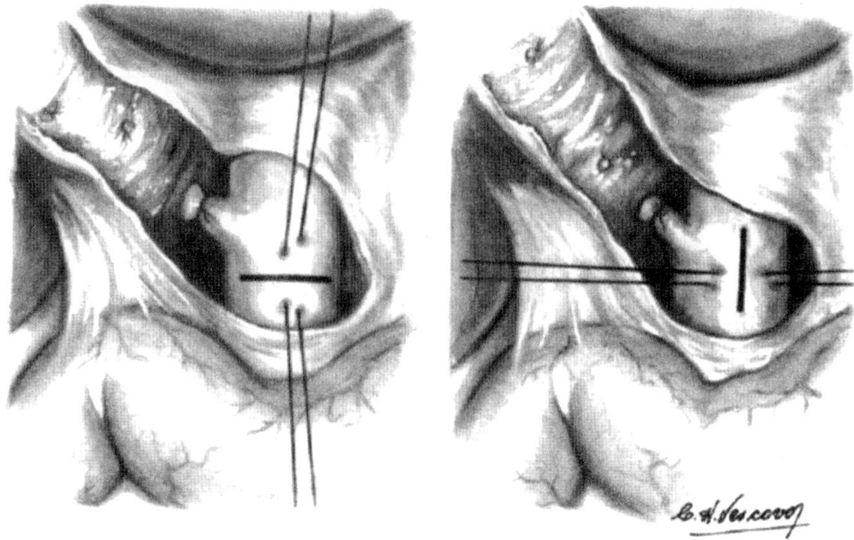

FIGURE 4.21

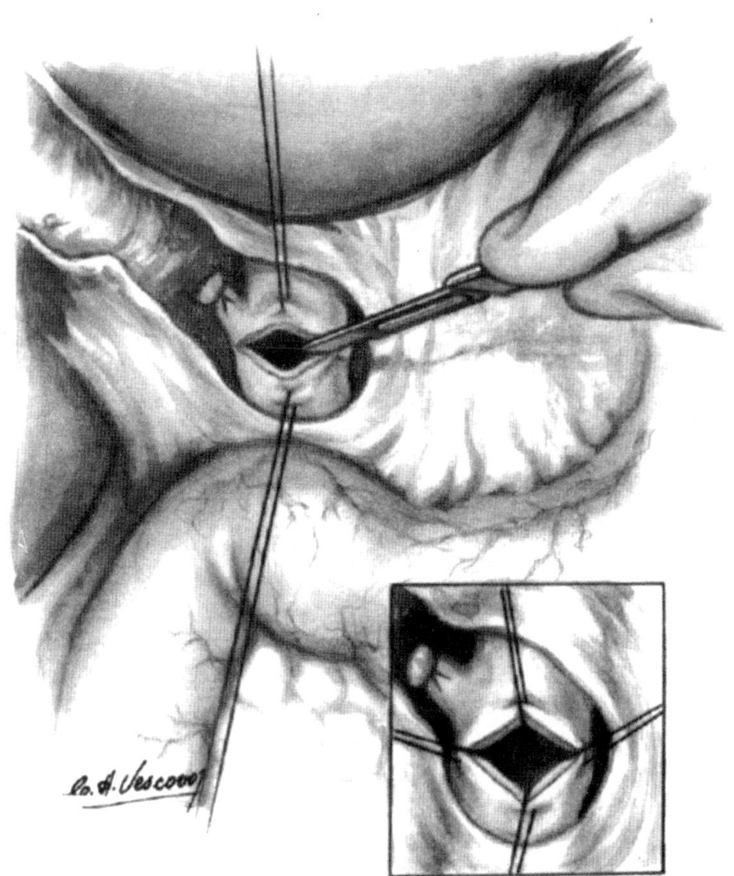

FIGURE 4.22

FIGURE 4.23
The transverse choledochotomy allows the removal of all the calculi in the common bile duct, no matter their size. The drawing reveals the removal of a large calculus of the common bile duct through the transverse choledochotomy. The calculus has been grasped by a Desjardins clamp. To facilitate the removal of calculi from the common hepatic duct it is useful to push them toward the choledochotomy by grasping the common hepatic duct between the index and thumb of the left hand. When the calculi appear at the choledochotomy, they are then grasped with a Desjardins clamp.

Choledochotomy and Instrumental Exploration of the Common Bile Duct

FIGURE 4.24
The drawing shows the removal of a calculus from the papilla using a malleable spoon. If the calculus in the papilla is not impacted, it is generally possible to remove it through the supraduodenal choledochotomy. The spoon is held with one hand and the fingers of the other hand so that the calculus can be removed by catching it in the concavity of the spoon. This same technique is used to remove other calculi in the distal common bile duct. If the calculi are located in the proximal common bile duct, they are pushed with the thumb and index finger of the left hand until they appear at the choledochotomy, where they are grasped with a Desjardins clamp.

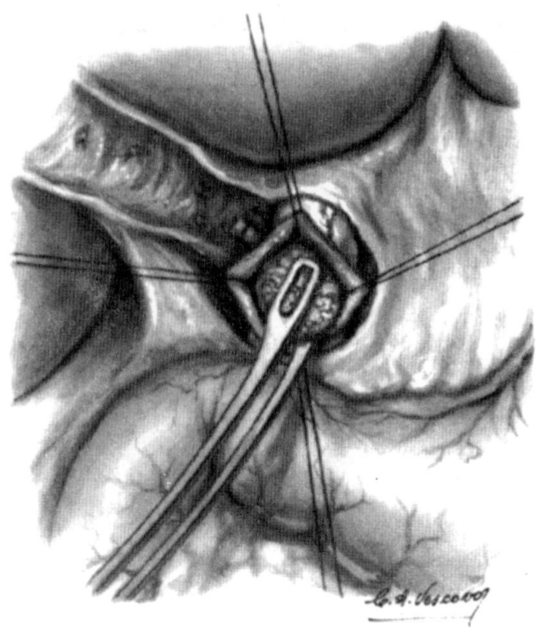

FIGURE 4.23

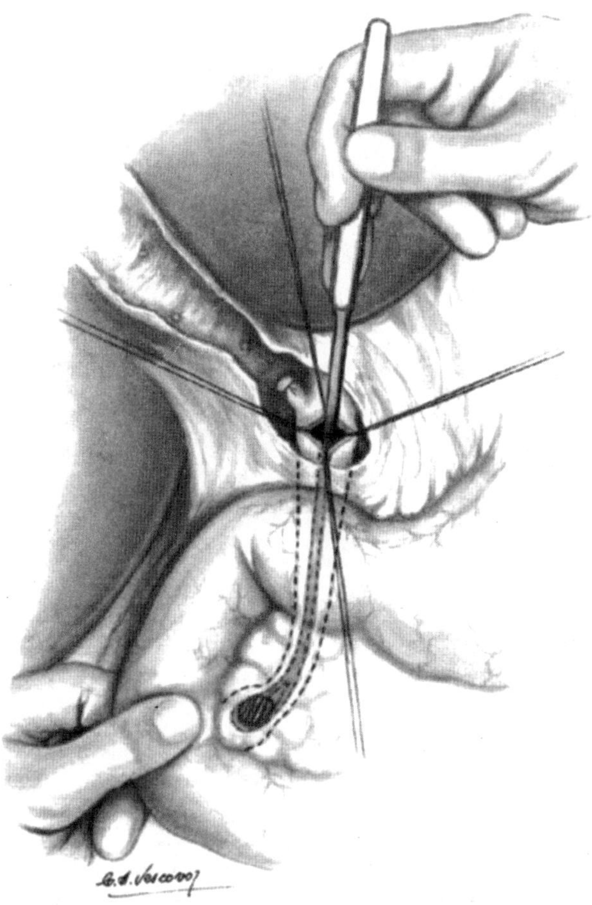

FIGURE 4.24

FIGURE 4.25
Some intrahepatic calculi can be removed using malleable spoons, as shown in the drawing.

Choledochotomy and Instrumental Exploration of the Common Bile Duct

FIGURE 4.26
Some other intrahepatic calculi can be removed using Dormia catheters, as shown in the drawing.

FIGURE 4.27
In other cases, to remove intrahepatic calculi, one has to recur to modified Fogarty catheters designed for removal of calculi in the biliary tract, as shown in the drawing.

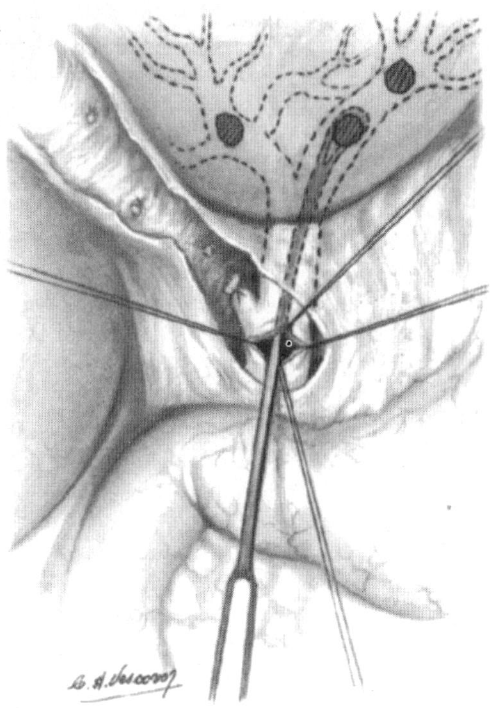

FIGURE 4.25

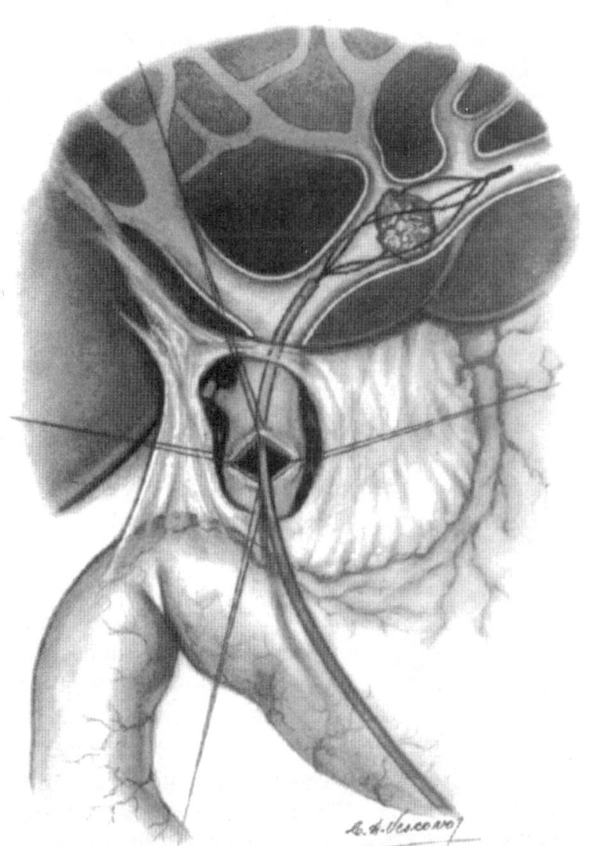

FIGURE 4.26

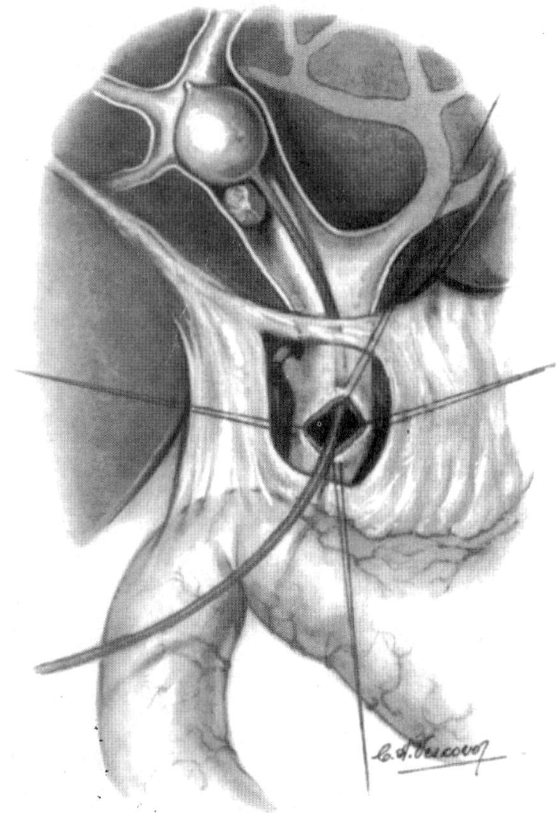

FIGURE 4.27

FIGURE 4.28

As much as possible of the exploration of the papilla should be performed with tapering olive-shaped semirigid plastic or silk tissue explorers. Metallic explorers should only be used in exceptional situations. If the operative cholangiogram has shown that the common bile duct is normal in caliber without images of calculi and the radiopaque substance passes into the duodenum normally, instrumental exploration of the papilla is unnecessary. With or without an operative cholangiogram, it is common for surgeons to perform instrumental exploration of the common bile duct. In this case it is enough that a 3 mm explorer be passed through the papilla. It is not necessary to pass explorers of greater caliber to show that the papilla presents a normal lumen. As a matter of fact, if there is some difficulty in passing a 3 mm explorer it does not mean that there is a stricture of the sphincter of Oddi, since this problem may appear in normal papillae. If metallic Bakes dilators are used these should not be used as dilators and only as explorers (which was the original reason why the Czech surgeon designed them). It is enough to pass a No. 3 Bakes explorer. Dilation of the papilla is completely unnecessary, useless, and traumatizing, and can cause false tracts with grave consequences. All exploring maneuvers of the papilla should be performed with extreme care. Recognition that the explorer has passed through the papilla is easily proven. In this case the end of the explorer is freely palpable within the lumen of the duodenum some 3 to 4 cm below the papilla and generally pushes the opposite wall of the duodenum giving the impression that it is going to perforate. If a metallic explorer is used, a typical metallic shine, described by the German surgeon Walzel, is seen as may be observed in the drawing.

Exploration of the Papilla

FIGURE 4.29

Metallic explorers can traumatize the papilla, producing lacerations of the papilla and false tracts. If a false tract is made toward the duodenal lumen it can be overlooked, but a false tract made into the pancreatic parenchyma can be much more serious, especially if the surgeon does not recognize it during the operative procedure. The present drawing reveals that the end of the explorer is about to enter the duodenum at a point above the papilla, producing a false tract.

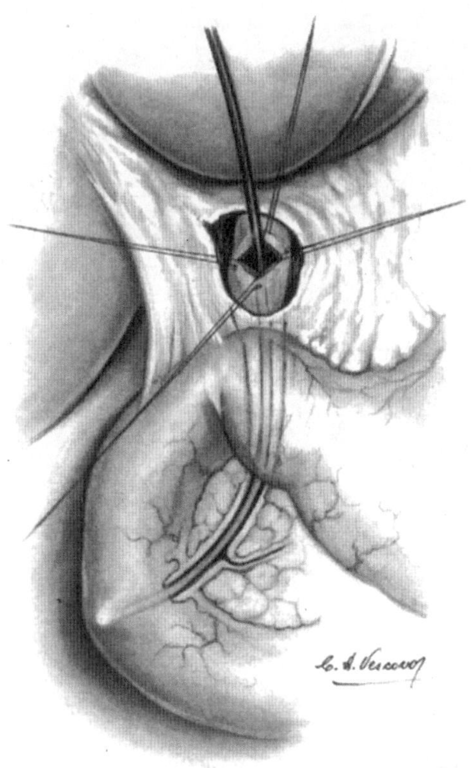

FIGURE 4.28

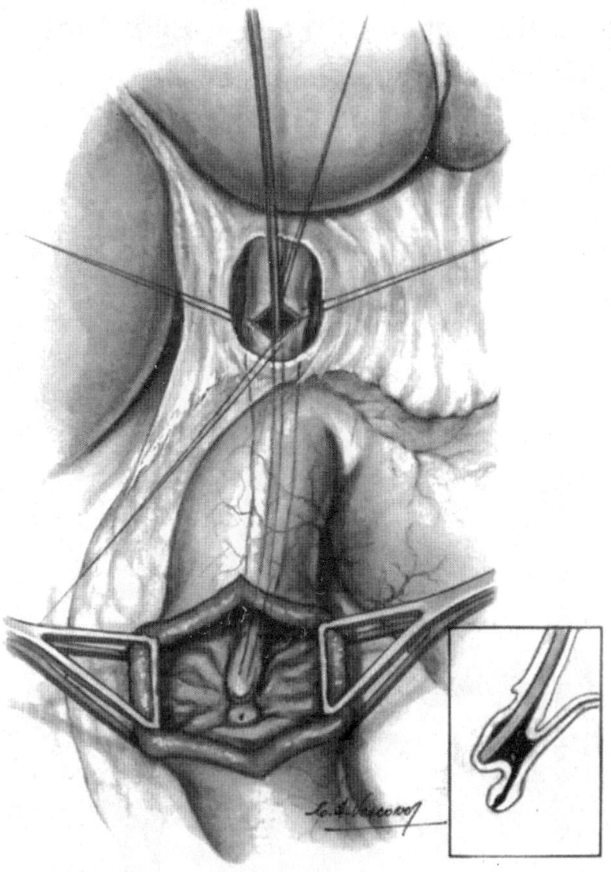

FIGURE 4.29

Exploration of the Common Bile Duct by Means of Choledochoscopy

FIGURE 4.30
It is useful to examine the interior of the common bile duct with a choledochoscope after instrumental exploration of the common bile duct and removal of calculi has been performed. This is useful as a method of control before placing the T-tube and performing the operative cholangiogram through the T-tube. Even though choledochoscopy is used it does not mean that one should not perform the operative control cholangiogram through the T-tube. The drawing reveals an exploration of the common bile duct with a rigid choledochoscope. Flexible choledochoscopes can also be used that are narrow and permit a more complete examination than that performed with a rigid choledochoscope, especially in the areas of the papilla and the intrahepatic ducts.

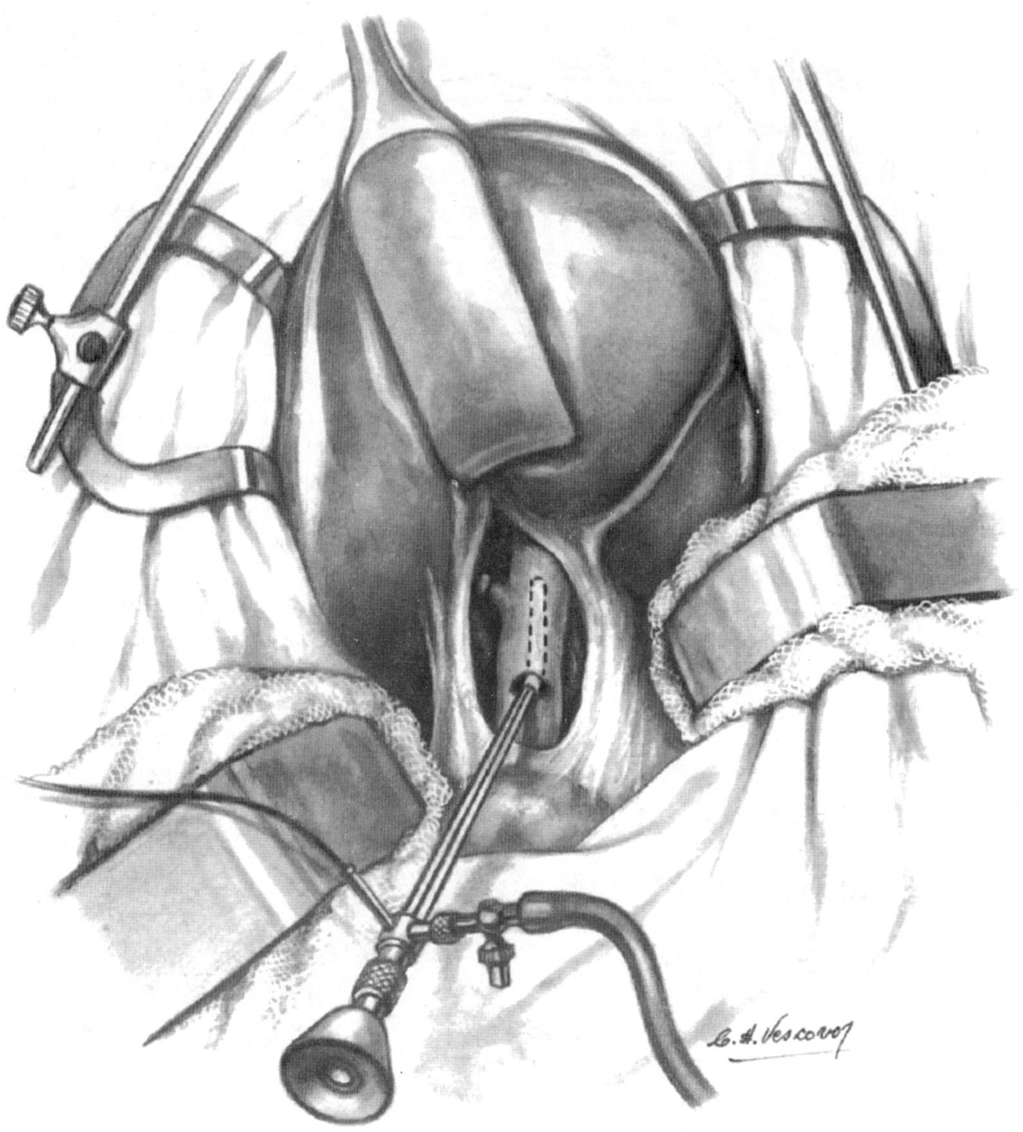

FIGURE 4.30

FIGURE 4.31
The T-tube should be selected according to the diameter of the common bile duct. One should choose T-tubes with the short limb being of smaller caliber than the long limb. The posterior surface of the short limb should be removed, transforming the short limb into a canal to facilitate its removal. At the same time the length of the short limb should be adapted to the length of the common bile duct. It should not be too short, because this would facilitate its spontaneous expulsion, nor too long, because that can lead to serious inconveniences as we will note later. The drawing shows an easy way of introducing the T-tube into the common bile duct. One side of the short limb is grasped with toothed forceps and introduced in the direction of the common hepatic duct.

Technique of Placement of the T-Tube

FIGURE 4.32
Once a short limb has been placed in the direction of the common hepatic duct it is very easy to direct the other segment of the short limb downward, toward the common bile duct, as can be appreciated in the insert.

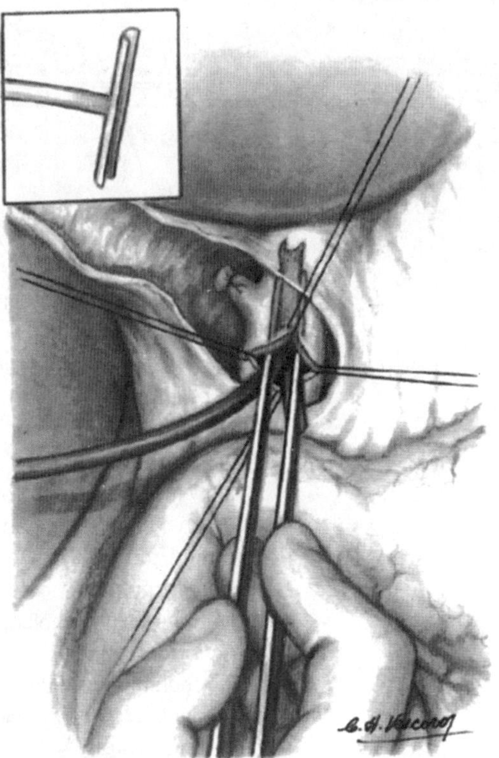

FIGURE 4.31

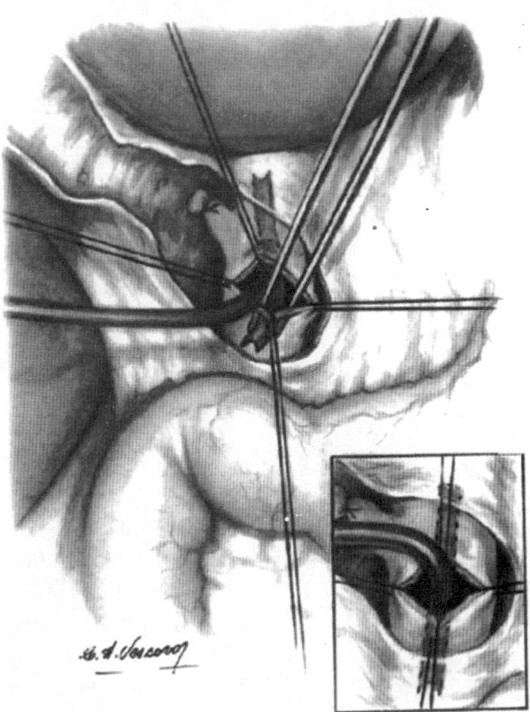

FIGURE 4.32

FIGURE 4.33

The choledochotomy is closed with interrupted sutures of 3-0 chromic catgut. The final control cholangiography is then obtained through the T-tube. A clamp is placed on the long limb of the T-tube, where bile has begun to flow, and the T-tube is punctured and dye injected slowly. The operative cholangiogram through the T-tube, if performed correctly, does not allow for the entrance of air bubbles. On the other hand, doubtful images of the papilla attributed to cholangiography performed through the T-tube are not caused by this procedure but by trauma inflicted on the papilla during explorations and dilations of the papilla, or by the production of false tracts. If a control cholangiogram has been obtained revealing that the common bile duct does not contain calculi and the dye passes readily into the duodenum, the closure of the choledochotomy is completed by suturing the peritoneum of the hepatoduodenal ligament over the closure of the common bile duct to make it more water-tight.

Technique of Placement of the T-Tube

FIGURE 4.34

After the choledochotomy has been closed the gall bladder bed is peritonealized with interrupted sutures. In some cases a precautionary measure can be taken fixing the T-tube with one suture of chromic catgut as seen in the drawing. On the other hand, if the closure of the choledochotomy was satisfactory and the surgeon was able to cover it with peritoneum, this additional step is not necessary.

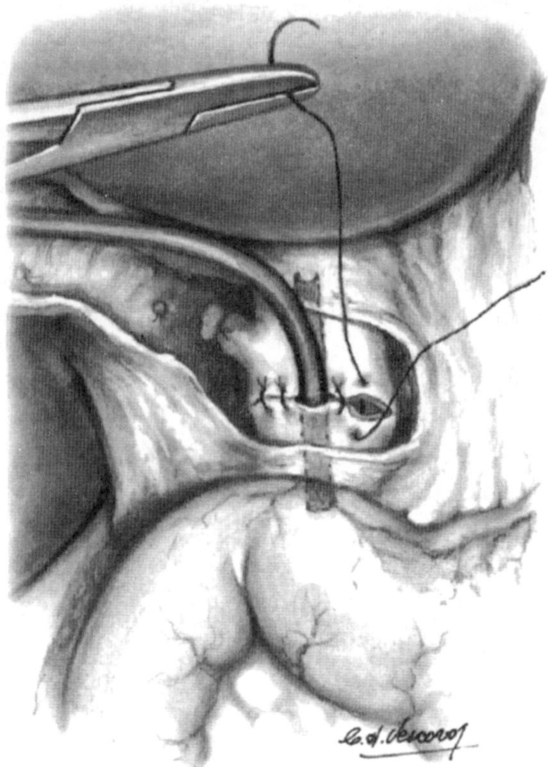

FIGURE 4.33

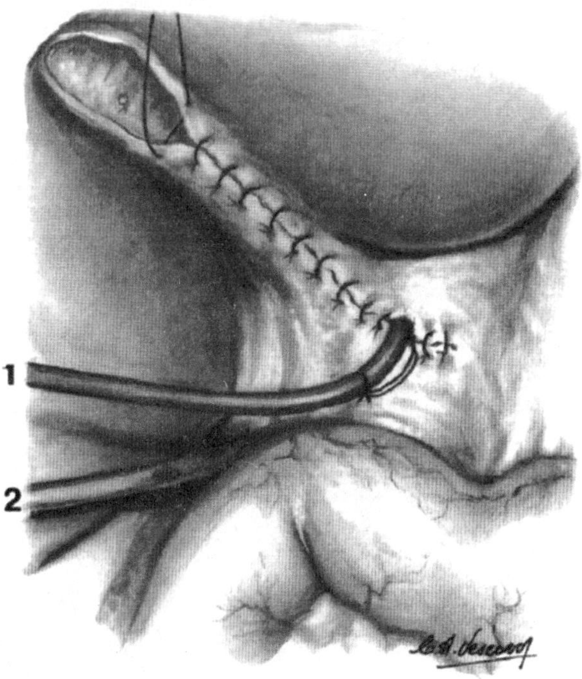

FIGURE 4.34

Errors that are Committed in Placing the T-Tube

FIGURE 4.35

1. Superior limb of the T-tube too long, touching the bifurcation of the common hepatic duct.
2. Superior limb of the T-tube too long, entering the right hepatic duct.
3. Superior limb of the T-tube too long, which upon touching the bifurcation of the common hepatic duct has doubled back on itself.
4. Superior limb of the T-tube has been introduced into the cystic duct, which has been left long.
5. The inferior limb of the T-tube is too long, producing an obstruction of the papilla.
6. The T-tube introduced too deeply. The short limb is placed at the bifurcation of the common hepatic duct.

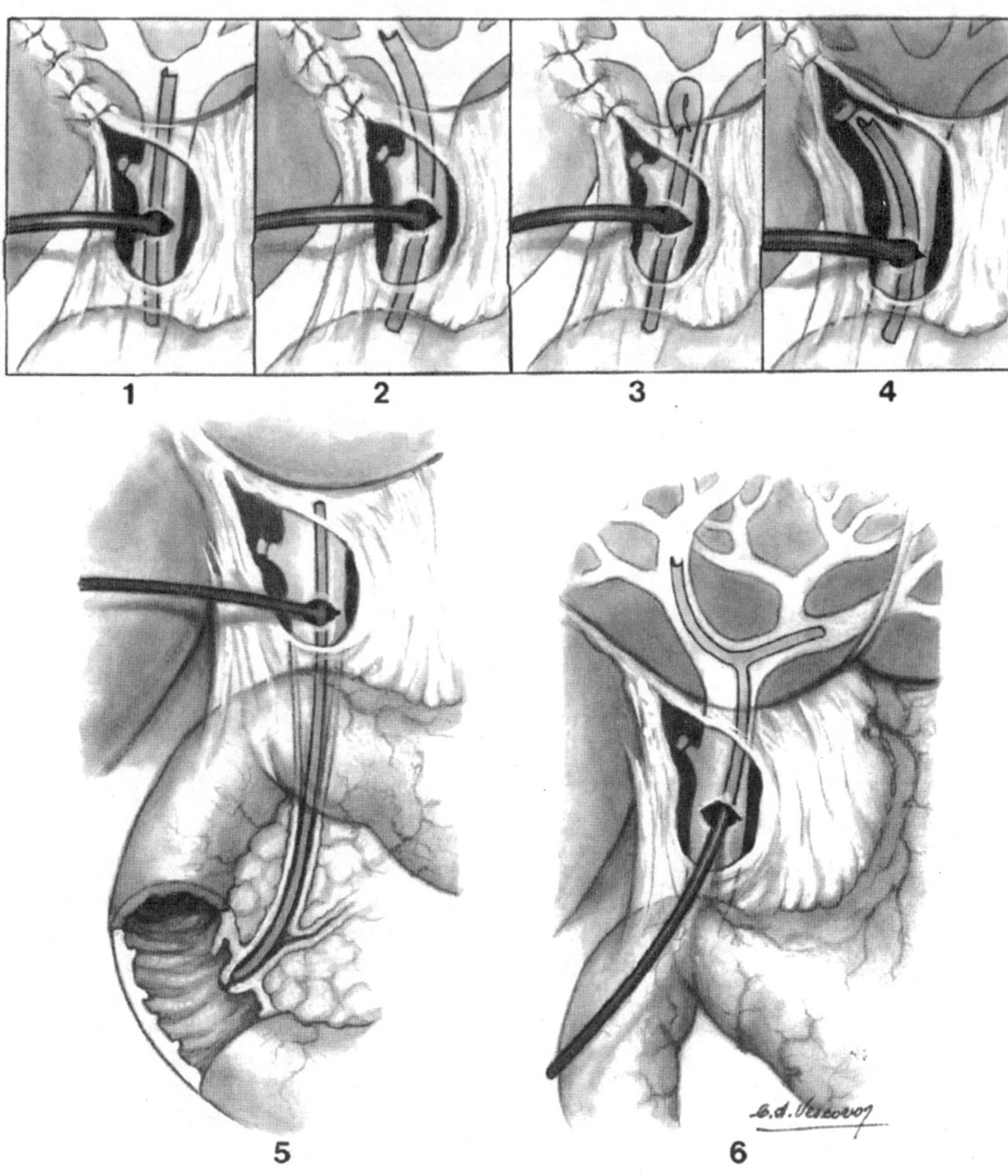

FIGURE 4.35

Technique for Removal of a Calculus Impacted in the Papilla Through a Transduodenal Sphincterotomy

FIGURE 4.36
When a calculus is impacted in the papilla that could not be easily removed through the supraduodenal choledochotomy, one should remove it through a transduodenal sphincterotomy. For this purpose a longitudinal incision is made on the external border of the duodenum. This incision should begin some 2 cm proximal to the papilla and extend 3 to 4 cm below it. The papilla can easily be localized by introducing an exploring catheter through the supraduodenal choledochotomy. The point of entrance of the right gonadal vein into the inferior vena cava is an excellent indicator of the location of the papilla (John L. Madden).

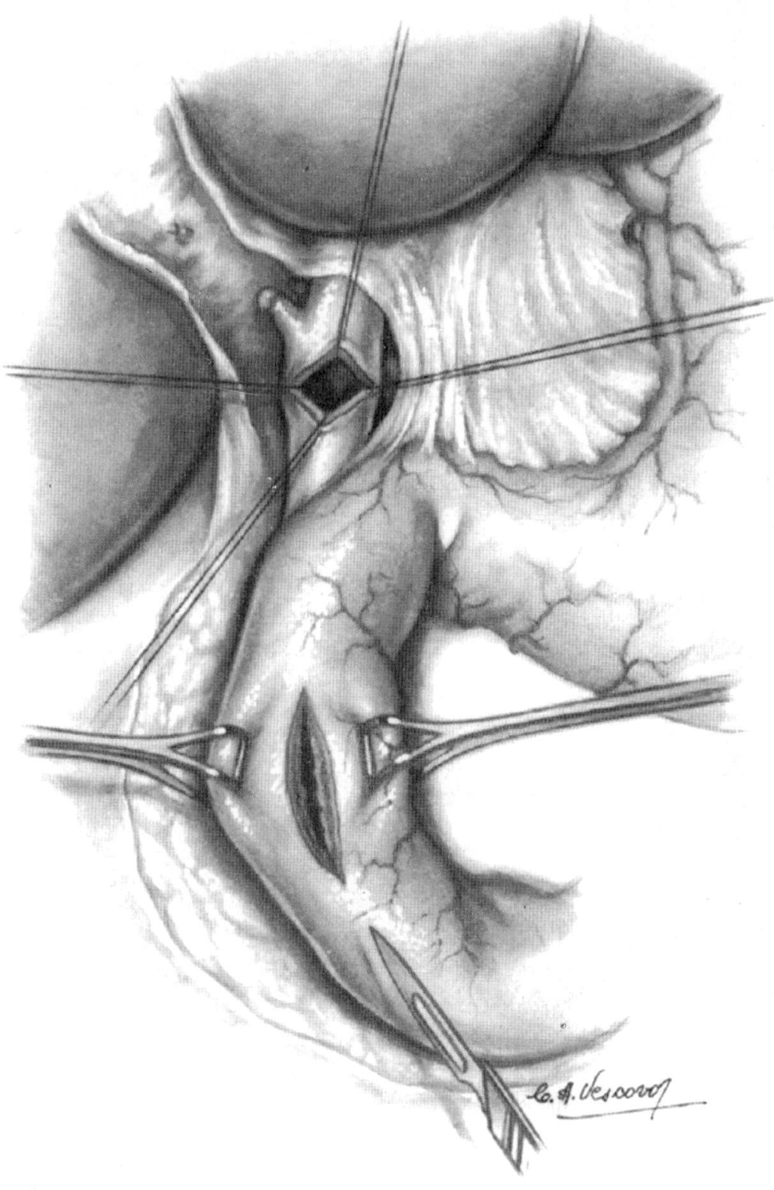

FIGURE 4.36

FIGURE 4.37
Once the duodenum is open, the edges of the incision are grasped with large triangular atraumatic Duval clamps. Gentle traction on the clamps helps expose the interior of the duodenum and at the same time attain temporary hemostasis of the duodenal wall. Once the papilla is identified, two sutures are placed into it, one at 11 o'clock and the other at 12 o'clock. Gentle traction is exerted on the ends of these sutures to facilitate sectioning the papilla between them, as can be seen in the drawing.

Technique for Removal of a Calculus Impacted in the Papilla Through a Transduodenal Sphincterotomy

FIGURE 4.38
Transection of the papilla has allowed the irregular impacted calculus to be removed. The calculus has been grasped with a fine-toothed clamp.

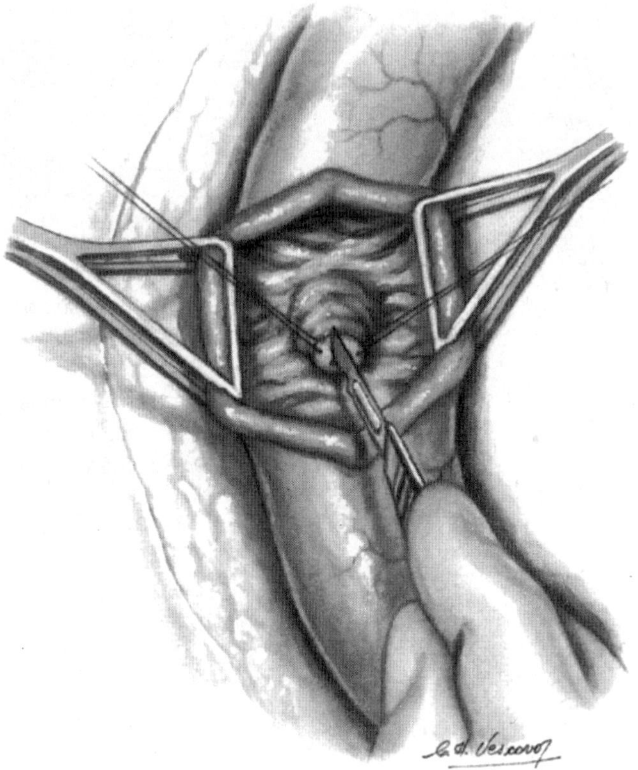

FIGURE 4.37

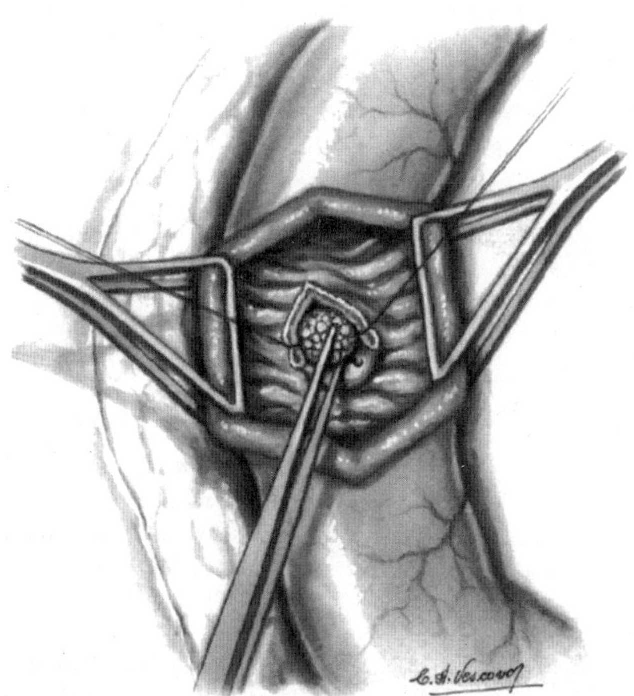

FIGURE 4.38

FIGURE 4.39
The incision in the papilla should be long enough to remove the calculus. It is not necessary to perform a more ample sphincterotomy. Many surgeons do not use any sutures after the calculus is removed. The author favors suturing the mucosa of the common bile duct with the mucosa of the duodenum as a method of attaining hemostasis. To perform this suture it is convenient to place the first stitch between the mucosa of the common bile duct and the duodenal mucosa leaving the ends long to apply traction to it and facilitate the placement of the stitch on the opposite side. Traction on these sutures facilitates the placement of the remaining sutures, as shown in the drawing. The drawing in addition reveals the location of the opening of the pancreatic duct which is generally at about 5 or 6 o'clock. One should not neglect placing a suture in the apex of the incision, as shown in the insert, to render the suture line more secure and avoid possible leakage of bile.

Technique for Removal of a Calculus Impacted in the Papilla Through a Transduodenal Sphincterotomy

FIGURE 4.40
After removal of the calculus and completion of the sphincteroplasty, the longitudinal duodenotomy is closed in two layers using interrupted sutures. The mucosal layer is closed with 3-0 chromic catgut or reabsorbable synthetic material. The seromuscular layer is closed with silk or nonabsorbable synthetic material. After the duodenum is closed, a T-tube is placed into the supraduodenal choledochotomy, as shown in the drawing, and the choledochotomy closed as previously described.

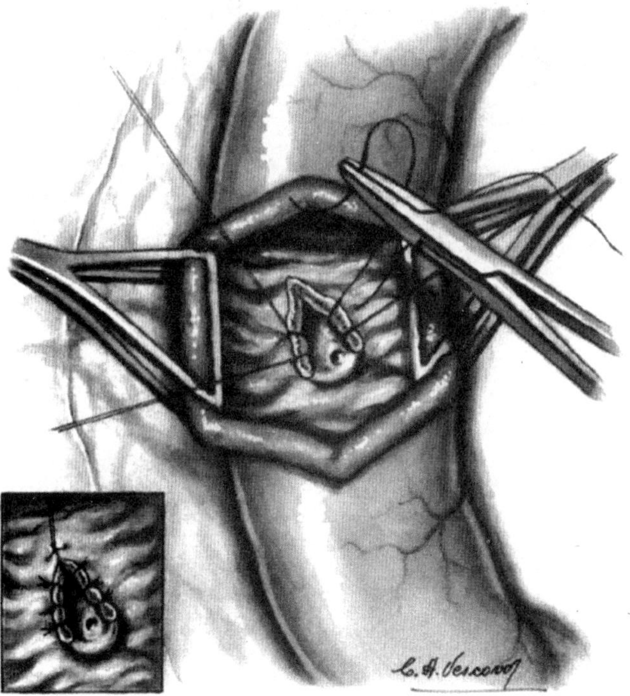

FIGURE 4.39

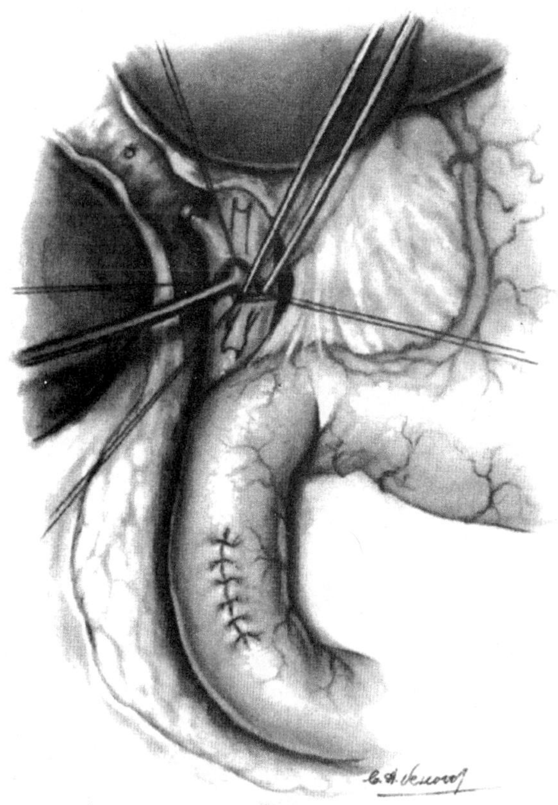

FIGURE 4.40

FIGURE 4.41
In this patient calculi in the common hepatic duct and the common bile duct were easily removed through a supraduodenal choledochotomy. It was impossible, however, to remove a moderate-sized calculus impacted in the left limb of the common hepatic duct. To facilitate the removal of this calculus, the "hilar plate" was incised following the Couinaud technique. This consists of incising Glisson's capsule at its site of union with the peritoneum of the hepatic hilus to make the left hepatic duct visible. The broken line illustrates where this incision will be made.

Removal of a Calculus Impacted in the Left Hepatic Duct

FIGURE 4.42
Once the "hilar plate" has been incised, the left branch of the common hepatic duct is visible revealing the site where the calculus is impacted. A transverse incision is made over the left branch of the common hepatic duct where the calculus presents itself.

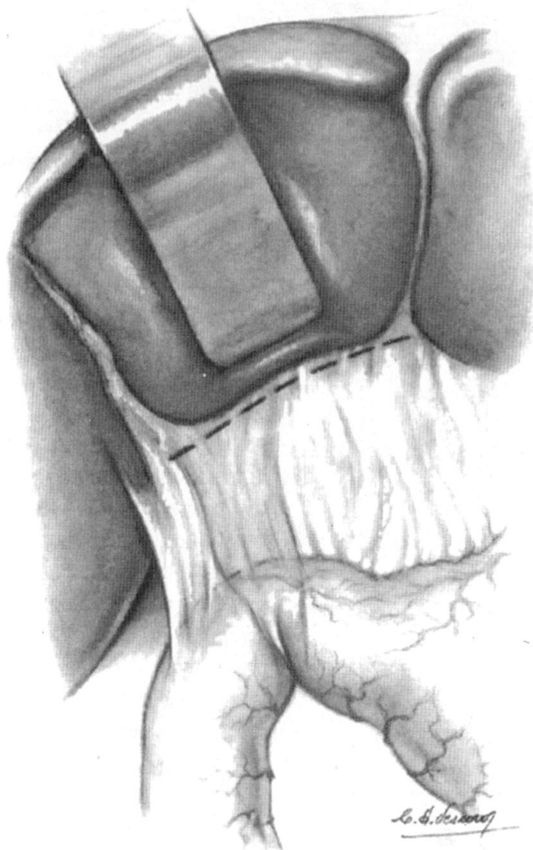

FIGURE 4.41

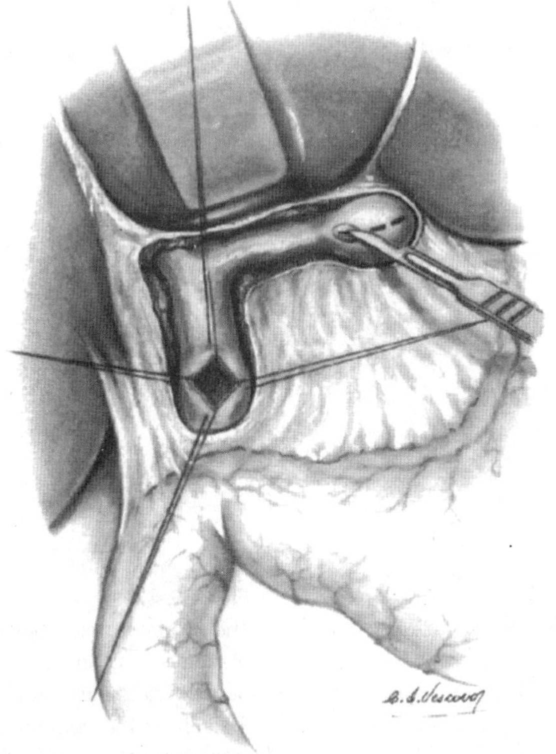

FIGURE 4.42

FIGURE 4.43

Impaction of a calculus in the retroduodeno-pancreatic common bile duct is very rare. If it occurs, the calculus can generally be removed through the supraduodenal choledochotomy. In some cases, however, it is not possible to remove the calculus through this choledochotomy and, to avoid traumatizing the common bile duct or the pancreas, it is advisable to perform a retroduodeno-pancreatic choledochotomy. This technique will be described as follows: A supraduodenal choledochotomy has been made and the impacted calculus could not be removed through this approach. The duodenum and the head of the pancreas are reflected to the left, and an attempt is made to reach the retropancreatic common bile duct through the posterior pancreatic groove. If this groove is not present, the pancreatic parenchyma should be incised until the common bile duct is exposed, directed by the prominence and consistency of the calculus, which is generally quite large. Upon arrival at the common bile duct, it is easy to separate the pancreas from it because the pancreas does not adhere to the common bile duct. Once the common bile duct and the calculus are visible a transverse incision is made in the common bile duct over the prominence of the calculus, as shown in the drawing.

Removal of a Calculus Impacted in the Retroduodeno-pancreatic Common Bile Duct

FIGURE 4.44

The common bile duct has been incised. Sutures have been placed in the angles of this incision to apply traction. If it is necessary to place sutures in the upper and lower edges of the incision in the common bile duct, these can be used to facilitate removal of the calculus. Once the calculus is mobilized it is removed using a Desjardins clamp.

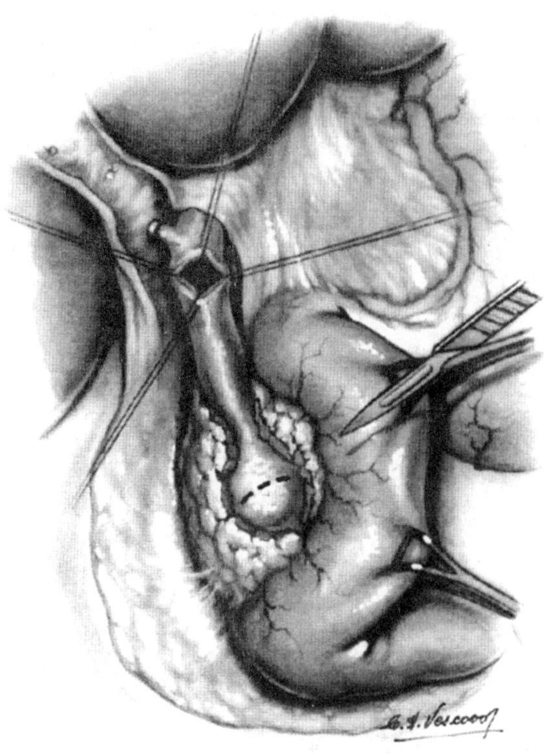

FIGURE 4.43

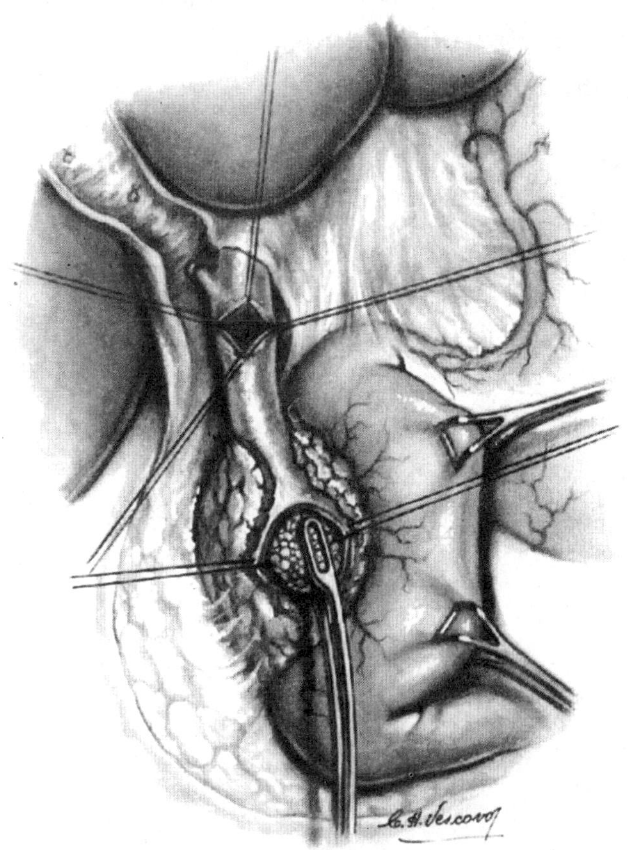

FIGURE 4.44

FIGURE 4.45
The incision in the common bile duct is closed using interrupted 3-0 chromic catgut sutures or synthetic reabsorbable sutures, as shown in the drawing.

Removal of a Calculus Impacted in the Retroduodeno-pancreatic Common Bile Duct

FIGURE 4.46
Once the common bile duct has been sutured the incision in the pancreas is closed with nonabsorbable suture material, either cotton or synthetic material. In addition to assisting with the closure of the common bile duct, these sutures make hemostasis in the pancreas.

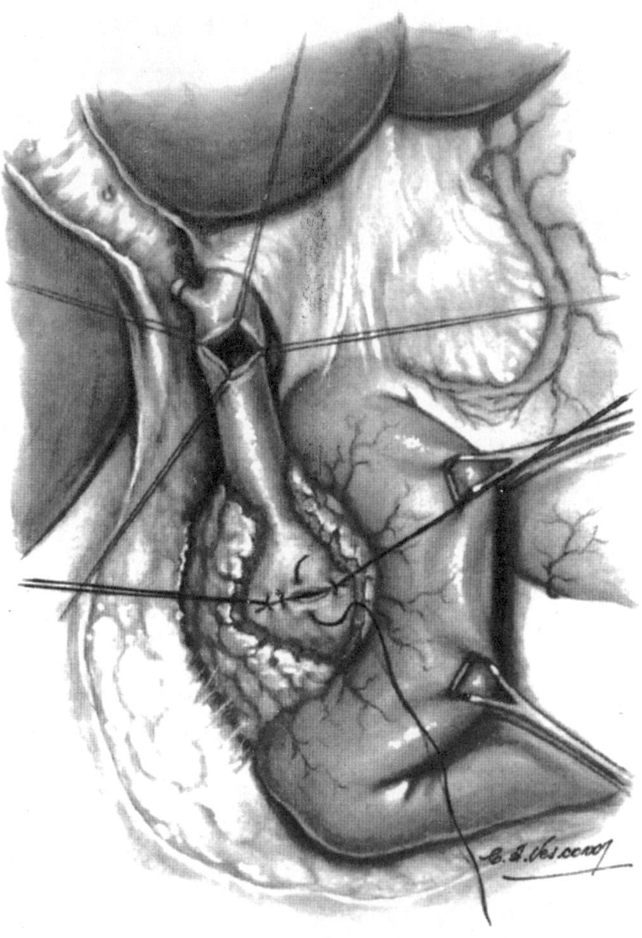

FIGURE 4.45

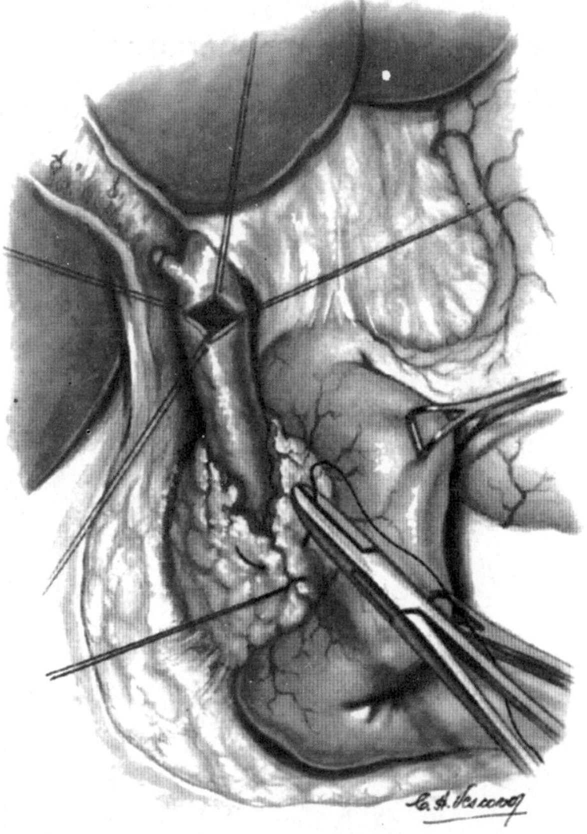

FIGURE 4.46

Removal of a Calculus Impacted in the Retroduodeno-pancreatic Common Bile Duct

FIGURE 4.47
The pancreas has been sutured, and a T-tube has been placed in the supraduodenal choledochotomy, which is then closed.

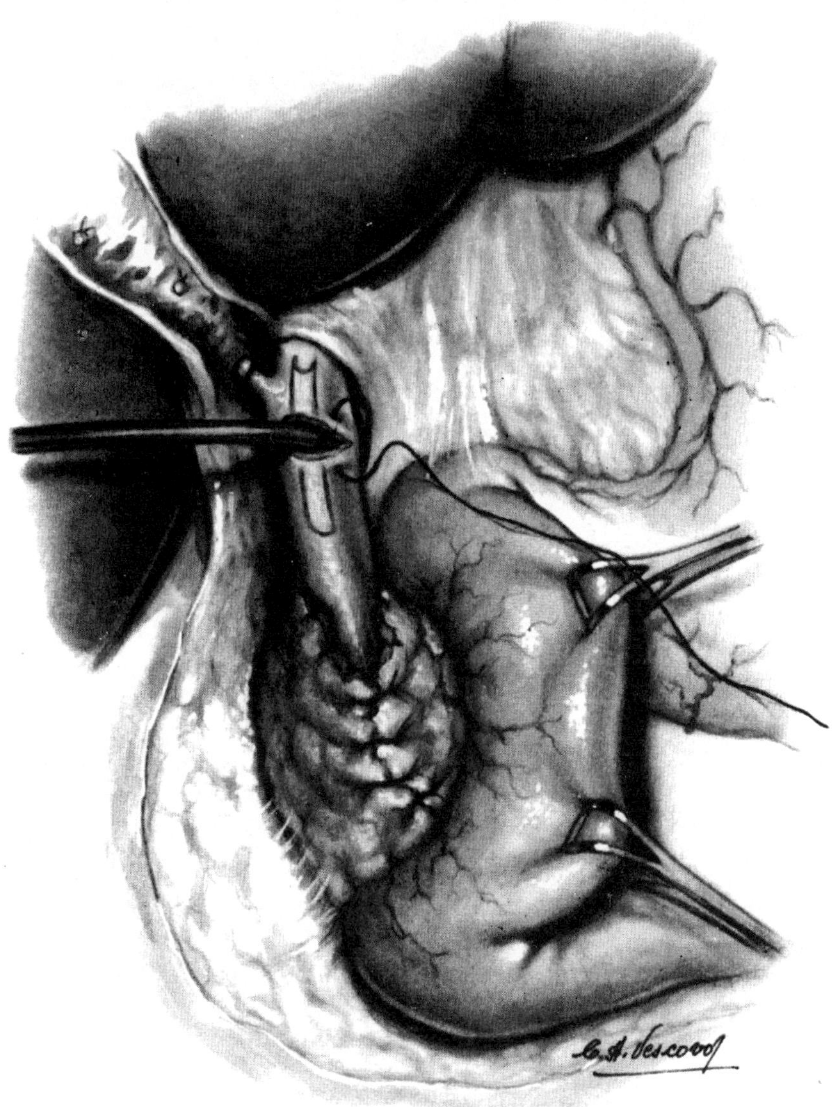

FIGURE 4.47

FIGURE 4.48
In some patients calculi in the common bile duct can become lodged in a diverticular dilation of the distal end of the common bile duct. The drawing reveals, in schematic form, gallbladder and common duct calculi as well as a diverticular dilation of the distal end of the common bile duct in which four calculi have become lodged in a 63-year-old patient with fever and jaundice.

Removal of Calculi Lodged in a Diverticular Dilation of the Distal End of the Common Bile Duct

FIGURE 4.49
Another patient with gallbladder calculi and three calculi lodged in a diverticular dilation of the end of the common bile duct. Exploring instruments pass readily into the duodenum. Operative cholangiography is the most adequate method of diagnosing these patients.

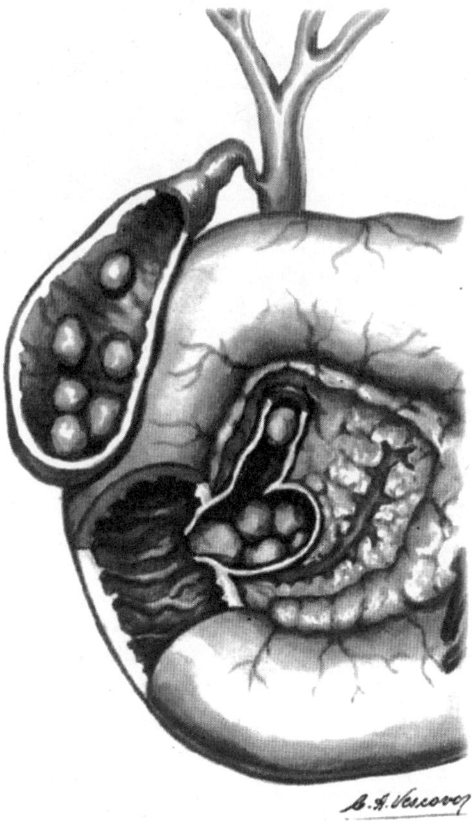

FIGURE 4.48

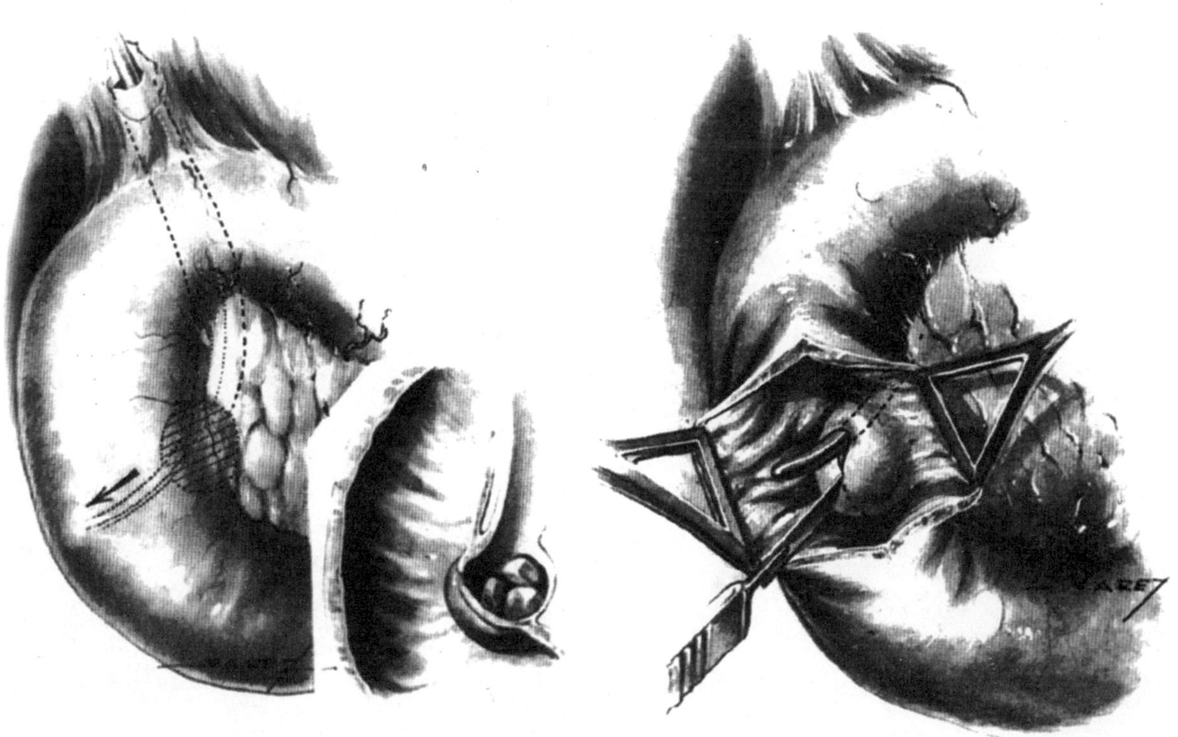

FIGURE 4.49

FIGURE 4.50

Attempts to remove these calculi through a supraduodenal choledochotomy exposes the patient to trauma and lesions of the common bile duct or the pancreas. The least traumatic way to remove these calculi is through a transduodenal sphincterotomy. In cases such as that shown in the drawing, if there is a sacciform dilation containing calculi that protrude into the duodenal lumen, an incision can be made over this dilation, the calculi removed, and the wall of the diverticular cavity sutured to the duodenum wall.

Removal of Calculi Lodged in a Diverticular Dilation of the Distal End of the Common Bile Duct

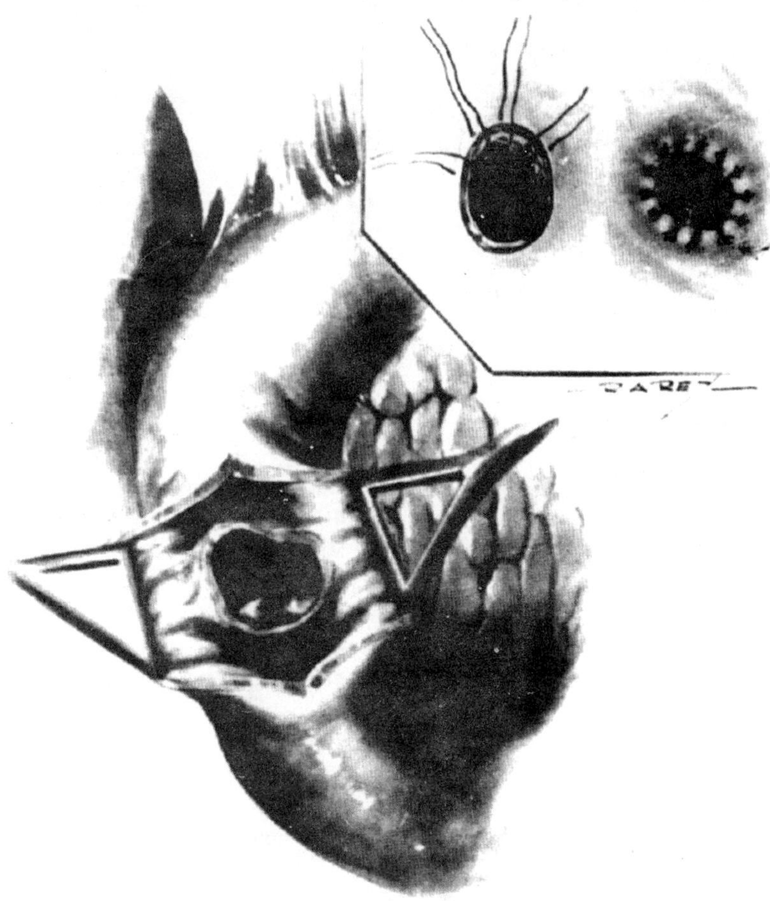

FIGURE 4.50

FIGURE 4.51
The Mirizzi hepatic duct syndrome is produced in this case by a cystic duct running in spiral fashion and passing in front of the common bile duct, emptying into the left border of the common bile duct. The gallbladder and cystic duct contain numerous calculi. The common hepatic duct is very dilated, as are the intrahepatic branches of the duct which contain many calculi. The common bile duct, on the contrary, is normal in diameter and does not contain calculi. This is due to the cystic duct compressing the common hepatic duct and not allowing calculi to enter the common bile duct.

The Mirizzi Hepatic Duct Syndrome

FIGURE 4.52
Since dense adhesions are present between the infundibulum of the gallbladder and the cystic duct, its liberation is started to demonstrate the anatomy of the region and proceed with resection of the gallbladder.

FIGURE 4.53
Once the gall bladder is removed and transected at the site of its junction of the infundibulum with the neck, liberation of the cystic duct, which is very adherent to the common hepatic duct, is continued. Complete removal of the cystic duct allowed the common hepatic duct to be freed of the obstruction caused by the cystic duct. A hepaticotomy is performed instead of a choledochotomy because the common bile duct is normal in caliber while the common hepatic duct is very dilated. The calculi are removed from the common hepatic duct and its branches and a T-tube placed in it.

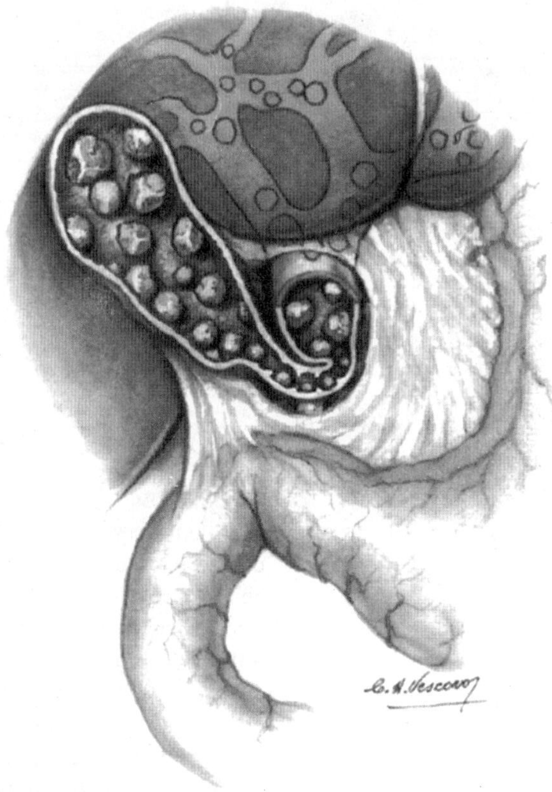

FIGURE 4.51

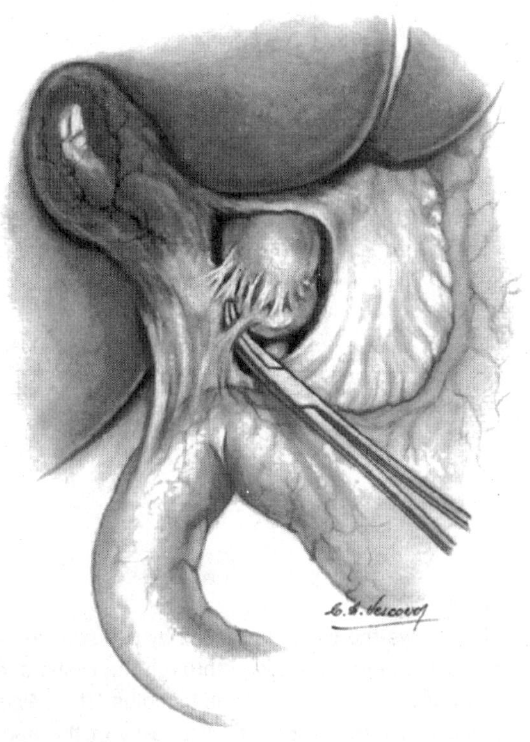

FIGURE 4.52

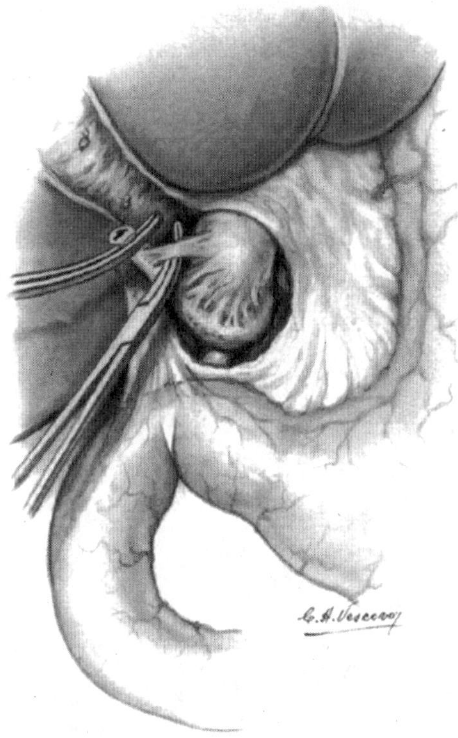

FIGURE 4.53

FIGURE 4.54
In patients with common bile ducts of normal caliber or slightly dilated that contain one or two calculi in the distal end of the common bile duct, removal of the calculi can be attempted through the cystic duct to avoid performing a choledochotomy. If the cystic duct is dilated, the removal of these calculi will be easier. If the cystic duct is normal in caliber, it can be dilated using a thin hemostatic clamp with fine ends. Using gentle movements of opening and closing this clamp, the valves of Heister are broken and the cystic duct dilated, allowing the introduction of a malleable spoon of the smallest caliber to remove the calculi from the common bile duct.

Removal of Calculi from the Common Duct Through the Cystic Duct

FIGURE 4.55
The drawing shows the cystic duct held by two sutures. A malleable spoon has been introduced through the cystic duct into the common bile duct to remove the calculus. The calculus is held in place and wedged into the concavity of the spoon so that it can be removed.

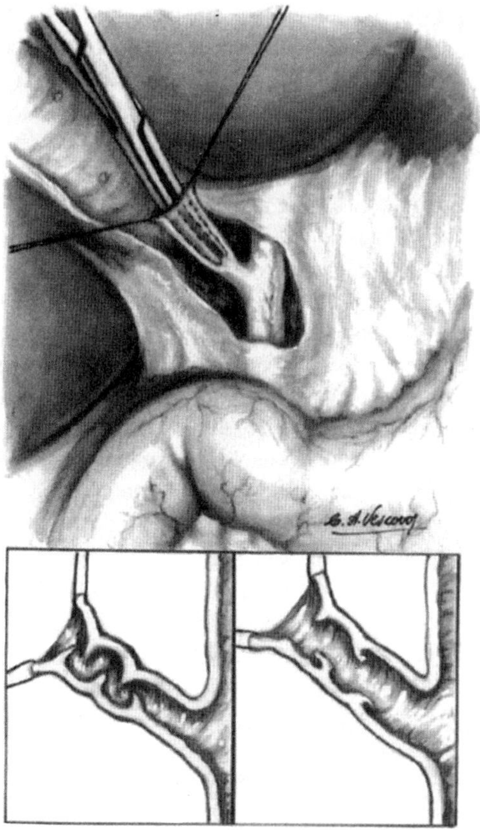

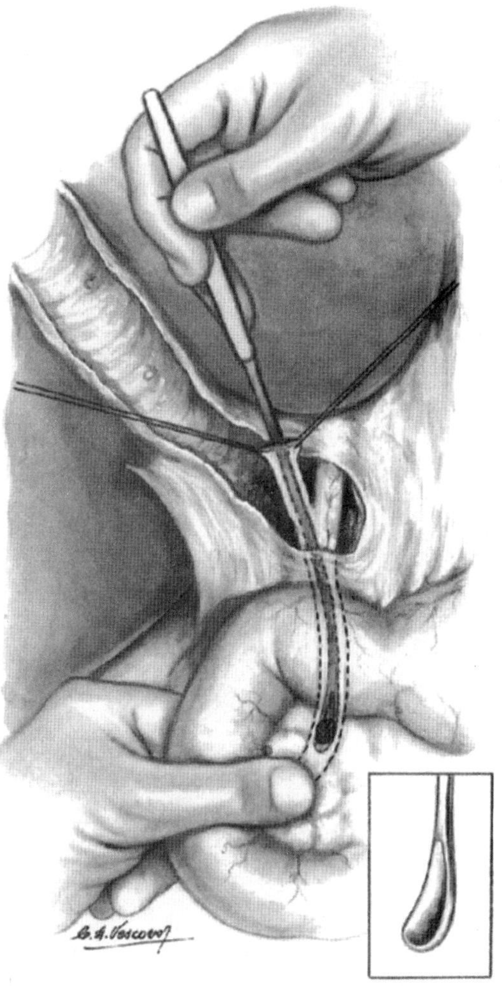

FIGURE 4.55

Removal of Calculi from the Common Duct Through the Cystic Duct

FIGURE 4.56

Once the calculus has been removed, a control cholangiogram is performed through the cystic duct to confirm that there are no other calculi and that dye passage into the duodenum is normal. Once this has been done and the common bile duct found to be normal, the cystic duct is sutured at its juncture with the common bile duct and a subhepatic suction drainage tube is left in place. Mirizzi, however, advises the introduction of a drain through the cystic duct using a fine catheter with several perforations into the common bile duct and fixed in place by a ligature on the cystic duct and two fixation sutures between the end of the cystic duct and the transcystic tube. This fixation is indispensable, since transcystic tubes have a tendency to come out spontaneously. The material to be used in fixing the transcystic tube should be synthetic reabsorbable suture material. It is not convenient to use chromic catgut because it can be rapidly absorbed and the tube extruded. This technique proposed by Mirizzi using a transcystic drainage tube after the calculi are removed has the object of preventing an increase in intracholedochal pressure postoperatively, which may lead to loosening of the ligature of the cystic duct. Some authors, instead of removing these calculi through the transcystic approach and in order not to perform a choledochotomy in a common bile duct of normal caliber, prefer to remove these calculi through a transduodenal sphincterotomy. In case the transcystic approach fails to remove the calculi the author prefers to remove the calculi through a transverse choledochotomy which has no tendency to lead to stenosis of the common bile duct as can occur with a longitudinal choledochotomy.

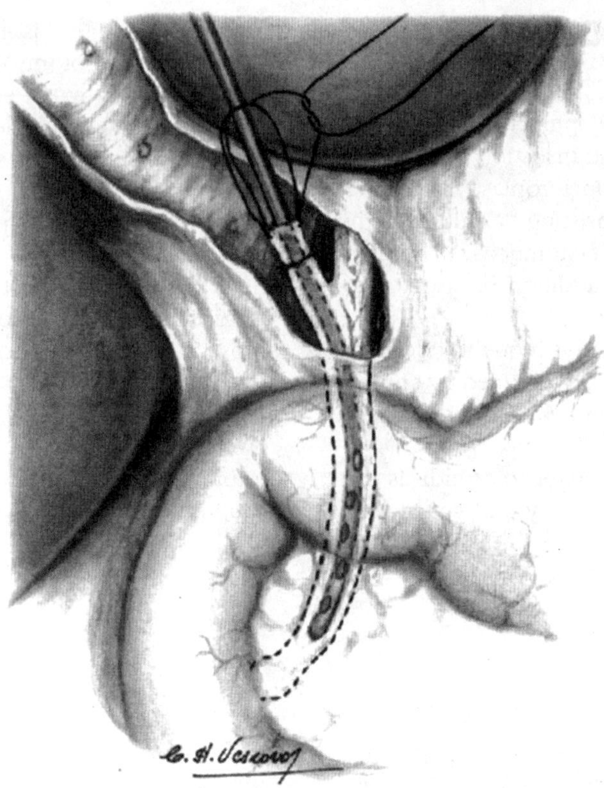

FIGURE 4.56 .

SPHINCTEROTOMY AND SPHINCTEROPLASTY

The term "sphincterotomy of the sphincter of Oddi," or simply "sphincterotomy," means transection of the muscular fibers of said sphincter. Sphincteroplasty is complementary to sphincterotomy, consisting of suturing the choledochal mucosa to the duodenal mucosa. The great majority of surgeons advise the addition of sphincteroplasty in all cases.

At present sphincterotomy is very frequently done by the endoscopic route and is not accompanied by sphincteroplasty. It is, however, associated with good immediate and late results.

Organic stenosis of the sphincter of Oddi is the principal indication for sphincterotomy and sphincteroplasty. This condition is, however, infrequently observed (24, 26). Sphincterotomy of the sphincter of Oddi used to be carried out in many surgical centers in patients with biliary calculi without clear documentation of its need (24, 72, 81). At present surgical sphincterotomy is performed, in the great majority of cases, to remove calculi that are impacted in the papillary or to facilitate postoperative passage into the duodenum of calculi that are lodged in the biliary ducts.

Endoscopic sphincterotomy is usually performed to remove a calculus that is impacted in the papilla, to remove calculi from the biliary duct using a Dormia basket, or to facilitate passage of calculi into the duodenum.

We will now describe the technique used in sphincterotomy and sphincteroplasty as performed surgically through the transduodenal approach.

Sphincterotomy and Sphincteroplasty

Sphincterotomy and Sphincteroplasty

FIGURE 4.57
Sphincterotomy and sphincteroplasty performed by the transduodenal approach. The gallbladder and its calculi have been removed. The operative cholangiogram revealed moderate dilation of the bile duct, which contained three calculi in it and the presence of stenosis of the sphincter of Oddi. A Vautrin-Kocher maneuver is performed to carry out visual and manual exploration of the biliary tract, pancreas, and duodenum. A transverse supraduodenal choledochotomy is performed and the common duct explored with instruments. The three calculi that were lodged in the duct are removed and exploration of the papilla, which showed stenosis on cholangiography, begun. Instrumental exploration confirms the presence of stenosis of the papilla, for which reason a longitudinal duodenotomy, some 5 cm long, is carried out. The midportion of the duodenotomy should coincide with the papilla. In case the papilla cannot be localized from the outside, it is advisable to make the duodenotomy beginning in the midpoint of its second portion. Once the papilla has been localized two fine sutures are placed, in its superior border, at the 11 and 12 o'clock positions, completely opposite the location of the terminal orifice of the pancreatic duct. Traction upward and laterally is applied with small clamps.

FIGURE 4.58
The papilla has been sectioned with a scalpel between the previously placed sutures in its superior border. On the right side a suture has been placed and tied joining the choledochal mucosa with the duodenal mucosa. On the left side a needle is being passed to carry out a suture similar to the one on the opposite side. A dotted line shows where the transection of the rest of the sphincter is to be carried out. The sutures are placed as the sphincter is transected, making the operation easier. The opening of the pancreatic duct can be seen in the inferior portion, far from where the sphincter is being sectioned.

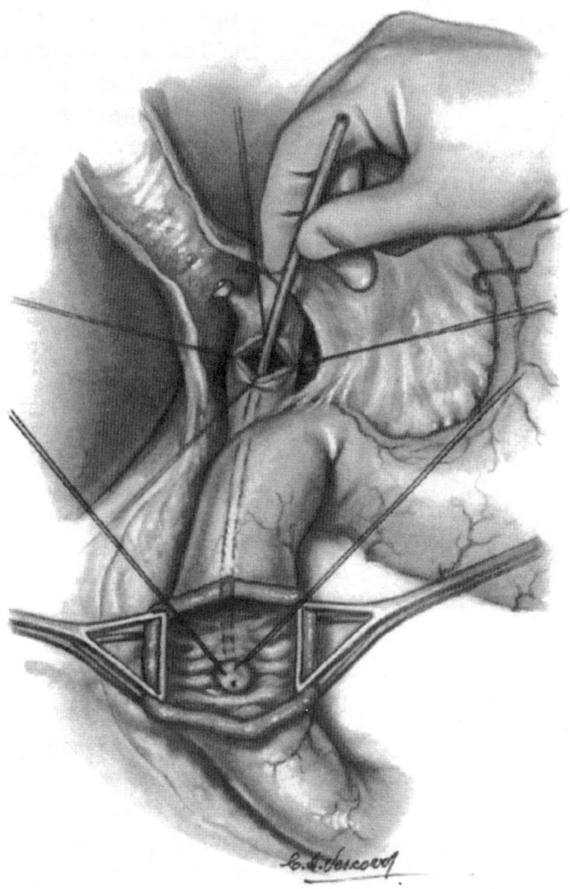

FIGURE 4.57

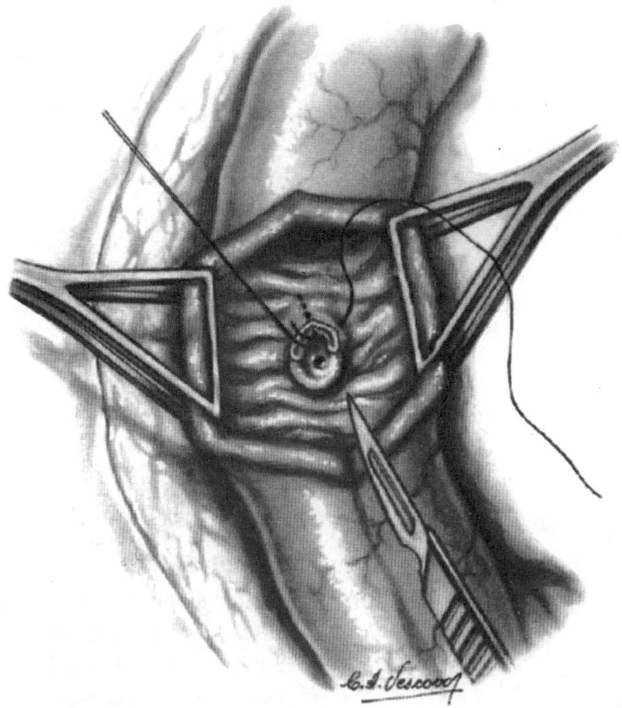

FIGURE 4.58

FIGURE 4.59

The drawing shows how traction on the previously inserted sutures makes transection of the rest of the sphincter, as well as suturing of the choledochal and duodenal mucosa, easier. The insert shows the completed sphincteroplasty. It is advisable to place a suture in the upper angle to prevent possible filtrations. The ends of the angle suture have been left long to make the suture more visible.

FIGURE 4.60

Once the sphincterotomy and sphincteroplasty have been completed the duodenotomy is closed in two planes of interrupted sutures. The mucosal plane is closed with 3-0 chromic catgut, and the seromuscular layer is closed with cotton, silk, or nonabsorbable synthetic sutures. A T-tube is then placed in the bile duct and the choledochotomy closed.

Sphincterotomy and Sphincteroplasty

FIGURE 4.61

The common bile duct has been closed with interrupted 3-0 chromic catgut sutures. If it has been possible to preserve the peritoneal layer of the area, it is closed with similar sutures to make the closure more water tight. The gallbladder bed is then closed with interrupted sutures.

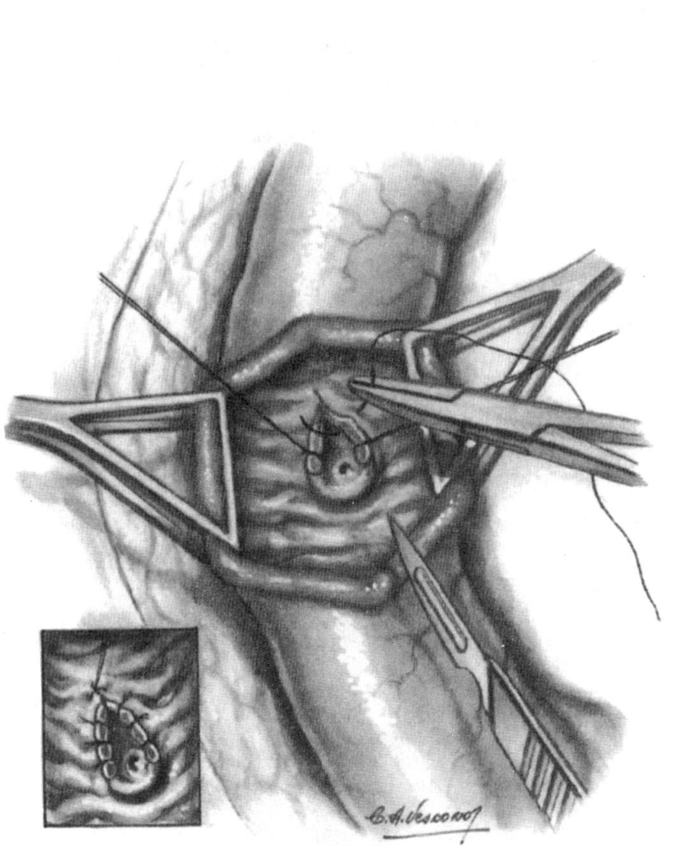

FIGURE 4.59

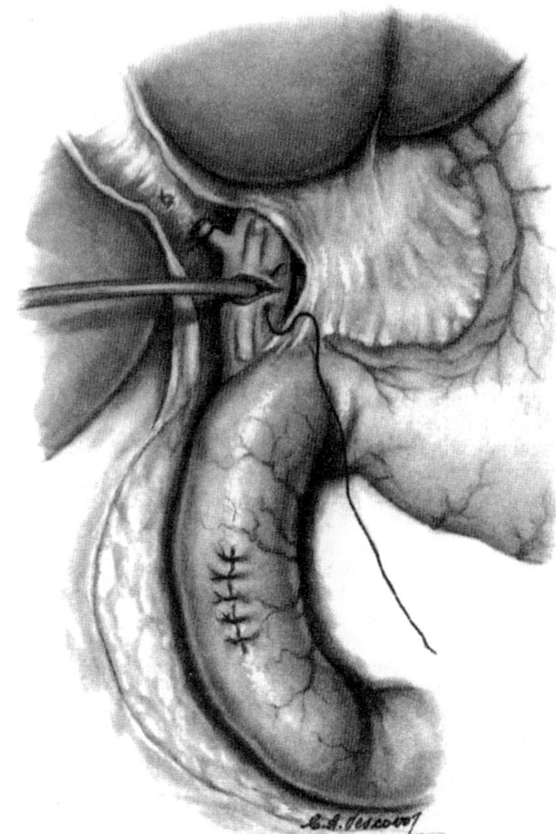

FIGURE 4.60

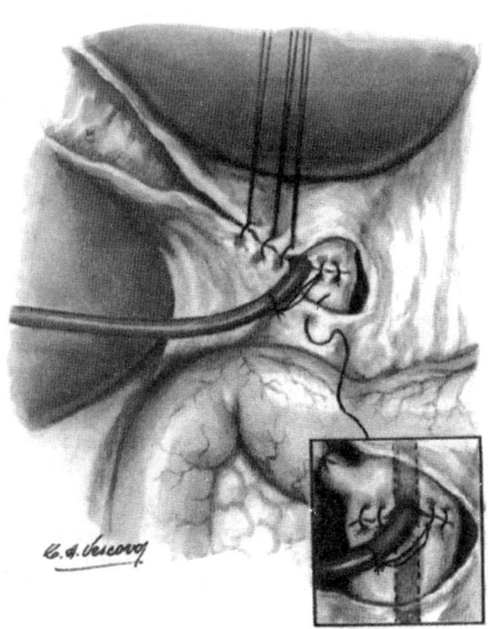

FIGURE 4.61

References

1. Alberro, J.M., Torino, F., Perera, S.G. Coledocoscopía intraoperatoria. Rev. Argent. Cir. 41:56, 1981.
2. Allen, B., Shapiro, H., Way, L.W. Management of recurrent and residual common duct stones. Am. J. Surg. 142:41, 1981.
3. Baker, A.R., Neoptolemos, J.P., Leese, T., Fossard, D.P. Choledochoduodenostomy transduodenal sphincteroplasty and sphincterotomy for calculi of the common bile duct. Surg. Gynecol. Obstet. 164:245, 1987.
4. Bartlett, M.K., Waddell, W.R. Indication for common duct exploration. Evaluation in 1000 cases. N. Engl. J. Med. 258:164, 1958.
5. Berci, G., Shore, J.M., Morgenstern, L., Hamlin, J.A. Choledochoscopy and operative fluorocholangiography in prevention of retained bile duct stones. World J. Surg. 2:411, 1978.
6. Berci, G. Intraoperative biliary diagnostic modalities: Present and future. Ital. J. Surg. Sci. 17:67, 1987.
7. Bernhoft, R.A., Pellegrini, C.A., Motson, R.W. Composition and morphologic and clinical features of common duct stones. Am. J. Surg. 148:77, 1984.
8. Bordley, J. IV, White, T.T. Causes for 340 reoperations on extrahepatic bile ducts. Ann. Surg. 189:442, 1979.
9. Burhenne, H.J. Non operative retained biliary stone extraction: A new roentgenologic technique. Am. J. Roentgen. 177:38, 1973.
10. Burhenne, H.J. Complication of non operative extraction of retained common duct stones. Am. J. Surg. 131:260, 1976.
11. Burhenne, H.J. Non operative instrument extraction of retained bile duct stones. World J. Surg. 2:439, 1979.
12. Casal, M. Secuencia de la exploración de la vía biliar principal. Rev. Argent. Cir. 23:39, 1972.
13. Cameron, J. Atlas of surgery. Vol. I, p. 10. B.C. Decker, Philadelphia, 1990.
14. Chardavogne, R., Subhaga, S.K., Auguste, L.J. et al. Comparison of intraoperative ultrasonography and cholangiography in detection of small common bile duct stones. Ann. Surg. 206:53, 1987.
15. Chassin, J.L. Operative Strategy in General Surgery. Vol. II, p. 83. Springer-Verlag, New York, 1984.
16. Chidyllo, S.A., Cordone, R.P., Reader, R. et al. Choledocholithiasis in Chinese immigrant with cholelithiasis. Surg. Gynecol. Obstet. 172:280, 1991.
17. Classen, M., Demling, L. Endoskopic sphincterotomie der papilli Vateri und steinextraktion aus dem ductus choledochus. Dtsch. Med. Wochenschr. 99:496, 1974.
18. DenBesten, L. Choledocholithiasis. In Way, L., Pellegrini, C.A. Eds. p. 283. W.B. Saunders, Philadelphia, 1987.
19. Dewar, G., Chung, S.C.S., Li, A.K.C. Operative strategy in Mirizzi syndrome. Surg. Gynecol. Obstet. 171:157, 1990.
20. Ellman, B.A., Berman, H.L. Treatment of common bile duct stones. Gastroint. Radiol. 6:357, 1981.
21. Etala, E. Litiasis incipiente del colédoco. Importancia de la colangiografía operatoria. Pren. Méd. Argent. 48:2128, 1961.
22. Etala, E. Valor de la colangiografía operatoria para el áncer de la cabeza del páncreas y de la ampolla de Vater. Bull. Soc. Intern. Chir. p. 1198. Rome, 1963.
23. Etala, E. Pablo L. Mirizzi. Pren. Méd. Argent. 51:845, 1964.
24. Etala, E. Indicaciones y resultados de la esfinterotomía. Rev. Int. Hepatol. 15:875, 1965.
25. Etala, E., Romero, L.M. Operative cholangiography in the diagnosis of tumoral obstruction of the distal end of the common duct. Recent advances in gastroenterology. Proc. 3rd World Congr. Gastroenterol. Tokyo, Japan. Vol. IV, p. 537. 1966.
26. Etala, E. Exploración intraoperatoria del extremo distal del colédoco. Pren. Méd. Argent. 60:589, 1973.
27. Finnis, D., Rowntree, T. Choledochoscopy in exploration of the common bile duct. Brit. J. Surg. 64:661, 1977.
28. Fontana, J.J. Adelantos en el diagnóstico y tratamiento de la patología biliar benigna. Rev. Argent. Cir. Número Extraordinario. p. 1, 1989.
29. Glenn, R., Moody, F.G. Acute obstructive suppurative cholangitis. Surg. Gynecol. Obstet. 113:265, 1961.
30. Hartmann, H. Cirurgie des voies biliaires. p. 248. Masson et Cie., Paris, 1923.
31. Hermann, R.E., Hoerr, S.O. The value of the routine use of operative cholangiography. Surg. Gynecol. Obstet. 121:1015, 1965.
32. Hermann, R.E. Manual of surgery of the gallbladder bile ducts, and exocrine pancreas. p. 103. Springer-Verlag, New York, 1979.
33. Hess, W. Operative cholangiograpy. Thieme, Stuttgart, 1955.
34. Hicken, N.F., McAllister, A.J. Operative cholangiography as an aid in reducing the incidence of overlooked common bile duct stones. A study of 1293 choledocholithotomy. Surgery 55:753, 1964.
35. Jolly, P.C., Baker, J.W., Schmidt, H.M. Operative cholangiography: A case for its routine use. Ann. Surg. 168:551, 1968.
36. Jones, S.A. The prevention and treatment of recurrent bile duct stones by transduodenal sphincteroplasty. World J. Surg. 2: 473, 1978.
37. Kullenan, E., Borch, K., Tarpila, E., Liedberg, C. Endoscopic sphincterotomy in the treatment of choledocholithiasis and ampullary stenosis. Acta Chir. Scand. 151:619, 1985.
38. Kune, G.A. The elusive common bile duct stone. Med. J. Aust. 1:254, 1966.
39. Kune, G.A., Sali, A. The practice of biliary surgery. Ed. 2, p. 154. Blackwell Scientific Publications, Oxford, 1980.
40. Le Quesne, L.P. Choledocholithiasis. In Smith, R., Sherlock, S. (Eds.) Surgery of the gallbladder and bile ducts. p. 118. Butterworth, Washington, 1964.
41. Liguori, C., Léger, L. Traitement perendoscopique des calculs de la voie biliaire principale. Chirurgie 102:466, 1976.
42. Lingren, B., Obsson, S.A. et al. Selective or routine intraoperative cholangiography. A cost-effectiveness analysis. World J. Surg. 4:315, 1980.
43. Mc Cormick, J.S., Bremner, D.N., Thomson, J.W.W., Philp, T. The operative cholangiogram: Its interpretation, accuracy, and value in association with cholecystectomy. Ann. Surg. 180:902, 1974.
44. Madden, J.L., Vanderheyden, L., Kandalaft, S. The nature and surgical significance of common duct stones. Surg. Gynecol. Obstet. 126:3, 1968.
45. Madden, J.L. Common duct stones. Their origin and surgical management. Surg. Clin. North Am. 53:1095, 1973.
46. Madden, J.L. Primary common bile duct stones. World J. Surg. 2:265, 1978.
47. Maki, T., Sato, T., Matsushiro, T.A. A re-appraisal of surgical treatment for intrahepatic gallstones. Ann. Surg. 175:155, 1972.
48. Mazzariello, R. Removal of residual biliary tract calculi without reoperation. Surgery 67:566, 1970.
49. Mazzariello, R. Review of 220 cases of residual biliary tract calculi treated without re-operation: An 8 year study. Surgery 73: 299, 1973.
50. Mazzariello, R. A 14 year experience with non operative instrument extraction of retained bile duct stones. World J. Surg. 2: 447, 1978.
51. Mazzariello, R. Nonoperative treatment of residual biliary tract stones. In Nyhus, L.M., Baker, R.J. (Eds.) Mastery of surgery. Vol. I, p. 678. Little, Brown & Co., Boston, 1984.
52. Mazzariello, R. Actualizacíon y progresos en el tratamiento de las lesiones de las vías biliares. Rev. Argent. Cir. 58:28, 1990.
53. Mazzariello, R., Novas, O., Perrone, R., Barbella, J.C. Colecistolitotomía percutánea. Pren. Méd. Argent. 78:20, 1991.
54. Mazzariello, R., Novas, O. Extracción de cálculos coledocianos por vía transparietohepática. Pren. Méd. Argent. 78:111, 1991.
55. Merenda, R., Norberto, L., Lemmolo, M.R., et al. Coledocolitiasi: Trattamento combinato endoscópico e lilolítico con M.T.B.E. e monoctanoína. Chirurgia 4:105, 1991.
56. Mirizzi, P.L. La colangiografía durante las operaciones de las vías biliares. Bol. Soc. Cir. Buenos Aires 16:1133, 1932.
57. Mirizzi, P.L. Fisiopatología del hepatocolédoco. Colangiografía operatoria. El Ateneo, Buenos Aires, 1939.
58. Mirizzi, P.L. Sindrome del conducto hepático. Bull. Soc. Int. Chir. 8:731, 1948.
59. Mirizzi, P.L. La lithiasis de la voie biliaire principale. A propos de 520 cas opérés sous cholangiographie operatoire. Mem. Acad. Chir. Paris 81:834, 1955.
60. Mirizzi, P.L. Lithiase de la voie biliaire principale. Masson et Cie., Paris 1957.
61. Mirizzi, P.L. Chirurgie du système du canal hépatique. Masson et Cie., Paris 1962.

62. Mondet, A. Técnica de la extracción incruenta de los cálculos on la litiasis residual del colédoco. Bol. Soc. Cir. Buenos Aires 14: 276, 1962.
63. Morris, D.L., Harrison, J., Balfour, T., Whery, D.C. Operative choledochoscopy vía the cystic duct: a pilot study with an ultra-thin fiberoptic endoscope. Br. J. Surg. 74:613, 1987.
64. Morrissey, K.P., Mc Sherry, C.K. Cholecystocholedochal fistula, including the Mirizzi Syndrome. In Blumgart, L.H. (Ed.) Surgery of the liver and biliary tract. Vol. I, p. 785. Churchill Livingstone, New York, 1988.
65. Nagorney, D.M., Lohmuller, J.L. Choledochoscopy. A cost minimization analysis. Ann. Surg. 211:354, 1990.
66. Nora, P.F., Berci, G., Dorazzio, R.A. et al. Operative choledochoscopy. Am. J. Surg. 44:105, 1977.
67. Orloff, M.J. Retained and recurrent bile duct stones. Introduction. World J. Surg. 2:401, 1978.
68. Orloff, M.J. Importance of surgical technique in prevention of retained and recurrent bile duct stones. World J. Surg. 2:403, 1978.
69. Peel, A.L.G., Bourke, J.B., Herman Taylor, J. et al. How should common bile duct be explored? Ann. R. Coll. Surg. Eng. 56:124, 1975.
70. Perera, S.G. Litiasis de la vía biliar principal. Diagnóstico y tratamiento quirúrgico. Rev. Argent. Cir. Número Extraordinario, p. 71, 1981.
71. P-Figueras, J. Práctica quirúrgica. Ed. 2, Vol. II, p. 624. Salvat, Barcelona, 1986.
72. Rutledge, R.H. Sphincteroplasty and choledochoduodenostomy for benign biliary obstructions. Ann. Surg. 183:476, 1976.
73. Saharia, P.C., Zuidema, G.D., Cameron, J.L. Primary common duct stones. Ann. Surg. 185:598, 1977.
74. Schulenburg, C.A.R. Operative cholangiography. Butterworth, London, 1966.
75. Schulenburg, C.A.R. Operative cholangiography: 1,000 cases. Surgery 65:723, 1969.
76. Shore, J.M., Shore, E. Operative biliary endoscopy. Experience with the flexible choledochoscope in 100 consecutive choledocholithotomies. Ann. Surg. 171:269, 1970.
77. Siegel, B., Coelho, J.C.V., Myhus, L.M. et al. Comparison of cholangiography and ultrasonography in the operative screening of the common bile duct. World J. Surg. 6:440, 1982.
78. Siegel, B., Coelho, J.C.V., Macchi, J. et al. The application of real-time ultrasound imaging during surgical procedures. Surg. Gynecol. Obstet. 157:33, 1983.
79. Smith, T.D., Rosel, P.D., Hunter, C.W. Percutaneous transhepatic biliary procedure. Gastroint. Radiol. 12:144, 1987.
80. Stanten, R., Frey, F. Pancreatitis after endoscopic retrograde cholangiopancreatography. Arch. Surg. 125:1032, 1990.
81. Sugasti, J.A. Esfínteroplastia. p. 24. López Libreros Editores, Buenos Aires, 1976.
82. Thomas, C.G., Jr., Nicholson, C.P., Owen, J. Effectiveness of choledochoduodenostomy and transduodenal sphincteroplasty in the treatment of benign obstruction of the common duct. Ann. Surg. 173:845, 1971.
83. Warren, K.W., Jenkins, R.L., Steele, G.D., Jr. Atlas of surgery of the liver, pancreas and biliary tract. p. 18. Appleton-Lange, East Norwalk, CT, 1991.
84. Way, L.W., Admirand, W.H. and Dunphy, J.E. Management of choledocholithiasis. Ann. Surg. 176:347, 1972.
85. White, T.T. Cholecystostomy, cholecystectomy and intraoperative evaluation of biliary tree. In Nyhus, L.M., Baker, R. (Eds.) Mastery of surgery. Vol I, p. 671. Little Brown & Co., Boston, 1984.
86. Wildegans, H. Endoscopy of the biliary tract. Ger. Med. Monthly. 62:377, 1958.
87. Zollinger, R.M., Zollinger, R.M., Jr. Atlas of surgical operations. Ed. 4, p. 152. Macmillan, New York, 1975.

Section A

Surgery of the Biliary Tract

CHAPTER 5

Choledochoduodenal Anastomosis

Choledochoduodenal anastomosis, also known as latero-lateral choledochoduodenal anastomosis and external choledochoduodenal anastomosis, was first performed by Riedel, in Germany, in 1888 (46), but the technique was first published in 1891 (34, 35). The patient died a few hours after the operation. Sprengel did the first choledochoduodenal anastomosis with survival of the patient in 1891 (52). This operation was not well accepted by the surgeons of that era, until 1913, when Sasse (48) published his well-known paper and became the great proponent of choledochoduodenal anastomosis in Europe. Sasse's principal objective with this procedure was to establish a connection between the common bile duct and the duodenum allowing direct passage of bile from the common bile duct to the duodenum and avoiding the use of the Kehr T-tube used to drain the bile to the exterior, with its associated problems. As a consequence of this operation, if calculi had been left in the common hepatic bile duct, these could pass into the duodenum. Later, the publications of Flörcken (15), Jurasz (28), Finsterer (14), Haberer (20), Mallet-Guy (36, 37), Valdoni (54, 55), and Pi-Figueras (40, 45) appeared in the literature and gave a great impetus to this procedure. Mirizzi, in 1931 in Argentina, was already recommending this operation but with very precise indications avoiding its overuse (40, 41). Sanders (47) was the first to perform choledochoduodenal anastomosis in the United States, an operation later popularized by Madden (34, 35). Although Sasse was not the creator of this operation, but was its advocate, in many surgical centers it is known as the Sasse Procedure.

Flörcken (15), Jurasz (28), Finsterer (14), Mirizzi, and other surgeons (40, 41, 44, 45) introduced modifications to the surgical technique. The ample indications for this procedure during the time of Sasse, Flörcken, Jurasz, Finsterer, an so on became more limited as time passed. Some of the reasons for this follow.

1. The more and more frequent use of operative cholangiography, notably diminished the number of patients

with residual stones in the common hepatic duct following surgery.

2. The description, in 1926, by Del Valle and Dónovan of Argentina (10) of the condition known as fibrosis of the Sphincter of Oddi, which these authors labeled Sclerotic Odditis. This clinical problem was later reconfirmed by Del Valle in his 1939 book (11), which led to the performance of sphincterotomies and sphincteroplasties in the treatment of strictures of the papilla.
3. The bloodless removal of residual calculi from the common hepatic bile duct in 1964 (38, 39) through the fibrous tract left by the long arm of the T-tube constituted a great step forward. This was first done by Mazzariello of Argentina in 1964 (38, 39).
4. Endoscopic sphincterotomy, described by Classen and Demling in 1974 in Germany (8) and by Kawai in Japan in the same year (29) was a great step forward in facilitating the elimination of retained calculi from the common hepatic bile duct in patients without a T-tube. At present, endoscopic sphincterotomy is used with frequency in the daily practice of trained endoscopists.
5. In recent years, the extraction of calculi from the common hepatic bile duct has been done by the transcutaneal hepatic approach in patients who are high surgical risks. Mazzariello (39) has described his experience using this technique.

These procedures have led to a significant limitation in the indications of choledochoduodenal anastomosis, but this operation continues to have its indications, since it represents an excellent solution in certain cases. The important thing is that the anastomosis of the common bile duct to the duodenum be well indicated and be performed with the correct technique. In some surgical centers, this technique continues to be used with the same enthusiasm as many years ago (12, 13, 16, 21, 22, 35).

INDICATIONS FOR CHOLEDOCHODUODENAL ANASTOMOSIS

1. Choledochoduodenal anastomosis is usually indicated in patients with multiple stones in the hepatic bile ducts that are dilated and in which one cannot be sure that some calculi may remain following surgery.
2. The procedure is also indicated in patients who are being subjected to a reoperation for residual stones in the common hepatic duct.
3. A very precise indication is that of primary stones in the common hepatic duct (4, 6, 9, 34, 35, 42).
4. In patients with chronic pancreatitis with compression of the retropancreatic bile duct (6, 19, 51, 57, 58).
5. In patients with fibrosis of the sphincter of Oddi with a very dilated bile duct, it is preferable to do a choledochoduodenal anastomosis instead of a sphincteroplasty. Very dilated bile ducts empty better with choledochoduodenal anastomosis than with sphincteroplasty (27).
6. In older patients or those with high risk, it is preferable to perform a choledochoduodenal anastomosis than a sphincteroplasty because it is an easier operation, it is performed in a shorter period of time, it is well tolerated, and it carries a lower morbidity and mortality rate.
7. There are surgeons who believe that choledochoduodenal anastomosis is indicated in malignant obstructive lesions in the distal end of the common bile duct (6). The author, as well as other surgeons, believes that this is not a correct indication because the carcinoma, as it grows, will rapidly obstruct the anastomosis. A more adequate operation in these cases is that of hepaticojejunostomy.
8. Some surgeons believe that choledochoduodenal anastomosis is indicated in cases of periampullary duodenal diverticula (6) in order to avoid the risk of damage to the ampulla during the removal of the diverticulum. This author, on the other hand, believes that the best treatment for symptomatic duodenal periampullary diverticula is diverticulectomy. However, the sole presence of a periampullary diverticulum does not increase the diameter of the common bile duct to facilitate the performance of the anastomosis with the duodenum. It is important to point out that in numerous occasions the author, as well as other surgeons, has proven that many choledochoduodenal anastomoses have been done unnecessarily.

CONDITIONS THAT MUST BE MET IN THE COMMON BILE DUCT AND THE DUODENUM TO FACILITATE THE PERFORMANCE OF CHOLEDOCHODUODENAL ANASTOMOSIS WITH GOOD, LASTING RESULTS

It is a sine qua non requirement that the common bile duct be sufficiently dilated to facilitate an ample and lasting anastomosis. The great majority of surgeons agree that the minimal diameter of the common bile duct should be two centimeters (4, 12, 13, 17, 21–26, 30, 34, 35). Other surgeons require a diameter of 2.5 cm (17, 21, 23, 30). It is the opinion of the author that choledochoduodenal anastomosis should not be performed if the common bile duct is less than 2 cm in diameter. On the other hand, there are surgeons who admit that the anastomosis can be performed with success when the common bile duct presents a diameter of 1.4 or 1.5 cm (9, 18, 31). Other surgeons admit that a common bile duct of 1.5 cm in diameter is sufficient for the anastomosis, but point out that it is preferable that the common bile duct be 2 cm in diameter.(6) Some technical modifications with the object of increasing the diameter of the anastomosis have been proposed. It must be pointed out that it is necessary and important that the diameter of the common bile duct be adequate, which is what regulates the flow of bile.

The duodenum should also present certain features if it is to be anastomosed to the common bile duct. It should have normal consistency in its tissues to allow safe suturing without tension. One should take great care in performing the procedure if the duodenum is inflamed and its wall is fragile, fibrotic, or retracted.

For many years, it was believed that reflux of duodenal content into the common bile duct was the cause of cholangitis in patients with choledochoduodenal anastomoses. There is no doubt that duodenal contents pass into the common bile duct easily due to the contractions of the powerful duodenal musculature, but the refluxed material returns rapidly to the duodenum as is easily demonstrable by radiologic examinations. In experimental studies (35) it has been possible to show that if the common bile duct is anastomosed to the colon, which contains very septic material, cholangitis does not result if the anastomosis is not narrow. Narrowing of the anastomosis, and not the reflux of duodenal content into the common bile duct, is the cause of cholangitis. That is why it is so important to perform choledochoduodenal anastomosis in common bile ducts that are sufficiently dilated to prevent cholangitis. Cholangitis is rare in choledochoduodenal anastomoses with common bile ducts with a diameter of 2 cm or more.

CHOLEDOCHODUODENAL ANASTOMOSIS OR SPHINCTEROPLASTY?

These two procedures are presented in the literature as competing procedures, which is a mistake. Surgeons should be able to perform both procedures applying the criteria that are most convenient to the patient according to his or her general state of health, age, surgical risk, the type of lesion present, and the degree of dilation of the common bile duct. Sphincteroplasty is indicated in several situations:

1. Impacted calculus in the ampulla.
2. Fibrosis of the sphincter of Oddi.
3. Multiple stones in the common hepatic duct when there is fear of having left behind residual calculi in common bile ducts only slightly dilated. Sphincteroplasty should always be the procedure of choice over choledochoduodenal anastomosis because it is a more physiologic and a more anatomic procedure for the elimination of calculi. On the other hand, biliary drainage in sphincteroplasty comes about at the most dependent, point and there is no chance for the formation of a blind pouch. It can also be performed without the common duct being dilated.
4. Sphincteroplasty may be indicated in cases in which one suspects that the patient may have a small carcinoma in the ampulla, with the object of confirming the diagnosis. One should not perform sphincteroplasty in lesions, extending from the distal common duct. The procedure can also be done in patients with periampullary diverticula, with a formal indication for sphincteroplasty, being careful not to injure the ampulla.

In summary, sphincteroplasty is more indicated in patients that are young, in good general health, and with only slightly dilated ducts. Choledochoduodenal anastomosis is more indicated in elderly patients with considerable surgical risk in which the bile duct is no less than 2 cm in diameter.

SUMP-SYNDROME

"Sump-syndrome" is a rare complication of choledochoduodenal anastomosis. This complication is also called "blind pouch," "blind sump," and "blind loop." It is produced by the accumulation or impaction of food, fibrous material, debris, biliary calculi, and stagnant bile in the duct below the anastomosis. If accumulation of residual material is very severe, it can rise to the level of the anastomosis, where it can cause disfunction of the stoma. The presence of infected bile in the stoma can cause inflammatory swelling and even cholangitis. Habitually, the sump-syndrome produces nonspecific discomfort in the upper abdomen and is seen in one to two percent of the patients with choledochoduodenal anastomoses. The treatment of this complication is endoscopic sphincterotomy (1, 6, 49, 53).

FIGURE 5.1
The abdominal incision used to perform choledochoduodenal anastomosis may be subcostal, paramedian, or transrectal. The author prefers the Mirizzi incision, which has been previously described. In the drawing, one can observe that a longitudinal incision 2.5 cm in length has been made in the common bile duct. This longitudinal incision may be transformed into a transverse incision by placing sutures in the middle third of each one of the sides and then applying traction in opposite directions. In the duodenum, a longitudinal incision 2.5 cm in length has been made. The great majority of surgeons practice choledochoduodenal anastomosis with this or a similar technique. This is because they perform instrumental exploration of the common bile duct through a longitudinal incision in the duct. In case choledochoduodenal anastomosis is then indicated, the longitudinal incision in the common bile duct is extended, and through it the anastomosis with the duodenum is performed.

Technique of Choledochoduodenal Anastomosis

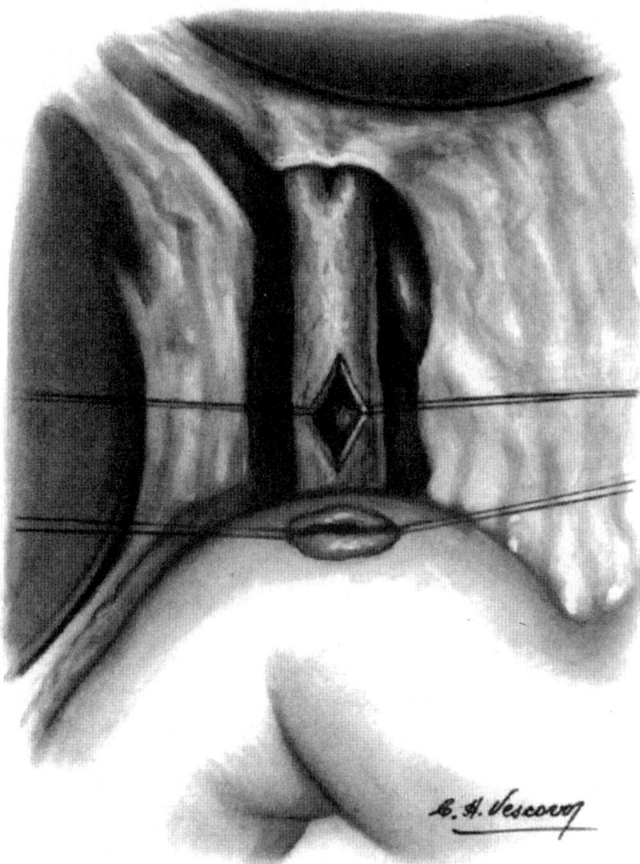

FIGURE 5.1

FIGURE 5.2

In this drawing, a transverse incision in the common bile duct has been performed to be used for the anastomosis with the duodenum and everything is ready to start suturing. The author prefers to perform a transverse incision in the common bile duct for the anastomosis with the duodenum for the following reasons:

1. The author always performs the instrumental exploration of the common bile duct through a transverse incision instead of a longitudinal incision.
2. The choledochotomy in transverse fashion allows one to perform a complete exploration of the common bile duct in a manner similar to that which is used with a longitudinal incision.
3. All calculi can be removed without difficulty through the transverse incision in the common bile duct.
4. In patients with common bile ducts of normal diameter, the closure of the transverse incision does not lead to narrowing, a complication that can occur with longitudinal incisions.
5. If choledochoduodenal anastomosis is indicated after the instrumental exploration, the same transverse incision is used as was used for the exploration of the duct.
6. The transverse incision of the common bile duct allows for a better conservation of the peritoneum over the hepatoduodenal ligament, which makes possible the performance of a more watertight closure of the choledochoduodenal anastomosis by including in the closure the serosa of the hepatoduodenal ligament.
7. The transverse incision of the common bile duct allows the performance of the suturing without tension in all cases, in contrast with the anastomosis in which a longitudinal incision in the common bile duct is used which can lead to tension in the suture line. In all cases, before suturing the anastomosis, the Vautrin-Kocher maneuver should be completely performed to avoid tension on the suture line.

Technique of Choledochoduodenal Anastomosis

The longitudinal incision in the duodenum should be made near the superior border of the duodenum, on the posterior aspect of the postbulbar segment. In order to do this, it is generally necessary to divide some loose adhesions that join the duodenum to the common bile duct (44, 45). Some surgeons, before starting choledochoduodenal suturing, place a row of sutures between the common bile duct and the duodenum so as to create a second layer of sutures. This is considered unnecessary since normally at this level, the common bile duct is adherent to the duodenum. One should take the precaution, before performing the incision in the common bile duct, of visualizing the localization of the cystic duct so as not to include it in the sutures. Once the incision is made in the duodenum, it is advisable to introduce the index finger and feel the ampulla so that a small carcinoma in this location will not be inadvertently missed.

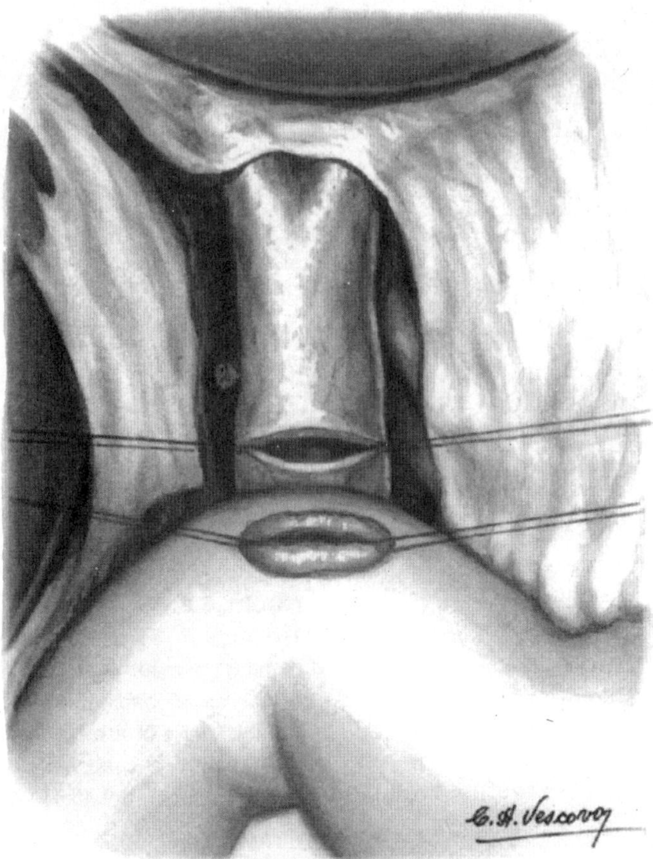

FIGURE 5.2

FIGURE 5.3
The surgeon is performing the sutures posteriorly between the common bile duct and the duodenum using interrupted sutures of 4-0 reabsorbable synthetic material. The sutures include the full thickness of the common bile duct and of the duodenum. One should take special care in the suture of the angles to avoid postoperative leakage.

Technique of Choledochoduodenal Anastomosis

FIGURE 5.4
Once having finished the posterior layer of sutures, the anterior layer is then performed in similar fashion. In the majority of patients, it is not possible to perform more than one row of sutures except in patients with very dilated common bile ducts and with thickened walls in which it can be possible to add another row of sutures anteriorly, including the adventitial layer of the common bile duct and the serosa of the hepaticoduodenal ligament with the seromuscular wall of the duodenum. Before closing the wall of the abdomen, a drainage tube is left in place for continuous suction in Morrison's pouch.

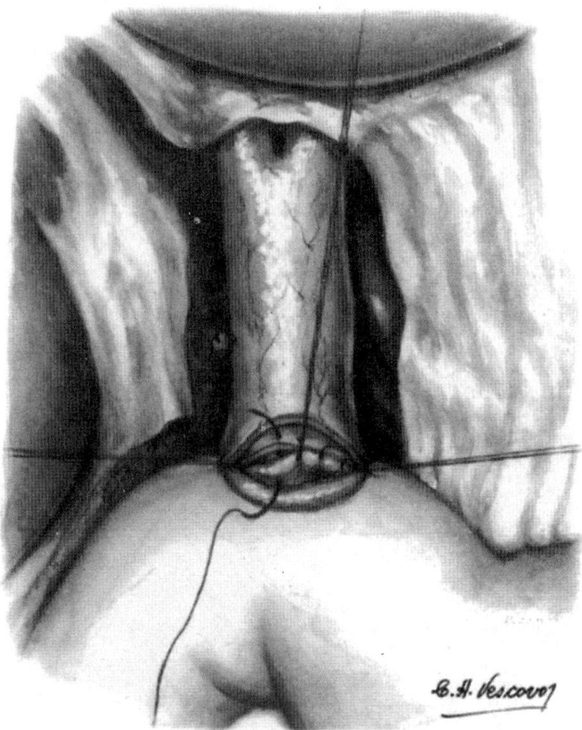

FIGURE 5.3

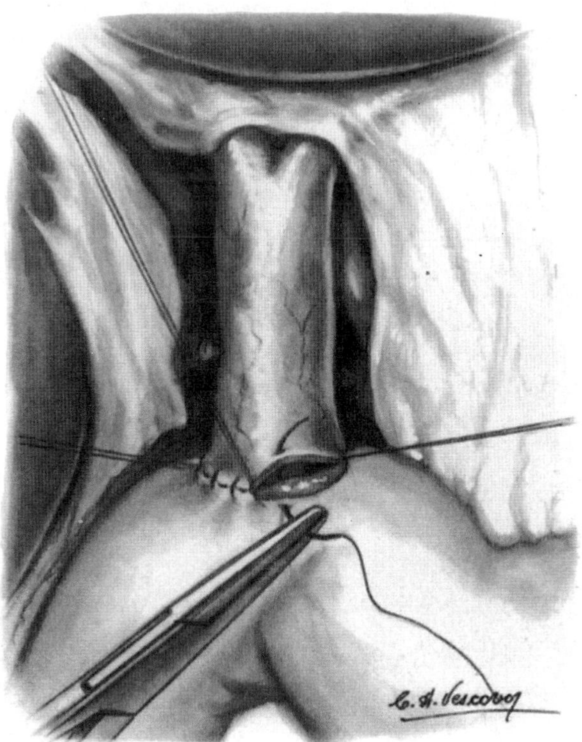

FIGURE 5.4

FIGURE 5.5 SUMP-SYNDROME

In 1 or 2 percent of patients with choledochoduodenal anastomoses, the complication of "sump-syndrome" may arise due to the accumulation of food, calculi, biliary mud, and septic bile in the duct, below the anastomosis. This may lead to a clinical picture of nonspecific discomfort in the upper abdomen. The drawing shows in semischematic fashion an anastomosis with accumulation of debris in the common bile duct, below the anastomosis.

If the anastomotic stoma remains completely permeable, cholangitis does not generally occur. If the sump-syndrome is complicated by a stricture of the anastomotic stoma or by an accumulation of septic bile, conditions will then be ideal for the occurrence of cholangitis. Treatment of the sump-syndrome is endoscopic transduodenal sphincterotomy.

Technique of Choledochoduodenal Anastomosis

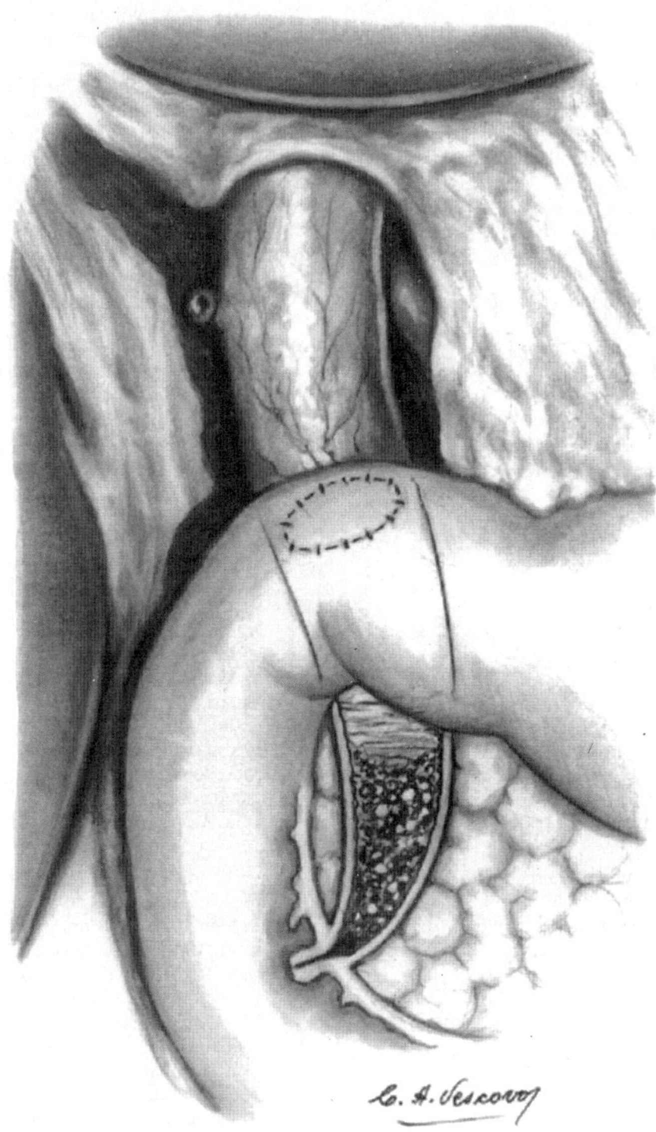

FIGURE 5.5 SUMP-SYNDROME

References

1. Akiyama, H., Ikezawa, H., Kameya, S., Iwasaki, M. Unexpected problems of external choledochoduodenostomy: Fibroscopic examination in 15 patients. Am. J. Surg. 140:660, 1980.
2. Baker, A.R., Neoptolemos, J.P., Carr-Locke. D.L., Fossard. D.P. Sump-Syndrome following choledochoduodenostomy and its endoscopic treatment. Br. J. Surg. 72:433, 1985.
3. Baker, A.R., Neoptolemos, J.P., Leese, T., Fossard, D.P. Choledochoduodenostomy, transduodenal sphincteroplasty and sphincterotomy for calculi of the common bile duct. Surg. Gynecol. Obstet. 164:245, 1987.
4. Berlatzky, Y., Freund, H. Choledochoduodenostomy in the treatment of benign biliary tract diseases. Am. J. Surg. 141:90, 1981.
5. Bismuth, H., Franco, D., Corlette, M.B., Hepp, J. Long term results of Roux-en-Y hepaticojejunostomy. Surg. Gynecol. Obstet. 146:161, 1978.
6. Cameron, J.L. Atlas of surgery. Vol. I, p. 28. B.C. Decker, Philadelphia, 1990.
7. Capper, W.M. External choledochoduodenostomy: An evaluation of 125 cases. Br. J. Surg. 49:292, 1961.
8. Classen, M., Demling, L. Endoskopische sphinterotomie der papilli Vateri und steinextrakion aus dem ductus choledocus. Dtsch. Med. Wochenschr.
9. Chassin, J.L. Operative strategy in general surgery. Vol. II, p. 121. Springer-Verlag, New York, 1984.
10. Del Valle, D., Dónovan, R. Colédoco. Odditis retráctil crónica. Concepto clínico-quirúrgico. Arch. Argent. Ap. Digest 1:141, 1926.
11. Del Valle, D. Patología y cirugía del esfínter de Oddi. El Ateneo, Buenos Aires, 1939.
12. Degenshein, G.A., Hurwitz, A. The techniques of side-to-side choledochoduodenostomy. Surgery 61:972, 1967.
13. Degenshein, G.A. Choledochoduodenostomy: An 18 years study of 175 consecutive cases. Surgery 76:319, 1974.
14. Finsterer, H. Die berentung der fur choledocoduodenostomie externa. Arch. Klin. Chir. 156:417, 1930.
15. Flörcken, H., Steden, E. Die nah-und fernergebnisse der choledocoduodenostomie. Arch. Klin. Chir. 124:59, 1923.
16. Fontana, J.J. Adelantos en el diagnóstico y tratamiento de la patología biliar benigna. Rev. Argent. Cir. No. Extraordinario, p. 26. Buenos Aires, 1989.
17. Freund, H., Charuzi, I., Granit, G., Berlatzky, Y. Choledochoduodenostomy in the treatment of benign biliary tract diseases. Arch. Surg. 112:1032, 1977.
18. Gliedman, M.L. Surgical techniques. p. 160. McGraw-Hill, New York, 1990.
19. Gregg, D.A., Carr-Locke, D.L., Gallagher, M.M. Importance of common bile duct stricture associated with chronic pancreatitis. Am. J. Surg. 141:199, 1981.
20. Haberer, H. Zurfrage der choledocus drainage nach dem duodenum. Zentralbl. F. Chir. 50:1138, 1923.
21. Hermann, R.E. Manual of surgery of the gallbladder, bile ducts and exocrine pancreas. p. 145. Springer-Verlag, New York, 1979.
22. Hoerr, S.O., Hermann, R.E. Choledochoduodenostomy. In Way L., Pellegrini, C.A. Surgery of the gallbladder and bile ducts, p. 367. W.B. Saunders, Philadelphia, 1987.
23. Johnson, A.G., Stevens, A.E. Importance of the size of the stoma in choledochoduodenostomy. Gut 10:68, 1969.
24. Johnson, A.G., Rains. A.J.H. Choledochoduodenostomy. Br. J. Surg. 59:277, 1972.
25. Johnson, A.G., Rains, A.J.H. Prevention and treatment of recurrent bile duct stones by choledochoduodenostomy. World J. Surg. 2:487, 1978.
26. Jones, S.A. The prevention and treatment of recurrent bile duct stones by transduodenal sphincteroplasty. World J. Surg. 2:473, 1978.
27. Jones, S.A. The choice between transduodenal sphincteroplasty and lateral choledochoduodenostomy for distal common duct obstruction. In Nyhus, L.M., Baker, R.J. (Eds.) Mastery of surgery. Vol. I, p. 695. Little, Brown & Co., Boston, 1984.
28. Jurasz, A. Die choledocoduodenostomie als method der wahl zur drainage der tiefen gallanwege. Zentralbl. Chir. 50:1000, 1923.
29. Kawai, K., Akasaka, Y., Murakami, K., Tada, M., Koh, L., Nakayima, M. Endoscopic sphincterotomy of the ampulla of Vater. Gastrointest. Endoscopy 20:148, 1974.
30. Kraus, M.A., Wilson, S.D. Choledochoduodenostomy: Importance of common duct size and occurrence of cholangitis. Arch. Surg. 115:1212, 1980.
31. Kune, G.A., Sali, A. The practice of biliary surgery. Ed. 2, p. 383. Blackwell Scientific Publications, Oxford, 1980.
32. Lygidakis, N.J. Surgical approaches to recurrent choledocholithiasis. Choledochoduodenostomy versus T tube drainage after choledochotomy. Am. J. Surg. 145:636, 1983.
33. McSherry, C.K., Fischer, M.G. Common bile duct stones and biliary intestinal anastomoses. Surg. Gynecol. Obstet. 153:669, 1981.
34. Madden, D.L., Gruwez, J.A., Tan, P.Y. Obstructive (surgical) jaundice: An analysis of 140 consecutive cases and a consideration of choledochoduodenostomy in its treatment. Am. J. Surg. 109:89, 1965.
35. Madden, J.L., Chung, D.Y., Kandalast, S., Parekh, M. Choledochoduodenostomy; an injustly maligned surgical procedure? Am. J. Surg. 119:45, 1970.
36. Mallet-Guy, P., Jeanjean, R., Marion, P. Le chirurgie biliaire sous contrôle manométrique et radiologique peropératoire. Masson et Cie., Paris, 1947.
37. Mallet-Guy, P., Descotles, J. Enquête sur les resultats éloignés de 100 choledocoduodenostomies d'indication relative. Lyon Chir. 50:659, 1955.
38. Mazzariello, R. Removal of residual biliary tract calculi without reoperation. Surgery 67:566, 1970.
39. Mazzariello, R. Extracción de cálculos por vía transparietohepática. Pren. Méd. Argent. 78:11, 1991.
40. Mirizzi, P.L. Colangiografía operatoria. Bol. Soc. Cir. Buenos Aires 16:1135, 1932.
41. Mirizzi, P.L. Lithiase de la voie biliaire principale. p. 149. Masson et Cie., Paris, 1957.
42. Moesgaard, F., Nielsen, M.L., Pedersen, T., Hansen, J.B. Protective choledochoduodenostomy in multiple common ducts: Stones in the aged. Surg. Gynecol. Obstet. 154:232, 1982.
43. Oría, A., Alvarez Rodríguez, J., Paladino, A., Epizzamiglio, N., Chiappetta Porrás, L., Fontana, J.J. La coledocoduodenoanastomosis en el tratamiento de la litiasis de la vía biliar principal. Rev. Argent. Cirug. 51:237, 1986.
44. Pi-Figueras, J. Technique de l'anastomose cholédocoduodenale pour la lithiase de la voie biliaire principale. Iconographia Chirurgica, Encyclopédie Médicochirurgicale, Paris, 1958.
45. Pi-Figueras, J. Práctica quirúrgica. Ed. 2, Vol. II, p. 640. Salvat, Barcelona, 1986.
46. Riedel, B.M.C.L. Erfahrungen über die gallensteinkrankeit mir und ohne icterus. Berl. Hirschwald p. 116, 1892.
47. Sanders, R.L. Indications for and value of choledochoduodenostomy. Ann Surg. 123:847, 1946.
48. Sasse, F. Ueber choledocoduodenostomie. Sintzung der mitteldheinischen churirgenvereiniung. Zentralbl. Chir. 40:91, 1913.
49. Scott, A.J., Khan, G.A. Partial biliary obstruction with cholangitis producing a blind loop syndrome. Gut 9:187, 1968.
50. Schein, C.J., Gliedman, M.L. Choledochoduodenostomy as an adjunct to choledocholithotomy. Surg. Gynecol. Obstet. 152:797, 1981.
51. Schwartz, F., Benshimol, A., Hurwitz, A. Choledochoduodenostomy in the treatment of stenosis of lower portion of the common bile duct. Surgery 46:1020, 1959.2
52. Sprengel, O. Ueber einen fall von exstirpation der gallanblase mit anlegung einer communication zwischen ductus choledochus und duodenum. Arch. Klin. Chir. 42:550, 1891.
53. Tanaka, M., Ikeda, S., Yoshimoto, H. Endoscopie sphincterotomie for the treatment of biliary sump-syndrome. Surgery 93:264, 1983.
54. Valdoni, P. Comunicación personal, 1957.
55. Valdoni, P. Abdominal surgery. An atlas of operative techniques. p. 79. W.B. Saunders Co., Philadelphia, 1976.
56. Walzel, P. Die widergutnachung nach unzweckmasig ausgeführten gallen operationen. Dtsch. Z. Chir. 195:954, 1926.
57. Warren, K.W., Jenkins, R.L., Steele, G.D., Jr. Atlas of surgery of the liver, pancreas and biliary tract. p. 28. Appleton-Lange, East Norwalk, CT, 1991.
58. Warshaw, A.L., Schapiro, R.H., Ferrucci, J.T., Galdabinni, J.J. Persistent obstructive jaundice, cholangitis and biliary cirrhosis due to common bile duct stenosis in chronic pancreatitis. Gastroenterology 70:562, 1976.
59. White, T.T. Indication for sphincteroplasty as opposed to choledochoduodenostomy. Am. J. Surg. 126:165, 1973.

Section A

Surgery of the Biliary Tract

CHAPTER 6

Repair of Surgical Lesions of the Common Bile Duct

Surgical lesions of the common bile duct usually constitute the beginning of a drama. The damage produced in one second by the end of a scissors may be so grave that its repair may last for the rest of the life of the patient. The repair of lesions of the biliary tract is a thankless surgery of unpredictable evolution and at times very disappointing. Even though these lesions are benign, their behavior is usually very similar to that of a malignant lesion because of the frequent recurrences and complications, which make repeated repairs necessary that are more and more complex each time. Surgical lesions of the biliary tract become more dramatic when they occur in young patients.

It is very important that the surgeon have the absolute conviction that the great majority of surgical lesions of the biliary tract can be avoided if correct surgical technique is used. This means that the surgeon must be prepared to avoid transformation of a simple well controlled benign procedure, as is a cholecystectomy, into a dangerous surgical act of grave consequences for the patient.

The author firmly believes that in a surgical atlas, besides describing the various techniques of repair of surgical lesions of the common bile duct, one should also point out the common causes that tend to produce these lesions with the object of avoiding them. It is also important to point out how one arrives at the diagnosis of these lesions, what is the proper conduct once these lesions are produced, according to various circumstances, and the moment at which one should intervene, be it to treat a complication or to perform the repair of the lesion. It is also important to point out the need for the surgeon to know the various surgical procedures for repair in order to be able to choose the most appropriate one after performing a thorough study of the individual patient, the type of lesion, its localization and extent, the presence of complications, the time interval since surgery, the number of previous procedures, the general condition of the patient, and so on. Since it is impossible to present all the possible situations that can occur as a consequence of surgical lesions of the biliary tract, the surgeon must frequently rely exclusively on his experience and his criteria to resolve the different situations that present themselves.

FREQUENCY

It is very difficult to have exact figures on the frequency with which lesions of the common bile duct occur during cholecystectomy. Frequently the surgeon is not aware that he has damaged the common bile duct during cholecystectomy, and in the cases in which he or she is aware of the damage will generally hide it or offer a false diagnosis, the most frequent of which is that of diffuse sclerosing cholangitis. The more experienced the surgeon, the less probability of damaging the common bile duct.

In a review of international literature the conclusion has been arrived at that, at centers of great experience in biliary surgery, lesions of the common bile duct occur once every five hundred cholecystectomies (20, 26, 32, 39, 44, 50).

FACTORS THAT FAVOR THE OCCURRENCE OF LESIONS OF THE COMMON BILE DUCT DURING SURGERY

The factors that may favor the production of lesions of the common bile duct are numerous and may be grouped in the following manner:

1. Errors in surgical technique
2. Pathologic factors
3. Variations of the normal anatomy

Errors in Surgical Technique

The most frequent cause of lesions of the common bile duct during cholecystectomy is errors committed by the surgeon. It is much less frequent that the lesions are caused by instrumental exploration of the common bile duct. Gastrectomy for penetrating duodenal ulcer is a more rare cause of lesions. Lesions produced during cholecystectomy are usually localized in the proximal segments of the common bile duct, and lesions produced by instrumental exploration or during a gastrectomy are usually localized in the distal section of the common bile duct.

Within the group of technical errors that may be committed by the surgeon, the most common one is failure to correctly identify the anatomic structures during cholecystectomy, before ligating or sectioning these structures.

The most common error is that of mistaking the hepatic duct for the cystic duct, particularly when the hepatic duct is small in diameter. The surgeon proceeds to ligate the hepatic duct or to resect it together with the cystic duct. This mistake explains why the majority of the lesions of the common hepatic duct are localized in the proximal segment, in the junction of the cystic with the hepatic duct and the common bile duct. The lesions occur in the common hepatic duct or with less frequency at the site of junction of the right and left hepatic duct (7, 26, 50).

There are other contributing factors for the surgeon to commit errors of technique such as insufficient exposure of the operative field, due to small incisions, poor illumination, untrained assistants, rough maneuvers, and so on.

In some cases lesions of the common bile duct occur because the surgeon does not keep calm when facing a hemorrhage, as may occur for example with the rupture of the cystic artery when it is being dissected prior to its ligation. Rupture of the cystic artery usually produces a profuse hemorrhage that obscures the operative field completely. The surgeon, who desires to perform hemostasis as rapidly as possible, places clamps blindly, which may lead to lesions of the common hepatic duct. When facing this critical situation the surgeon must remain very calm and transmit this serenity to the operative team, proceeding immediately to perform temporary hemostasis by means of the Pringle maneuver. This consists in compression of the hepatic artery between the index finger and thumb of the left hand within the hepatoduodenal ligament. Once temporary hemostasis is achieved, all the blood that spilled in the operative field is aspirated, a better anesthetic relaxation is requested, the laparotomy packs are better placed to obtain a more ample operative field, and the digital hemostasis is replaced by an atraumatic vascular hemostatic clamp. Only after performing these maneuvers should the surgeon turn to investigation and search for the end of the bleeding cystic artery, proceeding to clamp and ligate it. One must bear in mind that frequently the proximal end of the cystic artery has retracted and is now behind the common hepatic duct, which makes hemostasis more difficult and dangerous.

Another error that is occasionally made by the surgeon is that of placing excessive traction on the fundus of the gallbladder. This traction may lead to two accidents:

1. Rupture of the cystic artery when its walls have been altered by the inflammatory process. One must have in mind that the cystic artery is short and runs a straighter course than the cystic duct.
2. Excessive traction on the gallbladder may lead to

kinking of the common bile duct at the site of its junction with the cystic duct, specially if the common bile duct is thin in diameter. The surgeon, in trying to ligate the cystic duct, may include the kinked common bile duct in the ligature.

Cholecystectomy should not be considered an easy operation and should not be left in inexperienced hands. The surgeon who is in the learning stage should always operate under the supervision of an experienced surgeon. The biliary tract surgeon should have a good knowledge of the normal anatomy of the biliary tract and its more important anatomic variations and should not ligate or cut any anatomic structure without previously identifying it. There is no more dangerous instrument in the hepatic pedicle than the ends of a scissors. Before proceeding with the cholecystectomy the surgeon must identify the hepatic and common bile duct in their entire length. The cystic duct must also be identified in its entire length from the neck of the gallbladder to its junction with the common hepatic duct. During cholecystectomy the cystic artery must be identified from its origin to its entrance in the gallbladder, whether it is at the gallbladder neck or at the infundibulum. It should not be ligated at its origin and should be ligated in the vicinity of the gallbladder.

The surgeon should not insist on performing a cholecystectomy from the cystic duct toward the fundus of the gallbladder in cases in which it is impossible to clearly identify the triangle of Calot. Biliary tract surgery should always be associated with operative cholangiography because it contributes a very significantly the diagnosis of pathologic lesions of the common hepatic duct. It is also of great use in preventing lesions and in recognizing lesions that may have been produced. At present it is common for patients with jaundice to arrive at surgery with a transparietohepatic cholangiogram or with an endoscopic retrograde pancreatocholangiogram.

Easy Cholecystectomies

International statistics show that surgical lesions of the common bile duct are produced more frequently in "easy" cholecystectomies generally performed by surgeons with less experience. This is the origin of Maingot's assertion, "Easy cholecystectomy and an inexperienced surgeon constitute a sinister combination." Experienced surgeons may also damage the common bile duct in "easy" cholecystectomies but undoubtedly with much less frequency. The cause of injury in these cases may be overconfidence, lack of concentration, fatigue, trying to hurry the operation, and so on.

On some occasions surgeons of great experience have damaged the common bile duct during a surgical demonstration in front of surgical colleagues in their desire to show off their ability and speed. A surgeon's only consideration should be concentration on the operation that the surgeon is performing on the patient whose life is in his or her hands, and the opinions of spectator colleagues should be completely ignored.

Pathologic Factors

Severe alterations in the anatomy may be due to the pathology in the area leading to swelling, friability, repeated attacks of acute cholecystitis, and fibrosis of the hepatic hilum (27, 49, 50). These may substantially alter the anatomy of the biliary tract, favoring the production of surgical lesions of the common bile duct. On the other hand, the proportion of lesions caused by pathologic factors is much less than those caused by technical error. Generally the surgeon who is operating on a biliary tract with important pathologic alterations acts with great prudence to avoid error. This may explain the fact that the frequency of lesions in these cases is not so numerous. The less experienced surgeon who does not feel capable of performing a cholecystectomy in cases with very complex pathology always has the option of performing a cholecystostomy.

Severe pathologic alterations may be observed in acute processes (acute cholecystitis) or in chronic processes such as Hartmann's pouch, biliobiliary fistulas with disappearance of the cystic duct, and so on.

Variations

Anomalies of the biliary tract are very numerous, and the surgeon should always be prepared to encounter some of them. Lesions of the common bile duct owing to anatomic variation are evidently less frequent than those that occur due to errors in technique.

DIAGNOSIS

Surgical lesions of the common bile duct may be diagnosed during surgery, in the immediate postoperative period, or in the late postoperative period.

Surgeons notice that they have damaged the common bile duct during surgery in only 20% of cases. In the remaining 80%, surgeons do not notice that they have damaged the common bile duct (26, 50).

In the immediate postoperative period the existence of a lesion of the common bile duct is generally suspected when a biliary fistula appears or when the patient develops biliary peritonitis, choleperitoneum, or progressive jaundice. Symptoms that complicate the post-operative period generally appear between the second and seventh day following the surgical procedure. In some cases symptoms appear even later, making the diagnosis more difficult. One must point out that rarely can one obtain precise data from the surgeon who performed the cholecystectomy because in the great majority of cases that surgeon attributes the complications to some cause other than the possibility of having damaged the common bile duct.

In patients with a biliary fistula, cholangiography through the fistulous tract may show the existence of a lesion of the common bile duct. In patients with jaundice, be this due to ligature or to transection and ligature of a segment of the common bile duct, a transparietohepatic cholangiogram may show the level and the grade of obstruction. Endoscopic retrograde cholangiopancreatography is less efficient in arriving at an exact diagnosis because generally the radiopaque substance does not pass above the level of the lesion. In patients who present biliary peritonitis or bile in the peritoneal cavity, an abdominal tap may be of great diagnostic value. Ultrasonography or computed tomography may contribute to the diagnosis in some cases.

The certainty and the exact extent of a lesion of the common bile duct, its localization, and its type and extension will only be evident by surgical exploration, instrumental exploration, and operative cholangiography.

WHEN SHOULD ONE PROCEED TO REPAIR A LESION OF THE COMMON BILE DUCT?

The opportune moment to repair a surgical lesion of the common bile duct depends on several factors. Some of these will be analyzed as follows. In cases in which a surgeon realizes that he or she has damaged the common bile duct during the surgical procedure, the surgeon should proceed to repair it in the same surgical procedure if he or she is capable of doing so. If the surgeon is not capable of performing the repair he or she should immediately call an experienced surgeon to perform the repair of the lesion. If no experienced surgeon is available to solve the problem, the surgeon should end the operation, leaving a drainage tube in the proximal common bile duct to drain bile to the exterior of the abdomen. The repair of the common bile duct will then be performed later by a competent surgical team.

It has been shown that the best results in the repair of the lesions of the common bile duct are obtained when the repair is performed in the same surgical procedure. Delayed reoperations give a less satisfactory result because the tissues are changed by fibrosis, retraction, and infection.

In cases in which diagnosis of the surgical lesion of the common bile duct is made in the postoperative period, the proper moment to reoperate on the patient and repair the lesion will depend on several factors:

1. The presence of biliary peritonitis or choleperitoneum. In these cases the patient should be operated upon to save his or her life and drain bile to the outside. In a second stage, repair of the common bile duct can be undertaken.
2. The presence of an infectious clinical picture, subphrenic or intraperitoneal abscess. In these patients the infectious process will be treated and the common bile duct will be repaired when the infection has completely disappeared.
3. Patients with biliary fistula. In these cases expectant treatment can be undertaken. After a few weeks the fistula may close and consequently the patient becomes jaundiced and the common bile duct dilates above the site of the lesion. If at all possible repair of the lesion of the common bile duct should be performed in this stage—that is to say, with the infection controlled, the fistula closed, and a dilated common bile duct.
4. Patients with jaundice caused by ligation of the common bile duct. In these cases patients should be operated upon to repair the lesion but not necessarily urgently, although the operation should always be done before hepatic insufficiency sets in with infection, fibrosis, or portal hypertension.

Many patients come to surgery after having been subjected to several unsuccessful surgical procedures to repair the common bile duct. These patients should not be denied another attempt because in some cases success has been obtained after several previous failures. These circumstantial successes should not lead one to forget that as a patient has been operated on repeatedly for the repair of the common bile duct, the bile duct will become shorter, more fibrotic, and retracted as well as surrounded by adhesions. This will make the surgical procedure more difficult and the functional liver status more compromised.

PROCEDURES TO REPAIR SURGICAL LESIONS OF THE BILIARY TRACT

There are multiple procedures that can be used to repair surgical lesions of the common bile duct. Selection of the procedure to be used in an individual case depends on several factors:

1. Type, localization and extension of the lesion
2. Time when the lesion was recognized.
3. The presence and seriousness of complications of the lesion.
4. The patient has been subjected to previous repairs.
5. General condition of the patient.
6. Functional status of the liver, and so on.

We will now proceed to review surgical procedures that can be used to repair common bile duct lesions in accordance with the circumstances and later we will give a detailed description of the more commonly used techniques in surgical practice. The selection of the surgical procedure will vary according to the lesion and the moment in which the lesion is recognized.

As has been mentioned previously, surgical lesions of the common bile duct can be recognized in the same surgical procedure, in the immediate postoperative period and in the late postoperative period and well as in repeated repairs.

SURGICAL PROCEDURES USED FOR THE REPAIR OF LESIONS RECOGNIZED IN THE ORIGINAL INTERVENTION

End to end anastomosis is the procedure most used in lesions of the common bile duct due to ligation, complete transverse section, or transection with resection of a length of less than 10 mm.

In patients in which a transection with resection of the common bile duct of a length of more than 10 mm, end to end anastomosis can rarely be performed with success. In end to end anastomosis one should always perform the Vautrin-Kocher maneuver to elongate the common bile duct with the object in mind of avoiding tension on the suture line. One should note that the Vautrin-Kocher maneuver can increase the length of the common bile duct by only some 10 mm.

Small parietal transections of the common bile duct, 5 mm or less in diameter, may be treated by transverse suturing with placement of a T-tube either above or below the site of the lesion.

Defects of the common bile duct localized in the vicinity of the entry of the cystic duct may be treated by means of a plastic procedure performed using the posterior wall of the cystic duct which is then sutured to close the defect. A T-tube is placed above or below the site of the plastic closure.

In cases in which the lateral defect of a common bile duct of normal caliber is oriented longitudinally and not more than 10 mm in length, it can be closed in transverse fashion imitating the technique of the Heinecke-Mikulicz pyloroplasty, previously performing a Vautrin-Kocher maneuver to avoid tension on the suture line. This procedure is finalized by placing a T-tube through the site of the repair.

In patients that have lateral defects more than 15 mm long, it is not advisable to repair the defect by the Heinecke-Mikulicz technique because the suture line will have too much tension and will fail in spite of the previously performed Vautrin-Kocher maneuver. In these cases the lateral defect can be covered with a patch of saphenous vein (4, 7, 17, 27, 33, 34, 50). Saphenous vein patches are rapidity epithelialized (4, 34). In cases with similar defects, other authors (7) use serosal patches to close the defect, as we will see later on.

In patients in whom resection of the common bile duct has been performed and this defect is more than 10 mm long, reestablishment of biliary flow should be performed by means of a biliary jejunal anastomosis.

CONDITIONS THAT MUST BE MET TO PERFORM AN END TO END ANASTOMOSIS TO THE COMMON BILE DUCT

End to end anastomosis of the common bile duct must meet certain conditions in order to perform it with success.

1. The ends to be anastomosed must have a similar diameter.
2. The anastomosis must be performed in strict mucosa to mucosa fashion to avoid a later stricture.
3. There should be no tension on the suture line, otherwise it will be exposed to failure.
4. To avoid tension of the suture line the Vautrin-Kocher maneuver should be performed.
5. Patients who have undergone a resection of the common bile duct of more than 10 mm in length should not be treated by end to end anastomosis.
6. In end to end anastomosis of common bile ducts of normal caliber it is not advisable to place more than 8 to 10 sutures.
7. The sutures should not be tied to tightly to avoid ischemia of the edges of the anastomosis.
8. In order to be exact in the placement of the sutures, particularly in common bile duct of normal caliber, one should use a magnifying loupe or a surgical microscope.
9. The suture should be watertight to avoid filtration of bile, which may lead to fibrosis, retraction and stricture.
10. The water tightness of the suture line may be obtained by closing the peritoneum of the hepatoduodenal ligament, if available, over the suture line or using a plastic procedure to transpose the greater omentum.
11. The suture material should be interrupted synthetic reabsorbable 3-0 sutures. On the other hand many surgeons continue to use chromic catgut and others linen or silk. Some authors (27) affirm that the suture material used in performing the end to end anastomosis is not as important as it was thought to be for many years.

Although the great majority of surgeons leave a T-tube in place in end to end anastomoses as a stent (1–3, 7, 8, 10, 11, 21, 29, 47, 50), other authors of great experience (28, 31) do not advise against the use of a stent based on clinical and experimental studies. Still other surgeons (27) leave a T-tube in place not as a stent but simply to drain bile to the outside, and there are authors who leave a T-tube in place as a stent when the caliber of the common bile duct is normal but not in cases in which the common bile duct is dilated, allowing for the performance of a mucosa to mucosa anastomosis.

According to international bibliography, the T-tubes are frequently used after end to end anastomosis for the following reasons:

1. In addition to acting as a stent, the T-tube reduces the intraluminal pressure in the common bile duct, reducing the possibility of bile leakage through the suture line, which could lead to fibrosis and stricture.
2. The T-tube will permit irrigations with physiologic saline to be carried out to prevent obstruction caused by biliary mud.
3. The T-tube will also allow cholangiograms to be performed to evaluate the end to end anastomosis.

Surgeons who prefer transhepatic drainage place a drainage tube of this type in end to end anastomoses of the common bile duct (8, 22, 24, 36–38, 40, 50).

The length of time a T-tube should be left in place in end to end anastomoses has been discussed extensively. It is generally accepted that, if the end to end anastomosis was performed satisfactorily, the T-tube should be left in place for 6 weeks. If the anastomosis has not been entirely satisfactory, the T-tube is left in place for at least 12 weeks (1, 3, 7, 10, 11, 26, 29, 48–50).

Statistics have shown that end to end anastomosis of the common bile duct leads to recurrence of stricture in 30 to 50% of cases (7, 26, 50). It is possible that this high incidence of recurrence is caused by too much tension on the suture line or an unsatisfactory mucosa to mucosa layer. In other cases it is possible that there was bile leakage through the suture line postoperatively. Bile stimulates the formation and retraction of fibrous tissue.

SURGICAL PROCEDURES USED TO REPAIR LESIONS RECOGNIZED IN THE IMMEDIATE POSTOPERATIVE PERIOD

These patients generally have a complicated postoperative course with biliary fistula, bile peritonitis, abscesses, jaundice, and so on. Except for patients with obstructive jaundice caused by ligation of the common bile duct, other patients should be operated on in stages. An end to end anastomosis in these cases can only rarely be performed. Reestablishment of biliary transit can only be achieved by means of a hepaticojejunal anastomosis in the great majority of these cases.

SURGICAL PROCEDURES USED TO REPAIR LESIONS RECOGNIZED IN THE LATE POSTOPERATIVE PERIOD OR AFTER REPEATED SURGICAL PROCEDURES

In this group of patients there is less probability than in the previous group that an end to end anastomosis of the common bile duct can be performed. There are several reasons that prevent an end to end anastomosis from being carried out:

1. The distal segment of the traumatized duct is generally sclerosed, occluded, and retracted.
2. There is frequently great disparity between the ends, the proximal end being much larger in diameter, preventing a correct anastomosis from being carried out.
3. Some of these patients have had a segment of the common bile duct removed, which, together with the fibrosis and retraction, makes an end to end anastomosis impossible.
4. The main object of performing an end to end anastomosis is the conservation of the sphincter of Oddi to prevent cholangitis by conserving normal anatomy and function. It has been shown, however, that cholangitis can occur with a normal sphincter of Oddi.
5. A Vautrin-Kocher maneuver is performed to elongate the common bile duct. The duct can usually be elongated some 10 mm by this maneuver. Occasionally the elongation can be 15 mm. Some surgeons transect the pancreas where the duct passes through it to attain greater length. It has been shown, however, that very little is gained by these combined maneuvers, since the complications that they give rise to amply negate the short increase in length obtained.

For these reasons, patients reoperated for surgical lesions of the common bile duct can hardly ever have an end to end anastomosis. In the great majority of cases bile flow can only be reestablished by means of a hepaticojejunostomy. In patients with a common hepatic duct more than 15 mm in diameter in which a satisfactory mucosa to mucosa anastomosis can be performed, this is the procedure of choice. If the common hepatic duct is less than 15 mm in diameter, the hepaticojejunostomy will probably fail.

In these cases the procedure proposed by Hepp and Couinaud (25) in 1958, based on Couinaud's anatomic investigations and later popularized by Bismuth (5, 6), Blumgart (7) and others (49, 50) should be used (49, 50).

This procedure is based on lowering the hilar plate and using the left hepatic duct to widen the diameter of the anastomosis. According to French authors the hilar plate is made up of Glisson's capsule fused to the peritoneum of the hepatogastric ligament at the level of the posterior border of the quadrate lobe (segment IV of the liver). Lowering the hilar plate lowers the left hepatic duct, which normally runs for about 4 to 5 cm without being covered by hepatic parenchyma. By extending the incision onto the left hepatic duct you increase the diameter of the anastomosis. In addition to increasing the anastomotic opening, this technique uses a segment of the left hepatic duct that is generally not compromised by the fibrosis and retraction.

A mucosa to mucosa anastomosis of good diameter performed with healthy tissue is the best prophylaxis for recurrences of lesions of the common bile duct. If the surgical lesion involves the bifurcation of the common hepatic duct, reestablishment of biliary flow will be more frequently exposed to failure, no matter what technique is used in its repair.

In some patients it is impossible to perform a mucosa to mucosa hepaticojejunostomy due to the great proliferation of fibrous tissue covering the edges and part of the lumen of the common hepatic duct. In these cases one can resort to the Lord Smith of Marlow procedure (3, 27, 40–42), which consists of bringing jejunal mucosa up to the highest possible point inside the common hepatic duct, placing it in contact with the duct's healthy mucosa. In this way both mucosas are apposed far from the fibrotic process.

Patients that are not in condition to tolerate surgical repair of the common bile duct can be subjected to palliative dilations by the transcutaneohepatic or endoscopic retrograde approach performed by physicians experienced in these methods using adequate instruments.

FIGURE 6.1

Parietal defect of the common bile duct produced by a surgical lesion recognized during the same surgical procedure with its greatest diameter oriented longitudinally. This defect can be closed transversely as long as its diameter is not over 10 mm. A complete Vautrin-Kocher maneuver should be performed before beginning the suturing in order to increase the length of the common bile duct to avoid tension on the suture line. Closure of the defect is carried out with interrupted 5-0 synthetic reabsorbable material. This transverse closure is somewhat similar to the Heinecke-Mikulicz pyloroplasty. After closing the duct a small incision is made in it, distal to the closure, to insert a thin T-tube into the duct to drain bile to the outside.

Repair of Parietal Defects of the Common Bile Duct

FIGURE 6.2

Parietal defect of greater extent with a longitudinal defect 16 mm long. A defect this long, if closed transversely, will result in tension on the suture line which will fail in spite of the Vautrin-Kocher maneuver. These defects can be covered with a saphenous vein patch or a serosal patch. The drawing shows the placement of a vein patch. The edges of the venous patch are being sutured to the edges of the defect with synthetic reabsorbable 5-0 sutures. Once the patch is in place, the duct is drained with a thin T-tube.

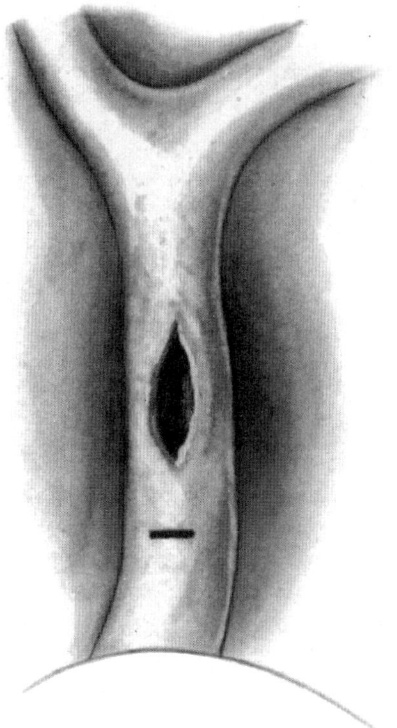

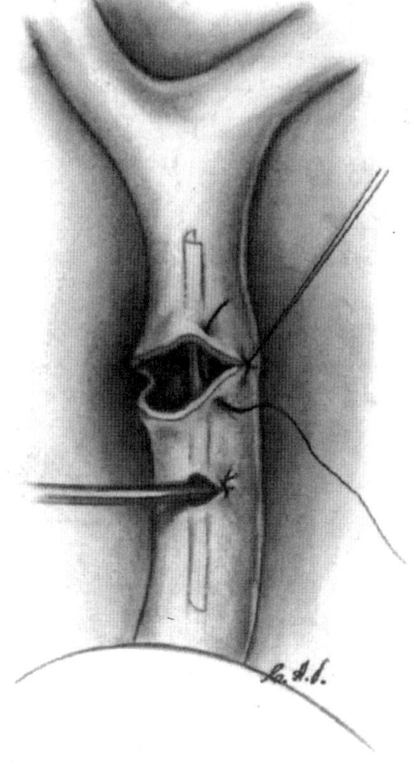

FIGURE 6.1

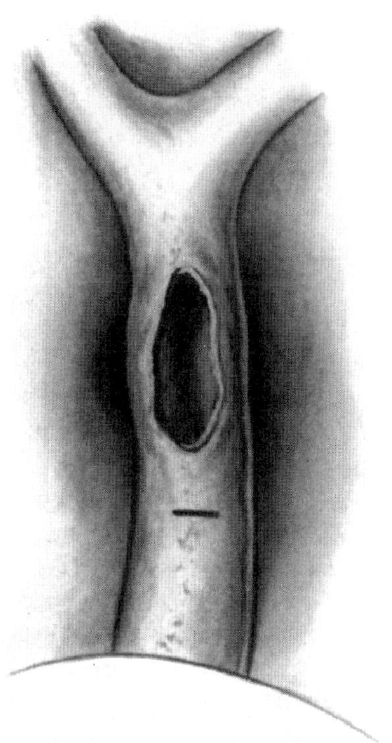

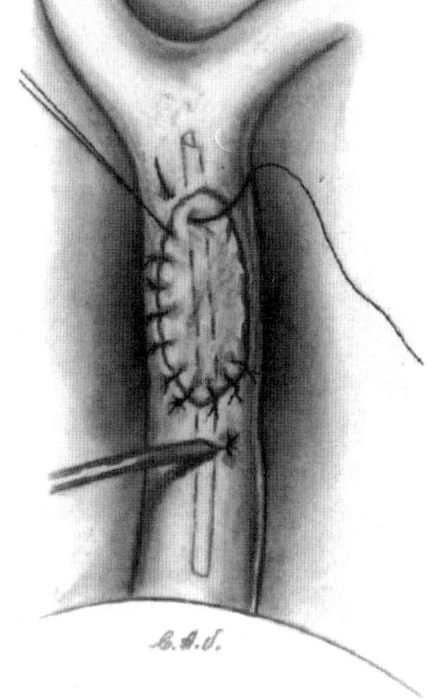

FIGURE 6.2

FIGURE 6.3
Parietal defect of the common bile duct similar to the one in the previous figure. In this case the parietal defect will be covered with a patch of serosa at the expense of the wall of a jejunal loop oriented in Roux-en-Y fashion. The ascending or anastomotic limb of the Roux-en-Y, whose end has been closed in two layers of sutures, is placed parallel to the common bile duct. As shown in the drawing, the seromuscular layer of the jejunum is sutured to the wall of the choledochus. This is done placing the sutures away from the edge of the defect, including the wall of the duct, near the edge, using 5-0 synthetic reabsorbable material (2).

Repair of Parietal Defects of the Common Bile Duct

FIGURE 6.4
Once the posterior suture line is completed, a T-tube is introduced into the common duct through the parietal defect so that the short limb of the T-tube is considerably longer than the defect. The long limb of the T-tube is then passed through the posterior and anterior walls of the jejunum using small openings, which are then hermetically closed with one or two sutures. The next step will consist of rotating the jejunal loop to cover the entire defect by suturing the loop to the bile duct using interrupted sutures similar to those used in the posterior suture line (7).

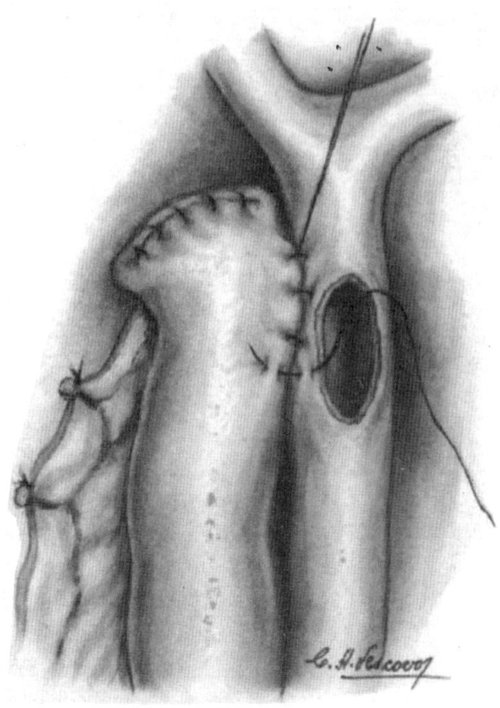

FIGURE 6.3

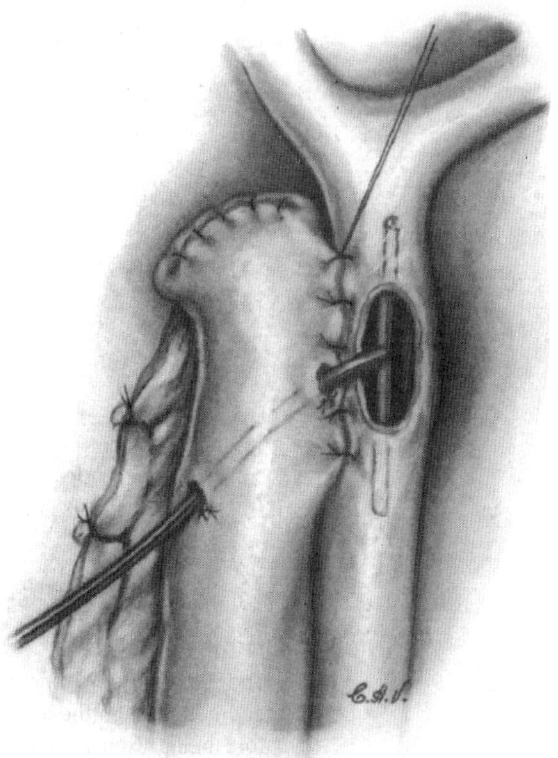

FIGURE 6.4

FIGURE 6.5
The jejunal loop has been rotated and applied to the common duct to cover the defect. The anterior suture line is being completed by placing the sutures between the seromuscular jejunal wall and the common bile duct. The long limb of the T-tube is brought out of the abdomen after going through the anastomotic jejunal limb.

Repair of Parietal Defects of the Common Bile Duct

FIGURE 6.6
The procedure is completed. The long limb of the T-tube courses through the jejunal wall using the Witzel technique before being fixed to the abdominal wall. Postoperative cholangiographic control will determine the time when the tube can be removed. Removal of the T-tube leaves a temporary fistula between the common bile duct and the jejunum.

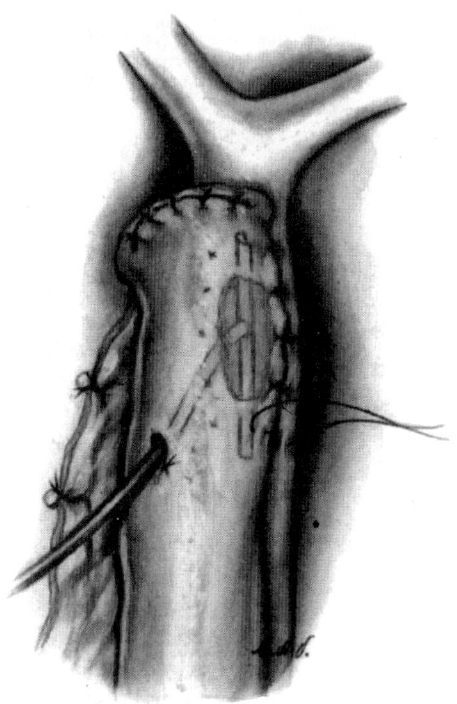

FIGURE 6.5

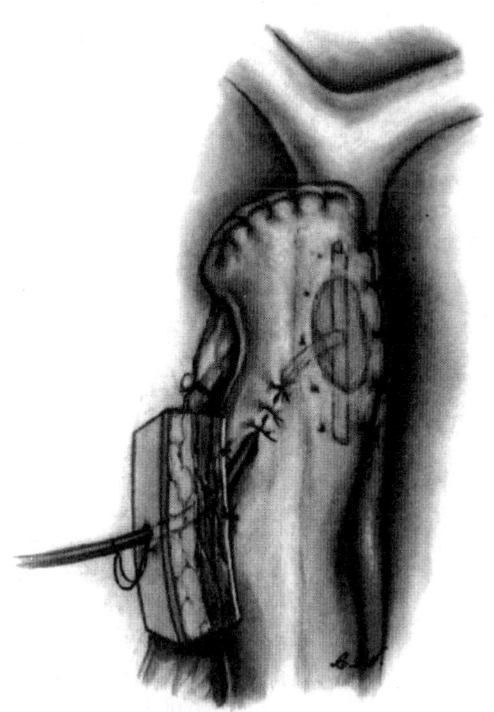

FIGURE 6.6

FIGURE 6.7
The drawing shows a case in which the common bile duct was ligated during cholecystectomy. If the surgeon recognizes the injury, he or she should repair it during the same operation. Lesions of the common bile duct due to ligature or the placement of a hemostatic clamp are not corrected by removing the ligature or the clamp and placing a T-tube in the duct. This course of action leads to a residual fibrous stricture making reoperation necessary. The repair should be performed by resecting the damaged segment, which usually is no longer than 5 to 6 mm, and then reestablishing continuity of the duct by means of an end to end anastomosis. To increase the length of the duct, a Vautrin-Kocher maneuver should be performed before beginning the suturing. The short damaged segment is then resected transversely to begin the end to end anastomosis, as will be shown later. This anastomosis will probably be successful if more than 10 mm of length have been resected. The Vautrin-Kocher maneuver can lengthen the duct some 10 mm, rarely more.

End to End Anastomosis of the Common Bile Duct

FIGURE 6.8
The Vautrin-Kocher maneuver has been carried out and the damaged segment of common bile duct resected. The ends to be anastomosed are approximated without tension. The angles of these ends have been grasped with sutures to facilitate the anastomosis. A satisfactory mucosa to mucosa suture of common bile ducts that are normal in diameter should be performed using a magnifying loop or surgical microscope. These drawings are made as visualized through a loop or microscope.

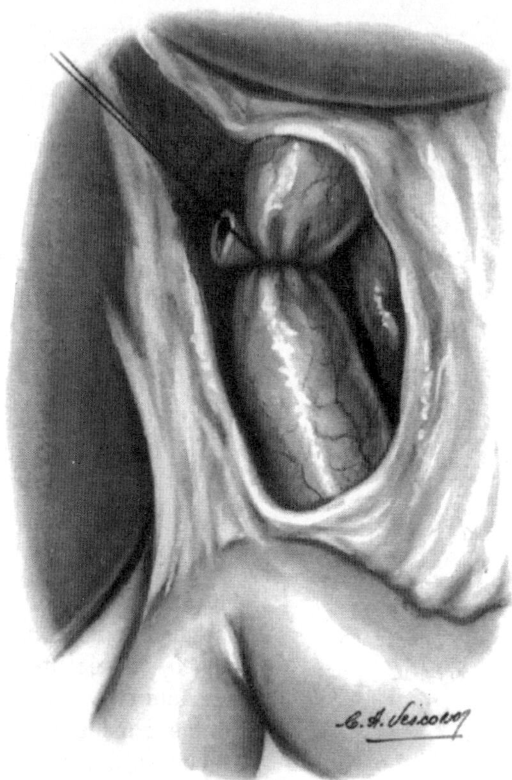

FIGURE 6.7

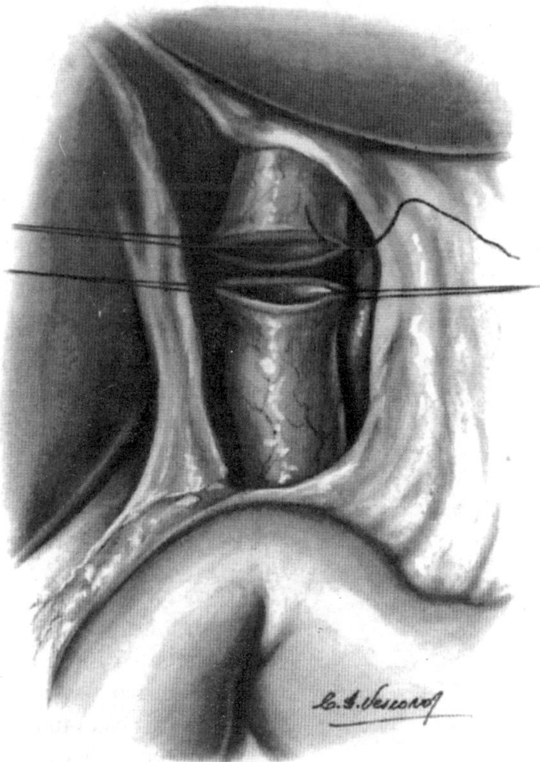

FIGURE 6.8

FIGURE 6.9
The guide sutures in the angles of the ends to be anastomosed are kept taut, and the posterior row of sutures has been started, including the entire thickness of the duct wall. Synthetic reabsorbable 5-0 suture material is being used. In common bile ducts of normal caliber one should not use more than eight or ten sutures. These sutures should not be tied too tightly to avoid ischemia of the ends to be anastomosed.

End to End Anastomosis of the Common Bile Duct

FIGURE 6.10
Once the posterior row of sutures are in place a small transverse incision is made below the anastomosis and the short limb of a thin T-tube is introduced so that the upper end is above the suture line to act as a stent for the anastomosis. The T-tube can come out either below (as shown in this case) or above the suture line, but never through the suture line.

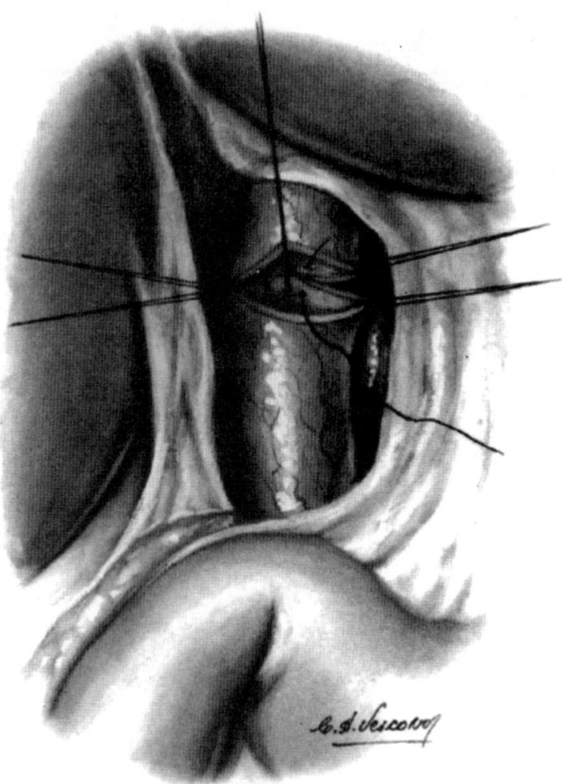

FIGURE 6.9

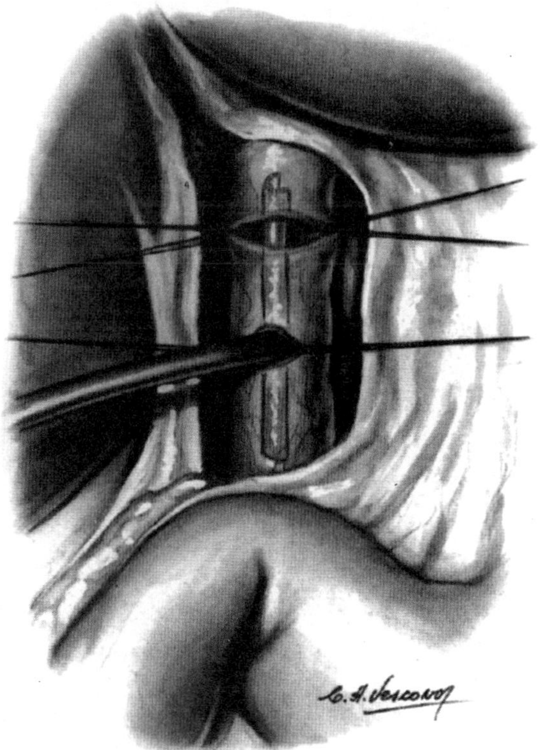

FIGURE 6.10

FIGURE 6.11
Once the T-tube is in place the anterior row of sutures is made in a similar manner as the posterior row.

End to End Anastomosis of the Common Bile Duct

FIGURE 6.12
The last suture of the anterior row is being placed and has been fixed with a suture at the site of exit of the long limb of the T-tube. Before closing the abdominal wall a drainage suction tube is left in place in Morrison's pouch.

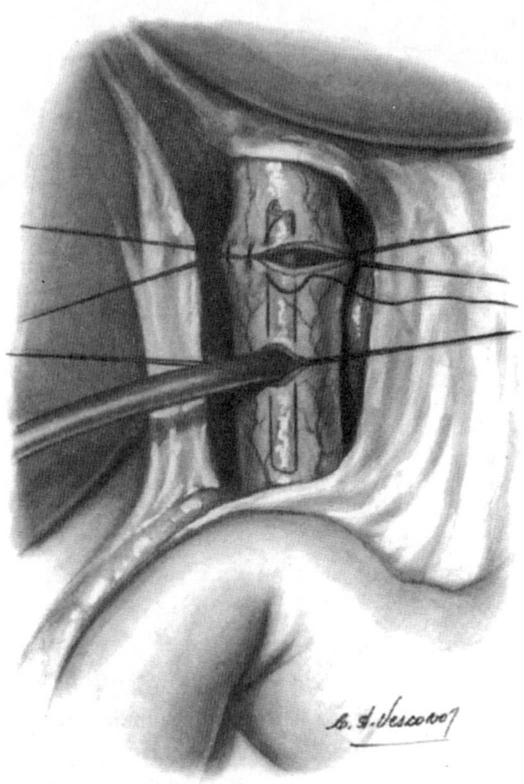

FIGURE 6.11

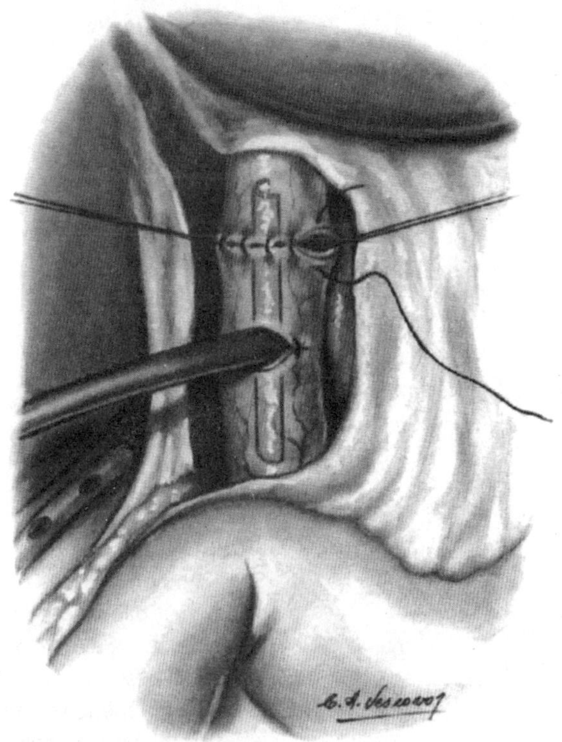

FIGURE 6.12

FIGURE 6.13
Some authors do not use a T-tube as a stent in end to end anastomoses because they believe it acts as a foreign body and would favor the production of a stricture at the site of the suture line. In this drawing one can see that the suture line is being finished without having placed a T-tube as a stent.

End to End Anastomosis of the Common Bile Duct

FIGURE 6.14
Some authors leave a T-tube not as a stent but with the object of draining bile to the outside and diminishing the intraductal pressure, thereby avoiding the possibility of leakage of bile through the suture line. The T-tube also allows for cholangiographic postoperative examination of the area. When a T-tube is left with the only object of draining bile to the outside, the short arm should not go through the anastomotic suture line as shown in the drawing.

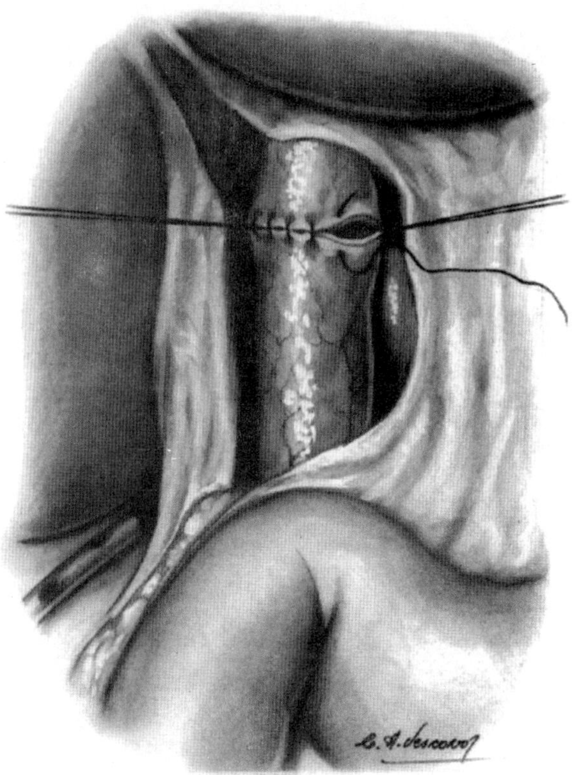

FIGURE 6.13

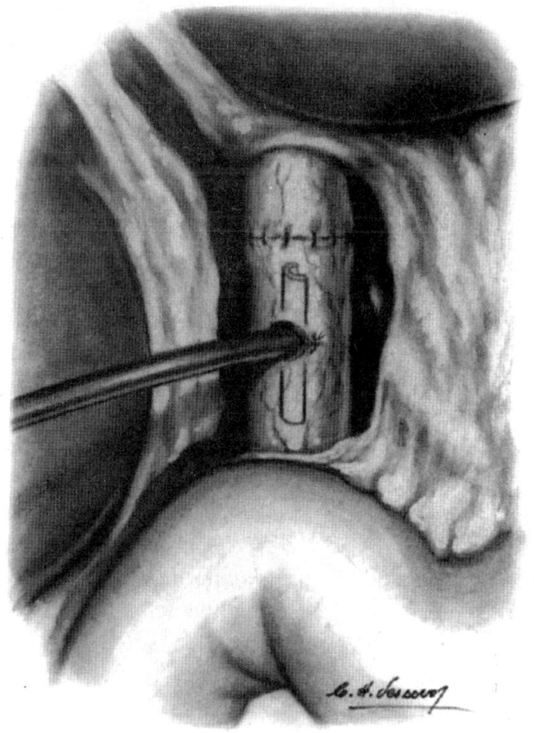

FIGURE 6.14

FIGURE 6.15

The most appropriate incisions to reoperate on the damaged biliary tract with the object of repairing them are the longitudinal incisions. These can be paramedian or right transrectal. Longitudinal incisions, besides providing an ample operative field, make possible the mobilization of the stomach, the duodenum, the hepatic flexure of the colon, ligament of Treitz, and so forth. These incisions also allow the abdominal cavity to be opened in the lowermost segment of the incision, where adhesions due to previous surgical procedures are less severe. Once the abdominal cavity is open, one usually sees, as is shown in the drawing, that all the supramesocolic organs are joined between themselves and the parietal peritoneum by numerous fibrous adhesions, which make the development of an adequate cleavage plane difficult. The adhesions are abundant not only because of previous surgical procedures but because there was spillage of bile, fistulas, or infection.

In reoperations on the biliary tract it is common to find the transverse colon, the hepatic flexure and the greater omentum fixed to the inferior surface of the right lobe of the liver. The surgical procedure is begun by freeing the loops of small bowel from the parietal peritoneum, sectioning adhesions that join them to the parietal peritoneum, using scissors, as shown in the drawing. One must be careful, during this freeing of adhesions, not to open the intestinal lumen. Once the small bowel is separated from the parietal peritoneum, the colon and the greater omentum are then freed from the parietal peritoneum and the adherent loops are also separated from each other.

Surgical Exposure of the Biliary Tract Following a Period of Time After the Primary Operation

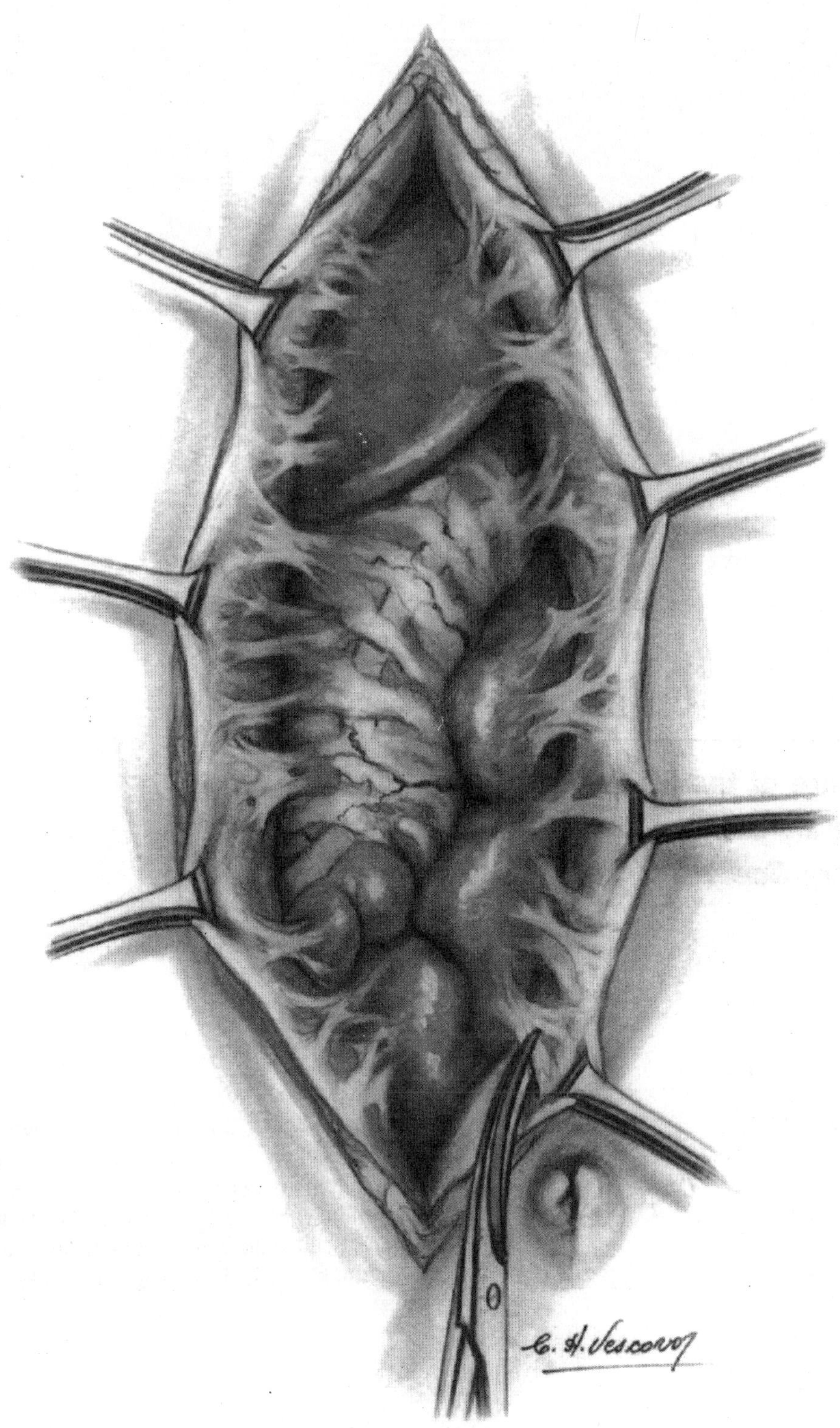

FIGURE 6.15

Surgical Exposure of the Biliary Tract Following a Period of Time After the Primary Operation

FIGURE 6.16
Once adhesions to the parietal peritoneum are divided, the greater omentum, adherent to the undersurface of the right lobe of the liver, is separated. In order to separate the greater omentum from the undersurface of the liver, traction is applied to it with the left hand or with a Babcock clamp, while the right hand cuts the adhesions right at the level of Glisson's capsule. Using this technique bleeding is generally minimal.

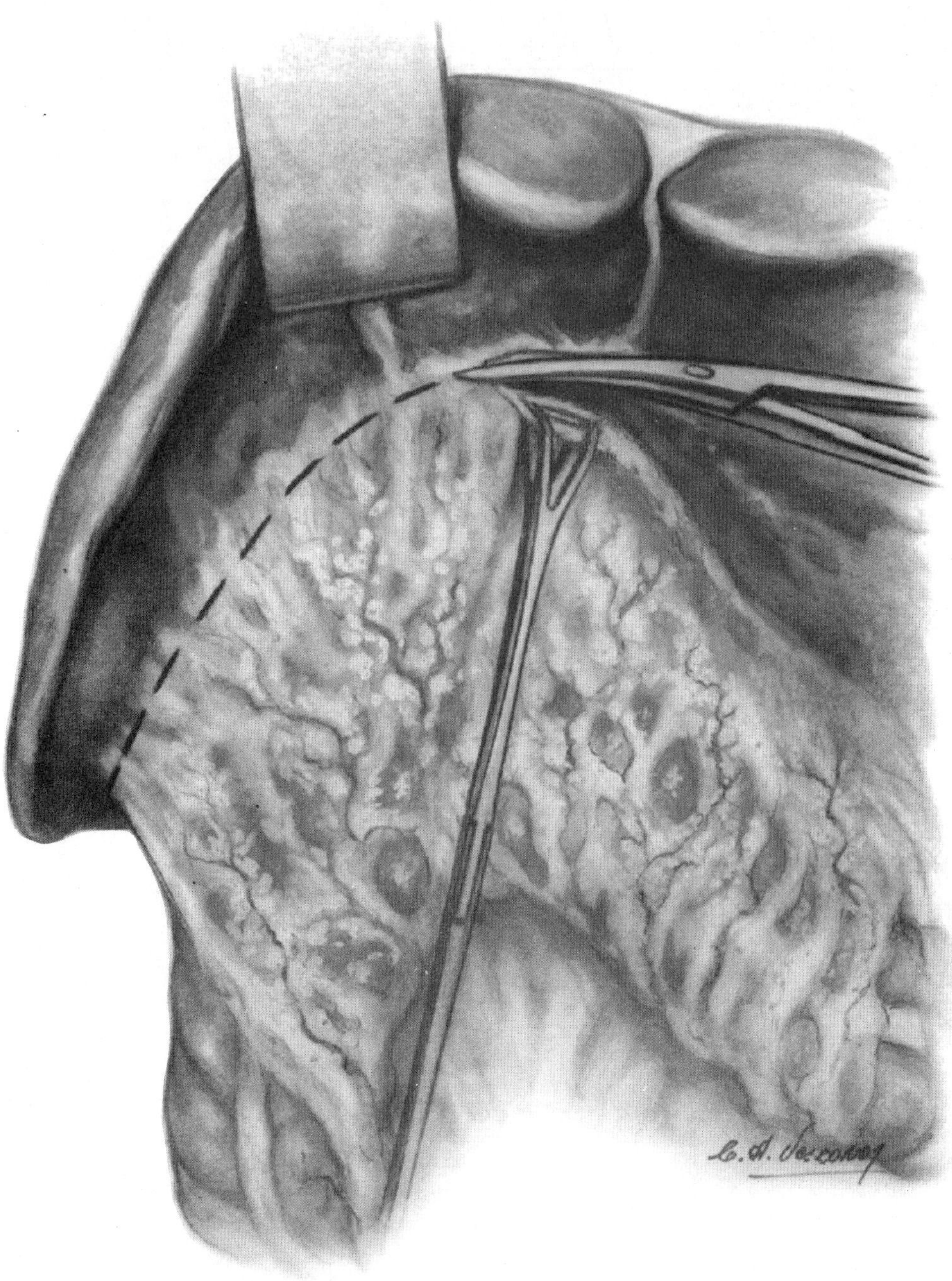

FIGURE 6.16

Surgical Exposure of the Biliary Tract Following a Period of Time After the Primary Operation

FIGURE 6.17
Once the greater omentum is freed and lowered, the next step consists of freeing the hepatic flexure of the colon and the right side of the transverse colon. To perform this mobilization adequately it is necessary to cut the lateral peritoneum of the right colon beginning at its lowermost portion where there are less adhesions. The dissection is then carried upward. To mobilize the hepatic flexure of the colon the phrenicolic ligament is sectioned. In cases in which the colon is very adherent to Glisson's capsule it is preferable to cut Glisson's capsule instead of opening the colon, even though some bleeding may be produced.

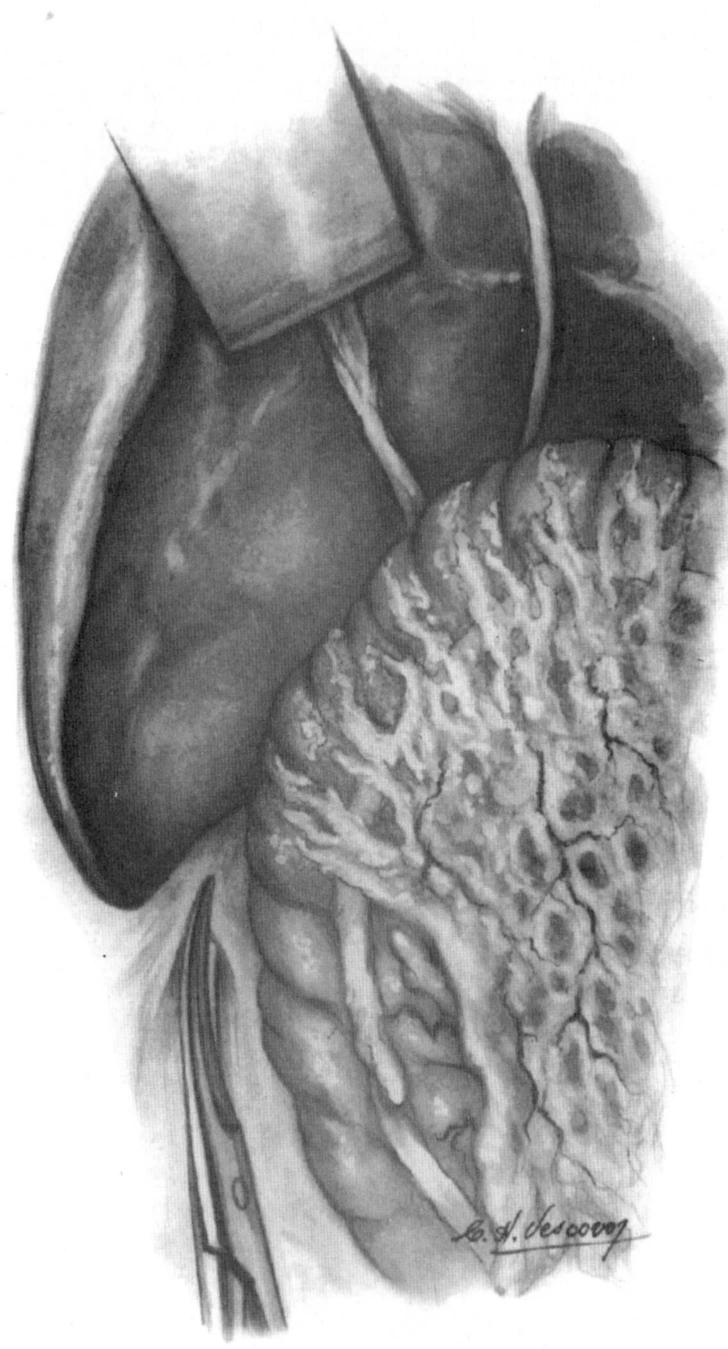

FIGURE 6.17

FIGURE 6.18

The stomach pylorus and duodenum are generally adherent to the posterior wall of the abdomen, to the hepatoduodenal ligament, and to the undersurface of the liver, making its liberation very difficult. The duodenum is usually found very retracted, against the undersurface of the liver. The less morbid technique to free the duodenum is by means of a Vautrin-Kocher maneuver, beginning at the third portion of the duodenum, where adhesions are usually less severe, later mobilizing the second portion of the duodenum together with the head of the pancreas. The Vautrin-Kocher maneuver makes it possible to identify the distal segment of the common bile duct. The common bile duct lymph node constitutes a valuable anatomic landmark that in the majority of cases is situated to the right and behind the lower end of the common bile duct.

Surgical Exposure of the Biliary Tract Following a Period of Time After the Primary Operation

FIGURE 6.19

Once the distal segment of the common bile duct is identified, the proximal portion of the hepatic hilus is dissected. In reoperations for surgical lesions of the common bile duct this constitutes the most important stage, since can the distal segment only can be used to perform an end to end reconstruction a few times. The identification of the common hepatic duct is carried out by dissecting the hepatic hilus outside and in front of the visible or palpable pulsations of the hepatic artery. In some patients the hepatic duct can be identified rapidly and easily because it is dilated, because of the presence of the ligating suture, or by following the remnants of the fistulous tract which leads to the bile duct. In the majority of cases identification of the hepatic duct is difficult owing to the presence of intense fibrosis surrounding the hepatic hilus due to previous repairs, bile drainage, or owing to the development of biliary cirrhosis and so forth. In difficult cases intraoperative ultrasonography may be of help in identifying the hepatic duct. Transcutaneohepatic cholangiography and the passage of the transhepatic catheters preoperatively facilitate the identification of the hepatic duct. These catheters can be replaced by Silastic tubes and left in place postoperatively. Puncture and aspiration of the hepatic duct during the surgical procedure is also a valuable maneuver. This is done using a 23 gauge needle, with a 10 mL syringe angled in relation to the hepatic hilus, as shown in the drawing, and not entering perpendicularly—to avoid perforation of the posterior wall of the hepatic duct and entering the portal vein with aspiration of blood, which usually leads to great confusion. Once the common bile duct is punctured, a few milliliters of bile are obtained for culture and sensitivity studies and a radiopaque substance is injected to obtain an operative cholangiogram, which will have very significant value.

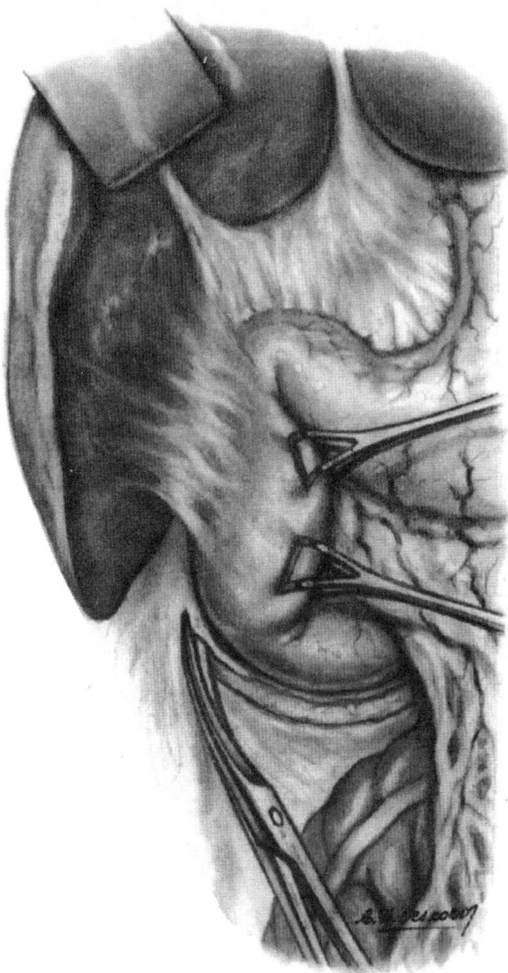

FIGURE 6.18

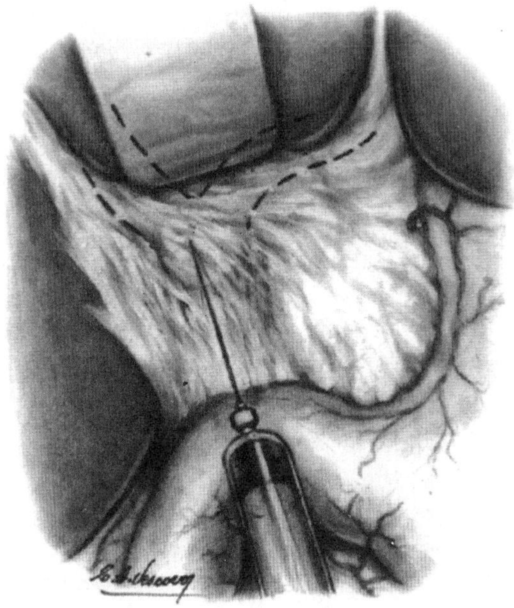

FIGURE 6.19

FIGURE 6.20
Localization of the common hepatic duct by means of puncture will facilitate its dissection. In cases in which puncture does not contribute to the localization of the duct, identification can only be carried out by dissection. Dissection should begin 2 to 3 cm to the right of the hepatic artery, which should not be lost from sight at any moment. Fibrous tissue should be sectioned longitudinally with a scalpel, as shown in the drawing. Later, the right edge of the common hepatic duct is freed completely using scalpel, scissors, or gauze dissectors interchangeably.

Surgical Exposure of the Biliary Tract Following a Period of Time After the Primary Operation

FIGURE 6.21
Once the right border of the hepatic bile duct is freed, the dissection is continued in order to free part of its anterior wall and later, with extreme care, some 10 mm of its posterior wall are also freed. It is not necessary to dissect more than 10 mm of the posterior wall, since this is sufficient to allow the performance of an anastomosis with the jejunum avoiding damage to the portal vein, which can be densely adherent to the hepatic bile duct. However, the portal vein is rarely seen during the dissection because it is generally well covered by fibrous tissue. If the portal vein is damaged the surgeon should be prepared for its repair, which is not an easy matter. Once the right edge and anterior wall and 10 mm of the posterior wall of the hepatic duct have been freed, the bottom of the duct is grasped with a Babcock clamp and gentle traction applied toward the right to permit freeing the left border of the hepatic duct, cutting fibrous tissue surrounding it with scissors, as can be seen in the drawing. In this part of the dissection one should not forget the dangerous presence of the hepatic artery. Once the hepatic duct is freed, one should be certain that the duct that has been dissected receives bile from all segments of the liver.

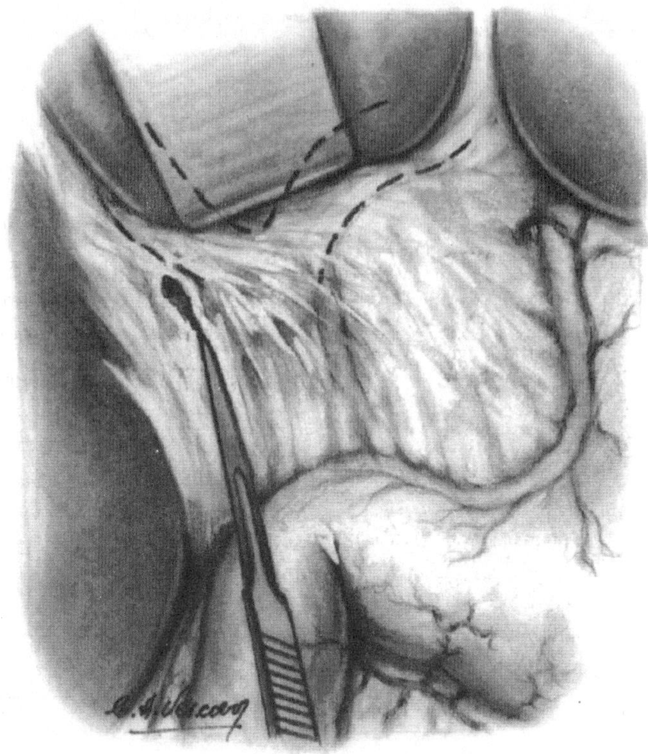

FIGURE 6.20

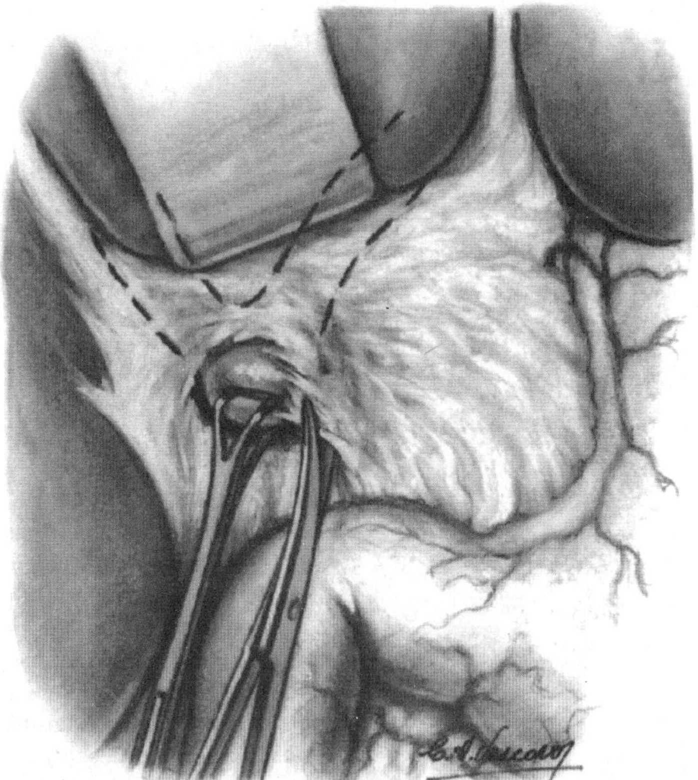

FIGURE 6.21

FIGURE 6.22

An anastomosis of the hepatic duct with the jejunum will give good immediate and late results if two conditions are met:

1. The duct is more than 15 mm in diameter.
2. The mucosa to mucosa anastomosis is performed without interposition of fibrous tissue.

In cases in which these conditions cannot be met one should resort to the Hepp-Couinaud or the Lord Smith of Marlow techniques, which will be described later. A jejunal loop has been prepared and placed in Roux-en-Y fashion. The anastomotic end of the loop Y has been closed in two layers and is placed so as to allow for an anastomosis using the terminal end of the hepatic duct with the lateral border of the jejunum. Suturing is performed with interrupted sutures in only one layer. In patients with a very dilated duct the possibility of performing two layers of sutures exists. The drawings show that the posterior layer is being performed. Synthetic 3-0 reabsorbable material is used.

Hepaticojejunostomy

FIGURE 6.23

The posterior layer has been performed and we are performing the anterior layer. If the duct presents a diameter greater than 15 mm and it was possible to perform a satisfactory mucosa to mucosa anastomosis, it is not necessary to leave a tube as a stent. In case the hepaticojejunal suture line has not been realized in a completely satisfactory fashion one can leave a transhepatic Silastic or latex tube, No. 16 F, in place. In some places it may be necessary to leave a U-shaped transhepatic tube in place. This tube can be replaced in case it becomes necessary to leave it in place for a long period of time. Besides, the U-shaped tube allows for the possibility of introducing dilators if a stricture of the anastomosis were to develop.

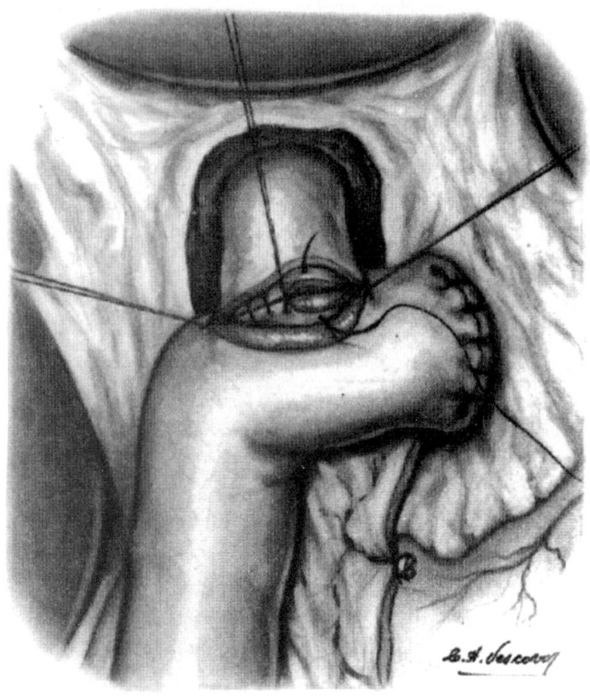

FIGURE 6.22

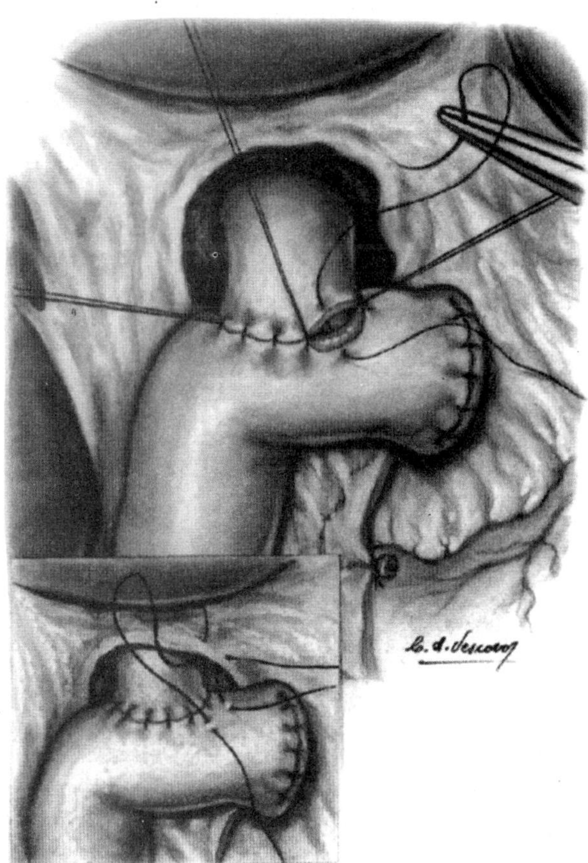

FIGURE 6.23

FIGURE 6.24
In patients in whom the common hepatic duct has a diameter under 15 mm, it is preferable to resect a segment of this duct to make it possible to extend the incision toward the left hepatic duct to increase the caliber of the anastomosis. The extension of the incision toward the left hepatic duct is made easier if one performs a lowering of the Hilar plate by the Hepp-Couinaud technique, which will be described later. In the drawing one can see that the common hepatic duct has been transected near the junction of the hepatic ducts to allow for the extension of the incision toward the left hepatic duct. The dotted line points out the extent of the incision. The ascending limb of the Roux-en-Y jejunal loop, whose end has been closed in two layers of sutures, has been placed next to the hepatic duct to proceed with the anastomosis.

Hepaticojejunal Anastomosis with Extended Incision into the Left Hepatic Duct

FIGURE 6.25
The posterior layer of the anastomosis is being performed, suturing the common hepatic duct and the left hepatic duct to the jejunum with interrupted reabsorbable 3-0 sutures of synthetic material. If the anastomosis is performed in a satisfactory fashion it is not necessary to leave a transhepatic tube in place.

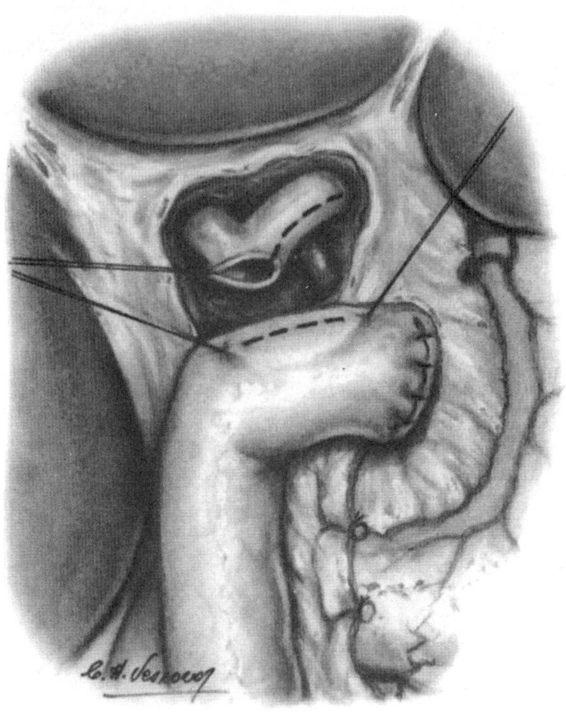

FIGURE 6.24

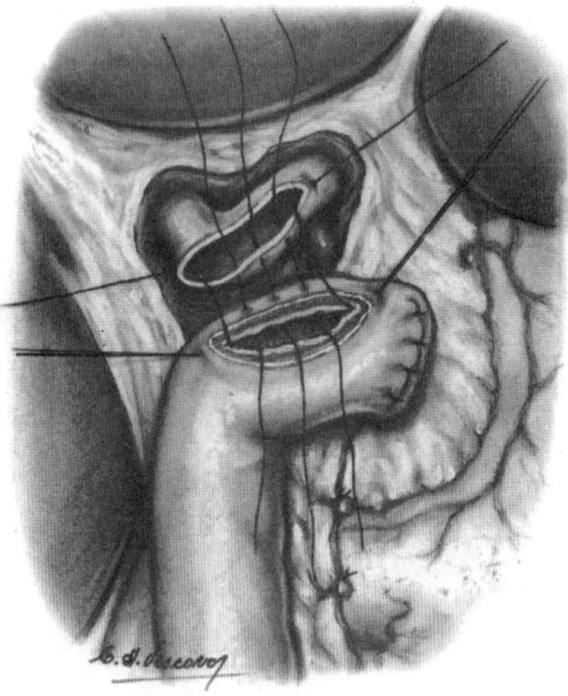

FIGURE 6.25

Hepp-Couinaud Technique

FIGURE 6.26

Using a wide Doyen retractor the liver is retracted upward. The posterior border of the quadrate lobe (segment IV of the liver) is identified. The hepatogastric ligament is sectioned with a scalpel at the site of its insertion into the inferior surface of the liver, as shown in the drawing by a broken line.

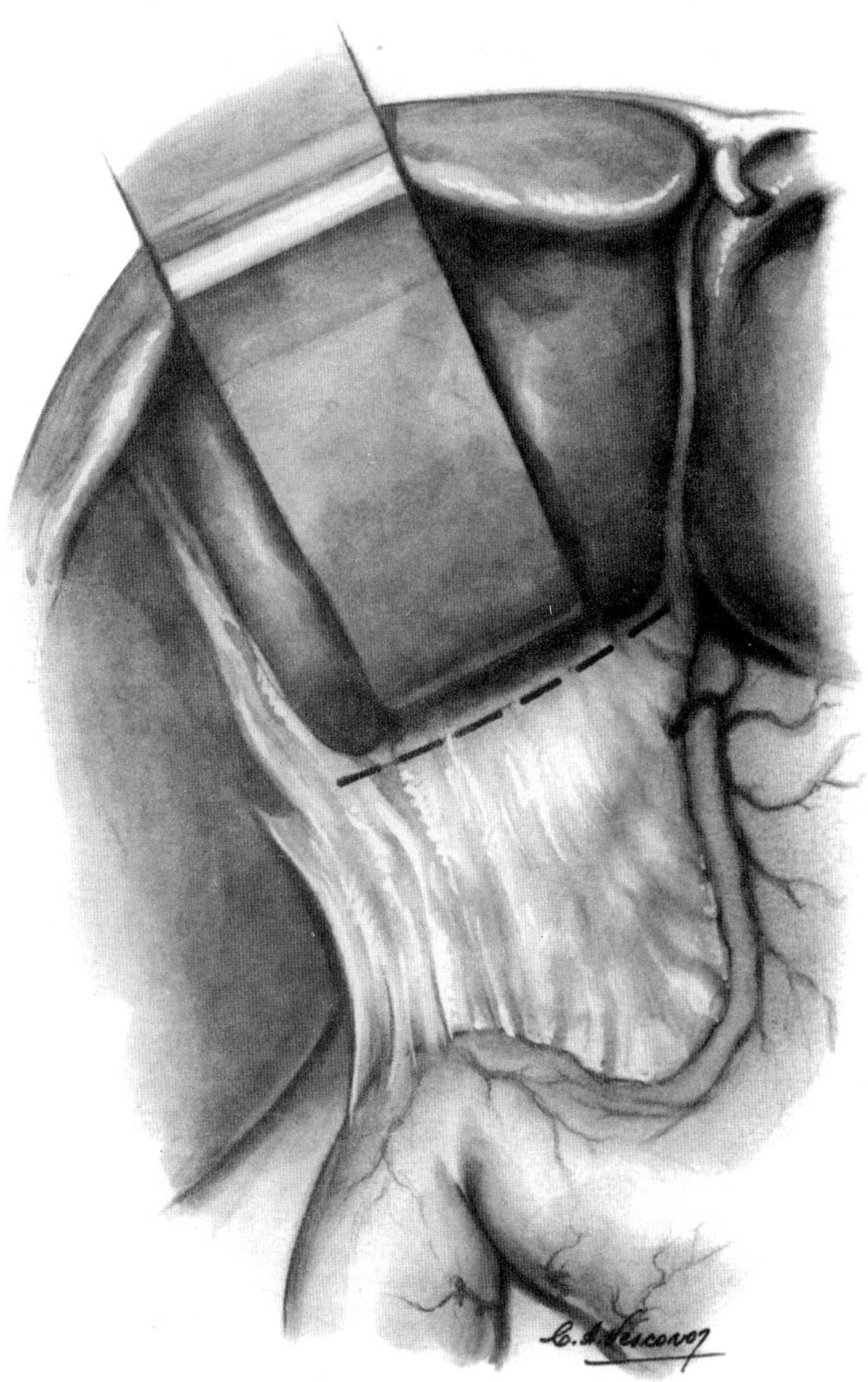

FIGURE 6.26

Hepp-Couinaud Technique

FIGURE 6.27
Once the hepatogastric ligament has been sectioned, you can see the base of the quadrate lobe. At this site, according to Couinaud's investigations, Glisson's capsule is welded to the hepatogastric ligament, constituting what the author calls the hilar plate. Glisson's capsule is then sectioned with a scalpel at this level, in the same direction as the hepatogastric ligament was sectioned. Using a gauze pledget Glisson's capsule is dissected in retrograde fashion, as shown in the drawing.

Proceeding in this manner it is possible to lower the left hepatic duct without bleeding, since this duct is not joined to the hepatic parenchyma.

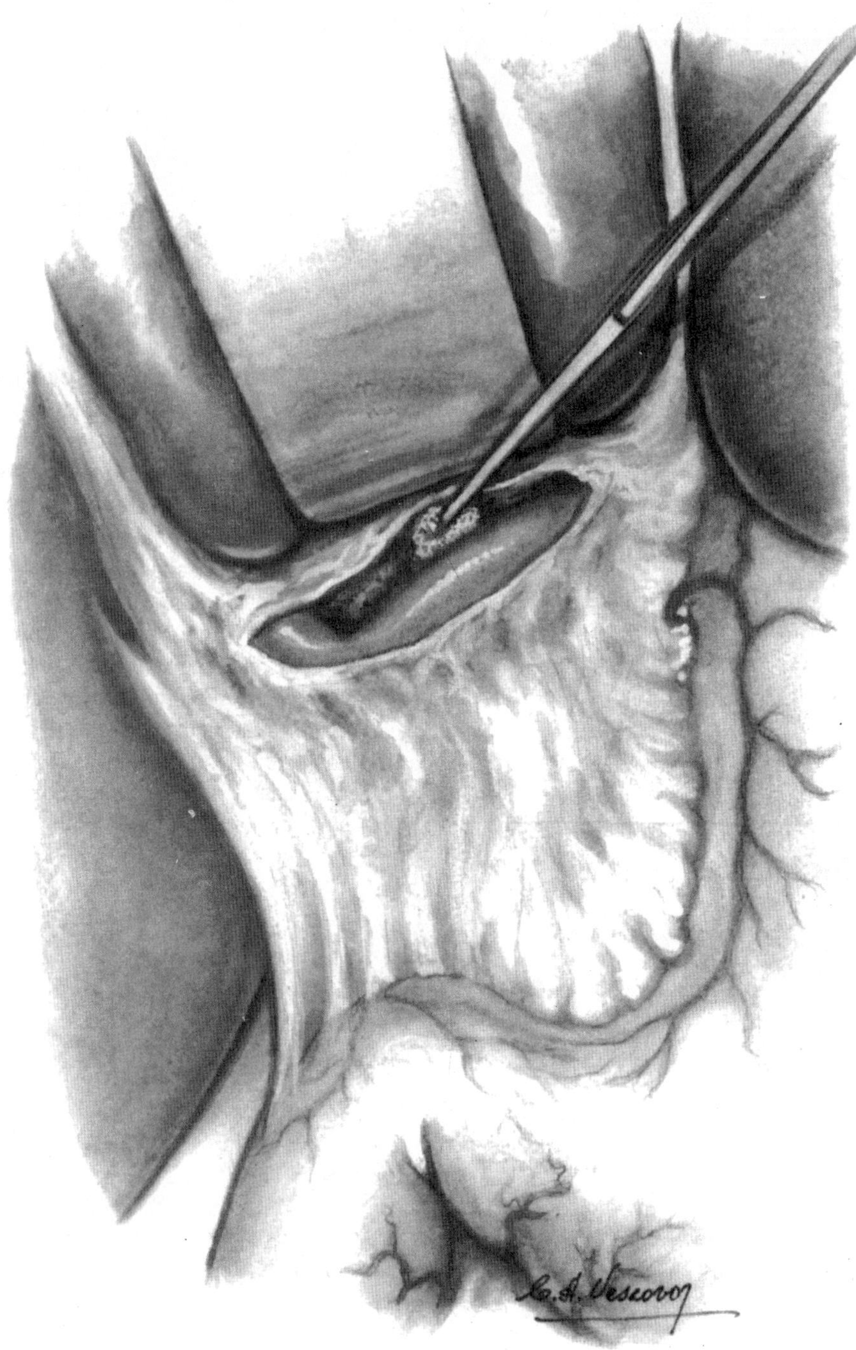

FIGURE 6.27

FIGURE 6.28
Once the hilar plate has been lowered together with the left hepatic duct, the dissection is completed toward the confluence of the ducts. Frequently, in repeated operations, the common hepatic duct is found to be stenosed. Dissection of this segment of the hepatic hilus has to be performed with extreme care using a scalpel, alternating with gauze pledgets and scissors, as previously described. The drawing shows dissection with a scalpel. In cases in which it is difficult to recognize the left hepatic duct owing to the presence of fibrosis or hypertrophy of the liver, and so on, one can resort to the Petersen maneuver, which consists in introducing a metallic probe through the common hepatic duct into the left hepatic duct, where it can be easily felt by the surgeon. The actual identification of the hepatic ducts is made easier by passing transhepatic catheters preoperatively. These catheters can be replaced by Silastic or latex tubes and left in place after surgery.

Hepp-Couinaud Technique

FIGURE 6.29
Once the left hepatic duct has been exposed an incision is made in it extending up to the junction with the right hepatic duct. A jejunal loop has been brought up previously in Roux-en-Y fashion with the ascending anastomotic limb closed at its end in two layers and placed parallel to the left hepatic duct. This limb of jejunum is held in place by an atraumatic triangular Duval clamp in order to perform the side to side anastomosis between the left hepatic duct and the jejunal loop. An incision has been made in the antimesenteric border of the jejunum of the same length as the incision performed in the left hepatic duct. Before beginning to perform the posterior layer of sutures between the bile duct and jejunum it is convenient to place the sutures in the anterior plane through the superior border of the common hepatic duct without passing them through the jejunal wall and without removing the needles. Gentle traction upward is placed on these sutures by an assistant. They are so placed in order to facilitate the suturing of the anterior layer.

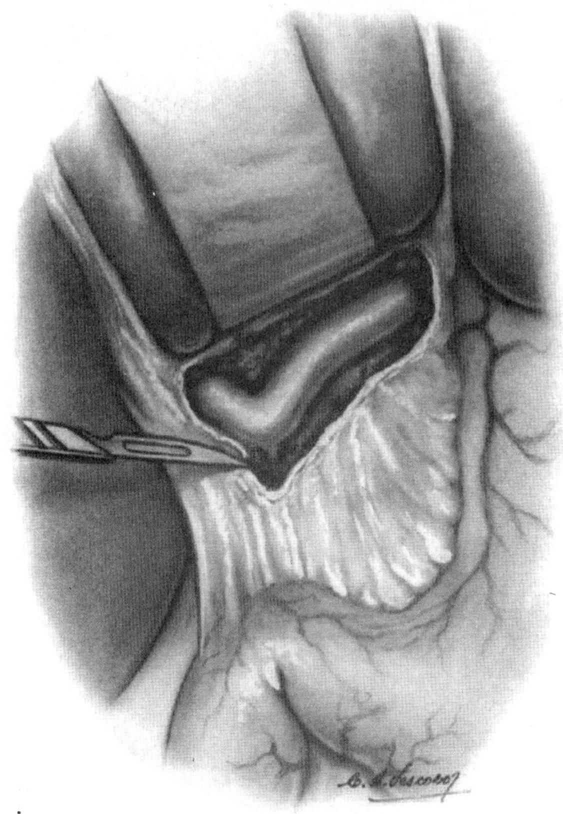

FIGURE 6.28

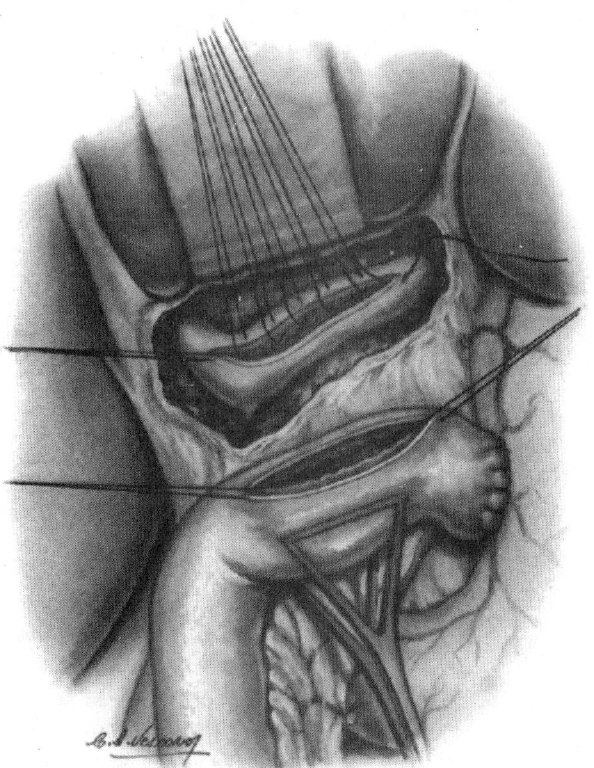

FIGURE 6.29

FIGURE 6.30
Sutures are being placed in the posterior row using interrupted synthetic reabsorbable 3-0 material. The sutures previously placed in the superior border of the left hepatic duct continue to serve as retractors by gentle traction applied by the assistant. In performing the anastomosis the surgeon must be sure that both hepatic ducts flow into the anastomosis.

Hepp-Couinaud Technique

FIGURE 6.31
Once the posterior anastomotic row has been finished the anterior row is then completed. The previously placed sutures in the superior border of the left hepatic duct are now used. These same sutures are the ones that will be used to perform the anterior plane of sutures passing them through the edge of the jejunum. If these sutures are not previously placed it can be very difficult to find the superior border of the hepatic duct to perform the anterior row of sutures.

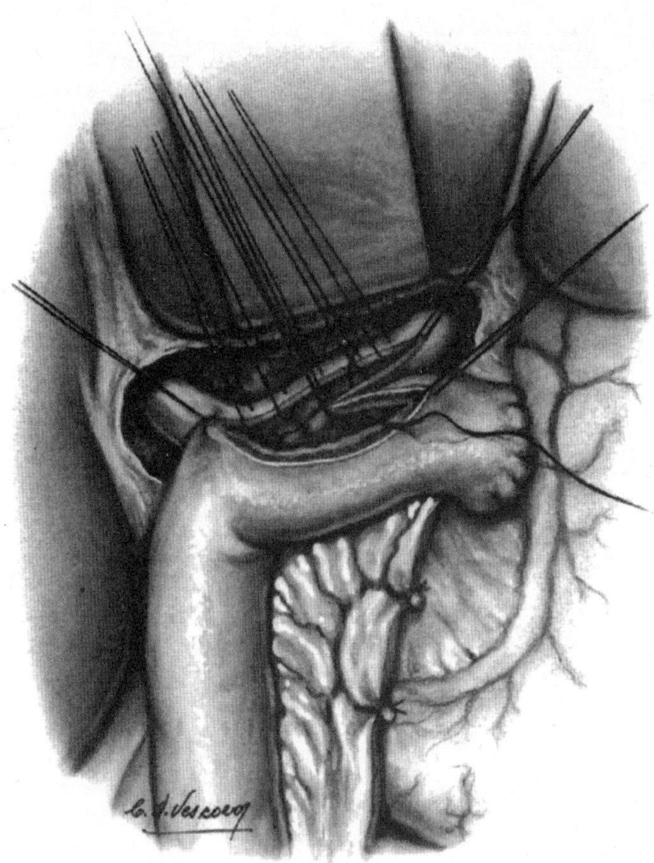

FIGURE 6.30

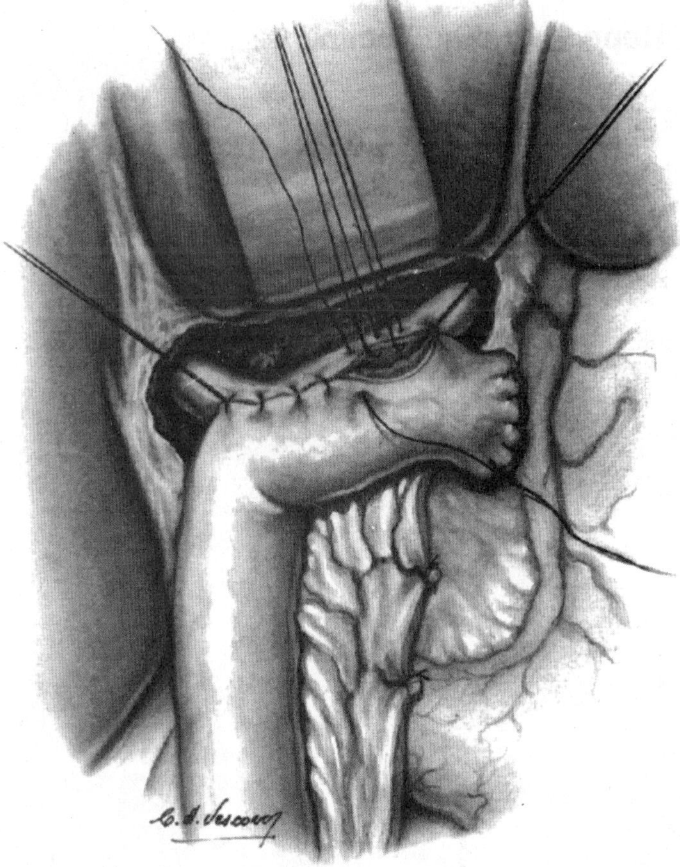

FIGURE 6.31

Hepp-Couinaud Technique

FIGURE 6.32
The anastomosis of the hepatic duct with the jejunum has been completed. To avoid traction on the jejunal loop several sutures are placed between Glisson's capsule and the seromuscular layer of the jejunum. The anastomosis of the jejunum to the left hepatic duct has the advantage of being able to perform an ample anastomosis of 2 to 3 cm in length in an area where there is generally no fibrosis.

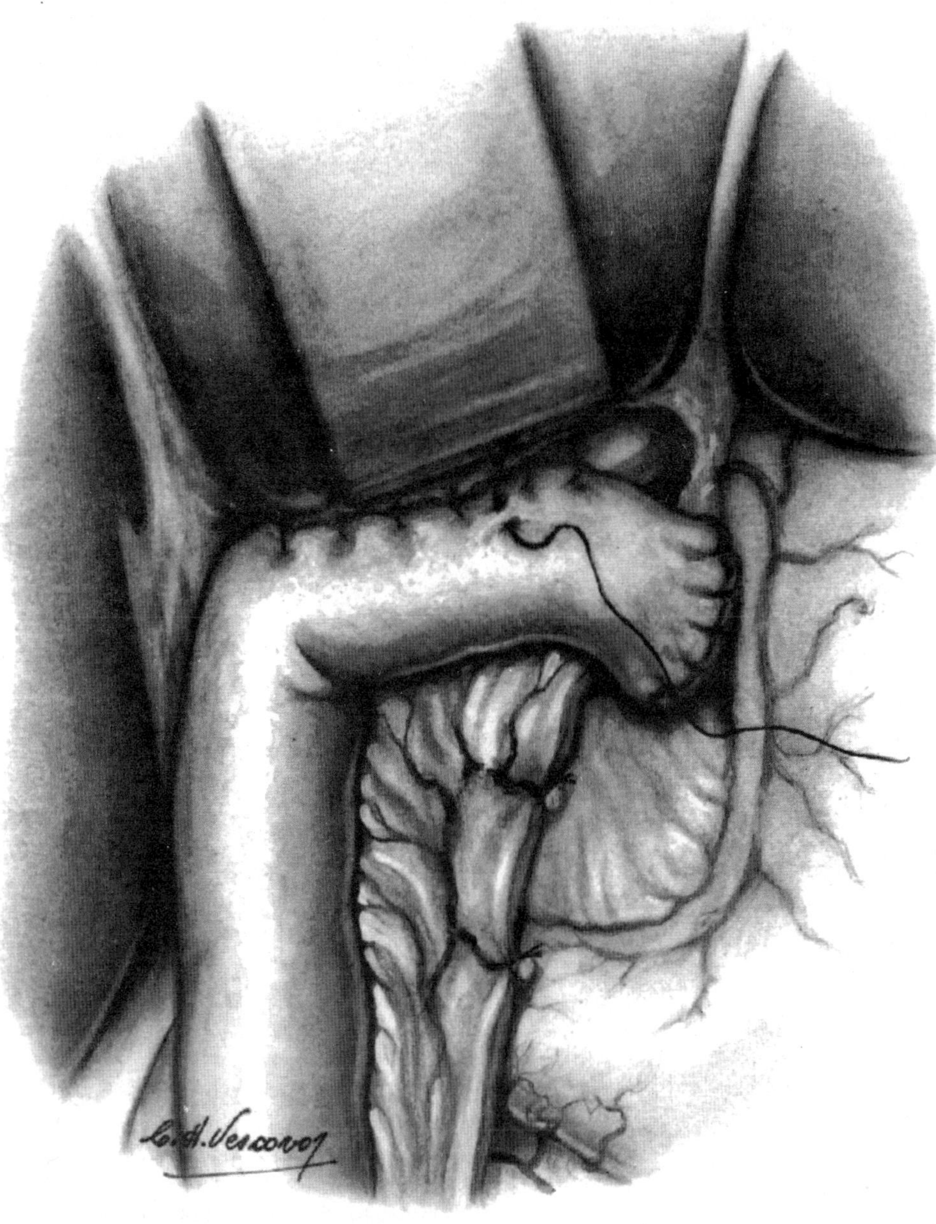

FIGURE 6.32

Hepp-Couinaud Technique

FIGURE 6.33
The drawing shows the completed surgical procedure using the Hepp-Couinaud technique. The ascending or anastomotic Roux-en-Y jejunal loop had been previously passed through the transverse mesocolon where it was fixed with several sutures to prevent the occurrence of internal hernias. The jejunal anastomosis, performed in end to side fashion, was placed some 50 cm from the hepaticojejunal anastomosis to prevent reflux of food. Some authors prefer to bring the jejunal ascending loop in front of the transverse colon, feeling sure that if there were a need for reoperation, this could be performed with greater ease. If the hepaticojejunal anastomosis performed by the Hepp-Couinaud technique is satisfactory, it is not necessary to leave a tube as a stent. In cases in which the anastomosis cannot be performed in a completely satisfactory fashion a stent can be left in place. The author, in these cases, prefers to leave a transhepatic tube. If the tube has to be left for a long time it is preferable to place a U-shaped transhepatic tube to be able to replace it if it were necessary. Figures 34 and 35 show both possibilities.

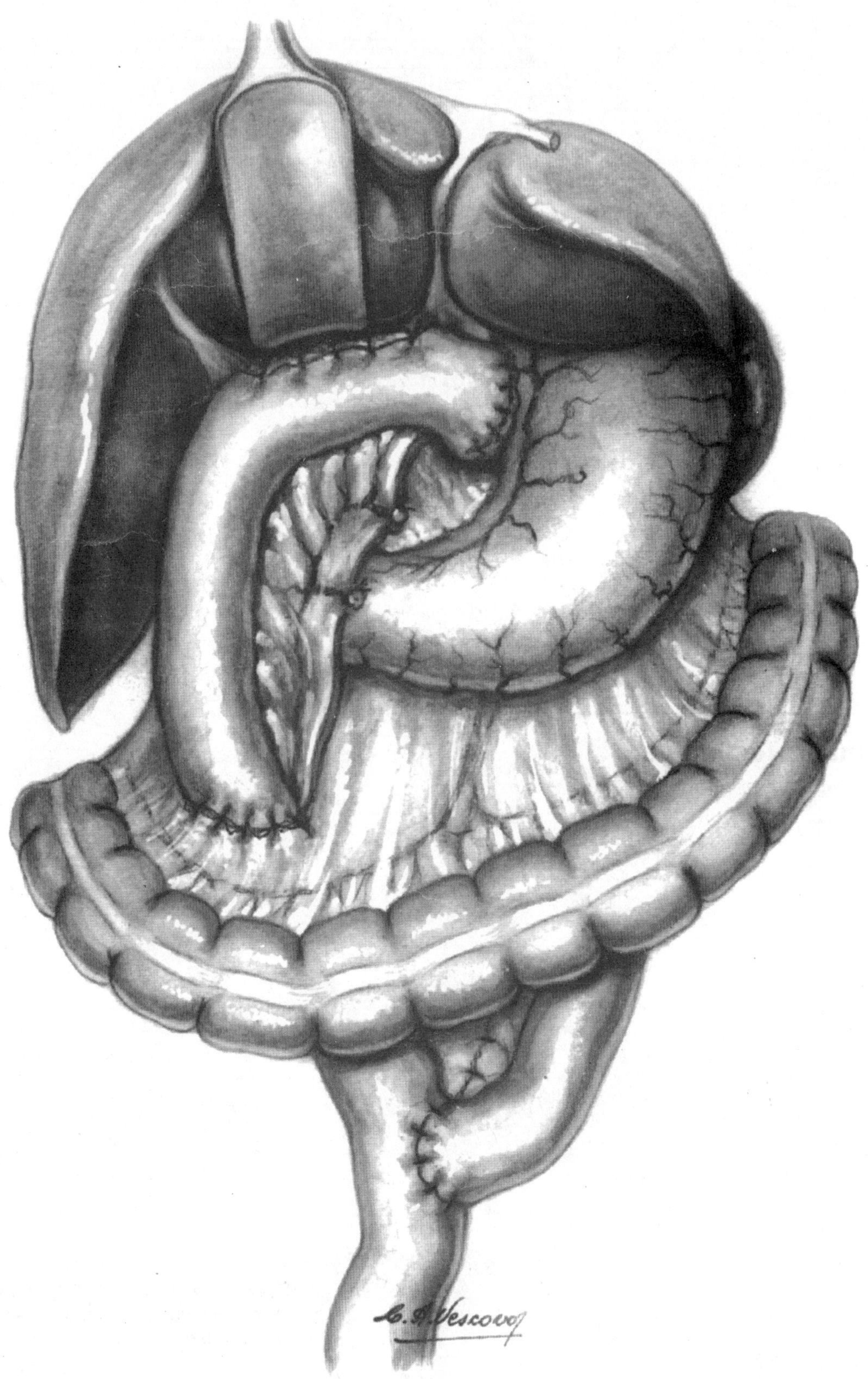

FIGURE 6.33

Hepp-Couinaud Technique

FIGURE 6.34
The drawing represents a surgical procedure performed using the Hepp-Couinaud technique in which a transhepatic No. 16 F Silastic tube has been left in place.

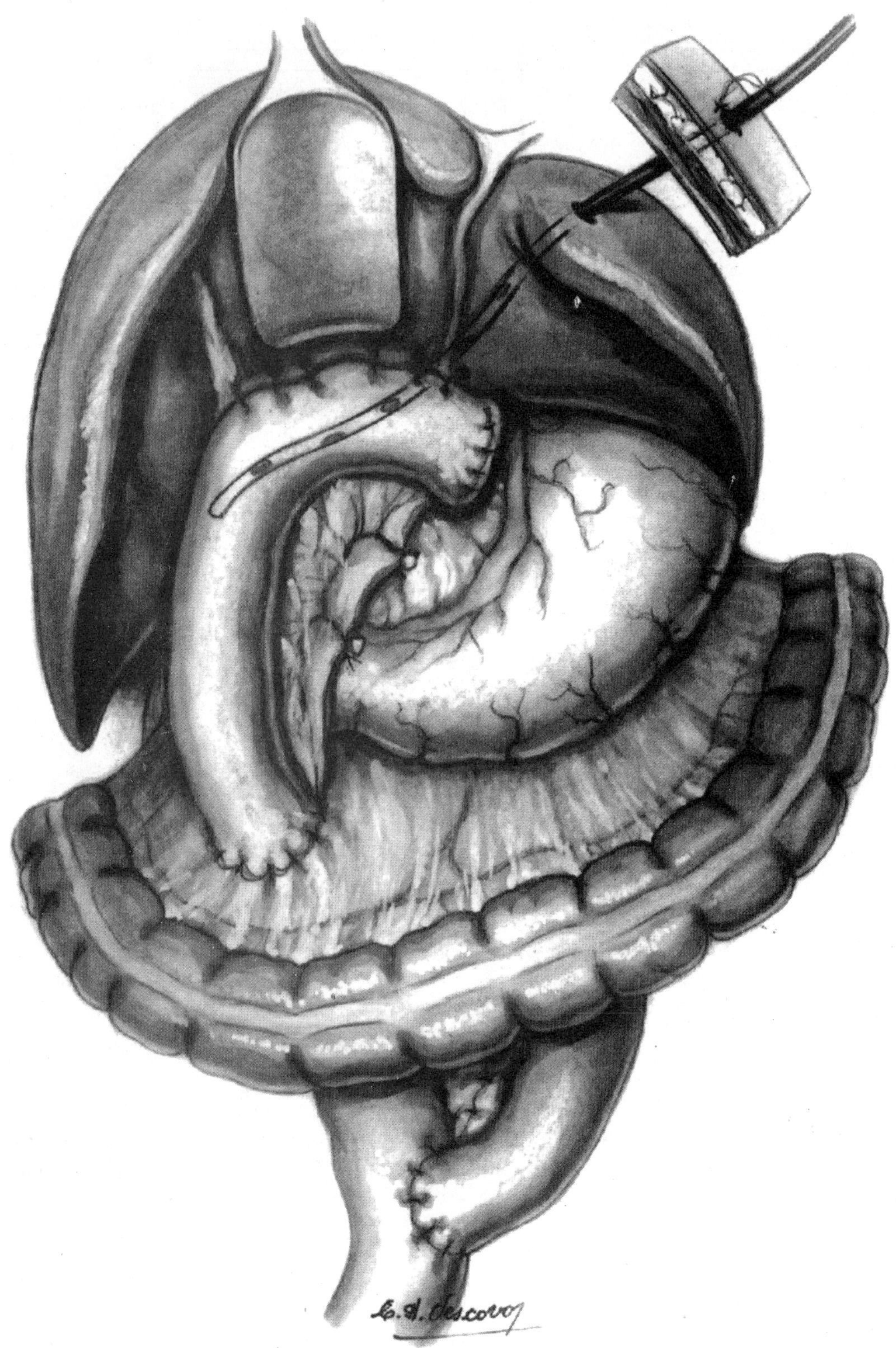

FIGURE 6.34

Hepp-Couinaud Technique

FIGURE 6.35
If a transhepatic tube has to be left in place over a long period of time it should be placed in U-fashion, as shown in this drawing. Besides serving as a stent and for drainage purposes this tube can be replaced if it becomes occluded by biliary mud, without the need of reoperating on the patient.

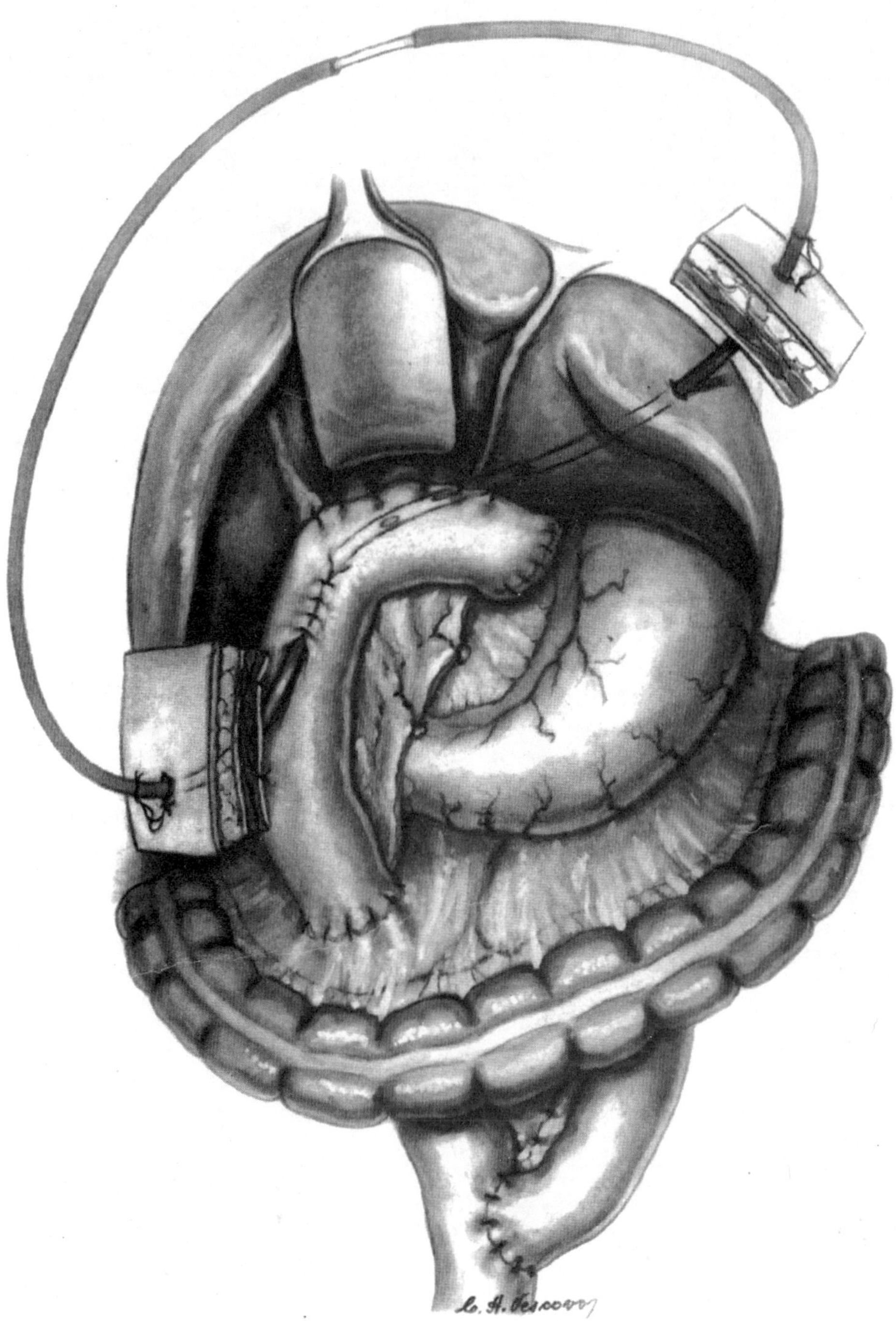

FIGURE 6.35

FIGURE 6.36

Some surgeons prefer to leave a drainage tube through the anastomosis instead of a transhepatic tube. Once the posterior layer of the anastomosis has been finished, a latex No. 16 F tube with several perforations is introduced, as seen in the drawing. The tube is fixed in the correct position, in the hepatic duct, using 2 or 3 sutures of reabsorbable synthetic 5-0 material. After the latex tube runs in the jejunal loop for a few centimeters it is passed through a tunnel in the wall of the jejunal, using the Witzel technique, finally bringing it out to the outside of the abdomen.

Hepp-Couinaud Technique

FIGURE 6.37

This drawing shows the complete Hepp-Couinaud procedure with an transanastomotic catheter in place. The jejunal loop through which the catheter passes is fixed with a few sutures to the parietal peritoneum. The tube is later fixed to the skin of the abdomen. In cases in which it is necessary to leave a drainage tube the author prefers to use a transhepatic tube, as mentioned previously.

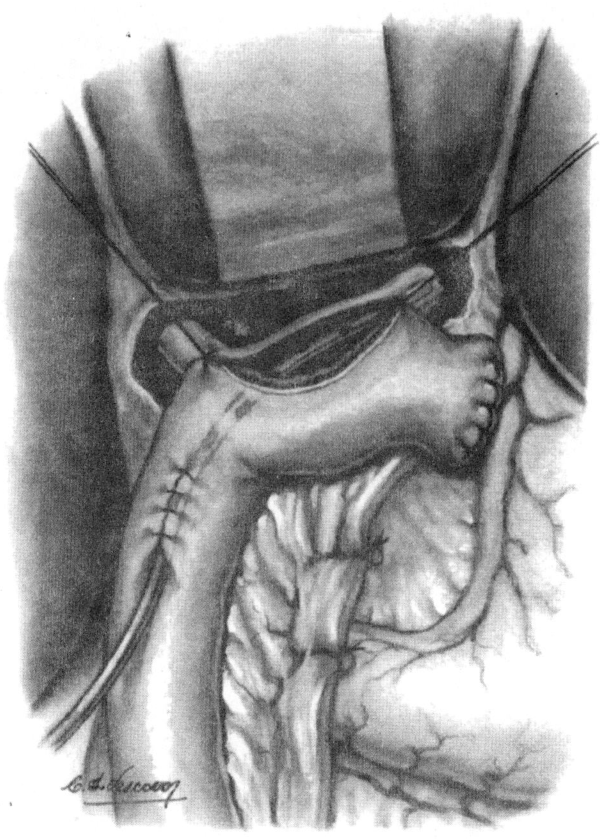

FIGURE 6.36

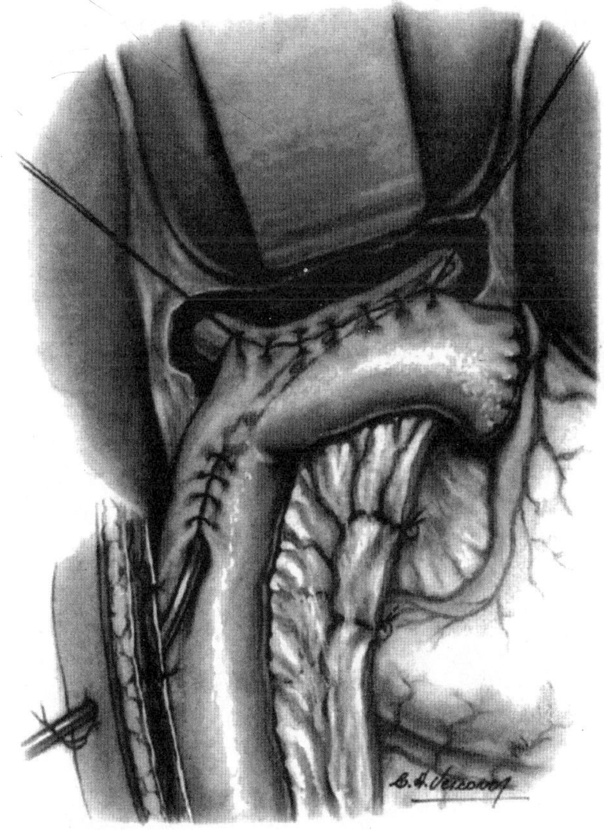

FIGURE 6.37

Lord Smith of Marlow Technique

FIGURE 6.38
In some patients the common hepatic duct is so infiltrated by fibrous and granulation tissue that it is impossible to perform a mucosa to mucosa anastomosis with the jejunum. In these cases healthy mucosa of the hepatic duct is usually found at a higher level. The operation is begun resecting the fibrous tissue of the common hepatic duct, as shown in the drawing. In this stage of the operation one must be sure that the duct that is being dissected receives bile from all segments of the liver.

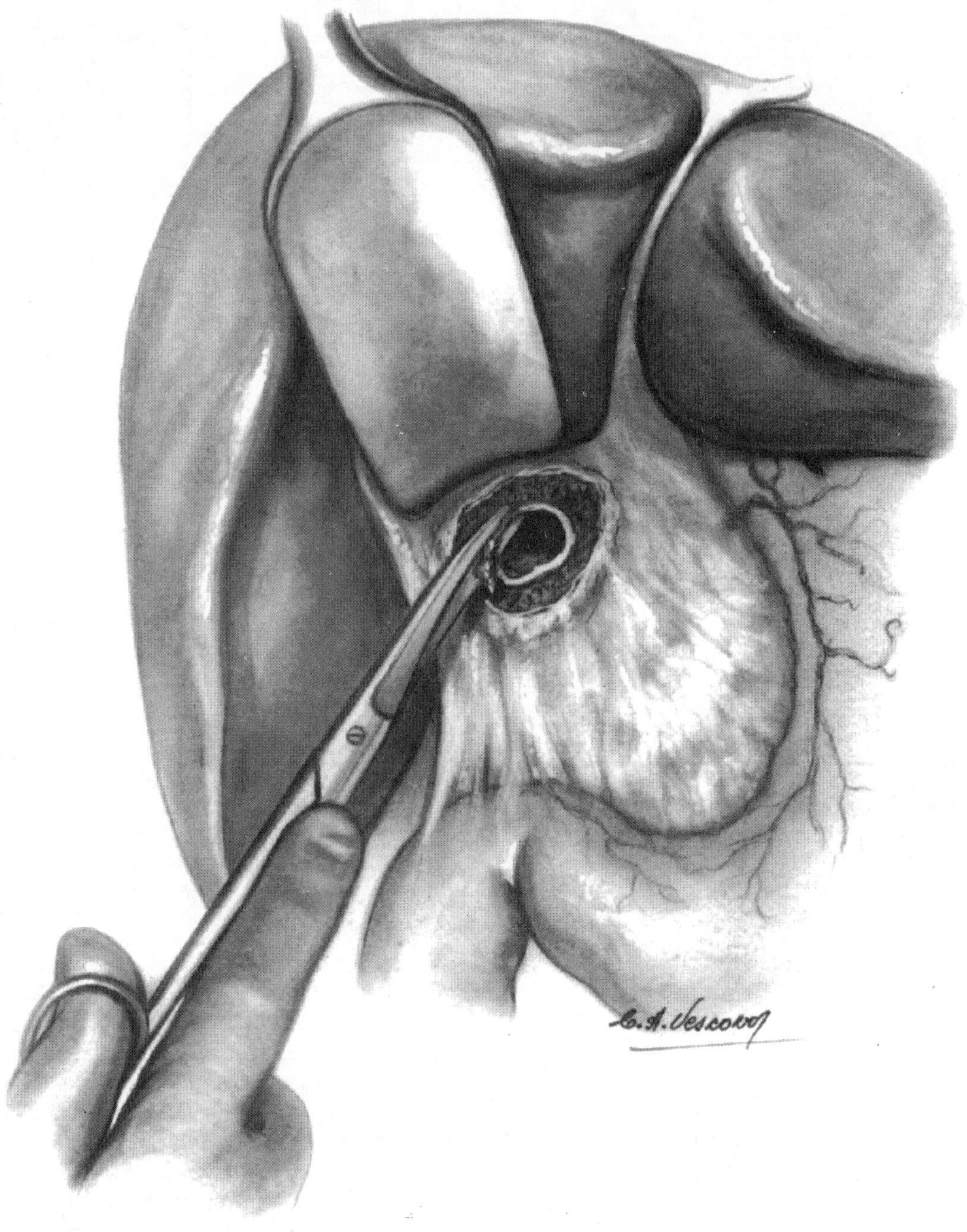

FIGURE 6.38

Lord Smith of Marlow Technique

FIGURE 6.39

The edges of the common hepatic duct are dissected and the borders resected beyond the point of invasion by fibrous tissue. A Silastic or latex No. 16 F tube is then passed through the abdominal wall. This tube has several perforations and is introduced immediately into the common hepatic and left hepatic ducts using a long curved clamp with blunt ends. The tube is then advanced until it perforates the hepatic parenchyma and Glisson's capsule. The end of the tube is then grasped and introduced through the abdominal wall, creating a transhepatic tract by traction on the clamp. Instead of the clamp described, as shown in the drawing, one can use a Randall clamp for the transhepatic passage of the tube. A bile duct explorer or a Bakes dilator can also be used.

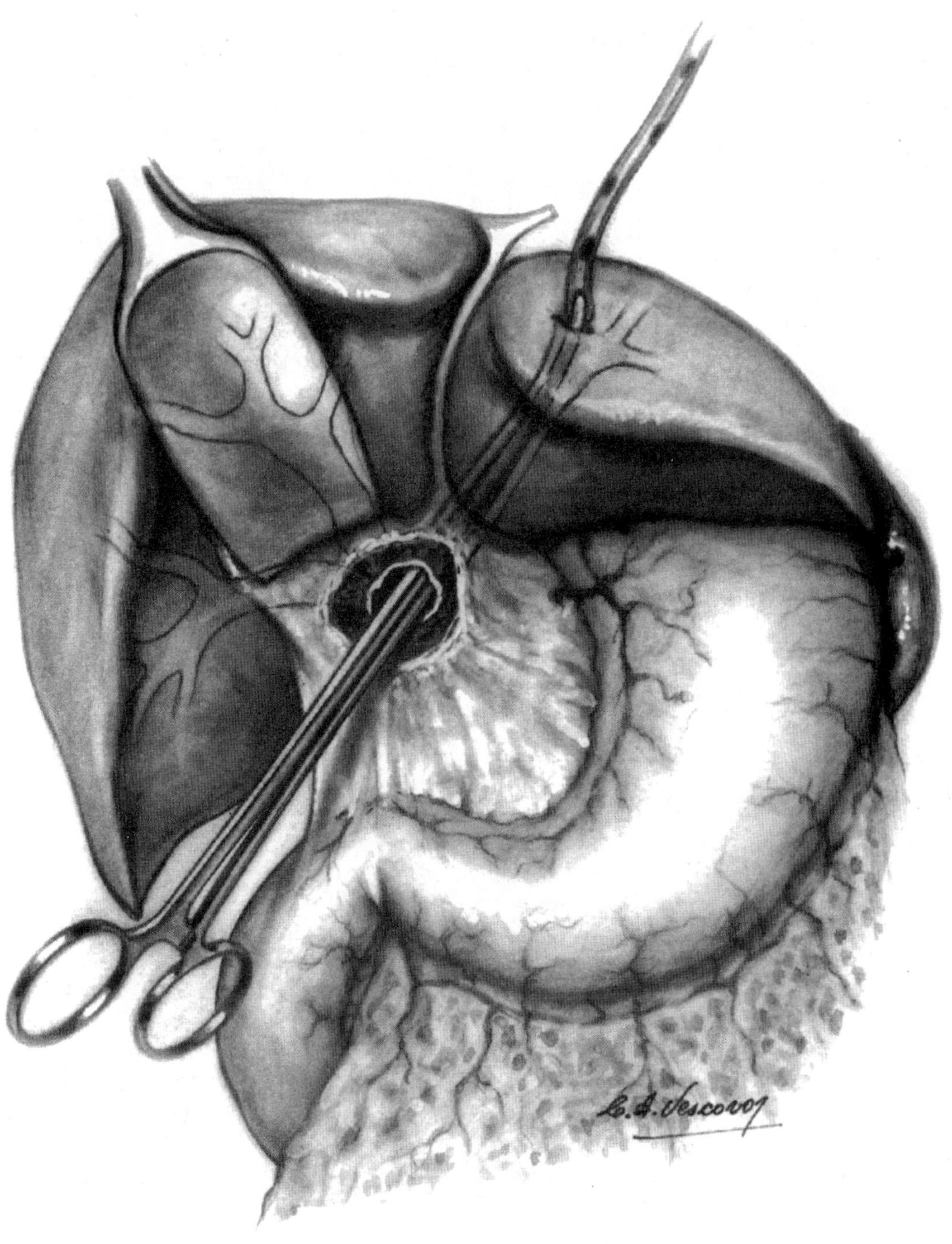

FIGURE 6.39

Lord Smith of Marlow Technique

FIGURE 6.40
The transhepatic tube has been passed, as seen in the drawing. A jejunal loop has been prepared and brought up in Roux-en-Y fashion. The anastomotic limb of the Roux-en-Y jejunal loop has been closed with two layers of sutures. About 3 cm from the end of the jejunal loop, which is being grasped by an atraumatic Duval clamp, an ellipse of the serosal layer is being removed about 15 mm long and 10 mm wide, leaving the mucosa intact.

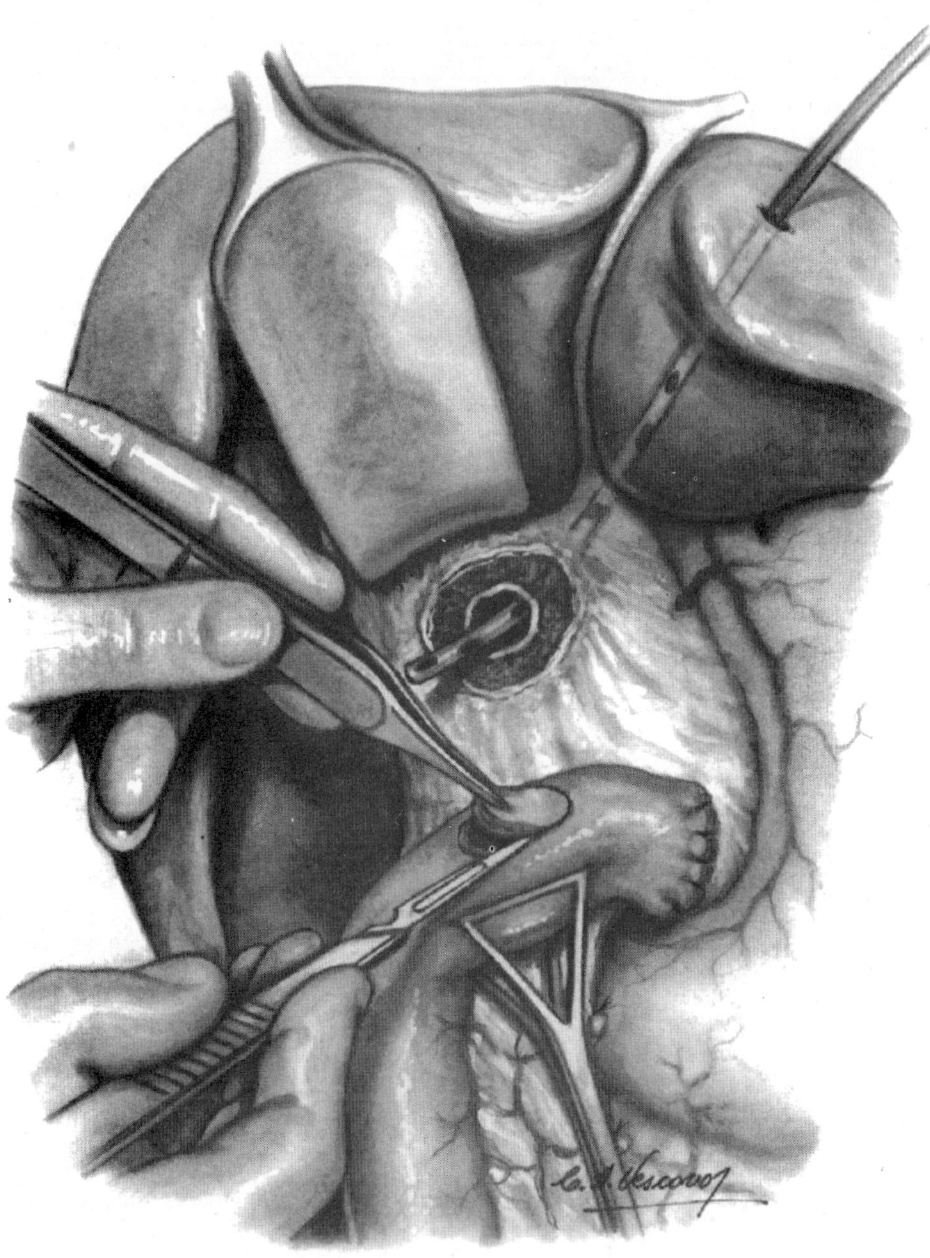

FIGURE 6.40

Lord Smith of Marlow Technique

FIGURE 6.41

At the site of the removal of this seromuscular ellipse a small incision is made in the mucosa, big enough to allow the distal end of the transhepatic tube to pass into the anastomotic jejunal loop where it is fixed with two sutures of 2-0 chromic catgut, as shown in the drawing. The mucosa of the jejunum is then fixed to the tube with two purse string sutures of 3-0 chronic catgut, as high as possible. It may be necessary to produce a ballooning of the mucosa of the jejunum by squeezing the jejunal loop with your hand. Once the transhepatic tube has been fixed to the wall of the jejunal loop and the jejunal mucosa by means of the purse string sutures, traction is applied to the tube, as shown in the drawing in the direction of the arrow until one can feel some elastic resistance. The tube is then fixed to the abdominal wall through which it had been introduced. In the insert one can observe the jejunal mucosa entering the interior of the common hepatic duct and coming in contact with its normal mucosa at a level where there is no fibrosis or granulation tissue. These two apposed mucosas will later unite. This junction is, therefore, by apposition and not by suturing.

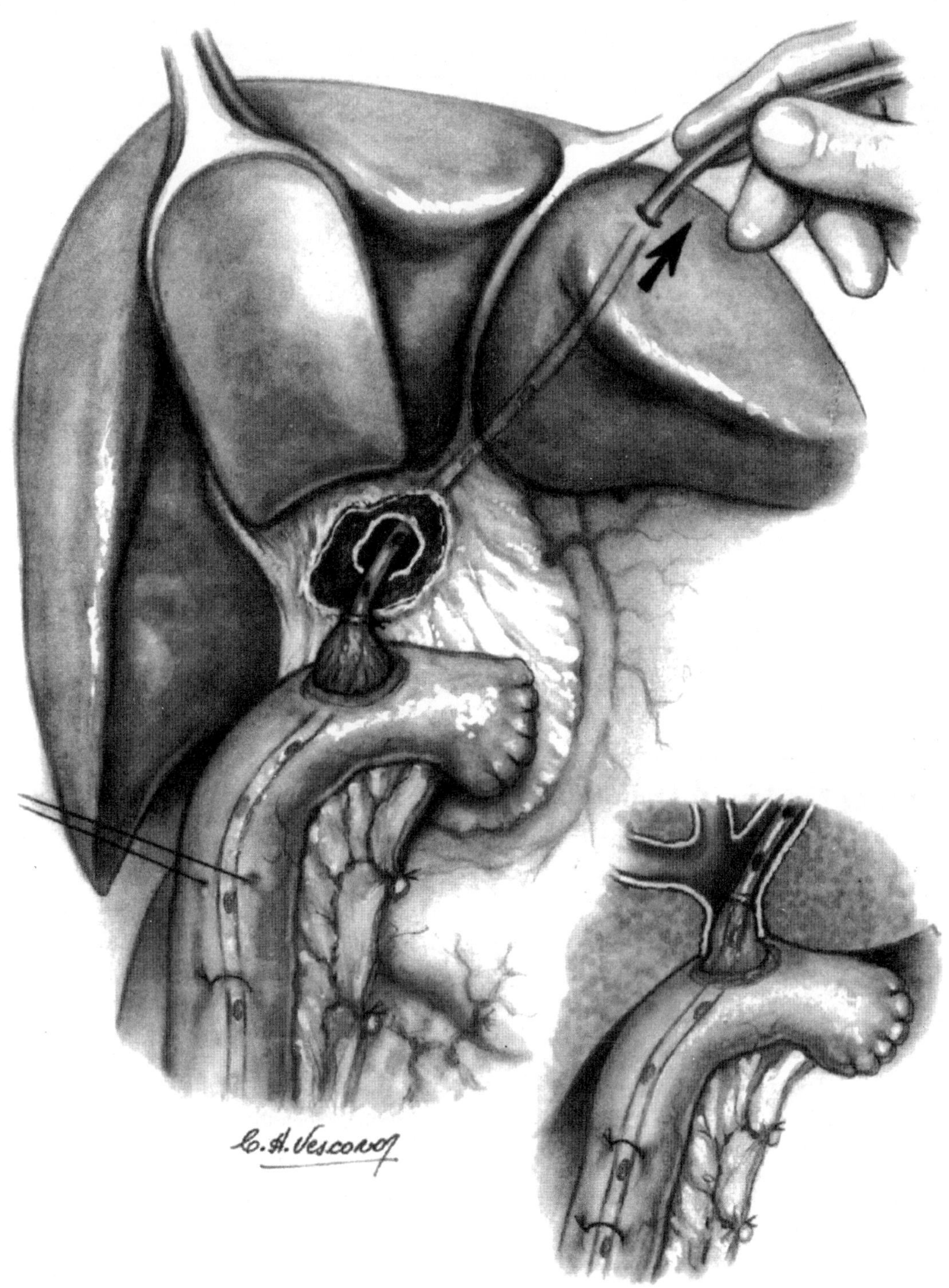

FIGURE 6.41

Lord Smith of Marlow Technique

FIGURE 6.42

The drawing shows the Lord Smith of Marlow procedure completed. The anastomotic jejunal loop has been fixed to Glisson's capsule with some sutures to avoid traction downward. One can also observe the Silastic tube fixed to the jejunal wall with two sutures. The jejunojejunal anastomosis has been performed some 50 cm below the hepaticojejunal anastomosis to avoid reflux. The ascending jejunal limb has been passed through the transverse mesocolon to the right of the middle colic artery, where it has been fixed with some sutures to prevent internal herniations. In this procedure the transhepatic tube is usually left in place between 3 to 6 months. In some patients the transhepatic tube should be left longer and at times for up to one or more years. In cases in which one believes that the transhepatic tube has to be left in place for a long period of time it is convenient to use a transhepatic tube in U fashion. Before closing the abdomen, a suction type of drainage tube is left in Morrison's pouch. About 2 to 3 weeks later a control cholangiogram should be performed, which can be repeated later to follow the postoperative evolution of the anastomosis.

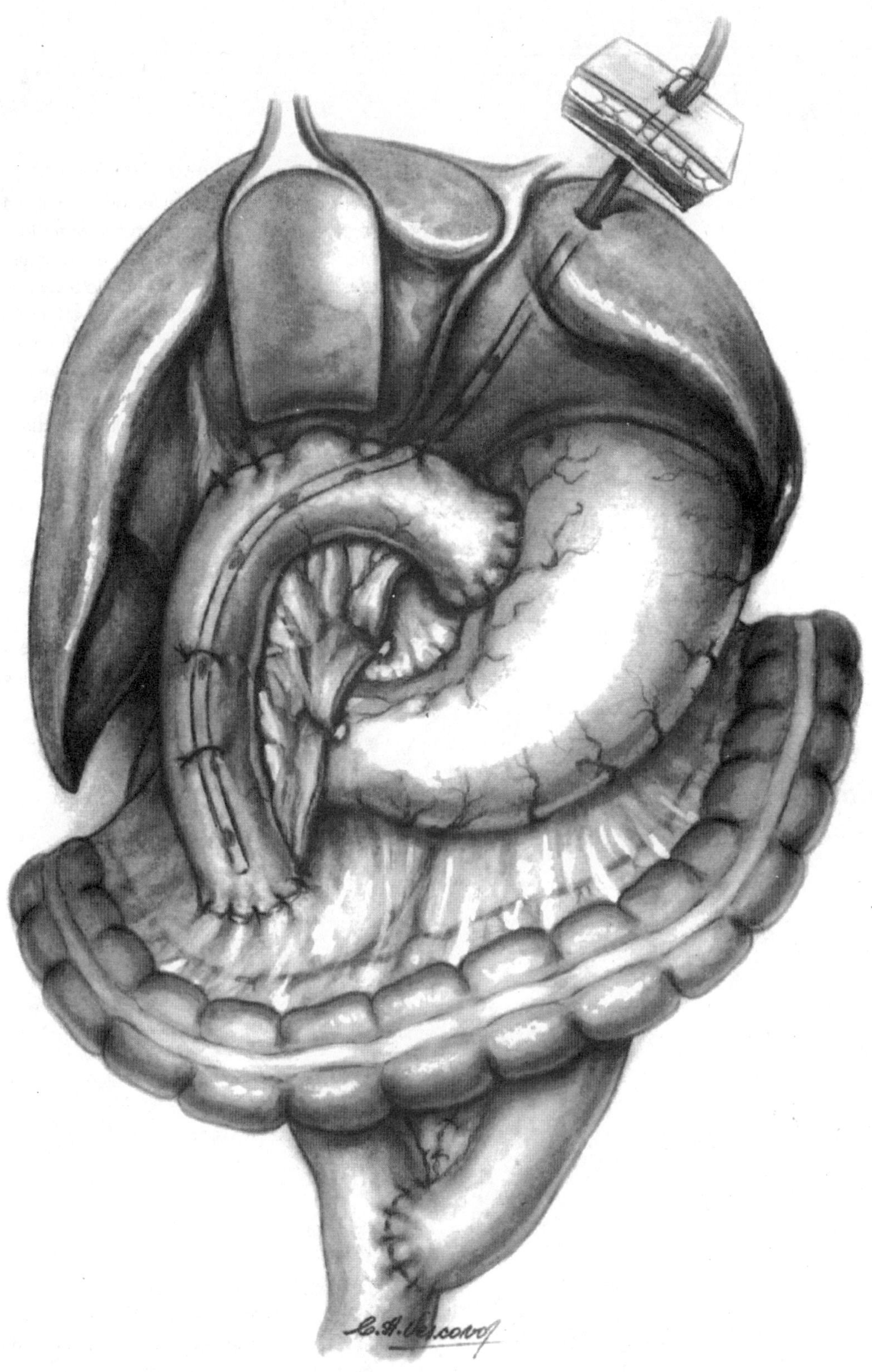

FIGURE 6.42

FIGURE 6.43
In cases in which the surgical lesion is localized at the junction of the right and left hepatic ducts and both ducts have become separated by the absence of the common hepatic duct, reestablishment of biliary continuity is a very complex problem and fraught with uncertain results. To attempt to improve this difficult situation one can use the Cattell technique. This technique consists of suturing both ducts in partial fashion by means of two rows of suture of silk or cotton, one row above and the other underneath, with a later sectioning, with a scissors, of the septum between both ducts in order to perform a single anastomosis with the jejunum. In the drawing one can see that the right hepatic duct has been sutured to the left hepatic duct and with a straight scissors the septum is being sectioned. It is extremely difficult preoperatively to pass transhepatic catheters, which besides helping identify the hepatic ducts (right and left) can be replaced during the operation by long Silástic or latex tubes to act as drainage and stents postoperatively. In this surgery the use of a loupe or surgical microscope is indispensable.

Lesions of the Confluence of the Hepatic Ducts

FIGURE 6.44
In the drawing one can observe that the septum joining both hepatic ducts has been sectioned. This undoubtedly increases the diameter, facilitating suturing to the jejunum. Traction is being applied to the angles of the new hepatic duct by means of the guide sutures. The previously prepared ascending limb of the Roux-en-Y jejunal loop, with its closed end, has been approximated to the joined hepatic ducts. This jejunal loop is held in place by an atraumatic Duval clamp. This incision to be used in the anastomosis has been drawn on the antimesenteric border of the loop, using a dotted line.

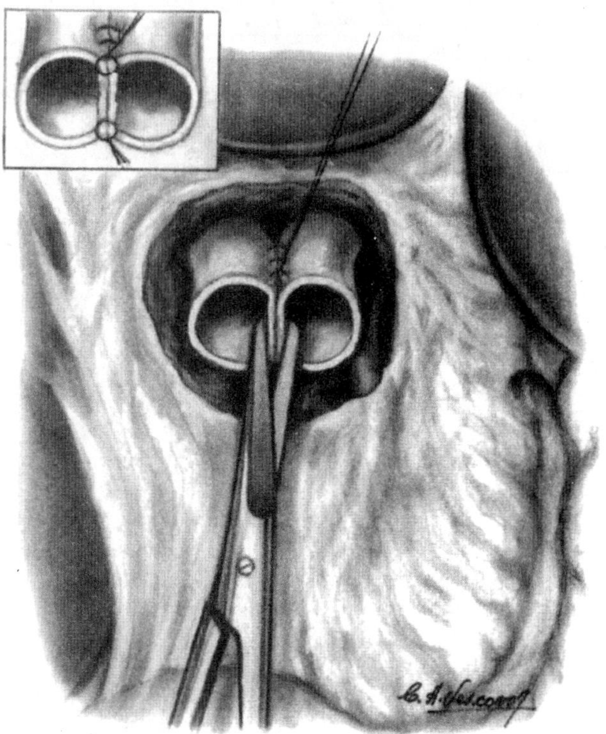

FIGURE 6.43

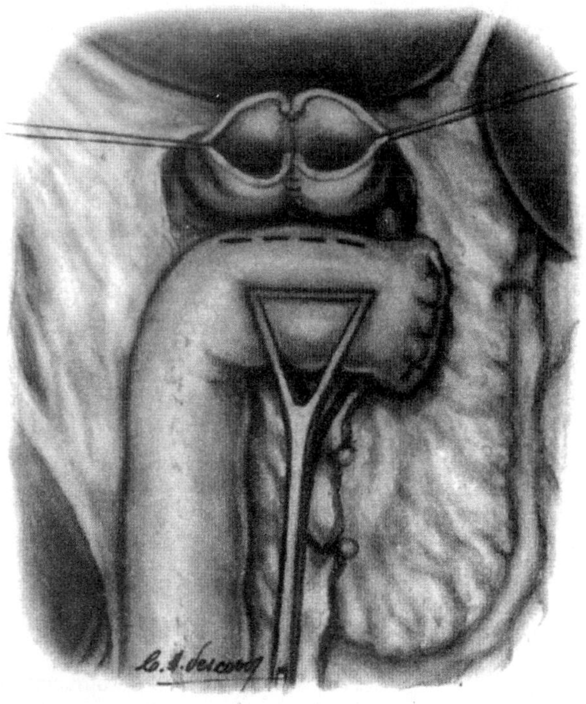

FIGURE 6.44

FIGURE 6.45
The posterior suture line has been completed and the anterior suture line has been started. Synthetic reabsorbable 3-0 sutures are being used. Some surgeons prefer silk or linen.

Lesions of the Confluence of the Hepatic Ducts

FIGURE 6.46
The anterior row of sutures is being finished. Once the anastomosis is completed, some sutures should be placed between the seromuscular layer of the jejunum and Glisson's capsule. These will give support to the intestinal loop and diminish the traction on the suture line.

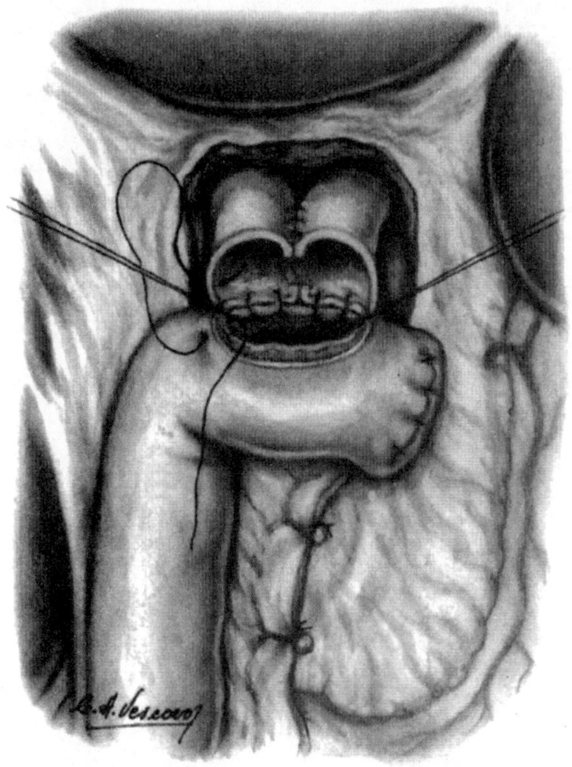

FIGURE 6.45

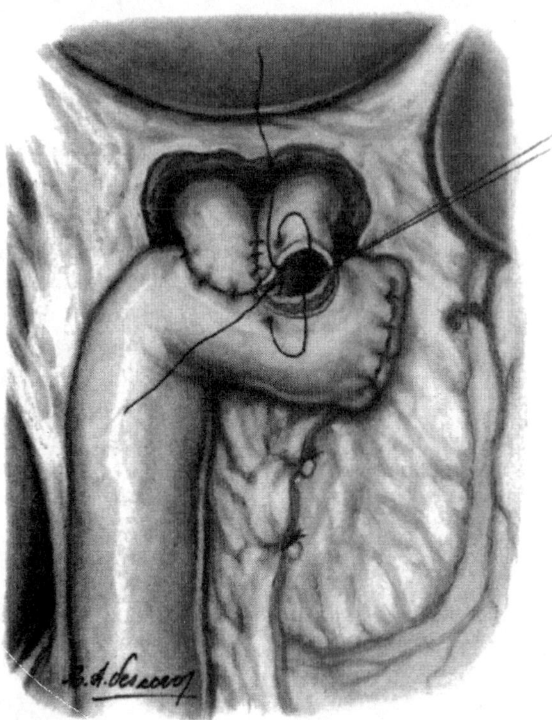

FIGURE 6.46

Lesions of the Confluence of the Hepatic Ducts

FIGURE 6.47

In cases in which it is not possible to join the left and right hepatic duct to perform a single anastomosis to the jejunum, as previously shown, each of the ducts must be anastomosed separately to the jejunum. To facilitate these anastomoses it is necessary to dissect the hepatic ducts from the hepatic parenchyma, a very difficult task. The anastomosis of each duct to the jejunum is performed in a manner similar to that described in previous drawings. In these cases it is extremely important to pass transhepatic catheters preoperatively. These catheters should be replaced by latex or Silastic tubes to be left in place postoperatively as stents, as shown in the drawing.

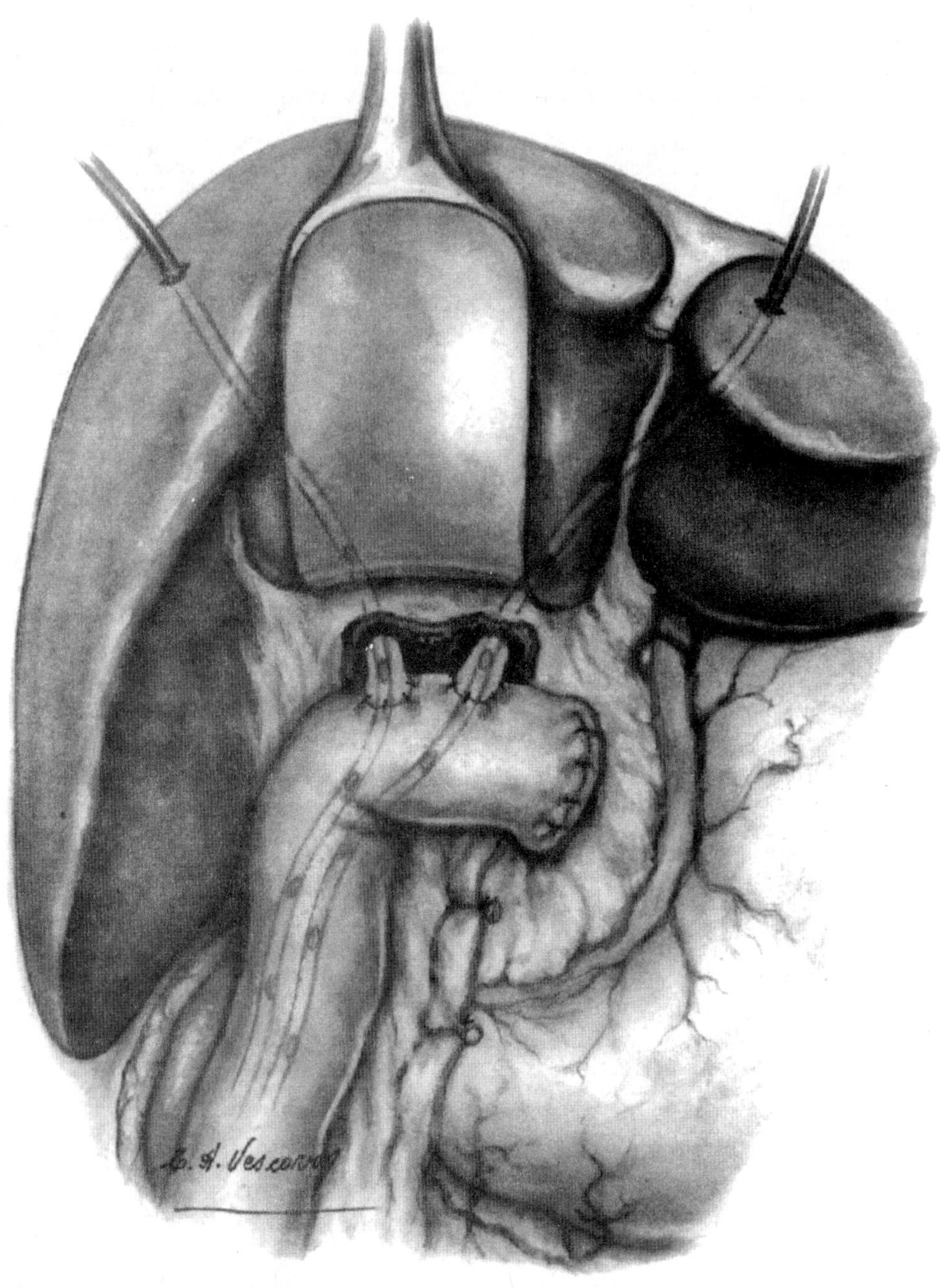

FIGURE 6.47

References

1. Almasqué Dedeu, R. Lesiones quirúrgicas de las vías biliares. Pren. Méd. Argent. 54:1490, 1967.
2. Aust, J.B., Root, H.A., Urdaneta, L., Varco, R. Biliary stricture. Surgery 62:601, 1967.
3. Braasch, J.W. Reconstruction of the biliary tract. In Nora, P.F. (Ed.) Operative surgery. Ed. 2, p. 571. Lea & Febiger, Philadelphia, 1980.
4. Belzer, F.O., Watts, J., Ross, H.B., Dunphy, J.E. Autoreconstruction of the common bile duct after venous patch graft. Ann. Surg. 162:346, 1965.
5. Bismuth, H, Lazorthes, F. Les traumatismes opératoires de la voie biliaire principle. Vol. 1. Masson et Cie., Paris, 1981.
6. Bismuth, H. Postoperative strictures of the bile duct. In Blumgart, L.H. (Ed.). The biliary tract. Clinical surgery international. Vol. 5, p. 209. Churchill Livingstone, Edinburgh, 1982.
7. Blumgart, L.H. Bile duct strictures. In Fromm, D. (Ed.) Gastro-intestinal surgery. Vol. 2, p. 755. Churchill Livingstone, New York, 1985.
8. Cameron, J.L., Skinner, D.B., Zuidema, G.D. Long-term trans-hepatic intubation for bilar hepatic duct strictures. Ann. Surg. 183:488, 1976.
9. Cameron, J.L. Atlas of surgery. Vol. I, p. 38. B.C. Decker, 1990.
10. Cattell, R.B., Braasch, J.W. Primary repair of benign strictures of the bile duct. Surg. Gynecol. Obstet. 109:531, 1959.
11. Cattell, R.B., Braasch, J.W. General considerations in the management of benign strictures of the bile duct. N. Engl. J. Med. 261: 929, 1959.
12. Cinelli, A.P. Contribución de la colangiografia operatoria en la profilaxis de las heridas accidentales operatorias y en la cirugía reparadora de las vias biliares. Pren. Méd. Argent. 54:1081, 1967.
13. Couinaud, C. Les envelopes vasculo-biliaires du fois en capsule de Glisson. Lyon Chir. 49:589, 1954.
14. Couinaud, C. Lobes et segments hépatiques, notes sur la architecture anatomique et chirugicale du fois. Presse Méd. 62:709, 1954.
15. Couinaud, C. Recherches sur la chirurgie du contluent biliair supérieur et des canaux hépatiques. Presse Méd. 1955;63:669.
16. Doutre, L., Perissat, J., Goutfiant, J., Bobois, J. A propos de réinterventions biliaires. J. Chir. 107:131, 1974.
17. Ellis, H., Hoile, R.W. Vein patch repair of the common bile duct. J. R. Soc. Med. 73:635, 1980.
18. Fernández Puente M. Reparación de la via biliar principal. Pren. Méd Argent. 62:269, 1975.
19. Fretheim, B., Flatmark, A. Treatment of Benign and Malignant Proximal Biliary Tract Stenosis. In Nyhus, L.M., Baker, R.J. eds. Mastery of surgery. Vol. 1, p. 715. Little, Brown & Co., Boston, 1984
20. Freund, H.R., Beriatzky, Y. Choledochojejunostomy. In Nyhus, L.M., Baker, R.J. eds. Mastery of surgery. Vol. 1, p. 728. Little, Brown & Co., Boston, 1984.
21. Glenn, F. Postoperative strictures of the extrahepatic bile duct. Surg. Gynecol. Obstet. 120:560, 1965.
22. Goëtze O. Die transhepatizche danedrainage der hollen gausstenose. Arch. Klin. Chir. 270:97, 1951.
23. Gouma, D.J., Wesdorp, R.I.C., Oostenbroek, R.J., et al. Percutaneous transhepatic drainage and insertion of an endoprosthesis for obstructive jaundice. Am. J. Surg. 145:763, 1983.
24. Grindlay, J.H., Eberle, J., Walters, W. Technique for external drainage of the biliary tract which leaves duct intact. Arch. Surg. 67:289, 1953.
25. Hepp, J., Couinaud, C. L'abord et l'utilisation du canal hépatique gauche dans les réparations de la voie biliare principale. Presse Méd. 64:94, 1953.
26. Kune, G.A., Saii, A. The practice of biliary surgery. Ed. 2, p. 192. Blackwell Scientific Publications, Oxford, 1981.
27. Kune, G.A. Acute and chronic repair of common hepatic duct injury. In Nyhus, L.M., Baker, R.J. (Eds) Mastery of surgery. Vol. 1, p. 710. Little, Brown & Co., Boston, 1984.
28. Lary, B.C., Scheibe, J. The effect of rubber tubing on the healing of common duct anastomosis. Surgery 32:789, 1952.
29. Lasaia, A., Moimenti, L. Reoperaciones en vias biliares por lesiones quirúrgicas. López Libreros Editores, Buenos Aires, 1966.
30. Lindenauer, M. Surgical treatment of the bile duct strictures. Surgery 73:875, 1976.
31. Madden, J.L., McCann, W.J. Reconstruction of the common bile duct by end-to-end anastomosis without the use of an internal splint or stent support. Surg. Gynecol. Obstet. 112:305, 1961.
32. Madsen, C.M., Sorensen, H.R., Truelsen, F. The frequency of operative bile duct injuries illustrated by a Danish county survey. Acta Chir. Scand. 119:110, 1960.
33. Mainetti, J.M., Soria, N. Coledocoplastia con vena sáfena. Pren.Méd. Argent. 56:810, 1969.
34. Michie, W., Gunn, A. Bile duct injuries. A new suggestion for their repair. Br. J. Surg. 51:96, 1964.
35. Moosa, R., Block, G., Skinner, D., Hall, H. Reconstruction of high bilary tract strictures employing transheptic intubation. Surg. Clin. North Am. 56:73, 1976.
36. Praderi, R. Coledocotomia transhepática. Bol. Soc. Ciru. Uruguay 32:237, 1961.
37. Praderi, R. Lesiones por el acto operatorio en la colecistectomía. Pren. Méd. Argent. 52:1989, 1965.
38. Praderi, R. Twelve years' experience with transhepatic intubation. Ann. Surg. 179:937, 1974.
39. Rosenquist, H., Myrin, S.O. Operative injuries to the bile ducts. Acta Chir. Scand. 119:92, 1960.
40. Smith, R. Hepaticojejunostomy with transhepatic intubation: A technique for very high stricture of the hepatic ducts. Br. J. Surg. 51:186, 1964.
41. Smith, R. Personal communication, 1971.
42. Smith, R. Lord of Marlow obstructions of the bile duct. Br. J. Surg. 66:69, 1979.
43. Tompkins, R.K., Pitt, H.A. Surgical management of benign lesions of the bile ducts. Curr. Probl. Surg. 1982;19:321.
44. Viikari, S.J. Operative injuries to the bile ducts. Acta Chir. Scand. 119:83, 1960.
45. Way, L., Dunphy, E.J. Biliary strictures. Am. J. Surg. 124:28, 1972.
46. Warren, K.W., Poulantzas, J.K., Kune, G.A. Use of Y-tube splint in the repair of biliary strictures. Surg. Gynecol. Obstet. 122:785, 1966.
47. Warren, K.W., McDonald, W.M. New concept in the management of an old problem. In Irvine, W.T. (Ed.) Modern trends in surgery. Ed. 2. Butterworth, London, 1966.
48. Warren, K.W., Christophi, C., Armendaria, R. The evolution and current perspectives of the treatment of benign bile duct strictures. A review. Surg. Gastroenterol. 1:141, 1982.
49. Warren, K.W., Jenkins, R.L., Steele, G.D. Jr. Atlas of surgery of the liver, pancreas and biliary tract. p. 42. Appleton-Lange, East Norwalk, CT, 1991.
50. Wilks, A.E., Berri, R.A. Lesiones quirúrgicas de las vías biliares. Rev. Argent. Cir. No. Extraordinario XLIX. Congr. Argent. Cir., p. 89, 1978.

Section A

Surgery of the Biliary Tract

CHAPTER 7

Cystic Dilation of the Common Bile Duct

Cystic dilation of the common bile duct appears in the medical literature under different names. Some of these are cysts of the common bile duct, congenital cysts of the common bile duct, biliary cysts, idiopathic aneurysmal or sack-shaped dilation, and so on. This anomaly has the external appearance of a cyst, but from a structural point of view it is not a cyst because it neither has its own walls nor is it lined interiorly by a mucosa. The designation of cysts or cystic dilation of the common bile duct is also inexact, since the cyst is not always limited to the common bile duct but extends into the common hepatic duct, compromising it either partially or completely. A more correct designation could be "segmental dilations of cystic appearance of the common bile duct." We will, however, continue to use the classical nomenclature.

In describing cysts of the common bile duct, authors frequently refer to only one of the varieties of these cysts, the one described at the beginning of this chapter. This variety is undoubtedly the most common, but there exist other varieties of these cysts that have very little similarity between them and should be treated by different surgical procedures. This shows the importance of classifying these cysts before describing the surgical technique, since there are profound topographic, morphologic, and structural differences between the different varieties.

The Alonso-Lej clinicopathologic classi cation proposed in 1959 (1) is the one used more frequently because of its simplicity. Alonso-Lej divides cyst of the common bile duct into three types, described as follows:

Type I. This is the most common variation and represents 93% of all common bile duct cysts. It is characterized by a sack-like dilation of a segment of the duct, involving its entire circumference, and beginning and ending suddenly. Above and below the dilated segment the bile duct is normal. The size of the cystic dilation is very variable, ranging from 300 to 1000 mL. In some patients the dilated segment may contain several liters (23). The cyst contains concentrated bile; because of this, it is dark in color (1, 15).

Culture of the contents of the cyst is usually positive for bacteria of intestinal origin (15). The interior of the cyst is usually devoid of mucosa except for some isolated areas with islands of mucosa. The thickness of the wall may vary from 3 to 10 mm (14, 21, 23, 24). The wall of the cyst is made of fibrous tissue, rich in collagen fibers, and frequently densely infiltrated by polymorphonuclear cells and lymphocytes. Cysts of the common bile duct are more common in women than in men in a proportion of 4:1. The gallbladder and cystic duct are normal. The opening of the cystic duct is frequently located at or near the junction of the common hepatic duct and the cyst. In a few cases the cystic duct empties directly into the cyst. Because of its fibrous structure and its lack of mucosa the cystic dilation is not a satisfactory structure to be anastomosed to the bowel.

Until a few years ago it was thought that cysts of the common bile duct were usually diagnosed in infancy or adolescence, but it is now proven that they can be diagnosed at any time. The latest statistics show an undoubted increase in the incidence of this problem in adults. Therefore, cysts of the common bile duct have ceased to be part of the patrimony of pediatricians and pediatric surgeons. Most investigators agree that cysts of the common bile duct are congenital in origin, observable in fetuses, newborns, and breastfeeding infants as well as older children. Some authors, however, maintain their opinion that the dilation can be acquired owing to a structural alteration or a congenital malformation of the wall (2). In 1969 Babbitt (2) pointed out the frequency with which patients with Type I Alonso-Lej choledochal cysts have an abnormally high junction of the pancreatic and common bile duct, with this junction outside the limits of the duodenal wall. Babbitt suggested this anomaly as the cause of the cystic dilation. Later, other investigators confirmed Babbitt's interesting observation (11–14), but did not believe the anomaly was the cause of the dilation. Recent studies in Japan, where cysts of the common bile duct are more frequent than in Europe or America, have shown that this high junction of the pancreatic duct with the common bile duct is found in almost 90% of patients with choledochal cysts (12, 18, 19). These authors have shown that the high junction of the pancreatic duct with the common bile duct favors the occurrence of reflux of pancreatic juice into the common bile duct due to lack of sphincter control. This increase in reflux of pancreatic juice is the cause of the hyperamylasemia that these patients usually have (19). Some authors believe that reflux is an important factor in the production of structural changes in the common duct that favor the development of malignant changes of the cystic as well as other segments of the biliary tree (14, 19, 26). It has been shown that patients with choledochal cysts are more prone to developing malignancies of the biliary tree and at an earlier age (10, 13, 14). The high junction of the pancreatic duct with the common bile duct has surgical importance because, as can be seen later, in dissecting the inferior end of the cyst and in identifying the common bile duct one must transect the duct very close to the dilation. If this is done too far down, one runs the risk of damaging the junction of the pancreatic duct to the common bile duct, which, in these patients, is frequently abnormally high.

Cysts of the common bile duct are not very frequent, but their prognosis is fatal if they are not treated surgically before the condition produces serious deterioration of the patient. The complications that a cyst of the common bile duct may produce are multiple: rupture of the cyst due to trauma or during pregnancy, hepatomegaly, biliary cirrhosis caused by stasis, portal hypertension, cholangitis, pancreatitis, duodenal compression by the cyst with the production of duodenal obstruction, and carcinoma of the cyst or other segments of the biliary tract.

The diagnosis of cysts of the common bile duct can be suspected by the symptomatology that the patient may present. More commonly, however, it is an incidental operative finding, especially in adults. Rarely, patients present the classic triad of pain, palpable mass, and jaundice. It is more common that patients will present one or two symptoms of the triad or no symptoms at all. This is most common in adults, who generally present nonspecific symptoms. There are various methods of diagnosing cysts of the common bile duct: intravenous cholecystocholangiography, ultrasonography, computerized tomography, endoscopic retrograde cholangiopancreatography, and transparietohepatic cholangiography.

The surgical treatment of cysts of the common bile duct, Type I, consists in the resection of the cyst and the reestablishment of biliary continuity by means of an anastomosis of the common hepatic duct with the jejunum brought up in Roux-en-Y fashion. Years ago a simple anastomosis of the cyst with the bowel was used. However, this is not used at present except in patients whose general condition will not tolerate resection or in patients in whom the cyst is densely fixed, making resection too dangerous or impossible. Simple anastomosis of the cyst to the bowel is a fast and easy procedure, but does not generally give good results because postoperative cholangitis and the formation of calculi as well as carcinomatous degeneration may occur. Anastomosis of the cyst to the bowel is not a mucosa to mucosa anastomosis. The anastomosis of the cyst to the jejunum in Roux-en-Y fashion should be preferred to the cystoduodenal anastomosis, even though it is somewhat more complex, because the cystoduodenal anastomosis produces more frequent complications, such as narrowing of the anastomosis and cholangitis. The gallbladder should always be resected, even if the cyst is not resected. It has been shown that when the gallbladder is not resected, the occurrence of cholecystitis postoperatively is more frequent (16, 19, 26, 27). Resection of the cyst of the common bile duct and anastomosis of the hepatic duct to the jejunum in Roux-en-Y fashion is a much more complex operation than simple cystojejunal anastomosis. At present, however, this operation in the hands of expert biliary surgeons, carries a very low mortality.

Type II. The Type II choledochal cyst is the least frequent of the choledochal cysts and represents only 2.1% of all cysts (21, 24). It is characterized by the presentation of a lateral diverticulum joined to the common bile duct by a pedicle. This pedicle is generally thin and only rarely wide. In the majority of the patients the diverticulum is generally to the right of the common hepatic duct, but in some it can be to the left. The pedicle of the diverticulum may be connected with the common bile duct, with the common hepatic bile duct in some cases, or rarely with one of the hepatic ducts. The surgical treatment of these diverticula consists in simple resection, ligating the pedicle at its junction with the bile duct if it is thin. In cases in which the pedicle is wide, it should be resected near the bile duct and sutured with interrupted sutures of synthetic reabsorbable 4-0 material. The operation is then completed using a T-tube above or below the pedicle suture, through a small transverse incision of the bile duct, to diminish internal pressure and protect the suture line.

Type III. Type III of the Alonso-Lej classification has very little in common with the two previous groups. Its frequency, although greater than Type II, represents only 5.2% of all choledochal cysts (1, 21, 24). Type III is characterized by the presentation of an ampullary dilation of the intraduodenal segment of the common bile duct, which dilation projects itself into the lumen of the duodenum like a terminal herniation of the common bile duct (21). In some cases, the ampullary dilation may be of great size and cause duodenal obstruction (9, 25). Wheeler, of England (31), proposed naming this anomaly choledochocele because of its similarity to ureterocele. Abraham Vater was the first to describe this ampullary dilation of the inferior end of the common bile duct in 1723 (28). The description that Vater made of this pathologic anomaly lead to the present designation of Ampulla of Vater when one mentions the interior of the normal Ampulla of Vater. Vater had described the dilation of the ampulla in a case corresponding to what is actually known as Type III in the Alonso-Lej classification of choledochal cyst and not of a normal anatomic structure. From this erroneous interpretation the name of Ampulla of Vater was used to designate the interior of the normal papilla which in reality is not an ampulla nor was it what Vater described in the year 1723.

Type III of the Alonso-Lej classification presents itself in two forms. It is important to distinguish between these two forms during surgical exploration because they must be treated by different surgical procedures. The first and most frequent is the form already described and consists of a cystic dilation of the intraduodenal portion of the common bile duct. This cystic dilation presents an opening in its surface through which the biliopancreatic secretion passes into the duodenum. The second variety is known as the lateral papillary variety and is constituted by a lateral diverticulum of the common bile duct very near the papilla that does not present an opening in its surface, the biliary pancreatic secretion passing through the papilla, which is in its normal position. Bass and Cremin (3) have called attention to a curious fact. This is that the first variety is similar to what is normally found in some animals such as guinea pigs and marsupials and the second variety is found in another group of animals, such as elephants, whales, seals, and so on (21).

FIGURE 7.1
Classification of the Alonso-Lej cystic dilations of the common bile duct.

Type I: This is the most common of the cystic dilations of the common bile duct.
Type II: This is the least common type. It is characterized by the presence of a diverticulum that communicates with the common bile duct through a narrow pedicle.
Type III: This is characterized by the presence of an ampullary dilation of the intraduodenal segment of the common bile duct (choledochocele). There are two varieties of choledochocele: (a) terminal choledochocele and (b) the lateral papillary choledochocele.

Cystic Dilation of the Common Bile Duct

FIGURE 7.2
In this drawing, we can see the most prominent characteristics of the cystic dilations of the common bile duct, Type I of Alonso-Lej, which have been described previously. One can see the abnormally high junction of the pancreatic duct with the common bile duct. In insert No. 1, the pancreatic duct joins the common bile duct in its normal position at the level of the papilla while in insert No. 2, the pancreatic duct joins the common bile duct at a higher level, above the limits of the duodenal wall as occurs in about 90% of the cysts of the common bile duct of Type I Alonso-Lej.

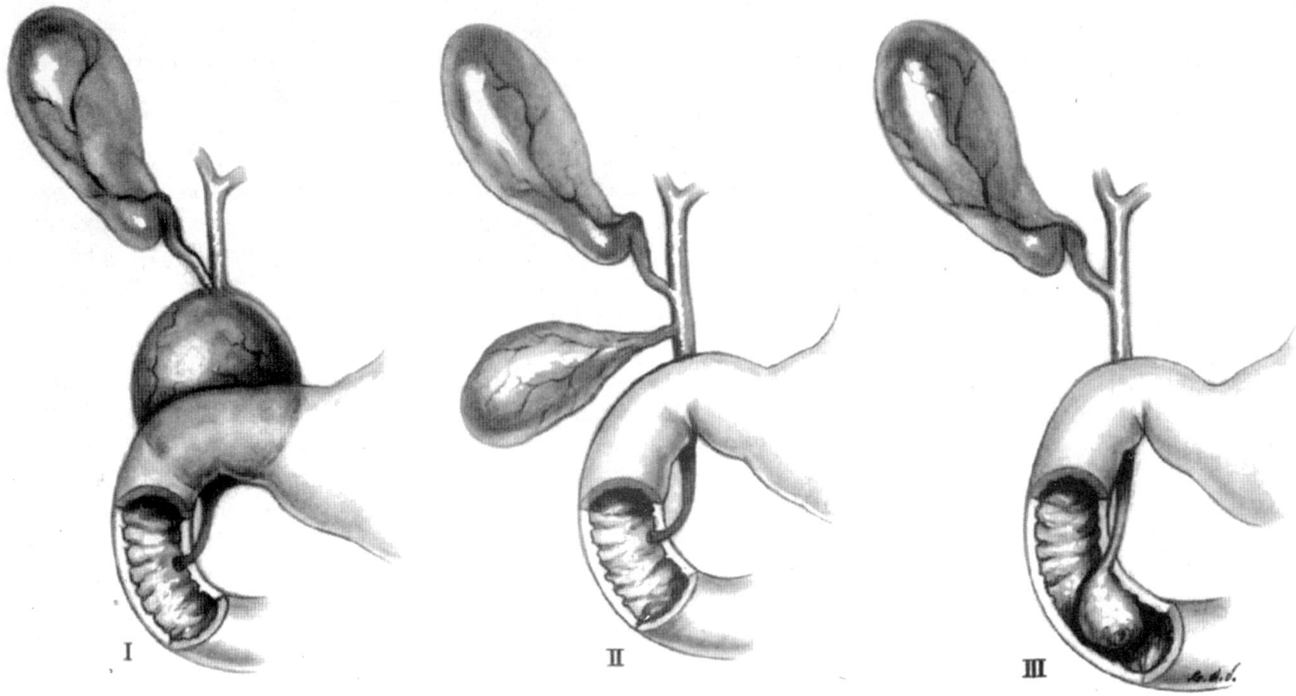

FIGURE 7.1

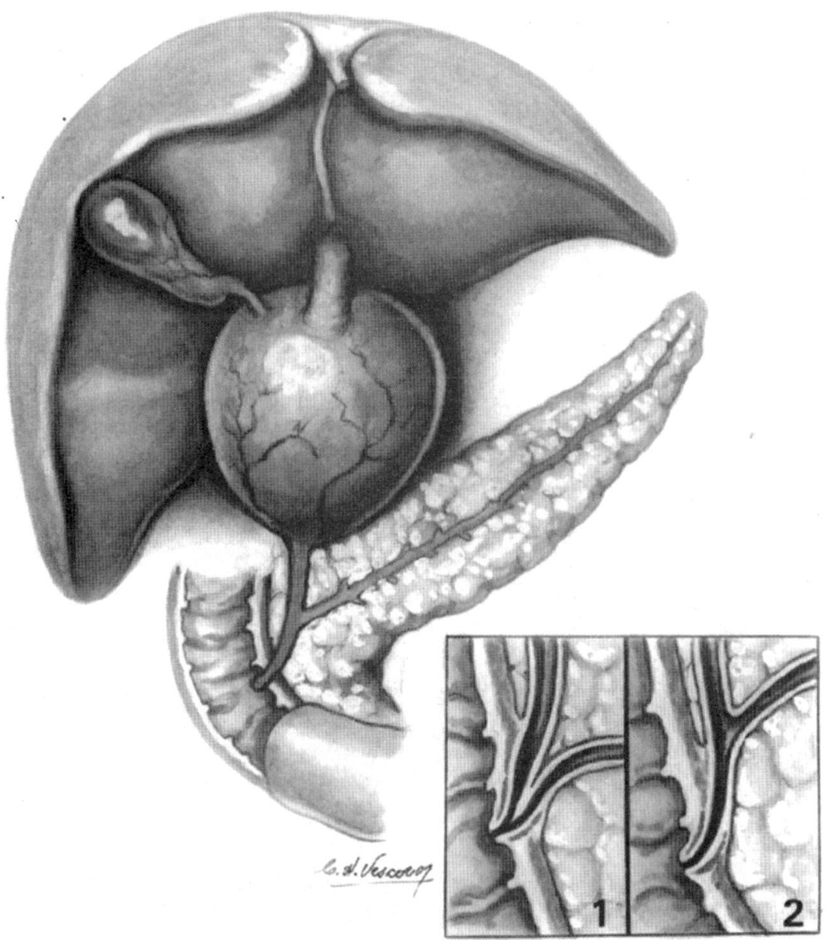

FIGURE 7.2

FIGURE 7.3
The surgical procedure of choice to treat cysts of the common bile duct of Type I of Alonso-Lej in resecting the cyst with the gallbladder and reestablishing the transit of the bile anastomosing the common hepatic duct with a loop of jejunum brought up in Roux-en-Y fashion. The abdomen is opened either through a transrectal incision or a right paramedian incision. Some surgeons use an extended subcostal incision. The operative diagnosis of cysts of the common bile duct is generally made easily because when cysts of the common bile duct change from silent to symptomatic they are generally well developed. During the asymptomatic phase the biliary tract is permeable. Decompensation begins when there are difficulties with the passage of bile. Surgical exploration usually reveals a well-localized dilation with very precise limits and easily distinguishable from the rest of the biliary tract. Its aspect is that of a bluish bag that usually extends laterally as well as posteriorly behind the first and second portions of the duodenum, ending suddenly in a common bile duct of small caliber that is easily identified. In order to inspect the entire surface of the cyst it is necessary to preform a Vautrin-Kocher maneuver. In this exploration, one should pay special attention to the degree of fixation of the cyst to its neighboring structures, especially on its posterior surface. It is of extreme importance to perform cholangiography through a puncture of the gallbladder, injecting sufficient dye to opacify the cyst and the rest of the biliary tract to obtain a complete picture of the biliary tree, which will be useful in deciding on the operative technique. To obtain adequate visualization of the entire biliary tree, one has to tilt the operating table because the cystic bag full of radiopaque dye generally makes visualization of some segments of the biliary tract difficult. The first surgical step will be to resect the gallbladder as shown in the drawing. The resection of the gallbladder is being performed starting at the cystic duct toward the fundus of the gallbladder. The stump of the cystic duct is visualized on the outer surface of the cystic dilation.

Cystic Dilation of the Common Bile Duct

FIGURE 7.4
The gallbladder bed has been sutured. The Vautrin-Kocher maneuver has made possible the dissection of the lateral segment and the inferior portion of the cystic dilation together with the beginning of the common bile duct of normal caliber. Scissors are being used to divide adhesions that join the anterior surface of the cyst with the first portion of the duodenal wall and the gastric antrum. Once the adhesions have been sectioned, the peritoneum has to be incised over the cyst to allow for its liberation.

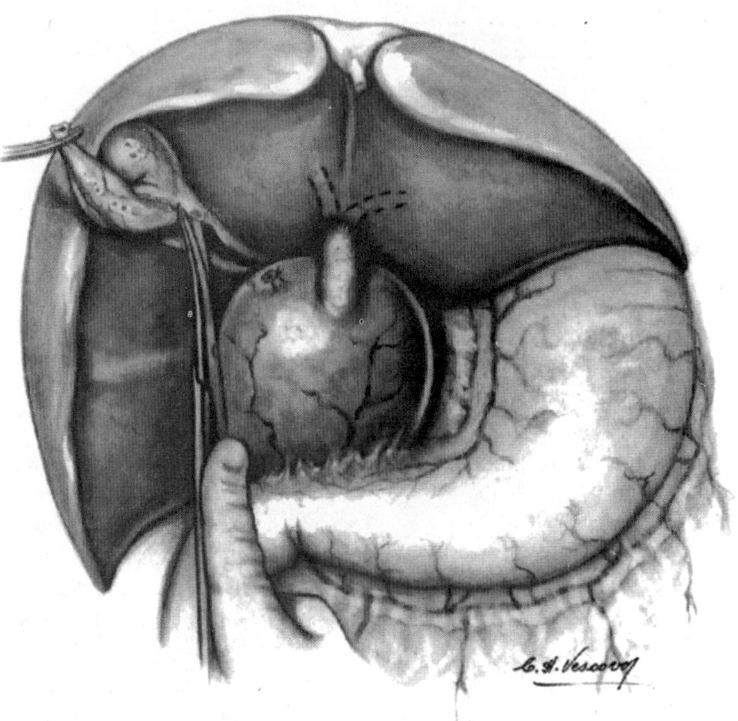

FIGURE 7.3

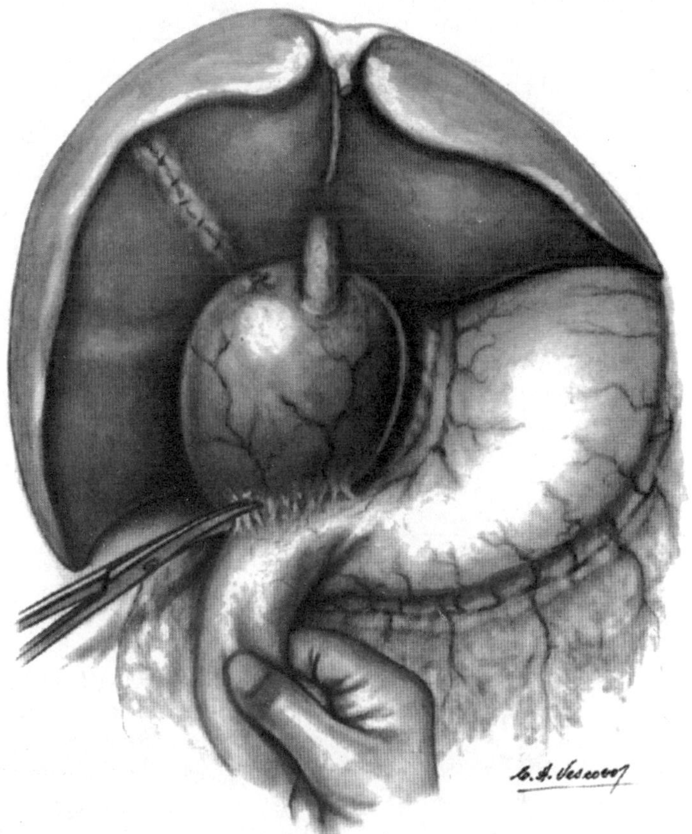

FIGURE 7.4

FIGURE 7.5
The inferior pole of the cyst has been dissected and the common bile duct immediately below it has been identified. One should not dissect the common bile duct too far beyond the cystic dilation because one then runs the risk of damaging the junction of the pancreatic duct to the common bile duct, which in patients with cysts of the common bile duct occurs in an abnormally high position in 90% of patients. The common bile duct has been clamped immediately below the cyst, and two traction sutures have been placed below the clamp. One then proceeds to transect the common bile duct with a scalpel. This common bile duct is generally somewhat narrow. The distal stump of the common bile duct is then closed with interrupted sutures of synthetic reabsorbable 4-0 material.

Cystic Dilation of the Common Bile Duct

FIGURE 7.6
After sectioning the common bile duct it is retracted upward placing traction on the hemostatic clamp and the cyst is then dissected in its posterior aspect using scissors. This is usually an easy dissection, but in some patients the posterior wall of the cyst is densely adherent to neighboring structures making its liberation difficult or impossible. In this case the operation is finished by performing an anastomosis of the anterior portion of the cyst to the jejunum.

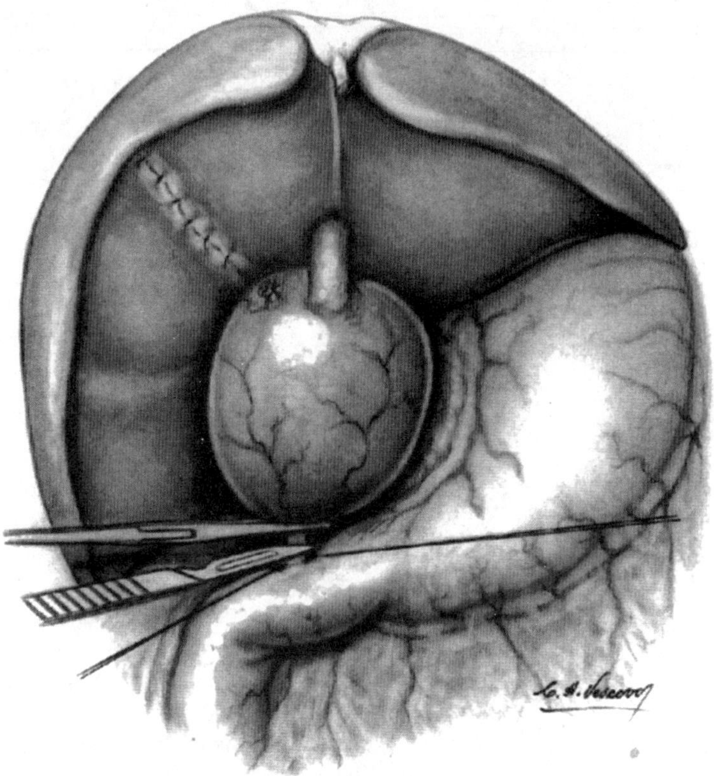

FIGURE 7.5

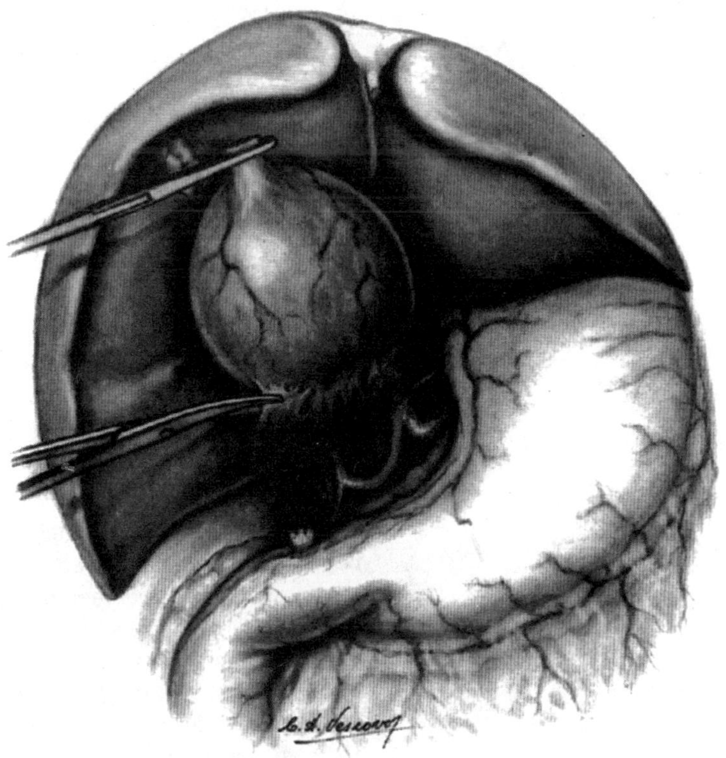

FIGURE 7.6

FIGURE 7.7
Once the entire surface of the cyst has been freed, one proceeds to transect the common hepatic bile duct just above the cyst. To perform this maneuver, two traction sutures are placed above the line of transection and two sutures are placed below this same line and the common hepatic duct is transected. If the common hepatic duct has a diameter of 15 mm or more, the hepaticojejunal terminolateral anastomosis is performed with interrupted sutures using synthetic reabsorbable 3-0 sutures. If the common hepatic duct has a smaller diameter, it will be necessary to increase this diameter using the left hepatic duct and lowering the hilar plate by the Hepp-Couinaud. In the insert we are showing in a dotted line the enlargement of the common hepatic duct at the expense of the left hepatic duct.

Cystic Dilation of the Common Bile Duct

FIGURE 7.8
The lowering of the hilar plate has been completed and the diameter of the common hepatic duct at the expense of the left hepatic duct has been increased. Two Silastic tubes with multiple perforations have been passed through the transhepatic route. A jejunal loop has been prepared using the Roux-en-Y technique and an incision has been made in the anastomotic limb to correspond with the diameter of the biliary duct. Several traction sutures have been applied in the biliary opening. The same has been done in the angles of the incision in the jejunum. It is advisable to preform this part of the technique and those in Figures 7.9 and 7.10 using a magnifying loupe.

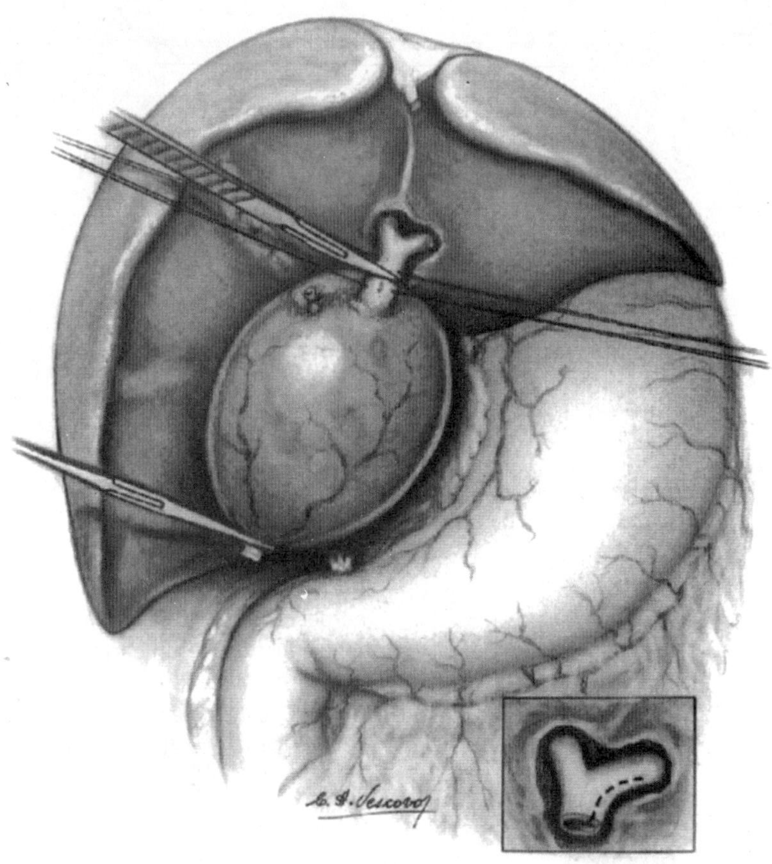

FIGURE 7.7

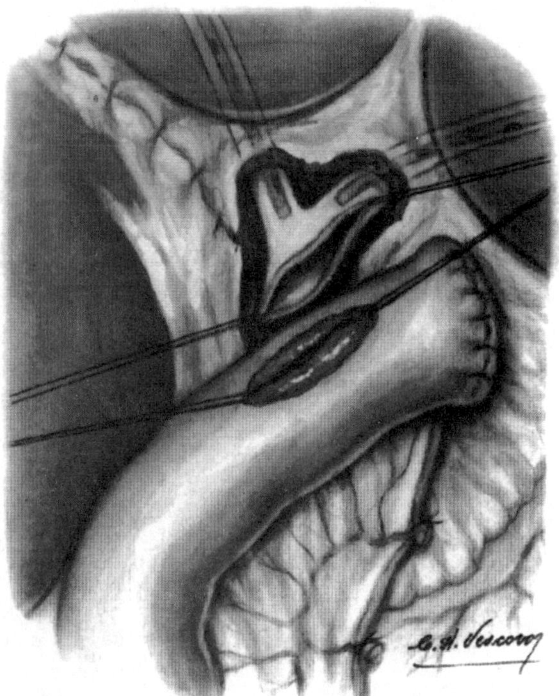

FIGURE 7.8

FIGURE 7.9
The posterior row of sutures between the biliary opening and the jejunum has been performed using interrupted sutures of synthetic reabsorbable 3-0 material. The ends of the transhepatic Silastic tubes have been passed into the jejunum, and the anterior row of sutures is being performed.

Cystic Dilation of the Common Bile Duct

FIGURE 7.10
The anterior row of sutures of the biliojejunal anastomosis is almost complete. Once the anastomosis has been completed, one proceeds to fix the jejunal anastomotic limb to Glisson's capsule with several sutures in order to diminish traction on the suture line, as shown in the insert. A drainage tube with continuous suction is placed in Morrison's pouch before closing the abdominal wall.

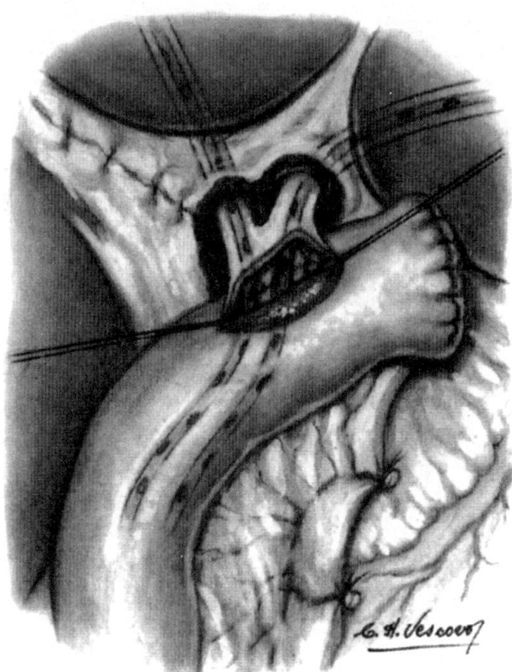

FIGURE 7.9

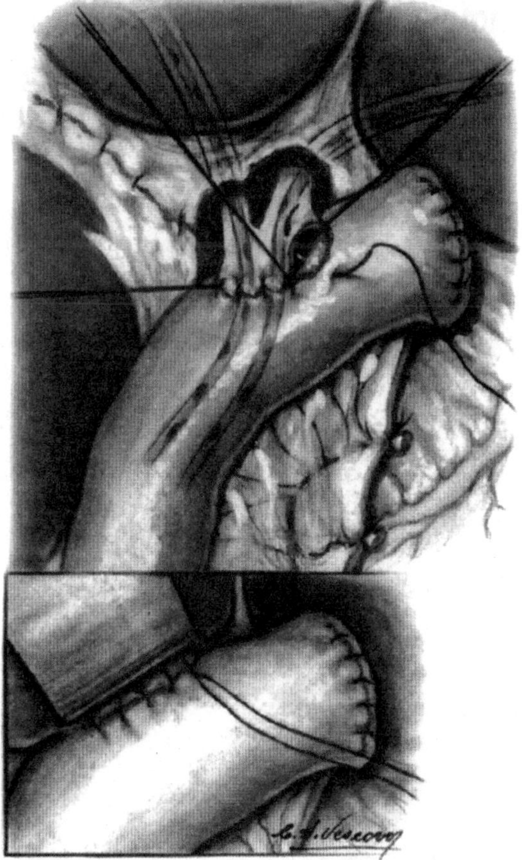

FIGURE 7.10

Cystic Dilation of the Common Bile Duct

FIGURE 7.11

In some patients, it is not possible to perform the resection of the cyst owing to the patient's poor general condition or because the cyst is fixed to neighboring structures. In these cases, an anastomosis is performed using interrupted sutures of synthetic 3-0 absorbable material between the most dependent portion of the cyst and the jejunum, as shown in the drawing. In some cases it is possible to perform this anastomosis in two planes, a full-thickness inner row of sutures using synthetic reabsorbable 3-0 sutures and an outer row of sutures, which on one side includes the peritoneum covering the cyst and on the other side includes the seromuscular jejunal tissue. This second row is performed with cotton or silk. This cystojejunal anastomosis may be permanent or temporary. Patients may improve their general condition, and this would allow, in a second operation, resection of the cyst. In the drawing one can observe that the resection of the gallbladder has been performed and its bed has been sutured. All patients who are subjected to a cystojejunal anastomosis should have the gallbladder resected because it has been shown that, if the gallbladder is left in place, cholecystitis will develop in the postoperative period. It should be noted that cystointestinal anastomosis will expose the patient to several complications and to the possibility of developing malignancy in the cyst and other segments of the biliary tract.

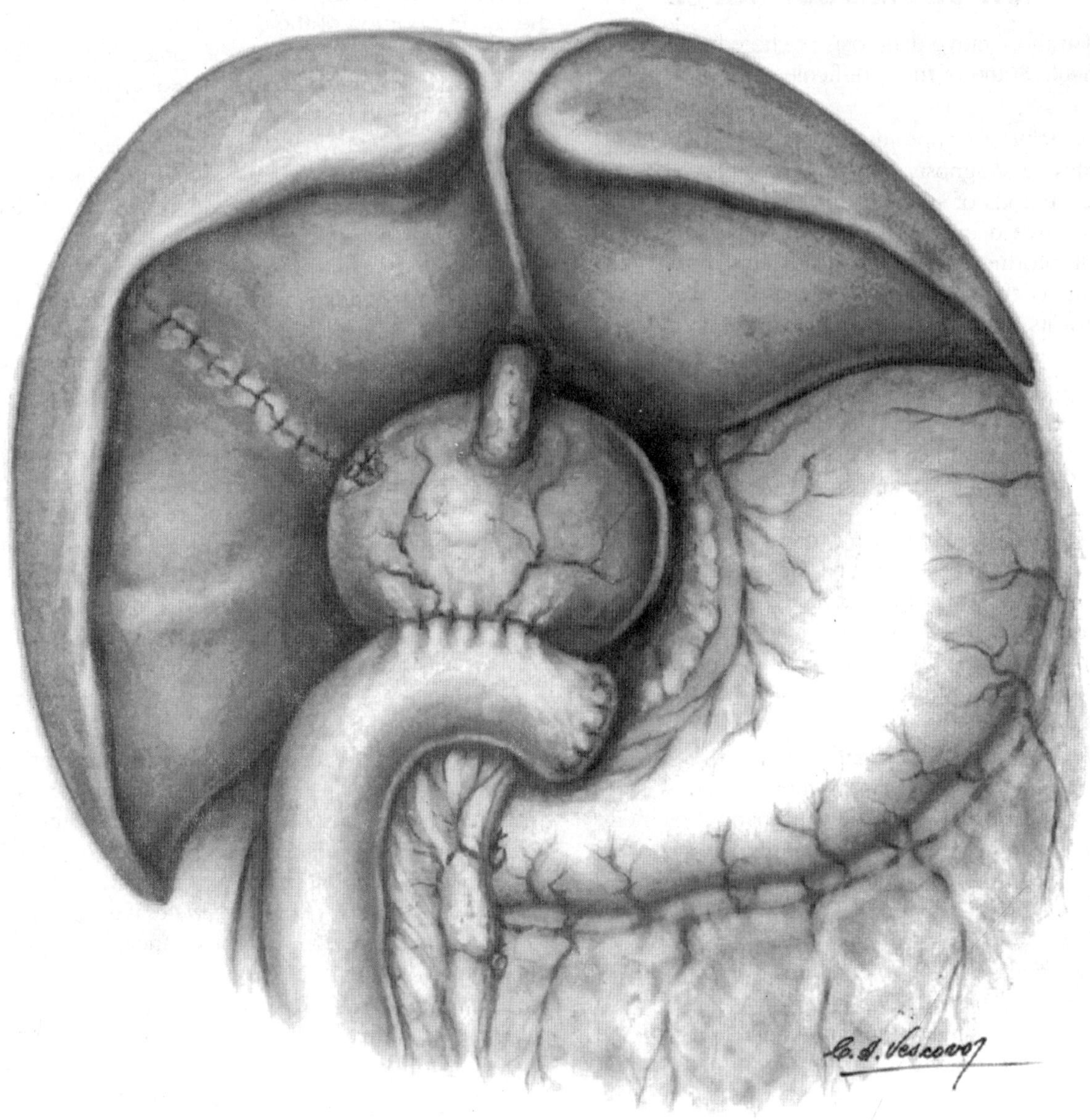

FIGURE 7.11

SURGERY FOR CHOLEDOCHOCELE

The clinical and operative diagnosis of choledochocele is usually difficult. Some of these difficulties are as follows:

1. Nonspecificity of symptoms presented by patients.
2. A conclusive diagnosis is rarely possible with the present methods of study at our disposal.
3. The operative diagnosis is difficult if the surgeon is not well informed on the characteristics of this condition and of the surgical maneuvers that must be realized for its identification.
4. Before resecting a choledochocele, it is important to determine exactly which variety is present and its relation with the common bile duct and the pancreatic duct because the surgical procedure to be employed is very different in each case. Choledochocele is a very rare affliction, and no surgeon can accumulate a very extensive experience with it. On the other hand, it is important to provide the greatest amount of information about this anomaly to facilitate its recognition and to perform adequate surgery for it. More than 50% of patients with choledochocele are under 30 years of age.

Some of the clinical manifestations that these patients present are vague dyspepsia; common hepatic biliary symptoms that improve with symptomatic treatment; right upper quadrant pain, usually moderate; and occasionally vomiting. Some patients may have intermittent jaundice; more rarely, some patients present a clinical picture of duodenal obstruction when the choledochocele is very large. Some patients may present bleeding due to erosions of the mucosa (25), and in some patients; one can see acute recurrent pancreatitis due to intermittent obstruction of the pancreatic duct (9, 15) and so on.

If the choledochal cyst is large, radiographic studies of the stomach and duodenum may show a tumorlike formation in the second portion of the duodenum that may lead to a diagnosis of a benign tumor of the second portion of the duodenum.

Endoscopic examination usually shows a smooth mass covered by duodenal mucosa of normal appearance, and this picture may be interpreted as a benign tumor. In cases in which it is possible to cannulate the common bile duct and perform retrograde endoscopic cholangiography, the diagnosis is more probable. Intravenous cholecystocholangiography is not usually adequate for a precise diagnosis, but at times it may show a cavity full of radiopaque material with the gallbladder and common hepatic duct normal in appearance.

Surgical procedures are generally performed through a longitudinal or subcostal incision in the right upper quadrant. One must always begin by performing an ample Vautrin-Kocher maneuver and a very careful palpation of the second portion of the duodenum. This careful palpation may detect the presence of something abnormal inside the duodenum, when the choledochal cyst is well developed. If the choledochal cyst is small, palpation of the duodenum is usually negative. To make an exact diagnosis, it is indispensable to perform a longitudinal duodenotomy in the second portion of the duodenum. The choledochocele presents itself as an ovoid mass of elastic consistency, covered by normal duodenal mucosa. This mass clearly protrudes into the duodenal lumen. The size of the mass is variable, varying generally from 2 to 15 cm in length and 2 to 12 cm in width. Duodenal mucosa constitutes the external wall of the choledochocele and is continuous with the mucosa of the rest of the duodenum. The interior wall of the choledochocele is made up of a mucosa that histologically may have the characteristics of duodenal mucosa, biliary mucosa, or a mixture of both.

Once the diagnosis of choledochal cyst has been confirmed, the next step is to determine which variety of choledochal cyst is present because the surgical procedure is different if the choledochal cyst is terminal, or lateral papillary. The general appearance of both varieties is very similar, but if a more detailed examination is performed one can note the differences that must be recognized. The choledochocele of the terminal variety presents on its surface an opening from which bile and pancreatic secretions flow. If the cyst is compressed, a few drops of bile will generally appear. If the gall bladder is compressed, bile usually comes out of the opening on the surface of the choledochocele. If a rubber catheter is introduced through the biliopancreatic opening, it generally stops because it gets rolled up in the cystic mass. In some cases, the choledochal cyst, instead of presenting one orifice that includes both the common bile duct and the pancreatic duct, presents two separate orifices, one corresponding to the common bile duct and the other to the pancreatic duct. In 40 to 50% of published cases, the cystic sac contains biliary calculi, generally of the stasis type. It is of utmost importance to perform operative cholangiography to obtain more exact information about the status of the biliary tract and of the relations of the biliary duct and the common bile duct with the choledochocele.

In the lateropapillary variety of choledochocele no opening is visible in its surface through which biliary and pancreatic secretions may come out, since these secretions pass through the papilla which is in its usual anatomic position. If a catheter is passed through the papilla, it will advance without obstruction into the common hepatic duct.

Once the exact diagnosis of the choledochal cyst and its variant is made, one can then proceed to its resection adapting the technique for each case, described as follows.

Surgery for Choledochocele

FIGURE 7.12
This semischematic drawing showing a choledochocele of the terminal variety projecting into the duodenal lumen. The exterior surface of the cyst is covered by normal duodenal mucosa. Its internal surface is covered by a mucosa that may be duodenal, biliary, or mixed. On the surface of the choledochal cyst, there is an opening through which biliary and pancreatic secretions flow. In other cases, there are two openings, one for biliary secretions and the other for pancreatic secretions.

Surgery for Choledochocele

FIGURE 7.13
The choledochocele is being resected by incising the duodenal mucosa covering its external surface.

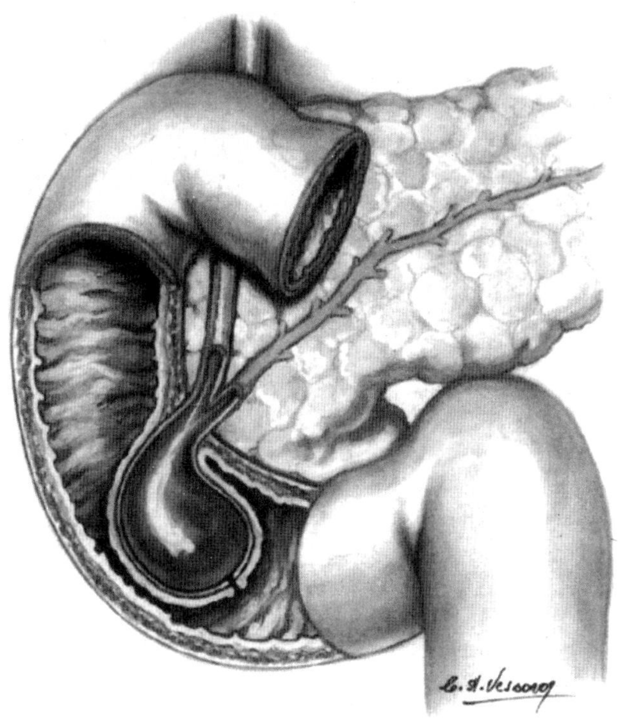

FIGURE 7.12

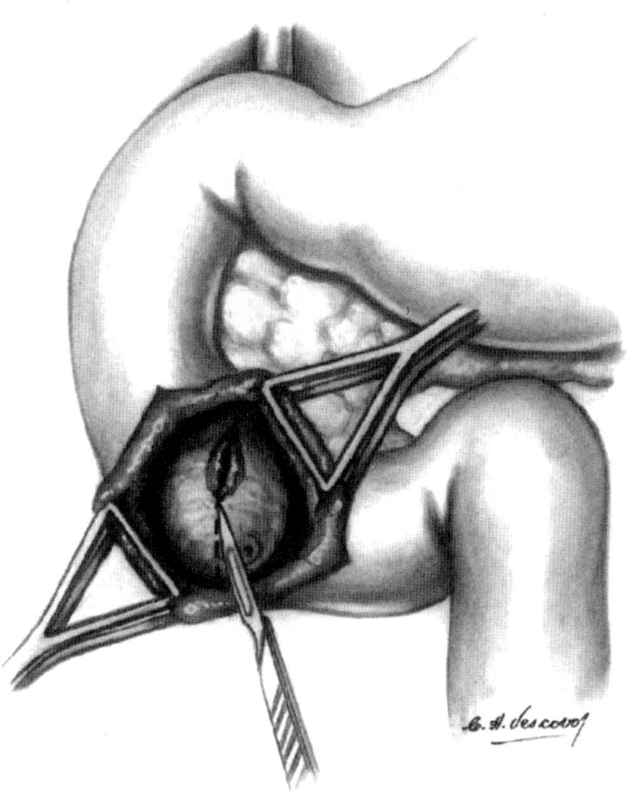

FIGURE 7.13

FIGURE 7.14
Seventy percent of the choledochocele is being removed. One must preserve the segment of the internal mucosa that surrounds the papilla and that will be sutured to the duodenal mucosa.

Surgery for Choledochocele

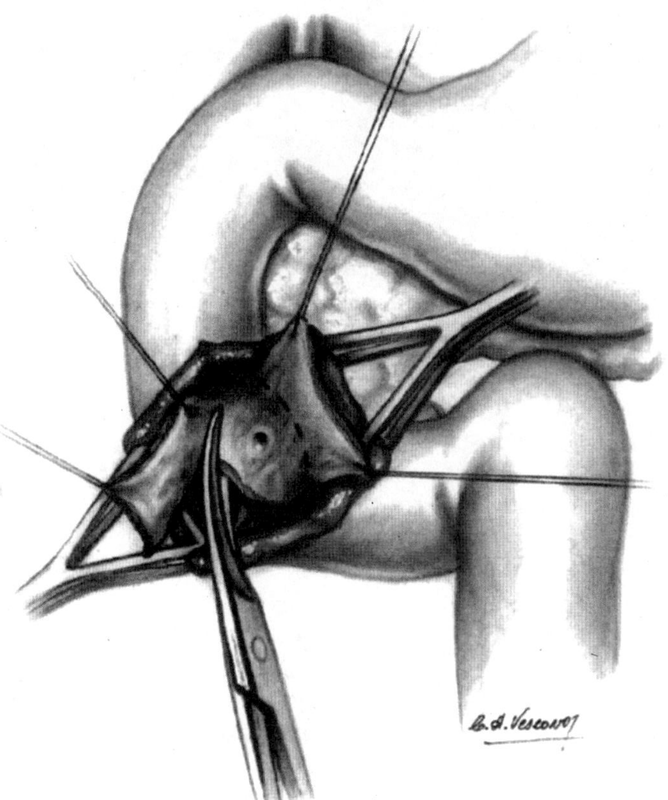

FIGURE 7.14

FIGURE 7.15
Once most of the choledochocele has been resected, the procedure is ended by performing an anastomosis between what remains of the internal mucosa surrounding the papilla and the duodenal mucosa using interrupted synthetic reabsorbable 3-0 sutures. Once the mucosal sutures are closed, the longitudinal duodenotomy is then closed in two layers, the internal plane with 2-0 chromic catgut, and the seromuscular suture line with cotton or silk. All of these are interrupted sutures.

Surgery for Choledochocele

FIGURE 7.16
Resection of a lateral papillary choledochocele. These choledochoceles are true diverticula of the common bile duct arising in the vicinity of the papilla. The diverticulum is joined to the common bile duct by a pedicle that is usually very thin. Resection of a choledochocele of this variety is much more simple than that of the terminal variety and consists in ligation and sectioning of the neck of the diverticulum near the common bile duct, as shown in the drawing. Some authors, fearing a residual stenosis of the papilla, add a sphincterotomy to this procedure.

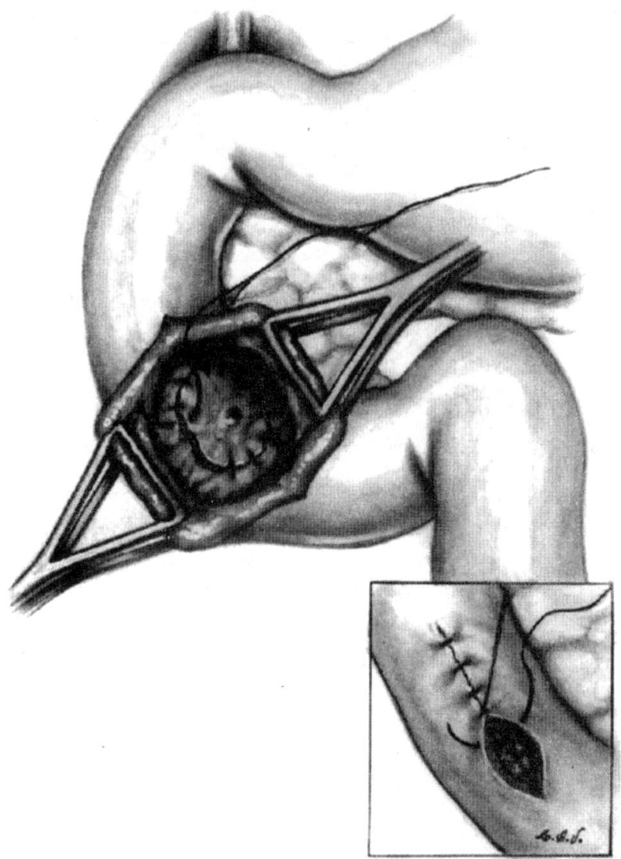

FIGURE 7.15

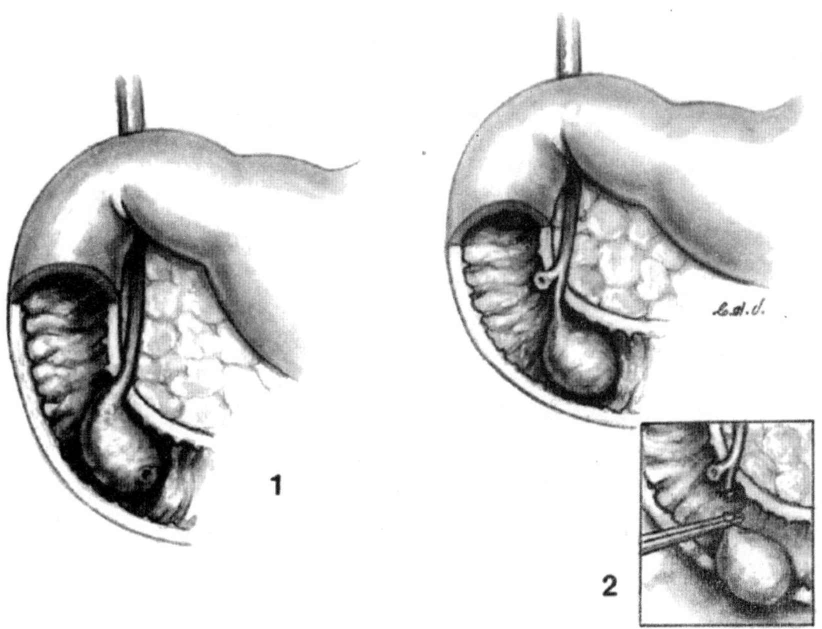

FIGURE 7.16

References

1. Alonso-Lej, F., Rever, W.B., Pessagno, D.J. Congenital choledochal cyst with a report of 2 and analysis of 94 cases. Int. Abstr. Surg. 108:1, 1959.
2. Babbitt, D., Sharshak, R., Clenimett, A. Choledochal cyst: A concept of etiology. Am. J. Roentgenol. 119:57, 1973.
3. Bass, E.M., Cremin, B.J. Choledochal cysts, a clinical and radiological evaluation of 21 cases. Pediatr. Radiol. 5:81, 1976.
4. Cameron J.L. Atlas of surgery. Vol. I., p. 116, B.C. Decker, Toronto, 1990.
5. Flanagan, D.P. Biliary cysts. Ann. Surg. 182:635, 1975.
6. Fonkalsrud, E.W., Boles, E.T. Choledochal cysts in infancy and childhood. Surg. Gynecol. Obstet. 121:733, 1965.
7. Fonkalsrud, E.W. Choledochal cysts. Surg. Clin. North Am. 58:1275, 1973.
8. Glenn, F., McSherry, C.K. Congenital segmental dilatation of the biliary ductal system. Ann. Surg. 177:705, 1973.
9. Greene, F.L., Brown, J.J., Rubinstein, P., Anderson, M.C. Choledochocele and recurrent pancreatitis. Diagnosis and surgical management. Am. J. Surg. 149:306, 1985.
10. Iwai, N., Deguchi, E., Yanagihara, J., et al. Cancer arising in a choledochal cyst in a 12 year old girl. J. Pediatr. Surg. 25:1261, 1990.
11. Iwai, N., Yanagihara, J., Tokiwa, K., Shimotake, T., Nakamura, K. Congenital choledochal dilatations with emphasis on pathophysiology of the biliary tract. Ann. Surg. 215:27, 1992.
12. Kimura, K., Ohto, M., Ono, T., et al. Congenital cystic dilatation of the common bile duct: Relationship to anomalous pancreatico-biliary ductal union. Am. J. Roentgenol. 128:571, 1977.
13. Kimura, K., Ohto, M., Saisho, H., et al. Association of gallbladder carcinoma and anomalous pancreatico-biliary ductal union. Gastroenterology 89:1258, 1985.
14. Kinoshita, H., Nagata, E., Hirohashi, K., Sakai, K., Kobayashi, Y. Carcinoma of the gallbladder with an anomalous connection between choledochus and the pancreatic duct. Report of ten cases and review of the literature in Japan. Cancer 54:762, 1984.
15. Kune, G.A., Sali, A. The practice of biliary surgery. Ed. 1, p. 275, Blackwell Scientific Publications, Oxford, 1980.
16. Longmire, W.P., Jr., Mandiola, S.A., Gordon, H.E. Congenital cystic disease of the liver and biliary system. Ann. Surg. 174:711, 1971.
17. Madding, G.F. Congenital cystic dilatation of the common bile duct. Ann. Surg. 154:288, 1961.
18. Miyano, T., Suruga, K., Suda, E. Abnormal choledocho-pancreatico ductal union related to the etiology of infantile obstruction disease. J. Pediatr. Surg. 14:16, 1979.
19. Nagata, E., Sakai, K, Kinoshita, H., Hirohashi, K. Choledochal cyst: Complications of anomalous connection between the choledochus and pancreatic duct and carcinoma of the biliary tract. World J. Surg. 10:102, 1986.
20. Nagorney, D.M., McLlrath, D.C., Adson, M.A. Choledochal cysts in adults: Clinical management. Surgery 96:656, 1984.
21. Pi-Figueras, J. Practica quirúrgica. Ed. 2, Vol. II, P. 744. Salvat, Barcelona, 1986.
22. Powell, S.C., Reynolds, H.V. Management of adult choledochal cysts. Ann. Surg. 193:666, 1981.
23. Roux, M., Debray, C., Le Canuet, R., Laumonier, R. Pathologie chirurgicale des voies biliarires extrahépatiques. p. 70. Masson et Cie., Paris, 1961.
24. Sherlock, S. Diseases of the liver and biliary system. Ed. 8, p. 500. Blackwell Scientific Publications, Oxford, 1989.
25. Simi, M., Carotenuto, F., Miceli, F. The so-called choledochocele: Report of a case. Chir. Ital. 3:160, 1973.
26. Todani, T., Tabuchi, K., Watanabe, Y., Kobayashi, T. Carcinoma arising in the wall of congenital bile duct cysts. Cancer 44:1134, 1979.
27. Trout, H.H., Longmire, W.F. Long term follow-up study of patients with congenital cystic dilatation of the common bile duct. Am. J. Surg. 121:68, 1971.
28. Vater, A. Dissertation in Auguralis Medica Proes. Diss quascirrhis viscerum dissert c.s. exlerus. 70:19, 1723.
29. Warren, K.W., Kune, G.A., Hardy, K.J. Biliary duct cysts. Surg. Clin. North Am. 48:567, 1968.
30. Warren, K.W., Jenkins, R.L., Steele, G.D., Jr. Atlas of surgery of the liver, pancreas and biliary tract. p. 54 Appleton-Lange, East Norwalk, CT, 1991.
31. Wheeler, W.I., DeCourcey, J. An unusual case of obstruction to the common duct (Choledochocele). Br. J. Surg. 27:446, 1940.

Section A

Surgery of the Biliary Tract

CHAPTER **8**

Caroli's Disease

Caroli's disease is a rare anomaly of congenital origin characterized by the presence of cystic dilations of the intrahepatic biliary ducts. These dilations are communicated between themselves by intrahepatic ducts that are of normal caliber or may be strictured. The dilations of the intrahepatic ducts in Caroli's disease produce a great alteration of the architecture of the liver and give rise to a substantial modi cation of the relation between parenchymatous tissue and ductal mass. It is a characteristic of these cystic dilations that they do not alter the smooth surface of the liver because they do not protrude outside of Glisson's capsule. Caroli's disease frequently manifests itself in localized form, but on some occasions, it can be accompanied by brosis of the liver or renal changes (2, 8, 11). Simultaneously with the cystic dilation of the intrahepatic ducts, one can observe in some patients a cystic dilation of the common bile duct (12). This association of cystic dilation of the intra- and extrahepatic ducts is seen frequently in oriental countries. More than 30% of the reports of these cystic dilations are by Japanese authors (15, 16).

According to Longmire and Tompkins (11), this disease was already known at the beginning of this century. The Englishmen Vachell and Stevens described this illness in 1906 (17), but this description was not remarked. It is probable that this poor repercussion of the discovery of this illness was due to the title of the publication, which was "A Case of Intrahepatic Stone." Jacques Caroli and his group wrote two papers in 1958 (3, 4) in which they describe the cystic dilations of the intrahepatic ducts including its clinical and pathologic aspects. Caroli was quite exact in describing the differences between this disease and polycystic disease of the liver. It was the excellent description made by the French gastroenterologist that led to the designation of this disease as Caroli's disease, and it is by this name that it is well known in international medical literature (5, 7, 10, 11, 18–20).

In the majority of cases, Caroli's disease presents in a diffuse form extending throughout the entire intrahepatic ductal system but it can also be limited to one of the hepatic lobes. It is six to seven times more frequent in the left lobe than the right lobe (19). There are very few reports in which Caroli's disease is strictly limited to a segment of the liver (11).

The symptoms of Caroli's disease are not very characteristic, and it is this lack of specificity together with the limited diagnostic methods available until the year 1973 that led to multiple operations in some patients in which the exact cause of the illness could not be determined and who were negative on surgical exploration.

The symptoms that these patients may present are pain in the right upper quadrant of the abdomen, sometimes with referral to the back, fever, chills, nausea, vomiting, intermittent jaundice, and so on. In some patients, Caroli's disease presents with a very grave clinical picture of a septic process.

The diagnosis of Caroli's disease is much easier now than before the year 1973. Technologic progress has allowed us to study these patients by ultrasonography, computerized endoscopic retrograde tomography, and transhepatic cholangiography.

Actually, patients with Caroli's disease are generally diagnosed preoperatively. If the diagnosis has not been made preoperatively, it can be made during the operation if cholangiography is included. Many cases of Caroli's disease have been missed because cholangiography was not performed during surgery. Operative cholangiography in these cases should be performed by puncture of the common hepatic duct and injecting the radiopaque substance with a certain pressure in a significant amount so that the intrahepatic ductal dilations can be shown. To ensure that the radiopaque material flows proximally into the intrahepatic ducts, the common hepatic duct should be obstructed distal to the site of puncture.

If the cholangiography is negative because there is no Caroli's disease, one should not forget to place a suture at the sight of the puncture to prevent leakage of bile postoperatively. If the diagnosis of Caroli's disease is made, the cholangiography will show the cystic dilations characteristically joined by ducts of normal caliber or ducts that are strictured. With some frequency operative cholangiography can demonstrate the presence of a variable number of calculi inside the cystic dilations. Sometimes it is possible to show some of the calculi that have migrated into the narrow strictured ducts blocking the passage of bile and leading to sepsis (8).

TREATMENT

The treatment of Caroli's disease varies according to the localization and the extension of the pathologic process. In patients in which the disease is localized to one of the hepatic lobes, the treatment of election is a left or a right hepatectomy. The removal of the affected lobe definitely cures the illness. Patients with diffuse Caroli's disease have a very poor chance of being treated adequately. The surgical treatment that is sometimes indicated in some patients with Caroli's disease is the anastomosis of the common hepatic duct to a loop of jejunum brought up in Roux-en-Y fashion, as will be detailed later. In the same operative procedure, transhepatic Silastic catheters are placed in each lobule that are later passed through the anastomosis and are connected to each other in a U-fashion. These will be used to continue postoperative treatment, to assist in dilating strictured ducts, in the removal of residual calculi as well as in performing endoscopic studies using flexible choledochoscopes of very small caliber to perform biopsies in areas that are suspicious for malignancy. It has been proven that Caroli's disease in some patients is a precursor of cholangiocarcinoma (1, 7, 9, 14–16). Some of the symptoms of Caroli's disease can improve temporarily following surgery. These may be disappearance of fever, diminution or disappearance of pain, disappearance of jaundice and cholangitis, and so on. This improvement of symptoms, however, in most cases is only partial and temporary, as is shown in the majority of new cases.

Patients that present a severe septic clinical picture should be treated intensively with antibiotics before surgery. If the treatment with antibiotics should fail, one can resort to transcutaneohepatic catheters. These catheters are left in place and joined in a U-fashion during surgery to continue treatment postoperatively.

Some surgeons, even without the patient presenting a septic clinical picture, place transhepatic catheters preoperatively (6). In cases in which Caroli's disease is associated with a cystic dilation of the common bile duct, resection of this cystic dilation of the common duct together with hepaticojejunal anastomosis should be performed in the same original surgical procedure (11, 12, 19).

Treatment

FIGURE 8.1
This drawing shows a case of diffuse Caroli's disease extending throughout the entire liver. The multiple sack-like dilations of the intrahepatic biliary ducts are communicated by strictured biliary ducts. Inside these cystic dilations one can observe multiple calculi. In addition, the drawing shows that the gallbladder has been removed and the gallbladder bed has been peritonealized. One can also see that the common hepatic duct is being transected by means of a scalpel in order to perform the anastomosis of this duct with a loop of jejunum brought up in Roux-en-Y fashion. The diagnosis of Caroli's disease at present should be made preoperatively. On the other hand, one should always perform operative cholangiography in order to confirm the diagnosis and determine the presence and localization of calculi, the location and caliber of strictured ducts and in order to facilitate the passage of catheters through the liver and the strictured areas. Cholangiography during surgery should be repeated after the removal of calculi to determine if any calculi remain, to remove them if it were possible and to try to identify them so that they can be removed postoperatively (6, 19, 20).

Treatment

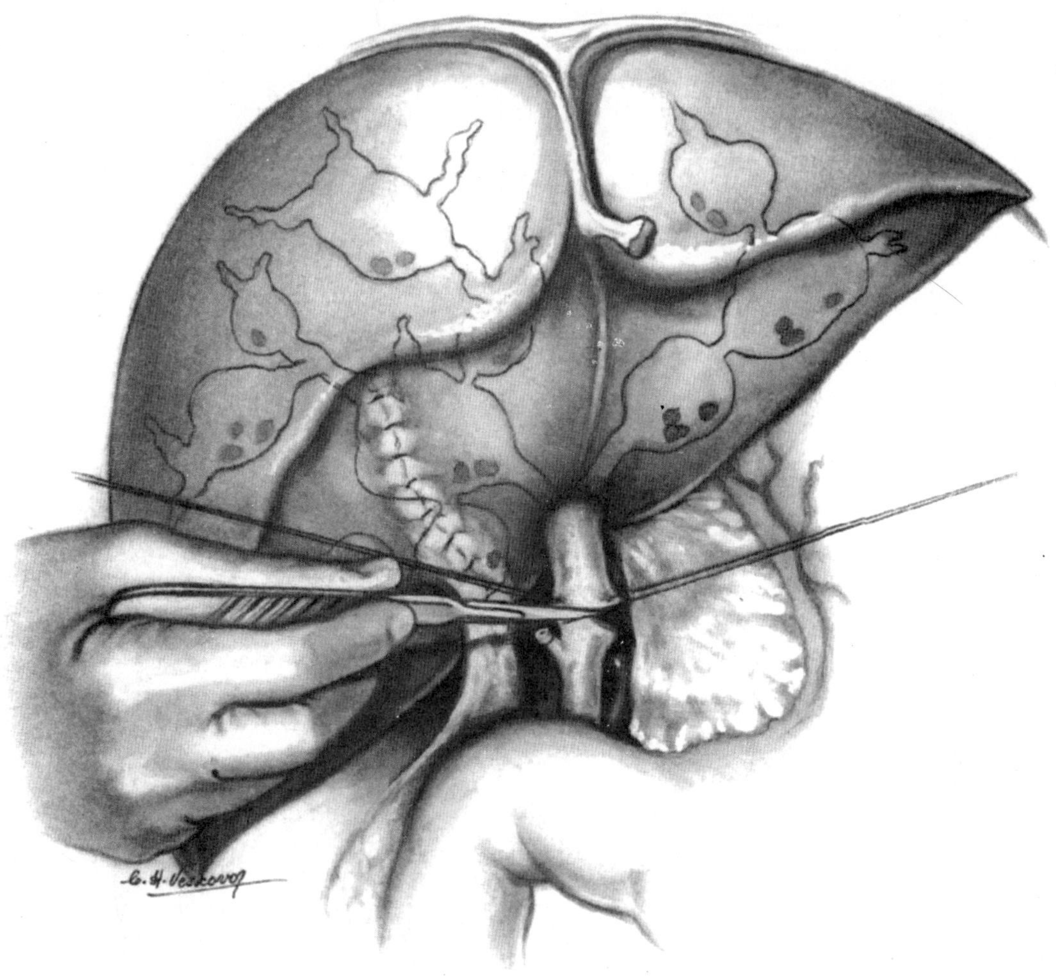

FIGURE 8.1

FIGURE 8.2

The common hepatic duct has been transected, revealing it to be somewhat dilated and being held open by two sutures on which traction is place in opposite directions. Through this common hepatic duct, a malleable spoon has been introduced to remove the multiple calculi that are lodged in the cystic dilations. The malleable spoon is reaching one of the calculi lodged in a cystic dilation. This maneuver must be repeated until the greatest number of calculi are removed. The distal portion of the common hepatic bile duct beyond the point of transection including the entire supraduodenal common bile duct have been resected. The distal stump of the common bile duct has been sutured with interrupted sutures of synthetic reabsorbable 4-0 material.

Treatment

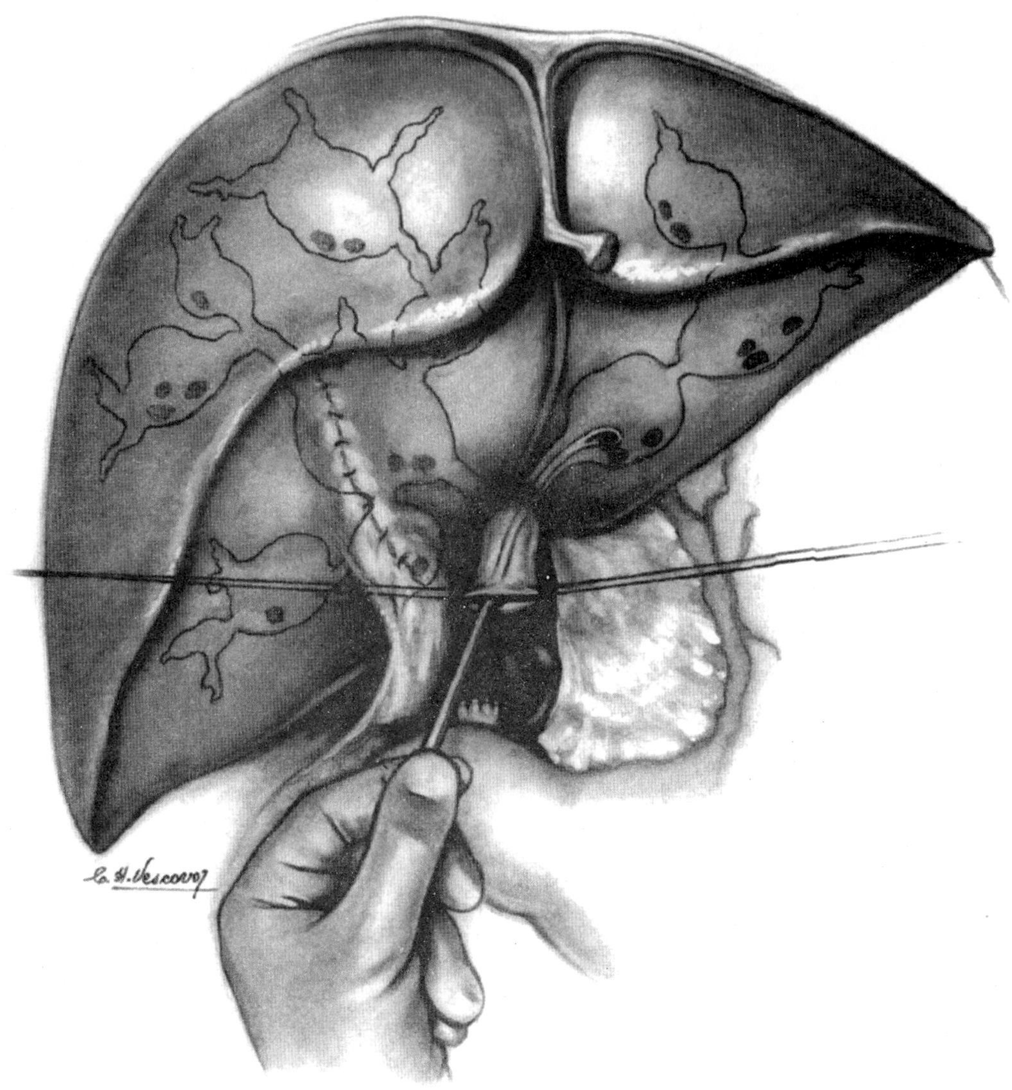

FIGURE 8.2

Treatment

FIGURE 8.3
Once all the calculi or most of them are removed, one proceeds to introduce a catheter through each lobe of the liver. These catheters are substituted by Silastic catheters with several perforations. In the drawing, one can observe that one of the transhepatic catheters placed in the right lobe is being substituted by a Silastic catheter. One then proceeds to do the same thing in the left lobe of the liver. One can observe in the drawing that not all of the calculi have been removed. One will attempt to remove these postoperatively (6, 18).

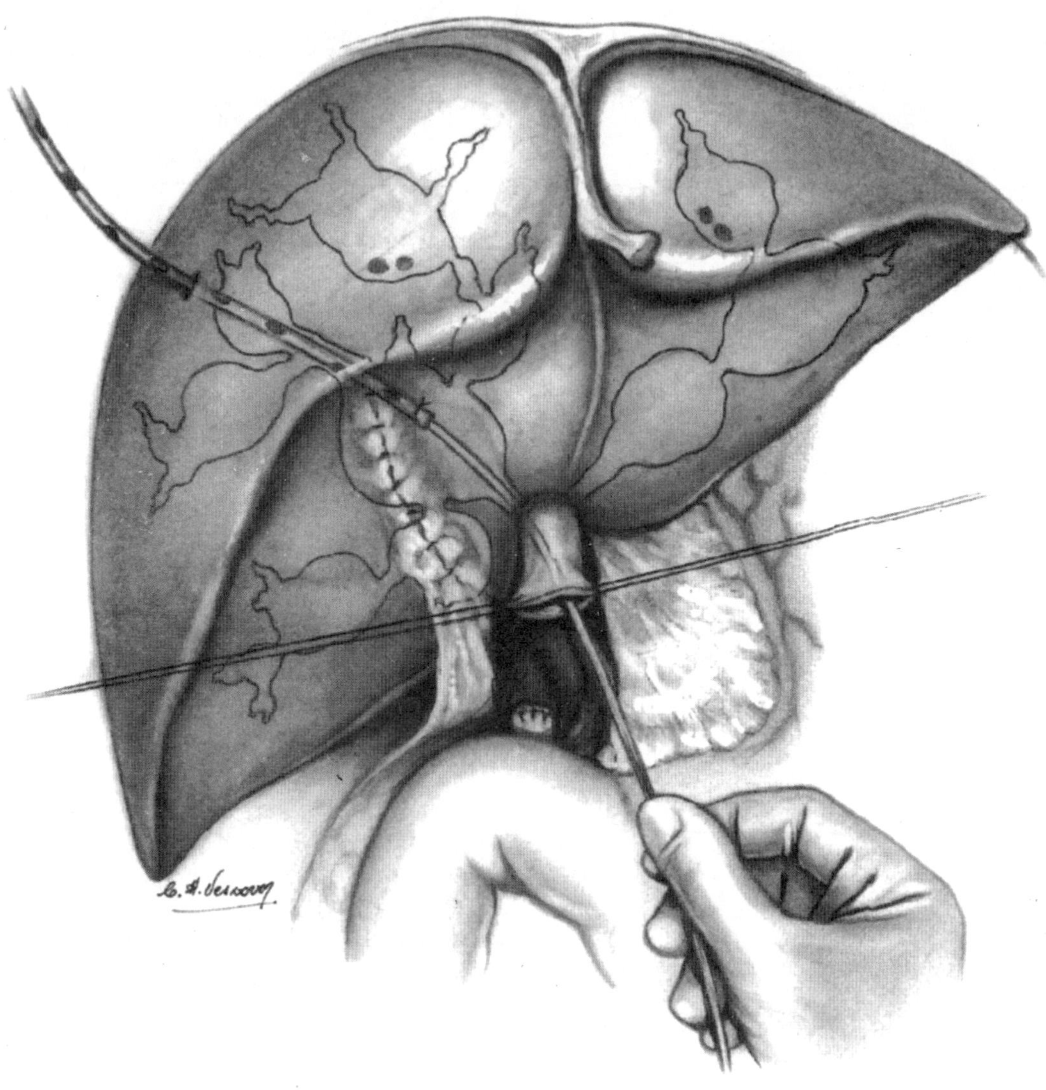

FIGURE 8.3

Treatment

FIGURE 8.4

The procedure has been completed. The dilated common hepatic duct has been anastomosed to the loop of jejunum brought up in Roux-en-Y fashion. The anastomosis has been performed in a terminolateral fashion with one row of sutures using interrupted reabsorbable 3-0 sutures. One can also observe the disposition of the transhepatic catheters in U-fashion. The ascending or anastomotic jejunal loop has been brought up through the transverse mesocolon and fixed to the mesocolon with a few sutures to avoid internal herniations. Postoperatively, one can complete the removal of calculi and dilate the strictured intrahepatic segments, and the possibility then exists for the introduction of a flexible choledochoscope of fine caliber in order to do biopsies of suspicious areas if this proves necessary (6, 18).

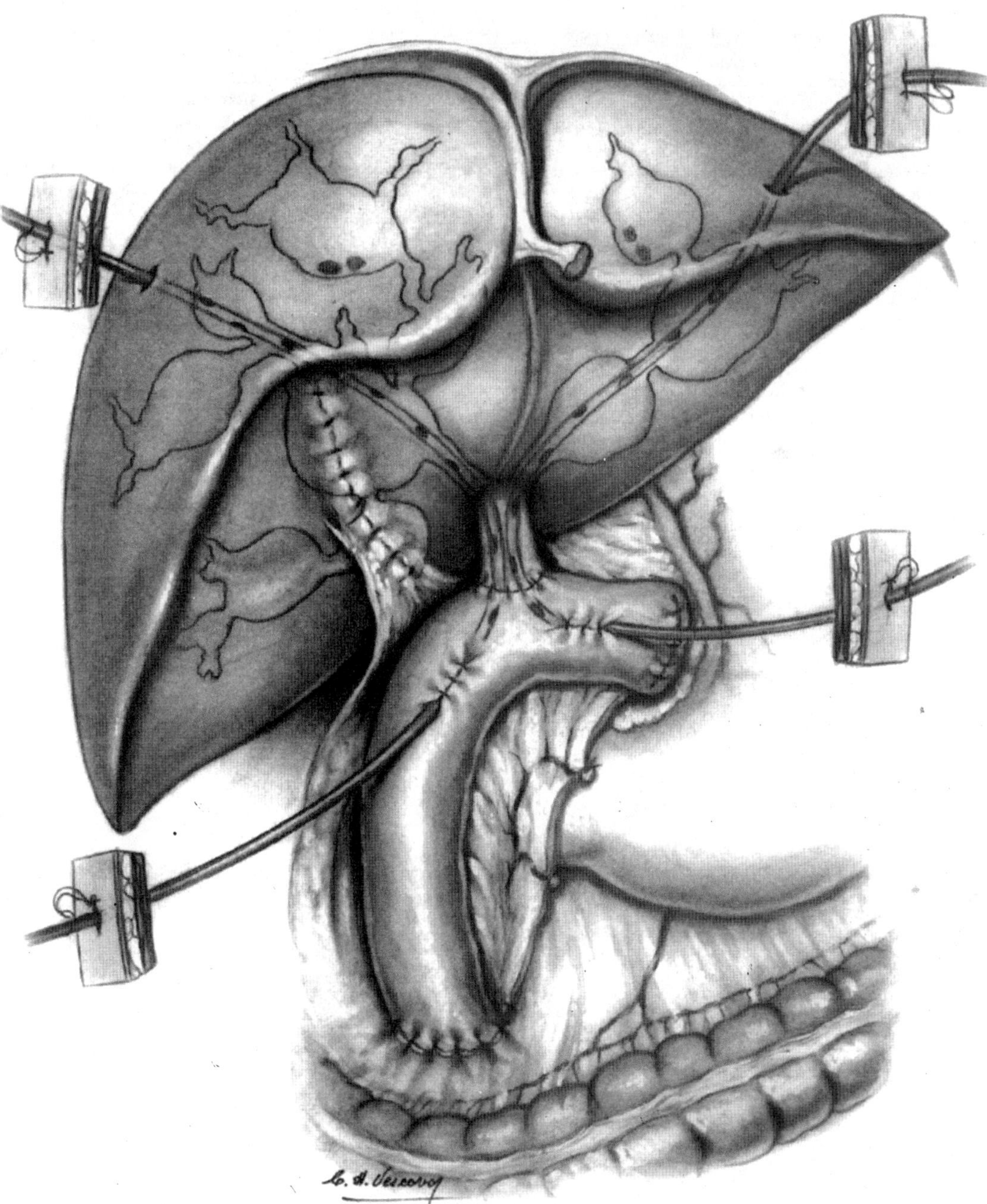

FIGURE 8.4

References

1. Bloustein, P.A. Association of carcinoma with congenital cystic conditions of the liver and bile ducts. Am. J. Gastroenterol. 67:40, 1977.
2. Cacchi, R., Ricci, V. Sur une rare maladie kistique multiple des pyramides rénales, le rein éponge. J. Urol. Med. Chir. 55:497, 1949.
3. Caroli, J., Soupault, R., Kossakowski, L., Plocker, L., Paradowska, M. La dilatation polykistique congénitale des voies biliaires intrahépatiques. Essai de classification. Semin. Hôp. Paris. 34:488, 1958.
4. Caroli, J., Couinaud, C. Une affection nouvelle, sans doute congénitale, des voies biliaires: La dilatation kystique unilobaire des canaux hépatiques. Semin. Hôp. Paris. 34:496, 1958.
5. Caroli, J., Laverdant, C., Moine, D., Hepp, J., Hadchouel, P. La dilatation kistique unilobaire des canaux biliaires segmentaires. Mal. J. Caroli Méd. Chir. Dig. 3:371, 1974.
6. Cameron, J.L. Atlas of surgery. Vol. I, p. 128. B.C. Decker, Toronto, 1990.
7. Dayton, M.T., Longmire, W.P., Tompkins, R.K. Caroli's disease: A premalignant condition? Am. J. Surg. 145:41, 1983.
8. Facciuto, E.M., Secchi, M.A., Todeschini, F. Dilatación congénita y litiasis de la vía biliar intrahepática. Enfermedad de Caroli. Rev. Argent. Cir. 55:7, 1988.
9. Jones, A.W., Shreeve, D.R. Congenital dilatation of the intrahepatic biliary ducts with cholangiocarcinoma. Br. Med J. 2:277, 1970.
10. Longmire, W.P., Mandiola, S.A., Gordon, H.E. Congenital cystic disease of the liver and biliary sister. Ann. Surg. 174:711, 1971.
11. Longmire, W.P., Tompkins, R.K. Manual of liver surgery. p. 138. Springer-Verlag, New York, 1981.
12. Loubeau, J.M., Steichen, F.M. Dilatation of intrahepatic bile ducts in choledochal cyst. Arch. Surg. 111:1384, 1976.
13. Mercadier, M., Chigot, J.F., Clot, J.P., Langlois, F., Lausiaux, P. Caroli's disease. World J. Surg. 8:22, 1984.
14. Mitchinson, M.J. Congenital dilatation of the intrahepatic bile ducts with cholangiocarcinoma. J. Clin. Pathol. 25:804, 1972.
15. Nagasue, N. Successful treatment of Caroli's disease by hepatic resection. Report of six patients. Ann. Surg. 200:718, 1984.
16. Tsuchida, Y., Ishida, M. Dilatation of intra-hepatic bile ducts in congenital cystic dilatation of the common bile duct. Surgery. 69:776, 1971.
17. Vachell, H.R., Stevens, W.M. Case of intrahepatic calculi. Br. Med. J. 1:434, 1906.
18. Warren, K.W., Jenkins, R.L., Steele, G.D., Jr. Atlas of surgery of the liver, pancreas and biliary tract. p. 64. Appleton-Lange, East Norwalk, CT, 1991.
19. Watts, D.R., Lorenzo, G.A., Beal, J.M. Congenital dilatation of the intrahepatic biliary ducts. Arch. Surg. 108:592, 1974.
20. Way, L.W. Current surgical diagnosis and treatment. Ed. 9, p. 554. Appleton-Lange, East Norwalk, CT. 1991.

Section A

Surgery of the Biliary Tract

CHAPTER 9

Laparoscopic Cholecystectomy

The first resection of the gallbladder was carried out by Langenbuch, of Berlin, on 15 July 1882. This operation was seriously criticized at that time, owing to the many complications that it caused, among which were biliary fistula and hemorrhage, for which reason it fell into disrepute. Several years later, Jean François Calot, of Paris, carried out extensive anatomic investigations of the biliary tract, especially the hepatic and cystic arteries and their relation to the cystic and common bile ducts. Calot published the results of his investigations in 1890. These were an important contribution to knowledge of the surgical anatomy of the hepatic hilus and were a valuable factor in diminishing the elevated morbidity and mortality of the cholecystectomy propounded by Langenbuch. Since then the mortality and morbidity of cholecystectomy progressively diminished to the low present figures. This is clear evidence that so-called open or conventional cholecystectomy is a very safe procedure (22, 26, 27). Many surgeons in many surgical centers around the world contributed to this progress. Among them were Ludwig Courvoisier, of Switzerland (1843–1918), who was the first surgeon to remove a calculus from the common duct, making an incision in the duct, and Hans Kehr, of Germany (1862–1916), who proposed exploration of the common bile duct through a choledochotomy to search for and remove any calculi in it. Kehr also proposed external drainage of the common bile duct after the choledochotomy and removal of calculi using a T-tube. Pablo Luis Mirizzi, of Argentina, in 1931, proposed the use of operative cholangiography. This is a radiographic examination of the common bile duct after the injection of radiopaque material. This diagnostic tool avoided an excess of choledochotomies and common duct explorations, which, according to Kehr, occurred in 50% of surgeries for biliary calculi. The operative cholangiography, proposed by Mirizzi, was used to observe the anatomy of the biliary tract, the presence of calculi in it, and the function of the sphincter of Oddi. The procedure identified which ducts should be explored. Mirizzi also proposed the use of control cholangiography to determine if all the calculi had been removed. The cholangiography that Mirizzi proposed in 1931 led to good results in surgery of the biliary tract and continues to be worthwhile today.

The first cholecystectomy by the laparoscopic route was performed by Muhe, of Boblingen, Germany, in 1985 (32). Two years later, in March 1987, Mouret of Lyon, France started to carry out this procedure. In addition to being a general surgeon, Mouret was also a gynecologic surgeon, used to doing surgical procedures via the laparoscope. François Dubois, of Paris (9, 10), in February 1988, stopped performing the minilaparotomy, which he favored greatly, and began to practice laparoscopic cholecystectomy. Périssat, of Bordeaux, France, started to perform laparoscopic cholecystectomy in November 1988, using his own technique (26, 27). Simultaneously, laparoscopic cholecystectomy was begun by McKerman and Saye, in Marietta, Georgia, using laser for the dissection of the gall bladder. Also in 1988, Reddick, of Nashville, Tennessee, began to perform laparoscopic cholecystectomy. This technique was also used by Berci, of Los Angeles, by Zucker, in Baltimore, by Cuschieri, in Dundee, England, by Testas, in Paris, and by many other surgeons (8, 9, 19, 21, 26, 27).

The great contributions made by engineers, builders of microcameras and of many endoscopic instruments, contributed greatly to the development and spread of this technique. In 1990, Reddick and Olsen published the first series of cases operated by the laparoscopic approach (34).

Laparoscopy is not a new procedure, having been described in 1901 but then used only for diagnostic purposes. Laparoscopy gained momentum in 1970, when it was first used in gynecologic surgery. Development of fiber optics, the transmission of light by means of optic fibers, and the addition of video contributed greatly to the development of this technique. The video made it possible for all the members of the surgical team to see the procedure.

As more experience with the procedure has been acquired by surgeons and patients have been correctly selected, the early very high rate of severe complications has been diminished (7, 14, 23, 28, 37, 38).

Surgeons who practice laparoscopic cholecystectomy should be experienced in open biliary surgery and be able to repair the biliary tree if it is injured. They should also be flexible enough to convert laparoscopic surgery into an open procedure if difficulties or complications should develop. Patients and their relatives should be clearly warned before the surgery of the possibility of having to convert to an open procedure.

The advantages of laparoscopic cholecystectomy are (a) less hospitalization time, (b) diminution of time before return to work, (c) better cosmetic results, and (d) less postoperative pain and less possibility of infections and eviscerations.

Laparoscopic cholecystectomy does have some disadvantages when compared to open surgery:

1. Vision is not tridimensional.
2. The surgeon cannot carry out manual or digital palpation.
3. Inflammatory edema may lead to an error in visual appreciation.
4. Laparoscopic surgery cannot be performed in 100% of cases with biliary calculi. According to the surgeon's experience, a larger or smaller proportion of cases will have to be converted to open surgery.
5. In some patients laparoscopic cholecystectomy is either contraindicated or impossible.
6. In some patients the laparoscopic surgery should be converted to open surgery owing to complications or technical difficulties.
7. Removal of calculi by the transcystic approach or through a choledochotomy during a laparoscopic cholecystectomy can only be carried out in selected cases owing to technical difficulties. There is no doubt that it is necessary to perfect the system to make it more efficient and safer in removing calculi from the common duct. On the other hand, the instruments now available are imperfect, fragile, and expensive.
8. Opening and closing the bile duct and the introduction of a T-tube are not easy and expose the patient to complications, some of them serious (16, 17, 23, 30, 35, 42).

CONTRAINDICATIONS OF LAPAROSCOPIC SURGERY

Cholecystectomy is contraindicated in patients in poor condition who cannot tolerate general anesthesia or in cardiac patients unable to tolerate pneumoperitoneum. Patients with serious hepatic conditions or with coagulation defects cannot be subjected to this technique. Careful selection should be made of patients with previous upper abdominal surgery, such as pancreatic, hepatic, or gastroduodenal procedures. Patients with calculi in the common duct that have not been resolved prior to surgery should be subjected to the open approach. Patients with severe changes in the gallbladder wall, such as marked thickening and increased consistency, should generally be excluded. Patients with biliary-biliary or biliary-enteric fistula, acute gangrenous or perforated cholecystitis, or porcelain cholecystitis (37) and patients with pacemakers should not be subjected to laparoscopic cholecystectomy. When laparoscopic cholecystectomy was first undertaken it was felt to be contraindicated in acute cholecystitis due to the high risk for the patient. At present, however, in experienced hands, 80% of these patients are operated by laparoscopy (5, 38, 41). In spite of this, the patient should be advised that acute cholecystitis is a frequent cause for conversion to open surgery.

There is a learning curve and the greater the experience of the surgeon, the lesser the contraindications.

POSITION OF THE PATIENT AND THE SURGICAL EQUIPMENT

The patient is placed in the dorsal decubitus position for both the laparoscopic or open procedure, if the latter becomes necessary. Local preparation is carried out as usual, with special care to clean and disinfect the umbilicus to prevent omphalitis. The surgeon is on the patient's left, with the second assistant on the surgeon's left to handle the laparoscope. The first assistant is to the right of the patient with the instrument nurse and the instrument tray to the right. The television screen, the videocassette player, the camera controls, the light source, and the electronically controlled CO_2 source are placed to the right of the patient's head. The surgeon and the second assistant will be facing the television images. The first assistant can observe the televised images in another television placed at the head of the left side of the operating table.

In France, as well as in some European and Latin-American countries, the patient's lower limbs are abducted and the surgeon stands between them. This is known as the French position (8, 9, 10, 26, 27).

PNEUMOPERITONEUM

Pneumoperitoneum is necessary for the laparoscopy. CO_2 gas is insufflated to produce the pneumoperitoneum for the following reasons: (a) It is innocuous. (b) It is soluble in blood. (c) It diffuses readily. (d) It is not combustible. (e) It does not irritate the peritoneum. (f) It is cheap (30). It is indispensable that the CO_2 concentration be monitored during the procedure.

The Veress needle is usually used to carry out the pneumoperitoneum (36). There are two Veress needles, a reusable metallic one and a disposable one. The latter is used more frequently, has an external diameter of 2 mm, and varies from 70 to 120 mm in length. It has an obturator with a blunt end that is fired by a trigger. The blunt end of the obturator is designed to cover the bevel of the needle as it passes through the peritoneum. The object of the blunt obturator is to prevent injury to an abdominal viscera or blood vessel. Some surgeons prefer to perform the pneumoperitoneum by a so-called open method, using the Hasson trocar (15).

Insufflation of carbon dioxide through a Veress needle may cause hypercapnia and acidosis, for which reason continuous, rigorous monitoring of cardiovascular and respiratory activity during the entire procedure is essential. If cardiovascular or respiratory complications occur, the carbon dioxide should be evacuated. Precautions should be taken to avoid injuries to viscera or blood vessels upon introduction of the Veress needle.

TECHNIQUE OF INTRODUCTION OF THE VERESS NEEDLE

An incision 10 mm long is made in the fold of skin just above the umbilicus to introduce the Veress needle and the following 10-11 mm trocar. The subcutaneous tissue is then dissected by blunt technique with the finger or a gauze pledget down to the fascia. Some surgeons place the incision in the fold below the umbilicus and others through the umbilicus itself. The patient is placed in the Trendelenburg position with 15 to 20 degrees of tilt. On both sides of the umbilicus Backhaus gauze clamps are placed so that they grasp the skin, the subcutaneous layer, and the anterior fascia of the rectus abdominis muscles. The clamps are pulled upward to pull the anterior abdominal wall away from the intraperitoneal viscera, diminishing the possibility of injuring the viscera when the Veress needle is introduced. In order to accomplish this, it is important that the clamps grasp the anterior fascia of the rectus abdominis muscles as well as the skin and subcutaneous tissue. Once this maneuver has been performed, the Veress needle is then introduced through the incision in the umbilical fold. Experienced surgeons do not place the patient in slight Trendelenburg nor do they orient the needle toward the pelvis. At the moment that the Veress needle perforates the peritoneum, the clear click of the needle's protective mechanism is heard.

Before insufflation of the carbon dioxide, it must be ascertained that the end of the Veress needle is free in the abdominal cavity. In order to confirm this, about 5 mL of saline solution are injected through the needle. This solution will very easily enter the abdominal cavity, and it will be impossible to recover the fluid by aspiration through the same needle. Aspiration through the needle should not yield gas bubbles indicative of a perforated hollow viscus. Further assurance of correct placement of the end of the needle is obtained as follows: A drop of normal saline is placed on the upper end of the needle and rapid passage of the drop into the peritoneal cavity is observed when the Backhaus clamps are pulled upward.

Once the position of the end of the Veress needle in the peritoneal cavity is confirmed, insufflation of CO_2 is begun, using moderate flow at first and using percussion to confirm the disappearance of hepatic dullness. Insufflation is gradually increased until a pressure of 14 mm of Hg in the abdominal cavity is attained, which usually requires 3 to 5 liters of CO_2. During insufflation, the insufflator should show a low intraabdominal pressure, insuring free flow of the gas. The alarm should not go off. The patient should be well relaxed.

PLACEMENT OF THE TROCARS

Placement of the first trocar is always blind, which makes trauma to a viscus or a blood vessel a distinct possibility. To diminish this risk, some precautions should be taken, particularly by inexperienced surgeons. The patient should be kept in the 15 to 20° Trendelenburg position. Traction should again be applied upward to the Backhaus clamps placed to separate the intraperitoneal viscera from the abdominal wall.

The first trocar to be introduced is 10 to 11 mm in diameter and will be passed through the small incision in the superior umbilical fold used to insert the Veress needle. The trocar is inserted making rotatory movements with the end directed toward the pelvic cavity. Once the trocar is in place, the obturator is removed and the CO_2 source is connected and inserted through the cannula of the laparoscope, to which the camera and the light source have already been coupled. The surgeon should first explore all visible parts of the abdominal cavity and verify if any lesions occurred during insertion of the Veress needle and the first trocar. Next, the anterior auxiliary 5-mm catheter is placed in the right flank at the level of the umbilicus. Through this channel an atraumatic grasper will be introduced. This grasper will grasp the fundus of the gallbladder, at the same time as it will produce an upward luxation of the liver exposing its inferior surface and the gallbladder. The third 5 mm trocar is then inserted in the midclavicular line, about 4 or 5 cm below the costal margin. Another atraumatic grasper is then passed through this channel and applied to the infundibulum of the gallbladder exposing the triangle of Calot. A fourth trocar, 10 to 11 mm in diameter, is inserted in the epigastrium, some 4 or 5 cm from the xiphoid process, slightly to the right of the midline. Through this channel special instruments will be passed, such as dissection hoods, spatulas, portaclips, aspirator-irrigators, scissors, and so on. The actual site of insertion of the various trocars can be varied according to the actual location of the anterior edge of the liver and the location of the gallbladder.

LAPAROSCOPIC CHOLECYSTECTOMY

Prior to starting the removal of the gallbladder, the position of the patient is changed from the original Trendelenburg with 15 to 20° of tilt to a reverse Trendelenburg with 15 to 20° of tilt with the addition of about 15° of tilt to the left to allow the abdominal viscera to fall away from the operative area, leaving the undersurface of the liver free. An atraumatic grasper is passed through the anterior axillary channel grasping the gallbladder. Traction is then applied upward displacing the liver and exposing the gallbladder and the undersurface of the liver. Another grasper is introduced through the midclavicular channel and the infundibulum of the gallbladder is grasped, starting the dissection of the gallbladder with the dissection of the cystic duct near the infundibulum. The cystic duct is freed circumferentially at this level, and it is then occluded with a clip near the infundibulum. When the area near the common bile duct and the hepatic artery is dissected, a cautery should not be used to avoid damaging these structures. A microscissors is introduced through the midclavicular channel, and a small transverse incision is made in the anterior wall of the cystic duct distal to the previously placed clip. This incision has the objective of allowing a thin catheter to be introduced into the duct with the help of an Olsen clamp, designed by this author to facilitate carrying out the cholangiography (1, 4, 12, 22, 29, 35, 42). Through the cystic duct catheter, held in place by the Olsen clamp, 5 mL of radiopaque solution, diluted to 35%, are injected under radiologic control with the image intensifier. This first injection has the objective of determining the diameter of the common duct, the presence of calculi, and the functional behavior of the sphincter of Oddi. An additional 5 mL of radiopaque solution are then injected to fill the hepatic ducts completely and see if there are variations, anomalies, or calculi, using at least two films.

If the bile duct is dilated, more radiopaque solution may have to be injected. If there is no Olsen clamp available for the operative cholangiogram, the surgeon can use a 4F ureteral catheter introduced into the cystic duct no more than 3 cm and held in place by means of a clip to prevent the reflux of dye without occluding the lumen of the catheter. Many catheters are available to facilitate laparoscopic operative cholangiography. The surgeon can select the most adequate one according to his or her experience and the condition of the cystic duct. Laparoscopic operative cholangiography is not difficult when the cystic duct is ample or normal in caliber and empties into the right edge of the common duct at an acute or right angle. There is also no great problem with small cystic ducts that can be dilated. Cholangiography can be difficult or impossible in strictured, sclerotic, retracted ducts that cannot be dilated. Cystic ducts with multiple valves of Heister can also present difficulties. Cystic ducts that run parallel or in spiral fashion in relation with the common duct, and that, instead of emptying into the right edge of the common duct, run behind or in front of it and empty into its left border, may be impossible to catheterize. (See "Surgical Anatomy of the Biliary Tract.")

In order to correctly perform the operative cholangiogram, the position of the patient has to be modified from a Trendelenburg position with 15 to 20° of tilt. The patient is placed horizontally and then tilted to the right some 15° to avoid superimposing the shadow of the duct on the vertebral column. Further superimposition of radiopaque shadows can be avoided by removing the laparoscope. Additionally, it is advisable to use disposable trocars that, in contrast with reusable ones, are made of plastic and are therefore radiolucent. If reusable metallic trocars are used, they should be oriented so that they do not obstruct complete visualization of the cholangiogram.

If the cholangiogram shows a common bile duct of normal caliber, without shadows of calculi and with passage of dye into the duodenum without difficulty, the catheter is removed from the cystic duct and the duct it is occluded with two clips placed on the common duct side. The cystic duct is then transected between the original clip on the infundibular side and the two clips placed near the common duct. After the cystic duct is transected, traction should be avoided on the gallbladder to prevent rupture of the cystic artery, which may lead to severe bleeding and having to convert to an open procedure at once. Once the cystic duct is divided, the cystic artery is dissected. It is usually in the triangle of Calot. Two clips are placed proximally and two additional clips distally, as near as possible to the infundibulum, and the artery is transected with scissors. It is necessary to clearly identify the cystic artery so as not to commit the error of ligating and transecting only one of its branches, most commonly the anterior branch as it enters the gallbladder wall.

After the cystic duct and artery have been transected, the gallbladder is dissected, separating it from its bed. This is carried out using hooks, spatulas, and other instruments connected to the electrocautery. Dissection is performed in retrograde fashion, from cystic duct to fundus. Hemostasis in the liver bed must be carried out with extreme care. Attention must be given to any bile leakage, which is generally from an aberrant bile duct in the liver bed. When the gallbladder has been almost completely dissected from its bed, it is still held by the graspers, to be able to see the liver bed and irrigate it with normal saline, in order to be sure there are no sites of bleeding or bile leakage. Aspiration should be limited to the gallbladder bed. Care should be taken with suction in the vicinity of the cystic duct or artery stumps, since the clips may be pulled off, leading to hemorrhage or bile leakage. Irrigation and aspiration of the subphrenic and subhepatic spaces should be carried out to prevent the development of septic collections, which may alter the postoperative course of the patient.

Once bleeding has been controlled, the laparoscope is transferred from the umbilical to the epigastric channel, in order to facilitate the removal of the gallbladder through the new work channel, the umbilical channel. The gallbladder has been completely freed but is still held by the graspers. A strong "claw clamp" or "crocodile" clamp is introduced through the umbilical channel, and after grasping the infundibulum of the gallbladder with it, the original graspers are removed. Traction is applied to the claw clamp to remove the gallbladder, following every move with the camera to confirm that the gallbladder enters the work channel. If CO_2 was being insufflated through this cannula, it should be changed to another cannula because the gallbladder will completely obstruct the lumen of the cannula, which is also removed with the cannula. The infundibulum is partially exteriorized, opened, and the calculi removed. If the calculi are larger than 1 cm. they should be crushed to remove them. Once the umbilical cannula has been removed, the fascia is sutured with interrupted Vicryl. Closure is completed with subdermal sutures. The 5-mm cannulas are then removed under laparoscopic vision. The gas is then removed from the abdomen, and the 10 to 11 mm epigastric channel and the two 5-mm channels are closed subdermally. The nasogastric tube is removed and the patient is allowed to take oral liquids, once he has woken from anesthesia. If there have been no complication, the patient can be discharged in a few hours or 24 to 48 hours after surgery.

Laparoscopic Cholecystectomy in Patients with Acute Cholecystitis

Acute cholecystitis is not an absolute contraindication to cholecystectomy by the laparoscopic approach. As previously stated, 80% of cases of acute cholecystitis can be operated by the laparoscopic approach in centers with experience in this surgery. The development of many instruments to facilitate laparoscopic surgery, and the experience gained by surgeons have, undoubtedly, contributed to this progress (40, 41).

Acute cholecystitis, however, continues to be the cause of many conversions (13, 19, 32, 41). Surgical resection of the acutely inflamed gallbladder should be performed by surgeons with experience in laparoscopic and open surgery. Some special measures should be taken in these patients. It must be remembered that frequently there are distended small bowel loops, which present a greater risk of perforation during the introduction of the Veress needle and the first trocar, which is done blindly. In these patients the gallbladder may be distended and its walls thickened, making it difficult to apply the graspers (41). In order to grasp a very distended gallbladder, a suture can be applied to the fundus, leaving the ends long so that traction can be exerted with an atraumatic grasper (41). In other cases, it may be necessary to puncture and aspirate the gallbladder, removing part of its contents, making it easier to grasp its wall with an atraumatic grasper. When a distended gallbladder is grasped, it can be perforated. This perforation can sometimes be closed with another grasper. If these maneuvers are not successful, an attempt can be made to close the perforation using a pretied laparoscopic suture. Rupture of the gallbladder should be controlled as soon as possible. If calculi fall into the abdominal cavity, some surgeons resort to the use of baskets introduced into the abdomen following atraumatic graspers holding the calculi. These maneuvers are not always successful, and several articles have pointed out that calculi abandoned in the abdominal cavity can give rise to complications. If the perforation of the gallbladder allows passage of calculi and septic contents into the peritoneum, the surgeon should not hesitate to convert the laparoscopic cholecystectomy to open surgery.

Conversion of Laparoscopic Cholecystectomy to Open Surgery

Many events can make conversion of laparoscopic surgery to open surgery necessary. The incidence of conversion is related to the surgeon's experience. Some surgeons have a 1 to 4% conversion rate; others have higher conversion rates, even over 10%. The acceptable conversion rate varies between 4 to 8% (3, 8, 13, 27, 31). The most frequent causes of conversion are acute cholecystitis and inability to clearly identify the surgical anatomy of the biliary tract. Other, less frequent, causes of conversion are the following:

1. Sclerotic, atrophic gallbladders with fibrous retraction and adhesion to the common duct.
2. Patients in whom carcinoma of the gallbladder is suspected or has been confirmed during laparoscopic exploration.
3. Patients with other unsuspected abdominal problems.
4. In patients whose common duct has been injured.
5. Hemorrhage that cannot be controlled laparoscopically.
6. Injury to a hollow viscus by burns caused by the electrocautery or perforations produced by introduction of the Veress needle or the trocars.
7. Choledocholithiasis that could not be resolved preoperatively or during the operation.
8. Patients with large Hartmann pouch adherent to the common duct.
9. Mirizzi syndrome.
10. In patients in whom the gallbladder, after being liberated, has been dropped into the abdominal cavity, where it cannot be found and removed.

Conversion to open surgery can be decided upon at various moments: (a) immediately after laparoscopic exploration, (b) shortly after beginning to dissect the gallbladder, (c) at the time of injury to the common duct, and (d) at the moment hemorrhage has occurred that could not be controlled laparoscopically.

The surgeon should be flexible enough to convert the laparoscopic cholecystectomy to an open procedure when he or she realizes the operation is not progressing in satisfactory manner, without waiting for an accident to happen before deciding on conversion.

Some surgeons believe that, if the laparoscopic procedure is not advancing well after an hour, conversion to an open procedure should be done (35).

Complications of Laparoscopic Cholecystectomy

Laparoscopic surgery may give rise to complications, some of minor importance, others very grave. Among the first group is shoulder pain due to diaphragmatic distension caused by CO_2 insufflation. This usually subsides in a few days. Another complication is vomiting, which usually subsides spontaneously. The serious complications are injury to the common duct, injury to hollow viscera, hemorrhage from the cystic artery due to loosening of the clip, hemorrhage from the gallbladder bed, hemorrhage from the trocar puncture sites, leakage of bile, omphalitis caused by inadequate preoperative cleansing and disinfection or contamination as the gallbladder is extracted, and development of subphrenic or subhepatic suppurative collections (7, 11, 14, 24, 36, 41).

REMOVAL OF CALCULI FROM THE COMMON DUCT

Removal of calculi from the common duct by laparoscopy is undoubtedly more complicated and has a higher risk than in open surgery. Even though laparoscopic surgery has progressed greatly, it has proved impossible to remove all the calculi from the common duct. For this reason, it should be considered that removal of calculi by the laparoscopic approach is still in evolution.

Calculi in the common duct can sometimes be removed though the cystic duct and through a choledochotomy in other cases.

Removal of calculi by the transcystic route should be tried, before opening the common duct. It should be admitted, however, that there are great limitations to this approach. Some of these limitations are the following:

1. Only small, free-lying calculi can be removed by this route.
2. The cystic duct has to be ample enough to permit extraction of calculi.
3. If not ample enough, the cystic duct should be dilatable.
4. It is difficult or impossible to remove calculi from the common duct through a strictured, fibrotic, nondilatable cystic duct.

5. The presence of numerous valves of Heister may make it difficult or impossible to remove calculi.
6. It is impossible or very difficult to remove impacted calculi through this route.
7. Only one or two calculi can be removed through the cystic duct, rarely more.
8. Only calculi in the common bile duct can be removed and not the calculi in the common hepatic duct or its branches.
9. In order to remove calculi from the common duct through the cystic duct, the cystic duct must empty at an acute or right angle into the right border of the common duct.
10. It is difficult or impossible to remove calculi from the common duct if the cystic duct empties into the left side of the common duct, running parallel or spiral fashion or passing in front or behind the common duct.

Extraction of calculi from the common duct by means of a choledochotomy during laparoscopic surgery also has its limitations. Some of these are as follows:

1. The supraduodenal common duct has to be clearly visible.
2. The common duct should be at least 10 mm in diameter.
3. It should not be surrounded by inflammatory tissue.
4. It should not be surrounded by an overdeveloped venous plexus.
5. Impacted calculi can be very difficult or impossible to remove, even with an embolectomy catheter.
6. Large calculi can rarely be extracted.
7. Hermetic closure of the choledochotomy with placement of a T-tube is usually difficult and carry an increased risk of very serious complications, such as common duct strictures and biliary fistula.
8. The use of instruments such as the fine flexible choledochoscope, with angled end, is very useful, but does not replace tactile sensation of the surgeon.

REMOVAL OF CALCULI FROM THE COMMON DUCT BY THE LAPAROSCOPIC APPROACH

Removal of Calculi Through the Cystic Duct

Calculi can be removed from the common duct, through the cystic duct by means of a Dormia basket with radiologic control, using an image intensifier. Extraction of calculi with the Dormia basket has led to serious complications, however, such as injury to the common duct and the papilla of Vater. Exploration and extraction of calculi with the Dormia basket should be done with extreme care and by very experienced surgeons (15, 17, 31, 33).

Before catching the calculus with the Dormia basket, one should be sure it will pass through the cystic duct and not get stuck in it. In order to replace the Dormia basket, a helical stone basket has been developed (Model G.U. 6354, Baxter, Deerfield, Ill.) 4-5 F, which will be described later.

The use of flexible choledochoscopes with angled ends has been popularized. A Dormia basket is passed through the choledochoscope to extract calculi under visual control (35, 40, 42).

Extraction of Calculi Through a Choledochotomy

Frequently it is not possible to extract calculi from the common duct through the cystic duct. In these cases the calculi should be extracted through a supraduodenal choledochotomy. In order to perform the choledochotomy, it is necessary to maintain the traction on the gallbladder originally applied to keep the liver displaced and be able to see the supraduodenal choledochus. A better view of the duct can be attained by using a laparoscope with a 30 to 45° angle. Before the choledochotomy is carried out, a 12 to 15 mm segment of the supraduodenal portion of the duct should be dissected, then a 10-mm longitudinal incision is made in its anterior wall with a No. 11 scalpel mounted on a laparoscopic needle holder (29, 30), or with a microscissors (30, 35, 40–42).

The calculi can be extracted through the choledochotomy with a Dormia basket, a helical stone basket 4–5 F, or by means of a Dormia basket introduced through a flexible choledochoscope. In contrast with the transcystic approach, a choledochotomy makes it possible to extract calculi from the common bile duct, from the common hepatic duct, and, at times, from its branches. It is logical to assume that only small calculi can be removed with a Dormia basket introduced through a choledochoscope. When a choledochoscope is used, it is very useful to have two video cameras available, one for the laparoscopic image and another for the choledoscopic image. Closure of the choledochotomy and placement of the T-tube can be quite difficult. It is very helpful to use a T-tube introducer (Gerald Medical, Charlton, Mass.) to place the T-tube. The choledochotomy is closed with 4-0 Vicryl sutures, using a laparoscopic needle holder. Patient subjected to choledochotomy and placement of a T-tube should have a subhepatic drain connected to continuous suction left in place.

ALGORITHM

Patients with suspicions or with clinical evidence of having calculi in the common bile duct, confirmed by endoscopic retrograde cholangiopancreatography (E.R.C.P.)

are usually treated, prior to operation, by means of endoscopic sphincterotomy and removal of the calculi. If endoscopic sphincterotomy cannot be done or has failed in trying to remove all the calculi, open surgery should be resorted to.

In patients in whom the presence of calculi in the common duct was not suspected preoperatively, but proven by laparoscopic cholangiography, experienced surgeons will attempt to remove the calculi during the surgery, by the transcystic approach or through a choledochotomy. If unsuccessful, open surgery is used. Surgeons without experience in removing calculi from the common duct during laparoscopy will opt for conversion to open surgery. It is not advisable, as recommended by some surgeons, to extract calculi from the bile duct by means of postoperative endoscopic sphincterotomy.

Operative Technique

Operative Technique

FIGURE 9.1

The patient is placed in the dorsal decubitus position. The patient, the operating room, and all the instruments should be ready to convert the procedure to open surgery, if this becomes necessary. The surgeon, 1, stands to the left of the patient. The second assistant, 2, who will be in charge of handing the laparoscope, stands at the surgeon's left. On the right side of the patient the first assistant, 3, stands with the instrument nurse, 4, and the instruments, 5, to the right. To the right of the head of the operating table, 7, are placed the television screen, the video cassette, the camera controls, the light source, and the source of carbon dioxide. The surgeon, 1, and the second assistant, 2, face the televised image, 7. The first assistant, 3, can observe the televised images in another television placed to the left of the head of the operating table, 7^1. The anesthesiologist is at the head of the table, 6. Some surgeons prefer the so-called French position, that is, in dorsal decubitus, with the lower limbs abducted and the surgeon between the abducted legs.

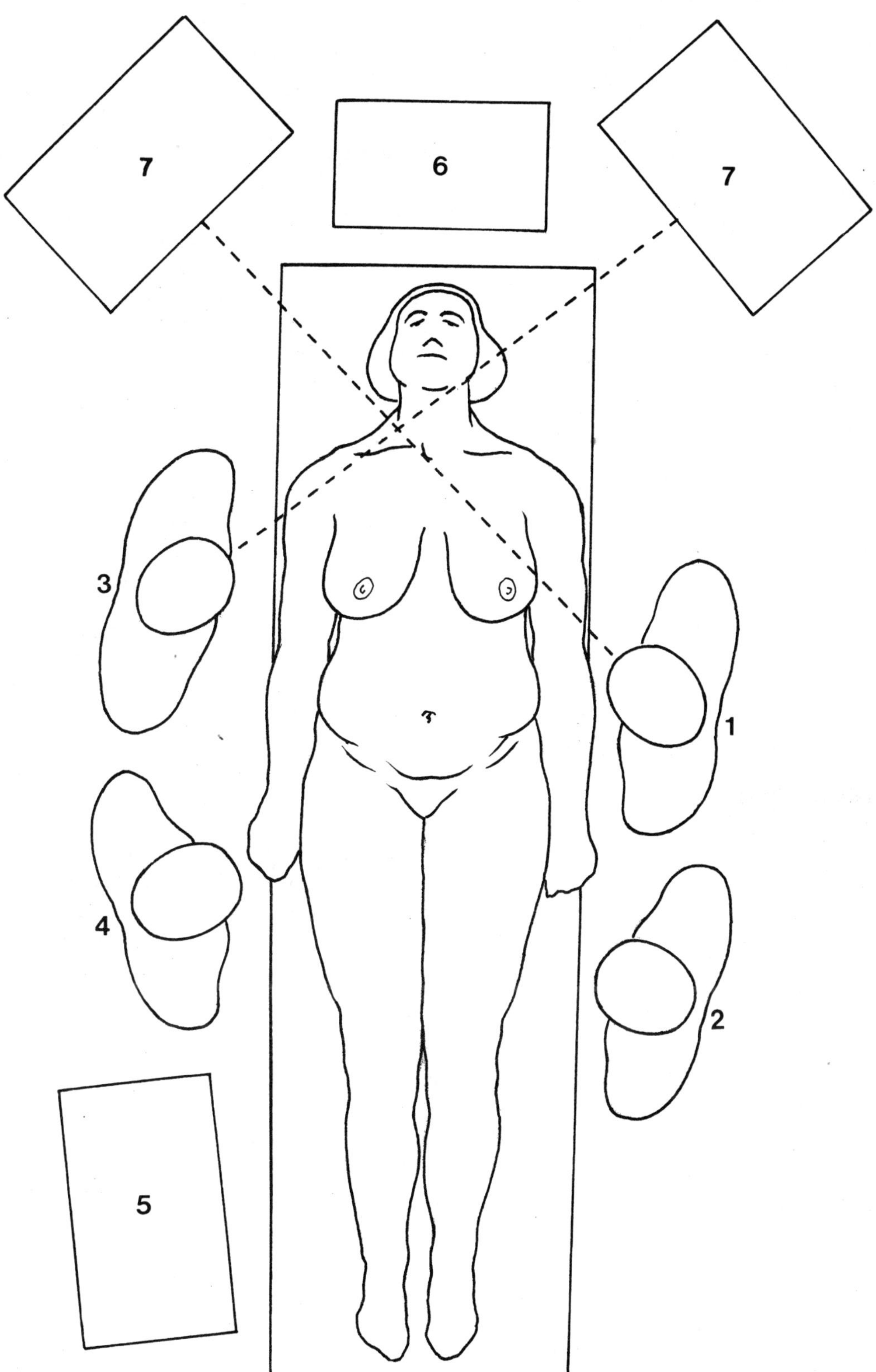

FIGURE 9.1

FIGURE 9.2

Prior to the laparoscopy, the abdominal cavity should be insufflated with CO_2, using a Veress needle with a blunt obturator, that is fired by a spring. The blunt obturator has the object of covering the bevel of the needle while it passes through the peritoneum, 3 and 4. The patient is placed in Trendelenburg position with 15 to 20° of tilt, as seen in the drawing. This slight Trendelenburg position is not essential for the introduction of the Veress needle and the production of the pneumoperitoneum, but it is advisable for inexperienced surgeons to reduce to a minimum any accidents that may occur. The needle puncture is carried out at the level of the umbilicus, either in its superior or right lateral fold.

Operative Technique

Before the needle is inserted, a 10 mm-long incision is made in the superior fold of the umbilicus, 1. The skin and the subcutaneous tissue is divided down to the fascia. The subcutaneous tissue is dissected with the finger or with a blunt instrument. Using two Backhaus clamps, the skin, the subcutaneous tissue and the fascia of the rectus abdominis muscles on both sides of the umbilicus is grasped. Traction is then applied upward to separate the abdominal wall from the intraperitoneal viscera. The Veress needle is then introduced through the small incision in the superior edge of the umbilicus, with its end directed down, toward the pelvis, as seen in the drawing, 2. At the moment the needle enters the peritoneum, the distinct protection click of the needle is heard, 3 and 4. Before beginning to insufflate the CO_2, the tip of the needle should be proven to be free in the abdominal cavity by carrying out the precautions previously described.

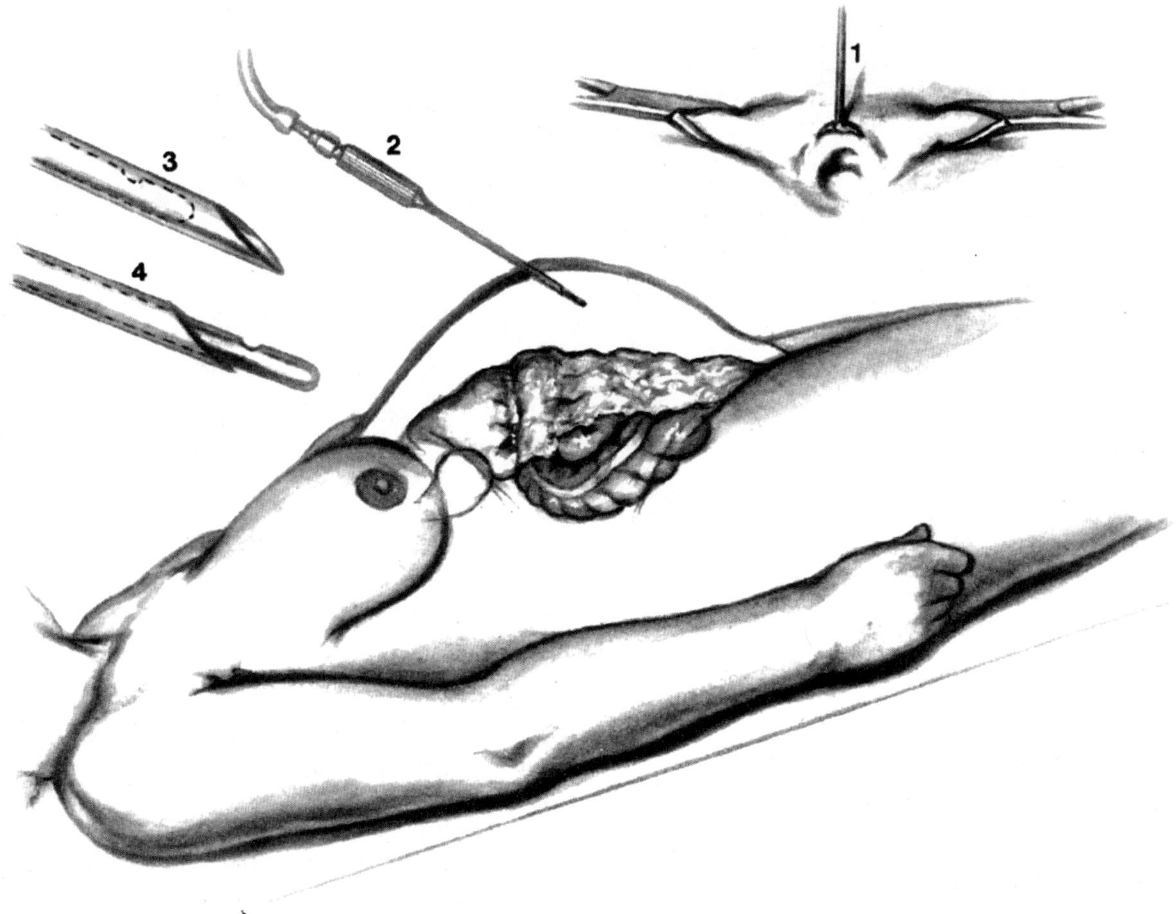

FIGURE 9.2

FIGURE 9.3
Laparoscopic cholecystectomy is usually performed by introducing four trocars through the abdominal wall, two 10 to 11 mm in diameter, and two 5 mm in diameter. The first 10 to 11-mm trocar is inserted through the small incision in the superior fold of the umbilicus. The laparoscope is introduced through this port, 1, once the trocar is removed. A 5-mm trocar is then introduced in the right flank, at the anterior axillary line, 2. Through this port an atraumatic grasper will be inserted to grasp the fundus of the gallbladder, and by applying traction, produce upward displacement of the liver, allowing the undersurface of the liver and the gallbladder to be visualized. A third trocar, 5 mm in diameter, is then inserted about 5 cm from the right costal arch, in the midclavicular line, 3. Through this port another grasper will be inserted to apply traction to the infundibulum, exposing the triangle of Calot. Finally, a fourth trocar, 10 to 11 mm in diameter, is inserted in the epigastrium, about 4 or 5 cm below the xiphoid process, and slightly to the right of the midline, 4. Through this port, dissecting clamps, hooks, spatulas, portaclips, scissors, aspirator-irrigators, and so on will be introduced.

Operative Technique

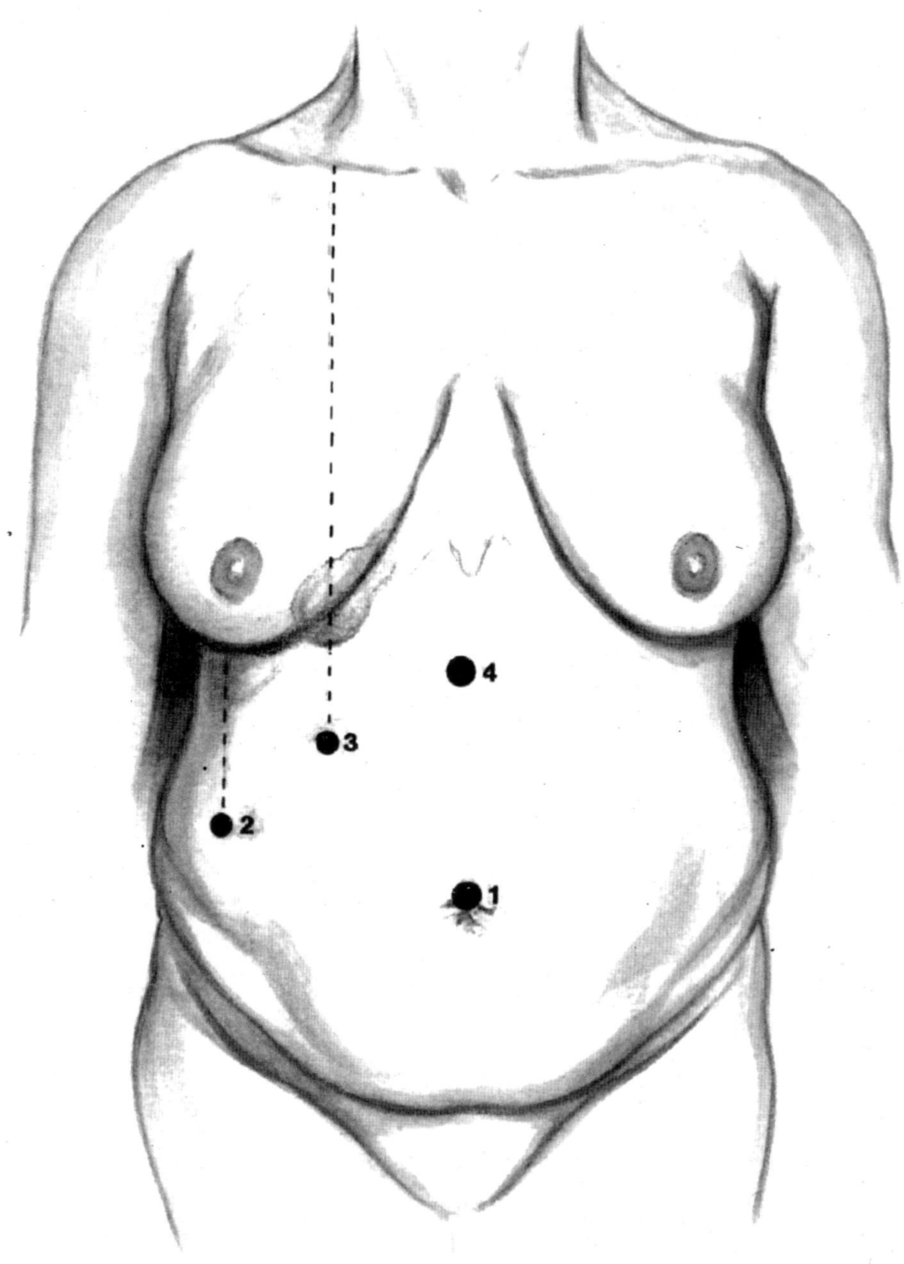

FIGURE 9.3

FIGURE 9.4

Placement of the first trocar is always dangerous, since it is inserted blindly. It is advisable to keep the patient in the Trendelenburg position with a tilt of 15 to 20° in order to diminish the possibility of injuring an intraperitoneal organ or blood vessel. In addition the Backhaus clamps are pulled upward in the same fashion as when the Veress needle was introduced in order to distance the abdominal wall from the viscera, 1. The first trocar is then introduced through the 10 mm incision in the superior umbilical fold, 2.

Operative Technique

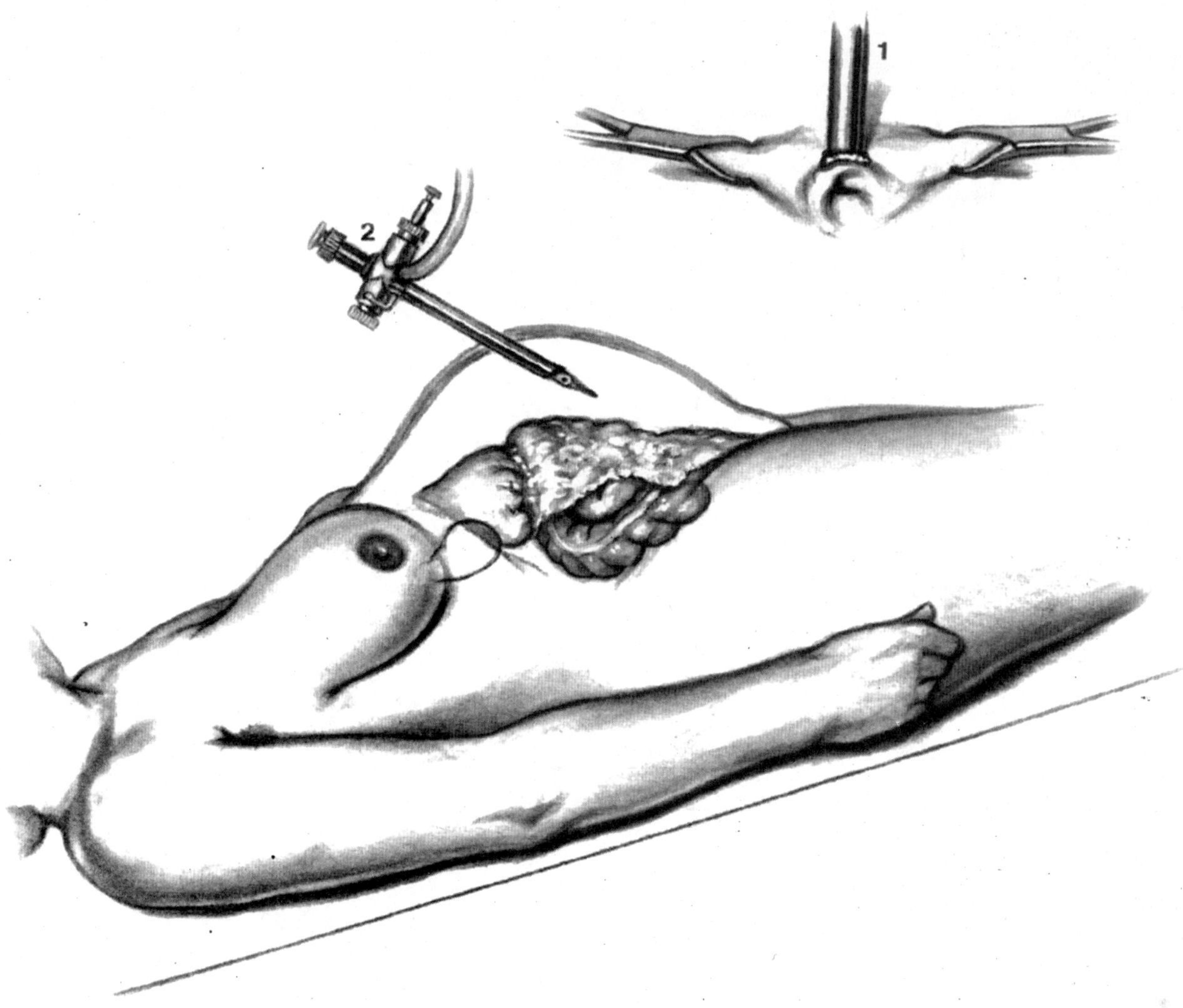

FIGURE 9.4

Operative Technique

FIGURE 9.5

Once the first 10 to 11 mm trocar, 1, is inserted, the obturator is removed, the CO_2 source (B) is attached, and the laparoscope (A), to which the light source (C) and the camera (D) have been coupled, is introduced. The position of the patient is then changed from a 15 to 20° Trendelenburg position to a reverse Trendelenburg ot 15 to 20°, so as to provoke a descent of the transverse colon and the greater omentum. In addition, the operating table is tilted to the left to separate the abdominal viscera from the operative area. The abdominal cavity is then explored under videolaparoscopic control and the three remaining trocars are inserted. An atraumatic grasper has been introduced through the 5 mm anterior axillary cannula, 2, and applied to the fundus of the gallbladder. Another grasper has been introduced through the 5-mm midclavicular trocar to grasp the infundibulum of the gallbladder, 3. A dissecting instrument has been passed through the 10 mm epigastric cannula, 4.

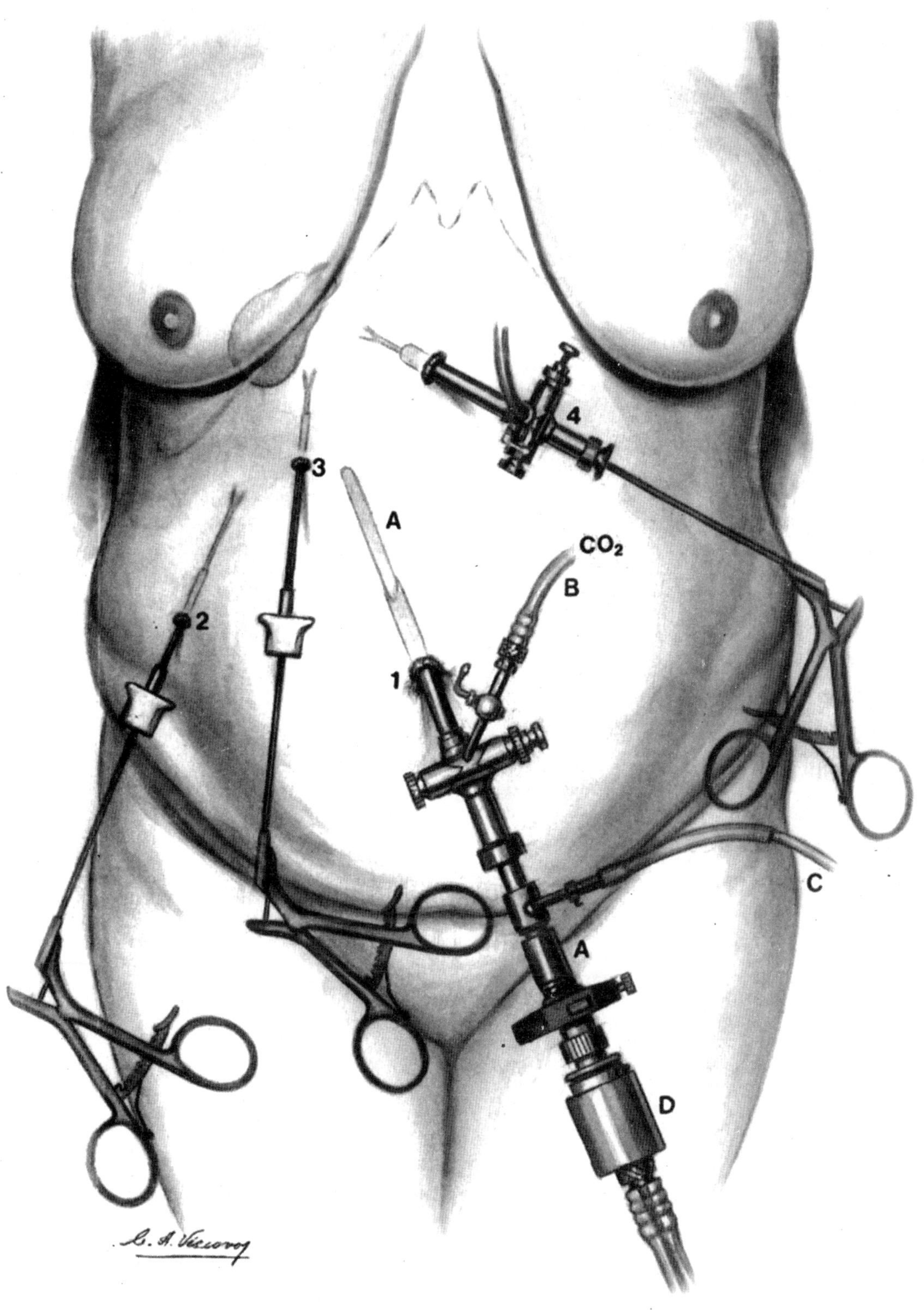

FIGURE 9.5

FIGURE 9.6
The atraumatic grasper introduced through the 5 mm anterior axillary cannula is applying traction to the gallbladder, displacing the liver upward, exposing the inferior surface of the liver and the gallbladder. The other grasper, in the 5 mm midclavicular cannula, is applying traction downward to the infundibulum of the gallbladder, exposing the triangle of Calot.

Operative Technique

FIGURE 9.7
The infundibulum and the cystic duct have been dissected with instruments passed through the 10- to 11-mm epigastric channel. The cystic duct has been freed circumferentially.

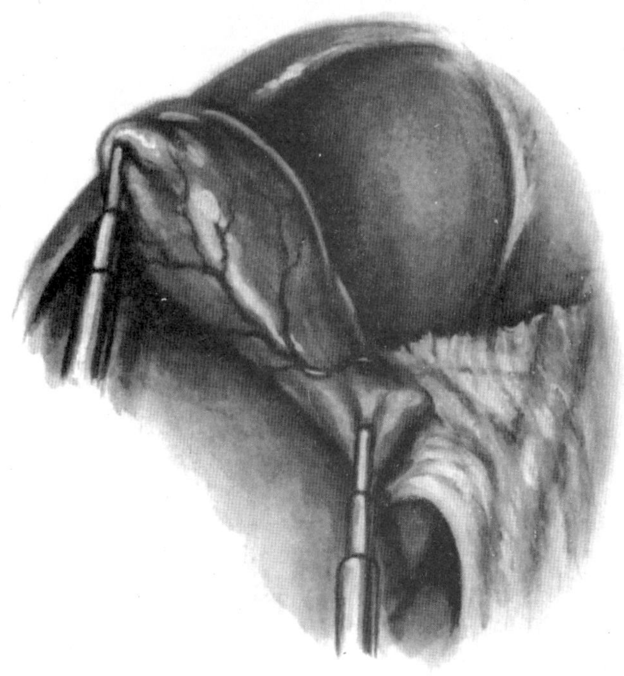

FIGURE 9.6

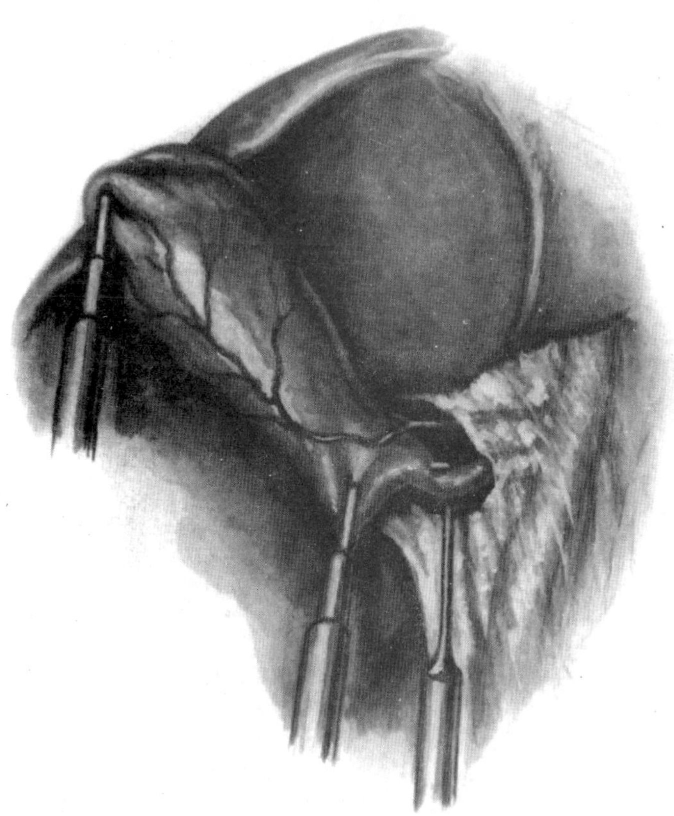

FIGURE 9.7

FIGURE 9.8
The cystic duct has been occluded with a clip near its junction with the infundibulum. A small transverse incision has been made in the anterior wall of the cystic duct, distal to the clip, using a microscissors. A catheter will be introduced through this incision in order to perform the cholangiogram.

Operative Technique

FIGURE 9.9
A 4 F ureteral catheter has been passed into the cystic duct. This is being held in place by a clip, taking care not to occlude its lumen, but avoiding reflux of the radiopaque substance. The catheter should not be introduced more than 3 cm. Actually, many catheters and clamps have been developed to facilitate performance of the operative cholangiogram.

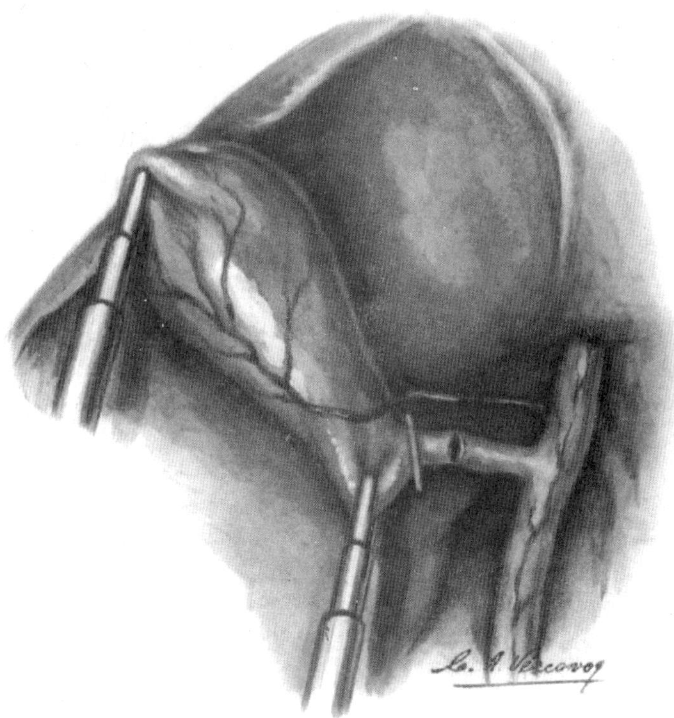

FIGURE 9.8

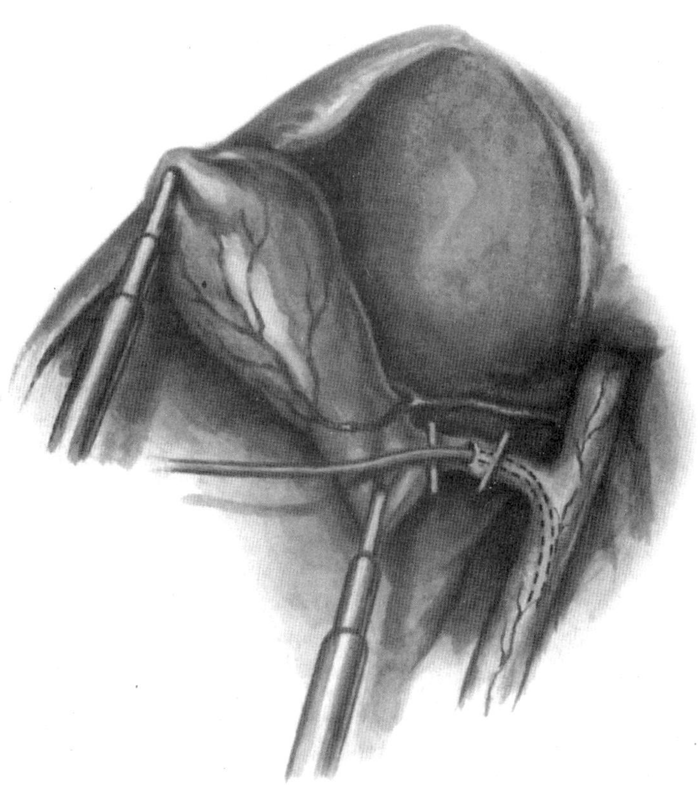

FIGURE 9.9

FIGURE 9.10
The operative cholangiogram is about to be performed by means of a catheter directed by an Olsen clamp, designed for this purpose (Olsen Clamp. Model No 20378 CH, Karl Storz, Culver City, Calif.).

Operative Technique

FIGURE 9.11
The catheter has been introduced through the cystic duct using the Olsen clamp. The Olsen clamp has been adjusted to the cystic duct, as shown, to proceed with the injection of the radiopaque substance. Before the injection, the patient should be removed from the Trendelenburg position. In addition, the operating table should be tilted some 15° to the right to prevent superimposition of the cholangiographic image on the vertebral column. The laparoscope should also be removed to prevent superimposition of other radiopaque shadows. The position of reusable metallic trocars should be modified, or disposable radiolucent metallic trocars should be used. Once all these precautions have been taken, 5 mL of radiopaque substance, diluted to 35%, are injected under radiologic control with the image intensifier. This will opacify the common duct and allow observation of the function of the sphincter of Oddi. An additional 5 mL of radiopaque substance are then injected to opacify the rest of the common duct. If the duct is dilated it may be necessary to inject more radiopaque solution.

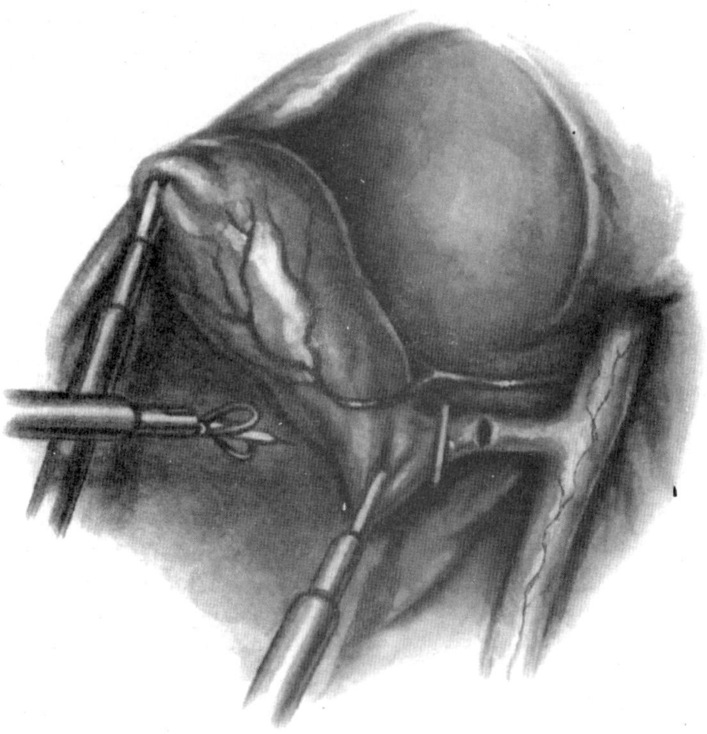

FIGURE 9.10

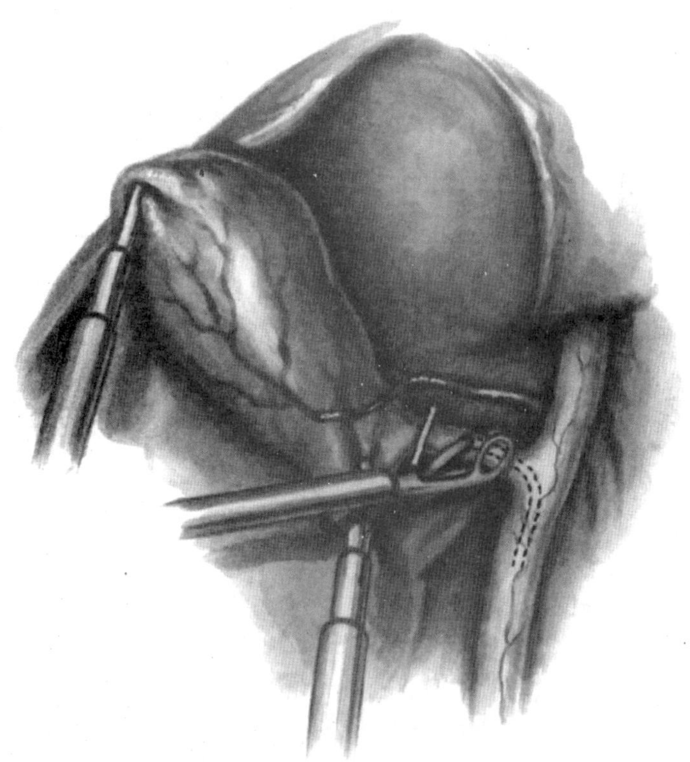

FIGURE 9.11

FIGURE 9.12

If the cholangiographic image shows a normal duct, without shadows of calculi or other pathology, and with good passage of the radiopaque solution into the duodenum, the cystic duct is transected, after the application of two clips on the common duct side of the incision. The cystic duct should be divided along the dotted line.

FIGURE 9.13

Once the cystic duct has been transected, care should be taken to avoid exerting traction on the gallbladder so as to avoid possible rupture of the cystic artery and its resulting hemorrhage. The cystic artery is then dissected in the area of the triangle of Calot. Two clips are placed proximally, and two other clips are placed distally, transecting the artery along the dotted line. The ligature and transection of the artery should be carried out as close to the gallbladder as possible unless the artery can be clearly seen, as in the drawing, in which the transection is to be performed farther from the gallbladder.

Operative Technique

FIGURE 9.14

Once the cystic duct and artery have been transected, dissection of the gallbladder from its bed is begun, using dissecting instruments (hooks, spatulas, etc.) connected to the electrocautery. Dissection is begun at the infundibulum and continued to the body and the fundus.

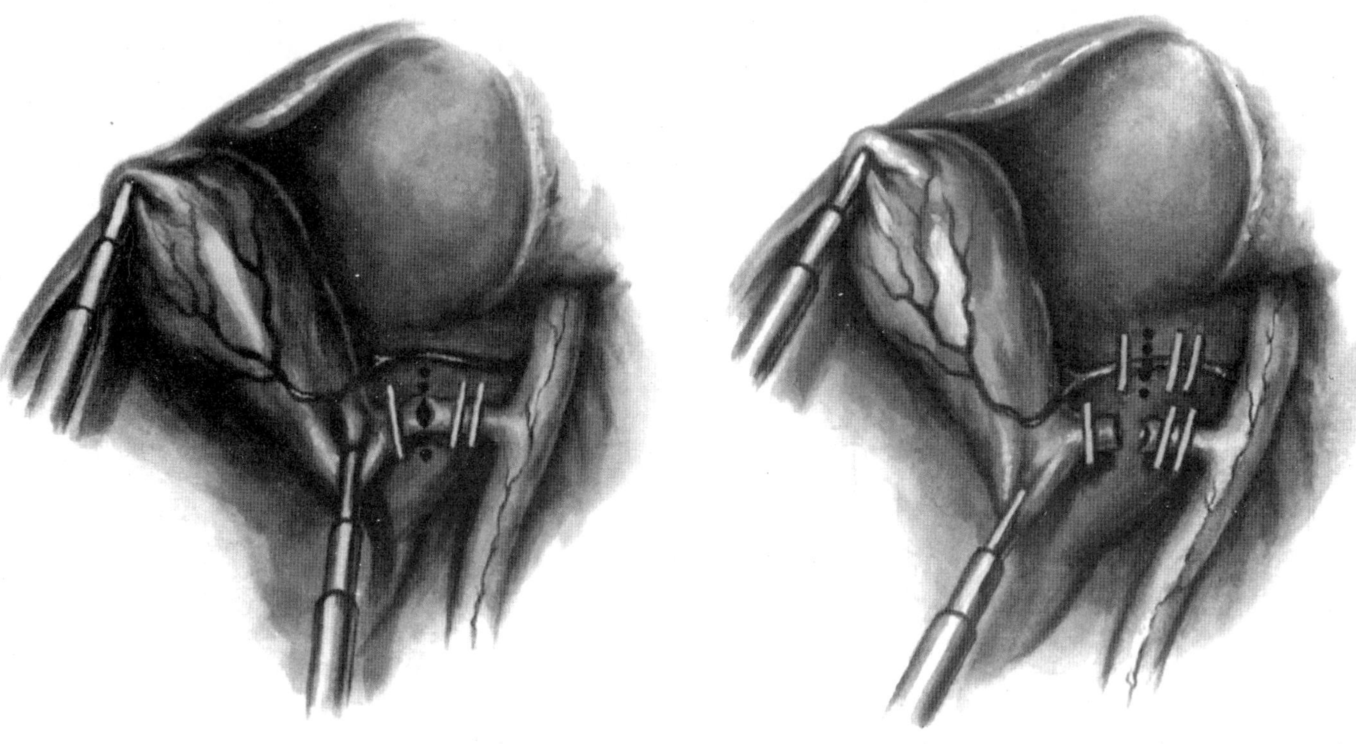

FIGURE 9.12

FIGURE 9.13

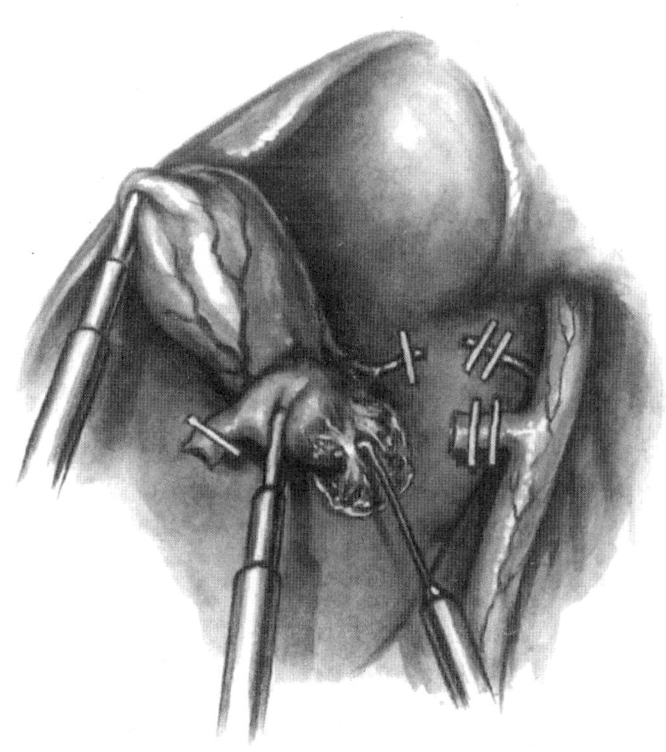

FIGURE 9.14

FIGURE 9.15
The drawing shows dissection of the body of the gallbladder from its bed. Hemostasis should be carried out with great care using the electrocautery. The presence of bile from ruptured aberrant ducts must be controlled.

Operative Technique

FIGURE 9.16
The gallbladder has been almost completely dissected, but must still be held by the graspers to continue to see the liver bed. The liver bed is irrigated with isotonic saline that is then aspirated in order to search for bleeding points or bile leakage, so they can be electrocoagulated. Irrigation and aspiration should be limited to the liver bed. It is not advisable to irrigate and aspirate near the stumps of the cystic duct or artery because of the danger of loosening the clips that clamp them. The subphrenic and subhepatic spaces are then aspirated to prevent postoperative accumulations of fluid.

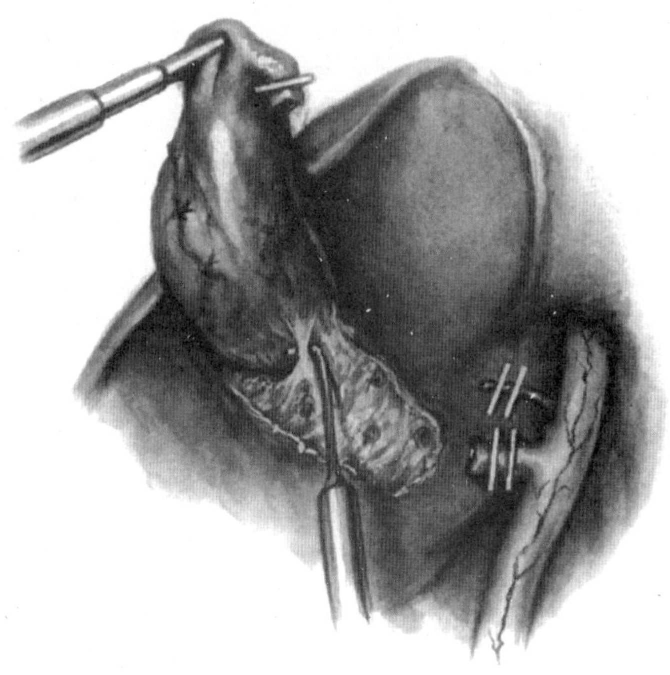

FIGURE 9.15

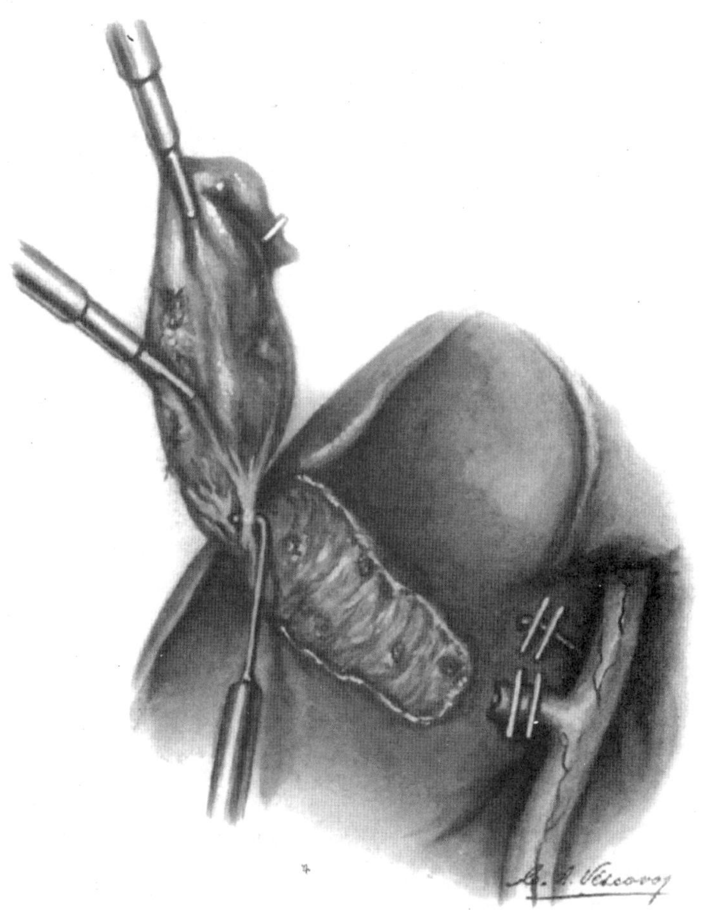

FIGURE 9.16

FIGURE 9.17

Once bleeding from the liver bed is controlled, the laparoscope is transferred from the umbilical to the epigastric channel, both 10 to 11 mm in diameter. The transfer of the laparoscope is done with the object of removing the resected gallbladder through the umbilical channel. The gallbladder is completely freed but still held with a grasper. A claw clamp or crocodile clamp is introduced through the umbilical port and the infundibulum of the gallbladder is grasped with it. The grasper that was holding the gallbladder is then removed. Traction is then applied to the claw clamp to exteriorize the gallbladder. All the maneuvers performed to extract the gallbladder should be controlled with the laparoscope to be sure the gallbladder enters the umbilical channel. If CO_2 was being insufflated through the umbilical channel, it should be changed to another channel because the umbilical channel will be obstructed during the extraction of the gallbladder and the umbilical cannula is also removed. If the gallbladder is thin walled and contains small calculi, it does not have to be opened. If the gallbladder cannot be removed through the umbilical port, it is partially exteriorized, the calculi are removed, and its contents aspirated to facilitate its extraction. If the calculi are over 10 mm in diameter, they can be crushed so they can be removed. In some patients with thick walled gallbladders, it may be necessary to amplify the umbilical channel. The drawing shows the gallbladder as it is being exteriorized by traction on the claw clamp.

Operative Technique

FIGURE 9.18

Extraction of calculi from the common duct can be carried out with a Dormia basket, through the cystic duct, under radiologic control, using an image intensifier. Complications have arisen due to the Dormia basket, some of them serious. There is less risk with a helical stone basket (Model G.U. 6354, Baxter, Ill.) 4–5 F, which is shown in the drawing. The drawing on the left shows the closed helicoidal basket. The dark areas in the middle and lower end are radiopaque and are used to determine the position of the basket. The drawing on the right shows an open basket. The basket is opened by applying traction slowly as the catheter is rotated in clockwise fashion. This allows the calculus to enter into the basket so that it can be extracted. The lower portion of the catheter is pliable, allowing it to pass through the sphincter of Oddi without damaging it.

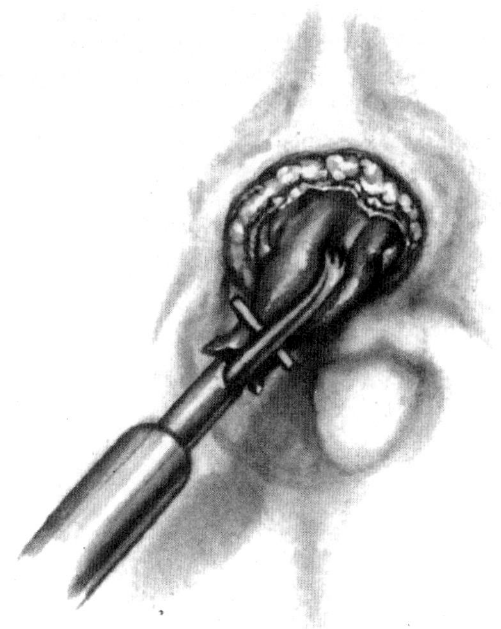

FIGURE 9.17

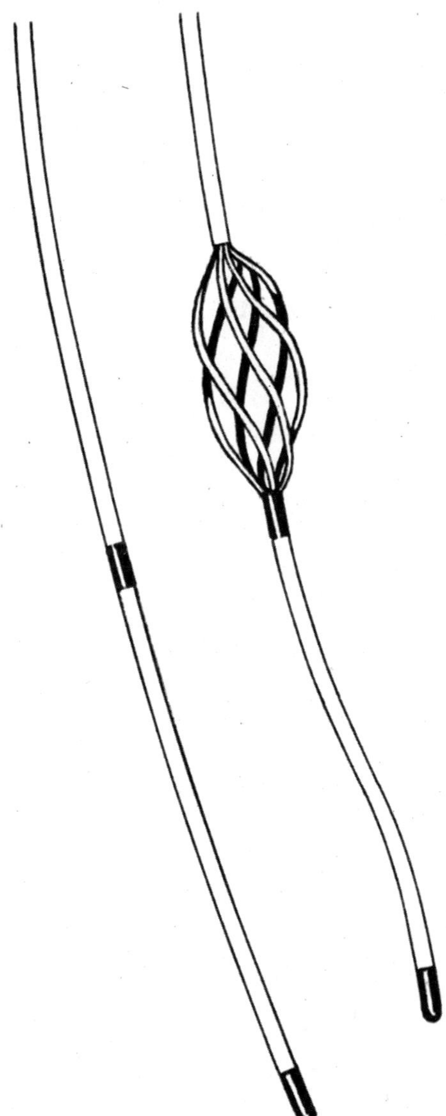

FIGURE 9.18

FIGURE 9.19

This drawing, and No. 20, which follows, show how a free-lying, faceted calculus in the common duct is trapped and extracted with the helicoidal basket. The catheter has been introduced through the cystic duct, and the closed basket has been advanced beyond the calculus in the common bile duct. The radiopaque area at the level of the basket is at the papilla, and the distal radiopaque area at the tip of the catheter is in the duodenum. The catheter is being rotated, and slow traction is being applied to it so as to open the helicoidal basket.

Operative Technique

FIGURE 9.20

Slow traction with added clockwise rotation is applied to the proximal end of the catheter. This has opened the basket and trapped the stone. When the stone is at the level of the cystic duct, the basket is closed to allow it to pass through the cystic duct. Removal of calculi from the common bile duct, through the cystic duct, is quite difficult and can only be carried out in favorable cases. In patients with spasm of the sphincter of Oddi, it is advisable to use 1 mg of glucagon intravenously to relax the sphincter.

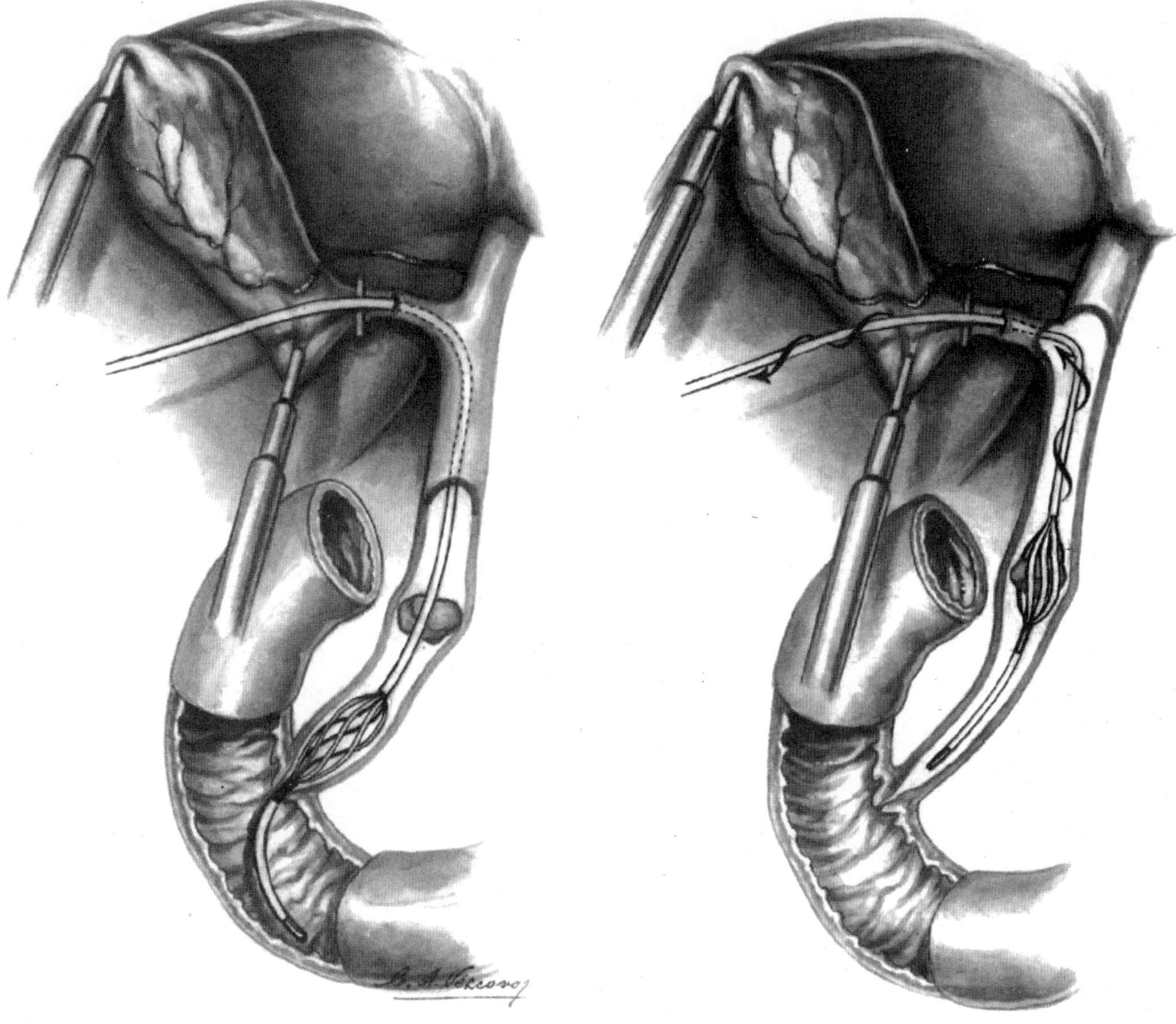

FIGURE 9.19

FIGURE 9.20

Operative Technique

FIGURE 9.21

A free-lying common duct calculus can be removed, under direct vision, by means of a thin, flexible choledoscope, with angled end and a Dormia-type basket. The figure shows a basket with a trapped calculus being extracted under laparoscopic control. In order to be removed through the cystic duct, the calculi must be small and lying free in the common duct. It is generally possible to remove only one calculus, occasionally two or three.

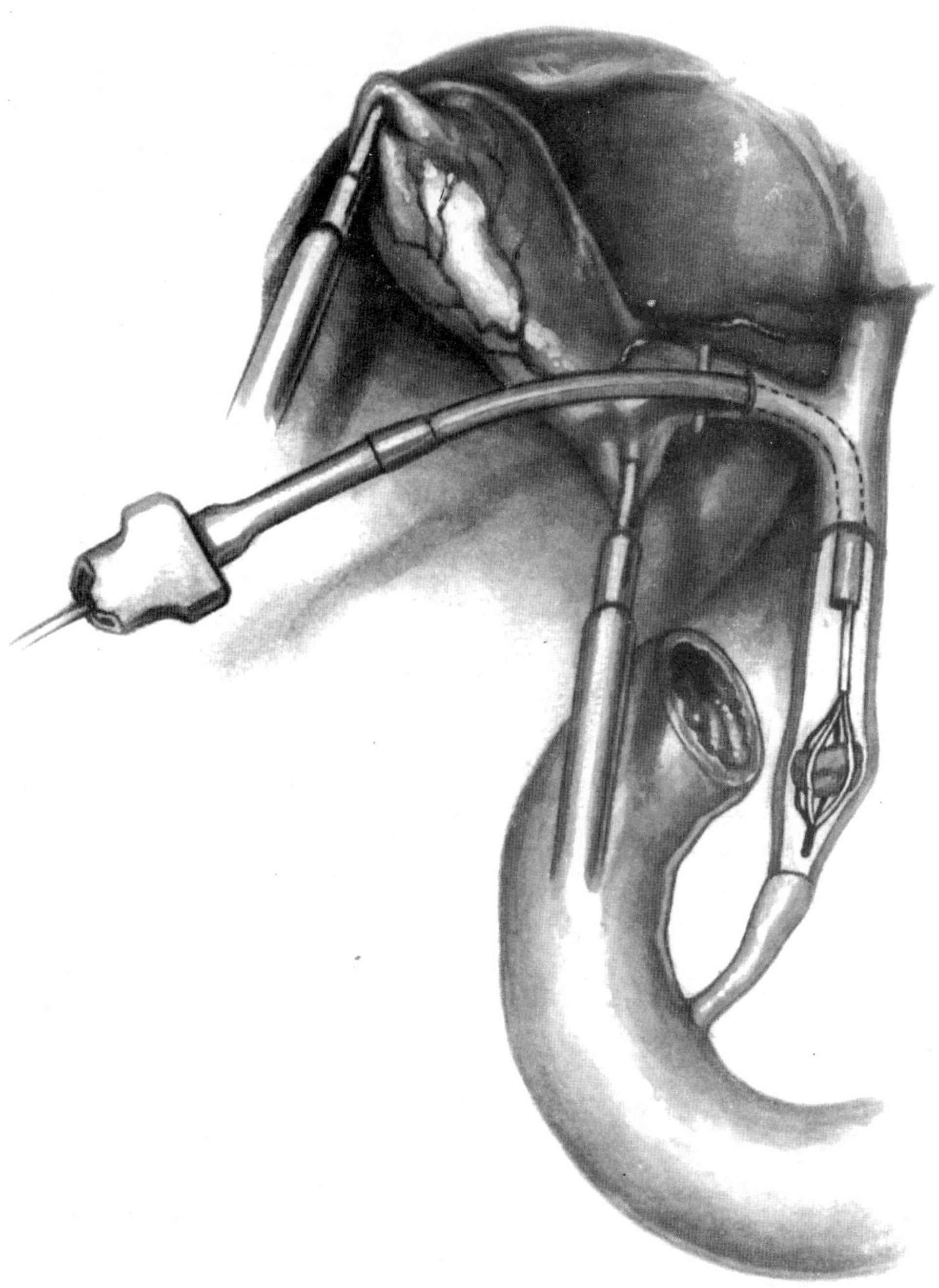

FIGURE 9.21

FIGURE 9.22

In favorable cases, calculi can be removed laparoscopically, from the common duct, through a choledochotomy. For this purpose a longitudinal incision about 10 mm long should be made in the anterior wall of the supraduodenal common duct. The incision can be made with a No. 11 scalpel mounted on a laparoscopic needle holder or with microscissors. A thin, flexible choledochoscope, with an angled end, and including a Dormia-type basket is used.

Operative Technique

FIGURE 9.23

The basket in the choledoscope has trapped a stone and it is being extracted. Through a choledochotomy it is possible to remove calculi from the common bile duct and the common hepatic duct. It should be pointed out, however, that only small calculi can be removed in this way.

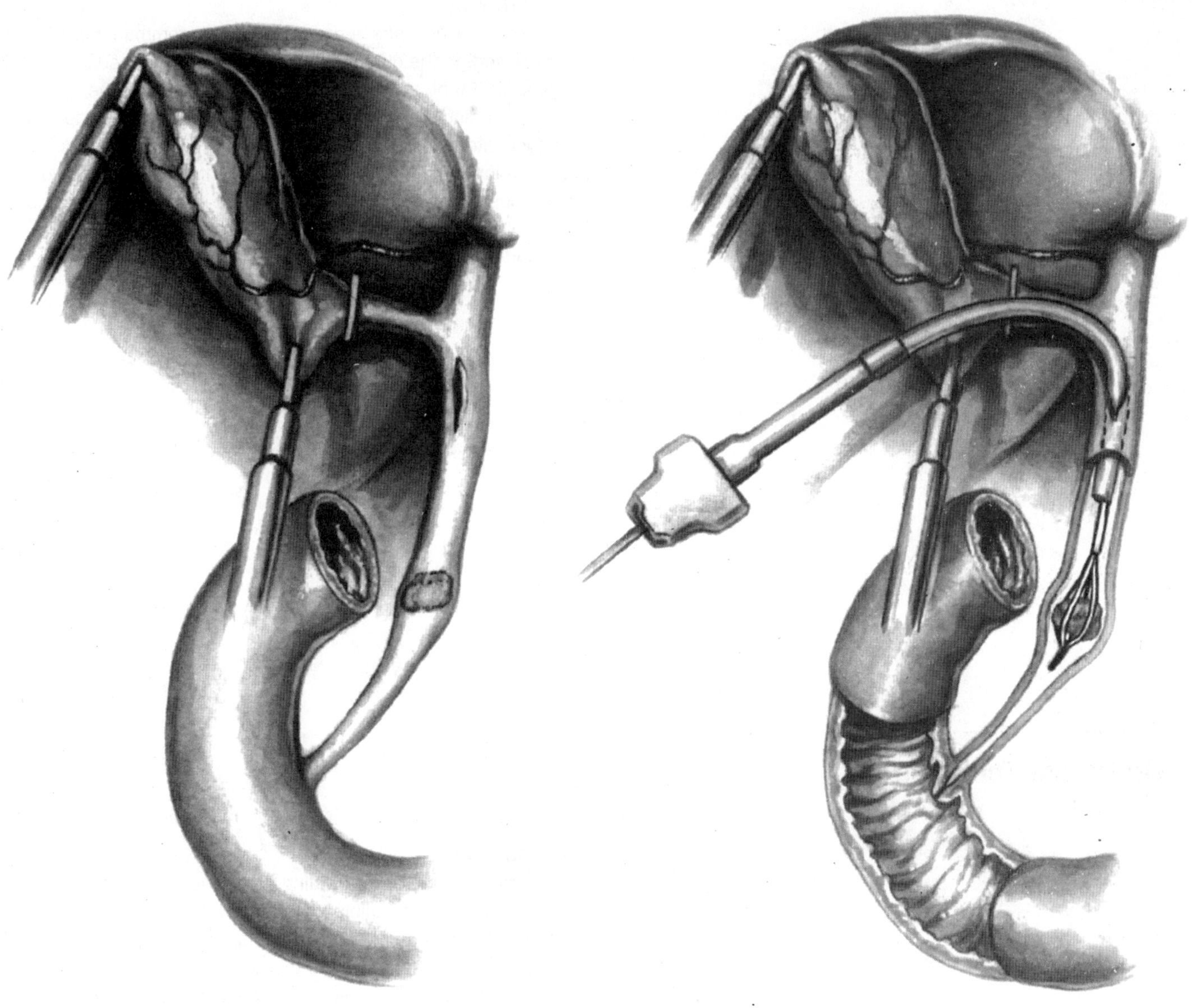

FIGURE 9.22

FIGURE 9.23

FIGURE 9.24
Once the calculus has been extracted, the common duct should be drained, to the outside, by placing a previously selected and prepared T-tube in the common duct. Insertion of the T-tube is usually difficult. The surgeon can use an instrument designed to facilitate placement of the T-tube, called a T-tube introducer (T-tube introducer, Gerald Medical, Charlton, Mass.). The drawing shows the T-tube being introduced into the common bile duct. Once the T-tube is in place, the common duct is closed around the T-tube with several absorbable sutures.

Operative Technique

FIGURE 9.25
Surgery is continued by dividing the cystic duct and artery and then resecting the gallbladder from cystic duct to fundus, as previously described. The long limb of the T-tube is exteriorized through the 5 mm channel in the right subcostal, midclavicular line. A subhepatic drainage tube connected to continuous suction should be left in place in patients in whom a choledochotomy has been performed.

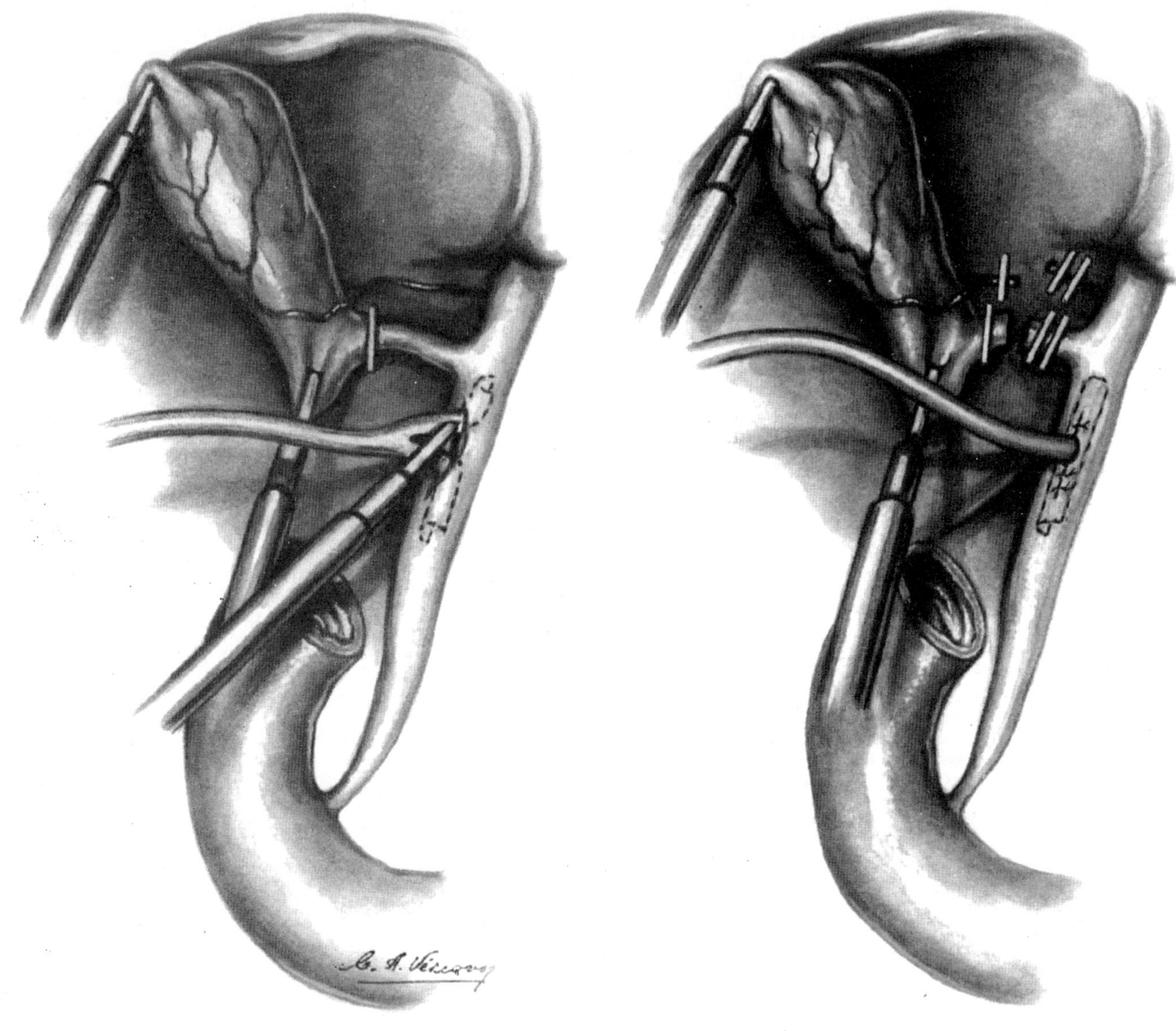

FIGURE 9.24

FIGURE 9.25

References

1. Bagnato, V.J., McGee, G.E., Halten, L.E., Varner, J.E., Culpeper, J.P. Justification for routine cholangiography during laparoscopic cholecystectomy. Surg. Laparosc. Endosc. 1:89, 1991.
2. Bailey, R.W., Imbembo, A.L., Zucker, K.A. Establishment of a laparoscopic cholecystectomy training program. Am. Surg. 57: 231, 1991.
3. Bruhat, M.A., Dubois, F. La chirurgie abdomino-pelvienne par coelioscopie. p. 89. Springer-Verlag, Paris, 1992.
4. Bruhn, E.W., Miller, F.J., Hunter, J.G. Routine fluoroscopic cholangiography during laparoscopic cholecystectomy: An argument. Surg. Endosc. 5:111, 1991.
5. Cameron, J.L. Atlas of biliary tract surgery. p. 17. Churchill Livingstone, New York, 1993.
6. Cooperman, A.M. Laparoscopic cholecystectomy. Difficult cases and creative solutions. p. 19. Quality Medical, St. Louis, 1992.
7. Csendes, A., Burdiles, P. Período postoperatorio normal y complicaciones de la colecistectomía laparoscópica. In Sepúlveda, A., Lizana, C. (Eds.) Cirugía laparoscópica. Ediciones Video Cirugía, Santiago, Chile, 1993.
8. Cuschieri, A., Dubois, F., Mouil, J., Mouret, P., et al. The European experience with laparoscopic cholecystectomy. Am. J. Surg. 161:385, 1991.
9. Dubois, F., Berthelot, G., Levard, H. Cholecistectomie per coelioscopie. Presse Med. 18:980, 1989.
10. Dubois, F., Icard, P., Berthelot, G., Levard, H. Coelioscopic cholecystectomy. Preliminary report of 36 cases. Ann. Surg. 211: 60, 1990.
11. Ferguson, C.M., Rattner, D.W., Warshaw, A.L. Bile duct injury in laparoscopic cholecystectomy. Surg. Laparosc. Endosc. 2:1, 1992.
12. Flowers, J.L., Zucker, K.A., Graham, S.M., Scovill, W.A., Imbembo, A.L., Bailey, R.W. Laparoscopic cholangiography. Results and indications. Ann. Surg. 215:209, 1992.
13. Fried, G.M., Barkun, J.S., Sigman, H.H., Joseph, L., Clas, D., Garzon, J., Hinchey, E.J., Meakins, J.L. Factors determining conversion to laparotomy in patients undergoing laparoscopy. Am. J. Surg. 167:35, 1994.
14. Gouma, D.J., Go, P.M.N. Bile duct injury during laparoscopic and conventional cholecystectomy. J. Am. Coll. Surg. 178:229, 1994.
15. Hasson, H.M. Open laparoscopy vs. closed laparoscopy. A comparison of complication rates. Adv. Planned Parenthood 13: 41, 1978.
16. Hunter, J.G. Laparoscopic transcystic common bile duct exploration. Am. J. Surg. 163:53, 1992.
17. Hunter, J.G., Soper, N. Laparoscopic management of bile duct stones. Surg. Clin. North Am. 72:1077, 1992.
18. Itoh, Y., Idozuki, Y., Noie, T., Nayeem, S.A., Abe, H. Experience with laparoscopic cholecystectomy. Reference to indications and methods. Surg. Laparosc. Endosc. 1:122, 1991.
19. Kleiman, A.S. Una historia de la colecistectomía laparoscópica. In Sepúlveda, A., Lizana, S. (Eds) Cirugía laparoscópica. p. 19. Ediciones Video Cirugía, Santiago, Chile, 1993.
20. Ko, S.T., Airan, M.C. Therapeutic laparoscopic suturing techniques. Surg. Endosc. 6:41, 1992.
21. Lizana, C., Sepúlveda, A. Colangiografía intraoperatoria en colecistectomía laparoscópica. In Sepúlveda, A., Lizana, C. (Eds.) Cirugía laparoscópica. p. 175. Ediciones Video Cirugía, Santiago, Chile, 1993.
22. McSherry, C.K. Cholecystectomy: The gold standard. Am. J. Surg. 158:174, 1989.
23. Mooney, M.J., Deyo, G.A., O'Reilly, M.J. T-tube placement during laparoscopic cholecystectomy. Surg. Endosc. 6:32, 1992.
24. Moossa, A.R., Easter, D.W., Van Sonnenberg, E., Casola, G., D'Agostino, H. Laparoscopic injuries to the bile duct. A cause for concern. Ann. Surg. 215:203, 1992.
25. Mouret, G. From the first laparoscopic cholecystectomy to the frontiers of laparoscopic surgery. The prospective surgery. Dig. Surg. 8:124, 1991.
26. Périssat, J., Collet, D., Belliard, R. Gallstones: Laparoscopic treatment cholecystectomy, cholecystostomy, and lithotripsy, our own technique. Surg. Endosc. 4:1, 1990.
27. Périssat, J., Collet, D., Belliard, R., et al. Laparoscopic cholecystectomy: the state of the art. A report on 700 consecutive cases. World J. Surg. 16:1074, 1992.
28. Phillips, E.H., Berci, G., Carroll, B., Daykhovsky, L., Sackier, J., Paz-Pathlow, M. The importance of intraoperative cholangiography during laparoscopic cholecystectomy. Am. Surg. 56:792, 1990.
29. Rossi, R.L., Schirmer, W.J., Braasch, J.W., Sander, L.B., Munson, J.L. Laparoscopic bile duct injuries: Risk factors, recognition, and repair. Arch. Surg. 127:596, 1992.
30. Sackier, J.M. Laparoscopic cholecystectomy. In Hunter, J.G., Sackier, J.M. (Eds.) Minimal invasive surgery. p. 213. McGraw-Hill, New York, 1993.
31. Sepúlveda, A., Lizana, C. Cirugía laparoscópica. Ediciones Video Cirugía, Santiago, Chile, 1993.
32. Sherman, S., Ruffolo, T.A., Hawes, R.H., Lehman, G.A. Complications of endoscopic sphincterotomy. Gastroenterology 101:1068, 1991.
33. Soper, N.J., Odem, R.R., Clayman, R.V., McDougall, E.M. Essentials of laparoscopic surgery. p. 48. Quality Medical, St. Louis, 1994.
34. Spaw, A.T., Reddick, E.J., Olsen, D.O. Laparoscopic laser cholecystectomy: Analysis of 500 procedures. Surg. Laparosc. Endosc. 1:2, 1991.
35. Swanstrom, L.L. Common bile duct exploration. In Hunter, J.G., Sackier, J.M. (Eds.). Minimal invasive surgery. p. 231. McGraw-Hill, New York, 1993.
36. Veress, J. Neues instrument zue ausfuhrung von brust oder bauchpunktionen. Dtsch. Med. Wochenschr. 41:1480, 1938.
37. Welch, V.T., Fitzgibbons, R.J., Hinder, R.A. Beware of the porcelain gallbladder during laparoscopic cholecystectomy. Surg. Laparosc. Endosc. 1:202, 1991.
38. Wilson, R.G., Macintyre, I.M.C., Nixon, S.J., Saunders, J.H., Varma, J.S., King, P.M. Laparoscopic cholecystectomy as a safe and effective treatment for severe acute cholecystitis. Br. Med. J. 305:394, 1992.
39. Woods, M.S., Traverso, W., Kosarek, R., Tsao, J., Rossi, R.L., Gaugh, D., Donahue, J.H. Characteristics of biliary tract complications during laparoscopic cholecystectomy: A multi institutional study. Am. J. Surg. 167:27 1994.
40. Zucker, K.A., Bailey, R.W., Gadarz, T.R., Imbembo, A.L. Laparoscopic guided cholecystectomy: A plea for cautious enthusiasm. Am. J. Surg. 161:36, 1991.
41. Zucker, K.A., Bailey, R.W. Laparoscopic management of acute cholecystitis. In Zucker, K.A. (Ed.) Surgical laparoscopy update. p. 109. Quality Medical, St. Louis, 1993.
42. Zucker, K.A., Bailey, R.W. Laparoscopic cholangiography and management of choledocholithiasis. In Zucker, K.A. (Ed.) Surgical laparoscopy update. p. 145. Quality Medical, St. Louis, 1993.

Section B

Surgery for Portal Hypertension

CHAPTER **10**

Portal Hypertension

Portal hypertension originates from the existence of an obstacle in the portal venous system that keeps blood that comes from the gastrointestinal tract, spleen, and pancreas from passing freely through the liver on the way to its return to the systemic circulation. The obstacle may be localized at the entrance to the liver, inside the liver, or at the exit from the liver. Normally the portal blood in the liver comes into an intimate relation with the parenchymal cells of the liver, later passing through the sinusoids to the central lobular hepatic veins and from there to the systemic circulation through the hepatic veins to the inferior vena cava.

The veins of the portal system do not have any valves. This permits venous flow to change direction according to the pressure gradient. Under normal conditions the venous flow is toward the liver (hepatopedal). In patients who present an obstruction to the portal circulation the venous flow may be reversed, and portal blood may then flow toward the systemic circulation through the development of a venous collateral circulation, which allows blood to be diverted to the system circulation without passing through the liver (hepatofugal). The most dangerous collateral is that which develops between the gastric veins and in particular between the coronary (left gastric) and the esophageal veins.

The esophageal veins empty into the azygos vein. Reversal of the blood flow in the coronary vein and in the short gastric veins produces a dilation of the submucous venous plexus of the inferior esophagus, producing esophageal varices, the rupture of which leads to very serious hemorrhages. Rupture of these varices is generally caused by an increase in hydrostatic pressure produced during effort, nausea, or vomiting. The development of collateral circulation allows the passage of neurotoxic substances into the systemic circulation, making the development of hepatic encephalopathy possible because the blood does not flow through the liver, where it can be detoxified.

ANATOMY OF THE PORTAL VENOUS SYSTEM

The portal vein is formed by the confluence of the superior mesenteric and the splenic veins. The union of these two veins is at the same level as the posterior surface of the head of the pancreas. From its origin up to its division in the hepatic hilus, the portal vein measures about 8 cm in length. In 75% of the cases the portal vein receives blood from the coronary or left gastric vein. It also receives blood from other tributaries that carry venous blood from the duodenum and the pancreas. The inferior mesenteric vein empties into the splenic vein a few centimeters from its junction with the superior mesenteric vein. Less frequently the inferior mesenteric vein empties into the confluence itself or into the superior mesenteric vein. The portal vein carries 75% of the blood supply of the liver with an oxygen saturation of 85%.

CLASSIFICATION OF PORTAL HYPERTENSION

Whipple (60–62) recognized three types of portal hypertension: *prehepatic*, *hepatic*, and *posthepatic*. Sheila Sherlock (46, 47) completed this classification relating portal hypertension with the hepatic sinusoids. The most used classification is as follows:

1. *Portal prehepatic presinusoidal hypertension*, generally produced by thrombosis of the portal vein.
2. *Portal hepatic hypertension* (also called intrahepatic hypertension), which is produced by
   A. Presinusoidal block, frequently originated by schistosomiasis, in endemic zones.
   B. Postsinusoidal block, generally produced by alcoholic cirrhosis of Laennec and, less frequently, by postnecrotic or biliary cirrhosis.
3. Posthepatic portal hypertension caused by postsinusoidal block originated by the Budd-Chiari syndrome, thrombosis of the hepatic veins caused by occlusion of the inferior vena cava above the entrance of the hepatic veins, obstruction of the inferior vena cava near the diaphragm, constrictive pericarditis, tumor, and so on (33, 34).

The resistance to portal blood flow in the sinusoids of patients with cirrhosis is due to various causes, among which are

1. Necrosis of the hepatic cells.
2. Fibrous reaction.
3. Neoformation of hepatic nodules as a consequence of regenerative process in the hepatic parenchyma.
4. Inflammatory infiltration.
5. Fatty deposits.
6. The formation of arteriovenous and venovenous shunts (60, 62).

The increase in portal pressure in cirrhosis is due to compression of small portal veins, sinusoids, central lobular veins, and the fibrous tissue surrounding the portal spaces and penetrating the lobules, all of which produces great structural changes. Another cause of compression of small veins is the development of nodules, which are of hepatic regeneration (20, 42, 47).

Evaluation of Patients

Patients who have suffered a hemorrhage caused by esophageal varices must be evaluated by specialized teams to determine the most adequate treatment for each patient. These patients must be classified according to their functional hepatic state, using the Child-Pugh classification. In addition, their general status, their nutritive status, and their cardiorespiratory and renal status must be evaluated. If possible, a liver biopsy should be obtained to determine the status of the hepatic parenchyma and thereby the existence of hepatic cellular necrosis, leucocytic polynuclear infiltration, and the presence of Mallory bodies (9, 42, 62).

Group C of the Child-Pugh classification presents the most serious hepatic alterations (9, 38). The risk in this group of patients is much greater no matter what therapy is used.

Measurement of Portal Pressure

The wedge hepatic venous pressure is measured by catheterizing the inferior vena cava. Pressure in the splenic pulp can be measured percutaneously. Portal pressure can also be measured by transcutaneohepatic catheterization and through the umbilical vein.

The ultrasonographic duplex method is a noninvasive method that provides a good correlation. With this examination it is possible to quantify and know the direction of venous flow through the portal vein. In cases in which, through the duplex ultrasonographic exploration, it is shown that there is no blood flow through the portal vein there is no object in carrying out a splenorenal shunt by the Warren technique. Under these conditions, if a surgical indication exists, a portocaval shunt should be performed (17, 29, 42, 47, 57, 62).

Selective Angiography

Evaluation of patients with portal hypertension should be completed with an angiographic study of the celiac trunk and the superior mesenteric artery, observing the venous phase with the object of determining the permeability, caliber, and localization, as well as the possible existence of an anatomic variations either in the portal vein or the splenic and superior mesenteric veins. By catheterizing the vena cava through the femoral vein, the left renal vein can be opacified to determine its length and caliber, with the object of knowing if a distal splenorenal shunt is possible (6, 20, 42, 47, 57).

Treatment of Portal Hypertension

In 1980 the use of endoscopic sclerotherapy for the treatment of esophageal varices began to be popularized. Sclerotherapy may be used during hemorrhage or after hemorrhage. At present the treatment of choice for esophageal varices is endoscopic sclerotherapy. Portosystemic shunts are used less and less frequently and are actually only indicated when endoscopic sclerotherapy has failed (4–6, 20, 26, 39, 40, 45, 57).

In the treatment of portal hypertension one has to distinguish between two distinct situations:

1. Emergency treatment for acute hemorrhage from esophageal varices.
2. Elective treatment of patients who are not bleeding but have bled from their varices. These patients have great probabilities of recurrence of bleeding with great danger to life (20, 39, 40, 42, 57).

Emergency treatment of patients with portal hypertension and bleeding esophageal varices

The great majority of acute hemorrhages caused by esophageal varices occur in patients with alcoholic cirrhosis of Laennec. In these patients the gravity of the hemorrhage is added to the organic alterations, which compromises the patient's situation even more. These patients commonly have a deficient state of nutrition, severe functional alterations of the liver, poor coagulation of the blood, infections, renal and cardiorespiratory and renal insufficiency, and so on. It must be kept in mind that, even though patients undoubtedly have hepatic cirrhosis, hemorrhage is not always caused by esophageal varices. In some 50% of patients with hepatic cirrhosis hemorrhage is caused by erosive gastritis and gastric or duodenal ulcer. Therefore, an upper gastrointestinal hemorrhage in patients with cirrhosis must be investigated to determine the cause of the hemorrhage. The most efficient procedure for this diagnosis is esophagogastroscopy. During endoscopic examination the esophageal varices are observed in the submucosa of the distal esophagus, forming three, and sometimes four, longitudinal columns, of dilated and tortuous bluish color caused by thinning of the mucosa over the varices. If the patient bleeds from the varices and the amount of blood is not profuse, it is generally possible to identify the vessel that is bleeding and start injections of sclerosing solutions immediately. In about 70 to 90% of cases sclerotherapy stops the bleeding. Sclerosing injections are repeated 48 to 72 hours later, or sooner if necessary. Later injections should be done once a week, sometimes twice a week, until hemostasis is assured.

In 20 to 30% of cases, hemorrhage recurs while the patient is hospitalized. In patients in whom the flow is blood is so profuse that it does not allow an acceptable view of the site of the hemorrhage, one can use injections of Vasopressin simultaneously with the administration of nitroglycerin. Vasopressin produces a contraction of the splanchnic arterioles, reducing the portal pressure and favoring hemostasis. However, it may produce cardiac arrhythmias, precordial pain, myocardial infarction, and, in some cases, intestinal necrosis. This effect may be prevented by the administration of nitroglycerin or Isoproterenol. Vasopressin is given in doses of 0.4 units per minute in an intravenous infusion. The nitroglycerin can be given sublingually in doses of 0.4 mg every 30 minutes, or by intravenous infusion at 0.4 units per minute.

At present, Terlipressin is frequently used. This is an analogous synthetic Vasopressin that is slowly changed in the body into Vasopressin, causing less noxious effects on the heart. Terlipressin is given as an injectable bolus using 2 mg every 6 hours.

Some endoscopists, when they cannot get a good view of the bleeding vein, because of excessive flow of blood, administer sclerotic injections blindly. This practice is extremely dangerous and may lead to ulceration or perforating lesions of the esophagus much more frequently than when the injections are performed with good observation of the bleeding vein. In this situation, it is preferable to use the pharmaceutical products previously mentioned. If these are not effective or produce severe collateral effects, one can then recur to the placement of the Sengstaken-Blakemore tube to stop the bleeding, even though momentarily, and allow the use of sclerosing injections with greater precision (4, 5, 14, 39, 40, 45, 48, 57).

Direct surgical approach to esophageal varices by various procedures, be it by the thoracic or abdominal route, has been practically abandoned because of numerous complications and frequent recurrences. The same inconvenience occurs with the azygoportal disconnection procedures initiated by Norman Tanner, in London, in the year 1950. These have been modified frequently without improving the results (1, 3, 7, 28, 35, 37, 38, 49, 54).

Portocaval Shunt

In patients in whom sclerosing injections with the help of pharmaceutical products and the Sengstaken-Blakemore balloon have failed to stop the bleeding, a portocaval shunt can still be resorted to. A terminolateral portocaval shunt is very efficient in stopping bleeding from esophageal varices because it produces very good decompression of the porta venous system and, particularly, of the sinusoidal circulation (29–32, 42, 52, 57).

The patient who is to be subjected to an emergency portocaval shunt must be in satisfactory condition to tolerate this intervention because it carries a high mortality. However, it has been shown that with sclerosing injections, the mortality of patients in Group C of the Child-

Pugh classification is very similar to the mortality of the portocaval shunt.

Laterolateral portocaval shunting is indicated in cases of uncontrollable hemorrhage from esophageal varices associated with massive ascites and with Budd-Chiari syndrome (31–34, 52, 57).

Portocaval shunts are very efficient in stopping acute hemorrhage that has been uncontrollable by other means. Portocaval shunts have, however, two great inconveniences:

1. Its elevated mortality when it is performed as an emergency.
2. It increases the deterioration of the functional status of the liver, leading to an aggravation of the encephalopathy or producing it, if it has not already manifested itself. This complication occurs because all the portal circulation is shunted to the systemic circulation (11–13). To diminish the frequency of hepatic encephalopathy several partial shunts have been proposed:

H portocaval shunt

H mesocaval shunt in which a Gore-Tex prosthesis, 10 to 12 mm in diameter and 4 cm long, is interposed between the portal vein and the vena cava (6, 43, 44).

Shunts with an interposed prosthesis between the superior mesenteric vein and the vena cava are indicated when the portal vein is thrombosed (6, 10). These shunts are undoubtedly less efficient than direct portocaval shunts and thrombose on an average of 30%. Distal splenorenal shunt should not be used in patients with active bleeding from varices.

Elective treatment of portal hypertension

Patients with hepatic cirrhosis who have bled once have a 70% probability of recurrence of bleeding, which leads to a very elevated mortality, varying between 50 to 70%. The most used procedure for the treatment of patients with portal hypertension that have bled once or more is endoscopic sclerotherapy of the esophageal varices. This procedure produces good results with fewer complications and sequelae than the shunts (39, 48, 50, 57, 58). In cases in which sclerosing injections have failed, the most used shunt is the distal splenorenal shunt, using the Dean Warren technique (6, 36, 55–57). The distal splenorenal shunt changes the circulation of the esophagus, stomach, and spleen toward the left renal vein, keeping portal flow intact. For this reason, the procedure produces a lower incidence of hepatic encephalopathy. However, it has been shown that, with the passage of time, the results are similar to those obtained with portocaval shunt because of the development of collaterals. For this reason, at present the entire splenic vein should be dissected up to the hilus of the spleen to ligate the great majority of affluent veins. Undoubtedly this leads to an increase in operative time, but it slows up the appearance of collaterals (6, 20, 56).

The Warren procedure should not be used in patients with ascites because this procedure tends to increase existing ascites or even to produce it, if it did not exist (17, 18, 19, 20).

Hepatic Transplant

The possibility of a hepatic transplant must be considered in all young patients with severe cirrhosis of the liver who have bled from esophageal varices. For this reason, in patients in this condition, one should try to avoid portacaval shunt or a surgical procedure in the hepatic hiatus because this can constitute an obstacle to the performance of a transplant and, at times, prevent it. A specialized surgical team of great experience should evaluate the condition of the patient to be submitted to a liver transplant and study its feasibility. There exists reports of survival of more than five years in 70% of transplanted patients belonging to the Group C of the Child-Pugh classification (20, 24).

Operative Technique

Distal Splenorenal Shunt

FIGURE 10.1

The patient is placed in the horizontal position with the left flank slightly elevated (some 15 cm) by means of a pillow. The most frequently used incision is a left subcostal incision extended into the right rectus abdominis muscle and passing some 3 cm below the left costal margin, as shown in the drawing. The incision is extended to the left rectus muscle, which is cut transversely, later extending the incision into the muscles of the left flank. Some surgeons use a midline supraumbilical incision starting at the xiphoid process and prolonged some 6 cm below the umbilicus. In cutting the deep planes of the abdominal wall one commonly encounters the falciform ligament and the recanalized umbilical vein, which receives several collateral veins. The umbilical vein and all collateral veins are cut and ligated.

Once the abdomen is open, it is not advisable to explore the organs of the abdominal cavity without previously confirming that the greater omentum is not adherent to the capsule of the spleen. For this reason special care should be taken to avoid traction on the stomach or the greater omentum toward the right or upward as well as placing traction on the colon and its mesocolon downward. In case there are adhesions between the greater omentum and the capsule of the spleen, traction on these may produce rupture of the capsule at the sites of adhesion, which is the cause of hemorrhage. This is difficult to control, especially in diseased spleens, which may lead to the need for a splenectomy. It is well known that splenectomized patients cannot undergo a distal splenorenal shunt. When adhesions to the splenic capsule exist, these must be ligated and divided carefully before beginning the exploration. Once the danger of rupture of the splenic capsule is avoided, one must search for ascitic fluid. The presence of ascitic fluid contraindicates the performance of a distal splenorenal shunt.

The liver is then completely inspected, noting its appearance, size, surface, configuration, nodularity, and consistency. Nodules of alcoholic cirrhosis are generally small whereas nodules of postnecrotic cirrhosis are larger in size. Palpation of both hepatic lobes must be complete, searching for the possible presence of a hepatoma. In patients with hepatic cirrhosis, it is frequently observed that the gallbladder is diseased, generally larger in size, distended, and with thickened walls. The serosa of the gallbladder is frequently opaque and dull, as if the patient had an acute cholecystitis. However, this pathologic appearance is apparent and not real, a fact that is usually seen in all patients with hepatic cirrhosis. Because of this appearance of the gallbladder, the surgeon is sometimes tempted to perform a cholecystectomy, which is absolutely unnecessary in patients in poor general condition and those with hepatic deficiency. The resection of the gallbladder would only add one more risk to a difficult and prolonged operation, such as the distal splenorenal shunt.

If a hepatic biopsy has not been performed in the preoperative period, it is advisable to do one before beginning the shunt. The liver biopsy is generally performed by taking tissue from the right lobe of the liver using a Travenol Tru-Cut disposable needle. Frequently the site of the biopsy bleeds, sometimes abundantly. Hemostasis is obtained by placing two or three sutures using chromic catgut. The lack of blood loss from the site of the biopsy should be controlled at the end of the procedure. This is why it is advisable to perform the biopsy at the beginning of the surgical procedure and not at the end. Once exploration of the abdomen has been performed and the liver biopsy has been obtained, a self-retaining retractor is placed to obtain a good operative field. It is of great use to place a retractor on the upper side of the wound to get a more ample view.

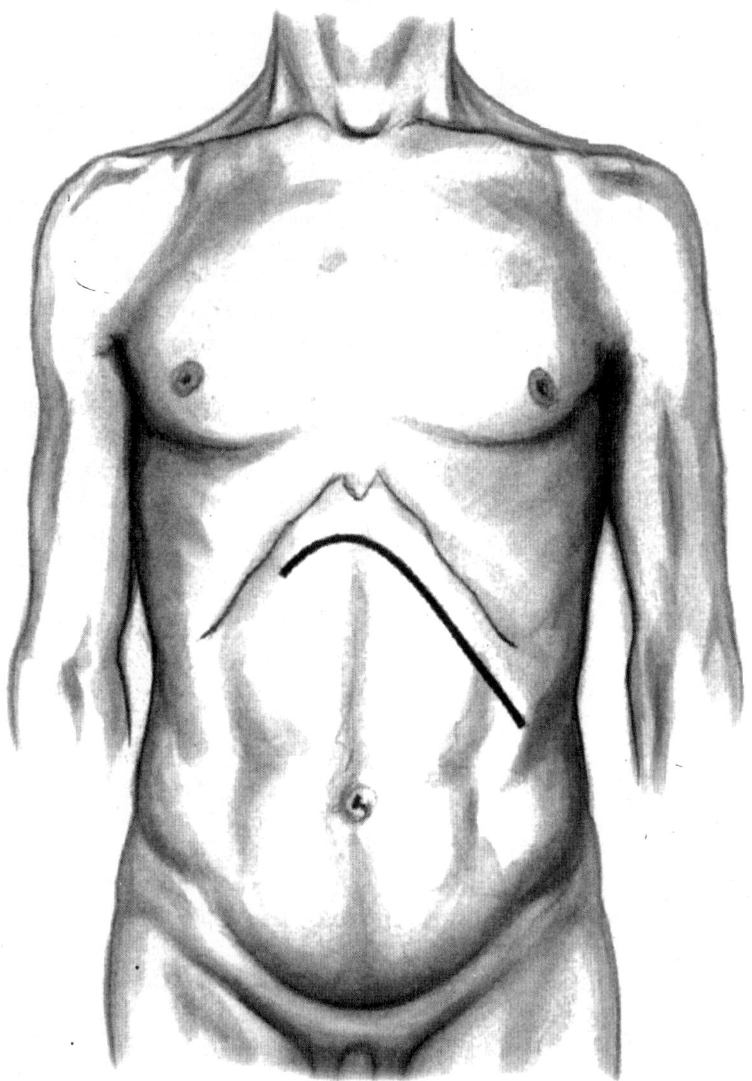

FIGURE 10.1

FIGURE 10.2

The surgical procedure is begun by sectioning the gastrocolic ligament below the gastroepiploic vessels. Sectioning of this ligament is begun below the short vessels, avoiding the inclusion of any short vessels in the ligature because these will constitute an important route for the flow of venous blood from the stomach to the splenic vein and the left renal vein. Ligation and section of the gastrocolic ligament should end at the level of the pylorus. The drawing shows the technique that is usually used to ligate the gastrocolic ligament before cutting it. With an angled clamp sutures of cotton or other material that is not absorbable are passed. The first assistant takes the suture and leads it toward the side of the stomach, where it is tied below the gastroepiploic vessels.

Through the same opening made in the gastrocolic ligament another suture is passed, which the surgeon takes and lowers in the direction of the transverse colon, where it is tied. The surgeon then cuts the gastrocolic ligament between the sutures. These bites into the gastrocolic ligament should not be too bulky. Upon nearing the zone of the pylorus, the right gastroepiploic vein should be identified, ligated, and sectioned. In some patients it can be very difficult to isolate the right gastroepiploic vein from the right gastroepiploic artery. In cases that present this problem the vein and artery may be ligated together (42). The right gastroepiploic vein, as it nears the vicinity of the pylorus, has a curved course and joins the right superior colic vein and the inferior and anterior pancreatic duodenal veins, forming Henle's trunk, which empties in the right side of the superior mesenteric vein at the level of the interior border of the neck of the pancreas. On the left side adhesions frequently exist between the greater omentum and the spleen. If these adhesions have not been ligated and sectioned before beginning the exploration of the abdomen, they should be ligated at this time. Ligation and section of these adhesions will allow the mobilization of the transverse colon downward without danger of damaging the splenic capsule. Ligation and section of the splenocolic ligament will complete this liberation.

Distal Splenorenal Shunt

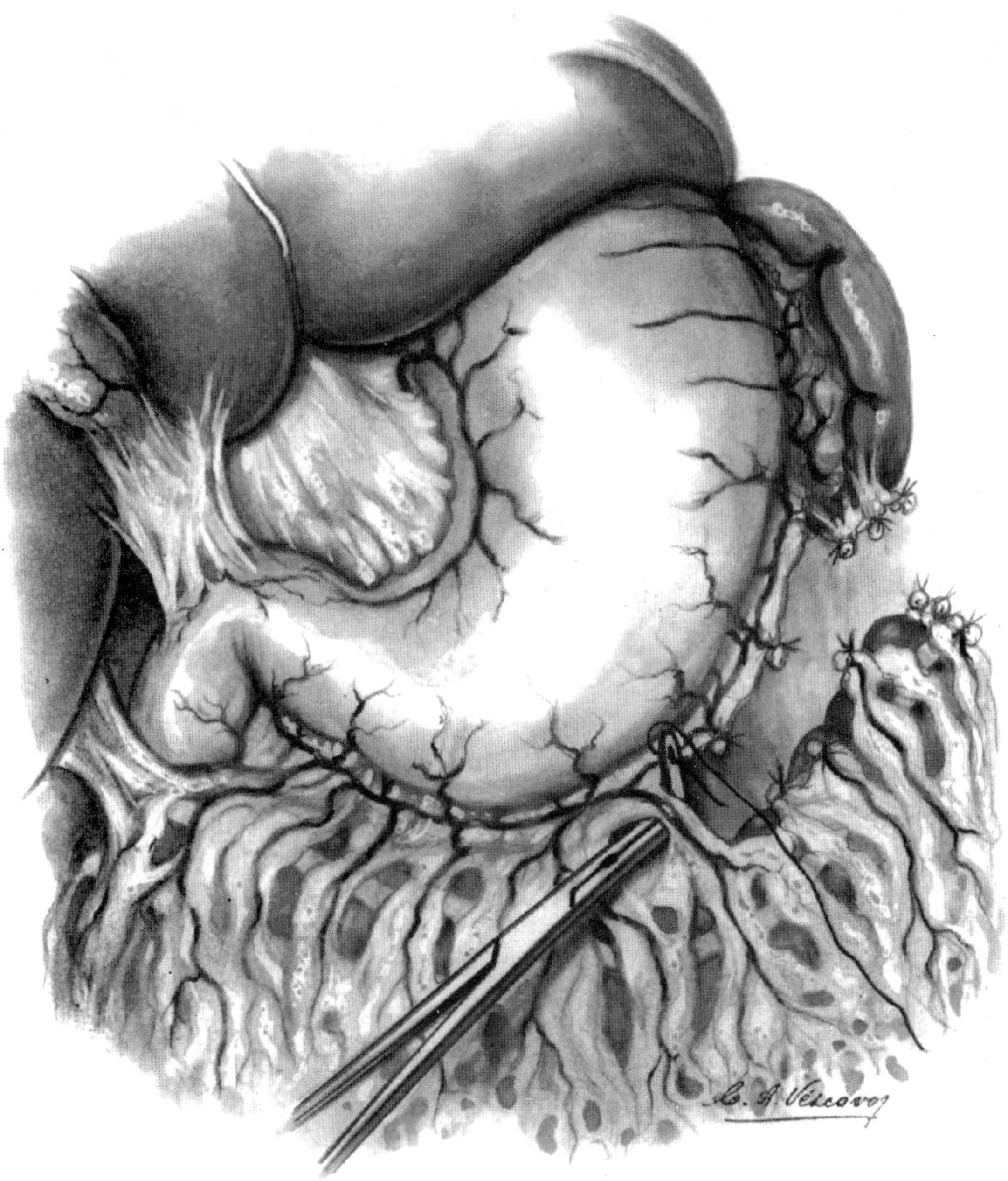

FIGURE 10.2

Distal Splenorenal Shunt (55)

FIGURE 10.3
Once the division of the gastroepiploic ligament has been completed, the first assistant applies traction to the stomach, upward, using both hands, as shown in the drawing. The second assistant applies traction to the transverse colon and its mesocolon downward, uncovering the anterior surface of the pancreas. In the Dean Warren procedure (55), in addition to carrying out the distal splenorenal shunt, the right gastroepiploic vein, the coronary or left gastric vein, and the pyloric or right gastric vein should be ligated. All these vessels should have been ligated before starting to perform the shunt so as not to have to ligate them after a long, tedious, difficult operation (42).

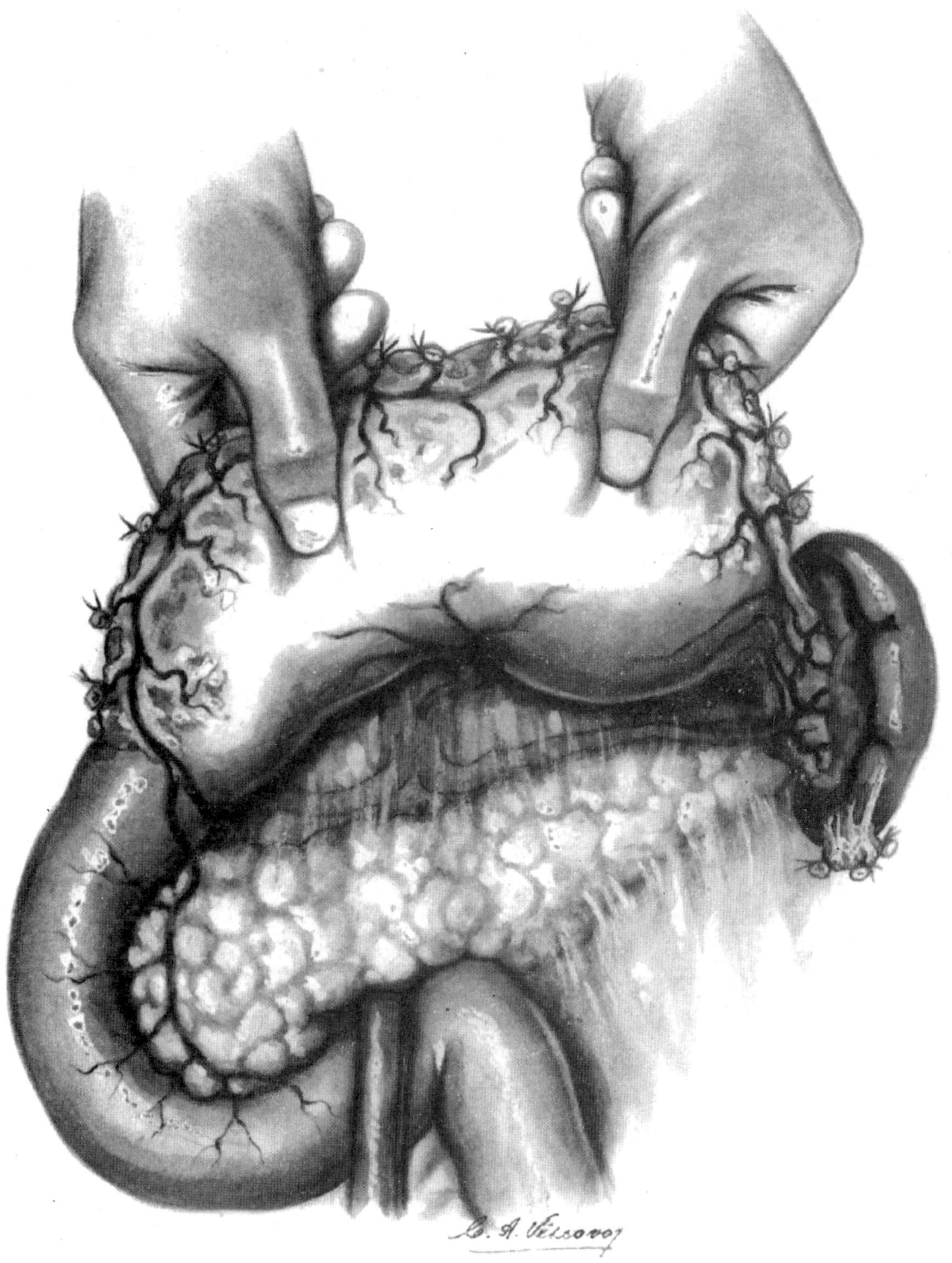

FIGURE 10.3

FIGURE 10.4

In order to mobilize the pancreas so as to identify and dissect the splenic vein, the peritoneum along the inferior border of the pancreas has to be divided as shown in the figure. An avascular portion is selected, usually at the junction of the tail and body of the pancreas. The peritoneum is sectioned, using scissors, continuing to the head of the pancreas. The pancreas is immobilized upward after the peritoneum is divided, exposing the splenic vein. It is usually possible to recognize the inferior mesenteric vein running obliquely upward to empty into the splenic vein. The inferior mesenteric vein is a good reference in identifying the splenic vein. In some cirrhotic patients it is not easy to recognize the inferior mesenteric vein because of severe engorgement of the retroperitoneal lymphatics, development of collateral venous circulation, and intense edema and thickening of the posterior peritoneum.

If identification of the inferior mesenteric vein is considered to be very important, the following maneuver can be resorted to: The transverse colon is pulled upward together with its mesocolon, and a longitudinal incision is made in the posterior peritoneum to the left of the ligament of Treitz, the site where the inferior mesenteric vein usually runs in its ascending course to join the splenic vein behind the pancreas. Once the splenic vein is identified, the inferior mesenteric vein is ligated where it empties into the splenic vein. In some patients the inferior mesenteric vein empties into the splenic vein at its confluence with the superior mesenteric vein; in others it empties directly into the superior mesenteric or into the portal vein. In the latter cases it is not necessary to ligate it. The incision in the posterior peritoneum, to the left of the ligament of Treitz, can be used to identify the left renal vein, which runs from the hilus of the left kidney to the inferior vena cava, passing in front of the aorta (15).

Distal Splenorenal Shunt

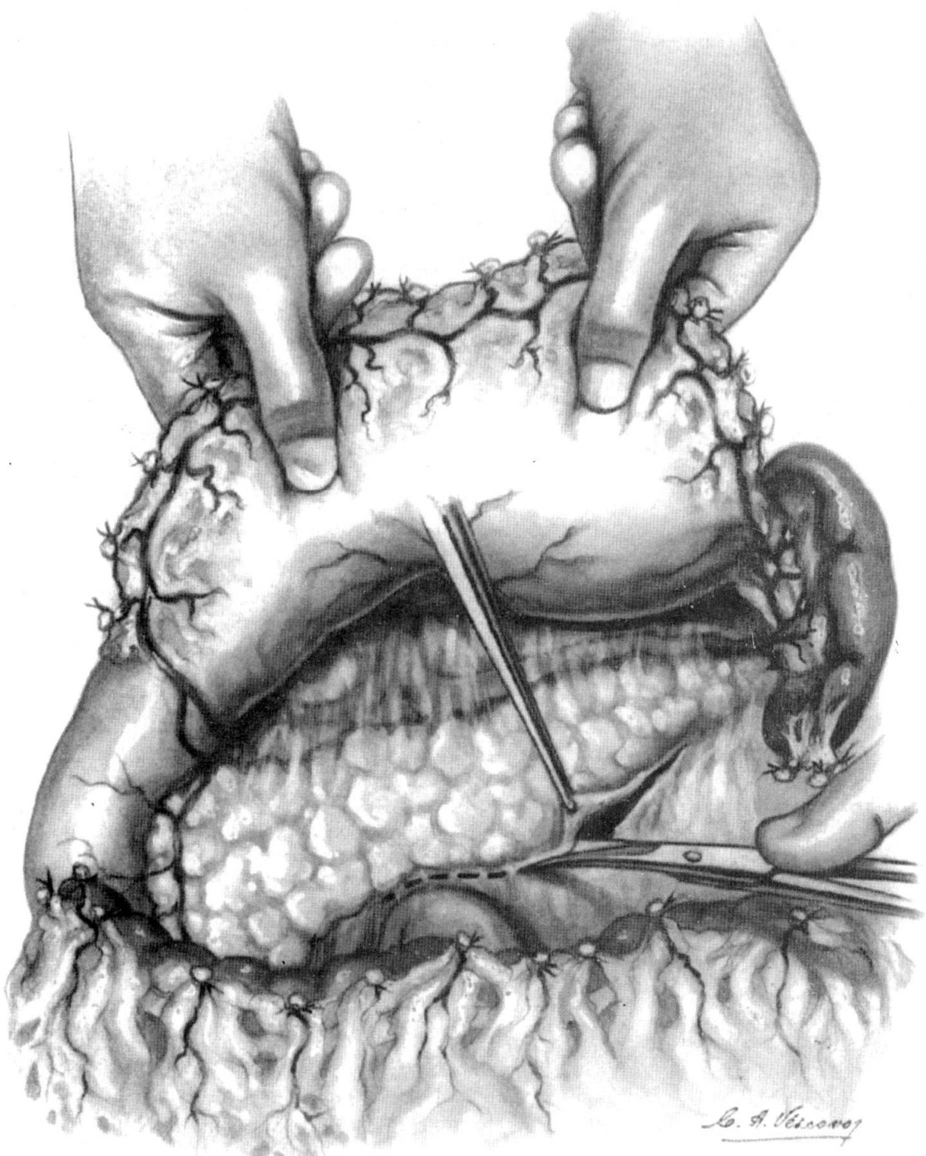

FIGURE 10.4

FIGURE 10.5

Once the inferior border of the pancreas has been dissected free, it is raised and held in place by two retractors, by the first assistant, to expose the posterior surface of the pancreas and be able to dissect the splenic vein. The splenic vein runs transversely along the middle of the posterior surface of the pancreas, but occasionally it runs along its upper third. Dissection of the splenic vein is begun near the site where it empties into the superior mesenteric vein. This is done with scissors, following the plane of areolar tissue between the adventihia and the sheath. If the surgeon does not enter the correct plane, the dissection can become very difficult. The drawing shows the dissection of the splenic vein with the scissors in the correct cleavage plane. In addition, the site of junction of the coronary vein with the superior border of the splenic vein near its confluence with the superior mesenteric vein. In 25% of patients, the coronary vein empties into the splenic vein (57). When this is the case, the coronary vein is ligated if possible (6).

Distal Splenorenal Shunt (55)

FIGURE 10.6

Once the splenic vein has been dissected free near its junction with the superior mesenteric vein and several pancreatic veins as well as the coronary vein have been ligated, a rubber loop is passed around it to exert mild traction downward to facilitate the dissection and ligation of the many affluent branches toward the caudal zone of the pancreas (6). These pancreatic veins are very thin walled and fragile, making them easy to rupture and producing copious bleeding. This may obscure the operative field, obliging the surgeon to make maneuvers that may injure the splenic vein. This may oblige the surgeon to suture or even tie off the splenic vein, which may make it necessary to carry out some other type of portosystemic shunt, and not a distal splenorenal shunt. Dissection of the splenic vein and ligation of its affluent branches is the most prolonged and difficult stage of this procedure (18–20). In order to be able to perform this shunt, the splenic vein must be freed for about 5 to 7 cm (42). The present tendency is to dissect the splenic vein all the way to the splenic hilus in order to ligate as many pancreatic veins as possible to delay the development of collateral veins, which, with the passage of time, is inevitable (6, 20). Ligation of pancreatic veins should be carried out by using a fine curved clamp to surround the vein and pass a suture around them to perform the ligation.

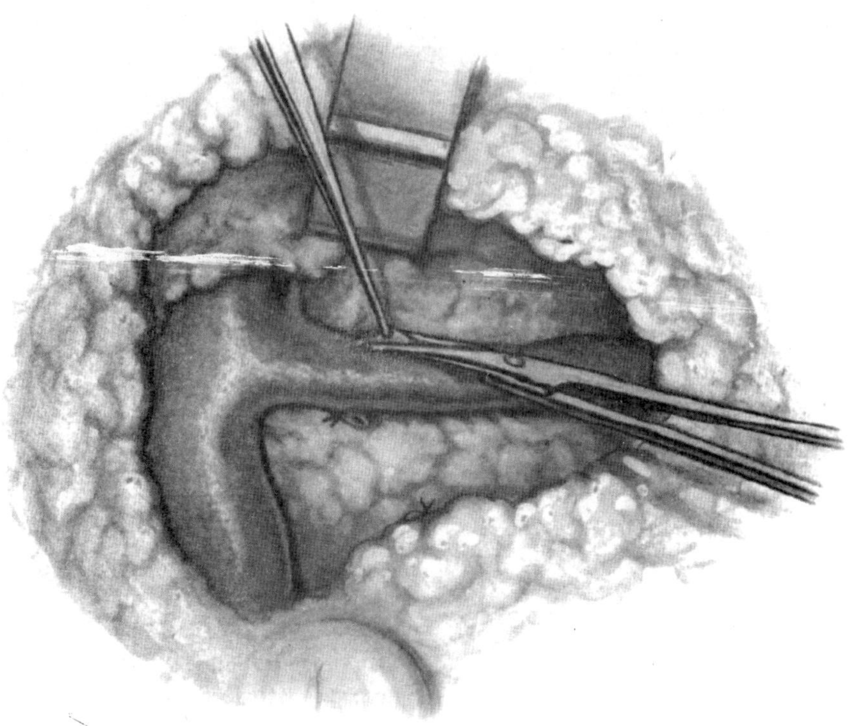

FIGURE 10.5

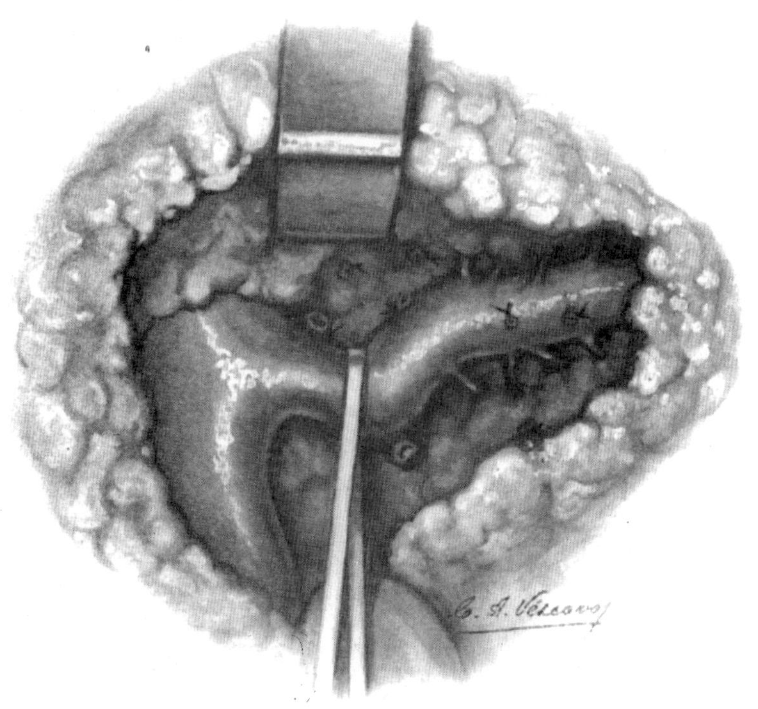

FIGURE 10.6

Distal Splenorenal Shunt

FIGURE 10.7

Once the splenic vein has been adequately liberated, a Satinsky clamp is placed near its junction with the superior mesenteric vein. About 3 or 4 cm distally, a vascular clamp (DeBakey, Cooley, Angled Potts, or a bulldog clamp, if the others are not available) is placed. Before transecting the splenic vein, two Prolene 6-0 sutures are placed on its inferior border, as shown. These serve to avoid torsion or rotation of the vein after it is divided (20, 55, 56). The splenic vein is transected using a scalpel or a Potts scissors, leaving enough of the vein on the splenic side to carry out a suture ligation of the vein with a 6-0 running Prolene suture, back and forth, to attain a watertight closure. The closure of the distal end of the splenic vein should not leave a stump, as used to happen when the stump was tied off instead of being suturing as described. Thrombosis is a complication of residual stumps (20).

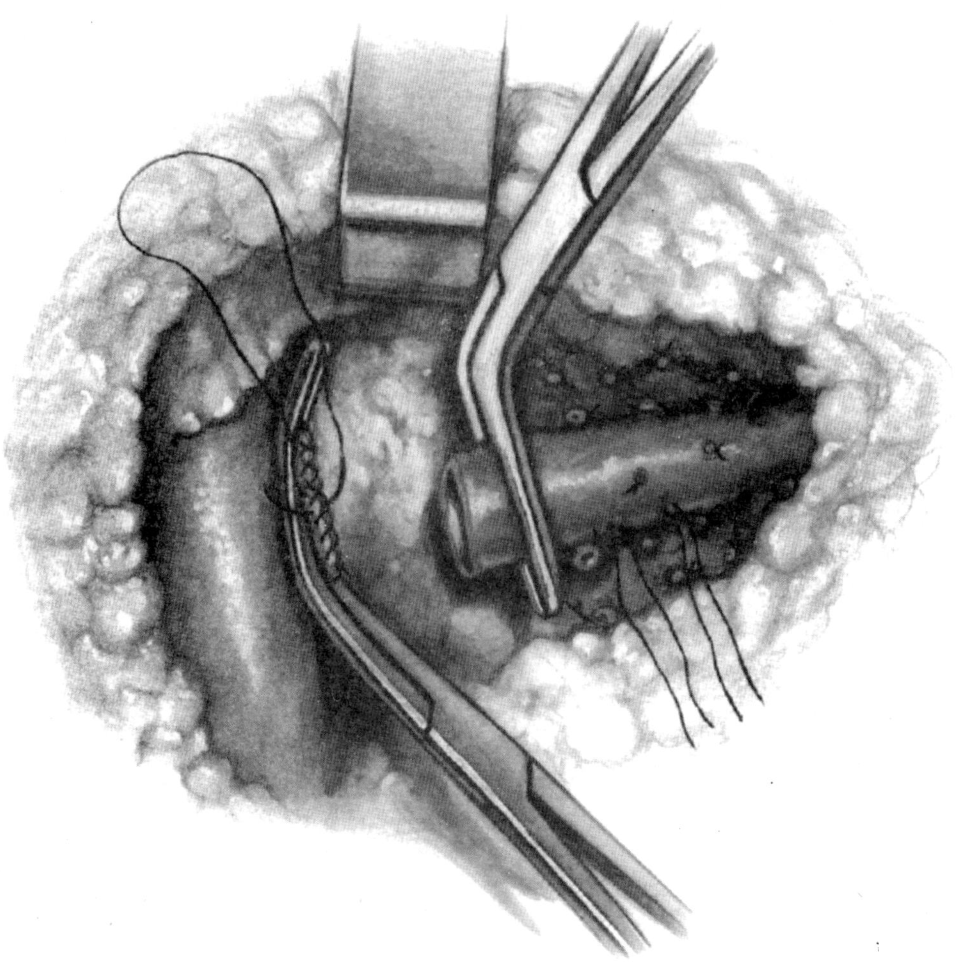

FIGURE 10.7

Distal Splenorenal Shunt (55)

FIGURE 10.8

The Satinsky clamp on the splenic vein is removed, and the left renal vein is identified. Its adequacy for anastomosis should have been determined preoperatively. The left renal vein, which is retroperitoneal, should be dissected from the left renal hilus to the aorta. In some cases identification of the left renal vein may be difficult because of severe thickening of the posterior parietal peritoneum and massive congestion of the retroperitoneal lymphatics. This engorgement of lymphatics makes it necessary for the surgeon to have to carry out multiple ligatures and divisions of the retroperitoneal tissues to prevent accumulation of ascitic fluid postoperatively. Several landmarks are useful in the identification of the left renal vein: the left renal pelvis, the vertebral column, the left renal artery, and the left gonadal vein, which empties into the left renal vein (42). If identification of the left renal vein continues to be difficult, the previously described maneuver used to find the inferior mesenteric vein in complex cases can be used. This consists of a longitudinal incision to the left of the ligament of Treitz (15).

The left renal vein courses horizontally in front of the aorta to empty into the inferior vena cava. During the dissection of the left renal vein it is frequently necessary to ligate and divide the left gonadal (ovarian or spermatic) vein, which empties into the inferior border of the left renal vein. The inferior adrenal vein, which empties into the superior border of the left renal vein, should also be ligated. Both of these veins can be ligated without any consequences to the patient. If the gonadal vein does not interfere with the shunt, it does not have to be ligated. From the practical point of view, the renal vein has been sufficiently liberated when two fingers can be passed around it together (42). Once the left renal vein has been liberated, the splenic vein is approximated to it to select the most appropriate site for the performance of the terminolateral splenorenal anastomosis. A Satinsky clamp is then placed on the renal vein, so as to partially occlude the vein, and a lozenge similar in length to the diameter of the splenic vein is removed from the anterior and superior aspect of the vein.

If the splenic vein does not have a large enough diameter, its end can be sectioned obliquely to make the lumen of the anastomosis larger. Another angled DeBakey clamp is applied to the splenic vein, nearer to the pancreas, and the DeBakey clamp that had been placed near the end of the splenic vein in order to transect it is removed. The splenorenal anastomosis is begun. To make suturing easier, stay sutures are placed in the angles of the splenic and renal veins, so that the knots are outside the lumen of both veins. Care should be taken to make the curve of the splenic vein smooth as the anastomosis is made. If the splenic vein is too long after it is dissected, the excess should be resected. There should be no traction or redundancy. Rotation and/or kinking of the splenic vein should be avoided. In order to avoid this, two 6-0 Prolene sutures have been inserted in the inferior border of the splenic vein before it is transected.

The posterior aspect of the anastomosis is performed using a continuous over and over 6-0 Prolene suture. The ends of this posterior running suture are tied to the traction sutures that had been placed in the angles so that the knots are outside the lumen of the veins. The drawing shows the stumps of the adrenal and gonadal veins. The insert shows the completion of the anterior portion of the anastomosis using interrupted 6-0 Prolene sutures to avoid narrowing of the anastomosis by avoiding a purse-string effect. Before inserting the last two anterior sutures, the DeBakey clamp should be opened to allow air, blood, and clots to come out. The clamp is then replaced and the anastomosis completed. Once the suturing is finished, the Satinsky clamp is removed and the DeBakey clamp is then removed.

If blood is coming out through the suture line, the line should be gently compressed with gauze and a few minutes allowed for hemostasis. In case blood continues to flow through the suture line, complementary sutures may be placed to assure hemostasis. In placing these sutures one must be careful not to narrow the lumen of the anastomosis.

If the ligature of the gastric veins has not been done prior to freeing the splenic vein, ligation and section of these veins should be performed at the end of the shunt. Ligation of the coronary, right gastroepiploic, and right gastric veins is an important part of this procedure.

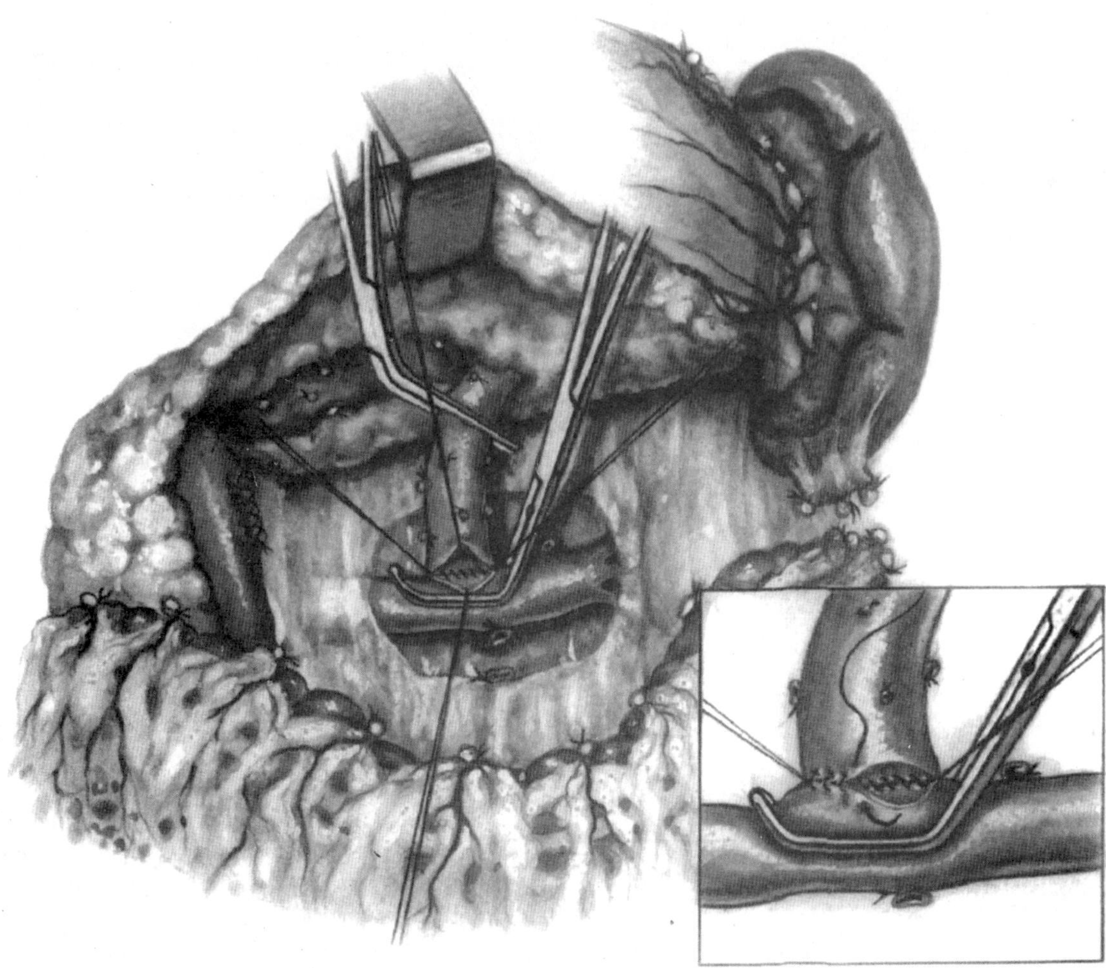

FIGURE 10.8

FIGURE 10.9
Schematic drawing showing the completed distal splenorenal shunt (6, 56). 1, Splenic vein. 2, Left renal vein. 3, Vena cava. 4, Portal vein with intact flow. 5, Ligated coronary vein. 6, Ligated right gastroepiploic vein. 7, Short vessels. 8, Spleen. 9, Left kidney. 10, Henle's trunk.

The gastric veins remain disconnected from the portal venous pressure. The esophageal varices are decompressed through the short vessels and the left gastroepiploic vein, which carry vomit blood to the splenic vein and from there to the systemic circulation through the shunt.

Distal Splenorenal Shunt

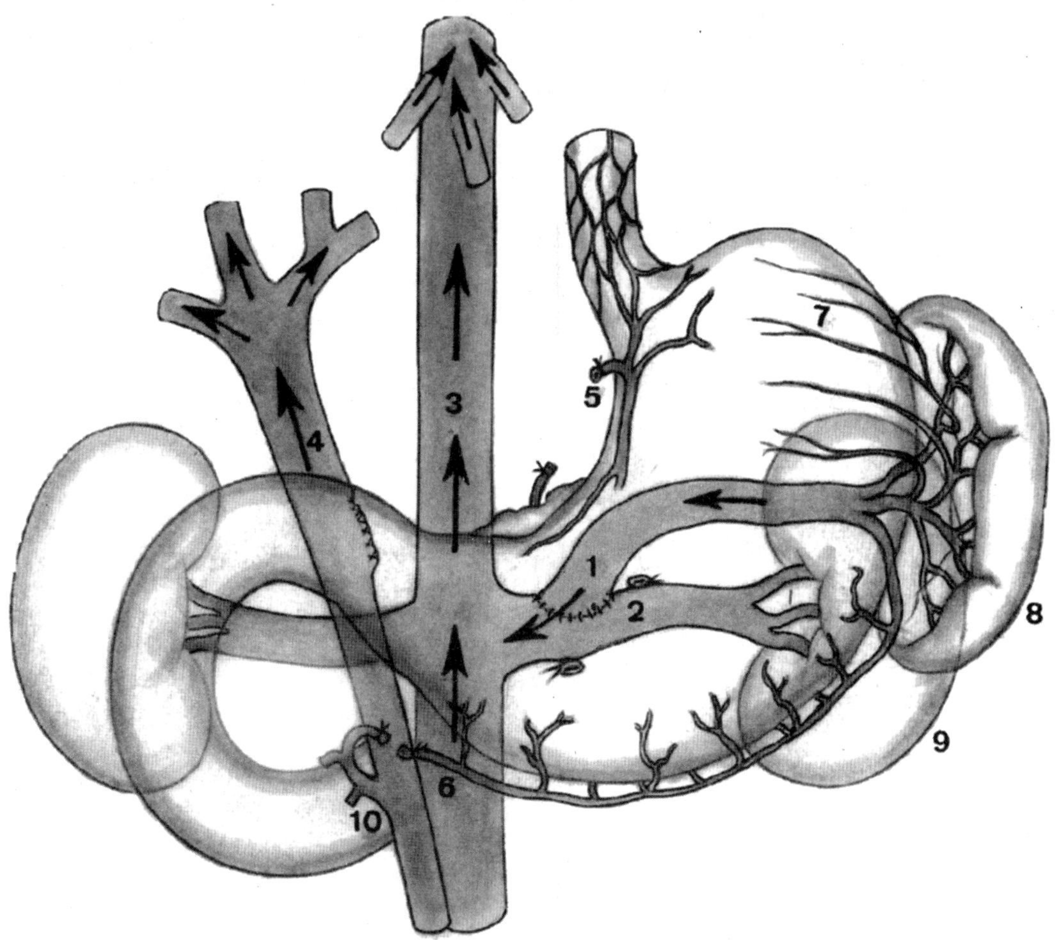

FIGURE 10.9

FIGURE 10.10
Subcostal incision some 3 cm below the costal margin and the xiphoid process. Half of the left anterior rectus muscle of the abdomen and the entire right anterior rectus muscle and the muscles of the right flank must be transected. The right side of the patient should be elevated some 15 cm from the horizontal plane. This incision provides a good operative field, making it unnecessary to enter the thorax. The abdominal incision should be widely opened by means of a large self-retaining retractor complemented with an "upper hand" type of retractor to raise the anterior wall of the abdomen. Exploration of the abdominal cavity and biopsy of the liver are performed using the same technique as described in the distal splenorenal shunt. Patients who present a very large gallbladder that interferes with the operative field can have the gallbladder diminished in size by manually compressing it. If this maneuver is not successful, the fundus of the gallbladder may be punctured with a syringe and a 22 F needle. The opening of the needle should be closed with two Prolene 6-0 sutures or a small pursestring suture.

Terminolateral Portocaval Shunt

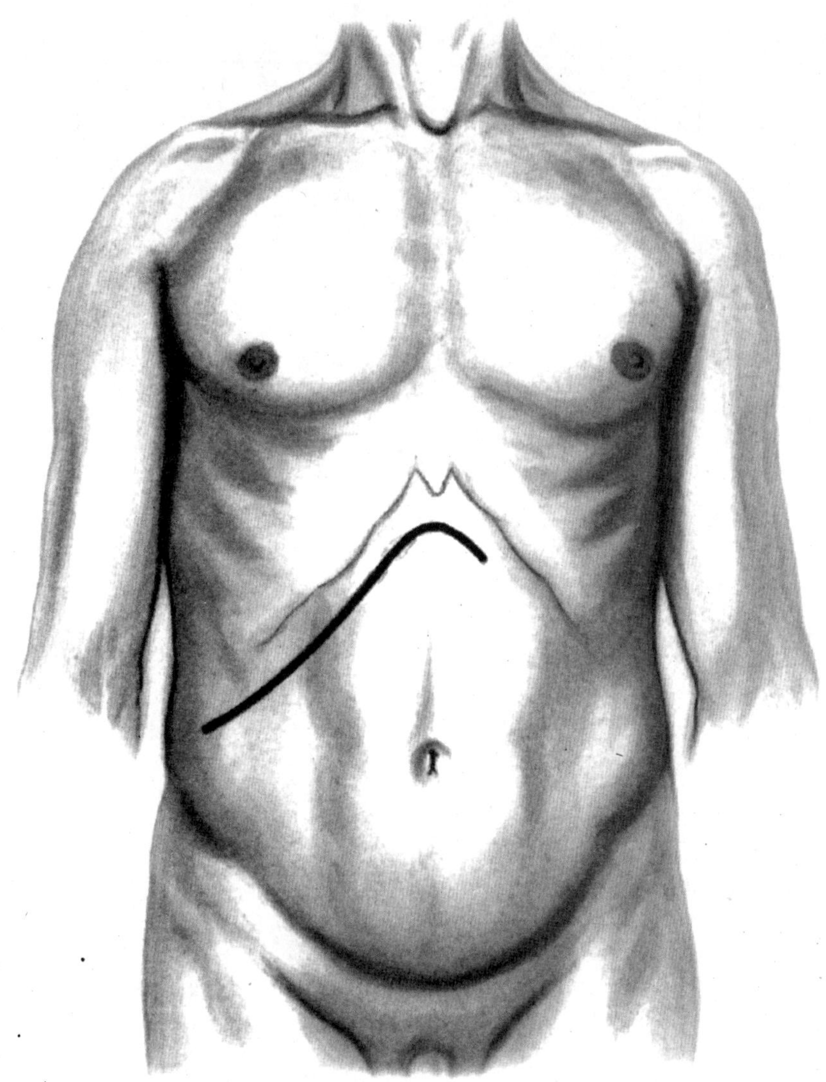

FIGURE 10.10

Terminolateral Portocaval Shunt

FIGURE 10.11

After exploration of the whole abdominal cavity, a Vautrin-Kocher maneuver is performed. This maneuver is begun by liberating the transverse colon, with its mesocolon, and keeping it retracted in the inferior portion of the incision with a moist compress held in place by a Deaver retractor. In some cases, it may be necessary to bring down the hepatic flexure of the colon. The inferior surface of the liver is retracted upward using a moist compress held in place by a Doyen or other similar retractor, as shown in the drawing. The peritoneum over the lateral border of the duodenum is incised and then sectioned upward to include the anterior portion of the peritoneum of the hepaticoduodenal ligament (broken line), and downward, along the lateral edge of the third portion of the duodenum, up to the superior mesenteric vessels (broken line). In order to perform the mobilization of the duodenum, it is easier if the assistant grasps it with two hands and applies traction to it upward and to the left. Manual traction is preferable to the use of atraumatic clamps because there is less possibility of tearing the duodenal wall. There is no doubt that the Vautrin-Kocher maneuver facilitates exposure of the inferior vena cava and the portal vein. Patients with cirrhosis frequently develop extensive venous collaterals, which make it necessary to use hemostatic clamps when the peritoneum along the lateral duodenal border is incised. This is in contrast to the practically bloodless incision of this area in patients without cirrhosis.

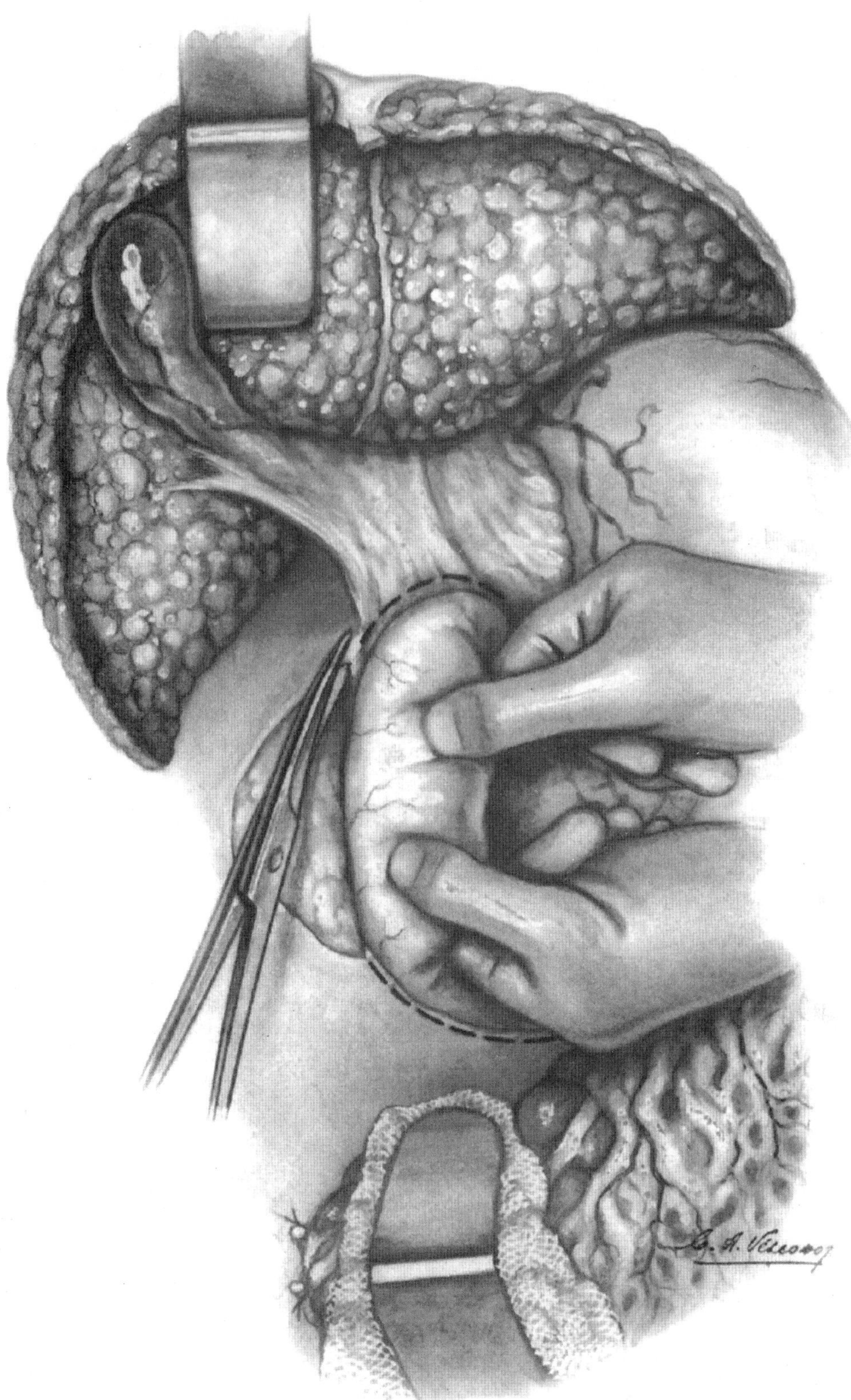

FIGURE 10.11

End to Side Portocaval Shunt

FIGURE 10.12

The Vautrin-Kocher maneuver has been completed. The duodenum and the head of the pancreas have been mobilized to the left, exposing the inferior vena cava covered with retroperitoneal tissue, the dissection of which is being completed with scissors. Liberation of the vena cava, in cirrhotic patients, can be very difficult owing to engorgement of the net of retroperitoneal lymphatics and the development of dense venous collateral circulation. This lymphatic and venous tissue has to be ligated and divided in several places to prevent the development of postoperative ascites. It is not necessary to mobilize the vena cava circumferentially. It is only necessary to dissect and expose its anterior and lateral aspects from the renal veins to the caudate lobe.

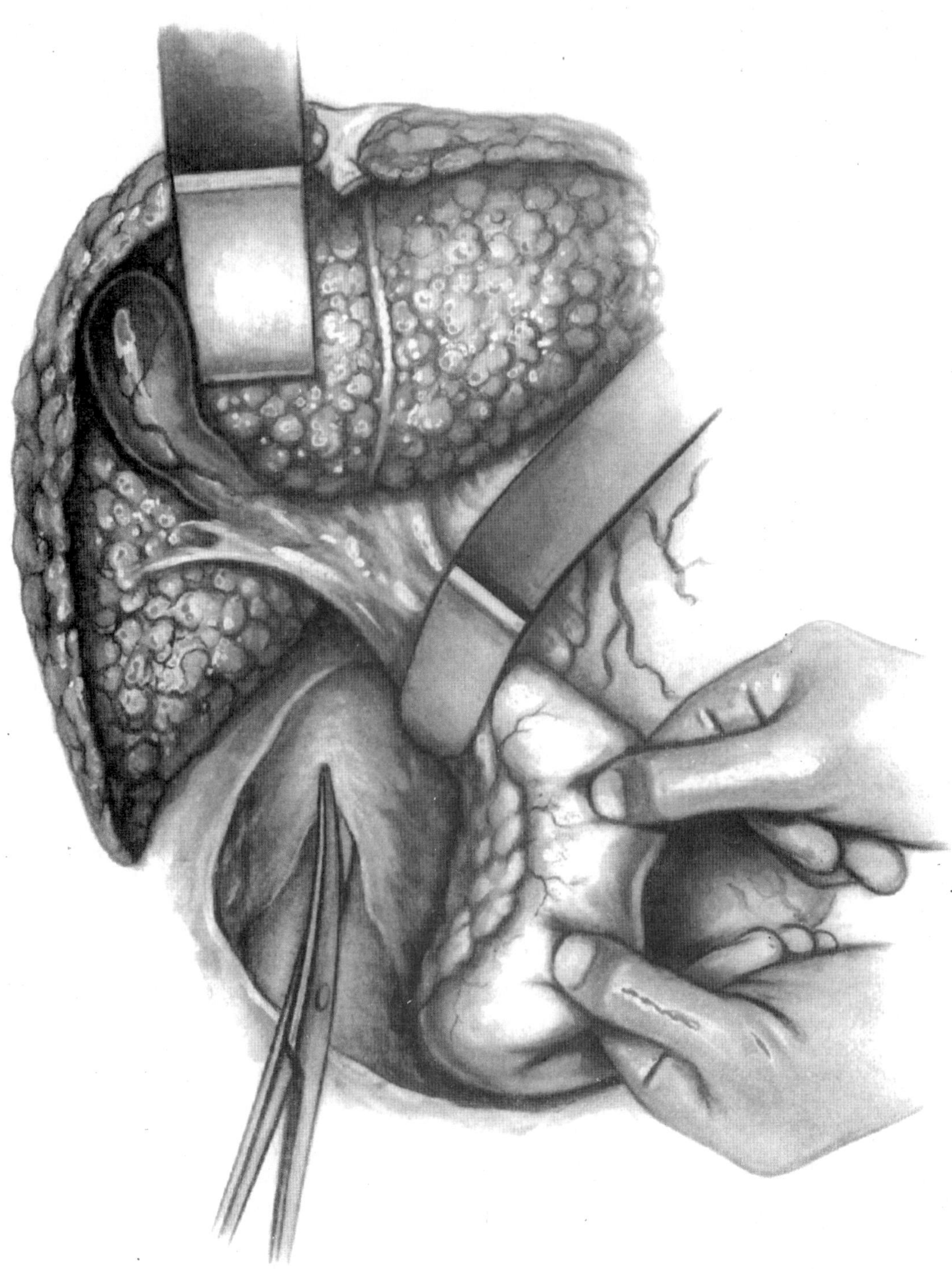

FIGURE 10.12

FIGURE 10.13

The portal vein should be dissected free and mobilized after the inferior vena cava has been cleared. The portal vein is located in the hepaticoduodenal ligament, in a plane posterior to the common bile duct and the hepatic artery, which are in an anterior plane. The hepaticoduodenal ligament with its contents forms the anterior border of the foramen of Winslow. Liberation of the portal vein is begun by performing a longitudinal incision in the posterolateral border of the hepaticoduodenal ligament over the portal vein, as shown in the insert (broken line). After the peritoneum is incised, the portal vein is freed, first posteriorly, then laterally, and finally on its medial side. In cirrhotic patients two or more lymph nodes can be seen, very adherent to the hepaticoduodenal ligament, which should be removed very carefully, unless they can be avoided during the dissection of the portal vein.

End to Side Portocaval Shunt

To completely dissect the portal vein, the common bile duct should be separated to the left and held in place with vein retractors. This will reveal several affluent veins entering the portal vein medially or posteriorly. These veins should be carefully dissected and ligated, since their rupture may make a terminolateral portocaval shunt impossible. The portal vein should be completely exposed, from its origin behind the pancreas to its bifurcation near the inferior surface of the liver. While the portal vein is being dissected, the full extension of the common bile duct and the hepatic artery should be exposed. Both of these may present numerous anatomic variations, which should be recognized to avoid injuring them.

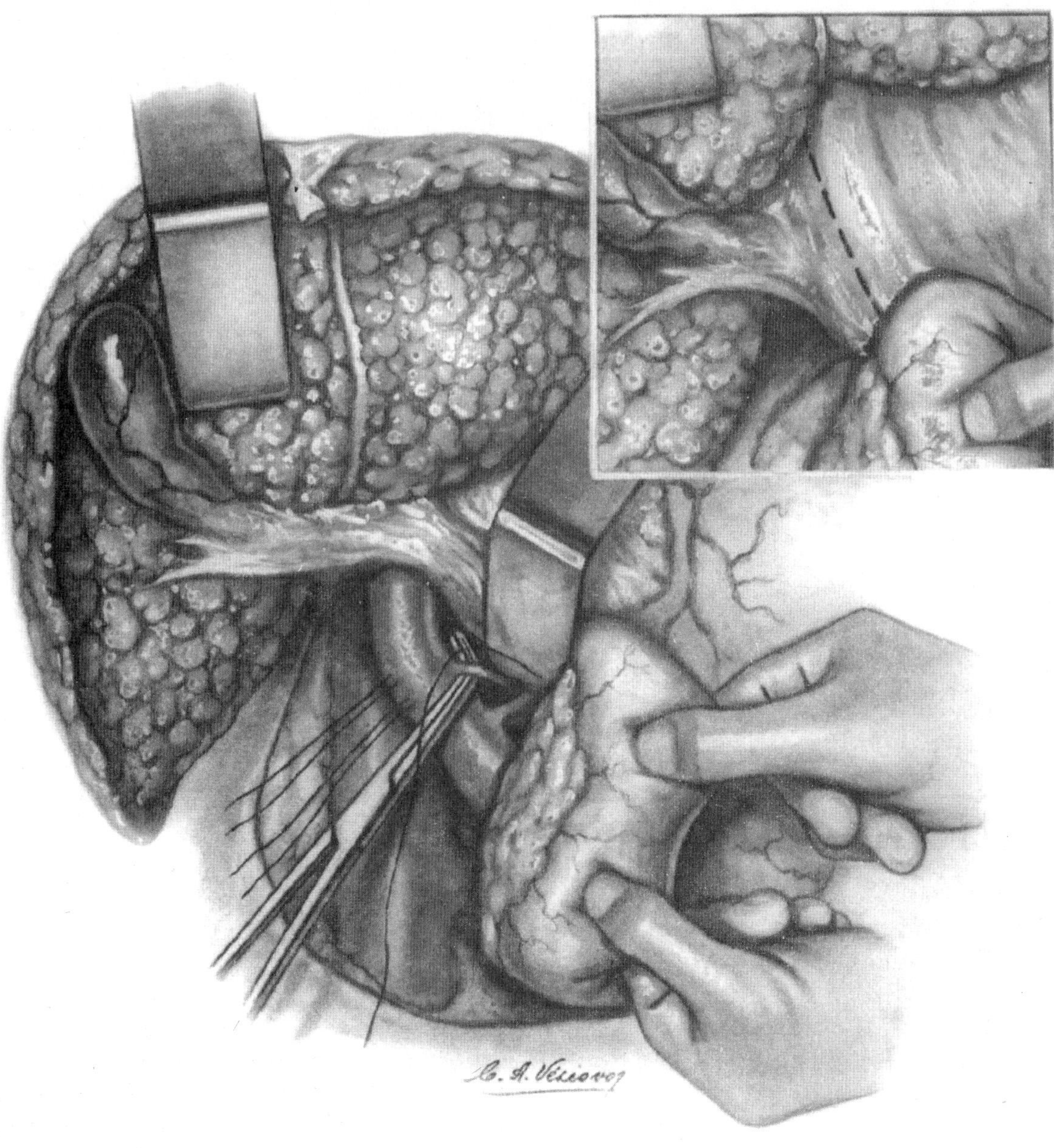

FIGURE 10.13

End to Side Portocaval Shunt

FIGURE 10.14

Once the portal vein has been completely liberated, two Cooley clamps are inserted, one at each end, in order to proceed with its transection. Two 6-0 Prolene sutures should be applied to the right border of the portal vein, as guide sutures, to prevent torsion or rotation of the vein after it is transected. Using a Potts scissors, the portal vein is transected below the upper Cooley clamp. The drawing shows the closure of the vein stump with a back and forth continuous 6-0 Prolene suture. In cases where a longer segment of portal vein is necessary, the branches of the portal vein can be sectioned beyond the bifurcation of the vein.

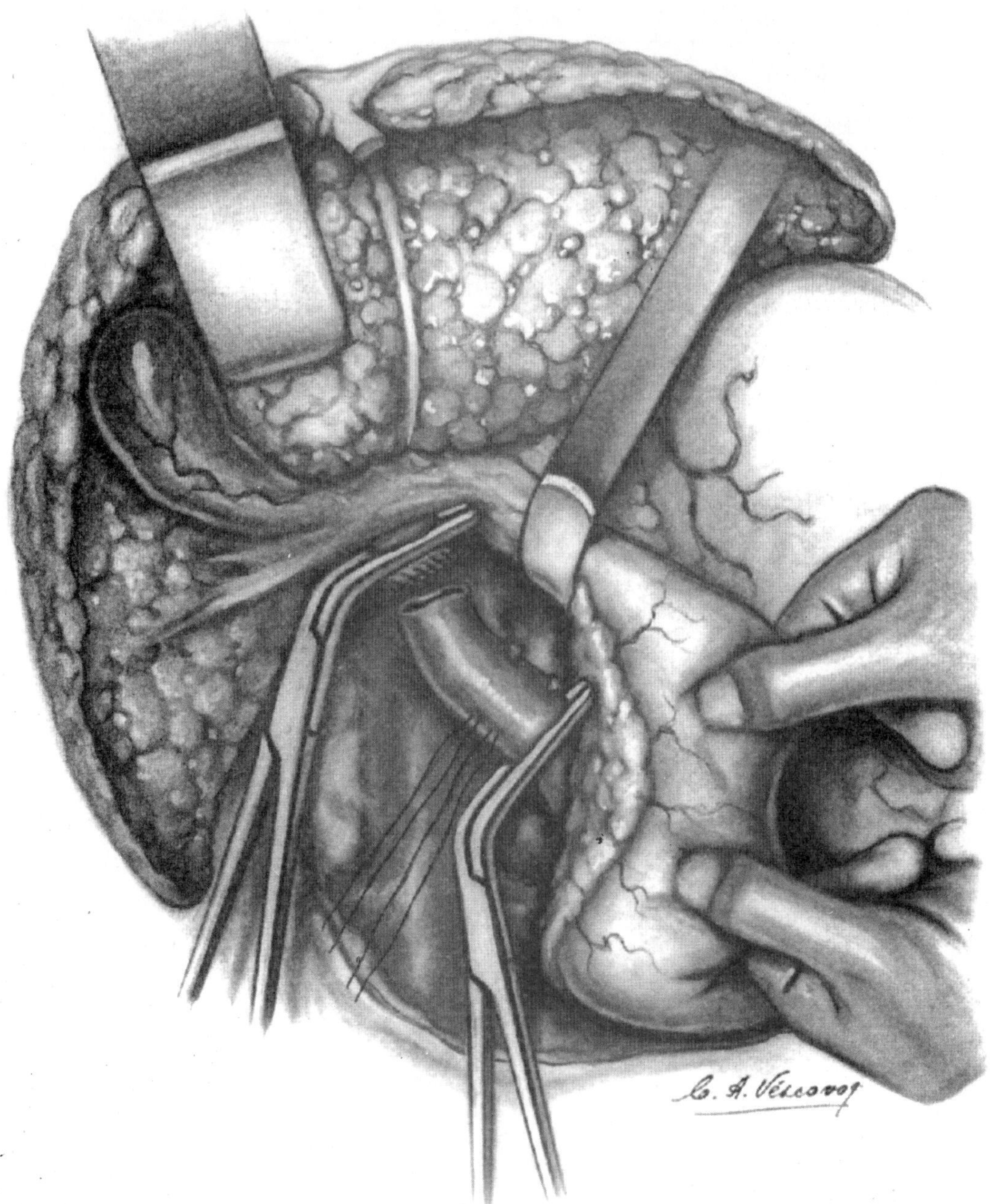

FIGURE 10.14

End to Side Portocaval Shunt

FIGURE 10.15
A Satinsky clamp has been placed on the segment of the vena cava selected for the anastomosis. This is placed to include its anterior and medial aspects to facilitate the anastomosis. A lozenge of vena cava the size of the diameter of the portal vein is excised from within the Satinsky clamp. Some authors have achieved the same results without excising this lozenge (42). Traction sutures have been placed in the angles and the lateral borders of the vena cava.

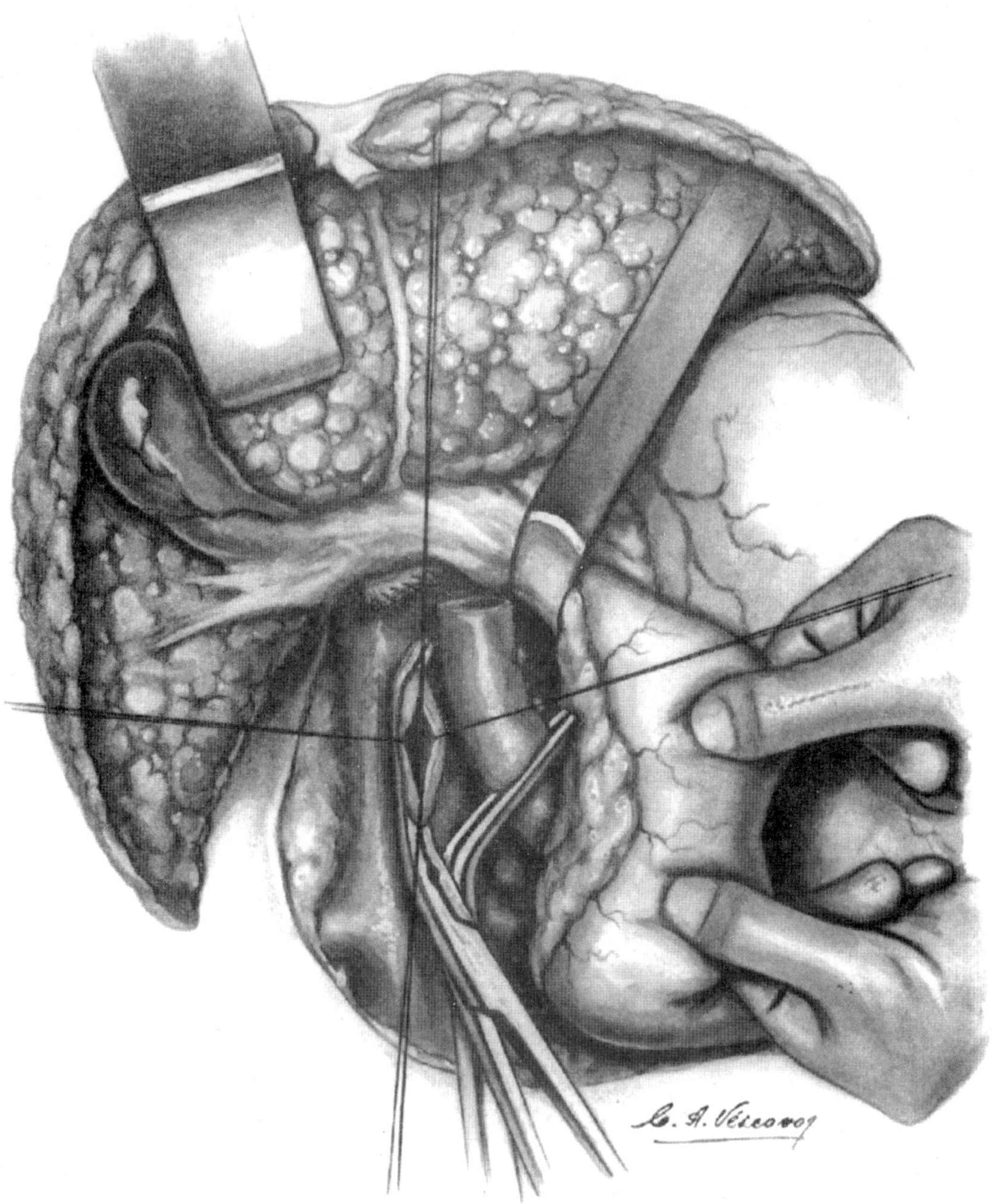

FIGURE 10.15

End to Side Portocaval Shunt

FIGURE 10.16
The transected end of the portal vein is approximated to the site where the vena cava has been opened. The anastomosis of the portal vein to the vena cava should make a gentle curve. Torsion and kinking should be avoided at all costs. Sutures of 5-0 Prolene should be placed at the angles of both veins, with the knots on the outside, before starting the anastomosis, as shown. A traction suture should also be placed on the lateral border of the opening in the vena cava.

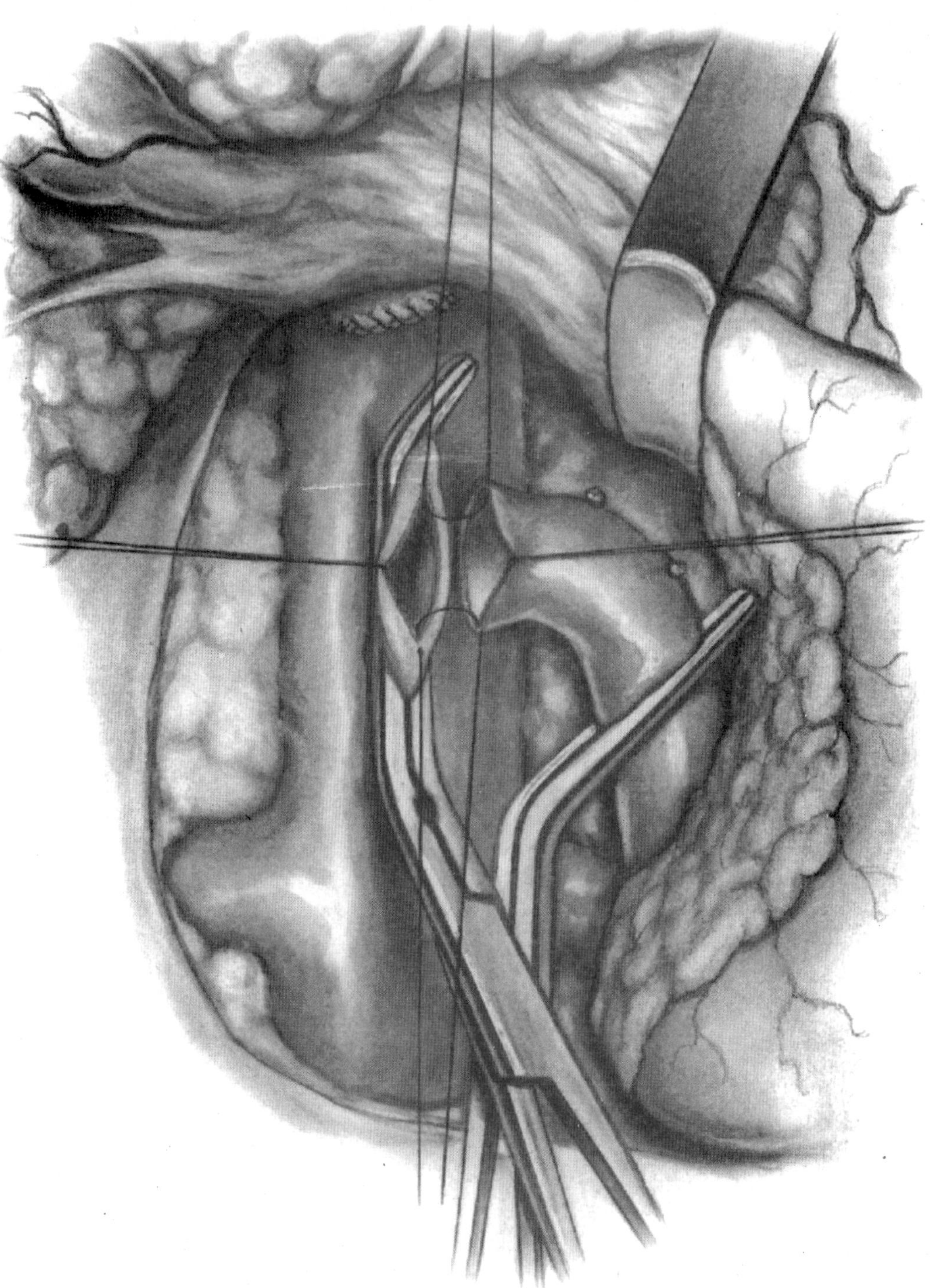

FIGURE 10.16

End to Side Portocaval Shunt

FIGURE 10.17
The over and over suture of the posterior plane has been begun, using 5-0 Prolene. When the angles are reached, the ends of the posterior suture are tied to the traction angle sutures that were previously placed with the knots on the outside of the venous lumen.

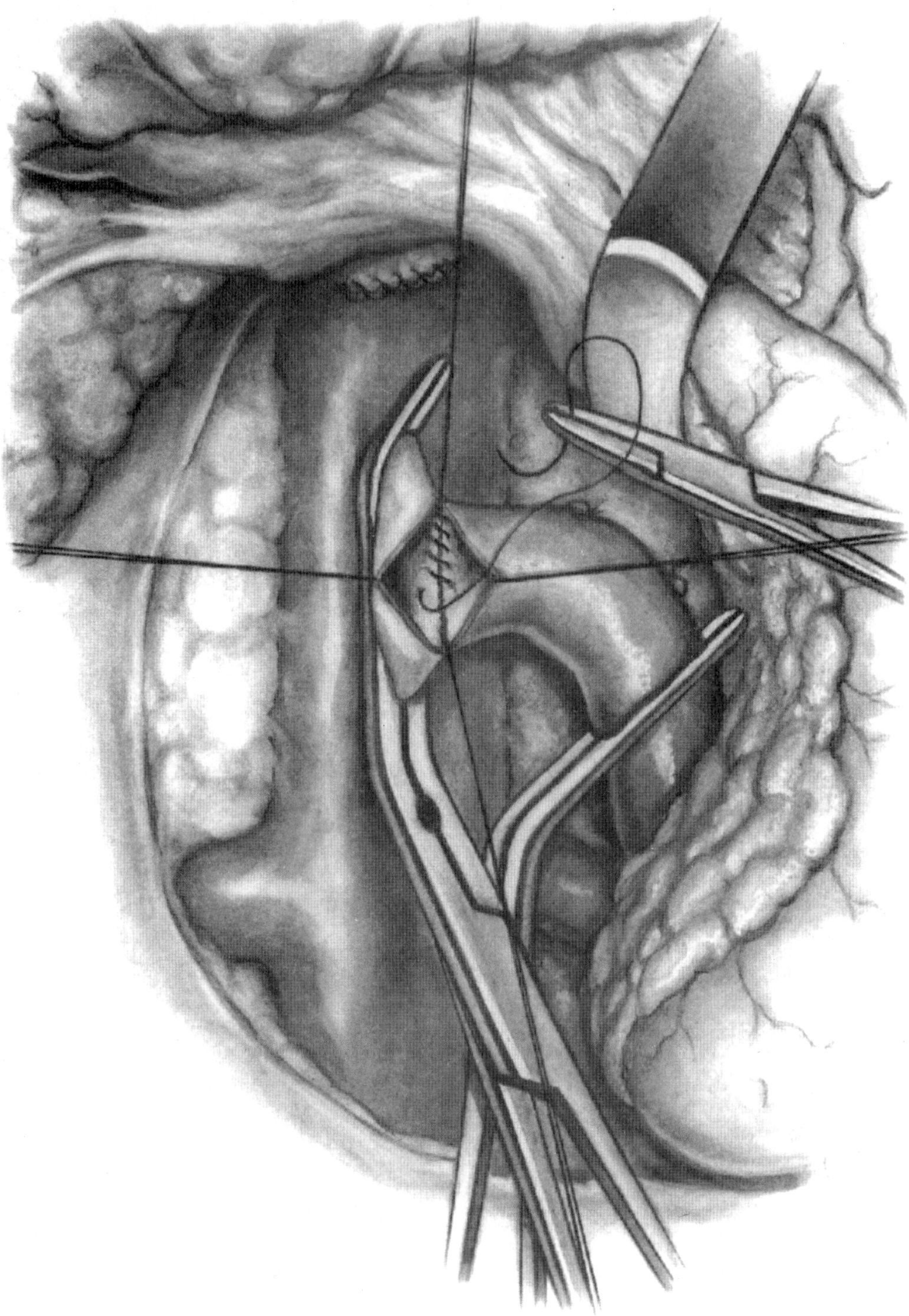

FIGURE 10.17

End to Side Portocaval Shunt

FIGURE 10.18

The anterior plane is then sutured in similar fashion, using a continuous 5-0 Prolene suture. A purse-string effect should be avoided, inserting the suture so as to avoid narrowing the lumen. When two or three sutures are still to be inserted, the Cooley clamp on the portal vein is loosened so as to allow any air, blood, or clots that may have formed to come out. The clamp is then reapplied, and the anterior suture line is completed. If some blood continues to ooze after clamps are removed, gentle compression with gauze is applied. This compression will usually control the bleeding. If it doesn't, one or more sutures can be placed where the blood is flowing, being careful not to narrow the lumen of the anastomosis.

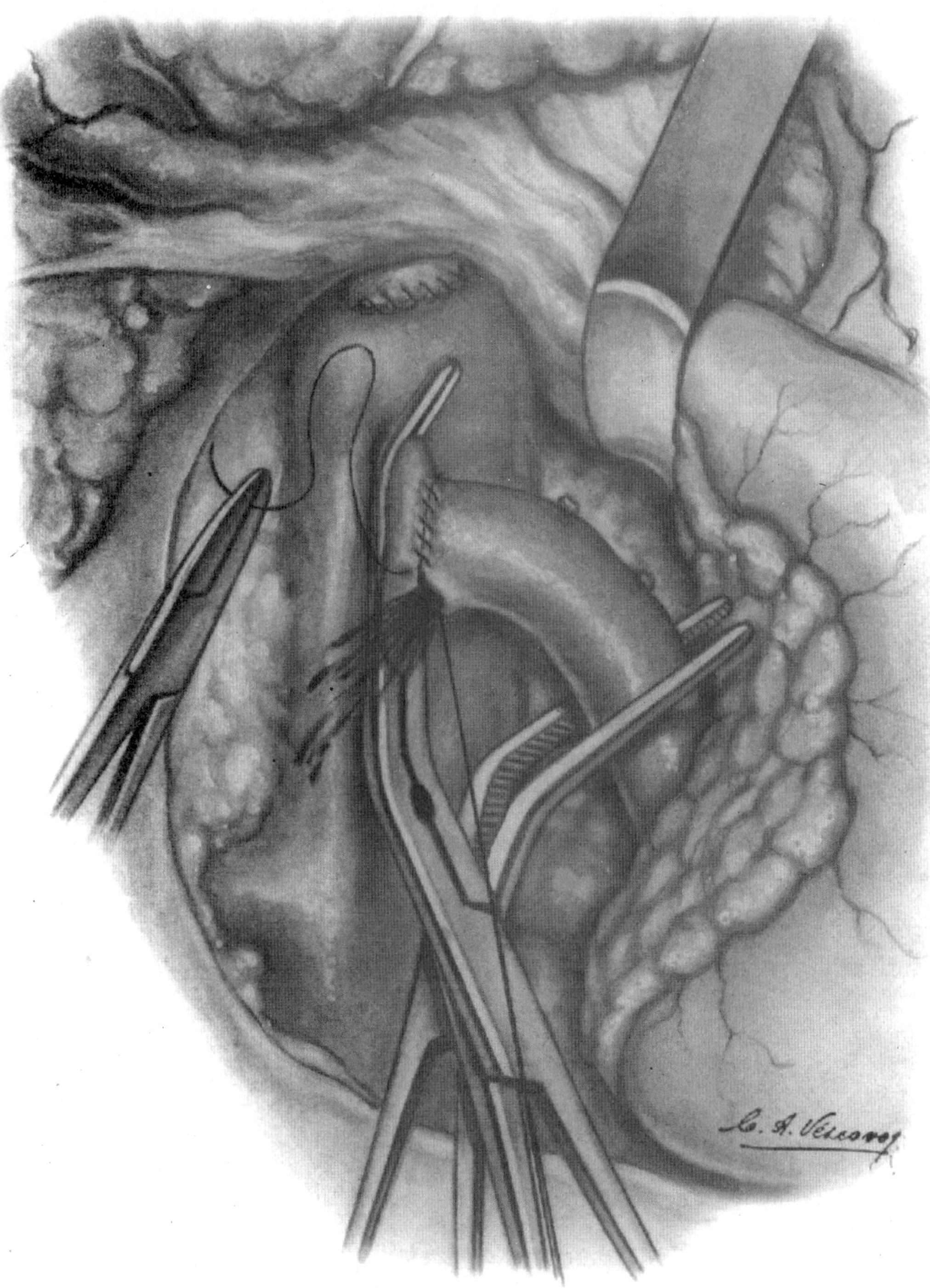

FIGURE 10.18

Side to Side Portocaval Shunt

FIGURE 10.19

A right subcostal incision is made 3 cm below the right costal border and the xiphoid process, extending upward to the middle of the left anterior rectus muscle and downward to include the right flank. The base of the right thorax should be elevated about 15 cm by using a small pillow. Identification and dissection of the inferior vena cava and the portal vein are similar to that carried out in the end to side portocaval shunt, except that it is necessary to mobilize the vena cava and the portal vein more extensively. If the portal vein lies in close proximity to the vena cava, it may be possible to carry out the anastomosis without great mobilization of the vena cava. In cases in which the veins are somewhat distant from each other, it becomes necessary to ligate some lumbar affluent veins to mobilize the vena cava enough to carry out the anastomosis without any tension. In patients with an enlarged caudate lobe, a common occurrence in Budd-Chiari Syndrome, approximation of both veins may be very difficult, even with ligation of several lumbar veins. This may make resection of a part of the caudate lobe necessary, or the side to side portocaval anastomosis may have to be substituted for an end to side procedure. In patients with massive ascites the side to side anastomosis should not be changed to an end to side procedure. It should again be pointed out that portocaval anastomoses lead to hepatic encephalopathy in 15 to 45% of patients. Encephalopathy may appear immediately or months, and even years, following surgery (12, 31, 33, 42). If there has been encephalopathy before surgery, it very frequently becomes worse after surgery.

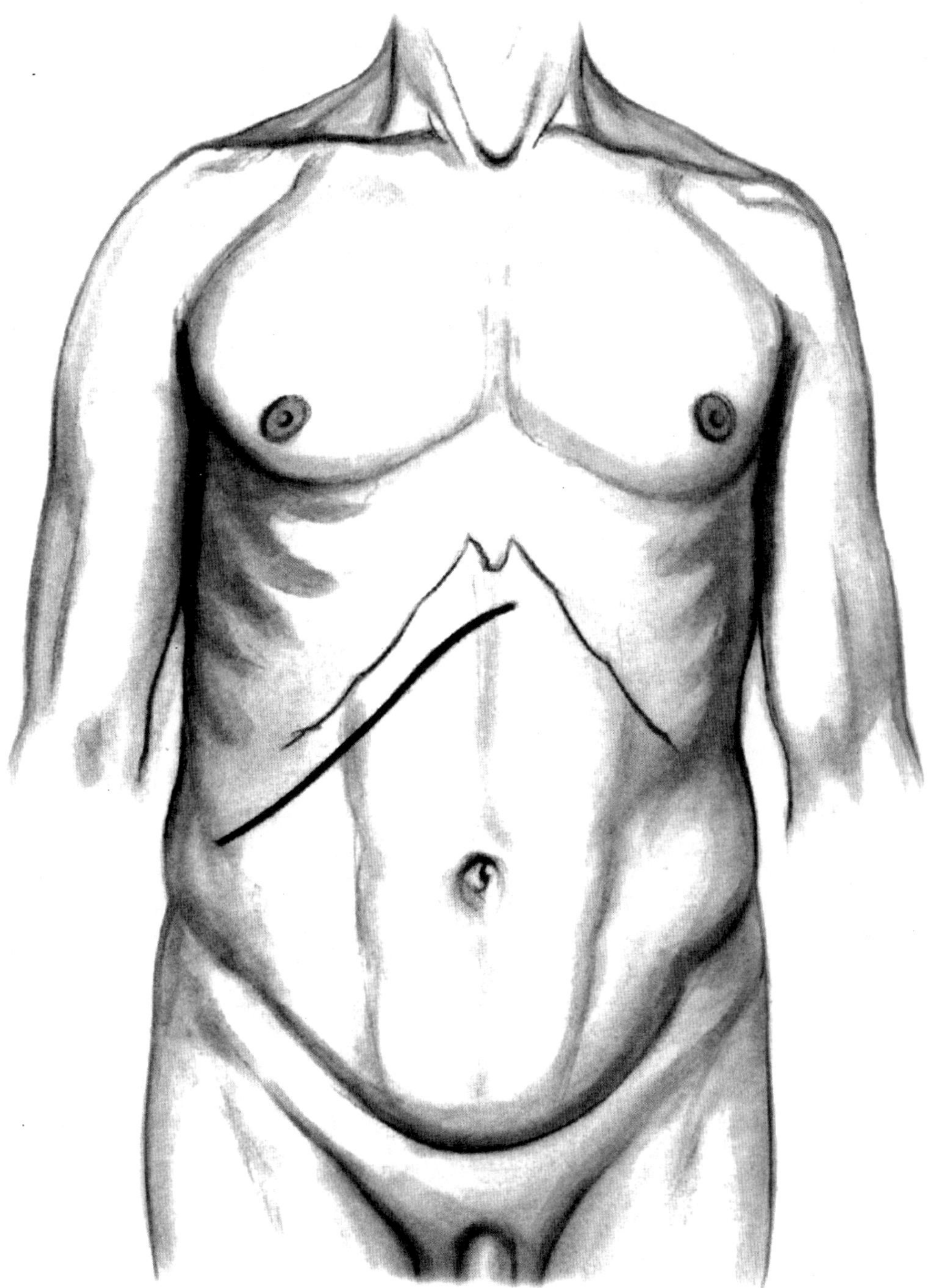

FIGURE 10.19

Side to Side Portocaval Shunt

FIGURE 10.20

The drawing shows that the inferior vena cava has been adequately mobilized and a Satinsky clamp has been applied, grasping the anteriomedial wall of the vena cava. A 2.0 to 2.5 cm. lozenge of vena cava is then removed. Some surgeons do not consider it necessary to remove a lozenge of vein wall from either the portal vein or the vena cava (42). The liberated portal vein has been clamped using two Cooley clamps, one near its bifurcation and the other near the pancreas. Both Cooley clamps are held by the first assistant and rotated 40 to 50° upward and to the left to facilitate removal of a lozenge of tissue from the posterior wall of the portal vein. This lozenge should be similar in size to the one removed from the vena cava, so as to facilitate the anastomosis (21).

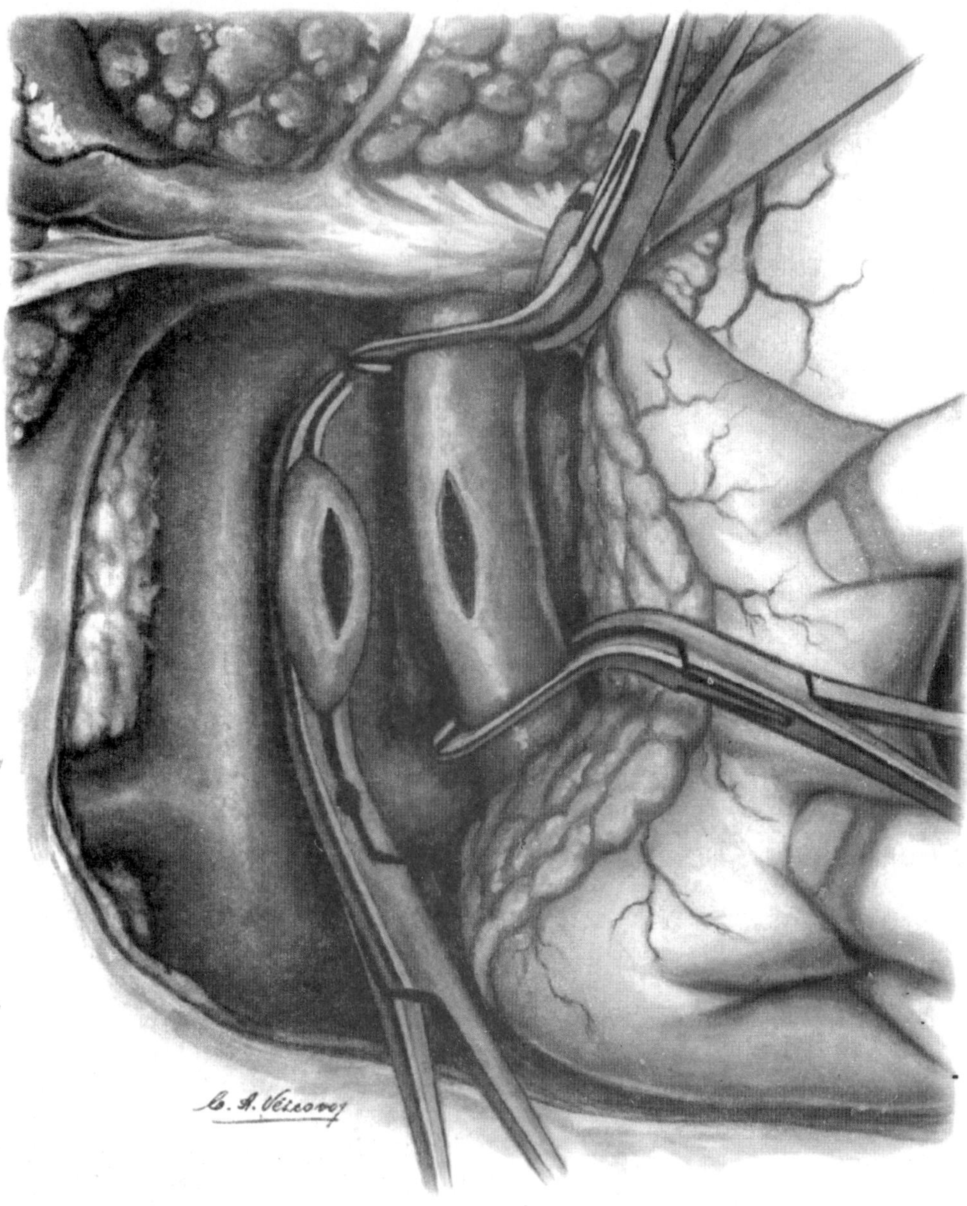

FIGURE 10.20

Side to Side Portocaval Shunt

FIGURE 10.21
The portal vein has been placed in contact with the inferior vena cava, traction sutures having been placed in its angles, with the knots on the outside of the venous lumen. The posterior suture line has begun, from below upward, using a continuous 5-0 Prolene suture. The initial stitch of the posterior suture is tied to the inferior angle suture, leaving the knot on the outside. When the upper angle is reached, the continuous suture is tied to the traction suture previously placed in this angle, again leaving the knot outside.

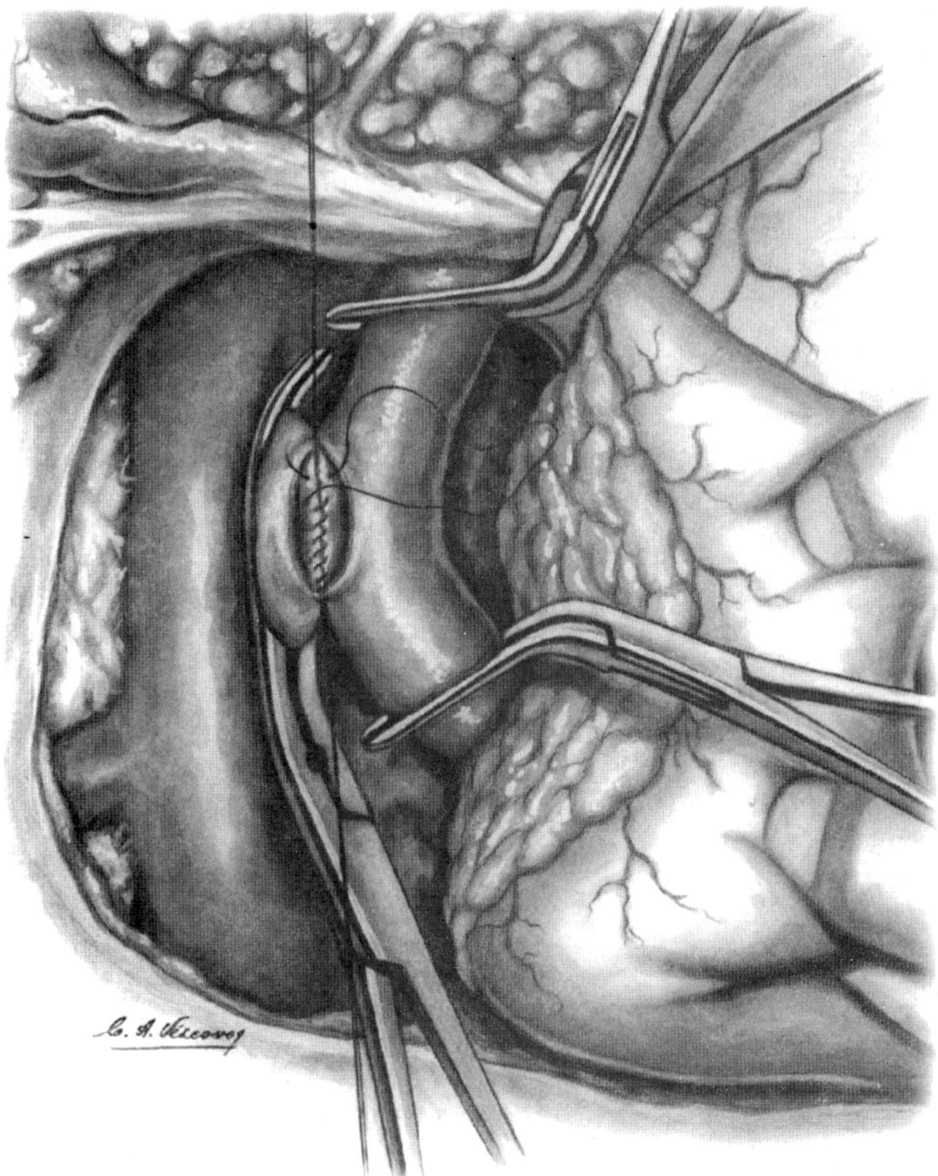

FIGURE 10.21

Side to Side Portocaval Shunt

FIGURE 10.22

Once the continuous posterior suture is completed, the anterior suture is performed, as seen in the drawing. When the anterior row is about to be completed, the Cooley clamp on the portal vein is temporarily loosened to allow blood, air, and clots that may have formed to come out. After this maneuver the Cooley clamp is replaced, allowing the completion of the anastomosis. It is advisable to remove the clamps in the following order: first, the Satinsky clamp from the vena cava, followed by the Cooley clamp on the upper portal vein, and finally the inferior Cooley clamp.

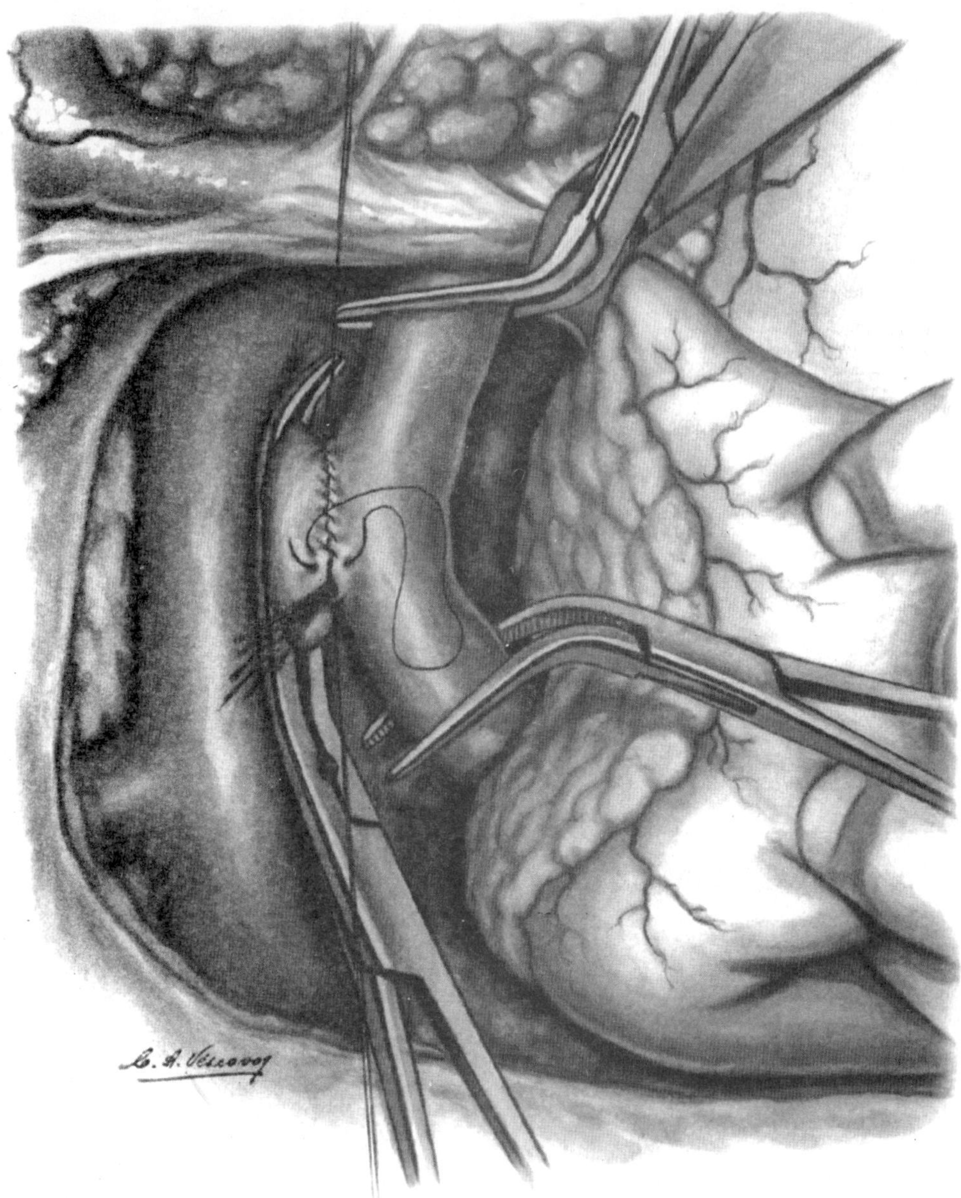

FIGURE 10.22

Side to Side Portocaval Shunt

FIGURE 10.23
A completed laterolateral portacaval anastomosis. Please note that the suturing of both veins is performed without tension.

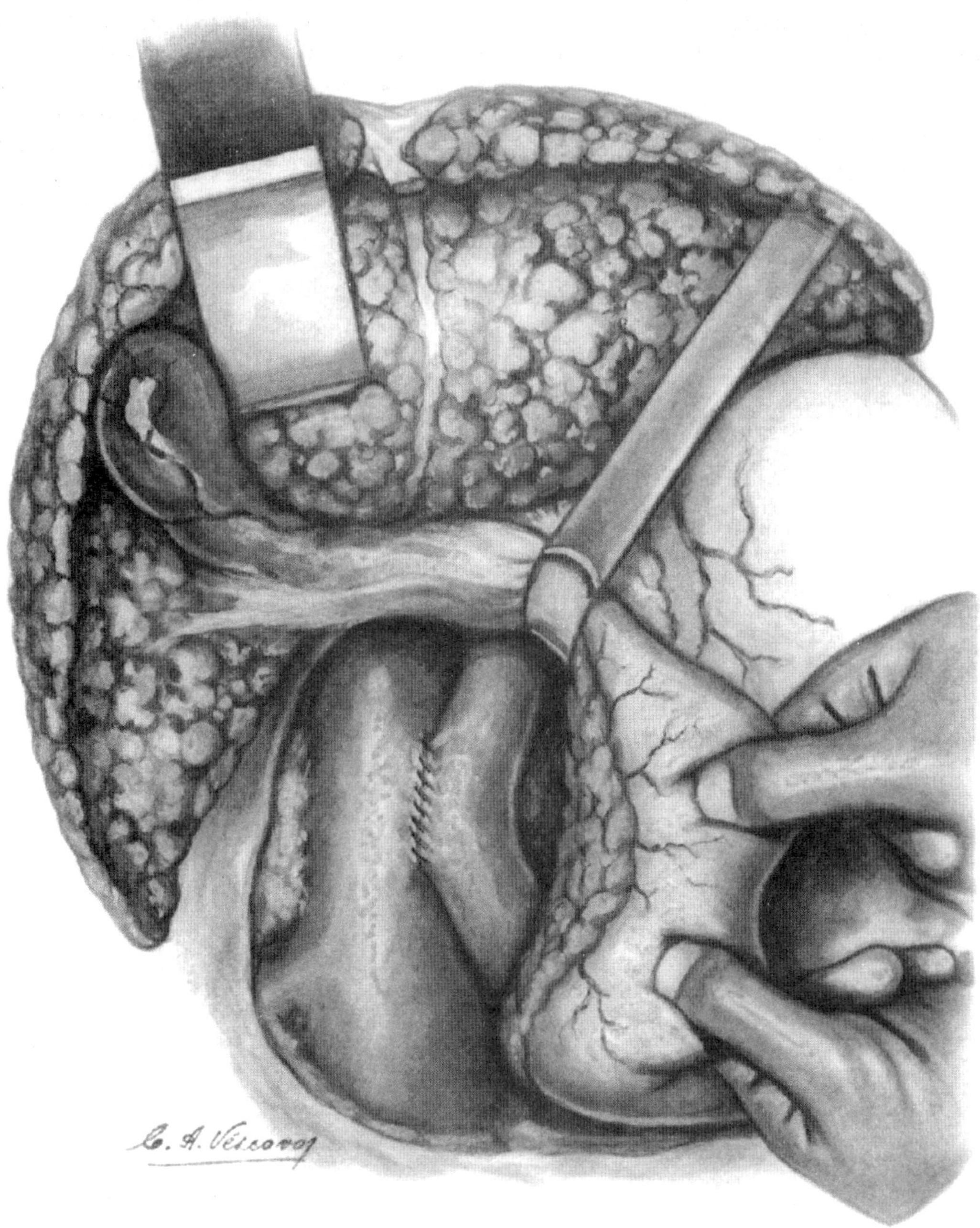

FIGURE 10.23

Portacaval Anastomosis with Interposition of Prosthesis (Portocaval H Graft)

In patients in whom it is not possible to perform a side to side portocaval anastomosis and in those in whom we are trying to diminish the possibility of hepatic encephalopathy, one can perform a portocaval anastomosis by interposing a polytetrafluoroethylene (Gore-Tex) prosthesis 12 mm in diameter and 4 to 5 cm long. The Gore-Tex tube should not be more than 5 cm long. The H portacaval shunt with Gore-Tex tube interposition leads to less frequent hepatic encephalopathy but has the serious inconvenience of a 30% incidence of thrombosis. At present it is possible in some cases, to successfully perform percutaneous dilation of the thrombosed segment.

Portocaval Anastomosis with Interposition of Prosthesis (Portocaval H Graft)

Portocaval Anastomosis with Interposition of Prosthesis (Portocaval H Graft)

FIGURE 10.24

The Gore-Tex tube is first anastomosed to the vena cava. To do this a Satinsky clamp is placed on the anteromedial aspect of the vena cava and the Gore-Tex tube is grafted to the vena cava using a running 5-0 Prolene suture. Once the Gore-Tex tube is sutured to the vena cava, two Cooley vascular clamps are placed on the portal vein, one superiorly near its bifurcation, and another inferiorly, near the pancreas. The Cooley clamps must be held by the first assistant rotating them upward and to the left to be able to perform the anastomosis of the Gore-Tex tube to the posterior aspect of the portal vein.

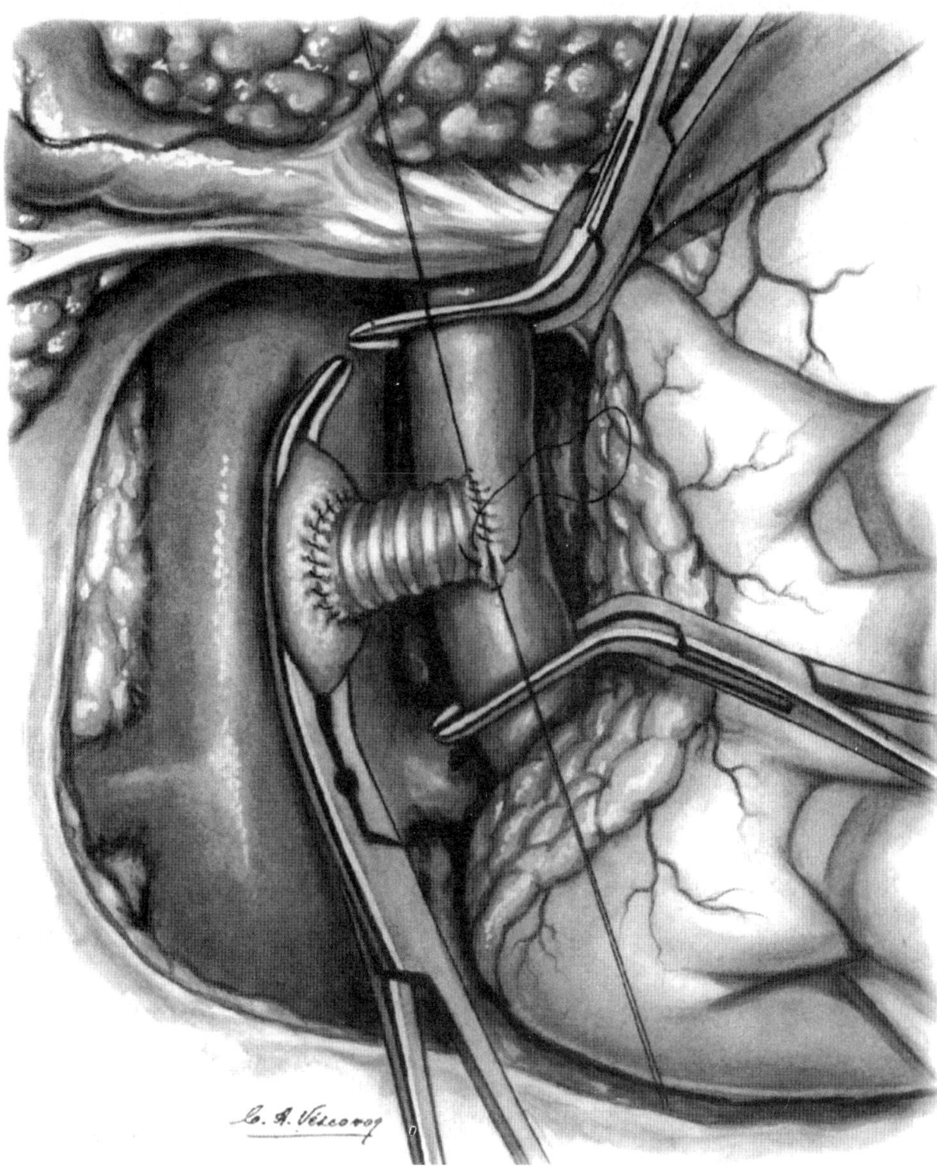

FIGURE 10.24

Anastomosis of the Superior Mesenteric Vein to the Inferior Vena Cava by the Interposition of a Gore-Tex Graft (H Mesocaval Shunt)

Shunts between the superior mesenteric vein and the vena cava are performed when a portacaval anastomosis is indicated but cannot be done due to thrombosis of the portal vein, or in patients who have had a surgical procedure in the hepatic hilus, making portocaval anastomosis very difficult (6, 10, 42, 57).

Anastomosis of the Superior Mesenteric Vein to the Inferior Vena Cava by the Interposition of a Gore-Tex Graft (H Mesocaval Shunt)

Anastomosis of the Superior Mesenteric Vein to the Inferior Vena Cava by the Interposition of a Gore-Tex Graft (H Mesocaval Shunt)

FIGURE 10.25
Midline incision extending from the midpoint of the xyphoumbilical line and further down, to midway from umbilicus to pubis.

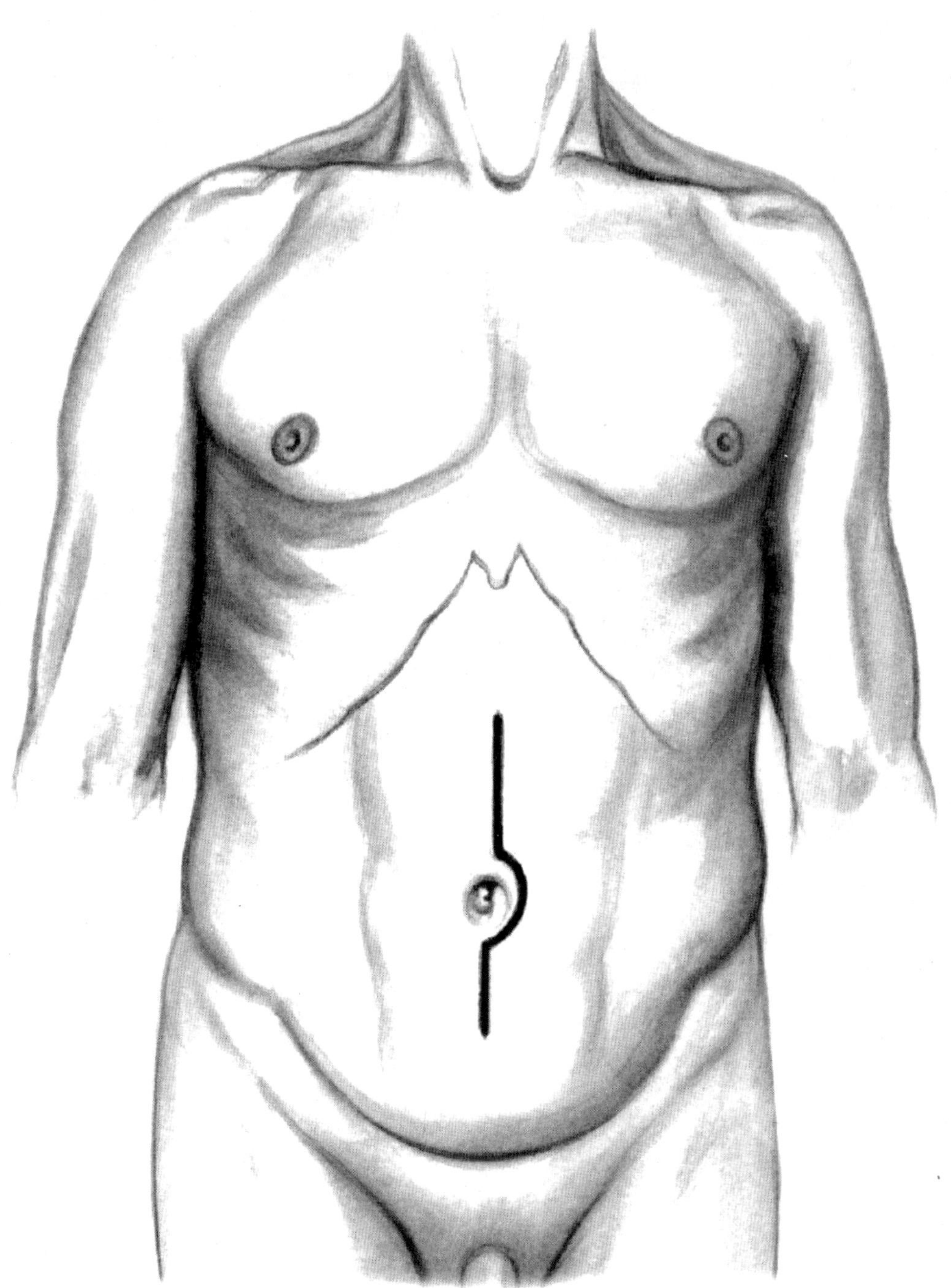

FIGURE 10.25

Anastomosis of the Superior Mesenteric Vein to the Inferior Vena Cava by the Interposition of a Gore-Tex Graft (H Mesocaval Shunt)

FIGURE 10.26
The transverse colon and its mesocolon are lifted and held upward by the first assistant. Through the mesocolon the third portion of the duodenum can be identified. It is also possible to identify the superior mesenteric vein guided by the pulsating superior mesenteric artery, which lies to the left, in a more posterior plane. As it is necessary to free the third portion of the duodenum and reflect it upward with a retractor, a horizontal incision should be made immediately inferiorly, as shown by the broken line. This incision will be used to identify and mobilize the inferior vena cava. In order to dissect the superior mesenteric vein longitudinally, an incision is made vertically over it, extending upward to the middle colic vessels and inferiorly to the ileocolic vessels, as shown by the vertical broken line.

FIGURE 10.27
The third portion of the duodenum and the superior mesenteric vein have been dissected, as shown in the drawing, where one can observe that the right colic vein is being ligated. Later, the right colic artery and other affluent veins of the superior mesenteric vein are ligated in order to liberate 4 to 6 cm of the vein circumferentially.

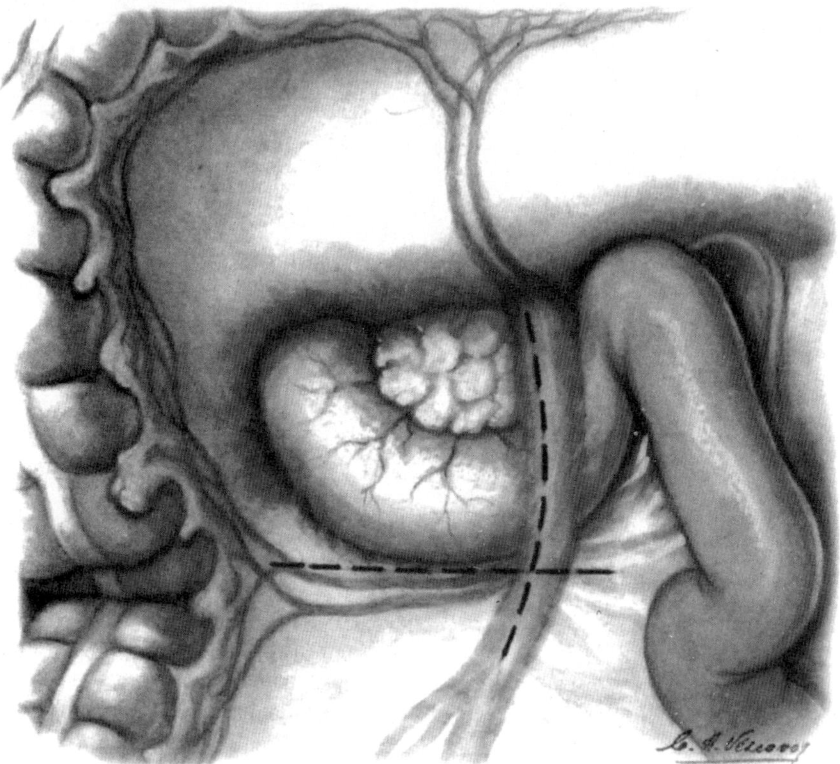

FIGURE 10.26

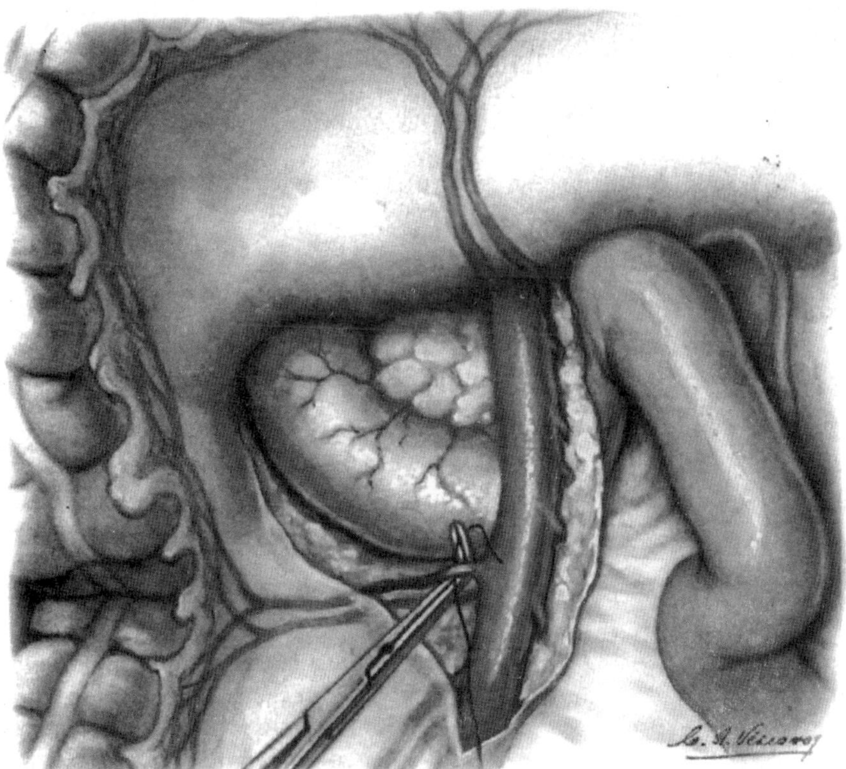

FIGURE 10.27

FIGURE 10.28
The mobilized third portion of the duodenum is retracted upward, exposing the inferior vena cava, which does not need to be freed circumferentially, only exposing its anterior and lateral aspects. The drawing shows that the superior mesenteric vein has been sufficiently mobilized to allow its anastomosis to the vena cava by interposing a Gore-Tex graft.

Anastomosis of the Superior Mesenteric Vein to the Inferior Vena Cava by the Interposition of a Gore-Tex Graft (H Mesocaval Shunt)

FIGURE 10.29
The vena cava has been grasped by a Satinsky clamp, a small lozenge of its anteromedial wall, 12 mm long, has been removed, and a Gore-Tex graft has been sutured in place with 5-0 Prolene. After the Gore-Tex tube has been sutured to the inferior vena cava, the superior mesenteric vein is grasped with two Cooley clamps, which are then rotated some 40 to 50 degrees upward and to the left to permit the performance of the anastomosis to the posterolateral wall of the superior mesenteric vein. The drawing shows the completed posterior suture between the Gore-Tex tube and the vein. The Gore-Tex tube should be 4-5 cm long and 12 mm wide.

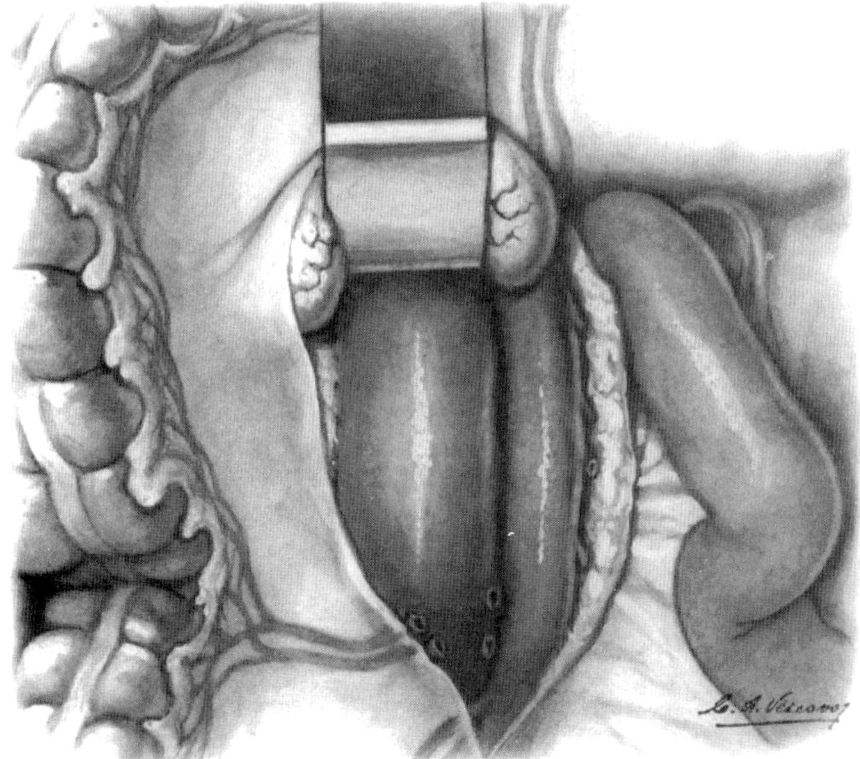

FIGURE 10.28

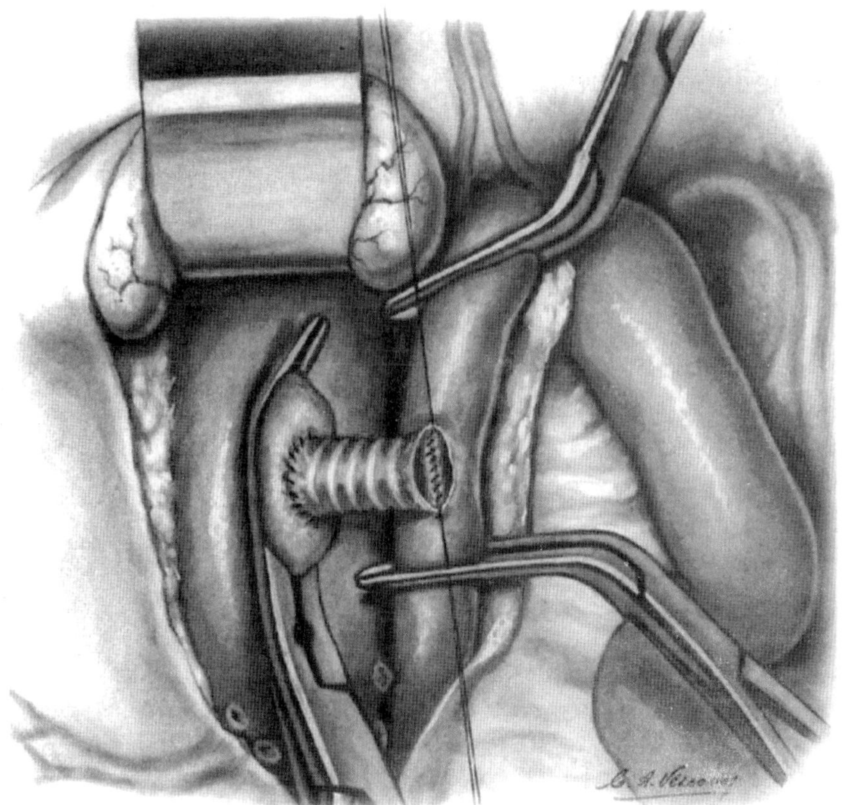

FIGURE 10.29

Anastomosis of the Superior Mesenteric Vein to the Inferior Vena Cava by the Interposition of a Gore-Tex Graft (H Mesocaval Shunt)

FIGURE 10.30
The drawing shows the almost completed suture line between the Gore-Tex tube and the superior mesenteric vein.

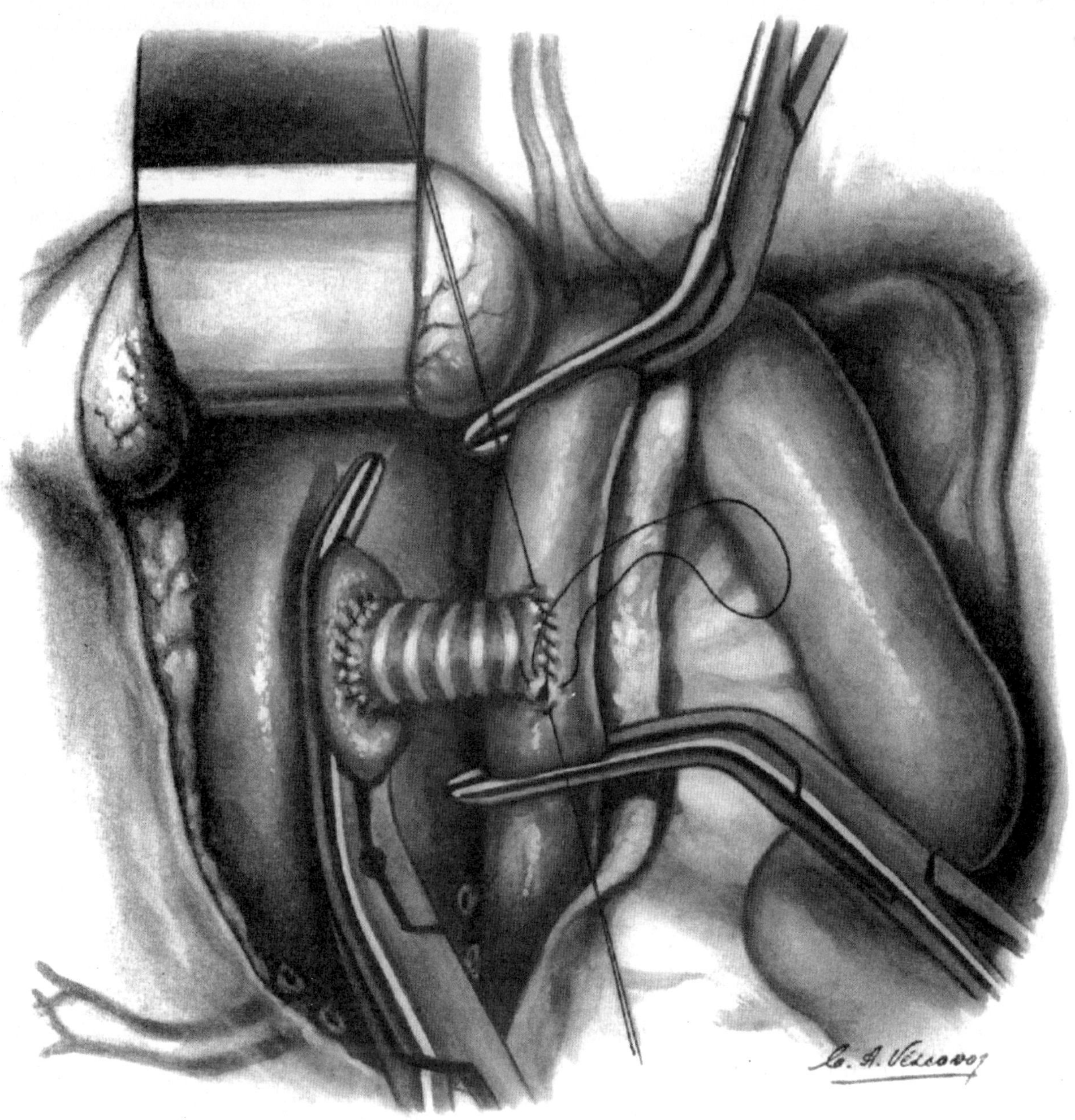

FIGURE 10.30

References

1. Barbot, D.J., Rosato, E.F. Experience with the esophagogastric devascularization procedure. Surgery 101:658, 1987.
2. Benhamon, J.P., Lebrec, D. (Eds.) Portal hypertension. Clin. Gastroenterol. 14:1, 1985.
3. Boerema, J., Klopper, F., Holcher, A. Transabdominal ligation of the esophagus in cases of bleeding esophageal varices. Surgery 67:409, 1970.
4. Burnett, D.A., Rikkers, L.F. Non operative emergency treatment of variceal hemorrhage. World J. Surg. 8:291, 1985.
5. Burnett, D.A., Rikkers, L.F. Non operative emergency treatment of variceal hemorrhage. Surg. Clin. North Am. 70:291, 1990.
6. Cameron, J.L. Atlas of surgery. Vol. I, p. 251. B.C. Decker, Toronto, 1990.
7. Crile, G. Transesophageal ligation of bleeding esophageal varices: A preliminary report of seven cases. Arch. Surg. 61:654, 1950.
8. Chesmar, J.L., Bernardino, M.E. Mesoatrial shunt for the treatment of Budd-Chiari syndrome: Radiologic evaluation in eight patients. A. J. R. 149:707, 1987.
9. Child, C.G. III The liver and portal hypertension. In Dunphy, J.E. (Ed.) Major Problems in Clinical Surgery Vol. I, p. 56 W.B. Saunders, Philadelphia, 1964.
10. Drapanas, T., LoCicero, J. III, Dowling, J.B. Hemodynamics of the interposition mesocaval shunt. Ann. Surg. 181:523, 1975.
11. Ericksson, L.S. Hepatic encephalopathy and treatment of esophageal varices. Scand. J. Gastroenterol. 23:641, 1988.
12. Fischer, J.E. Hepatic coma in cirrhosis, portal hypertension and following portacaval shunt. Arch. Surg. 108:325, 1974.
13. Fraser, C.L., Arieff, A.I. Hepatic encephalopathy. N. Engl. J. Med. 313:865, 1985.
14. Gimson, A.E., Estably, D., Hegarty, J., et al. A randomized trial of vasopressin and vasopressin plus nitroglycerin in the control of acute variceal hemorrhage. Hepatology 6:410, 1986.
15. Gliedman, M.L. Atlas of surgical techniques. p. 206. McGraw-Hill, New York, 1990.
16. Grace, N.D. Prevention of recurrent variceal bleeding. Is surgical rescue the answer? Ann. Intern. Med. 112:242, 1990.
17. Henderson, J.M., Warren, W.D. Portal hypertension. Curr. Probl. Surg. 25:155, 1988.
18. Henderson, J.M. The distal splenorenal shunt. Surg. Clin. North Am. 70:405, 1990.
19. Henderson, J.M., Millikan, W.J., Galloway, J.R. The Emory perspective of the distal splenorenal shunt in 1990. Am. J. Surg. 160:54, 1990
20. Henderson, J.M., Zeppa, R. Gastroesophageal varices. In Scott, H.W. Jr., Sanyers, J.L. (Eds.) Surgery of the stomach, duodenum and small intestine. Ed. 2, Blackwell Scientific Publications, Boston, 1991.
21. Hermann, R. End-to-side and side-to-side portacaval shunts. In Nyhus, L.M., Baker, R.J. (Eds.) Mastery of surgery. Vol. II, p. 841, Little, Brown & Co., Boston, 1984.
22. Holman, J.M., Rikkers, L.F. Success of medical and surgical management of acute variceal hemorrhage. Am. J. Surg. 140:816, 1980.
23. Hosking, S.W., Johnson, A.G., Chir, M. What happens to esophageal varices after transection and devascularization? Surgery 101:531, 1987.
24. Iwatsuki, S., Starzl, T.E., Todo, S., et al. Liver transplantation in the treatment of bleeding esophageal varices. Surgery 104:697, 1987.
25. Jones, E.A., Gammal, S.H., Martin, P. Hepatic encephalopathy. New light on an old problem. Q. J. Med. 69:851, 1988.
26. Johnson, G.W., Rodgers, H.W. A review of 15 years' experience in the use of sclerotherapy in the control of acute hemorrhage from esophageal varices. Br. J. Surg. 60:797, 1975.
27. Langer, B., Taylor, B.R., Greig, P.D. Selective or total shunts for variceal bleeding. Am. J. Surg. 75:160, 1990.
28. Liard, W., Balboa, O., Puig, R., Perdomo, R. Una nueva endoprótesis para la operación de Vosschulte. Rev. Cir. Uruguay 46:229, 1976.
29. Lillemol, K.D., Zuidema, G.D., Cameron, J.L. Portacaval anastomosis. In Nora, P.F. (Ed.) Operative surgery. Ed. 3, p. 809. W.B. Saunders, Philadelphia, 1990.
30. Orloff, M.J., Thomas, H.S. Pathogenesis of esophageal varix rupture. Arch. Surg. 87:301, 1963.
31. Orloff, M.J. Effect of side-to-side portacaval shunt on intractable ascites, sodium excretion and aldosterone metabolism in man. Am. J. Surg. 112:287, 1966.
32. Orloff, M.J. Emergency portacaval shunt:A comparative study of shunt, varix ligation and non surgical treatment of bleeding oesophageal varices in unselected patients with cirrhosis. Ann. Surg. 45:165, 1967.
33. Orloff, M.J., Girard, B. Long-term results of treatment of Budd-Chiari syndrome by side-to-side portacaval shunt. Surg. Gynecol. Obstet. 33:168, 1989.
34. Orloff, M.J., Daily, P.O., Girard, B. Treatment of Budd-Chiari Syndrome due to inferior vena cava occlusion by combined portal and vena cava decompression. Am. J. Surg. 137:163, 1992.
35. Orozco, H., Mercado, M.A., Takahashi, T., Hernández Ortiz, J., Capellán, J.F., García Tsao, G. Elective treatment of bleeding varices with the Sugiura operation over 10 years. Am. J. Surg. 163:585, 1992.
36. Paquet, K.L., Mercado, M.A., Koussouris, P., et al. Improved results with distal splenorenal shunt in a highly selected patient population. A prospective study. Ann. Surg. 184:210, 1989.
37. Prioton, J., Michel, H., Blanc, F. Long-term results after partial disconnection of the esophagus using an anastomotic button for bleeding esophageal varices in cirrhosis. Surg. Gynecol. Obstet. 121:162, 1986.
38. Pugh, R.N.H., Murray-Lyon, I.M., Dawson, J.L., Pietroni, M.C., Williams, R. Transection of the oesophagus for bleeding oesophageal varices. Br. J. Surg. 60:646, 1973.
39. Rikkers, L.F., Burnett, D.A., Volentine, G.D., et al. Shunt surgery versus endoscopic sclerotherapy for long-term treatment of variceal bleeding. Ann. Surg. 206:261, 1987.
40. Rikkers, L.F. Bleeding esophageal varices. Surg. Clin. North Am. 67:475, 1987.
41. Rikkers, L.F. Is the distal splenorenal shunt better? Hepatology 8:1705, 1988.
42. Rocko, J.M., Swan, K.G. Portal hypertension. In Fromm, D. (Ed.) Gastrointestinal surgery. Vol. 2, p. 853, Churchill Livingstone, New York, 1985.
43. Rypins, E.B., Sarfeh, I.J. Small-diameter portacaval H graft for variceal hemorrhage. Surg. Clin. North Am. 70:395, 1990.
44. Sarfeh, I.J., Rypins, E.B., Mason, G.R. A systemic appraisal of portacaval H graft diameters. Ann. Surg. 204:356, 1986.
45. Schiff, E.R. Nonsurgical management of emergency hemorrhage from esophageal varices. World J. Surg. 8:646, 1985.
46. Sherlock, S. Extrahepatic portal venous hypertension in adults. Clin. Gastroenterol. 14:1, 1985.
47. Sherlock, S. Diseases of the liver and biliary system. Ed. 8, p. 119. Blackwell Scientific Publications, London, 1989.
48. Snady, H. The role of sclerotherapy in the treatment of esophageal varices: Personal experience and a review of randomized trial. Am. J. Gastroenterol. 82: 813, 1987.
49. Sugiura, M., Futugawa, S. Esophageal transection with paraesophagogastric devascularization (the Sugiura procedure) in the treatment of esophageal varices. World J. Surg. 8:673, 1984.
50. Terblanche, J. The surgeon's role in the management of portal hypertension. Ann. Surg. 209:381, 1989.
51. Terblanche, J., Burroughs, A.K., Hobbs, K.E.F. Controversies in the management of bleeding esophageal varices. N. Engl. J. Med. 320:1469, 1989.
52. Valdoni, P. Abdominal surgery. An atlas of operative techniques. p. 115 W.B. Saunders, Philadelphia, 1976.
53. Voorhees, A.B. Jr., Price, J.B. Jr., Britton, R.C. Portasystemic shunting procedures for portal hypertension: Twenty six year experience in adults with cirrhosis of the liver. Am. J. Surg. 199:501, 1970.
54. Vosschulte, K. Place de las section par ligature de l'oesophage dans le traitement de l'hypertension portale. Lyon Chir. 53:519, 1957.
55. Warren, W.D., Zeppa, R., Fomon, J.J. Selective transsplenic decompression of gastroesophageal varices by distal splenorenal shunt. Ann. Surg. 166:437, 1967.
56. Warren, W.D., Henderson, J.M., Millikan, W.J. et al. Distal splenorenal shunt versus endoscopic sclerotherapy for long-term management of variceal bleeding. Preliminary report of a prospective randomized trial. Ann. Surg. 203:454, 1986.

57. Way, L.W. Current surgical diagnosis and treatment. Ed. 9, p. 510. Lange Medical Book, Norwalk, 1991.
58. Westaby, D., MacDougall, B.R.D., Williams, R. Improved survival following injection sclerotherapy for esophageal varices: Final analysis of a controlled trial. Hepatology 5:827, 1985.
59. Westaby, D., Williams, R. Injection sclerotherapy for the long-term management of variceal bleeding. World J. Surg. 8:667, 1985.
60. Whipple, A.O. The problem of portal hypertension in relation to the hepato-splenopathies. Ann. Surg. 122:449, 1945.
61. Whipple, A.O. Rationale of portacaval anastomosis. Bull. N. Y. Acad. Sci. 22:251, 1946.
62. Zeppa, R., Hutson, D.G., Levi, J.U., Livingstone, A.S. Factors influencing survival after distal splenorenal shunt. World J. Surg. 8:733, 1985.

Section B

Surgery for Portal Hypertension

CHAPTER 11

LeVeen Peritoneovenous Shunt

Until a few years ago the only therapeutic modality available to treat ascites caused by cirrhosis of the liver refractory to medical treatment was the portocaval shunt. However, the portocaval shunt carried a high mortality with frequent complications due to encephalopathy and aggravation of hepatic insufficiency.

At present, due to the efficient action of modern diuretics and of antialdosterone medications together with a low salt dietary regimen (1), the great majority of patients with ascites caused by cirrhosis respond to treatment. Before starting a more aggressive treatment of ascites caused by cirrhosis, one should always attempt to use a rigorous medical regimen for at least two weeks. In 1974, Harry LeVeen (4) designed a peritoneovenous shunt that included a unidirectional valve that allowed the flow of ascitic fluids from the peritoneal cavity to the venous system. This valve is designed to open when the abdominal pressure is over 3 cm of water, this pressure being higher than the intrathoracic and central venous pressures. The valve closes when central venous pressure becomes elevated (4–7).

There is no doubt that the LeVeen shunt is an ingenious innovation and has contributed to alleviate the symptoms of ascites. On the other hand, when patients who are under medical treatment cease to respond to diuretics, the danger of tubular necrosis arises. In this situation, patients will not respond to placement of the shunt. On the other hand, patients with hepatorenal syndrome may develop tubular necrosis if a shunt is not used. At times these two situations are difficult to distinguish from one another. On the other hand, the concentration of sodium in the urine may be an important distinguishing factor (5, 6).

In spite of its simple design, the peritoneovenous shunt may lead to numerous complications, be they during its placement or in the postoperative period. These complications may be infection, thrombotic lesions, diffuse intravascular clotting, air embolism, and so on (6, 12). The incidence of these and other complications diminishes substantially if the instructions of LeVeen and his collaborators are followed strictly since they have accumulated a vast experience (6, 7). Other peritoneovenous valves are used for the same purpose as the LeVeen valve, one of which is the Denver shunt. A comparative study between the LeVeen and Denver valves performed by Fulenwider and colleagues (2) come to the conclusion that the LeVeen valve is superior to the Denver valve, even though both lead to the same patient survival times. This author's experience has been exclusively with the LeVeen shunt. The peritoneovenous shunt has also been used to treat ascites due to other causes, such as ascites caused by malignant tumors. However, the placement of a peritoneovenous valve in patients with carcinoma is performed on rare occasions, save in some select cases of carcinomas of the ovary. The ascitic fluid produced by carcinomas frequently contains neoplastic cells that are capable of becoming colonized leading to the shunt being a factor in the dissemination of these neoplastic cells through the blood stream.

The only therapeutic alternative to cirrhosis of the liver and its complications is a liver transplant. In cases in which the transplant cannot be done, the peritoneovenous shunt can be a temporary solution to alleviate the bothersome symptoms that patients suffer making their remaining time more tolerable. The shunt improves the nutritive state and the respiratory problems produced by the increased abdominal pressure with its hemodynamic consequences. The shunt also facilitates the mobilization of the patient, and so on.

CONTRAINDICATIONS TO THE USE OF PERITONEOVENOUS SHUNTS

For obvious reasons, a shunt should not be placed in patients with peritonitis. On the other hand, it is necessary to point out that the clinical picture of peritonitis is not always evident in patients with ascites. To confirm this diagnosis it is indispensable to perform an abdominal tap to remove ascitic fluid and do a cytologic and bacteriologic examination of this fluid. The presence of cloudy fluid should be suspicious of the presence of peritonitis even though the patient presents no symptoms of this disease (5–7). Patients with esophageal varices that are bleeding or have bled recently should not have a shunt if their varices have not been previously treated. Patients with tubular necrosis may not be candidates for the placement of a shunt. On the other hand, as mentioned earlier, patients with hepatorenal syndrome are generally benefitted by the placement of a shunt. In general, a shunt should not be used in patients with a bilirubin greater than 10 mg/dL (2, 5–7).

PREOPERATIVE PREPARATION OF THE PLACEMENT OF A PERITONEOVENOUS SHUNT

A cirrhotic patient with refractory ascites has to be subjected to a complete evaluation prior to the placement of the shunt. Any hydroelectrolytic alterations must be corrected and a complete examination for possible bleeding problems as well as a measure of urinary sodium over a period of 24 hours and a study of renal and cardiorespiratory function must be performed. It is indispensable that the ascitic liquid be proven to be sterile. Twenty four hours before the placement of the shunt, the patient should be started on wide spectrum antibiotics. The surgical preparation of the skin of the abdomen, chest and neck must be started 24 hours before surgery with the object of diminishing infectious complications, which can produce serious problems in the postoperative course of the patients (2, 5–7).

It is advisable to use local anesthesia for the abdominal incision as well as for the cervical incision. On the other hand, during the time that the subcutaneous tract for the passage of the venous tube is being done from the abdomen to the neck, it is convenient to use mild general anesthesia, since this part of the procedure is usually painful (12).

Technique for the Implantation of the LeVeen Peritoneovenous Shunt

Technique for the Implantation of the LeVeen Peritoneovenous Shunt

FIGURE 11.1

This photograph shows a LeVeen shunt apparatus. The shunt consists of three parts:

A. A tube with multiple perforations called an abdominal tube that is introduced into the abdominal cavity and will allow the exit of ascitic fluid.
B. A unidirectional valve that allows the passage of ascitic fluid picked up by the venous tube toward the superior vena cava.
C. A venous tube that comes from the valve and will transport the ascitic fluid from the valve to the venous system.

Ascitic fluid passes through the shunt when the pressure gradient between the interperitoneal pressure and the central venal pressure is over 3 cm of water (4–7).

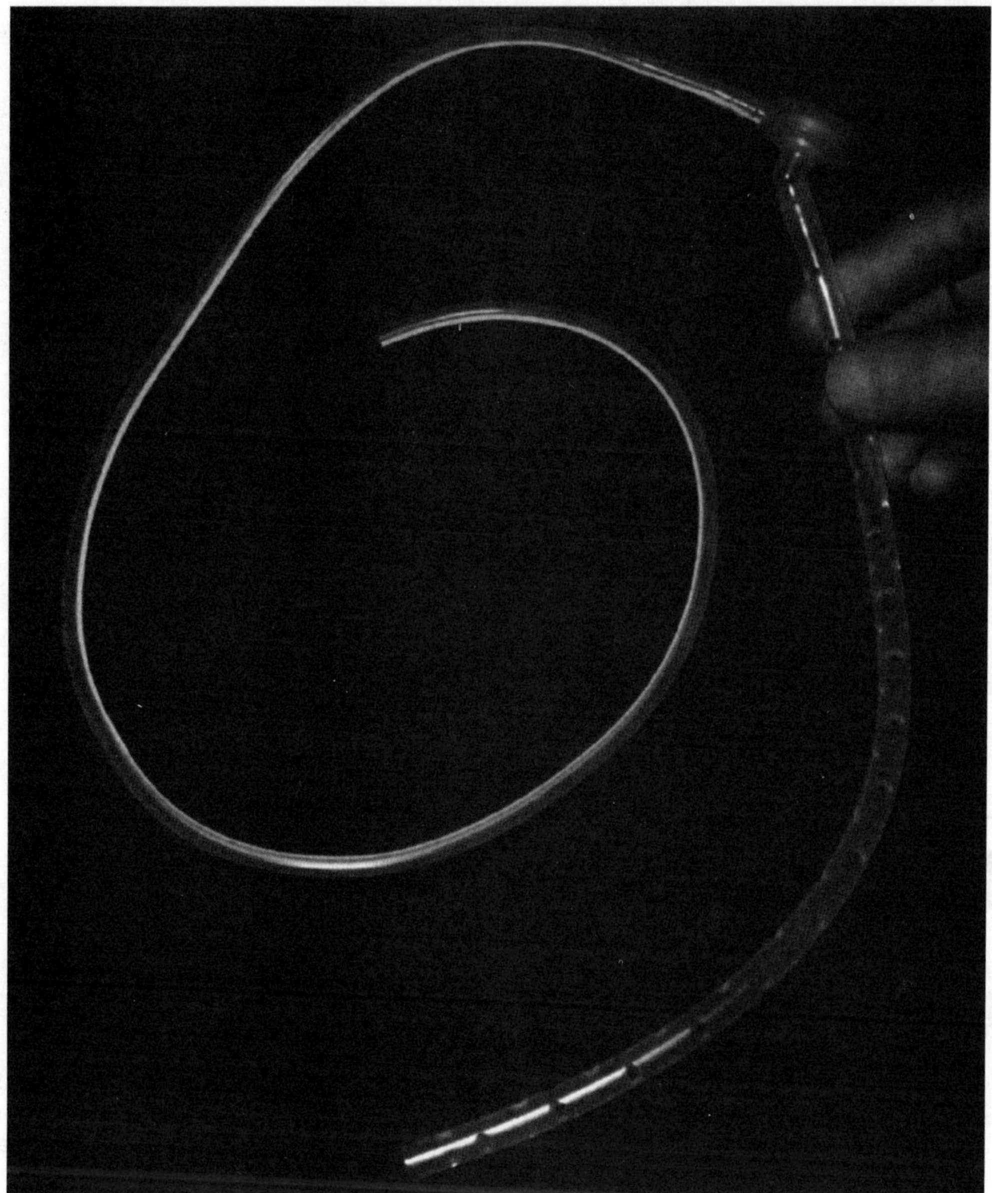

FIGURE 11.1

Technique for the Implantation of the LeVeen Peritoneovenous Shunt

FIGURE 11.2

This is a semischematic drawing to show the function of the LeVeen shunt. The arrows indicate the direction in which ascitic fluid flows from the abdominal cavity to the superior vena cava.

A. Abdominal tube
B. Unidirectional valve
C. Venous tube
D. Segment of the venous tube introduced into the jugular vein and the superior vena cava.

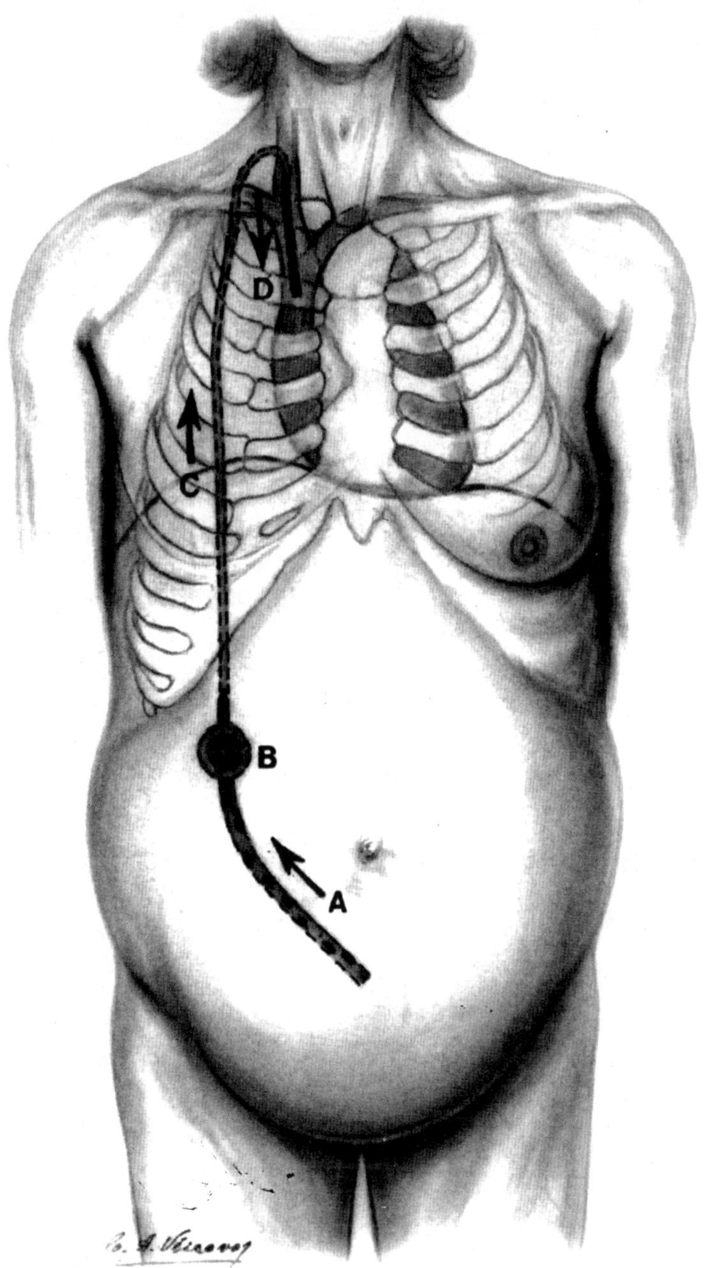

FIGURE 11.2

FIGURE 11.3

This drawing shows a patient with severe ascites caused by cirrhosis of the liver of alcoholic origin. The patient is rotated to the left with the neck extended and rotated to the same side. A line has been drawn to show where the incisions will be made for the implantation of the LeVeen shunt (4–7).

1. An incision 8 cm long is made at a point 6 cm below the right costal margin, lateral to the rectus abdominis muscle. At this site, the LeVeen valve will be placed (4). The incision should not be made close to the costal margin because this may cause kinking of the venous tube and pain (4, 5).
2. An incision 6 cm long is made in the neck, horizontally, about three finger breadths above the right clavicle with its center located between the sternal and clavicular heads of the sternocleidomastoid muscle (4, 5, 11). The abdominal tube should not be any longer than 20 cm. The end of the tube introduced into the jugular vein should reach the distal end of the superior vena cava just above the right auricle (4–7, 11). The length of the venous tube introduced into the deep jugular and superior vena cava should be 11.5 cm. Any extra length should be cut and discarded (4, 11). The distance between the site of introduction of the tube into the deep jugular vein and the second rib is the length of the tube that should be introduced into the venous system. In children, it is preferable to introduce the tube through the subclavian vein, preferably the left one, instead of the deep jugular vein because the incidence of kinking is very high (4–6, 11).

Technique for the Implantation of the LeVeen Peritoneovenous Shunt

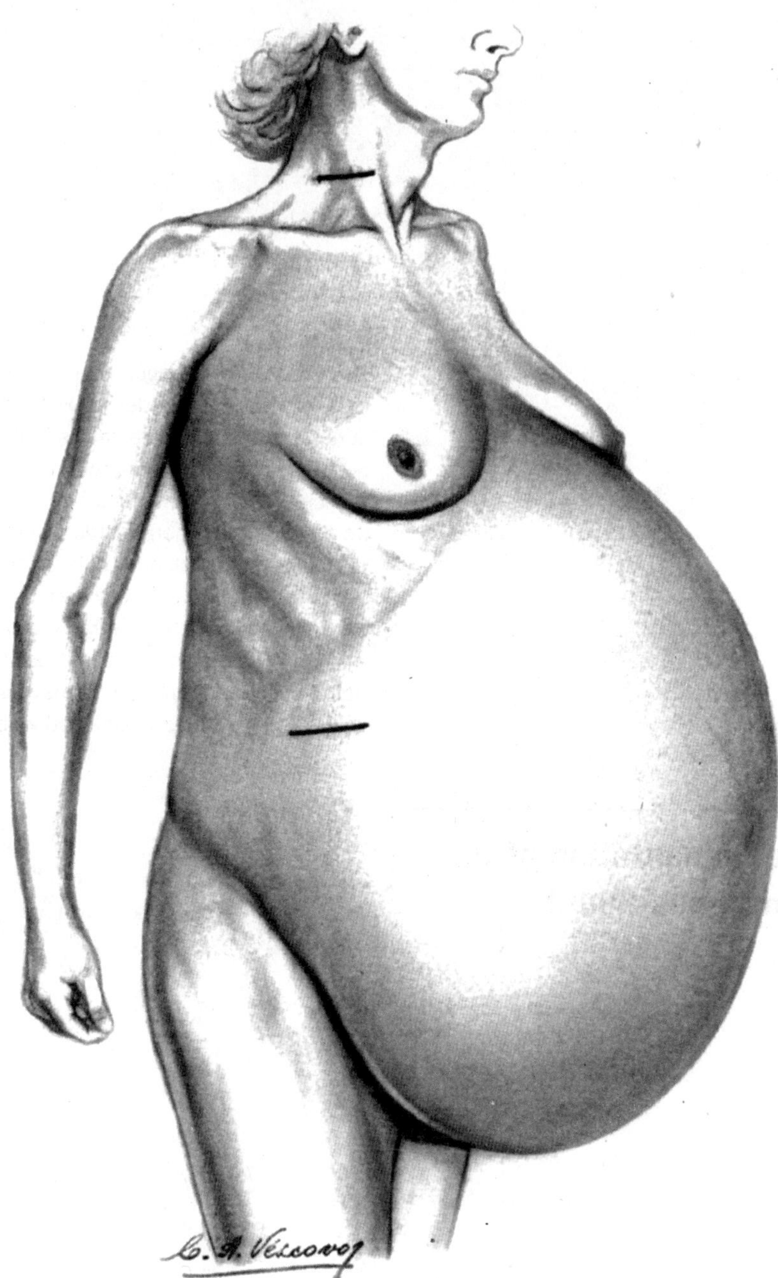

FIGURE 11.3

FIGURE 11.4
The procedure is begun by making the abdominal incision at the site described under Figure 3. Once the skin and the subcutaneous tissues are incised, one arrives at the external oblique muscle. The aponeurotic facial portion of this muscle is incised and the muscular portion is split in the direction of its fibers. With a hemostatic clamp the internal oblique (2) is also split. It is not advisable to incise the transversus abdominis muscle (3) or the transversalis fascia. In the drawing, one can observe that retractors are separating the external oblique allowing one to see that the internal oblique is being split. In the bottom, the transversus abdominis can be observed and should not be sectioned.

Technique for the Implantation of the LeVeen Peritoneovenous Shunt

FIGURE 11.5
In the drawing, one can see that two concentric purse string sutures have been placed using synthetic nonabsorbable sutures. These purse string sutures include the transversus abdominis, the transversalis fascia, and the peritoneum. It is not advisable to perform these purse string sutures on the peritoneum only because it is usually very thin and fragile owing to the distension caused by the ascites and the passage of needles through this thin peritoneum to perform the purse string suture may leave openings through which ascitic fluid will leak (7).

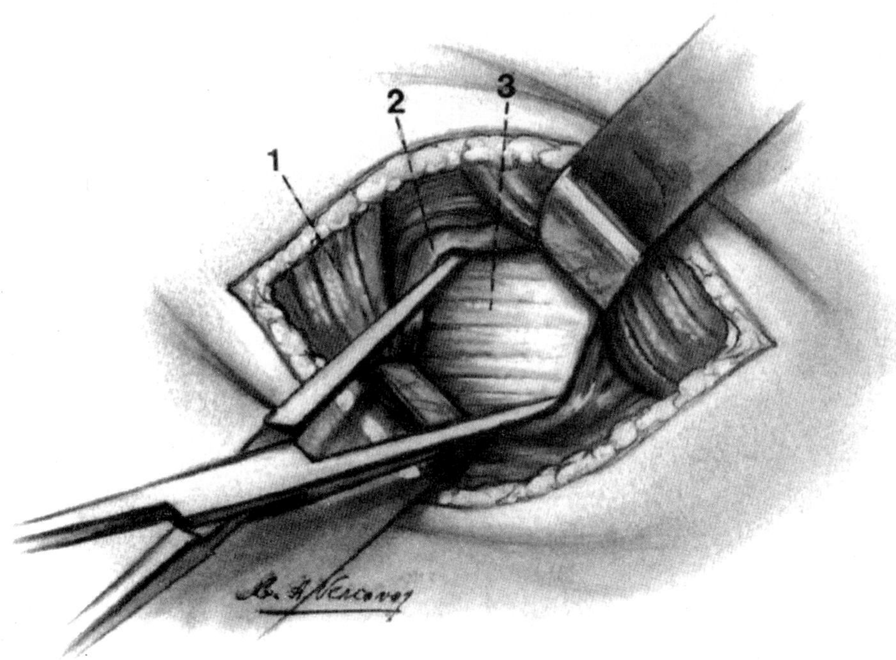

FIGURE 11.4

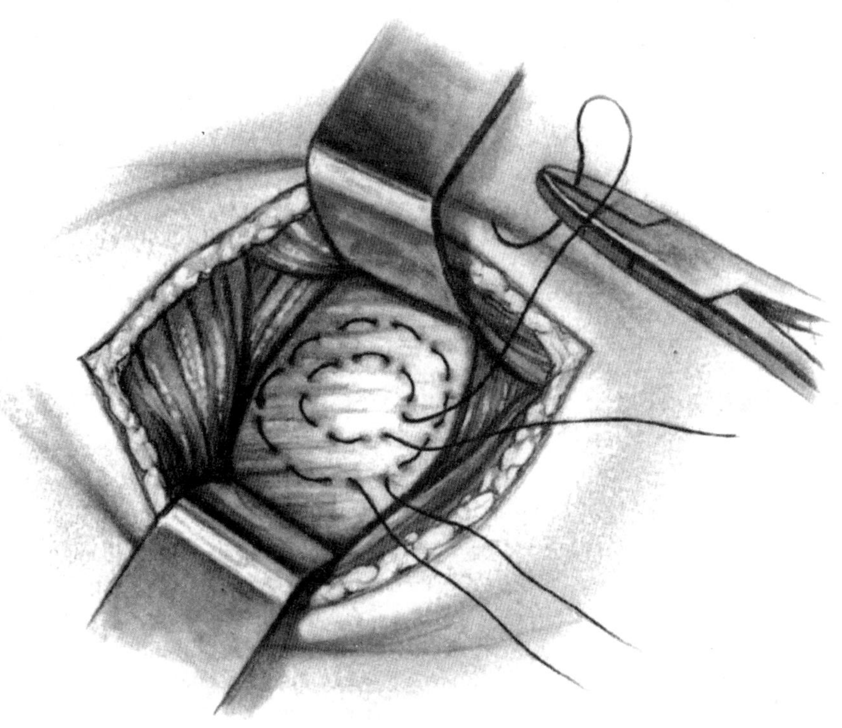

FIGURE 11.5

FIGURE 11.6
In the center of the internal purse string suture a small incision is made, using the tip of a cataract knife, sufficiently large for the introduction of a suction trochar. Since the patient is rotated to the left the opening of the peritoneum will not lead to any great leakage of ascitic fluid because the incision will be in the highest part of the abdomen (7).

Technique for the Implantation of the LeVeen Peritoneovenous Shunt

FIGURE 11.7
Through the peritoneal opening a suction catheter is introduced to remove a great part of the ascitic fluid, in this way preventing the passage of great quantities of fluid into the circulation leading to overhydration and a great diuresis with great loss of sodium and potassium. The possibility of acute pulmonary edema and the production of diffuse intervascular clotting may also occur because ascitic fluid contains substances that enhance coagulation (7, 12).

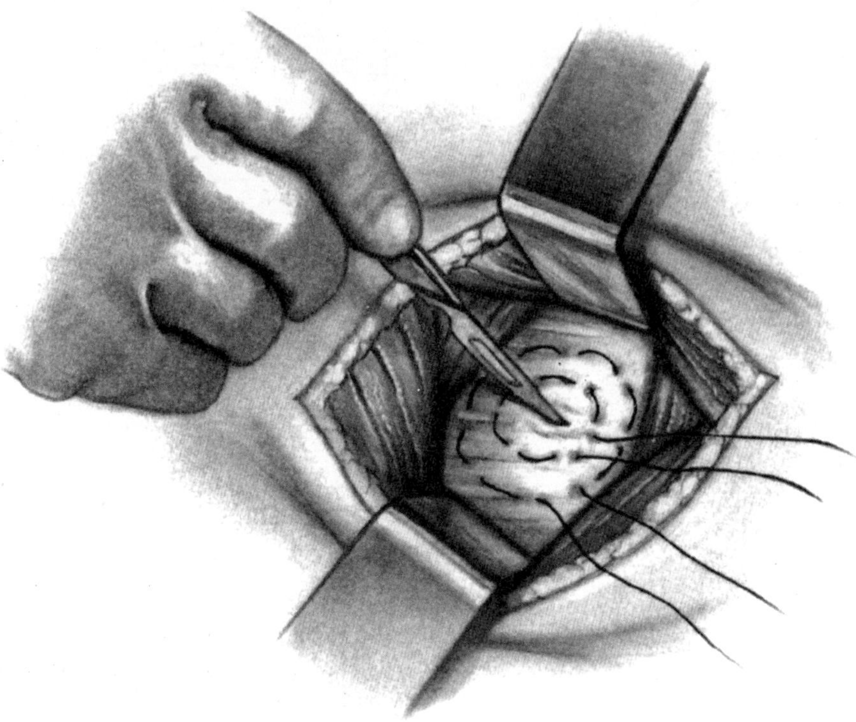

FIGURE 11.6

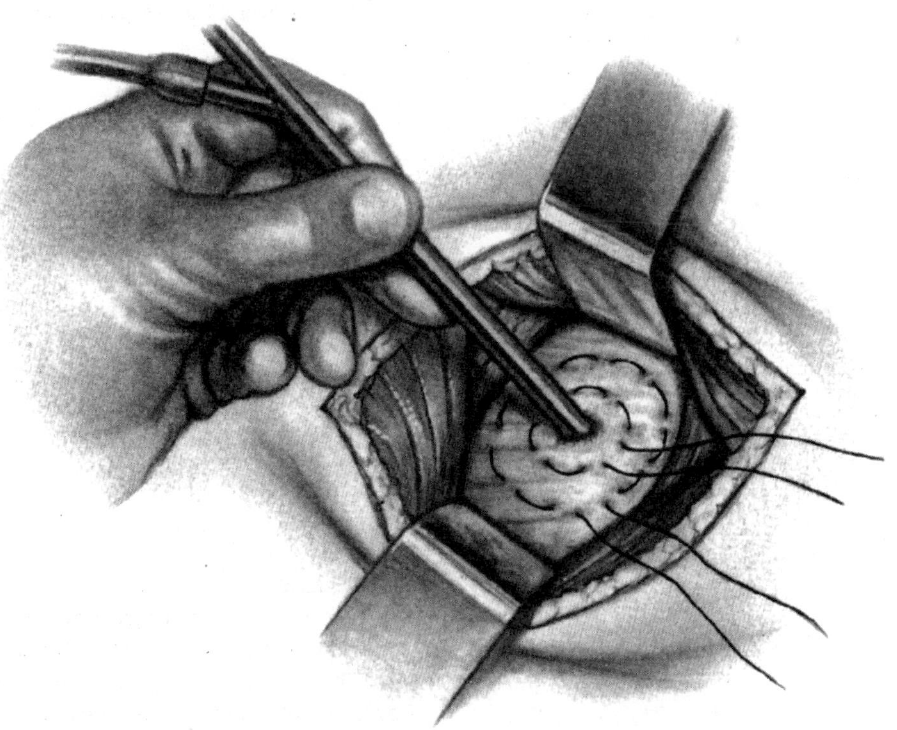

FIGURE 11.7

FIGURE 11.8
The aspirating trochar has been removed and the interior of the peritoneal cavity has been filled with warm saline solution to displace air that may have gotten in while the abdomen was open.(12) Intraperitoneal air may lead to air embolism. After the introduction of warm saline, the abdominal tube with multiple perforations that comes with the LeVeen shunt is introduced into the abdomen directing it to the lower portion of the abdomen. The length of tube introduced into the abdomen should not exceed 20 cm except in very tall patients. The excess tube should be cut and discarded prior to its introduction. If the tube is over 20 cm long, it may cause discomfort (7, 11).

Technique for the Implantation of the LeVeen Peritoneovenous Shunt

FIGURE 11.9
The tube has been introduced into the abdominal cavity and the purse string sutures, central and peripheral, have been tied. This is done leaving the valve outside of the abdominal cavity. To better fix the valve in place, after the purse string sutures are tied the loose ends of these are tied around the venous tube as observed in Figure 11.10 (1).

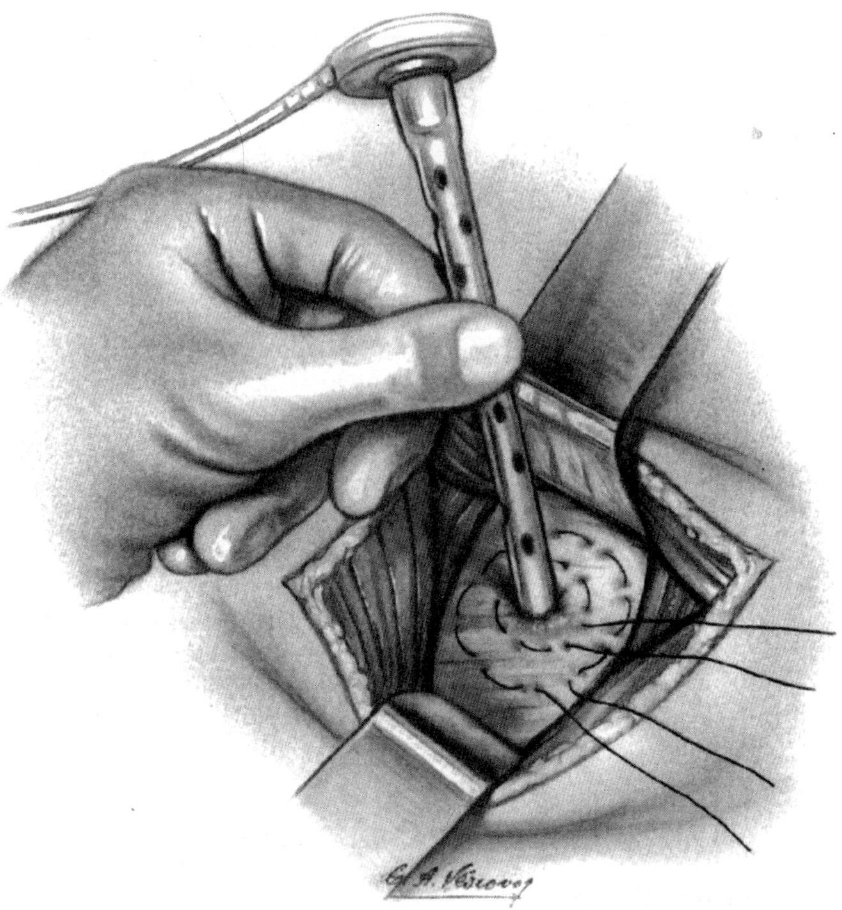

FIGURE 11.8

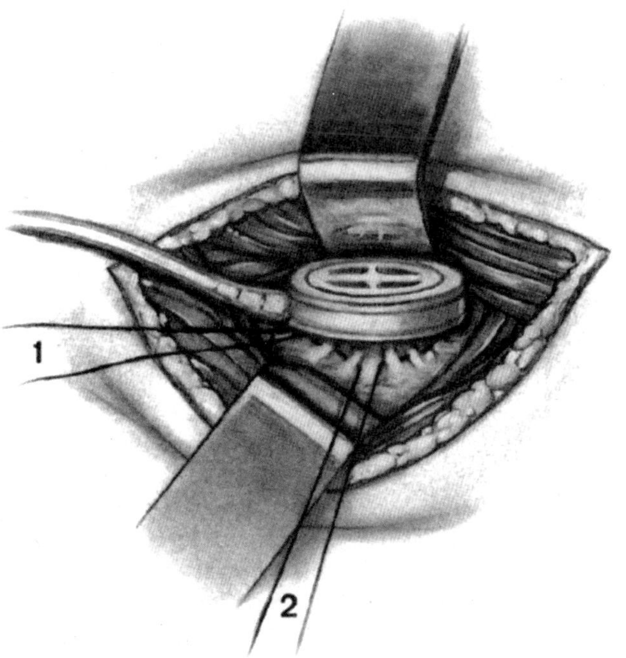

FIGURE 11.9

FIGURE 11.10
In the drawing, one can see that the loose ends of the purse string sutures are being tied around the venous tube at its exit from the valve. The ends of the internal purse string suture have already been tied and the ends of the external purse string suture are yet to be tied.

Technique for the Implantation of the LeVeen Peritoneovenous Shunt

FIGURE 11.11
With a curved hemostat, a perforation is made in the internal and external oblique muscles some 4 cm above the line where these muscles were split. The end of the venous tube is then grasped by the clamp to pass it through the muscles and place it in the subcutaneous tissue layer towards the upper part of the wound. This venous tube will later be passed through the subcutaneous tract toward the neck.

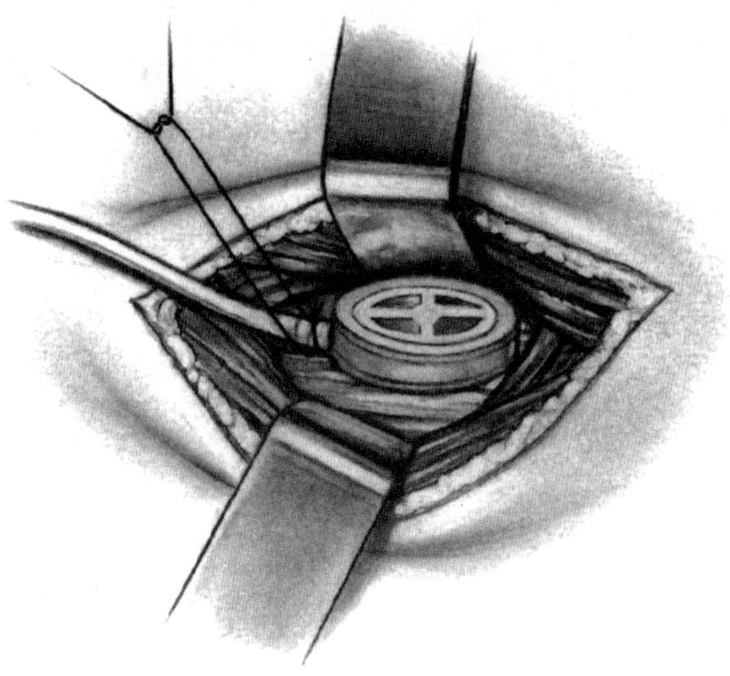

FIGURE 11.10

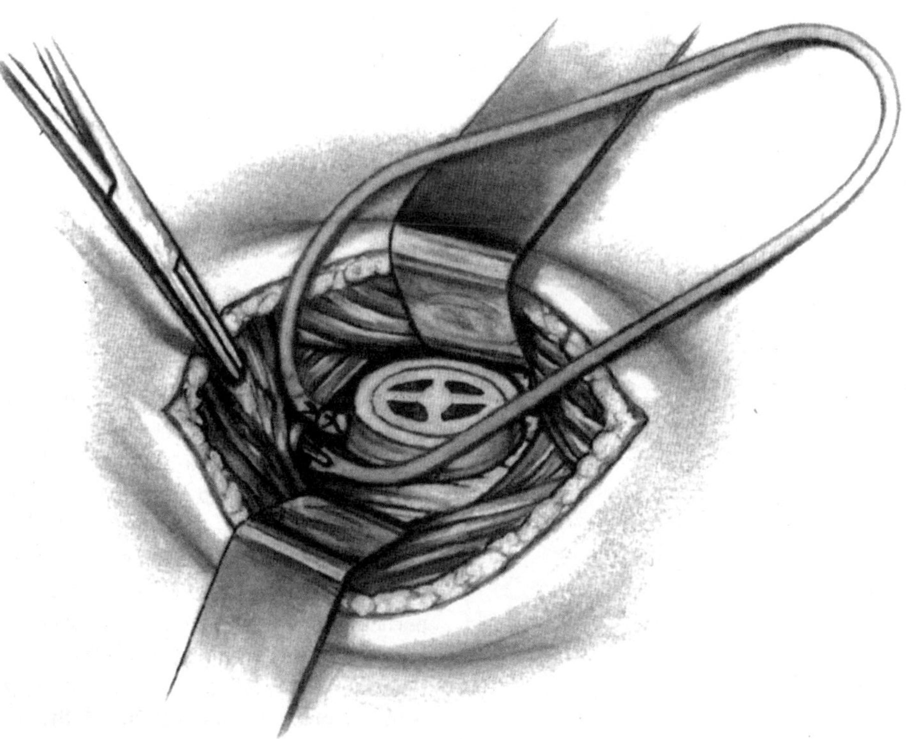

FIGURE 11.11

Technique for the Implantation of the LeVeen Peritoneovenous Shunt

FIGURE 11.12
The valve of the LeVeen shunt is then completely covered suturing the external and internal oblique muscles over it. The suturing should be water tight and performed with synthetic reabsorbable material of 2-0 caliber to prevent leakage of ascitic fluid.

FIGURE 11.13
This is a diagram showing the abdominal wall transected through the sight of the surgery to illustrate the location of the LeVeen valve. The valve is located outside the peritoneal cavity between the deep layer constituted by the peritoneum, transversalis fascia and transversus abdominis muscle and the more superficial plane composed of the internal and external oblique muscles (7). At the end of the procedure, the superficial plane will be covered by subcutaneous tissue and skin as shown in the drawing. Label No. 1 shows skin and subcutaneous tissue; No. 2 the venous tube; No. 3 the internal and external oblique muscles; No. 4 the transversus abdominis muscle, transversalis fascia and peritoneum; No. 5 the unidirectional valve; and No. 6 the abdominal tube.

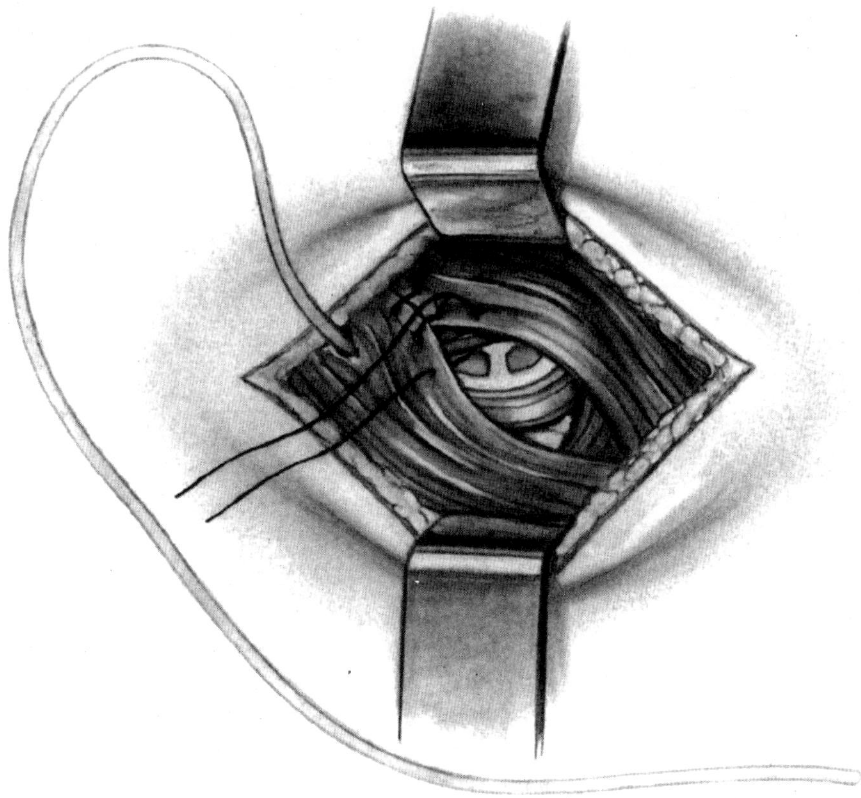

FIGURE 11.12

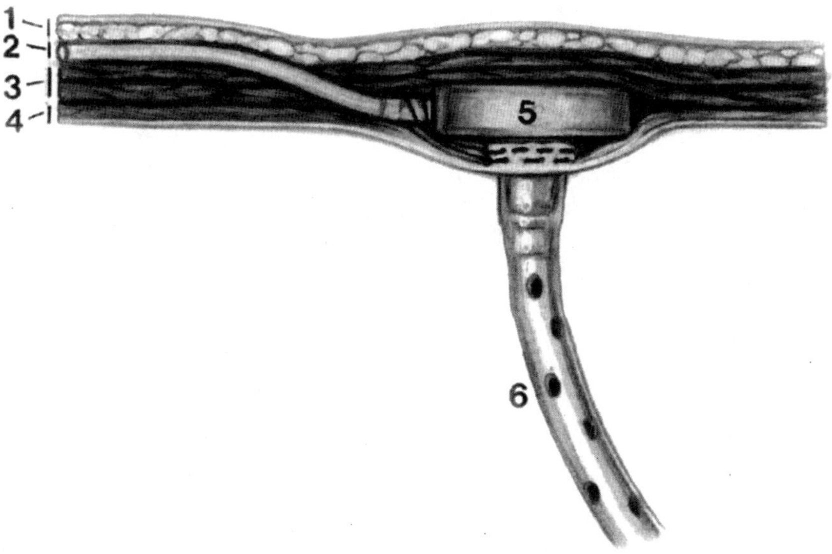

FIGURE 11.13

FIGURE 11.14
This illustrates the transverse incision in the neck at a level three finger breadths above the clavicle as described under Figure 3. The surgeon has cut the skin, the subcutaneous tissue, and the Platysma muscle of the neck. The internal jugular vein has been identified and dissected free in its usual position in front of the carotid artery. Two heavy sutures have been passed under the internal jugular vein, one in the upper portion and one in the lower portion.

Technique for the Implantation of the LeVeen Peritoneovenous Shunt

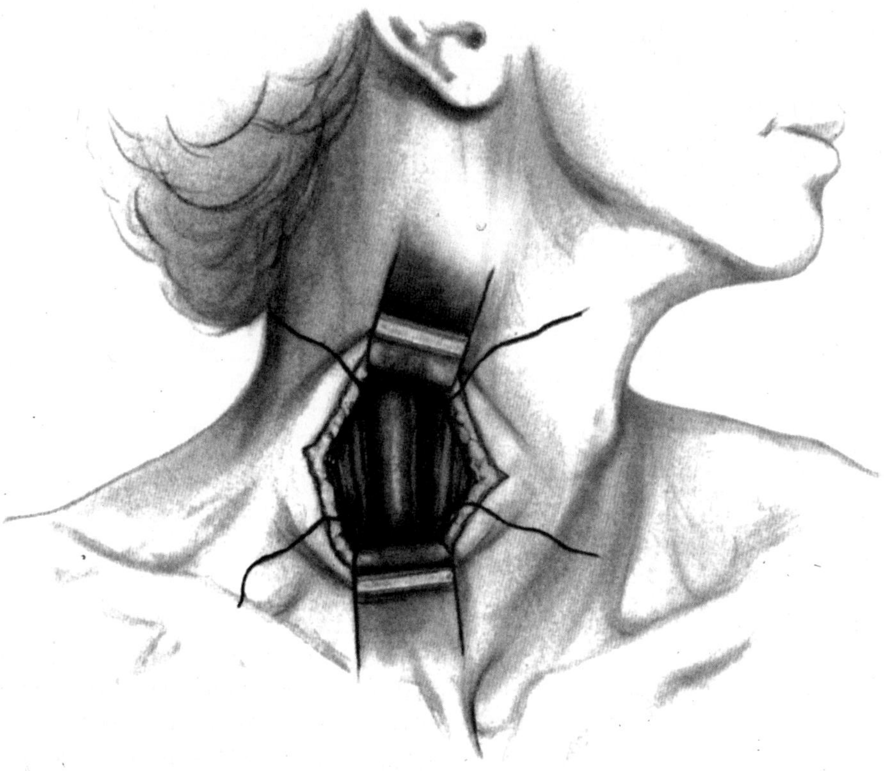

FIGURE 11.14

FIGURE 11.15
To pass the venous tube from the abdominal incision to the cervical incision, it is necessary to construct a narrow subcutaneous tract uniting both incisions. To construct this tract, one uses an esophagoscopic or bronchoscopic biopsy forceps that is passed subcutaneously from the abdominal to the cervical incision. This subcutaneous tunnel should be barely wide enough to allow the passage of the venous tube, avoiding accumulation of ascitic fluid. In the drawing the biopsy forceps have been passed to the neck and are grasping a heavy thread. In the insert, one can observe the detail of the thread being grasped by the biopsy forceps.

Technique for the Implantation of the LeVeen Peritoneovenous Shunt

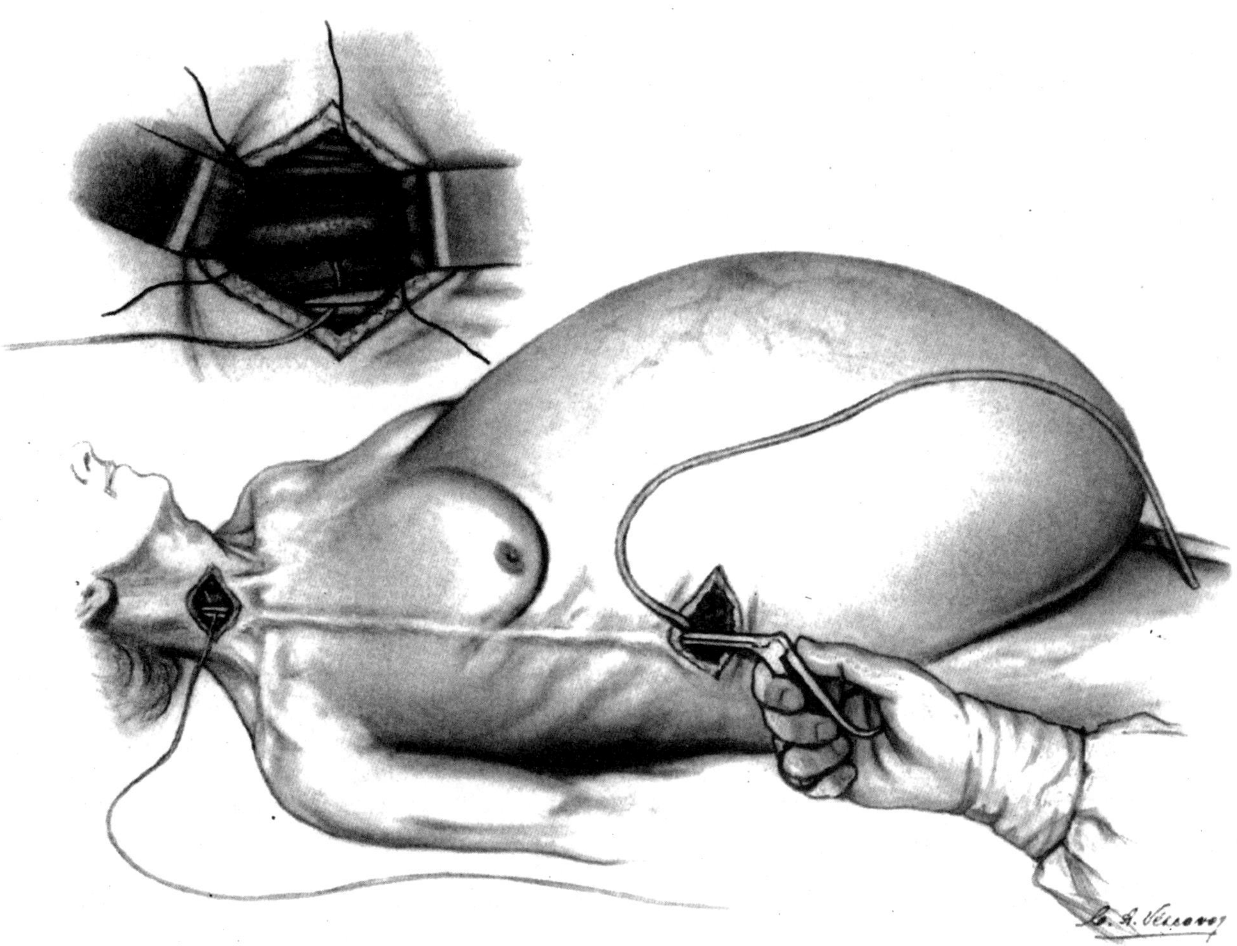

FIGURE 11.15

FIGURE 11.16

The heavy suture material is grasped by the biopsy forceps and pulled through the subcutaneous tunnel until it protrudes through the abdominal incision. The lower end of this suture material is tied to the venous tube while the upper end remains in the surgical incision. By pulling on the upper end of the suture in the neck the venous tube is passed through the subcutaneous tunnel from the abdominal to the cervical incision. In the insert, one can observe that the venous tube has been passed to the neck through the subcutaneous tunnel.

Technique for the Implantation of the LeVeen Peritoneovenous Shunt

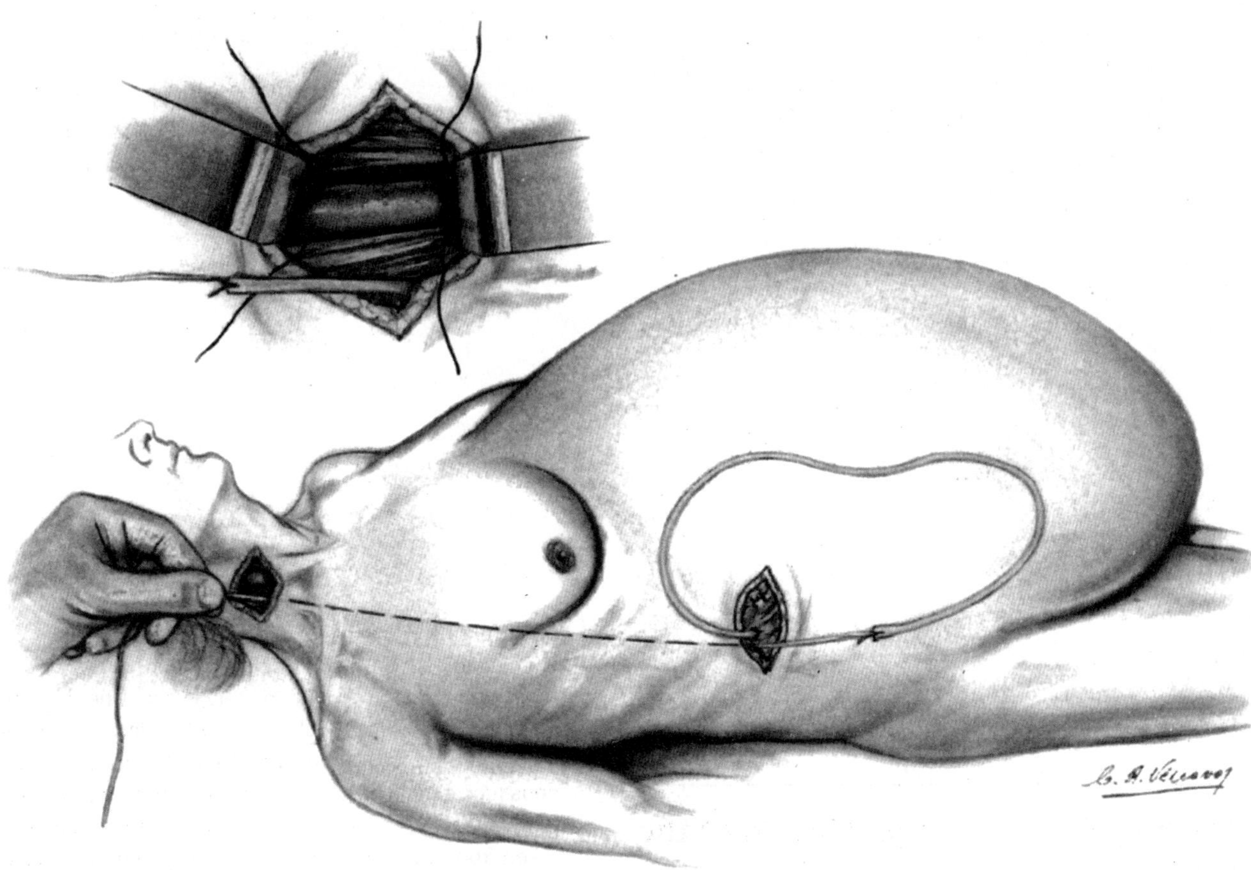

FIGURE 11.16

FIGURE 11.17
The venous tube that has been passed to the neck is being measured to determine the distance from where the tube is to be introduced in the jugular vein to the right second rib, a distance that is usually about 11.5 cm. The lower end of this venous tube should be placed in the superior vena cava just above the right auricle. The figure shows that the measure is being taken from the point where the tube is to be introduced in the jugular vein to the level of the second rib on the right side.

Technique for the Implantation of the LeVeen Peritoneovenous Shunt

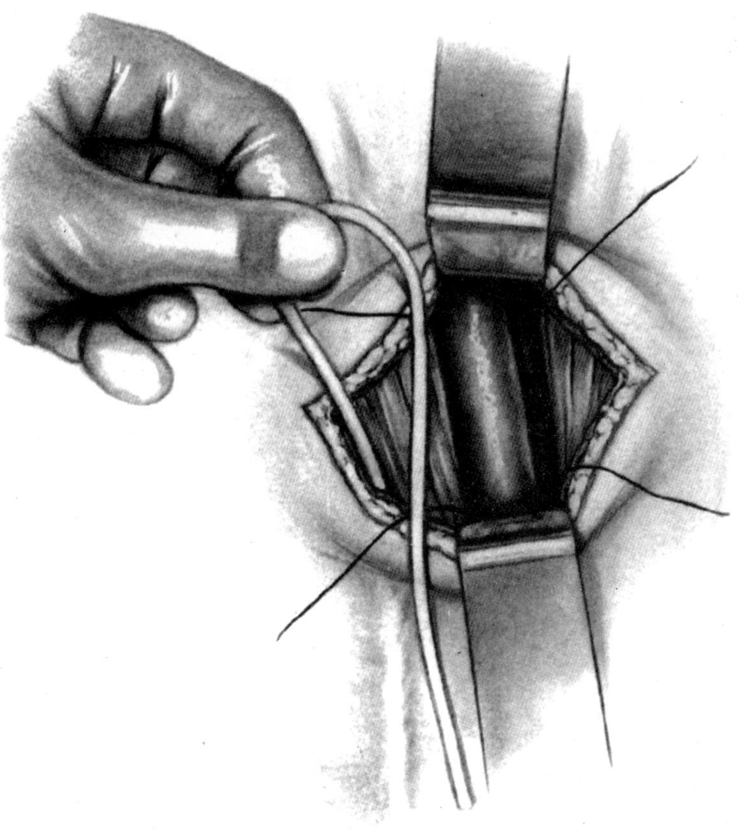

FIGURE 11.17

Technique for the Implantation of the LeVeen Peritoneovenous Shunt

FIGURE 11.18

The upper suture that had been previous passed around the internal jugular vein has been tied. Two fine sutures are placed in the jugular vein below this point to place traction on the anterior wall of the vein at the site where the tube is to be introduced. A small incision is made in the internal jugular vein just large enough to introduce the venous tube and to direct it toward the superior vena cava, locating its tip just above the right auricle. Once the venous tube had been passed to the appropriate site, the lower suture around the internal jugular vein is tied and this suture is then tied to hold the venous tube in place. The venous tube should enter the internal jugular vein in a gentle curving fashion. Precautions should be taken so that the tube will not kink. At the site of entrance of the venous tube at the internal jugular vein, one can place one or two fine sutures to close the venous opening completely.

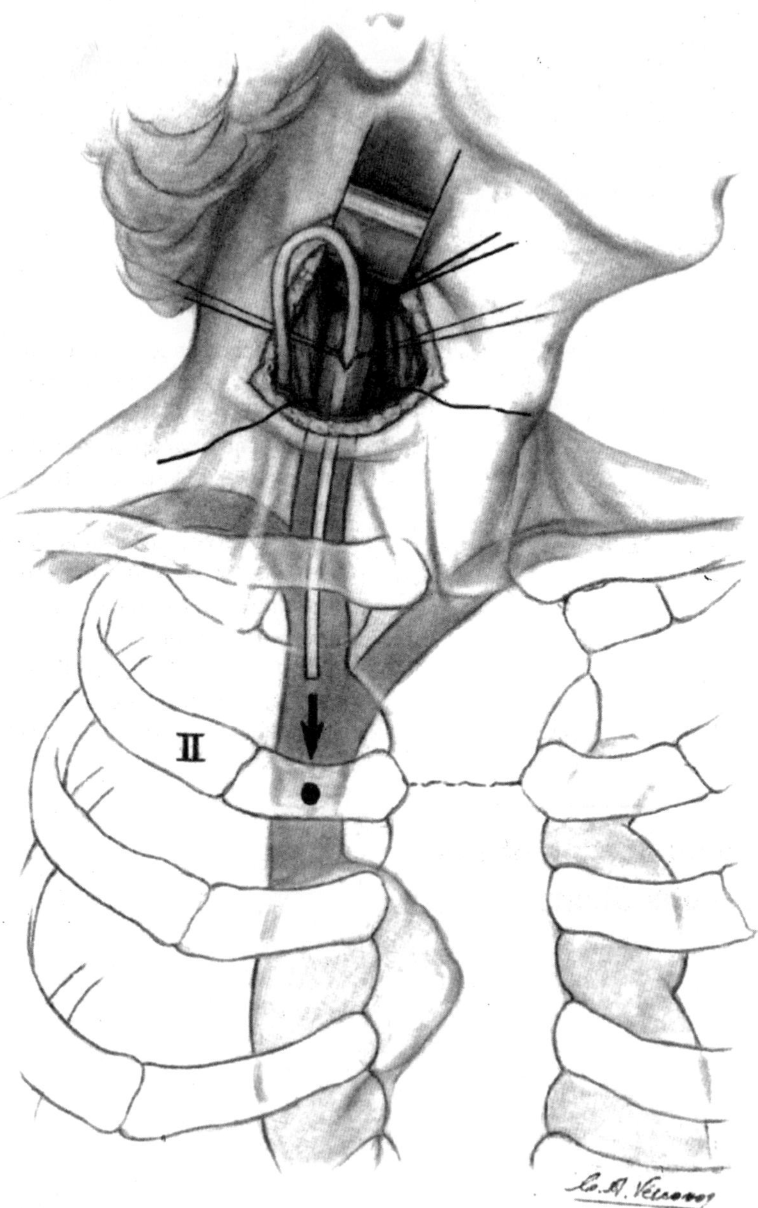

FIGURE 11.18

FIGURE 11.19
The surgical procedure has been completed. One can observe the gentle curve that the venous tube has as it enters the internal jugular vein. The venous tube has been passed into the superior vena cava up to a point near the right auricle. The upper and lower sutures that have been passed around the internal jugular vein have been tied fixing the venous tube in place. The cervical incision is closed in two planes. The first is a muscular plane in the neck including subcutaneous tissue using synthetic absorbable 3-0 interrupted sutures. The skin is closed with interrupted sutures. The abdominal wound should be carefully closed so that it is watertight. The subcutaneous tissue is closed with a continuous suture of absorbable material. The skin is closed with a continuous subcuticular suture.

Technique for the Implantation of the LeVeen Peritoneovenous Shunt

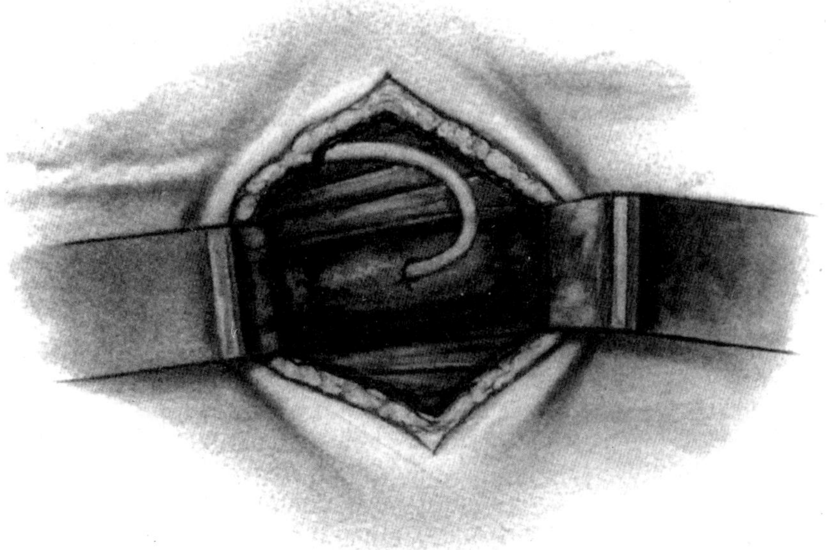

FIGURE 11.19

Complications of Peritoneovenous Shunt

Some of these complications have been previously mentioned:

1. Air embolism.
2. Diffuse intervascular clotting.
3. Occlusion of the valve.
4. Infection.
5. Leakage of ascitic fluid at the site where the valve was located and up the subcutaneous tunnel where the venous tube was passed.
6. Too long a venous tube or too short a venous tube.
7. Too long an abdominal tube.
8. The ascitic fluid was not aspirated, allowing its massive introduction into the circulation.
9. The ascitic fluid was not studied for infection.
10. Warm saline solution was not introduced into the abdominal cavity after the removal of the fluid to displace and diminish the amount of intraperitoneal air.
11. The abdominal incision was made too close to the costal margin, which may kink the venous tube and produce discomfort.
12. The abdominal incision was not closed in a water tight fashion.

Postoperative Follow-up of Patients with Peritoneovenous Shunts

In the postoperative period, one should continue the administration of wide spectrum antibiotics. A strict balance of intake and output of fluids, including electrolytes, must be observed. It is extremely important to reestablish diuresis in the postoperative period to avoid acute pulmonary edema. This diuresis will be directly proportional to the amount of ascitic fluid that has passed into the circulation. Diuretics should be used every 4 to 6 hours. If an excessive excretion of potassium is encountered, it will be necessary to administer Spirolactone. Patients should be weighed every 12 hours and their waist measurement taken every 24 hours for the first 3 to 4 days. The urinary output should be measured every 24 hours for at least 10 postoperative days. A hematocrit should be performed every 4 hours; the urea and creatinine levels in the serum must be observed daily, and one should also measure the aldosterone level. The patient should remain in the supine position for the first 3 days. If the hematocrit falls below 20, it will be necessary to place the patient in a sitting position.

After the third day, moderate compression of the abdomen by abdominal elastic support should be continuous. After the third day, respiratory exercises should begin. One should be alert for the appearance of acute pulmonary edema or disseminated intravascular clotting. In the latter case, purpura or hemorrhages may appear and should be immediately treated with heparin. Some patients will have a moderate fever. This fever will occur without the presence of infection and usually disappears in a few days. In case the valve becomes obstructed, this is easily recognized by the reappearance of ascites which is manifested by weight gain, rapid growth of the abdomen, respiratory difficulty, oliguria, hyponatremia, and so on. If this situation arises, it will be necessary to remove the valve together with the peritoneal tube and replace it with another. It is usually not necessary to remove the venous tube. Patients who have cirrhosis and ascites in which a LeVeen valve has been placed begin to notice a decrease in their waist size and body weight within 24 to 48 hours. This is usually accompanied by an increase in diuresis and a reduction of the retention of aldosterone. Patients with hepatorenal syndrome usually improve, and their abnormal physiopathology is reversed. A few days later, patients usually show an improvement in their general condition, with a better state of nutrition, and relief of symptoms as the ascites disappears. Patients are usually discharged from the hospital from 8 to 15 days following placement of the LeVeen shunt.

References

1. Cameron, J.L. Atlas of surgery. Vol. I, p. 312. B.C. Decker, Toronto, 1990.
2. Fulenwider, J.T., Galambon, J.D., Henderson, J.N., Smith, R.B., III, Dean, W.W. LeVeen vs. Denver peritoneovenous shunts for intractable ascites of cirrhosis: A randomized, prospective trial. Arch. Surg. 121:351, 1986.
3. Greenlee, H.B., Stanley, M.M., Reinhardt, G.F. Intractable ascites treated with peritoneovenous shunts (LeVeen): A 24 to 64 month follow-up of results in 52 alcoholic cirrhotics. Arch. Surg. 116:518, 1981.
4. LeVeen, H.H., Christoudias, G., Moon, I.P., Luft, R., Falk, M.S., Grosberg, S. Peritoneo-Venous shunting for ascites. Ann. Surg. 180:580, 1974.
5. LeVeen, H.H., Wapmick, S., Grosberg, S., Kinney, M.J. Further experience with peritoneo-venous shunt for ascites. Ann. Surg. 184:574, 1976.
6. LeVeen, H.H., Wapnick, S., Guinto, R., Kinney, M.J. Indications for peritoneo-venous shunt for ascites. World J. Surg. 2:367, 1978.
7. LeVeen, H.H., Piccone, V.A. The LeVeen shunt for intractable ascites. In Nyhus, L.M., Baker, R.J. (Eds.) Mastery of surgery. Vol. II, p. 873. Little, Brown & Co., Boston, 1984.
8. Perez, R.A., Rypins, E.B., Lazaro, E. Revision of the peritoneovenous valve. Surg. Gynecol. Obstet. 156:81, 1983.
9. Stanley, M.M. Treatment of intractable ascites in patients with alcoholic cirrhosis by peritoneovenous shunting (LeVeen). Med. Clin. North Am. 63:523, 1979.
10. Straus, A.K., Roseman, D.L., Shapiro, T.H. Peritoneovenous shunting in the management of malignant ascites. Arch. Surg. 114:489, 1979.
11. Wapnick, S., Grosberg, S., Kinney, M., LeVeen, H.H. LeVeen continuous peritoneal-jugular shunt. JAMA 237:131, 1977.
12. Warren, K.W., Jenkins, R.L., Steele, G.D. Atlas of surgery of the liver, pancreas and biliary tract. p. 326. Appleton-Lange, East Norwalk, CT, 1991.
13. Wormser, G.P., Hubbard, R.C. Peritonitis in cirrhotic patients with LeVeen shunt. Am. J. Med. 71:358, 1981.

Section B

Surgery for Portal Hypertension

CHAPTER 12

Transjugular Intrahepatic Portosystemic Shunts (T.I.P.S)

The most frequently used treatment to control bleeding from esophageal varices is endoscopic sclerotherapy. However, sclerotherapy of esophageal varices is not always effective and, even when it is effective, reoccurrence of bleeding may be frequent. In this situation, portosystemic shunts, as previously described, are habitually undertaken. It should be pointed out that these shunts are not easy and are associated with high morbidity and mortality, specially if performed during acute bleeding.

The inconveniences that have been mentioned have stimulated researchers to look for an effective solution for this serious problem with lower morbidity and mortality. In 1969, Rosch, Hanofee and Snow (5) attempted, experimentally, in dogs, to establish a communication between the hepatic veins and the portal vein, using dilators and plastic stents through a transjugular approach. These authors were able to establish intrahepatic portosystemic shunts. These shunts were all rapidly occluded, probably due to their small diameter. The same authors (6) insisted on this technique, using tubes of greater diameter, without better results. With the development of balloon catheters used in angioplasties, interest in these procedures was renewed.(2) According to Barton and colleagues (1), the most precise indication for this technique is in patients with acute hemorrhage as an emergency procedure when endoscopic sclerotherapy has failed and the patient cannot tolerate a portocaval shunt. This procedure can be used in patients who can be transplanted in the future, since it does not represent an inconvenience to transplantation, because the shunt is entirely intrahepatic, and a laparotomy is not done. It is well known that extrahepatic porto-systemic shunts usually are an impediment to hepatic transplantation.

Briefly, intrahepatic portosystemic shunts are carried out as follows: A catheter is placed through the jugular vein, then introduced into the right hepatic vein, and then passed through the hepatic parenchyma into the portal vein. This tract is progressively dilated with balloon catheters. Later, a stent is left in place communicating the entire intrahepatic tract. Some authors use the Gianturco-Rosch Z-stent, others use the Palmaz stent (3), still others the Wallstent stent (1).

It has been shown that these shunts lower the portal pressure and therefore have been proven effective in controlling esophageal variceal bleeding.

It is premature, however, to form a definitive opinion on the results of this procedure since more experience and longer follow-up of these patients is necessary. It should be realized that this procedure is still experimental and not easy to carry out, and those who are doing it should first acquire more experience (1).

References

1. Barton, R.E., Rosch, J.R., Keller, F.S., Uchida, B.T. Transjugular intrahepatic portosystemic shunts. In Hunter, J.G., Sackier, J.M. (Eds) Minimally invasive surgery. p. 269. McGraw-Hill, New York, 1993.
2. Coapinto, R.F., Stronell, T.D., Birch, S.J. et al. Creation of an intrahepatic portosystemic shunt with Gruntzig balloon catheter. Can. Med. Assoc. 126:267, 1982.
3. Palmaz, J.C., Garcia, F., Sibbit, R.R. et al. Expandable intrahepatic portacaval shunt stents in dogs with chronic portal hypertension. Am. J. Roentgenol. 147:1251, 1986.
4. Richter, G.M., Noeldge, G., Palmaz, J.C. et al. Transjugular intrahepatic portacaval stent shunt. Preliminary clinical results. Radiology 174:1027, 1990.
5. Rosch, J.R., Hanofee, W.N., Snow, H. Transjugular portal venography and radiologic portacaval shunt. An experimental study. Radiology 92:1112, 1969.
6. Rosch, J.R., Hanofee, W.N., Snow, H. et al. Transjugular intrahepatic portacaval shunt. Am. J. Surg. 121:588, 1971.
7. Rosch, J.R., Uchida, B.T., Putnam, J.S. Experimental intrahepatic portacaval anastomosis. Use of expandable Gianturco stents. Radiology 162:481, 1987.
8. Uchida, B.T., Putnam, J.S., Rosch, J.R. "Atraumatic" transjugular needle for portal vein puncture in swine. Radiology 163:580, 1987.

Section C

Surgery of the Pancreas

CHAPTER **13**

Surgery of the Pancreas

SURGICAL ANATOMY OF THE PANCREAS

The pancreas is an organ of both exocrine and endocrine secretion, with multiple functions, some of which are not completely known. This organ is located deep in the abdominal cavity applied to the superior portion of the posterior wall of the abdomen, extending from the internal border of the second portion of the duodenum to the hilus of the spleen, running a slightly oblique course upward and to the left. The average weight of the pancreas is 80 g, and its length varies between 14 and 22 cm. Its median height, at the level of the head, is 7 cm and its thickness at this same level is from 20 to 25 mm.

The endocrine secretion of the pancreas is produced by the cells of the islets of Langerhans, whose number approximates one million. The total weight of the islets is approximately 1 g.

The pancreas is a fixed organ, and only its tail moves slightly in a craniocaudal direction.

Surgical Anatomy of the Pancreas

FIGURE 13.1
In an arbitrary fashion, the pancreas is usually divided into four sections: 1, head, 2, neck, 3, body, 4, tail. Some anatomists divide the pancreas into five segments, adding the uncinate process to the above four segments. In reality, the uncinate process is part of the head of the pancreas, in spite of presenting some peculiarities which we will later describe.

From the surgical anatomy point of view, the concept proposed by Couinaud (2, 8), who asserts that, since the pancreas is an elongated organ oriented transversely, two sections can be distinguished, one a right section and the other a left section (right pancreas and left pancreas), which can be mobilized surgically with different approaches, joined by a section that would correspond to the hilus of the pancreas where the major arteries enter and then distribute themselves to the left or to the right. The same thing occurs with the nervous elements, which enter the pancreas as thick nerve layers.

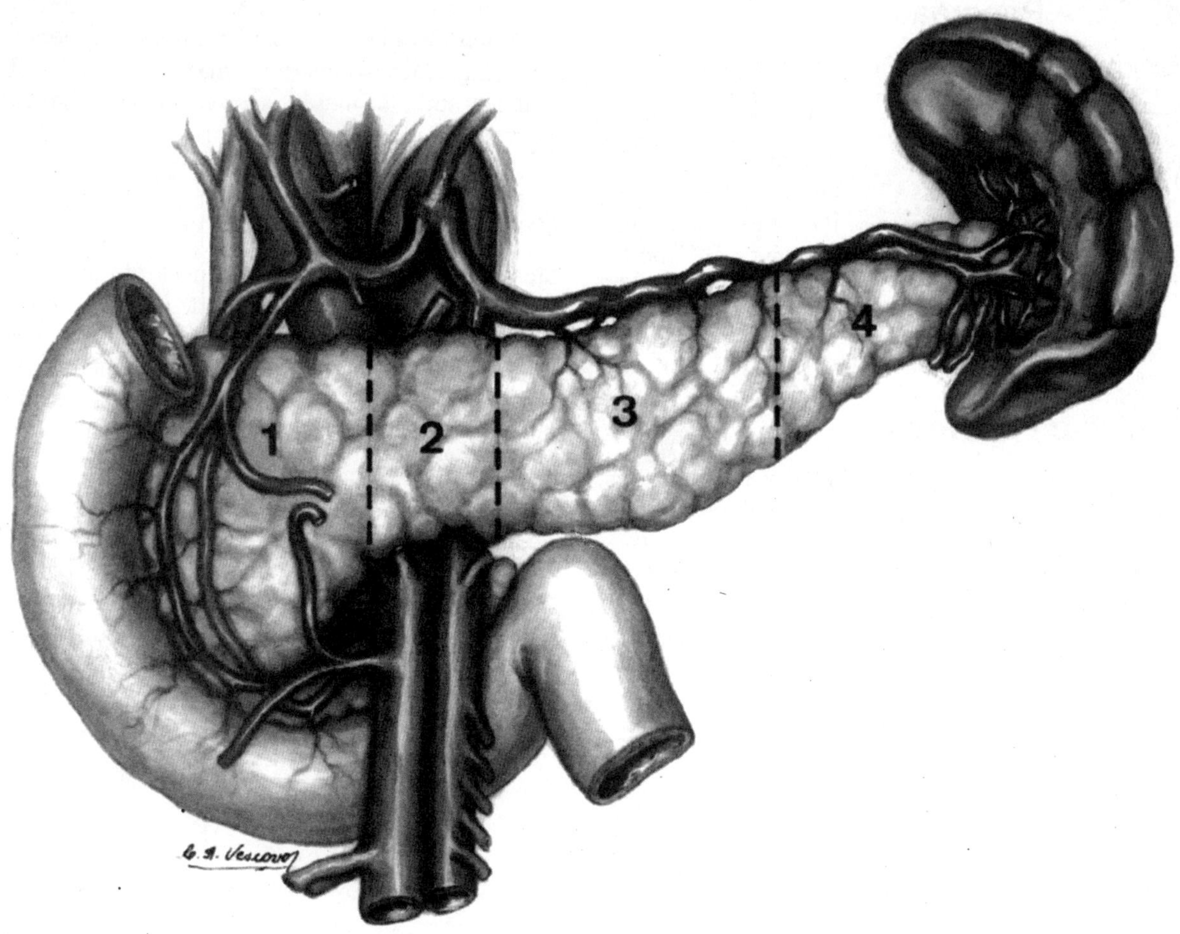

FIGURE 13.1

Head of the Pancreas

This segment extends from the inner border of the duodenum to the right edge of the superior mesenteric vein. Some authors consider the left limit as the groove which the gastroduodenal artery makes on the anterior and superior border of the pancreas (7). The uncinate process, which we have said forms a part of the head of the pancreas, has the form of a hook directed downward and to the left, passing behind the superior mesenteric vessels while the rest of the pancreas passes in front of these vessels.

Neck of the Pancreas

This is the segment that joins the head of the pancreas with the body. Its diameter is generally smaller than that of the head. Very frequently, the neck of the pancreas is described as a line that separates the head from the body. This is not exact, and we must consider that the neck is a segment of pancreas covering the superior mesenteric vessels whose width varies between 2 to 6 cm, its average being 4 cm (15). The posterior surface of the neck of the pancreas does not have any efferent vein draining in the anterior wall of the portal vein or the superior mesenteric vein. These veins drain into the lateral walls of the portal or superior mesenteric veins (14). There can, however, be some exceptions to this.

Body of the Pancreas

This segment extends from the neck of the pancreas (left border of the superior mesenteric artery) to the tail. The boundary between the body and the tail is probably the most arbitrary of the segments of the pancreas. The body of the pancreas is prominent anteriorly in the lesser omenta bursa owing to the forward protrusion of the vertebral bodies of the first and second lumbar vertebrae.

Tail of Pancreas

This is the narrowest and most mobile segment of the pancreas. Its end contacts the hilus of the spleen. In some cases, however, the tail of the pancreas does not reach the hilus of the spleen.

Surgical Anatomy of the Pancreas

Surgical Anatomy of the Pancreas

FIGURE 13.2 UNCINATE PROCESS

This forms part of the head of the pancreas and is located in a plane posterior to the superior mesenteric vessels. Because of its location and its relations with the superior mesenteric vessels and owing to its arterial and venous supply, it constitutes the portion of the head of the pancreas that is most difficult to explore and to free when a pancreaticoduodenectomy is being performed. The extent of development of the uncinate process is variable. In some patients, it is poorly developed or may even be absent, which greatly facilitates resection of the head of the pancreas. In other cases, the uncinate process extends to the posterior wall of the superior mesenteric vein, and in others, it may extend behind the superior mesenteric artery and even go beyond it and become adherent to its adventitia. There exists a layer constituted of fibrous tissue, lymphatic vessels, and nervous fibers (2, 8, 16, 17) that extends from the uncinate process and divides into two retropancreatic portions, one that joins the semilunar ganglion and is called the uncolunar layer, the other, which joins the adventitia of the superior mesenteric artery, called the uncomesenteric layer. When these layers are well developed, liberation of the uncinate process during resection of the head of the pancreas is more difficult.

In some patients, the ligament extending from the adventitia of the superior mesenteric artery should be separated or divided. Several very fragile small veins go from the uncinate process to the superior mesenteric vein. These veins must be carefully ligated and divided individually during the liberation of the uncinate process. The uncinate process receives several arterial vessels, which arise from the superior mesenteric artery and which also must be ligated and divided individually during the liberation of the uncinate process (7–11). All surgeons accept that resection of the pancreatic segment to the right of the aorta is much more difficult to perform than resection of the segment to the left of the aorta. For this reason Couinaud (2) believes it is useful to divide the pancreas from the surgical point of view into two segments—the right pancreas and the left pancreas—considering the segment that joins them as the hilus of the pancreas (2). In the drawing, the different degrees of development of the uncinate process are shown. 1, Poorly developed uncinate process. 2, Uncinate process extending to the superior mesenteric vein. 3, Uncinate process extending beyond the posterior wall of the superior mesenteric artery.

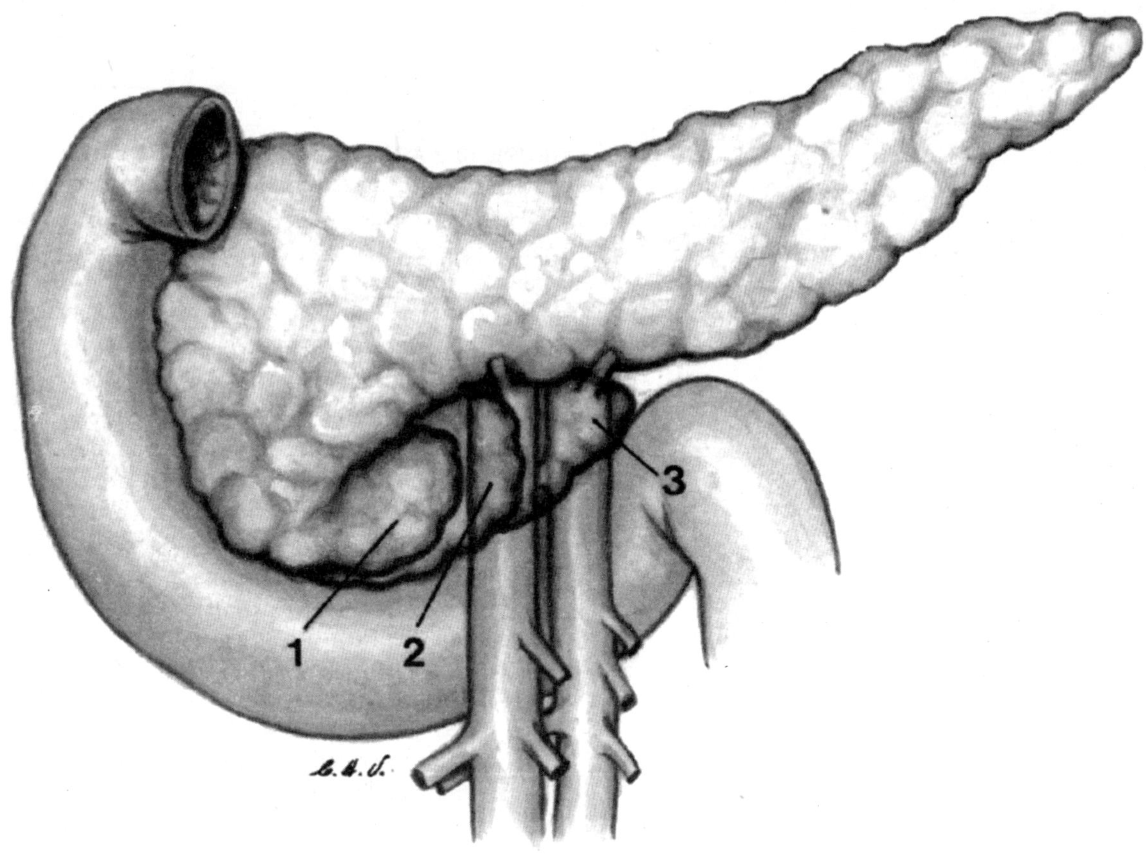

FIGURE 13.2 UNCINATE PROCESS

FIGURE 13.3 ARTERIES OF THE PANCREAS
The pancreas is a very profusely irrigated organ. In the drawing we are showing the principal arteries of the pancreas and some arteries of the region which have some relation with the organ (2, 6, 9–11). 1, Coronary gastric artery or left gastric artery. 2, Common hepatic artery. 2', Hepatic artery. 3, Gastroduodenal artery. 4, Superior and posterior pancreaticoduodenal arteries, the first branch arising from the gastroduodenal artery. 5, Right gastroepiploic artery. 6, Superior and anterior pancreaticoduodenal artery. The right gastroepipl[illegible] and superior and anterior pancreaticoduodenal arteries are the terminal branches of the gastroduodenal artery, which arise from the common hepatic artery. 7, Common trunk of the inferior pancreaticoduodenal arteries arising from the superior mesenteric artery. From this common trunk the inferior posterior pancreaticoduodenal artery arises and the inferior anterior pancreaticoduodenal artery also arises. These two arteries may arise separately from the superior mesenteric artery. In some cases the common trunk of the inferior pancreaticoduodenal and the inferior anterior pancreaticoduodenal may pass in front of the superior mesenteric vein. 8, Superior mesenteric artery. 9, Splenic artery. 10, Dorsal pancreatic or superior pancreatic artery. 11, Transverse pancreatic artery. 12, Great pancreatic artery. 13, Caudal pancreatic artery (5, 7, 9, 12).

Surgical Anatomy of the Pancreas

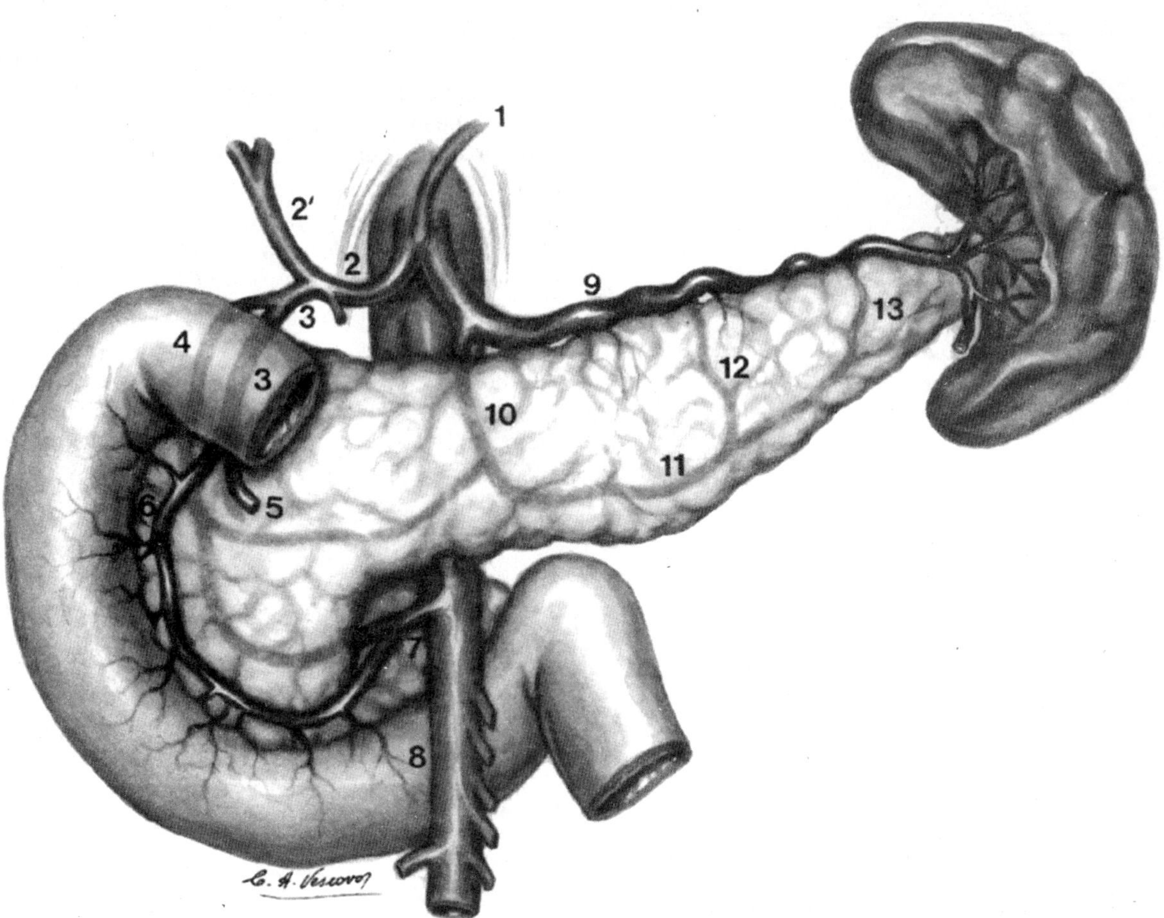

FIGURE 13.3 ARTERIES OF THE PANCREAS

FIGURE 13.4 ANOMALIES OF THE HEPATIC ARTERY

The hepatic artery may present numerous anomalies in its origin and in its course. The surgeon must be alert to these possibilities during the surgical procedure. The most frequent anomaly of the hepatic artery is its origin from the superior mesenteric artery. The common hepatic artery and the right hepatic artery arise from the superior mesenteric artery in slightly more than 20% of patients (5, 7, 11). The left hepatic artery much less frequently arises from the superior mesenteric artery, but this is only important in surgery of the pancreas, when it arises from the right side of the superior mesenteric artery, and this is very infrequent. Generally, the common hepatic artery or the right hepatic artery, when they arise from the superior mesenteric artery, run behind the pancreas, but in some cases they can run through the head of the pancreas or the uncinate process, which would make pancreaticoduodenectomy a contraindication. The operative abdominal angiography is useful to determine the presence of an anomalous hepatic artery but can only demonstrate its origin and course, not whether it passes through the pancreatic parenchyma or not. The experienced surgeon, even without angiography, can determine the existence of this anomaly and take the necessary precautions. The drawing shows a common hepatic artery arising from the superior mesenteric artery and passing behind the head of the pancreas.

Surgical Anatomy of the Pancreas

FIGURE 13.5 VEINS OF THE PANCREAS

This drawing shows the principal efferent pancreatic veins, which generally run the same course as the arteries (5, 6, 12). 1, Portal vein. 2, Superior mesenteric vein. The superior mesenteric vein and portal veins form what is usually known as the mesentericoportal axis. 3, Splenic vein. 4, Inferior mesenteric vein. This vein may empty into the splenic vein or in the angle formed by the splenic vein with the portal vein. Rarely, the inferior mesenteric vein empties into the portal vein. 5, Gastrocolic trunk or venous Trunk of Henle. In 60% of cases, Henle's Trunk is formed by the junction of the right gastroepiploic vein, the right superior colic vein, and the inferior and anterior pancreaticoduodenal veins (12). 6, Right gastroepiploic vein. 7, Right superior colic vein. 8, Inferior and anterior pancreaticoduodenal veins. 9, Inferior and posterior pancreaticoduodenal veins. 10, Superior and posterior pancreaticoduodenal veins. 11, Superior and anterior pancreaticoduodenal veins. 12, Middle colic vein.

Ligation of Henle's Trunk is an important step in pancreaticoduodenectomy because it permits the bloodless separation of the mesogastrium, mesoduodenum, and mesocolon. Ligation of Henle's Trunk prevents troublesome hemorrhage, which is difficult to control owing to rupture of some of its constituting branches, particularly the inferior anterior pancreaticoduodenal vein.

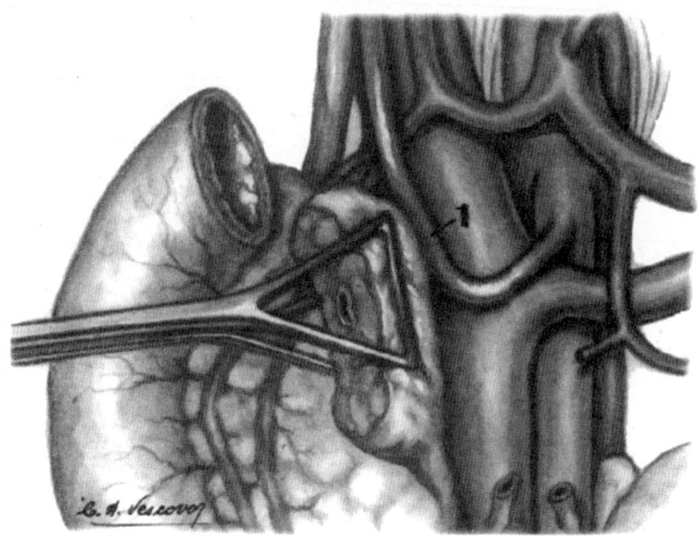

FIGURE 13.4 ANOMALIES OF THE HEPATIC ARTERY

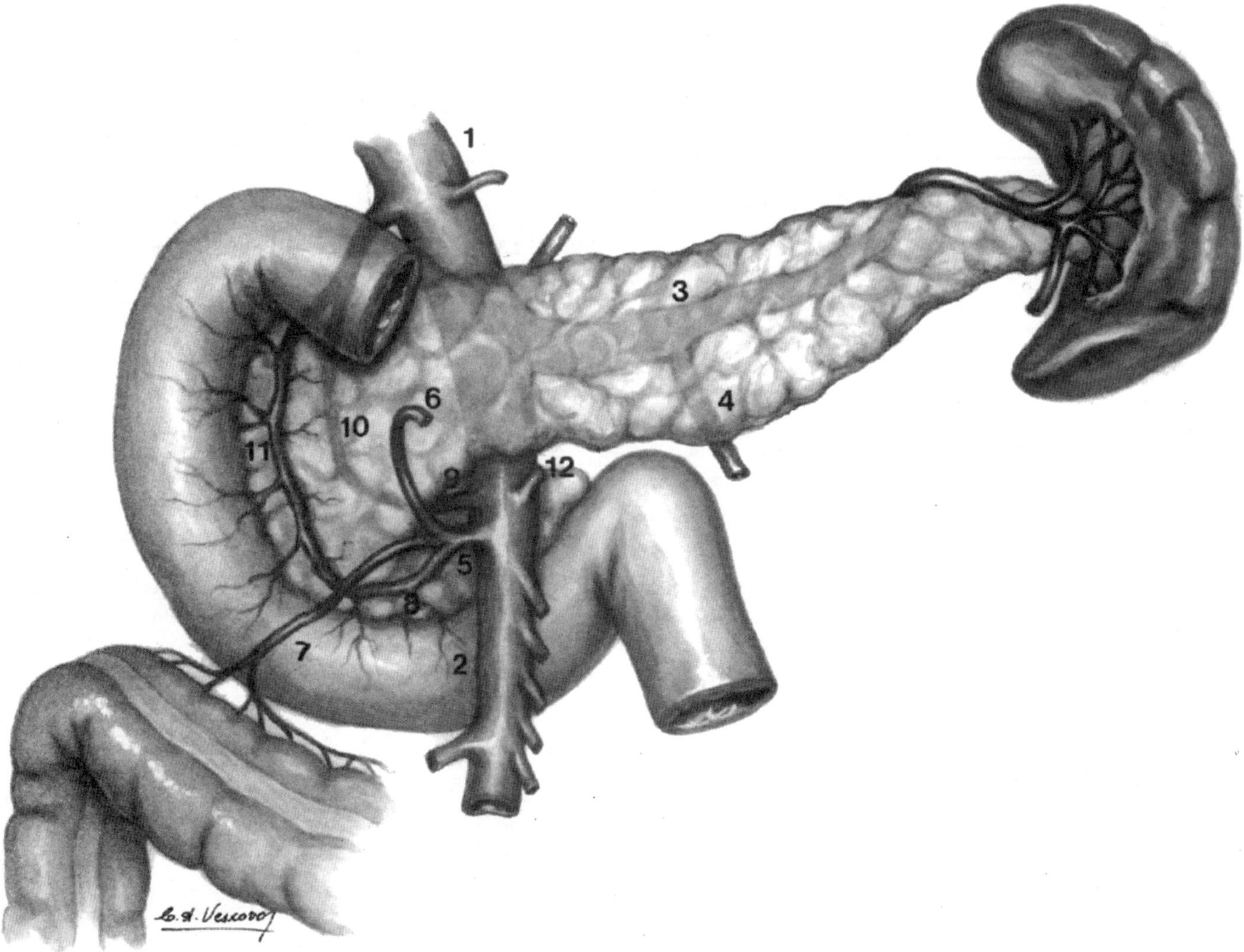

FIGURE 13.5 VEINS OF THE PANCREAS

Surgical Anatomy of the Pancreas

FIGURE 13.6 LYMPHATICS OF THE PANCREAS

The principal lymphatic groups of the pancreas are as follows: 1, Hepatic nodes. 2, Celiac nodes. 3, Coronary nodes. 4, Superior pancreatic nodes. 5, Inferior pancreatic nodes. 6, Splenic nodes. 7, Subpyloric nodes. 8, Anterior pancreaticoduodenal nodes. 9, Mesenteric nodes (3, 4, 6, 12, 13).

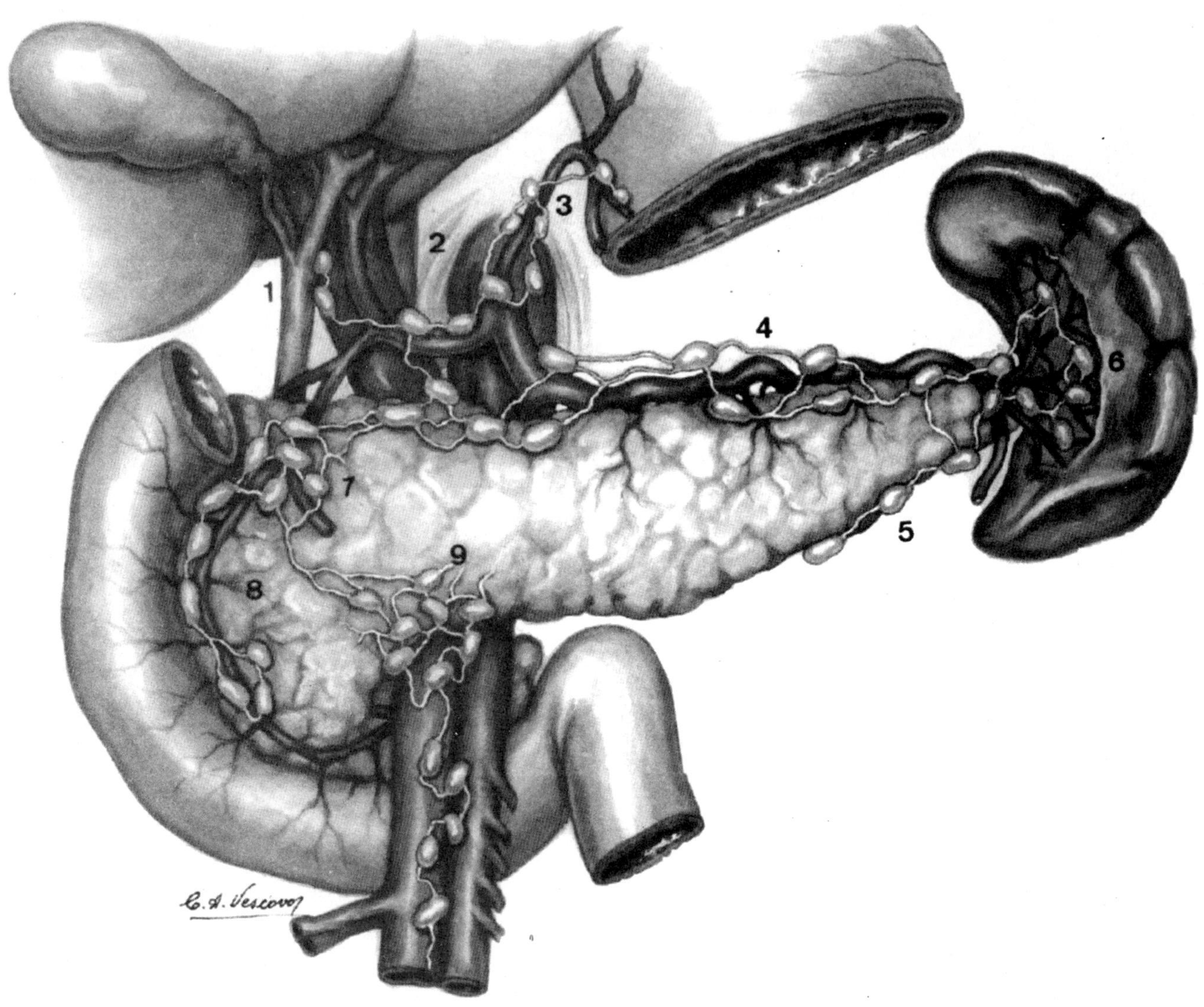

FIGURE 13.6 LYMPHATICS OF THE PANCREAS

References

1. Cattell, R.B., Warren, K.W. Surgery of the pancreas. p. 261. W.B. Saunders Co., Philadelphia, 1953.
2. Couinaud, C., Huguet, C. Le temps d'exérèse dans la duodéno-pancréatectomie totale. J. Chir. 91:181, 1966.
3. Cubilla, A.L., Fortner, J., Fitzgerald, P.J. Lymph node involvement in carcinoma of the head of the pancreas area. Cancer 41:880, 1978.
4. Evans, B.P., Ochsner, A. The gross anatomy of the lymphatics of the human pancreas. Surgery 36:177, 1954.
5. Flint, E.R. Abnormalities of the right hepatic cystic and gastroduodenal arteries and of the bile ducts. Br. J. Surg. 10:509, 1923.
6. Hermann, R.E. Manual of surgery of the gallbladder, bile ducts and exocrine pancreas. p. 155. Springer-Verlag, New York, 1979.
7. Hollinshead, W.H. Anatomy for surgeons. Vol. 2, p. 355. Hoeber Harper, New York, 1956.
8. Marchal, G., Hureau, J. Les tumeurs oddiennes. p. 122. Masson S.A., Paris, 1978.
9. Marchal, G., Balmes, M., Vergues, J., Grynfelt, E., Sellami, A. Le problème vasculaire en rapport avec la chirurgie d'exérèse pancréatique. Montpelier Chir. 17:407, 1971.
10. Michels, N.A. The hepatic, cystic and retroduodenal arteries and their relations to the biliary ducts. Ann. Surg. 133:503, 1951.
11. Michels, N.A. Blood supply of the liver and the upper abdominal organs. J.P. Lippincott, Philadelphia, 1969.
12. Moosa, A.R., Lewis, M.H., Mackie, C.R. Surgical treatment of pancreatic cancer. Mayo Clin. Proc. 54:468, 1979.
13. Rouvière, H. Anatomie des lymphatiques de l'homme. p. 203. Masson et Cie., Paris, 1932.
14. Silen, W. Surgical anatomy of the pancreas. Surg. Clin. North Am. 44:1253, 1964.
15. Skandalakis, J.E., Gray, S.W., Rowe, J.S., Jr., Skandalakis, L.J. Anatomical complications of pancreatic surgery. Contemp. Surg. 15:17, 1979.
16. Yoshioka, H., Wakabayashi, T. Traitement de la douleur des pancréatites chroniques par la neurectomie de la tête du pancréas. Lyon Chir. 53:836, 1957.
17. Yoshioka, H., Wakabayashi, T. Therapeutic neurotomy on head of pancreas for relief of pain due to chronic pancreatitis. Arch. Surgery 76:546, 1958.
18. Woodburn, R.T. Essentials of human anatomy. Ed. 6, Oxford University Press, New York, 1978.

Section C

Surgery of the Pancreas

CHAPTER **14**

Surgical Treatment of Pseudocysts of the Pancreas

There are many surgical procedures used in the treatment of pseudocysts of the pancreas. The procedure to be used in any one case depends on the anatomy and pathology present as well as the general condition of the patient. Several factors must be considered in determining what procedure to use: size and location of the pseudocyst, condition of its wall, its relation to the stomach or duodenum, the presence of complications such as rapid growth with threatening rupture or with rupture into the peritoneal cavity, active hemorrhage caused by arterial erosion or rupture of a pseudoaneurysm, pseudoaneurysm without hemorrhage, massive suppuration of the pseudocyst, age and general condition of the patient, and so on.

The surgical procedure most frequently used and that gives the best results is an anastomosis between the cyst and the digestive tract, be it the stomach, the jejunum, or the duodenum (1–4). Other procedures are employed with less frequency, such as external drainage of the pseudocyst, percutaneous aspiration of the pseudocyst with sonographic control or with computerized tomography, marsupialization, pancreatic resection, the combination of medical procedures with surgical procedures such as embolization of the bleeding artery or its occlusion by arterial catheterization, followed by surgical intervention, and so on. All these emphasize the importance of complete preoperative studies of patients with pancreatic pseudocysts in order to be able to plan the surgical procedure most convenient to each case.

PREOPERATIVE STUDIES OF PANCREATIC PSEUDOCYSTS

A chest x-ray is indispensable, since there is frequently left or bilateral pleural effusion. An upper gastrointestinal x-ray study must be performed to determine the relation of the pseudocyst with the stomach, the duodenum, and the rest of the bowel. Ultrasonography is important, not only to diagnose the pseudocyst, but also to follow its evolution, its variations in size, the condition of its wall, the presence of biliary calculi, or dilation of the biliary tract. If possible, a computed tomographic study should be performed, since this will add more precise data than that given by ultrasonography. Cholecystography can, in some cases, be a complementary study together with the ultrasonogram for the diagnosis of biliary calculi. A transparietohepatic cholangiogram can be done, particularly if there is dilation of the biliary tract or jaundice. Endoscopic retrograde cholangiopancreatography can be a useful procedure (10), but it should be performed with maximal precautions, since it can lead to infection in the biliary tract. Sometimes endoscopic retrograde cholangiopancreatography may lead to opacification of the pancreatic duct and the pseudocyst. It is presumed that this communication is present in all cases of pancreatic pseudocyst, but it is not always demonstrable, possibly because the communication acts like a valve (15).

Performance of selective arteriography of the celiac trunk and of the superior mesenteric artery before surgery is very important when the pseudocyst is complicated by active hemorrhage to determine the site of the hemorrhage with the object of adopting the most adequate surgical procedure for the anatomy present. Some authors believe that all cases of pseudocysts of the pancreas should undergo selective angiography even if there is no bleeding, with the objective of investigating the presence of an arterial pseudoaneurysm, which can bleed postoperatively (13). It is important to remember that the wall of the pseudocyst requires some six weeks to mature and to be strong enough to hold a suture (1, 3, 6). Sometimes the wall of the pseudocyst matures earlier, but it is hard to be absolutely sure of this, and many suture failures have occurred because the pseudocyst wall is not mature. In addition to the clinical picture, the time of evolution of the pseudocyst, computed tomography, ultrasonography, and the "old amylase" blood level can help to establish if the wall of the pseudocyst is or is not mature prior to the operation (2, 4, 20).

Between 30 and 40% of pseudocysts of the pancreas resolve spontaneously within 6 weeks of their appearance and therefore will not need surgical treatment. After 6 weeks it is very difficult for pseudocysts to resolve spontaneously, and they will be more prone to present complications.

SURGICAL PROCEDURES USED TO TREAT PSEUDOCYSTS OF THE PANCREAS

External Drainage of the Pseudocyst

Drainage of pseudocysts of the pancreas to the outside of the abdomen is indicated when the cyst grows rapidly and rupture into the abdominal cavity is imminent. Since the cyst wall is not mature, it is not possible to anastomose it to the digestive tract. To drain the cyst to the outside, a midline incision is made between the xiphoid and the umbilicus. The cyst is aspirated with syringe and a No. 16 needle, and the fluid in it is aspirated in order to rule out the presence of blood and an intracystic hemorrhage. The fluid is studied for bacteria, enzyme levels, and cytology. The cyst is then punctured with a trocar, and all of its contents are removed. A drainage tube for continuous suction is placed in the pseudocyst and held to the wall of the pseudocyst with a pursestring suture, if possible. The drainage tube is brought out through a small incision in the abdomen and is connected to continuous suction. The wall of the abdomen is closed in layers, using nonabsorbable material. If the pseudocyst is ruptured before surgery, a similar procedure to the one described is performed.

Drainage of the pseudocyst to the outside is not a procedure of choice. It only serves to resolve an emergency and is exposed to complications such as fistulas, lesions of the skin due to the action of enzymes, and frequent recurrences with elevated mortality and morbidity (1, 4, 5, 7).

Pseudocysts that increase dangerously in size can also be drained by the percutaneous route with ultrasonographic or computerized tomographic control. Percutaneous drainage should be performed in an institution where considerable experience has been had with this procedure (1, 2, 10, 19). It has been shown that the incidence of recurrence of pseudocysts treated by percutaneous drainage is much higher than those treated surgically (2, 4, 5).

Pseudocysts of the Pancreas with Hemorrhage

Pseudocysts of the pancreas can become complicated by active hemorrhage caused by the erosion of an artery or the rupture of a pseudoaneurysm in the wall of the cyst. Selective preoperative angiography can determine the site of the hemorrhage and can also demonstrate the presence of a pseudoaneurysm of an artery in the wall of the cyst such as the splenic artery, the gastroduodenal artery, or a pancreaticoduodenal artery.

Even though localization of the new vessel or demonstration of the presence of a pseudoaneurysm is not always possible, it is convenient to perform selective angiography in all cases (1, 18). It is sometimes possible to achieve hemostasis by means of arterial embolization. In some cases, it may be possible to obtain temporary hemostasis preoperatively by placing a catheter with an inflatable balloon in its end in the proximal side of the bleeding vessel and thus continue the surgical procedure under better control (1, 14).

In cases of pseudocysts with massive hemorrhage, pancreatic resection together with the pseudocyst, be it by means of a distal pancreatectomy or by pancreatoduodenectomy with ligature of the bleeding vessel proximally outside the pseudocyst, is the procedure of choice (6). Pancreatic resection under these conditions carries a high mortality and morbidity, and for this reason, the surgeon who undertakes this procedure should be very experienced in pancreatic surgery (1, 18).

Some surgeons, before performing pancreatic resection, prefer to attempt to place a suture ligature in the bleeding artery from within the pseudocyst. The ligature, under these conditions, even if performed with polypropylene No. 1 suture, including the artery together with neighboring tissues, is prone to failure because the tissues are friable and the sutureligature may cut the tissues as it is tied. Some surgeons (2), however, advise that, before proceeding with pancreatic resection, one should attempt to obtain hemostasis with a sutureligature, which may give good results in some cases. If the patient does not bleed but presents an arterial pseudoaneurysm, the procedure to be performed is the same, since the pseudoaneurysm may rupture postoperatively with grave consequences (1, 6, 18).

Marsupialization of Pancreatic Pseudocysts—Gussenbauer (1883)

Marsupialization of pancreatic pseudocysts was frequently used in years past but at present has only few indications. It is logical to deduce that, if a pseudocyst has mature enough walls to allow it to be sutured to the wall of the abdomen, it can be advantageously sutured to the digestive tract. Indications for marsupialization of a pseudocyst are at present reduced to cases of a pseudocyst with mature walls, adequate for anastomosis to the digestive tract, but whose contents are massively infected, this having been confirmed by bacteriologic examination. In this situation, it is preferable to drain the septic contents of the cyst to the outside instead of emptying it into the digestive tract.

Pancreatic Resections

Resection of the pancreas with a pseudocyst may be indicated, as mentioned previously, in very critical situations when hemostasis has been impossible in the face of an active hemorrhage of one of the arteries in the cyst wall. Resection of the pancreas in these cases carries a very high mortality and morbidity (4, 5, 6, 18).

Pancreatic Pseudocysts Complicated by Biliary Tract Problems

Pancreatitis of alcoholic origin is infrequently associated with biliary lithiasis. The opposite is true in pancreatitis secondary to biliary problems. If the patient with the pancreatic pseudocyst has biliary lithiasis, it is advisable during surgery to remove the gallbladder first, and then proceed to treat the pseudocyst. If operative cholangiography reveals the presence of calculi in the biliary ducts, these are removed and a new cholangiogram performed to be sure all calculi have been removed and the biliary tract is not obstructed. If the common bile duct is compressed by the pseudocyst, a condition that produces a very typical cholangiographic image, this obstruction is usually relieved after the cyst is treated. If the common bile duct is compressed by a chronic pancreatitis of the head of the pancreas, a biliary bypass to the digestive tract may be necessary.

Cystogastrostomy by the Transgastric Route—Jurasz (1929)

Cystogastrostomy through the transgastric approach is indicated in cases in which the pseudocyst of the pancreas has mature walls and the anterior wall of the cyst is solidly adherent to the posterior wall of the stomach.

FIGURE 14.1
The abdomen is entered through a midline, upper abdominal incision. The adhesion of the pseudocyst to the posterior wall of the stomach and the presence of mature cyst wall able to hold a suture are confirmed. The diagram shows the presence of a large pancreatic pseudocyst occupying the lesser sac and displacing the stomach anteriorly. The line drawn near the greater curvature of the stomach indicates the site where an incision about 5 to 6 cm long is going to be performed in the anterior gastric wall. It is convenient to avoid the antrum in performing this incision.

Surgical Procedures Used to Treat Pseudocysts of the Pancreas

FIGURE 14.2
The drawing shows the gastric wall being incised. As the wall of the stomach is incised, its edges are grasped with Duval forceps which, besides holding the gastric wall, give temporary hemostasis.

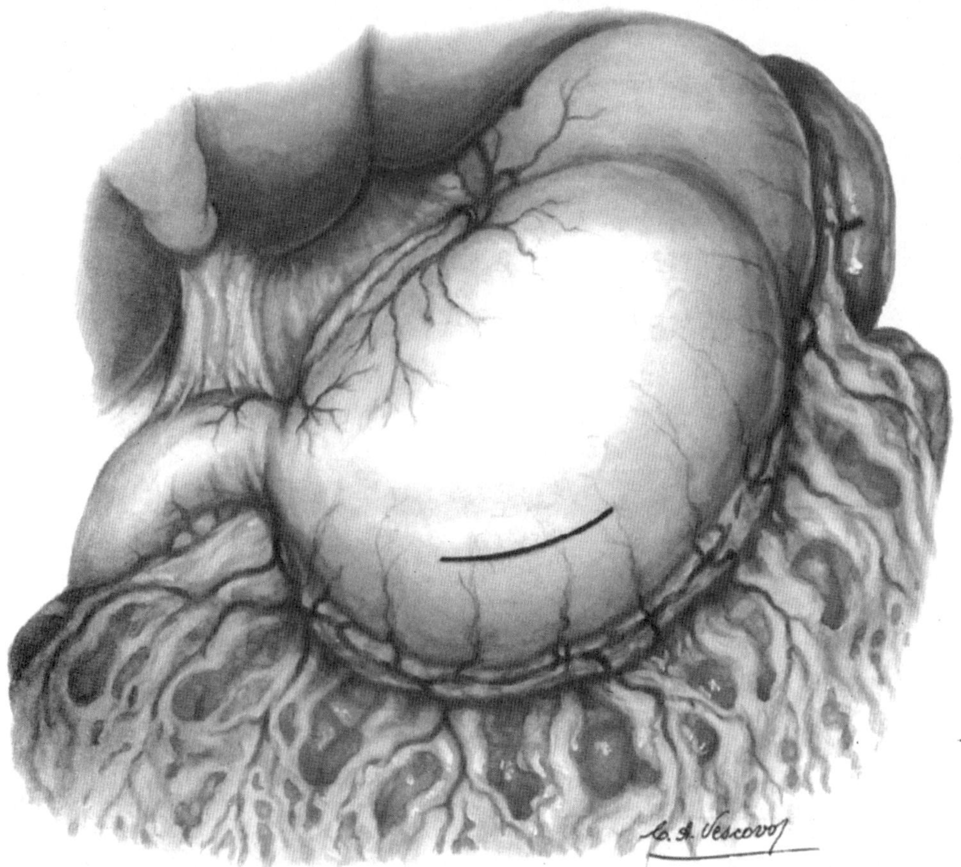

FIGURE 14.1

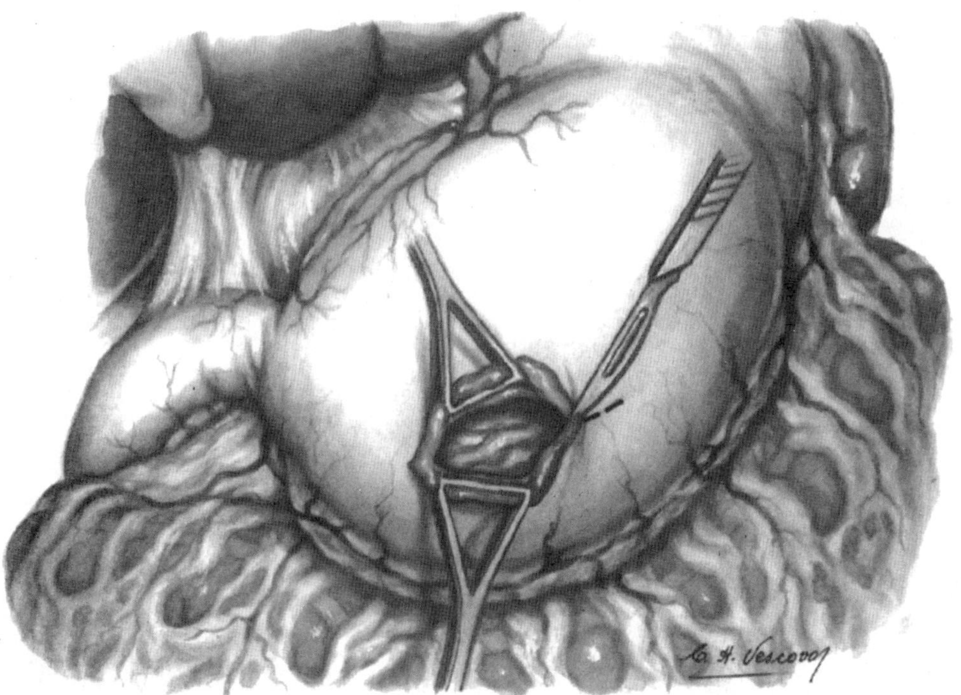

FIGURE 14.2

FIGURE 14.3
The posterior gastric wall is punctured with a syringe and a No. 16 needle, entering the pseudocyst and removing a few cubic centimeters of its contents in order to examine its visual characteristics. The removed material will be used for a Gram stain, to determine the presence of bacteria, and for enzymatic levels and cytologic studies.

Surgical Procedures Used to Treat Pseudocysts of the Pancreas

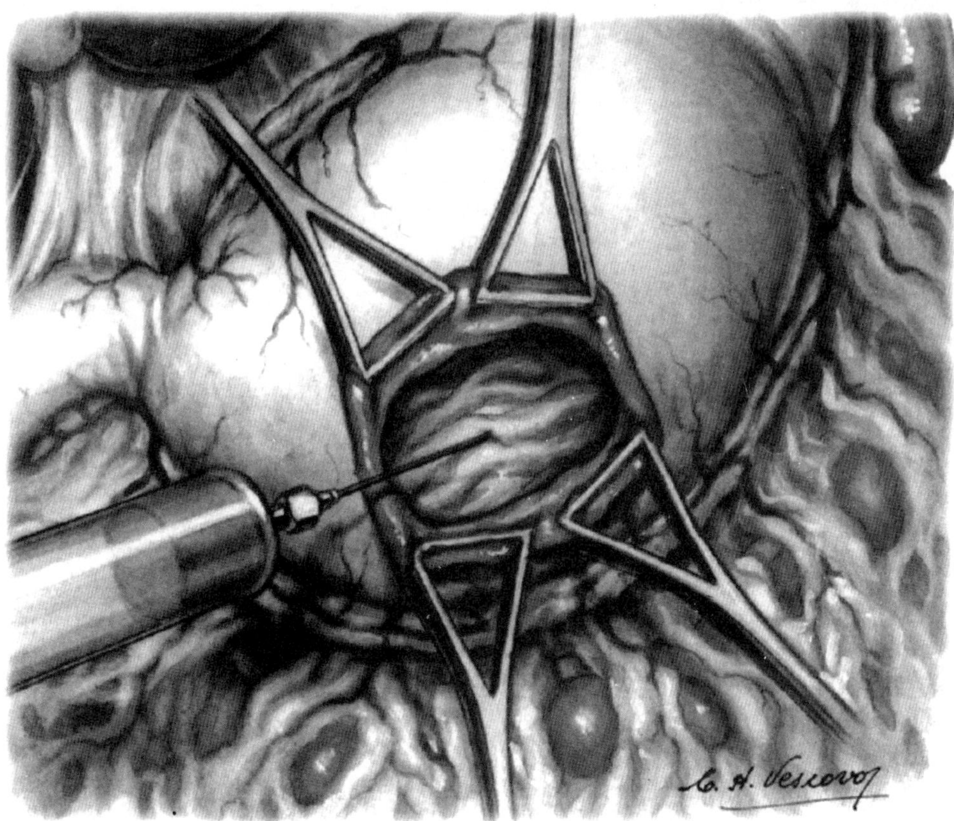

FIGURE 14.3

Surgical Procedures Used to Treat Pseudocysts of the Pancreas

FIGURE 14.4

Once the presence of fluid is confirmed by the puncture, a trocar is introduced through the same opening made by the needle and all the cyst's contents are removed, as shown in 1. Once the contents of the cyst are removed, a catheter with several perforations is introduced through the same opening and the inside of the pseudocyst is irrigated with physiologic solution as shown in 2. With the cyst full of physiologic solution, a laparoscope or fiberoptic choledochoscope is introduced in order to inspect the inside of the pseudocyst (16), as shown in 3. Visualization with the laparoscope or the fiberoptic choledochoscope of the interior of the pseudocyst may allow for the observation of a possible arterial pseudoaneurysm, formation of compartments, or the presence of papillary growths, which may complicate later evolution of the pseudocyst or establish that we are facing a cystic tumor.

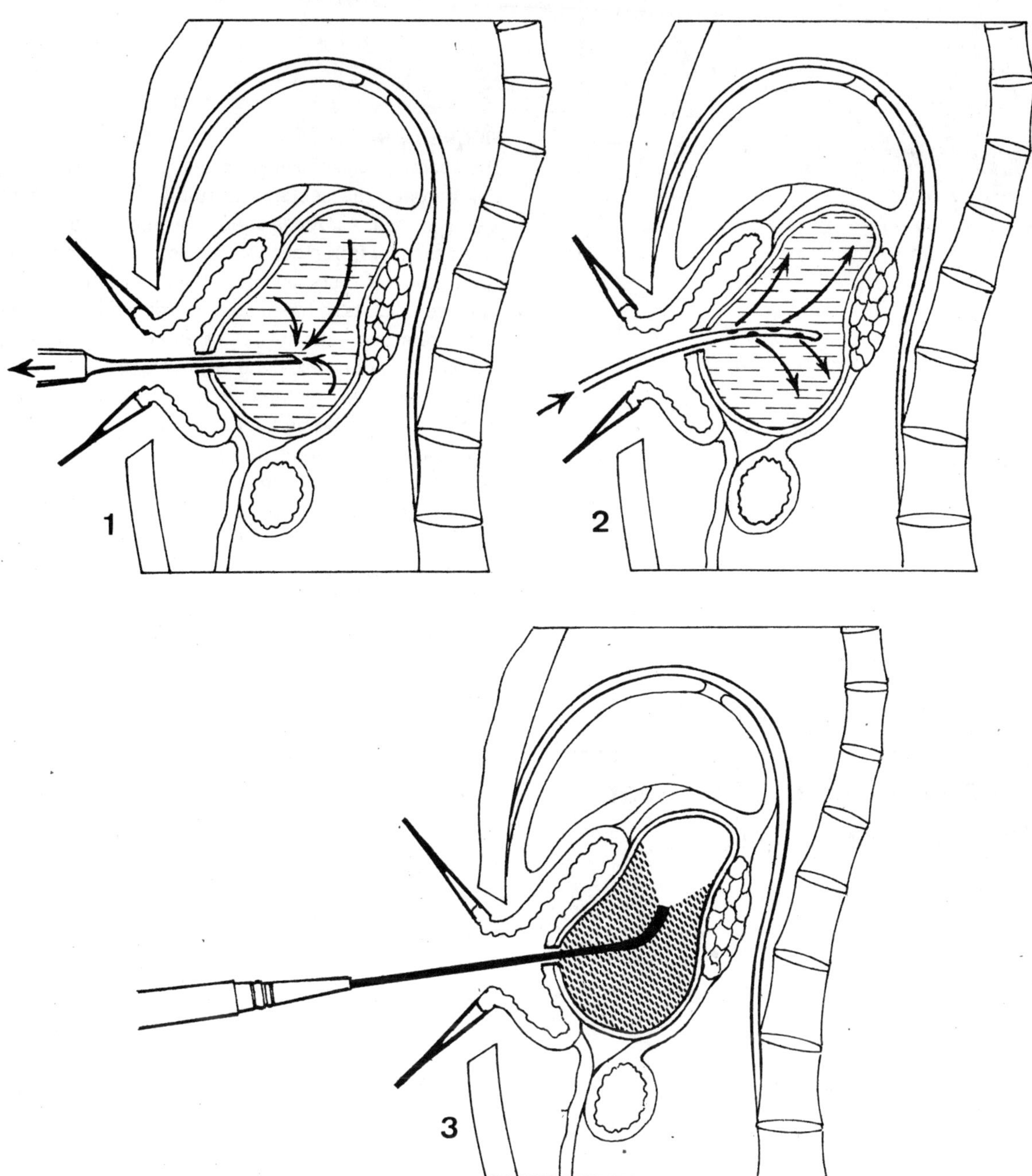

FIGURE 14.4

FIGURE 14.5
The fiberoptic choledochoscope is removed, and the common wall between the posterior gastric wall and the anterior cyst wall is incised. A lozenge-shaped segment of the common wall is removed for frozen section histologic study, since there have been cases of cystadenocarcinoma that have been confused with pseudocysts of the head of the pancreas. Histologic study of the removed segment is not always definitive to eliminate the presence of a cystadenocarcinoma, since malignant zones may be irregularly distributed on the internal surface of the neoplasm. It should be kept in mind that only pseudocysts of the pancreas that have no epithelium can be anastomosed. Cystadenocarcinomas are always lined by epithelium and should not be anastomosed, but should be resected. The inside of the pseudocyst should be emptied of all solid material, but its removal must be performed very gently. The contents should be easy to remove. One should not force the removal by using curettes or clamps, since they can traumatize the inside of the pseudocyst and lead to hemorrhages that are difficult to control.

Surgical Procedures Used to Treat Pseudocysts of the Pancreas

FIGURE 14.6
The anterior wall of the pseudocyst is sutured to the posterior wall of the stomach using interrupted sutures of nonabsorbable material. It is extremely important to perform excellent hemostasis of the edges of the stomach and the pseudocyst to prevent postoperative hemorrhage. Hemorrhages of the gastric wall or of the pseudocyst have been confused with hemorrhage caused by the rupture of a pseudoaneurysm of the cyst wall. Some surgeons, instead of performing the anastomosis with interrupted sutures, perform it with continuous suture. Other surgeons do not perform an anastomosis and simply perform hemostasis. They believe an anastomosis to be unnecessary, since both structures are densely adherent (4).

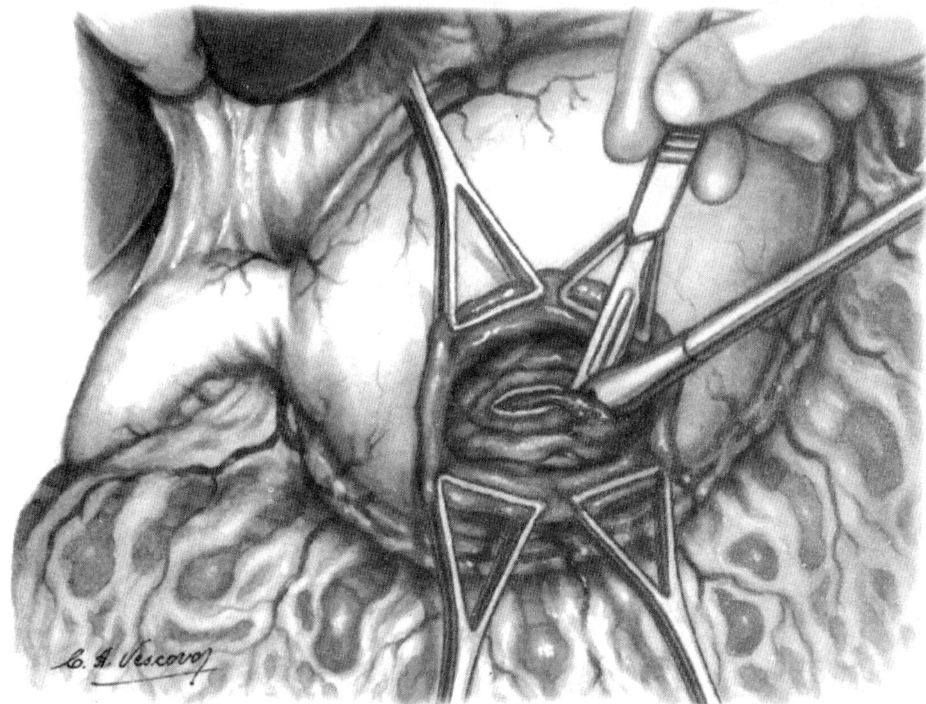

FIGURE 14.5

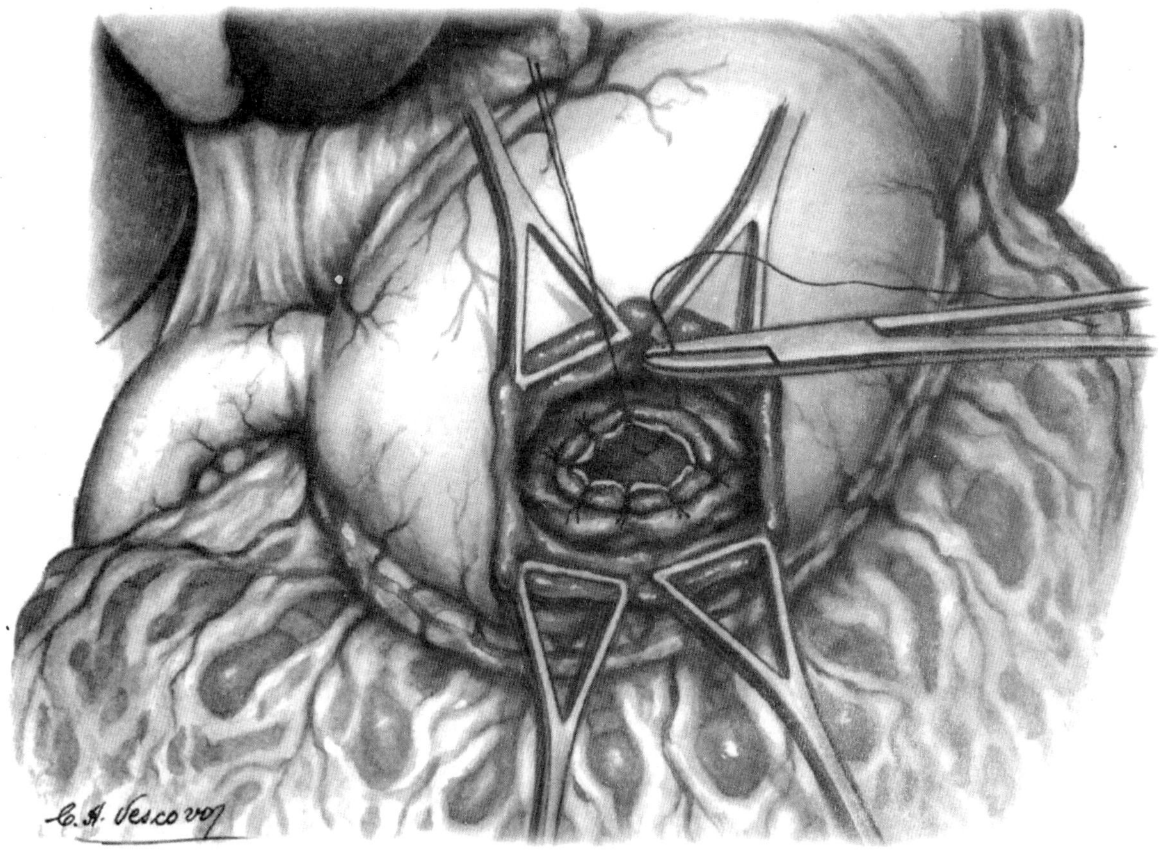

FIGURE 14.6

FIGURE 14.7

Once hemostasis is obtained of the cystogastric anastomosis, the anterior wall of the stomach is closed in two layers, an inner mucosal layer with 2-0 chromic catgut and an external layer with cotton. If radiographic control with the ingestion of a radioopaque substance three to four weeks postoperatively is performed, one can observe that the pseudocyst is generally completely obliterated. Ultrasonographic examination will also show in the same period of time complete disappearance of the pseudocyst. If gastroscopic serial studies are performed, it can be shown that about 4 to 6 weeks postoperatively no trace of the cystogastrostomy can be seen.

Regurgitation of gastric contents into the pseudocyst occurs in all the cases, a fact that does not prevent disappearance of the pseudocyst. The low pH of gastric contents inhibits enzymatic activity of the pancreatic fluid.

Surgical Procedures Used to Treat Pseudocysts of the Pancreas

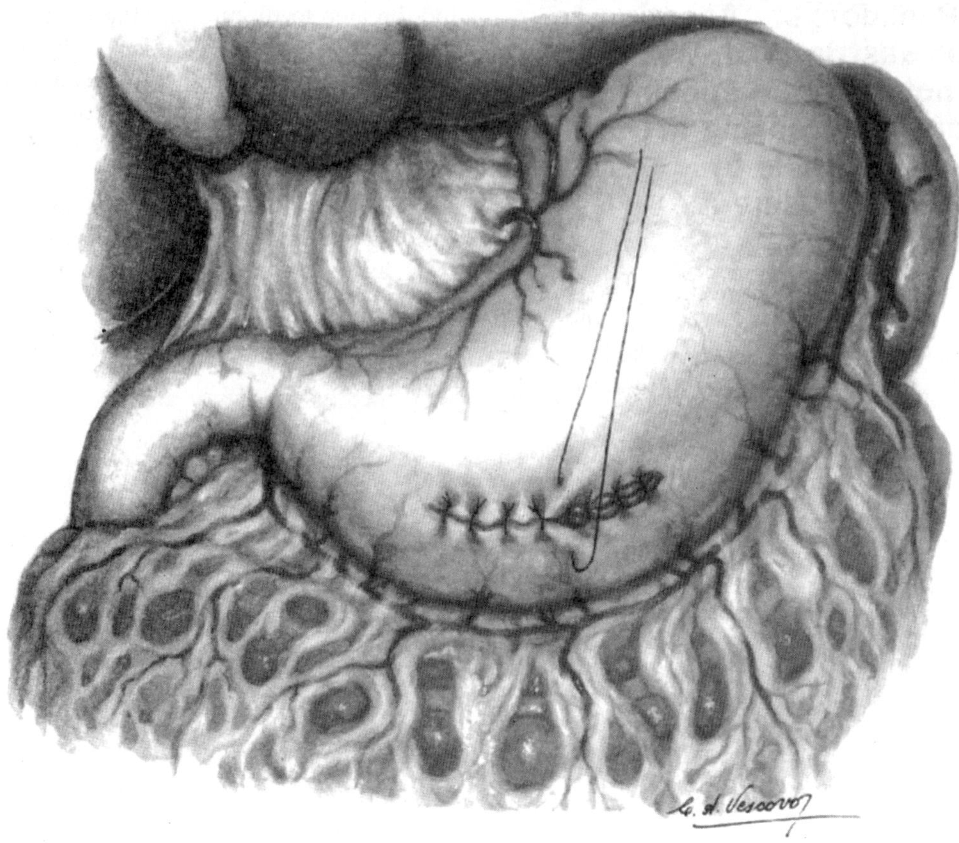

FIGURE 14.7

Pancreatic Pseudocysts Adhering to the Posterior Gastric Wall, Whose Walls Have not Matured Enough but are Dangerously Increasing in Size. Drainage to the Outside by Transgastric Route Using a Foley Catheter.

We have observed patients with pseudocysts of the pancreas of 3 to 4 weeks evolution that rapidly and dangerously increase in size and whose walls have not matured enough to permit suturing to the gastric wall and threaten to rupture into the peritoneal cavity or into abdominal viscera. When it is possible to confirm, during the surgical procedure, that the pseudocyst was adherent to the posterior wall of the stomach, although not densely, we proceeded to divert the contents of the pseudocyst to the outside through the stomach as we will describe, with the object of preventing its rupture and avoiding external drainage and its serious problems.

If, during the surgical intervention, one cannot establish that the pseudocyst is adherent to the posterior gastric wall, the procedure we are going to describe should not be performed, and drainage to the outside should be performed as previously described.

Surgical Procedures Used to Treat Pseudocysts of the Pancreas

Surgical Procedures Used to Treat Pseudocysts of the Pancreas

FIGURE 14.8

Pseudocysts of the pancreas of 3 weeks' evolution that in the last 24 hours have increased dangerously in size. The pseudocyst located in the lesser sac displaces the stomach forward. It is presumed that the cyst walls are not mature enough. The patient is operated on because of the danger of rupture of the pseudocyst. In the drawing one can observe the large volume of the pseudocyst and the anterior displacement of the stomach. The line indicates the site of the incision in the anterior wall of the stomach.

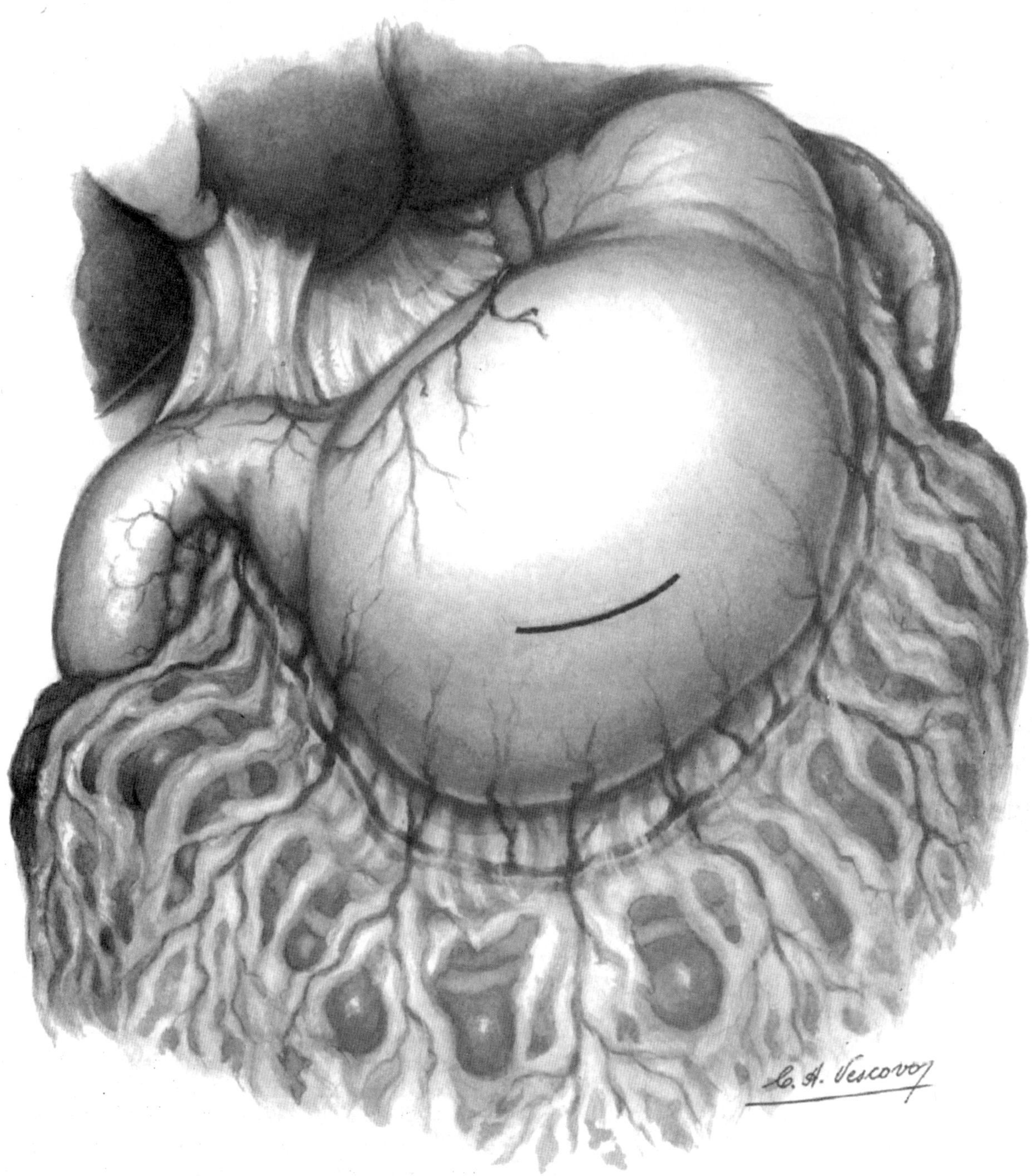

FIGURE 14.8

Surgical Procedures Used to Treat Pseudocysts of the Pancreas

FIGURE 14.9
The anterior gastric wall has been incised for a length of about 4 to 5 cm, and its borders are held with Duval clamps, which, at the same time, control hemorrhage temporarily. The pseudocyst is punctured through the posterior gastric wall, removing fluid that will be submitted with bacteriologic, enzymatic, and cytologic studies. The color of the removed fluid proves that it is not fresh blood, thereby excluding intracystic bleeding as a cause of the sudden increase in size.

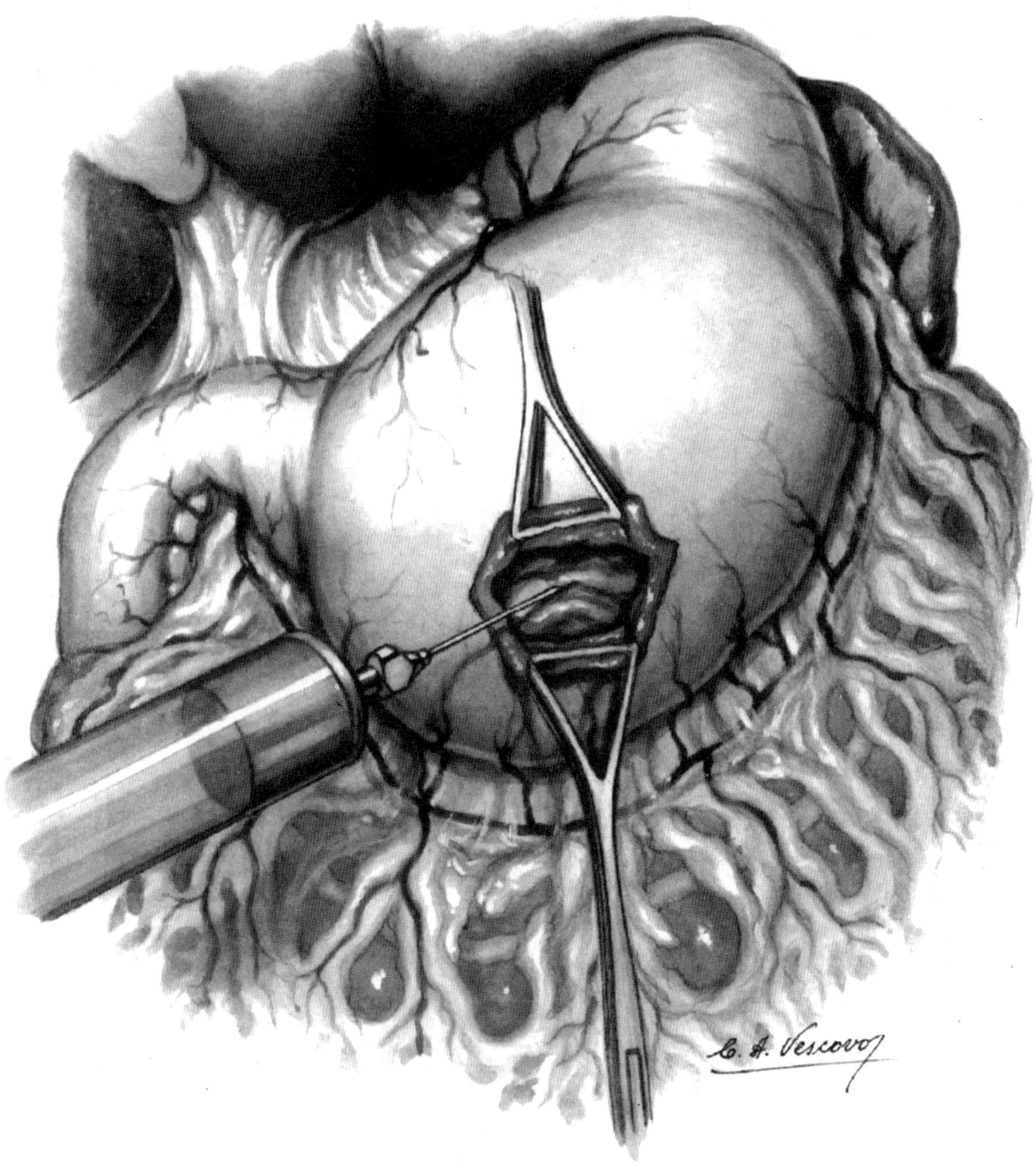

FIGURE 14.9

Surgical Procedures Used to Treat Pseudocysts of the Pancreas

FIGURE 14.10

At the same site as the needle puncture, using a cataract knife, an incision is made to allow for the introduction of a No. 16 Foley with a 5 mL bag, which, once introduced into the cyst, is gently pulled toward the entry wall of the cyst, as shown in the lower diagram. The catheter is then fixed with two sutures of 4-0 polyglactin to the wall of the stomach, as shown in the insert.

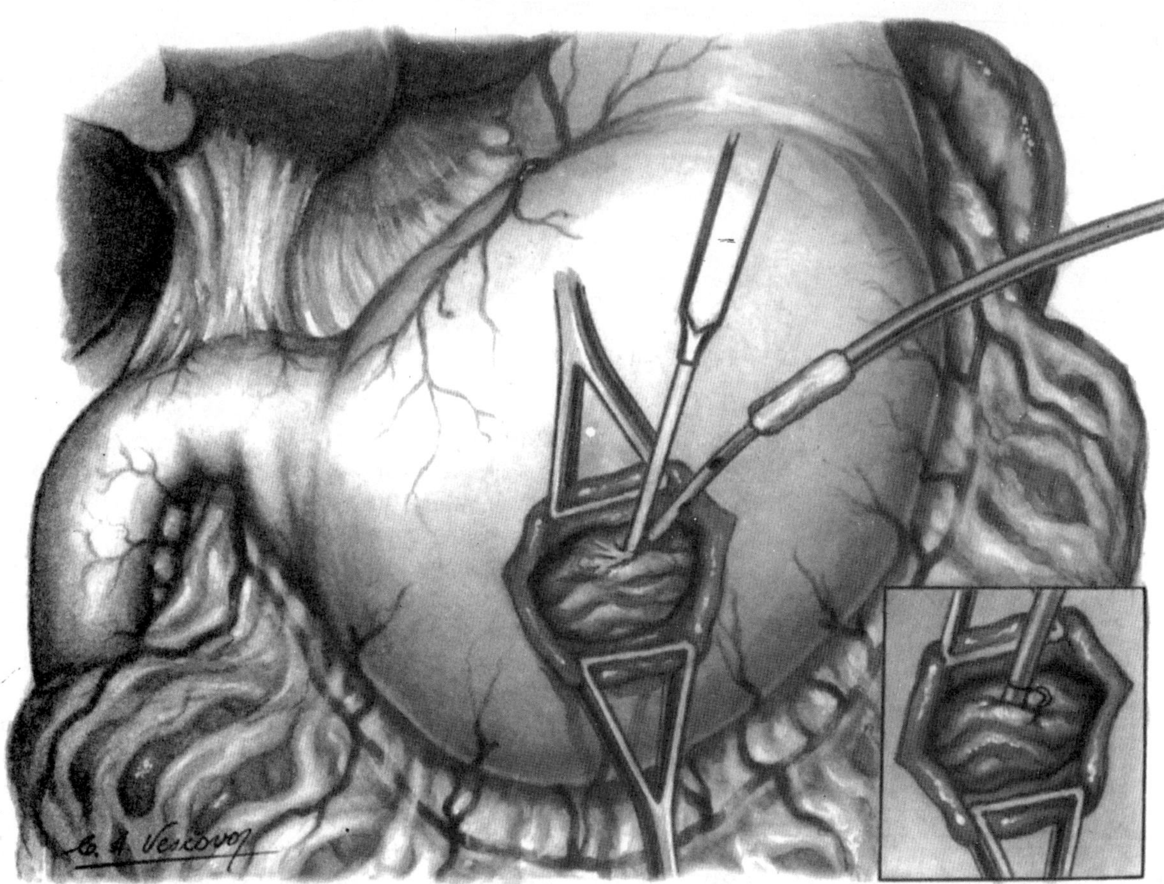

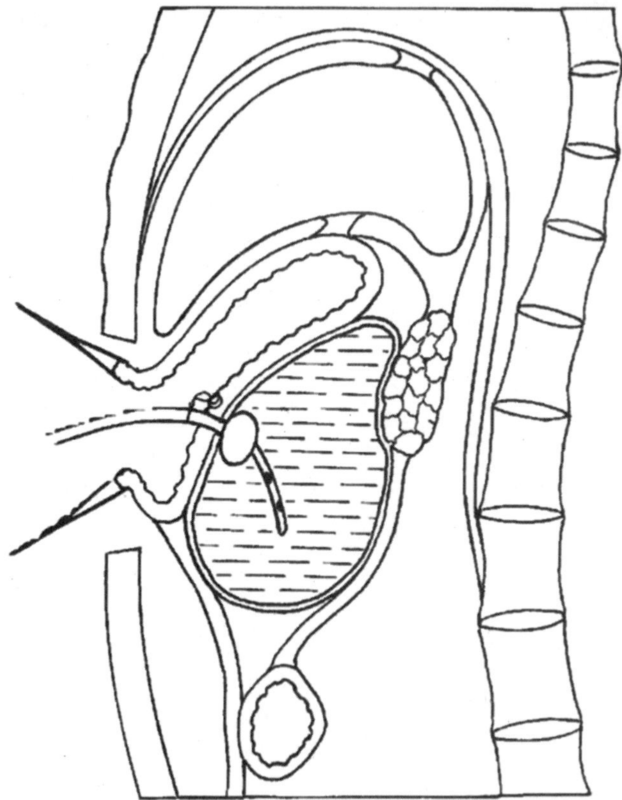

FIGURE 14.10

FIGURE 14.11
The Foley catheter is passed through the anterior wall of the stomach, where it is fixed with a 4-0 polyglactin suture. The incision of the anterior wall of the stomach is closed in two planes. Before closing the abdominal wall, the Foley catheter is brought out of the abdomen through a small incision and the neighboring gastric wall is sutured to the parietal peritoneum with several interrupted sutures around the Foley catheter. The pseudocyst should be studied postoperatively by ultrasonography. If the pseudocyst continues to increase in size, fluid is allowed to come out through the tube in adequate amounts. If the pseudocyst does not increase in size, drainage of its contents is performed intermittently and in small amounts by closing the Foley catheter on and off. The object of this is to avoid sudden emptying of the cyst when its walls are still not mature and solidly adherent to the gastric wall, which may lead to separation of the pseudocyst from the gastric wall. About a week or two after the operation, the Foley catheter is left permanently open until the pseudocyst disappears on ultrasonographic examination, which is usually between 2 and 4 weeks following the surgical procedure.

In patients who are in very poor general condition in whom a surgical intervention may be too risky, one can try to perform a cystogastrostomy endoscopically if one can establish that the pseudocyst wall is adherent to the stomach.

Surgical Procedures Used to Treat Pseudocysts of the Pancreas

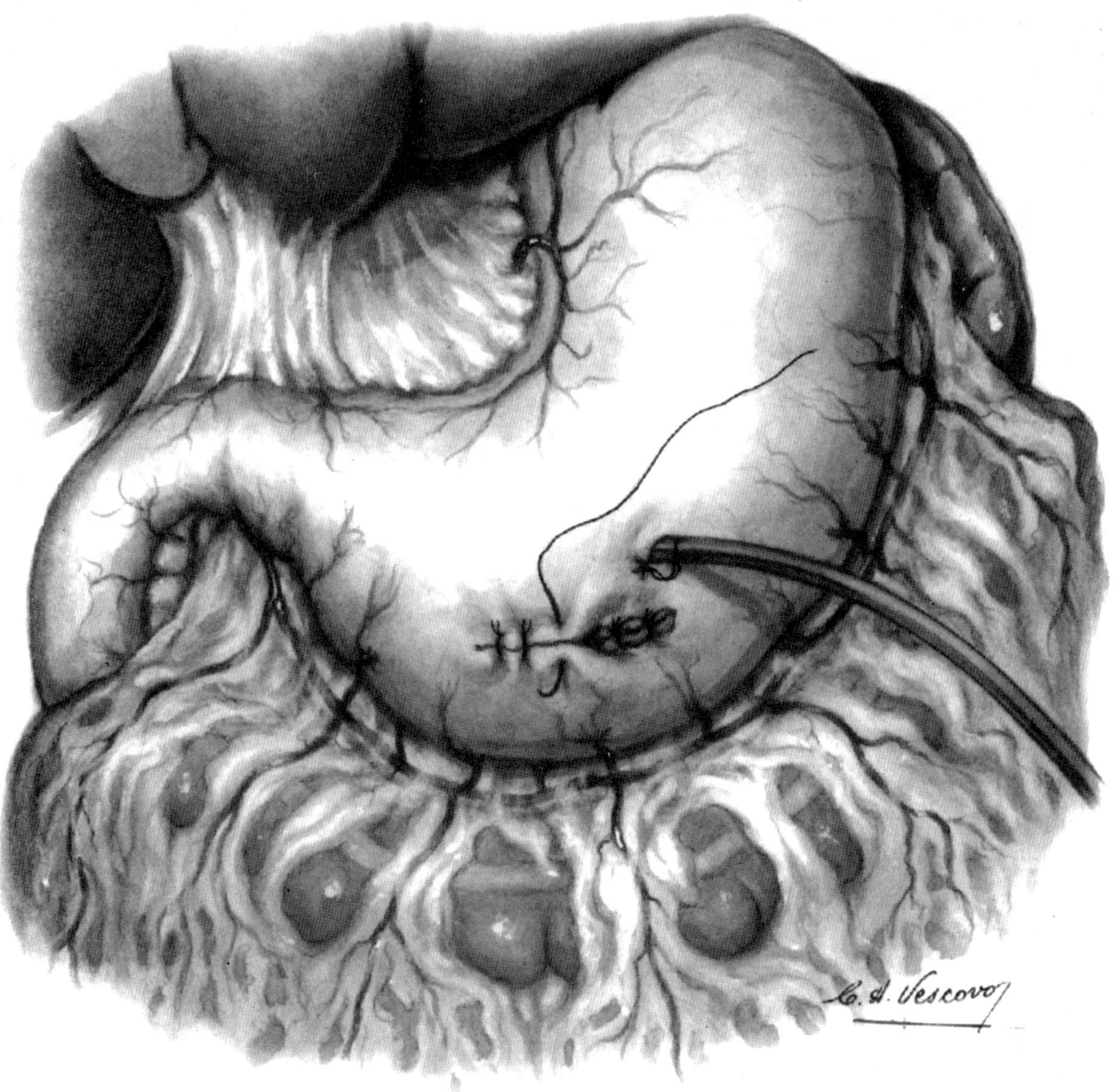

FIGURE 14.11

Cystoduodenostomy—Kerschner (1929)

Cystoduodenostomy may be indicated in pseudocysts of the head of the pancreas that are firmly adherent to the internal wall of the duodenum in its second or third portion.

Surgical Procedures Used to Treat Pseudocysts of the Pancreas

Surgical Procedures Used to Treat Pseudocysts of the Pancreas

FIGURE 14.12

Pseudocyst of the head of the pancreas firmly adherent to the second portion of the duodenum, with mature walls proper for the performance of a cystoduodenal anastomosis. A Vautrin-Kocher maneuver has been performed, and a line showing the extent of the incision of the second portion of the duodenum can be seen in the diagram. The extension of the duodenal incision may vary in accordance to the localization of the pseudocyst, and for this reason, it is advisable to perform a longitudinal incision of the duodenum, which can be extended if necessary.

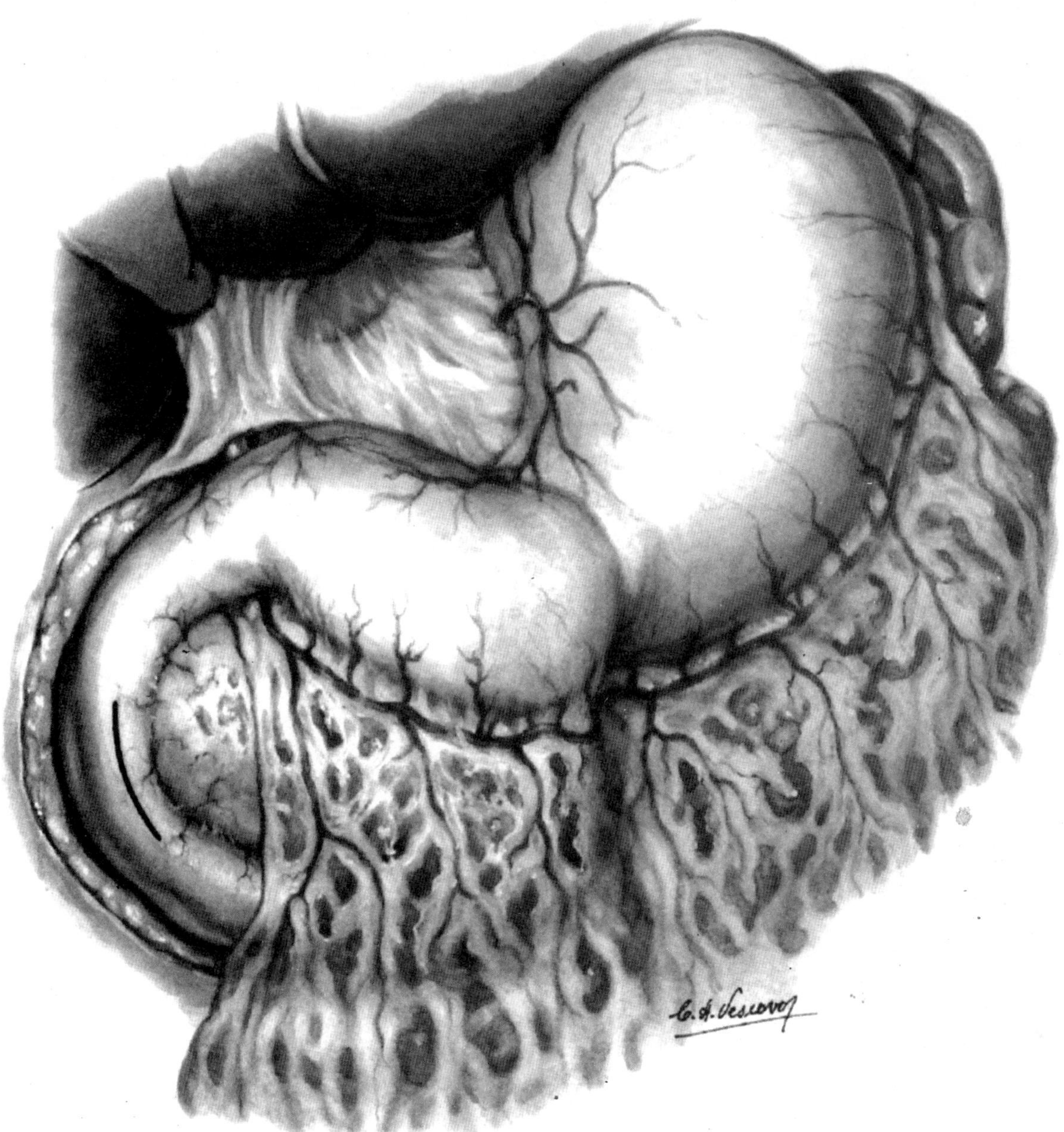

FIGURE 14.12

FIGURE 14.13
The anterior wall of the duodenum has been incised and its edges held by Duval clamps to apply traction and provide temporary hemostasis. Once the duodenum is open, the exact location of the papilla and its relation to the pseudocyst has to be investigated. The same investigation must be made of its relation with the biliary tract. If there is any doubt about these relations, it will be necessary to catheterize the common bile duct before incising the internal duodenal wall. In this patient, the pseudocyst is most prominent distal to the papilla. With a syringe and No. 16 needle, the interior duodenal wall is punctured, and the pseudocyst entered, aspirating several cubic centimeters of fluid for bacteriologic, enzymatic, and cytologic study.

Surgical Procedures Used to Treat Pseudocysts of the Pancreas

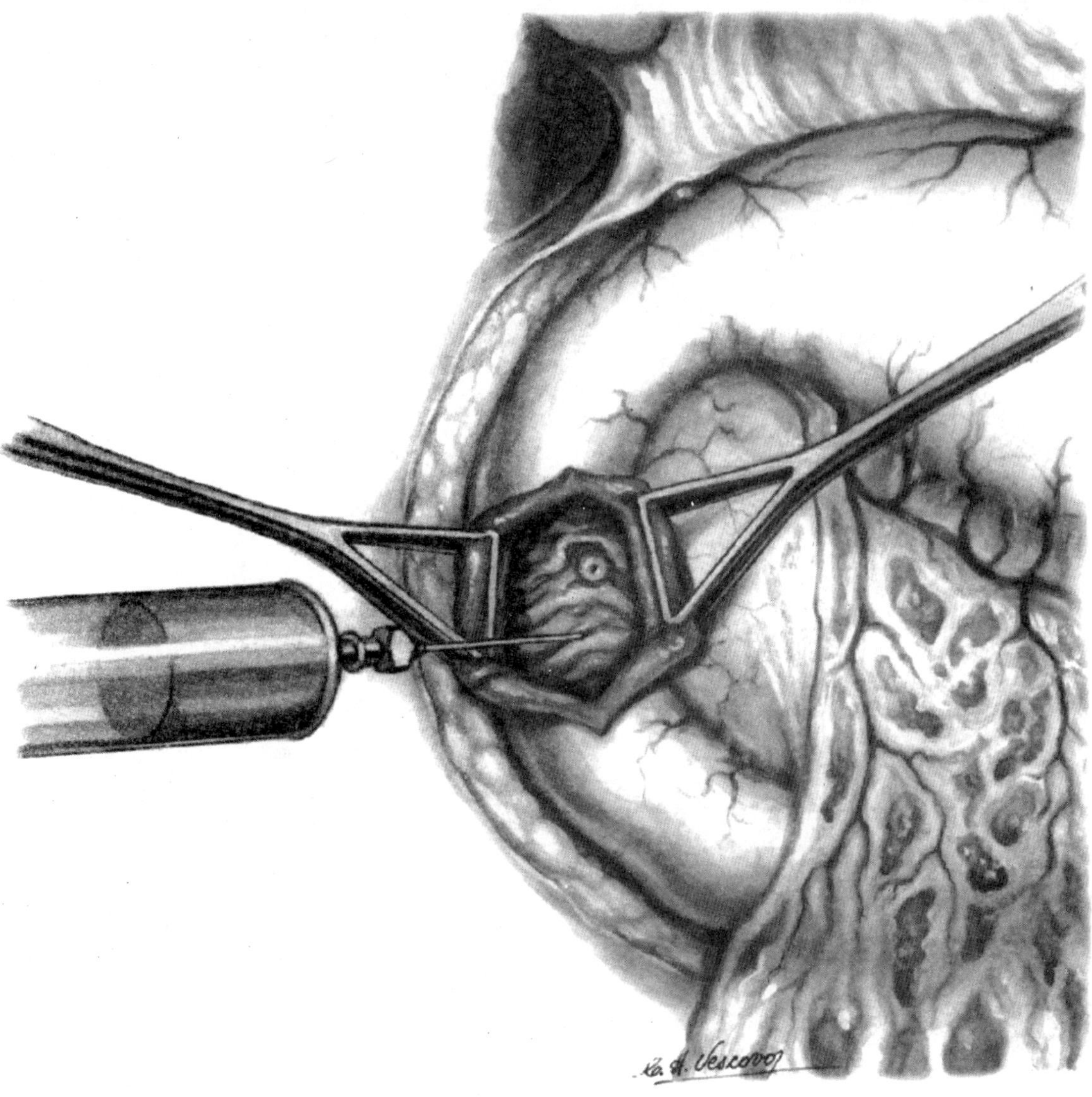

FIGURE 14.13

Surgical Procedures Used to Treat Pseudocysts of the Pancreas

FIGURE 14.14
At the site of the puncture, a cataract knife is introduced and its contents are aspirated, as shown in the drawing.

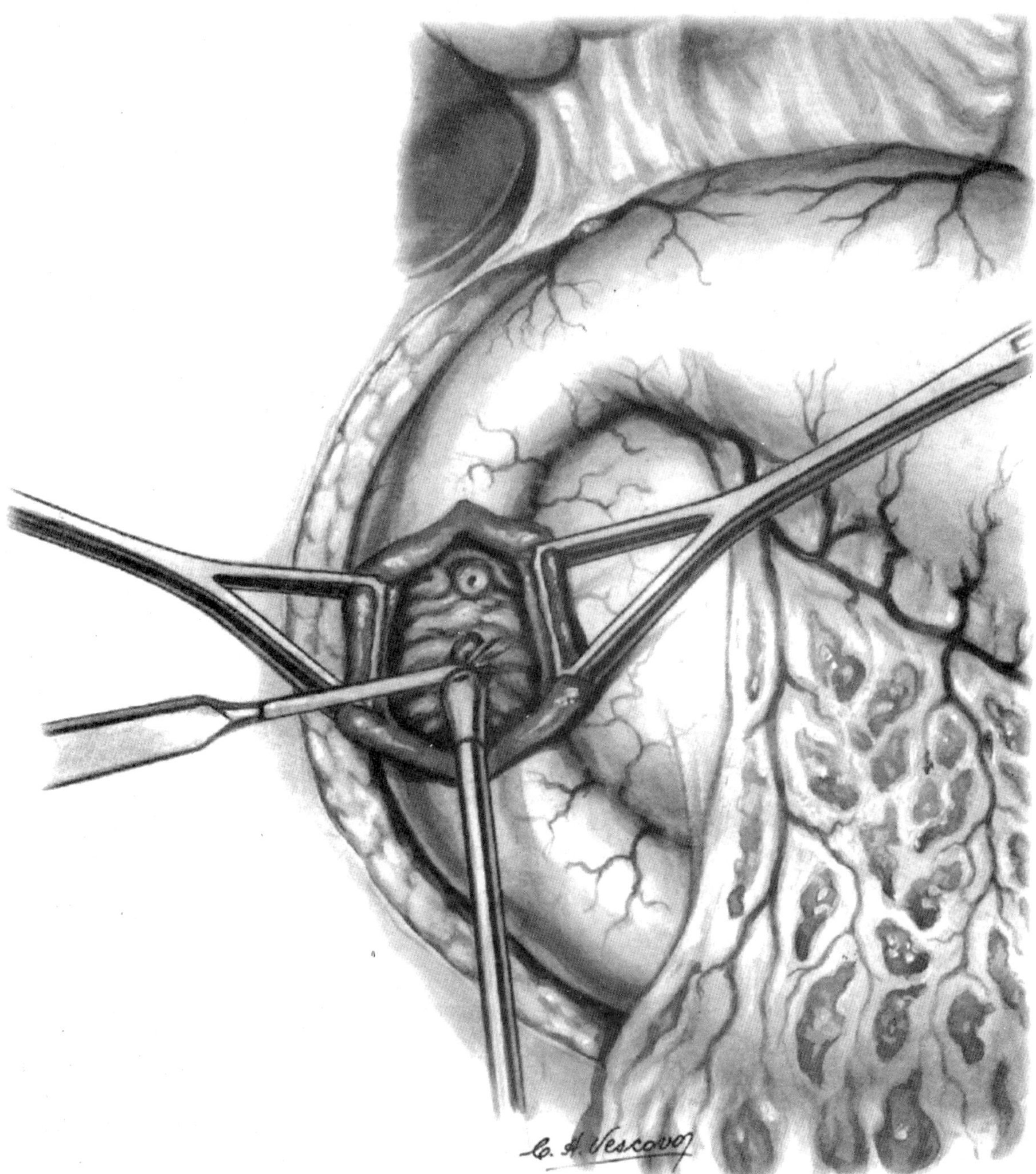

FIGURE 14.14

Surgical Procedures Used to Treat Pseudocysts of the Pancreas

FIGURE 14.15

The small incision performed with the cataract knife is widened with a hemostatic clamp, which is introduced with its jaws closed and then opened to widen the communication between the pseudocyst and the duodenum. This communication should measure 1 to 2 cm in diameter. All the contents of the pseudocyst are then aspirated.

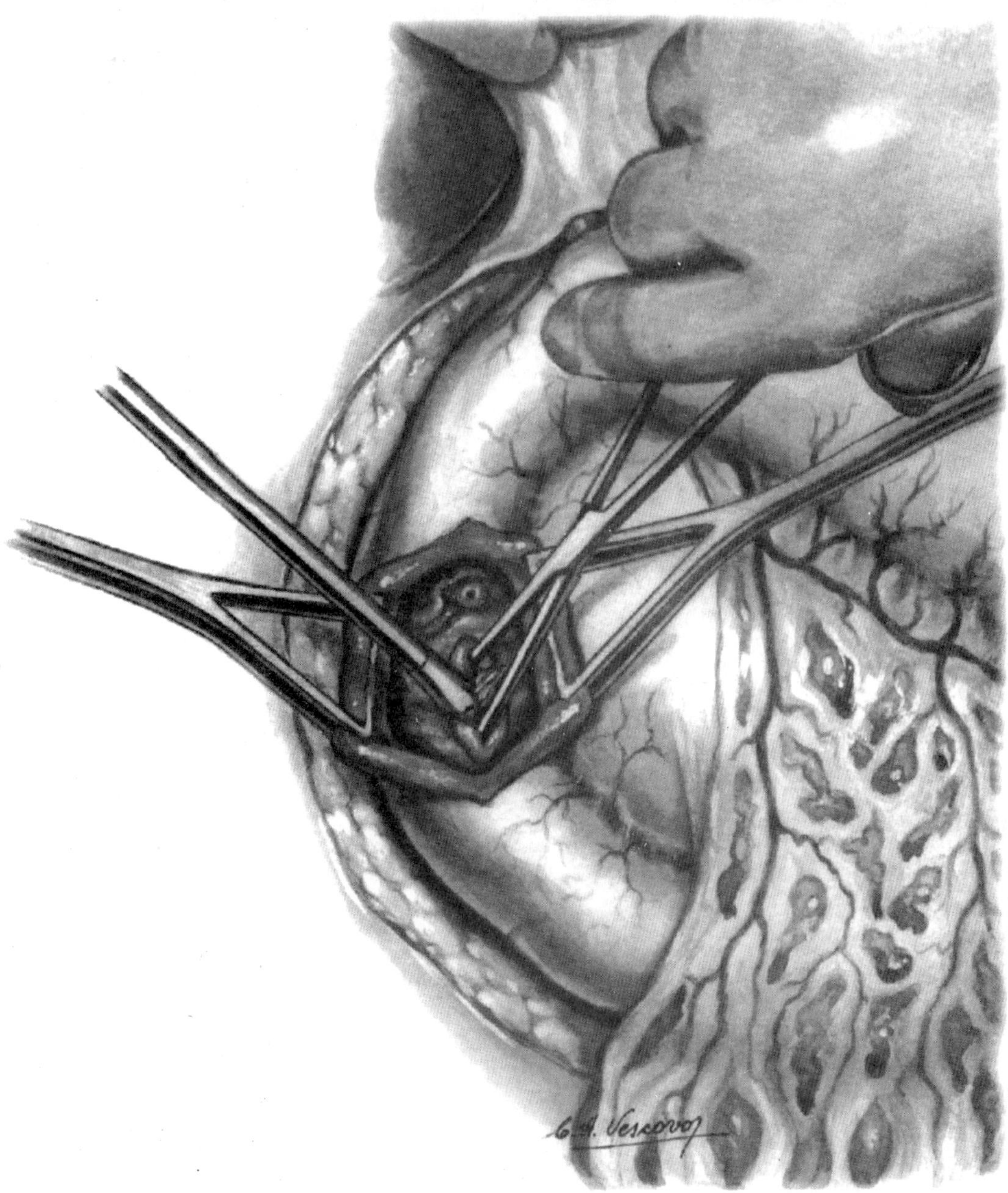

FIGURE 14.15

Surgical Procedures Used to Treat Pseudocysts of the Pancreas

FIGURE 14.16

The anterior duodenal wall and the wall of the pseudocyst are sutured with interrupted, nonabsorbable material. Hemostasis of the edges should be carefully obtained to avoid postoperative hemorrhage. The gastric wall and the duodenal wall are rich in blood supply, and this blood supply is usually increased by the proximity of the inflammatory process. Some surgeons do not suture the wall of the pseudocyst to the duodenum (4).

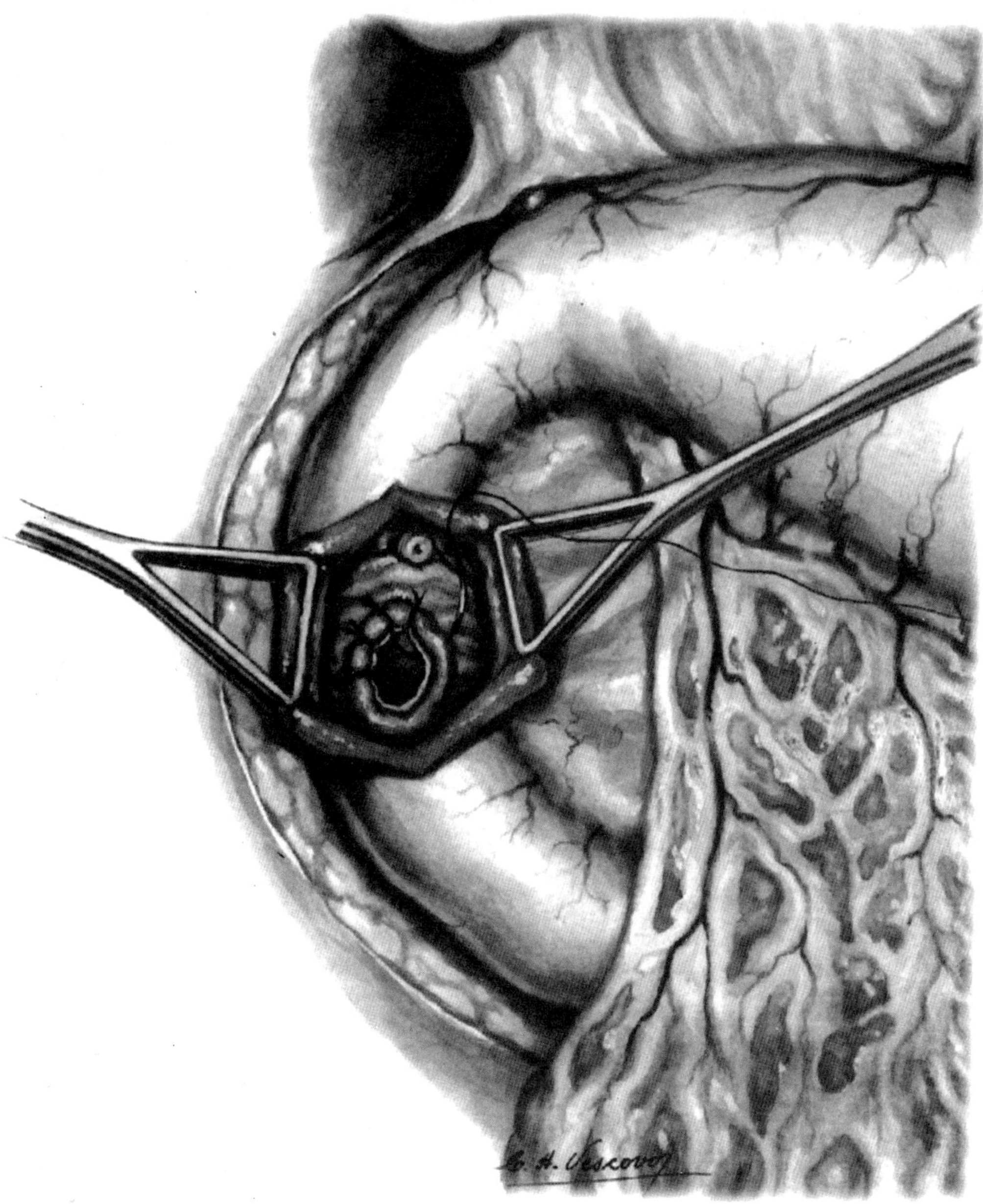

FIGURE 14.16

Surgical Procedures Used to Treat Pseudocysts of the Pancreas

FIGURE 14.17

The anterior duodenal wall is closed in two layers, using interrupted sutures. The inner layer is closed with 3-0 chromic catgut, the outer layer with silk or cotton. For greater security the greater omentum may be included in the suture fixed to the duodenum, as shown in the diagram on the right.

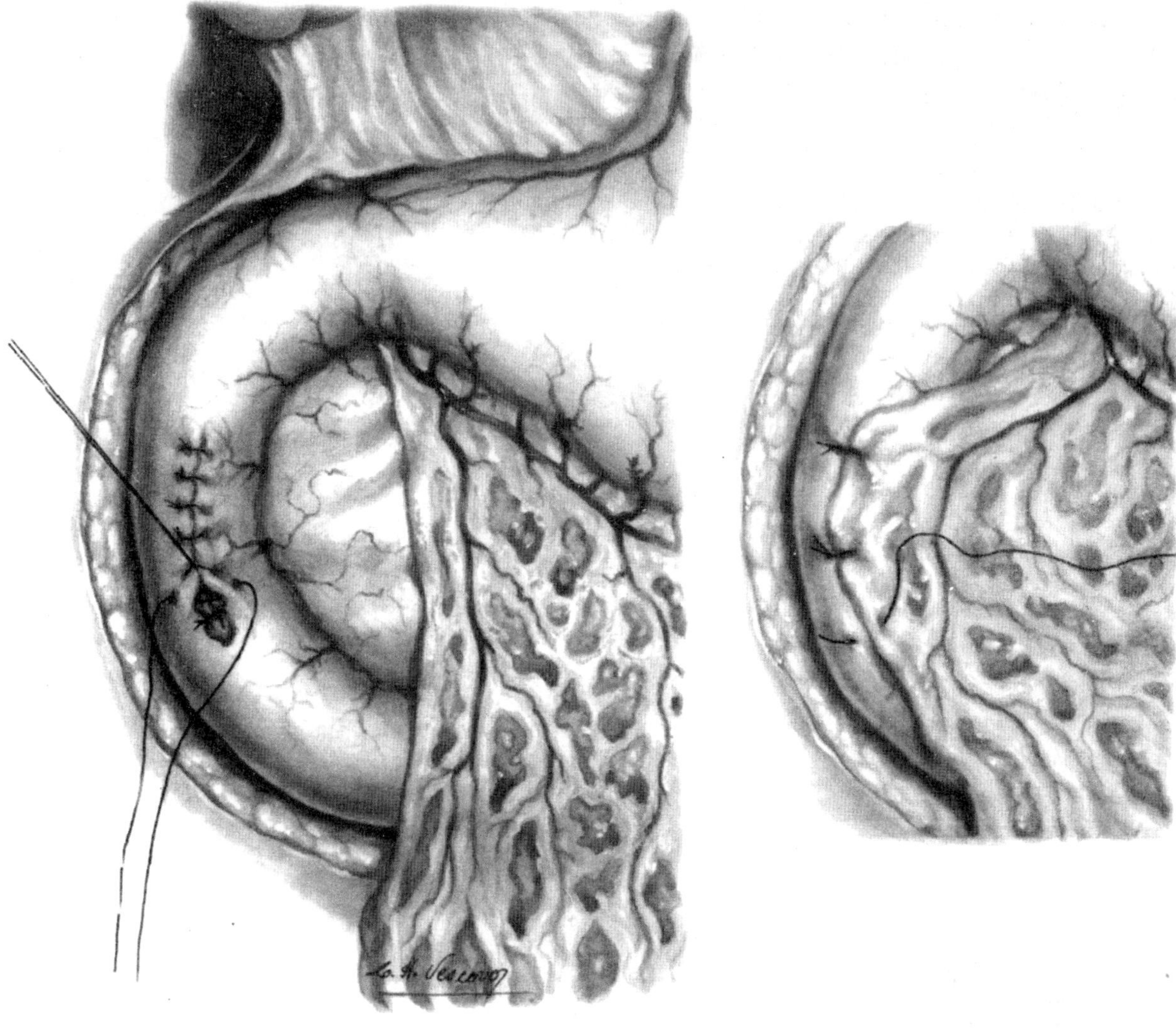

FIGURE 14.17

Cystojejunostomy (Simple Loop, Henle and Hahn 1927; Roux-en-Y, König 1946)

If the pseudocyst is not adherent to the stomach or the duodenum, but its walls are mature and capable of holding sutures safely, the cyst can be anastomosed to a jejunal limb disposed in Roux-en-Y fashion (1, 4, 13). Once the abdomen is open, the condition of the cyst wall has to be confirmed. The pseudocyst is then punctured with syringe and needle, removing fluid for bacteriologic, enzymatic, and cytologic study. The puncture should be performed in the most dependent portion of the anterior wall of the pseudocyst. A trocar is then introduced at the same site and the entire contents of the pseudocyst removed. A horizontal incision is made in the pseudocyst as extensive as possible on its anterior lower wall. A lozenge of the wall of the pseudocyst is removed for histologic study by frozen section. Since an ample incision has been made in the pseudocyst, it is possible to examine the interior of the cyst by direct vision before anastomosing it to the jejunum.

Surgical Procedures Used to Treat Pseudocysts of the Pancreas

FIGURE 14.18

The distal limb of the Roux-en-Y anastomosis is brought up in front of the transverse colon to be anastomosed to the pseudocyst in side to side fashion, with one layer of nonabsorbable material. Some surgeons, however, perform this anastomosis in two layers. The end of the anastomotic loop has been previously closed in two layers. Some 50 to 60 cm from the cystojejunal anastomosis, the jejunojejunal anastomosis is performed. If a dehiscence of the cystojejunal suture line occurs, it is less serious than a dehiscence of a cystogastrostomy or a cystoduodenostomy because the jejunal loop has been defunctionalized. In the late postoperative period of the cystojejunal anastomosis in Roux-en-Y fashion, complications may occur that should be known. The pseudocyst disappears 2 to 3 weeks postoperatively, and the jejunal anastomotic loop, once it ceases to function, atrophies, remaining in place as a dangling loop. In some cases, the jejunal loop separates from its original suture to the pseudocyst and becomes adherent to some abdominal viscera or to the abdominal wall, possibly leading to bowel obstruction caused by the traction of the atrophic loop on the jejunojejunal anastomosis (1, 4).

Some pseudocysts with their mature walls that are very adherent to the posterior gastric wall, but owing to their size extend well below the greater curvature of the stomach, should be sutured to the jejunum rather than to the stomach because if they are sutured to the stomach, they leave a deep, hanging sack, making healing of the cyst difficult.

Surgical Procedures Used to Treat Pseudocysts of the Pancreas

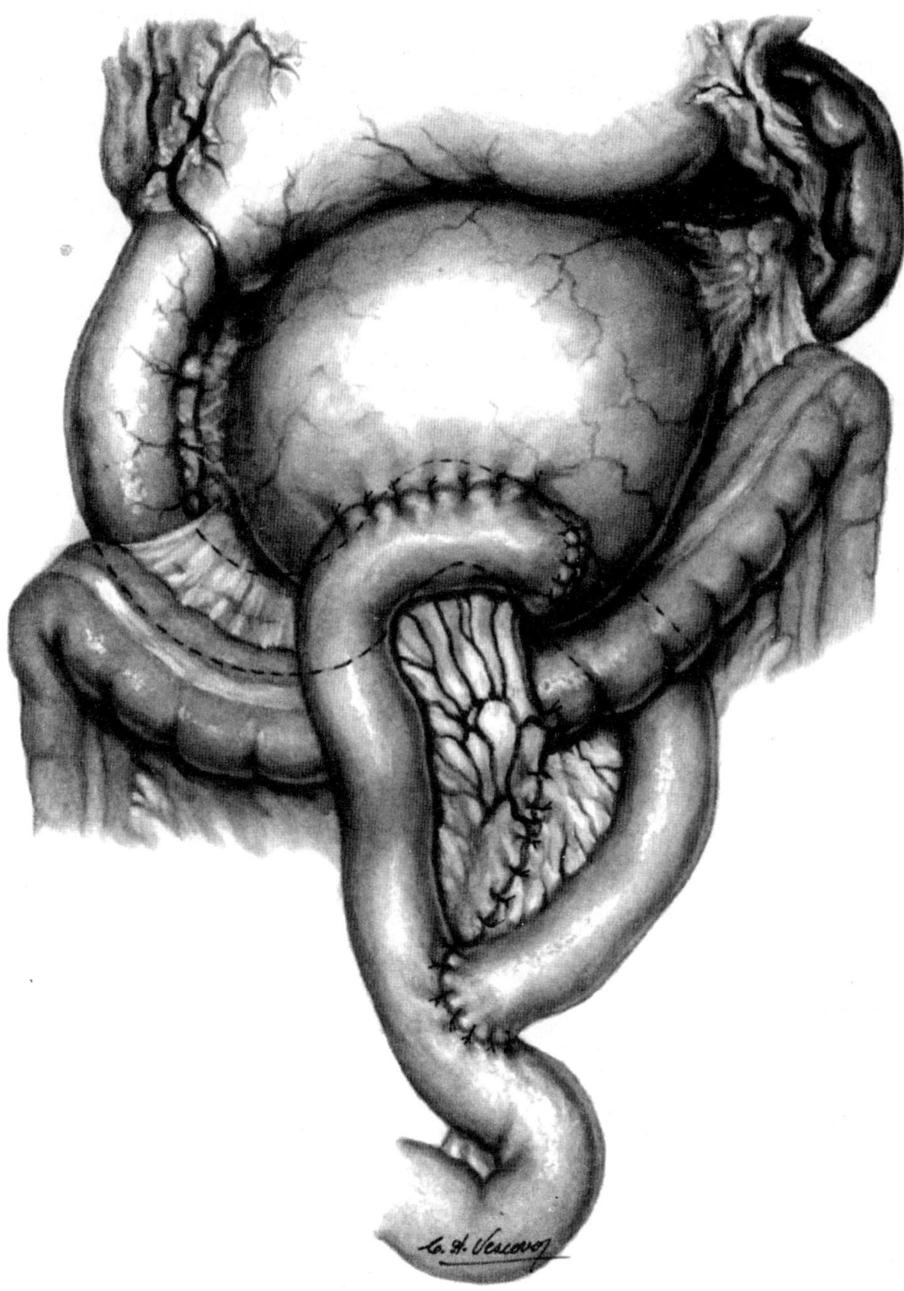

FIGURE 14.18

References

1. Anderson, M.C., Chapman, W.C. Pseudocysts of the pancreas. In Howard, J.M., Jordan, G.L. Jr., Reber, H.A. (Eds.), Surgical diseases of the pancreas. p. 564. Lea & Febiger, Philadelphia, 1987.
2. Becker, J.M. Pancreatic pseudocyst. Post-graduate course. Diseases of the liver, biliary tract and pancreas. p. 119. Clinical Congress, American College of Surgeons, Chicago, 1988.
3. Bradley, E.L., II, Clements J.L., Jr., González, A.C. The natural history of pancreatic pseudocysts: A unified concept of management. Am. J. Surg. 137:135, 1979.
4. Carey, L.C., Ellison, E.C. Pancreas. In Fromm D. (Ed.), Gastrointestinal surgery. Vol. 2, p. 871, Churchill Livingstone, New York, 1985.
5. Corbelle, J.L., Sugasti, J.A. Patología del páncreas exócrine y endócrino. In Michans, J.R. Patología quirúrgica. Ed. 4, p. 680. El Ateneo, Buenos Aires, 1987.
6. Frey, C.F. Pancreatic pseudocyst, operative strategy. Ann. Surg. 188:652, 1978.
7. Grace, R.R., Jordan, P.H., Jr. Unresolved problems of pancreatic pseudocyst. Ann. Surg. 184:16, 1976.
8. Gussenbauer, C. On the operative treatment of pancreatic cysts. Langenbeck's Archiv. 29:355, 1883.
9. Jurasz, A. Zur Frage der operativen behandlung der pankreascysten. Arch. Klin. Chir. 164:272, 1931.
10. Karlson, K.B., Martin, E.C., Fankuchen, E.I., et al. Percutaneous drainage of pancreatic pseudocysts and abscesses. Radiology 142:619, 1982.
11. Kerschner, F. Transduodenale anastomosierung einer pankreascyste mit dem duodenum. Beitr. Klin. Chir. 147:28, 1929.
12. Kohler, H. et al. Surgical treatment of pancreatic pseudocyst. Br. J. Surg. 74:813, 1987.
13. Madden, J.L. Atlas of technics in surgery. Ed. 2, Vol. 1, p. 522, Appleton-Century-Crofts, New York, 1964
14. Martin, E.W., Jr., Catalano, P., Cooperman, M., et al. Surgical decision making in the treatment of pancreatic pseudocysts. Am. J. Surg. 138:821, 1979.
15. O`Connor, M., et al. Preoperative endoscopic retrograde cholangiopancreatography in the surgical management of pancreatic pseudocysts. Am. J. Surg. 151:18, 1986.
16. Scott-Connor, C.E.H., Coil, J.A. The fiberoptic choledochoscope in the operative management of pancreatic pseudocysts. Surg. Gynecol. Obstet. 165:445, 1987.
17. Shatney, C.H., Lillehei, R.C. Surgical treatment of pancreatic pseudocysts. Analysis of 119 cases. Ann. Surg. 189:386, 1979.
18. Stroud, W.H., Cullom, J.W., Anderson, M.C. Hemorrhagic complication of severe pancreatitis. Surgery 90:657, 1981.
19. Torres, W.E., et al. Percutaneous aspiration and drainage of pancreatic pseudocysts. Am. J. Roentgenol. 147:1007, 1986.
20. Warshaw, A.L., Lee, K.H. Aging changes of pancreatic iso-amylases and the appearance of "old amylase" in the serum of patients with pancreatic pseudocysts. Gastroenterology 79:1246, 1980.

Section C

Surgery of the Pancreas

CHAPTER 15

Surgery for Chronic Pancreatitis

LONGITUDINAL PANCREATICOJEJUNAL ANASTOMOSIS (MODIFIED PUESTOW-GILLESBY OPERATION)

Several surgical procedures have been proposed for the treatment of severe chronic pancreatitis associated with persistent severe pain, but in actual practice, only two procedures are used frequently and have led to superior results. It should be recognized, however, that neither of the two are universally efficient. They are:

1. Longitudinal anastomosis of the pancreatic duct with a jejunal loop disposed in Roux-en-Y fashion (modified Puestow-Gillesby procedure).
2. Partial, subtotal, or total pancreatic resection.

Indication for one or the other procedure depends on the caliber of the pancreatic duct and the condition of the pancreatic parenchyma. Pancreaticojejunal anastomosis can only be used in cases in which the pancreatic duct is at least 8 mm in diameter. If the pancreatic duct is not dilated because the chronic pancreatitis is principally localized to the parenchyma and the small pancreatic ducts, the anastomotic procedure is not indicated and a resection should be performed.

It has been proven that surgery may be needed in chronic pancreatitis of alcoholic origin, whereas in chronic pancreatitis of biliary origin, improvement is generally obtained with removal of the gallbladder, removal of calculi from the bile ducts where they may be present, or anastomosis of the biliary tract to the intestinal tract if compression of the common bile duct were present due to a thickened pancreas or peripancreatic fibrosis. In the latter cases the bile duct is usually dilated.

It should be pointed out that the only object of surgical treatment for chronic pancreatitis of alcoholic origin is to relieve the intense abdominal or back pain which these patients usually have owing to their illness. The anatomic changes and the functional changes of the pancreas, both exocrine and endocrine, will not improve.

Deterioration of the pancreas will continue and be progressive due to the invasion of the pancreatic tissue by fibrosis (13, 14, 16, 18, 23). This invasion will make pancreatic insufficiency worse and the insufficiency will inexorably continue to get worse during the passage of time. Pancreaticojejunal anastomosis is a simple procedure, leading to minimum mortality and morbidity (13, 14, 17, 18, 22, 24, 25, 29). Pancreatic resections, on the other hand, are procedures that carry a greater risk of mortality and morbidity and compromise pancreatic function more.

The pancreatic resection that is more frequently performed is pancreatoduodenectomy (Whipple Procedure) (13–15, 17, 18, 22, 23). Resection of the distal 80 to 95% of the pancreas (9, 10) or total pancreatectomy (1, 11, 15) have very limited indications.

Resection of more than 70% of a normal pancreas leads to both exocrine and endocrine pancreatic insufficiency in normal pancreas. If the pancreas is anatomically and functionally deteriorated because of chronic alcoholic pancreatitis, postoperative insufficiency will be markedly worse. Therefore, when pancreatic resection is indicated for further treatment of pain associated with chronic alcoholic pancreatitis, the surgeon should consider resecting 80 to 95% or a complete resection of the pancreas. These operations produce a diabetes that is very difficult to control, especially in alcoholic and drug-dependent patients. Resection of the tail and part of the body of the pancreas has not been efficacious in relieving pain in chronic alcoholic pancreatitis patients (15, 16, 22).

Pancreatoduodenectomy in cases of chronic pancreatitis is safer to perform than in the case of tumors because the fibrosis of the pancreas makes it considerably easier to carry out a good suture anastomosis. On the other hand, morbidity and mortality are definitely lower. The only difficulty that the surgeon may encounter in freeing up the neck of the pancreas is the portomesenteric venous axis and the liberation of the uncinate process because of peripancreatic fibrosis. Pancreatoduodenectomy can be carried out as in the classical Whipple procedure with resection of the distal half of the stomach or, preferably, using the pylorus preserving technique of Traverso and Longmire. This technique can also be used in cases in which a total pancreatectomy is performed (11, 28, 30).

Laterolateral pancreaticojejunal anastomosis and pancreatic resections do not bring relief of pain in all cases. About 60 to 70% of patients improve with some of these procedures. In the rest, the pain continues in spite of the surgical intervention. There is no satisfactory explanation of why this happens. Pancreaticojejunal anastomosis may fail even though the pancreatic duct is well dilated and anastomosis perfectly permeable. If after failure of the pancreaticojejunal anastomosis a pancreatic resection is performed, it too may fail (13, 14, 16–18, 23).

PREOPERATIVE STUDY OF PATENTS

Before advising the performance of surgery to treat patients with chronic pancreatitis, a complete study of the patient should be performed to make an exact diagnosis and be oriented about the surgical procedure to be carried out. It is extremely important to determine the diameter of the pancreatic duct, the predominant location of the inflammatory process, its stage of evolution, and the functional status of the pancreatic parenchyma. The existence of diabetes or exocrine insufficiency and with the presence of pancreatic calcifications and calculi in the pancreatic duct or in the secondary duct will be determined prior to the operation. The condition of the gallbladder and the biliary ducts or the probable presence of calculi and/or dilation of the common bile duct by compression of the thickened or fibrotic pancreatic head, as well as compression of the duodenum or the stomach, will also be determined (2, 3, 7, 8, 14, 20, 26). It is indispensable to verify if a pseudocyst of the pancreas is present. The nutritional state of the patient has to be evaluated and the existence of a pathology such as cirrhosis of the liver, which would contraindicate the operation has to be evaluated.

In order to carry out these studies, in addition to the clinical history and the laboratory examinations, it is necessary to perform an x-ray of the abdomen (calcifications and pancreatic calculi); a gastroduodenal x-ray to determine the presence of obstruction or compression of the stomach and duodenum; ultrasonography or computed tomography for a pancreatic mass, pseudocysts, and in some cases to determine the diameter of the pancreatic duct and the presence of biliary lithiasis or dilation of the biliary tree. The most important study to determine the diameter of the pancreatic duct is retrograde endoscopic cholangiopancreatography. If this examination cannot be carried out preoperatively, it should be performed during surgery by means of a puncture of the pancreatic duct (with ultrasonography). When the pancreatic duct is dilated, it frequently shows several areas of stenosis interspersed between areas of dilation. This gives it the "chain of lakes" configuration (21, 25, 26). In these cases a lateral anastomosis of the pancreatic duct to the jejunum is indicated, with the conviction that the pain is caused by an increase in pressure in the duct of Wirsung, although this has not been completely confirmed (28). This is the technique that we will describe here. The techniques of pancreatic resection are similar to those for resections for pancreatic tumors or periampullary tumors, for which reason they will not be described here.

Modified Puestow-Gillesby Procedure

FIGURE 15.1
Semischematic drawing with the object of showing the image of a Wirsungraphy with a dilated duct and interspersed zones of dilation (chain of lakes). Some calculi can be seen in the duct of Wirsung and in some of the secondary branches.

Modified Puestow-Gillesby Procedure

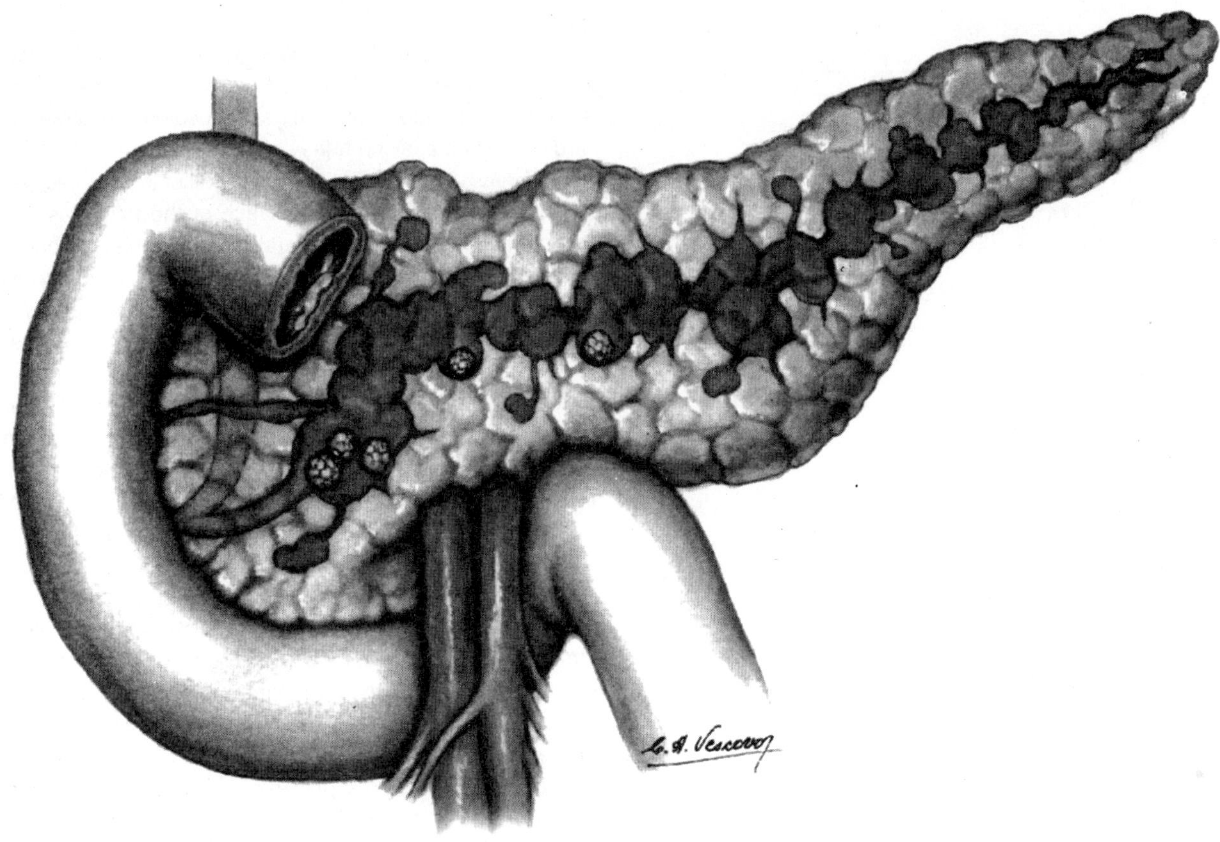

FIGURE 15.1

FIGURE 15.2

The greater omentum has been separated from the transverse colon and the stomach reflected upward by the second assistant. The transverse colon with its mesocolon is reflected downward by the first assistant, leaving the entire anterior surface of the pancreas exposed. The posterior wall of the stomach is usually adherent to the anterior surface of the pancreas by peripancreatic fibrosis, which generally accompanies chronic alcoholic pancreatitis. These adhesions should be carefully divided with scissors in the vicinity of the pancreatic surface. A thorough exploration is then carried out of the entire pancreas and an attempt is made to identify the pancreatic duct.

When the pancreatic duct is well dilated throughout its entire extension, it is usually visible and palpable and it is a simple task to puncture it with a syringe and a 22 F needle. About 2 mL of pancreatic fluid, which will be used for chemical, enzymatic, and bacteriologic studies and investigation for neoplastic cells, is removed. If an endoscopic retrograde cholangiopancreatography has not been performed, the needle puncture is used to inject 2 mL of radiopaque material to obtain an operative Wirsungraphy and confirm that the pancreatic duct is sufficiently dilated, showing the number and the extent of the narrow zones. In some cases it is difficult to identify the pancreatic duct even though cholangiopancreatography may have shown that it was dilated. This may be owing to the inflammatory process, edema, fibrosis of the pancreatic parenchyma that covers the duct, or the existence of rather extensive narrow segments in addition to the dilated zones. In these cases, it is sometimes necessary to carry out several punctures with needle and syringe to find the duct. If after several punctures the duct has not been localized, one can recur to the Greenlee maneuver (14), which consists in performing an oblique incision in the anterior surface of the pancreas near the juncture of the body and tail. This is where the duct is supposed to be found and the incision is carried out until the duct is found.

Modified Puestow-Gillesby Procedure

If operative ultrasonography is available, identification of the pancreatic duct is greatly simplified. If, before or during the operation the presence of biliary pathology such as gallstones, stones in the common bile duct, or dilation of the biliary tree caused by a pancreatic compression or peripancreatic fibrosis is found, it should be treated in the same operative procedure. Compression of the common bile duct with proximal dilation caused by chronic alcoholic pancreatitis occurs in 10 to 15% of cases. Preoperative cholangiography or operative cholangiography is of great importance in diagnosing chronic pancreatitis with obstruction of the bile ducts caused by predominance of the pancreatitis in the head of the pancreas. This produces a very characteristic image of a smooth or irregular elongated stenosis of the transpancreatic biliary duct. In case of compression of the duct owing to pancreatitis, there is generally passage of the radiopaque material into the duodenum. Passage is rarely present in obstruction of the common bile duct caused by carcinoma of the head of the pancreas. In these cases, the obstruction is easily complete and occurs in a portion of the duct proximal to the papilla. If, during preoperative or operative exploration, the presence of a pseudocyst is demonstrated, it should be also treated in the same operative procedure.

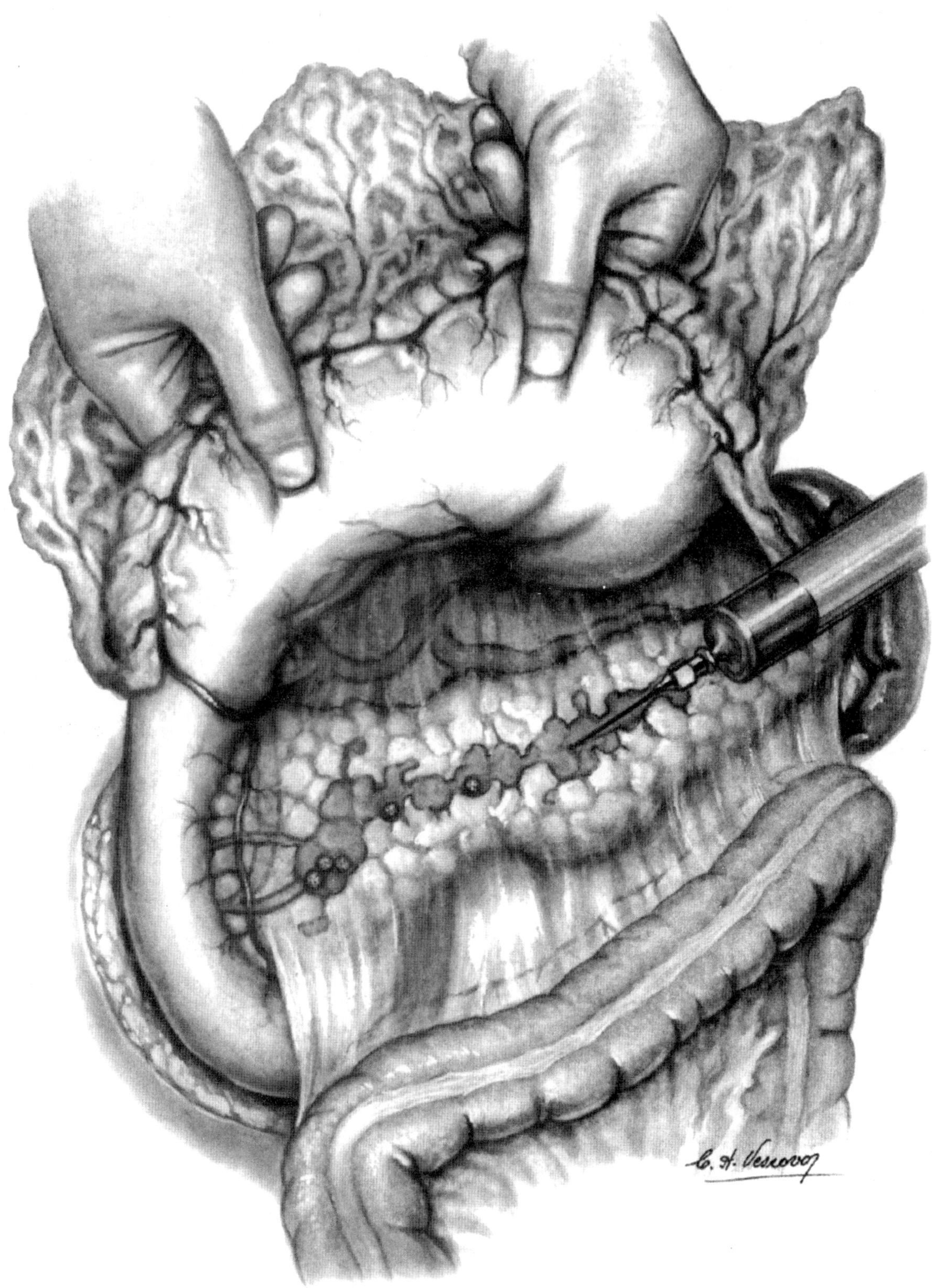

FIGURE 15.2

FIGURE 15.3

If the dilated pancreatic duct has been identified, a small incision is made at the site of the puncture. One of the branches of the Potts scissors is then introduced with the purpose of incising the pancreatic duct longitudinally together with the layer of pancreatic tissue that covers it. This incision should extend to the entire length of the duct.

Modified Puestow-Gillesby Procedure

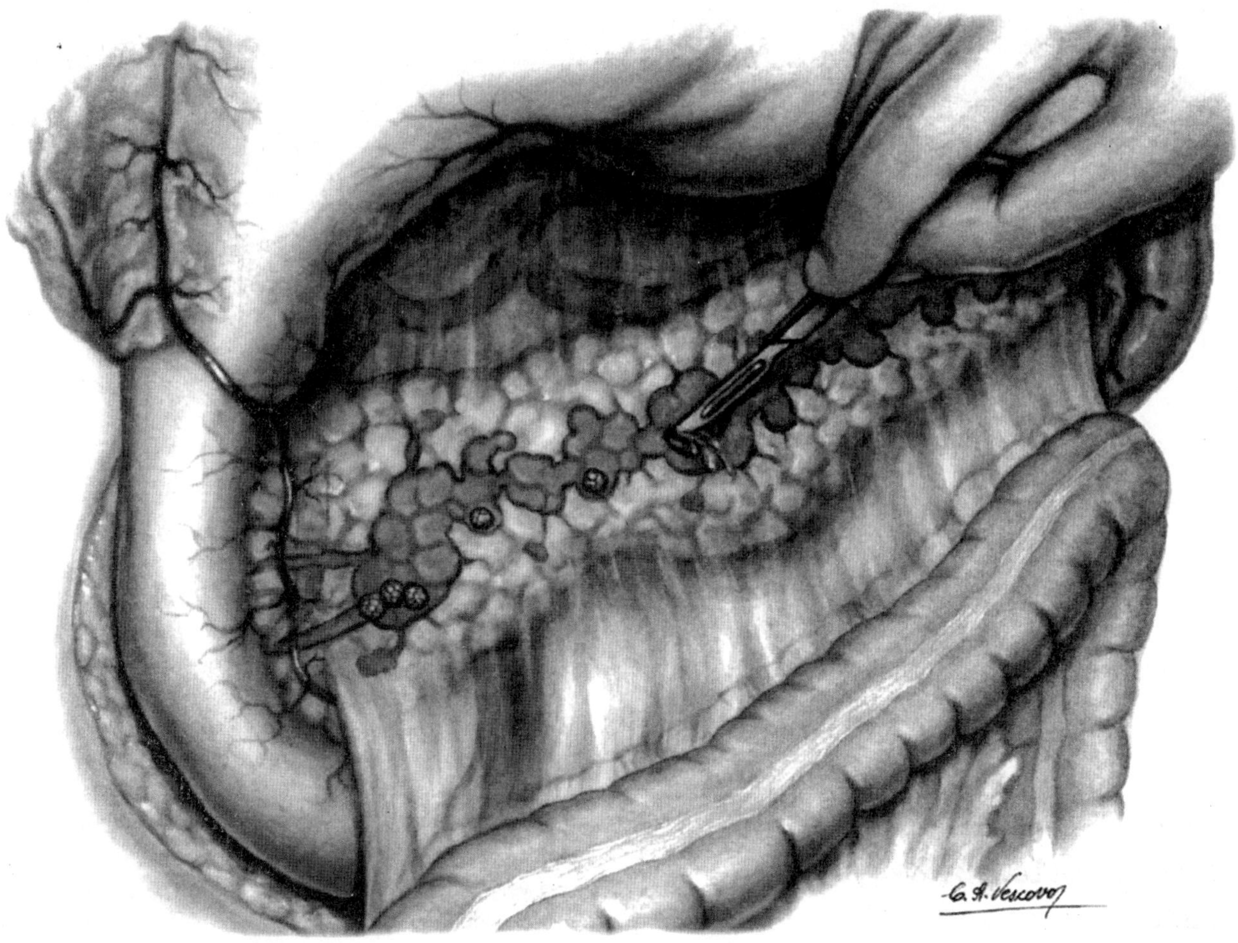

FIGURE 15.3

FIGURE 15.4
The Potts scissors has been introduced through the small incision, and the pancreatic duct is being incised together with the fibrotic parenchyma covering it. This division of the duct should be extended from the tail of the pancreas to about 2 or 3 cm from the internal curve of the duodenum. In order to divide the duct at the sites of the interspersed dilated zones, it is convenient to use a biliary duct explorer, a malleable Mayo-Robson spoon, in order to remove the calculi and, if the narrowing is very severe, a lacrimal explorer. Hemostasis of the divided pancreatic tissue is carried out with electrocautery or using suture ligatures. This fibrotic tissue does not usually bleed very much because it is not very vascularized, except near the duodenum where there are some larger vessels. If suspicious areas are found during the division of the duct, biopsies should be performed in order to eliminate the presence of carcinoma of the pancreas.

Modified Puestow-Gillesby Procedure

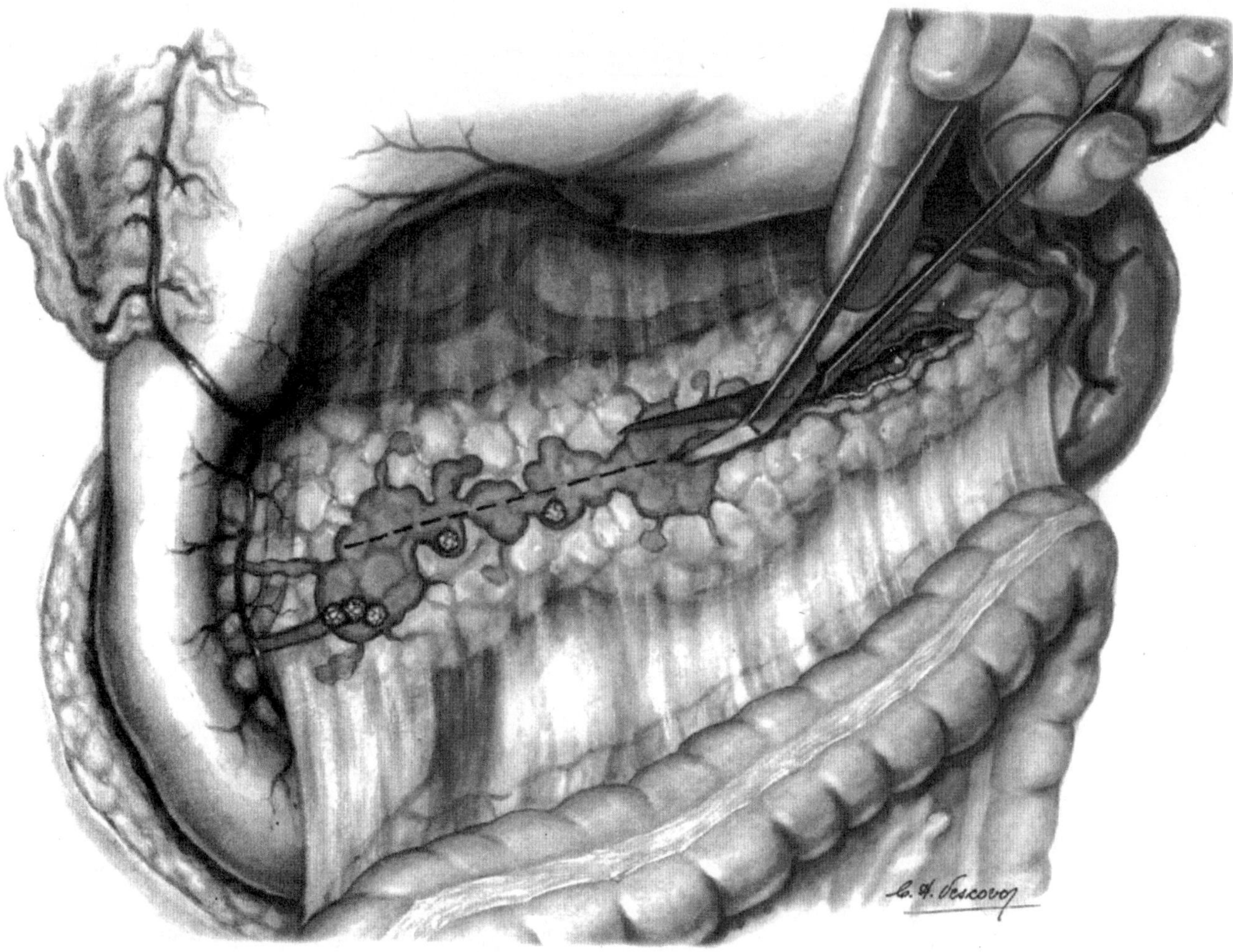

FIGURE 15.4

Modified Puestow-Gillesby Procedure

FIGURE 15.5
During division of the duct, it is occasionally useful to introduce the index or little finger if possible, to have a more exact idea where to continue the division of the duct in the narrow zones. Introduction of the finger will also allow the surgeon to feel free or wedged calculi in the principal duct or the secondary ducts.

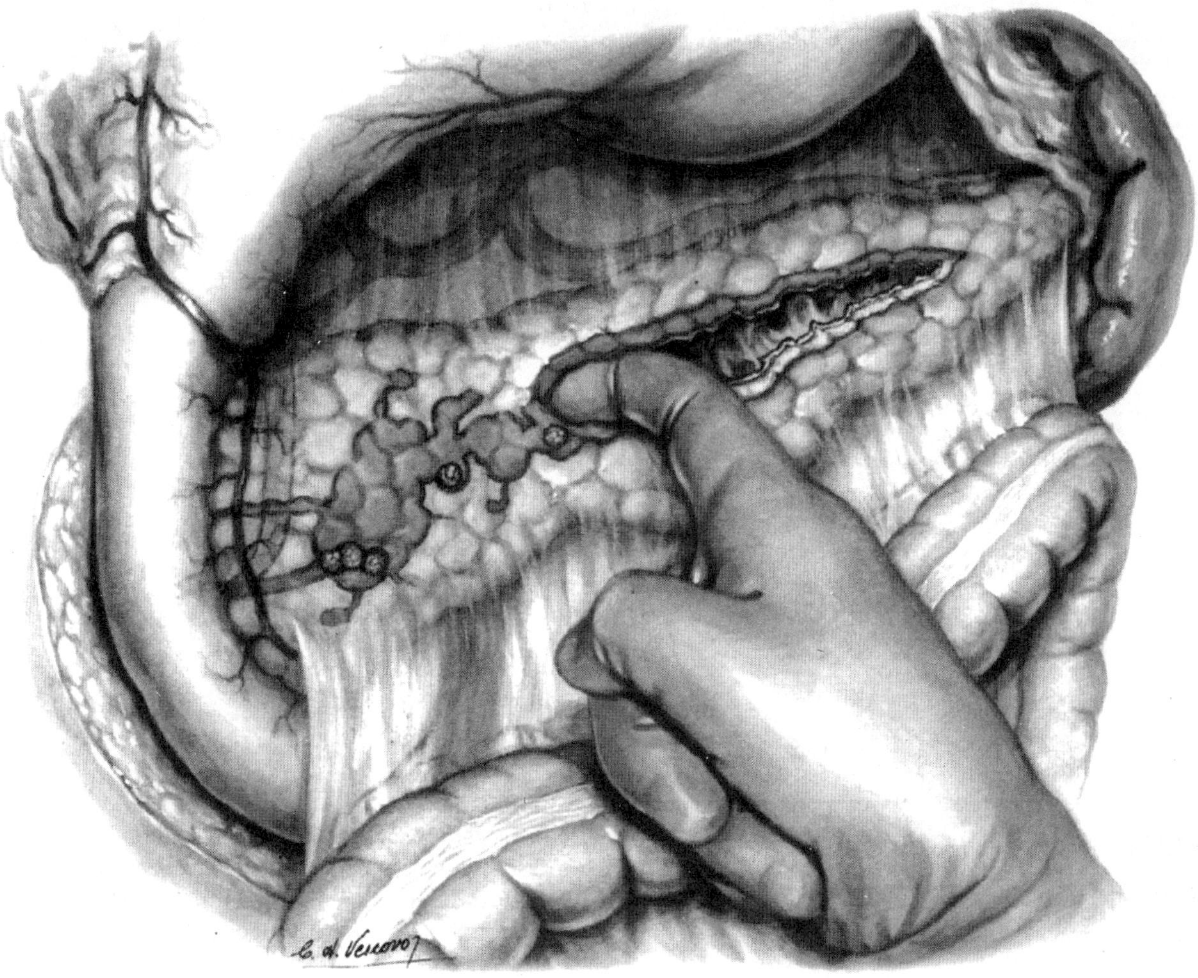

FIGURE 15.5

Modified Puestow-Gillesby Procedure

FIGURE 15.6

If the finger cannot be introduced in the narrow zones, a biliary explorer, a malleable Mayo-Robson spoon or a lacrimal explorer can be used as a guide for the longitudinal incision of the duct. The Mayo-Robson spoon serves for the removal of calculi, as can be seen in the drawing.

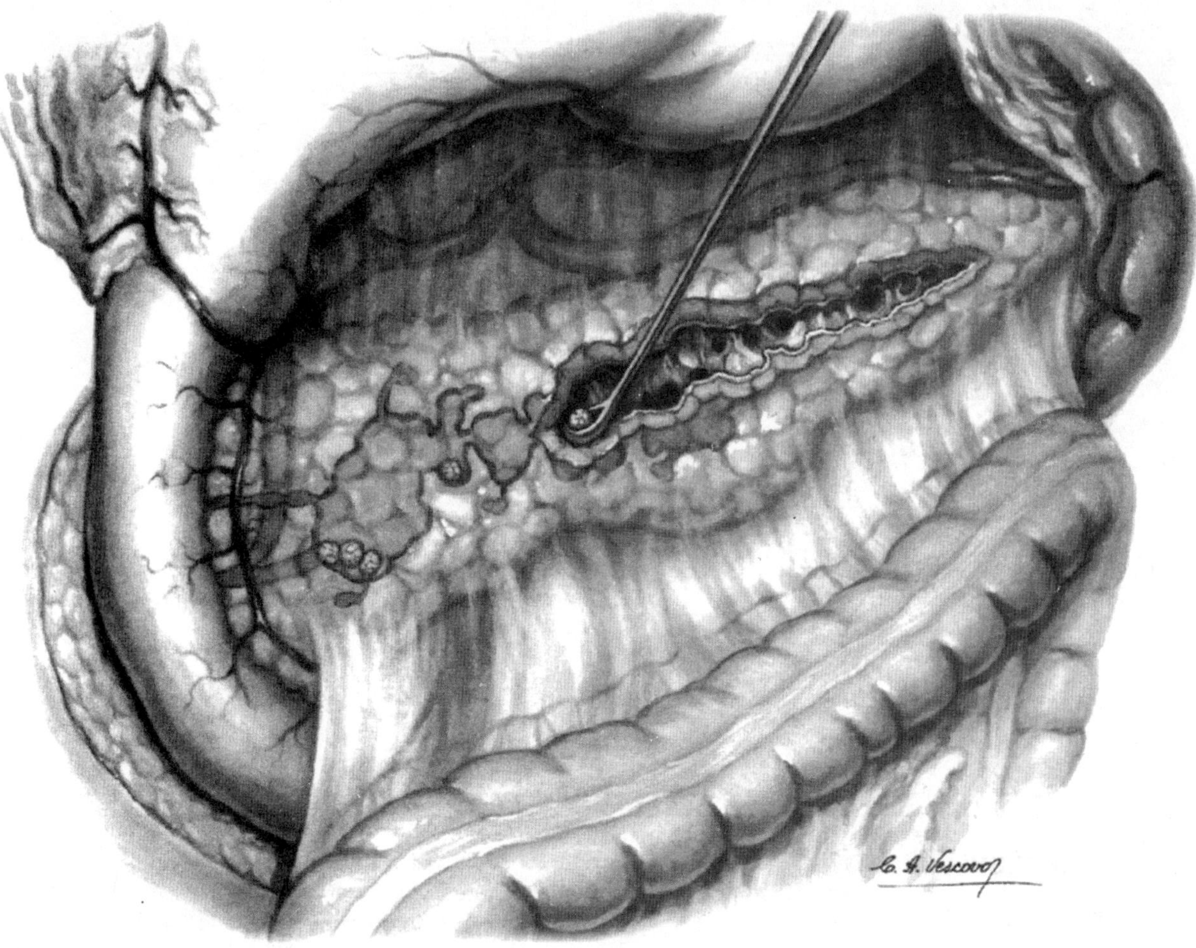

FIGURE 15.6

FIGURE 15.7
The pancreatic duct has been incised from the tail to about 2 to 3 cm in from the internal border of the duodenum. The interior of the duct has been cleaned of debris, and all calculi that were easy to remove have been removed. The pancreatic duct is prepared for anastomosis to the jejunum. The drawing demonstrates that the duct wall is thickened and covered by fibrotic pancreatic parenchyma.

Modified Puestow-Gillesby Procedure

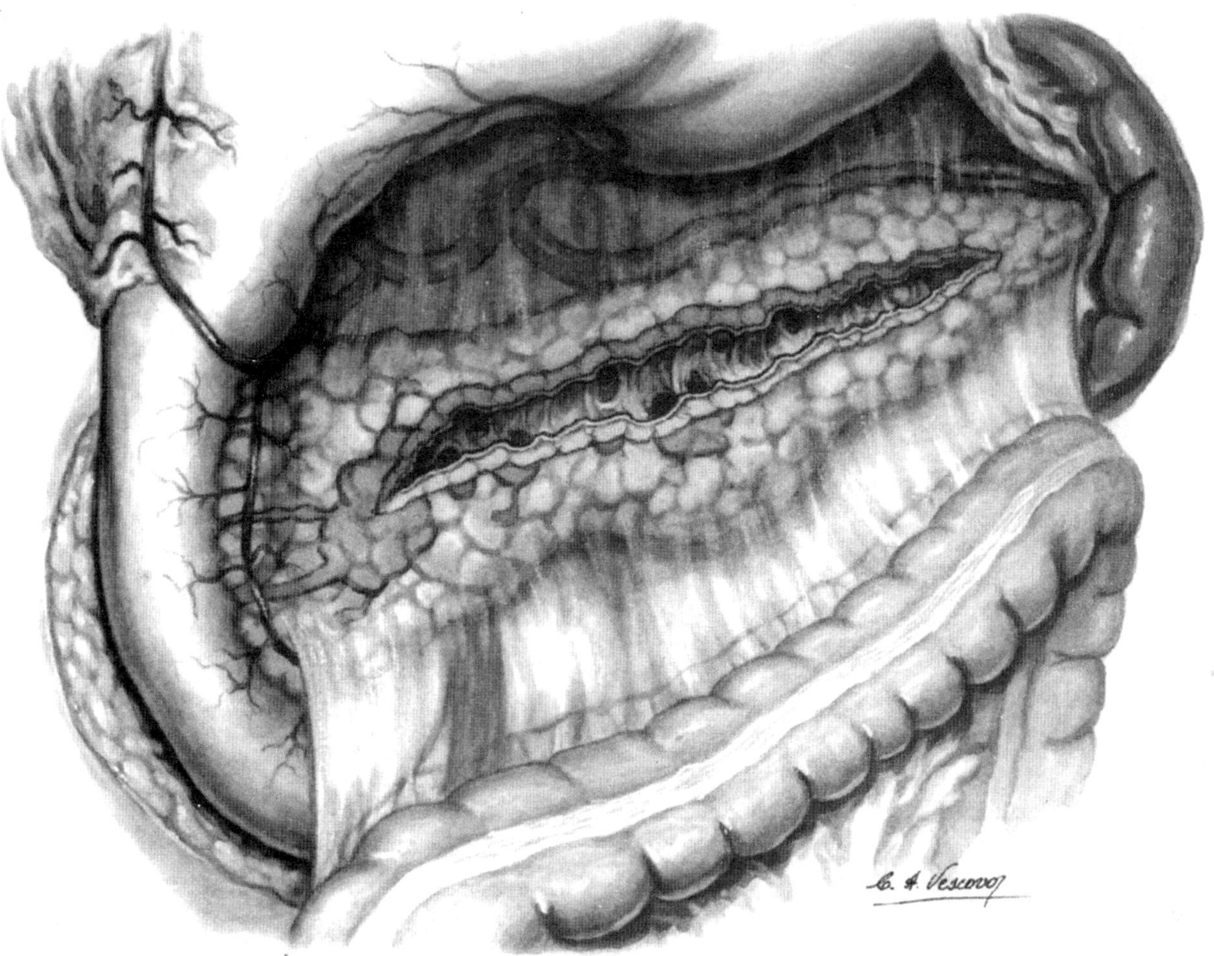

FIGURE 15.7

Modified Puestow-Gillesby Procedure

FIGURE 15.8
This shows the line of division of the mesentery and the jejunum in order to prepare the Roux-en-Y limb. Division is usually carried out between the third and fourth arterial arches. The jejunum is transected and the distal end closed in two layers in order to bring it up through the transverse mesocolon to the right of the mesocolic vessels (avascular zone). The adequate blood supply of the anastomotic limb should be confirmed.

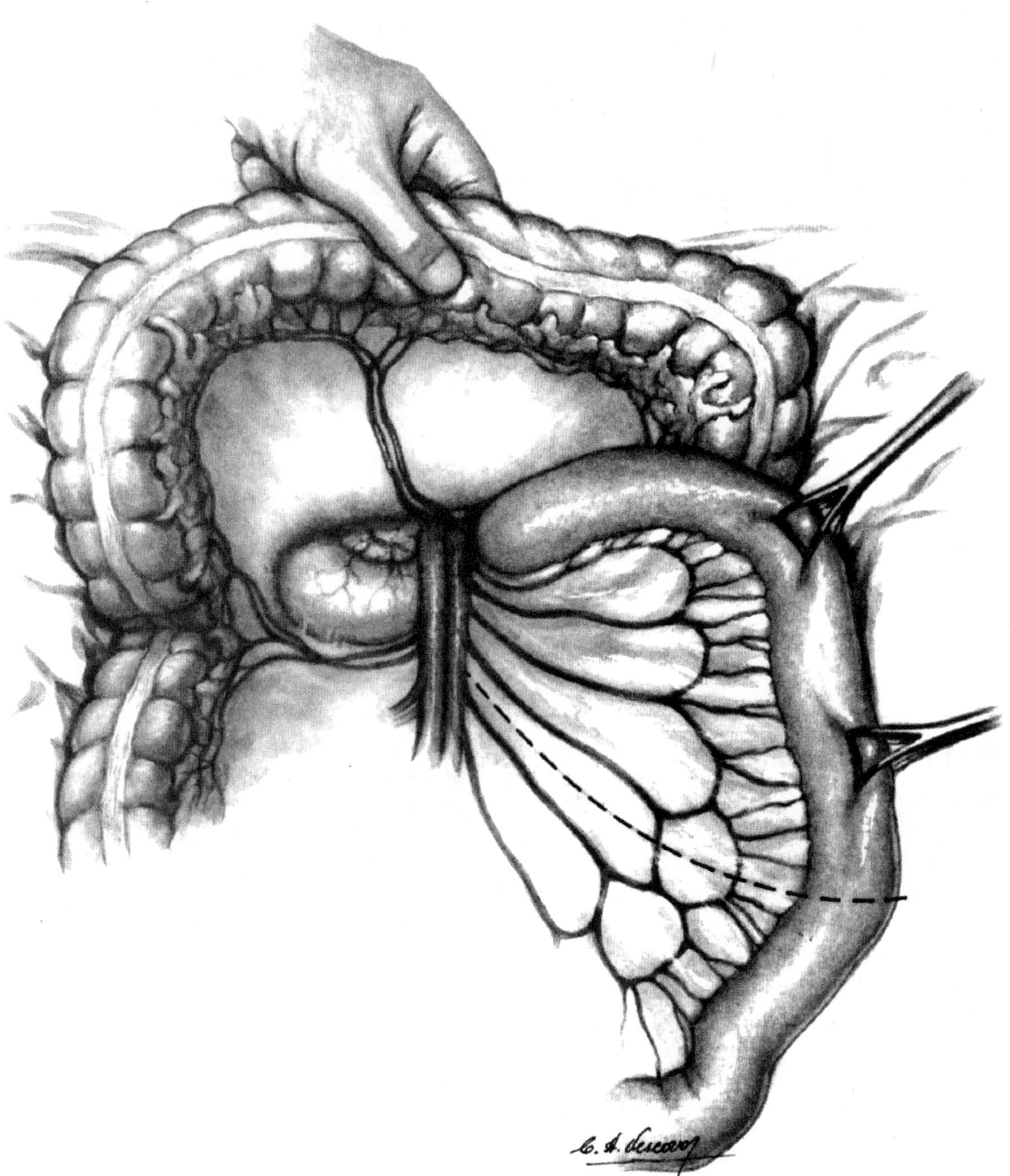

FIGURE 15.8

Modified Puestow-Gillesby Procedure

FIGURE 15.9
The distal jejunal limb, which has been brought up through the transverse mesocolon, has been placed parallel to the open pancreatic duct without any traction. A broken dotted line demonstrates the line of incision of the jejunum along its free border.

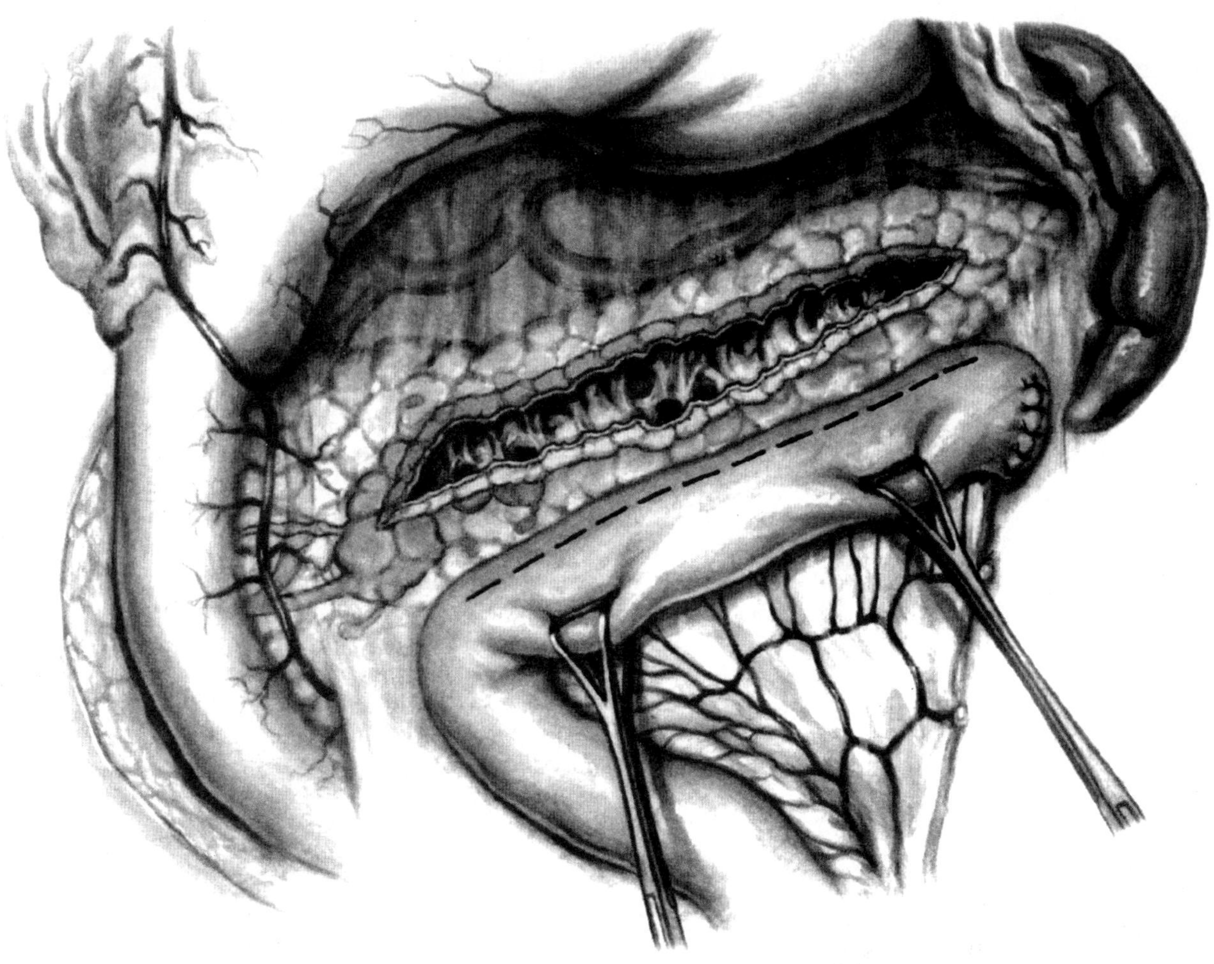

FIGURE 15.9

FIGURE 15.10

Suturing of the pancreatic duct to the wall of the jejunum has begun using interrupted nonabsorbable sutures. On one side the sutures include the wall of the pancreatic duct together with fibrotic pancreatic tissue covering it, and on the other side the jejunal wall. The sutures can get a good hold on the duct and the pancreas covering it because their consistency is increased and they offer resistance to the suture. It is not convenient to perform this suture using reabsorbable material, either catgut or synthetic, because these are easily disintegrated by the action of the pancreatic trypsin. Some surgeons carry out this anastomosis without including the edge of the pancreatic duct in the sutures or the edge of the jejunum, including only the thickened pancreatic capsule near the duct and the seromuscular layer of the jejunum (14). This means they do not perform a mucosa to mucosa suture. Other surgeons perform this anastomosis in two layers. One layer is extramucosal, between the pancreatic capsule and the seromuscular layer of the jejunum, and the other includes the entire wall of the pancreatic duct and the entire wall of the jejunum. Generally, one layer of sutures is sufficient to carry out a secure anastomosis.

Modified Puestow-Gillesby Procedure

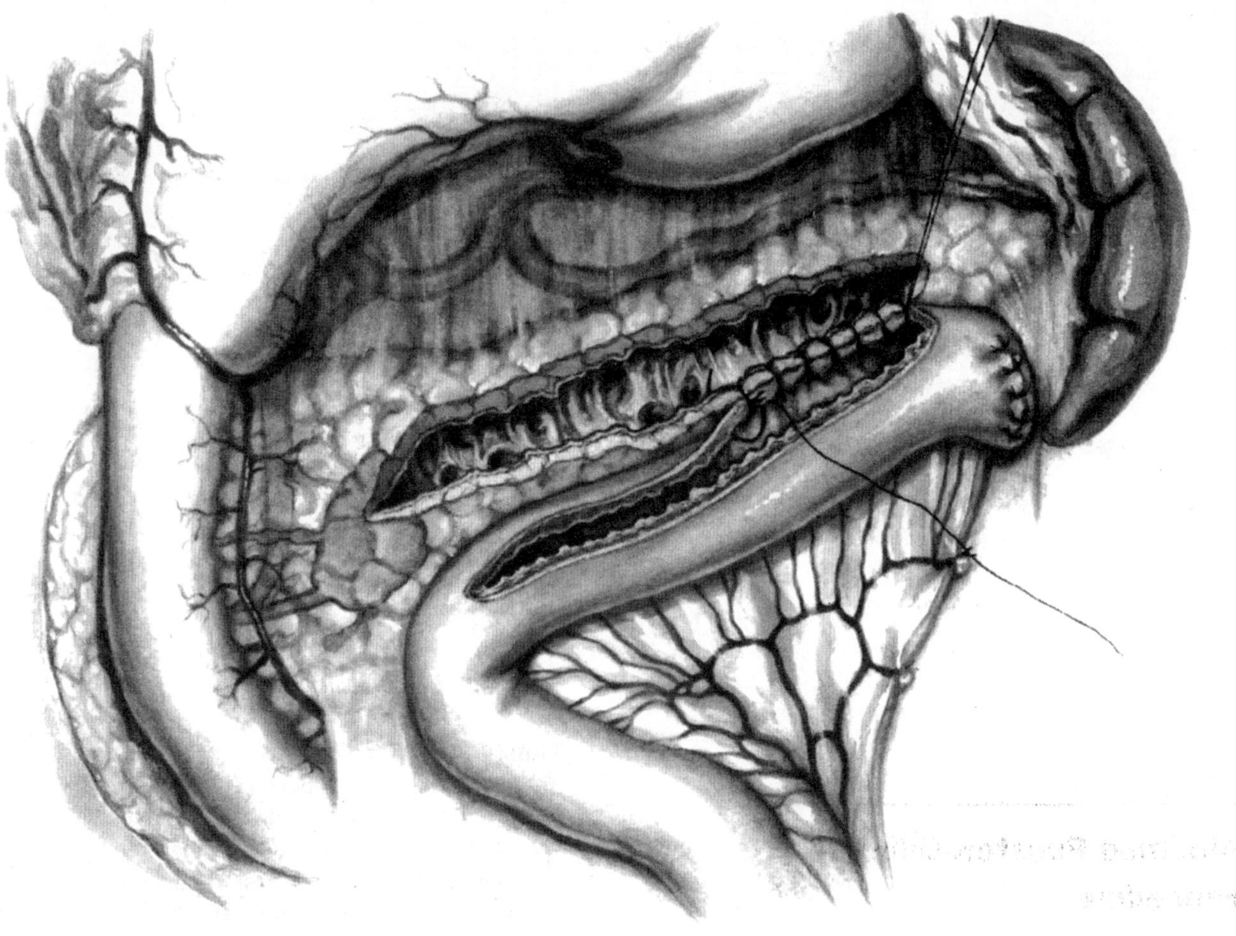

FIGURE 15.10

FIGURE 15.11
The posterior layer has been completed and the anterior layer is being sutured. The drawing demonstrates the adequate bite that has to be taken in the pancreatic duct and the parenchyma covering it in order to attain a good anastomosis. The insert shows a transverse section of the pancreaticojejunal anastomosis.

Modified Puestow-Gillesby Procedure

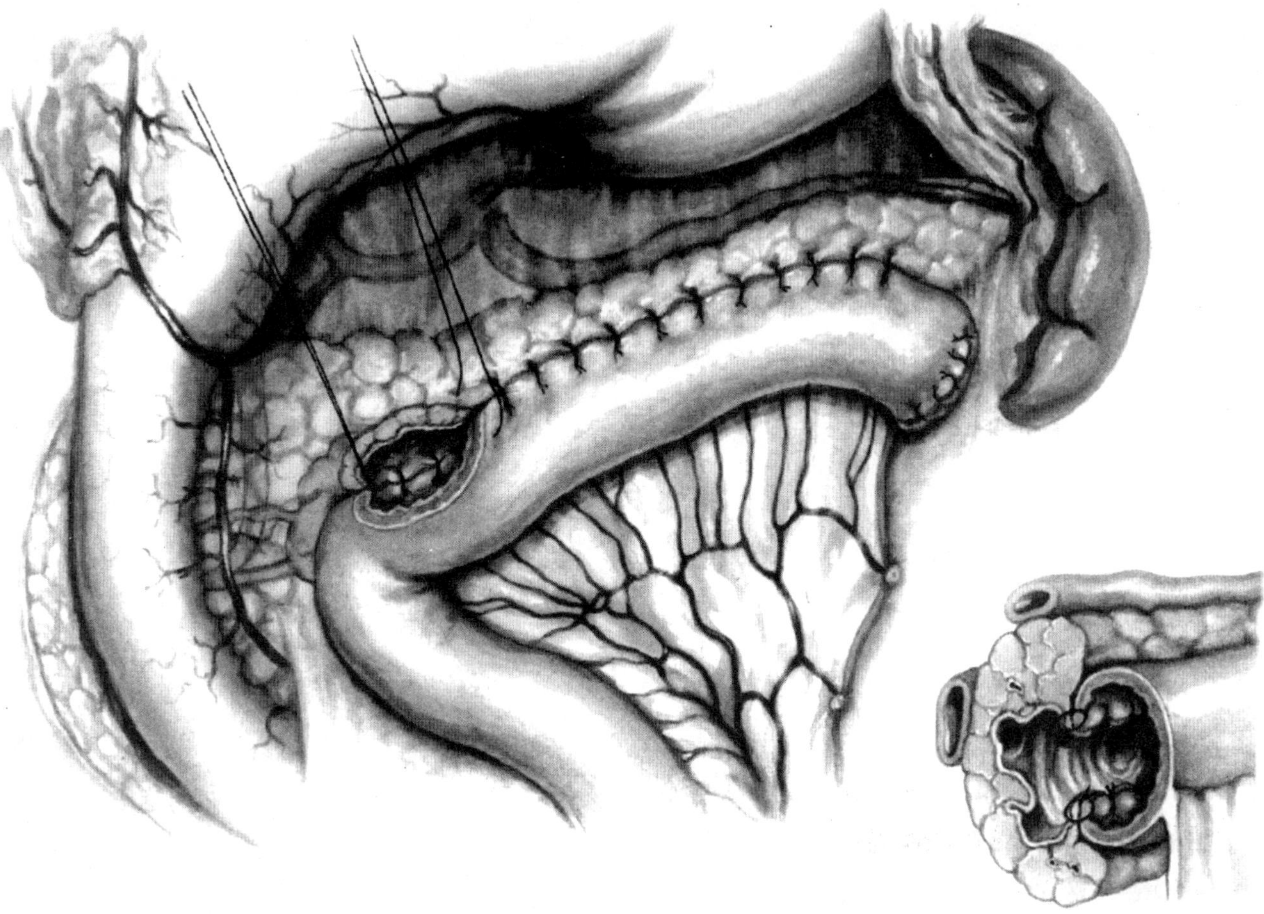

FIGURE 15.11

FIGURE 15.12

This shows the anastomosis of the pancreatic duct to the jejunum which has been disposed in Roux-en-Y fashion. The proximal end of the jejunum has been anastomosed in end to side fashion to the free border of the distal jejunal limb, about 40 to 50 cm from the pancreaticojejunal anastomosis. One can also see that the distal jejunal limb, which was anastomosed to the pancreatic duct, was passed through the transverse mesocolon to the right of the middle colic vessels and fixed with several sutures to the mesocolon to avoid internal hernias. Suction drainage should be left in the vicinity of the pancreas and brought out through a counterincision. The abdominal wall is closed with nonabsorbable material.

Modified Puestow-Gillesby Procedure

Postoperatively, it is possible to confirm the adequacy of the pancreaticojejunal anastomosis by means of endoscopic retrograde cholangiopancreatography. If the anastomosis is proven to be patent and the pains disappear, the operation was a success. If the pains disappear after surgery but recur after a variable period of time and one finds that an obstruction has developed in the anastomosis, the patient should be reoperated to perform a new anastomosis or a pancreatic resection. If the anastomosis remains patent postoperatively but the pains have not disappeared, the operation has failed. One can then undertake a pancreatic resection without guaranteeing disappearance of pain. In general it has been shown that the anastomosis is more effective when the duct is very dilated, or when there are pancreatic calcifications or calculi in the duct of Wirsung or in its branches (14, 16–18, 23). Pancreatic resection may fail to relieve pain in chronic pancreatitis in the same proportion as a pancreaticojejunal anastomosis. It has been shown that resection cases are more apt to relieve pain when the duct is well dilated and there are calcifications and calculi present. Both resection and anastomosis are effective in 60 to 70% of cases, failing in 30 to 40%.

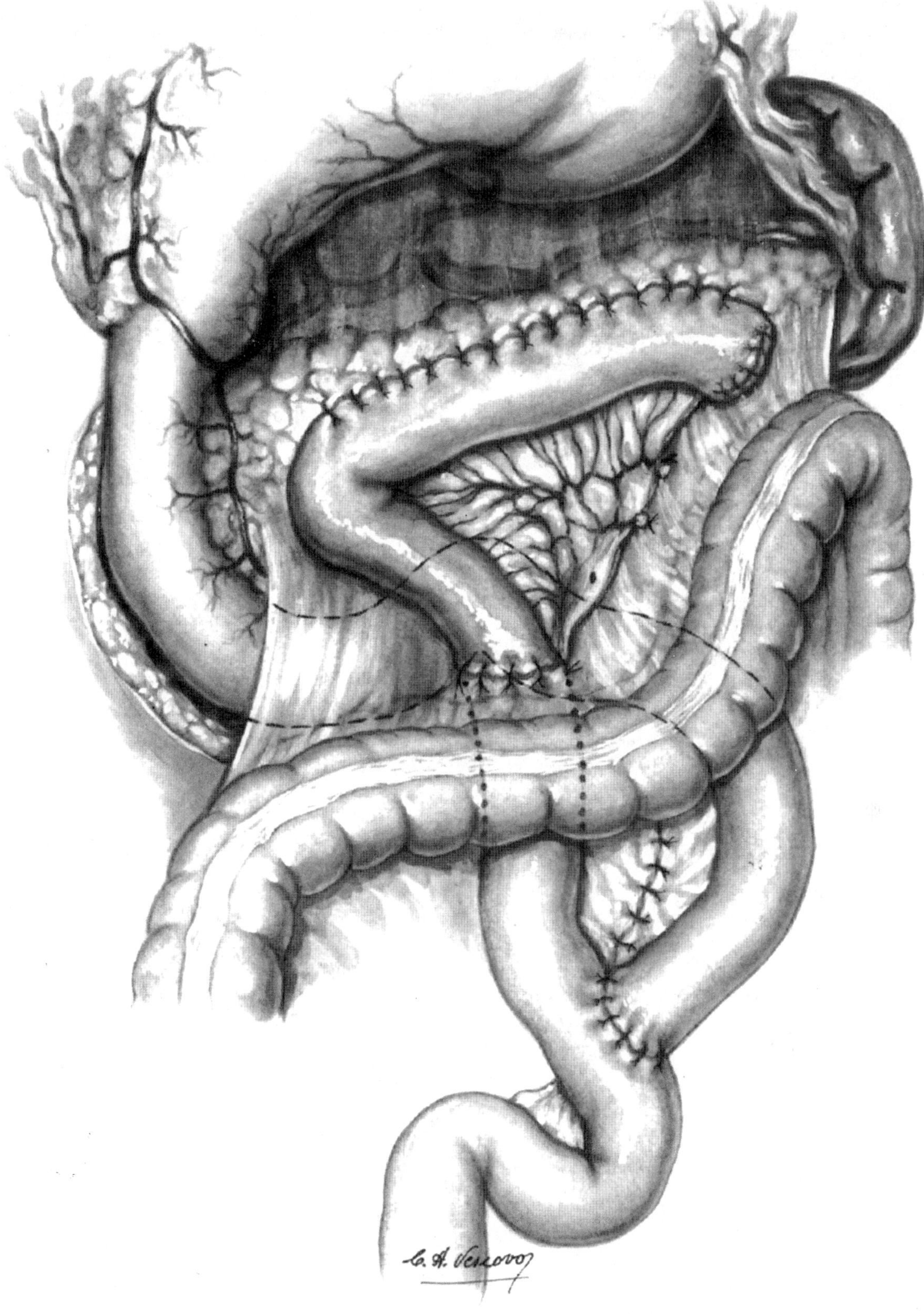

FIGURE 15.12

References

1. Braasch, J.W., Vito, L., Nugent, F.W. Total pancreatectomy for end stage chronic pancreatitis. Ann. Surg. 188:317, 1978.
2. Bradley, E.L., Clements, J.L., Jr. Idiopathic duodenal obstruction:An unappreciated complication of pancreatitis. Ann. Surg. 193:638, 1981.
3. Caroli, J., Nora, J. L'hépato-cholédoque dans les pancréatites. III Congrès Européen de Gastroentérologie. Bologna 20–26 April. p. 609. Licinio Cappelli, Bologna, 1952.
4. Child, C.G., Frey, C.F., Fry, W.J. A reappraisal of removal of 95% of the distal portion of the pancreas. Surg. Gynecol. Obstet. 129:49, 1969.
5. Duval, M.K. Caudal pancreaticojejunostomy for chronic pancreatitis. Ann. Surg. 140:775, 1954.
6. Etala, E. Valor de la colangiografía operatoria para el diagnóstico del cáncer de la cabeza del páncreas y de la ampolla de Vater. Comptes Rendus de la Société Internationale de Chirurgie. p. 1198. Roma, 1963.
7. Etala, E., Russo, R. Diagnóstico operatorio del cáncer de la ampolla de Vater. Soc. Cir. Buenos Aires 50:334, 1966.
8. Etala, E. Exploración operatoria del extremo distal del colédoco. Pren. Méd. Argent. 60:589, 1973.
9. Frey, C.F., Child, C.G. Pancreatectomy for chronic pancreatitis. Ann. Surg. 184:403, 1976.
10. Frey, C.F. Role of subtotal pancreatectomy and pancreaticojejunostomy in chronic pancreatitis. J. Clin. Res. 31:361, 1981.
11. Gall, F.P., Muhe, E., Gebhart, G. Results of partial and total pancreaticoduodenectomy in 117 patients with chronic pancreatitis. World J. Surg. 5:269, 1981.
12. Gillesby, W.J., Puestow, C.B. Pancreaticojejunostomy for chronic relapsing pancreatitis: An evaluation. Surgery 50:859, 1961.
13. Greenlee, H.B. Role of surgery for chronic pancreatitis, its complications. Surg. Annu. 15:283, 1983.
14. Greenlee, H.B. Roux-en-Y pancreaticojejunostomy for chronic pancreatitis. In Nyhus, L.M., Baker, R.J. (Eds.) Mastery of surgery. Vol. II, p. 774, Little, Brown & Co., Boston, 1984.
15. Guillemin, G. Chronic pancreatitis. Surgical management including 63 cases of pancreatoduodenectomy. Am. J. Surg. 122:802, 1971.
16. Hart, M.J., Miyashita, H., Marita, N. Pancreaticojejunostomy. Report of 25 years experience. Am. J. Surg. 145:567, 1983.
17. Howard, J.M. Surgical treatment of chronic pancreatitis. In surgical diseases of the pancreas. p. 496. Howard, J.M., Jordan, G.L., Reber, H.A. (Eds.) Lea & Febiger, Philadelphia, 1987.
18. Jordan, G.I., Jr., Strug, B.S., Crowder, W.E. Current status of pancreaticojejunostomy in the management of chronic pancreatitis. Am. J. Surg. 133:46, 1977.
19. Léger, L., Lenriot, J.P., Lemaigres, G. Five to twenty-five years followup after surgery for chronic pancreatitis in 148 patients. Ann. Surg. 180:185, 1974.
20. Littenberg, G., Afroudakis, A., Kaplowity, N. Common bile duct stenosis from chronic pancreatitis: A clinical and pathological spectrum. Medicine 58:385, 1979.
21. Partington, P.F., Rochelle, R.P. Modified Puestow procedure for retrograde drainage of the pancreatic duct. Ann. Surg. 152:1.037, 1960.
22. Prinz, R.A., Greenlee, H.B. Pancreatic drainage in 100 patients with chronic pancreatitis. Ann. Surg. 194:313, 1981.
23. Prinz, R.A., Aranha, G.V., Greenlee, H.B., Kruse, D.M. Common duct obstruction in patients with intractable pain of chronic pancreatitis. Am. Surg. 48:373, 1982.
24. Proctor, H.J., Mendes, O.C., Thomas, C.G., Jr. et al. Surgery for chronic pancreatitis. Drainage versus resection. Ann. Surg. 189: 664, 1979.
25. Puestow, C.B., Gillesby, W.J. Retrograde surgical drainage for chronic relapsing pancreatitis. Arch. Surg. 76:898, 1958.
26. Puestow, C.B., Gillesby, W.J. Pancreaticojejunostomy for chronic relapsing pancreatitis: an evaluation Surgery 50:859, 1967.
27. Sarles, H., Sehel, I. Cholestasis and lesions of the biliary tract in chronic pancreatitis. Gut 19:851, 1978.
28. Traverso, L.W., Tompkins, R.K., Urrea, P.T., Longmire, W.P., Jr. Surgical treatment of chronic pancreatitis. 22 years experience. Ann. Surg. 190:312, 1979.
29. Warshaw, A.L. et al. Persistent obstructive jaundice, cholangitis and biliary cirrhosis due to common bile duct stenosis in chronic pancreatitis. Gastroenterology 70:502, 1976.
30. Way, L.W., Gadacz, T., Goldman, L. Surgical treatment of chronic pancreatitis. Am. J. Surg. 127:202, 1974.

CHAPTER **16**

Pancreaticoduodenectomy

Section C

Surgery of the Pancreas

Pancreaticoduodenectomy (Whipple procedure) is indicated for exocrine cancer of the pancreas, for periampullary cancers, and for some cases of chronic pancreatitis (alcoholic), predominantly in the head. It may also be indicated in less common situations of the head of the pancreas such as cystadenocarcinoma, endocrine cancer, mucous cystadenoma, serous cystadenoma, and so on.

The surgical technique is similar in these situations. We portray the pancreaticoduodenectomy for cancer of the head of the pancreas as the model operation. We describe the technique of the surgery, the surgical exploration prior to resection, the technique of operative cholangiography and its contribution to the differential diagnosis of chronic pancreatitis (particularly in the head), and its contribution in cases of carcinoma of the ampulla and in cases of calculi impacted in the distal choledochus. Operative biopsy of the head of the pancreas with discussion of its contribution shall be presented. We shall also show some instances of operative cholangiography in chronic pancreatitis of the head to demonstrate specific differences from cancer of the head of the pancreas. The very valuable operative cholangiography in cases of small and soft papillary cancers will also be demonstrated.

After describing the classic (Whipple) pancreaticoduodenectomy, the technique with pyloric sphincter preservation (Traverso and Longmire) will be described. The description of total pancreatectomy will follow.

Pancreaticoduodenectomy

FIGURE 16.1 INCISION

The incision should conform to the habitus of the patient. We commonly use a supraumbilical midline incision extending some 8 cm below the umbilicus. This may be further extended by removing the xiphoid. Once the abdominal cavity has been opened, complete and careful exploration follows, searching for metastases in the liver, greater omentum, root of the mesentery, cul de sac, and so on. Lymphatic ganglia about the hepatic artery, celiac axis, subpyloric and duodenopancreatic nodes are evaluated. Suspicious tissues and ganglia should be biopsied and studied by frozen section. If there are no metastases, the diagnosis of cancer of the head is to be confirmed. This must include biopsy and operative cholangiography. Determination of resectability follows.

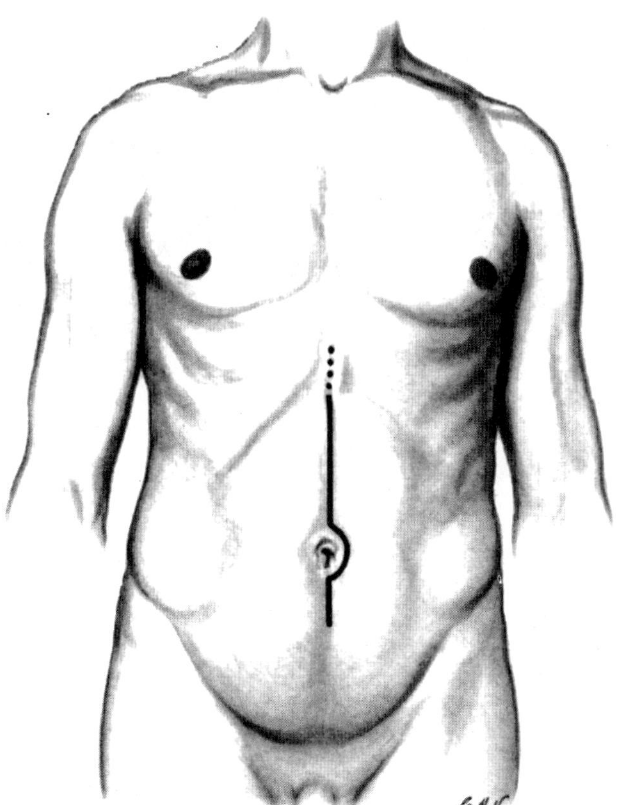

FIGURE 16.1 INCISION

OPERATIVE CHOLANGIOGRAPHY

Operative cholangiography contributes very significantly not only to the diagnosis of lithiasis but also to the diagnosis of cancer of the head of the pancreas and to the diagnosis of chronic pancreatitis of the head of the pancreas that obstructs the retropancreatic choledochus. It can also contribute to the diagnosis of cancer of the papilla of Vater.(19–24, 39, 40, 50, 70)

Cholangiography protrays the caliber of the bile ducts, the level and degree of obstruction, and the radiologic morphology of the lesion. It also indicates the presence and course of the cystic duct and the relation of the cystic duct to the tumor. It establishes or rules out whether there is a stone in the distal choledochus. Marked dilation of the biliary tree with complete and blunt obstruction of the common duct is very suggestive of malignancy. Preoperative cholangiography, either transhepatic or endoscopic, may render intraoperative cholangiography unnecessary but not always so.

Technique of Operative Cholangiography in Cancer of the Head of the Pancreas and Other Obstructions of the Distal Choledochus

Technique of Operative Cholangiography in Cancer of the Head of the Pancreas and Other Obstructions of the Distal Choledochus

FIGURE 16.2
We perform the operative cholangiography in cases of distal tumoral choledochal obstruction as follows (19–21):

A pursestring suture is laid down at the fundus of the gallbladder. The suture is untied. A trocar is thrust through the center of the pursestring. The contents are aspirated with a suction machine, as the thick and gelatinous and tenacious contents of the gallbladder cannot be readily aspirated with needle and syringe (to attempt to do so enhances the possibility of wound soiling).

FIGURE 16.3
Once aspiration of the gallbladder and biliary tree has been accomplished, 60 to 80 mL of water-soluble radiopaque material is injected through the same puncture access. The purse-string suture is closed by traction without cutting the suture ends. These are retracted upwards and to the right of the patient to avoid superimposition of the now opaque gallbladder over the choledochus being studied.

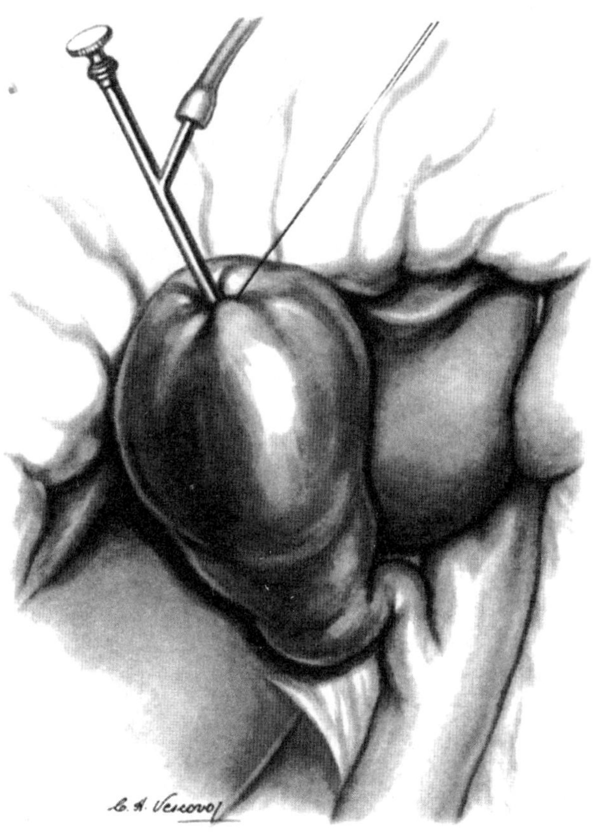

FIGURE 16.2

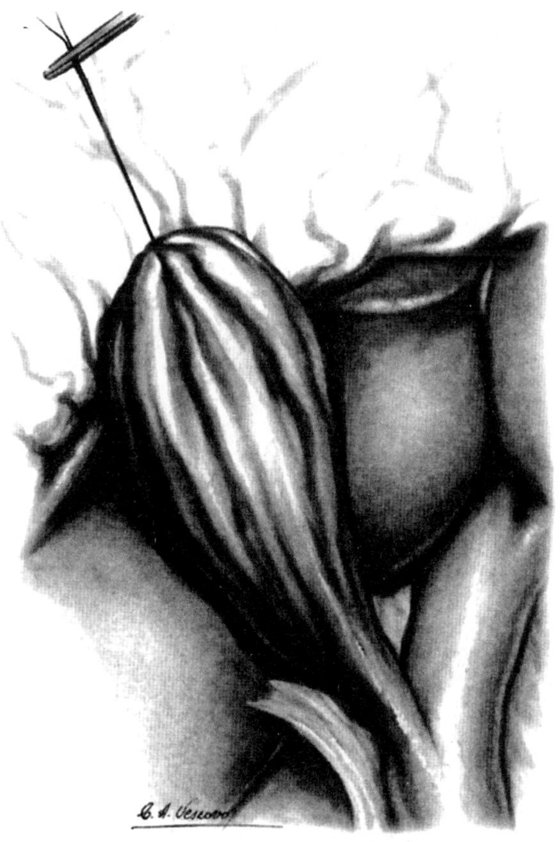

FIGURE 16.3

Technique of Operative Cholangiography in Cancer of the Head of the Pancreas and Other Obstructions of the Distal Choledochus

FIGURE 16.4
This semischematic drawing shows the effect of a cancer of the head of the pancreas on the biliary tree. Usually there is total obstruction of the choledochus and the gallbladder and biliary tree are markedly dilated. In general the obstruction is proximal to the papilla and gives the impression as of an amputation of the choledochus. The blockage is complete, convex, and smooth. It is caused by compression of the choledochus by tumor. If the cancer is very advanced, it may invade the wall of the choledochus and produce a lacunar image such as is illustrated under D.

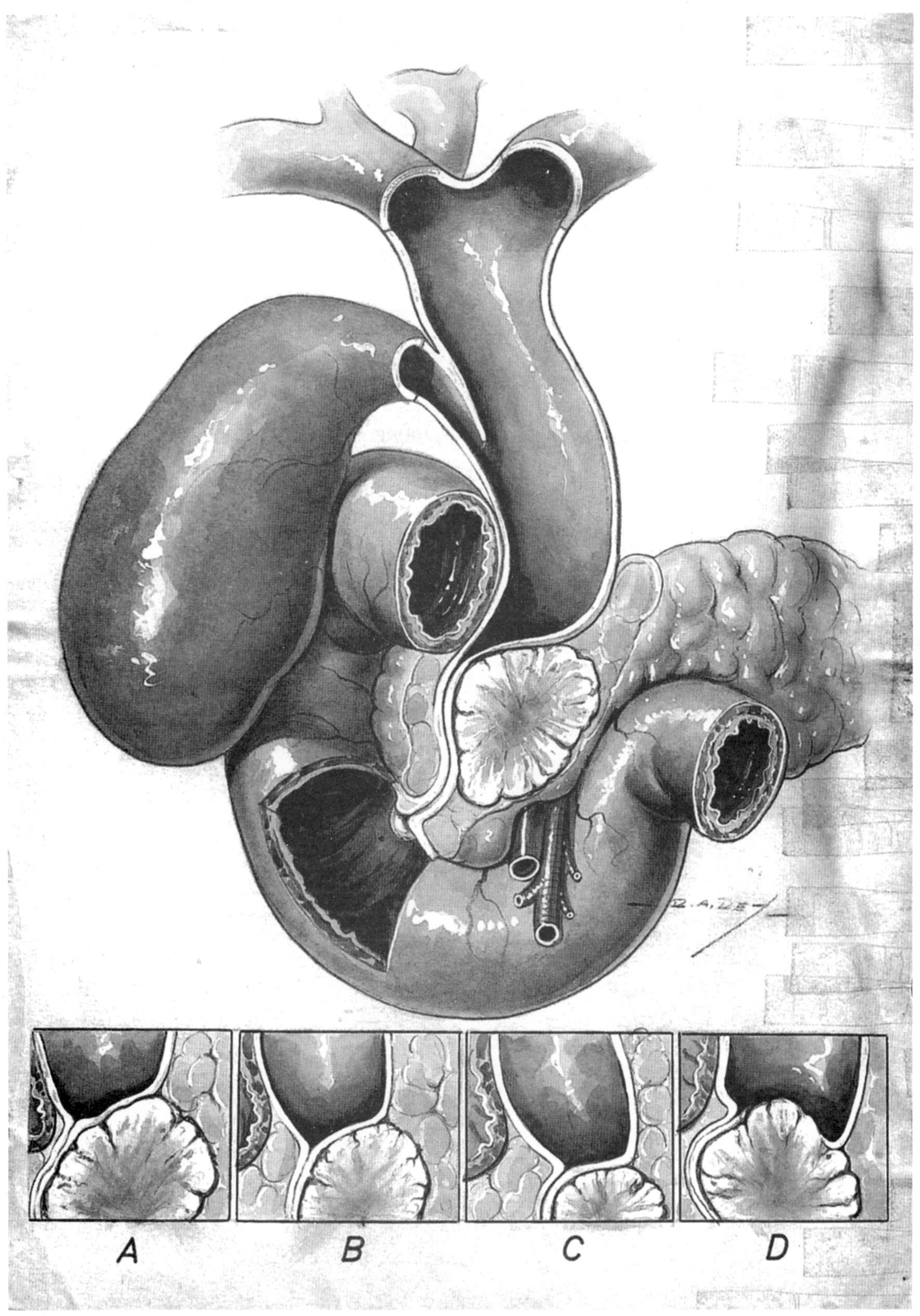

FIGURE 16.4

FIGURE 16.5
Schematic drawing obtained from cholangiography in a case of cancer of head of pancreas. The characteristic findings include very marked dilation of the gallbladder and of the extra and intrahepatic bile ducts. The obstruction is complete, convex, and smooth, as if the choledochus had been amputated at the superior border of the pancreas. The axis of the hepatocholedochus has assumed a more horizontal posture; this is frequent in cancers of the head of the pancreas ("horizontalization" of the hepatocholedochus). The finding suggesting amputation of the choledochus is not constant and varies with the localization and size of the tumor and with the extent of peritumoral pancreatitis.

Technique of Operative Cholangiography in Cancer of the Head of the Pancreas and Other Obstructions of the Distal Choledochus

FIGURE 16.6
Operative cholangiography in a patient with cancer of the head of the pancreas. Noteworthy are the marked dilation of the gallbladder and of the biliary tree from a site proximal to the papilla. Horizontalization of the hepatocholedochus is observed. The cystic duct enters the common duct well away from the tumor.

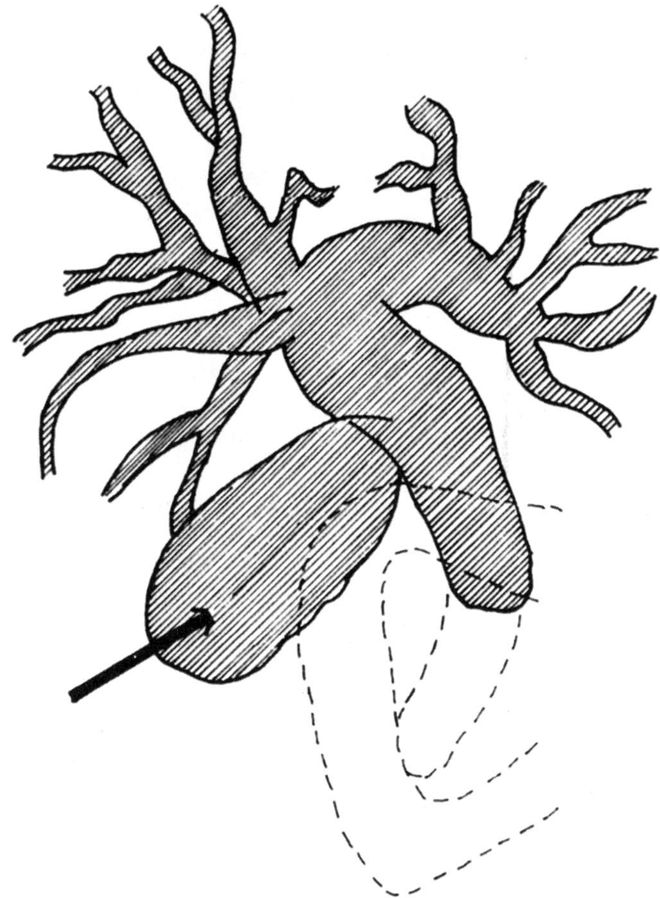

FIGURE 16.5

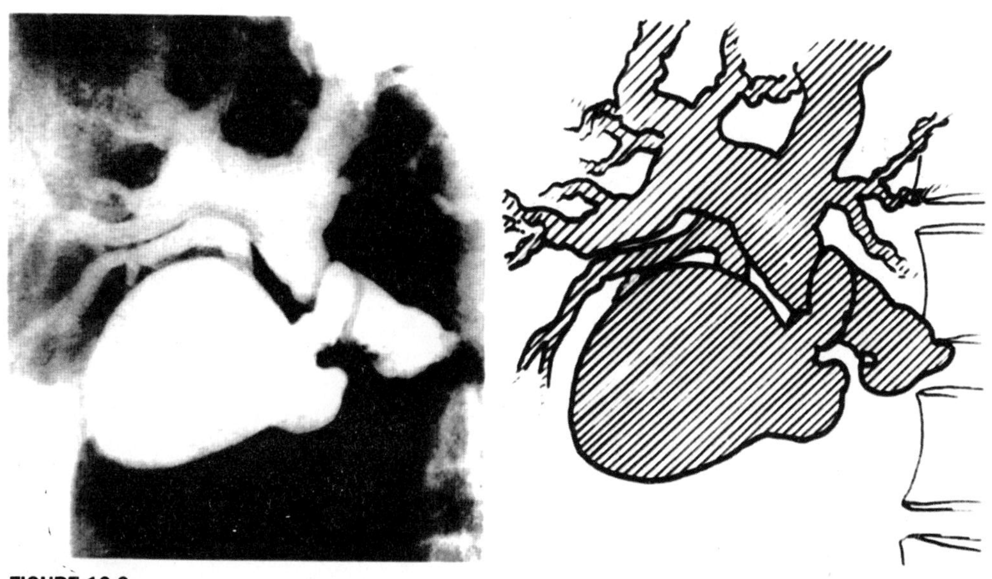

FIGURE 16.6

FIGURE 16.7
Cholangiographic images of carcinomas of the head of the pancreas are quite similar. Here again we note marked dilation of the gallbladder and of the intra- and extrahepatic biliary tree, and complete and blunt obstruction of the common bile duct proximal to the papilla of Vater. Horizontalization of the hepatocholedochus is also present. The cystic duct enters the common duct very near to the tumor, and this would contraindicate using the gallbladder for bile flow diversion.

Technique of Operative Cholangiography in Cancer of the Head of the Pancreas and Other Obstructions of the Distal Choledochus

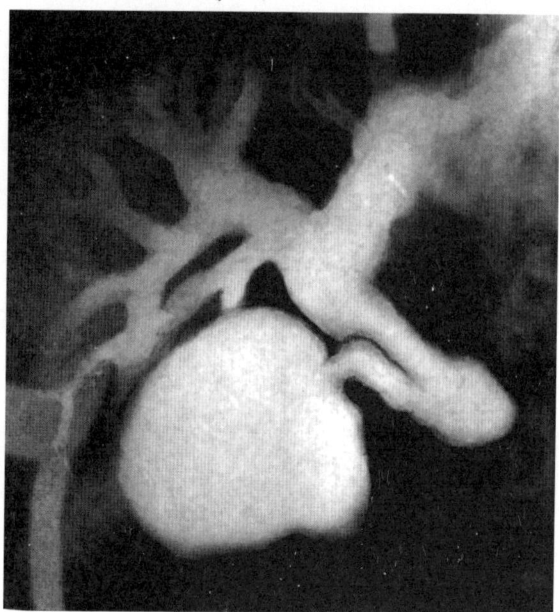

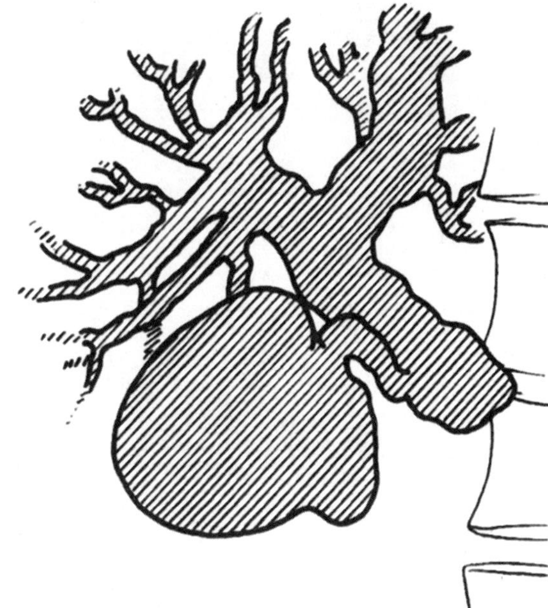

FIGURE 16.7

Technique of Operative Cholangiography in Cancer of the Head of the Pancreas and Other Obstructions of the Distal Choledochus

FIGURE 16.8

This semischematic drawing illustrates the usual cholangiographic image in cases of chronic pancreatitis with involvement of the head of the pancreas, obstructing the choledochus. The choledochal obstruction is caused by the inflammation of the pancreas and by the accompanying peripancreatic fibrosis. The choledochal obstruction is usually incomplete and elongated, and can be regular or irregular. Only rarely does chronic pancreatitis produce total choledochal obstruction.

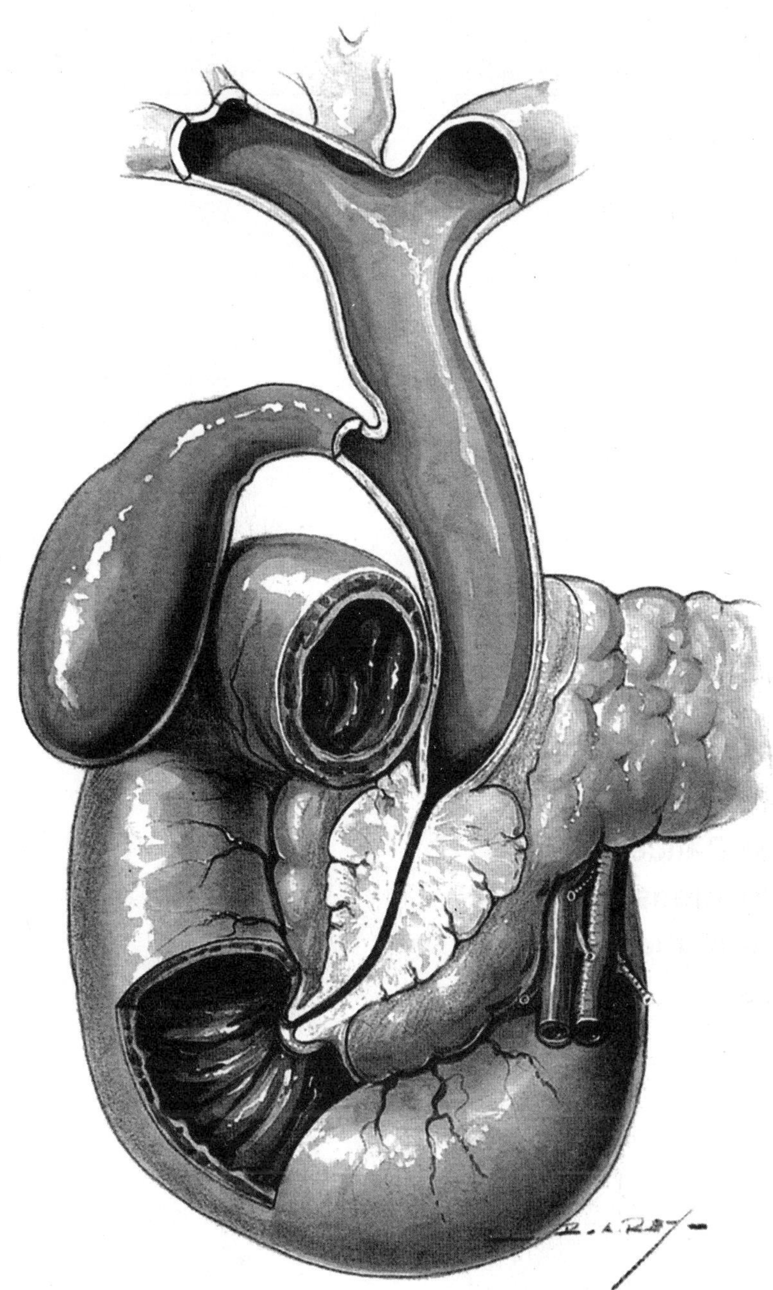

FIGURE 16.8

Technique of Operative Cholangiography in Cancer of the Head of the Pancreas and Other Obstructions of the Distal Choledochus

FIGURE 16.9
Operative cholangiogram in a case of chronic pancreatitis, partial obstruction of retropancreatic choledochus, elongated narrowing, and moderate biliary tree dilation.

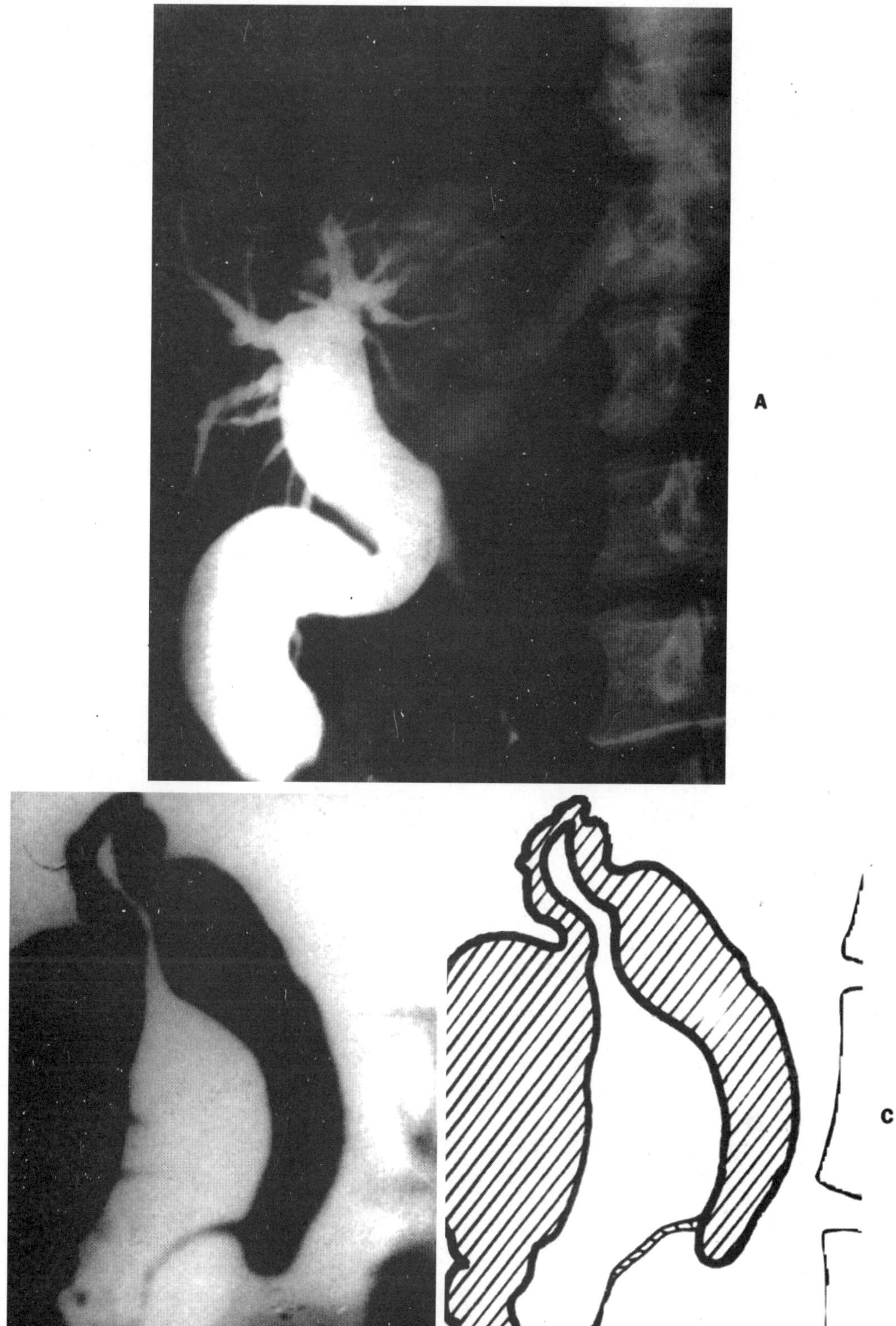

FIGURE 16.9

FIGURE 16.10
Operative cholangiogram in patient with alcoholic chronic pancreatitis. There is retropancreatic compression of the common bile duct and elongated narrowing, which permits dye to pass to the duodenum. The gallbladder and the common duct are dilated.

Technique of Operative Cholangiography in Cancer of the Head of the Pancreas and Other Obstructions of the Distal Choledochus

FIGURE 16.11
Operative cholangiography 1 year after previous surgery at which cholecystectomy for lithiasis had been performed together with removal of two calculi from the common bile duct. The T-tube was removed 29 days later, after cholangiography was negative for residual stones. Two months later, the patient developed pains and recurrent jaundice for which she was referred to us. At surgery we established the diagnosis of chronic pancreatitis, predominantly of the pancreatic head. This compressed the retropancreatic choldedochus. Operative cholangiography shows choledochal distension with an elongated and smooth narrowing of the retropancreatic choledochus. All symptoms abated after choledochoduodenostomy was done proximal to the stenotic choledochus.

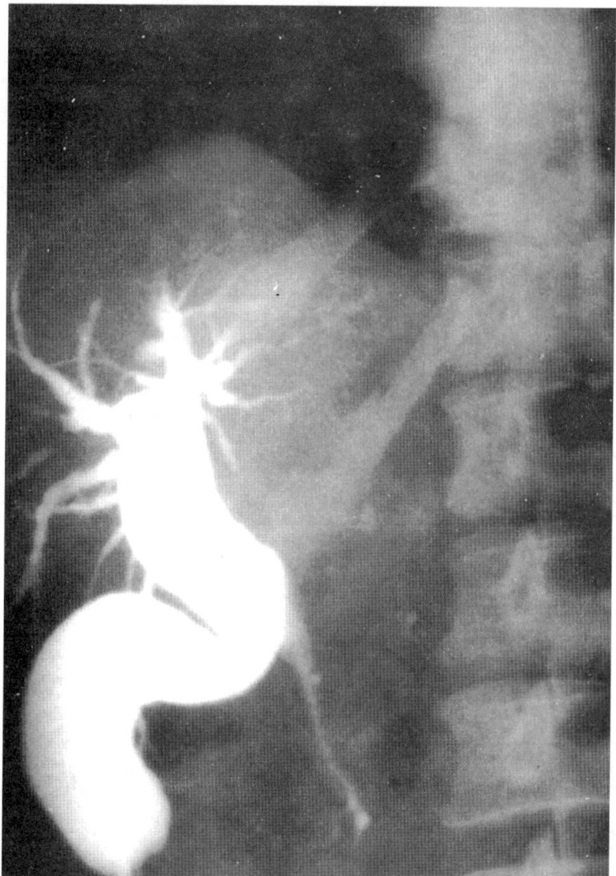

FIGURE 16.10

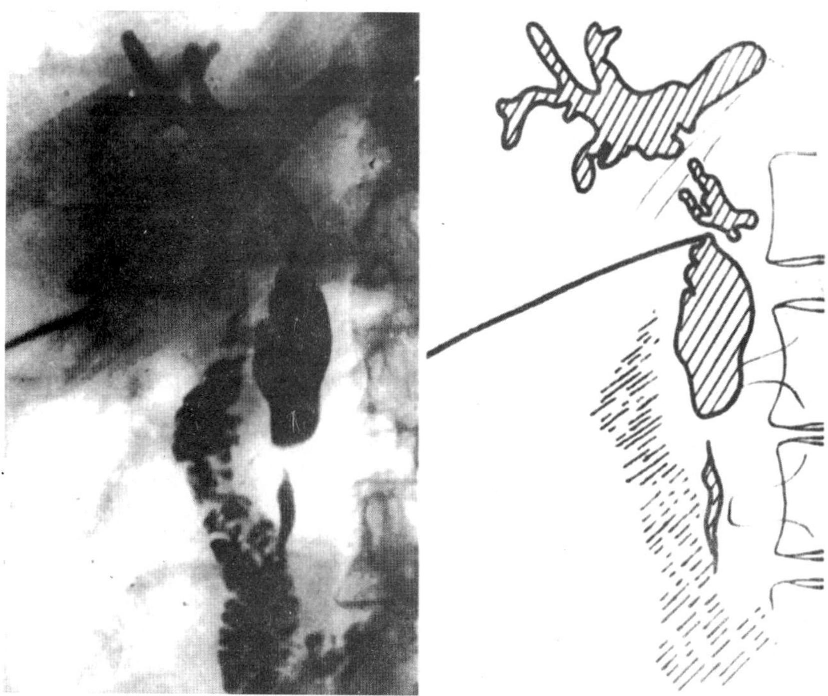

FIGURE 16.11

Technique of Operative Cholangiography in Cancer of the Head of the Pancreas and Other Obstructions of the Distal Choledochus

FIGURE 16.12

This is a semischematic image of the cholangiography picture more frequently found in cancer of the papilla of Vater. (19, 20) The gallbladder and the common duct are dilated. The obstruction at the level of the papilla (internal border of the second portion of the duodenum) is blunt and complete. The obstruction is complete in 85% of such cases. In 15% it is incomplete, and the image is irregular, lacunar, or punched out, suggesting neoplasia and calculus. In 20% of cases the obstruction is proximal to the papilla, and this usually indicates an advanced carcinoma. Operative cholangiography is particularly useful in small and soft cancers of the papilla; these are difficult to palpate. Operative cholangiography reveals distal obstruction and indicates duodenotomy and biopsy. The diagnosis of ampullary carcinoma can be established preoperatively by radiology, hypotonic duodenography, endoscopy, and biopsy.

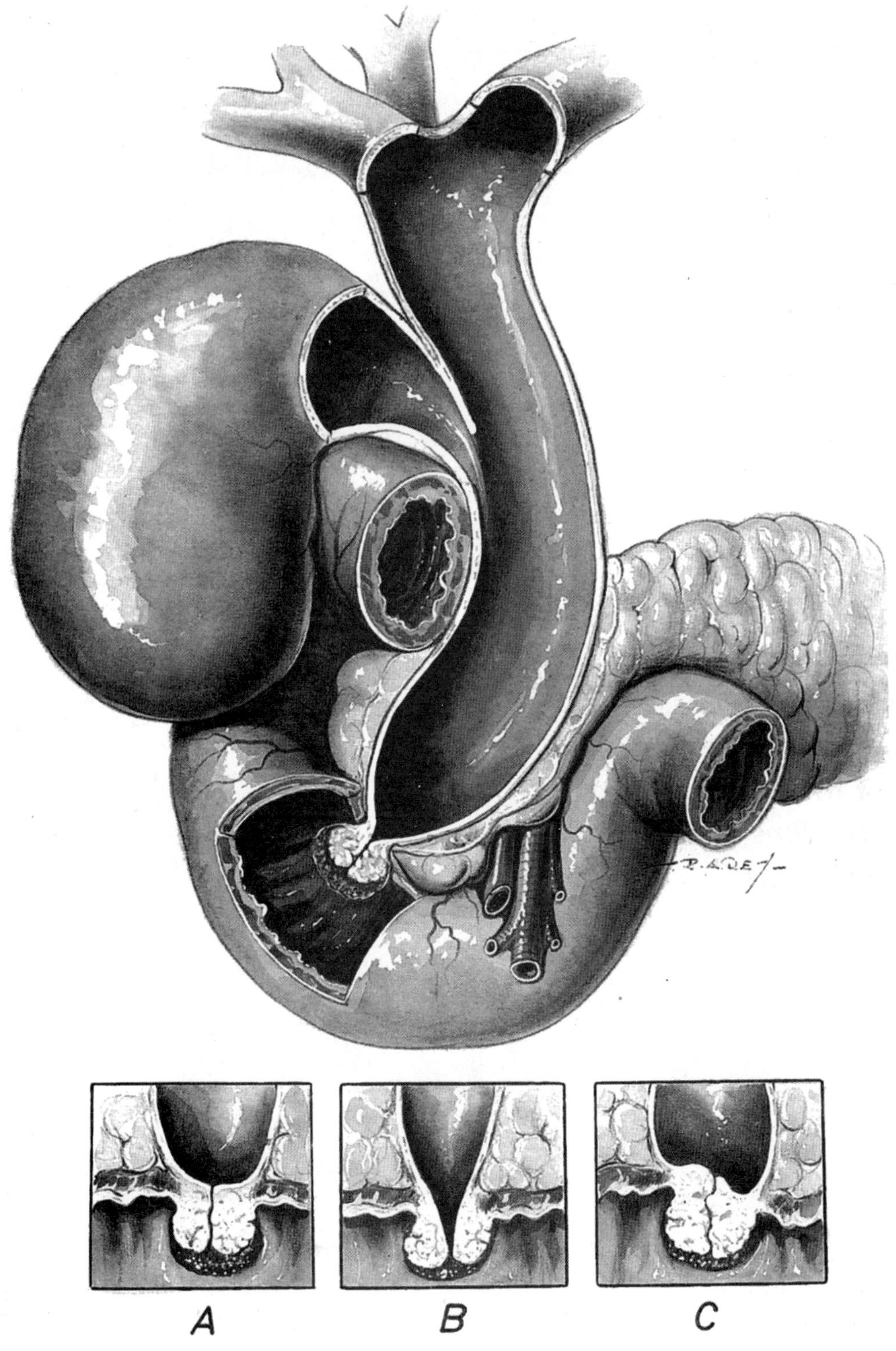

FIGURE 16.12

FIGURE 16.13
Semischematic drawing from operative cholangiography in a case of cancer of the papilla of Vater. The gallbladder and choledochus are distended. There is complete and blunt blockage at the level of the papilla (internal border of the second portion of the duodenum). The distal portion of the choledochus does not appear amputated, as is the case in cancer of the head of the pancreas. The hepatocholedochal axis is normal; it has not assumed a horizontal plane as seen so frequently in cancers of the head of the pancreas.

Technique of Operative Cholangiography in Cancer of the Head of the Pancreas and Other Obstructions of the Distal Choledochus

FIGURE 16.14
Operative cholangiogram in cancer of the papilla of Vater with distention of biliary tree and complete and blunt blockage at level of the papilla.

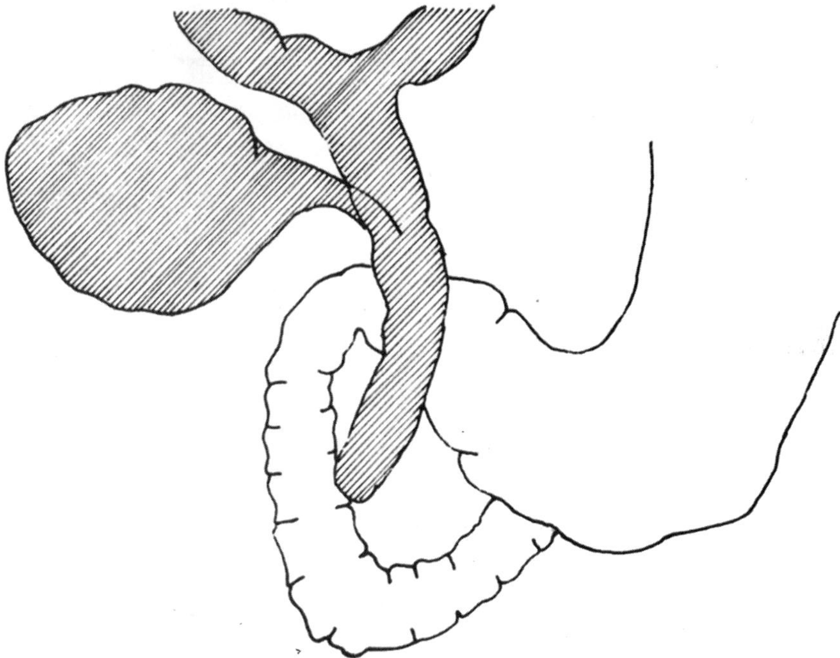

FIGURE 16.13

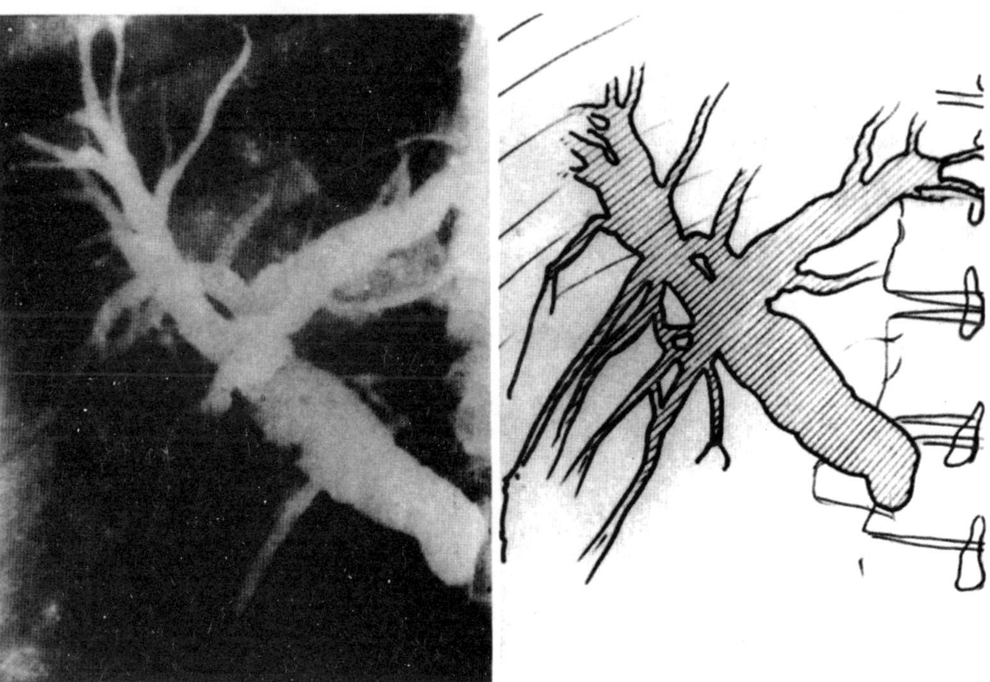

FIGURE 16.14

FIGURE 16.15
Operative cholangiogram in case of cancer of papilla of Vater showing a dilated hepatocholedochus and complete blockage at the level of the papilla with a lacunar image produced by growth of the tumor.

Technique of Operative Cholangiography in Cancer of the Head of the Pancreas and Other Obstructions of the Distal Choledochus

FIGURE 16.16
Operative cholangiogram in case of cancer of papilla of Vater, with the biliary tree very distended and blockage complete and blunt at level of papilla. This cancer was very small, soft, and not palpable, and readily admitted probing of the duodenum. Biopsy through duodenotomy established the diagnosis.

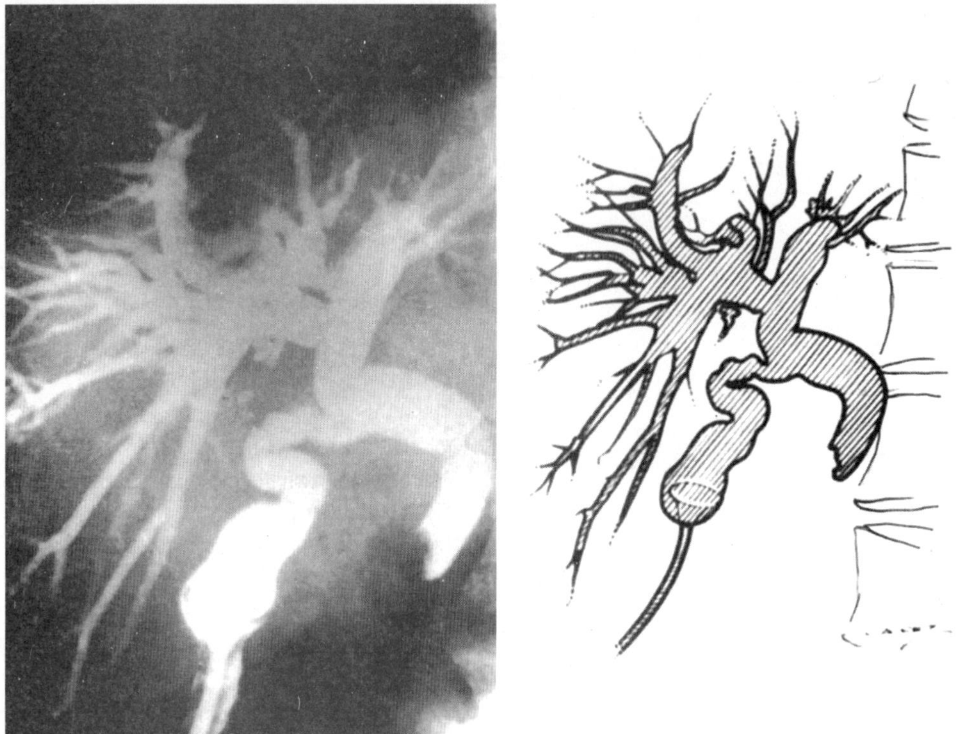

FIGURE 16.15

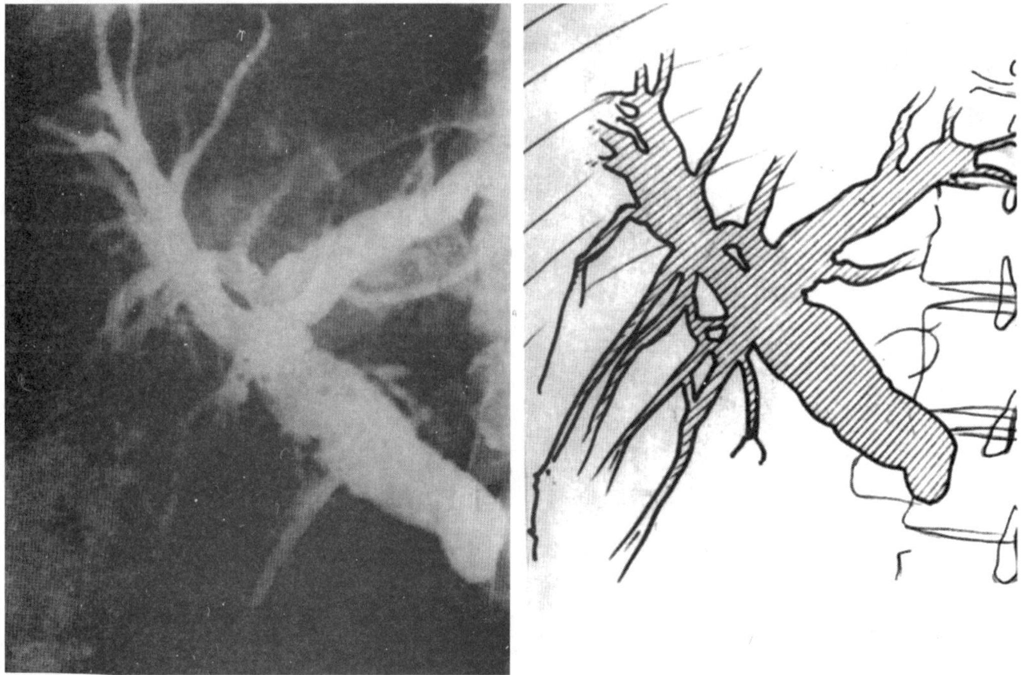

FIGURE 16.16

FIGURE 16.17
Operative cholangiography of a female patient with a very dilated choledochus with complete and blunt obstruction at the level of the papilla. Two prior surgical interventions had been performed elsewhere without operative cholangiography. The surgeon at these surgeries reported having found no calculi and no tumor, and that probing had been done easily and without detecting obstruction. At the patient's third surgery we found the operative cholangiogram as shown. The duodenotomy is shown in the next figure.

Technique of Operative Cholgangiography in Cancer of the Head of the Pancreas and Other Obstructions of the Distal Choledochus

FIGURE 16.18
This is a picture of the duodenotomy on the patient shown in Figure 16.17. The small tumor of the papilla is seen; it is soft, not palpable through the intact duodenum, and barely palpable with the duodenum open. Much more visible than palpable. Biopsy established the diagnosis of carcinoma and pancreaticoduodenectomy was performed.

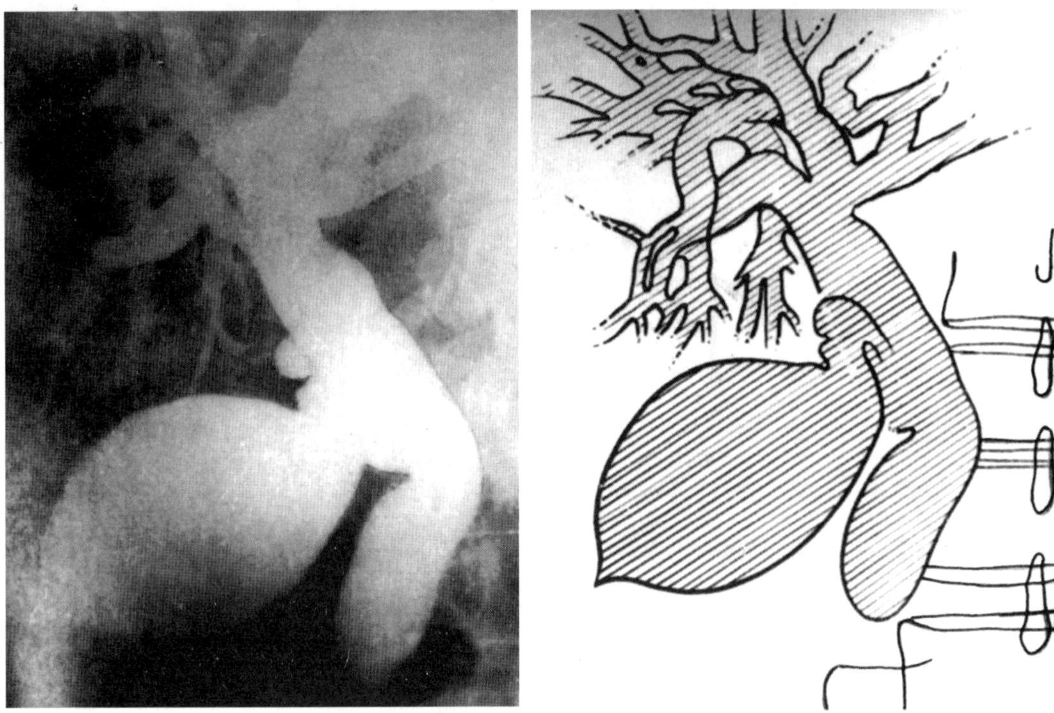

FIGURE 16.17

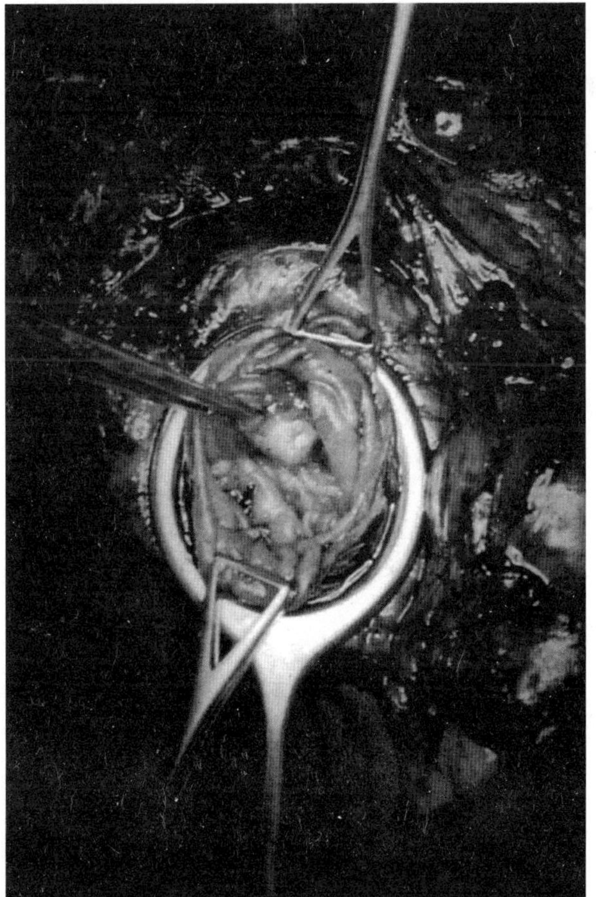

210

FIGURE 16.18

FIGURE 16.19
A 46-year-old female who had had biliary surgery for lithiasis plus removal of two choledochal stones. Operative cholangiography had not been performed. The surgeon found no other stones, and his dilators passed easily into the duodenum. The patient subsequently developed intense pains, which were relieved by opening the T-tube for drainage. We received her in transfer. Cholangiography through the T-tube was done together with gastroduodenography. One of these films is shown here. Complete and blunt blockage of the choledochus is seen at the level of the papilla. The gastroduodenography carried out simultaneously confirms this. Duodenostomy at surgery revealed a small, soft cancer of the papilla that permitted passage of dilators. Pancreaticoduodenectomy was performed.

Technique of Operative Cholangiography in Cancer of the Head of the Pancreas and Other Obstructions of the Distal Choledochus

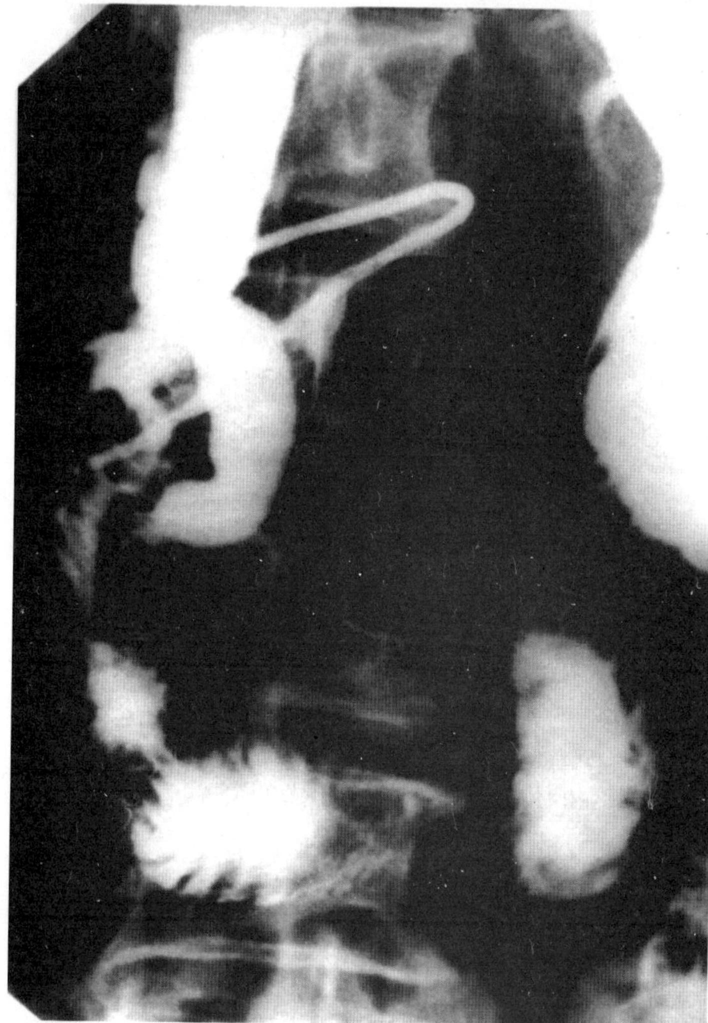

FIGURE 16.19

Vautrin-Kocher Maneuver

FIGURE 16.20 VAUTRIN-KOCHER MANEUVER
After scrupulously exploring the abdomen for metastatic disease, attention is directed to the biliohepatic duodenal area. To this purpose the Vautrin-Kocher maneuver is applied. This is done in two stages. The first stage takes down the transverse colon with its mesentery as portrayed in the drawing. This exposes all of the second portion of the duodenum plus the lateral aspect of the third portion. This takedown is done sharply with scissors (Fig. 16.21).

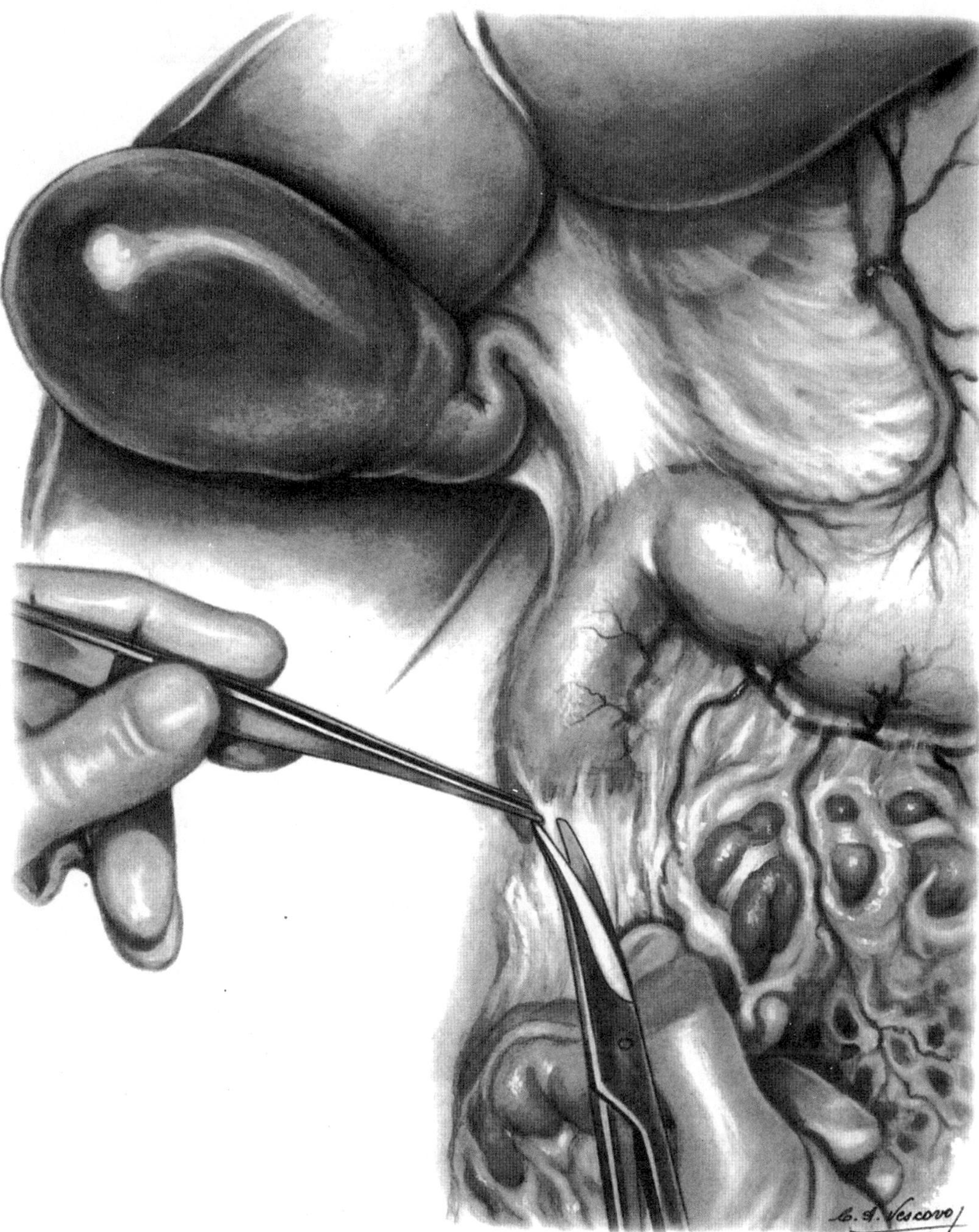

FIGURE 16.20 VAUTRIN-KOCHER MANEUVER

Vautrin-Kocher Maneuver

FIGURE 16.21
The transverse colon and its mesocolon are packed and retracted inferiorly. Stage 2 of the Vautrin-Kocher maneuver is then performed. All the length of the peritoneum at the lateral border of the second portion of the duodenum is incised to (include) the lateral segment of the third portion of the duodenum and the anterior leaf of the hepaticoduodenal ligament.

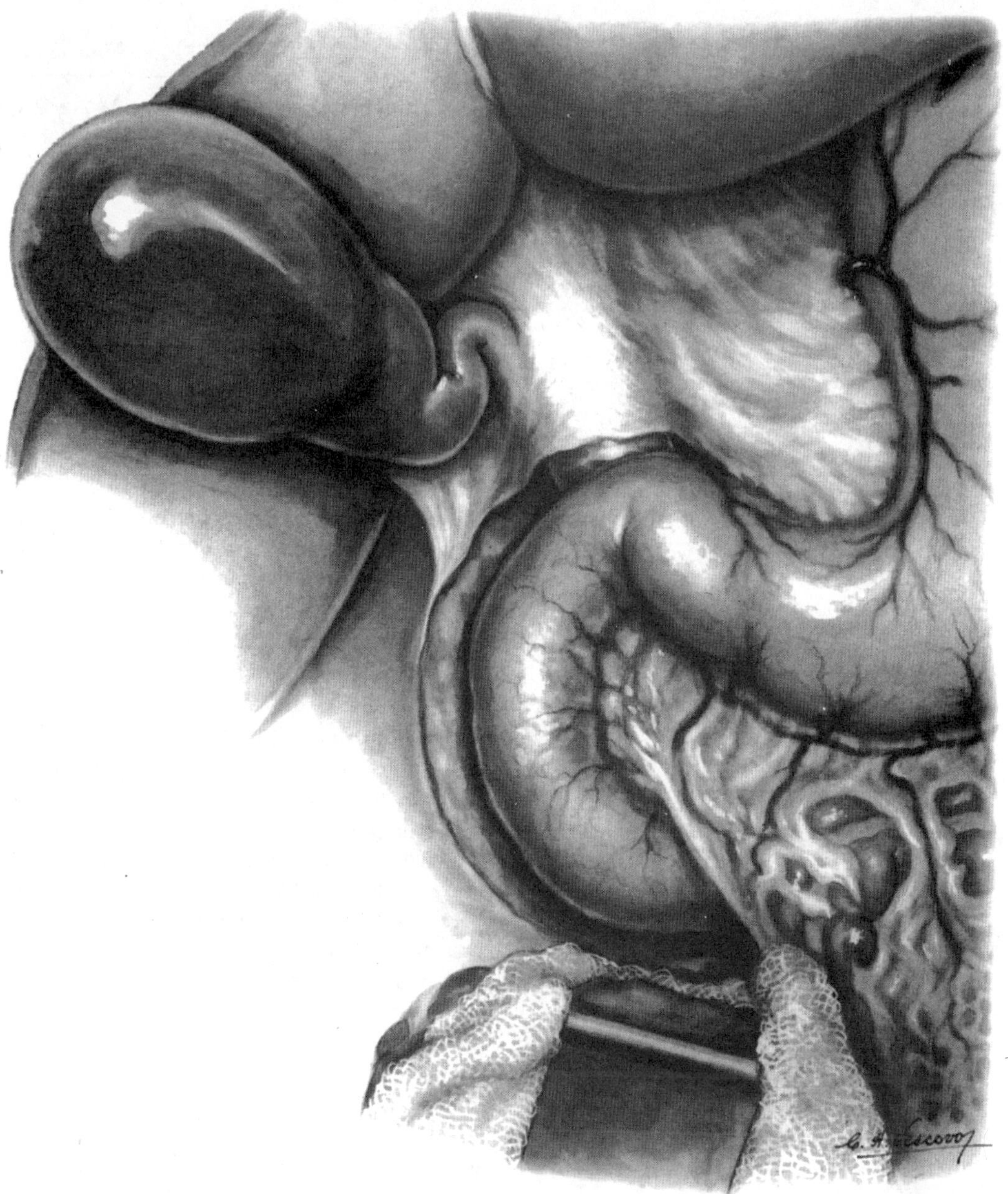

FIGURE 16.21

Vautrin-Kocher Maneuver

FIGURE 16.22

The lateral border of the second portion of the duodenum is retracted upward and to the left; this can be done either by the hand of the first assistant or with an atraumatic Foerster or Babcock type of instrument. This retraction has as its purpose to present to the surgeon that the surgeon may simply mobilize the duodenum and the head of the pancreas using the practically avascular plane of the fascia of Treitz. Correctly performed, the Vautrin-Kocher maneuver will display the inferior portion of the common duct, the superior posterior portion of the head of the pancreas, the inferior vena cava, part of the right renal vein (R), the internal portion of the perirenal fat with the kidney and right ureter (U), the right gonadal vein (G), the aorta (A), and the origin of the superior mesenteric artery. The Vautrin-Kocher maneuver will facilitate all subsequent surgical maneuvers and will permit determining whether the cancer of the head of the pancreas invades posterior tissues and the inferior vena cava. If the inferior vena cava is invaded, the tumor should be considered nonresectable.

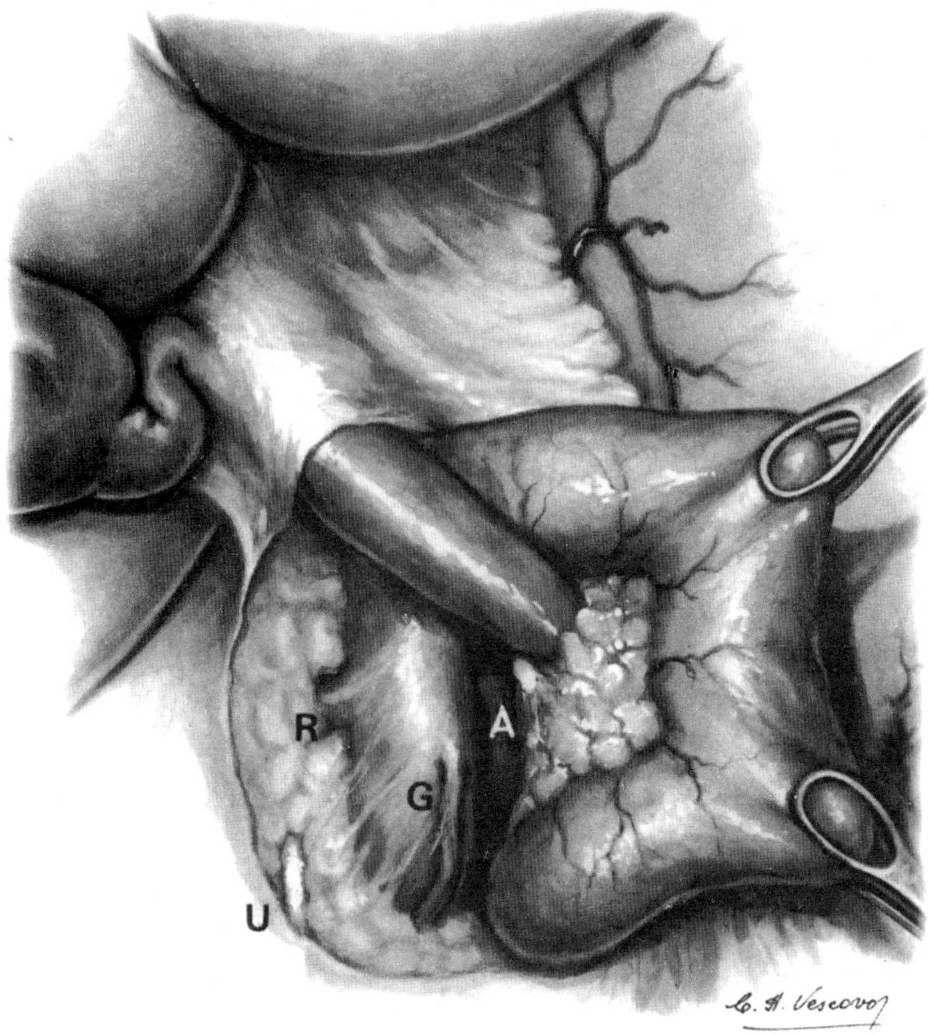

FIGURE 16.22

Surgical Exploration of the Pancreas

FIGURE 16.23

Upon completion of the Vautrin-Kocher maneuver, the gastrocolic ligament is divided under the vascular gastroepiploic arcade.

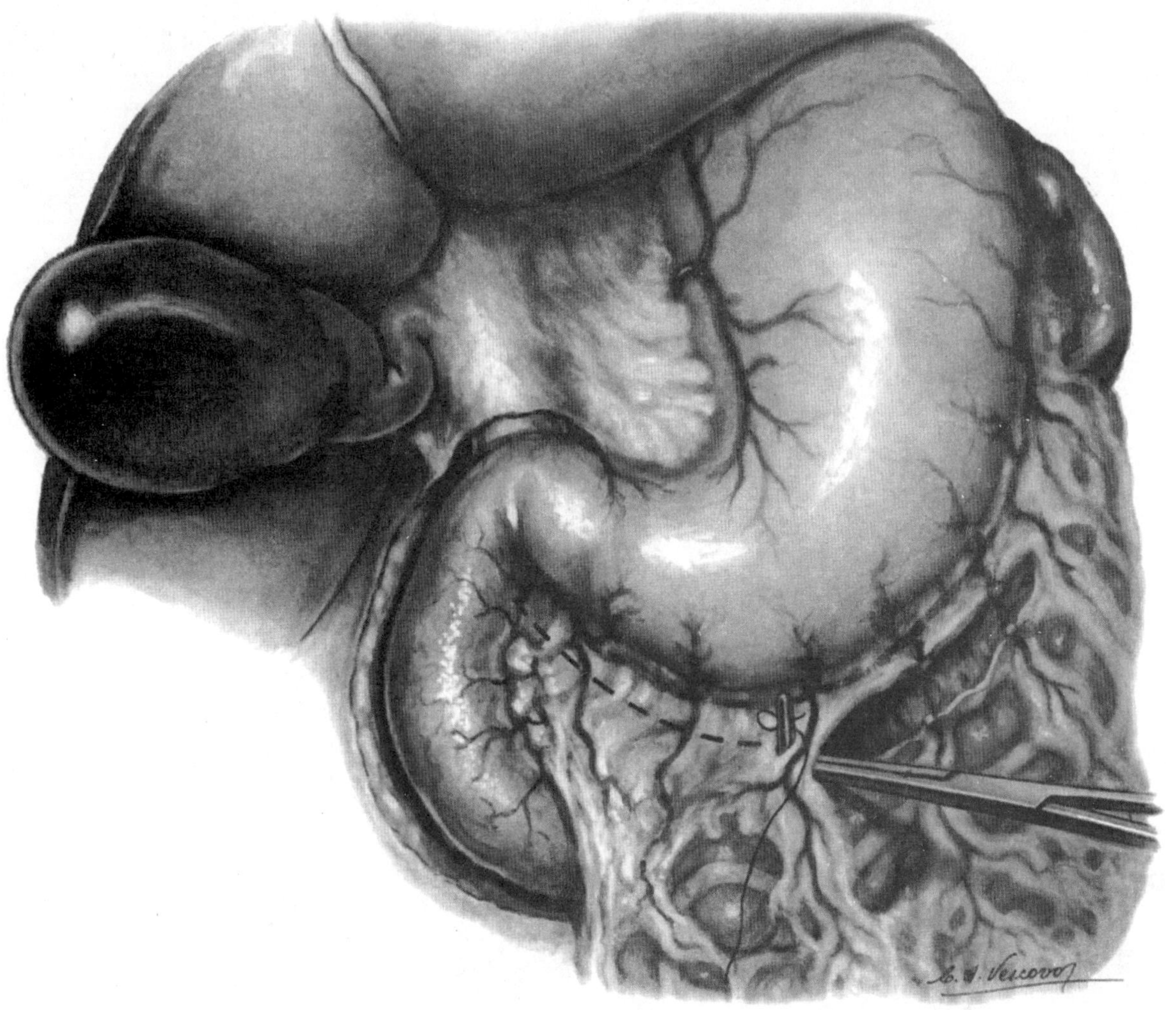

FIGURE 16.23

Surgical Exploration of the Pancreas

FIGURE 16.24
Once the gastrocolic ligament has been divided, traction is applied to the stomach upward and the transverse colon, with its mesocolon downward, exposing the entire anterior surface of the pancreas, as seen in the drawing.

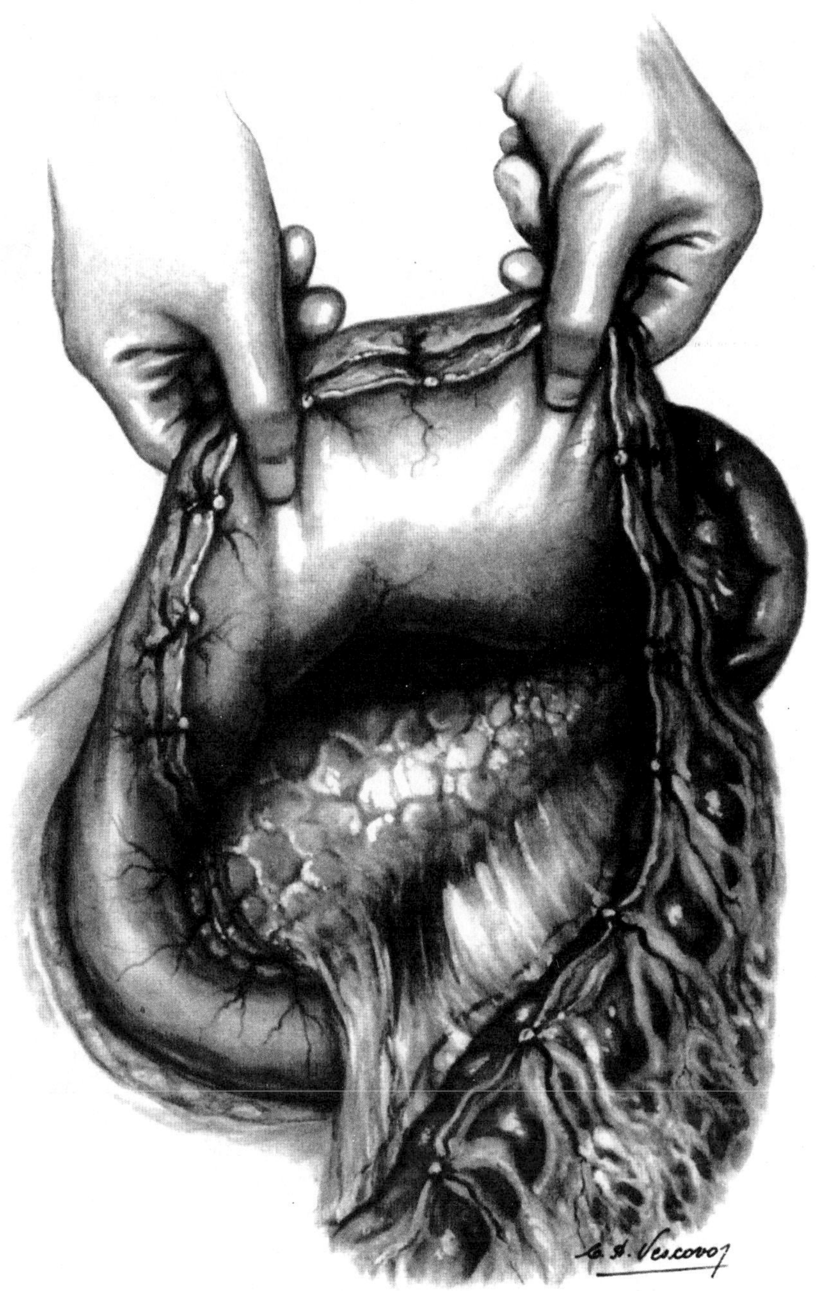

FIGURE 16.24

Surgical Exploration of the Pancreas

FIGURE 16.25

These maneuvers permit an adequate examination of the head of the pancreas anteriorly and posteriorly as well as the anterior surface of the body and tail of the pancreas. To palpate the head of the pancreas, the left thumb is placed anteriorly and the index and middle fingers of the left hand are placed posteriorly, as seen in the drawing. This maneuver permits one to determine if there is a mass in the head of the pancreas as well as its characteristics such as size, shape, consistency, softness, and limits. If the pancreatic duct is very dilated, it can also be felt by running the thumb along toward the left of the tumor, revealing a difference in consistency between the hard, irregular pancreatic mass and the elastic yielding consistency of the dilated pancreatic duct. The insert reveals a semischematic section of the details of this maneuver.

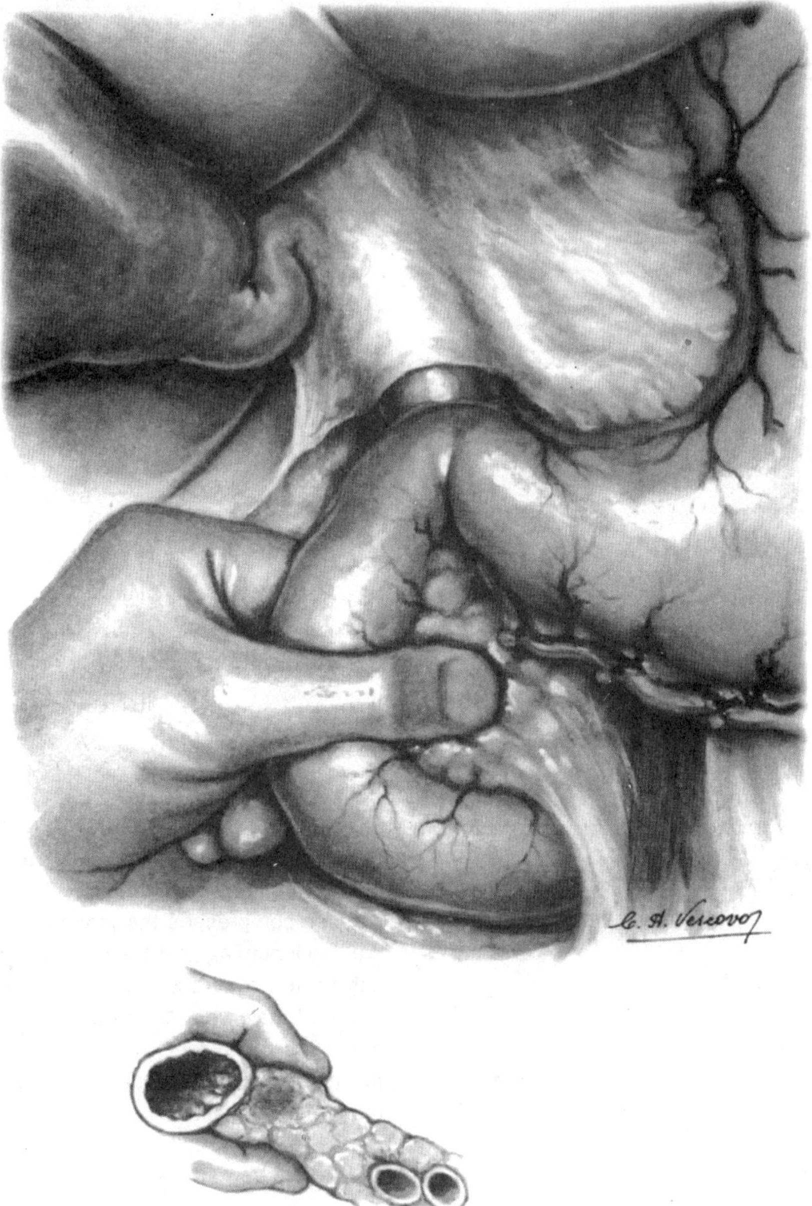

FIGURE 16.25

Surgical Exploration of the Pancreas

FIGURE 16.26 PALPATION OF THE PAPILLA

To feel a tumor of the papilla of Vater the maneuver shown in the drawing may be useful.(19, 20, 23) The right thumb of the surgeon compresses the antimesenteric or external border of the duodenum against the mesenteric or internal border. An exophytic tumor of the papilla is easily palpable with this maneuver. Small, soft tumors and small intrapapillary tumors are more difficult to feel. Some other maneuvers described later for the detection of these tumors will be necessary. (See "Tumors of the Papilla.")

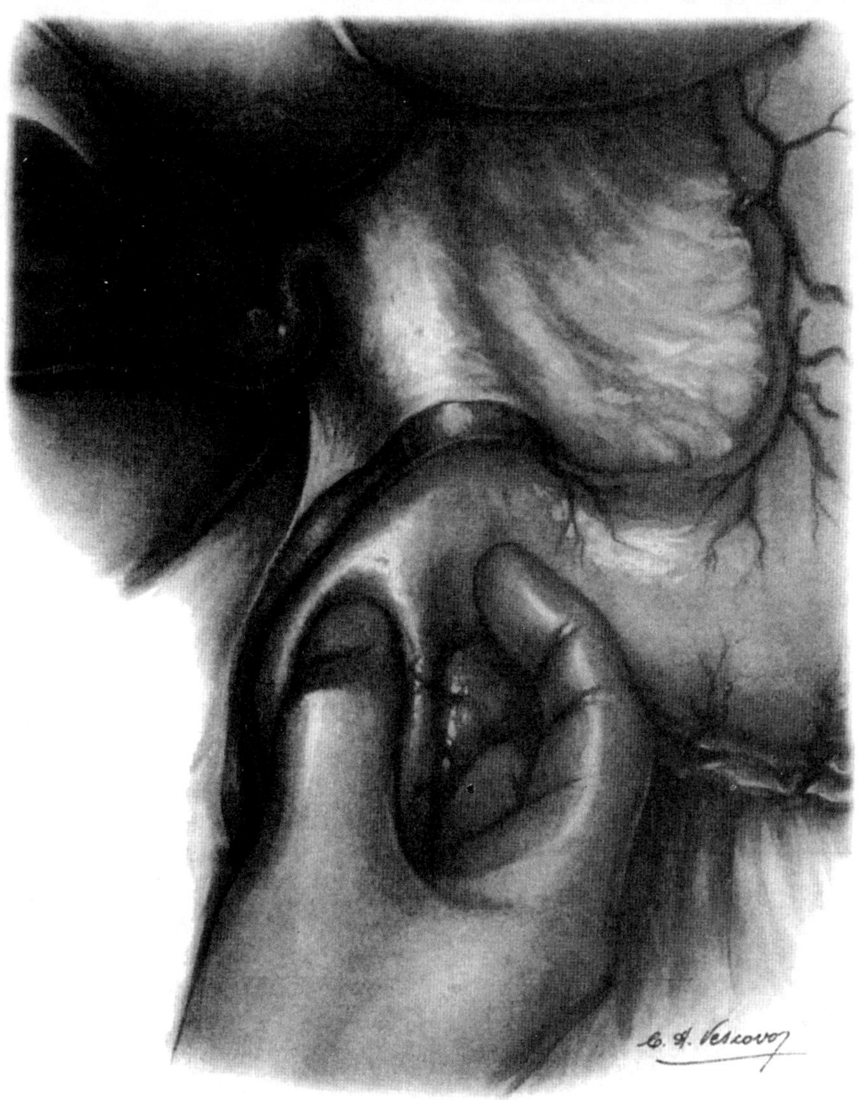

FIGURE 16.26 PALPATION OF THE PAPILLA

Surgical Exploration of the Pancreas

FIGURE 16.27 PALPATION OF THE UNCINATE PROCESS
During the fulfillment of these preresectional maneuvers, one should try to feel the uncinate process. A useful maneuver is that which is observed in the drawing. To perform it, the peritoneum over the interior border of the pancreas at the level of the neck is transected. The surgeon should then place the palm of his or her left hand behind the head and neck of the pancreas, and the pulp of his right index finger underneath the neck, attempting to feel the uncinate process, which is located behind the superior mesenteric vessels.

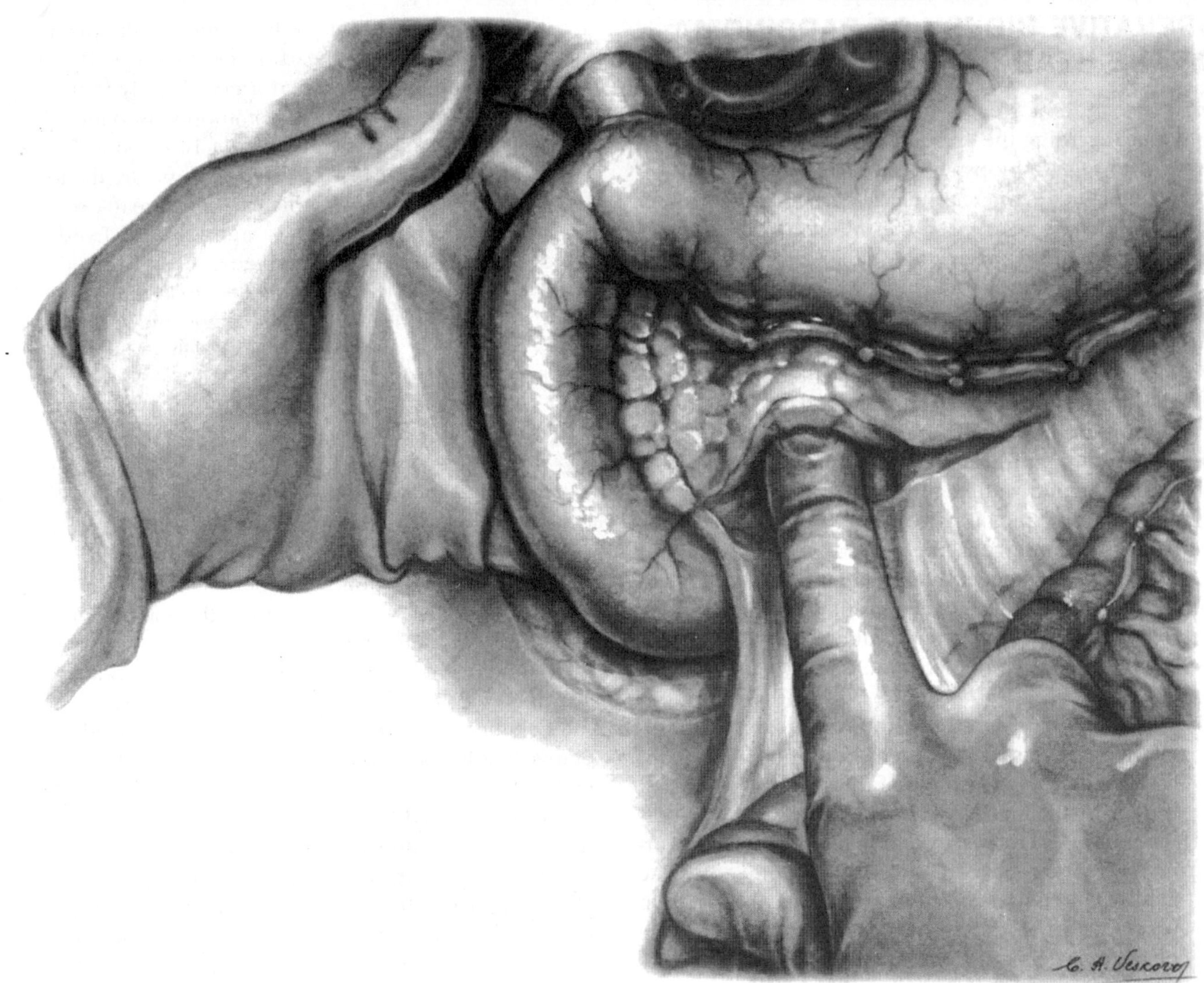

FIGURE 16.27 PALPATION OF THE UNCINATE PROCESS

OPERATIVE BIOPSY OF CARCINOMA OF THE HEAD OF THE PANCREAS

For many years a great controversy has existed among surgeons regarding the convenience and value of operative frozen section biopsy for the diagnosis of carcinoma of the head of the pancreas. It has been stated that frozen section biopsy is insecure in the differentiation of carcinoma from chronic pancreatitis.(19, 20, 31, 53, 90) Other complications have also been attributed to operative biopsy of the pancreas, such as pancreatic fistulas, hemorrhages, and acute pancreatitis.(7) There are surgeons who believe that the fear of complications due to pancreatic biopsy has been exaggerated.(6, 23, 31, 41, 44, 88) At present biopsies are frequently performed preoperatively using a fine needle with ultrasonographic control and computerized axial tomography, as well as by means of endoscopic biopsy.(102)

Before performing a pancreaticoduodenectomy for carcinoma of the pancreas, it is convenient to have a histologic diagnosis. This, however, is not always possible.

Operative biopsy of a pancreatic mass can be performed by three different techniques:

1. *Direct Biopsy:* This is only practical in large, superficial tumors, especially when the tumor mass is located in the neighborhood of the superior or inferior border of the pancreas. Direct biopsy can be performed by excision or preferably with a Vim-Silverman or a Travenol "Tru-cut" disposable needle. The latter is preferable because excisional biopsy can lead to complications. Besides, carcinoma of the pancreas is generally surrounded by an inflammatory process (peritumoral pancreatitis) and excisional biopsy may not be representative.(6, 18, 19, 21, 22, 44, 48, 52, 63, 70, 88)
2. *Transduodenal Biopsy:* This can be performed through the duodenum, either closed or open using a Vim-Silverman or "Tru-cut" needle as shown in Figure 16.28. Transduodenal biopsy has a much lower chance of leading to pancreatic fistula and is especially indicated in small, deep tumors of the pancreas.(6, 21, 22)
3. *Fine Needle Aspiration Biopsy:* Aspiration biopsy with a fine needle, to obtain cytologic examinations, is being used more and more frequently in the diagnosis of carcinoma of the head of the pancreas. Puncture and aspiration may be performed directly or through the duodenum. The most commonly used technique is as follows: a 23 needle with a 10 mL syringe containing 3 to 4 mL of air is used to puncture the tumor and aspirate material, which is then spread on a sterile slide. The material is immediately fixed and stained. The air in the syringe is used to be able to completely empty the aspirated material in the syringe and the needle. It is indispensable to obtain the services of an experienced cytologist to interpret the preparation.(13, 102)

A positive result, either histologic or cytologic, has great value. If the result is negative, it should be ignored and a diagnosis of probable carcinoma of the head of the pancreas made if the following conditions are met: solid, hard, irregular mass of the head of the pancreas in a nonalcoholic patient with deep obstructive jaundice and great dilation of the gallbladder and biliary tree. Operative cholangiography can add to these findings of a very dilated biliary tree both extra- and intrahepatic, and a complete blunt obstruction of the common bile duct at a level above the papilla. Operative cholangiography adds to the diagnosis by exclusion of the presence of an impacted calculus in the end of the dilated bile duct.(18, 22, 39, 40, 50, 70) The most difficult problem for the surgeon is differentiating between carcinoma of the head of the pancreas and chronic pancreatitis with a predominant location in the head of the pancreas obstructing the common bile duct and producing jaundice, which is present in 10 to 30% of cases. If the pancreatitis does not obstruct the common bile duct and therefore does not produce jaundice, the diagnosis is easier. Retropancreatic obstruction of the common bile duct in the great majority of cases of chronic pancreatitis is only partial with the characteristics we have mentioned in our description of the cholangiography. On the other hand, if the chronic pancreatitis of alcoholic origin and predominant localization in the head of the pancreas presents a pancreatic duct of normal caliber, the indicated treatment is also pancreaticoduodenectomy as the condition is not controllable by medical treatment.

Operative Biopsy of Carcinoma of the Head of the Pancreas

FIGURE 16.28
Biopsy of a mass in the head of the pancreas with a Travenol "Tru-cut" needle through the closed duodenum. With this technique a pancreatic fistula only rarely occurs. With a similar technique an aspiration biopsy of the pancreatic mass using a fine needle can be performed for cytologic examination.

Operative Biopsy of Carcinoma of the Head of the Pancreas

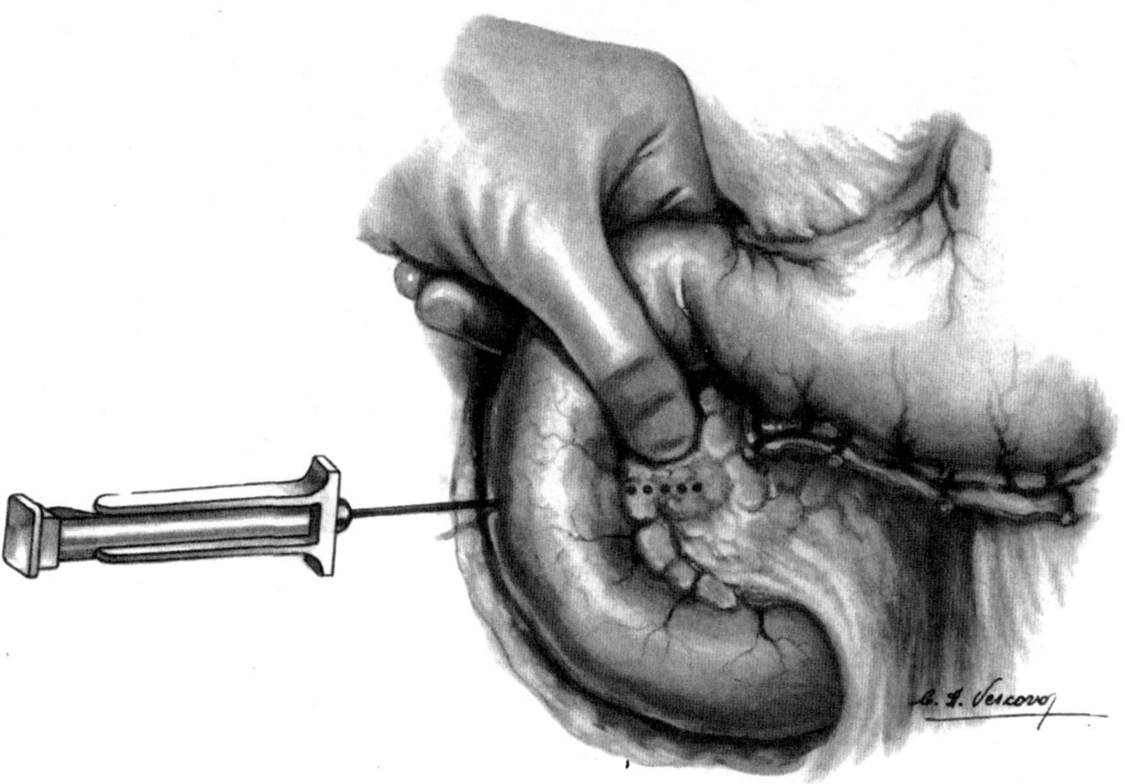

FIGURE 16.28

Determination of Local Resectability of Carcinoma of the Head of the Pancreas

FIGURE 16.29

A dissection of the horizontal portion of the common hepatic artery is performed beginning at its origin in the celiac axis, removing some areolar tissue and 2 or 3 lymph nodes, which should be submitted for frozen section study. Once the common hepatic artery has been dissected, the gastroduodenal and pyloric (right gastric) arteries are ligated. Ligature of the gastroduodenal artery should be very carefully performed to avoid its slippage, which can lead to severe hemorrhage.

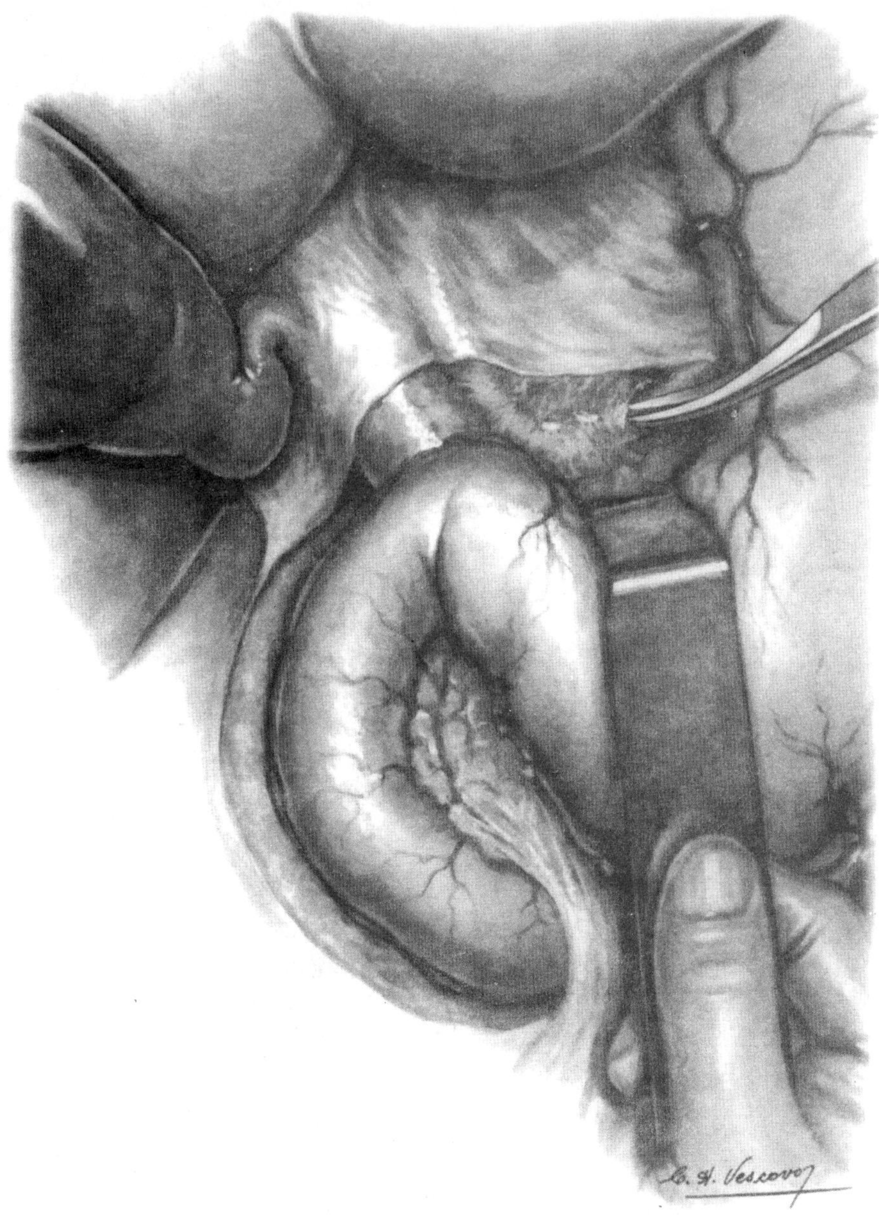

FIGURE 16.29

Determination of Local Resectability of Carcinoma of the Head of the Pancreas

FIGURE 16.30

The drawing shows the stumps of the gastroduodenal and pyloric arteries. A Penrose has been passed around the common bile duct, which is very dilated, and traction is applied to the Penrose toward the right, exposing the portal vein in a more posterior plane.

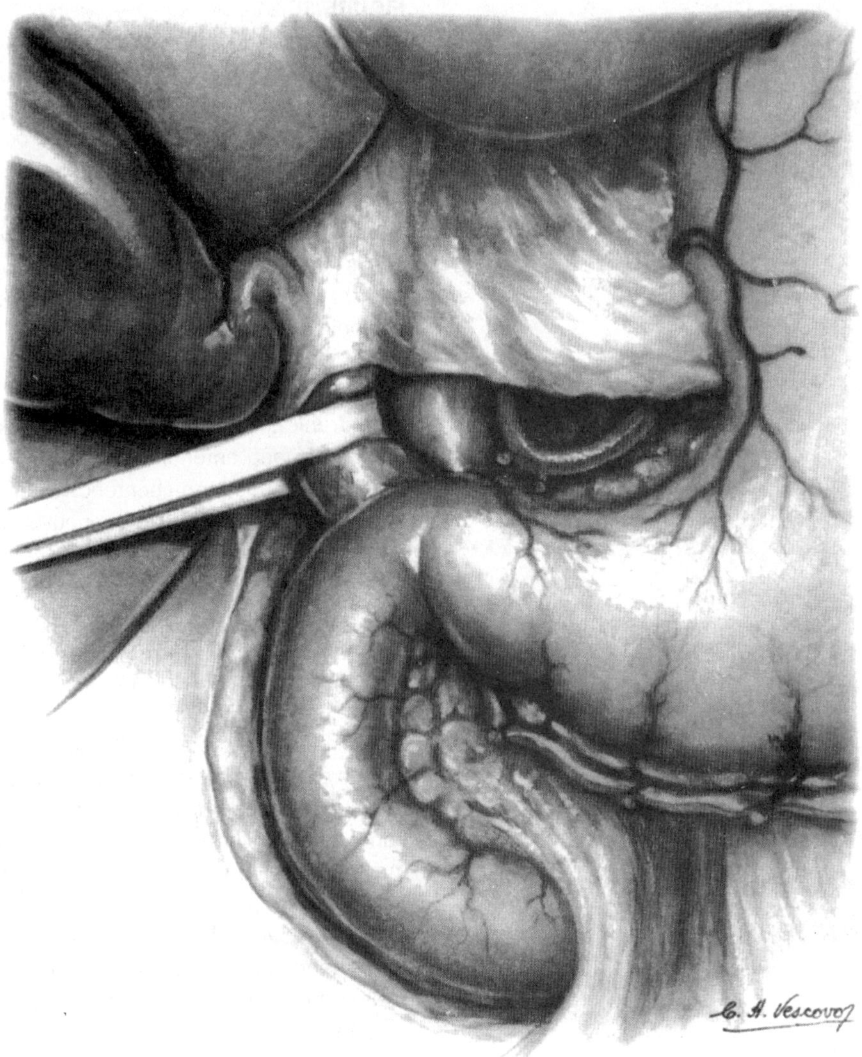

FIGURE 16.30

FIGURE 16.31

The previously performed maneuvers permit the introduction of the left index finger of the surgeon from above downward between the portal vein and the posterior surface of the neck of the pancreas. The surgeon then introduces the right index finger under the inferior border of the neck of the pancreas, whose peritoneum has been transected, as can be seen in the superior or inferior inserts of the drawing. The right index finger is directed upward between the superior mesenteric vein and the posterior surface of the neck of the pancreas. Before beginning this maneuver the middle colic vessels, Henle's trunk, and the inferior pancreaticoduodenal arteries should be identified to avoid injuring them. Occasionally, the common arterial trunk of the inferior pancreaticoduodenals or the individual inferior and anterior pancreaticoduodenal arteries pass in front of the superior mesenteric vein in their course toward the head of the pancreas. The maneuver of passing the left index and the right index fingers between the venous of the portomesenteric axis and the posterior surface of the neck of the pancreas should be performed with extreme care trying to get the pulp of the index fingers to touch. If this can be attained, it means that the carcinoma does not infiltrate the wall of the portomesenteric venous axis. If the fingers cannot be approximated because there is interposed hard, irregular tissue, it means that the patient has an inoperable, unresectable carcinoma of the head of the pancreas. In some cases of chronic pancreatitis of the pancreatic head, passage of these fingers may be quite difficult due to narrowing caused by the chronic pancreatitis.

Determination of Local Resectability of Carcinoma of the Head of the Pancreas

Both in carcinoma of the head of the pancreas infiltrating the anterior wall of the venous axis, as well as in narrowing caused by chronic pancreatitis, insistence on passing the fingers may lead to severe bleeding that is very difficult to control. Usually the pulp of the fingertips can be joined without difficulty because the efferent pancreatic veins empty into the side and not into the anterior surface of the portomesenteric venous axis. For this reason, the fingers of the surgeon should remain on the anterior wall of the venous axis.

It should also be kept in mind that in some patients, the carcinoma may not invade the anterior wall of the venous axis but its lateral walls. This can only be confirmed after sectioning the pancreas. It is therefore advisable not to perform any maneuver that will not allow one to discontinue the procedure until the pancreas has been transected and it has been shown that the portomesenteric venous axis has not been infiltrated laterally. Palpation of the uncinate process as previously described, has great importance, since, if it is infiltrated, it should be considered that the patient has an unresectable carcinoma of the head of the pancreas.

Once resectability of the carcinoma of the head of the pancreas has been confirmed, one can proceed with pancreaticoduodenectomy.

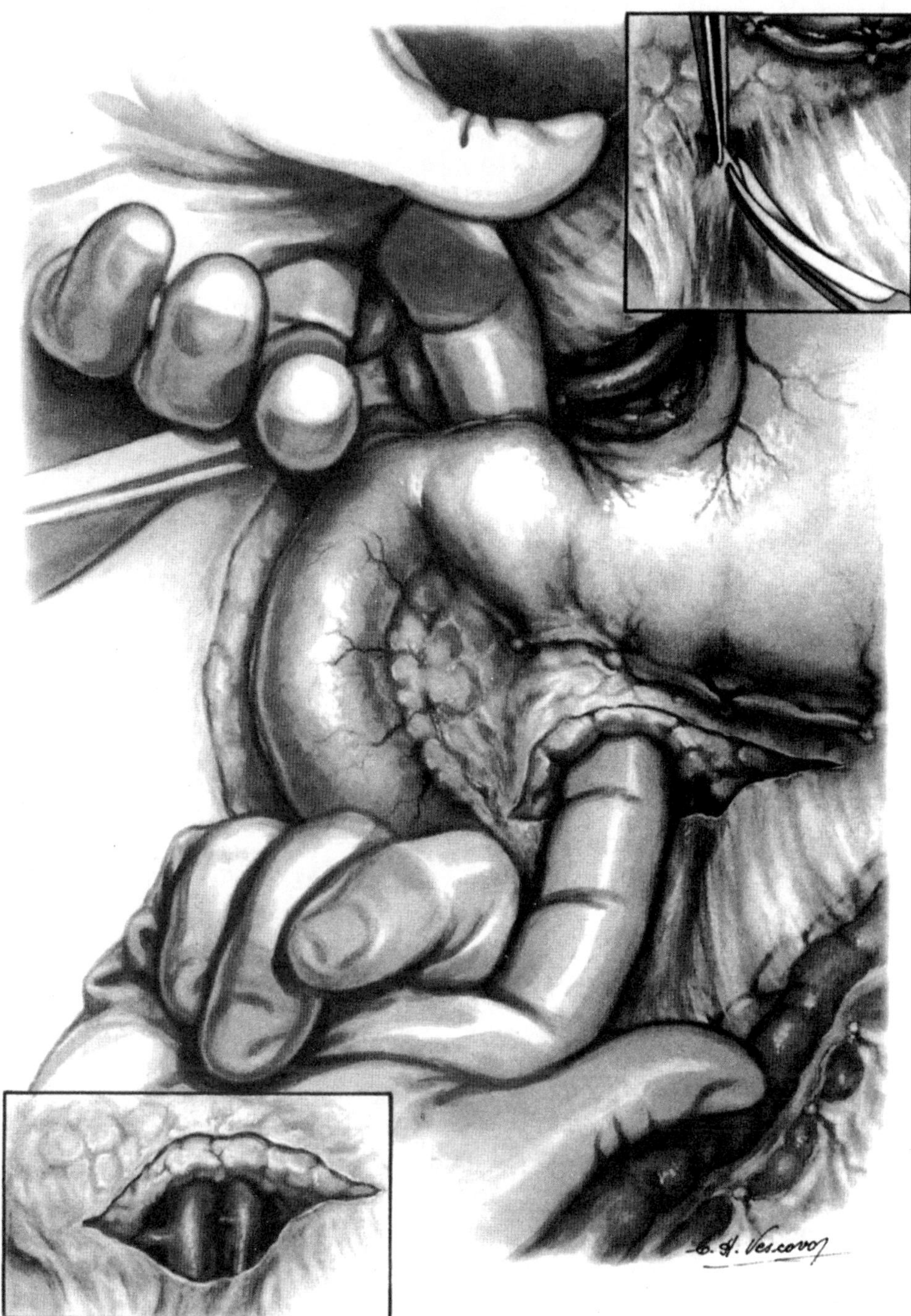

FIGURE 16.31

Technique of Resection of Carcinoma of the Head of the Pancreas

FIGURE 16.32
Semischematic drawing showing the extent of resection in a classical pancreaticoduodenectomy. The lined areas represent what should be resected: head, neck, and proximal segment of the body of the pancreas, distal end of the stomach, the entire duodenum, some 12 to 15 cm of the proximal jejunum, the gallbladder, and the distal common bile duct. One generally adds a truncal bilateral vagotomy to the hemigastrectomy to diminish the complications of ulcer or postoperative hemorrhage.

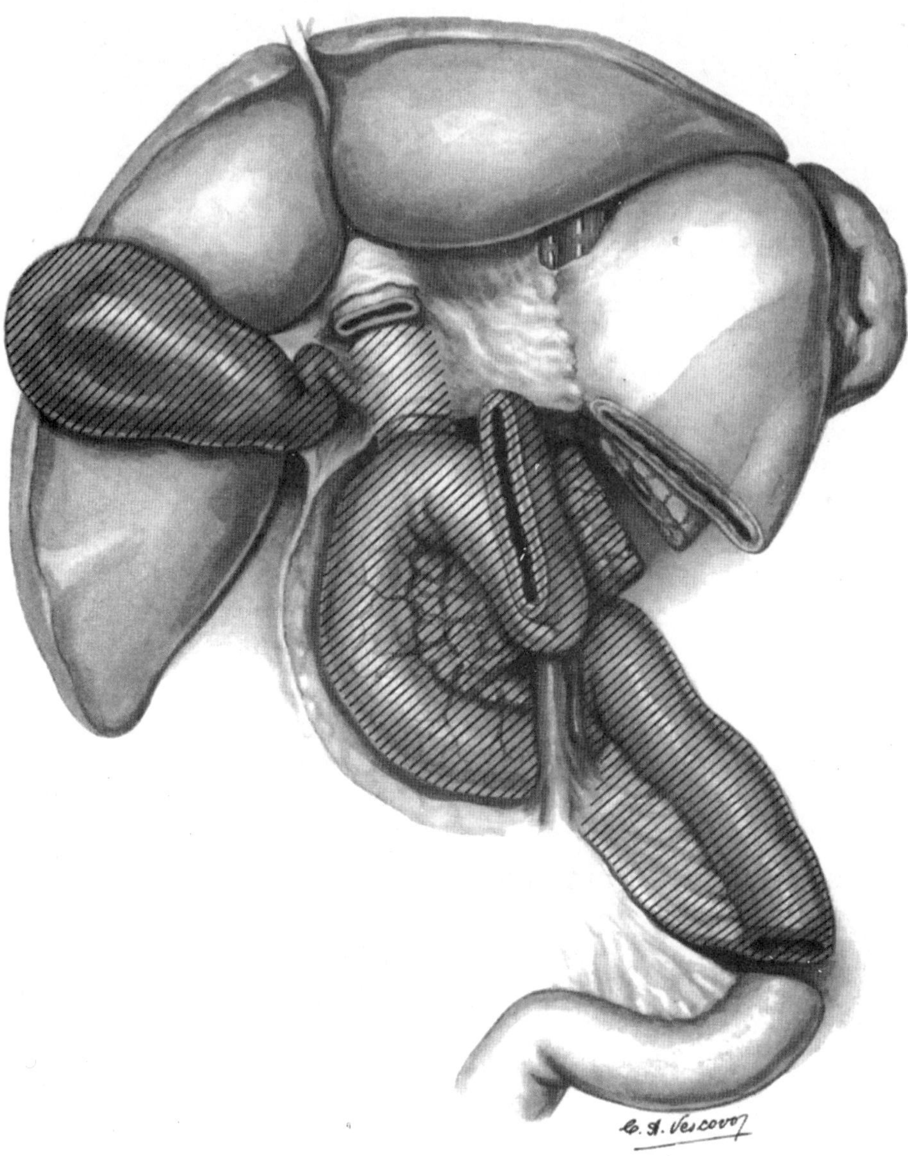

FIGURE 16.32

Technique of Resection of Carcinoma of the Head of the Pancreas

FIGURE 16.33
The drawing shows a preparation for a hemigastrectomy. Prior to the transection of the stomach the coronary artery has been ligated some 2 to 3 cm below the level at which this artery enters the lesser curvature. The gastroepiploic arcade along the greater curvature has been ligated approximately at the point of junction of the right gastroepiploic and left gastroepiploic arteries. Two elastic Finochietto or similar clamps are placed across the stomach and the stomach transected between them, using straight scissors.

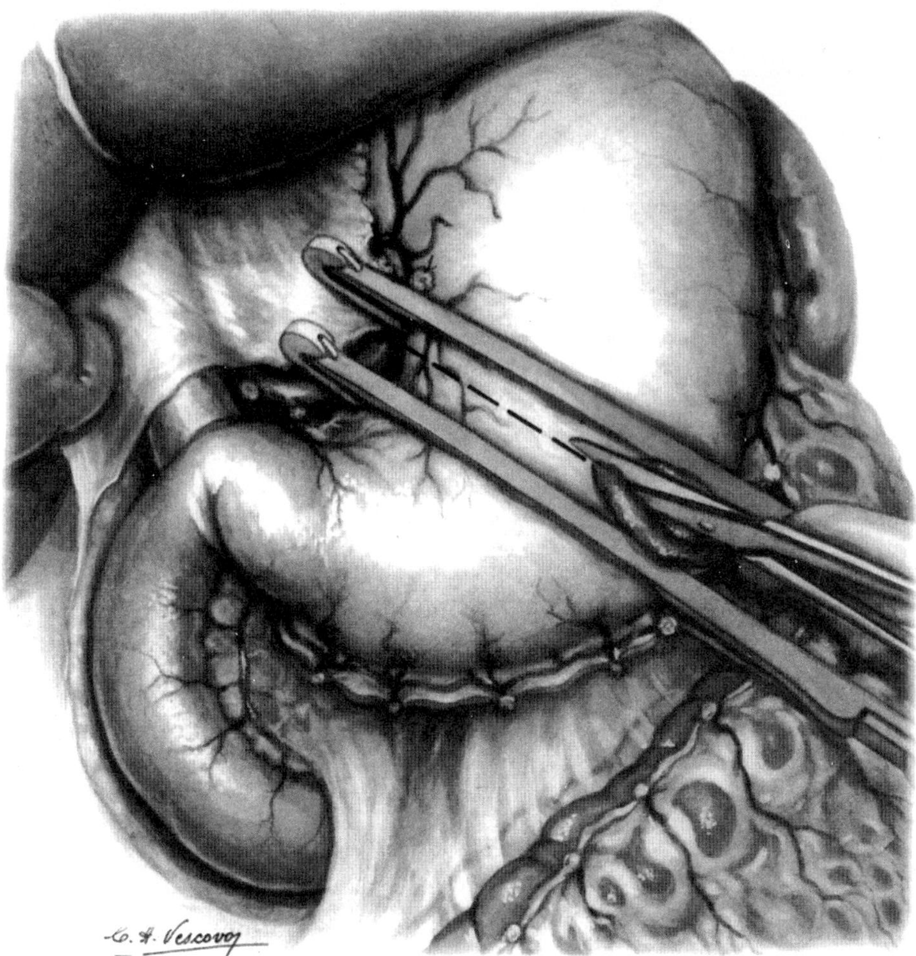

FIGURE 16.33

Technique of Resection of Carcinoma of the Head of the Pancreas

FIGURE 16.34
Once the stomach has been divided, the distal gastric segment is drawn to the right while the proximal gastric segment is left in place covered with a gauze pad. Both segments should remain clamped. The anterior surface of the pancreas is now clearly exposed.

FIGURE 16.35
We prefer to perform the transection of the pancreas about 4 to 6 cm to the left of the superior mesenteric artery and not at the level of the superior mesenteric vein as is frequently performed. For this purpose it is necessary to ligate 3 or 4 tributary veins entering the splenic vein. To perform these ligatures the peritoneum over the superior border of the pancreas is divided and the previous incision over the peritoneum over the inferior border is extended. The first assistant, using two hands, grasps the inferior border of the pancreas and reflects it upward, allowing the surgeon to perform the ligature of the tributary veins and allowing his index and middle fingers to grasp behind the pancreas without causing hemorrhage.

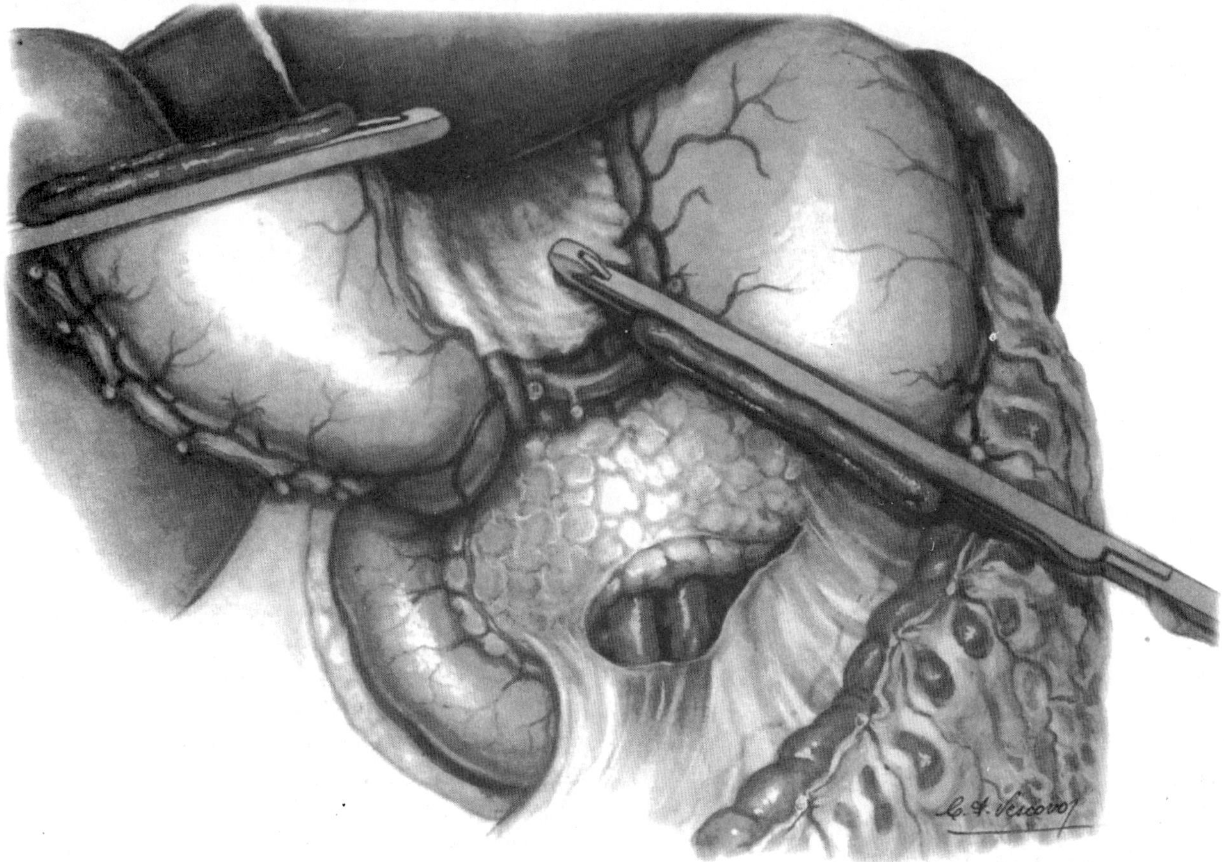

FIGURE 16.34

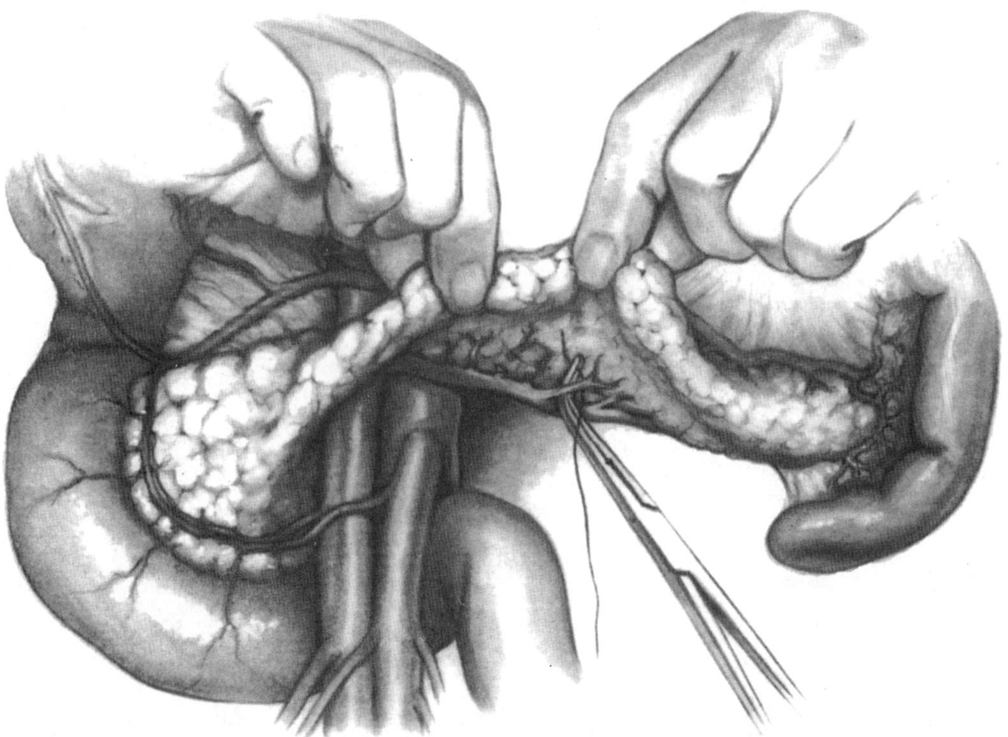

FIGURE 16.35

FIGURE 16.36
The tributary veins of the splenic vein have been divided and the surgeon can introduce the right index and middle fingers behind the pancreas to facilitate transection. This transection is performed 4 to 6 cm to the left of the superior mesenteric artery. This has some advantages over transecting the pancreas as is usually done at the level of the neck. Transection of the pancreas at the level of the body takes one further away from the primary tumor located in the head and therefore is performed in normal pancreatic tissue. On the other hand, if one has plans to perform a pancreaticojejunostomy by intussusception, the diameter of the pancreas at this level is usually smaller, making introduction of the pancreatic stump into the jejunum easier. Finally, if the pancreaticojejunal anastomosis were complicated by a fistula formation, it would have greater possibilities of closing faster. Transection of the pancreas at the indicated level does not produce any endocrine or exocrine insufficiency.

Technique of Resection of Carcinoma of the Head of the Pancreas

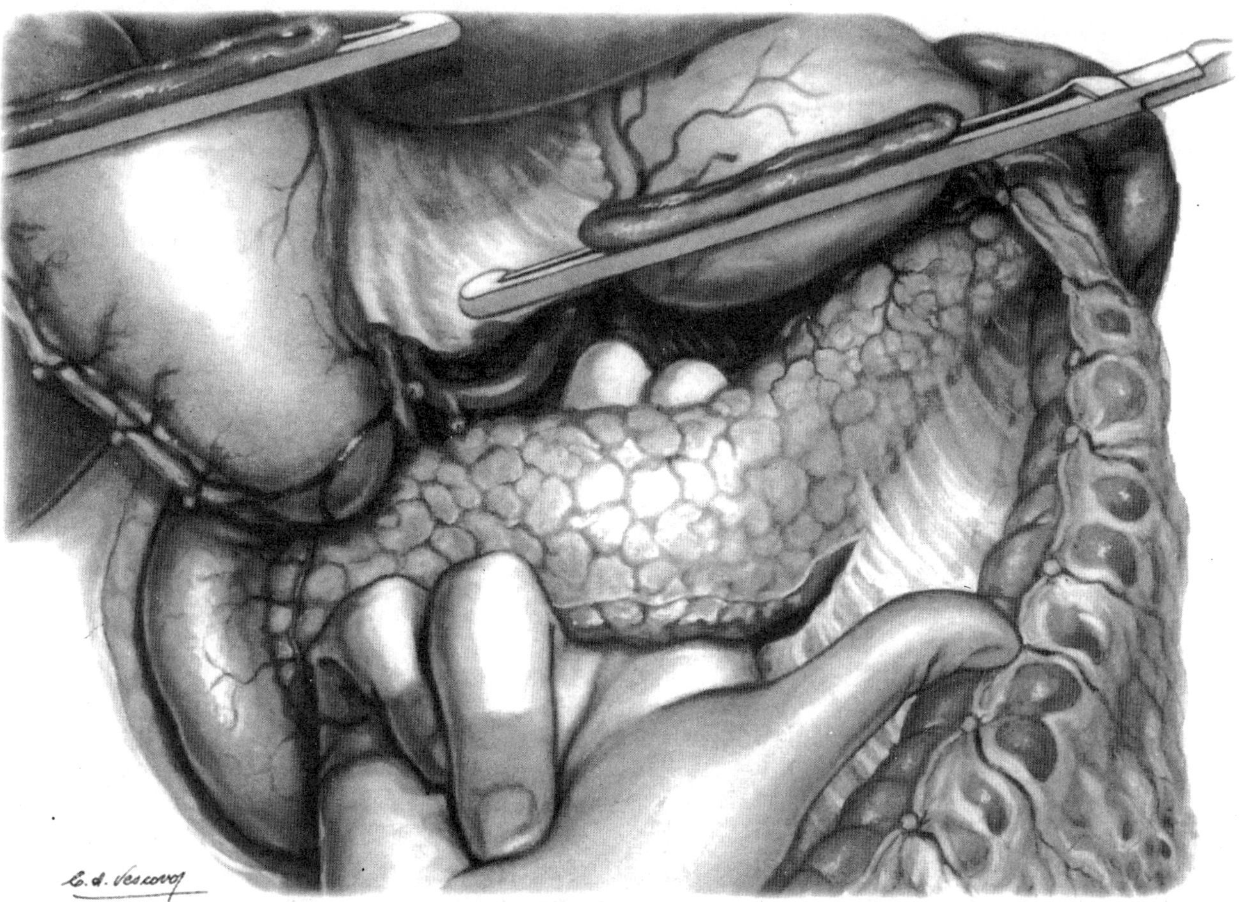

FIGURE 16.36

Technique of Resection of Carcinoma of the Head of the Pancreas

FIGURE 16.37

Once the level at which the pancreas is to be transected has been selected, large, straight atraumatic vascular clamps are placed with the object of diminishing blood loss from the transected pancreas and preventing spillage of pancreatic fluid, which would contain neoplastic cells that can be implanted and colonized. One must protect the abdominal cavity with compresses before transecting the pancreas. As shown, the section of the pancreas is done with a scalpel.

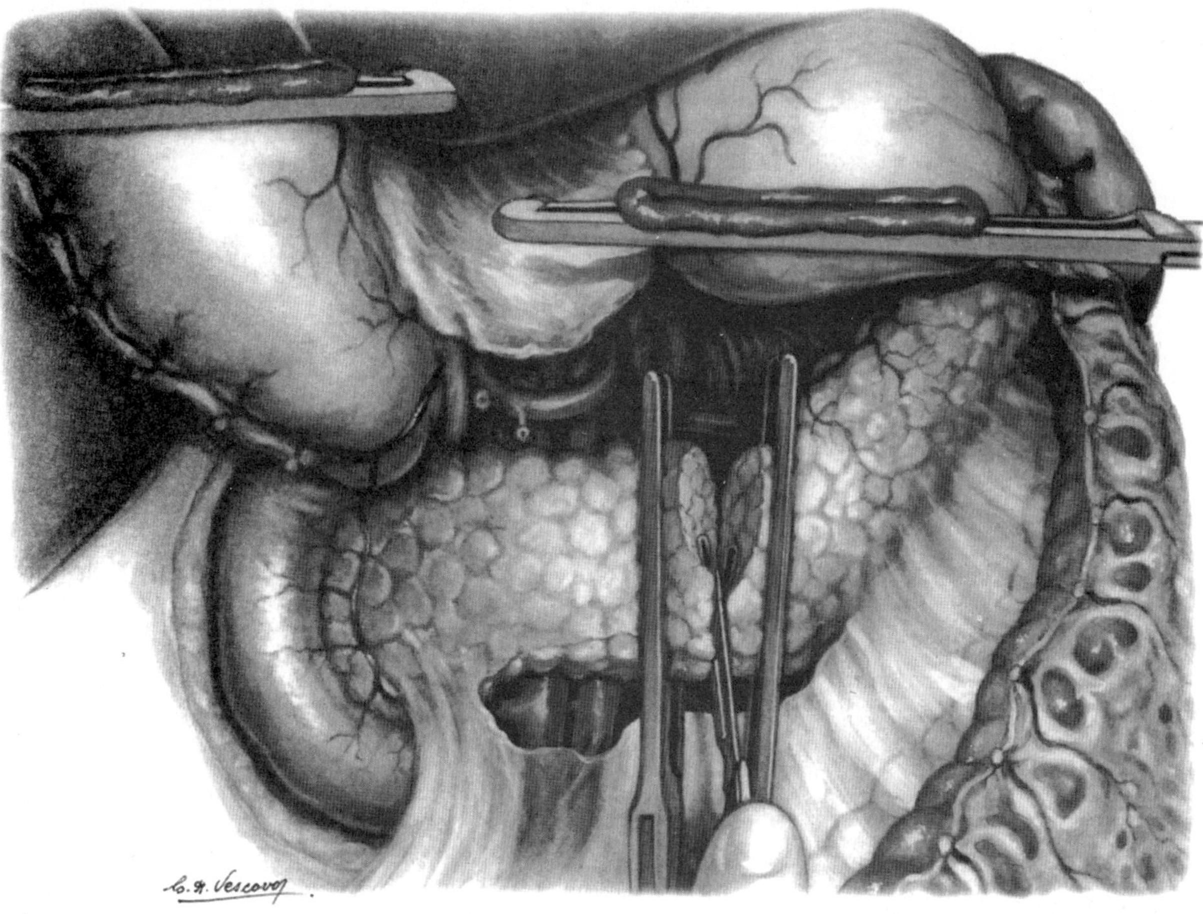

FIGURE 16.37

FIGURE 16.38

The pancreas has been transected, and the pancreatic duct of the segment to be resected has been closed with interrupted cotton or silk sutures to prevent spillage of pancreatic fluid. The distal segment of the pancreas is protected with gauze compresses, which are not shown in the drawing. Immediately after transecting the pancreas, it is possible to confirm if the carcinoma is invading the portomesenteric venous axis laterally. If the venous axis has been invaded, resection is interrupted, as the case is considered to be inoperable.

Technique of Resection of Carcinoma of the Head of the Pancreas

If the venous axis is not invaded laterally, resection of the pancreas is continued, removing the gallbladder as the next step and then transecting the hepatic duct immediately above the entrance of the cystic duct. Henle's venous trunk is then ligated and the inferior pancreaticoduodenal arteries are then tied and divided. The next step is to transect the jejunum some 12 to 15 cm from the ligament of Treitz. Finally a bilateral truncal vagotomy is performed. The drawing shows the transected pancreas with its proximal segment reflected to the right, revealing the head of the pancreas joined to the superior mesenteric vessels by a series of small veins and arteries that have to be ligated individually with great care. One can also observe the transected hepatic duct obstructed by a bulldog clamp to avoid spillage of bile into the peritoneal cavity. Resection of the gallbladder is being performed from the neck toward the fundus. Here, after transection of the pancreas, if the venous portomesenteric trunk is found to be invaded laterally, the operation is finished, resecting the distal pancreatic segment together with the spleen and re-establishing gastric continuity, suturing both gastric segments in two planes. The abdominal wall is closed in layers, leaving a suction drainage in the pancreatic bed.

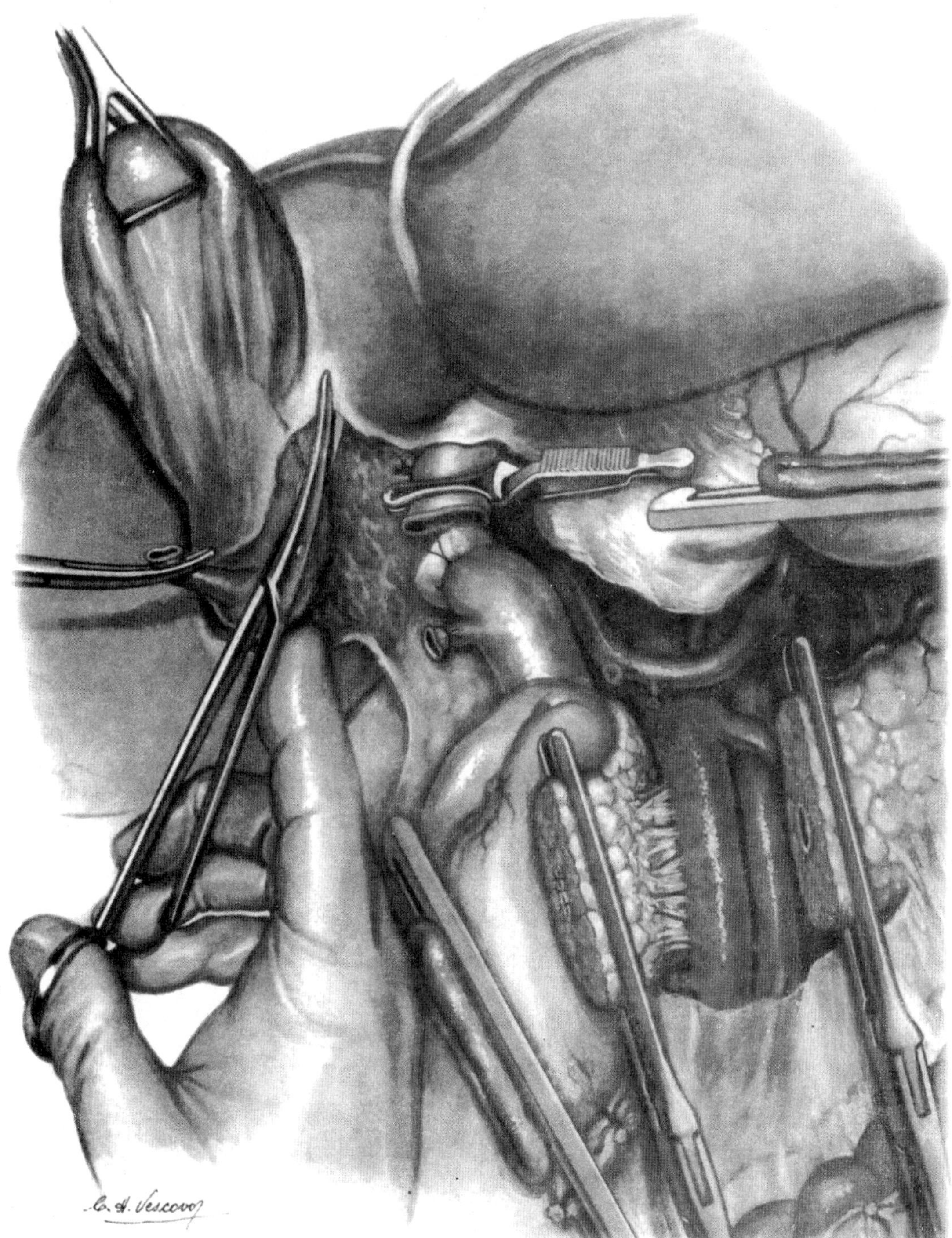

FIGURE 16.38

Technique of Resection of Carcinoma of the Head of the Pancreas

FIGURE 16.39

After the pancreas is transected and no lateral infiltration of the portomesenteric venous axis is demonstrable, one proceeds to transect the jejunum. To perform this, the transverse colon with its mesocolon is elevated and the jejunum grasped with a Foerster clamp, as shown in the drawing, applying smooth traction toward the right and upward. Using a scissors, the fibromuscular ligament of Treitz is transected and the entire duodenal jejunal flexure freed.

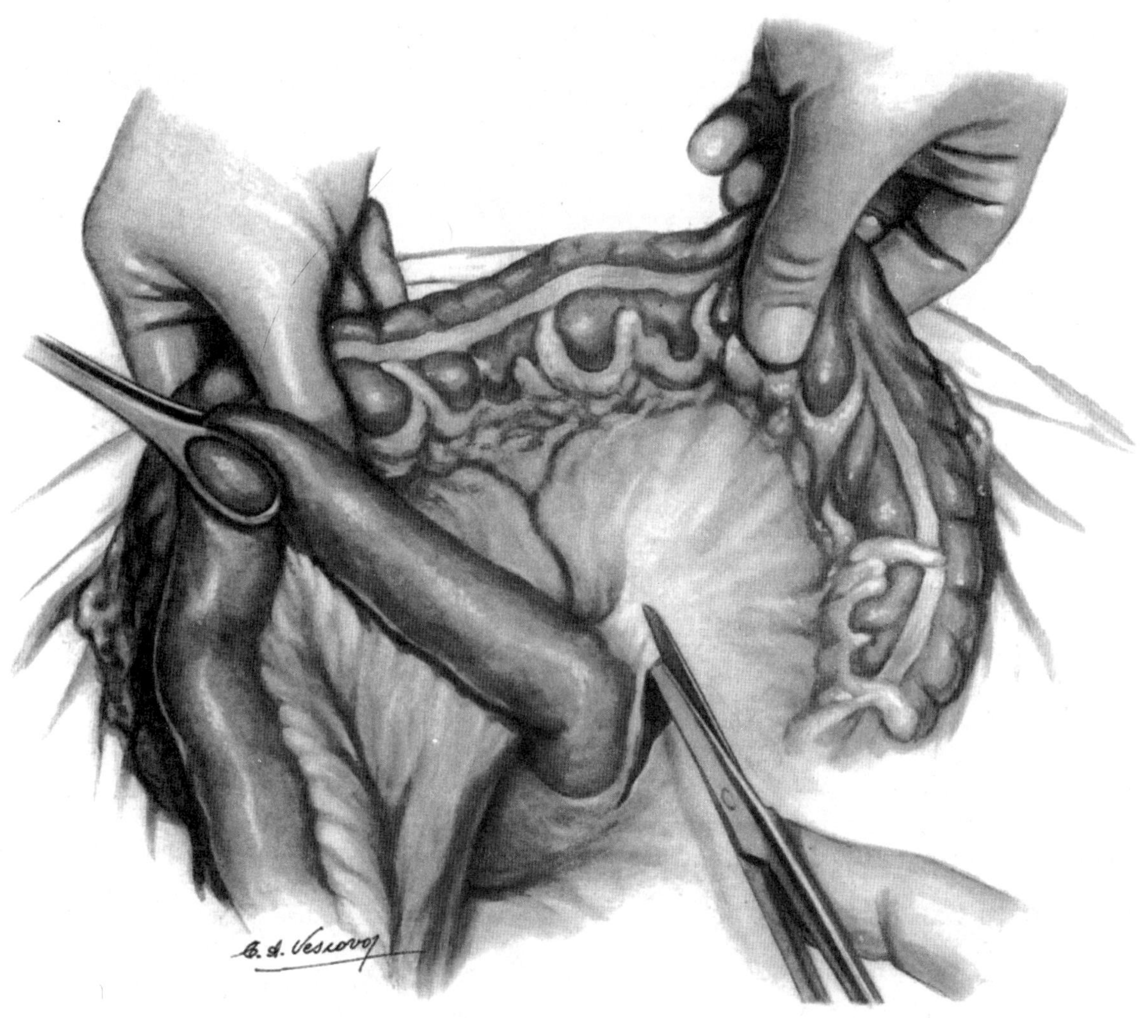

FIGURE 16.39

Technique of Resection of Carcinoma of the Head of the Pancreas

FIGURE 16.40
The jejunum is transected together with its mesentery at a point 12 to 15 cm beyond the ligament of Treitz, taking care that the distal jejunal segment does not lose its vascular supply. The proximal jejunal segment is occluded with a ligature, completing the liberation of the third portion of the duodenum and additionally freeing the fourth portion of the duodenum, going on to the proximal jejunum behind the superior mesenteric vessels, leading to the right supramesocolic area. The distal jejunal end is occluded with an elastic clamp. This end is to be anastomosed to the pancreatic stump if one is to perform a pancreaticojejunal anastomosis with intussusception. If a terminolateral mucosa to mucosa anastomosis is to be performed between the pancreatic duct and the jejunal mucosa, the distal jejunal stump is closed in two layers. Transection of the jejunum and the transposition of the proximal jejunal segment to the supramesocolic area, as well as liberation of the third and fourth portions of the duodenum, will facilitate liberation of the head of the pancreas and the uncinate process from the superior mesenteric vessels, as we will show in the next stages.

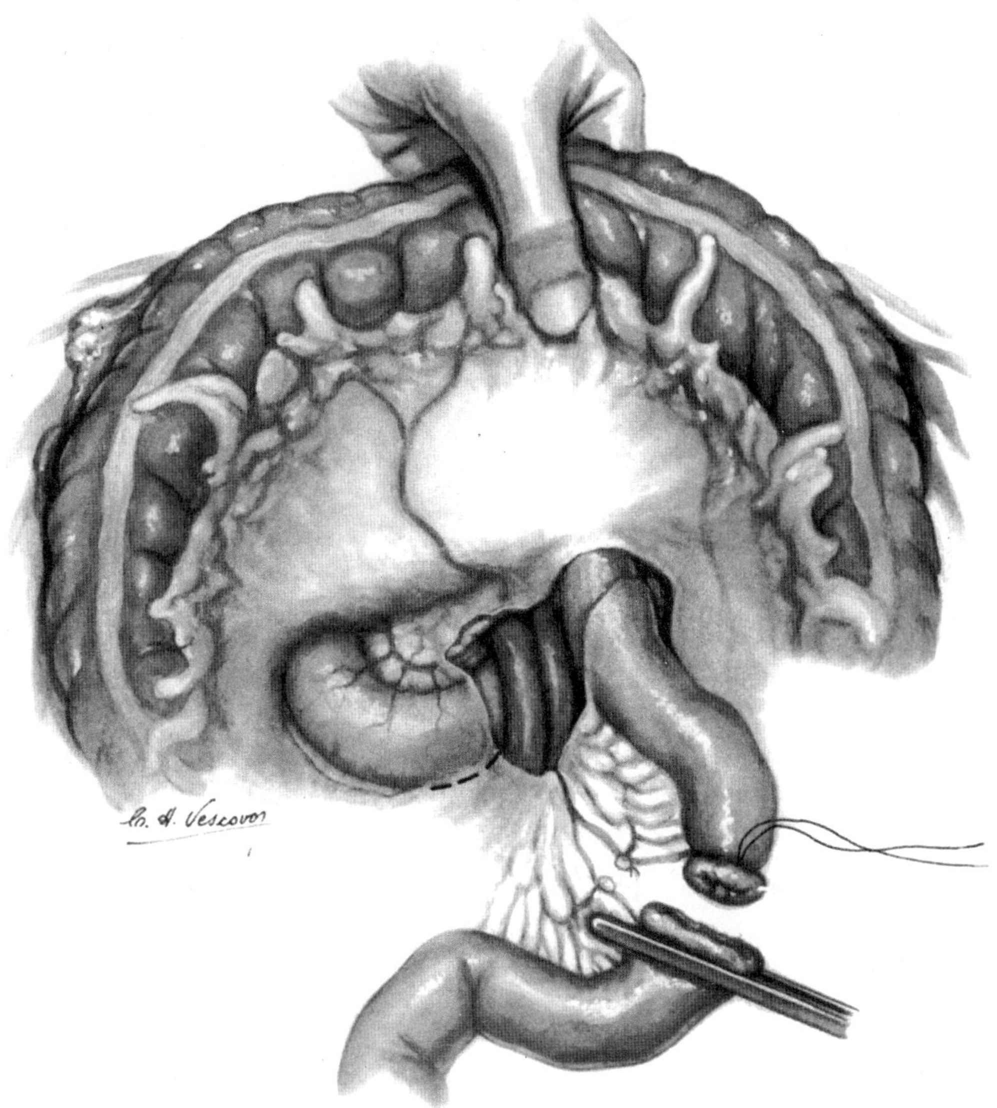

FIGURE 16.40

Technique of Resection of Carcinoma of the Head of the Pancreas

FIGURE 16.41

Liberation of the head of the pancreas has begun by ligating and transecting 6 to 8 veins from the head of the pancreas, which empty laterally into the superior mesenteric vein. To facilitate liberation of the head of the pancreas and the uncinate process from the superior mesenteric vessel, it is advisable to grasp the head of the pancreas with the left hand, as shown in the drawing, applying gentle traction to the right to expose the posterior surface of the head of the pancreas with the object of ligating the vessels. Mobilization of the head of the pancreas to the right is greatly facilitated if, in addition to the action mentioned earlier by the left hand on the pancreas, the ligature of Henle's trunk has been performed, the common bile duct has been transected, and the inferior and anterior pancreaticoduodenal arteries have been ligated and transected. In addition, the proximal jejunal segment has been transposed to the right, as shown in the drawing.

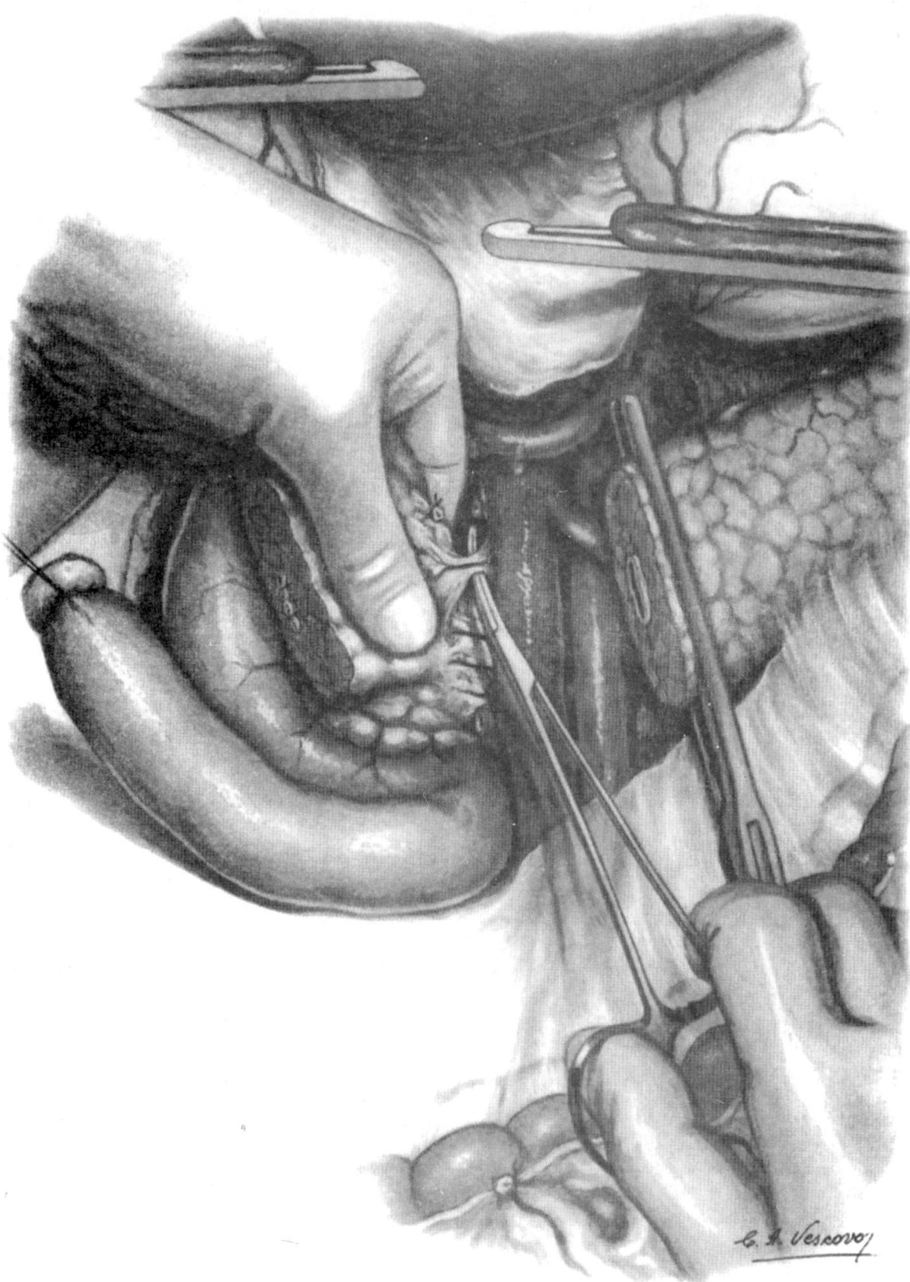

FIGURE 16.41

Technique of Resection of Carcinoma of the Head of the Pancreas

FIGURE 16.42
The efferent veins of the head of the pancreas have been ligated and we are proceeding to ligate the arteries that enter the head of the pancreas from the superior mesenteric artery, generally situated in a more posterior plane than the veins. Some of the arteries that have to be ligated are of small caliber, but others are larger in diameter. In some cases these small arteries are not clearly separated from the veins. During ligature of the arteries that enter the head of the pancreas, the left hand of the surgeon should be kept in the same position, and it is additionally helpful to gently raise the superior mesenteric vein with a vein retractor as shown in the drawing.

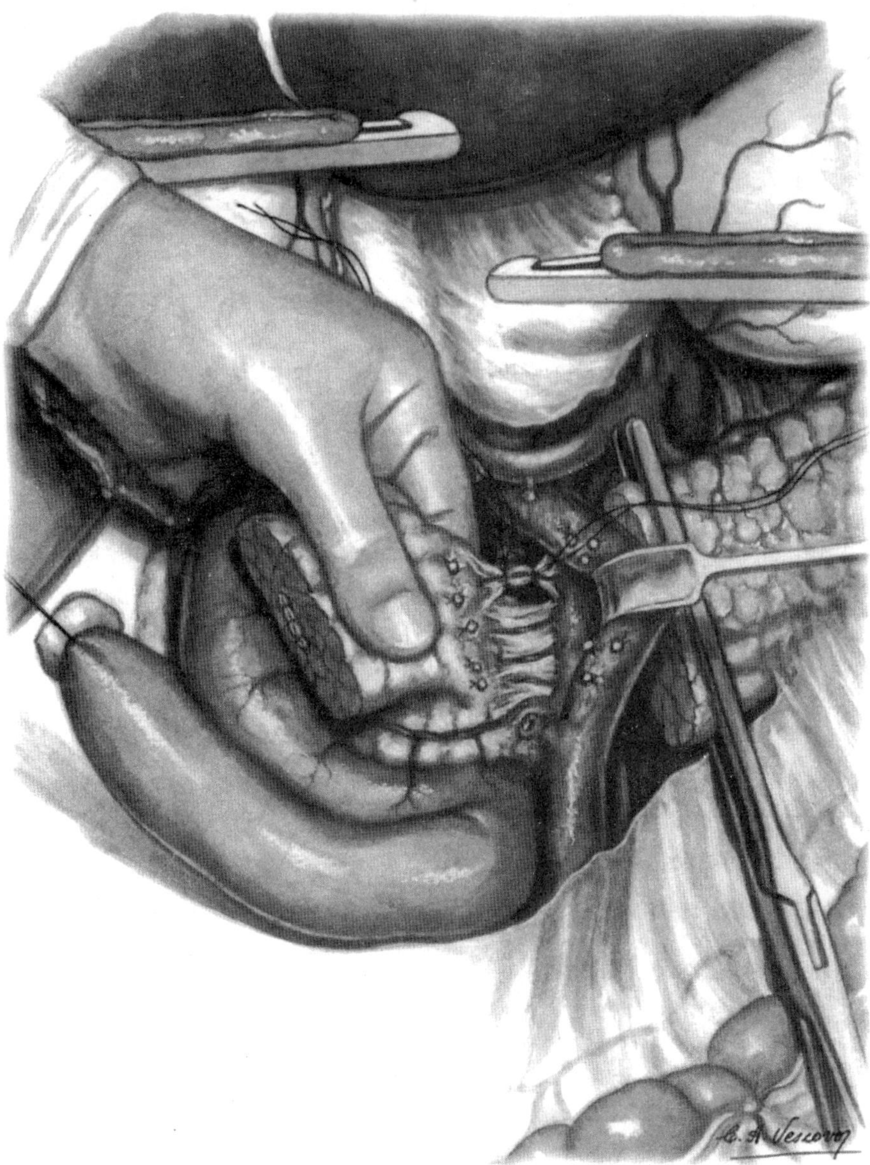

FIGURE 16.42

Technique of Resection of Carcinoma of the Head of the Pancreas

FIGURE 16.43

Once the veins and arteries of the head of the pancreas are tied, the uncinate process is freed. This is the most complex stage of pancreaticoduodenal resection. As the uncinate process is situated in a plane posterior to the superior mesenteric vessels, it is convenient to elevate the superior mesenteric vein with one or two vein retractors and carefully ligate all venous branches exiting the uncinate process toward the superior mesenteric vein. It is not always possible to distinguish between the venous plane and the arterial plane, which is more posterior. In this case, vessels are ligated as they are being identified.

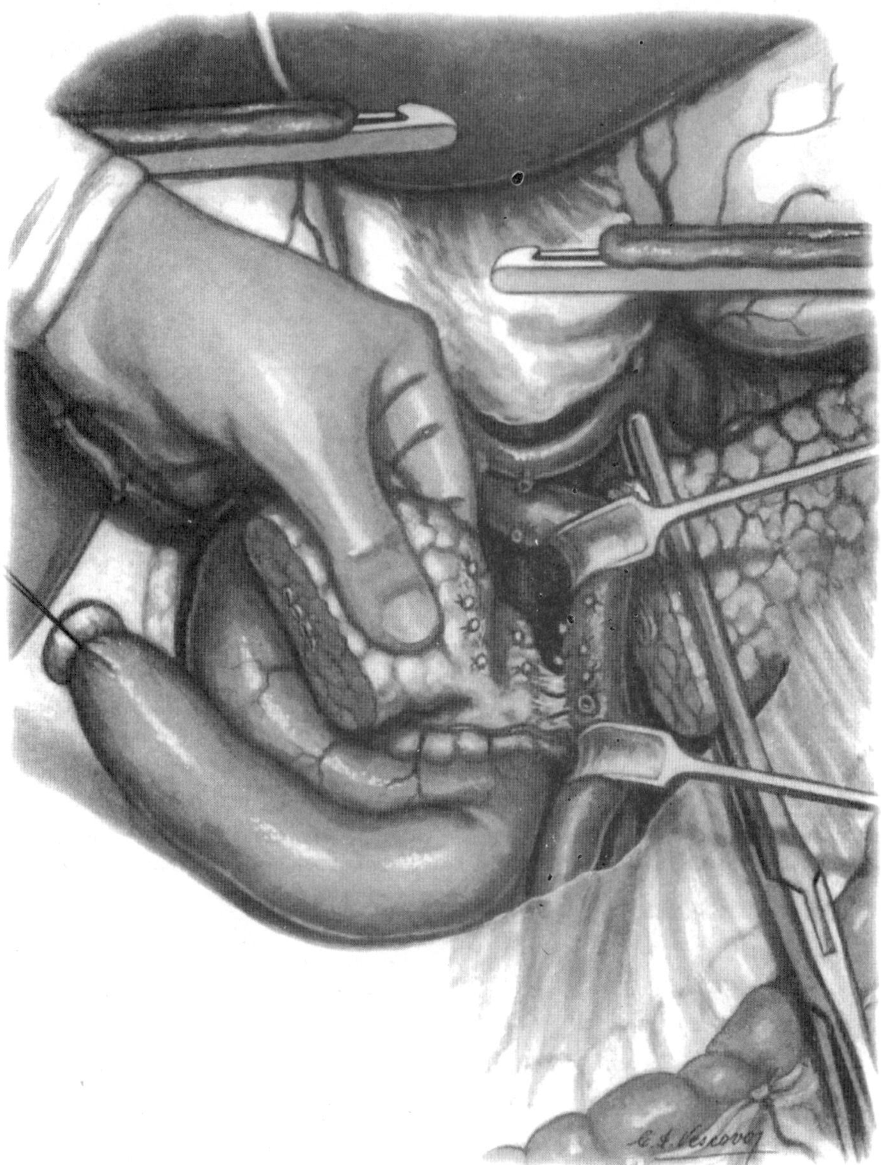

FIGURE 16.43

Technique of Resection of Carcinoma of the Head of the Pancreas

FIGURE 16.44

Once the venous plane of the uncinate process has been divided, the arterial plane is ligated where the vessels enter the uncinate process from the superior mesenteric artery. In some patients, the uncinate process is poorly developed, which makes its resection easier. In others, on the contrary, it is very well developed and intimately related to the superior mesenteric artery, making its liberation and resection more difficult. In some patients, one can observe a dense membrane made up of fibrous tissue, nerve fibers from the solar plexus, and retroperitoneal lymphatic collecting channels, which run from the uncinate process to the right uncolunar node. This segment of this membrane has been designated with the name of uncolunar ligament; another segment of the membrane runs from the superior mesenteric artery, being intimately adherent to the adventitia of this artery. This segment of the membrane has been designated the uncomesenteric ligament (see "Surgical Anatomy of the Pancreas"). When the uncomesenteric ligament is well developed, it becomes necessary to apply a vascular clamp prior to dividing it and ligating it.

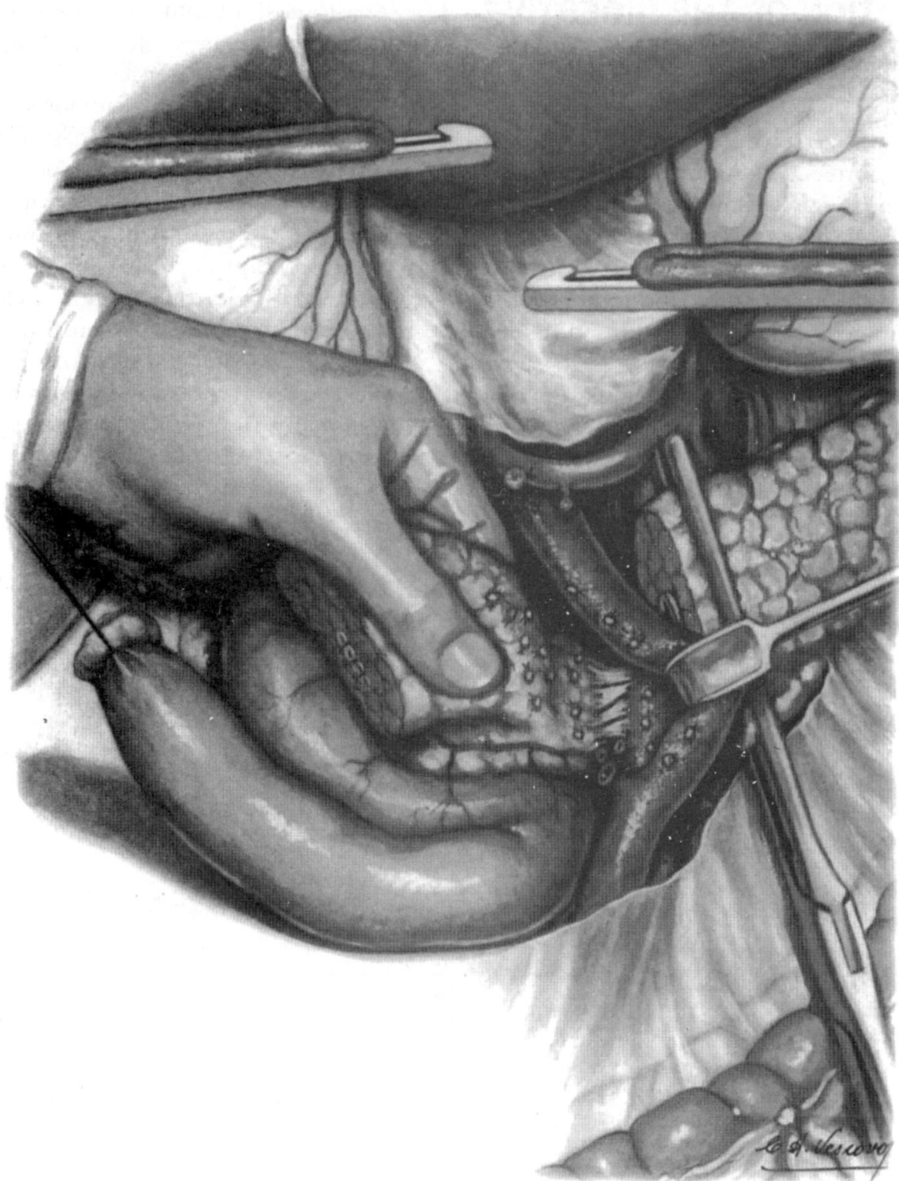

FIGURE 16.44

RECONSTRUCTION OF THE DIGESTIVE TRACT AFTER PANCREATICO-DUODENAL RESECTION

Once the resection is done reconstruction of the digestive tract should be performed. There are numerous techniques and many variations used in reconstruction of the digestive tract, but we will only describe procedures that we have used in our practice. The first stage of the reconstruction of the digestive tract is the anastomosis of the pancreatic stump to the jejunum or the stomach. Pancreaticojejunal anastomosis or pancreaticogastric anastomosis may be performed in two ways: (a) by intussusception or implantation and (b) by anastomosis of the pancreatic duct to the jejunal or gastric mucosa (mucosa to mucosa anastomosis).

Anastomosis by intussusception is indicated in cases in which the pancreas is soft with a fragile capsule and with a pancreatic duct of normal caliber.

Mucosa to mucosa anastomosis between the pancreatic duct and the jejunal or gastric mucosa may be indicated when the pancreatic duct is very dilated, with thickened walls and the pancreatic parenchyma is increased in consistency owing to chronic pancreatitis and a thickened capsule. We will first describe pancreaticojejunostomy by intussusception, followed by mucosa to mucosa anastomosis between the pancreatic duct and the jejunal mucosa. We will follow that with a description of the pancreaticogastric anastomosis by implantation and later mucosa to mucosa anastomosis between the posterior wall of the stomach and the pancreatic duct.

Pancreaticojejunal Anastomosis By Intussusception

FIGURE 16.45
Before beginning this anastomosis, one must be sure that hemostasis has been assured by means of suture ligatures in the transected end of the pancreas. U stitches are then placed through the transected edge, as shown in the drawing, being careful not to compromise the lumen of Wirsung's duct. Hemostasis of the transected pancreas must be complete to prevent postoperative hemorrhages, which can be quite severe. The anastomotic jejunal limb is brought to the supramesocolic region, passing it through an opening in the transverse mesocolon to the right of the midcolic vessels. Some surgeons prefer to bring this loop in front of the transverse colon, since it would be more difficult for it to become invaded in cases of recurrence of the tumor. The jejunal anastomotic limb must easily reach the pancreatic stump without traction. The ends of the jejunal limb and the transected pancreas are held with two guide sutures to facilitate anastomosis. Nonabsorbable suture material is used between the posterior surface of the pancreas and the seromuscular portion of the jejunum some 3 cm away from the transected end of both organs. The pancreatic sutures should include the capsule and a substantial portion of the pancreatic parenchyma to give the sutures consistency. One should always be careful of not compromising the lumen of the pancreatic duct.

Pancreaticojejunal Anastomosis By Intussusception

FIGURE 16.46
The posterior plane of the pancreaticojejunostomy is completed by suturing the free edge of the jejunum with the posterior surface of the lining of the section of the pancreas. These sutures should include the entire jejunal wall and the capsule as well as some of the parenchyma of the pancreas.

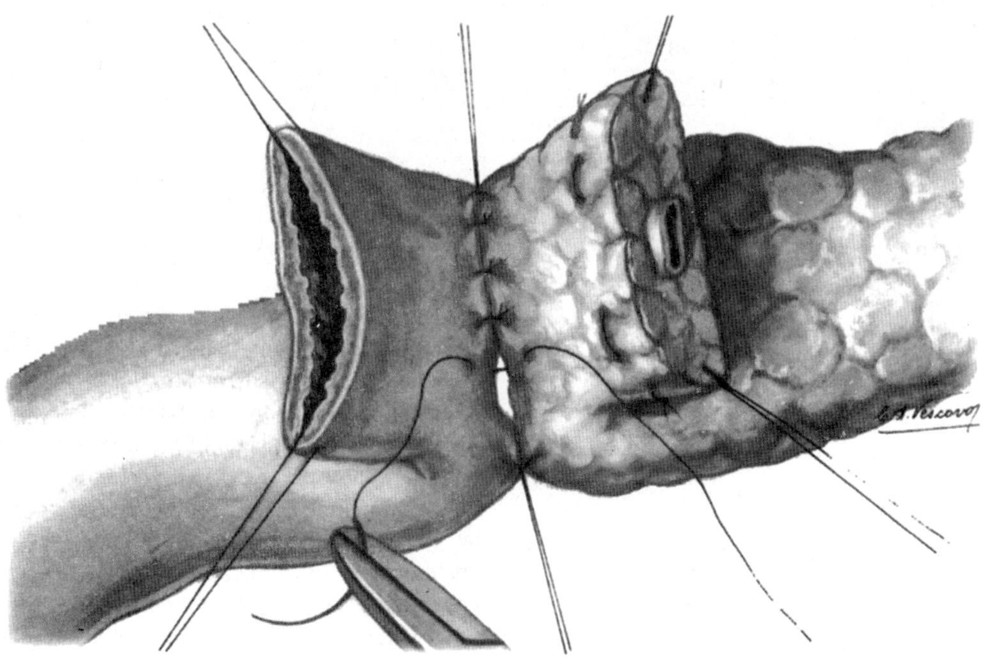

FIGURE 16.45

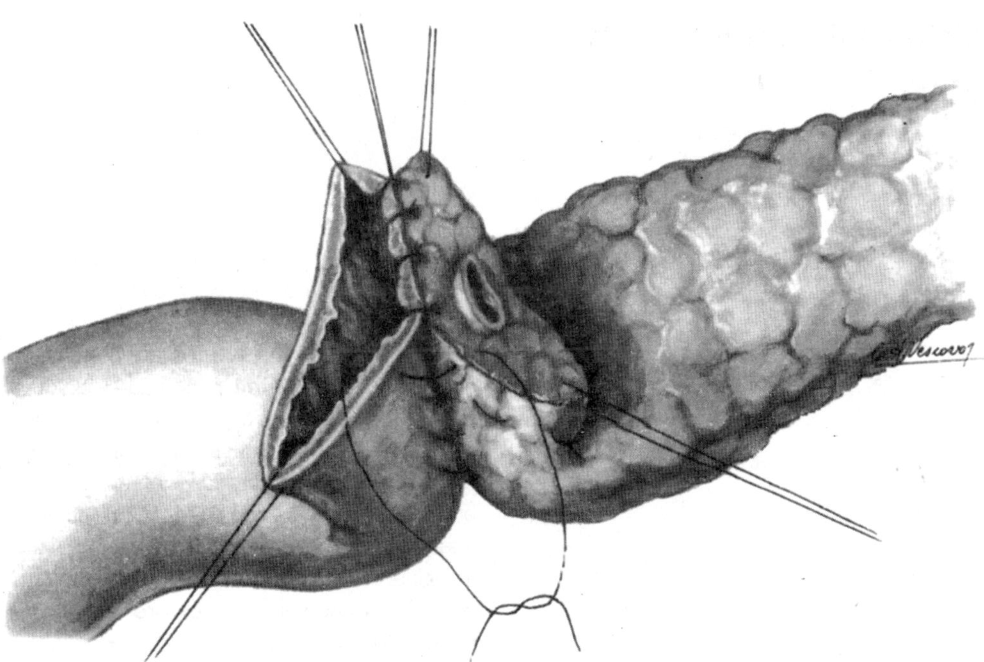

FIGURE 16.46

FIGURE 16.47

Once the posterior layer of the pancreaticojejunostomy has been completed, a fine Silastic tube with several perforations in the segment that is to be introduced into the pancreatic duct is placed in its lumen. The Silastic tube should not fit tightly into the pancreatic duct, but there should be space between it and the wall of the duct. This tube is then fixed to the end of the pancreatic duct with two sutures of nonabsorbable material. Reabsorbable material, be it catgut or synthetic material, should not be used because it will be rapidly disintegrated by pancreatic juice. Once the tube has been fixed in place, the anterior sutures are performed between the wall of the jejunum and the capsule and part of the pancreatic parenchyma.

Pancreaticojejunal Anastomosis By Intussusception

FIGURE 16.48

Once the edge of the jejunum has been sutured to the capsule and parenchyma of the pancreas, the anterior suture is completed so as to produce an intussusception of the pancreas into the jejunum. The sutures are placed some 3 cm from the edge of the transected pancreas—including the capsule and part of the pancreatic parenchyma on one side, and on the other side, the seromuscular layer of the jejunum. Three sutures are placed in this layer at each end and in the middle, and these are then tied down at the same time while the first assistant gently pushes the pancreatic stump, to facilitate its invagination into the lumen of the jejunum. Once this is obtained, intermediate sutures are placed to make the anastomosis more secure.

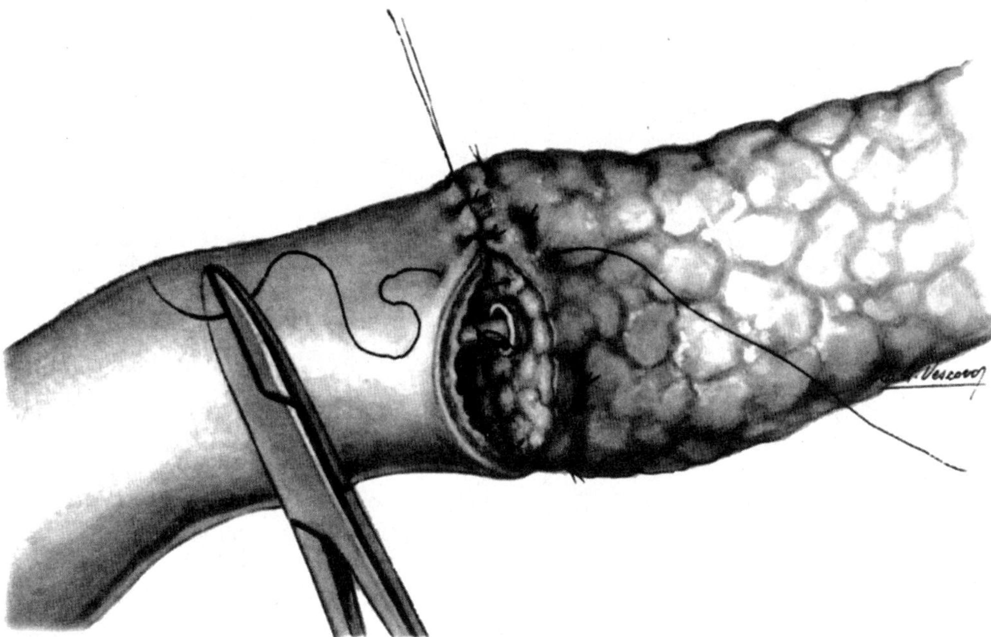

FIGURE 16.47

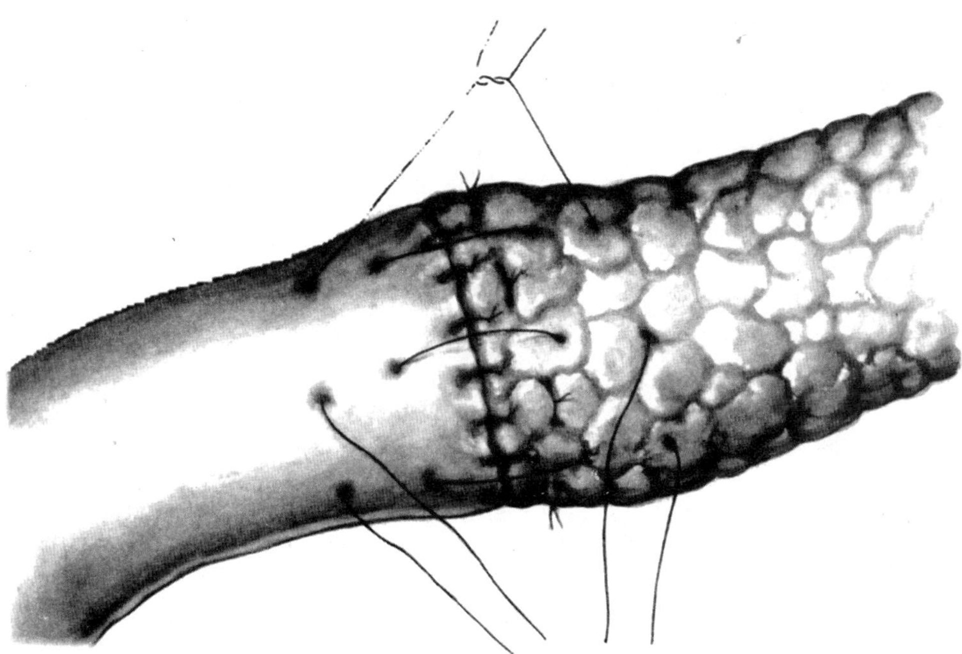

FIGURE 16.48

FIGURE 16.49
Semischematic drawing showing in one section the pancreaticojejunal anastomosis by intussusception. One can observe the pancreatic stump introduced in the jejunal lumen. The Silastic tube, in which several openings have been made, has been fixed at the end of the pancreatic duct, and after running some 10 to 12 cm within the jejunum, it is brought out of the jejunal wall all the way to the outside with the object of diverting pancreatic secretions from the body. This diversion to the outside considerably diminishes the incidence of pancreatic fistulas by disruption of the pancreaticojejunal anastomosis.(1, 2, 12, 13, 25, 26, 30, 32, 39, 48, 92) The drawing also shows a portion of the hepatic duct ready to be anastomosed to the jejunum in terminolateral fashion once the pancreaticojejunostomy is completed.

Pancreaticojejunal Anastomosis By Intussusception

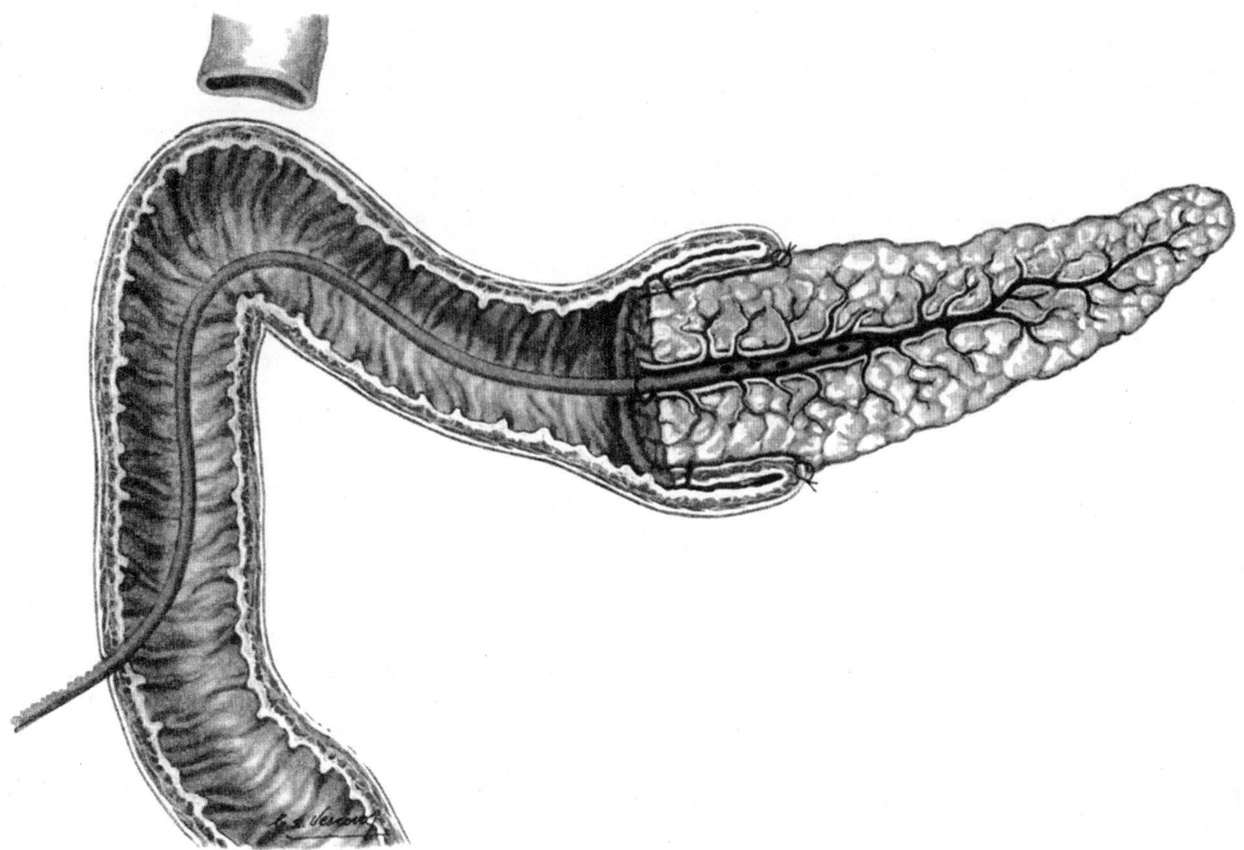

FIGURE 16.49

FIGURE 16.50
The drawing shows the completed pancreaticojejunostomy by intussusception. The Silastic tube, after running for a short distance in the jejunal lumen, is brought out of the wall of the jejunum and passed through a tunnel made in the seromuscular layer of the jejunum to bring it to the outside of the abdominal wall through a small stab incision. The hepatic duct is being sutured to the jejunum in terminolateral fashion using one layer of slow absorbing synthetic material. A Silastic tube has been placed in the hepatic duct which, after running through the jejunum for a distance of 8 to 10 cm is brought out the jejunal wall through a seromuscular tunnel and later brought out of the abdominal cavity through a small stab wound.

Pancreaticojejunal Anastomosis By Intussusception

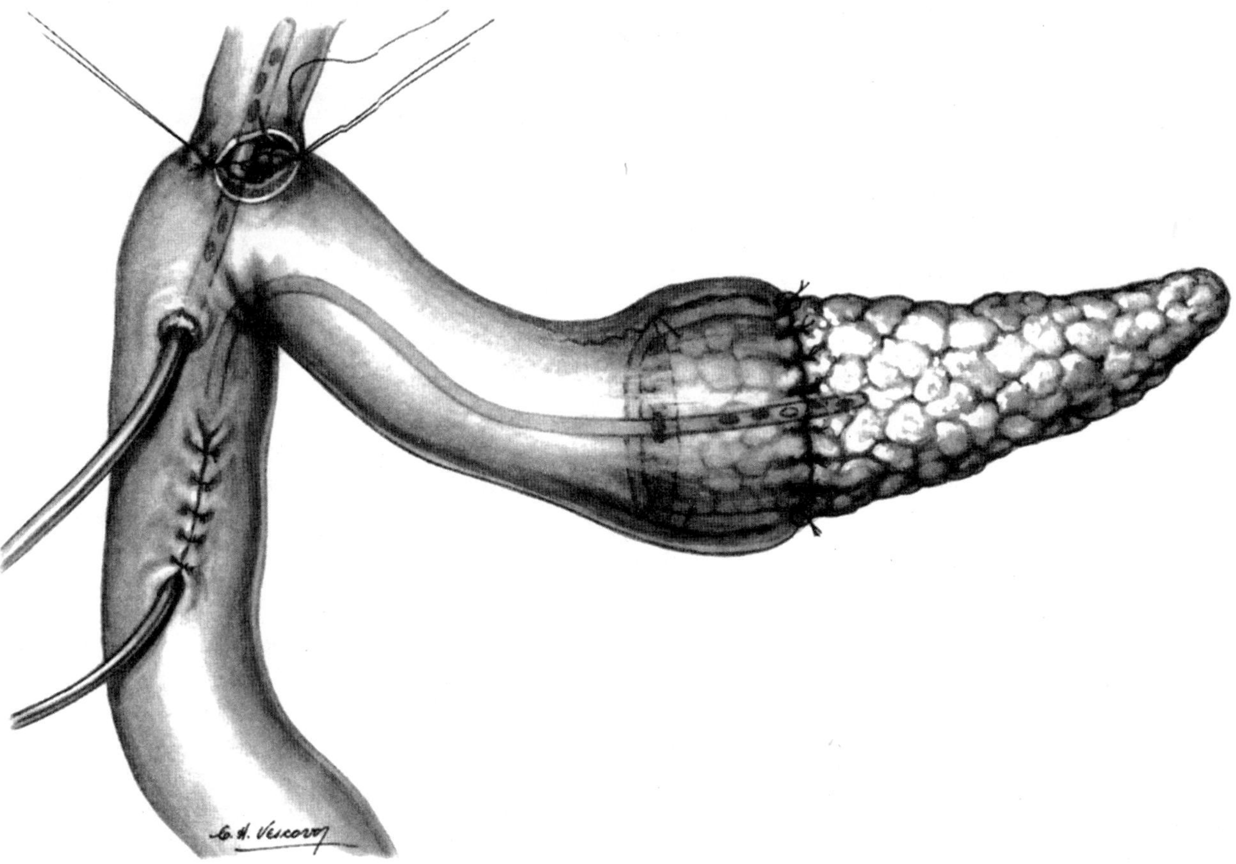

FIGURE 16.50

FIGURE 16.51
The pancreaticojejunal and the hepaticojejunal anastomosis have been completed. The hepaticojejunal anastomosis is placed some 12 cm distal to the pancreaticojejunal anastomosis. Kinking of the jejunum between both sutures should be avoided. The drainage tubes from the pancreas and the biliary tract are brought out separately. The jejunal loop through which these drainage tubes run should be sutured to the abdominal wall around the exit of these tubes. The tubes should also be sutured to the skin. It is convenient to test the hepaticojejunal anastomosis for leaking once it is completed. For this purpose, the jejunum is obstructed a few cm beyond the anastomosis and about 50 mL of physiologic solution is injected. If leakage occurs through a suture line, it can be corrected immediately and biliary fistulas avoided postoperatively.(6)

Pancreaticojejunal Anastomosis By Intussusception

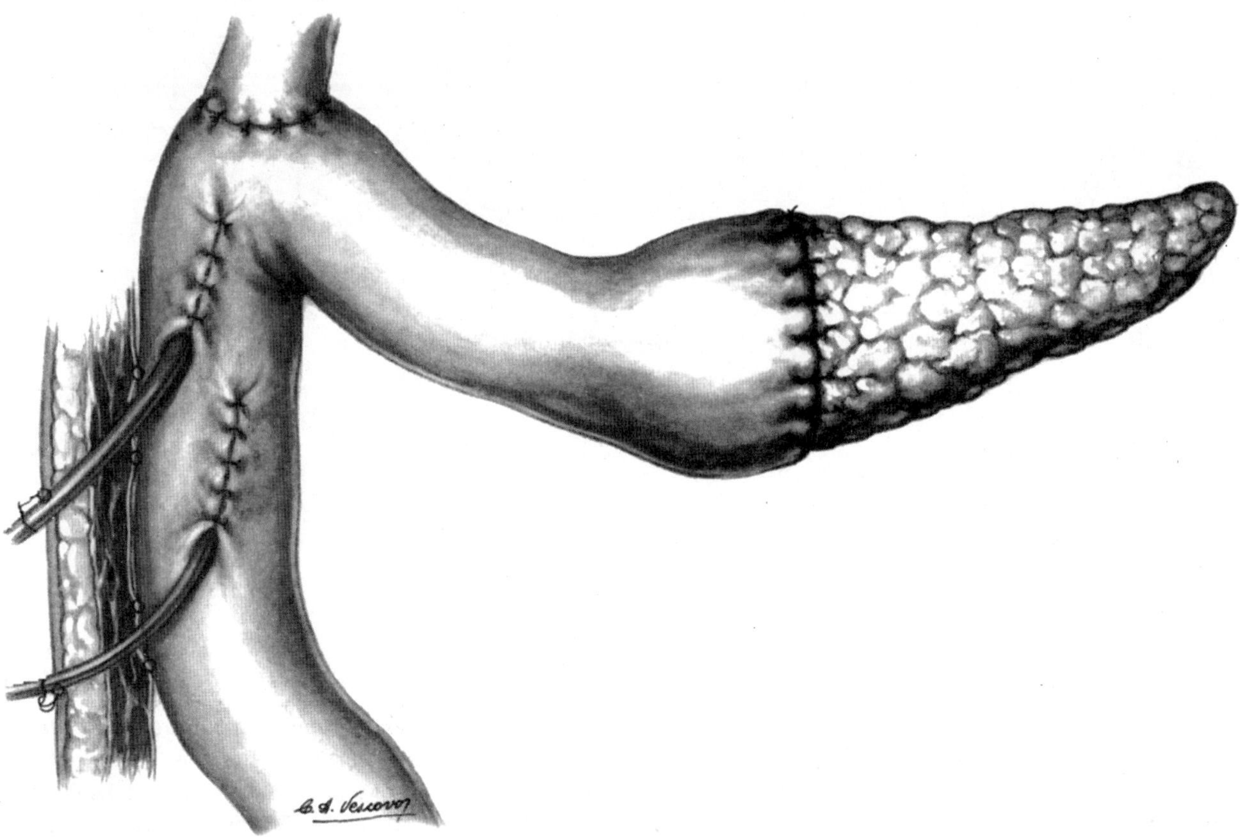

FIGURE 16.51

FIGURE 16.52

This drawing reveals the completed pancreaticoduodenectomy with complete re-establishment of the digestive tract. The gastrojejunal antecolic anastomosis can be seen using the Polya-Hofmeister technique. The hepaticojejunal anastomosis is located some 12 cm distal to the pancreaticojejunal anastomosis. It is rarely possible to perform the hepaticojejunal anastomosis further away from the pancreaticojejunostomy because it would then lead to kinking of the jejunal limb. The gastrojejunal anastomosis is located about 45 cm distal to the hepaticojejunal anastomosis. A hemigastrectomy with a bilateral truncal vagotomy has been performed to prevent ulcerations and postoperative hemorrhage. However, some surgeons of great experience in pancreatic surgery do not perform vagotomy.(39) The jejunal limb has been brought up through an avascular zone in the mesocolon to the supramesocolic region. The jejunal limb is fixed to the mesocolon with several sutures to prevent internal herniation. The insert reveals details of the jejunal limb anastomosed to the hepatic duct held in place with several sutures to the hepatogastric ligament.

Pancreaticojejunal Anastomosis By Intussusception

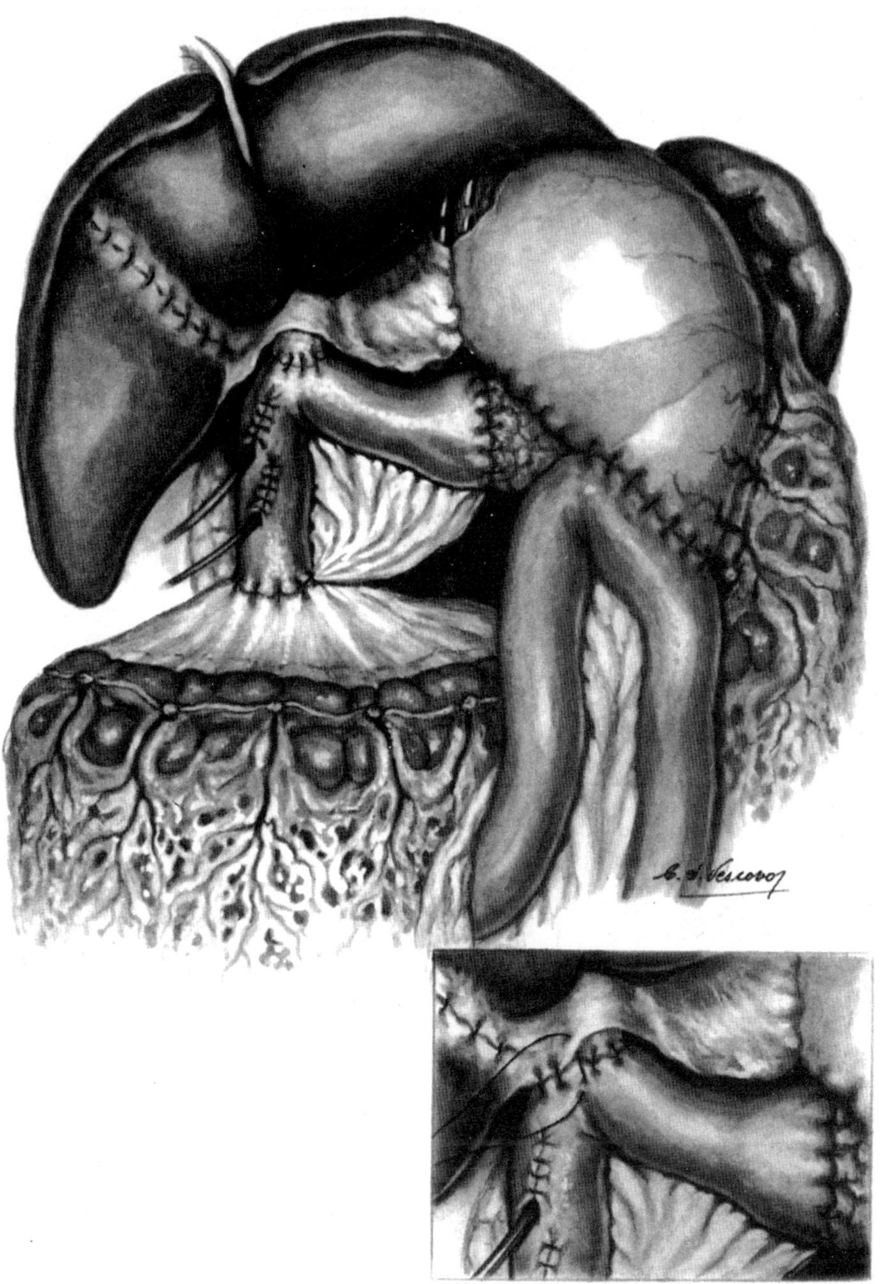

FIGURE 16.52

FIGURE 16.53
The end of the jejunal limb has been closed in two layers. Some 3 cm above the end of the jejunal limb, the anastomosis has begun by placing a row of interrupted sutures, using nonabsorbable material, between the posterior portion of the transected pancreas and the seromuscular layer of the jejunum. Pancreatic sutures should include the capsule and part of the pancreatic parenchyma, avoiding compromising the lumen of the pancreatic duct.

Pancreaticoduodenectomy With Pancreaticojejunal Terminolateral Anastomosis (Mucosa To Mucosa Suture)

FIGURE 16.54
Once this posterior layer is finished, a small incision is made in the jejunal wall of the same diameter and level with the pancreatic duct. The end of the pancreatic duct and the opening of the jejunum are grasped with two sutures as shown in the picture. Gentle traction on these sutures amplifies both openings, facilitating the anastomosis.

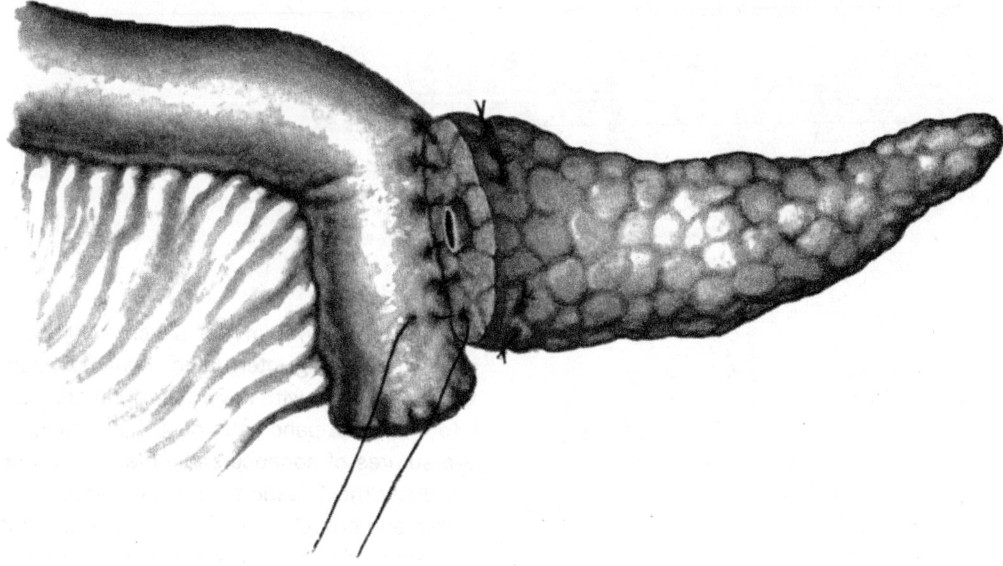

FIGURE 16.53

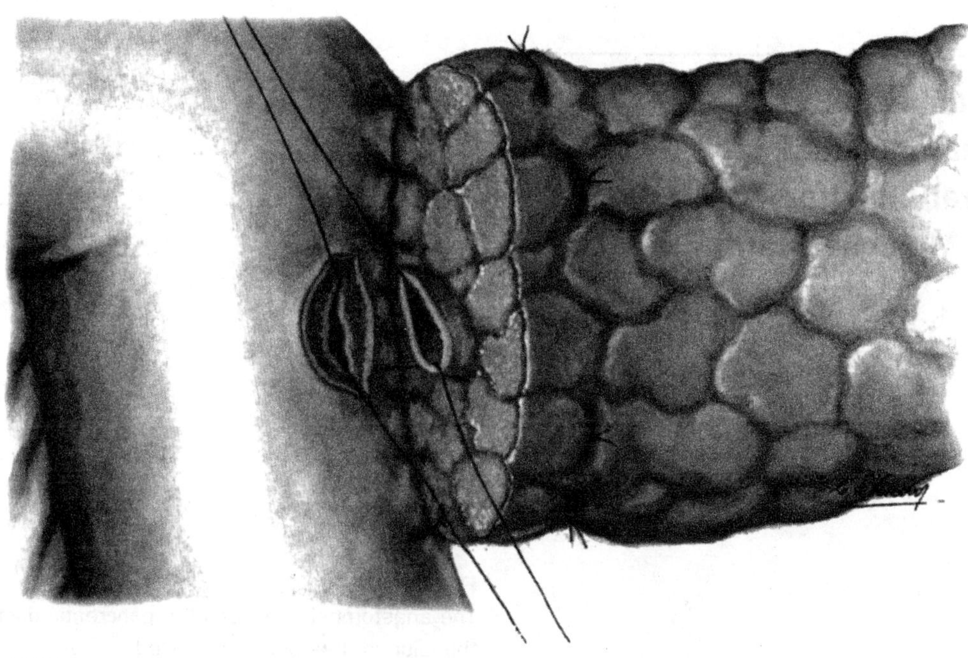

FIGURE 16.54

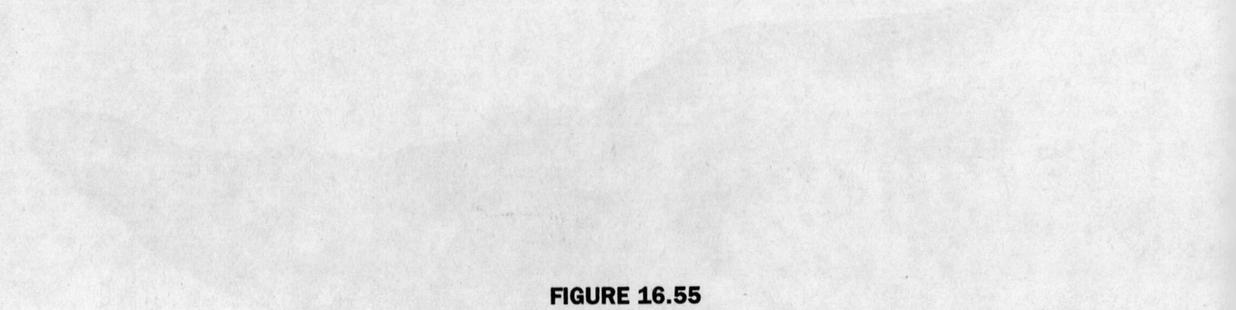

FIGURE 16.55
The posterior layer of the pancreaticojejunostomy has been completed, using interrupted, nonabsorbable sutures. A fine Silastic catheter with several perforations has been introduced into the distal pancreatic duct. The Silastic tube is fixed with two sutures of nonabsorbable material to the posterior end of the duct. The Silastic tube is then introduced into the jejunal lumen and brought out to the outside with the object of draining pancreatic secretions. One can observe in the drawing that the first anterior layer suture between the pancreatic duct and the jejunal wall is being placed.

Pancreaticoduodenectomy With Pancreaticojejunal Terminolateral Anastomosis (Mucosa To Mucosa Suture)

FIGURE 16.56
The anastomosis between the pancreatic duct and the wall of the jejunum has been completed.

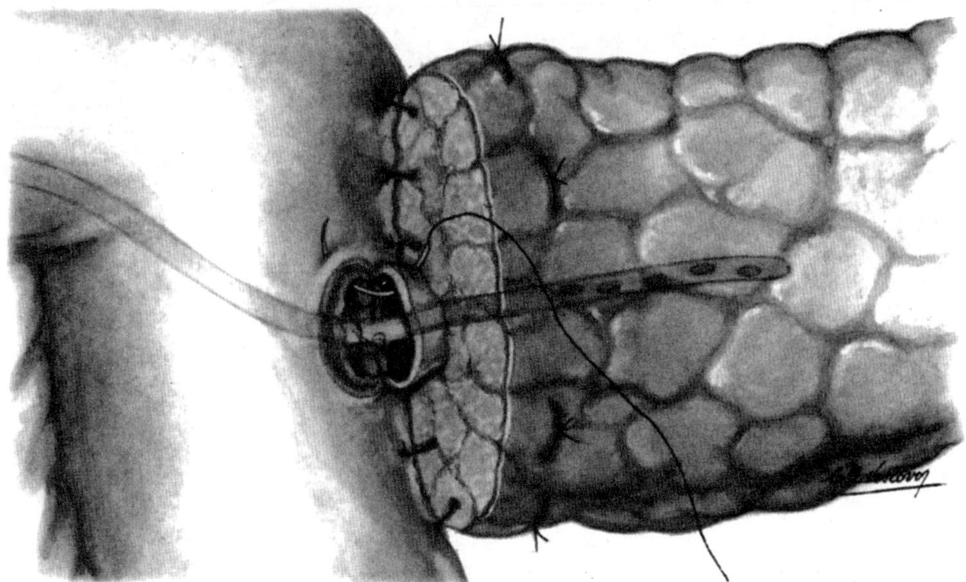

FIGURE 16.55

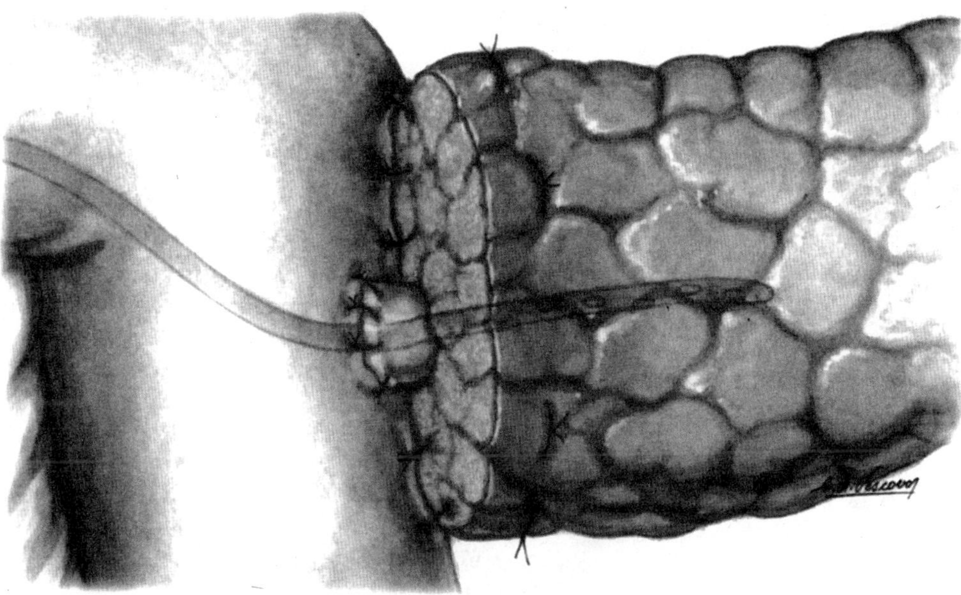

FIGURE 16.56

FIGURE 16.57
The surface of the transected pancreas anteriorly is being sutured to the seromuscular layer of the jejunum.

Pancreaticoduodenectomy With Pancreaticojejunal Terminolateral Anastomosis (Mucosa To Mucosa Suture)

FIGURE 16.58
The anastomosis of the pancreatic duct to the jejunal wall has been completed. Some 12 cm distal to this anastomosis, the hepaticojejunal anastomosis has been performed in one layer, using synthetic material of slow absorption and this anastomosis has been tested for leakage. Within the lumen of this anastomosis, another Silastic tube has been placed to drain bile to the outside. Both tubes, after running through the jejunal lumen for a short distance, have been brought out the jejunum and passed through a seromuscular tunnel to the outside through two small stab wounds in the abdominal wall. The jejunal wall is then fixed to the parietal peritoneum around the exit of the tube to partially separate the tubes from the peritoneal cavity.

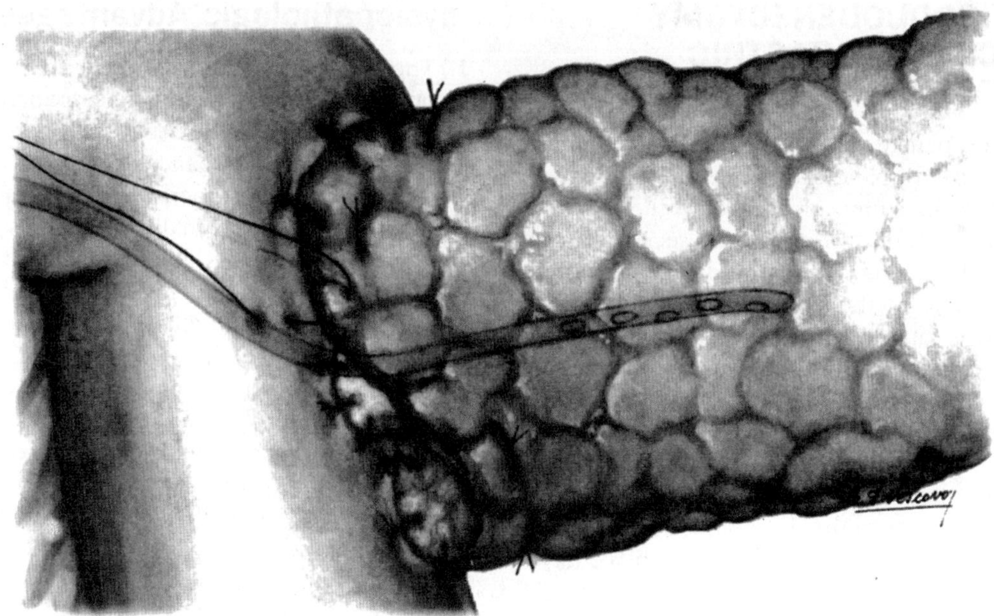

FIGURE 16.57

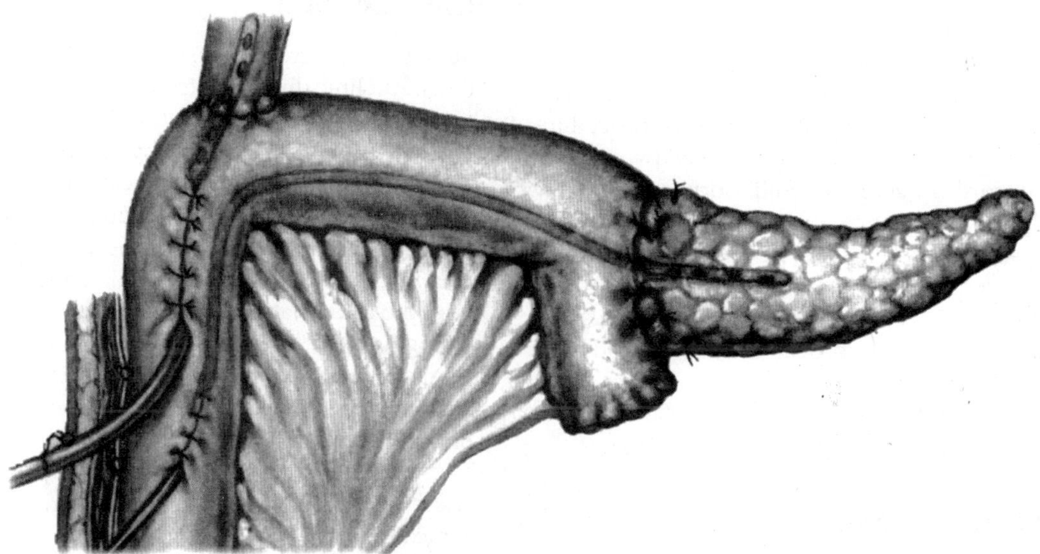

FIGURE 16.58

PANCREATICODUODENECTOMY WITH PANCREATICOGASTRIC ANASTOMOSIS

In previous pages, pancreaticoduodenectomy with re-establishment of transit of pancreatic secretions by anastomosing the pancreatic stump or its duct to the jejunum has been described. Transit of pancreatic secretions can also be obtained by anastomosing the pancreatic stump or the pancreatic duct to the stomach. The pancreaticogastric anastomosis can be performed by implantation of the pancreatic stump into the gastric wall, a technique that is similar to the pancreaticojejunal anastomosis by intussusception previously described. In addition, the pancreaticogastric anastomosis can be performed by suturing the pancreatic duct to the gastric wall (mucosa to mucosa suture) in a form similar to the anastomosis of the pancreatic duct to the wall of the jejunum, which we have also described.

The particular technique to be selected also depends on the degree of dilation and thickening of the pancreatic duct and the consistency of the parenchyma of the pancreas and its capsule. Pancreaticogastric anastomosis has been proposed and performed for many years. However, it has not been greatly accepted by surgeons in spite of its excellent qualities.(17, 43, 62, 68, 75, 77, 83, 100, 101) We began to perform pancreaticogastric anastomosis in the year 1966 (25) as an alternative procedure to pancreaticojejunal anastomosis, influenced by publications of the Swedish surgeon Erik Millbourn (62), who up to 1959 had performed pancreaticogastric anastomosis in seven patients, with good results. At present, greater enthusiasm is evident for this technique, according to recent publications.(25, 28, 42, 54, 78, 89) Pancreaticogastric anastomosis is a simple procedure, secure and easy to control postoperatively.

Some of the advantages of pancreaticogastric anastomosis can be outlined as follows (25, 28, 68, 89):

Technical Advantages

1. There is a close relation between the pancreas and the posterior wall of the stomach.
2. The gastric wall is well qualified for the acceptance of sutures owing to its thickness, flexibility, and excellent blood supply.
3. The wide lumen of the stomach does not present problems for the implantation of the pancreas, as sometimes occurs with intussusception of the pancreas into the jejunum.
4. The wide lumen of the stomach allows for the performance of an external suture, and an internal suture from within the gastric lumen, which reinforces the anastomosis, making it more secure.

Physiopathologic Advantages

1. The gastric pH is not the most adequate for activation of trypsinogen and other pancreatic enzymes, which, in order to be active, need an alkaline pH.
2. The alkaline pH of pancreatic secretions protects the stomach from postoperative ulceration.
3. If a pancreaticojejunal anastomosis were to become obstructed, it is inevitable that a blind loop, with all its consequences, would develop, a fact that cannot occur with a pancreaticogastric anastomosis.(28, 29)
4. In pancreaticojejunal anastomosis, accumulation of a large amount of pancreatic and biliary secretions in the anastomotic jejunal loop may occur. This may even weigh up to 1 kg, which, together with postoperative intestinal ileus, may lead to the dehiscence of the pancreaticojejunal anastomosis, particularly when the pancreatic and biliary fluid is not drained to the outside.(25, 28, 29, 68, 89) In pancreaticogastric anastomosis, this is not a possibility.

Patency of Pancreaticogastric Anastomosis

Patency of pancreaticogastric anastomosis has been established clinically and experimentally by numerous authors.(25, 28, 29, 43, 54, 62, 77, 78, 89, 100) Patency can be established clinically and by examining fecal material in the same fashion as in pancreaticojejunal anastomosis. However, in pancreaticogastric anastomosis, patency can also be established by the amount of pancreatic secretions in the gastric contents and fundamentally by gastroscopic examination, which allows one to visualize and photograph the anastomosis. Even in the cases in which this communication is not clearly visualized due to the thickness of the gastric folds, one can recur to intravenous injection of secretin, 1 unit per kilogram of weight, which will rapidly increase the flow of pancreatic secretion, revealing the pancreaticogastric communication.

We will now describe pancreaticogastric anastomosis by implantation and pancreaticogastric anastomosis between the pancreatic duct and the wall of the stomach.

PANCREATICOGASTRIC ANASTOMOSIS BY IMPLANTATION

Pancreaticogastric anastomosis by implantation is indicated in patients with a soft pancreas and with a pancreatic duct that is not dilated. It can also be used as an alternative process when the pancreatic stump, because of its great diameter, is too difficult for invagination into the jejunum.

Pancreaticogastric Anastomosis By Implantation

FIGURE 16.59
The pancreatic stump has been approximated to the posterior wall of the stomach to begin the pancreaticogastric anastomosis by implantation. In the superior and inferior borders of the transected surface of the pancreas, large sutures have been placed as guide sutures to apply traction to the pancreatic stump as it is introduced into the gastric cavity. The gastric stump has been occluded by an elastic clamp.

Pancreaticogastric Anastomosis By Implantation

FIGURE 16.60
An external layer of sutures has been applied posteriorly between the seromuscular layer of the stomach and the anterior surface of the pancreas some 2 cm from its cut edge, using nonabsorbable material. With a scalpel, the posterior wall of the stomach is incised for a length of approximately the same diameter as the pancreatic stump at a distance some 5 to 6 cm from the edge of the transected stomach.

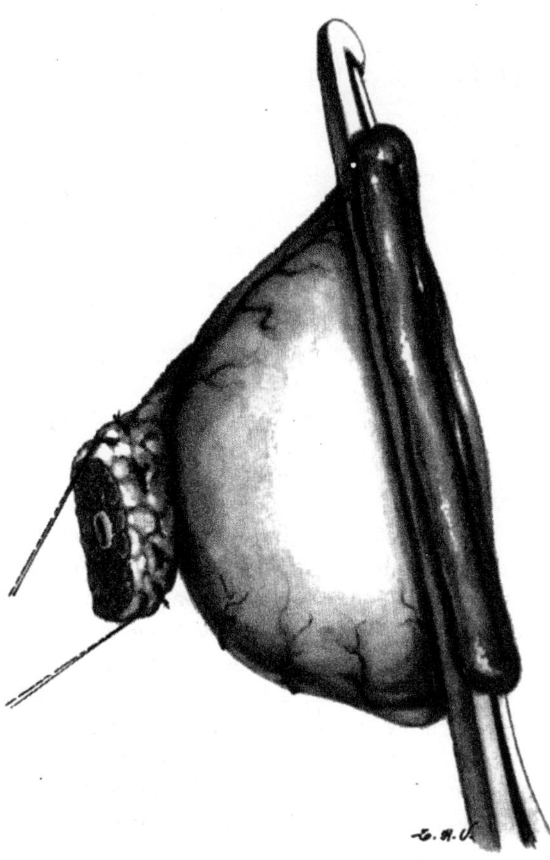

FIGURE 16.59

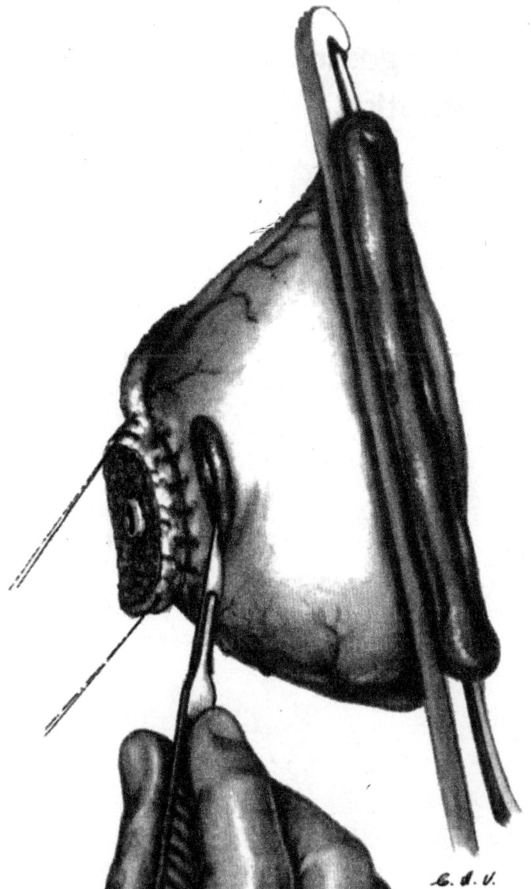

FIGURE 16.60

FIGURE 16.61
The elastic clamp of the stomach has been temporarily removed from the gastric stump, and the edges of the stomach have been grasped by two pairs of Duval atraumatic clamps, which, at the same time as they provide hemostasis for the gastric wall, allow the stomach to be opened so that the internal suture between the pancreatic stump and the gastric wall can be performed. With the stomach open, the guide traction sutures previously placed in the gastric stump are pulled and the pancreatic stump introduced for a distance of some 2 cm into the inside of the stomach, as can be seen in the drawing.

Pancreaticogastric Anastomosis By Implantation

FIGURE 16.62
The drawing shows the internal suture between the pancreatic stump and the wall of the stomach being performed, using nonabsorbable material. The needle passes through the entire thickness of the gastric wall on one side and through the capsule and part of the pancreatic parenchyma on the other side. The amount of pancreatic parenchyma to be included in the suture should be substantial to give the suture consistency, always avoiding compromising the lumen of the pancreatic duct. Once the internal suture between the pancreas and the gastric wall has been performed, the next stage will be to complete the external suture between the pancreas and the seromuscular layer of the gastric wall.

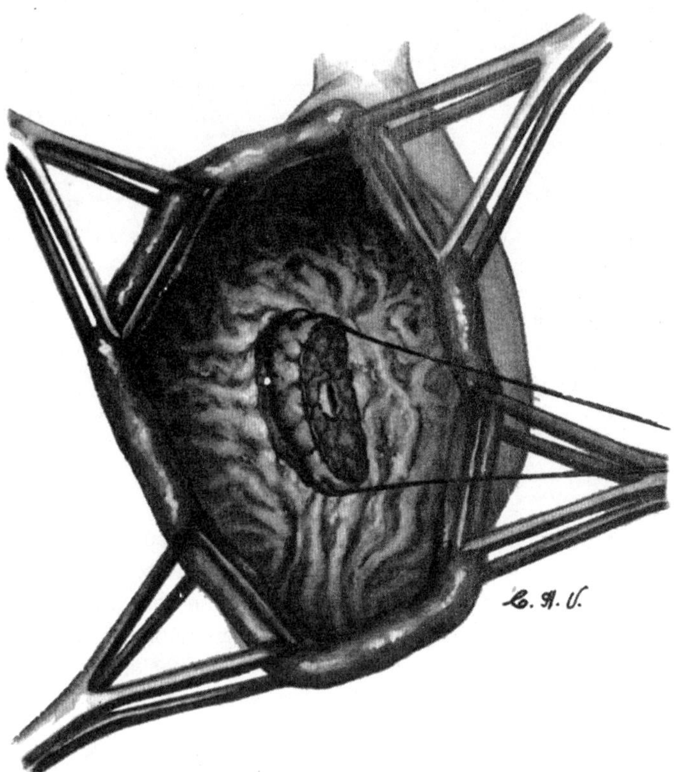

FIGURE 16.61

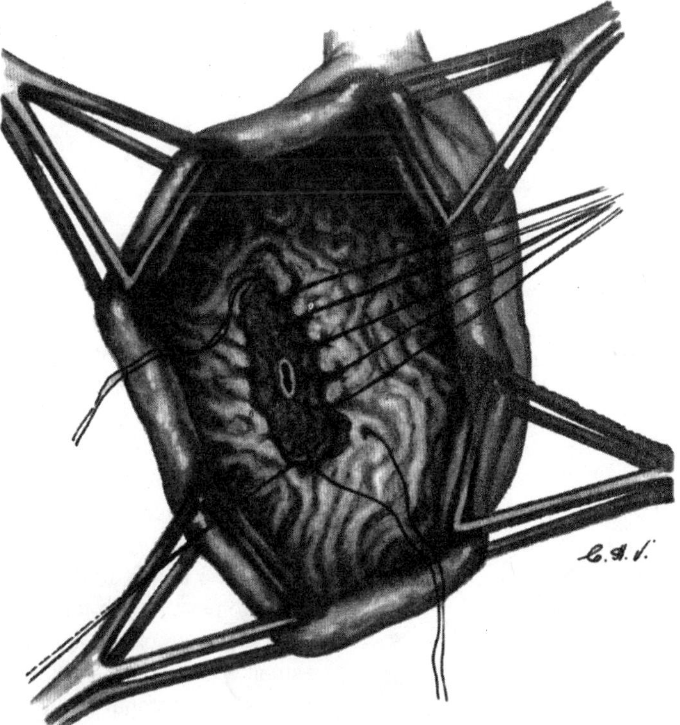

FIGURE 16.62

FIGURE 16.63
The external suture between the posterior surface of the pancreas and the seromuscular layer of the stomach is being completed. The double suture, external and internal, between the pancreatic stump and the gastric wall lends great security to the anastomosis, this being one of the advantages of pancreaticogastric anastomosis.

Pancreaticogastric Anastomosis By Implantation

FIGURE 16.64
Once the pancreaticogastric anastomosis has been completed, a fine Silastic tube with several perforations is introduced into the pancreatic duct. This tube is fixed with two sutures of nonabsorbable material to the end of the pancreatic duct. The Silastic tube is brought out through the anterior wall of the stomach. The small opening in the anterior wall of the stomach through which the Silastic tube passes is closed by a purse-string suture of nonabsorbable material, the ends of which should not be tied to the Silastic tube to facilitate the later removal of the tube. Once the pancreaticoduodenectomy has been completed, the Silastic tube is brought out through a small opening in the anterior abdominal wall, as shown in the insert. The anterior wall of the stomach is fixed to the parietal peritoneum by means of some sutures placed around the Silastic tube.

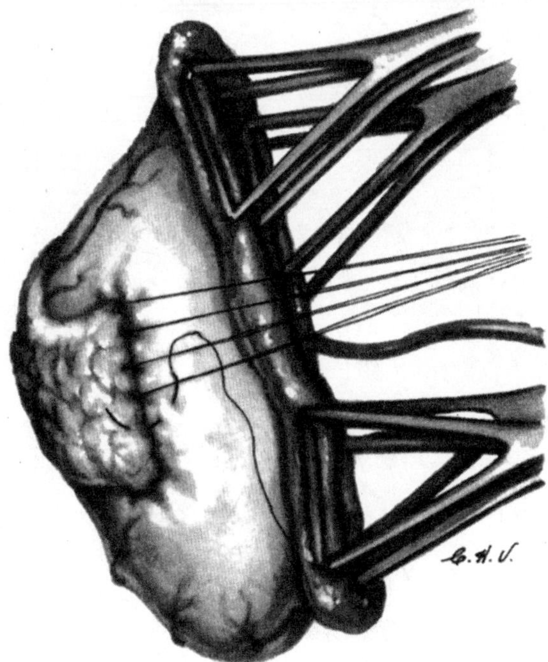

FIGURE 16.63

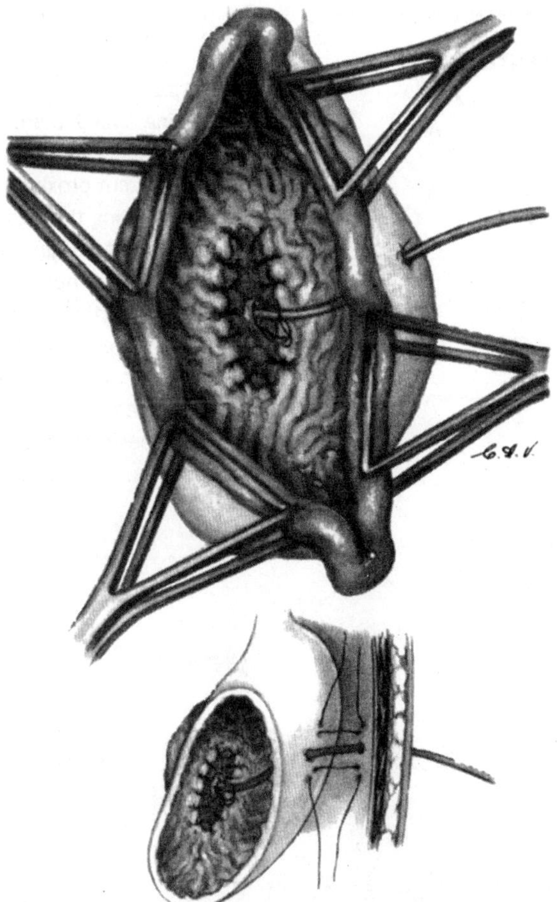

FIGURE 16.64

Pancreaticogastric Anastomosis By Implantation

FIGURE 16.65

The drawing shows the completed operation. One can observe the pancreaticogastric anastomosis by implantation located some 5 to 6 cm proximal to the gastrojejunostomy. The Silastic tube is exiting through the anterior wall of the stomach and to the outside to drain pancreatic secretions. In addition, one can observe the hepaticojejunal terminolateral anastomosis draining bile to the outside through a separate Silastic tube. The drawing reveals that a hemigastrectomy with bilateral truncal vagotomy has been performed and an antecolic gastrojejunal anastomosis, using the Polya-Hofmeister technique, has been performed some 45 cm from the hepaticojejunal anastomosis.

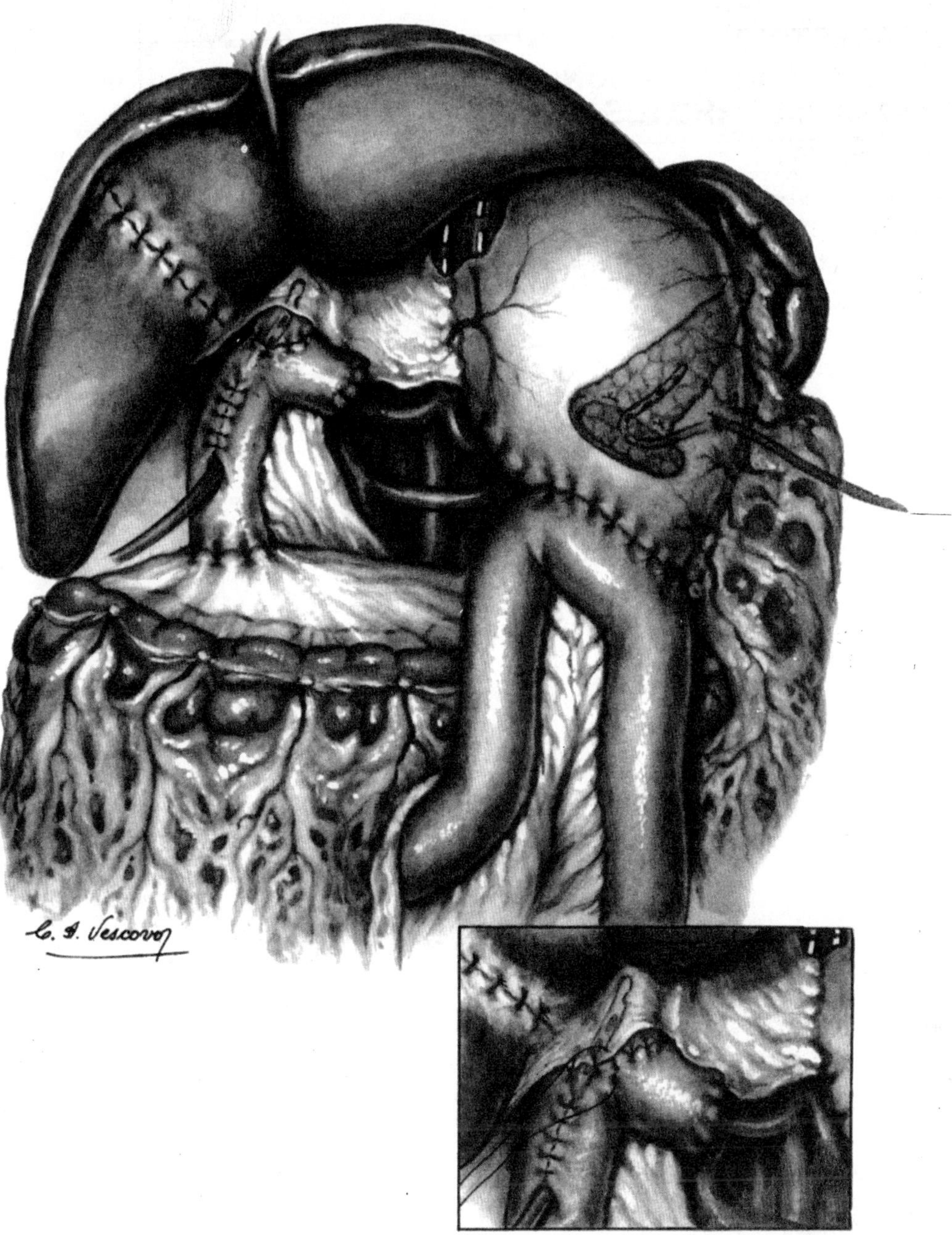

FIGURE 16.65

PANCREATICOGASTRIC ANASTOMOSIS BY IMPLANTATION USING THE JONATHAN RHOADS TECHNIQUE (54, 68)

The Rhoads technique is a variation of the previously described technique and has, as its object, making the pancreaticogastric anastomosis by implantation easier. It consists in performing the external pancreaticogastric layer first and then performing the internal layer.

Pancreaticogastric Anastomosis By Implantation Using the Jonathan Rhoads Technique (54, 68)

FIGURE 16.66
A row of nonabsorbable sutures has been placed between the anterior surface of the pancreas and the seromuscular layer of the posterior gastric wall. An incision has been made in the posterior gastric wall about the diameter of the pancreatic stump, some 5 to 6 cm proximally to the level of transection of the stomach. Through the anterior gastric wall a Reverdin or Doyen needle or a fine curved clamp is passed, as seen in the drawing. The end of the clamp is then passed through the incision in the posterior wall in the stomach. The guide sutures previously placed in the pancreas are grasped by the clamp and traction is applied upward and to the left to introduce some 2 cm of the pancreatic stump into the stomach. While traction is maintained on these sutures, the anastomosis of the posterior surface of the pancreas to the seromuscular layer of the gastric wall is performed, as will be shown in the next figure. This is the maneuver that makes this procedure different from that previously described.

Pancreaticogastric Anastomosis By Implantation Using the Jonathan Rhoads Technique (54, 68)

FIGURE 16.67
While the first assistant maintains traction on the sutures, the surgeon completes the external layer. Once the external layer is complete, only the internal layer is yet to be completed, as shown in the following figure. This is in no way different from the previously described technique.

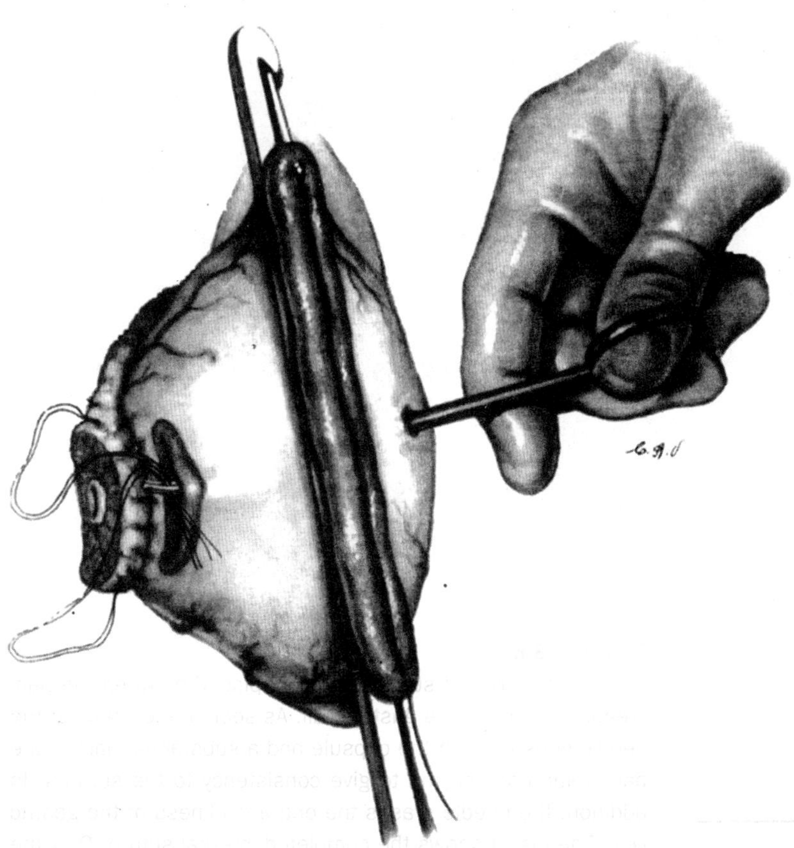

FIGURE 16.66

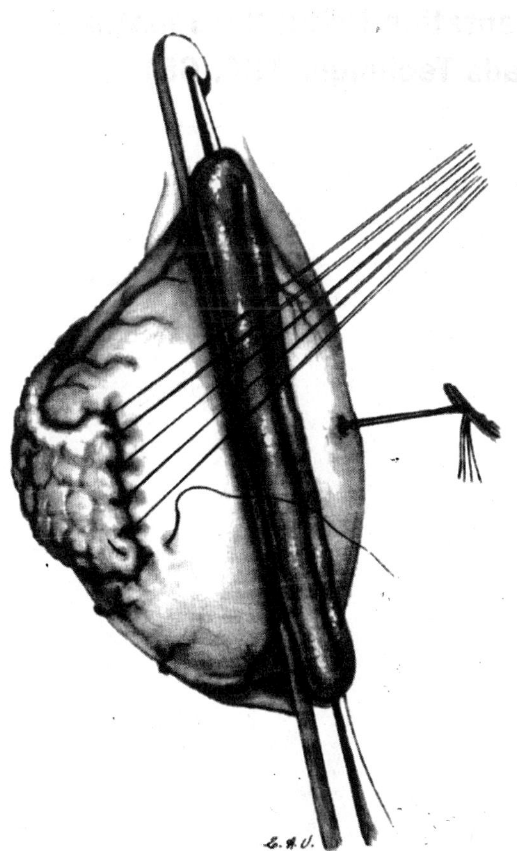

FIGURE 16.67

FIGURE 16.68
The internal layer of sutures is being placed between the pancreatic stump and the gastric wall. As seen in the drawing, the needle goes through the capsule and a substantial part of the pancreatic parenchyma to give consistency to the sutures. In addition, the needle grasps the entire thickness of the gastric wall. The insert shows the completed internal suture. Only the placing of the Silastic tube in the pancreatic duct is yet to be done, together with its later being brought out the anterior wall of the stomach.

Pancreaticogastric Anastomosis By Implantation Using the Jonathan Rhoads Technique (54, 68)

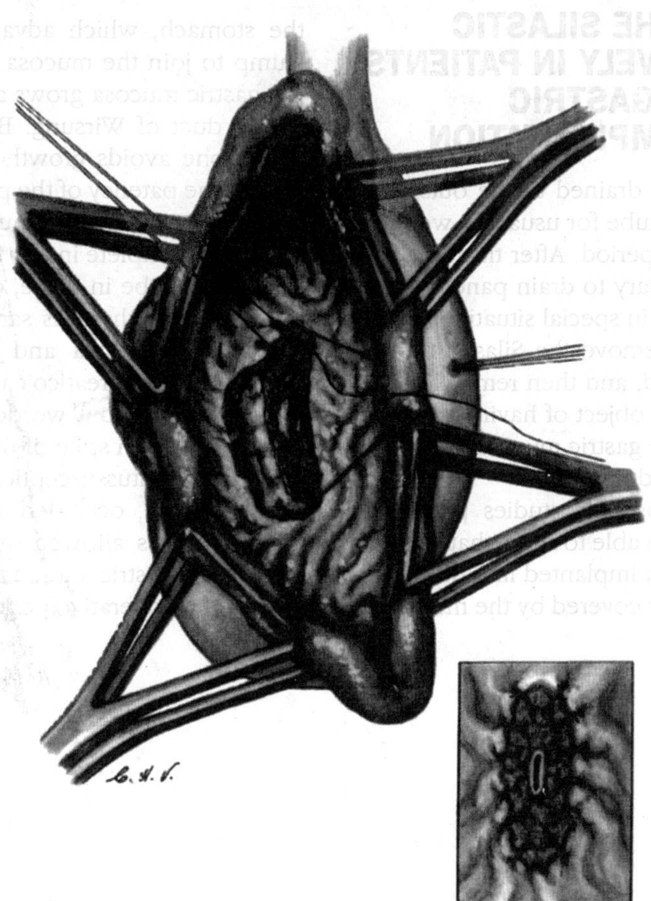

FIGURE 16.68

MANAGEMENT OF THE SILASTIC TUBE POSTOPERATIVELY IN PATIENTS WITH PANCREATICOGASTRIC ANASTOMOSIS BY IMPLANTATION

The pancreatic secretions are drained to the outside of the body through the Silastic tube for usually 2 weeks in the immediate postoperative period. After this length of time it is generally not necessary to drain pancreatic secretions to the outside except in special situations. However, it is not advisable to remove the Silastic tube. It should be left in place, closed, and then removed some 10 to 12 weeks later, with the object of having the Silastic tube act as a stent until the gastric mucosa has joined the mucosa of the pancreatic duct.

By means of serial gastroscopic studies performed postoperatively, we have been able to show that the pancreatic stump, which has been implanted into the lumen of the stomach, is aggressively covered by the mucosa of the stomach, which advances as projections over the stump to join the mucosa of the duct of Wirsung. Only the gastric mucosa grows and advances, not the mucosa of the duct of Wirsung. By leaving the Silastic tube in place, one avoids growth of the gastric mucosa, maintaining the patency of the pancreatic duct. Junction of the gastric mucosa and the mucosa of the duct of Wirsung is generally complete in 6 to 8 weeks. That is why we leave the Silastic tube in place, occluded, for 10 to 12 weeks. It is probable that this same process of union between the jejunal mucosa and the mucosa of the duct of Wirsung in pancreaticojejunal anastomosis by intussusception occurs, but we do not have any objective evidence of this. In spite of this, in pancreaticojejunal anastomosis by intussusception, we also leave the Silastic tube in place, occluded, during 10 to 12 weeks. This procedure has allowed us to establish permeability of pancreaticogastric and pancreaticojejunal anastomosis in the late postoperative period.

Management of the Silastic Tube Postoperatively in Patients with Pancreaticogastric Anastomosis By Implantation

FIGURE 16.69
This is a gastroscopic photograph of a patient in whom a pancreaticogastric anastomosis by implantation was performed taken 10 years after a pancreaticoduodenectomy for endocrine carcinoma (nonfunctional) of the head of the pancreas. In the endoscopic photograph, one can see the communication as well as the exit of pancreatic fluid. In some patients, thickened gastric folds may make visualization of the communication difficult. In those cases it is usually useful to give intravenous secretin (1 unit per kilogram of weight). Immediately after injection pancreatic secretion increases, allowing the patency of communication to be demonstrated.

Management of the Silastic Tube Postoperatively in Patients with Pancreaticogastric Anastomosis By Implantation

FIGURE 16.70
Gastroscopic photograph of a patient who was subjected to pancreaticoduodenectomy with pancreaticogastric anastomosis by implantation 2 years previously. Permeability of the anastomosis can be observed.

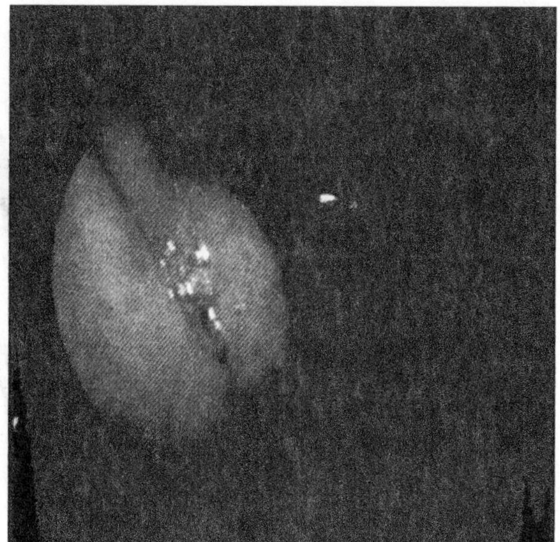

FIGURE 16.69

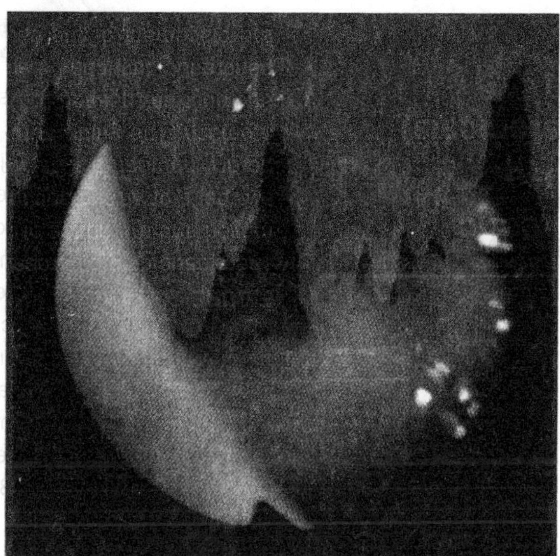

FIGURE 16.70

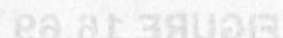

Management of the Silastic Tube Postoperatively in Patients with Pancreaticogastric Anastomosis By Implantation

FIGURE 16.71
Semischematic drawings interpreted by the illustrator that show the growth process of the gastric mucosa in covering the pancreatic stump and joining the mucosa of the duct of Wirsung, such as is observed in serial gastroscopic examinations. 1, The gastric mucosa grows in the form of digitations to cover the pancreatic stump and join the mucosa of the duct of Wirsung. The Silastic tube acts as a stent to prevent excessive growth of the gastric mucosa and obstruction of the pancreatic duct. 2, A view of the pancreaticogastric junction in a section. 3, A frontal view of the pancreaticogastric anastomosis. 4, The junction of the gastric mucosa and the pancreatic duct is almost completed. However, the Silastic tube should be left in place an additional 2 to 3 weeks so that the junction of the mucosas will be complete.

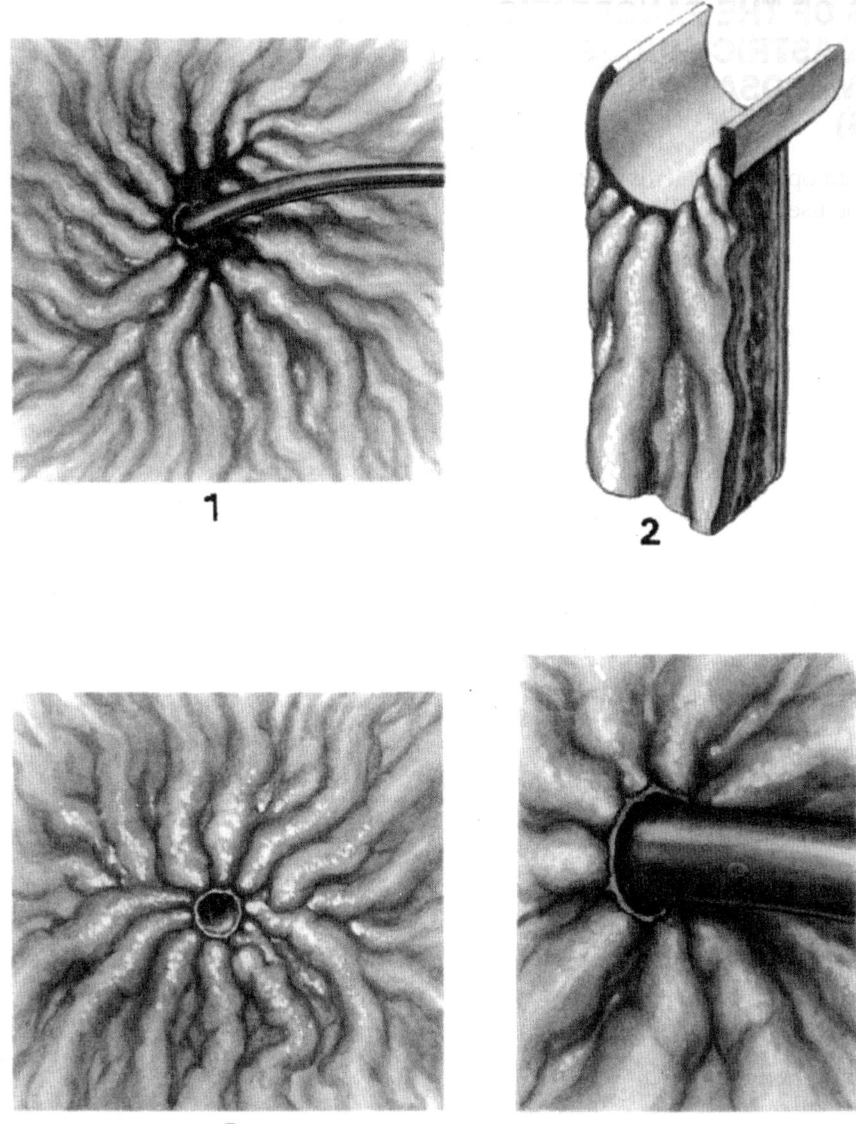

FIGURE 16.71

ANASTOMOSIS OF THE PANCREATIC DUCT TO THE GASTRIC MUCOSA (MUCOSA TO MUCOSA ANASTOMOSIS)

For this anastomosis, an operating microscope or a magnifying glass should be used.

Anastomosis of the Pancreatic Duct to the Gastric Mucosa (Mucosa to Mucosa Anastomosis)

Anastomosis of the Pancreatic Duct to the Gastric Mucosa (Mucosa to Mucosa Anastomosis)

FIGURE 16.72
The pancreatic stump has been approximated to the posterior wall of the stomach. The pancreatic duct is observed to be very dilated and having thickened walls, making it adequate for a mucosa to mucosa anastomosis.

FIGURE 16.73
A series of interrupted sutures using nonabsorbable material have been placed between the anterior border of the transected surface of the pancreas and the seromuscular layer of the stomach. The pancreatic sutures should include the capsule and a substantial portion of the pancreatic parenchyma to give adequate support to the suture. A small incision has been made in the posterior gastric wall the same diameter as the pancreatic duct. Guide sutures, which will be used to exert gentle traction and introduce the duct into the gastric lumen to facilitate the internal suture, have been placed in the ends of the pancreatic duct.

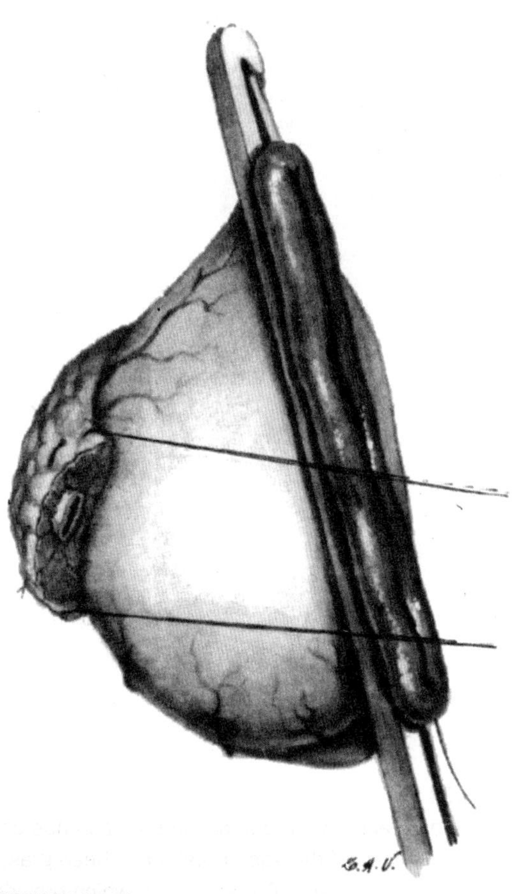

FIGURE 16.72

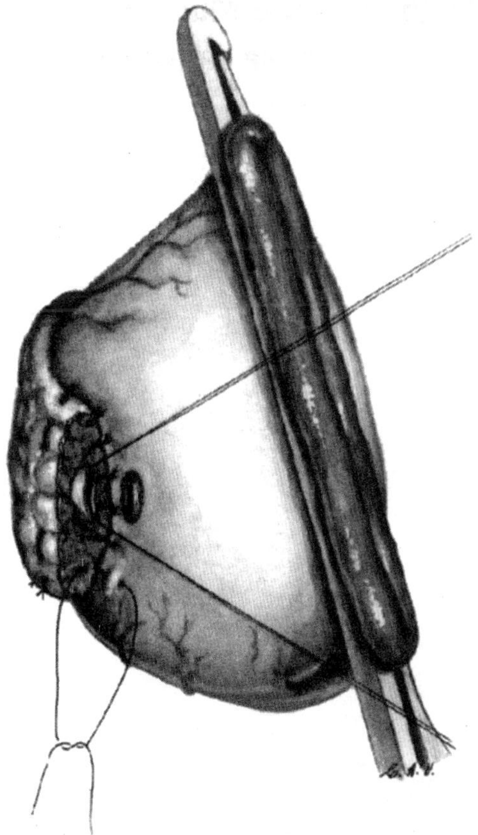

FIGURE 16.73

FIGURE 16.74
The elastic clamp across the end of the stomach has been removed and the edges of the gastric wall have been grasped by two pairs of atraumatic large Duval clamps, which provide temporary hemostasis as well as exposure of the cavity in the stomach. The guide sutures placed in the end of the pancreatic duct are passed to the interior of the stomach so that the pancreatic duct can be sutured to the gastric wall. Additionally, the placement of the catheter in the lumen of the pancreatic duct facilitates performance of the suture line.

Anastomosis of the Pancreatic Duct to the Gastric Mucosa (Mucosa to Mucosa Anastomosis)

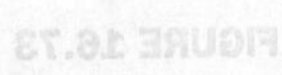

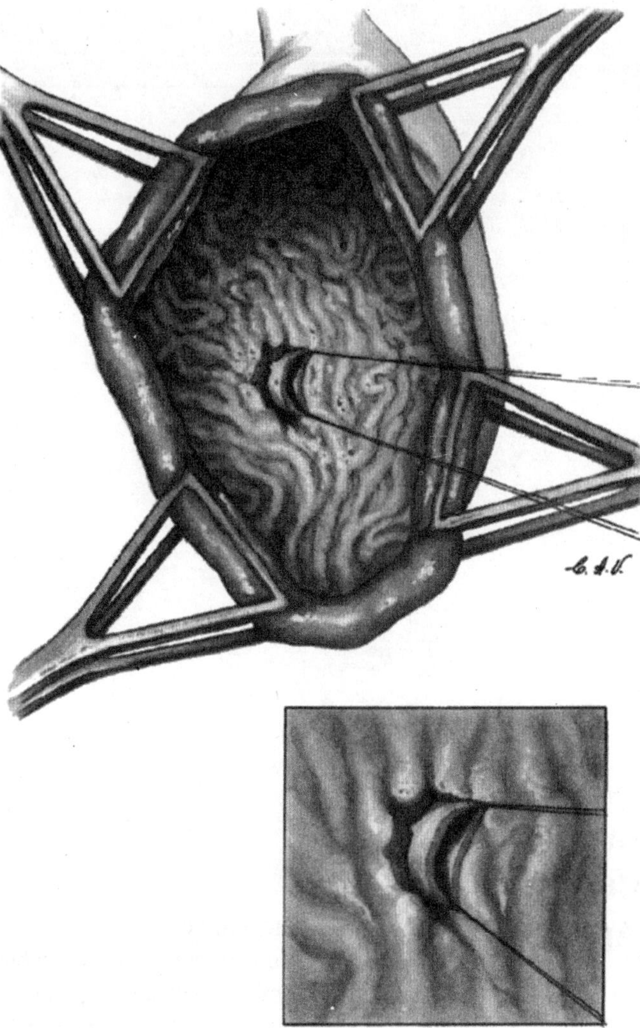

FIGURE 16.74

Anastomosis of the Pancreatic Duct to the Gastric Mucosa (Mucosa to Mucosa Anastomosis)

FIGURE 16.75
Sutures are being placed between the pancreatic duct and the entire thickness of gastric wall. The insert shows the same step seen through a magnifying lens.

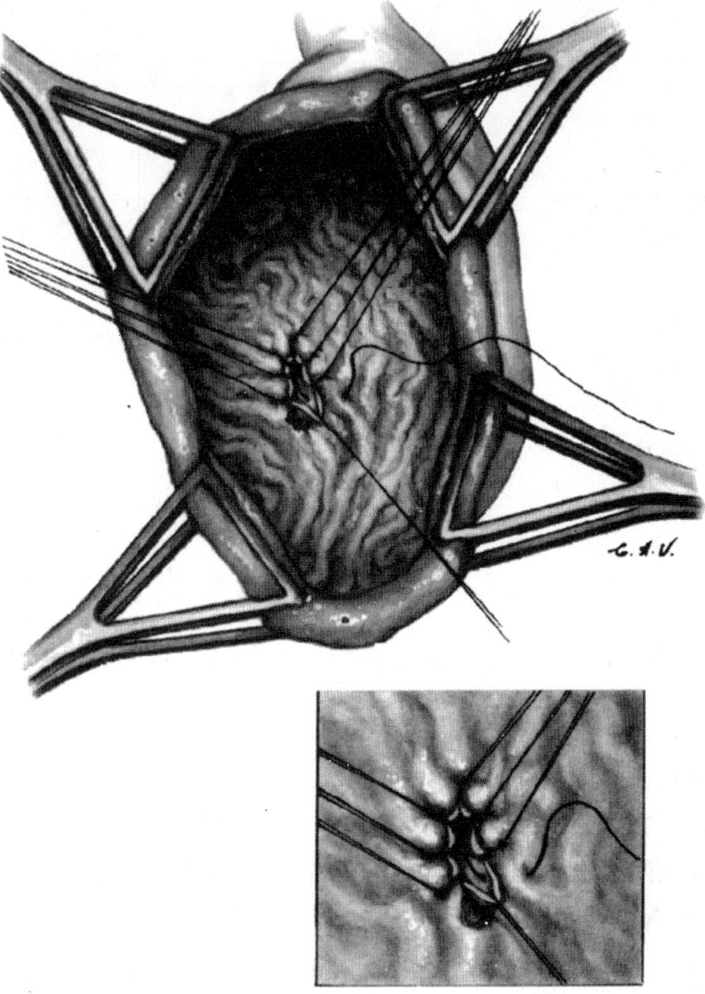

FIGURE 16.75

Anastomosis of the Pancreatic Duct to the Gastric Mucosa (Mucosa to Mucosa Anastomosis)

FIGURE 16.76
The anastomosis of the pancreatic duct and the gastric wall has been completed, and a Silastic tube with several perforations has been placed in the pancreatic duct. This tube is fixed to the pancreatic duct with two sutures of nonabsorbable material. The tube is passed through the anterior gastric wall to drain pancreatic secretions to the outside. The insert reveals this step using a magnifying lens.

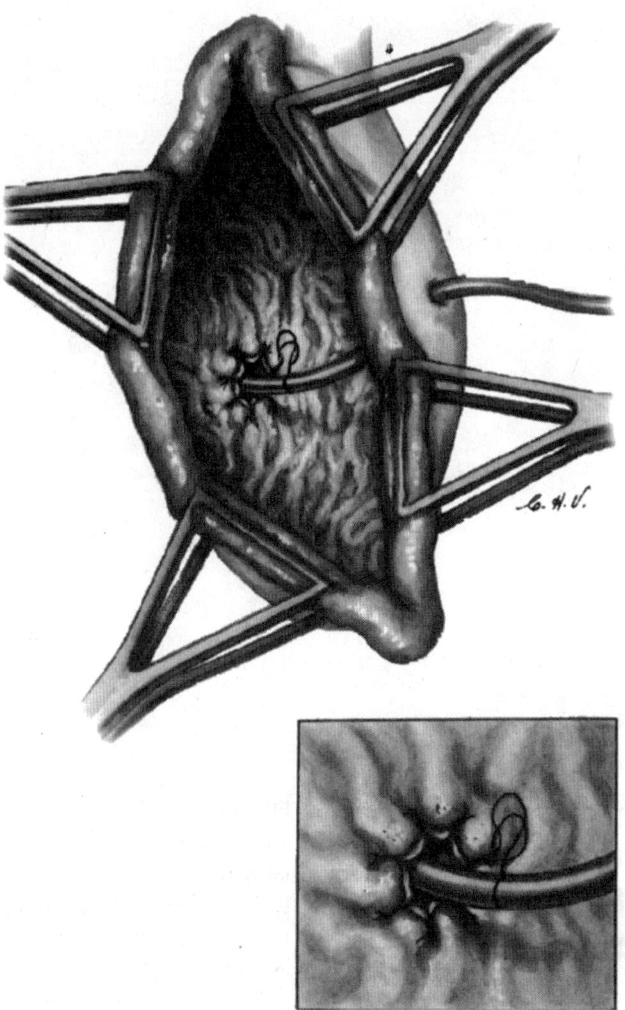

FIGURE 16.76

Anastomosis of the Pancreatic Duct to the Gastric Mucosa (Mucosa to Mucosa Anastomosis)

FIGURE 16.77
The external suture of the pancreas and the seromuscular layer of the stomach is completed. Once re-establishment of the digestive tract following pancreaticoduodenectomy is complete the Silastic tube is brought out the wall of the stomach and to the outside. The gastric wall is sutured to the parietal peritoneum of the anterior abdominal wall around the Silastic catheter to locally isolate the tube from the peritoneum.

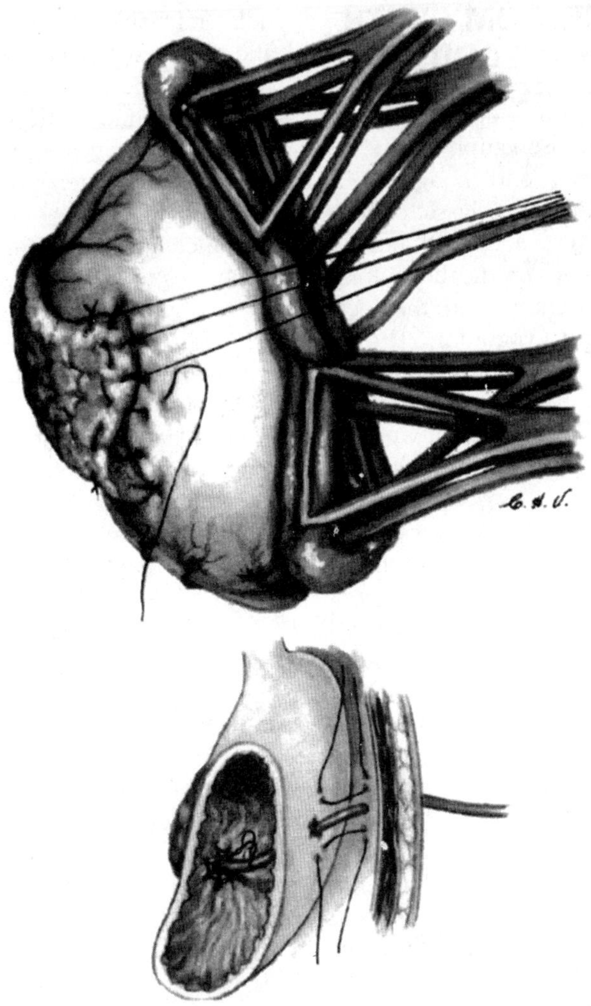

FIGURE 16.77

PANCREATICODUODENECTOMY WITH PRESERVATION OF THE PYLORUS (TRAVERSO-LONGMIRE TECHNIQUE)

Pancreaticoduodenectomy with conservation of the pylorus was described by Traverso and Longmire in 1978.(91) This technique differs from the classic pancreaticoduodenectomy or Whipple procedure by not including a gastric resection and conserving the pylorus and the first 2 to 3 cm of the duodenum. With this technique, it is not necessary to perform a vagotomy. The authors proposed this procedure for benign pancreatic conditions (chronic pancreatitis of the head of the pancreas) and for malignant lesions of the duodenum that were localized and far from the second portion of the duodenum. However, indications for this procedure were later expanded and the procedure applied in cases of carcinoma of the head of the pancreas and carcinoma of the papilla.(2, 45, 65, 86, 95) The procedure is considered contraindicated in carcinomas of the proximal portion of the second segment of the duodenum and in carcinomas of the distal third of the common bile duct.(2) In spite of the enthusiasm with which some surgeons use this procedure, others with great experience in pancreatic surgery believe that preservation of the pylorus can only be practiced in benign pancreaticoduodenal lesions.(28, 63)

It is of interest to record that pioneers in duodenal surgery such as Codevilla, Krausch, Herschel, Tenani, Denck, and Whipple (2, 25, 30, 45, 85, 91), used to conserve the pylorus and part of the duodenum but would re-establish gastric transit by means of a gastrojejunostomy. In the technique of Traverso and Longmire, transit is re-established by performing an anastomosis between the short duodenal stump and the jejunum in terminolateral fashion. In medical literature, there exists the precedent of the British surgeon Watson (99) who, in the year 1943, performed a pancreaticoduodenectomy with conservation of the pylorus and 2.5 cm of the proximal duodenum in a patient with carcinoma of the papilla of Vater, who had a good late survival. Watson differed from Traverso and Longmire, however, performing the operation in two stages, anastomosing the gallbladder to the jejunum and the duodenal stump to the jejunum in terminolateral fashion. In addition, Watson ligated the pancreatic duct, excluding pancreatic secretions. In 1975, Adson, from the Mayo Clinic, performed two pancreaticoduodenectomies with pyloric preservation.(2)

The advantages attributed to this technique over the classical technique are as follows:

1. Since no gastrectomy is performed, the stomach continues to act as a reservoir for foods and as a mixer and grinder, favoring digestion.
2. With this technique some postoperative problems owing to the gastrectomy and the vagotomy are avoided.
3. Preservation of at least 2 cm of the proximal duodenum is enough for patients to continue producing secretin, which inhibits hydrochloric and peptic secretions, lowering the frequency of ulcers and hemorrhages.
4. In addition, the small remaining duodenal segment continues to act as a pacemaker for antropyloric motility.

Postoperatively, the Traverso-Longmire procedure may cause retardation of gastric emptying for 2, 3, or more weeks before returning to normal. (97) For this reason, it is convenient to decompress the stomach by means of a gastrostomy rather than a nasogastric tube. This gastrostomy tube should be left in place until gastric function is normalized. Delayed gastric emptying may be caused by:

1. Edema of the duodenojejunostomy.
2. Injury to the prepyloric vagal branches.
3. Inclusion of the pylorus in sutures of the duodenojejunostomy, interfering with the sphincteric mechanism.
4. As a consequence of ischemia of the duodenal stump, without actual necrosis. (13)

The operative steps of pancreaticoduodenectomy with preservation of the pylorus are similar to the classic operation except for preservation of the stomach, pylorus, and 2 cm of proximal duodenum. Following, we will describe the steps that differ from the classical procedure.

Pancreaticoduodenectomy with Preservation of the Pylorus (Traverso-Longmire Technique)

Pancreaticoduodenectomy with Preservation of the Pylorus (Traverso-Longmire Technique)

FIGURE 16.78

The greater omentum has been separated from the colon and retracted upward with the stomach. The lined areas are the parts to be resected. The site where the right gastroepiploic artery is to be ligated, as close to the pylorus as possible, is shown, 1. The point of ligation of the pyloric arterty should be as close as possible to the lesser curvature, 2, and the site where the gastroduodenal artery should be ligated where it arises from the hepatic artery, 3, is also seen. This latter ligature should be performed with great care to avoid slippage.

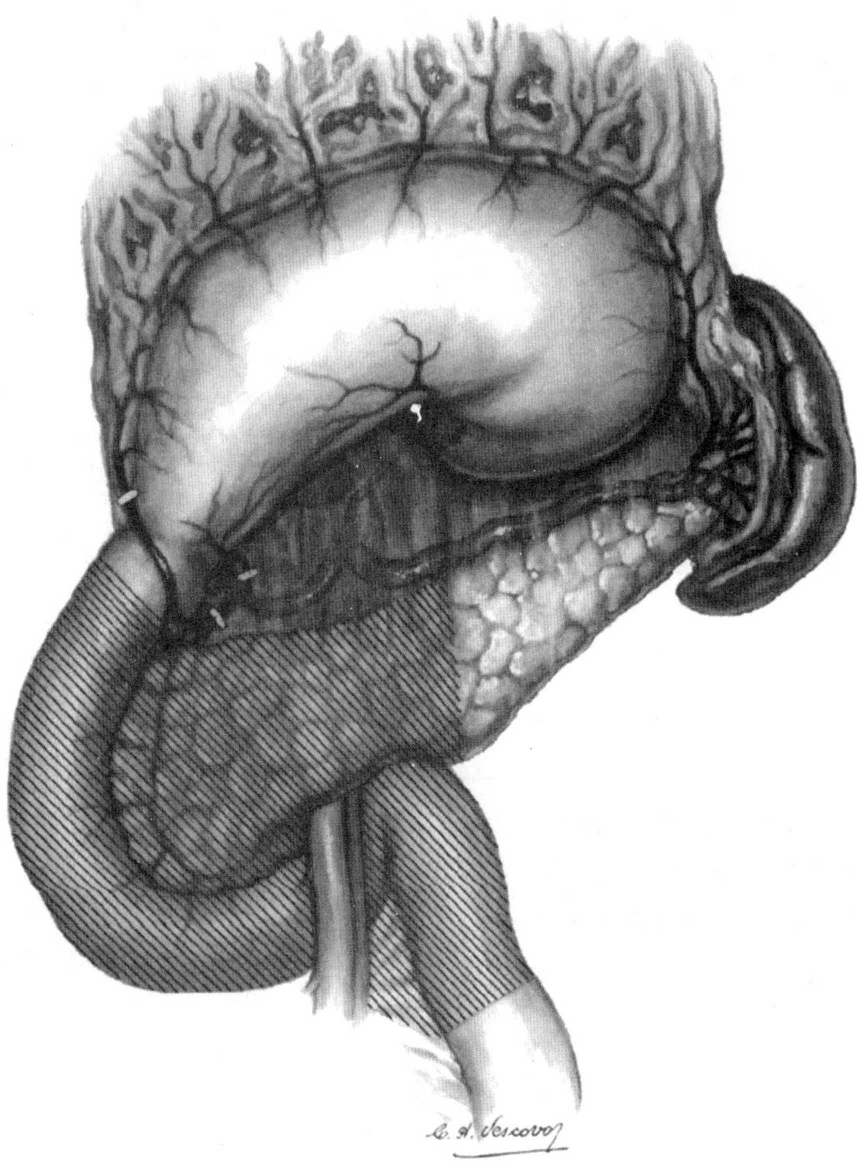

FIGURE 16.78

FIGURE 16.79
The drawing shows the ligated right gastroepiploic, 1, pyloric, 2, and gastroduodenal, 3, vessels. The duodenum has been divided about 2 cm from the pylorus. The distal duodenal segment is grasped with a Duval clamp. The end of the proximal duodenal segment is tagged with two guide sutures, taking care to observe its blood supply, which must be preserved for later completion of a successful anastomosis. The blood supply of this small duodenal segment depends almost exclusively on intramural circulation through the coronary or left gastric artery and the left gastroepiploic artery. It should be borne in mind that the first 3 cm of the duodenum correspond to the duodenal bulb, which is surrounded by peritoneum and is free and mobile, while the distal or "postbulbar" segment is attached to the posterior wall of the stomach by the parietal peritoneum.

Pancreaticoduodenectomy with Preservation of the Pylorus (Traverso-Longmire Technique)

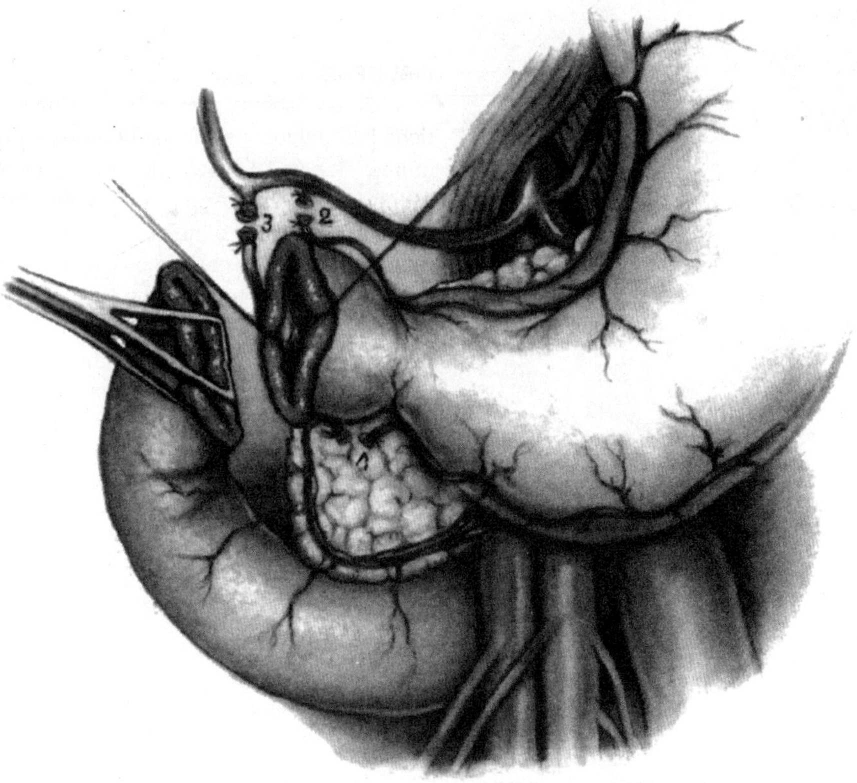

FIGURE 16.79

FIGURE 16.80
The surgeon should always bear in mind the numerous variations in the duodenal blood supply as he or she carries out ligatures of blood vessels during a pancreaticoduodenectomy with pyloric preservation, with the object of preserving an adequate blood supply to the duodenal stump so that the success of the procedure is not compromised. This figure and the next four figures show some of the multiple variations of the arterial blood supply of the first portion of the duodenum. This figure shows the blood supply of the first portion of the duodenum from the pyloric or right gastric artery, arising from the common hepatic artery, 1, from the supraduodenal artery, arising in the common hepatic artery, 2, and from a retroduodenal artery arising from the right gastroepiploic artery, 3.

Pancreaticoduodenectomy with Preservation of the Pylorus (Traverso-Longmire Technique)

FIGURE 16.81
In this case the blood supply of the first portion of the duodenum is from the pyloric or right gastric artery arising from the hepatic artery, 1, from the supraduodenal artery arising from the gastroduodenal artery, 2, and by several small arteries from the right gastroepiploic artery, 3.

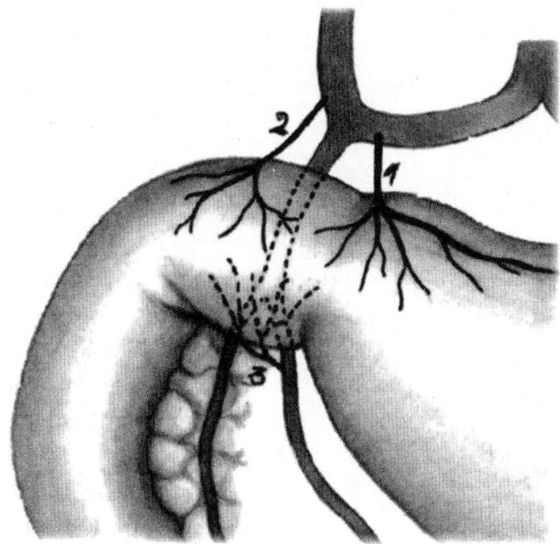

FIGURE 16.80

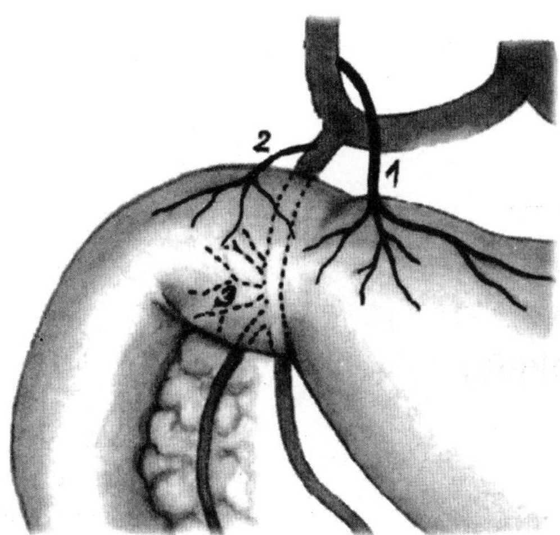

FIGURE 16.81

FIGURE 16.82
Posterior view of the blood supply of the first portion of the duodenum. The pyloric artery can be seen arising from the hepatic artery, 1. The supraduodenal artery arises in the gastroduodenal artery, 2. Small retroduodenal arteries arise from the gastroduodenal artery, 3, the gastroepiploic artery and the superior posterior pancreaticoduodenal artery.

Pancreaticoduodenectomy with Preservation of the Pylorus (Traverso-Longmire Technique)

FIGURE 16.83
In this case the pyloric (right gastric) artery arises from the common hepatic artery, 1. The supraduodenal artery is absent, replaced by small arteries arising from the pyloric, 2, the gastroduodenal, 3, and the right gastroepiploic, 4, arteries.

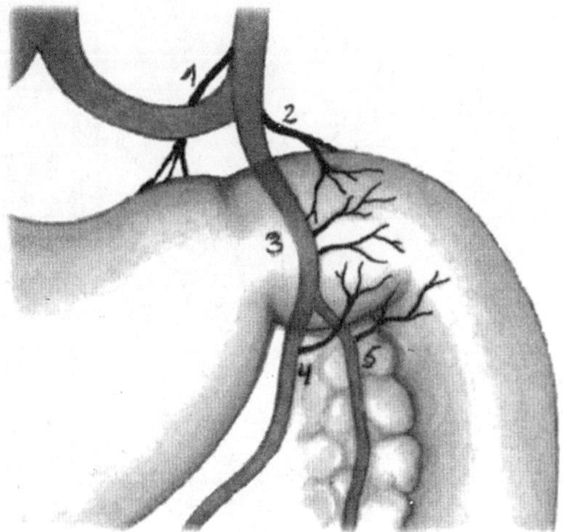

FIGURE 16.82

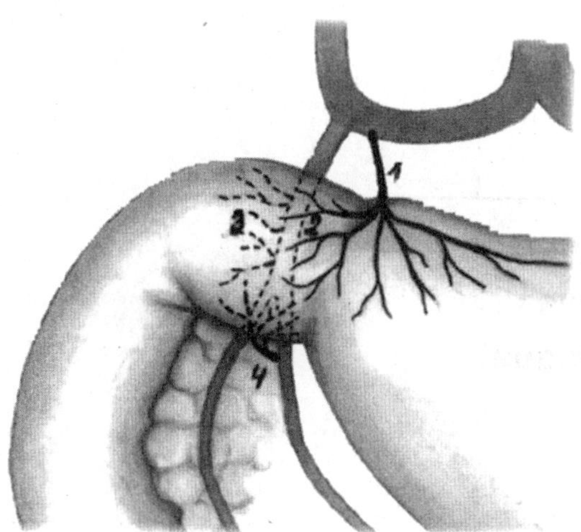

FIGURE 16.83

FIGURE 16.84
In this case the pyloric artery is absent, being replaced by the supraduodenal artery, 1, which anastomoses with branches of the coronary (left gastric) artery, 2. The supraduodenal artery irrigates part of the lesser curvature of the stomach and the duodenum. Some retroduodenal small branches arise from the right gastroepiploic artery, 3.

Pancreaticoduodenectomy with Preservation of the Pylorus (Traverso-Longmire Technique)

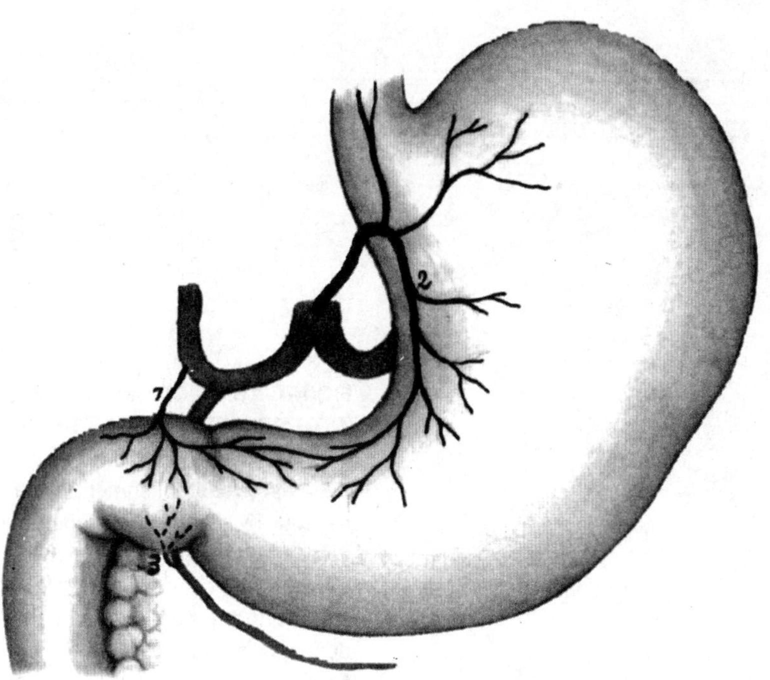

FIGURE 16.84

FIGURE 16.85 COMPLETED PANCREATICODUODENECTOMY WITH PRESERVATION OF THE PYLORUS

The pancreaticoduodenectomy has been completed and, in this case, reestablishment of pancreatic transit has been carried out by means of a pancreaticojejunal anastomosis by intussusception, using technique similar to that described in the classic pancreaticoduodenectomy. The pancreatic secretion is drained to the outside by means of a Silastic tube. The small duodenal stump has been anastomosed to the jejunum about 15 to 20 cm distal to the hepaticojejunal anastomosis, using two layers of sutures. In order to perform this anastomosis without risk, care must be taken to be sure the duodenal stump has an adequate intramural blood supply. It is also important to avoid putting sutures into the pylorus to avoid postoperative problems with emptying. Suturing should be carried out using fine needles and suture material to diminish postoperative edema. It is convenient to decompress the stomach by means of a gastrostomy using a Foley catheter instead of by means of a Levine tube, since gastric decompression may be needed for 2 or more weeks.

Pancreaticoduodenectomy with Preservation of the Pylorus (Traverso-Longmire Technique)

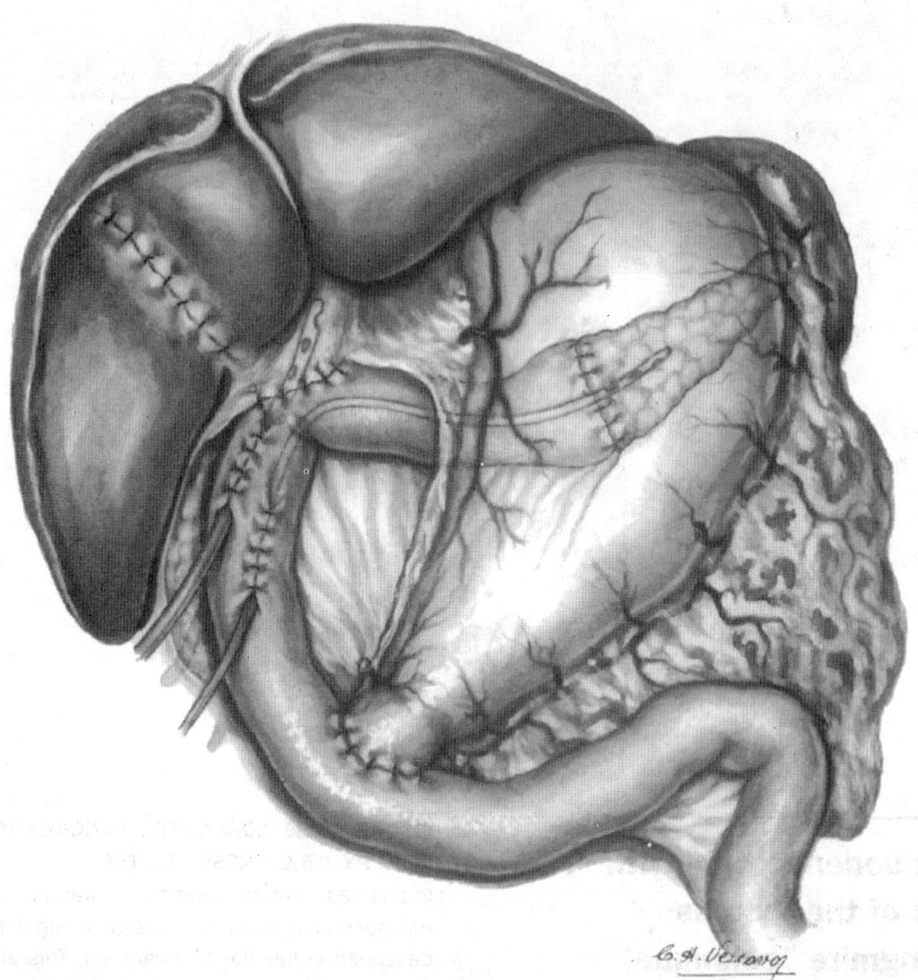

FIGURE 16.85 COMPLETED PANCREATICODUODENECTOMY WITH PRESERVATION OF THE PYLORUS

Pancreaticoduodenectomy with Preservation of the Pylorus (Traverso-Longmire Technique)

FIGURE 16.86 COMPLETED PANCREATICODUODENECTOMY WITH PYLORIC PRESERVATION

In this case the pancreatic duct was anastomosed to the jejunal mucosa (mucosa to mucosa) using the same technique as described in the classic operation. This anastomosis can only be carried out when the pancreatic duct is very dilated and its walls thickened. The other anastomoses are similar to those in the previous figure.

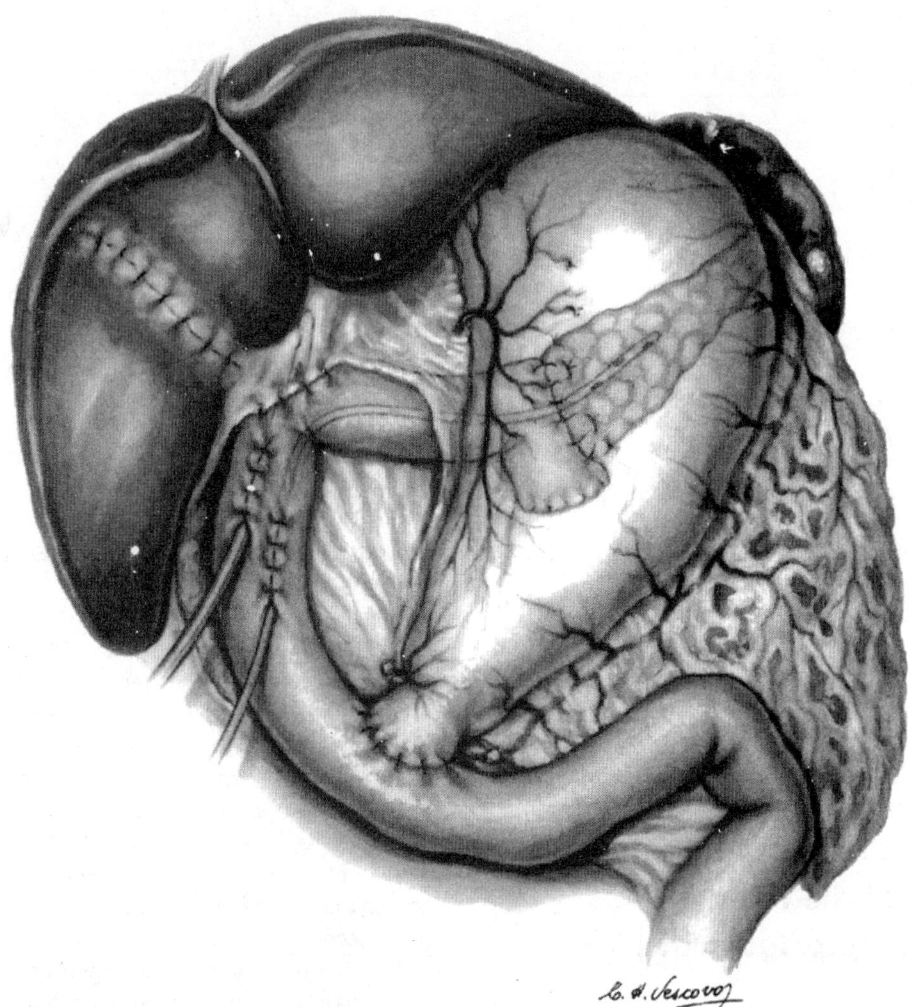

FIGURE 16.86 COMPLETED PANCREATICODUODENECTOMY WITH PYLORIC PRESERVATION

FIGURE 16.87 COMPLETED PANCREATICODUODENECTOMY WITH PYLORIC PRESERVATION

In this case, the anastomosis of the pancreatic stump has been carried out by implantation of the stump into the posterior gastric wall. As in the classic operation, the pancreas can be anastomosed to the jejunum or the stomach by implantation or by mucosa to mucosa anastomosis of the pancreatic duct to the posterior gastric wall. Anastomosis of the pancreatic stump of the pancreatic duct to the gastric wall may be performed by means of a single row of sutures from the outside of the stomach, or by means of two rows of sutures, one on the outside and the other on the inside of the stomach. Either technique is used, depending on the circumstances. If a second row of sutures is to be used inside the stomach, it can only be applied through an incision in the anterior gastric wall, since, in the Traverso-Longmire technique, there is no gastric resection.

Pancreaticoduodenectomy with Preservation of the Pylorus (Traverso-Longmire Technique)

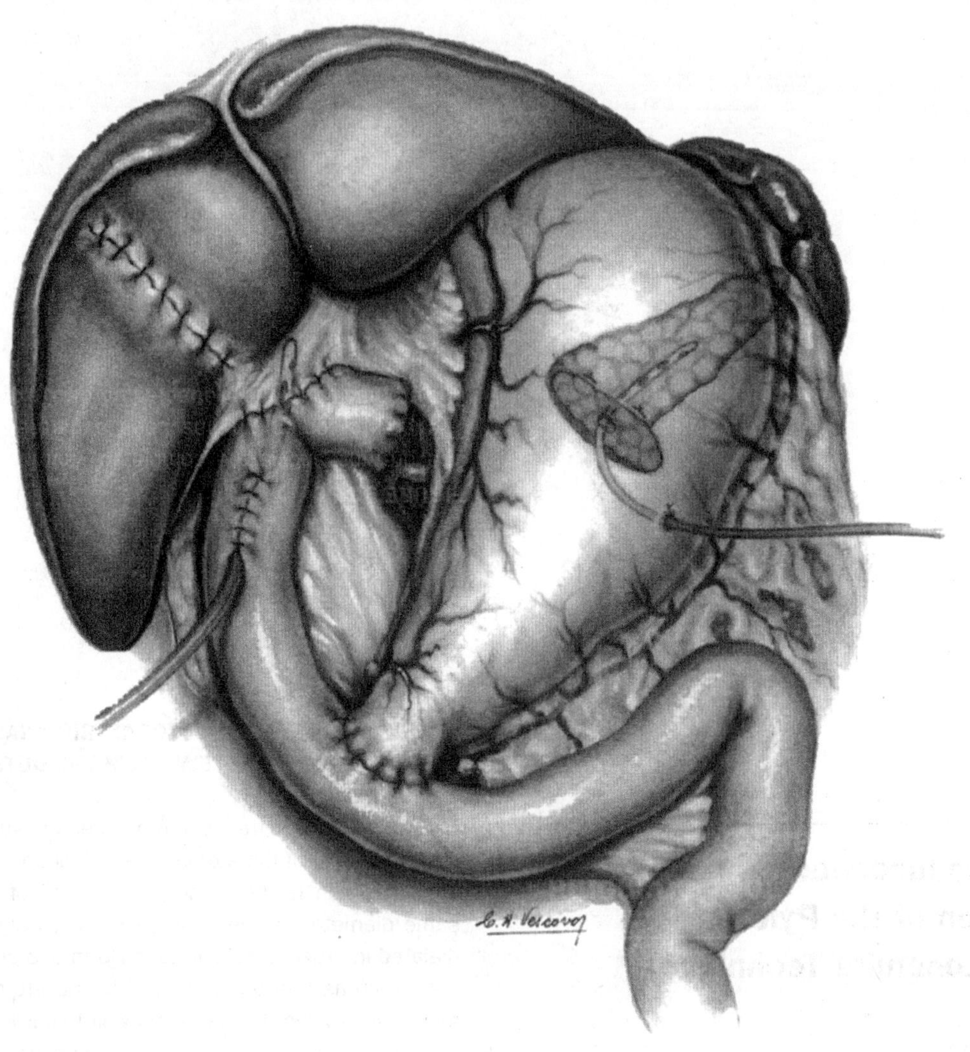

FIGURE 16.87 COMPLETED PANCREATICODUODENECTOMY WITH PYLORIC PRESERVATION

FIGURE 16.88 PANCREATICOGASTRIC ANASTOMOSIS PERFORMED COMPLETELY FROM THE OUTSIDE OF THE STOMACH

The surface of the transected pancreas is sutured to the seromuscular layer of the stomach using nonabsorbable sutures. A small incision is then made in the wall of the stomach the same diameter as the pancreatic duct, which should be very dialated in order to be able to perform this anastomosis. Once the pancreas has been sutured to the stomach, the anastomosis of the duct to the gastic wall is carried out using interrupted nonabsorbable sutures, 1. A Silastic catheter is then introduced into the pancreatic duct and fixed in place with two nonabsorbable sutures. The anastomosis of the duct is then completed, 2. A magnifying loop should be used in this anastomosis. The anastomosis is then completed by suturing the surface of the pancreatic stump to the seromuscular layer of the stomach on the opposite side, 3.

Pancreaticoduodenectomy with Preservation of the Pylorus (Traverso-Longmire Technique)

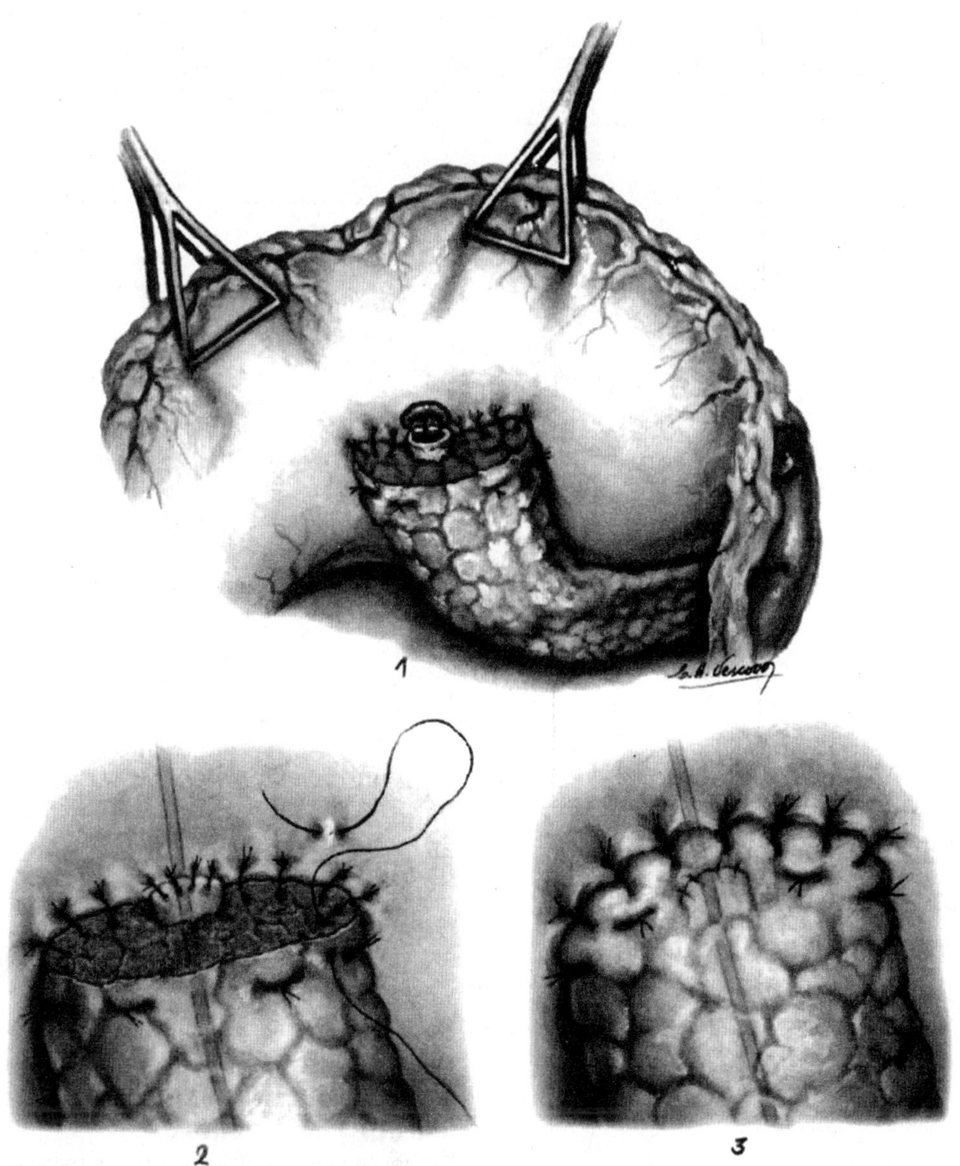

FIGURE 16.88 PANCREATICOGASTRIC ANASTOMOSIS PERFORMED COMPLETELY FROM THE OUTSIDE OF THE STOMACH

Pancreaticoduodenectomy with Preservation of the Pylorus (Traverso-Longmire Technique)

FIGURE 16.89 ANASTOMOSIS OF THE PANCREATIC STUMP OR DUCT TO THE STOMACH USING EXTERNAL AND INTERNAL SUTURES

The technique is very similar to the technique described in the classic operation. Since the Traverso-Longmire procedure does not include gastrectomy, an 8 to 10 cm incision has to be made in the anterior gastric wall to carry out the internal portion of the anastomosis. 1, Anastomosis of the pancreatic stump to the posterior gastric wall by implantation. 2, Anastomosis of the pancreatic duct to the gastric wall (mucosa to mucosa). 3, Completed anastomosis with a Silastic tube brought to the outside through the anterior gastric wall.

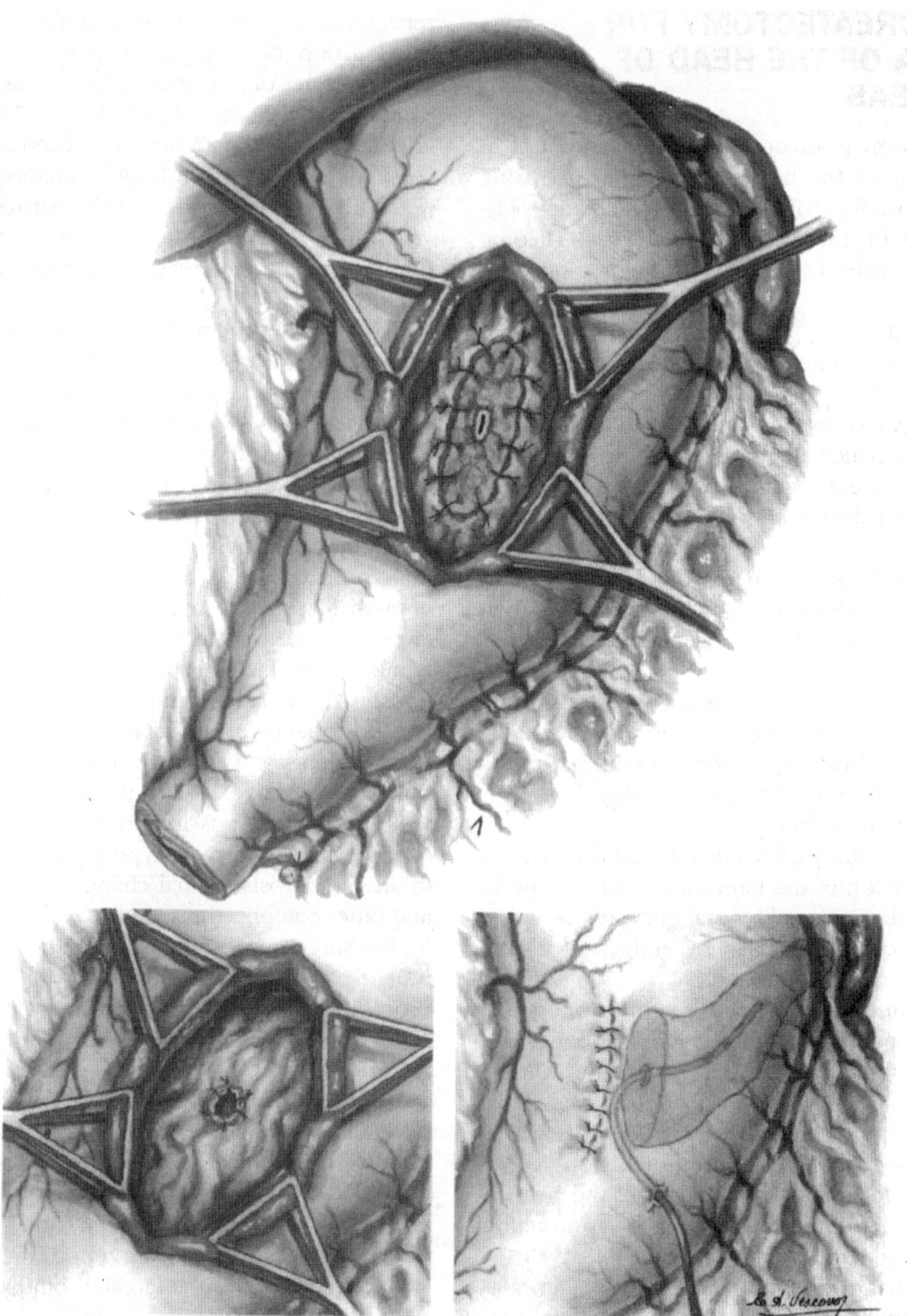

FIGURE 16.89 ANASTOMOSIS OF THE PANCREATIC STUMP OR DUCT TO THE STOMACH USING EXTERNAL AND INTERNAL SUTURES

TOTAL PANCREATECTOMY FOR CARCINOMA OF THE HEAD OF THE PANCREAS

Total pancreatectomy is advocated by many surgeons in treating carcinoma of the head of the pancreas, using the Whipple procedure only in extrapancreatic periampullary tumors. (4, 13, 51, 63, 79, 80, 81, 92–94) Some of the arguments used by those who favor total pancreatectomy are

1. Carcinoma of the pancreas is frequently multicentric in origin. (4, 79)
2. Partial pancreatectomy may leave residual tumor in the line of the pancreatic transection. (4, 79)
3. Resection of the entire pancreas eliminates the possibility of direct dissemination of the tumor to more distal areas.
4. Since the pancreatic duct is not divided, spillage of pancreatic fluid, which may contain tumor cells that can be implanted into the peritoneal cavity, is avoided.
5. In total pancreatectomy there is no need for anastomoses of the duct or stump into the digestive tract, avoiding a possibility of dehiscence with its consequent increase in morbidity and mortality.
6. Operating time is shorter.
7. Proponents of total pancreatectomy affirm that the exocrine secretion of the pancreas is not indispensable and can be replaced by oral enzymes.
8. The ensuing diabetes caused by endocrine insufficiency can be easily controlled.
9. Total pancreatectomy is a more complete operation, since it includes a more complete lymphadenectomy.
10. Acute pancreatitis of the residual pancreatic stump is avoided.

In spite of these advantages, some more theoretic than real, total pancreatectomy for carcinoma of the head of the pancreas has not diminished morbidity or mortality, nor has it improved survival rate.

On the other hand, operative morbidity or mortality of the Whipple operation has decreased considerably in recent years, in experienced surgical centers where a small group of surgeons practice pancreatic surgery. Mortality rates of 5%, or even 2% or less, have been published. (2, 12, 26, 32, 39, 42, 48, 61, 72, 89, 92, 98) The argument that the Whipple procedure, according to some authors, carries a high morbidity and mortality is not valid at present. Additionally, survival for 5 or more years after pancreaticoduodenectomy for carcinoma of the head of the pancreas has increased in recent years. (12, 26, 32)

The most important disadvantage of total pancreatectomy is that it leads to a very difficult to control diabetes, of unpredictable evolution, with daytime or, even more serious, nightime hypoglycemias that may cause death. The diabetes in these patients needs permanent adjustments, even several years later. Though it is true that these patients rarely need more than 15 to 25 units of insulin daily, sensitivity to this hormone can be so severe that an increase of 2 or 3 units of insulin in one day is enough to provoke hypoglycemic shock. Patients who are subjected to total pancreatectomy, as well as their families, must face this problem and be alert to it continuously. These patients must be managed in the early and late postoperative period by experienced endocrinologists. Patients with total pancreatectomy should have a blood sugar above 2% as a preventative measure, to prevent, as much as possible, dangerous hypoglycemias or even death. This forced hyperglycemica frequently leads to arteriosclerosis, retinal changes, cataracts, fatty livers, and other complications.

The surgeon planning a total pancreatectomy must be more rigorous in making the diagnosis than in a Whipple procedure because the operation will cause a diabetic state that is difficult to control and of unpredictable evolution.

In the following, we will describe the stages of total pancreatectomy that differ from the classic pancreaticoduodenectomy, since both procedures are similar, except that the total resection involves removal of the body and tail of the pancreas, the spleen, and the entire greater omentum, because, in ligating both the splenic and gastroduodenal artery, the greater omentum will lose its blood supply.

Total Pancreatectomy for Carcinoma of the Head of the Pancreas

Total Pancreatectomy for Carcinoma of the Head of the Pancreas

FIGURE 16.90
The drawing shows the completed Vautrin-Kocher maneuver. The greater omentum has been separated from the colon. The stomach has been retracted upward, exposing the anterior surface of the pancreas

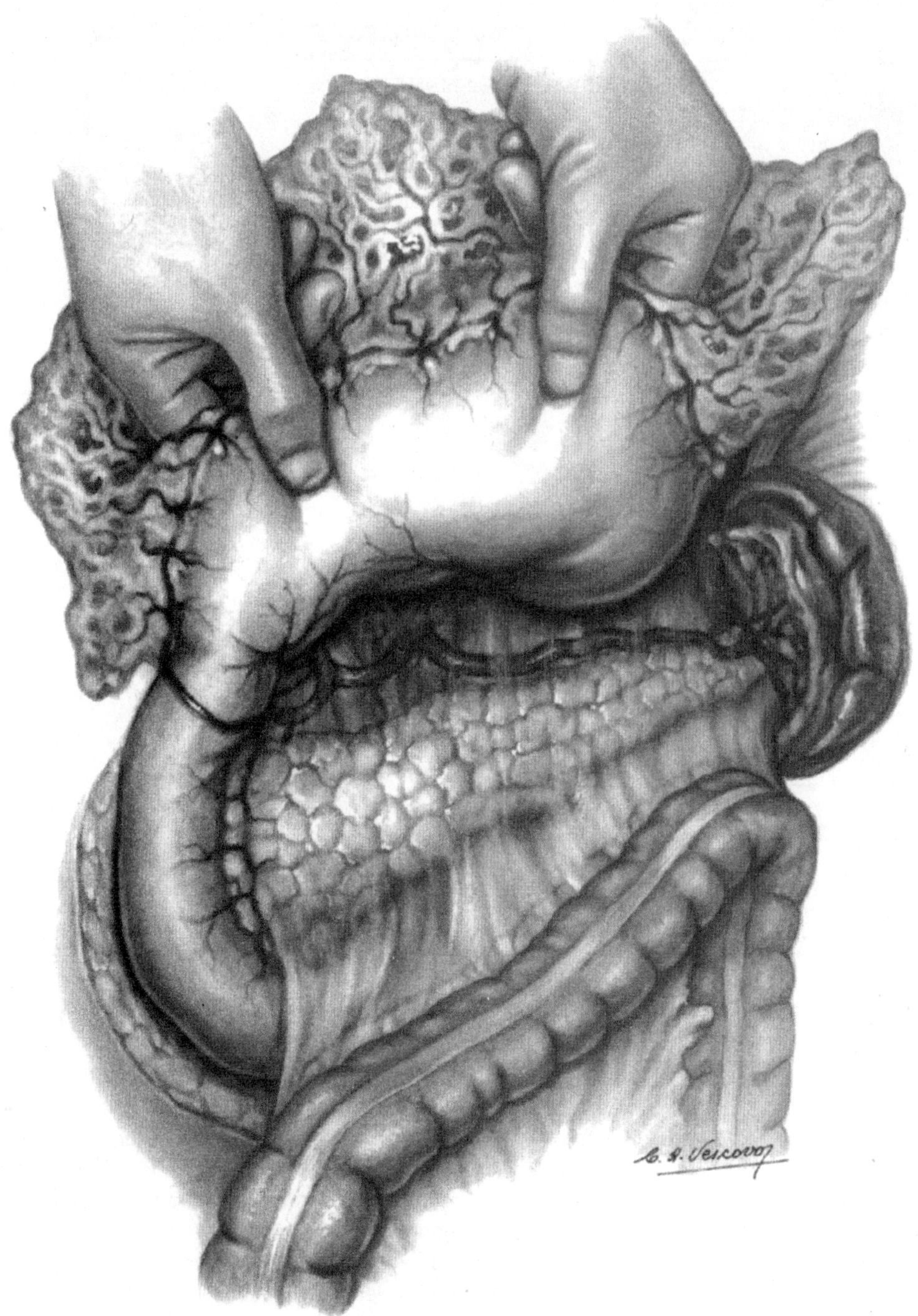

FIGURE 16.90

Total Pancreatectomy for Carcinoma of the Head of the Pancreas

FIGURE 16.91
The short vessels have been ligated and divided. The left gastroepiploic artery has been ligated and divided. The left half of the greater omentum has been removed. The right half will be removed with the surgical specimen. The phreno-splenic, splenocolic, and splenorenal ligaments have been ligated and divided, allowing the spleen to be mobilized. Section of the peritoneum over the inferior border of the pancreas has begun. The peritoneum over the superior border will then be divided. This will allow retraction of the pancreas, together with the spleen, toward the right.

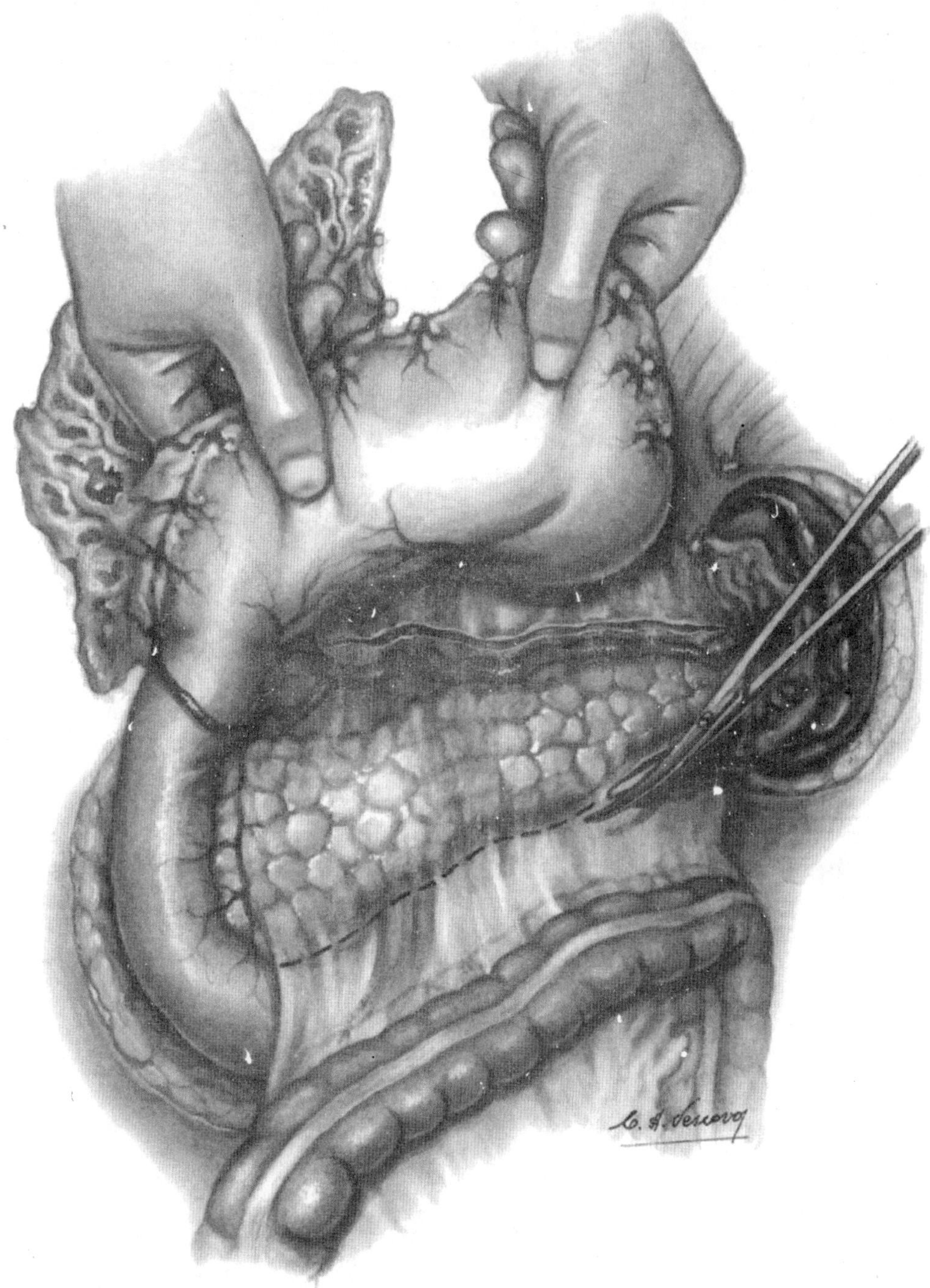

FIGURE 16.91

Total Pancreatectomy for Carcinoma of the Head of the Pancreas

FIGURE 16.92
The drawing shows that a bilateral truncal vagotomy has been done. The stomach has been divided at the correct site for a hemigastrectomy. The proximal gastric segment, which is free of omentum, is closed by an elastic clamp. The distal stomach has been reflected to the right, together with the pancreas and spleen. It is important to point out that the proximal gastric segment, which is to be anastomosed to the jejunum, will be supplied with blood only by the cardioesophageal artery. Retraction of the spleen and the body and tail of the pancreas allows the splenic artery to be doubly ligated and divided at its origin in the celiac axis. In addition, the splenic vein has been doubly ligated and divided at its junction with the superior mesenteric vein.

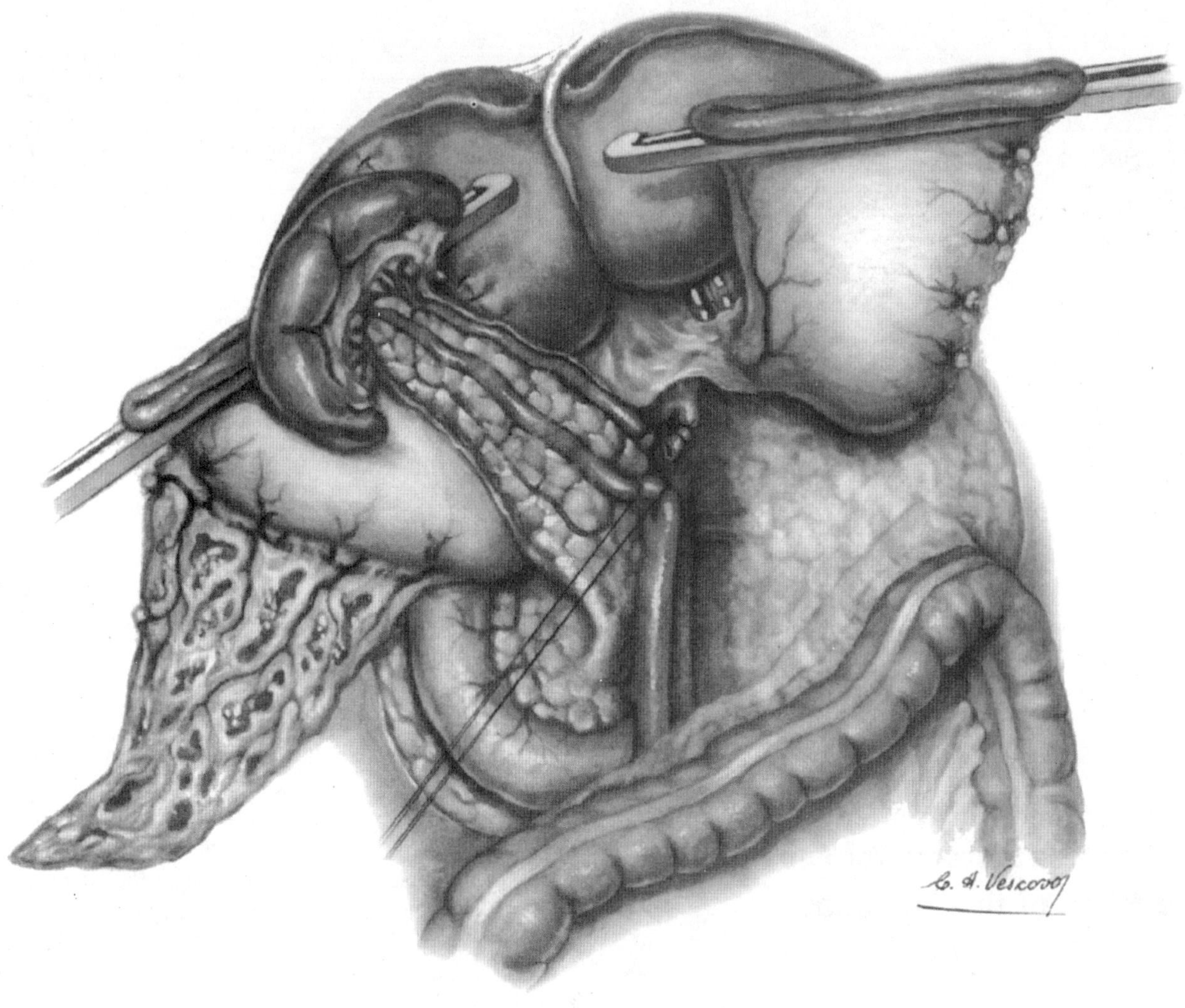

FIGURE 16.92

FIGURE 16.93
The reflected pancreas is held toward the right by the left hand of the surgeon while the head of the pancreas and the uncinate process are liberated using the same technique as in the classic pancreaticoduodenectomy. This means that the hepatic duct is divided and the gallbladder resected, Henle's trunk is ligated, and the jejunum is transected about 10 to 12 cm beyond the angle of Treitz, carrying it toward the right side of the patient. These maneuvers facilitate liberation of the head and neck as well as the uncinate process of the pancreas. The surgeon, using the left hand, holds the pancreas rotating it slightly to the right, in order to ligate and divide the veins that run from the head of the pancreas to the superior mesenteric vein. The superior mesenteric vein is gently retracted to the left, using a vein retractor, so as to begin ligating the arteries that run from the superior mesenteric artery to the head of the pancreas. The uncinate process is then freed and the surgical specimen removed.

Total Pancreatectomy for Carcinoma of the Head of the Pancreas

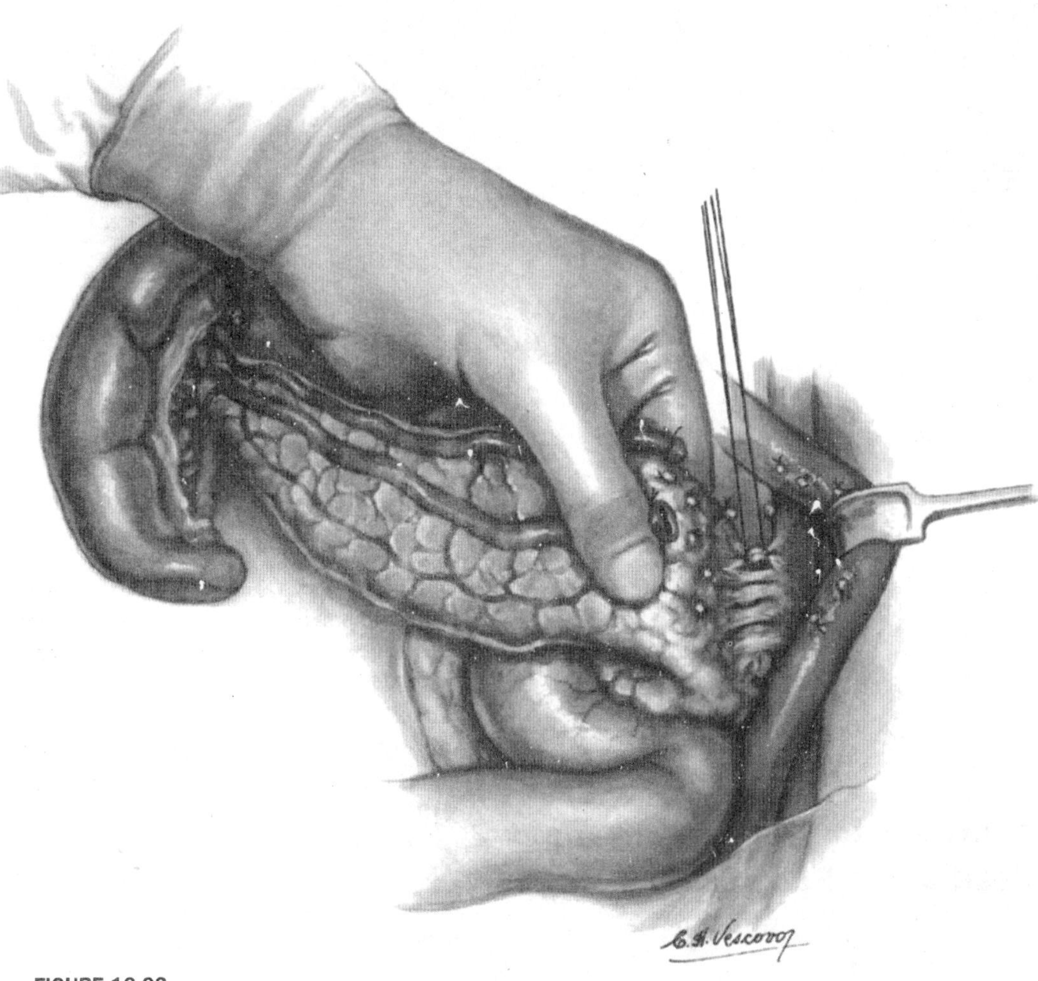

FIGURE 16.93

FIGURE 16.94
This drawing shows the completed total pancreatectomy. The terminolateral one layer anastomosis of the bile duct to the jejunum, using sutures of slow reabsorption, can be seen. Biliary secretions are drained to the outside by means of a Silastic tube. This anastomosis should be tested for leakage. In order to carry out this test, an elastic clamp is placed across the jejunal loop about 5 or 6 cm from the anastomosis to the hepatic duct. The Silastic tube is then occluded and about 50 mL of physiologic saline is injected into it with a syringe and needle. If leakage is detected, it is repaired at that time. The drawing shows the truncal vagotomy and the hemigastrectomy with antecolic gastrojejunal anastomosis.

Total Pancreatectomy for Carcinoma of the Head of the Pancreas

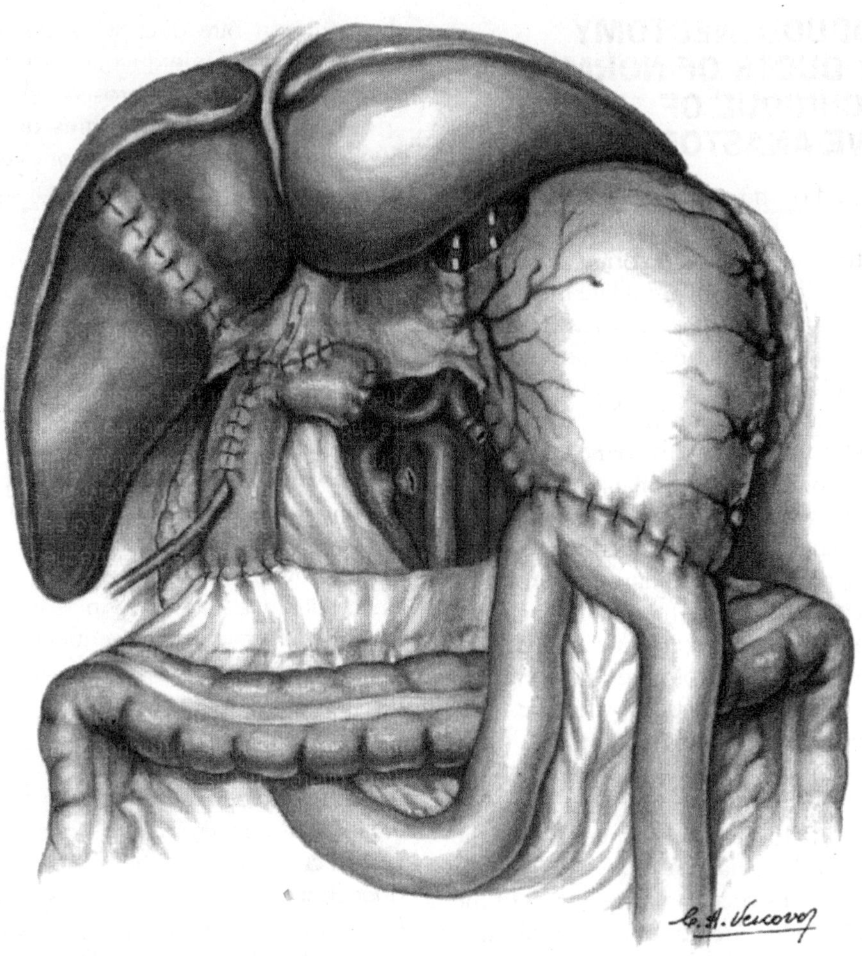

FIGURE 16.94

PANCREATICODUODENECTOMY WITH BILIARY DUCTS OF NORMAL CALIBER—TECHNIQUE OF BILIODIGESTIVE ANASTOMOSIS

Carcinomas of the head of the pancreas and the papilla of Vater usually obstruct the choledochus, producing marked dilation of the biliary duct, favoring its anastomosis to the jejunum with good early and late results. On the other hand, if the tumors do not obstruct the biliary duct and the diameter of the duct remains normal (6–8 mm), anastomosis with the jejunum becomes difficult and late results are unsure. This means that a factor of uncertainty is added to the complex pancreaticoduodenectomy, since anastomosis of a normal biliary duct to the jejunum may lead to stricture of the anastomosis, with its consequent complications and need for reoperations. The number of patients with biliary tracts of normal caliber that have to be subjected to pancreaticoduodenectomy is limited, but does constitute a group of patients with definite possibilities of cure and long survival. This group is composed of patients who present a very heterogeneous pathology. Among the conditions that involve the duodenum without compromise of the papilla are carcinoma of the duodenum; some patients with chronic pancreatitis located predominantly in the pancreatic head who do not have a dilated pancreatic duct and do not have an obstruction of the lumen of the bile duct; patients with endocrine nonfunctional or functional tumors of the head of the pancreas, which, due to its soft consistency, may not obstruct the common bile duct; some patients with serous or mucous cystademonas, cystadenocarcinomas, or cystopapillary carcinomas; lymphomas of the head of the pancreas or the duodenum; carcinoid tumors of the head of the pancreas or the duodenum; some cases of trauma to the pancreas; and so on.

Some surgeons with great experience in biliary and pancreatic surgery maintain that, for an anastomosis of the common bile duct to the digestive tract to be successful, the duct should have a minimal diameter of 2.5 cm.(6, 16, 34, 35, 46, 49, 50, 57–59, 70) Another group of surgeons maintain that if the common bile duct has a diameter of 2 cm or even 1.5 cm, this is enough to perform an adequate anastomosis. There are also surgeons who maintain that the caliber (diameter) of the common bile duct is not important in this anastomosis and that the only factor that should be considered is the normal or pathologic state of the walls of the common bile duct.(10, 50, 96) If the common bile duct has fibrosed walls or if there is fibrosis in the surrounding tissues, as occurs in surgical strictures of the biliary tract, the diameter of the common bile duct must be very ample or the patient will be exposed to stenosis and its sequelae.

Experience, however, shows that an anastomosis of the common bile duct with the digestive tract should have a common bile duct at least 2 cm in diameter, be it with normal walls or fibrosis of the walls.

Several surgical procedures have been described in the literature with the object of overcoming the problem of an anastomosis of the normal diameter common bile duct to the digestive tract. Results of these different procedures have not been obtained as far as we know.(34, 35, 50, 70)

When the first resections of the pancreas and duodenum were performed, it was a common occurrence that the surgeon re-establish biliary drainage by anastomosing the gallbladder to the digestive tract after ligating and transecting the common bile duct. This technique was later abandoned because of bad results. Anastomosis of the biliary tract to the digestive tract leads to obstruction to the passage of bile from the hepatic duct to the gallbladder owing to the presence of the valves of Heister in the cystic duct, leading to increased pressure in the common bile duct which is frequently followed by infection in the biliary tract (cholangitis) and sometimes rupture of the tied or sutured end of the common bile duct.

The valves of Heister regulate passage of bile from the common bile duct to the gallbladder and in the opposite direction. We began to realize in 1969 that following pancreaticoduodenectomy with normal diameter of the biliary tract, rupture of the valves of Heister in the cystic duct should be done by means of the technique we will show later to allow free passage of bile and then perform the anastomosis of the gallbladder to the jejunum. This technique has given good results be it in the early or late postoperative period. Destruction of the valves of Heister to facilitate passage of bile through the cystic duct is based on anatomic, histologic, and physiologic facts:

1. Anatomic basis: The cystic duct, when seen from the outside, presents its characteristic appearance as an irregular structure with a twisted appearance owing to the presence of a series of depressions or narrowings separated by dilations. The depressions present an oblique disposition, maintaining a certain parallelism that gives the cystic duct a spiral appearance. If examined from within, the cystic duct presents the valves of Heister, which are classically described as mucosal folds within the cystic duct disposed in semilunar fashion with one edge, called the adhesive edge, applied to the wall of the duct and a free edge that projects into the lumen of the duct. The free edges of the semilunar configuration of the valves of Heister are oriented obliquely and may occupy from 25 to 75% of the circumference of the duct. The semilunar valves give the cystic duct a spiral appearance.(90) The valves are separated from each other, maintaining their individuality, but since they are ultimately disposed in different directions,

they give the impression of a continuous spiral. They do not lead to complete obstruction because between the free edge of the valve and the opposite wall of the cystic duct, there is always room through which it is possible to introduce the end of a curved, fine hemostatic clamp. This space must be sought individually, since it varies from one valve to the next according to the direction of the valve. To advance the end of the clamp placed within the cystic duct, the semilunar valves of Heister must be broken up one by one, separately.

2. *Histologic basis:* Histologic study of the cystic duct reveals that it is composed of a mucosal layer of cylindrical epithelium with a tunica propia containing mucous glands and possessing a weak submucosal layer that is not present in the gallbladder. This submucosal layer is composed of connective tissue. In this submucosal layer the cystic duct has a thin longitudinal muscular layer. The cystic duct does not contain oblique or circular muscle fibers. The thin muscular longitudinal layer of the cystic duct is located on the surface of the duct, covered only by the peritoneum, which surrounds the entire cystic duct.(90)

   Two facts catch our attention in the structure in the cystic duct: (a) The valves are not erased by distending the cystic duct either with air or fluid, and (b) the base or adherent border of each of the valves exactly coincides with the groove on the external surface of the cystic duct and presents a similar oblique direction.

   Histologic studies of the cystic duct have shown that studies of the valves of Heister reveal that the base of the valves extends beyond the mucosa of the cystic duct and partially penetrates the thin, longitudinal muscle layer. Penetration of the base of the valves of Heister in the muscular layer coincides with the external grooves of the cystic duct, suggesting that the external groove of the cystic duct may be produced by the penetration of the valve into the muscular layer of the duct. When the valve of Heister is ruptured, a tear occurs in the thin, muscular layer of the cystic duct. Rupture of all the valves of the cystic duct changes this spiral duct into a cylindrical duct, smooth, of greater diameter and thinner walls, making it similar to the hepatic duct and with the same ability for the free passage of bile. Changes produced in the cystic duct by rupturing the valves of Heister are not temporary, but permanent.

3. *Physiologic basis:* The difference between the physiologic pressure existing between the gallbladder and the common bile duct is produced by the simultaneous action of the musculature of the neck of the gallbladder and the valves of Heister.(37) In this manner, the valves of Heister regulate filling and emptying of the gallbladder. As said before, the valves of Heister allow the passage of bile in either direction, but in a regulated fashion, not in a free fashion. Rupture of the valves of Heister eliminates regulation of the passage of bile.

We will now show the anatomy of the cystic duct from without and within, the technique of rupture of the valves of Heister, and anastomosis of the gallbladder to the jejunum.

FIGURE 16.95

Cystic duct seen from the outside. The cystic duct has a variable length, but usually is between 3 and 5 cm long. Its medium diameter, near the gallbladder, is 2.5 mm and its distal diameter, near the common bile duct, is 3 mm. Its external aspect is one of a twisted tube owing to the presence of grooves oriented obliquely and separated by dilations, giving the duct a spiral appearance. This spiral appearance, however, is limited to the proximal half or two-thirds of the duct, since the duct in its distal end is cylindrical. This is because the proximal portion of the duct has valves of Heister, while the distal portion does not. The figure shows the normal diameter of the common bile duct, which is 6 to 8 mm, and the diameter of the hepatic branches, which are 3 mm.

Pancreaticoduodenectomy with Biliary Ducts of Normal Caliber—Technique of Biliodigestive Anastomosis

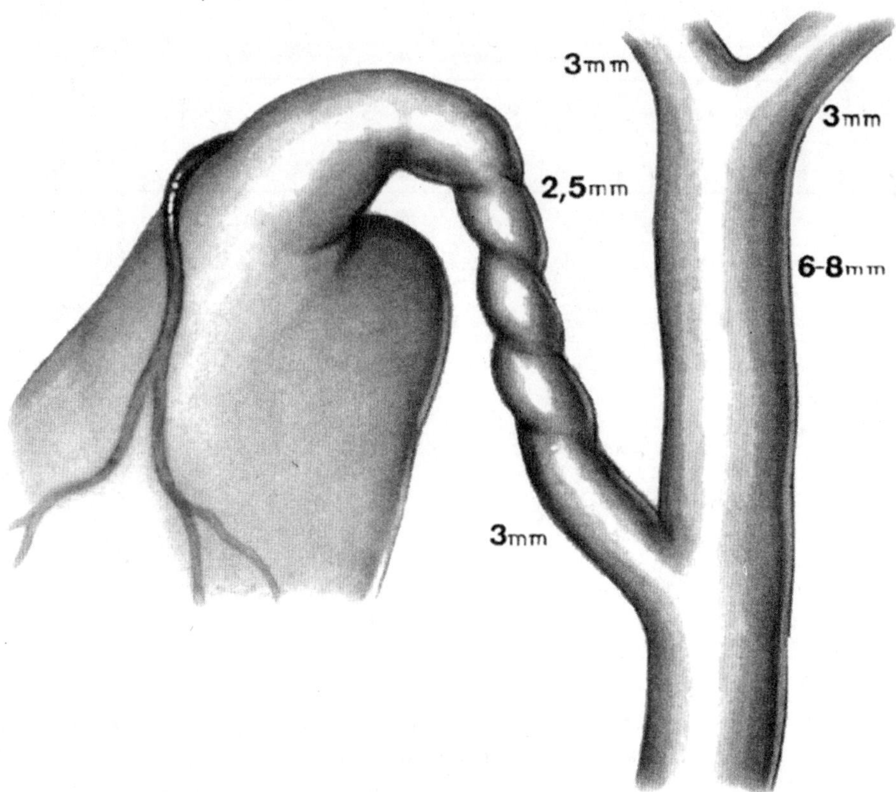

FIGURE 16.95

FIGURE 16.96 CYSTIC DUCT SEEN FROM WITHIN
The cystic duct seen from within presents an irregular aspect produced by the folds in the mucosa or valves of Heister, which are limited to the proximal half or two-thirds of the duct (pars spiralis), while the distal end (pars glabra) does not have valves. Heister's valves present a semilunar aspect with one border applied to the wall of the cystic duct and a free border which projects into the lumen of the duct following an oblique direction similar to the direction of the grooves on its external surface. In spite of the fact that the conjunction of semilunar valves gives the cystic duct a spiral appearance from within, they do not constitute a continuous spiral. Each valve maintains its individuality because they have different directions alternating in a spiral continuous fashion.(90)

Pancreaticoduodenectomy with Biliary Ducts of Normal Caliber—Technique of Biliodigestive Anastomosis

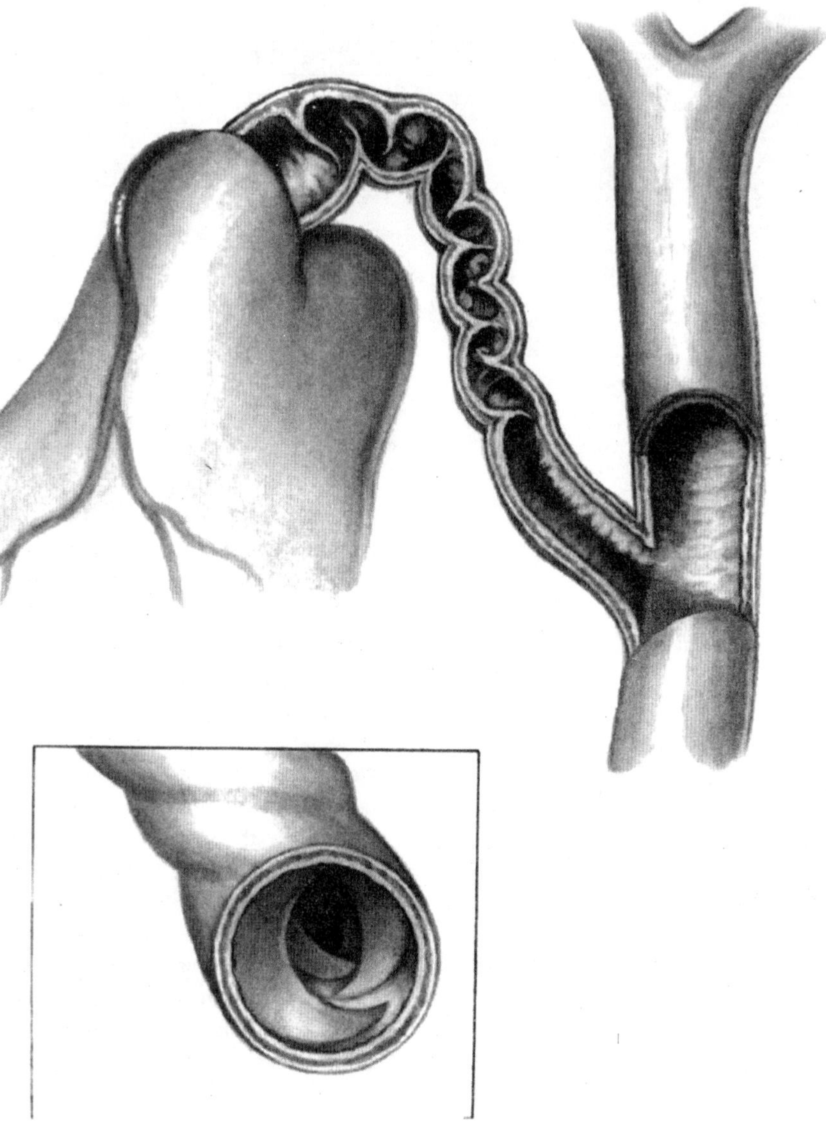

FIGURE 16.96 CYSTIC DUCT SEEN FROM WITHIN

Operative Technique

FIGURE 16.97

In these patients, pancreaticoduodenectomy should be performed without resecting the gallbladder and by sectioning the common bile duct some 10 mm from the entrance of the cystic duct, as shown in the upper figure. Through the short stump of common bile duct a fine, curved, closed hemostat is introduced into the cystic duct as shown in the figure in the center. This clamp generally passes without difficulty through the pars glabra up to the most distal valve of Heister in the pars spiralis. To make the clamp progress it is necessary to introduce its end into the space between the free border of the valve and the opposite wall of the cystic duct. With gentle opening and closing of the clamp, the most distal valve is ruptured. The surgeon can feel valve rupture and can see that the cystic duct is more dilated in this sector. Once the most distal valve is ruptured, the clamp is introduced further up to the next valve, which has a direction different to the previous valve. Rupture of this valve is then carried out, and successively all the valves in the cystic duct are ruptured using the same technique and obtaining a smooth, cylindrical cystic duct of greater diameter and thinner walls.

If the gallbladder is too attached to the inferior surface of the liver, it may be necessary to separate the gallbladder from its bed, partially or completely, as shown in this case, to perform the anastomosis with the jejunum. If the cystic artery and its most important branches are protected, no alterations of the blood supply of the gallbladder will occur. If this should occur the problem is easily solved by resecting the fundus and part of the body of the gallbladder, anastomosing the rest of the gallbladder to the jejunum.

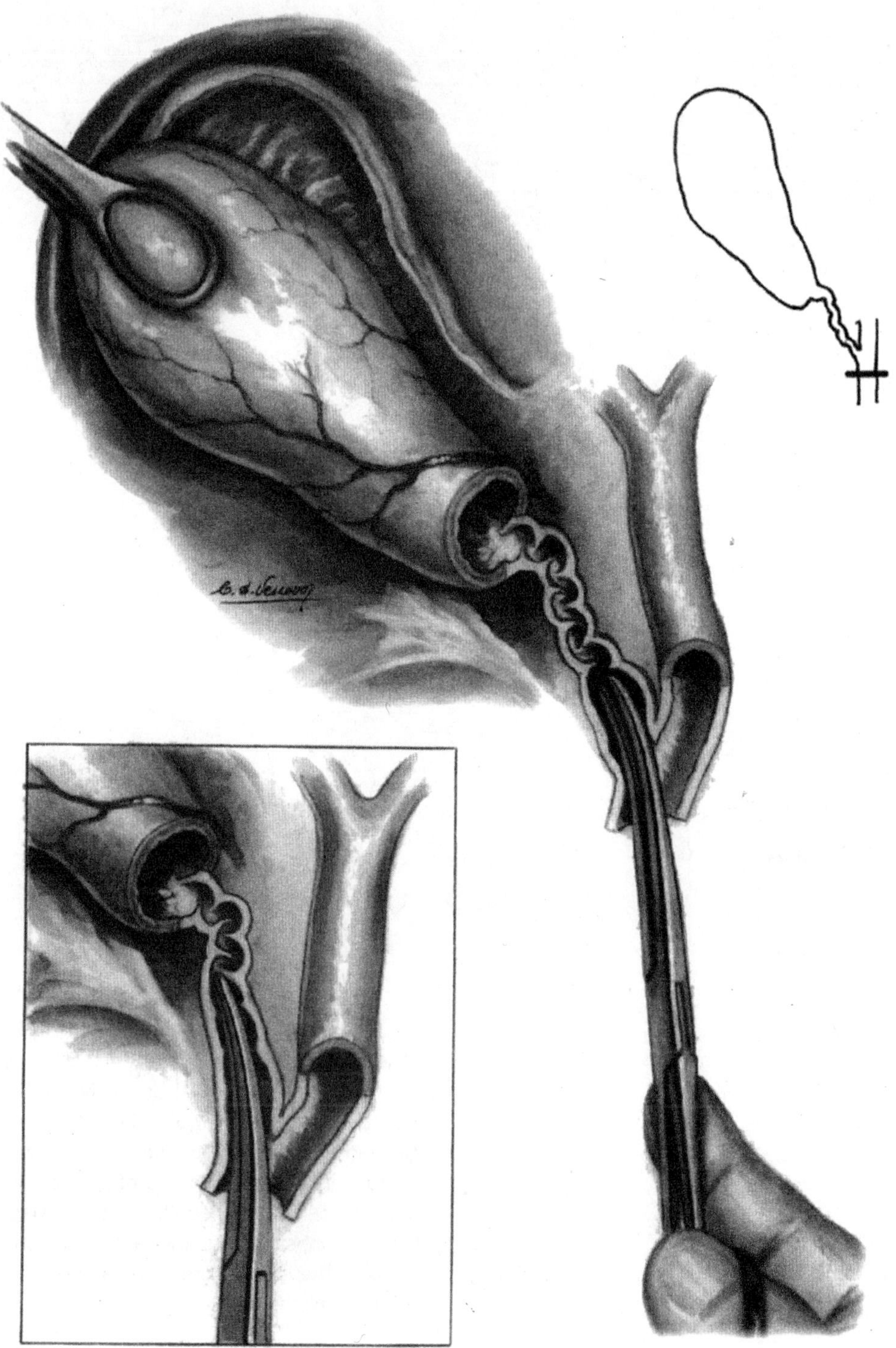

FIGURE 16.97

Operative Technique

FIGURE 16.98
Rupture of all of the valves of the cystic duct has been attained, and the end of the clamp can be introduced into the gallbladder. The cystic duct has been transformed into a cylindrical duct, smooth and of greater diameter, of the same appearance as the hepatic duct, allowing the free flowing of bile. The upper figure shows a dilated cystic duct seen from the outside. The lower figure shows a dilated cystic duct seen in a longitudinal section.

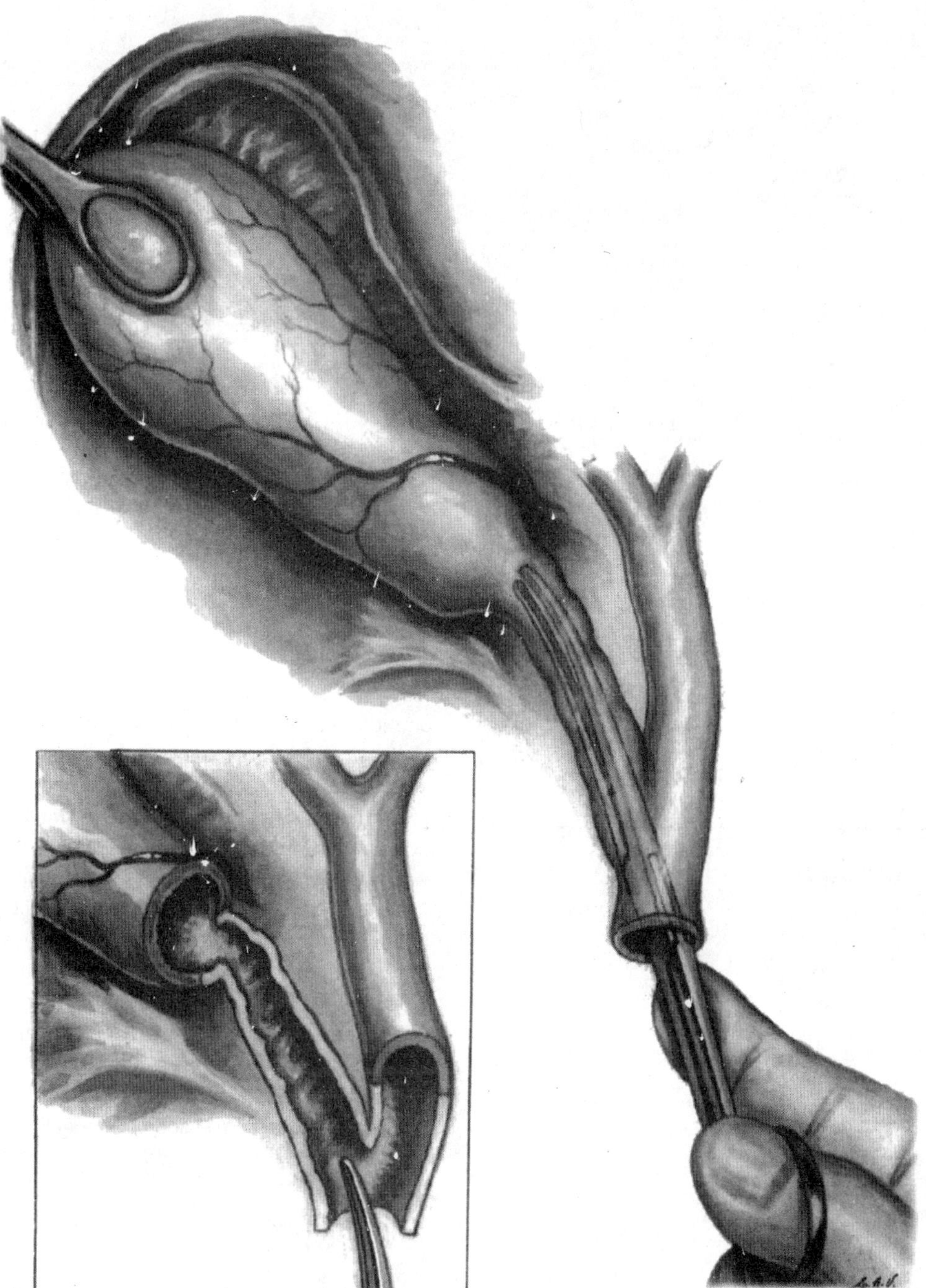

FIGURE 16.98

Operative Technique

FIGURE 16.99

Once all of the valves of Heister of the cystic duct have been ruptured, one proceeds to hermetically close the stump of common bile duct without leaving a blind stump, as shown in the drawing. Anastomosis of the fundus of the gallbladder in a terminolateral fashion is then performed to the jejunal loop using two layers of suture. The inner or mucosal layer should be sutured with 4-0 chromic catgut and the external layer, between the serosa of the gallbladder and the seromuscular layer of the jejunum, should be sutured with silk, cotton, or nonabsorbable synthetic material. It is not necessary that the diameter of the anastomosis be more than 3 cm, since biliary flow will be regulated by the diameter of the hepatic and cystic ducts. The lower drawing will show that the cholecystojejunal anastomosis has been performed in the distal portion of the body of the gallbladder owing to having resected the fundus and part of the proximal body of the gallbladder. This variation may be used when there is doubt about the blood supply of the gallbladder. This is an exceptional occurrence. On the other hand, it is occasionally necessary to separate the gallbladder from its entire bed.

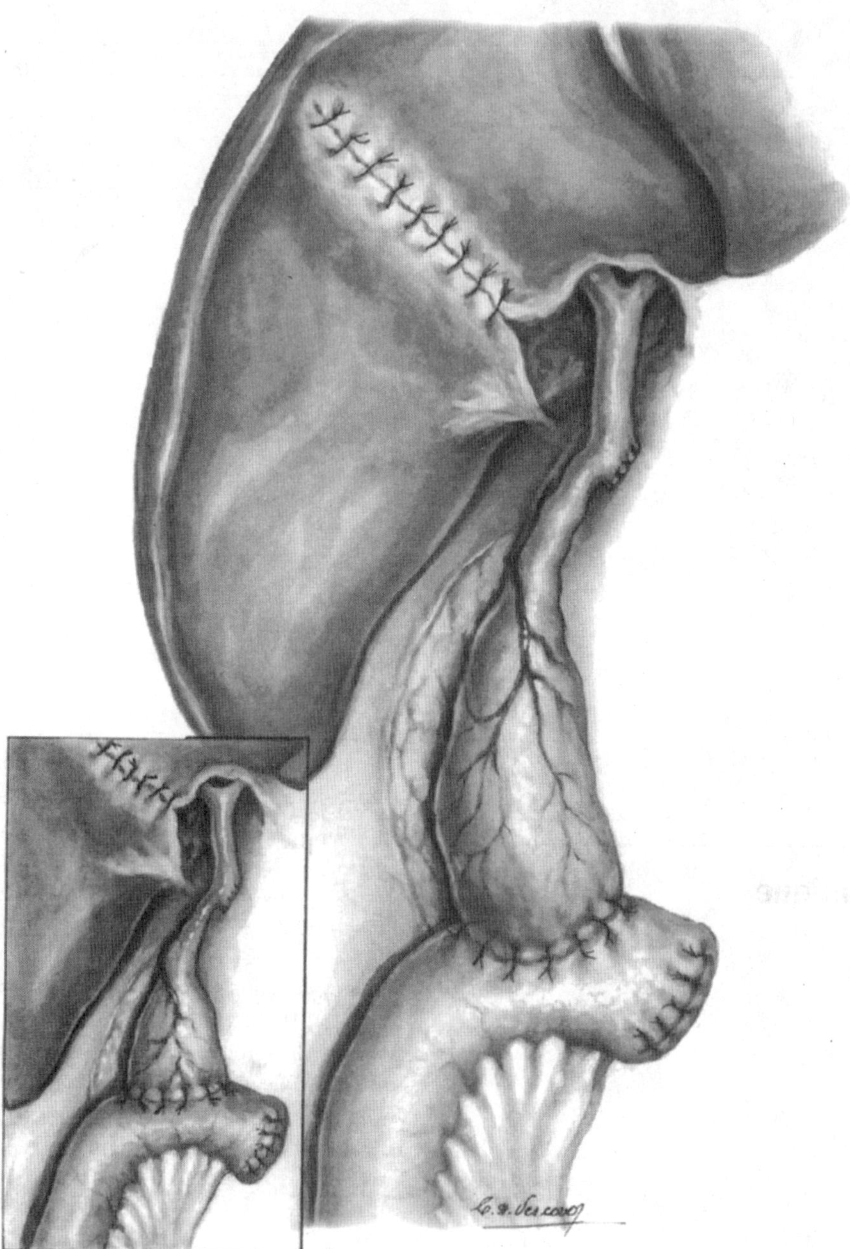

FIGURE 16.99

Operative Technique

FIGURE 16.100
This drawing shows the completed pancreaticoduodenectomy with biliary tract of normal caliber. As can be seen, a hemigastrectomy with bilateral truncal vagotomy and an antecolic gastrojejunostomy has been performed. The pancreatic stump has been anastomosed to the posterior wall of the stomach by implantation. A Silastic tube drains pancreatic secretions to the outside. Biliary drainage has been re-established by a cholecystojejunal anastomosis with previous rupture of the valves of Heister in the cystic duct. The jejunal loop has been brought up through the transverse mesocolon to the right of the mid-colic vessels. Some sutures have been placed between the jejunal loop and the mesocolon to prevent the occurrence of an internal hernia.

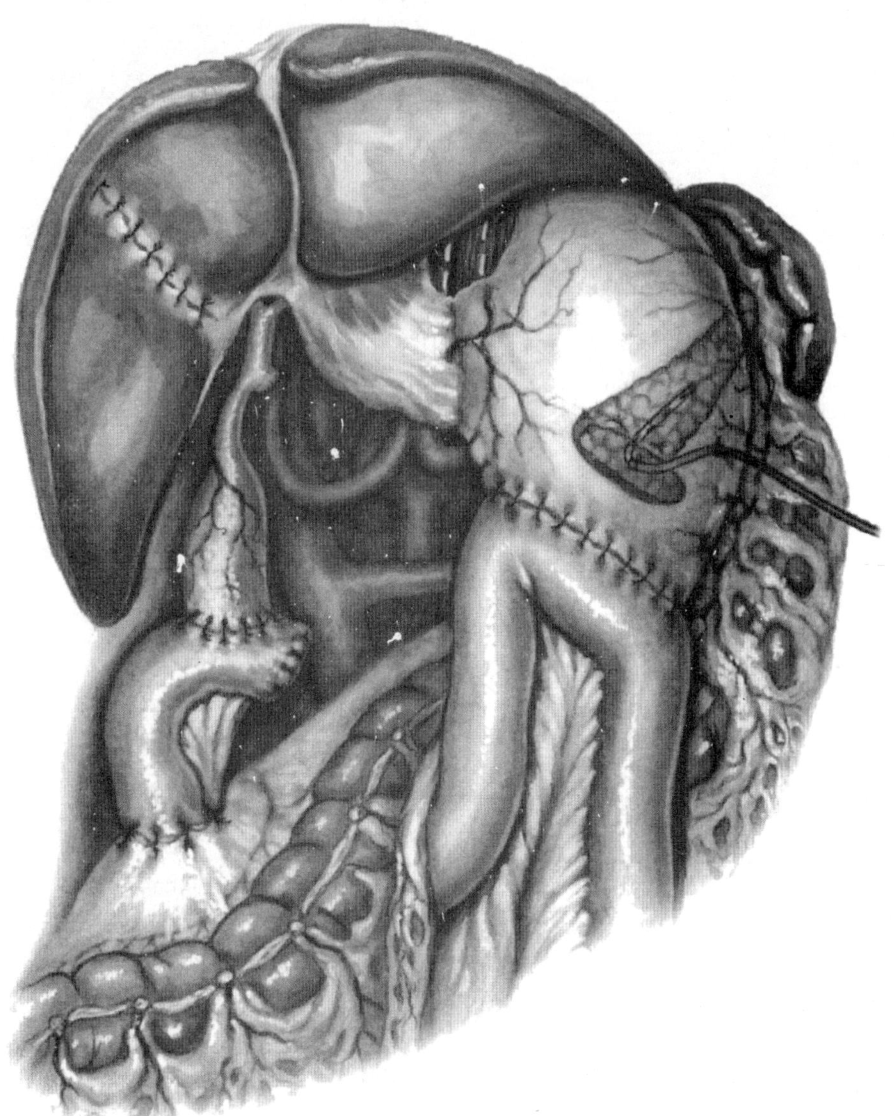

FIGURE 16.100

FIGURE 16.101
Pancreaticoduodenectomy with preservation of the pylorus in a patient with biliary tract of normal caliber. The short duodenal stump has been anastomosed in terminolateral fashion to the jejunum some 15 to 20 cm from the cholecystojejunostomy. The pancreatic stump has been anastomosed to the posterior wall of the stomach. A fine Silastic tube has been fixed within the pancreatic duct and brought out the anterior wall of the stomach to be brought out of the body to drain pancreatic secretions. Anastomosis of the gallbladder to the jejunum with previous rupture of the valves of Heister of the cystic duct has been performed with the techniques described earlier.

Operative Technique

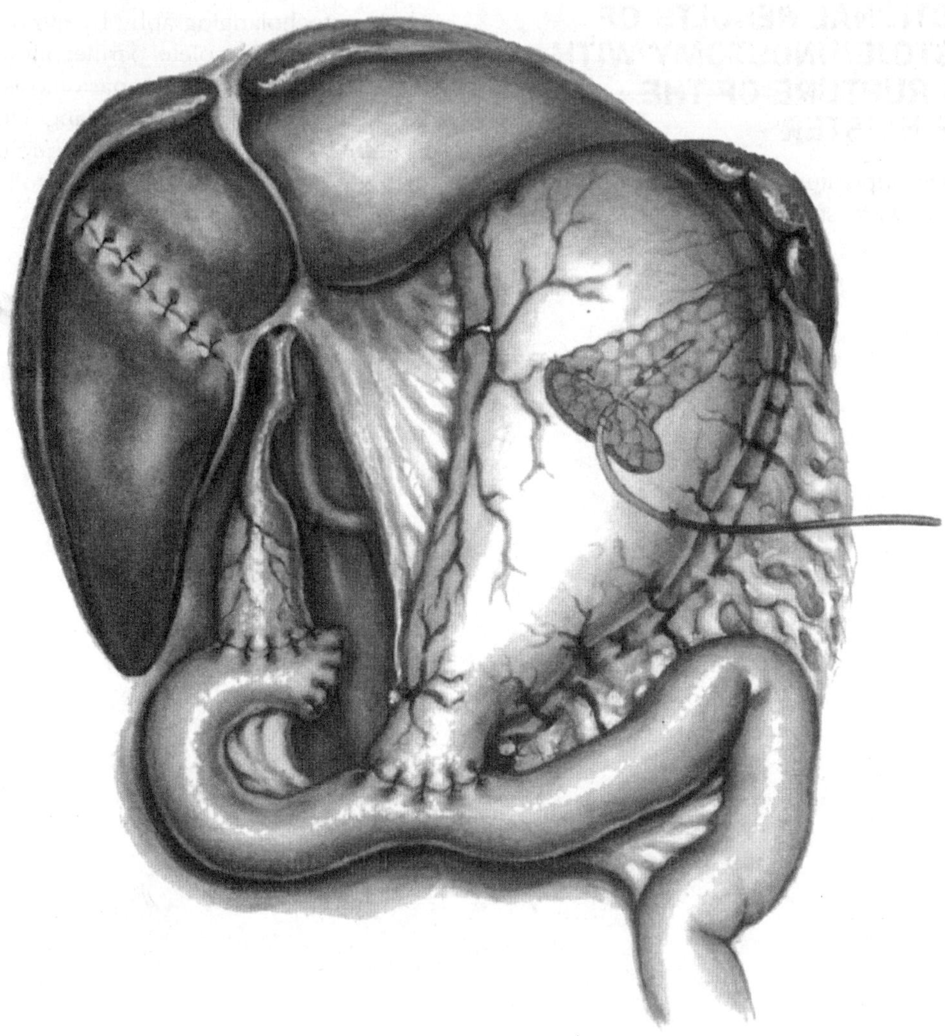

FIGURE 16.101

LATE FUNCTIONAL RESULTS OF CHOLECYSTOJEJUNOSTOMY WITH PREVIOUS RUPTURE OF THE VALVES OF HEISTER

Patients who were operated on by means of the procedure given here were studied clinically by means of cholecystocholangiography by intravenous drip in periodic fashion. Complete permeability of the cystic duct and the cholecystojejunal anastomosis was demonstrated. We will show cholecystocholangiograms in one of the operated cases for endocrine carcinoma of the head of the pancreas, which was controlled during 18 years postoperatively.

Late Functional Results of Cholecystojejunostomy with Previous Rupture of the Valves of Heister

FIGURE 16.102
Cholecystocholangiogram in a patient who survived 18 years following a pancreaticoduodenectomy with cholecystojejunostomy and previous rupture of the valves of Heister. One can observe that the radiopaque substance has opacified the gallbladder, 1.

Late Functional Results of Cholecystojejunostomy with Previous Rupture of the Valves of Heister

FIGURE 16.103
X-ray obtained 30 minutes after the preceding. One can observe that about 50% of the gallbladder contents have emptied, 1 showing part of the radiopaque liquid in the small bowel, 2.

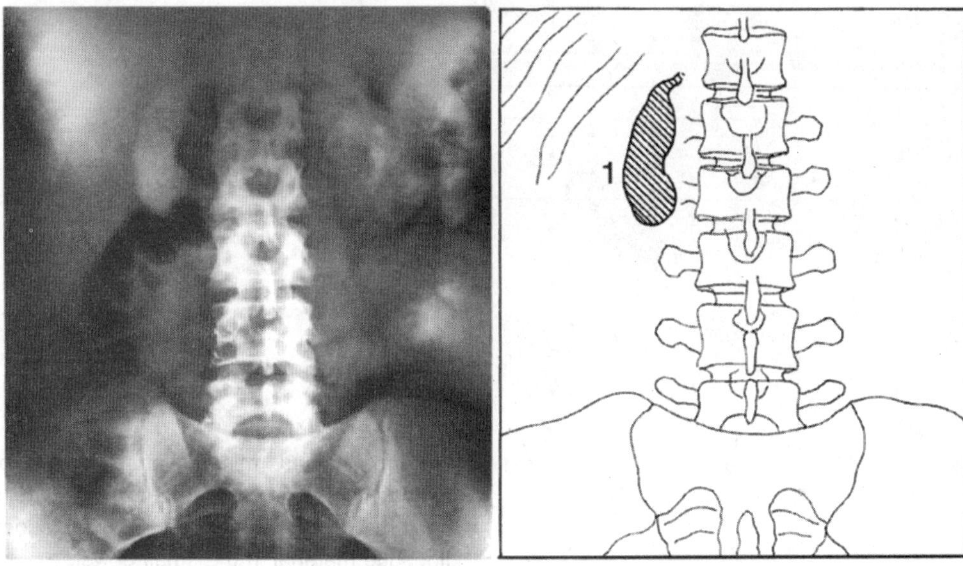

FIGURE 16.102

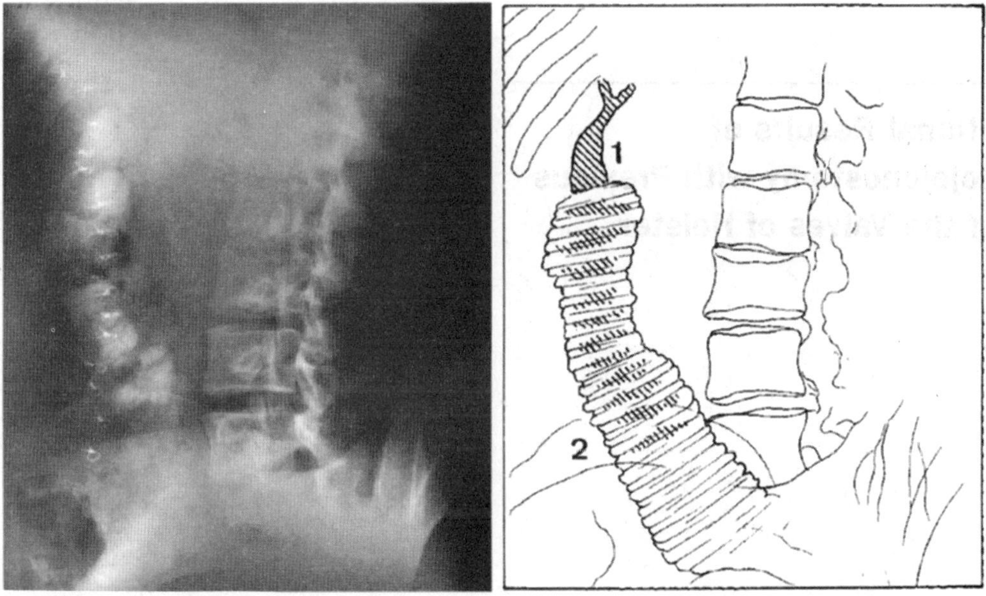

FIGURE 16.103

FIGURE 16.104
X-ray obtained 60 minutes after the previous one. The gallbladder has practically emptied all of its contents into the small bowel. 1. Traces of the gallbladder. 2 and 2′, Radiopaque material in the small bowel.

Late Functional Results of Cholecystojejunostomy with Previous Rupture of the Valves of Heister

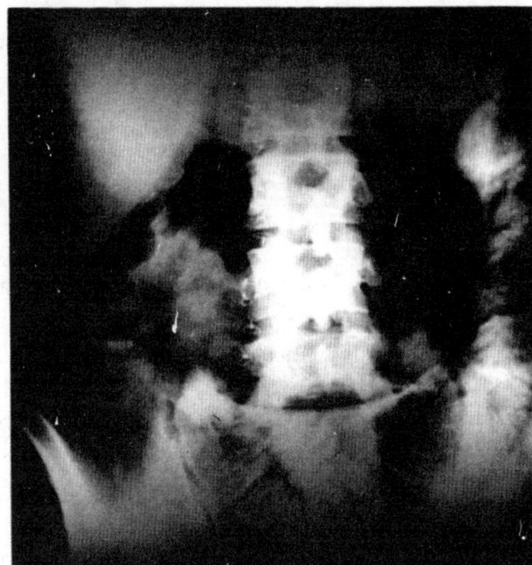

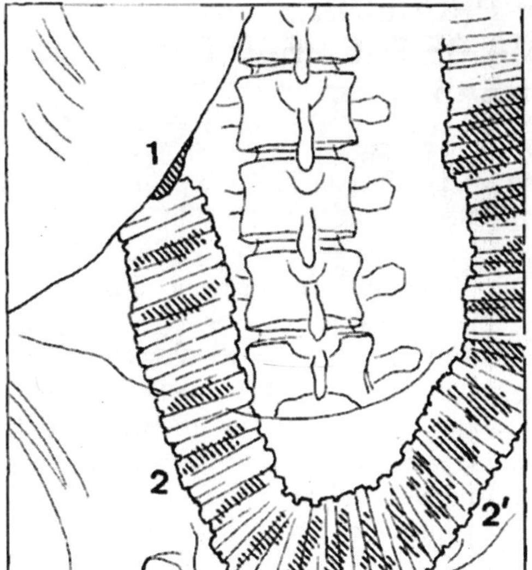

FIGURE 16.104

PALLIATIVE PROCEDURES IN CARCINOMA OF THE HEAD OF THE PANCREAS

Many surgeons perform pancreaticoduodenectomy for carcinoma of the head of the pancreas as a palliative procedure. In our practice this procedure is only performed when there is hope for cure. Even though it has been proven statistically that palliative pancreaticoduodenectomies for carcinoma of the head of the pancreas result in a slight increase in survival when compared with palliative procedures, it is no less certain that resections lead to greater mortality and morbidity with a more complicated postoperative course, which does not compensate for the slight increase in survival. Palliative bypass procedures will solve the deep jaundice and itching even though the bilirubin is not always returned to normal levels.

At present there are two procedures to decompress biliary tracts obstructed by carcinoma: (a) nonsurgical procedures and (b) surgical procedures. The former consist of placement of an endoluminal prosthesis by transparietal hepatic or transduodenal endoscopic route. We will only describe surgical procedures used most frequently for biliary bypass.

Cholecystojejunostomy

Cholecystojejunostomy is a good procedure, easy to perform, and anastomosis of the gallbladder to the jejunum is quite secure. However, cholecystojejunostomy requires certain conditions (40, 50):

1. The opening of the cystic duct into the common bile duct must be far away from the carcinoma. To determine exactly the course of the cystic duct and its relation with the carcinoma, it is extremely useful to perform an operative cholangiogram. (19, 21, 25)
2. The gallbladder should be healthy.
3. Cholecystojejunostomy should only be performed when the patient survival is short. If the patient survives longer than had been thought, invasion of the cystic duct by the tumor and invalidation of the cholecystojejunal anastomosis may occur. It is well known that carcinomas of the pancreas and periampullary carcinomas tend to grow upward in the hepatic pedicle.
4. If the patient lives longer than originally thought, infection of the biliary tract by bile stasis in the common duct may occur owing to obstruction by the valves of Heister in the cystic duct. It is advisable that cholecystojejunal anastomosis be performed with a simple jejunal loop and not with the jejunal loop disposed in Roux-en-Y fashion, since the latter is a more complex operation and does not give better results.

Cholecystojejunostomy

FIGURE 16.105
This drawing presents a cholecystojejunostomy using a simple antecolic loop. Anastomosis between the gallbladder and the jejunum is performed in two layers of sutures using interrupted sutures. The external serosal layer of the gallbladder and the seromuscular layer of the jejunum are sutured together with nonabsorbable fine material using a fine needle. The internal mucosal layer is sutured with 3-0 chromic catgut. The drawing shows the completed posterior plane between the gallbladder and jejunum together with the beginning of the anterior mucosal plane. The mucosal plane really includes the entire thickness of the wall of the gallbladder and the jejunum. It is not necessary that the anastomosis have a diameter of more than 2.5 to 3 cm, since biliary flow will be regulated by the cystic duct.

Cholecystojejunostomy

In some patients it is necessary to separate part of the gallbladder from its bed to facilitate its suture as can be seen in the drawing. Once the cholecystojejunal anastomosis has been completed, we habitually place some sutures that include the seromuscular layer of the jejunum distal to the anastomosis and Glisson's capsule, as shown in the insert. These sutures have the object of protecting the cholecystojejunal suture line from traction which may be exerted by the jejunal loop. We usually place a jejunojejunal anastomosis some 50 cm from the cholecystojejunal anastomosis (Braun anastomosis) to prevent reflux of intestinal contents with its ensuing cholangitis. Some authors (50, 57) consider the jejunojejunal anastomosis unnecessary, since the occurrence of cholangitis is improbable because this complication only occurs when there is a stricture of the biliary tree or in the anastomosis between the biliary tree and the digestive tract.

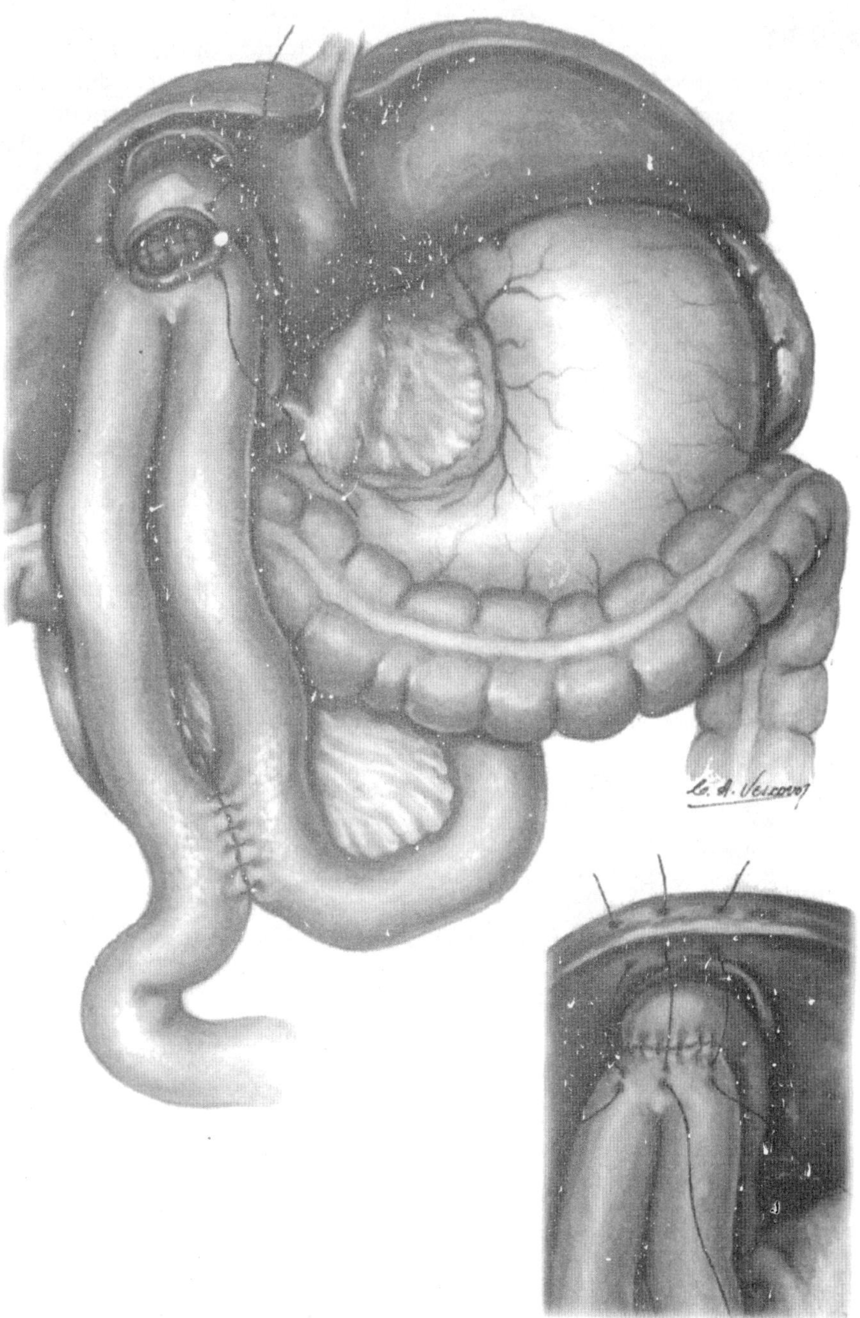

FIGURE 16.105

Hepaticojejunostomy

Hepaticojejunostomy is the best of the bypass biliary procedures in cases of carcinoma of the head of the pancreas and other malignant obstructions of the distal common duct. The hepaticojejunal anastomosis results in a direct derivation of the biliary tract in a location generally far from the tumor causing the obstruction. There are several techniques for the performance of the hepaticojejunostomy. We will briefly describe the most frequently used techniques.

Hepaticojejunostomy

Hepaticojejunostomy

FIGURE 16.106 HEPATICOJEJUNAL ANASTOMOSIS WITH A ROUX-EN-Y LOOP

Anastomosis of the common bile duct with the jejunum should be performed using a jejunal loop brought up in Roux-en-Y fashion. The end of the anastomotic loop is closed in two layers, and the loop is brought upward, placing it in contact with the hepatic duct to perform a laterolateral anastomosis between the duct and the antimesenteric edge of the jejunal loop. The drawing shows that the posterior suture line between the wall of the hepatic duct and the wall of the jejunum has been completed, using interrupted sutures of nonabsorbable material. Some surgeons use synthetic sutures of slow absorption, either continuous or in interrupted fashion, for this anastomosis, and some surgeons use two suture planes. However, it has been very difficult for us to perform this anastomosis in two layers. In the insert, one can observe that the anastomosis in one suture line between the hepatic duct and the jejunum has been completed. The terminolateral anastomosis between the jejunal loops of the Roux-en-Y are performed some 50 cm distal to the hepaticojejunal anastomosis. In this procedure we do not usually remove the gallbladder because these patients usually present a poor general condition and the procedure should be abbreviated. On the other hand it has not been shown that patients who have a short life span following the diverting procedure have presented complications owing to not having had the gallbladder removed. If the general state of the patient allows it and it is felt that postoperative life span will be somewhat more prolonged, one can perform the procedure described as follows.

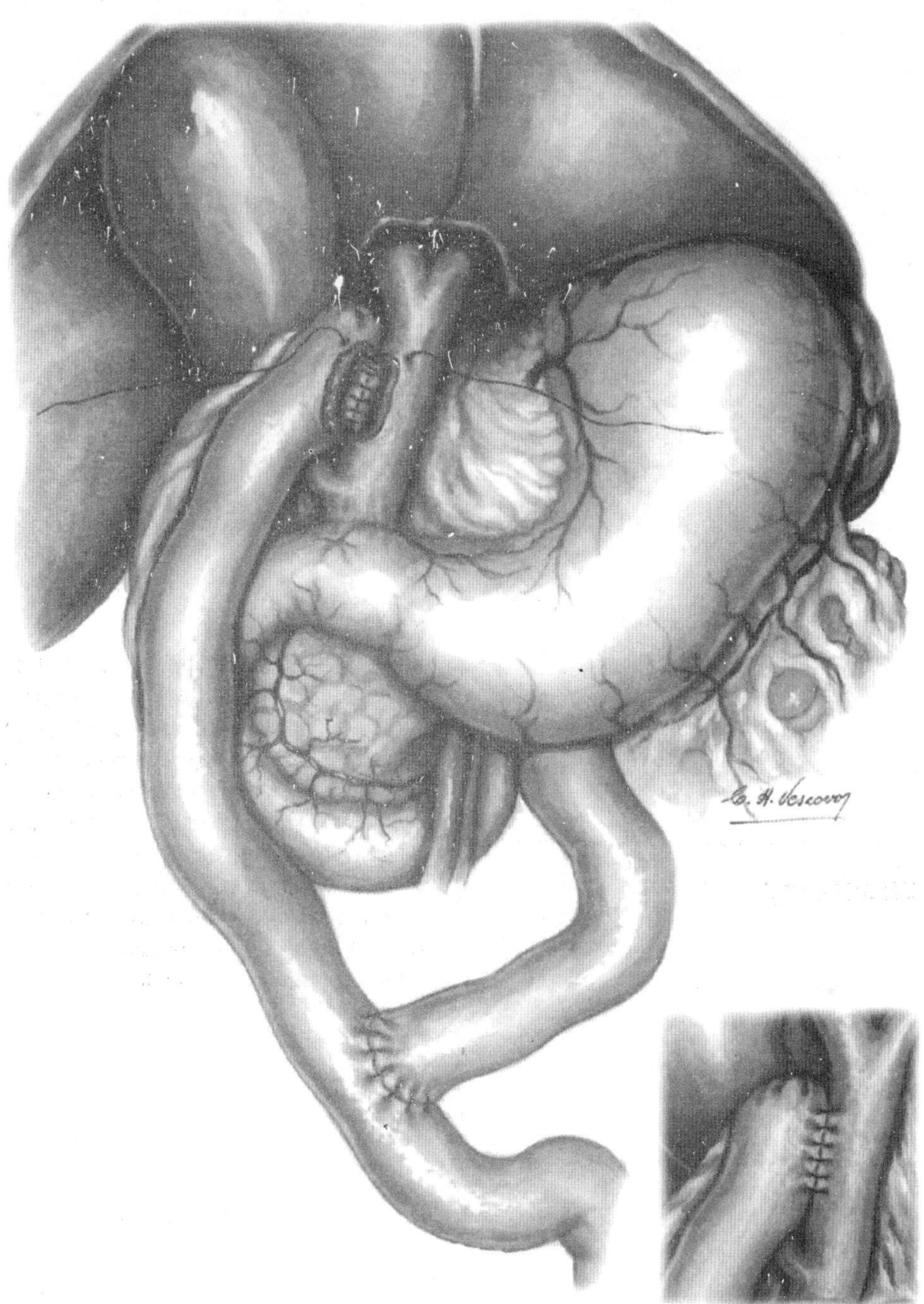

FIGURE 16.106 HEPATICOJEJUNAL ANASTOMOSIS WITH A ROUX-EN-Y LOOP

Hepaticojejunostomy

FIGURE 16.107
The drawing shows marked dilation of the gallbladder and the common bile duct caused by a carcinoma of the head of the pancreas. Since the general condition of the patient was not too bad, the gallbladder was resected and the common hepatic duct transected above the entrance of the cystic duct. The distal end of the common hepatic duct was closed with a continuous suture reinforced by a few interrupted sutures, using nonabsorbable materials. The proximal end of the common hepatic duct was anastomosed to the ascending loop of the Roux-en-Y in a terminolateral fashion using one layer of sutures as shown in the following figure.

FIGURE 16.108
This figure shows the completed anastomosis of the common hepatic duct with the ascending loop of the jejunum in terminolateral fashion. The anastomosis was performed in one layer with synthetic suture material of slow absorption and a very fine atraumatic needle. It is important that the hydraulic test be performed once the anastomosis is finished. For this purpose, an elastic clamp is placed across the jejunum some 5 to 6 cm from the anastomosis and about 50 mL of physiologic solution is injected into the jejunum above the clamp using needle and syringe. If any loss through the suture line is observed, this should be corrected before closing the abdomen.

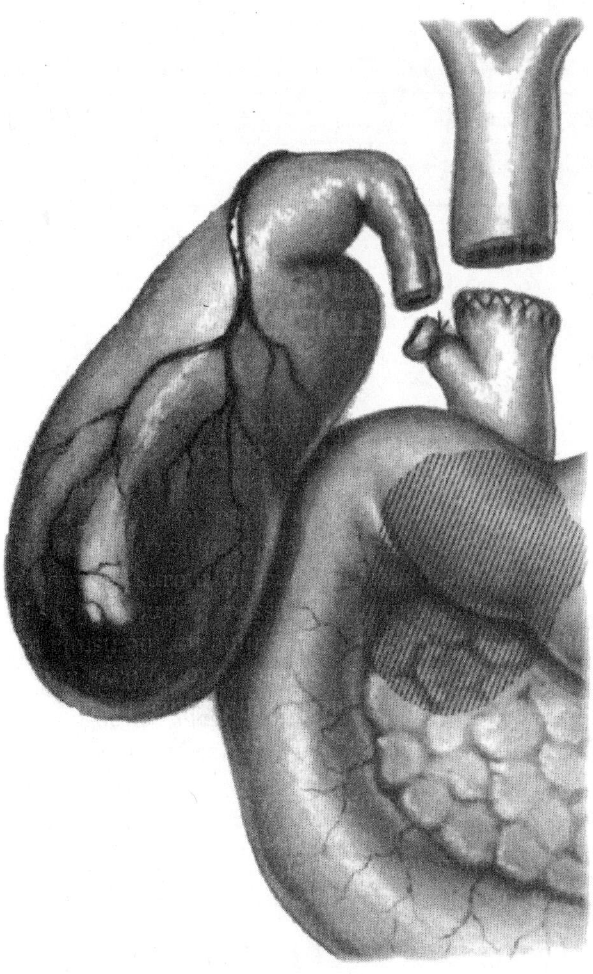

FIGURE 16.107

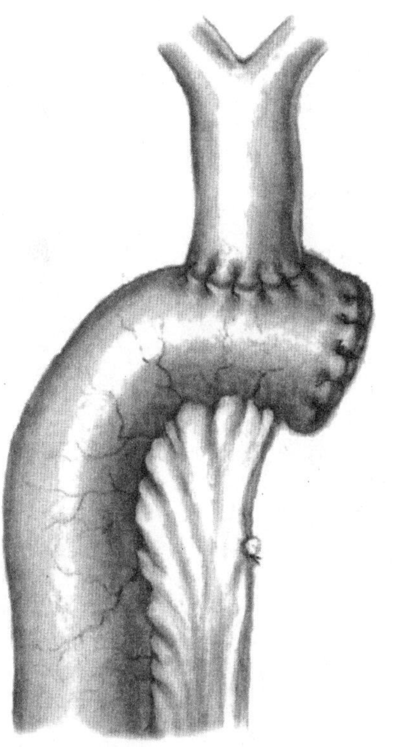

FIGURE 16.108

FIGURE 16.109
In some patients with carcinoma of the head of the pancreas a palliative bypass can be performed as shown in this and the next drawing (50, 70, 75). The procedure is begun by performing a one layer anastomosis between the infundibulum of the gallbladder and the hepatic duct using synthetic suture material of slow absorption. The drawing shows that the posterior suture line has been performed.

Hepaticojejunostomy

FIGURE 16.110
The short limb of a T-tube is placed in the hepatic duct, passing the long limb through the gallbladder and removing it through the fundus of the gallbladder. In the insert one can observe that the anterior layer of sutures is being placed between the common hepatic duct and the infundibulum of the gallbladder. The fundus of the gallbladder is then anastomosed with the ascending jejunal loop of the Roux-en-Y in terminolateral fashion using two layers of suture, the outer one with nonabsorbable material and the internal or mucosal layer with 3-0 chromic catgut. The long limb of the T-tube is passed to the inside of the jejunal loop and advanced for some 8 to 10 cm, then brought out of the jejunal lumen through a tunnel made with seromuscular sutures in the jejunum. The T-tube is then passed through the abdominal wall to drain bile to the outside. The jejunal limb is fixed with several sutures to the parietal peritoneum around the T-tube.

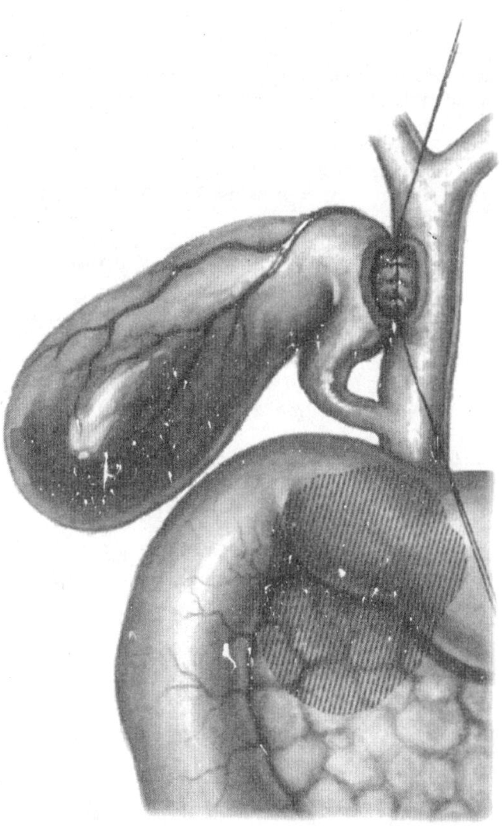

FIGURE 16.109

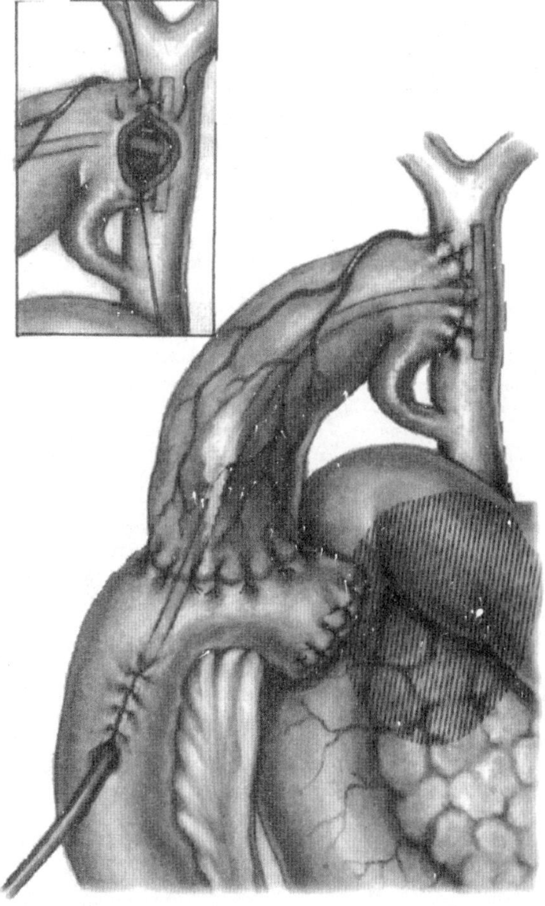

FIGURE 16.110

References

1. Astor, S.J., Longmire, W.F., Jr. Pancreaticoduodenal resection: Twenty years experience. Arch. Surg. 106:813, 1973.
2. Braasch, J.W., Deziel, D.J., Rossi, R.L., Watkins, E., Jr., Winter, P.F. Pyloric and gastric preserving pancreatic resection. Experience with 87 patients. Ann. Surg. 204:411, 1986.
3. Bodner, E., Schwamberger, K., Mikuz, G. Cytological diagnosis of pancreatic tumors. World J. Surg. 6:103, 1982.
4. Brook, J.R., Culebras, J.M. Cancer of the pancreas. Palliative operation, Whipple procedure or total pancreatectomy? Am. J. Surg. 131:516, 1976.
5. Brunschwig, A. Resection of head of pancreas and duodenum for carcinoma. Pancreaticoduodenectomy. Surg. Gynecol. Obstet. 65:681, 1937.
6. Carey, L.C., Ellison, E.C. Pancreas. In Fromm, D. (Ed.) Gastrointestinal surgery. Vol. 2, p. 902. Churchill Livingstone, New York, 1985.
7. Cattell, R.B., Warren, K.W. Surgery of the pancreas. p. 261. W.B. Saunders, Philadelphia, 1953.
8. Cohen, J.R., Kuchta, N., Geller, N., Shires, T., Dineen, P. Pancreaticoduodenectomy. A 40 year experience. Ann. Surg. 185:608, 1982.
9. Cooperman, A.M. Cancer of the pancreas: A dilemma in treatment. Surg. Clin. North Am. 61:107, 1981.
10. Copper, W.M. External choledochoduodenostomy. An evaluation of 125 cases. Br. J. Surg. 49:292, 1961.
11. Couinaud, C., Huguet, C. Le temps d'exérèse dans la duodénopancréatectomie totale. J. Chirurg. 91:2, 1966.
12. Crist, D.W., Switzman, A., Cameron, J.D. Improved hospital morbidity, mortality and survival after the Whipple procedure. Ann. Surg. 206:358, 1987.
13. Chassin, J.L. Operative strategy in general surgery. Vol. II, p. 159. Springer-Verlag, New York, 1984.
14. Child, C.G. Carcinoma of duodenum. One stage radical pancreaticoduodenectomy, preserving the external pancreatic secretion. Ann. Surg. 118: 838, 1943.
15. Decoud, J.A., Kaplan, J., Flejlejer, A., Bendersky, D., Rapela, R. Duodenopancreatectomía cefálica. Rev. Argent. Cir. 53:13, 1987.
16. Degenshein, G.A. Choledochoduodenostomy: An 18 year study of 175 consecutive cases. Surgery 76:319, 1974.
17. Dill-Russell, A.S. Pancreaticogastrostomy. Lancet 1:589, 1952.
18. Etala, E. Diagnóstico operatorio del cáncer de la cabeza del páncreas. Importancia de la biopsia extemporánea. Comptes Rendus de la Société Internationale de Chirurgie, 24:648, Roma, 1959.
19. Etala, E., Russo, R. Operative cholangiography in the diagnosis of tumoral obstructions of the distal end of the common duct. III World Congress of Gastroenterology. Tokyo, Japan. Abstracts of papers. 3:84, 1966.
20. Etala, E., Russo, R. Diagnóstico operatorio del cáncer de la ampolla de Vater. Soc. Cir. Bs. As. Bol. y Trab. 18:334, 1966.
21. Etala, E. Diagnóstico operatorio de las obstrucciones malignas del tercio distal del colédoco. Pren. Méd. Argent. 54:941, 1967.
22. Etala, E. Cirugía del páncreas. Tácticas y técnicas. XXI Congreso Uruguayo de Cirugía. Vol. I, p. 45. Montevideo, 1970.
23. Etala, E. Cáncer de la cabeza del páncreas. Diagnóstico y tratamiento. Actas de Cirugía Hépato-Bilio-Pancreática, p. 203. Dirección General de Publicaciones, Córdoba, Argentina, 1974.
24. Etala, E. Tumores de la cabeza del páncreas. Pren. Méd. Argent. Numero del 60 Aniversario, p. 145, 1974.
25. Etala, E. Anastomosis pancreatogástrica en la pancreatoduodenectomía. Pren. Méd. Argent. 75:174, 1988.
26. Etala, E., Juan, J.R. Pancreatoduodenectomía por carcinoma de la cabeza del páncreas. Morbilidad, mortalidad, sobrevida. Pren. Méd. Argent. 76:164, 1989.
27. Fink, A.S., De Souza, I.R., Mayer, E.A. et al. Long-term evaluation of pylorus preservation during pancreaticoduodenectomy. World J. Surg. 12:663, 1988.
28. Flautner, L., Tihangi, T., Szécsény, A. Pancreatogastrostomy: An ideal complement to pancreatic head resection with preservation of the pylorus in the treatment of chronic pancreatitis. Am. J. Surg. 150:508, 1985.
29. Flint, E.R. Abnormalities of the high hepatic cystic and gastroduodenal arteries and of the bile ducts. Br. J. Surg. 10:509, 1923.
30. Forrest, J.R., Longmire, W.P. Jr. Carcinoma of the pancreas and periampullary region. A study of 279 patients. Ann. Surg. 189:129, 1979.
31. George, P., Brown, C., Gilchrist, J. Operative biopsy of the pancreas. Br. J. Surg. 62:280, 1975.
32. Grace, P.A., Pitt, H.A., Tompkins, R.K., DenBesten, L., Longmire, W.P. Jr. Decreased morbidity and mortality after pancreatoduodenectomy. Am. J. Surg. 151:141, 1986.
33. Gray, S.W., Skandalakis, J.E. Atlas of surgical anatomy for general surgeons. p. 138. Williams & Wilkins, Baltimore, 1985.
34. Hepp, J., Couinaud, C. L'abord et utilisation du canal hépatique gauche dans les réparations de la voie biliaire principale après cholecystectomie. Mém. Acad. Chir. 81:274, 1955.
35. Hepp, J., Couinaud, C. L'abord et utilisation du canal hepatic gauche dans la réparation de la voie biliaire principale. Presse Med. 64:947, 1956.
36. Hermreck, A.S., Thomas, C.Y., Friesen, S.R. Importance of pathological staging in the surgical management of adenocarcinoma of the exocrine pancreas. Am. J. Surg. 127:653, 1974.
37. Hess, W. Enfermedades de la vías biliares y del páncreas. p. 10, Cientifico Medica, Barcelona, 1963.
38. Hollinshead, W.H. Anatomy for surgeons. Vol. 2, p. 355. Hoeber Harper, New York, 1956.
39. Howard, J.M. Pancreatico-duodenectomy: Forty-one consecutive Whipple resections without an operative mortality. Ann. Surg. 168:640, 1968.
40. Howard, J.M., Jordan, G.L. Jr., Reber, H.A. Eds. Surgical diseases of the pancreas. p. 666. Lea & Febiger, Philadelphia, 1987.
41. Hyland, C., Kheir, S.M., Kashlan, M.B. Frozen section diagnosis of pancreatic carcinoma. A prospective study of 64 biopsies. Am. J. Pathol. 5:179, 1981.
42. Icard, P., Dubois, F. Pancreaticogastrostomy following pancreatoduodenectomy. Ann. Surg. 207: 253, 1988.
43. Ingebrigtsen, R., Langfeldt, E. Pancreaticogastrostomy. Lancet 2:270, 1952.
44. Issacson, R., Weiland, L.H., McIllrath, D.C. Biopsy of the pancreas. Arch. Surg. 109:227, 1974.
45. Itani, K.M.F., Coleman, R.E., Meyer, W.C., Akuari, C.E. Pylorus preserving pancreatoduodenectomy. Ann. Surg. 204:655, 1986.
46. Johnson, A.G., Stevens, A.E. Importance of the size of the stoma in choledochoduodenostomy. Gut 10:68, 1969.
47. Jordan, G.J., Jr. Pancreatic fistula. Am. J. Surg. 119:200, 1970.
48. Jordan, G.L., Jr. Pancreatic resection for pancreatic cancer. In Howard, J.M., Jordan, G.L. Jr., Reber, H.A. Surgical diseases of the pancreas. p. 666. Lea & Febiger, Philadelphia, 1987.
49. Kraus, M.A., Wilson, S.D. Choledochoduodenostomy: Importance of common duct size and occurrence of cholangitis. Arch. Surg. 115:1212, 1980.
50. Kune, G.A., Sali, A. The practice of biliary surgery. Ed. 2, pp. 384–390. Blackwell Scientific Publications, Oxford, 1980.
51. Lawrence, A.G., Ghosh, B.C. Total pancreatectomy for carcinoma of the pancreas. Am. J. Surg. 133:244, 1977.
52. Lee, Y.T.N. Tissue diagnosis for carcinoma of the pancreas and periampullary structure. Cancer 49:1035, 1982.
53. Lightwood, R., Reber, H.A., Way, L.W. The risk and accuracy of pancreatic biopsy. Am. J. Surg. 132:189, 1976.
54. Mackie, J.A., Rhoads, J.E. Pancreatogastrostomy following pancreaticoduodenal resection. Bull. Soc. Int. Chir. 34:611, 1975.
55. Mackie, C.R., Moosa, A.R. Surgical anatomy of the pancreas. In Moosa, A.R. Tumors of the pancreas, p. 1. Williams & Wilkins, Baltimore, 1980.
56. Madden, J.L. Technique for pancreaticoduodenectomy. Surg. Gynecol. Obstet. 118:247, 1964.
57. Madden, J.L., Cruwez, J.A., Tan, P.Y. Obstructive (surgical) jaundice: An analysis of 140 consecutive cases and a consideration of choledochoduodenostomy in its treatment. Am. J. Surg. 109: 89, 1964.
58. Madden, J.L., Chun, J.Y., Kandalaft, S., Parekh, M. Choledochoduodenostomy. An injustly maligned surgical procedure. Am. J. Surg. 119:45, 1970.

59. Madden, J.L. Personal communication, 1989.
60. Mainetti, J.M. Duodenopancreatectomía oncológica. Pren. Méd. Argent. 57:1337, 1970.
61. Mason, G.R. Discussion of Crist, D.W., Switzman, A., Cameron, J.D. Improved hospital morbidity, mortality and survival after the Whipple procedure. Ann. Surg. 206:358, 1987.
62. Millbourn, E. Pancreaticogastrostomy in pancreaticoduodenal resection for carcinoma of the head of the pancreas or the ampulla of Vater. Acta Chir. Scand. 116:12, 1958.
63. Moosa, A.R., Lewis, M.H., Mackie, C.R. Surgical treatment of pancreatic cancer. Mayo Clin. Proc. 54:468, 1979.
64. Moroni, J.M. Cáncer del páncreas. 39 Cong. Argent. Cir. Buenos Aires, Argentina, 1979:1.
65. Mosca, F., Giulianotti, P.C., Arganini, M. et al. Pancreaticoduodenectomy with pylorus preservation. Ital. J. Surg. Sci. 14:319, 1984.
66. Papachristou, D.N., Fortner, J.G. Management of the pancreatic remnant in pancreatoduodenectomy. J. Surg. Oncol. 18:1, 1981.
67. Papachristou, D.N., Fortner, J.G. Pancreatic fistula complicating pancreatectomy for malignant disease. Br. J. Surg. 88:236, 1981.
68. Park, C.D., Mackie, J.A., Rhoads, J.E. Pancreaticogastrostomy. Am. J. Surg. 113:85, 1967.
69. Parson, I. Jr., Palmer, C.H. How accurate is fine-needle biopsy in malignant neoplasia of the pancreas? Arch. Surg. 124:681, 1989.
70. Patel, J., Patel, J.C., Léger, L. Nouveau traité de technique chirurgicale. Vol. XII, p. 219. Masson et Cie., Paris, 1969.
71. Patti, M.G., Pellegrini, C.A., Way, L.W. Gastric emptying and small bowel transit of solid food after pylorus preserving pancreaticoduodenectomy. Arch. Surg. 122:528, 1983.
72. Pellegrini, C.A., Heck, C.F., Raper, S., Way, L.W. An analysis of the reduced morbidity and mortality rates after pancreaticoduodenectomy. Arch. Surg. 124:778, 1989.
73. Pi-Figueras J. Práctica quirúrgica. Ed. 2, Vol. 2, p. 823. Salvat, Barcelona, 1986.
74. Praderi, R., Hormaechea, C., Delgado, B. Duodenopancreatectomía cefálica. Consideraciones técnicas a propósito de 18 casos. Cir. Uruguay 41:298, 1971.
75. Praderi, R. Personal communication, 1989.
76. Priestley, J.T., Comfort, M.W., Radcliffe, J., Jr. Total pancreatectomy for hyperinsulinism due to an islet cell adenoma. Survival and cure at 16 months after operation. Ann. Surg. 119:211, 1944.
77. Privitera, A., Moscato, V. Modificazioni della funzionalitá gastrica e pancreatica dopo l'abboccamento della testa del pancreas allo stomaco. Riforma Med. 65:600, 1951.
78. Reding, R. Die pancreato-gastrostomie als modifikation der Whippleschen operation. Zentralbl. Chir. 103:943, 1978.
79. ReMine, W., Priestley, J.T., Judd, E., King, J. Total pancreatectomy for ductal carcinoma. Surg. Gynecol. Obstet. 133:16, 1971.
80. Rockey, E.W. Total pancreatectomy for carcinoma. A case report. Ann. Surg. 118:603, 1943.
81. Ross, D.E. Cancer of the pancreas. A plea for total pancreatectomy. Am. J. Surg. 87:20, 1954.
82. Rossi, R.L., Braasch, J.W. Techniques of pancreaticojejunostomy in pancreatoduodenectomy. Problems in general. Surgery 2:506, 1985.
83. Sames, P.C. Pancreaticogastrostomy. Lancet 1:718, 1952.
84. Sarr, M.G., Gladen, H.E., Beart, R.W., Van Heerden, J.A. Role of gastroenterostomy in patients with unresectable carcinoma of the pancreas. Surg. Gynecol. Obstet. 152:597, 1981.
85. Sharp, K.W., Ross, C.B., Halter, S.A. et al. Pancreatoduodenectomy with pyloric preservation for carcinoma of the pancreas: A cautionary note. Surgery 105:645, 1989.
86. Siano Quirós, R., Linares, C., Chiesa, D., Gallo, E., Berbel, D. Duodenopancreatectomía cefálica. Conservación del píloro y oclusión del muñón pancreático. Rev. Argent. Cir. 45:198, 1983.
87. Smith, R. Cancer of the pancreas. J. R. Coll. Surg. Edinburgh 23:133, 1978.
88. Spjut, H.J., Ramos, A.J. An evaluation of biopsy-frozen section of the ampullary region and pancreas: A report of 68 consecutive patients. Ann. Surg. 146:923, 1957.
89. Telford, G.L., Mason, R.G. Pancreaticogastrostomy: Clinical experience with a direct pancreatic-duct-to-gastric-mucosa anastomosis. Am. J. Surg. 147:832, 1984.
90. Testut, L. Tratado de anatomía humana. Ed. 7, Vol. 4, p. 432. Salvat, Barcelona, 1923.
91. Traverso, L.W., Longmire, W.P., Jr. Preservation of the pylorus in pancreaticoduodenectomy. Surg. Gynecol. Obstet. 146:959, 1978.
92. Trede, M., Schwall, G., Saeger, H.D. Survival after pancreatoduodenectomy. 118 consecutive resections without an operative mortality. Ann. Surg. 211:447, 1990.
93. Van Heerden, J., ReMine, W., Weiland, L. et al. Total pancreatectomy for ductal adenocarcinoma of the pancreas. Am. J. Surg. 142:30, 1981.
94. Van Heerden, J.A.. Pancreatic resection for carcinoma of the pancreas: Whipple versus total pancreatectomy: An institutional perspective. World J. Surg. 8:880, 1984.
95. Viaggio, J.A., Sisco, P.J., Perrone, N.B. Duodenopancreatectomía cefálica con conservación del píloro y exclusión del páncreas. Rev. Argent. Cir. 50:277, 1986.
96. Warren, K.W., Kune, G.A., Poulantzas, J.K. Surgical treatment of chronic pancreatitis. Proceedings of the Third World Congress of Gastroenterology. Vol. 4, p. 385, Tokyo, 1966.
97. Warshaw, A.L., Turchiana, D.L. Delayed gastric emptying after pylorus-preserving pancreaticoduodenectomy. Surg. Gynecol. Obstet. 160:1, 1985.
98. Warshaw, A.L., Swanson, R.S. Pancreatic cancer in 1988. Possibilities and probabilities. Ann. Surg. 208:541, 1988.
99. Watson, K. Carcinoma of ampulla of Vater; successful radical resection. Br. J. Surg. 31:368, 1944.
100. Wells, C., Annis, D. Experimental pancreatogastrostomy. Lancet 1:97, 1949.
101. Wells, C., Shepherd, J.A., Gibbon, N. Pancreaticogastrostomy. Lancet 1:588, 1952.
102. Willems, J.S., Löwhagen, T. Aspiration biopsy cytology of the pancreas. Schweiz. Med. Wochenschr. 100:845, 1980.
103. Wilks, A.E., Miranda, N. Cirugía del cáncer de páncreas. Nuestra experiencia. Acad. Argent. Cir. 56:92, 1972.

Section C

Surgery of the Pancreas

CHAPTER 17

Surgical Treatment of Pancreatico-cutaneous Fistulas

Pancreatic fistulas are caused by loss of integrity of the pancreatic duct. The great majority of pancreatic fistulas are external or pancreaticocutaneous. Only rarely can internal fistulas to the stomach, duodenum, or transverse colon be seen.

External pancreatic fistulas usually have three main causes:

1. Penetrating or closed pancreatic trauma.
2. Surgical intervention on the pancreas or organs relating to it.
3. Acute pancreatic pathology and its complications.

Pancreatic trauma is usually accompanied by lesions to other abdominal viscera, which make surgical intervention urgent and then determine the procedure to be carried out.

Traumatic pancreatic lesions are variable: hematoma, lacerations, pancreatic transection, or the destruction of a part of the organ. Pancreatic fistulas can develop as a result of surgical intervention, acute pancreatitis, or a pseudocyst related to the trauma. Fistulas of traumatic origin through which pure pancreatic juice flows, without active enzymes, frequently close with medical therapy.

Surgical intervention on the pancreas may be complicated by a pancreatic fistula. Fistulas that develop after a distal resection of the pancreas, in general, close spontaneously. Fistulas that develop following pancreaticoduodenectomy (Whipple procedure) or pancreaticojejunostomy (modified Puestow-Gillesby operation) generally produce more severe changes and last longer because the pancreatic secretion is activated by intestinal or biliary secretions. Many of these fistulas close with medical treatment, but some may need to be reoperated. Pancreatic fistulas can be caused by pancreatic biopsy or following enucleation of an insulinoma. These generally close spontaneously. Some pancreatic fistulas that are very serious originate, not from surgical procedures of the pancreas, but from procedures practiced on neighboring organs, as occurs in gastrectomy for a penetrating duodenal ulcer be it bulbar or postbulbar. Fistulas may also appear as a result of incorrect surgical maneuvers resulting in disconnection of the papilla of Vater. An important source of origin of pancreatic fistulas is acute pancreatic pathology and its complications, abscesses, pseudocysts, and so on.

DEFINITION AND CHARACTERISTICS OF PANCREATICOCUTANEOUS FISTULAS

A pancreatic fistula exists when pancreatic secretion is proven to be coming out to the skin for more than 2 days. Some authors only accept the presence of a fistula of the pancreas when the amount of secretion is over 100 mL daily.

The diagnosis of a pancreatic fistula is relatively easy, owing to the characteristics of the fluid that flows and the amylase content, which is several times the amylase content of blood. The pH of pancreatic fluid is usually from 8 to 8.6.

Jordan (12, 13) classifies pancreatic fistulas in relation to the amount of loss:

1. Minor fistulas when there is a loss of less than 100 mL daily.
2. Moderate fistulas when daily loss is from 100–700 mL.
3. Major fistulas when the secretion is over 700 mL daily.

Some fistulas may have a daily loss of 1,800 mL. If the liquid is pure pancreatic fluid it usually contains between 20,000 and 50,000 Somogyi units of amylase. If the pancreatic juice is mixed with enteric secretions, biliary or lymphatic, it can have a concentration of only 1,000 to 5,000 Somogyi units. In normal persons pancreatic secretion varies between 600 and 1,500 mL daily. This secretion is continuous even though food is not ingested, because of vagal action and the stimulus of secretin produced by the passage of gastric juice into the duodenum. When food is ingested, the amount of secretin increases and the amount of pancreatic fluid also increases. Pancreatic juice should not be allowed to accumulate in the peritoneal cavity, even if it is pure, because its simple accumulation may lead to sepsis, digestion of tissues, hemorrhage, and so on. When this happens, particularly in the first days of the formation of a fistula, the aspiration tube should be cleared, since it could be occluded by debris or clots.

If the fistula is complete, it will drain the entire pancreatic secretion to the outside. These complete fistulas are caused by an obstruction of the cephalic portion of the pancreatic duct by stricture or calculus. Complete fistulas have very little tendency to close under medical treatment. Incomplete fistulas have a greater possibility of closing. This affirmation is not absolute, however, since fistulas have been observed with great loss, which decrease a few days later. On the other hand, fistulas with moderate loss may show a little tendency to close with medical treatment.

CONTROL OF THE FISTULA AND THE PANCREATIC SECRETION

Once the pancreatic fistula is established, its daily loss should be controlled as should the characteristics of the liquid that is draining. It is important to control the concentration of amylase and to keep strict track of the evolution time of the fistula with the object of determining the time at which fistulography can be carried out without risk. Periodically, cultures of the secretion should be performed with the object of determining the degree of sepsis and the type of germs present in order to be able to combat them with adequate antibiotics. It is important to obtain a fistulogram with both truncal and lateral profiles to determine its length and trajectory, as well as its direct or indirect communication with the pancreatic duct, and to establish if there is obstruction in some sector of the pancreatic duct or if it is completely open.

Fistulography will allow the determination of whether the radiopaque substance passes into the duodenum, if the fistula's tract is single or multiple. It will also allow determination of the possible presence of some cavity within the abdomen related to the fistula. Fistulography should not be performed before 20 to 30 days after the fistula's origin, in order to give time for the fistula to be well constituted with fibrous tissue. It is not always possible to see the pancreatic duct by means of fistulography. In that case retrograde endoscopic colangiopancreaticography will have to resorted to (16, 17). Some authors advise the performance of both examinations in every case (17). Others prefer not to perform the retrograde endoscopic colangiopancreaticography because of fear of infection (13).

MEDICAL TREATMENT OF PATIENTS WITH PANCREATICOCUTANEOUS FISTULAS

More than 70% of patients with pancreaticocutaneous fistulas are cured with medical treatment. Medical treatment should be tried in all cases before a decision to operate is made, even though closure may be delayed for months, and in some cases over a year. Surgical treatment is indicated only when it is obvious that medical treatment, correctly used, has failed.

The medical treatment usually employed is

1. Nasogastric intubation to diminish to a minimum the passage of gastric juice into the duodenum.
2. Administration of H_2 blockers to diminish acid secretion in the stomach.
3. Maintenance of electrolytic equilibrium.
4. The use of parenteral hyperalimentation to maintain the nutritional state of the patient until a fistula's tract with fibrous walls has been constituted. Only then can oral feeding be started, which at first would be an elemental diet, producing little stimulus for secretions, later going on to a more appetizing diet. It is not necessary to maintain parenteral alimentation very long because it has been shown that it does not contribute to closure of the fistula (13).
5. Permanent suction by means of a catheter placed in the fistulous tract.
6. The aspirated fluid can be returned to the body through the nasogastric tube in order to diminish the losses to the patient. Howard (8) recommends mixing the pancreatic juice with grape juice to improve its flavor when the nasogastric tube has been removed.
7. Some authors have used pharmacologic agents to diminish pancreatic secretion. One of these agents is somatostatin, in doses of 250 μg per hour intravenously (11, 18). Other authors have not established any advantages with the use of somatostatin because it has not shortened the period of time necessary for closure of the fistula (16). Somatostatin diminishes pancreatic secretion but only temporarily, and in some patients its discontinuation has led to an obvious increase in the amount of secretions (16). Other authors have reported serious complications by the administration of somatostatin (7). Williams and colleagues (20) assert that octreotide acetate, which is an analogue of somatostatin, is efficient in the treatment of pancreatic fistulas because it diminishes the secretion of pancreatic juice and may act as a preventive to the formation of pancreatic fistulas. Unlike somatostatin, which has a short life and therefore has to be given continuously intravenously, octreotide acetate has a much longer life, for which reason it can be administered three times a day subcutaneously. Other pharmacologic agents, such as glucagon, terbutaline (11), and acetazolamide (18), have also been used for the same purpose but with little success.
8. The skin of patients with pancreatic fistulas should be protected with karaya paste. This should not be discontinued until the fistula is cured, and the paste should be added as the fistula becomes smaller. It is extremely useful to attach an ileostomy bag to the cutaneous orifice of the fistula. Maceration of the skin of these patients should be avoided by all means.

As the fistula becomes established, the principal task of the physician is to control the patient's life, which is usually in danger. Once this time has passed, correct control of the fistula will be an essential task.

Surgical Treatment of Pancreaticocutaneous Fistulas

The indications for surgical treatment of pancreatic fistulas are

1. When the fistula shows no tendency to close.
2. When the fistula has caused serious metabolic alterations in the patient.
3. When the digestive action of the pancreatic fluid has caused destruction of the tissues surrounding the fistula.
4. When the skin lesions have become intolerable.

Surgical treatment of pancreatic fistulas is a complex problem with many aspects. For this reason, patients must be treated individually, since clinical and pathologic variations are numerous.

Surgical treatment of pancreaticocutaneous fistulas consists of redirecting the fistula to the digestive tract, either the jejunum or the stomach. In order to carry out these objectives, several operations have been proposed that consist in anastomosing the fistulized pancreas to the jejunum or the stomach. The anastomosis has to be performed directly to the surface of the pancreas and not to the fistulous tract, as proposed by many authors (1–3, 5, 14, 21). The tract is not suitable for suturing, since it does not have the necessary consistency to hold sutures because of its fragility. Because of this fragility it is also very difficult to dissect it without producing one or more perforations of the tract. Its deficient blood supply does not guarantee the duration or efficiency of its permeability. On the other hand, we believe that the fistulous tract should serve as a guide to the surgeon to rapidly localize the pancreatic opening of the fistula. It is very common that the surface of the pancreas around the fistula's opening has become more consistent and firm because of the fibrosis produced by the fistula. This allows safe suturing to perform the anastomosis with the jejunum or with the stomach.

Some surgeons, when faced with a distal pancreatic fistula caused by a pancreaticoduodenectomy, resect the segment of residual pancreas and perform a total gastrectomy. It is well known, however, how difficult it is to manage diabetes in a patient with total pancreatectomy.

Before continuing with the description of the operative technique in the treatment of pancreatic fistulas, it is useful to note that many pancreatic fistulas are produced by surgical errors of technique or of criteria in the treatment of pancreatic conditions. It should be remembered that the majority of pancreatic fistulas close with medical treatment and that surgical treatment should only be used in the case of failure of a well-conducted medical treatment.

In all pancreatic surgeries nonabsorbable material should be used because slow or rapid absorption material is immediately destroyed by the enzymes. After an operation on the pancreas is completed and before closing the abdomen, one or two draining suction tubes should be left in place postoperatively in case some of the sutures do not hold, so that the pancreatic secretion will not spread throughout the abdomen but will come to the outside through the continuous suction tubes, constituting a fistula which later, by the action of the fibrosis, will become more firm.

Surgical Treatment of Pancreatic Fistulas by Means of a Pancreaticogastric Anastomosis

FIGURE 17.1
X-rays of the fistulous tract of a patient 48 years old who had been operated upon for a pseudocyst of the pancreas that included the head and the body, but whose wall had not reached maturity so that an anastomosis could be carried out. One can observe that the pancreatic duct is dilated and the end of a drainage tube is located within the duct. The radiopaque material passes easily into the duodenum. The average daily loss from the fistula was 600 ml of pure pancreatic juice. After a period of observation of 4 months without showing any tendency to decrease, surgical intervention was recommended.

Surgical Treatment of Pancreatic Fistulas by Means of a Pancreaticogastric Anastomosis

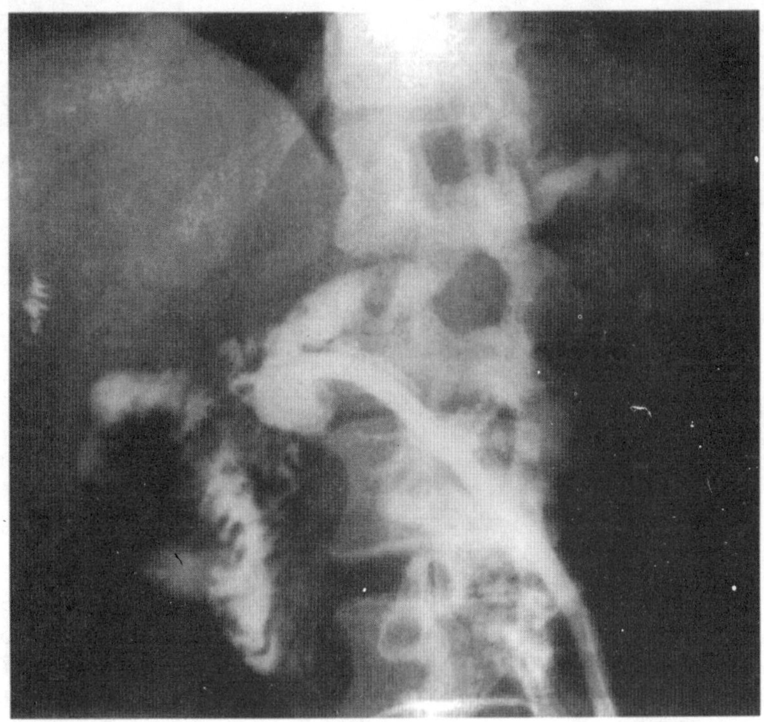

FIGURE 17.1

FIGURE 17.2

This drawing shows the fistulography study seen in the previous figure. The patient had a xyphoumbilical incision, and suction draining of the pseudocyst had been carried out through a small incision in the right side of the abdomen, lateral to the anterior rectus muscle, where the external opening of the fistula is located. Before preparing the abdomen for surgery it is advisable to remove the drainage tube located in the fistulous tract through which continuous suction was carried out. The abdominal skin is washed and cleaned with antiseptic solutions to prepare the operative field. A new sterile tube is inserted into the tract to serve as a guide during the intra-abdominal exploration and in order to facilitate dissection of the tract. A midline xyphoumbilical incision is carried out through the previous scar. extending some 5 cm below the umbilicus.

Surgical Treatment of Pancreatic Fistulas by Means of a Pancreaticogastric Anastomosis

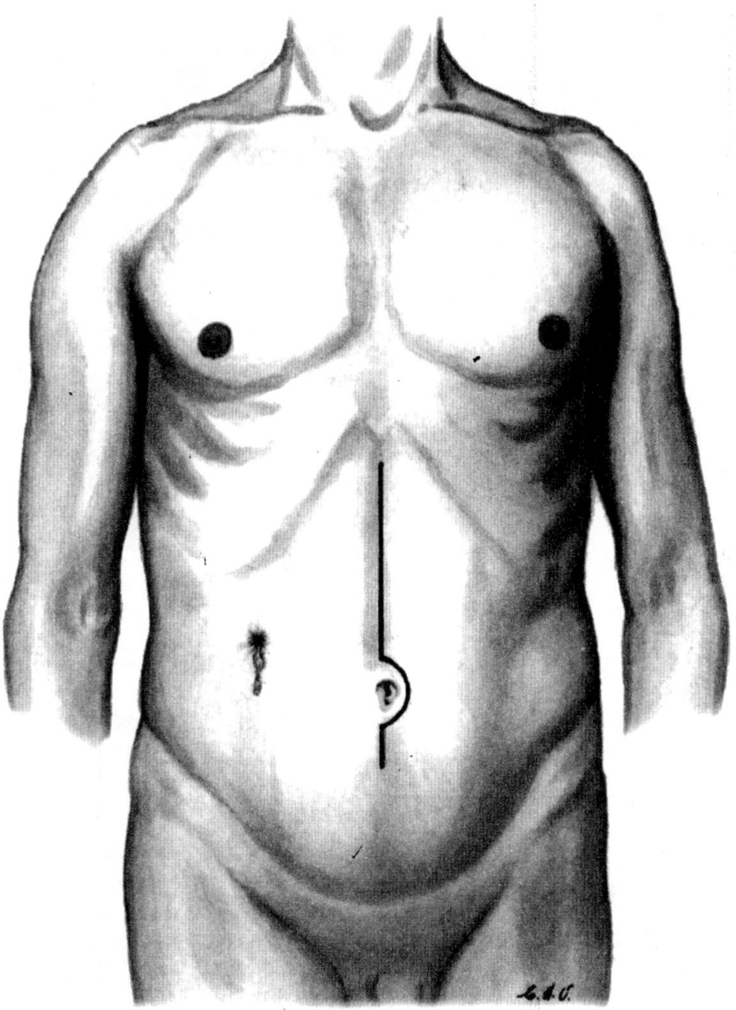

FIGURE 17.2

Surgical Treatment of Pancreatic Fistulas by Means of a Pancreaticogastric Anastomosis

FIGURE 17.3
Once the abdominal cavity is open, traction is applied to the right side of the wound toward the right, using two or more Allis clamps. At the same time, the stomach is retracted to the left, using two Foerster clamps. The fistulous tract is easily identified with the tube inside it. The tract runs obliquely toward the left and backward, densely adherent to the wall of the stomach, later turning backward toward the anterior surface of the pancreas. The drawing shows that the parietal peritoneum around the fistula is being incised to free it from the abdominal wall.

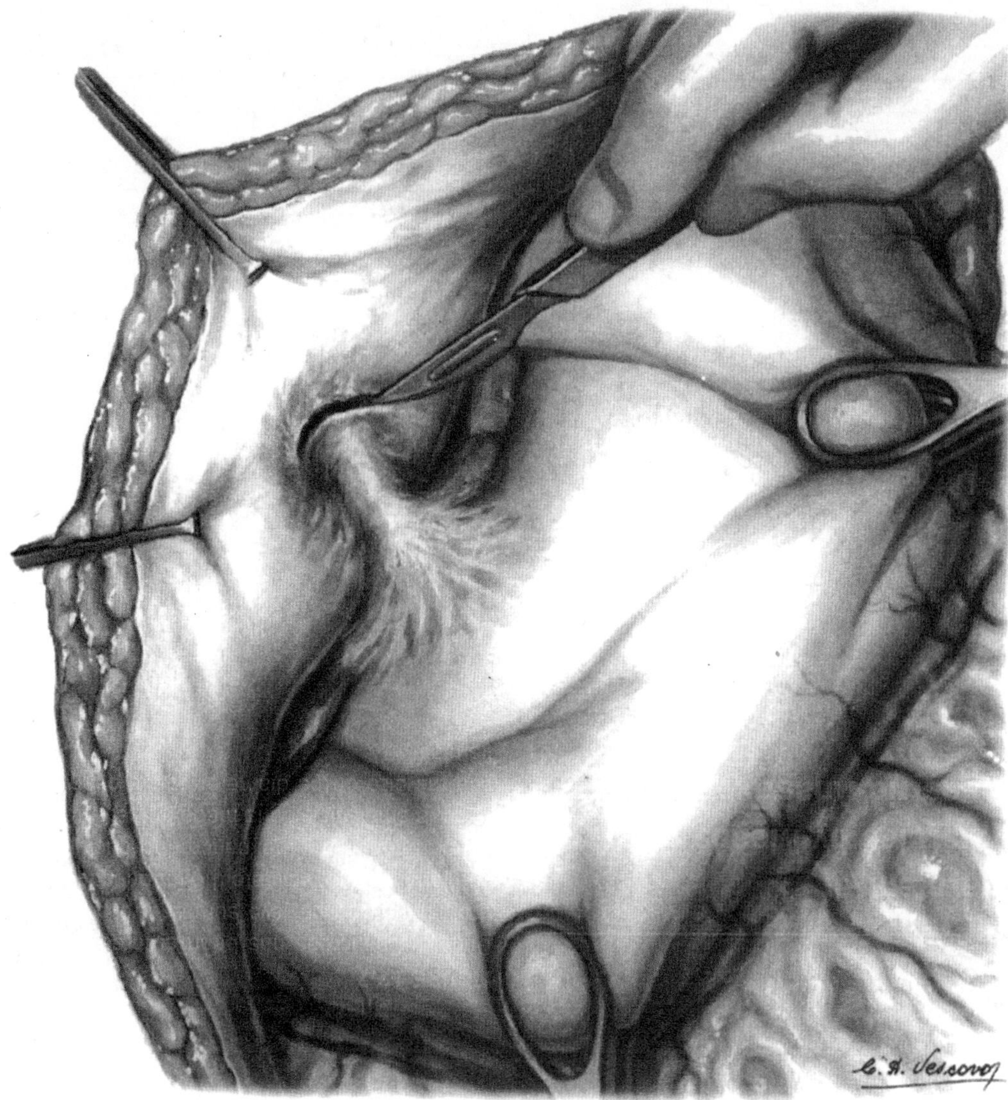

FIGURE 17.3

Surgical Treatment of Pancreatic Fistulas by Means of a Pancreaticogastric Anastomosis

FIGURE 17.4
The fistulous tract has been completely separated from the abdominal wall. The previously introduced tube is fixed to the tract with a cotton suture because it tends to come out. Dissection of the tract is continued, using scissors and passing through the tissues surrounding the fistula. The anterior surface of the pancreas, where the fistula originated, is arrived at, and it can be shown that an anastomosis between the pancreas and the posterior wall of the stomach is perfectly plausible.

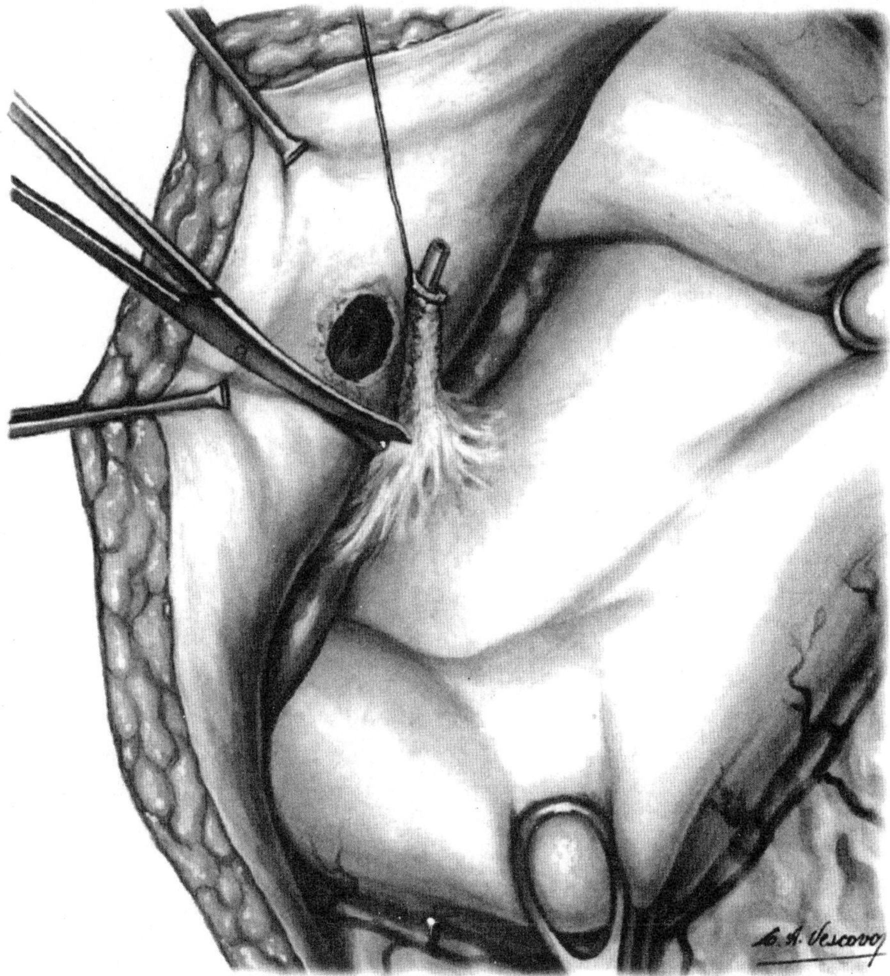

FIGURE 17.4

FIGURE 17.5
Operative photograph of the patient. One can notice that the fistulous tract has been separated from the abdominal wall. The tube in the tract will be fixed to the tract and dissection carried up to the anterior wall of the pancreas.

Surgical Treatment of Pancreatic Fistulas by Means of a Pancreaticogastric Anastomosis

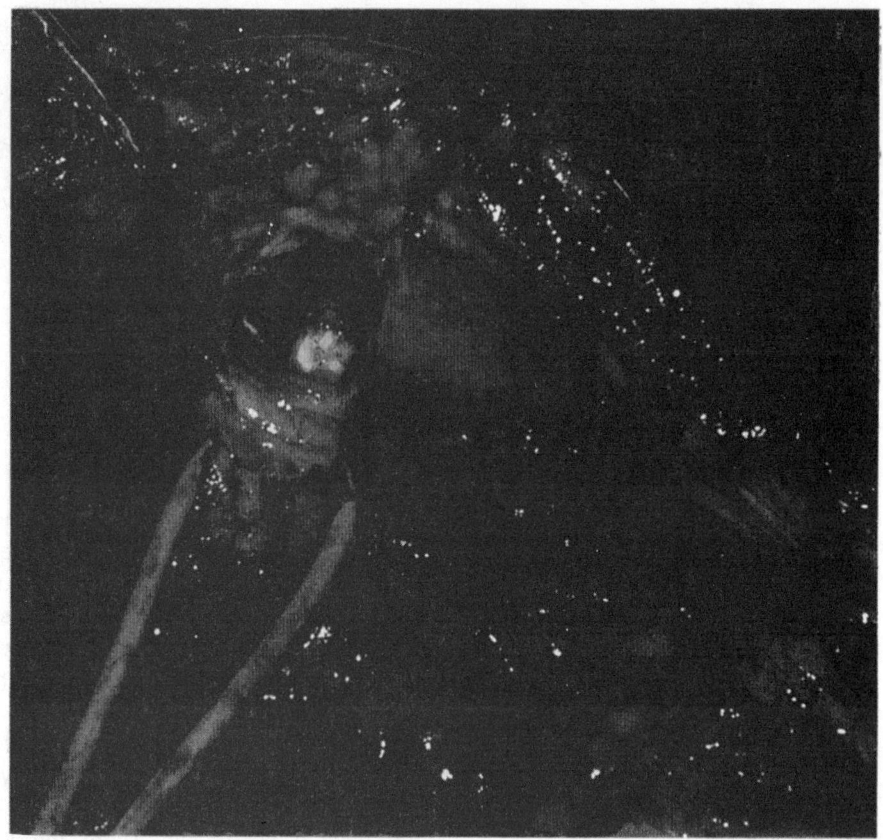

FIGURE 17.5

FIGURE 17.6
Dissection has been carried out up to the pancreas. The tract, together with the tube, has been divided, leaving only a few millimeters of tract projecting from the surface of the pancreas in order to facilitate placement of the sutures. Sutures have started to be placed in what used to be the external layer of the pancreaticogastric anastomosis. These sutures include the seromuscular layer of the stomach on one side and the capsule and part of the parenchyma of the pancreas on the other side, below the fistula's orifice. Two sutures have been placed, and a third one is being introduced. One can note that the parietal peritoneum where the fistula's tract passed through has been closed. The rest of the fistula is left to close by secondary intention.

Surgical Treatment of Pancreatic Fistulas by Means of a Pancreaticogastric Anastomosis

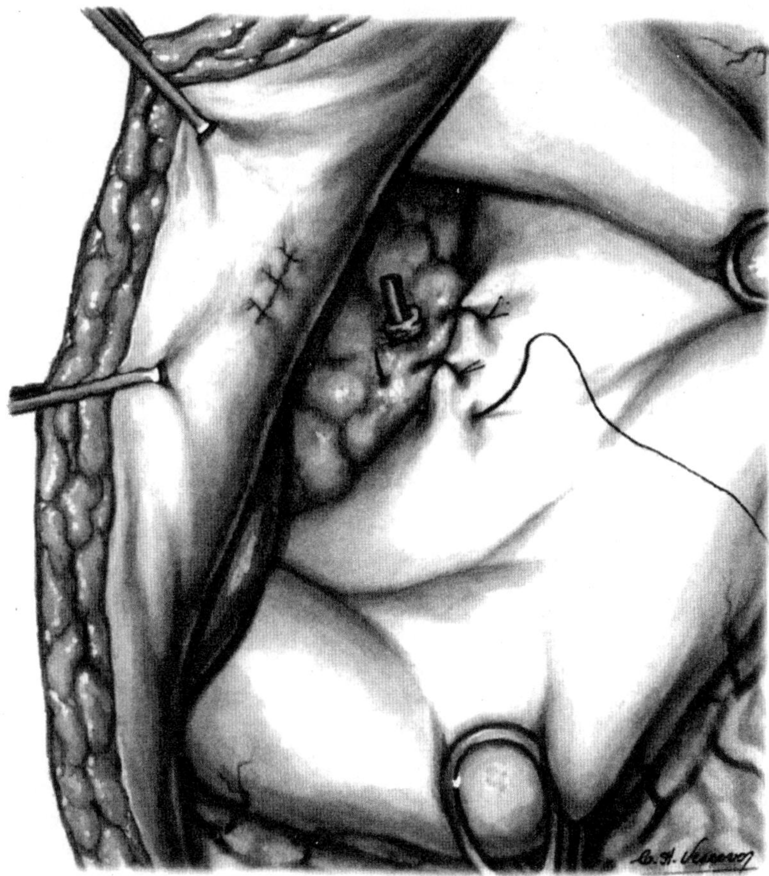

FIGURE 17.6

Surgical Treatment of Pancreatic Fistulas by Means of a Pancreaticogastric Anastomosis

FIGURE 17.7
Once the pancreas has been sutured to the stomach, below the fistula's orifice, two sutures are placed at the end of the fistulous tract to facilitate the introduction of a short branch of a fine T-tube into the pancreatic duct. Once this has been done, a small incision is made in the anterior wall of the stomach the size of the diameter of the opening of the pancreatic fistula.

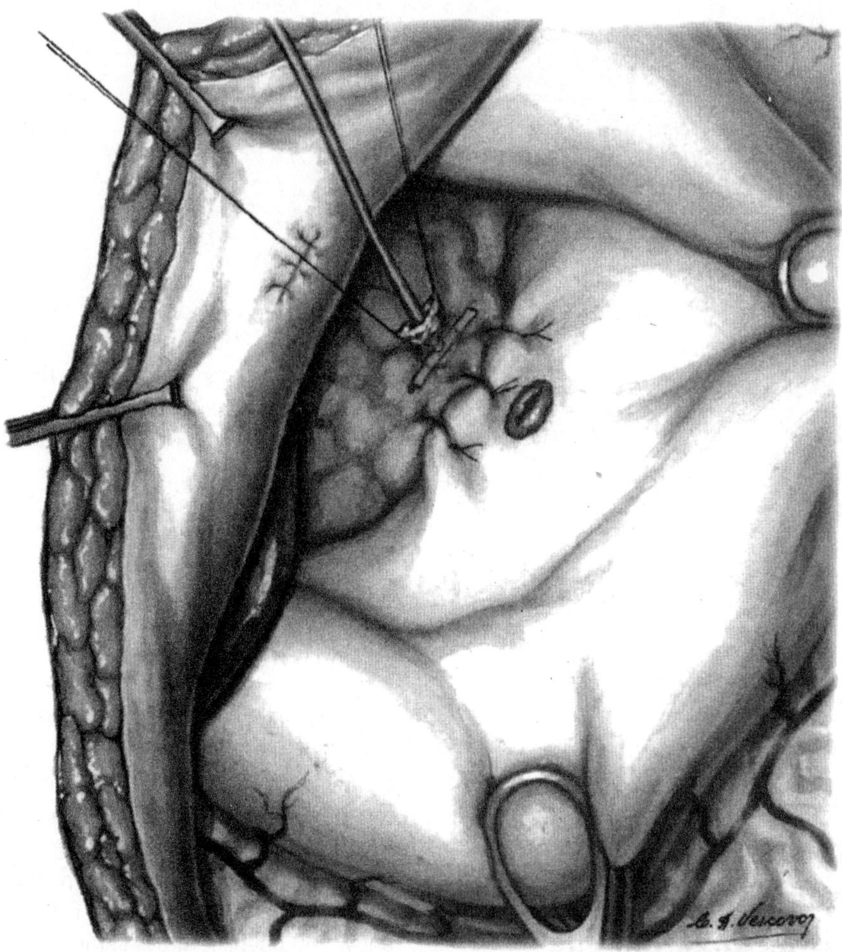

FIGURE 17.7

FIGURE 17.8

In order to facilitate the internal sutures between the border of the pancreatic orifice and the gastric wall, a small incision has been made in the anterior wall of the stomach, about 8 to 10 cm long. The long limb of the T-tube has been passed through this opening in the gastric wall and introduced into the cavity of the stomach. Sutures have started to be placed to include the seromuscular layer of the posterior stomach wall on one side and the capsule and part of the pancreatic parenchyma above the opening of the fistula on the other.

Surgical Treatment of Pancreatic Fistulas by Means of a Pancreaticogastric Anastomosis

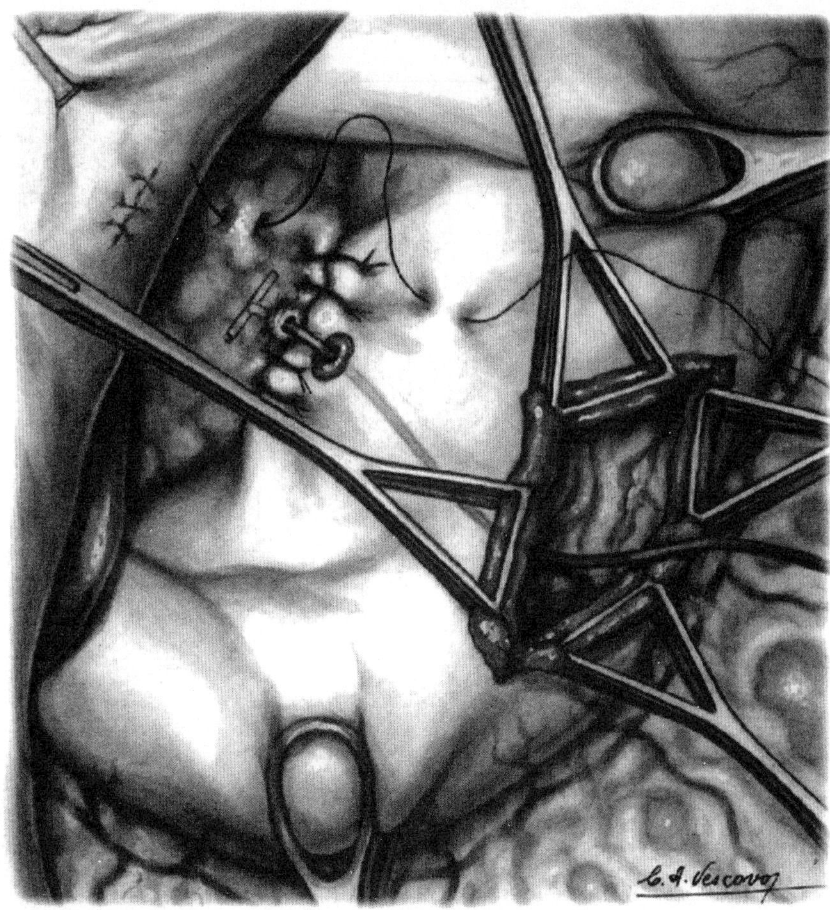

FIGURE 17.8

FIGURE 17.9
The suture line of the external pancreaticogastric anastomosis is being completed surrounding the fistulous opening. The next step is to carry out the internal suturing of the edges of the pancreatic opening with the posterior gastric wall.

Surgical Treatment of Pancreatic Fistulas by Means of a Pancreaticogastric Anastomosis

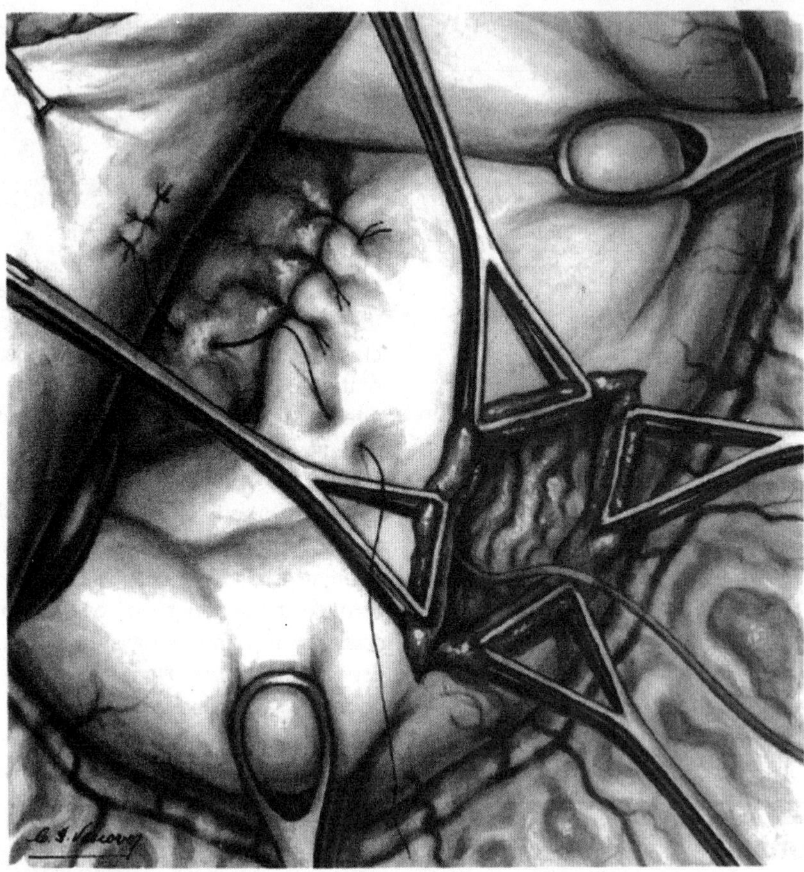

FIGURE 17.9

FIGURE 17.10
Atraumatic triangular Duval clamps are grasping the edges of the incision made in the anterior wall of the stomach. These clamps not only help the hemostasis, but they permit exposure of the inside of the stomach in order to be able to carry out the internal suture line between the gastric wall and the edges of the pancreatic opening. The suture material used in all the sutures of the pancreas is nonabsorbable material, cotton, silk, or synthetic. Three sutures have been introduced and a fourth is being placed between the edges of the pancreatic opening and the gastric wall. The T-tube has been passed through the anterior wall of the stomach where it is held in place by a purse string suture. The anterior stomach wall is then closed in two layers. The T-tube is brought out outside the abdomen through a small incision in the abdominal wall. The anterior gastric wall is fixed with several sutures to the parietal peritoneum, around the T-tube. The T-tube should be left in place at least 3 weeks.

Surgical Treatment of Pancreatic Fistulas by Means of a Pancreaticogastric Anastomosis

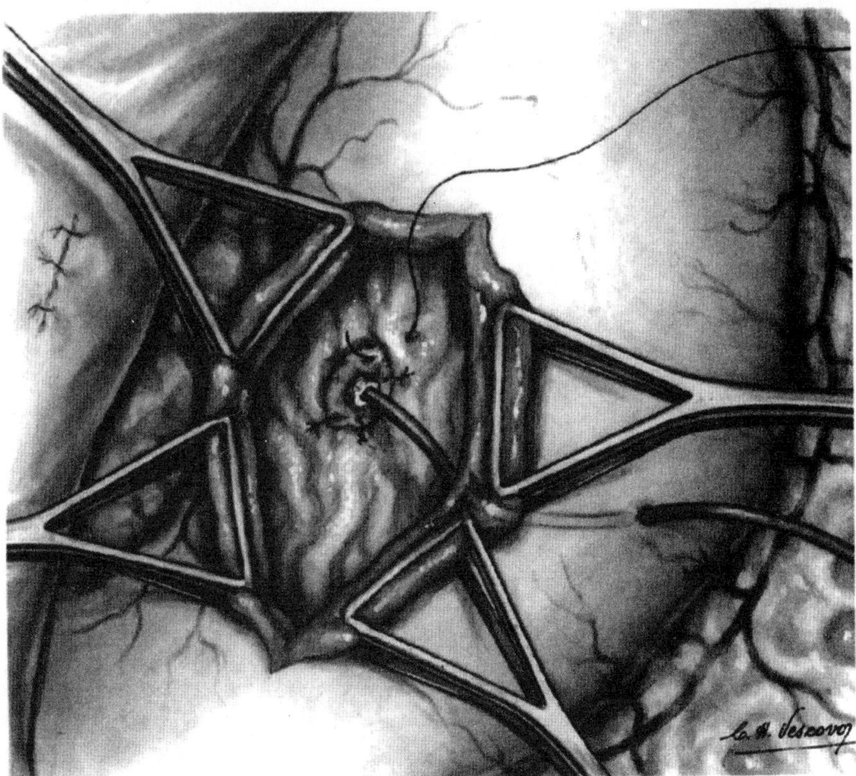

FIGURE 17.10

FIGURE 17.11

The fistulous tract is dissected in a fashion similar to that described in the pancreaticogastric anastomosis. Once the tract has been dissected and the pancreatic orifice has been identified, a jejunal loop is prepared in Roux-en-Y fashion. The end of the defunctionalized loop is closed in two layers. The anastomotic jejunal loop is placed below the pancreatic orifice and five sutures of nonabsorbable material are placed between the edge of the seromuscular layer and the capsule and part of the pancreatic parenchyma below the fistulous opening. The jejunal loop is held by an atraumatic triangular Duval clamp to afford exposure of the fistulous opening.

Surgical Treatment of Pancreatic Fistulas with Anastomosis to the Jejunum

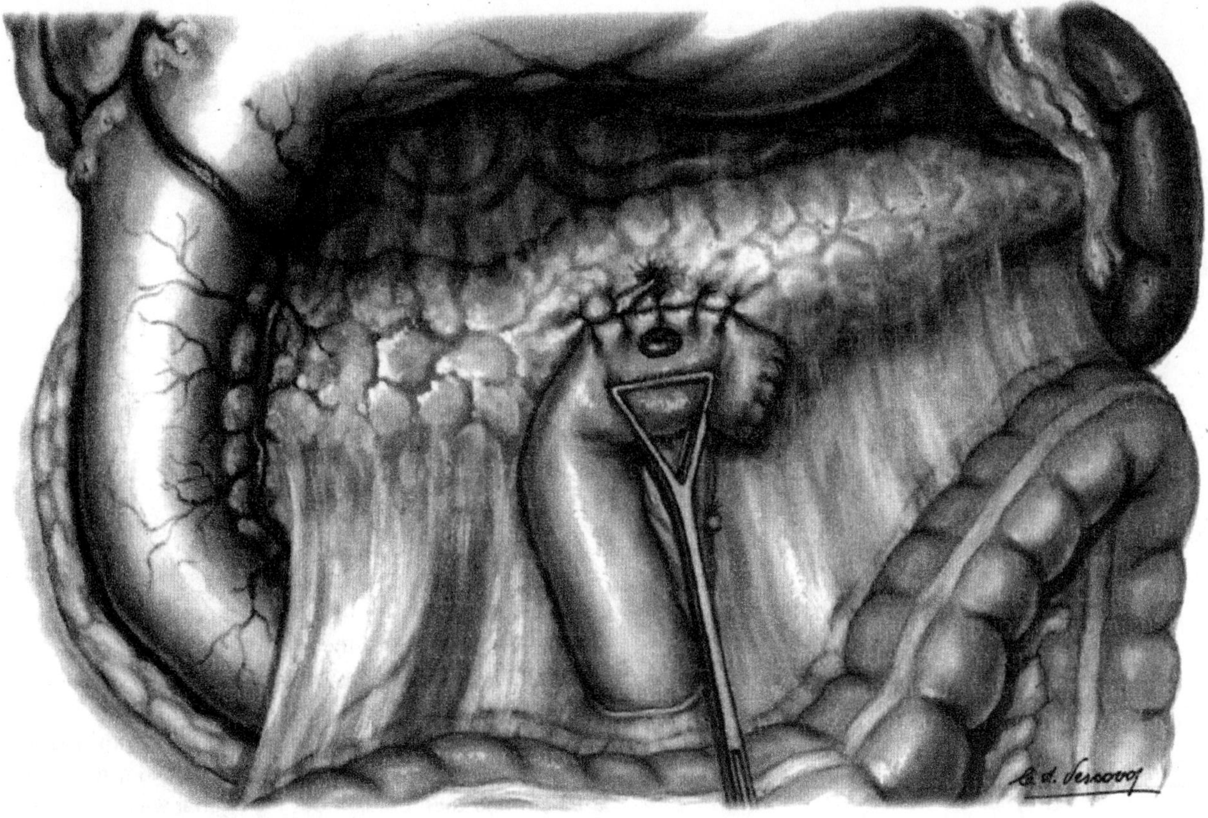

FIGURE 17.11

FIGURE 17.12
An opening is made in the jejunum, the same size as the opening of the fistulous tract. The short limb of a thin T-tube is placed in the pancreatic duct and the long limb is introduced through the small opening made in the jejunum. The long limb of the T-tube is passed through the jejunum for some 10 to 12 cm and then brought out the jejunal wall, as shown in the drawing. Sutures are being placed to include the seromuscular layers of the jejunum and the capsule and parenchyma of the pancreas.

Surgical Treatment of Pancreatic Fistulas with Anastomosis to the Jejunum

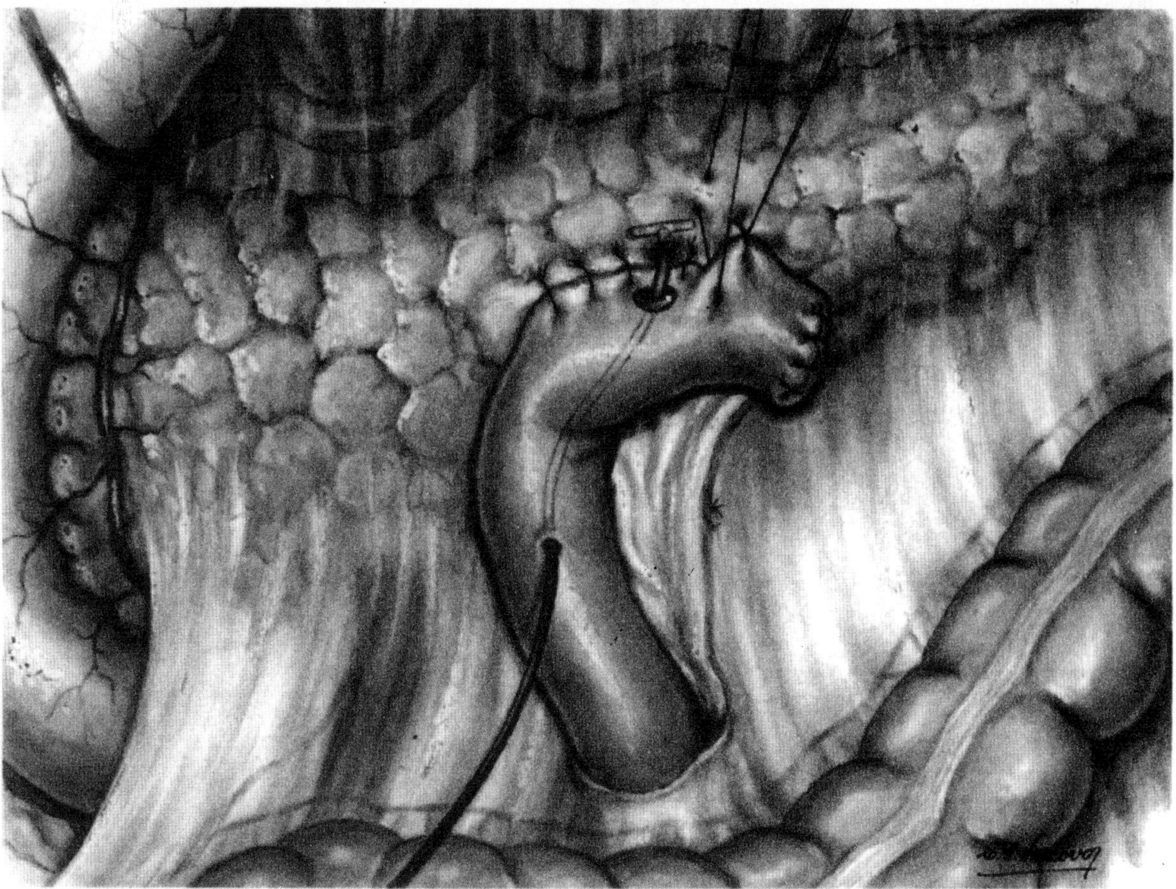

FIGURE 17.12

Surgical Treatment of Pancreatic Fistulas with Anastomosis to the Jejunum

FIGURE 17.13

The anastomosis between the jejunum and the pancreas has been completed. The long limb of the T-tube is brought out through a Witzel seromuscular tunnel 5 cm long. The long limb of the T-tube will be brought out of the abdomen through a small incision. At the end of the operation the anastomotic limb of the jejunum is fixed to the parietal peritoneum with several sutures around the point of exit of the T-tube. The drawing also shows the terminolateral jejunojejunostomy some 40 to 50 cm distal to the pancreaticojejunal anastomosis. The anastomotic jejunal limb has been passed through the transverse mesocolon, to which it has been fixed with several sutures.

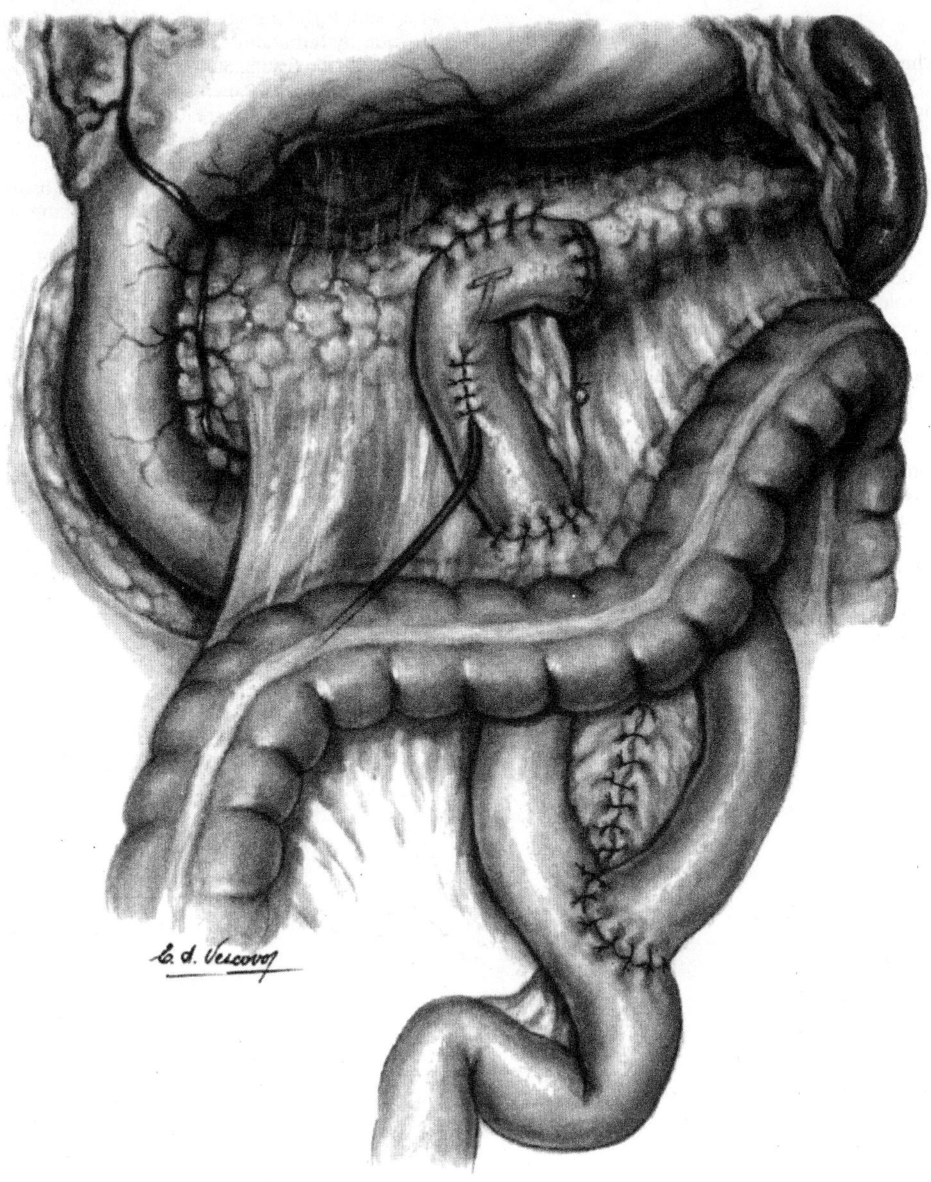

FIGURE 17.13

References

1. Antila, L.E. A technique for operative connection of pancreatic fístula. J. Int. Coll. Surg. 42:379, 1964.
2. Artigas, V. Fistulas pancreáticas. In Pi-Figueras (Ed.) Práctica quirúrgica. Ed. 2, Vol. II, p. 914 Salvat, Barcelona, 1986.
3. Bartlett, L.C., Thorlakson, P.H.T. The etiology and technique of surgical management of pancreatic fístula. Surg. Gynecol. Obstet. 102:413, 1956.
4. Bohlman, T.W., Katon, R.M., Lee, T.G., Eidemiller, L.R. Case report: Use of endoscopic retrograde cholangiopancreatography in the diagnosis of pancreatic fistula. A case report and review of the literature. Gastroenterology 70:582, 1976.
5. Coffey, R.J., Blumberg, J.J. Surgery in nonacute diseases of the pancreas. U.S. Armed Forces Med. J. 2:803, 1951.
6. Dudrick, S.J. Spontaneous closure of traumatic pancreatoduodenal fistula with total intravenous nutrition. J. Trauma 10:542, 1970.
7. Halma, C., Jancen, J.R. et al. Life-threatening water intoxication during somatostatin therapy. Ann. Intern. Med. 107:518, 1987.
8. Howard, J.M. Pancreatic fistula. Experiences in the management of 52 patients. In Howard, J.M., Jordan, G.L. (Eds.) p. 584 Lippincott, Philadelphia, 1960.
9. Huang, C.H., Kuyama, T., Takeda, J. Post-traumatic external pancreatic fistula. Am. J. Surg. 113:816, 1967.
10. Isaacson, R., Weiland, L.H., McIllarath, O.C. Biopsy of the pancreas. Arch. Surg. 109:227, 1974.
11. Joehl, R.J., Nahrwold, D.L. Inhibition of human pancreatic secretion by terbutaline as a potential agent for treating patients with pancreatic fistula. Surg. Gynecol. Obstet. 160:109, 1985.
12. Jordan, G.I., Jr. Pancreatic fistula. Am. J. Surg. 138:821, 1979.
13. Jordan, G.I., Jr. Pancreatic fistula. In Howard, J.M., Jordan, G.I., Jr. (Eds.) Surgical diseases of the pancreas. p. 898. Lea & Febiger, Philadelphia, 1987.
14. Lahey, F., Lium, R. Cure of pancreatic fistula by pancreatojejunostomy: Report of a case with review of the literature. Surg. Gynecol. Obstet. 64:79, 1937.
15. Lygidakis, N.J., van der Heyde, M.N. Early complications after pancreatic resection. In Lygidakis, N.J., Tytgat, G.N.J. (Eds.) Hepatobiliary malignancies. p. 304. Thieme Verlag, Stuttgart, 1989.
16. Martin, F.M., Rossi, R.L., Munson, J.L. et al. Management of pancreatic fistulas. Arch. Surg. 124:571, 1989.
17. Nardi, G.L. Discusión del trabajo: Martin, E.M., Rossi, R.L., Munson, J.L. et al. Management of pancreatic fistulas. Arch. Surg. 124:571, 1989.
18. Prinz, R.A., Pickleman, J., Hoffman, J.P. Treatment of cutaneous fistulas with a somatostatin analogue. Am. J. Surg. 155:36, 1988.
19. Stone, H.H., Fabian, T.C., Saliam, B., Turkleson, M.L. Experiences in the management of pancreatic trauma. J. Trauma 21:257, 1981.
20. Williams, S.T., Woltering, E.A., O'Dorisio, T.M. et al. Effect of octreotide acetate on pancreatic exocrine function. Arch. Surg. 157:476, 1989.
21. Wiper, T.B., Miller, J.M. Surgical aspects of pancreatic fistula. Ann. Surg. 120:52, 1944.

Section C

Surgery of the Pancreas

CHAPTER 18

Surgery for Carcinoma of the Papilla of Vater

Carcinoma of the papilla of Vater includes a group of carcinomas called periampullary. In addition to carcinoma of the papilla, carcinomas that originate in the distal end of the pancreatic duct and in the mucosa and submucosa of the duodenum in the vicinity of the papilla are included in this group. Although periampullary tumors constitute a heterogeneous group, they present several clinical evolutionary and diagnostic characteristics that are similar. In general they are well-differenciated tumors, slow in evolution, and with a great tendency to grow and spread locally before metastasizing to distal areas. These biologic characteristics of periampullary tumors, together with the development of early symptoms, are undoubtedly the reasons why they have better prognosis than carcinoma of the head of the pancreas. All statistical studies show that pancreaticoduodenectomy for periampullary carcinomas show more than 5 years of survival, definitely an improvement on the results for carcinoma of the head of the pancreas (4, 10, 21, 22, 25, 28, 34, 55, 56). This is the reason for establishing a clear distinction between periampullary carcinomas and carcinomas of the head of the pancreas.

On the other hand, there are authors that include carcinoma of the head of the pancreas in the group of periampullary tumors (4, 24). Even though this inclusion is correct from the topographic view, it is not correct from the point of view of their biologic behavior. To avoid confusion we have opted for the designation of extrapancreatic periampullary tumors instead of periampullary to differentiate tumors that originate in the head of the pancreas. In some cases, the exact origin of the tumor is difficult to establish—numerous mistakes in histologic diagnosis of resected specimens have been proven. For this reason it is advisable to review histologic preparations when a patient who has been subjected to pancreaticoduodenectomy with a diagnosis of carcinoma of the head of the pancreas survives more than 5 years. These preparations should be reviewed by a different pathologist from the one who made the original diagnosis. In some cases it has been shown that the supposed carcinoma of the head of the pancreas was in reality a periampullary extrapancreatic carcinoma, an endocrine carcinoma, or a case of chronic pancreatitis (2, 10). In order to facilitate the identification of the origin of periampullary extrapancreatic tumors, it has been advised that the common bile duct and the pancreatic duct be injected with a solution of 10% formalin immediately after resection of the surgical specimen in a pancreaticoduodenectomy before the mucosa of these ducts is destroyed.

Carcinoma of the papilla of Vater is the most frequent of the extrapancreatic periampullary tumors and presents in different ways pathologically making its surgical diagnosis rather difficult. For this reason before making a diagnosis of carcinoma of the papilla during surgery, we believe it is useful to describe the macroscopic findings. Since the diagnosis of carcinoma of the papilla is frequently made preoperatively we have felt it convenient to succinctly describe the available means to make this diagnosis since some of these are also used during the actual procedure.

PATHOLOGY OF CARCINOMA OF THE PAPILLA OF VATER

We consider it useful to establish three types of carcinoma of the papilla in relation to its size, its growth, localization and its consistency:

I. Exophytic papillary carcinomas grow into the duodenal lumen, are easy to diagnose because of their size and appearance, and represent about 75% of malignant tumors of the papilla.
II. Intrapapillary carcinomas grow into the ampulla.
III. Peripapillary carcinomas grow into the mucosa or submucosa in the vicinity of the papilla.

Types II and III may be small and soft, presenting some difficulty in making the diagnosis. Type I tumors are usually easily palpable during surgery with the duodenum closed and very visible with the duodenum open or during duodenal endoscopy. In order for biopsies of these tumors to be representative the bites should be deep, not superficial. A superficial biopsy may show a benign tumor even though benign tumors of this location are very rare.

Tumors of Type I may become ulcerated or vegetating during their evolution, and, in some cases, may become infiltrated and retractile. According to Williams and colleagues (59), vegetating carcinomas of the papilla with a diameter of 2 cm and without positive nodes have a good possibility of surviving more than 5 years following pancreaticoduodenectomy. Many authors admit that the size of the tumor or the presence of positive nodes does not exclude the possibility of cure even though it may be less frequent (2, 10, 28, 37).

CARCINOMA TYPE II. Intrapapillary carcinomas are usually small in size and originate in and grow within the papillary lumen. When they are small they may not deform or increase the size of the papilla. Intrapapillary carcinoma has been confused with papillitis with hypertrophy of the papilla. In some patients the carcinoma, which is small in size originally, grows and increases the size and consistency of the papilla, revealing it as a rigid, erect, thickened and sometimes very indurated, turning it downward and backward. This may make it necessary to elevate the papilla with a finger so as to be able to expose the tumor through the duodenotomy. In more advanced cases, the papilla, which is increased in size, becomes ulcerated or retracts. The diagnosis of intrapapillary carcinoma in its initial stage may offer difficulties and sphincterotomy may be necessary to make a histologic diagnosis. In cases where the lumen of the papilla permits it, a small curette can be introduced and material extracted for microscopic examination.

CARCINOMA TYPE III. Peripapillary carcinomas, on occasions, can also be small and may be soft in consistency making it difficult to palpate them with the duodenum closed.

These tumors, as already stated, may originate in the mucosa or submucosa, in the vicinity of the papilla. If they originate in the submucosa they may be covered by normal duodenal mucosa and are then designated as intraparietal or intramural. They have at times been confused with heterotopic pancreatic nodules, which, as is known, are located in the submucosa of the duodenum, but are generally situated over the papilla. Peripapillary tumors of small size and soft consistency may only be felt or seen with the duodenum open (14, 17, 20, 41, 42, 59).

Pathology of Carcinoma of the Papilla of Vater

FIGURE 18.1
Semischematic drawing to show the three types of carcinoma of the papilla that have just been described. A, Exophytic papillary or vegetating carcinoma of the papilla, growing into the duodenal lumen. This is the most common type of carcinoma of the papilla (75%) and is the easiest to diagnose, either in surgery or by preoperative endoscopy (12). B, Intrapapillary carcinoma. This tumor develops inside the papilla without producing any changes in the duodenal mucosa. In the course of time the papilla will increase in size, appearing like a uterine cervix. Later the papilla may ulcerate or retract owing to neoplastic infiltration. C, Peripapillary carcinoma. These tumors develop in the vicinity of the papilla, be it in the mucosa or submucosa, as seen in the drawing.

Pathology of Carcinoma of the Papilla of Vater

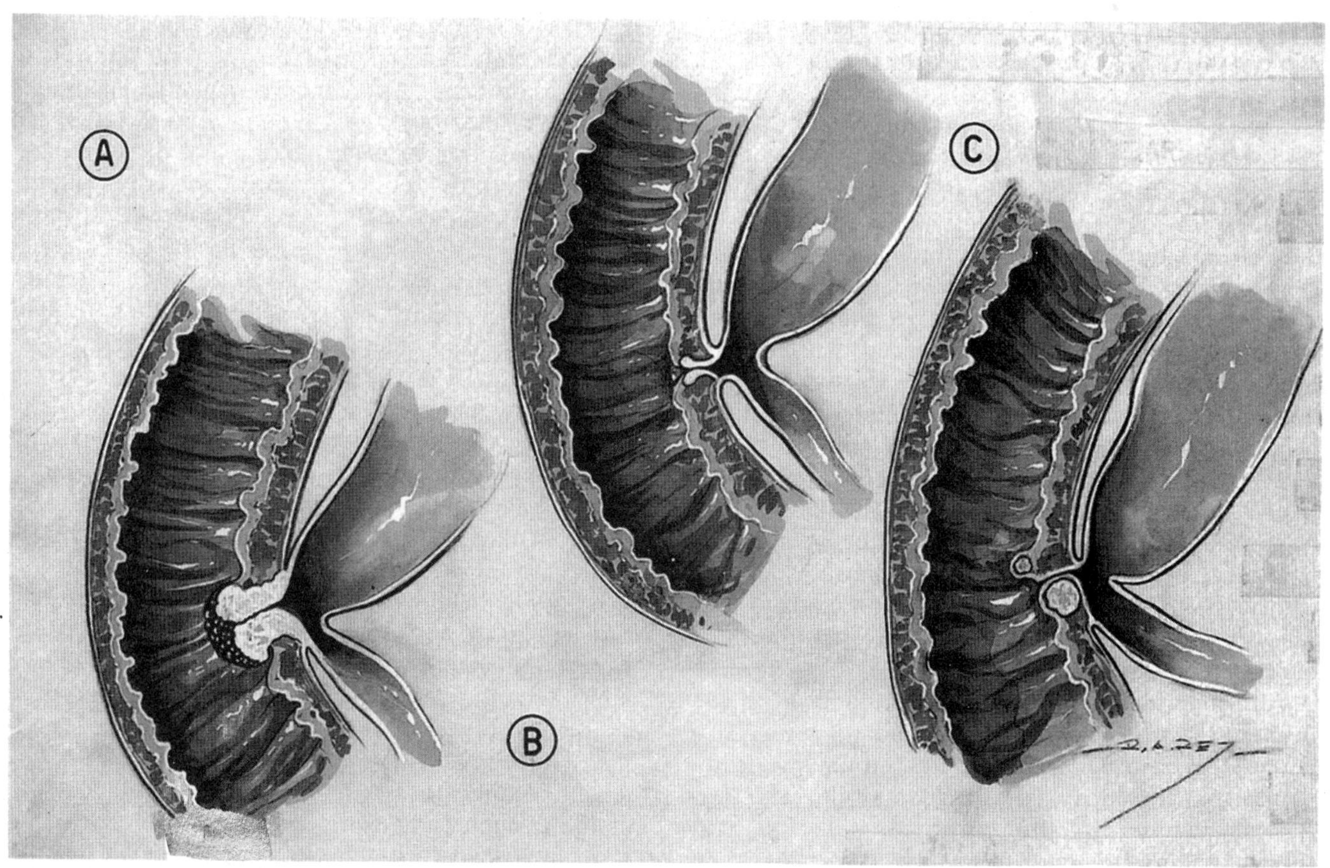

FIGURE 18.1

PREOPERATIVE DIAGNOSIS OF CARCINOMA OF THE PAPILLA OF VATER

Preoperative diagnosis of carcinoma of the papilla of Vater can be made in 60 to 70% of cases. In centers with considerable experience in pancreaticoduodenal surgery, the percentage of diagnoses can be higher (2, 12). The clinical picture can lead to a diagnosis of obstructive jaundice, confirmed by laboratory tests. Ultrasonography and computed axial tomography, in most cases, reveal dilation of the extra- and intrahepatic biliary tree. Dilation of the intrahepatic biliary tree is highly suggestive of neoplastic obstruction. Fiberoptic duodenoscopy is the most valuable method in diagnosing carcinoma of the papilla because it allows visualization of the lesion in 60 to 70% of the patients as well as the obtaining of biopsies to certify the microscopic diagnosis. The vegetating type of tumor can be seen more frequently proliferating into the duodenal lumen, as well as the ulcerating, vegetating tumors.

Small intrapapillary tumors are more difficult to see. In these cases endoscopic sphincterotomy may have to be used to remove neoplastic tissue from inside the papilla. Small peripapillary carcinomas can also present difficulty in diagnosis, particularly when they are submucosal. Diagnosis of carcinoma of the papilla by means of endoscopy and biopsy preoperatively precludes the necessity of having to repeat this during surgery. Retrograde endoscopic cholangiopancreatography may be necessary in some doubtful cases. This study permits visualization of the entire biliary tree, which in some cases, may be decisive in making the diagnosis. Ultrasonography and transhepatic cholangiography may confirm the presence of biliary and choledochal calculi, which tend to coexist with carcinoma of the papilla in 20% of cases. Even though not indispensable for confirmation of the diagnosis, gastroduodenal x-ray studies may supply data of interest, especially if hypotonic duodenography is carried out simultaneously (36, 52). This study generally shows some abnormality of the second portion of the duodenum in more than 70% of patients (6, 50). In spite of the methods we have at present to diagnose carcinoma of the papilla, an earlier diagnosis is still not possible (27).

OPERATIVE DIAGNOSIS OF CARCINOMA OF THE PAPILLA OF VATER

An early diagnosis is easy in cases in which the tumors of the papilla are large and exophytic, as stated previously, since they can be palpated with the duodenum closed and are very visible with the duodenum open. This type of neoplasm is very similar to carcinoma of the mouth (54). The tumors, which present some difficulty in diagnosis, are small, soft, intrapapillary or periampullary tumors. If endoscopy and biopsy were not carried out preoperatively, they can be done during the operation. The endoscopist introduces the fibroendoscope with the help of the surgeon. If the endoscopy and biopsy confirm the diagnosis of carcinoma of the papilla, it is not necessary to open the duodenum to make the diagnosis. In this manner possible dissemination of neoplastic cells into the peritoneal cavity is avoided (15, 16, 51).

In our practice we proceed as follows: after carrying out the abdominal incision, exploring all the viscera, and determining the presence of metastases, inspection and palpation of the extrahepatic biliary tree, the duodenum, and the pancreas is carried out. Before mobilization of the duodenum and pancreas, we always perform an operative cholangiogram through the gallbladder, if this has no calculi, or by direct injection of the common bile duct if calculi are shown (6, 13–15). The biliary tree is always dilated and contains thick bile in carcinomas of the papilla. For this reason the contents of the biliary tree should be aspirated and a sufficient amount of hydrosoluble, radiopaque material injected, no less than 40 mL (15, 16). While the x-rays are being developed, the Vautrin-Kocher maneuver is carried out, the gastrocolic ligament is divided, and the palpation of the head of the pancreas and the duodenum with exploration and possible biopsy of involved lymph nodes, in order to establish the resectability of the tumor, and so on.

Operative cholangiography is of importance because it shows much dilation of the common bile duct with obstruction at the papilla. When obstruction is found to be at the level of the papilla it becomes necessary to carry out a deeper exploration at that zone to investigate the cause of the obstruction. In some of these cases, we have established that the cause of the obstruction was a small tumor of the papilla that had not been suspected prior to operative cholangiography, since it was not palpable with a closed duodenum. Operative cholangiography pointed out the necessity of performing a duodenotomy and biopsy to confirm the existence of carcinoma of the papilla.

In 90% of cases of obstruction by carcinoma of the papilla operative cholangiography reveals the obstruction to be at the level of the papilla itself, that is, at the internal border of the second portion of the duodenum. In 10% of cases, obstruction is found to be proximal to the papilla, be it caused by neoplastic infiltration of the head of the pancreas or by coexisting chronic pancreatitis. In 80% of cases of carcinoma of the papilla the obstruction of the common bile duct is complete, and in 20% it is incomplete.

Once the operative cholangiography has been performed and the films studied, a supraduodenal choledochotomy is carried out with the object of exploring the common bile duct and the papilla of Vater by means of instruments. In the great majority of cases of carcinoma of the papilla there is complete obstruction at the papilla and instruments cannot be passed through it. In some cases instruments pass with some difficulty and in other cases the instruments are easily passed through the papilla. Ease of passage of instruments depends on the localization of the carcinoma and its consistency. Small peripapillary tumors usually allow the passage of explorers as easily as in soft carcinomas of the papilla, be they exophytic or intrapapillary.

Doubts may arise during the exploration as to whether the tumor is one of the papilla or of the common bile duct. A simple maneuver that is useful to make this differentiation is introducing the index finger into the common bile duct through the choledochotomy. Introduction of the finger is almost always possible because of dilation of the biliary tree. If the carcinoma is localized in the wall of the common bile duct, an irregular surface characteristic of malignant growths will be felt, whereas if the carcinoma is in the papilla, the internal surface of the common bile duct will be completely smooth.

Some patients are operated on for biliary and common duct calculi without any suspicion that they simultaneously harbor a carcinoma of the papilla. If the operative cholangiogram shows the presence of calculi in the common bile duct, these should be removed and another cholangiogram performed to show that all the calculi have been removed and that the radiopaque substance has passed through the papilla, presenting normal images. In some patients, it has been shown that, after removing all the calculi in the common bile duct, an obstruction remains at the level of the papilla owing to an unsuspected carcinoma, which is then confirmed by duodenotomy and biopsy. In other cases, the carcinoma was discovered a short time after the operation (6, 24, 44, 50).

DUODENOTOMY

Duodenotomy should be performed taking all precautions to prevent dissemination of neoplastic cells into the peritoneal cavity (15–17). The duodenotomy in cases of carcinoma of the papilla is usually performed vertically near the lateral border of the second portion of the duodenum. If the carcinoma is exophytic in type, its identification will be easy, and biopsies can then be taken to confirm the histology of the tumor. In cases in which the tumor is intrapapillary, it is necessary to carry out a sphincterotomy and removal of material for microscopic examination. If the tumor is small in size and peripapillary in location, be it in the mucosa or in the submucosa, it should be completely removed or partially removed in order to carry out the microscopic examination. When peripapillary tumors of small size are present, it is very useful to leave a biliary tract explorer in the common bile duct to make it easier to see and resect these small tumors for the histologic examination.

Once exploration of the duodenum is completed, the duodenum is closed with a running suture. All the abdominal compresses and the surgical instruments that have been used are removed from the operative field. All members of the operating team should change gloves and then proceed to carry out the pancreaticoduodenectomy, if the lesion is resectable. In rare cases in which a local resection of the tumor may be indicated, the operation will be continued with the duodenum open, changing only the instruments, the compresses, and the gloves after the endoduodenal procedure has been finished and the duodenal wall closed.

FIGURE 18.2
Operative photograph of a patient with carcinoma of the papilla of Vater, exophytic and papillary in growth. These are the carcinomas that are easily diagnosed.

Duodenotomy

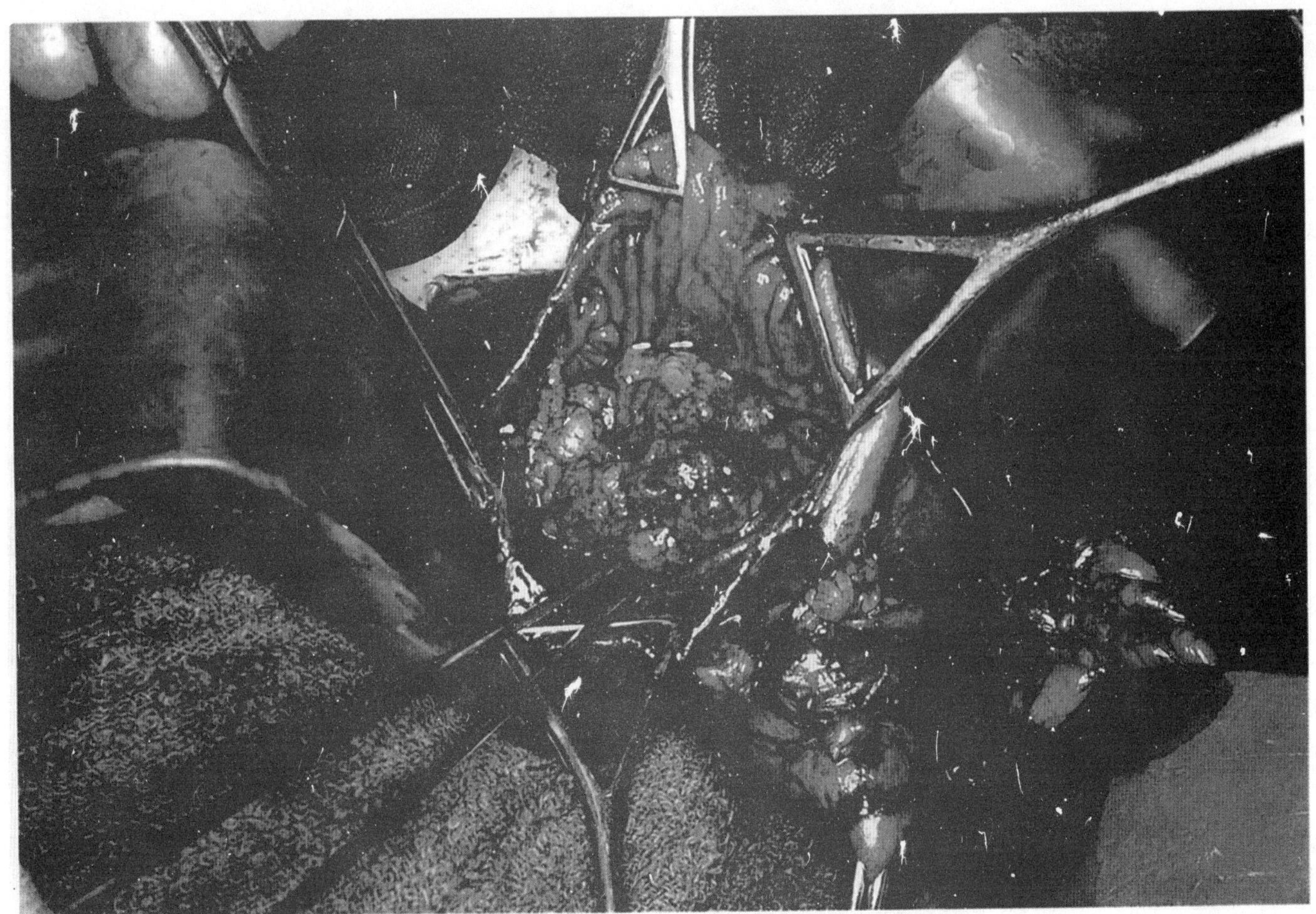

FIGURE 18.2

Duodenotomy

FIGURE 18.3
Operative photograph of a patient with a vegetating, ulcerated, and retractile carcinoma of the papilla.

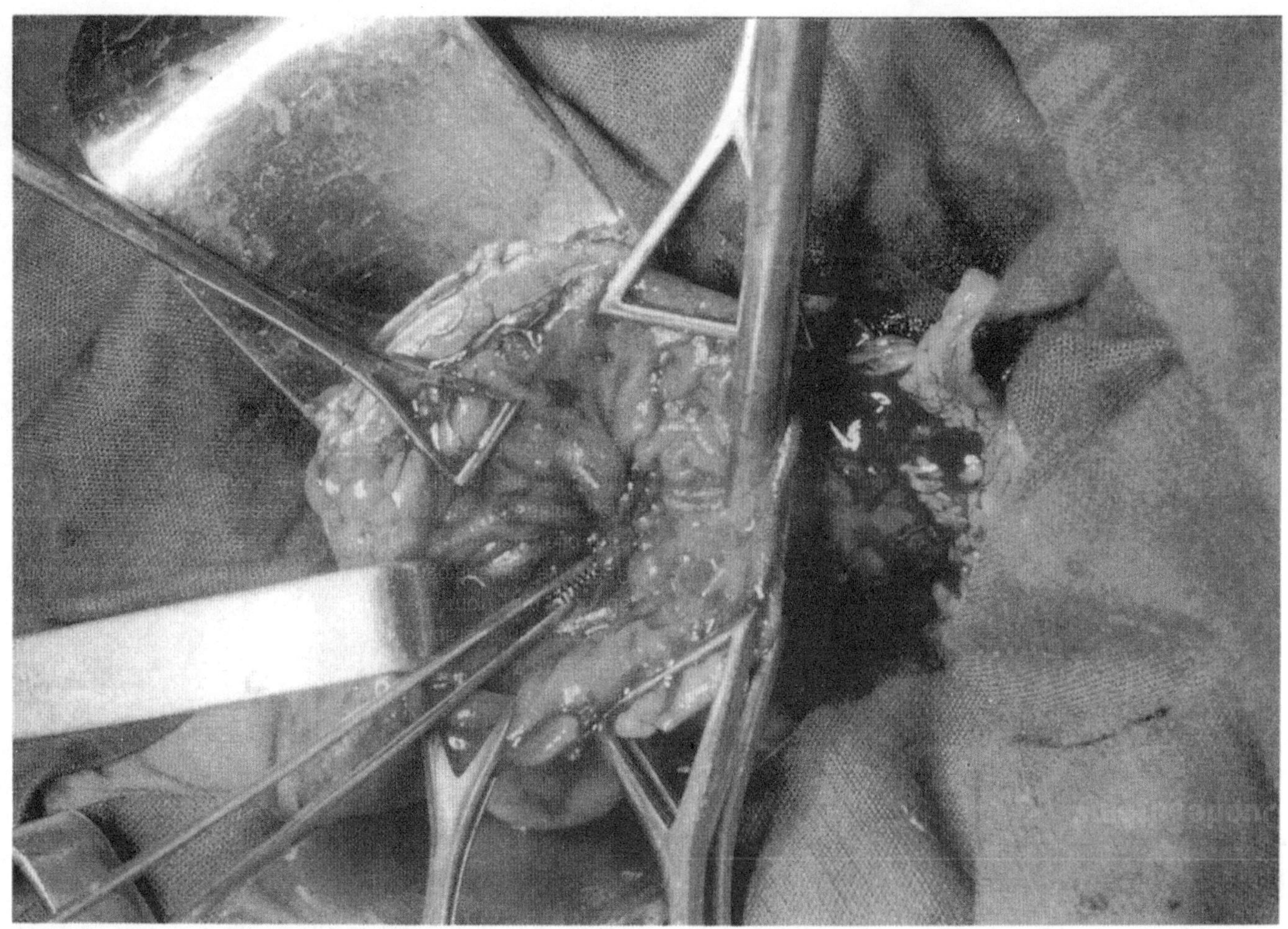

FIGURE 18.3

FIGURE 18.4
Operative photograph of an intrapapillary carcinoma. The papilla is slightly increased in size. With a very delicate malleable curette, material is being removed from the inside of the papilla for microscopic examination. Operative cholangiogram had shown a marked dilation of the biliary tree in its extra- and intrahepatic portion with a complete blunt-shaped obstruction at the level of the papilla. This made a duodenotomy and biopsy necessary.

Duodenotomy

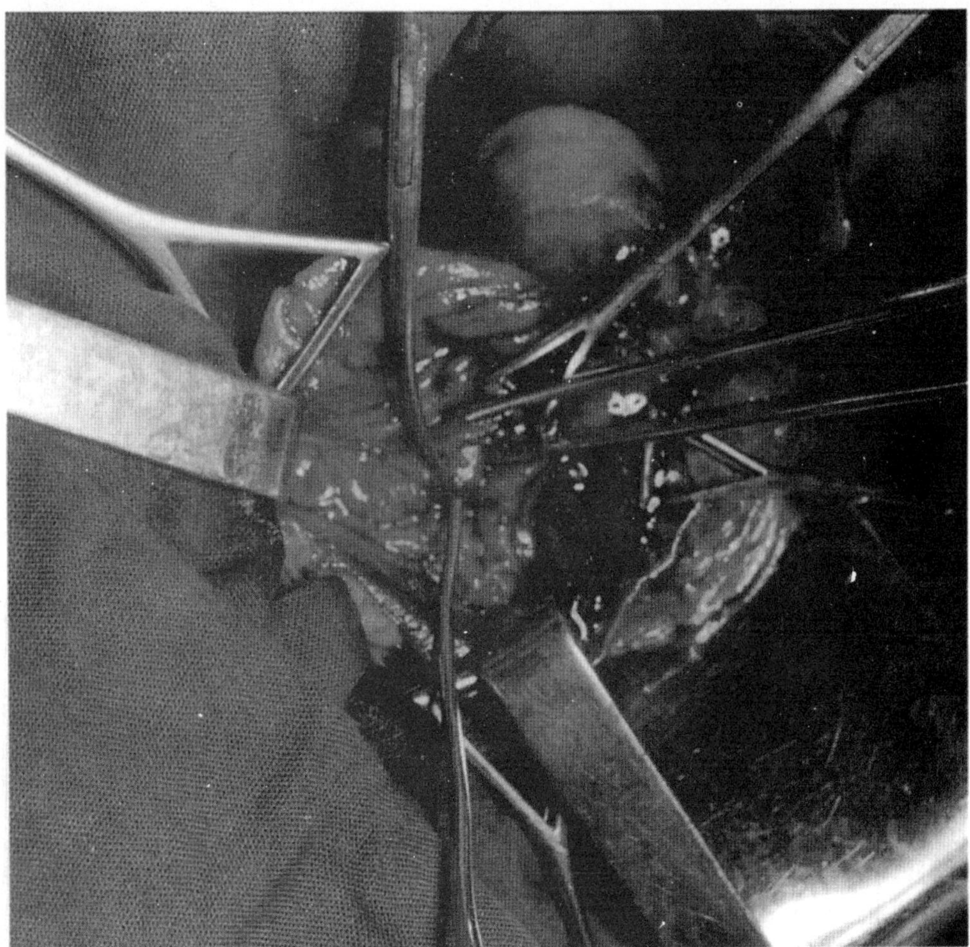

FIGURE 18.4

FIGURE 18.5
Operative photograph of a patient with an intrapapillary carcinoma of the papilla. The papilla is seen to be increased in size, erect, firm and somewhat rigid, covered by the normal duodenal mucosa. In order to expose the papilla to a full view, it was necessary to raise it with a finger. When the papilla was compressed, a small amount of bloodstained secretion exuded from the papillary opening. The appearance of the papilla was similar to that of a uterine cervix. Sphincterotomy and biopsy confirmed the diagnosis of carcinoma of the papilla. Operative cholangiography had shown a marked dilation of the intra- and extrahepatic biliary tree with a complete obstruction at the level of the papilla.

Duodenotomy

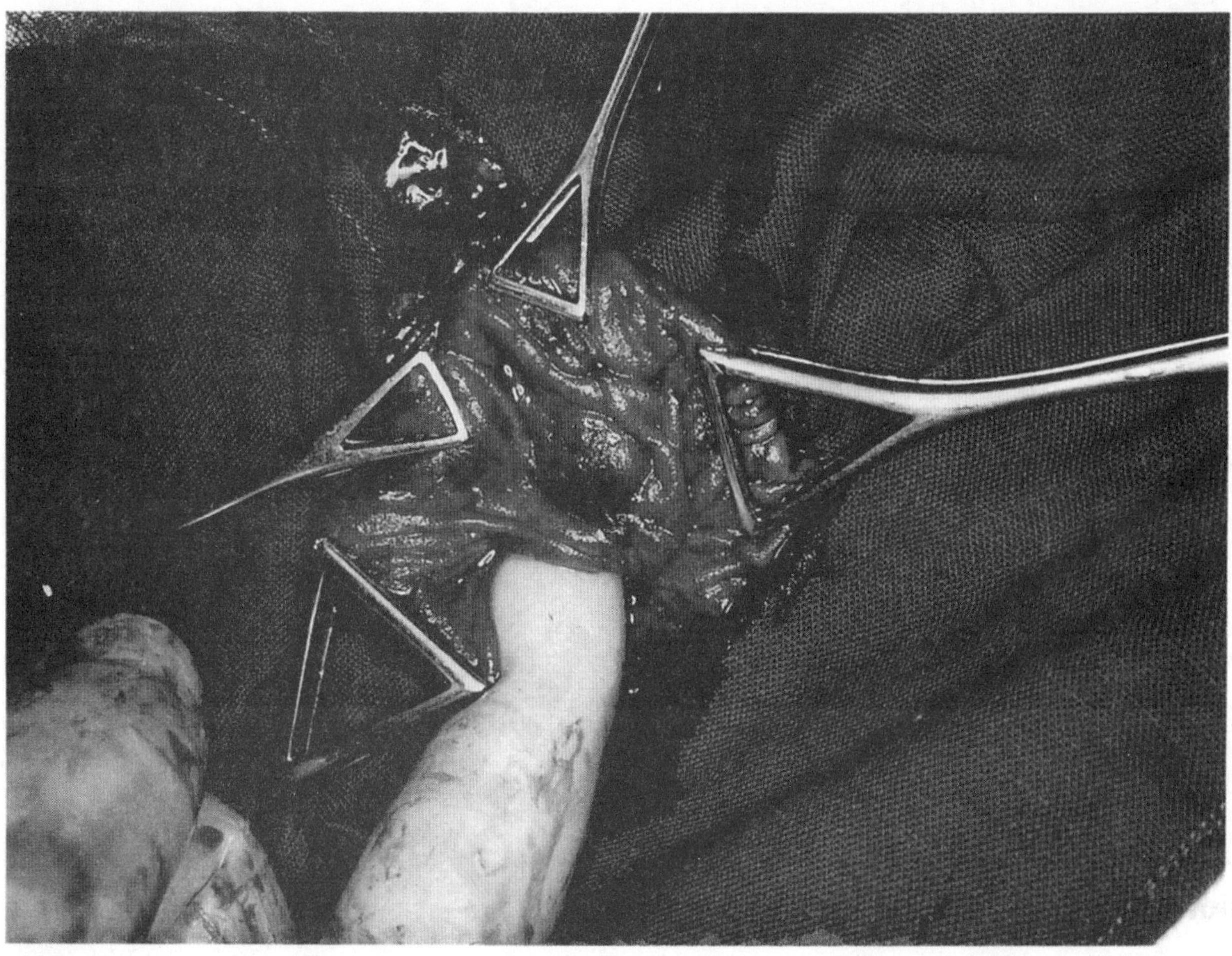

FIGURE 18.5

Duodenotomy

FIGURE 18.6
Operative photograph of an intrapapillary carcinoma of the papilla. The carcinoma has developed inside the papilla, increasing its size considerably and making it firm. The tumor has protruded into the duodenal surface through an ulceration with elevated border.

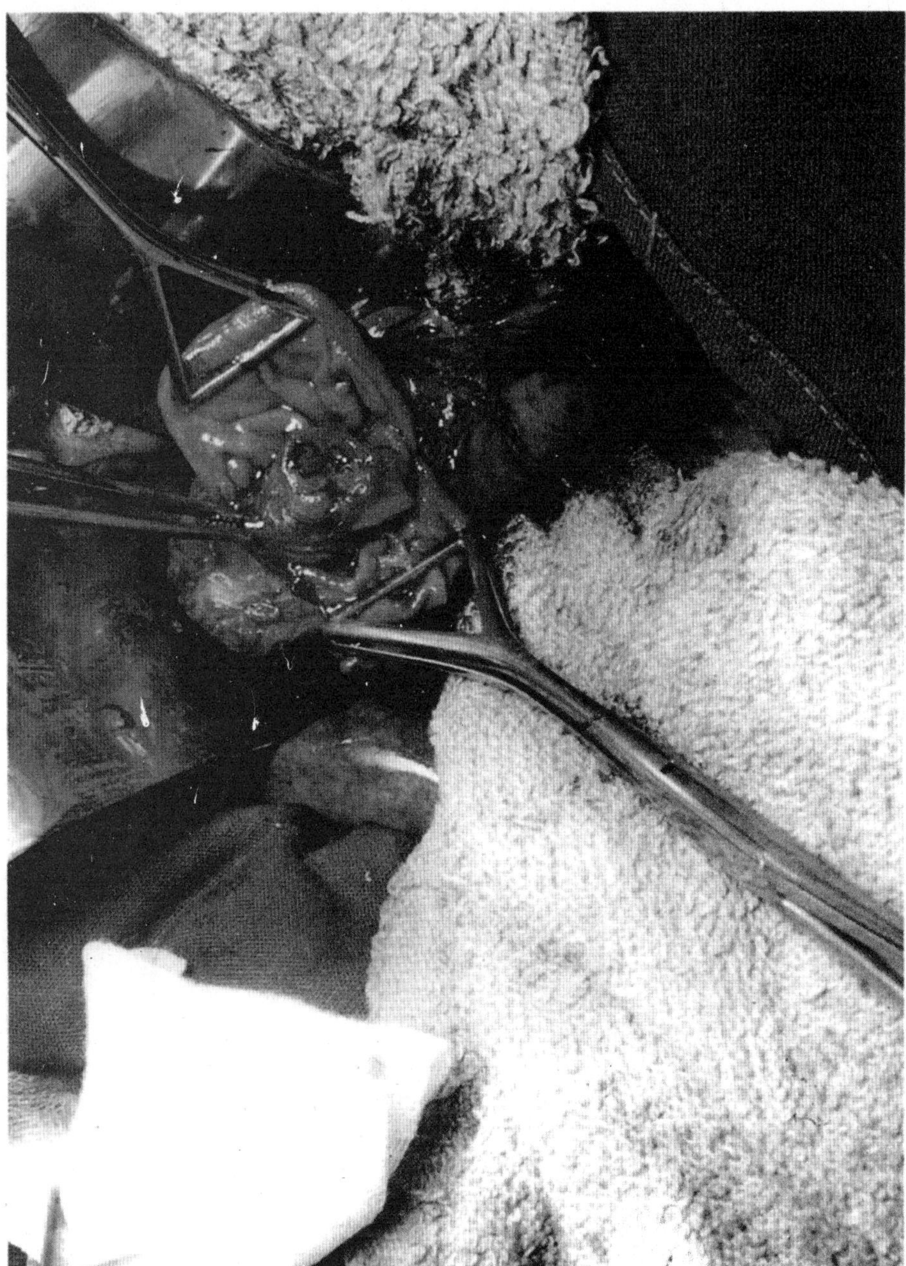

FIGURE 18.6

Duodenotomy

FIGURE 18.7
Operative photograph of a patient with a peripapillary carcinoma about 5 mm from the papilla, originating in the submucosa. Operative cholangiography revealed marked dilation of the common bile duct and a complete blunt obstruction at the level of the papilla. An explorer has been passed through the common bile duct and another through the pancreatic duct. A small (6 mm) tumor is being resected for microscopic examination.

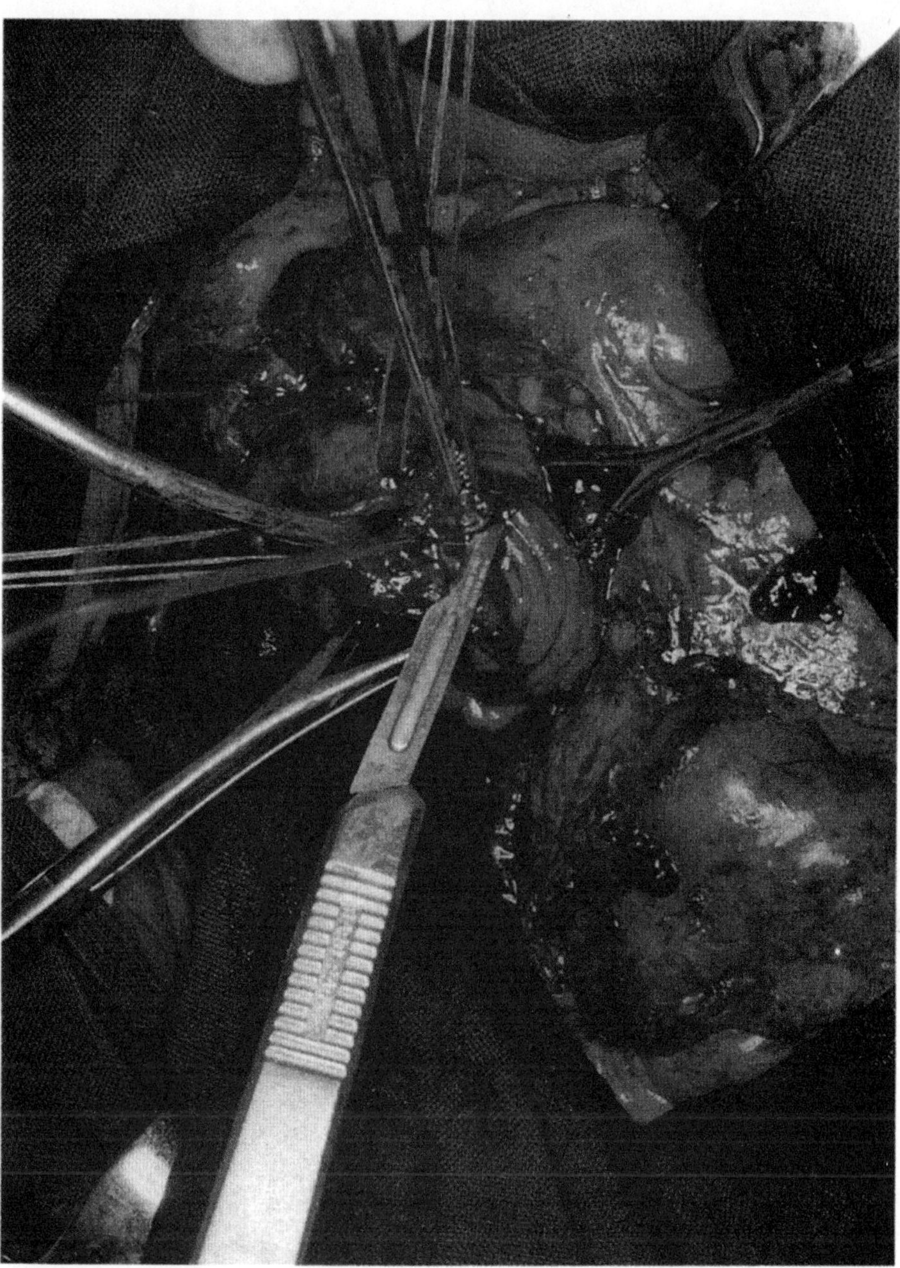

FIGURE 18.7

Duodenotomy

FIGURE 18.8
Microphotograph of an intrapapillary carcinoma of the papilla. To carry out the diagnosis it was necessary to perform a sphincterotomy and resect a small segment of the sphincter. In the inferior portion of the photograph the carcinoma of the papilla can be seen to be covered by duodenal mucosa, which is normal in appearance.

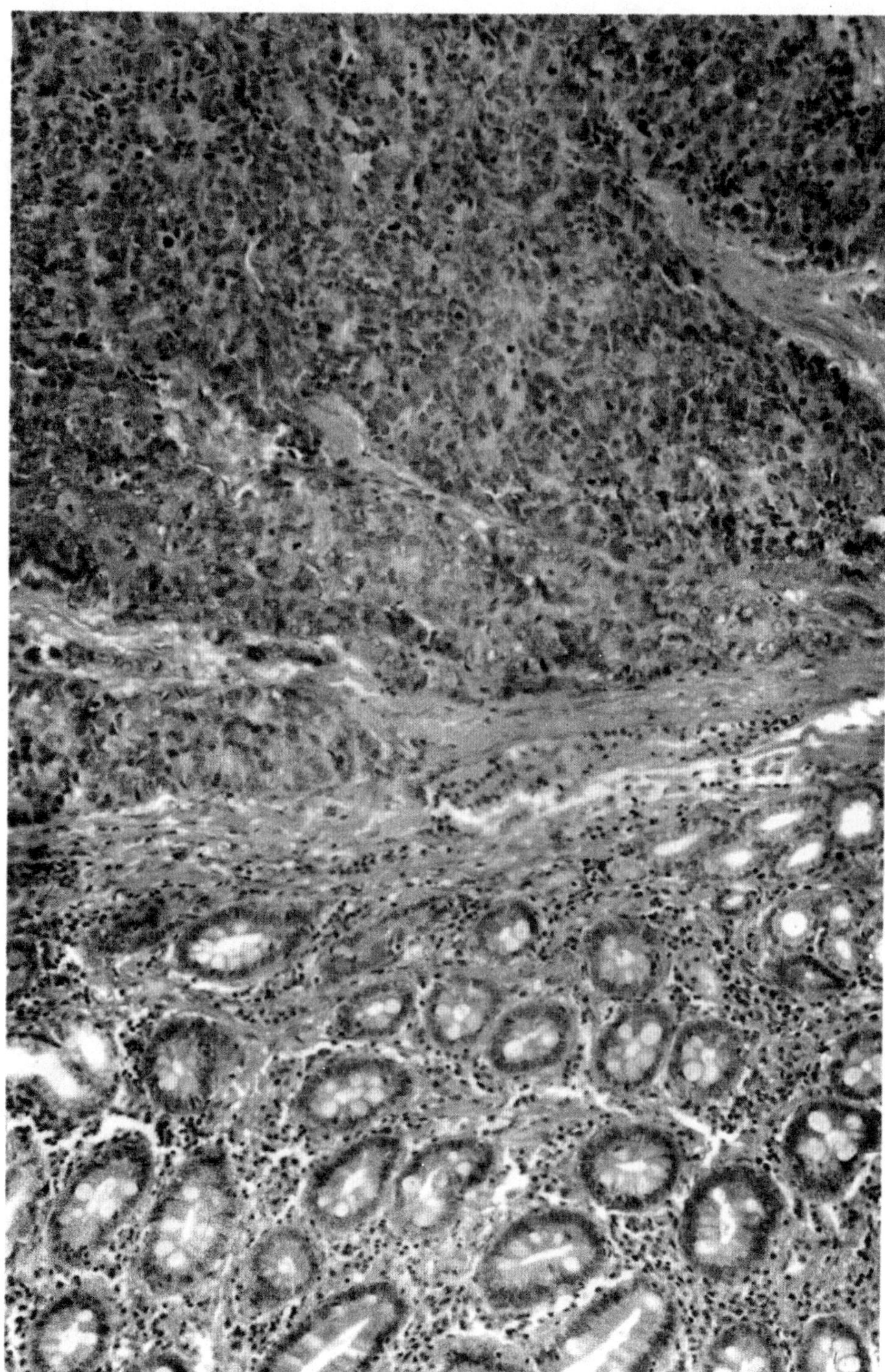

FIGURE 18.8

FIGURE 18.9
Microphotograph of a patient with a small peripapillary carcinoma, located about 8 mm from the inferior portion of the papilla, starting in the mucosa, and measuring 10 mm in diameter. The tumor can be observed to be completely intraparietal, covered by normal duodenal mucosa.

Duodenotomy

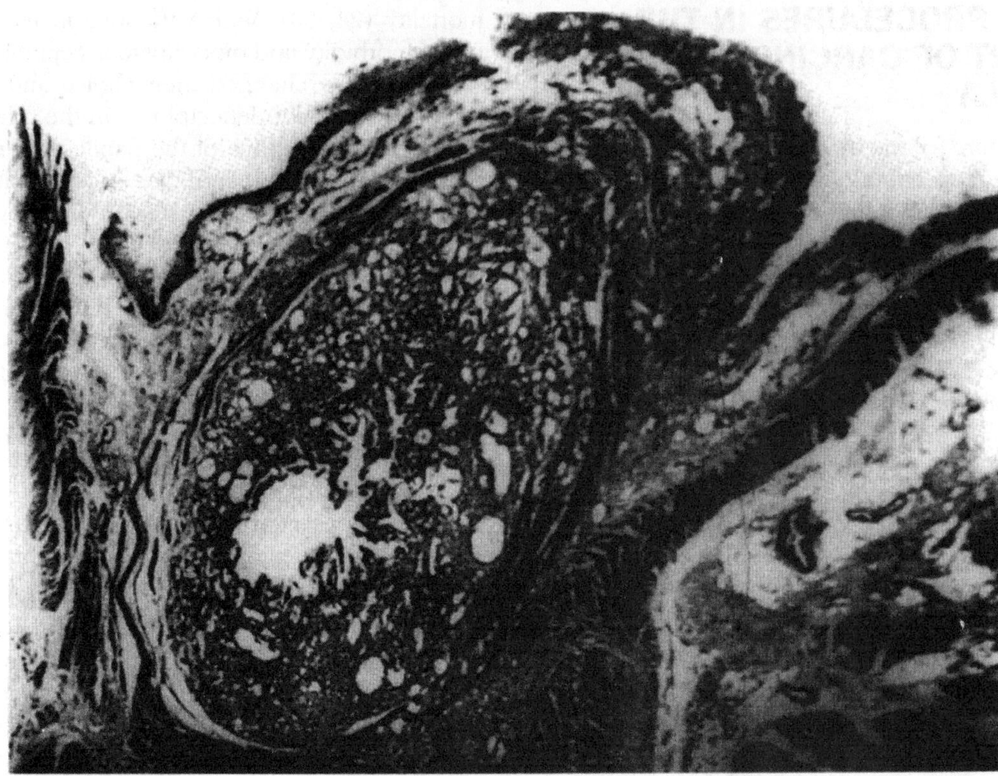

FIGURE 18.9

SURGICAL PROCEDURES IN THE TREATMENT OF CARCINOMA OF THE PAPILLA

The best procedure for the treatment of carcinoma of the papilla is pancreaticoduodenectomy (Whipple procedure). It has been shown that this procedure is the one with best late results (2, 10, 18, 19, 28, 37–39). In recent years, the morbidity and mortality of the Whipple procedure has decreased considerably (2, 10, 19, 20, 28, 56).

In 1978 Traverso and Longmire (53) presented a technique for pancreaticoduodenectomy with preservation of the pylorus. Since that time many surgeons have adopted this technique in the treatment of carcinoma of the papilla. The late results of this procedure have been very similar to those that are attained with the classic Whipple procedure (2, 18, 25, 53).

The technical details of the classic pancreaticoduodenectomy and of the technique with preservation of the pylorus have been described previously under the treatment for carcinoma of the head of the pancreas. We will only describe the technique of local resection for carcinoma of the papilla.

LOCAL RESECTION OF CARCINOMA OF THE PAPILLA OF VATER

Local resection of carcinoma of the papilla was performed by Halsted in 1889 (26). Hunt and Budd (29, 30) published an article in 1935 that had great influence on surgeons, leading them to choose local resection. In this same year, Whipple and colleagues (57) presented their classical work on pancreaticoduodenectomy to treat carcinoma of the papilla of Vater. For many years, local resection was preferred over the Whipple procedure because the latter technique produced high morbidity and mortality (24, 50). With variations in technique to improve morbidity and mortality to acceptable levels, many surgeons have changed their choice and now perform the pancreaticoduodenectomy. On the other hand, local resection of carcinoma of the papilla became less popular due to frequent recurrences, postoperative complications, and very low 5-year survival figures.

Local resection is considered an alternative to the Whipple procedure and is reserved for a few patients who, because of advanced age and poor general condition, are considered too great a risk for pancreaticoduodenal resection (11, 24, 31, 35, 44). In addition, it is necessary to establish that carcinomas of the papilla that can be resected locally should present certain conditions, which are indispensable for success with this procedure. In our opinion, carcinomas of the papilla that can be resected locally should be small, exophytic, and papillary in type, and should not present deep ulcerations, infiltration, or retraction. In addition, the tumor should not be fixed, should not invade the muscular layer of the duodenum, should not be invading neighboring organs, and the lymph nodes should not be involved by the carcinoma. On the other hand, the surgeon should be sure that, by means of local resection, he or she can resect all the neoplastic tissue, since incomplete resection leads to very poor results. In recent years, some articles on local resection of carcinoma of the papilla have been published with results comparable to those obtained by pancreaticoduodenectomy.

The technique of local resection, which we will describe in the following, consists of block resection of the papilla with the tumor, a segment of the duodenal wall, the inferior end of the common bile duct, and the inferior end of the pancreatic duct, with reimplantation of both ducts sutured to the duodenal wall.

Local Resection of Carcinoma of the Papilla of Vater

Local Resection of Carcinoma of the Papilla of Vater

FIGURE 18.10
Semischematic section of the pancreaticoduodenal region showing a small, exophytic, well-limited tumor of the papilla that does not infiltrate the deep levels of the duodenal wall. The line shows where the incision will be carried out using a scalpel. This incision should pass through completely healthy tissue.

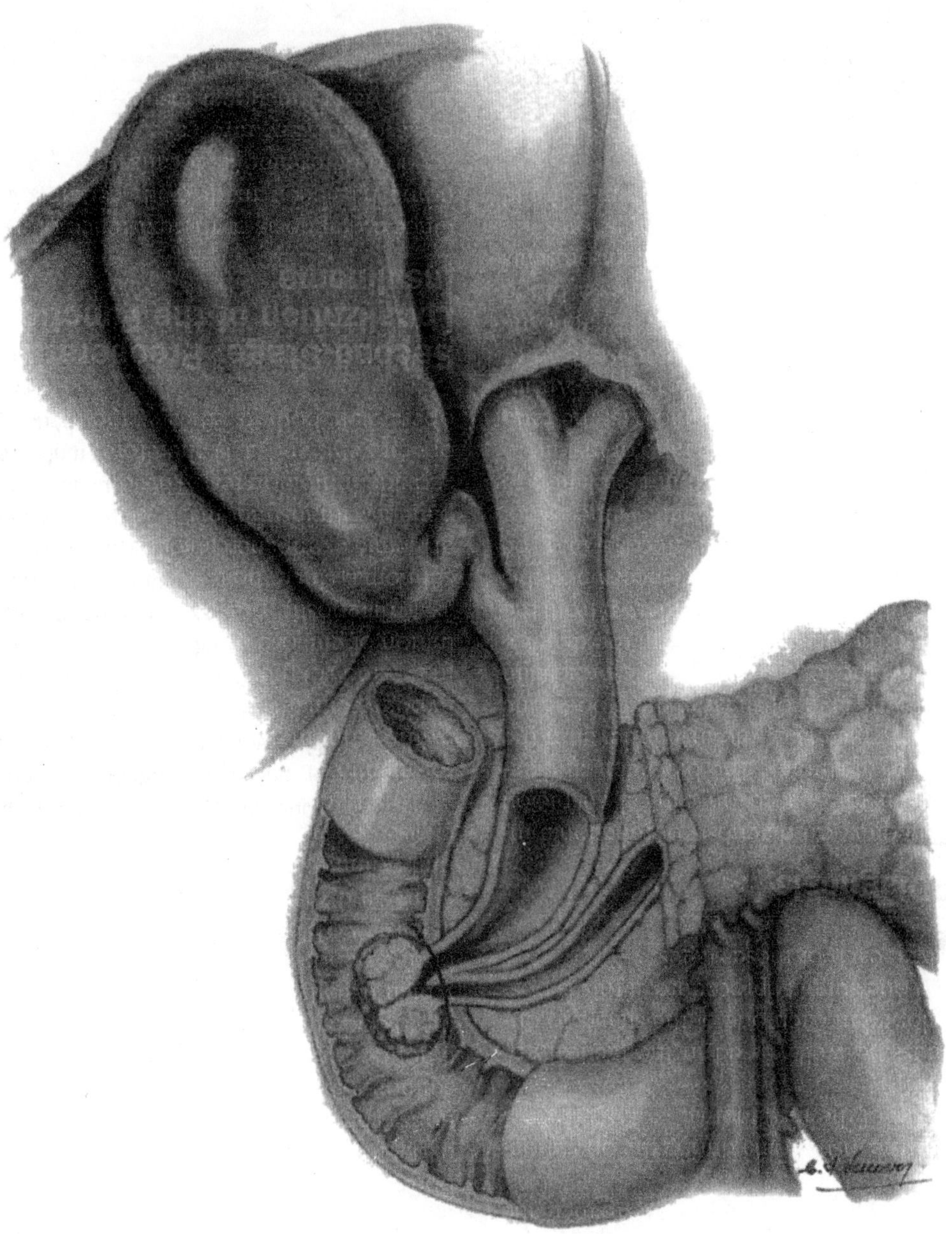

FIGURE 18.10

FIGURE 18.11
After mobilizing the duodenum and head of the pancreas by means of the Vautrin-Kocher maneuver and division of the gastrocolic ligament, the abdominal cavity is protected and the duodenum is surrounded with gauze pads. This is done before the duodenum is open, to avoid, as much as possible, spillage of neoplastic cells into the peritoneum. A longitudinal incision is made in the lateral border of the second portion of the duodenum, and the edges of the incision are grasped with atraumatic Duval clamps, which not only permit the duodenum to be opened and its interior examined but provide temporary hemostasis for the wall. Using an Allis clamp, traction is applied to the papilla with the tumor and the duodenal wall is transected through a completely healthy area. The dotted line shows where the transection is to be carried out. This is usually done with a scalpel, but some surgeons use an electric scalpel to carry out this incision (11, 29, 30, 35, 40).

Local Resection of Carcinoma of the Papilla of Vater

FIGURE 18.12
The resection in block of the papilla with the tumor as well as a segment of duodenal wall and the ends of the common bile duct and pancreatic duct is being completed. When the common bile duct is transected, it is convenient to grasp the proximal end with sutures. The same maneuver should be repeated when the pancreatic duct is divided. This maneuver and the increase in caliber of both ducts in cases of carcinoma of the papilla facilitates their reimplantation and suture into the duodenal wall.

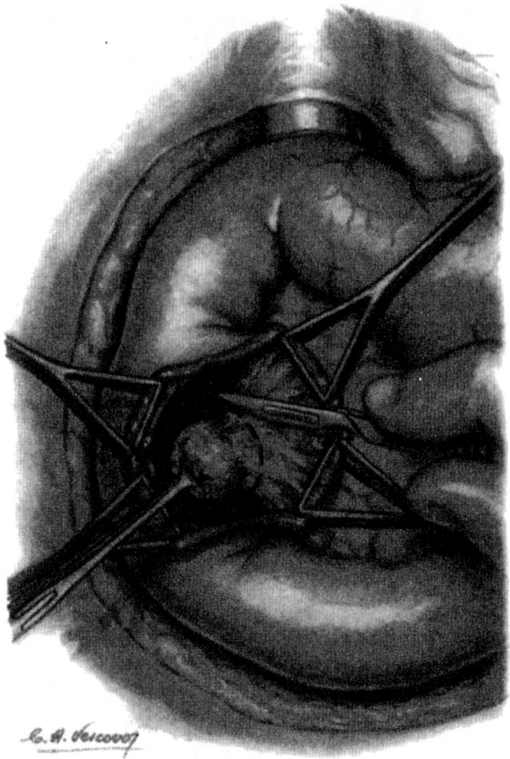

FIGURE 18.11

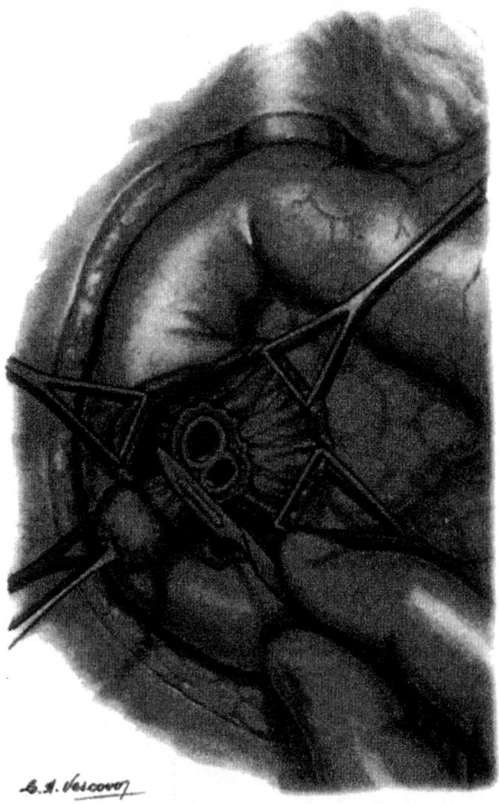

FIGURE 18.12

FIGURE 18.13

The resection of the tumor has been completed and the ducts have been reimplanted into the duodenal wall using interrupted sutures of nonabsorbable material.

The common bile duct is sutured first, followed by the end of the pancreatic duct. The sutures should have adequate bites into the duodenal wall and the ends of both ducts. The suturing of these ducts should be carried out near each other, as shown in the drawing. Some surgeons use a stent in the pancreatic duct, using a fine Silastic tube with multiple perforations introduced into the pancreatic duct. This stent is fixed to the pancreatic duct and the duodenal wall with two sutures. The stent is eliminated spontaneously some time later. The incision in the duodenal wall is closed in two layers of interrupted sutures. The mucosal layer is closed with 3-0 chromic catgut and the seromuscular layer with cotton or synthetic nonabsorbable material. If it is correctly carried out, longitudinal closure of the duodenal incision does not lead to stenosis or disruption. Once the duodenum has been closed, the abdominal compresses are removed, and all the instruments are changed together with the gloves. It is advisable to leave a T-tube in the supraduodenal common bile duct. In addition, some surgeons perform a biliary bypass, either with a Roux-en-Y hepaticojejunostomy or with a cholecystojejunostomy. The object of this anastomosis is to prevent biliary stasis, which occurs in some patients due to postoperative stricture of the inferior portion of the common bile duct (24, 50).

Local Resection of Carcinoma of the Papilla of Vater

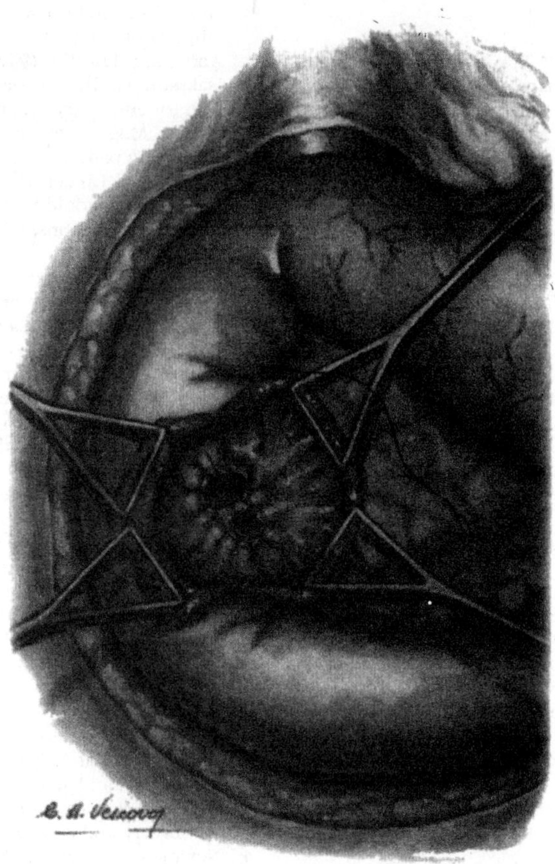

FIGURE 18.13

References

1. Akwari, O.E., van Heerden, J.A., Adson, E.A. et al. Radical pancreatoduodenectomy for cancer of the papilla of Vater. Arch. Surg. 122:451, 1977.
2. Braasch, J.W., Deziel, D.J., Rossi, R.L. et al. Pyloric and gastric preserving pancreatic resection. Experience with 87 patients. Ann. Surg. 204:411, 1986.
3. Blumgart, L.H., Kennedy, A. Carcinoma of the ampulla of Vater and duodenum. Br. J. Surg. 60:33, 1973.
4. Cameron, J. Atlas of Surgery. Vol. 1, p. 386. B.C. Decker, Toronto, Philadelphia, 1990.
5. Caroli, J. Diagnostique du cancer de l'ampoule de Vater. Semin. Hôp. Paris 25:1314, 1949.
6. Caroli, J. Les ictères par rétention. p. 41. Masson, Paris, 1956.
7. Cooperman, A.M. Cancer of the ampulla of Vater, bile duct and duodenum. Surg. Clin. North Am. 61:99, 1981.
8. Couinaud, C., Huguet, C. Le temps d'exérèse dans la duodénopancréatectomie total. J. Chir. 91:181, 1966.
9. Coutsoftides, T., Mac Donald, J., Shibata, H.R. Carcinoma of the pancreas and periampullary region: A 41 year experience. Ann. Surg. 186:730, 1977.
10. Crist, D.W., Sitzmann, V., Cameron, J.D. Improved hospital morbidity, mortality and survival after the Whipple procedure. Ann. Surg. 206:358, 1987.
11. Chatelin, C.L. Technique de l'ampullectomie. J. Chir. 97:465, 1969.
12. Chavy, A., Liguory, C. Duodénoscopie, cholangiographie at wirsungraphie rétrograde dans le cancer de l'ampoule de Vater. Ann. Gastroenterol. Hépat. 11:395, 1975.
13. Etala, E. Valor de la Colangiografía Operatoria para el diagnóstico del cáncer de la cabeza del páncreas y de la ampolla de Vater. Comptes Rendus de la Société Internationale de Chirurgie p. 1198. Roma, 1963.
14. Etala, E., Russo, R. Diagnóstico operatorio del cáncer de la ampolla de Vater. Valor de la Colangiografía operatoria. Soc. Cir. Buenos Aires. Bol. Trab. 50:334, 1966.
15. Etala, E., Russo, R. Operative cholangiography in the diagnosis of tumoral obstruction of the distal end of the common duct. Recent advances in gastroenterology. Vol. IV, p. 537. Tokyo, 1966.
16. Etala, E. Diagnóstico operatorio de las obstrucciones malignas del 1/3 distal del colédoco. Pren. Med. Argent. 54:941, 1967.
17. Etala, E. Exploración intraoperatoria del extremo distal de colédoco. Pren. Med. Argent. 60:589, 1973.
18. Etala, E. Anastomosis pancreatogástrica en la pancreatoduodenectomía. Pren. Med. Argent. 75:174, 1988.
19. Etala, E., Juan, J.R. Pancreatoduodenectomía por carcinoma de la cabeza del páncreas y periampulares. Morbilidad, mortalidad, sobrevida. Pren. Med. Argent. 76:164, 1989.
20. Feroldi, J. Les cancer de l'ampoule de Vater. En cancer primitif du foie et des voies biliaries. Citado por Marchal y Huneau en "Les tumeurs Oddiennes." p. 35. Masson, Paris, 1978.
21. Fish, J.C., Cleveland, B.R. Pancreaticoduodenectomy for periampullary carcinoma. Ann. Surg. 159:469, 1964.
22. Forrest, J.F., Longmire, W.P. Carcinoma of the pancreas and periampullary region. A study of 279 patients. Ann. Surg. 189, 129, 1979.
23. Gold, M.S., Bordley IV, J. Pancreatoduoenectomy for bleeding periampullary tumors. Arch. Surg. 125:675, 1990.
24. Goldberg, M., Zamir, A., Nissans, S. Wide local excision as an alternative treatment for periampullary carcinoma. Am. J. Gastroenterol. 82:1169, 1987.
25. Grace, P.A., Pitt, H.A., Tompkins, R.K. et al. Decreased morbidity and mortality after pancreatoduodenectomy. Am. J. Surg. 151:141, 1986.
26. Halsted, W.S. Contribution to the surgery of the bile passage, especially the common bile duct. Boston Med. Surg. 141:645, 1899.
27. Hayes, D.H., Bolton, J.S., Willis, G.W., Bowen, J.C. Carcinoma of the ampulla of Vater. Ann. Surg. 206:572, 1987.
28. Howard, J.M. Pancreaticoduodenectomy: Forty-one consecutive Whipple resections without an operative mortality. Ann. Surg. 168:640, 1968.
29. Hunt, V.C., Budd, J.W. Transduodenal resection of the ampulla of Vater; for carcinoma of the distal end of the common duct. Surg. Gynecol. Obstet. 61:651, 1935.
30. Hunt, V.C., Budd, J.W. Surgical management of carcinoma of the ampulla of Vater and of periampullary portion of the duodenum. Ann. Surg. 114:570, 1941.
31. Isaksson, G., Ihse, I., Sandberg, A., Evander, A. et al. Local excision for ampullary carcinoma. Acta Chir. Scand. 148:163, 1982.
32. Itani, K.M.F., Coleman, R.E., Meyer, W.C., Akwari, C.E. Pylorus preserving pancreatoduodenectomy. Ann. Surg. 204:655, 1986.
33. Jones, B.A., Langer, B., Taylor, B.R. et al. Periampullary tumors: Which ones should be resected? Am. J. Surg. 149:46, 1985.
34. Jordan, G.L., Simons, B.E. Carcinoma of the ampulla of Vater. Tex. Med. 66:70, 1970.
35. Lieber, M.N., Stewart, H.L., Lund, H. Carcinoma of the periampullary portion of the duodenum. Ann. Surg. 109:209, 1939.
36. Liotta, D. Pour le diagnostique des tumerus du pancréas: la duodénographie hypotonique. Lyon Chir. 50:455, 1955.
37. Lygidakis, N.J., van der Heyde, M.N. Subtotal duodenopancreatectomy for the management of pancreatic duct, distal common bile duct and ampullary carcinoma. In Lygidakis, N.J., Tytgat, G.N.J. Hepatobiliary and pancreatic malignancies. p. 261. Thieme Verlag, Stuttgart, 1989.
38. Madden, J.L. Technique for pancreatoduodenectomy. Surg. Gynecol. Obstet. 118:247, 1964.
39. Madden, J.L. Transduodenal excision of tumor about the papilla of Vater. In Madden, J.L. Atlas of techniques in surgery. Ed. 2, Vol. I, p. 538. Appleton-Century-Crofts, New York, 1964.
40. Maingot, R. Transduodenal excision of tumor of the ampulla of Vater. In Maingot, R. (Ed.) Abdominal operation. Ed. 7, Vol. 1, p. 932. Appleton-Century-Crofts, New York, 1980.
41. Marchal, G., Hureau, J. Les tumerus Oddiennes. p. 111. Masson, Paris, 1978.
42. Martin, E.D. Anatomie pathologique des tumeurs Oddiennes. Citado por Marchal, G., Hureau, J. In Les tumeurs Oddiennes. p. 35. Masson, Paris, 1978.
43. Moosa, A.R. Pancreatic cancer. Approach to diagnosis, selection for surgery and choice of operation. Cancer 50:2689, 1982.
44. Newman, R.J., Pitam, M.R. Local excision in the treatment of carcinoma of the ampulla of Vater. J. R. Coll. Surg. Edinburgh 27:154, 1982.
45. Nora, P.F. Gallbladder and biliary tract. In Nora, P.F. Ed. Operative surgery. Ed. 2, p. 541. Lea & Febiger, Philadelphia, 1980.
46. Outerbridge, G.W. Carcinoma of the papilla of Vater. Ann. Surg. 57:402, 1913.
47. Park, C.D., Mackie, J.A., Rhoads, J.E. Pancreatogastrostomy. Am. J. Surg. 113:851, 1967.
48. Ponka, J.L., Uthapa, N.S. Carcinoma of the ampulla of Vater. Am. J. Surg. 121:263, 1971.
49. Rettori, R. Etude morphologique du système musculaire de la fonction cholédoco-pancréatico-duodénale et bases anatomiques de la section du sphincter d'Oddi. Presse Med. 64:1208, 1956.
50. Schlippert, W., Lucke, D., Amuras, S., Christensen, J. Carcinoma of the papilla of Vater. A review of fifty-seven cases. Am. J. Surg. 135:763, 1978.
51. Sivak, M. Jr., Esselstyn, C.E., Owens, F.J. Intra-operative upper gastrointestinal endoscopy and biopsy. Cleveland Clin. Quart. 41:67, 1974.
52. Soria, F. (Córdoba, Argentina) Comunicación personal, 1956.
53. Traverso, L.W., Longmire, W.P. Jr. Preservation of the pylorus in pancreaticoduodenectomy. Surg. Gynecol. Obstet. 146:959, 1978.
54. Tudor, R. Long-term survival following local resection of carcinoma of ampulla of Vater. Br. J. Surg. 71:271, 1984.
55. Walsh, D.B., Eckhauser, F.E., Cronenwet, J.L. et al. Adenocarcinoma of the ampulla of Vater. Diagnosis and treatment. Ann. Surg. 195:152, 1982.
56. Warren, K.W., Choe, D.S., Plaza, J. et al. Results of radical resection for periampullary cancer. Ann. Surg. 181:534, 1975.
57. Whipple, A.O., Parson, W.B., Mullins, C.R. Treatment of carcinoma of the ampulla of Vater. Ann. Surg. 102:763, 1935.
58. Wilks, A.E., Gorostiague, N.P. Cáncer de la vesícula y de las vías biliares. In Deschamps, J.H. Grinfeld, D., Ortiz, F.E., Wilks, A.E. (Eds.) Cirugía. p. 876. El Ateneo, Buenos Aires, 1987.
59. Williams, J.A., Cubilla, A., Maclean, B., Fortner, J.G. Twenty-two year experience with periampullary carcinoma at Memorial Sloan-Kettering Cancer Center. Am. J. Surg. 138:662, 1979.

Section C

Surgery of the Pancreas

CHAPTER 19

Surgical Treatment of Functional Insulinomas

Insulinomas are tumors that originate in the beta cells of the islets of Langerhans, which compose the APUD system, the meaning of which is: A, Amino; P, Precursor; U, Uptake; D, Decarboxylation (47). The cells of the APUD system have common cytochemical characteristics, with the ability to synthesize, store, and secrete polypeptides and amines.

Insulinomas are not frequent tumors, but neither are they extremely rare (57). This fact, together with their protean symptomatology, has contributed to their recognition being fragmentary and incomplete, which has led to a correct diagnosis and treatment in many cases. Insulinomas represent 70 to 80% of endocrine tumors of the pancreas and were the first to be discovered.

Three important scientific discoveries have led to the investigation and historical development of insulinomas: First, the discovery of the islets of pancreas by Paul Langerhans, of Germany, in 1869 while still a student of medicine (33). These islets were designated islets of Langerhans, honoring their discoverer. Second, the revolutionary discovery of insulin by Banting and Best, in Canada, in 1922, while Best was still a medical student (4). Third, the discovery of the technique of radioimmunoassay by Yalow and Berson, in the United States, in 1959 (65, 66), which led to the determination of insulin levels by immunoreactive assays in plasma, making possible the unequivocal diagnosis of insulinoma. The introduction of the concept of hyperinsulinism by Harris, in 1925, in the United States and the recognition of the relationship between hyperinsulinism and hypoglycemia by Wilder, in 1927, in the United States must be added to these three concepts.

Surgeons who undertake the treatment of a functional insulinoma should not limit themselves to the performance of the surgical procedure. The surgeon has to know all the steps to be taken to arrive at the diagnosis and localization of the insulinoma, having clear criteria about the strategy to be followed in the surgical maneuvers to carry out an adequate pancreatic exploration, as well as other methods of exploration when the insulinoma cannot be identified by surgical palpation. Identification of an insulinoma is often simple but can be very complex, testing the criteria and experience of the surgeon in obtaining positive results and reducing mistakes to a minimum.

STAGES TO BE COMPLETED IN THE DIAGNOSIS AND TREATMENT OF FUNCTIONAL INSULINOMAS

These stages are four:

1. The unequivocal diagnosis of functional insulinoma.
2. Localization of the insulinoma in the pancreatic parenchyma.
3. Identification of the insulinoma during the operation.
4. Surgical resection of the insulinoma.

The surgeon must be well versed in the tactical approach to be developed in each one of the stages to obtain better results in one surgical procedure, if this is possible. We will analyze each of these stages.

First Stage: Diagnosis

In this stage, the unequivocal diagnosis of functional insulinoma should be made, based on clinical suspicion followed by biochemical studies. The biochemical diagnosis is established by means of the insulin level in the plasma together with the level of sugar in the blood. One should also determine the levels of plasmatic proinsulin and the C-peptides in the plasma to confirm the diagnosis. It is very important that blood be withdrawn from the patient during the hypoglycemic crisis, since, once this has passed, the levels of insulin and glucose may be within normal ranges. The most important value is not the absolute level of plasmatic insulin, but its relation to the blood sugar. In normal persons, the ratio of insulin to glucose is always less than 0.4. In insulinomas, the ratio of insulin to glucose is generally greater than 1. An insulin level of 10 to 20 μg per mL with a glucose level of 90 mg% has no diagnostic value, but is of diagnostic value if the same level of insulin accompanies a blood sugar lower than 45 mg%, as long as the patient presents symptoms of hypoglycemia. If the patient shows no symptoms, the diagnosis of functional insulinoma should be doubted.

Simultaneously with those of the plasmatic insulin, the levels of proinsulin and the peptides (C-peptides) should be obtained. In normal persons, the level of present proinsulin presents a concentration of 22% of the immunoreactive plasmatic insulin. In insulinomas, the concentration of proinsulin is higher than 25% of the concentration of immunoreactive plasmatic insulin. If the concentration of proinsulin is over 50% of the concentration of plasmatic immunoreactive insulin, one should suspect that the insulinoma is malignant. Normally, C-peptides are liberated in the blood in equimolar concentrations as insulin and therefore alterations in the concentration of C-peptides in the plasma reflect the concentration of insulin. In patients with insulinoma, the level of C-peptides is increased, and this is an important fact when you must perform a differential diagnosis between a functional insulinoma causing the hypoglycemia or hypoglycemia caused by injections of commercial insulin. In this case, the C-peptides are not increased or are at a very low level because commercial insulins do not contain C-peptides. In addition, these factitious hypoglycemias may be diagnosed by the presence of antibodies to insulin, which develop in patients who receive exogenous insulin 2 months after beginning the injections. The surest test to make a diagnosis of functional insulinoma is prolonged fasting, with blood samples every 6 hours, to determine the level of insulin and the level of the blood sugar until the hypoglycemic crisis develops, which usually appears within 72 hours of beginning the fasting period. At the moment of the hypoglycemic crisis, at least two blood samples should be taken 2 to 3 minutes apart, and then the test should be discontinued, giving oral or intravenous glucose to shorten the hypoglycemic crisis.

The triad of Whipple and Franz was very much used for many years after 1935 (62). This test is characterized by three findings: (a) The patients must have symptoms of hypoglycemia, (b) the blood sugar should be below 45 mg%, and (c) the symptoms disappear with the administration of glucose orally or intravenously. This test serves as a diagnostic presumption but is not specific for insulinoma, since the test can be positive in several hypoglycemic extrapancreatic illnesses. Before operating on a patient with insulinoma, it is advisable to perform the diazoxide inhibition test. This drug may be indicated postoperatively, and it is therefore necessary to know preoperatively both its efficacy and its tolerance (7, 10, 14).

Second Stage: Preoperative Localization of the Functional Insulinoma

Once a diagnosis of the existence of a functional insulinoma has been made with certainty, one should proceed to determine its localization either within the pancreas or in very rare case, in ectopic pancreatic tissue (1%). Many functional insulinomas are very small in diameter, between 5 and 25 mm, and of a density similar to that of normal pancreatic parenchyma, making their localization by means of ultrasonography, computed axial tomography, or magnetic resonance studies difficult. Recently, Böttger and colleagues (9) have obtained a good result combining computed tomography with an intravenous injection of a radiopaque substance.

The two methods that are used at present to localize insulinoma hypoglycemia are selective and supraselective angiography, and the method proposed by Ingemansson and colleagues in 1975 (31), which consists in transcutaneohepatic catheterization of the efferent pancreatic veins, taking samples of blood from different veins to determine the insulin level in these samples. It is not necessary to use both methods systematically. If localization by angiography is positive, it is not necessary to perform the transparietal hepatic catheterization.

If the angiogram is negative, transparietal hepatic catheterization is indicated, with the object of localizing, at least regionally, the insulinoma within the pancreatic parenchyma.

Third Stage: Identification of the Insulinoma During Surgery

If the localization of the insulinoma preoperatively is unequivocal, surgical treatment will be greatly facilitated. There is a group of patients in whom the diagnosis of insulinoma is certain, and its localization is determined preoperatively but cannot be identified during surgery. There is also another small group of patients with insulinomas diagnosed with certainty preoperatively that could not be located preoperatively nor identified during surgery. These latter two groups may give rise to therapeutic problems that are, at times, not easily solved. When the diagnosis of functional insulinoma is unequivocal, the patient should be operated upon and the surgeon should try to identify the insulinoma during surgery to remove it. At present, the identification of the insulinoma during the surgery is performed by the following methods:

1. Surgical exploration of the pancreas by inspection and palpation.
2. Exploration of the pancreas by means of operative ultrasonography.
3. Determination of plasmatic insulin levels by removal of blood from efferent pancreatic veins, using the rapid radioimmunoassay method.
4. Identification of the insulinoma by means of toluidine blue injection into the splenic artery or the gastroduodenal artery.
5. Serial progressive resection of the distal pancreas, removing sections oriented transversely from the pancreatic parenchyma every 5 mm, exploring the removed segment by visualization, palpation, and microscopic study of the surface and of the section of the pancreas.
6. Frozen section study of biopsy to confirm the histologic diagnosis of the enucleated insulinoma or the insulinoma found on the surface of the resected pancreas.

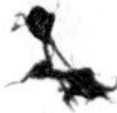

Surgical Exploration of the Pancreas

FIGURE 19.1 INCISION
A longitudinal midline incision above the umbilicus is the usual incision used, since it is easy to perform, easy to close, and gives excellent late results. In case it is necessary, it can be extended upward, resecting the xiphoid process, and downward some 6 to 8 cm below the umbilicus. In some cases, however, the incision should be adapted to the habitus of the patient. Once the peritoneum is opened, the entire abdominal cavity is explored to search for metastasis and then the entire pancreas is explored beginning with the Vautrin-Kocher maneuver.

FIGURE 19.2 VAUTRIN-KOCHER MANEUVER
The Vautrin-Kocher maneuver is performed in three stages. In the first stage, the transverse colon and its mesocolon are brought downward, exposing the entire second portion of the duodenum and the external portion of the third portion of the duodenum. Once the colon and its mesocolon have been brought down, they are covered by a gauze pad and held in place with a Deaver retractor.

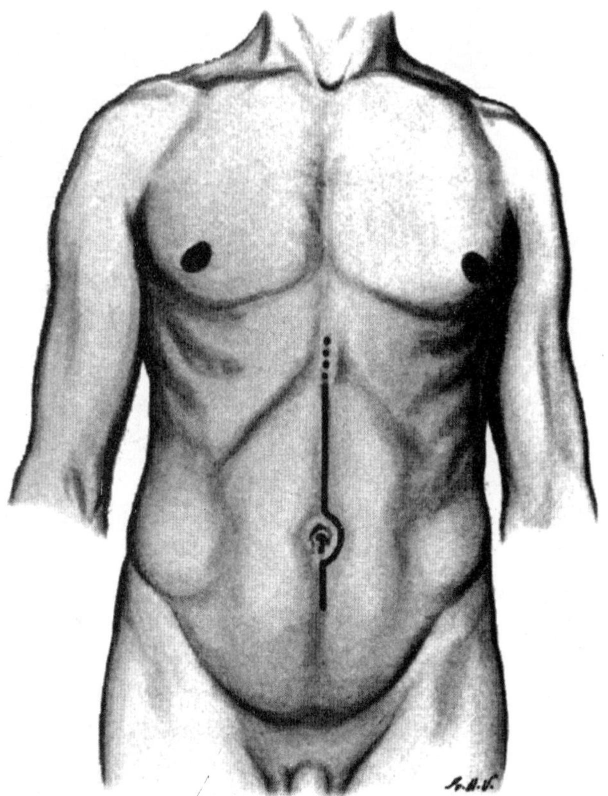

FIGURE 19.1 INCISION

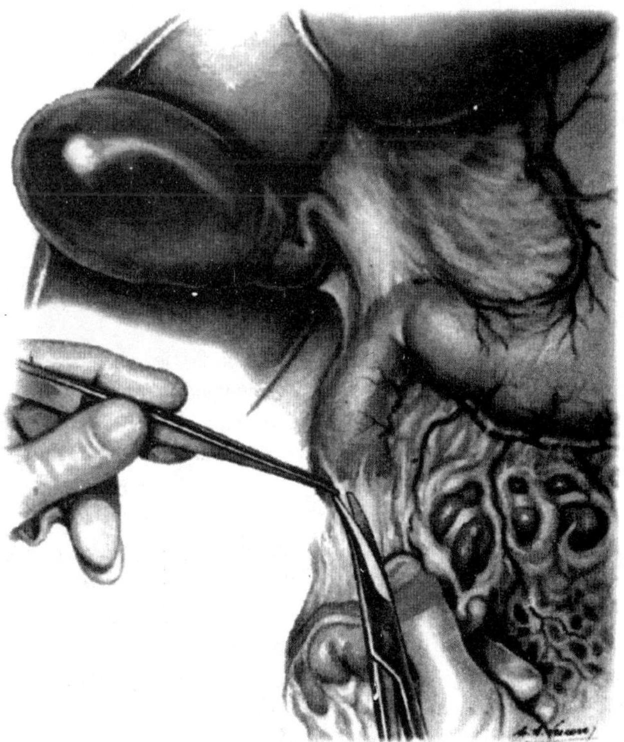

FIGURE 19.2 VAUTRIN-KOCHER MANEUVER

FIGURE 19.3

The second stage of the Vautrin-Kocher maneuver consists in transecting the peritoneum near the external border of the second and third portions of the duodenum and transecting the anterior peritoneal coverage of the hepaticoduodenal ligament.

Surgical Exploration of the Pancreas

FIGURE 19.4 THE THIRD STAGE OF THE VAUTRIN-KOCHER MANEUVER

The duodenum and the head of the pancreas are mobilized, including the uncinate process, up to the midline, exposing the inferior vena cava and the right gonadal vein entering the inferior vena cava. The papilla of Vater is found at the same level as the entrance of the right gonadal vein into the inferior vena cava (Madden). The Vautrin-Kocher maneuver, once completed, should clearly expose, in addition to the inferior vena cava and the right gonadal vein, the perirenal fat over the right kidney, the aorta, the superior mesenteric vessels, the right renal vein, and the left renal vein entering the inferior vena cava. One can note in the drawing that the posterior wall of the duodenum is completely covered by peritoneum, contrary to what most authors show in their drawings, in which it is possible to see the posterior wall of the duodenum without any peritoneum exposing the muscular layer, which is incorrect.

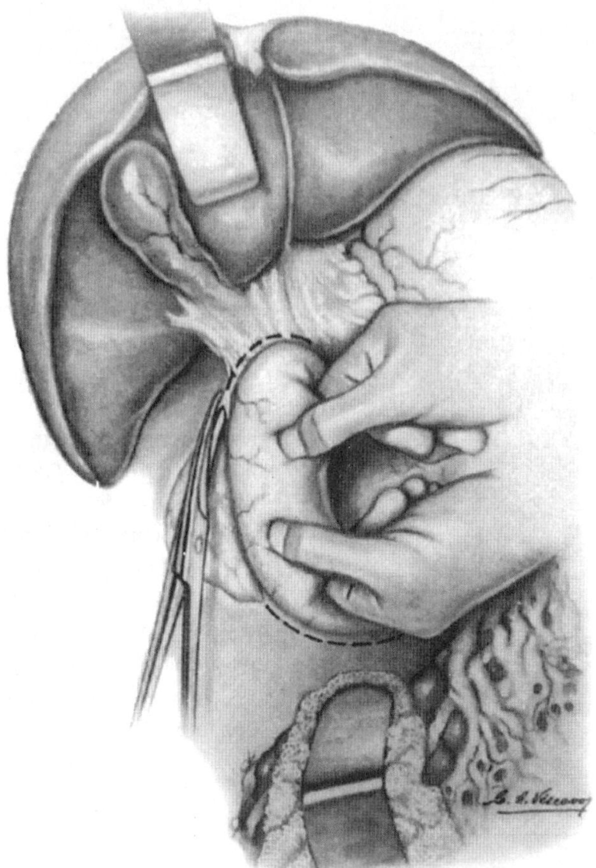

FIGURE 19.3

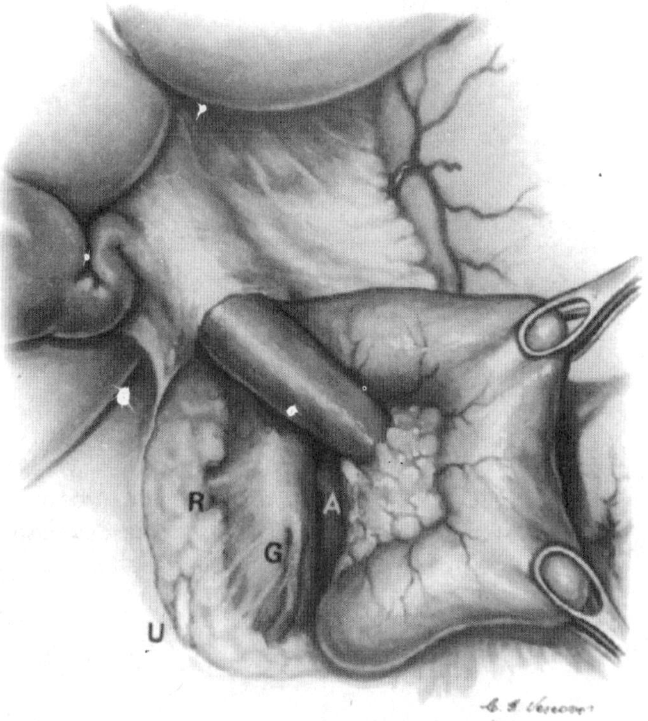

FIGURE 19.4 THE THIRD STAGE OF THE VAUTRIN-KOCHER MANEUVER

FIGURE 19.5
Photograph of a Vautrin-Kocher maneuver in an injected cadaver performed by Dr. John L. Madden of New York. This photograph forms part of an anatomic investigation that reveals three important facts: (a) that the duodenum is completely covered by peritoneum, in its anterior wall as well as its posterior wall, (b) that if a horizontal line is drawn from the entrance of the right gonadal vein into the inferior vena cava, one can see that it coincides with the level of the papilla of Vater, and (c) that one can also observe that the vessels which supply the second portion of the duodenum run clearly transversely.

Surgical Exploration of the Pancreas

FIGURE 19.6 PALPATION OF THE HEAD OF THE PANCREAS
The head of the pancreas should be felt very carefully and thoroughly, as well as repeatedly, since this is the thickest section of the pancreas, for which reason some insulinomas in this location are difficult to feel. It has been shown that it is in the head of the pancreas that insulinomas are more frequent. Palpation of the head of the pancreas is performed by placing the index and middle fingers of the left hand behind the pancreas and the thumb in front of the pancreas. The lower portion of the head of the pancreas can better be felt with the right hand in the same manner as was just described for the left hand.

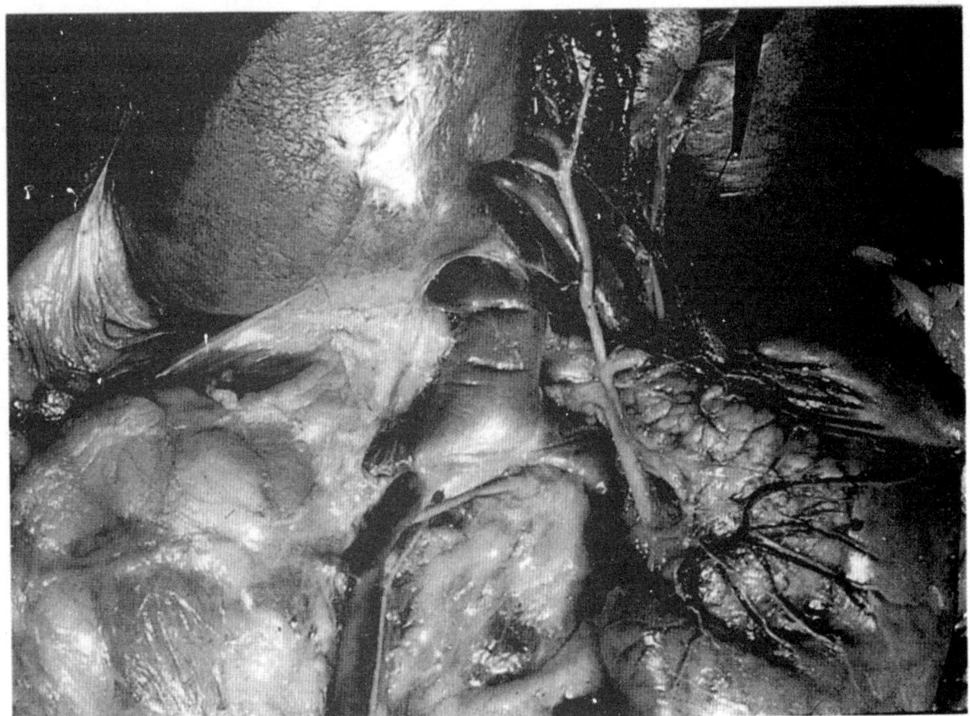

FIGURE 19.5

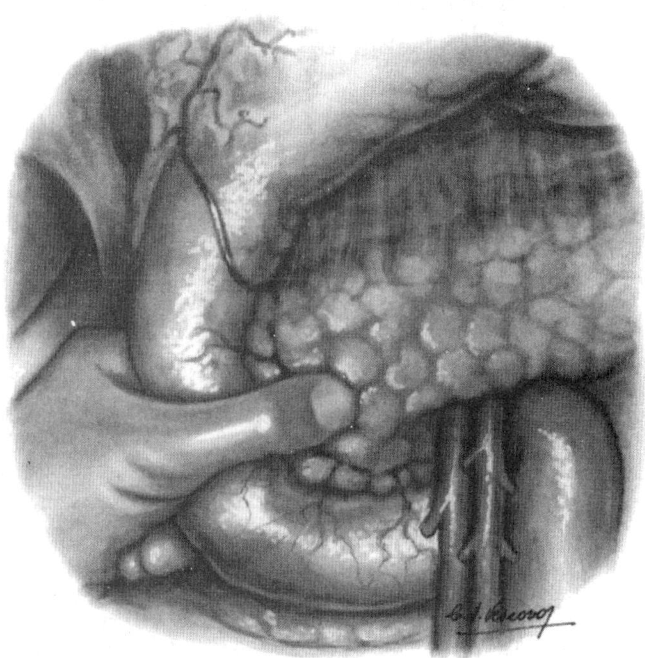

FIGURE 19.6 PALPATION OF THE HEAD OF THE PANCREAS

FIGURE 19.7 PALPATION OF THE UNCINATE PROCESS

The uncinate process is the most difficult segment of the head of the pancreas to palpate. Palpation of this segment should be performed very carefully, so as not to injure the parenchyma or the blood vessels that irrigate it, since hemostasis is very difficult to perform. If the pancreatic parenchyma is injured, resection of the uncinate process is very difficult. It is also very difficult to localize the pancreatic duct in the uncinate process in order to ligate it. A simple method of palpating the uncinate process is as shown in the drawing. The surgeon places the left hand behind the duodenum and pancreas with the palm facing forward, and the index finger of the right hand is gently introduced between the mesenteric vessels and the neck of the pancreas.

Surgical Exploration of the Pancreas

FIGURE 19.8 EXPLORATION OF THE BODY AND TAIL OF THE PANCREAS

To adequately explore the body and tail of the pancreas, it is necessary to divide the gastrocolic ligament below the gastroepiploic arcade, as shown in the drawing. Section of the gastrocolic ligament exposes the anterior surface of the pancreas. If the insulinoma is superficial in location, it can be seen before palpation is performed. It is necessary to point out that the color of the insulinoma depends on its degree of vascularization. Very well vascularized insulinomas have a reddish appearance, while poorly vascularized insulinomas have a color similar to that of normal pancreas. The usual description of an insulinoma, stating that it is a violaceous red color completely different from the yellow, rosy color of normal pancreas, is not completely exact.

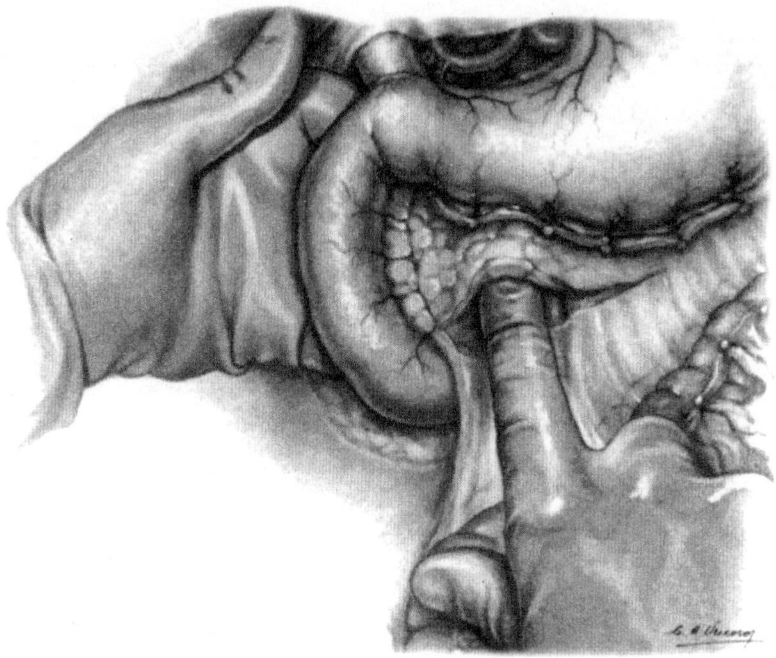

FIGURE 19.7 PALPATION OF THE UNCINATE PROCESS

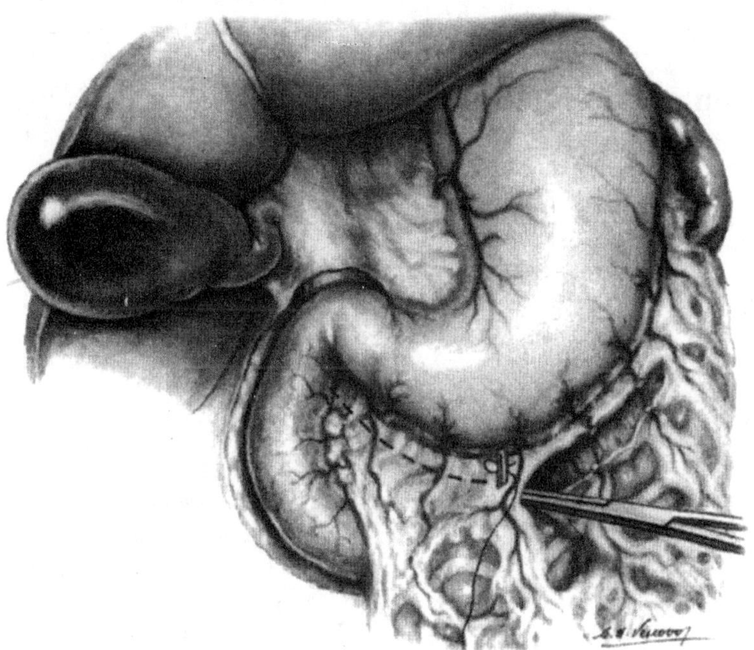

FIGURE 19.8 EXPLORATION OF THE BODY AND TAIL OF THE PANCREAS

Surgical Exploration of the Pancreas

FIGURE 19.9 PALPATION OF THE INFERIOR SEGMENT OF THE BODY AND TAIL OF THE PANCREAS

To explore the inferior segment of the body and tail of the pancreas, it is necessary to divide the peritoneum of the inferior and superior edges of the pancreas. The drawing shows the incision being made along the inferior border of the pancreas, using scissors.

FIGURE 19.10

After having sectioned the peritoneum over the inferior and superior borders of the pancreas, it is necessary to ligate several veins that run from the posterior surface of the pancreas into the splenic vein. This will allow a more adequate palpation of the posterior surface of the pancreas without the danger of producing hemorrhages owing to trauma to these veins caused by the surgeon's fingers. To ligate these veins, it is necessary for the first assistant to raise, using both hands, the inferior border of the pancreas, exposing its posterior surface as well as the splenic vein and its affluent branches. In some cases, with the object of better exposing the posterior surface of the body of the pancreas, it may be necessary to replace the assistant's hands by two malleable retractors. With the splenic vein exposed, one can then ligate the affluent branches as shown in the drawing.

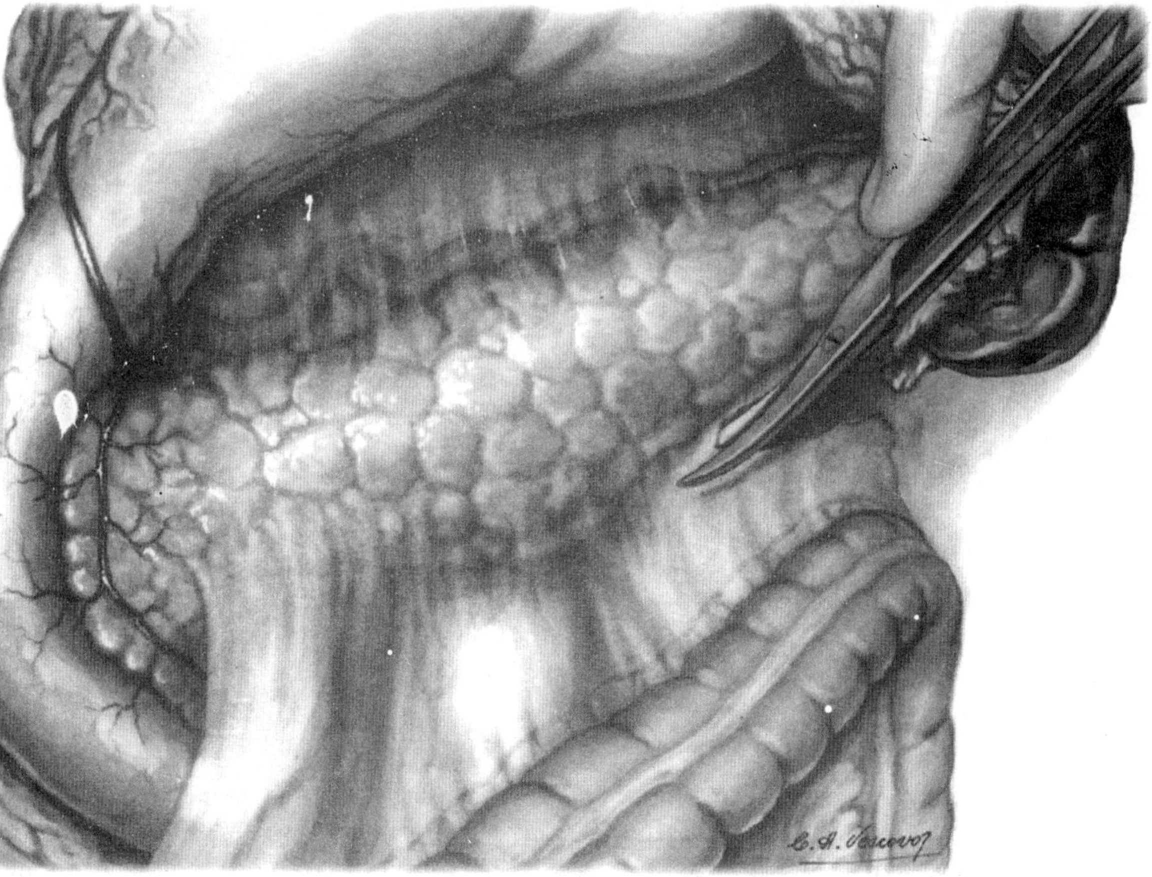

FIGURE 19.9 PALPATION OF THE INFERIOR SEGMENT OF THE BODY AND TAIL OF THE PANCREAS

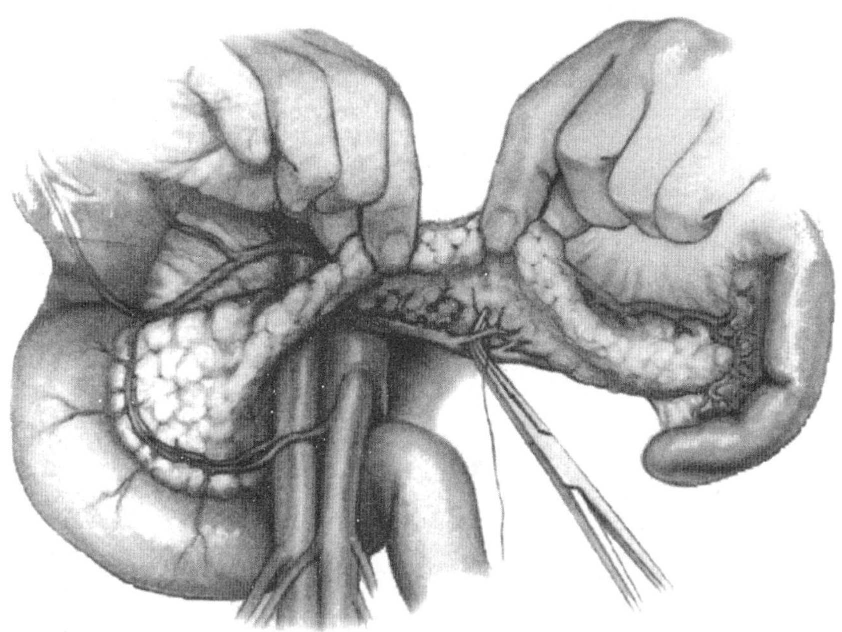

FIGURE 19.10

FIGURE 19.11
Palpation of the inferior segment of the body of the pancreas has begun. For this maneuver, the right thumb is placed in front and the right index finger behind the pancreas. The end of the thumb is pointing out the presence of a small superficial tumor corresponding to an insulinoma.

Surgical Exploration of the Pancreas

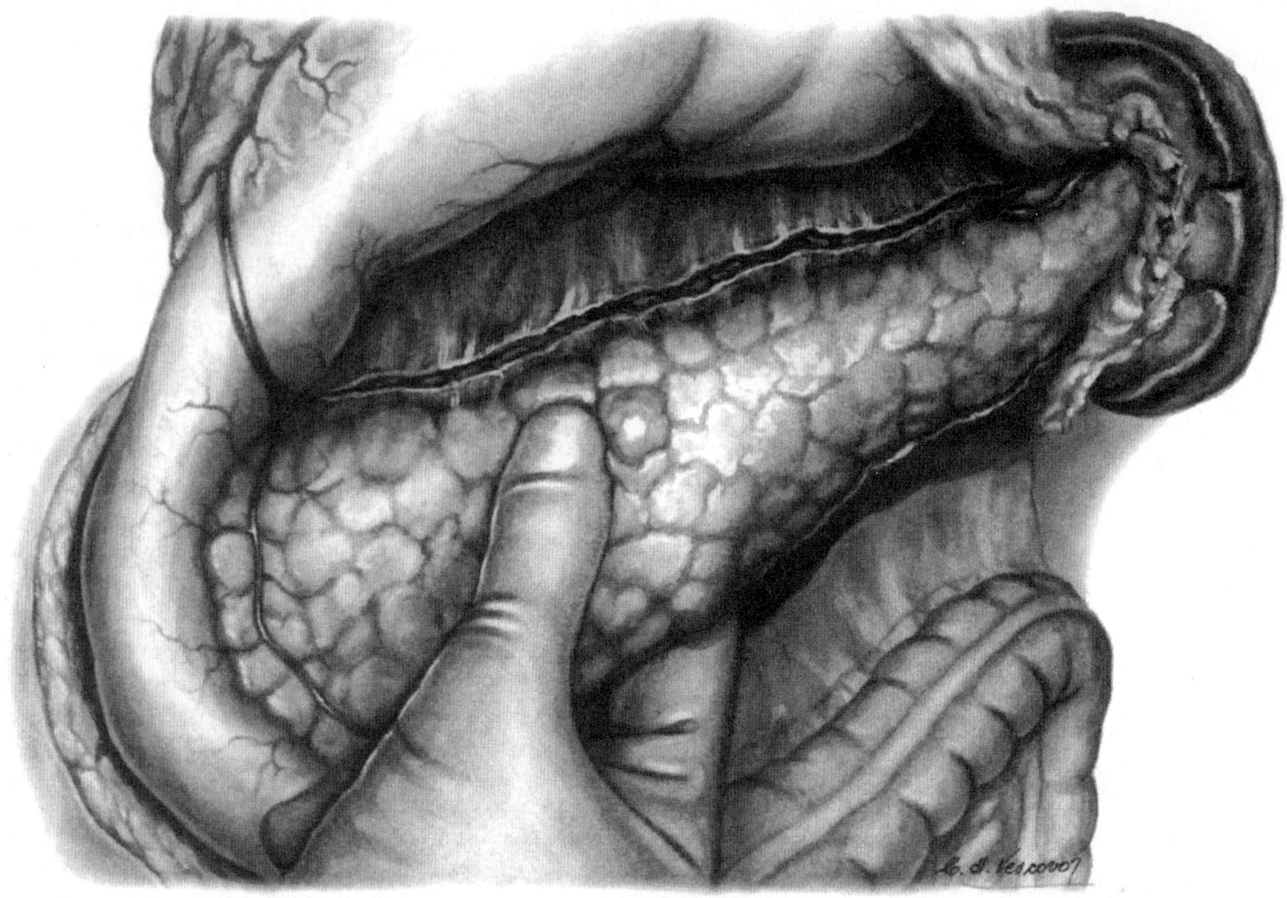

FIGURE 19.11

FIGURE 19.12

Once palpation of the inferior half of the body and tail of the pancreas has been completed, one proceeds to palpate the superior half. To perform this maneuver, the left index finger is placed behind the pancreas and the film in front of it. The pulp of the thumb is pointing out the presence of a rather superficial insulinoma.

Insulinomas are generally firmer than normal pancreatic tissue. However, there are many exceptions. The consistency of the insulinoma is related to its vascularity and to a greater or lesser abundance of connective tissue in its structure. The very well vascularized insulinomas, which are the most active, may present a softer consistency than normal pancreatic tissue. In other cases, the insulinoma may be firmer in consistency. This consistency, however, may be less than that of pancreatic parenchyma that has been affected by chronic pancreatitis. Insulinomas of less than 10 mm in diameter are difficult to palpate, especially if they are deep. Insulinomas that are more easily palpated are those that measure more than 15 mm in diameter.

Surgical Exploration of the Pancreas

Palpation of the pancreas for the identification of insulinomas should be performed completely, centimeter by centimeter. Palpation should be repeated several times before completing exploration.

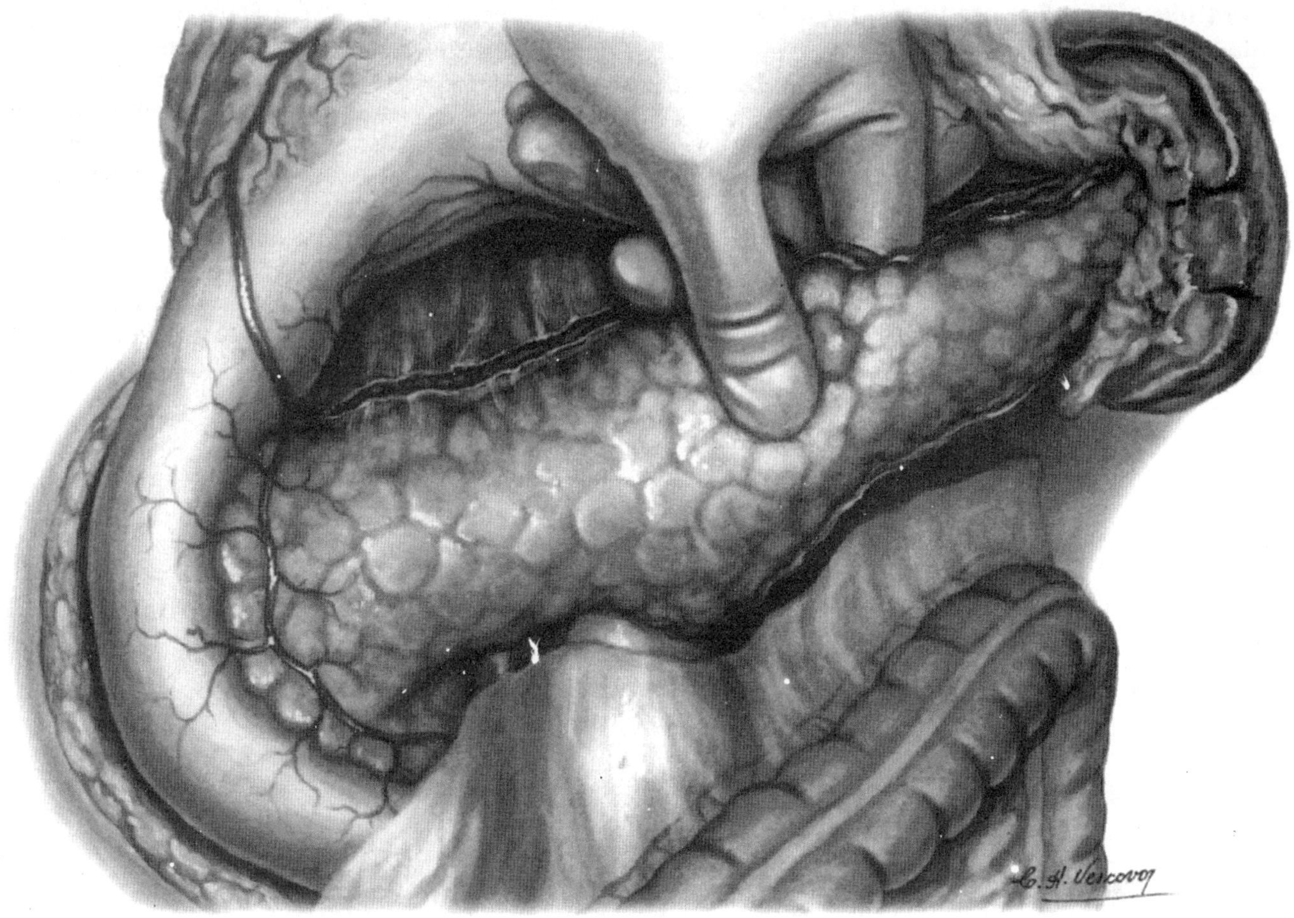

FIGURE 19.12

Exploration of the Pancreas by Operative Ultrasonography

In recent years operative ultrasonography is being used more frequently for the detection of insulinomas of small size. A high-frequency transducer is used, smaller than that used in percutaneous ultrasonography. The insulinoma manifests itself as a hypoechoic image when compared to the normal pancreatic parenchyma. There are authors who believe that ultrasonography during surgery is not better than a good palpation by an experienced surgeon (9, 32, 56). Other surgeons believe that operative ultrasonography is indicated in all cases, not only because of the good results obtained with it, but also because it is a noninvasive method that may make possible the detection of insulinomas that are not visible or palpable (2, 3, 16, 32, 44, 45, 51). It has been shown that ultrasonography can show the relation of the insulinoma with the pancreatic duct so that the surgeon can take all precautions to perform the enucleation of the tumor without injuring the duct. For best results, ultrasonography should be performed by the surgeon together with the invaluable collaboration of an experienced ultrasonographist (13).

Exploration of the Pancreas by Operative Ultrasonography

FIGURE 19.13
Drawing showing the technique of ultrasonographic exploration of the pancreas. To perform this exploration during surgery, a high-frequency transducer is used, which is smaller than that used in percutaneous ultrasonography. The insulinoma is usually seen as a hypoechoic image when compared to the normal pancreatic parenchyma.

Exploration of the Pancreas by Operative Ultrasonography

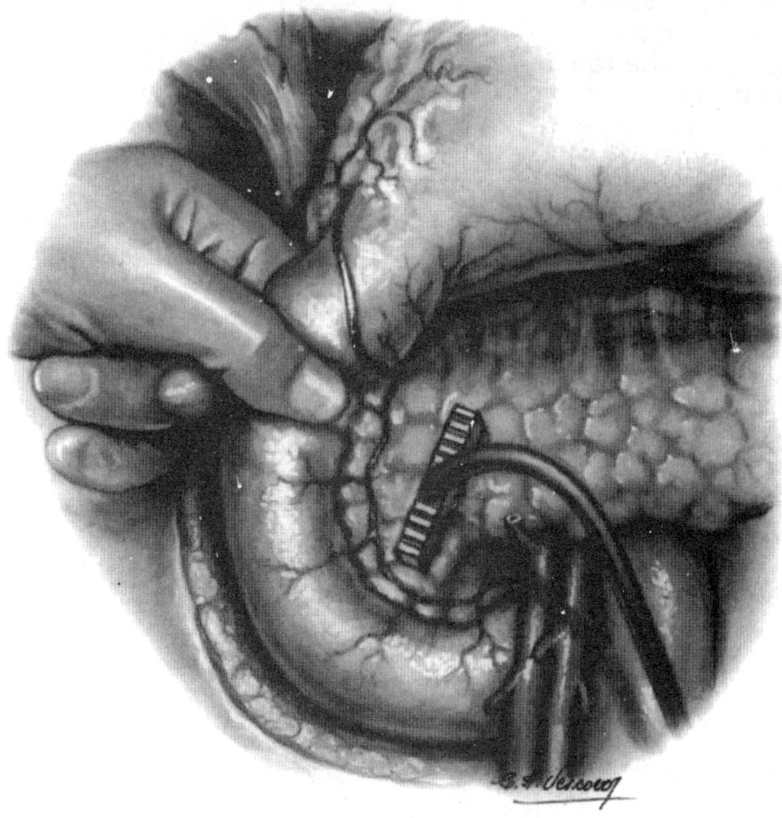

FIGURE 19.13

Selective catheterization of efferent pancreatic veins during surgery to determine insulin levels by the rapid radioimmunoassay method

This procedure is being used more and more frequently during surgery for the regional localization of occult insulinomas and is based on the technique of Ingemansson and colleagues (31), which we have previously described. During the surgical procedure, blood is removed from the efferent veins of the pancreas to determine the level of insulin by the rapid radioimmunoassay method, which takes some 30 minutes to perform. An elevated level of insulin will show the segment in which the insulinoma is located, which would avoid having to perform blind pancreatic resection in some patients. In addition, the region where the insulinoma is presumably located can be explored by means of operative ultrasonography, making it possible to identify the insulinoma and enucleate it in some patients (9, 13). In cases in which the Ingemansson and colleagues method is performed preoperatively, the results obtained can be compared with those obtained during surgery.

Toluidine blue coloration test

Some authors (9) recommend that a test for the localization of insulinomas intraoperatively be performed by injecting toluidine blue into the splenic or gastroduodenal arteries. In three cases in which we have performed this test, the results have not been very convincing.

Progressive distal resections of the pancreas

In cases of occult insulinomas, not identifiable by the previously described method, it may be necessary to resort to distal progressive resections of the pancreas, realizing serial transverse sections every 5 mm, with the object of identifying grossly, or by palpation or microscopic examination of the surfaces of the section removed, the presence of the insulinoma. By this method, we have been able to identify one insulinoma that we could not identify by the other methods. There is no doubt that using this procedure, it is possible to identify some 30 to 40% of occult insulinomas. Some authors, who disagree with progressive resections, prefer closing the abdomen and waiting 1 or 2 years to perform a second operative intervention, with the hope that the insulinoma will have increased in size and will be able to be identified. During this period of time, hypoglycemia is controlled by the administration of diazoxide (40). Arguments against this procedure are as follows:

1. As has been shown, in some 30 to 40% of cases of progressive pancreatic resections, the insulinoma has been identified.
2. Re-exploration of a pancreas that has been previously submitted to a meticulous exploration is always a difficult task, undoubtedly resulting in increased mortality and morbidity. For this reason, it is advisable that whenever possible, resection of the insulinoma should be performed in the first operative intervention.
3. Diazoxide is not an efficacious drug in all patients and carries with it frequent collateral and toxic side effects, especially with prolonged treatments.
4. In case the insulinoma is included in the resected segment were malignant, treatment has been completed. Some authors (21), based on the fact that the majority of occult insulinomas are localized in the head of the pancreas, have proposed that a pancreaticoduodenectomy (Whipple operation) be performed instead of distal pancreatic resection. No one doubts, however, that the Whipple procedure carries greater risk with greater morbidity and mortality and may result in remaining insulinomas that have not been found.

Frozen section biopsy

Diagnostic confirmation of the resected tumor must be proven microscopically. For this reason, the presence of a pathologist when a probable insulinoma is being operated upon is essential. An insulinoma may be confused microscopically with a lymph node, a nodule of chronic pancreatitis, and so on.

SURGICAL PROCEDURES FOR THE RESECTION OF INSULINOMAS

Enucleation of Insulinomas

Enucleation is the procedure of choice in the surgical treatment of insulinomas with the object of resecting as little normal pancreas as possible. Even though the term "enucleation" is used in removal of insulinomas, it is in reality not a real enucleation, since these tumors do not have a capsule and it is always necessary to remove some of the surrounding pancreatic tissue as it is necessary to perform several ligatures of blood vessels irrigating the insulinoma. Following enucleation, it is important to investigate if the pancreatic duct was injured. Insulinomas located in the head of the pancreas, near the duodenum, have to be investigated for possible injury of the transpancreatic common bile duct. Operative ultrasonography is of great help to determine the relation of insulinomas to the pancreatic duct and avoid injuring it. If there is some suspicion that the pancreatic duct has been injured, it is useful to inject secretin intravenously to stimulate pancreatic secretion and reveal the existence of a lesion to the pancreatic duct in order to take adequate measures to treat it. If the pancreatic duct has not been injured, the cavity left in the pancreas by enucleation should be sutured using nonabsorbable sutures, grasping both edges of the pancreatic capsule. Complete hemostasis should be performed within the cavity prior to closing it. A suction drain tube should be left in the abdomen and brought out a counter incision.

If the pancreatic duct was injured, a postoperative fistula will occur, which will usually take several weeks to close. Some surgeons recommend the administration of a somatostatin analogue of prolonged action subcutaneously three times a day to diminish pancreatic secretion and enhance closure of the fistula (64). If the pancreatic duct was injured in the distal portion of the pancreas, a distal resection of the pancreas is indicated to prevent the development of the fistula. If the pancreatic duct was severely injured in the region of the head of the pancreas, it is advisable to perform an anastomosis of the injured area of the pancreas with the jejunum in Roux-en-Y fashion or with the posterior wall of the stomach. Some surgeons prefer to treat injuries of the pancreatic duct by placing a fine Silastic tube within it brought out through the papilla of Vater and to the outside, together with a T-tube in the common bile duct. The pancreatic wound is closed with interrupted nonabsorbable sutures, leaving a suction drain brought out of the abdomen through a counter incision. If the transpancreatic bile duct has been injured, the wound in the common bile duct is closed using synthetic, slow-absorption sutures and the common bile duct is drained with a T-tube brought out of the abdomen. Enucleation of an insulinoma may lead to other complications, such as acute pancreatitis, pancreatic pseudocysts, and so on. It is necessary to point out, however, that complications are rare if the enucleation is performed with correct technique and adequate precautions.

Surgical Procedures for the Resection of Insulinomas

FIGURE 19.14 ENUCLEATION OF AN INSULINOMA IN THE HEAD OF THE PANCREAS

The capsule of the anterior surface of the pancreas has been incised and the insulinoma is being enucleated. The insulinoma does not have a capsule, so a true enucleation cannot be performed. However, this is the term that is commonly used. To resect the insulinoma it is necessary to ligate several vessels and incise part of the pancreatic parenchyma around it. Hemostasis is carried out as the tumor is being resected. Once the insulinoma has been resected, the bottom of the resulting depression should be explored to determine if the pancreatic duct has been injured and adopt the proper corrective measures. If some doubt still exists regarding possible injury of the pancreatic duct, it is useful to inject 2 units per kg of secretin intravenously to increase pancreatic secretion and show the injury to the duct. If the duct is not injured, hemostasis is completed and the excavation closed with two or three sutures that include the capsule and part of the pancreatic parenchyma. Before closing the abdomen, a suction drain tube is brought out through a counter incision in the abdominal wall.

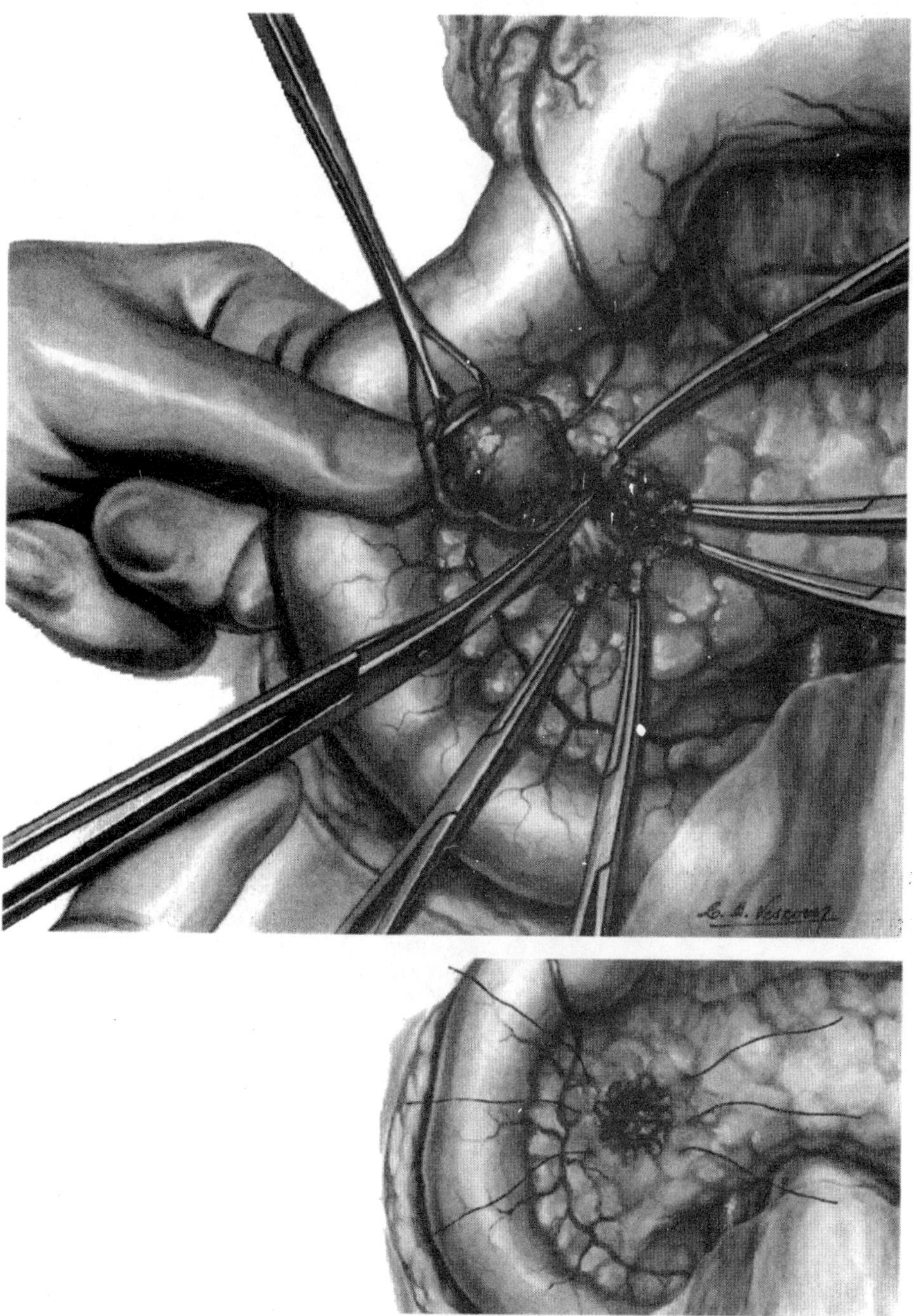

FIGURE 19.14 ENUCLEATION OF AN INSULINOMA IN THE HEAD OF THE PANCREAS

FIGURE 19.15
Operative photograph of an insulinoma 10 mm in diameter, pink in color, located in the anterior surface of the body of the pancreas, easily visible and palpable.

Surgical Procedures for the Resection of Insulinomas

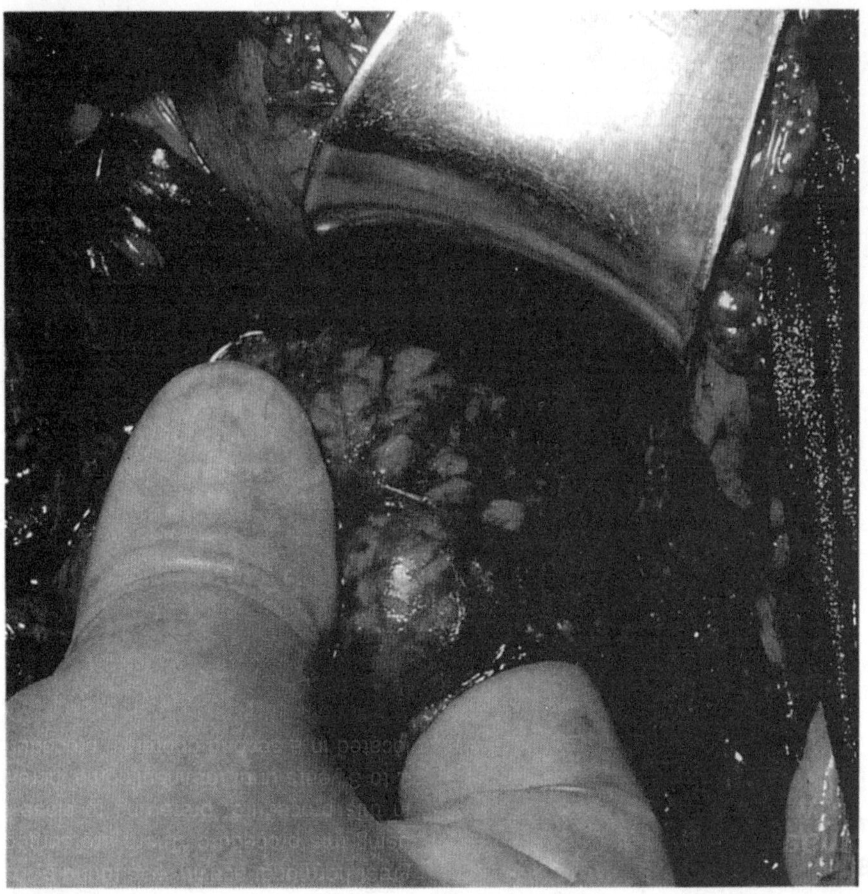

FIGURE 19.15

Surgical Procedures for the Resection of Insulinomas

FIGURE 19.16

Operative photograph of a patient with an insulinoma 14 mm in diameter, pale pink in color, of slightly increased consistency when compared to the pancreas, located in the anterior surface of the head of the pancreas near the internal border of the duodenum and deeply penetrating into the pancreatic parenchyma. As seen in the photograph, the insulinoma is being enucleated. It became necessary to use numerous hemostatic clamps during the course of the enucleation. The pancreatic duct was not injured.

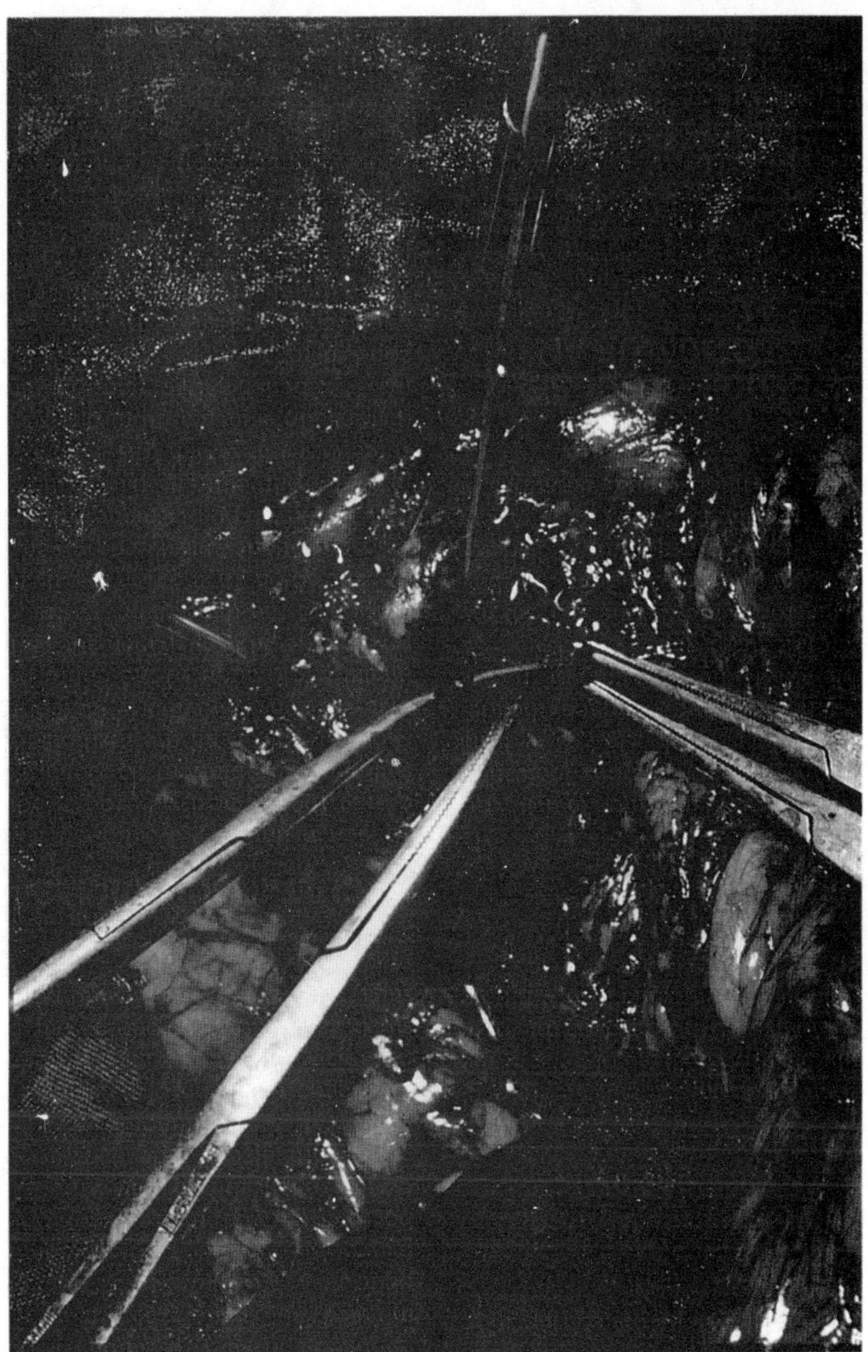

FIGURE 19.16

FIGURE 19.17
Operative photograph of an insulinoma of 7 mm in diameter, violaceous in color, soft in consistency, with a lobulated surface, hard to feel, which was located between the body and tail of the pancreas near its superior border. In addition to being soft in consistency, the small insulinoma was completely covered by a lymph node which was increased in size and consistency. First, it was felt that the lymph node was the insulinoma. Microscopic examination revealed the mistake. However, behind the resected lymph node, and completely hidden by it, was the insulinoma.

Surgical Procedures for the Resection of Insulinomas

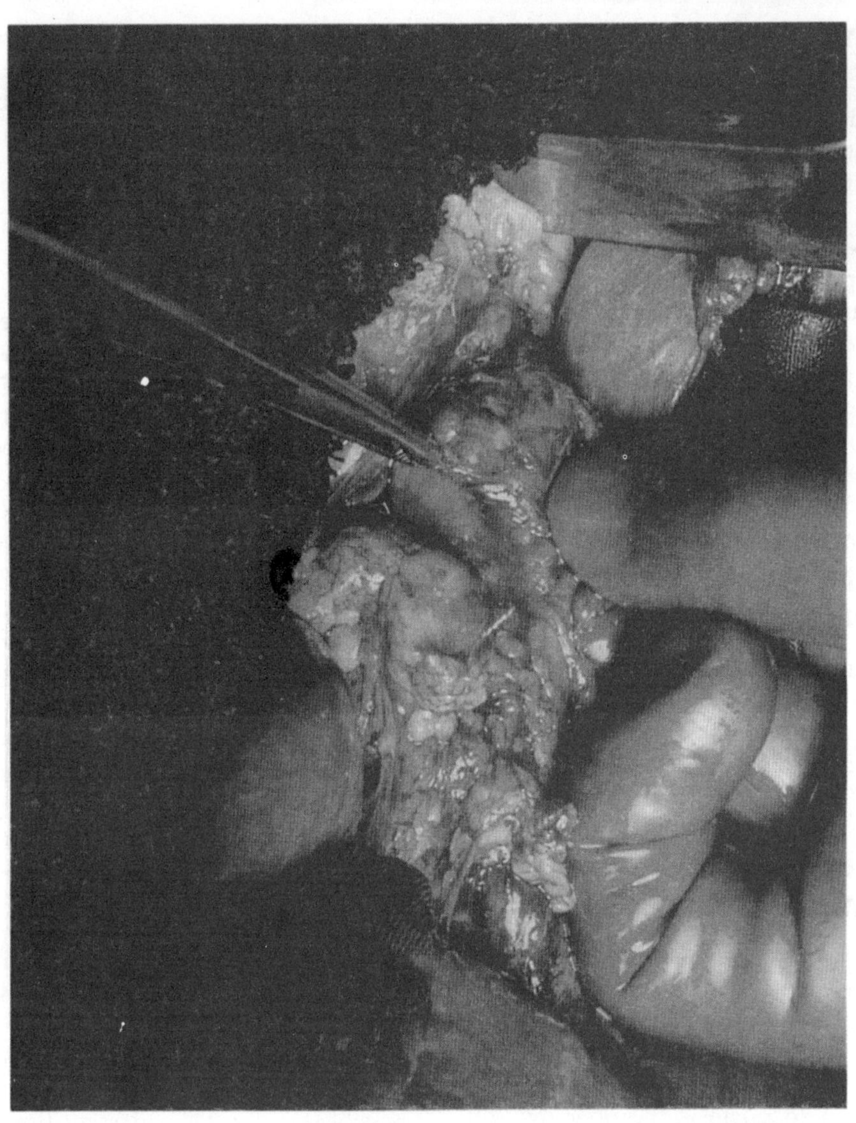

Resection of the Distal Pancreas

Distal resection of the pancreas may be indicated in insulinomas of the body or tail, of great size, in insulinomas located deep to the pancreatic duct, in multiple insulinomas in this location, and in malignant insulinomas. In some insulinomas of the tail of the pancreas it is at times preferable to perform resection instead of enucleation, even if this is possible, for technical reasons. Resection of the body and tail of the pancreas is indicated in the occasional case of polymicroadenomatosis of the islets of pancreas or hyperplasia of the beta cells. Resections of the distal pancreas should be performed as much as possible using technique that will permit conservation of the spleen, especially in young people.

Pancreaticoduodenectomy (Whipple Operation) in the Treatment of Functional Insulinomas

Pancreaticoduodenectomy is the precise indicated procedure in malignant insulinomas of the head of neck of the pancreas. Benign insulinomas of the head of the pancreas should only exceptionally be treated by a Whipple procedure.

Total Pancreatectomy in the Treatment of Insulinomas

Total pancreatectomy is only rarely indicated in the treatment of functional insulinomas. One serious indication would be in a patient previously subjected to a distal pancreatic resection without having obtained the desired results and unable to tolerate diazoxide or in case diazoxide has not been adequate in the operative test. Total pancreatectomy transforms these patients from hypoglycemic (with their usual severely symptomatic clinical picture) into hyperglycemics, acquiring a diabetes that is difficult to control, chaotic in evolution, and very sensitive to insulin even in small doses and variations of 2 to 3 units.

MONITORING OF BLOOD GLUCOSE LEVELS AFTER RESECTION OF AN INSULINOMA

Even though the monitoring of the blood sugar as proposed by McMillan and Scheibe in 1951 (41) is a rather controversial procedure, it is used in many surgical centers with good results (18, 20, 27, 28, 52, 53, 55, 61). Once the functional insulinoma has been resected, the blood sugar evidently rises after 30 minutes have passed. If this rise does not occur in the blood sugar, it should be suspected that another insulinoma is present. Some authors do not trust this test because of the possibility of false positives and false negatives (5, 8, 9, 13, 14).

In order to monitor the blood sugar level, it is necessary that the patient receive during the operation a constant amount of glucose, so that the level of glycemia is maintained at a fixed level in order to be able to observe the net rise in the glycemia 30 minutes after the insulinoma is resected. Administration of glucose during surgery is necessary to prevent the patient from going into hypoglycemia during the surgery, be it due to manipulation of the insulinoma or spontaneously. Before the insulinoma is resected, blood is removed every 15 minutes, and after resection, blood is removed every 5 minutes. Automatic analyzers are used that facilitate the performance of these tests. Administration of diazoxide may be suspended the day before surgery so that it will not interfere with the secretion of insulin. In general, elevation of the blood sugar after resection of the insulinoma normalizes rapidly. However, in some patients, resection of the insulinoma may lead to a marked and prolonged elevation of the blood sugar. It has become necessary at times to inject insulin to lower the blood sugar as occurred in one of our patients whose blood sugar went above 500 mg and persisted over a period of seven days.

OCCULT INSULINOMAS

Hidden insulinomas are those that could not be identified during the surgical procedure. Some 10 to 20% of insulinomas are hidden. To identify occult adenomas one should resort to all the methods of operative diagnosis that we have previously described. This includes bidigital exploration of the entire pancreas and zones of possible heterotopic pancreatic tissue such as the second portion of the duodenum, gastric antrum, hepatic pedicle, and so on. In addition to palpation, ultrasonography, whose efficiency has been proven, should be performed and the level of plasmatic insulin found in blood removed from efferent pancreatic veins determined. In some cases in which this latter procedure may indicate that insulin is increased in one sector of the pancreas, it may be beneficial to perform ultrasonography of this zone to try to identify the insulinoma and resect it by enucleation instead of by pancreatic resection (44, 45). When unable to identify the insulinoma, we can resort to progressive distal resection of the pancreas, realizing serial sections of the pancreatic parenchyma oriented transversely, every 5 mm, to attempt visual identification, palpation, or microscopic identification of the insulinoma. In patients suffering with polymicroadenomatosis of the islets of Langerhans, or hyperplasia of the beta cells, the only method available for diagnosis is microscopic examination. Monitoring of the blood sugar can be of great usefulness in these cases, as we have demonstrated.

Occult Insulinomas

FIGURE 19.18

If the insulinoma cannot be identified by bidigital palpation of the entire pancreas, by determining the blood sugar levels in the efferent veins of the pancreas by the rapid method, or by operative ultrasonography, one can resort to progressive distal resection of the pancreas, realizing serial transections of the pancreatic parenchyma every 5 mm as shown in the drawing, and performing a visual palpatory and microscopic examination of the sections. In some 30 to 40% of progressive pancreatic resections, it has been possible to find the insulinomas. In one of my cases, an insulinoma 3 mm in diameter of great hormonal activity was found by microscopic examination using this procedure. There are surgeons who do not believe in this procedure, preferring to close the abdomen and wait 1 to 3 years until the insulinoma increases in size and can be located in a second operative procedure.

Occult Insulinomas

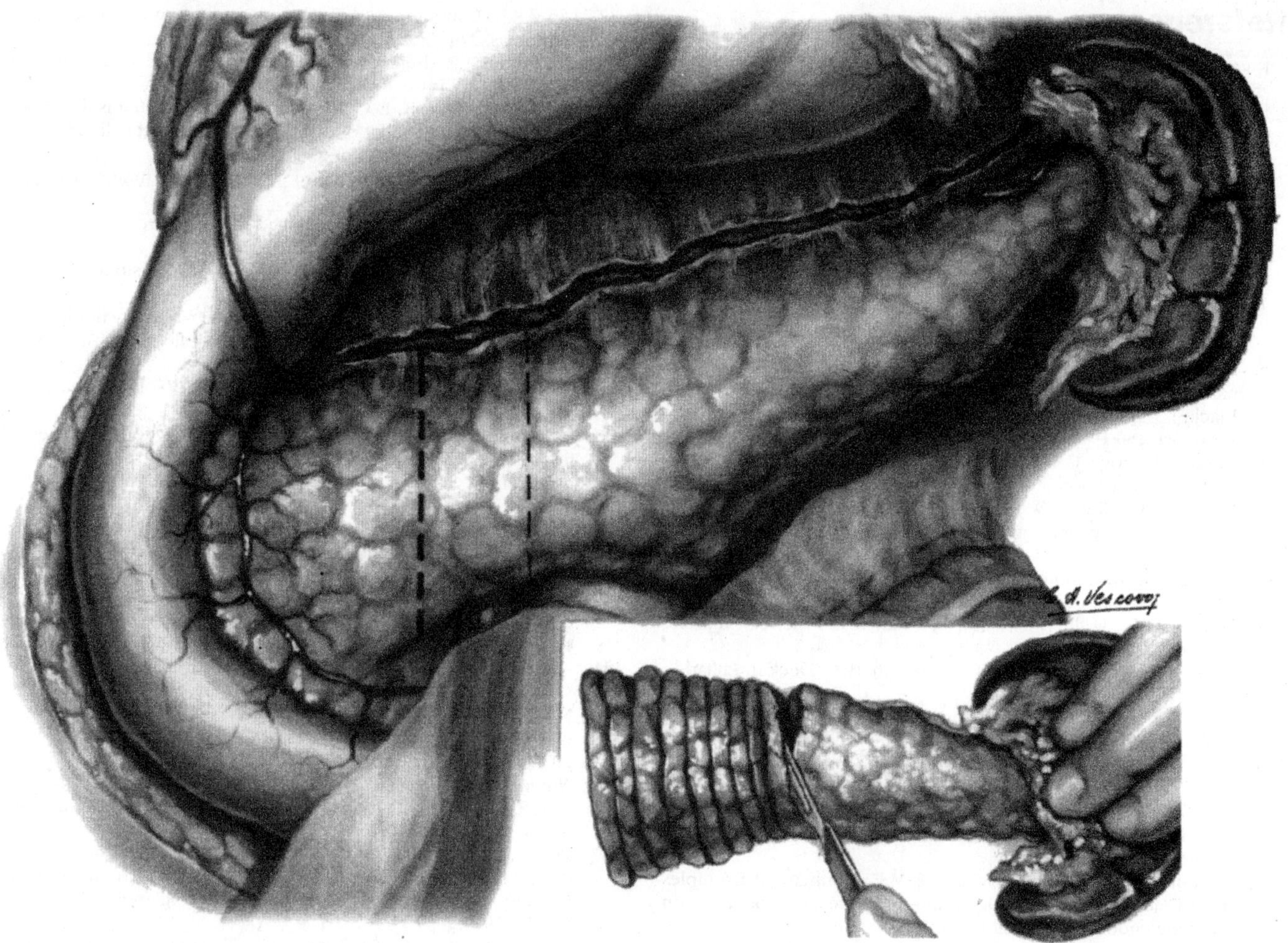

FIGURE 19.18

References

1. Alsever, R.N., Robert, J.P., Gerber, J.G., et al. Insulinoma with low circulating insulin levels: The diagnostic value of proinsulin measurement. Ann. Intern. Med. 82:347, 1975.
2. Angelini, L., Maceratini, R., Bezzi, M., et al. Intraoperative high resolution ultrasonography in the localization of occult endocrine pancreatic tumors. Ital. J. Surg. Sci. 13:209, 1983.
3. Avant, C.S., van Heerden, J. Insulinoma. The value of intraoperative ultrasonography. Arch. Surg. 123:843, 1988.
4. Banting, F.G., Best, C.H. The internal secretion of the pancreas. J. Lab. Clin. Med. 7:251, 1922.
5. Beger, H.G., Büchler, M. Endocrine tumors of the pancreas. In Lygidakis, N.J., Tytgat, G.N.J. 0Eds.) Hepatobiliary and pancreatic malignancies. p. 328. Thieme, New York, 1989.
6. Beveraggi, E.M., Sivori, E.A., Pietravallo, A. Híperplasias funcionantes del páncreas. Rev. Assoc. Med. Argent. 89:97, 1976.
7. Black, J. Diazoxide and the treatment of hypoglycemia. Ann. N.Y. Acad. Sci. 150:194, 1968.
8. Boissel, P., Proye, C. Les tumeurs endocrines du pancréas. 87 Congrès de l'Association Française de Chirurgie. Masson, Paris, 1985.
9. Böttger, T.C., Weber, W., Beyer, J., Junginger, T. Value of tumor localization in patients with insulinoma. World J. Surg. 14:107, 1990.
10. Brooks, J.R. Insulinoma. In Brooks, J.R. Surgery of the pancreas. p. 348. W.B. Saunders, Philadelphia, 1983.
11. Broughan, T., Leslie, J.D., Soto, J.M. Pancreatic islet cell tumors. Surgery 99:671, 1986.
12. Cameron, J. Atlas of surgery. Vol. I, p. 436. B. C. Decker, Philadelphia, 1990.
13. Carty, S.E., Norton, J.A. Comentarios por invitación. World J. Surg. 14:112, 1990.
14. Centarti, J.C., Martini, R.B., Rolfo, R.D. et al. Insulinomas. Cir. Esp. 42:857, 1987.
15. Creutzfeldt, W., Arnold, C., Creutzfeldt, C. et al. Biochemical and morphological investigations of 30 human insulinomas. Diabetologia 9:217, 1973.
16. Chapuis, Y., Hernigou, A., Plainfossé, M.C., Bonnette, P. Exemples d'application de la ultrasonographie—temps réel peropératoire en chirurgie endocrinienne. Chirurgie 110:97, 1984.
17. Doutre, L.P., Aubertin, J., Ponzo, J., Gin, H. La chirurgie des insulinomes sous pancréas artificial. Ann. Chir. 39:177, 1985.
18. Edis, A.J., Mellrath, D.C., van Heerden, J.A. et al. Insulinoma. Current diagnosis and surgical management. Curr. Probl. Surg. 13:1, 1976.
19. Etala, E. "Insulinomas" cuadernos Chilenos de cirugía. Congreso Anual del Capítulo Chileno del American College of Surgeons. p. 366. Santiago, Chile, 1977.
20. Etala, E. Insulinomas. Rev. Argent. Cir. 34:67, 1978.
21. Fonkalsrud, E.W., Dilley, R.B., Longmire, W.P., Jr. Insulin secreting tumors of the pancreas. Ann. Surg. 159:730, 1964.
22. Fraker, D.L., Norton, J.A. Localization and resection of insulinomas and gastrinomas. J.A.M.A. 259:3.601, 1988.
23. Friesen, S.R. Insulinomas pancreático:Una endocrinopatía entópica. Pren. Méd. Argent. 66:679, 1979.
24. Garriz, R.A. Discusión del trabajo: Etala, E. "Insulinomas" Rev. Argent. Cir. 34:67, 1978.
25. Harris. S. Hyperinsulinism and dysinsulinism. J.A.M.A. 83:729, 1924.
26. Harrison, T.S., Child, C.G., Fry, W.D. Current surgical management of functioning islet cell tumors of the pancreas. Ann. Surg. 178:485, 1973.
27. van Heerden, J.A., Edis. A.J., Service, F.J. Surgical aspect of insulinoma. Ann. Surg. 189:677, 1979.
28. van Heerden, J.A., Edis, A.J. Insulinoma. Diagnostic and management. Surg. Rounds. 3:42, 1980.
29. van Heerden, J.A. Comentario por invitación. World J. Surg. 12:689, 1988.
30. Howland, G., Campbell, W.R., Waltby, E.J., Robinson, W.L. Dysinsulinism. J.A.M.A. 93:674, 1929.
31. Ingemansson, S., Lunderquist, A., Lunderquist, I. Portal and vein catheterization with radioimmunologic determination of insulin. Surg. Gynecol. Obstet. 141:705, 1975.
32. Lane, R.J., Coupland, G.A.E. Operative ultrasonic features of insulinomas. Am. J. Surg. 144:585, 1982.
33. Langerhans, P. Beitrage zur Mikroskopischen. Anatomie der Bauchspeicheidruse. Gustav Lange, Berlin, 1869.
34. Laroche, G.P., Ferris, D.O., Prestley, J.T. Hyperinsulinism. Surgical results and management of occult functioning islet cell tumor. Review of 154 cases. Arch. Surg. 96:763, 1968.
35. Laurent, J., Debry, G., Floquet, J. Hypoglycemic tumors. Excerpta Medica. p. 9. Amsterdam, 1971.
36. Malamud, S.W., Kleiman, V., Emma, C.E. et al. Pren. Méd. Argent. 67:524, 1980.
37. Mammoni, O.H. Discusión del trabajo: Etala, E. "Insulinomas" Rev. Argent. Cir. 34:67, 1978.
38. Markowitz, A.M., Slanetz, C.A. Jr., Frantz, V.K. Functioning islet cell tumors of the pancreas: 25 years follow-up. Ann. Surg. 171:394, 1970.
39. Marks, V., Clifford, Rose F. Hypoglycaemia. p. 97 Blackwell Scientific Publications, Oxford, 1967.
40. Mengoli, L., Le Quesne, P. Blind pancreatic resection for suspected insulinoma: A review of the problem. Br. J. Surg. 54:749, 1967.
41. McMillan, F., Scheibe, J.R. Islet cell tumor of the pancreas. Am. J. Surg. 82:759, 1951.
42. Moosa, A.R., Dhorajiwala, J.M. Surgery of the endocrine pancreas. In Moosa, A.R. (Ed.) Tumors of the pancreas. Williams & Wilkins, Baltimore, 1980.
43. Moss, N.H., Rhoads, J.E. Hyperinsulinism and islet cell tumors of the pancreas. In Howard, J.M., Jordan, G.L. (Eds.) Surgical diseases of the pancreas. p. 321. Lippincott, Philadelphia, 1960.
44. Norton, J.A., Sigel, B., Baker, A.R. et al. Localization of an occult insulinoma by intraoperative ultrasonography. Surgery 97:381,1985.
45. Norton, J.A., Cromack, D.T., Shawker, T.H. et al. Intraoperative ultrasonographic localization of islet cell tumors. Ann. Surg. 207:160, 1988.
46. Nubiola, P., Badia, J.M. Treatment of 27 post-operative enterocutaneous fistulas with the long half-life somatostatine analogue. S.M.S. Ann. Surg. 210:56, 1989.
47. Pearse, A.G.E. The diffuse neuroendocrine system and the A.P.U.D. concept: Related "endocrine" peptides in brain, intestine, pituitary, placenta and anuran cutaneous glands. Med. Biol. 55:115, 1977.
48. Perrone, L., Silva, C., Chifflet, J. et al. Tumores insulares del páncreas. Cir. Uruguaya 57:12, 1987.
49. Proye, C., Fulla, Y., Fourlinerie, J.C., Cecat, P., Vergnes, R. Chirurgie des tumeurs pancréatiques hypoglycémiantes. Interêt des dosages per-opératoires de l'insulinémie portale. Lille Chir. 37:79, 1982.
50. Rubenstein, A.H., Kuyuya, H., Horwitz, D.L. Clinical significance of circulating C-peptides in diabetes mellitus and hypoglycemic disorders. Arch. Intern. Med. 137:625, 1977.
51. Rueckert, K.F., Klotter, Hans J., Kümmerle, Fritz. Intraoperative ultrasonic localization of endocrine tumors of the pancreas. Surgery 96:1.045, 1984.
52. Schwartz, S.S., Horwitz, D.L., Zehfus, E. et al. Continuous monitoring and control of plasma glucosa during operation for removal of insulinomas. Surgery 85:702, 1979.
53. Service, F.J., Dale, A.J.A., Elveback, L.R., Jiang, N.S. Insulinoma, clinical and diagnostic features of 60 consecutive cases. Mayo Clin. Proc. 51:417, 1976.
54. Service, F.J., Horwitz, D.L., Rubenstein, A.H. et al. C-peptide suppression test for insulinoma. J. Lab. Clin. Med. 90:180, 1977.
55. Shatney, C.H., Grage, T.B. Diagnostic and surgical aspect of insulinoma. A review of 27 cases. Am. J. Surg. 127:174, 1974.
56. Siegel, B., Guarte, B. et al. Localization of insulinoma of the pancreas by real-time ultrasound scanning. Surg. Gynecol. Obstet. 156:145, 1983.
57. Stefanini, P., Carboni, M., Patrassi, N. et al. The surgical treatment of occult insulinomas. A review of the problem. Br. J. Surg. 61:1, 1974.
58. Stefanini, P., Carboni, M., Patrassi, N., Basoli, A. Beta islet cell tumors of the pancreas. Results of a study on 1,067 cases. Surgery 75:597, 1974.
59. Teichmann, R.K., Spelsberg, F., Heberer, G. Intra-operative biochemical localization of insulinomas by quick radioimmunoassay. Am. J. Surg. 143:113, 1982.

60. Tseng, H.C., Wu, W.J., Chu, V., Liu, T.L. Insulinomas. Arch. Surg. 115:647, 1980.
61. Tutt, G.O., Jr., Edis, A.J., Service, F.J., van Heerden, M.B. Plasma glucose monitoring during operation for insulinoma. A critical reappraisal. Surgery 88:351, 1980.
62. Whipple, A.O., Frantz, V.K. Adenoma of the islet cell tumors of the pancreas. Ann. Surg. 101:1.299, 1935.
63. Wilder, R.M., Allen, F.N., Power, M.H., Robertson, H.E. Carcinoma of the island of the pancreas. Hyperinsulinism and Hypoglycemia. J.A.M.A. 89:348, 1927.
64. Williams, S.T., Woltering, E.A., O'Dorisio, T.M. et al. Effect of octreotide acetate on pancreatic exocrine function. Arch. Surg. 157:476, 1989.
65. Wilks, A. Discusión del trabajo: Etala, E. "Insulinomas" Rev. Argent. Cir. 34:67, 1978.
66. Yalow, R.S., Berson, S.A. Assay of plasma insulin in human subjects by immunological methods. Nature. 184:1648, 1959.
67. Yalow, R.S., Berson, S.A. Immunoassay of endogenous plasma insuln in man. J. Clin. Invest. 39:1157, 1960.
68. Zuckerberg, C., Etala, E. Microscopía electrónica en el insulinoma hipoglucemiante. Pren. Méd. Argent. 65:256, 1978.

PART II

Surgery of the Stomach and Duodenum

Section D

Anatomy

CHAPTER **20**

Surgical Anatomy of the Stomach and Duodenum

STOMACH

The stomach is the most ample segment of the digestive tract, located in the supramesocolic region of the abdomen, and forming a great reservoir between the esophagus and duodenum.

Before describing the surgical anatomy of the stomach and duodenum, we will quickly describe the embryologic development of these organs to make it easy to understand some anatomic variations and the reason for certain surgical maneuvers that are frequently used in gastroduodenal surgery.

The stomach, first portion of the duodenum, and proximal half of the second portion of the duodenum originate from the foregut. The distal segment of the second portion of the duodenum, as well as the third and fourth portions, together with the jejunum, the ileum, and the right colon, originate in the midgut. The stomach appears during the fourth week of embryonic life as a fusiform dilation of the foregut in which it is possible to distinguish a right and a left wall, an anterior border joined to the anterior wall of the abdomen by the ventral mesentery, and a posterior border or dorsal border joined to a posterior wall by the dorsal mesentery. The posterior border develops rapidly, becomes convex, and will constitute the greater curvature. The anterior border becomes concave and will constitute the lesser curvature. In its embryonic development the stomach rotates to the right in such a way that its left wall becomes the anterior wall and its right wall becomes the posterior wall. The anterior border or lesser curvature moves to the right, and the posterior border or greater curvature moves to the left. Due to this rotation the ventral and dorsal mesenteries also change position. The ventral mesogastrium will give rise to the gastrohepatic ligament, while the dorsal mesogastrium will give rise to the gastrocolic ligament, the greater omentum, and the gastrosplenic ligament. The spleen develops from the mesenchyma, and the dorsal pancreas develops from the endoderm. Both will develop between the leaves of the dorsal mesogastrium.

The duodenum originates in the more caudal position of the foregut and from the more cephalic portion of the midgut. It grows rapidly, forming a loop that remains joined to the posterior wall of the abdomen by the dorsal mesentery and to the anterior wall by the ventral mesentery. When the stomach rotates to the right, it is accompanied by the duodenum, and due to this rotation, the entire duodenum, except the proximal portion of the first portion, will be fixed to the posterior wall of the abdomen by the fusion of the right leaf of the mesoduodenum to the peritoneum of the posterior wall of the abdomen, forming the fascia of Treitz. To reproduce the primitive embryonic position of the duodenum it is necessary to mobilize the duodenum and pancreas, known as the Kocher maneuver, even though he was not the first surgeon to propose this maneuver (23, 25, 29, 48, 52).

Shape, Walls, Curvatures

Once the stomach has completed its embryologic development it acquires the shape of a sort of bagpipe or a capital J. The shape of the stomach, however, varies greatly according to several factors: constitutional body type of the patient, sex, tone of the gastric musculature, state of activity or rest of the stomach, degree of filling, and upright or prone position of the individual. The shape of the stomach in the cadaver differs from that in the live person. On the other hand, anatomic descriptions differ from radiologic descriptions, even though they do show some similarity.

The stomach is described classically as having two walls, anterior and posterior, and two borders, the right or superior border (known as the lesser curvature) and the left or inferior border (known as the greater curvature). The anterior wall of the stomach is located within the peritoneal cavity, and the posterior wall forms part of the lesser omental bursa (lesser sac). The anterior wall is in contact with the liver, diaphragm, and anterior wall of the abdomen. The posterior wall of the stomach is in contact with to the diaphragm, pancreas, spleen, left kidney, and left suprarenal gland (5, 19, 43–45).

The lesser curvature is concave and presents a superior segment, which runs vertically, and an inferior segment, which runs horizontally. The junction of these two portions of the lesser curvature forms an angle known as the incisura angularis. This angle is visible in asthenic individuals but tends to disappear in the hypersthenic person, when the person is lying down, or when the stomach is full. On the lesser curvature there is no clear demarcation visible from the outside between the esophagus and the stomach nor between the body and the antrum. The incisura, even if it is visible, does not represent the anatomic limits between the body and antrum of the stomach.

The greater curvature is convex, begins in the esophagogastric angle of His, and extends through the fundus, the gastric body, and the antrum, ending in the pylorus. The greater curvature is much longer than the lesser curvature and does not present any external demarcation between the gastric fundus and the body of the stomach or between the body and the antrum of the stomach. The esophagogastric angle of His, which appears to be the external point of separation between the esophagus and the stomach, does not correspond to the internal line of separation between the gastric mucosa and the esophageal mucosa, as we will show later.

Cardia

In some anatomic descriptions of the stomach it is said that the cardia of the stomach corresponds to the esophagogastric junction, but this is mistaken. The cardia of the stomach is a segment represented by some 15 to 40 mm of stomach surrounding the esophagogastric junction. The cardia is distinguished from the rest of the stomach by the microscopic structure of its mucosa, which differs from that of the fundus, body, and antrum. The cardia contains only mucus secreting cells. The apex of the angle of His from the outside apparently shows the line of junction of the mucosa of the esophagus and the stomach; however, seen from inside, the line of junction of these mucosas is situated a few millimeters higher (in some cases, even farther). The line of junction of both mucosas is not straight, but irregular, festooned and known as the ora serrata or Z line. In practice, the esophagogastric junction is represented from the point of view of endoscopists by the ora serrata. This is the line of junction of the epidermoid mucosa of the esophagus and the cylindric epithelium of the gastric mucosa. As the esophagoscope passes into the stomach, the pale pink mucosa of the esophagus changes to a reddish mucosa with thicker folds that is present in the stomach. As has been pointed out by several authors (16, 17), the point of junction of the esophageal and gastric mucosas as observed by endoscopists does not coincide with that of anatomists, who locate the esophagogastric junction at a horizontal line passing through the angle of His. As has been pointed out previously, this horizontal line does not coincide with the ora serrata, which is higher than this line. Radiologists, on the other hand, place the esophagogastric junction at an even lower level (16). Hitherto it has been impossible to show with either an optic or an electronic microscope, the presence of an anatomic, macroscopic, or microscopic structure with the characteristics of a sphincter. However, above the gastroesophageal junction, in the esophagus itself, the presence of a functional sphincter (high pressure zone), which under normal conditions prevents reflux of stomach contents into the esophagus, has been demonstrated. This sphincter is known as the inferior esophageal sphincter. Some authors maintain that the oblique fibers of the deep muscular layer of the esophagus form a sort of sling, which contracts and relaxes synchronously with the lower esophageal sphincter, reinforcing the latter's closure.

Pylorus

In contrast with the proximal end of the stomach, in the lower end of the stomach there is an anatomic and functional sphincter, called the pylorus (from the Greek for "doorkeeper"), which separates the stomach from the duodenum. The pyloric sphincter is composed of a ring of circular muscular fibers mixed with some longitudinal and oblique fibers (19, 44, 45). The pylorus is generally visible and palpable. In the groove that separates the pylorus from the duodenum runs a small vein that is quite constant and was described in the year 1908 by William J. Mayo, who named it the pyloric vein. Actually, this vein is known as the Mayo pyloric vein or simply as the Mayo vein to differentiate it from the right gastric vein, also known as the pyloric vein, which empties into the portal vein. The Mayo vein runs in the groove separating the pylorus from the duodenum. It generally runs a short course, and in some patients it is hardly visible (17, 44). The Mayo vein empties into the right gastroepiploic vein. In some cases this vein joins another small vein that empties into it or into the supraduodenal vein, which makes the Mayo vein more visible. The Mayo vein can be useful to the surgeon to determine the limit between the pylorus and duodenum in some cases of retractile ulcerating processes that have led to deformity of the duodenum (17, 19, 45).

Topographic Divisions

In medical literature there is no topographic division of the stomach with which everybody agrees. Anatomists, radiologists, and surgeons have never agreed on the designation of different areas of the stomach. The classic division of the stomach into cardia, fundus, body, antrum, and pylorus is not always interpreted uniformly by different authors. The difficulty rests in the lack of external demarcations of the stomach (except for the pylorus) that would make possible the differentiation of one area from another. This makes all topographic divisions of the stomach somewhat arbitrary. However, even though arbitrary, a universally accepted topographic division of the stomach would be very useful and would lead to greater uniformity in statistics as to the location of different lesions of the stomach. A short description will now be made of each one of the segments of the stomach except for the cardia and the pylorus, which have been already described.

Fundus or fornix

This is the highest portion of the stomach, located above a line passing through the vertex of the angle of His. The mucosa of the fundus is covered by secretory cells producing mucus and by parietal cells, which secrete pepsinogen and hydrochloric acid, respectively. The proportion of chief cells to parietal cells is lower than that in the gastric body (45).

Gastric body

This is the largest segment of the stomach, connecting the cardia above with the fundus and the antrum below. The mucosa of the gastric body is characterized by epithelial cells that secrete mucus but especially by containing an abundant number of principal and chief cells. The cardia and the fundus together with the body represent two thirds of the stomach (45).

Gastric antrum

This is the lowermost segment of the stomach and ends in the duodenum, from which it is separated by the pyloric ring. There is no clear demarcation visible to the naked eye between the body and the antrum. Only microscopic examination can reveal the structural differences between one and the other. The antral mucosa does not contain either principal or parietal cells and therefore does not produce pepsinogen or hydrochloric acid, but secretes a hormone called gastrin, which stimulates the secretion of parietal cells. Gastrin is a very potent polypeptide secreted by the G cells of the antral mucosa. The stimulating action of gastrin on acid secretion is some 30 times stronger than that of histamine (17). Gastrin exerts a tropic effect on gastric mucosa that clearly comes into play in the Zollinger-Ellison syndrome. The antral mucosa extends more proximally over the lesser curvature than over the greater curvature. It was long felt that the incisura angularis was the limit between the antrum and the gastric body, but at present it is known that this is erroneous, since the antral mucosa extends for several centimeters above the incisura. The antrum represents approximately one third of the entire gastric surface (5, 17, 19, 45).

Peritoneum and Ligaments

The stomach is completely covered by peritoneum except for a small area in the posterior wall of the stomach near the cardia, which has no peritoneum. The leaves of the peritoneum, after covering the anterior and posterior wall of the stomach, extend to the lesser and greater curvatures, where they join to form the gastrohepatic and gastrocolic ligaments. The gastrohepatic ligament arises on the lesser curvature of the stomach and extends into the inferior surface of the liver. The gastrocolic ligament arises in the greater curvature of the stomach to join the transverse colon. Arteries, veins, lymphatics, and nerves run along the curvatures between the two layers of the peritoneum. The vessels in the lesser curvature run within the gastric wall while the vessels of the greater curvature do so at a distance that varies from 1 to 3 cm from the greater curvature (5, 17, 35).

Gastrohepatic ligament

Classically this ligament is considered to be composed of three different parts: the dense portion (pars condensa); the flaccid portion (pars flaccida); and the hepatoduodenal ligament.

1. The pars condensa or highest portion, has the greatest consistency of the gastrohepatic ligament. Through this segment between 2 and 5% of aberrant hepatic arteries may run. These are known as left hepatic or hepatogastric arteries and arise from the left gastric or coronary artery. This artery will be described in greater detail when the arterial circulation of the stomach is described.
2. The pars flaccida of the gastrohepatic ligament is the largest portion of this ligament, located between the pars condensa and the hepatoduodenal ligament. This portion is formed by two leaves of peritoneum that form a translucent, thin, practically avascular layer that is easily broken with the fingers.
3. The hepatoduodenal ligament is the lowest portion of the gastrohepatic ligament and constitutes the anterior wall of the foramen of Winslow. Through this ligament run the elements of the hepatic hilus. In an anterior plane the common hepatic duct runs located to the right and the hepatic artery runs located to the left. The portal vein is found in a more posterior plane. The hepatoduodenal ligament joins the proximal or mobile portion of the first portion of the duodenum to the undersurface of the liver.

Gastrocolic ligament

This ligament arises from the greater curvature of the stomach and joins the transverse colon, later descending into the peritoneal cavity to form the greater omentum, which again rises to become adherent to the transverse colon. The gastrosplenic ligament is a prolongation of the gastrocolic ligament and joins the highest portion of the greater curvature of the stomach to the splenic hilus. The short vessels and the left gastroepiploic artery run through this ligament before entering the gastrocolic ligament. Another prolongation of the gastrocolic ligament is the splenocolic ligament, which joins the transverse colon to the inferior pole of the spleen. Within the highest portion of the greater curvature of the stomach, one can find the gastrophrenic ligament, which joins the fundus of the stomach to the diaphragm. This ligament may have a white fibrous aspect but can be very well irrigated by branches of the short vessels (45). Traction on the gastrocolic ligament or its prolongations may lead to a tear of the capsule of the spleen, producing a hemorrhage that may make splenectomy necessary.

The peritoneum covering the anterior wall of the stomach, upon arriving at the cardia, covers the anterior wall of the cardia applying the abdominal esophagus to the posterior abdominal wall, and afterward it covers the inferior surface of the diaphragm. The peritoneum of the posterior wall of the stomach, upon arriving at the cardia, is reflected posteriorly and downward to cover the posterior abdominal wall without covering the cardia and the abdominal esophagus. To free the abdominal esophagus it is necessary to divide the esophagodiaphragmatic peritoneum together with the pars condensa of the gastrohepatic ligament. Dividing the pars condensa frees the right border of the abdominal esophagus.

The peritoneum, which covers the anterior and posterior walls of the stomach, extends distally and completely covers the pylorus and the proximal or mobile portion of the first part of the duodenum. The distal segment of the first portion of the duodenum is fixed in a fashion similar to that of the second, third, and fourth portions of the duodenum, being attached to the posterior wall of the abdomen by the posterior parietal peritoneum.

Arterial Circulation

The arterial circulation of the stomach arises almost completely from the celiac trunk (celiac axis or celiac artery). A very small part of the gastric arterial supply comes from the superior mesenteric artery through its two inferior pancreaticoduodenal arteries, anterior and posterior, which anastomose with two superior pancreaticoduodenal arteries, anterior and posterior, which are branches of the gastroduodenal artery (17, 19, 45).

The celiac trunk arises from the anterior wall of the aorta very near its entrance into the abdomen. The celiac trunk has a short trajectory—8 to 20 mm long—and a diameter of 10 to 30 mm. After arising from the aorta the celiac trunk runs anteriorly and inferiorly, passing very close to the superior border of the pancreas. This is why, when it is necessary to expose the celiac trunk covered by the posterior peritoneum, the pancreas should be retracted downward and this peritoneum divided over the celiac trunk. The celiac trunk is surrounded by celiac lymph nodes and by the nodes and ganglia of the solar plexus. The classic description of the anatomy of the celiac trunk shows it dividing into three branches: the splenic artery, which is the largest; the hepatic artery, which is somewhat smaller; and the left gastric artery or coronary artery, which is the smallest. However, this division into three branches is only found in about 40% of cases (17, 19). In the rest of individuals there exists a great variation in the origin of the three arteries. Some of these variations will be described here.

The coronary artery usually rises from the superior border of the celiac trunk before it divides into splenic and hepatic branches. In some cases the celiac trunk is made up only of the splenic and hepatic arteries, the coronary artery arising directly from the aorta. In other cases the common hepatic artery or the right branch of the hepatic artery arises directly from the superior mesenteric artery. The splenic artery in some cases arises directly from the aorta or from the superior mesenteric artery. In some individuals the celiac trunk is made up of four branches: splenic artery, hepatic artery, left gastric (coronary) artery, and gastroduodenal artery. In some individuals the celiac trunk is not present and the splenic, hepatic, and coronary arteries rise independently from the aorta (5, 17, 19, 43–45).

Knowledge of the anatomy of the arterial circulation in the abdomen with its numerous variations has been enriched in recent years by the use of abdominal angiography.

Left gastric or coronary artery

Sylvius (11) was the first to call this artery the coronary artery whereas Usadel (11) labeled it the left gastric artery. Both names are used in world literature. The left gastric or coronary artery, when it arises from the celiac trunk, runs upward and to the left in a curving direction as a half-crown or arch (this is what made Sylvius give it the name "coronary"), with the concavity oriented downward, then runs forward and enters into the lesser curvature of the stomach about 3 cm below the esophagogastric juncture. In its trajectory toward the gastric curvature the coronary artery elevates the posterior parietal peritoneum, forming a fold called the gastropancreatic fold. The curve that the coronary artery takes is known as the sickle of the coronary. This sickle formed by the artery, which raises the posterior parietal peritoneum before entering into the lesser curvature, is very important because it is at this level that incision of the posterior parietal peritoneum is performed to identify the coronary artery, dissect the celiac trunk, and remove the lymphatic ganglia around the celiac artery and around the sickle of the coronary in order to ligate the coronary artery near its origin in the celiac trunk when the stomach is resected for carcinoma.

When the coronary artery arrives at the lesser curvature of the stomach, in 30% of cases it divides into an anterior and a posterior branch. Both branches run between the layers of the gastrohepatic ligament, close to the edge of the lesser curvature. Upon arriving near the antrum, these branches of the coronary artery anastomose with the right gastric or pyloric artery branches. In some patients, only the posterior branch of the coronary artery anastomoses with the pyloric artery. Anastomosis of these arteries is either direct, on the surface of the lesser curvature, or, in some cases, within the wall of the gastric antrum, in the submucosal layer (19, 45). Before entering the lesser curvature of the stomach the coronary artery gives off an ascending branch called the ascending esophageal or cardioesophageal branch, which irrigates the cardia and the inferior portion of the esophagus. This artery anastomoses with the inferior esophageal artery, which arises in the thoracic aorta. The caliber of this anastomosis is of great importance in extensive gastrectomies because in some cases irrigation of the gastric remnant may depend exclusively on this anastomosis. The ascending esophageal artery is usually designated in the literature as an esophagocardiotuberositary artery, which is self-explanatory. In some patients there may be two cardioesophageal arteries, one anterior and another posterior. The left inferior phrenic artery and the right inferior phrenic artery arise from the aorta immediately above the celiac trunk. In some 2% of cases the left inferior phrenic artery arises from the coronary artery.

Since the left inferior phrenic artery irrigates a section of the highest portion of the stomach, in cases in which this artery arises from the coronary artery, its ligature at the site of the sickle, as is performed in gastrectomies for cancer, may lead to ischemia of the residual gastric stump, especially if a splenectomy has been performed (15, 17).

An aberrant left hepatic artery may also arise from the coronary artery, as described originally by Walther (49). It was later designated by von Haller as the gastrohepatic artery. Rio-Branco (38) and Hyrtl (11, 47) studied this aberrant vessel years later. In European medical literature it is usually designated as the Rio-Branco artery and also as the Hyrtl artery (9, 11, 47), even though these authors were not its discoverers. This aberrant left hepatic artery may be the only arterial supply of the left lobe of the liver, or at least contribute substantially to its irrigation. In these cases ligation of the left hepatic artery, or of the coronary artery proximal to the origin of the left hepatic artery, may lead to complete or partial necrosis of the left lobe of the liver. In other cases the left hepatic artery contributes only a small proportion of the blood supply of the left lobe of the liver. Ligature of the left hepatic artery in the latter carries with it little or no alteration of the circulation of the left lobe of the liver. It is important that the surgeon performing a gastric resection for carcinoma, before proceeding to ligate the coronary artery at the sickle, investigate the presence of an aberrant left hepatic artery and try to establish if its caliber and course result from its being clamped, if it is a replacement left hepatic artery (19), which irrigates all or a grand portion of the left lobe of the liver, or if it is an accessory left hepatic artery whose ligature may not lead to important circulatory disturbances of the left lobe of the liver.

This distinction between a replacement left hepatic and an accessory left hepatic artery will explain in part the great differences in the statistics that exist in the literature about this aberrant artery. In gastric resections for carcinoma in which an aberrant replacement left hepatic artery is present, ligature of the coronary artery should be performed distal to the origin of the left hepatic artery (47). In patients with esophageal hiatus hernia in whom it is necessary to mobilize the distal esophagus to repair the hernia and the pars condensa of the gastrohepatic ligament has to be divided, the possibility of the presence of an aberrant replacement left hepatic artery has to be kept in mind. In this case the aberrant hepatic artery has to be carefully dissected and its ligature avoided.

Close to the lesser curvature of the stomach the coronary artery gives off numerous anterior and posterior collateral branches, which irrigate both walls of the stomach, anastomosing with the branches from the gastroepiploic arteries.

The coronary artery and the other arteries that supply the walls of the stomach anastomose in the submucosal layer through a very extensive arterial network. This permits maintenance of good circulation in the stomach wall even after three of the four principal arteries that supply the stomach have been ligated, allowing displacement of the stomach even up to the neck while still maintaining an adequate circulation. This fact also demonstrates the inadequacy of ligating one or two extrinsic gastric arteries to control gastric hemorrhage.

Some anatomists (17) describe the coronary artery as bifurcating as it approaches the lesser curvature into a superior ascending esophageal or cardioesophageal artery and a piece of the branch, which is the coronary artery.

Hepatic artery

The hepatic artery branch of the celiac trunk contributes considerably to the irrigation of the stomach by means of its branches. After its origin the hepatic artery runs to the right horizontally, later changing direction upward entering the hepatoduodenal ligament. Before changing direction, the hepatic artery gives off a branch known as the gastroduodenal artery, the name of which is immediately changed to hepatic artery proper. The gastroduodenal artery originates near the superior border of the first portion of the duodenum and runs downward, coursing on the anterior surface of the head of the pancreas behind the first portion of the duodenum between the proximal free and the distal fixed portions. Before the gastroduodenal artery passes behind the first portion of the duodenum, it gives out a collateral branch, the superior posterior pancreaticoduodenal artery, which runs to the posterior surface of the pancreas and later enters the latter's parenchyma and anastomoses with the inferior posterior pancreaticoduodenal artery, a branch of the superior mesenteric artery. Together these form the posterior pancreaticoduodenal arcade and supply the posterior surface of the head of the pancreas and the posterior wall of the second portion of the duodenum.

The gastroduodenal artery, as it runs behind the duodenum, gives out duodenal, retroduodenal, and pancreatic branches (17). In 60% of patients the gastroduodenal artery gives rise to the supraduodenal artery, which contributes to the irrigation of the anterior wall of the first portion of the duodenum. Upon nearing the vicinity of the inferior border of the duodenum, the gastroduodenal artery divides into its two terminal branches: the superior anterior pancreaticoduodenal and the right gastroepiploic. The superior anterior pancreaticoduodenal artery passes in front of the surface of the head of the pancreas to enter further down into the parenchyma and anastomose with the inferior anterior pancreaticoduodenal artery, a branch of the superior mesenteric artery. These pancreaticoduodenal arteries make up the anterior pancreaticoduodenal arcade, which contributes to the blood supply of the anterior surface of the head of the pancreas and the posterior wall of the second portion of the duodenum (7,19).

The right gastroepiploic artery, so named by von Haller (11, 18), runs into and enters the gastrocolic ligament bordering the greater curvature of the stomach at a distance between 1 and 3 cm, running all the way to anastomose with the left gastroepiploic artery, a branch of the splenic artery. The right gastroepiploic artery is greater in caliber and longer in extent than the left gastroepiploic artery. Both the right and left gastroepiploic arteries give off ascending or gastric branches, both anteriorly and posteriorly, which anastomose from the branches coming from the coronary artery and right gastric artery or pyloric artery. The gastroepiploic arteries, in addition, give off descending or epiploic branches that supply the greater omentum. The right gastroepiploic artery gives off 5 to 8 anterior epiploic arteries, which run vertically down between the two anterior leaves of the greater omentum (17). The first of these descending epiploic arteries (and at times the second) is the one of greatest importance and is designated as the right epiploic artery, running near the edge of the greater omentum. The right epiploic artery, upon reaching the distal third of the greater omentum, turns horizontally to the left to anastomose with the left epiploic artery, a branch of the left gastroepiploic artery, to form von Haller's major arch (11), also known as Barkow's arch (17). Barkow's arch is located between the two posterior leaves of the greater omentum.

The rest of the epiploic arteries that originate in the right gastroepiploic artery also run between the anterior leaves of the greater omentum, and upon reaching its inferior free border may change direction and ascend on the posterior surface of the greater omentum to empty into Barkow's arch. The left gastroepiploic artery also gives off epiploic branches but in lesser number than the right gastroepiploic. Generally only 2 to 4 arteries arise from it, and the first one is of greater importance, as it descends along the left edge of the greater omentum. It later changes direction and runs to the right to anastomose with the right epiploic artery to form Barkow's arch. The rest of the branches that arise from the left gastroepiploic artery run vertically, and upon arriving at the inferior free border of the greater omentum, they run on its posterior surface to empty into Barkow's arterial arch, which, as mentioned previously, is located between the posterior leaves of the greater omentum. Some of the these posterior epiploic arteries do not arise from the gastroepiploic arcade but may arise from other arteries such as the transverse dorsal pancreatic or the greater pancreatic artery (16, 17).

After the hepatic artery changes direction, running upward, it enters the hepatoduodenal ligament, where it gives off the right gastric or pyloric branch. This artery was called the right gastric artery by Bauhin (11), and the pyloric artery by Glisson (11). The right gastric or pyloric artery is smaller in caliber than the coronary artery, to which it anastomoses. The right gastric artery may also arise from the common hepatic artery before it gives off the gastroduodenal branch and upon occasion may arise from the branches of the bifurcation of the hepatic artery proper. In 25% of cases the supraduodenal artery may originate from the hepatic artery proper.

Splenic artery

This is the artery of greatest caliber arising from the celiac trunk. After its origin it runs to the left following the superior border of the pancreas or taking an anterior position on the posterior surface of this organ as it arrives at the tail of the pancreas, to later bifurcate in the splenic hilus. During its course the splenic artery gives off numerous collateral arteries such as the dorsal pancreatic, the greater pancreatic, and the posterior gastric. The posterior gastric artery is found in 50% of patients. After arising from the splenic artery, the posterior gastric artery runs upward to supply the higher portion of the posterior wall of the stomach (16, 18, 38, 42). This artery was originally described by von Haller in 1745 (18). It was later studied by Rio-Branco and Michels (31, 32, 38), and in recent years this artery has been studied by Suzuki, Didio, and others (31, 32, 38).

The left gastroepiploic artery is an important branch of the splenic artery. It can arise from the splenic artery or from its inferior bifurcation. After its origin the left gastroepiploic artery enters the gastrosplenic ligament, running downward and penetrating the gastrocolic ligament along the greater curvature of the stomach to anastomose with the right gastroepiploic artery. The region of the junction between the left gastroepiploic and the right gastroepiploic arteries is important as a point of reference to determine the extent of resection in cases of duodenal ulcer (17, 26). The splenic artery gives off, in addition to the short vessels (vasa brevia or short gastric arteries), other small vessels that irrigate the gastric fundus. The number of short vessels may vary from 2 to 10, between 4 and 6 being most common. The short vessels are of small caliber and may arise from the trunk of the splenic artery itself, from one or both of its branches, or from the left gastroepiploic artery before it enters the gastrocolic ligament. In some cases one or more short vessels may arise from the polar vessels of the spleen, which are also branches of the splenic artery.

Venous Circulation

The veins of the stomach, which originate in the submucous venous plexus, follow the course of the arteries parallel to them as they run along the curvatures of the stomach, but upon abandoning the curvatures they separate from the arteries (44, 45). The right gastroepiploic vein follows the course of the right gastroepiploic artery along the curvature of the stomach, but further on it abandons the greater curvature of the stomach and joins the superior right colic vein and the inferior and anterior pancreaticoduodenal vein to constitute Henle's trunk, which empties into the right border of the superior mesenteric vein, immediately below the inferior border of the neck of the pancreas. The right gastric or pyloric vein runs along the lesser curvature of the stomach together with the right gastric or pyloric artery but later separates from this artery and from the lesser curvature to empty into the portal vein. The left gastric or coronary vein runs together with the left gastric artery along the lesser curvature but later separates from it and passes in front of the artery in the neighborhood of the celiac trunk to empty into the portal vein. At the level of the abdominal esophagus the coronary vein anastomoses with the inferior esophageal veins, forming a portosystemic anastomosis.

In cases of hypertension in the portal system the direction of the venous current in the coronary vein reverses itself, and blood, instead of emptying into the portal vein, empties into the venous system of the superior vena cava through the azygos vein, leading to dilation of the inferior esophageal vein and thus forming esophageal varices, whose rupture may be significant, producing severe hemorrhage. The left gastroepiploic vein runs away from the greater curvature of the stomach to empty into the splenic vein. The short gastric veins, which accompany the short gastric arteries, empty into the splenic vein, but in some cases, these veins empty directly into the splenic parenchyma.

Lymphatics

The intramural lymphatics of the stomach are distributed throughout all of its layers. They originate in the mucosal network passing to the submucosa and then to the muscular layers and the subserosa. The submucosal lymphatics form a very rich plexus, and through this layer a gastric carcinoma may disseminate itself extensively. From the subserosal lymphatics arise intermediate collecting lymphatics, which transport lymph to the ganglionic chains that follow the course of the arteries in a direction opposite to that of the flow of blood.

Lymphatic drainage of the stomach is very complex, quite different from lymphatic drainage of the colon. There are no intramural lymphatic areas of the stomach independent one from the other, there is continuity between all the different areas. There is some intercommunication present between extragastric lymph node groups. The intramural lymphatics of the stomach as well as their course toward the extragastric lymphatic collection areas has been studied for many years by numerous investigators such as Delamère, Poirier, and Cunéo (13), Jamieson and Dobson (22), Coller, Kay, and McIntyre (10), Rouvière (39), and more recently by Japanese authors (26, 30, 33, 41).

As previously mentioned, gastric carcinomas spread easily through the submucosal layer. A carcinoma of the upper third of the stomach may extend extensively toward the esophagus, where there is no barrier to prevent this invasion. Carcinomas of the antrum may spread into the duodenum, although not as easily as carcinomas of the stomach spread into the esophagus. For a long time it was felt that carcinoma of the antrum could not extend through the pylorus, as if the pylorus were a barrier preventing the invasion of the duodenum. This erroneous concept is based on the macroscopic appearance of the surgical specimen and the radiographic images. It has been well demonstrated that carcinoma of the antrum may spread to the duodenum microscopically through the submucosal and subserosal routes (54). For this reason it has been advised that, when doing gastric resections for carcinoma, at least 3 cm of the proximal duodenum should be removed.

Knowledge of the lymphatic supply of the stomach is fundamental for the surgeon undertaking a gastric resection for carcinoma. The majority of surgical textbooks give considerable attention to the technique of gastrectomy but only mention a few details of the resection of the different groups of lymph nodes. Resection of the groups of lymph nodes has to be performed following a strict system, labeling each group so the pathologist can identify them during microscopic examination. Japanese surgeons have emphatically insisted on the systematization of the surgical resection of groups of lymph nodes of the stomach during gastric resection for carcinoma. It has been shown that the lymphatic current of all the gastric lymph nodes converges on the celiac nodes.

The different lymphatic areas of the stomach are described as follows (10, 13, 19, 22, 26, 30, 33, 36, 39, 41, 43–45, 50):

I. Coronary or Left Gastric Lymph Node Area
This area corresponds to the medial two thirds of the vertical portion and a segment of the horizontal portion of the stomach.

II. Splenic Lymph Node Area
This includes the portion of stomach to the left of the above mentioned area, from the fundus to the middle portion of the greater curvature.

III. Hepatic Artery Lymph Node Area
This corresponds to the rest of the gastric surface.

A. The lymph node area of the coronary or left gastric artery includes the following groups of nodes:
   1. Parietal nodes located against the gastric wall.
   2. Nodes located around the cardia: internal, external, and posterior cardiac nodes.
   3. Nodes of the lesser curvature of the stomach, which are 3 to 5 nodes located along the course of the coronary artery.
   4. Nodes of the sickle of the coronary artery, which include 2 to 6 nodes in the vicinity of the arch of the coronary.
   5. Celiac nodes surrounding the celiac trunk, which are not exclusively from the coronary area but constitute a lymph node area of great importance.

B. The lymph node area of the splenic artery includes the following groups of nodes:
   6. Nodes of the gastrosplenic ligament.
   7. Nodes of the pancreaticosplenic ligament
   8. Lymph nodes of the hilus of the spleen.
   9. Lymph nodes of the left gastroepiploic artery.
   10. Suprapancreatic nodes located around the superior border of the pancreas up to the celiac region.

C. Hepatic artery nodes include the following groups:
   11. Nodes located around the right gastroepiploic artery over the greater curvature of the stomach, usually 5 or 6 nodes.
   12. Intrapyloric nodes, numbering 3 to 6.
   13. Retropyloric nodes, numbering 2 or 3 and located along the gastroduodenal artery.

14. Nodes along the horizontal portion of the common hepatic artery.
15. Nodes along the vertical portion of the hepatic artery known as the proper hepatic artery.
16. Suprapyloric node (inconstant).
17. Anterior pancreaticoduodenal group of nodes located on the anterior surface of the pancreas along the anterior pancreaticoduodenal arcade.
18. Retroduodenal pancreatic group of nodes following the course of the posterior pancreaticoduodenal arcade. The anterior pancreaticoduodenal nodes and the nodes that follow the course of the right gastroepiploic vein are attached to the superior mesenteric vessels (2, 3, 16, 17).

Nerves

The stomach is innervated by the parasympathetic system through the vagus nerves and by the sympathetic system through the celiac plexus. The celiac plexus has little importance in gastric surgery, so we will only describe the parasympathetic system.

The vagus nerves are disposed as two trunks along the distal end of the esophagus, one right and the other left, located on both sides of the esophagus and in close contact to it. Upon arrival at the esophageal hiatus, the right vagus becomes posterior and the left vagus becomes anterior. There are numerous variations in the distribution of the vagus nerves, but the distribution as two trunks is the most frequent one found. The anterior vagus, after passing through the esophageal hiatus, gives off a hepatic branch that follows the gastrohepatic ligament to arrive at the hepatic hilus where it is distributed integrating the gallbladder, biliary ducts, liver, and pancreas. After giving off the hepatic branch, the anterior vagus nerve is called the anterior gastric nerve of Latarjet and follows the lesser curvature of the stomach, giving off several branches to integrate the anterior wall of the stomach. The nerve of Latarjet, after running along the lesser curvature, divides in the antrum into several branches, constituting what is known as the Crow's foot, which is located about 7 cm proximal to the pylorus. The Crow's foot innervates the antrum and the pylorus (27).

The posterior vagus nerve, after passing through the hiatus, gives off a celiac branch that innervates the small bowel and the right colon, that is, the midgut. The distal bowel, including the left colon and rectum, is innervated by the parasympathetic sacral plexus and not by the vagus (17). After giving off its celiac branch, the posterior vagal trunk changes its name to the posterior gastric nerve of Latarjet and runs along the lesser curvature of the stomach posteriorly, where it gives off gastric branches and ends in the posterior Crow's foot, innervating the antrum and pylorus.

DUODENUM

The duodenum is the first portion of the small bowel, starting at the pylorus and ending in the duodenal jejunal angle of Treitz. During its entire course, the duodenum is deep within the abdomen. The name duodenum arises from the Greek *dodekadaktylos,* meaning twelve fingers, related to its length, which undoubtedly is an erroneous appreciation. With the exception of the proximal segment of the first portion of the duodenum, which is mobile and is completed covered by visceral peritoneum, the rest of the duodenum, also covered by visceral peritoneum, is fixed to the posterior wall of the abdomen by the posterior parietal peritoneum, due to the fusion of the right leaf of the primitive mesoduodenum with the posterior parietal peritoneum, forming the fascia of Treitz. The average length of the duodenum is 25 cm, varying from 20 to 30 cm. The diameter of the duodenum is about 4 cm, although it may vary according to the segment that is studied. Its diameter, however, is always greater than the diameter of the jejunum and ileum (19, 44, 45). The duodenum has a very intimate connection with the head of the pancreas, which it surrounds and to which it is solidly fixed. Viewed as a whole, the duodenum has the form of a capital C with the open side directed upward and to the left. Sometimes the duodenal C is more closed than others, appearing as an O, and in other cases it is more open, appearing as a U (11, 43–45).

The proximal segment of the first portion of the duodenum, though closely related to the pancreas, is not joined to this viscera, nor does it share its circulation as does the rest of the duodenum.

In the majority of anatomic and surgical texts the posterior wall of the second portion of the duodenum is described and drawn as being free of visceral peritoneum, with the muscular layer visible, which is an error. This was shown in describing the embryology of the duodenum during its development before rotating and being attached to the posterior wall of the abdomen by the parietal peritoneum, since it was already covered by visceral peritoneum. The entire duodenum is covered by visceral peritoneum even though it is attached to the posterior portion of the abdomen by the parietal peritoneum. The only exception to this is the internal border of the duodenum, which is the hilus of the duodenum, where arteries enter and veins come out (43–45).

The duodenum may present many variations in its disposition due to rotation defects or due to its attachment to the posterior wall of the abdomen by the parietal peritoneum.

Classically and arbitrarily the duodenum is divided into four segments or parts. These divisions are more according to the changes in direction of the duodenum than due to anatomic reasons. A short description of each segment will follow.

1. *First Portion of the Duodenum:* This is about 5 cm long. It begins at the pylorus and runs backward and upward as well as somewhat to the right. This segment can be divided into two segments, presenting some differences: the proximal segment, some 3 cm long and completely covered by visceral peritoneum, is free and mobile. From its superior border arises the hepatoduodenal ligament. This portion of the duodenum corresponds to what is radiographically known as the duodenal bulb. More than 90% of duodenal ulcers are localized in this portion. The proximal segment of the first portion of the duodenum is followed by the distal segment, which is about 2 cm long and is attached to the posterior wall of the abdomen and therefore fixed in place. Usually the gastroduodenal artery marks the limit between these two segments.

   From a radiologic point of view the distal segment of the first portion of the duodenum corresponds to what is known as the postbulbar segment of the first portion of the duodenum. The anterior wall of the first portion of the duodenum is closely related to the infundibulum of the gallbladder, which explains why inflammatory processes of the gallbladder may extend to the first portion of the duodenum and give origin to cholecystoduodenal fistulas and the passage of calculi into the duodenum. On its interior the first portion of the duodenum shows longitudinal superficial folds that are collapsible and can be seen not only radiologically but endoscopically. These folds are made up of the duodenal mucosa and, as will be seen, will be differentiated from the Kerckring folds or valvulae conniventes that appear in the second portion of the duodenum. On the other hand the first portion of the duodenum contains Brünner glands, which diminish in the proximal half of the second portion of the duodenum and disappear in its distal half (17, 45).

   Because the first portion of the proximal segment of the duodenum is free and mobile it is easily freed surgically except in cases where a chronic perforating ulcer of the duodenum into the pancreas is present in this segment.
2. *Second Portion of the Duodenum:* This is the descending portion, which arises in the superior genu and runs downward to the right of the vertebral column. This portion of the duodenum surrounds and is completely fixed to the head of the pancreas. The median length of the second portion of the duodenum is 7.5 cm. This portion is transversely overlain by the transverse mesocolon, which divides it into supra- and inframesocolic portions. The posterior wall of the second portion is attached to the medial border of the kidney, the renal pedicle and right ureter, the inferior vena cava, and the gonadal vessels.

   The internal side of the second portion of the duodenum has Kerckring folds, which are oriented transversely, relatively thick and permanent, and made up of the mucosa and submucosa. These folds, which never involve the entire circumference of the duodenum, start in the junction of the first and second portion of the duodenum and become more evident distal to the papilla of Vater. They continue through the entire duodenum, jejunum, and ileum. In the middle of the second portion of the duodenum, over its medial border and posterior wall, is the papilla of Vater, into which the common bile duct and the pancreatic duct empty. The papilla is frequently covered by a Kerckring fold, and its inferior border is joined to the wall by another fold called the frenulum of the papilla. The papilla is usually between 8 and 11 cm from the pylorus, although many variations may exist, and in the presence of retractile ulcerating processes of the duodenum this distance may be very much reduced. Santorini's duct empties 2 to 3 cm above the papilla. In 7% of cases Santorini's duct may be the principal pancreatic duct, replacing the functions of the pancreatic duct. Duodenal diverticula are most frequently localized in the second portion of the duodenum, especially along its internal border, near the papilla. To explore the posterior wall of the second portion of the duo-denum and the distal end of the common bile duct as well as the posterior surface of the head of the pancreas, it is necessary to carry out the Vautrin-Kocher maneuver.
3. *Third Portion of the Duodenum:* Also known as the transverse portion, this forms the inferior genu in its angle with the second portion. From its origin it runs horizontally toward the left, crosses the vertebral column at the third lumbar vertebra (sometimes the fourth). It has a median length of 12.5 cm. This portion of the duodenum is crossed by the mesentery of the jejunum and ileum, which contains the superior mesenteric vessels. The superior mesenteric artery comes out of the inferior border of the neck of the pancreas and runs in front of the third portion of the duodenum together with the superior mesenteric vein (45). In rare patients of asthenic habitus the superior mesenteric artery may compress the third portion of the duodenum and give rise to an obstructed duodenal clinical picture. In order to explore the third portion of the duodenum, which is located to the right of the superior mesenteric vessels, it is necessary to carry out a Vautrin-Kocher maneuver, whereas to explore the segment of the third portion

of the duodenum located to the left of the superior mesenteric vessels, it is useful to carry out the maneuver of Cattell and Braasch (8), or make an incision in the transverse mesocolon. The retroperitoneal area behind the third portion of the duodenum contains the inferior vena cava and the aorta.

4. *Fourth Portion of the Duodenum:* From its origin this segment of the duodenum runs obliquely upward and upon reaching the body of the second lumbar vertebra, changes direction and runs forward and downward to continue with the jejunum, constituting the duodenal jejunal junction or duodenal jejunal angle of Treitz. The juncture of the duodenum and jejunum is fixed by the fibromuscular ligament of Treitz, which arises in the right crux of the diaphragm. The angle of Treitz is a point of reference that is of great importance in surgical exploration of the abdomen. The length of the fourth portion of the duodenum varies from 2.5 to 5 cm, and in some individuals this portion does not exist. To explore this segment of the duodenum one can resort to the maneuver of Cattell and Braasch or to division of the transverse mesocolon.

Anatomic Variations

The duodenum may present numerous variations according to its position, variations that are, in general, due to lack of rotation or fixation of the duodenum to the posterior plane. The surgeon, as well as the radiologist, should be alert to these possible variations. We will only refer briefly to the three most important ones:

1. The third portion of the duodenum is joined to the jejunum without forming the duodenojejunal angle of Treitz because the fourth portion of the duodenum does not exist.
2. A redundant duodenum due to lack of fixation of the duodenum to the posterior planes.
3. An inverted duodenal C, with the duodenojejunal angle to the right instead of the to the left of the vertebral column.

Arteries

The circulation of the first portion of the duodenum is independent of and less rich than the other three portions of the duodenum. The arteries irrigating the first portion of the duodenum are small in caliber and present numerous variations. The supraduodenal artery previously described irrigates the anterior wall of the first portion of the duodenum. In 60% of patients, this artery arises from the gastroduodenal artery, in 25% from the hepatic artery, and in 12% from the pyloric artery (7, 16, 19, 53). The posterior wall of the first portion of the duodenum is usually supplied by small retroduodenal arteries arising from the gastroduodenal artery and from several small branches from the pyloric or right gastric artery. The supraduodenal artery is not always present, and when it is absent, arterial supply of the anterior wall of the first portion of the duodenum comes from small branches arising in the right gastric or pyloric artery and from the gastroduodenal artery. The blood supply of the posterior wall of the first portion of the duodenum also presents numerous variations (4, 7, 19, 31, 32, 40, 53).

The remaining portions of the duodenum, on the contrary, are very well supplied by the anterior and posterior pancreaticoduodenal arcades. The anterior pancreaticoduodenal arcade generally runs near the internal border of the duodenum while the posterior pancreaticoduodenal arcade runs somewhat further away from the internal border of the duodenum.

The fourth portion of the duodenum also receives blood supply from the first jejunal artery.

Arteries

FIGURE 20.1 ARTERIES OF THE STOMACH AND GREATER OMENTUM

1. Aorta
2. Celiac trunk
3. Left gastric or coronary artery
4. Splenic artery
5. Common hepatic artery
6. Hepatic artery proper
7. Right gastric or pyloric artery
8. Gastroduodenal artery
9. Supraduodenal artery
10. Ascending esophageal or cardioesophageal artery
11. Short vessels
12. Right inferior phrenic artery
13. Left inferior phrenic artery
14. Left gastroepiploic artery
15. Right gastroepiploic artery
16. Superior posterior pancreaticoduodenal artery
17. Superior anterior pancreaticoduodenal artery
18. Superior mesenteric artery
19. Superior pancreatic artery
20. Inferior pancreatic artery
21. Transverse pancreatic artery
22. Pancreatic magna artery
23. Posterior gastric artery
24. Right epiploic artery
25. Left epiploic artery
26. Barkow's arch
27. Anterior epiploic artery
28. Posterior epiploic artery

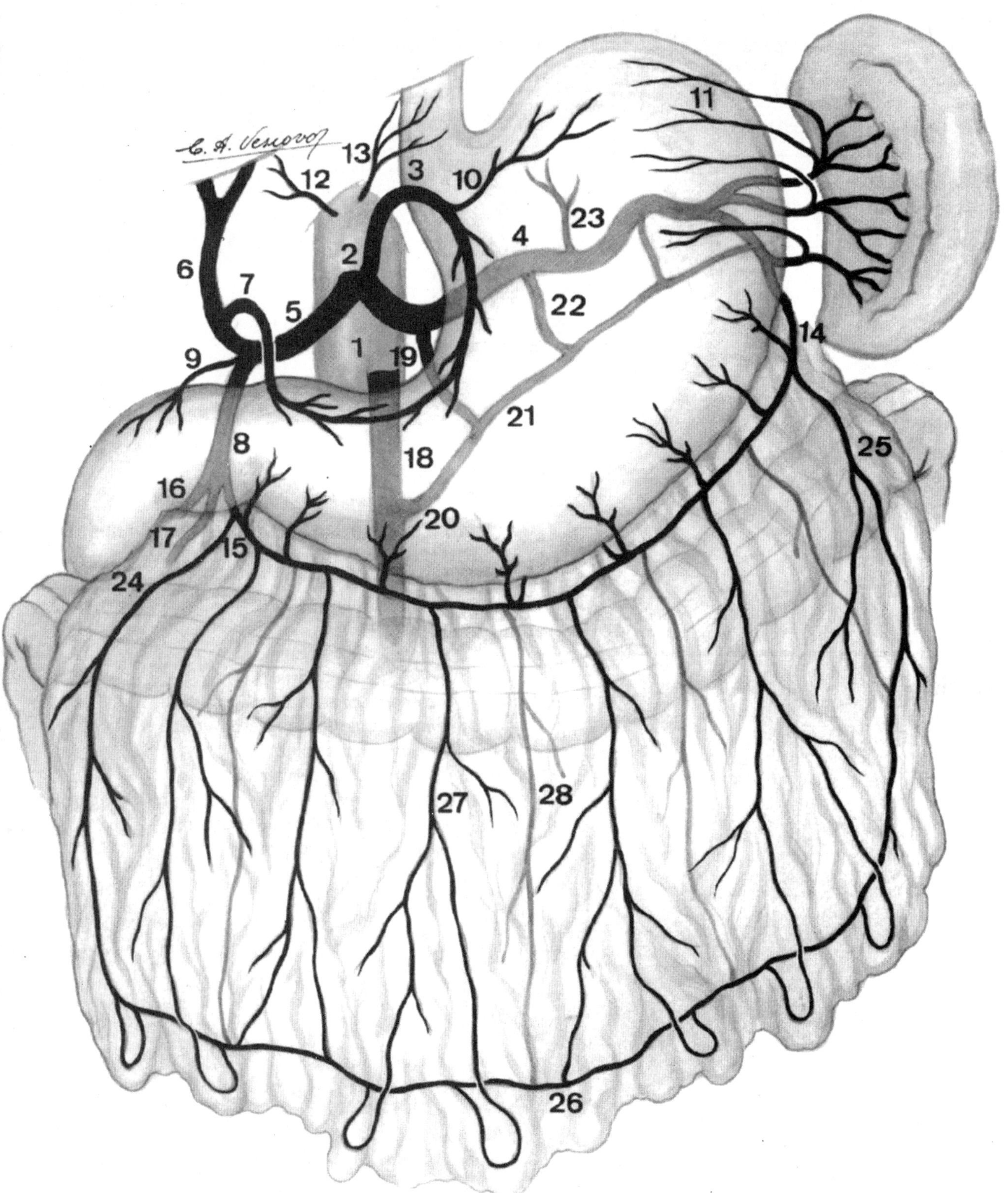

FIGURE 20.1 ARTERIES OF THE STOMACH AND GREATER OMENTUM

FIGURE 20.2 ARTERIES OF THE STOMACH AND DUODENUM

1. Left gastric or coronary artery
2. Hepatic artery
3. Splenic artery
4. Right gastric or pyloric artery
5. Gastroduodenal artery
6. Supraduodenal artery
7. Posterior pancreaticoduodenal arcade
8. Anterior pancreaticoduodenal arcade
9. Superior pancreatic artery
10. Transverse pancreatic artery
11. Gastroduodenal artery after giving off the superior and posterior pancreaticoduodenal artery
12. Right gastroepiploic artery

Arteries

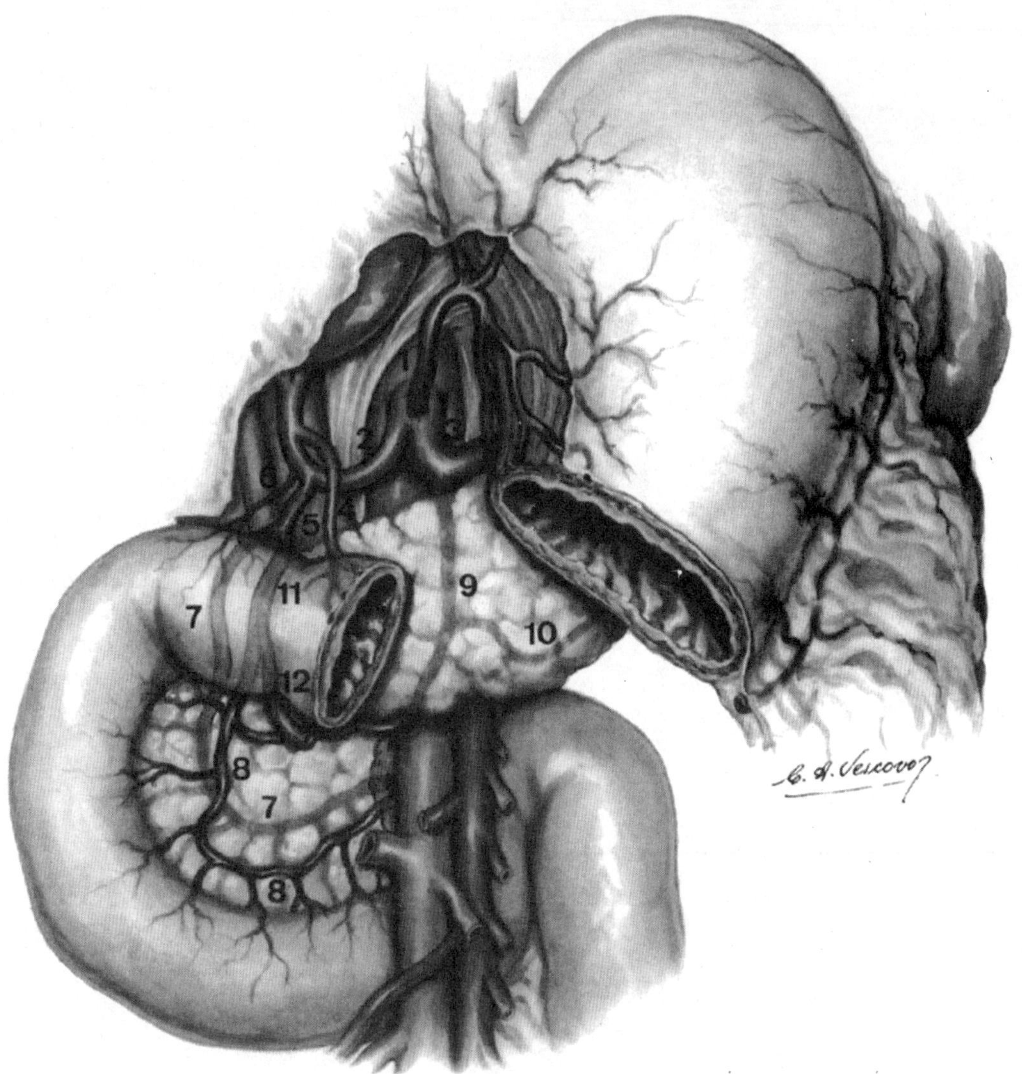

FIGURE 20.2 ARTERIES OF THE STOMACH AND DUODENUM

FIGURE 20.3
The drawing shows a left gastric or coronary artery from which arises an aberrant left hepatic artery (A), which, because of its caliber, appears to be a replacement left hepatic artery that can irrigate all or part of the left lobe of the liver.

The drawing on the right (B) shows a coronary artery from which the left inferior phrenic artery arises. The left inferior phrenic artery normally arises from the aorta immediately above the celiac trunk. The left inferior phrenic artery irrigates a segment of the highest portion of the stomach. In 2% of patients, the left phrenic artery arises, as shown in the drawing, from the coronary artery. Ligature of the coronary artery at its origin from the celiac trunk, in cases of carcinoma of the stomach, may lead to ischemic changes in the gastric remnant, particularly if a splenectomy has also been performed.

Arteries

FIGURE 20.4
In patients with carcinoma of the stomach who have an aberrant replacement left hepatic artery, one should avoid ligating the coronary artery at its origin in the celiac trunk due to the danger of producing necrosis of the left lobe of the liver. In these cases it is advisable to ligate the coronary artery distal to the origin of the aberrant artery, even though the operation may be less radical.

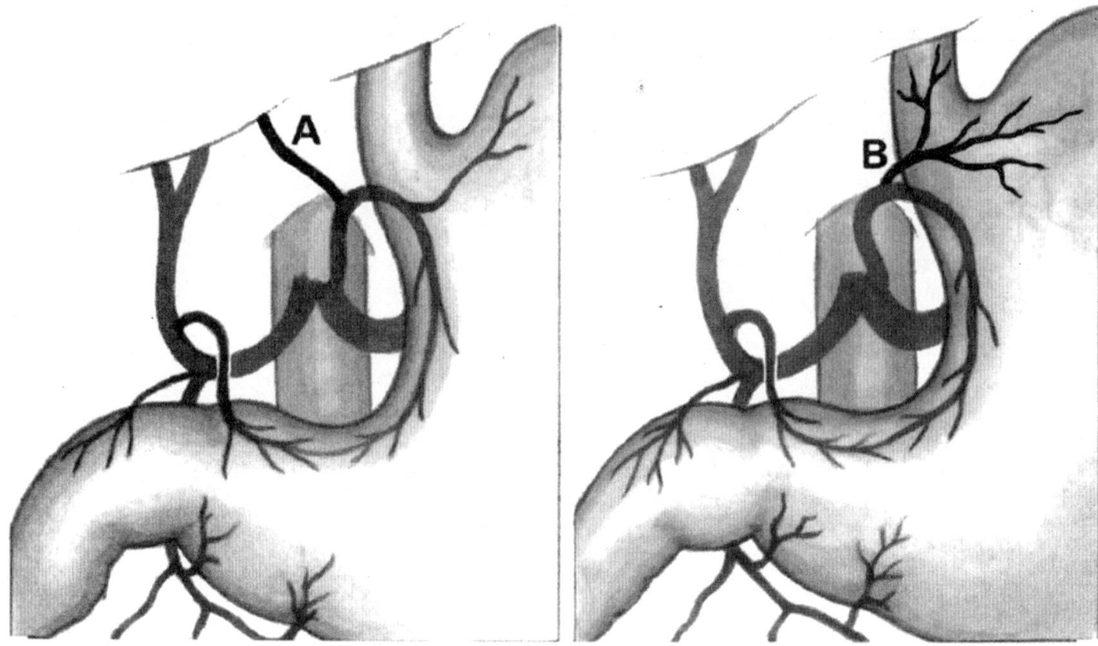

FIGURE 20.3

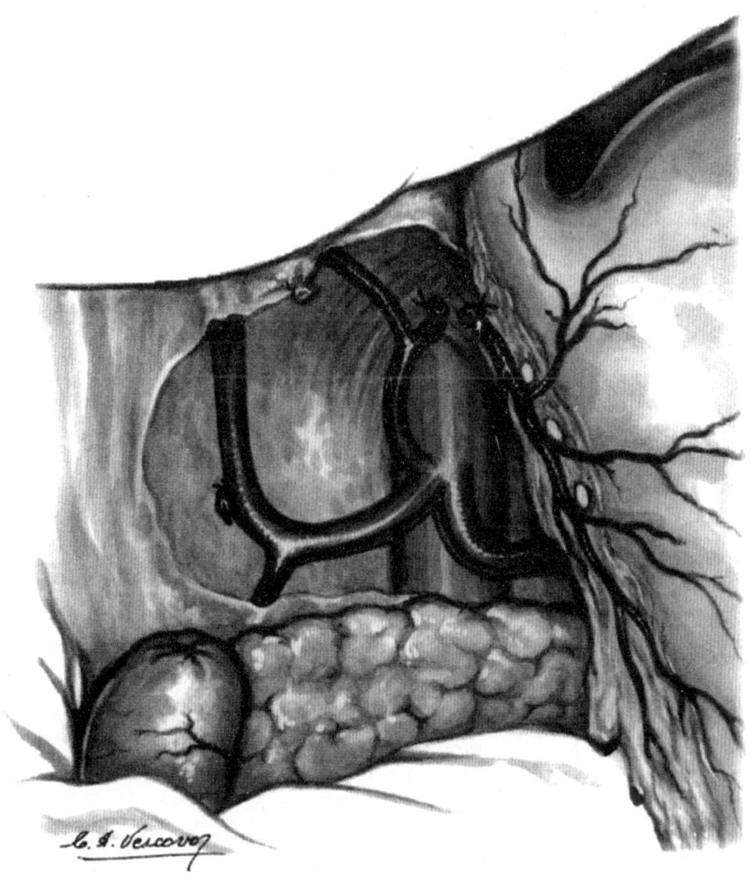

FIGURE 20.4

Arteries

FIGURE 20.5
In gastric resections, especially for duodenal ulcer, the point where the right gastroepiploic artery joins the left is a useful reference point as to the extension of the gastric resection to be carried out. The point of junction may be clearly visible (A), may appear as a narrow area in the gastroepiploic arch (A″), or may appear as if the left and right gastroepiploic arteries do not join (A′).

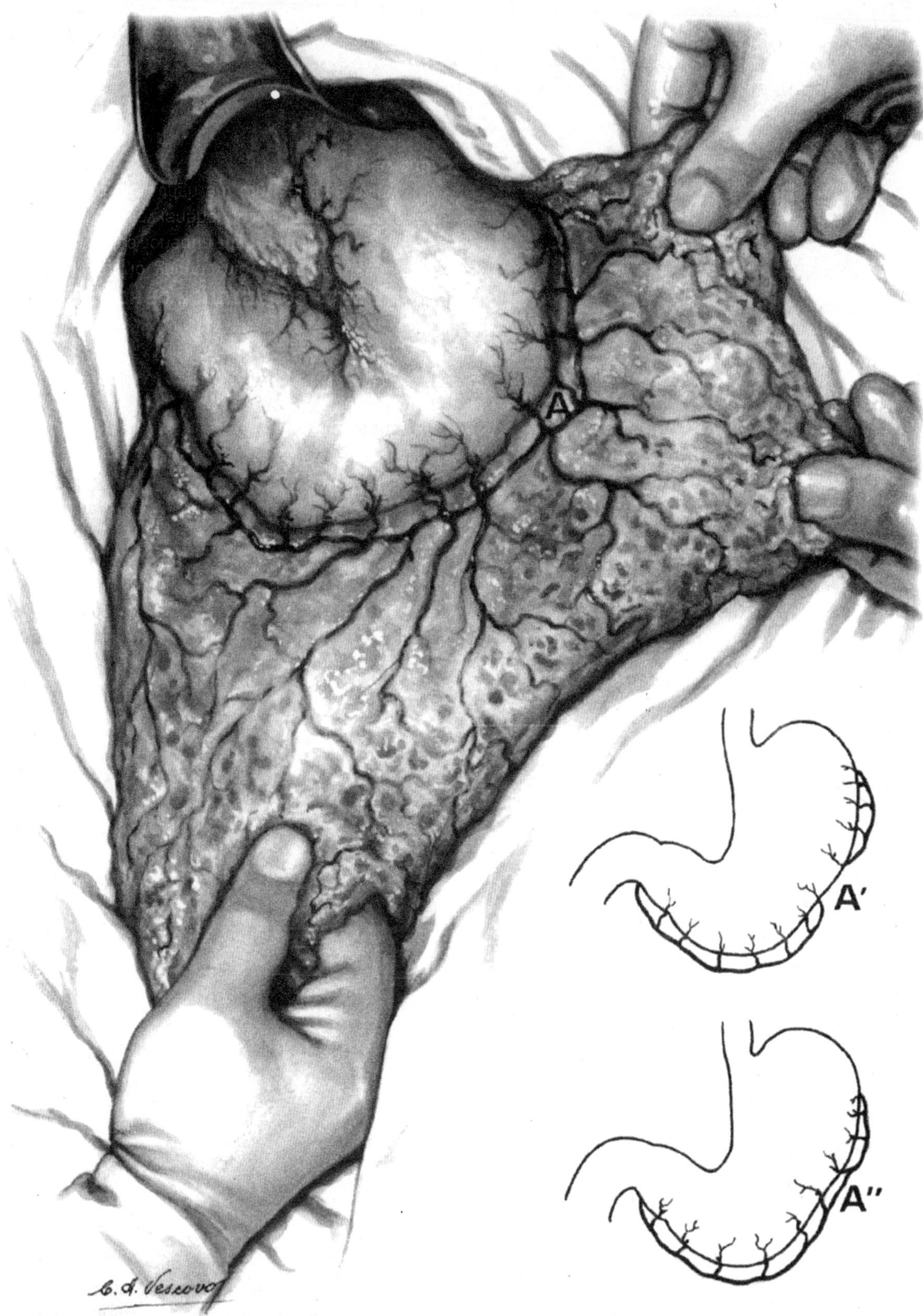

FIGURE 20.5

FIGURE 20.6
The right gastric artery, the left gastric artery, and the gastroepiploic arteries, short vessels, and other minor arteries give off numerous collaterals that irrigate the walls of the stomach, anastomosing extensively between each other within the wall, particularly in the submucosal layer, where a rich net of arterials of a relatively large caliber is formed. The importance of performing careful hemostasis of the vessels in the submucosa is due to these extensive anastomoses, since a small artery that bleeds can lead to the death of the patient even in a simple operation such as a gastrostomy.

Arteries

FIGURE 20.7
Ligation of the coronary artery in gastric resections for carcinoma should be carried out at the artery's exit from the celiac trunk, whereas ligation of the coronary artery in gastric resections for benign lesions of the stomach should be performed when the coronary artery has already entered the lesser curvature. The drawing is with the purpose of showing this difference.

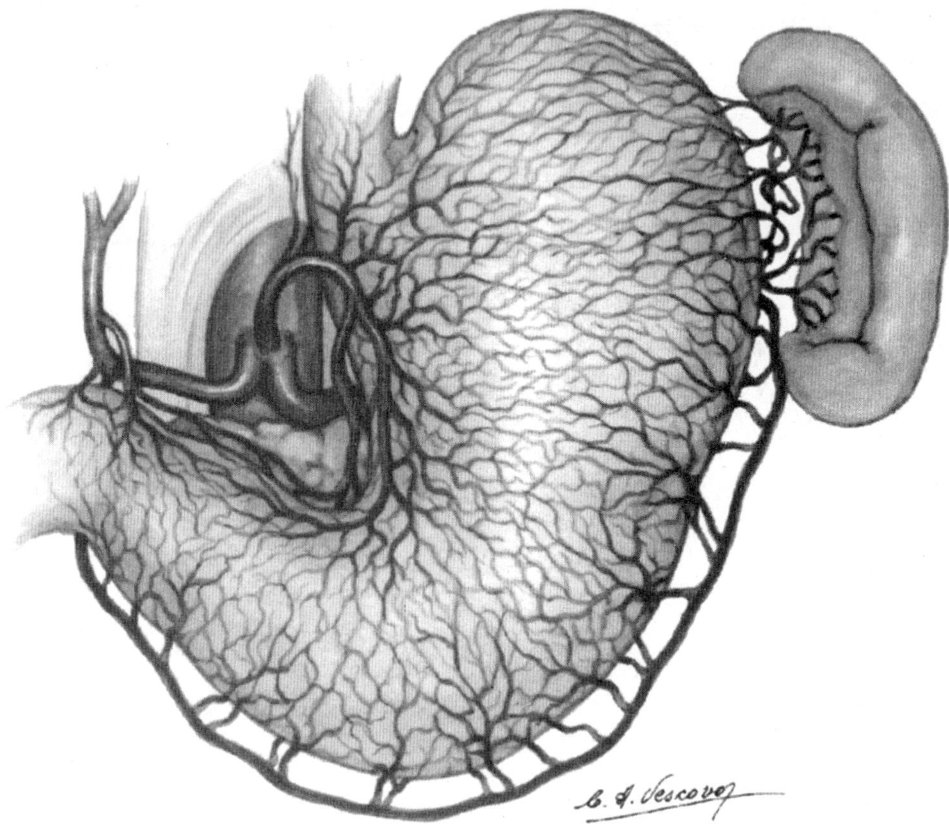

FIGURE 20.6

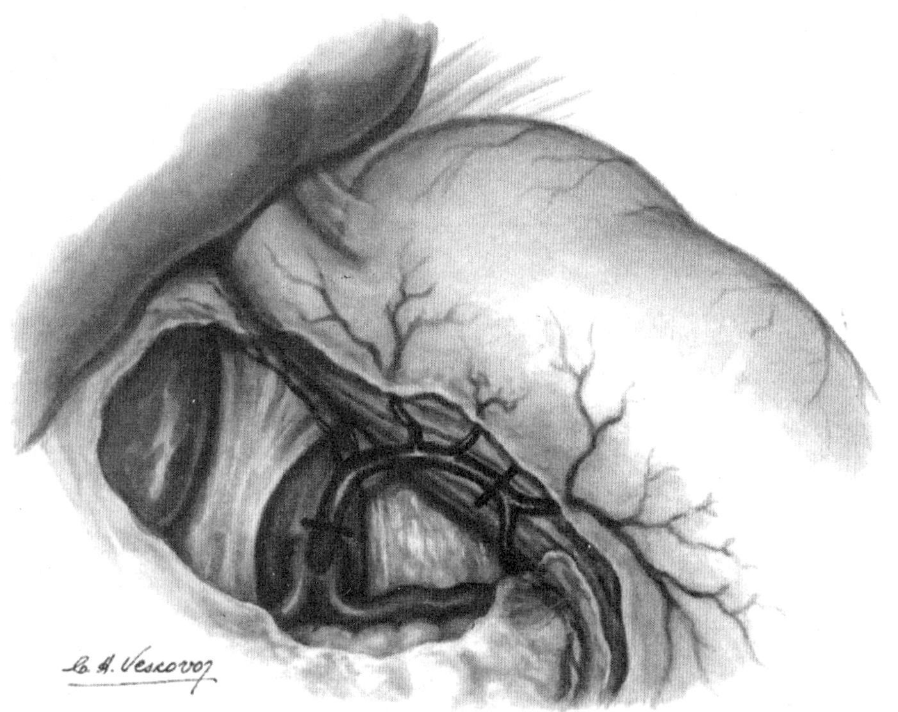

FIGURE 20.7

Arteries

FIGURE 20.8
In order to ligate the coronary artery at its exit from the aorta, it is convenient to lift the stomach upward as shown in the drawing and divide the posterior peritoneum at the level of the celiac trunk. Once the peritoneum has been divided, the coronary vein is found and should be ligated. The surgeon should then proceed to search for the celiac axis, dissect the lymph nodes, and ligate and divide the coronary artery near its origin.

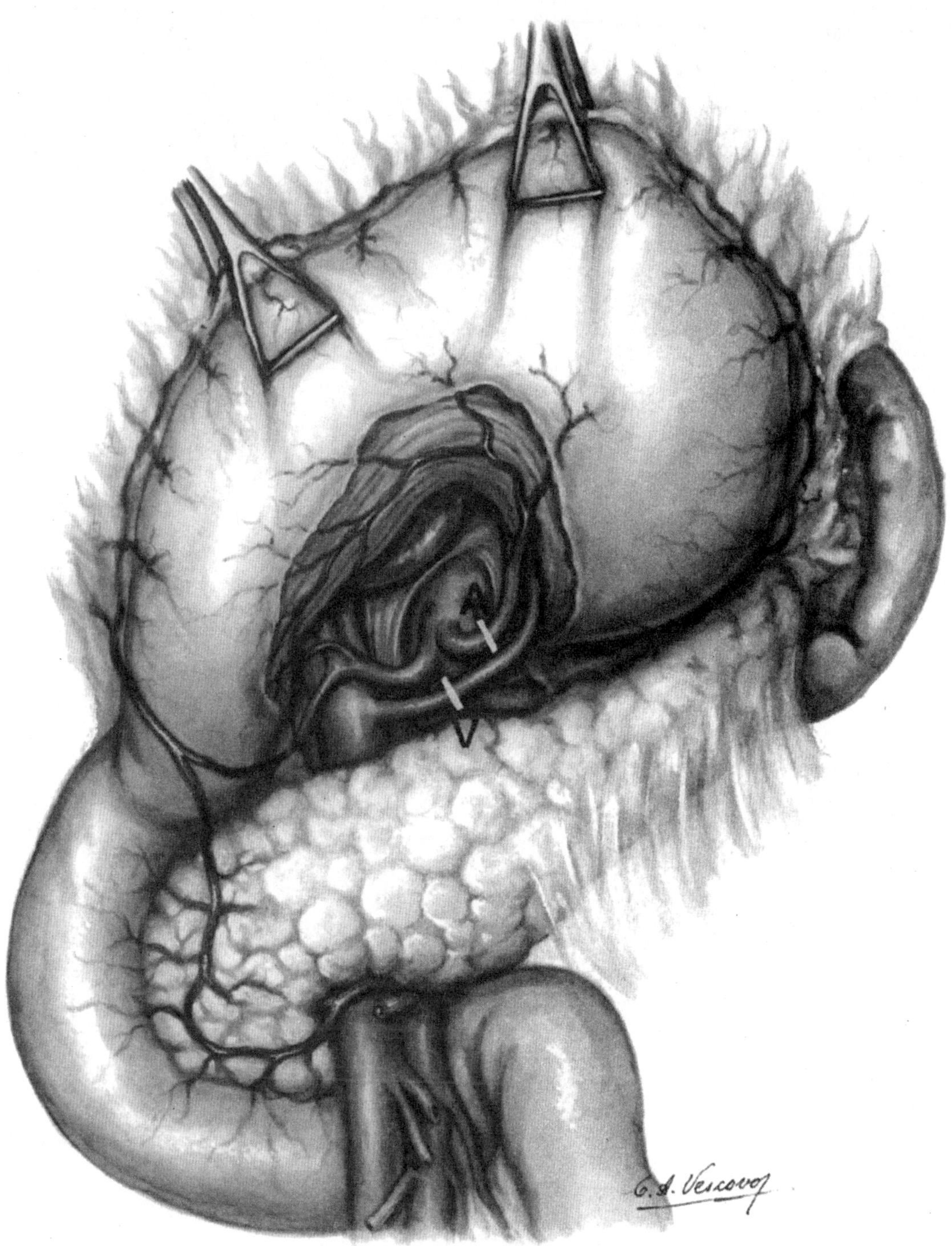

FIGURE 20.8

FIGURE 20.9
The transverse mesocolon is frequently somewhat adherent to the posterior wall of the antrum. In these cases, before ligating the vessels of the greater curvature, it is convenient to completely separate the posterior wall of the antrum to avoid committing the possible mistake of ligating the middle colic artery (CM).

Veins

FIGURE 20.10 VEINS OF THE STOMACH AND DUODENUM

1. Portal vein
2. Superior mesenteric vein
3. Splenic vein
4. Coronary vein
5. Pyloric vein
6. Right gastroepiploic vein
7. Left gastroepiploic vein
8. Inferior mesenteric vein
9. Henle's trunk
10. Anterior pancreaticoduodenal venous arch
11. Posterior pancreaticoduodenal venous arch
12. Right superior colic vein
13. Inferior anterior pancreaticoduodenal vein
14. Inferior posterior pancreaticoduodenal vein
15. Mayo vein

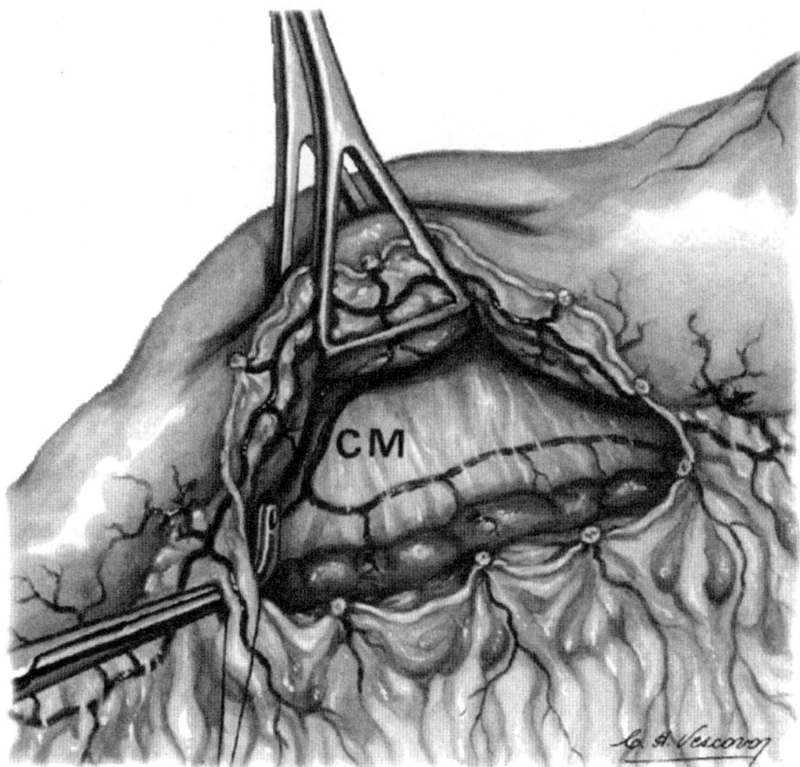

FIGURE 20.9

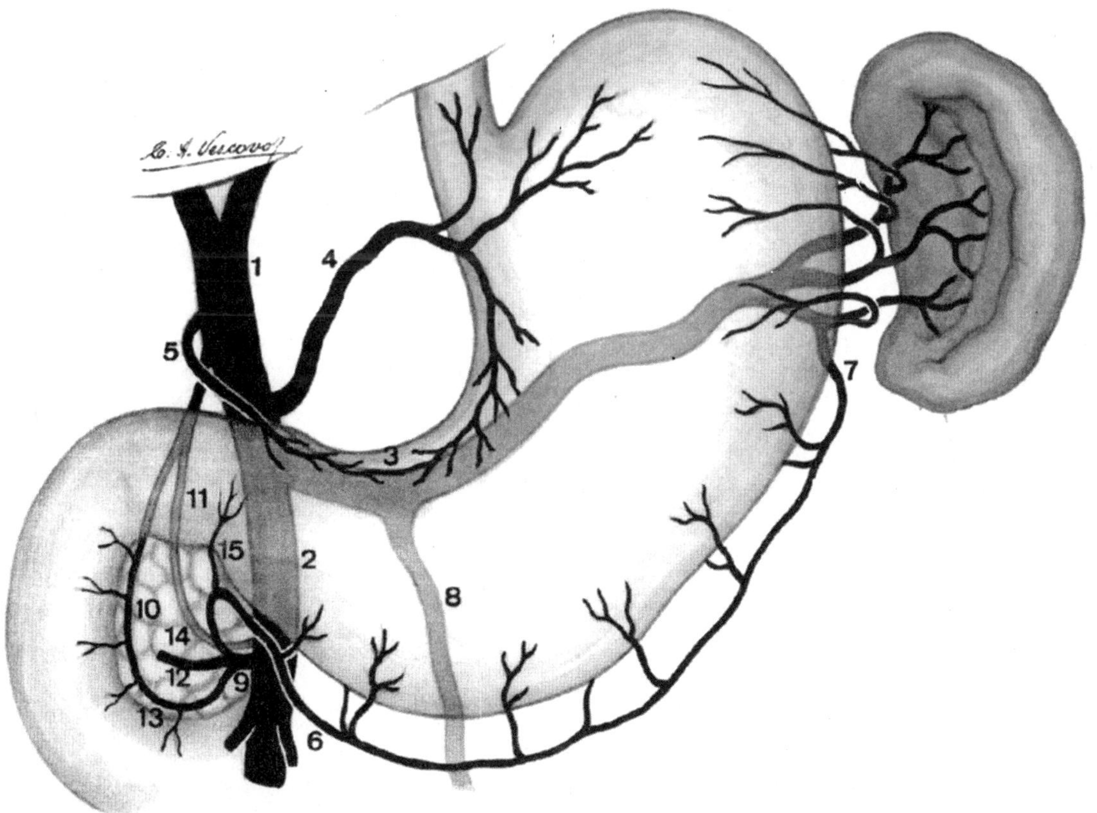

FIGURE 20.10 VEINS OF THE STOMACH AND DUODENUM

Veins

FIGURE 20.11 CONSTITUTION OF HENLE'S VENOUS TRUNK
Right gastroepiploic vein coming off the right gastroepiploic artery (A) to join the right superior colic vein (C) and the inferior anterior pancreaticoduodenal vein (P) to form Henle's trunk (H), which empties into the right edge of the superior mesenteric vein.

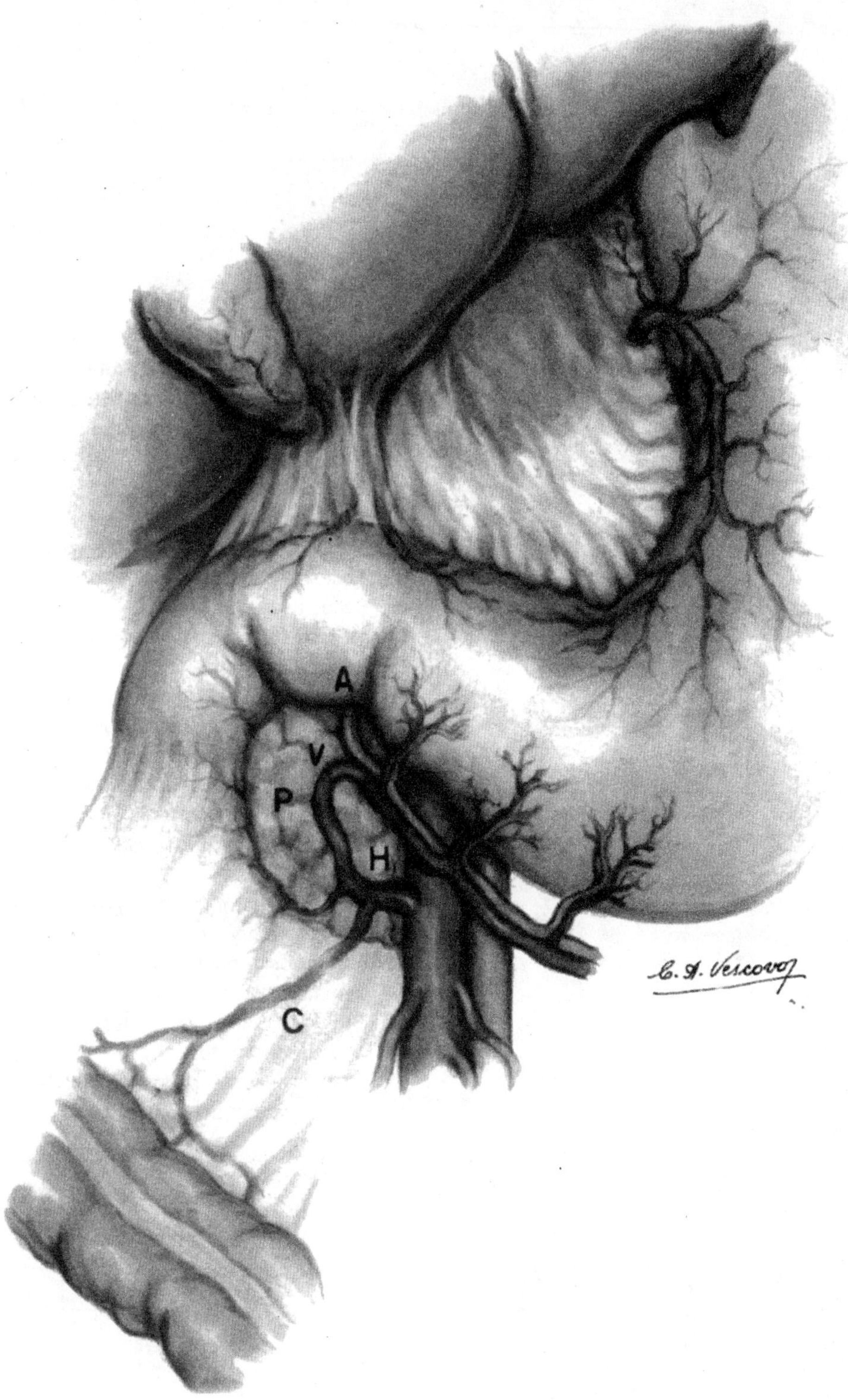

FIGURE 20.11 CONSTITUTION OF HENLE'S VENOUS TRUNK

FIGURE 20.12 LYMPH NODE AREAS AND LYMPH NODE GROUPS OF THE STOMACH (ANTERIOR VIEW)

A. Lymph node area of the coronary or left gastric artery
   Lymph node groups:
   1. Parietal nodes
   2. Cardiac nodes
   3. Nodes of the lesser curvature of the stomach
   4. Nodes of the sickle of the coronary artery
   5. Celiac nodes

B. Lymph node area of the splenic artery
   Lymph node groups:
   6. Nodes of the gastrosplenic ligament
   7. Nodes of the pancreaticosplenic ligament
   8. Nodes of the hilus of the spleen
   9. Nodes of the left gastroepiploic artery
   10. Suprapancreatic nodes

C. Lymph node area of the hepatic artery
   Lymph node groups:
   11. Lymph nodes of the right gastroepiploic artery
   12. Infrapyloric nodes
   13. Retropyloric nodes
   14. Common hepatic artery nodes
   15. Proper hepatic artery nodes
   16. Suprapyloric nodes
   17. Anterior pancreaticoduodenal nodes
   18. Retroduodenal pancreatic nodes

Lymphatics

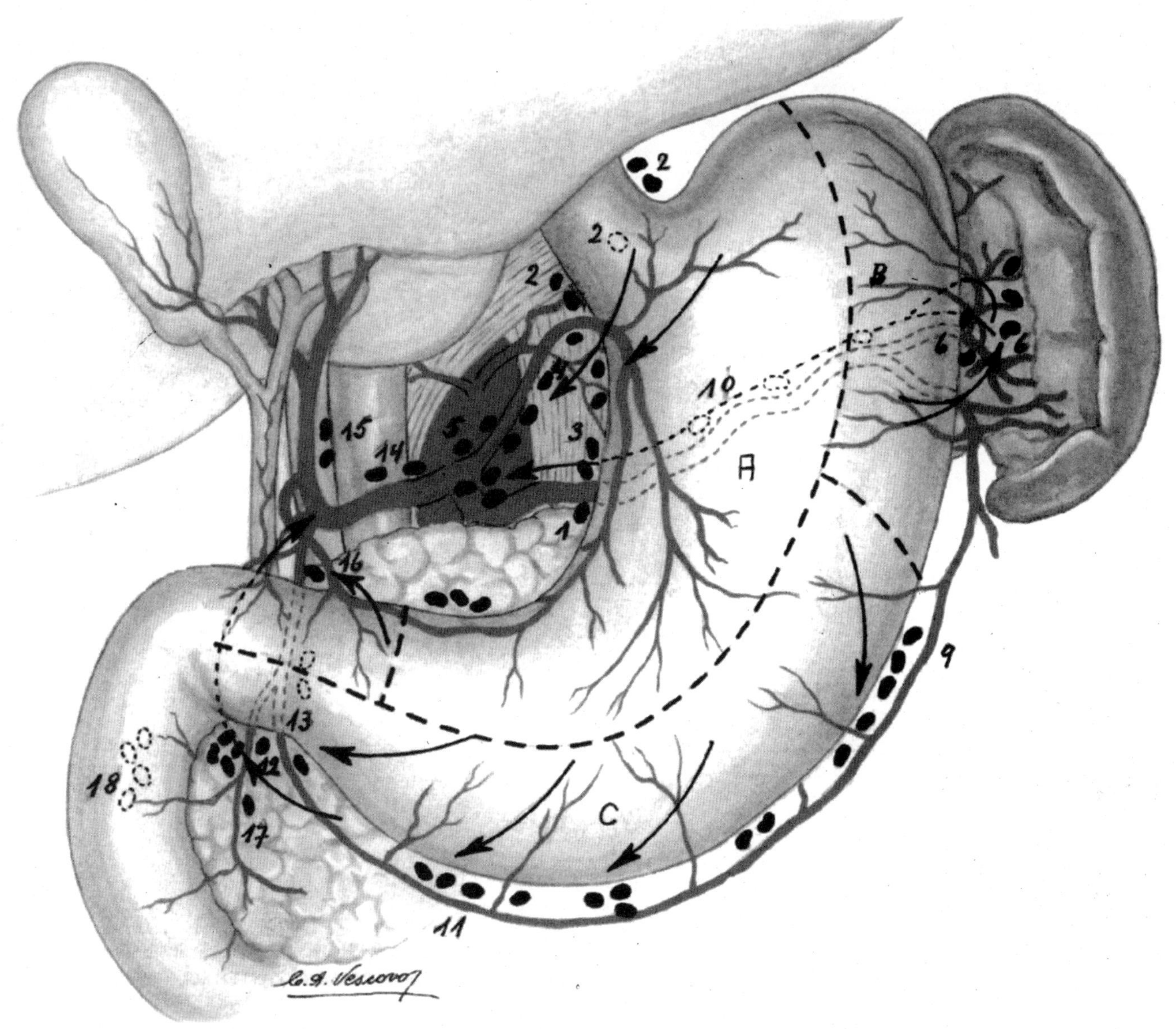

FIGURE 20.12 LYMPH NODE AREAS AND LYMPH NODE GROUPS OF THE STOMACH (ANTERIOR VIEW)

Lymphatics

FIGURE 20.13 LYMPH NODE AREAS AND LYMPH NODE GROUPS OF THE STOMACH (POSTERIOR VIEW)

5. Celiac nodes
7. Pancreaticosplenic ligament nodes
8. Lymph nodes of the hilus of the spleen
10. Suprapancreatic nodes
17. Anterior pancreaticoduodenal nodes
18. Retroduodenal pancreatic nodes
19. Superior mesenteric nodes

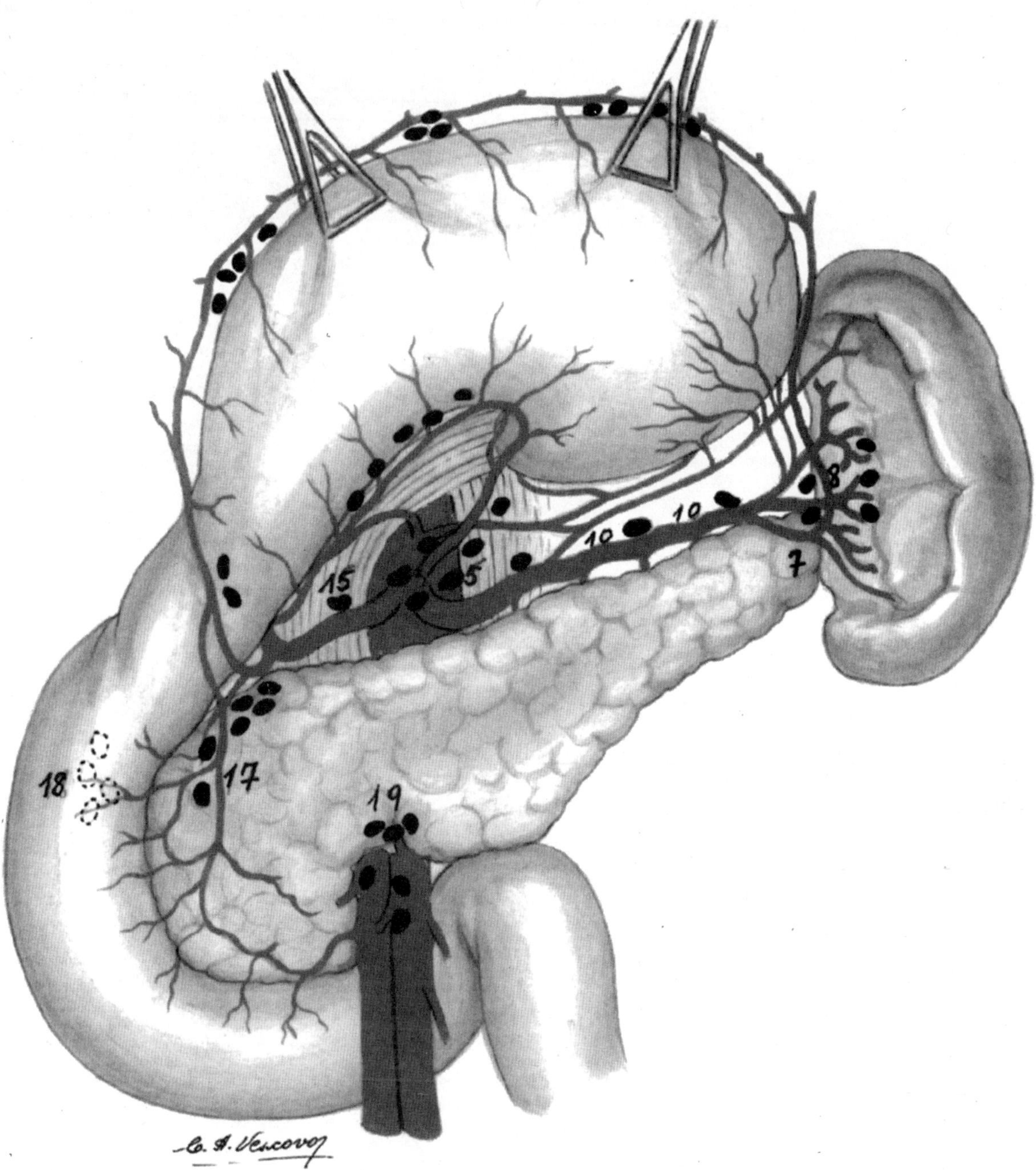

FIGURE 20.13 LYMPH NODE AREAS AND LYMPH NODE GROUPS OF THE STOMACH (POSTERIOR VIEW)

Ligaments

FIGURE 20.14 GENERAL ANTERIOR VIEW OF THE STOMACH WITH ITS LIGAMENTS AND THE GREATER OMENTUM

1. Gastrohepatic ligament
   - A. Pars condensa
   - B. Pars flaccida
   - C. Hepatoduodenal ligament
2. Gastrocolic ligament
3. Greater omentum
4. Gastrosplenic ligament
5. Gastrophrenic ligament
6. Right phrenocolic ligament

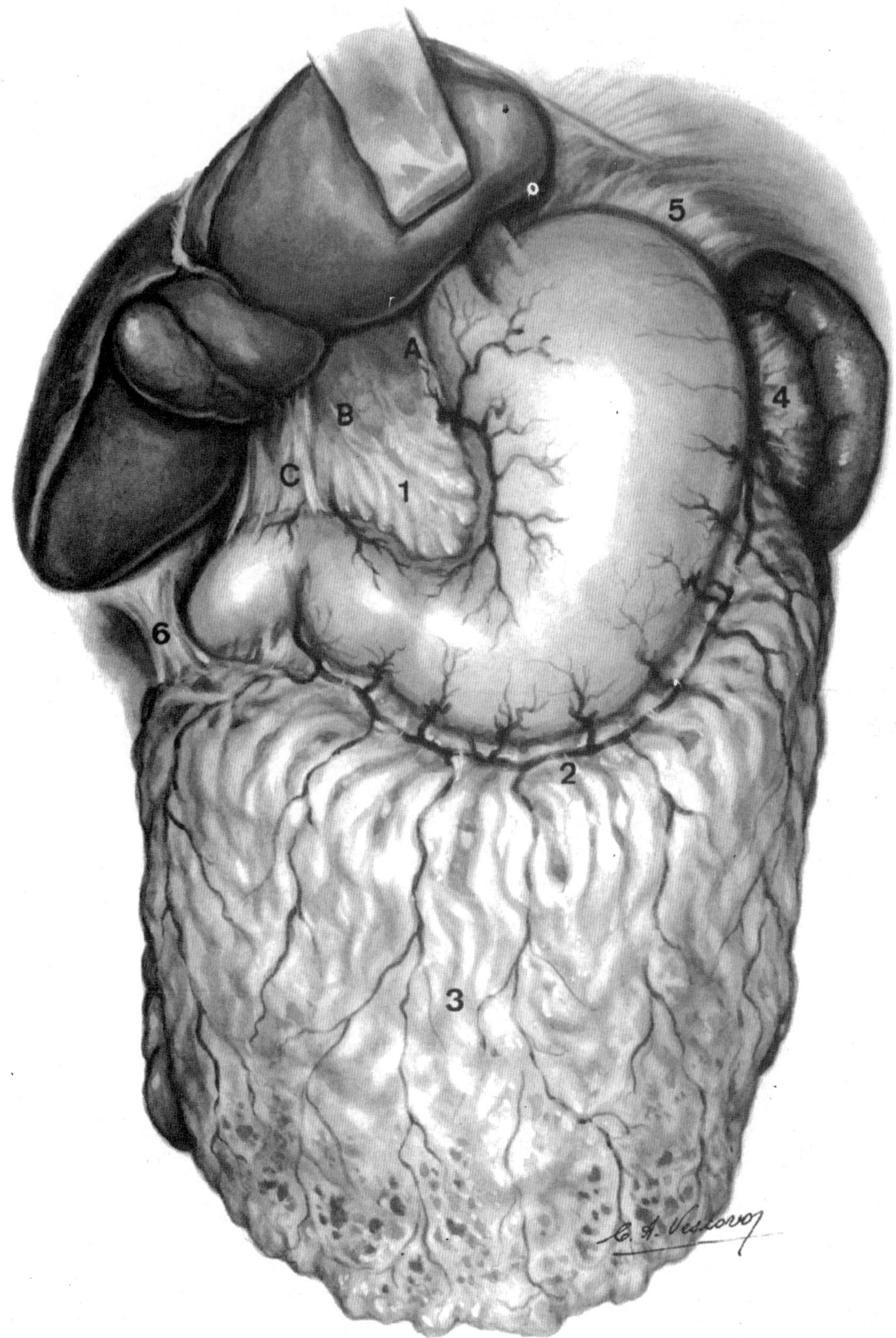

FIGURE 20.14 GENERAL ANTERIOR VIEW OF THE STOMACH WITH ITS LIGAMENTS AND THE GREATER OMENTUM

Ligaments

FIGURE 20.15
To explore the posterior wall of the stomach, it is necessary to enter the lesser sac. To do this, the gastrocolic ligament is divided below the gastroepiploic vascular arcade, at the level of the greater curvature in the region of the body of the stomach, as shown by the broken line.

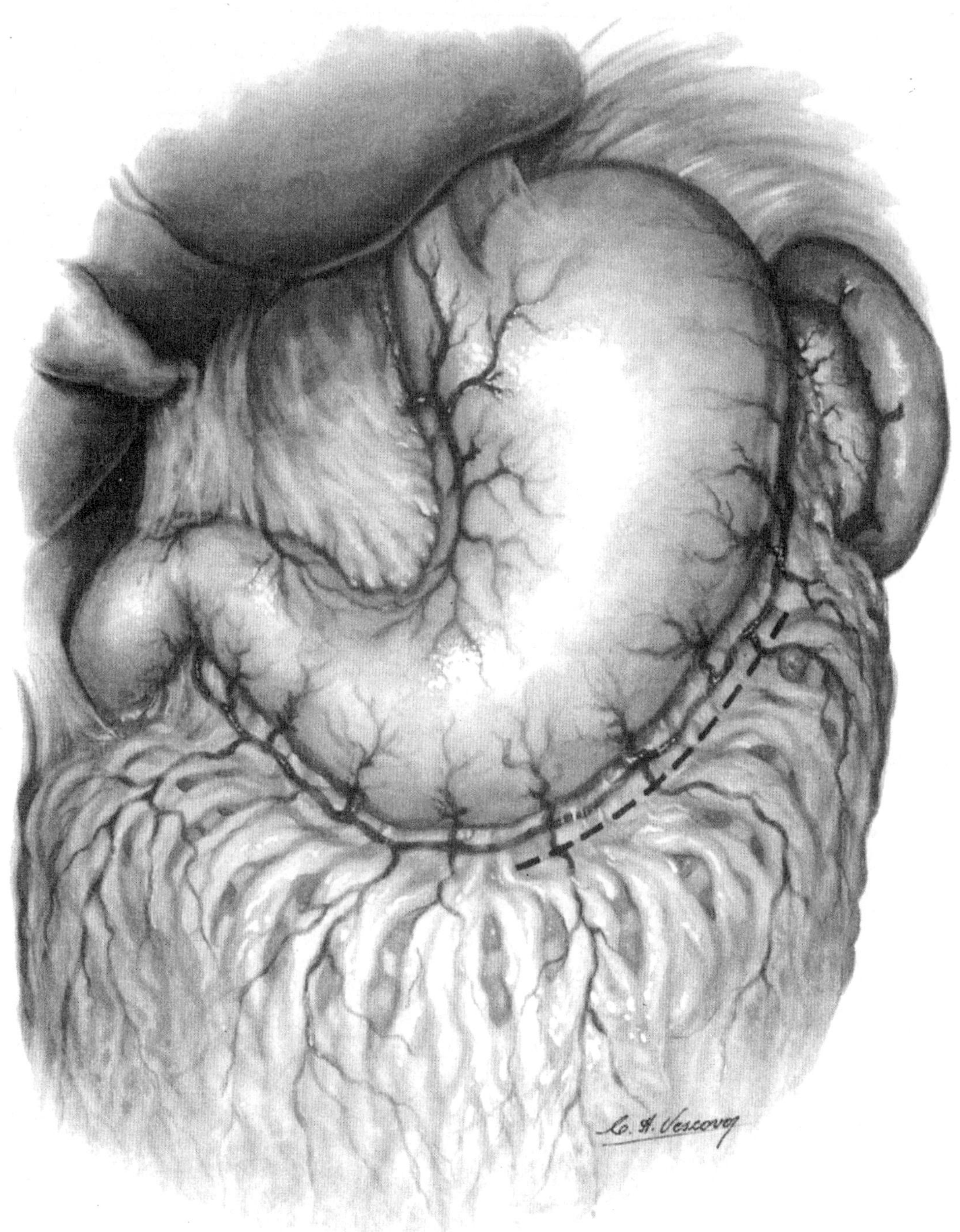

FIGURE 20.15

Ligaments

FIGURE 20.16
The gastrocolic ligament has been divided and exploration of the posterior wall of the stomach is being carried out.

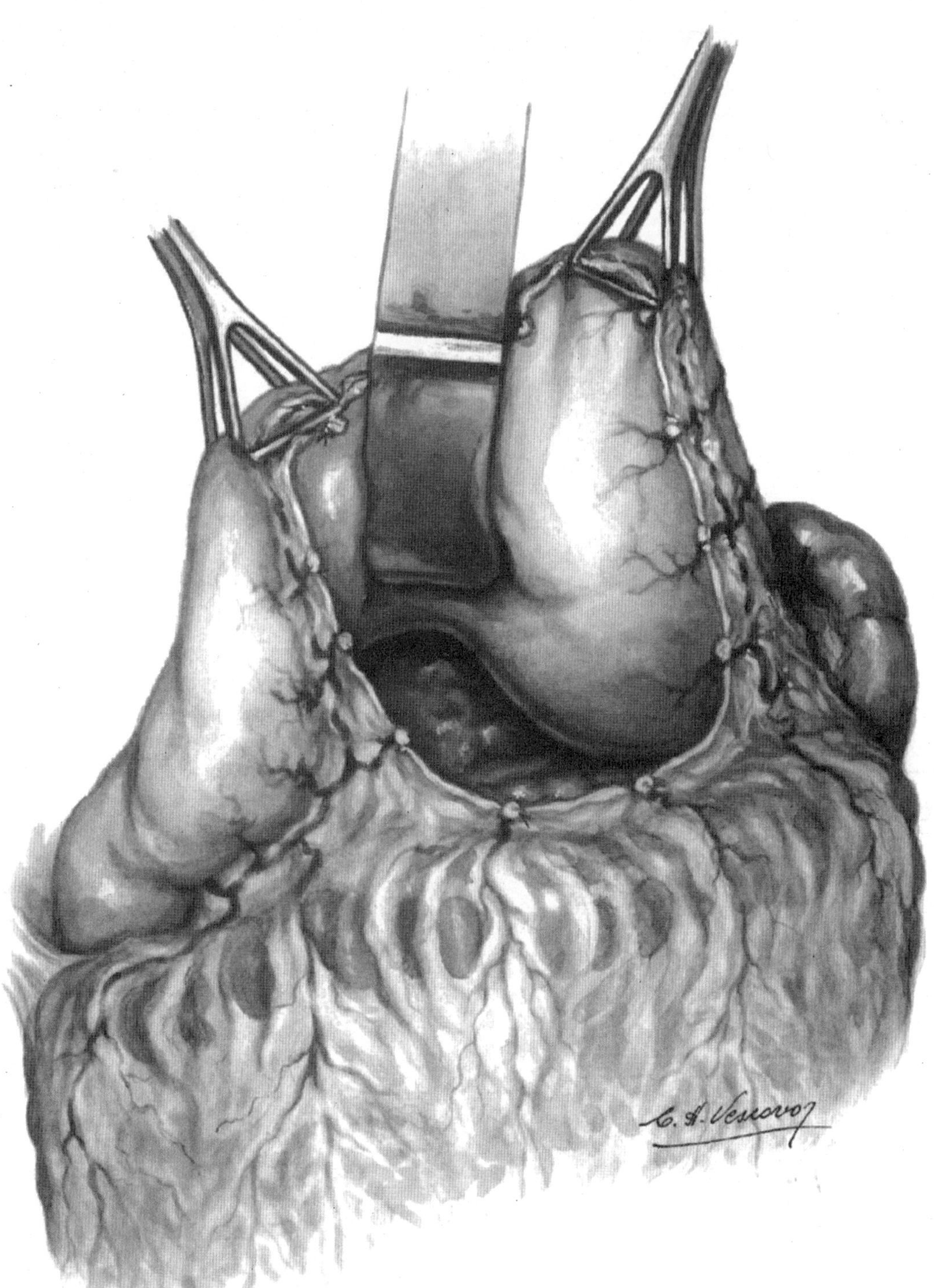

FIGURE 20.16

FIGURE 20.17 SEPARATION OF THE GREATER OMENTUM FROM THE TRANSVERSE COLON

Separation of the greater omentum from the transverse colon can be carried out without any loss of blood. The first assistant applies traction to the omentum upward, using both hands. The second assistant applies traction to the transverse colon downward, also with both hands. The surgeon divides the area of junction of the greater omentum to the transverse colon, which is practically avascular, using scissors. Separation of the greater omentum from the transverse colon is performed from the hepatic flexure to the splenic flexure.

Ligaments

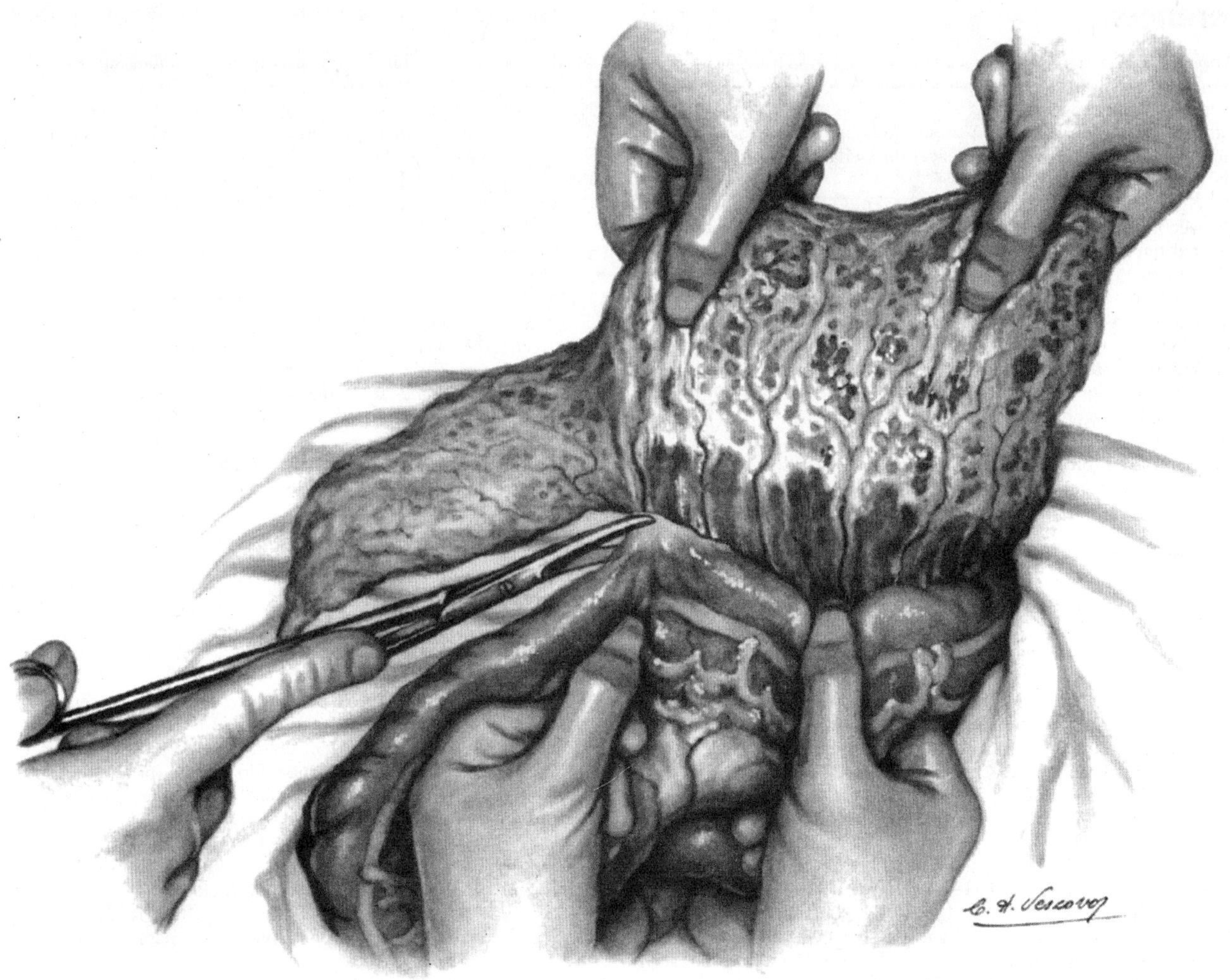

FIGURE 20.17 SEPARATION OF THE GREATER OMENTUM FROM THE TRANSVERSE COLON

References

1. Appleby, L.H. Removal of the celiac axis in gastrectomy for carcinoma of the stomach in selected cases: A ten year assessment. J. Int. Coll. Surg. 34:143, 1960.
2. Arhelger, S.W., Jenson, C.B., Wangensteen, O.H. Dissection of the hepatic pedicle and retropancreaticoduodenal area for cancer of the stomach. Surgery 38:675, 1955.
3. Arhelger, S.W., Jenson, C.B., Wangensteen, O.H. Current status of the second look procedure in the management of the gastrointestinal tract. Proc. Third National Cancer Conference. Lippincott, Philadelphia, 1957.
4. Darlow, T.E., Bentley, F.H., Walder, D.N. Arteries, veins and arteriovenous anastomoses in the human stomach. Surg. Gynecol. Obstet. 93:657, 1951.
5. Becker, H.D., Lierse, W., Schreiber, H.W. Topographic anatomy of stomach and duodenum. In Becher, H.D., Lierse, W., Schreiber, H.W. (Eds.) Surgery of the stomach. P. 1 Springer-Verlag, Berlin, 1986.
6. Brenier, J.L. Du problème ganglionnaire dans la gastrectomie pour cancer. Les curages de l'espace retroduodeno-pancréatique et du pédicule hépatique. J. Chir. 80:3, 1960.
7. Bronn, J.R., Derr, J.W. Arterial blood supply of human stomach. Arch. Surg. 64:616, 1952.
8. Cattell, R.B., Braasch, J.W. A technique for the exposure of the third and fourth portions of the duodenum. Surg. Gynecol. Obstet. 111:378, 1960.
9. Clarke, J.S. Hepatic necrosis following celiac artery ligation during gastric resection in man. Arch. Surg. 71:171, 1955.
10. Coller, F.A., Kay, E.B., McIntyre, R.S. Regional lymphatic metastases of carcinoma of the stomach. Arch. Surg. 43:748, 1941.
11. Corachan, M. Cirugía gástrica. Vol. I, p. 38. Salvat, Barcelona, 1934.
12. Csendes, A., Strauszer, T. Cáncer gastrico. P. 143. Andrés Bello, Santiago de Chile, 1984.
13. Delamère, G., Poirier, P., Cunéo, B. The Lympfatic. Constable and Co., London, 1913.
14. Devin, R., Carcassonne, M., Inglésakis, J. Chirurgie de l'estomac. In Devin, R., Lataste, J., Maillet, P. Nouveau Traité de Tecnique Chirurgicale. Vol. X, p. 196. Masson et Cie. Paris 1968.
15. Fell, S.C., Seindenberg, B., Hurwitt, E.S. Ischemic necrosis of the gastric remnant. An uncommon complication of radical subtotal gastrectomy. Surgery 43:490, 1950.
16. Gray, S.W., Skandalakis, J.E. Atlas of surgical anatomy for general surgeons. P. 110. Williams & Wilkins, Baltimore, 1985.
17. Griffith, C. Anatomy. In Nyhus, L., Wastell, C. (Eds.) Surgery of the stomach and duodenum. Ed. 3, p. 41. Little, Brown, Boston 1977.
18. Haller, A. Tabulae arteriae coeliacae. In Icones anatomicae partes corporis humani. Fasiculus VIII. Gottingae, Vandenhoeck, 1756.
19. Hollinshead, W.H. Anatomy for surgeons. Vol. 2, p. 382 A. Hoeber-Harper, New York, 1956.
20. Jackson, P.P. Ischemic necrosis of the proximal gastric remnant following subtotal gastrectomy. Ann. Surg. 150:1071, 1959.
21. Jaehne, J., Meyer, H.J. Maschek, H., Geerlings, H., Bruns, E., Pichlmayr, R. Lymphadenectomy in gastric carcinoma. Arch. Surg. 127:290, 1992.
22. Jamieson, J.K., Dobson, J.F. The lymphatic system of the stomach. Lancet 1:1061, 1907.
23. Jourdan, M. De la cholédocotomie. G. Steinheil, Paris 1895.
24. Kirschner, P.A., Garlock, J.H. The rationale of routine omentectomy in subtotal gastrectomy. Surgery 36:884, 1954.
25. Kocher, T. Mobilisierung des Duodenum and Gastroduodenostomy. Zentralbl. Chir. 30:34, 1903.
26. Kodama, Y., Sugimachi, K., Soejima, K., Matsusaka, T., Inokuchi, K. Evaluation of extended lymph node dissection for the carcinoma of the stomach. World J. Surg. 5:241, 1981.
27. Latarjet, A. Resection des nerfs de l'estomac. Bull. Acad. Natl. Med. 87:681, 1922.
28. Leriche, R., Villemin, F. Recherches anatomiques sur les artères de l'estomac. Bibl. Anat. 16:111, 1907.
29. Madden, J.L., Kandalaft, S., Eghrari, M. Mobilization of the duodenum: A surgical maneuver incorrectly credited to Kocher. Surgery 63:522, 1968.
30. Marugana, K., Okabayashi, K., Kinoshita, T. Progress in gastric cancer survey in Japan and its limits of radicality. World J. Surg. 11:418, 1987.
31. Michels, N.A. The variational anatomy of the spleen and splenic artery. Am. J. Anat. 70:21, 1942.
32. Michels, N.A. Blood supply and anatomy of the upper abdominal organs. Lippincott, Philadelphia, 1955.
33. Mishima, Y., Hírayama, R. The role of lymph node surgery in gastric cancer. World J. Surg. 11:406, 1987.
34. Okajima, K. Surgical treatment of gastric cancer with special reference to lymph node removal. Acta Med. Okayama 31:369, 1977.
35. Park, K.G.M., Chung, S.C., McGuire, L., Li, A.K.C., Crofts, T.J. Intraoperative assessment of lymph node involvement in gastric carcinoma. Ann. R. Coll. Surg. Engl. 11:127, 1981.
36. Pi-Figueras Badía, J. Fundamentos anatómicos y fisiológicos. In Pi-Figueras, J. Práctica quirúrgica. Ed. 2, vol. II, p. 3. Salvat, Barcelona, 1980.
37. ReMine, W.H., Payne, W.S., van Heerden, J.A. Manual of upper gastrointestinal surgery. P. 61. Springer-Verlag, New York, 1985.
38. Rio-Branco, B. Essai sur l'anatomie et la médicine opératoire du tronc coeliaque et de ses branches. De l'artère hépatique en particulier. G. Steinheil, Paris 1912.
39. Rouvière, H. Anatomy of the human lymphatic system. Edwards Brothers, Ann Arbor, Michigan, 1938.
40. Shapiro, A.L., Robillard, G.L. Morphology and variations of the duodenal vasculature: Relationship to the problem of leakage from a postgastrectomy duodenal stump, bleeding peptic ulcer and injury to the common duct. Arch. Surg. 52:571, 1946.
41. Soga, L., Kobayashi, K. Role of lymphadenectomy in curative surgery for gastric cancer. World J. Surg. 3:701, 1979.
42. Suzuki, K., Prates, J.C., Didio, L.J.A. Incidence and surgical importance of the posterior artery. Ann. Surg. 187:134, 1978.
43. Testus, L. Tratado de anatomía humana. (Spanish translation) vol. 4, p. 141. Salvat, Barcelona, 1923.
44. Testus, L., Jacob, O. Tratado de anatomía topográfica. (Spanish translation) vol. II, p. 105. Salvat, Barcelona, 1923.
45. Testus, L., Latarjet, A. Tratado de anatomía humana. (Spanish translation) ed. 9, vol. 4, p. 184. Salvat, Barcelona 1960.
46. Valdoni, P. Billroth II. Operation. In Cooper, Ph. Vol. II, p. 958. Little, Brown, Boston, 1964.
47. Valdoni, P. Abdominal surgery. An atlas of operative techniques. P. 63. W.B. Saunders, Philadelphia, 1976.
48. Vautrin, A. De l'obstruction calculeuse du cholédoque. Rev. Chir. 16:446, 1896.
49. Walther, A.F. De vena portae. Lipsiae, 1740.
50. Weinberg, J., Greany, E.M. Identification of regional lymph nodes by means of vital staining dye during surgery of gastric cancer. Surg. Gynecol. Obstet. 90:561, 1950.
51. Welch, C. Gastric resection for duodenal ulcer. In Scott, H.W. Jr., Sawyers, J.L. (Eds.) Surgery of the stomach, duodenum and small intestine. Ed. 2, p. 540. Blackwell, Boston, 1992.
52. Wiart, P. Recherches sur l'anatomie chirurgical et voie d'accès du cholédoque. Gynecol. Chir. 3:149, 1899.
53. Wilkie, D.P.D. The blood supply of the duodenum, with special reference to the supraduodenal artery. Surg. Gynecol. Obstet. 13:399, 1911.
54. Zinninger, M.M. Extension of gastric cancer in the intramural lymphatics and its relation to gastrectomy. Am. Surg. 20:920, 1954.

Section E

Hiatus Hernia

CHAPTER **21**

Sliding Hiatal Hernia and Gastroesophageal Reflux

There are two main types of esophageal hiatal hernia:

1. Sliding hiatal hernias
2. Paraesophageal hiatal hernias

The first type is by far the one most frequently seen, comprising 95% of all hiatal hernias. Paraesophageal hiatal hernias make up only 5% of all hiatal hernias. Some paraesophageal hernias develop a sliding component, making up a small group known as mixed or combined hernias.

Sliding hiatal hernias present anatomic characteristics and functional alterations that clearly distinguish them from paraesophageal hernias.

Sliding hiatal hernias are characterized by displacement of the stomach and the esophagogastric junction toward the thorax. Migration of the esophagogastric junction toward the thorax frequently leads to loss of competence of the esophagogastric junction, producing esophagogastric reflux and its frequent complication, reflux esophagitis. Displacement of the stomach into the thorax brings with it the parietal peritoneum of the abdomen in a fashion similar to sliding inguinal hernias. In these hernias one of the walls of the hernial sac is made up by the herniated viscous, the stomach in hiatal hernia, and the colon in inguinal hernia. About 85% of patients with gastroesophageal reflux have sliding hiatal hernias (79). About 15% of patients with hiatal hernia do not suffer from gastroesophageal reflux. There are undoubtedly some individuals who have gastroesophageal reflux without sliding hernia.

In paraesophageal hernias displacement of the stomach into the thorax is not accompanied by displacement of the esophagogastric junction, which remains below the diaphragm, anchored and fixed to the preaortic fascia and the median arcuate ligament. The lack of displacement of the esophagogastric junction into the posterior mediastinum generally does not lead to alteration of the competence of the reflux mechanism as is frequently seen in sliding hiatal hernias.

PHYSIOPATHOLOGIC BASIS OF SURGICAL TREATMENT

The surgeon who undertakes the surgical treatment of a sliding hiatal hernia that is complicated by reflux and esophagitis must have a good knowledge of the physiology of the esophagus and gastroesophageal junction so that he can carry out the correction of the functional alterations with the greatest possible precision. It is logical that anatomic repair of the hernia be carried out simultaneously with correction of the functional alterations. Adequate correction of the functional alterations that frequently accompany sliding hiatal hernias can be carried out as long as these changes are diagnosed and evaluated before surgery. These functional changes may be multiple, of varying importance, and very variable in different patients.

The diagnosis of functional alterations is made by carrying out a complete study of patients with hiatal hernia, reflux, and esophagitis. Besides the clinical history, a well performed radiologic study and an esophagoscopic examination, it is necessary to obtain a 24 hour manometric study with pH monitoring. Esophageal manometry permits the localization of the inferior esophageal sphincter, measurement of its pressure and evaluation of its response to deglutition, measurement of the length of the abdominal esophagus under positive abdominal pressure, and determination of the existence or not of coordination of peristaltic waves as well as the presence of anomalies in the progression of peristaltic waves, excessive contractions, weak waves, and the presence of spasm, nonpropulsive tertiary waves, diffuse spasm, "nutcracker," and so on (7, 46, 47). Alterations found and evaluated before surgery should be corrected during surgery. If correction is not possible, the surgical procedure should be selected that is best adapted to the changes seen in the patient. For example, a patient with strong, well-coordinated peristaltic waves can be successfully treated with a Nissen fundoplication. However, this operation is not advisable in patients with peristaltic disorders, lack of coordination, weak waves, or absence of peristalsis. The severity of peristaltic changes increases in direct relation to the severity of the esophagitis, leading in turn to a deterioration of esophageal clearance (47).

Monitoring of the pH for 24 hours is very useful in identifying the severity of reflux and when it occurs. It also makes possible the identification of slow clearance allowing for correlation of reflux with the symptoms presented by the patient (47).

Before entering into surgical indications in sliding hiatal hernias with reflux and esophagitis, as well as the surgical approaches and more commonly used techniques, a brief description of normal deglutition will be made. We will then refer to causal factors in reflux and esophagitis to facilitate the selection of the best surgical procedure in different situations.

Normal Deglutition

The normal act of deglutition is divided in three stages:

1. Oral stage of deglutition (voluntary)
2. Pharyngeal stage of deglutition (involuntary)
3. Esophageal stage of deglutition

During the oral stage the bolus of food is carried to the posterior part of the mouth, where it is pushed toward the pharynx by the tongue. During the pharyngeal stage the bolus is pushed into the esophagus. Passage of the bolus is assisted by relaxation of the superior esophageal sphincter. Once in the esophagus the bolus produces initiation of a great propulsive peristaltic wave, which carries the bolus of food through the entire esophagus. When the bolus nears the distal third of the esophagus, the inferior esophageal sphincter relaxes, allowing passage of the bolus into the stomach. Once this occurs the inferior esophageal sphincter closes until the next act of deglutition takes place. The peristaltic wave initiated with swallowing is the primary peristaltic wave. There is another peristaltic wave in the esophagus, of less propulsive strength than the previous one, called a secondary wave, which is not initiated with deglutition but takes place when there is reflux of gastric content into the esophagus or when there are food remnants in the esophagus after deglutition. In synthesis, deglutition gives origin to the primary wave. This primary wave takes place simply swallowing saliva. When gastroesophageal reflux takes place the secondary peristaltic wave originates with the purpose of clearing the esophagus.

A normal fasting person swallows saliva about 70 times per hour (21, 46). During meals swallowing can take place 180 to 200 times. During sleep swallowing of saliva diminishes considerably. During deep sleep there is practically no swallowing of saliva, and during light sleep only 7 to 8 deglutitions of saliva occur every hour. As said previously, swallowing of saliva is very important in clearing the esophagus by provoking a primary peristaltic wave of excellent propulsive power. In addition the swallowing of saliva makes saliva neutralize acid reflux, though only slightly.

Gastroesophageal Reflux

The lower esophageal sphincter (LES) constitutes the most important antigastroesophagic reflux barrier. This inferior esophageal sphincter is normally closed, opening when a primary peristaltic wave is near. The sphincter opens from below upward and closes from above downward. This sphincter is a physiologic sphincter, since up to the present nobody using optical, or electronic microscopy has shown conclusively, either in humans or primates, qualitative differences between the muscular fibers of the sphincter and the rest of the smooth muscle fibers of the esophagus (91, 93). It is accepted that the sphincter is kept closed while at rest under the control of myogenic and neurogenic stimuli modulated by neural and hormonal factors (21, 47, 89, 90, 95). The pressure of the inferior esophageal sphincter is greater than the pressure of the stomach and greater than the pressure of the segment of esophagus immediately above it.

The inferior esophageal sphincter corresponds to the high pressure zone of the esophagus (HPZ) (33). This zone is located below the phrenoesophageal membrane. The normal pressure of the lower esophageal sphincter varies between 8 and 25 mm Hg. Some authors give slightly different figures. If the pressure of the inferior esophageal sphincter is over 30 mm Hg one should suspect that the sphincter is hypertonic (47). When the pressure is below 8 mm Hg the presence of reflux should be suspected. This value is not absolutely certain, however, since some people with a pressure lower than 8 mm Hg do not show reflux. It is more probable that reflux exists if the pressure of the lower esophageal sphincter is lower than 5 mm Hg.

The lower esophageal sphincter is normally 2 to 3 cm long under the action of positive abdominal pressure, which in some cases may reach 4 cm or more. People with a lower esophageal sphincter less than 1 cm long under the action of positive abdominal pressure are believed to have an incomplete sphincter. When the total length of the lower esophageal sphincter is less than 2 cm it should be considered to be incompetent (20–23, 47, 89–93). The lower esophageal sphincter should be considered mechanically deficient when it presents the following alterations (21, 22, 24, 47):

1. Manometric pressure below 5 mm Hg.
2. Less than 1 cm long under positive abdominal pressure.
3. The total length of the esophageal segment within the abdomen is less than 2 cm.

Patients showing the above figures have a great probability of gastroesophageal reflux, and it is important to point out that these patients have little probability of improving with medical treatment (47). Patients with these conditions have an intragastric pressure higher than that of the inferior esophageal sphincter, favoring reflux (47). In some patients a low pressure in the sphincter may be compensated for by a sphincter over 4 cm long (25, 47). On the other hand, if the length of the lower esophageal sphincter exposed to positive abdominal pressure is less than 1 cm, it can be compensated for if the sphincter pressure is elevated (47). When surgery for sliding hiatal hernia with reflux is performed correctly, the minimal length that can be generally given to the abdominal esophagus is between 3 and 4 cm, and very frequently between 5 and 7 cm (45, 46). It has been shown that even though the presence of the sphincter may be normal, cyclic relaxations may take place in some individuals frequently enough to lead to gastroesophageal reflux and reflux esophagitis, which may occasionally be very severe in spite of normal manometric pressure readings in the lower esophageal sphincter.

The action of the positive intraabdominal pressure has its basis in the law of the Marquis de Laplace: "If a similar pressure is exerted on two tubes, one of large diameter and the other of small diameter, the first one to collapse is the tube with the smaller diameter." Positive intraabdominal pressure contributes very efficiently to reinforce the antireflux barrier (45, 46, 47). The level of insertion in the esophagus of the phrenoesophageal ligament is of great importance, since the zone of high pressure of the esophagus is located below the insertion of this membrane. It is in these 2 to 3 cm of esophagus located below the insertion of the phrenoesophageal ligament that the main antireflux barrier resides. For this reason people with a high insertion of the phrenoesophageal membrane have a greater manometric pressure in the esophagus, because the entire extension of the esophagus is within the membrane and exposed to the positive pressure of the abdomen. In people with a lower insertion of the phrenoesophageal membrane, the action of the positive abdominal pressure will be less. It is presumed that a sliding hiatal hernia without reflux is due to a higher insertion of the phrenoesophageal membrane. On the other hand, in cases of low insertion of the phrenoesophageal ligament, even in people without sliding hernia of the hiatus, there is a greater possibility of reflux (5, 6, 21, 23, 25, 47).

In cases in which the esophagus is replaced by a segment of small bowel, colon, or a gastric tube constructed from the greater curvature of the stomach, the positive pressure in the abdomen may have the same efficiency in controlling reflux as long as a segment of a certain length is located within the abdominal cavity (35, 61, 77, 92, 104).

Even though the oblique muscular fibers of the internal

layer of the stomach were described in 1731 by Thomas Willis, it is only recently that attention to their function has been given. These oblique muscular fibers have been compared to a collar, a tie (Swiss tie), or a sling, which upon contracting, makes the esophagogastric angle of His more acute. As the sling contracts, a gastroesophageal valve forms in the stomach, constituted by a muscular layer and a mucosal layer (46), which, resting upon the higher portion of the lesser curvature of the stomach, contributes to a greater sufficiency of the closure brought about by the lower esophageal sphincter (29, 30, 34, 46, 55, 56, 74, 101). Lucius Hill and his collaborators (46) have been able to prove this theory by the introduction of a gastroscope through a gastrostomy, which has allowed them to have a retrograde view of the closing and opening of the gastroesophageal valve. It has also been proven that when the sling contracts, in addition to developing the gastroesophageal valve, the intraabdominal esophagus becomes longer, contributing to increase the antireflux barrier (46). In 1951 Allison (1) affirmed that when the sling contracts, it produces an angulation of the esophagogastric junction in a form similar to the action of the puborectalis muscle, whose contraction produces a marked angulation of the rectum, favoring continence. Ellis and Olsen (30) had observed in 1969 that in patients subjected to a modified Heller procedure in cases of achalasia of the esophagus, if the incision of the muscular layers of the esophagus were extended to the stomach, cutting the fibers of the sling, gastroesophageal reflux would frequently originate postoperatively, whereas if only the esophageal fibers were transected, the development of gastroesophageal reflux was very rare.

Numerous investigations have been performed concerning the action of the sling and its importance in the closure of the esophagogastric junction (3, 5, 6, 34, 46, 47, 55, 56, 58, 87, 101). Siewert was able to prove that the muscular fibers of the sling contract and relax synchronously with the contractions and relaxations of the lower esophageal sphincter. This has great practical importance in its application to surgical procedures most frequently undertaken to correct gastroesophageal reflux. An example of this is the Nissen fundoplasty technique. The gastric wrapping that is performed around the lower esophagus should include only the gastric fundus. If, in this gastroplasty, more than the gastric fundus is used, such as part of the gastric body, it is probable that dysphagia will develop postoperatively (see Nissen technique), due to the fibers of the gastric body which do not relax synchronously with the lower esophageal sphincter during the act of swallowing as do the muscular fibers of the fundus (25, 58).

Reflux Esophagitis

Reflux esophagitis can be defined as a chemical inflammation of the esophageal mucosa produced by reflux material, gastric or duodenal (6). Reflux esophagitis is a complication of gastroesophageal reflux. This does not mean that all people with gastroesophageal reflux must suffer from esophagitis. On the other hand, the degree of inflammation of the esophageal mucosa differs from one person to the other in relation to aggressive factors and the resistance of the mucosa, as well as other still unknown factors (29). In addition, it is possible to find severe esophagitis in individuals who are absolutely asymptomatic. The magnitude of the esophageal lesions may be very mild or even not visible during esophagoscopy, when they can only be established by aspiration biopsy (49), or very severe, associated with fibrous stricture, ulcer, or a Barrett type of esophagus.

Several factors influence the origin, evolution, and severity of reflux esophagitis, some of which follow.

1. Frequency of reflux (6, 7)

   The insult to the esophageal mucosa is undoubtedly greater when reflux is more frequent. There are, however, exceptions. There are patients who have infrequent reflux but who develop severe esophagitis. On the other hand, patients with frequent reflux may not suffer changes of the esophageal epithelium.
2. Volume of refluxed material

   The greater the volume of gastric material that refluxes, the greater the damage to the esophageal mucosa, though numerous exceptions may occur. When the volume of reflux material is abundant, it will take longer to clear the esophagus, making the insult on the esophageal mucosa greater. The volume of refluxed gastric material may be related to a functional or organic change in the stomach.
3. Duration of contact of refluxed material with the esophageal mucosa

   The greater the duration of contact of the refluxed material with the esophageal mucosa, the greater the possibilities of producing esophagitis. The three factors that have been pointed out—greater frequency, greater volume, and greater duration of reflux—are present more frequently and generally simultaneously in patients with a mechanical deficiency of the lower esophageal sphincter (21, 25, 47). The sum of these three factors generally leads to an aggravation of the esophageal lesions.
4. Composition of refluxed material

   The degree of aggressiveness of the refluxed material is directly related to its composition. This is the way that hydrochloric acid exerts an aggressive action on the esophageal mucosa, but this aggressiveness increases greatly and becomes corrosive in the presence of pepsin and a pH less than 2.0 (27, 36). Bile and trypsin are very aggressive elements when they act on the esophageal mucosa (38, 51, 53, 85). It is not correct to designate esophagitis as alkaline when bile and trypsin are found in the reflux material because it has been shown that it is not alkalinity that is the important factor, but the aggressiveness of the reflux material, which can act upon an acid or neutral medium (7). Unconjugated biliary salts, be they taurocholic or glycocholic acids, combined with trypsin, may lead to very severe lesions of the esophageal mucosa in a neutral pH (27, 38, 51, 53). On the other hand, conjugated biliary salts have a corrosive action with an acid pH (10, 38, 53, 57). A mixture of hydrochloric acid and pepsin with conjugated biliary salts (taurocholic or glycocholic) has a destructive effect upon the esophageal mucosa. An acid pH and conjugated biliary salts increase the diffusion of the hydrogen ion through the esophageal mucosa (27, 32, 38, 78, 81). Reflux of bile and trypsin is generally secondary to a gastric operation or to duodenal gastroesophageal reflux, alterations that should be corrected with an antireflux operation.

5. Importance of Esophageal Clearance

In people with normal physiologic esophagus, when gastroesophageal reflux occurs, mechanisms immediately come into play to protect the esophagus from the insult. Secondary peristaltic waves appear, which are originated by the reflux itself to produce esophageal clearance. Other factors, such as the action of gravity, come into play. An upright position favors clearance of the esophagus, whereas a lying down position slows up clearance. Other factors such as salivation provoking the development of primary waves contribute very efficiently to clearance of the esophagus. Alterations of esophageal motility can notoriously affect esophageal clearance. Motor deficiencies may precede the appearance of reflux but are more frequent as the esophagitis provoked by the reflux develops, notably affecting the power of the esophagus to clear itself and making the insult on the esophagus more serious. It is a common observation that patients who have esophagitis complicated by fibrotic stricture or Barrett esophagus present a very altered motor activity of the esophagus. On the other hand, patients who have normal motor activity of the esophagus with a capacity to clear effectively may compensate for a mechanical deficiency of the lower esophageal sphincter. But in those patients in whom motor deficiency of the esophagus coexists with a mechanical deficiency of the lower esophageal sphincter with its serious consequences, an aggravation of the esophagitis will inevitably occur and surgical correction will frequently be necessary (47).

It has been shown that motor alterations of the esophagus can be produced by the simple migration of the lower esophageal sphincter into the thorax. Some cases of problems with esophageal motility may be due to the lack of fixation of the gastroesophageal junction in the abdomen, as if there were no point of support. In these cases, altered motility disappears when the esophagogastric junction is lowered and fixed to the preaortic fascia and the arcuate ligament below the diaphragm (46). It should be pointed out that there are patients with dysphagia that is not due to an esophageal stricture due to esophagitis but to the presence of a motor deficiency of the esophagus. The selection of the surgical procedure to be used in the presence of motor alterations of the esophagus has great importance.

6. Resistance of Esophageal Mucosa to Reflux

The resistance of esophageal mucosa to reflux varies greatly among different individuals. This fact has still not been understood. As affirmed by Donahue (29), several points in gastroesophageal reflux and esophagitis remain a mystery.

7. Alterations in Gastric Emptying

Functional or organic alterations of the stomach can lead to the production of gastroesophageal reflux even in the presence of a lower esophageal sphincter that is normal in function. Some of the gastric alterations that can lead to reflux are dilation of the stomach, alterations in gastric emptying, Zollinger-Ellison syndrome, duodenogastric reflux, delay in gastric emptying due to neuromuscular alterations, vagotomy, duodenal dysfunction, and so on.

Patients with sliding hiatal hernia usually swallow saliva very frequently. It has been shown that with each swallowing of saliva, 1 to 2 mL of air (47) enter into the stomach, which can lead to a great dilation of the stomach by air (aerophagia). This great dilation of the stomach leads to a shortening of the abdominal esophagus, making the lower esophageal sphincter less efficient and favoring reflux. This alteration must be kept in mind postoperatively following some antireflux procedures, especially the Nissen technique, since generally patients who continue to swallow saliva and air postoperatively develop "gas-bloat" syndrome. It is advisable to leave a nasogastric tube in these patients longer than usual.

A single operation should correct the various alterations that have been mentioned. An antireflux operation should be considered satisfactory when the patient has seen the symptoms that bothered him disappear and has preserved the physiologic possibility of burping and vomiting, when the lower esophageal sphincter has recovered its competency and normal manometric pressure in which the lower esophageal sphincter opens and closes with each swallowing motion, when the length of the esophagus within the abdomen has been reestablished so that abdominal positive pressure will be exerted upon it, and when monitoring of the pH for 24 hours reveals that the reflux has been reduced to physiologic levels and that there are no alterations of esophageal motility (5, 46, 47, 92, 93).

WHEN IS SURGERY INDICATED IN SLIDING HIATAL HERNIAS?

The great majority of patients with sliding hiatal hernias can be treated medically with good results. Medical treatment should be carried out during a minimum of 3 months. Surgical treatment should be recommended only in the group of patients in whom medical treatment has failed. In patients without hiatal hernia but with symptomatic reflux in which medical treatment was used without good results, a surgical antireflux procedure may also be indicated. As will be seen later, disappearance of symptoms with medical treatment does not always mean that the esophagitis has improved or disappeared. In some patients medical treatment leads to improvement in symptoms but the esophagitis diagnosed by esophagoscopy can persist and, in some cases, become worse.

Patients in whom surgical treatment is recommended should be shown to have symptoms that are definitely due to reflux and esophagitis and not to a coexisting condition. One must correct an error that some surgeons commit when they open an abdomen to operate for biliary calculi, gastroduodenal ulcer, or some other affection of the upper abdomen. When they explore the intraabdominal organs and find a sliding hiatal hernia which is generally asymptomatic, they reduce the hernia into the abdomen and place several sutures to close the esophageal hiatus. This mistaken conduct, in addition to revealing a lack of knowledge of the physiopathology of hiatal hernia and its treatment, improvises an unnecessary and incorrectly performed operation, exposing the patient to postoperative complications and, frequently, to a reoperation. Fortunately, in recent years, this tendency to repair a hiatal hernia because of its mere presence in the open upper abdomen has diminished considerably. Special care must be taken with patients with neuropathies who have a hiatal hernia. These patients frequently request surgery because they believe that their neuropathologic symptoms are due to the presence of the hernia.

Surgery for sliding hiatal hernia is correctly indicated in patients with severe esophagitis or persistent esophagitis in spite of well carried out medical treatment. Surgical treatment in these patients may prevent a future development of a fibrous stricture of the esophagus or a Barrett esophagus. The group of patients with mechanical deficiency of the lower esophageal sphincter have a surgical indication in the majority of their cases because very few of them improve with medical treatment. In spite of that, medical treament should be attempted before recommending surgery because many of these patients may compensate for their deficiency if they have a good capacity to clear the esophagus. Surgical treatment is unquestionably necessary in patients with fibrous stricture of the esophagus and in patients with esophageal ulceration or with a shortened esophagus and a Barrett esophagus.

Surgery may also be indicated in some patients with upper digestive hemorrhage due to gastric ulcer. These ulcers may be located in the supradiaphragmatic area or in the subdiaphragmatic area. In some cases the ulcer overrides the edge of the diaphragm (riding ulcer). Gastric hemorrhage may in some cases be due to stasis or due to compression of the diaphragm upon the gastric walls. Surgery may also be indicated in patients with recurrent aspiration pneumonia confirmed by radiologic examination and in patients with pulmonary fibrosis, asthmatic syndromes, or persistent laryngitis due to the same problem.

Abdominal or Thoracic Approach?

One cannot refer to an abdominal approach as opposed to a thoracic approach. The approach should be selected after an individual study of the patient, adapting it to each one. One should not use a predetermined approach, be it abdominal or thoracic, according to the preference of the surgeon or his specialty, but according to the needs of the patient. The surgeon who undertakes the responsibility of treating a hiatus hernia surgically should be capable of performing the procedure through either approach. A complete study of the patient will give the correct indication for which approach is more convenient for the patient. For example, is the patient thin or obese? Is this a first antireflux operation, or is it an operation to correct a recurrence? Does the patient present another surgical affliction of the upper abdomen? Does the patient present a chronic respiratory problem? Does the patient or has the patient ever suffered from upper gastrointestinal hemorrhage? Does the patient have severe esophagitis, fibrous stricture of the esophagus, shortening or ulceration of the esophagus, Barrett esophagus, diffuse spasm, or epiphrenic diverticulum? Is the motor activity of the esophagus normal, or is it deficient with weak waves and aperistalsis? and so on.

The abdominal approach is more frequently used in antireflux operations. The abdominal incision is easier to perform, allows the abdomen to be thoroughly explored, and permits treatment of coexisting diseases such as biliary calculi or duodenal ulcer. Upon occasion the abdominal approach allows the recognition of a diagnostic error when the patient has not been completely studied—for example, carcinoma of the right colon, chronic pancreatitis, and so on. This mistake cannot be discovered through a thoracotomy. The abdominal approach is better tolerated than the thoracotomy in patients at risk. On the other hand, postoperative thoracotomy pain is more severe, more persistent, and more frequent than the pain of an abdominal incision. The abdominal approach is preferable in patients with hernia and upper GI tract hemorrhage, as well as in patients with chronic pulmonary problems. The thoracic approach is indicated in patients in whom the stomach does not descend into the abdomen in the upright position, in patients with severe esophagitis, stricture of the esophagus, shortened esophagus, ulcerated esophagus, or Barrett esophagus, or when the hernia coexists with an esophageal affliction such as diffuse spasm of the esophagus, epiphrenic diverticulum, and so on. The thoracic approach is indispensable in cases in which it is necessary to mobilize the esophagus with ligation of the left superior and inferior bronchial arteries to bring the esophagogastric junction into the abdomen without traction. Mobilization of the esophagus through the thorax is safer because it is done by direct vision. On the other hand, in cases of shortening of the esophagus not due to fibrosis, it is possible, in the majority of cases, to free the esophagus and lower it into the abdomen. Liberation and lowering of the esophagus in these cases through the abdominal approach is generally insufficient and dangerous, because the esophagus may be traumatized and the vagus nerves injured. In very obese patients, it is more convenient to operate through the thoracic approach.

A special problem is frequently presented in patients who have previously been operated on for hiatal hernia with reflux that has recurred. In the first place, one should find out if the recurrence is due to unnecessary traction when the esophagus was lowered, or due to the presence of a shortening of the esophagus that was missed by the surgeon. In patients who are reoperated, surgical treatment is much more complicated, due to the presence of scar tissue and viability of the walls of the esophagus, which are easily perforated during dissection. In patients who are to be reoperated for recurrent hiatus hernia, the most convenient approach is the thoracic one, which frequently has to be enlarged to include the abdomen (thoracoabdominal incision). In some patients the surgery can be performed through the thoracotransdiaphragmatic approach. Some surgeons, however, prefer a thoracic incision with a separate abdominal incision without transecting the costal margin.

SURGICAL TECHNIQUE

The most frequently used techniques in the treatment of hiatus hernia with reflux and esophagitis are three:

1. Hill technique
2. Nissen technique
3. Belsey Mark IV technique

The first two techniques are performed by the abdominal approach, whereas the Belsey technique is performed through the thorax. The Nissen technique can be performed through the thorax, but due to many complications, the thoracic approach has been discontinued.

The three techniques have the same object: (a) Reconstruct the antireflux barrier. (b) Repair the hernia. The three techniques have several similarities, although these are obtained in different fashion. They all mobilize the lower esophagus in the posterior mediastinum and lower the esophagogastric junction below the diaphragm. In addition, the three techniques increase the pressure of the lower esophageal sphincter: The Nissen procedure does it with a fundoplication around the esophagus through 360°; the Belsey procedure attains this through a fundoplication through 240°; and the Hill procedure attains an increase in the lower esophageal sphincter pressure by calibrating the esophagogastric junction. The Hill technique also fixes the esophagogastric junction to the preaortic fascia and the medial arcuate ligament.

Lucius Hill Technique (Posterior Gastropexy)

The Hill technique (43, 45, 46) consists in performing through the abdominal route the following stages in the surgical treatment of sliding hiatal hernia:

1. Lowering the stomach and the esophagogastric junction into the abdomen.
2. Calibrating the esophagogastric junction to normalize the pressure in the lower esophageal sphincter.
3. Fixing the esophagogastric junction to the preaortic fascia and the median arcuate ligament.

Normally the preaortic fascia and the median arcuate ligament are fused to the phrenoesophageal ligament posteriorly, anchoring the esophagogastric junction to the posterior wall of the abdomen and constituting the posterior mesogastrium (46). This fixation is of great importance to keep the esophagogastric junction fixed below the diaphragm. In addition, this fixation constitutes an important point of support for normal esophageal peristaltic activity (46). The Hill technique has good immediate and late results with low morbidity and mortality. The greatest inconvenience that surgeons find in performing the Hill technique is difficulty in identifying the preaortic fascia and the medial arcuate ligament. These structures are not clearly visible, and the surgeon must search for them. Some surgeons have even denied the presence of these structures due to this difficulty (46). Both the preaortic fascia and the medial arcuate ligament are located in a deep position, in front of the anterior wall of the aorta, immediately above the celiac trunk and its branches. In addition, these structures are covered by the muscular fibers of the right crux of the diaphragm and its anterior and posterior bifurcations, which later form the esophageal hiatus. Difficulty in identifying these structures leads to problems in teaching the Hill technique. To facilitate identification of these structures and make the operative stages more practical, modifications of the original Hill technique have been made without logically changing its solid basis and with the object of facilitating its performance and its teaching (18, 45, 46, 100, 102).

Before describing the Hill technique, a brief description of the anatomy of the preaortic fascia and the medial arcuate ligament will be made in order to understand this technique and make its realization possible.

Anatomy of the preaortic fascia and the medial arcuate ligament

The preaortic fascia is a fibrous layer located beneath the diaphragm, on the anterior wall of the aorta, that is generally covered by muscular fibers of the right crux of the diaphragm and its bifurcation. The preaortic fascia is some 4 cm long and has a median width of 3 cm. The inferior border of the preaortic fascia is thickened, constituting the median arcuate ligament. The median arcuate ligament is located immediately above the celiac trunk and the inferior phrenic arteries. Identification of the median arcuate ligament and the preaortic fascia can be performed, as advised by Hill, beginning above the celiac trunk and the inferior phrenic arteries or, as advised by Vansant, Baker, and Ross (100), by freeing the preaortic fascia from above with the left index finger until the medial arcuate ligament is reached. At present, the Vansant technique is the one most frequently used to identify the preaortic fascia and the median arcuate ligament. Hill (46) advises using the Vansant technique if the surgeon has limited experience in this procedure.

Hill Posterior Gastropexy

Following is a description of the Hill procedure with the modifications introduced by Vansant and his co-workers in order to make identification of the preaortic fascia and the median arcuate ligament easier. Chassin (18) has added technical details that are of great practical use to make this excellent surgical procedure safer and easier to perform.

Hill Posterior Gastropexy

FIGURE 21.1

The most frequently used incision is a left paramedian incision. In case it may become necessary to obtain a wider operative field, the xiphoid process can be resected and the incision prolonged some 5 to 6 cm below the umbilicus. A Balfour self-retaining retractor is placed. It is advisable to have an upper-hand type of retractor to help lift the sternum and the costal cartridges to improve visualization of the esophageal hiatus. The peritoneum is opened, but before exploring the abdominal viscera the presence of adhesions between the greater omentum and the splenic capsule is determined so that they may be divided and sectioned before traction on the greater omentum or on the stomach or colon, which otherwise may lead to hemorrhage due to rupture of the splenic capsule. This would lead to sometimes difficult hemostatic procedures on the spleen, which are not always sure and may make a splenectomy necessary. Once hemorrhage from the spleen has been avoided, a complete exploration of the abdominal viscera is performed to investigate the possibility that there may be a simultaneous pathologic process that has not been detected preoperatively. Following this, attention must be directed to the stomach and duodenum to determine if there is some process that would disturb its normal function and favor gastroesophageal reflux, as may occur in the presence of dilation or gastric hypersecretion, functional alterations of the stomach, antropyloric ulcer, duodenal ulcer, pyloroduodenal sclerosis, pyloric hypertrophy of the adult, and so on.

Hill Posterior Gastropexy

Once exploration of the abdominal viscera has been performed, the left triangular ligament of the liver is sectioned with a scissors, as can be seen in the drawing, being careful not to damage the left hepatic vein or the inferior vena cava. Some surgeons, before sectioning the left triangular ligament, ligate it, because, in some cases, they have been able to show blood vessels and aberrant biliary ducts within it. Once the left triangular ligament has been divided, it is reflected upward with the left lobule of the liver, using a large pad and a Harrington retractor. In some patients it is not necessary to divide the left triangular ligament in order to get good visualization of the esophageal hiatus. In these cases it is only necessary to retract the left lobe upward with a Harrington retractor.

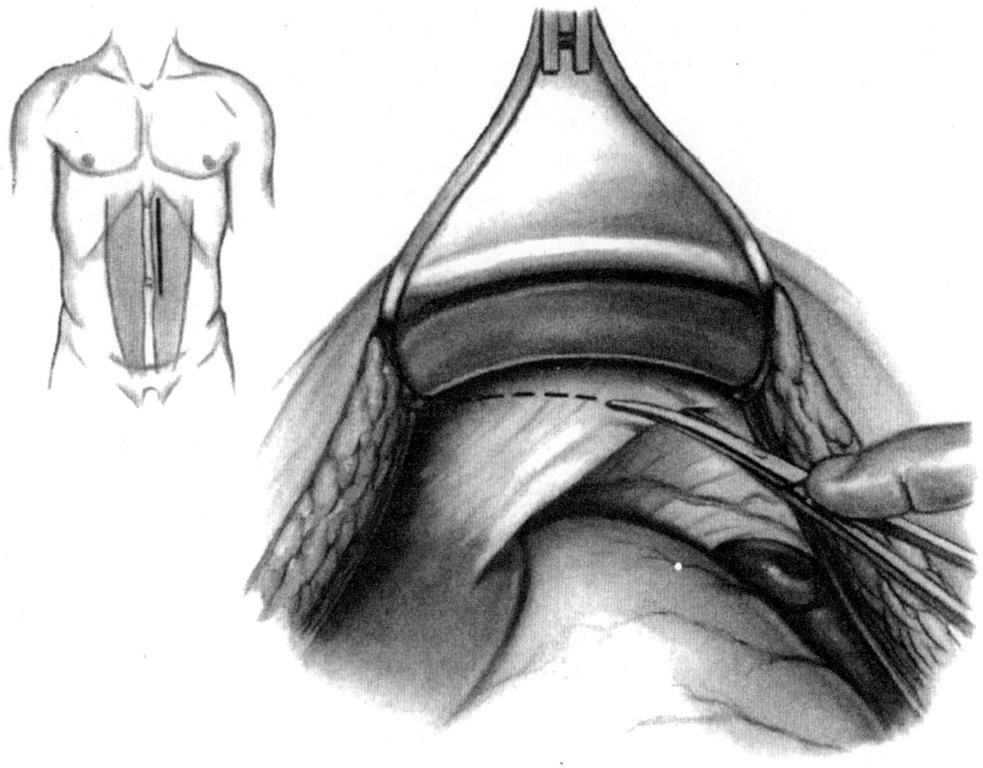

FIGURE 21.1

Hill Posterior Gastropexy

FIGURE 21.2
The stomach and the esophagogastric junction have been manually delivered into the abdomen. With a long toothed forceps, the peritoneum covering the diaphragm and the lower end of the esophagus is grasped. This peritoneal fold is incised together with the phrenoesophageal ligament, which is located behind it. The incision of the peritoneum and the phrenoesophageal membrane is completed so that the esophagus is completely free anteriorly.

FIGURE 21.3
Once the anterior wall of the lower esophagus has been freed, the proximal segment of the gastrohepatic ligament is tied and divided. This is begun in the thinnest and most transparent part of the ligament, going upward to the highest part. At this level, one may run into an accessory left hepatic artery (arising from the left gastric or coronary artery), which is generally small and whose ligature will not lead to any serious consequence. However, a small group of patients may present with an aberrant left hepatic artery arising from the left gastric or coronary artery but of greater caliber and comprising an important portion of the blood supply of the left lobe of the liver and whose ligature may lead to necrosis of the left lobe of the liver. In these cases this artery should be considered an aberrant replacement artery and not an accessory artery. The artery should not be ligated, but should be dissected and retracted to avoid necrosis of the left lobe of the liver.

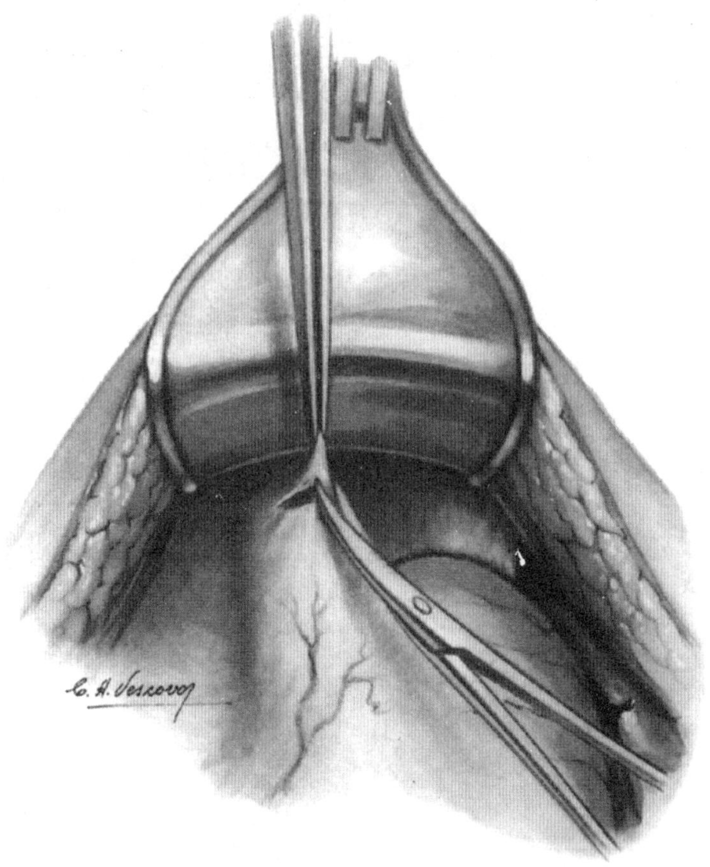

FIGURE 21.2

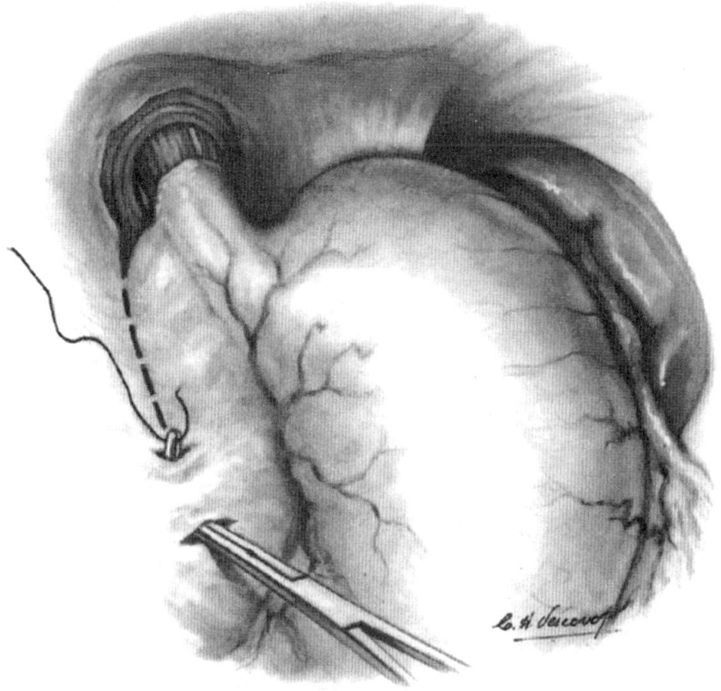

FIGURE 21.3

Hill Posterior Gastropexy

FIGURE 21.4

The lower esophagus has been freed in its entire circumference using the finger. Dissection of the lower esophagus should be performed carefully, especially in patients with severe esophagitis, since the fragile walls of the esophagus may be involuntarily opened. Damage to the esophagus is very serious, since it may require resection of the esophagus. The surgeon should be very alert in dissecting the esophagus posteriorly, since trauma to this wall may be missed by the surgeon. In performing this dissection and mobilization of the lower esophagus, damage to the vagus nerves or its branches should be avoided, particularly damage to the hepatic branch of the anterior vagal nerve or other branches, be they from the anterior or posterior vagus.

Once the lower esophagus has been freed, the gastric fundus is freed. To free the gastric fundus it is necessary to divide the gastrophrenic ligament, which fixes the gastric fundus to the diaphragm. Transection of this ligament is performed (see the figure) by placing the index and middle fingers of the left hand behind the gastric fundus, placing the gastrophrenic ligament under tension to facilitate its transection by means of a scissors in the right hand of the surgeon. The gastrophrenic ligament extends from the esophagogastric angle of His to the most proximal short vessel. Once the ligament has been divided, two or three proximal short vessels are ligated, taking care not to injure the spleen or the greater curvature of the stomach. Liberation of the gastric fundus by ligation of several short vessels will facilitate calibration of the esophagogastric junction. This calibration has the object of increasing the manometric pressure of the lower esophageal sphincter, an important step in the Hill procedure. It is important to deliver as much esophagus as possible to attain a better functional postoperative result. For this purpose the distal esophagus is freed digitally from the posterior mediastinum.

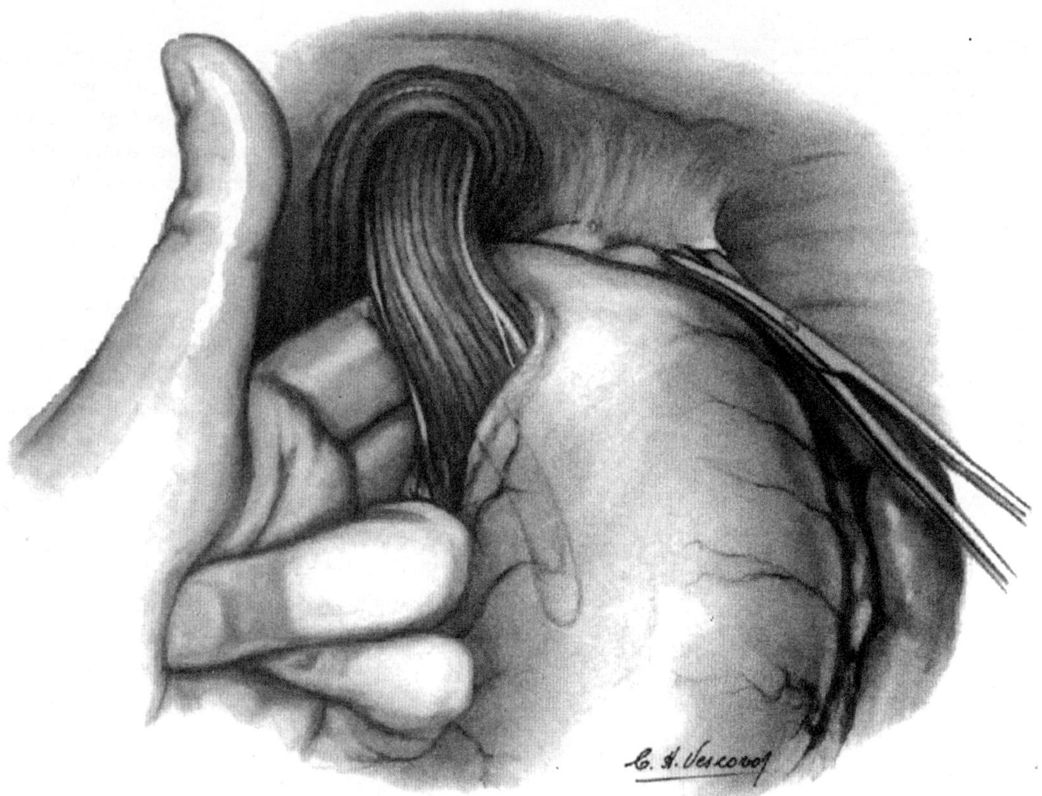

FIGURE 21.4

FIGURE 21.5

Liberation is adequate when it is possible to deliver 5 to 7 cm of distal esophagus into the abdomen. A Penrose drain is passed around the liberated esophagus with both ends held by a clamp. This is given to the first assistant so that gentle traction is applied downward and to the left. The surgeon then identifies the preaortic fascia and the medial arcuate ligament, which are fundamental structures in performing the Hill technique (18, 43, 45, 46, 100, 102). In order to identify these structures, the left index finger is introduced between bifurcation bundles of the right crux of the diaphragm, on the anterior wall of the aorta. At this site it is usually necessary to make a transverse incision just big enough to introduce the tip of the left index finger. The end of the finger is then directed caudally to separate the preaortic fascia from the anterior wall of the aorta. The preaortic fascia is usually covered by muscle fibers, which usually do not have to be dissected to show the fascia. The pulp of the left index finger is held up by the medial arcuate ligament, above the celiac trunk. This technique, used to identify the preaortic fascia and the medial arcuate ligament is that proposed by Vansant, Baker, and Ross (100), and is simpler and safer than the technique originally described by Hill.

Hill Posterior Gastropexy

FIGURE 21.6

This drawing shows the preaortic fascia and the medial arcuate ligament, key structures in the Hill posterior gastropexy technique. The drawing shows the right diaphragmatic crux, dividing shortly after its origin into two fascicles, one passing in front and the other behind the esophagus, forming the esophageal hiatus. At point 1 the site where the left index finger should be introduced is shown, in order to identify the preaortic fascia. In 1′ the preaortic fascia is shown, free of muscular fibers. The medial arcuate ligament makes up the base of the preaortic fascia, which is a fibrous thickening above the celiac trunk. During surgery these structures are not as clearly seen as in these drawings, but the drawings have didactic value in learning this technique.

In those patients in whom it is not possible to bring down into the abdomen an adequate segment of esophagus, be it due to severe esophagitis, esophageal shortening, or stricture, some other technique should be used with a thoracic or thoracoabdominal approach.

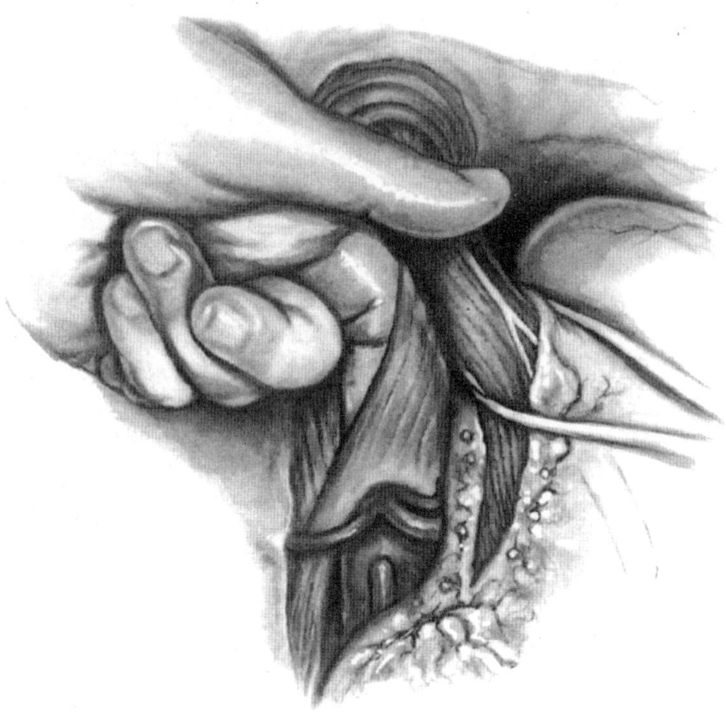

FIGURE 21.5

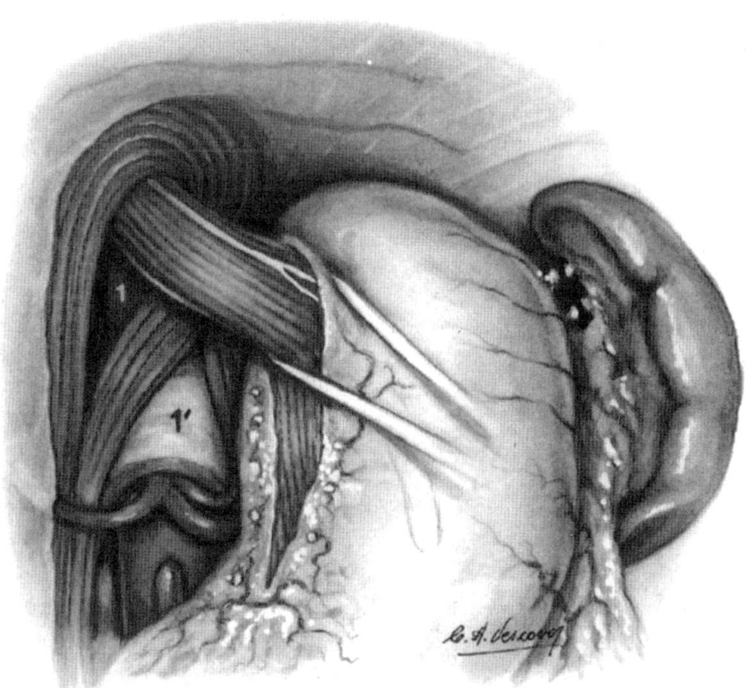

FIGURE 21.6

FIGURE 21.7
Once the medial arcuate ligament and the preaortic fascia have been identified, they are temporarily left alone while the sutures are placed in the esophageal hiatus, without tying them. The esophageal hiatus will be closed later. If the hiatal sutures are tied, it would be very difficult to re-identify the medial arcuate ligament and the preaortic fascia. The sutures placed to close the hiatus should include substantial bites in the edge of the hiatus, including no less than 15 mm of muscular tissue as well as the peritoneum and the fascia. These sutures should be 10 mm from each other. Usually, 5 or 6 sutures are necessary. Nonabsorbable sutures should be used. The suture closest to the esophagus should be precise, avoiding excess narrowing of the hiatus, with postoperative dysphagia, or too ample a space between the esophagus and the edge of the hiatus, which favors recurrence of the hernia. It is felt that the hiatus has been adequately closed when one can pass the tip of the right index finger between the esophagus (with an 18 F nasogastric tube within it) and the edge of the hiatus.

Hill Posterior Gastropexy

FIGURE 21.8
Insertion of the sutures into the esophageal hiatus, without tying them, has permitted re-identification of the preaortic fascia and the medial arcuate ligament. In A one can see the left index finger, which has been introduced between the anterior aortic wall and the preaortic fascia. The lower limit of the preaortic fascia, shown by using a darker tint, corresponds to the medial arcuate ligament. The sutures used to close the esophageal hiatus have not been tied and are being held toward the patient's right costal arch by clamps. In B the surgeon's left index finger has been replaced by a narrow malleable retractor so that the surgeon can place the sutures more precisely as he carries out the posteriogastropexy and so that he can use both hands for the next steps.

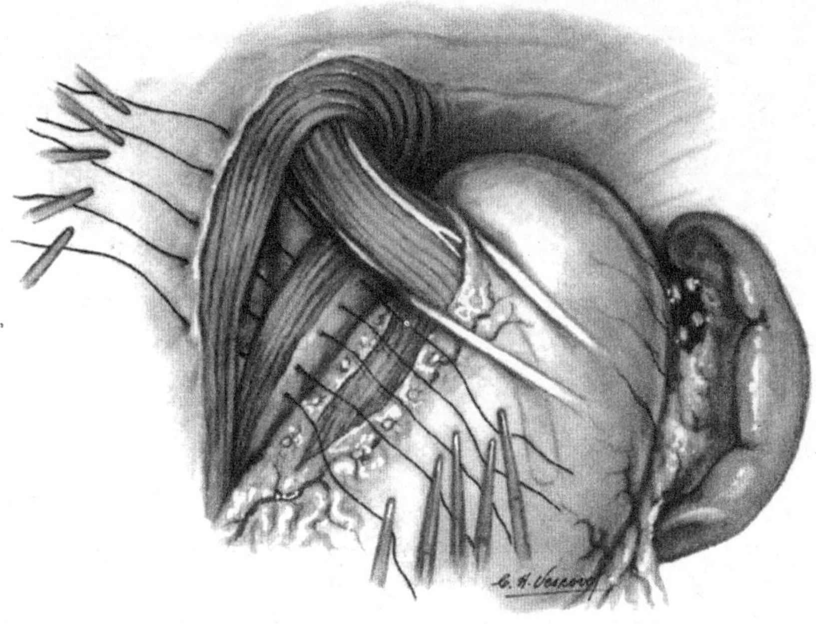

FIGURE 21.7

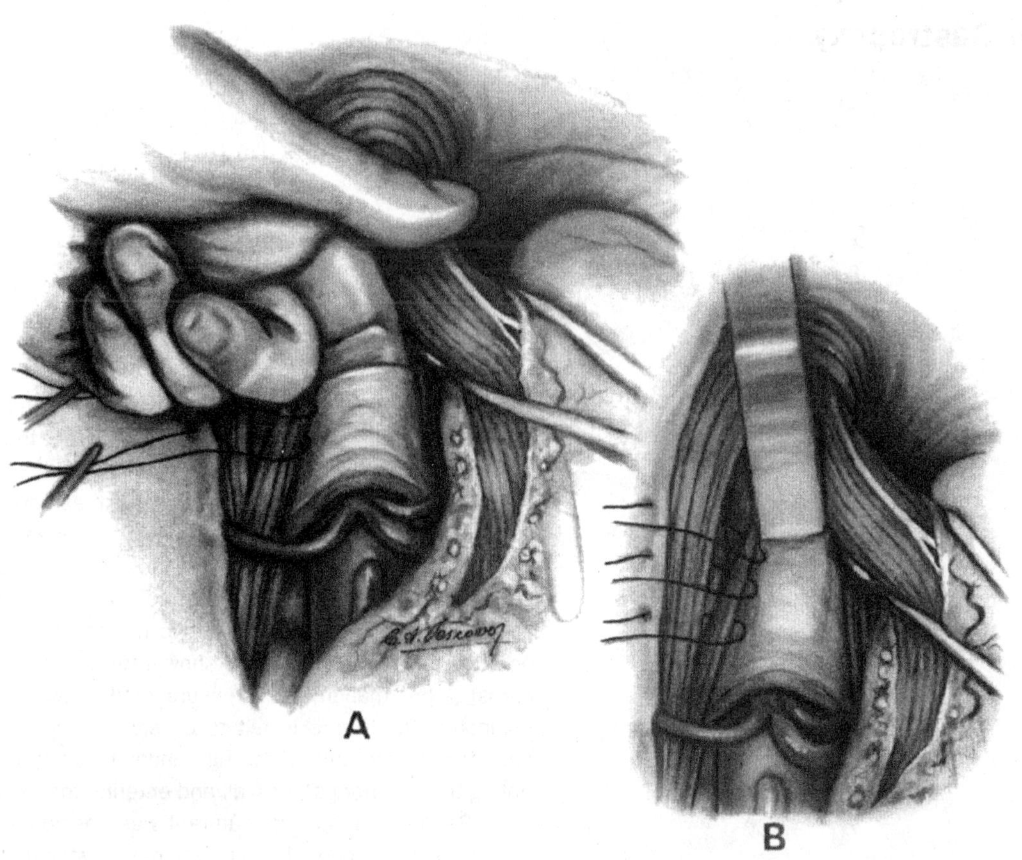

FIGURE 21.8

FIGURE 21.9
The preaortic fascia and the arcuate ligament have been re-identified, and closure of the esophageal hiatus can now be carried out. The previously placed sutures to close the hiatus are ready to be tied.

Hill Posterior Gastropexy

FIGURE 21.10
The esophageal hiatus has been closed by adjusting the sutures. To avoid necrosis of the muscular tissue, these sutures should not be tied too tightly. The stomach has been rotated so that the lesser curvature faces forward, as shown, in order to proceed with the calibration of the esophagogastric junction (18, 46). To do this the suture closest to the esophagus is crossed, without tying it, as shown, to confirm that it has been placed precisely, to show that it is not too tight, leading to postoperative dysphagia, or to show it to be inefficacious in increasing the manometric pressure of the lower esophageal sphincter. The suture is felt to be situated correctly when it only permits the pulp of the right index finger to pass, invaginating the anterior gastric wall and entering the esophageal lumen. Before tying the first suture it was possible to introduce the whole index finger (10). An 18 F nasogastric tube has been passed into the esophagus.

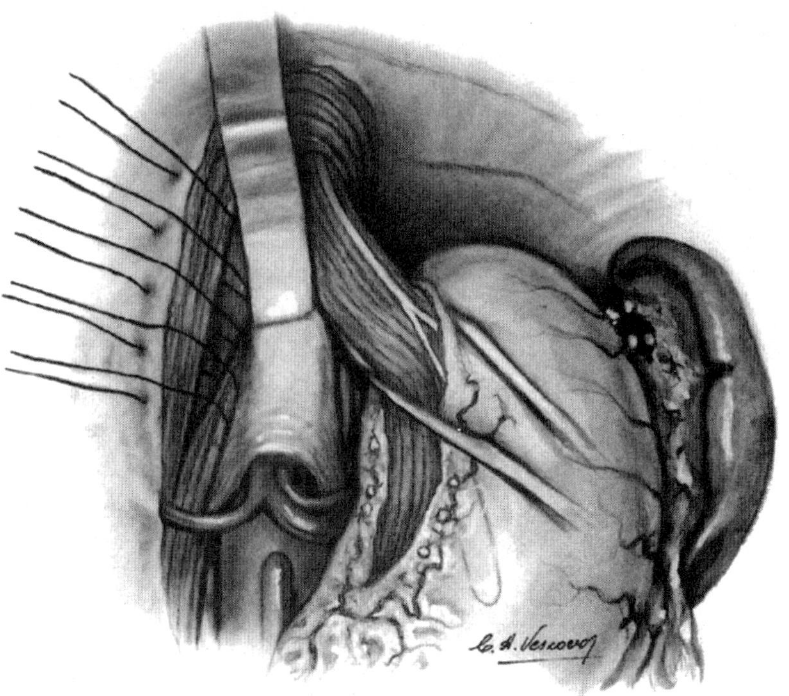

FIGURE 21.9

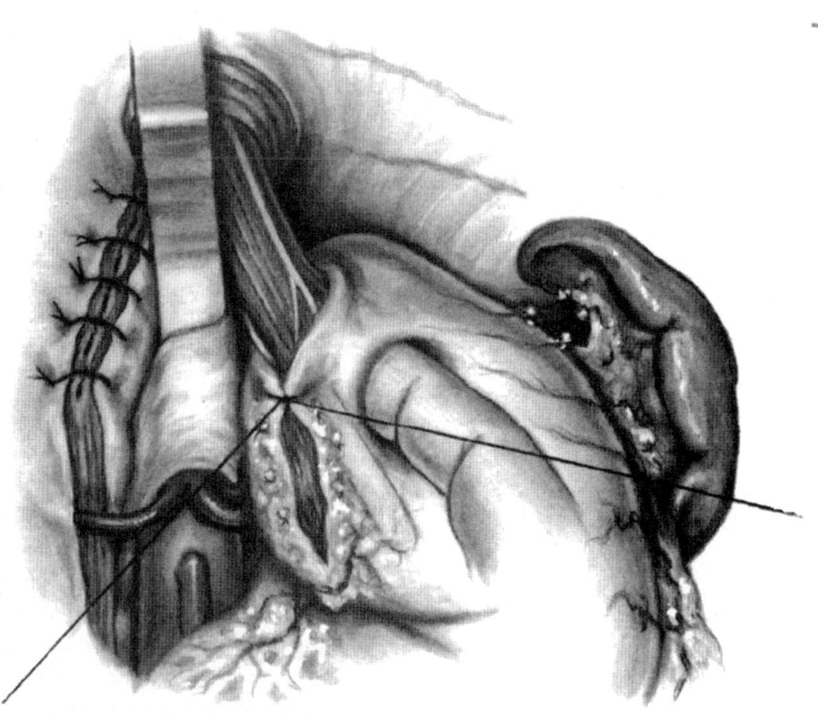

FIGURE 21.10

FIGURE 21.11
Once it has been shown that the suture closest to the esophagus has been placed correctly, three more sutures should be placed below it. The knotted sutures calibrate the esophagogastric junction, increasing the manometric pressure to normal levels (18, 46). These sutures should include both sides of the lesser curvature, taking up the seromuscular and submucosal layers of the stomach at the level of the esophagogastric junction.

Hill Posterior Gastropexy

FIGURE 21.12
The four previously placed sutures are adjusted simultaneously, without tying them, to confirm that the calibration they produce is correct. The sutures are then inserted into needles so they can be introduced through the arcuate ligament and the preaortic fascia to carry out the posterior gastropexy (43, 45, 46). When these needles are inserted they should come in contact with the malleable retractor so that they include a substantial amount of the tissue of these structures. It is important not to limit the bites to the muscular fibers covering the preaortic fascia, since they are not strong enough to assure a firm posterior gastropexy (18).

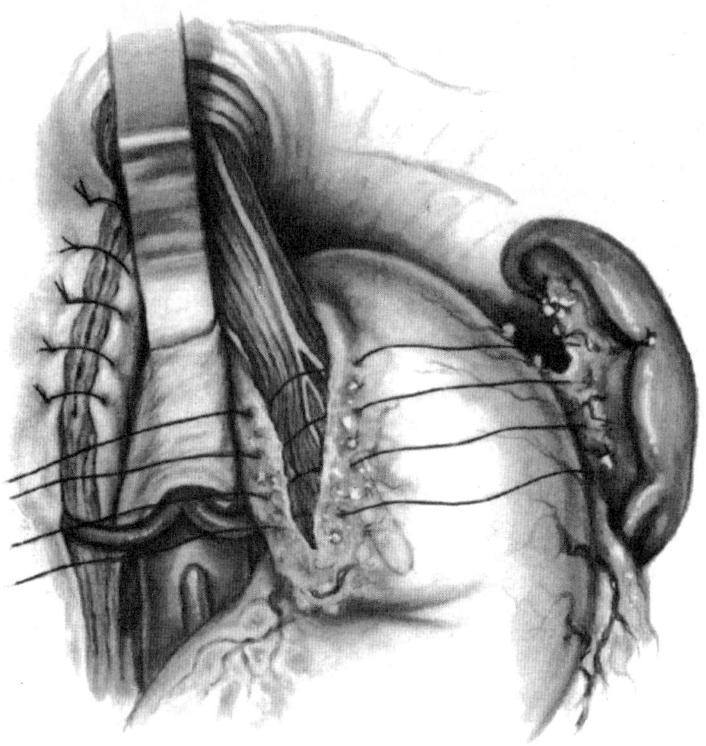

FIGURE 21.11

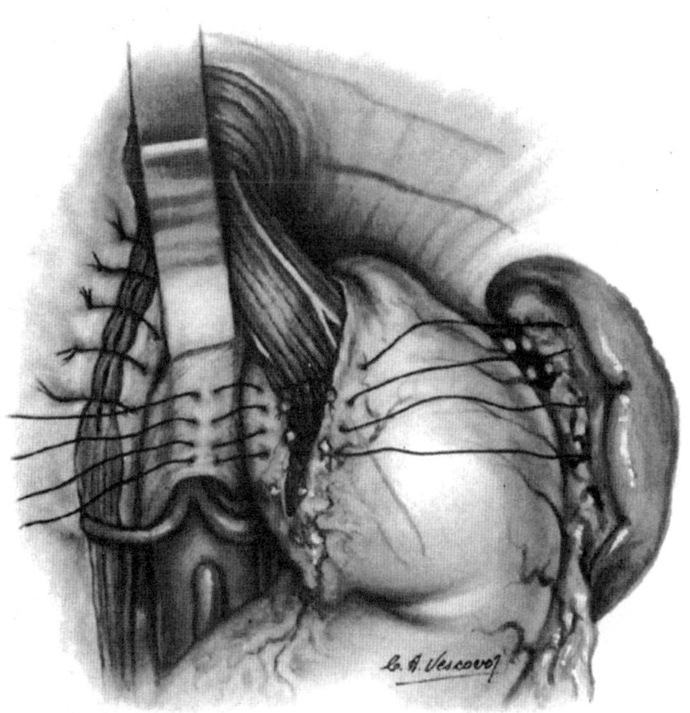

FIGURE 21.12

FIGURE 21.13

The four sutures have been tied, assuring the calibration and the posterior fixation of the esophagogastric junction to the median arcuate ligament and the preaortic fascia. The adequacy of the calibration is again confirmed by introducing the index finger through the gastric wall and into the esophageal lumen with its 18 F nasogastric tube. If the calibration is correct, only the pulp of the index finger can be inserted into the esophagus (18). For a more exact control, Hill carries out an intraoperative manometric measurement of the pressure of the lower esophageal sphincter (45, 46). Other authors (68) do not believe this pressure measurement to be reliable.

Before proceeding with the closure of the abdomen, it is advisable to carry out a hydraulic test to confirm the degree of esophagocardiac competence. This test is done by introducing 500 mL of warm saline through the nasogastric tube into the stomach. The nasogastric tube is then taken into the third portion of the esophagus, and an elastic clamp is applied to close the duodenum. The stomach is then squeezed with both hands; if the gastric fluid does not pass into the esophagus, it means the esophageal sphincter has recovered its competence.

The Hill procedure, with the modifications used to facilitate its being carried out, gives very good results.

Hill Posterior Gastropexy

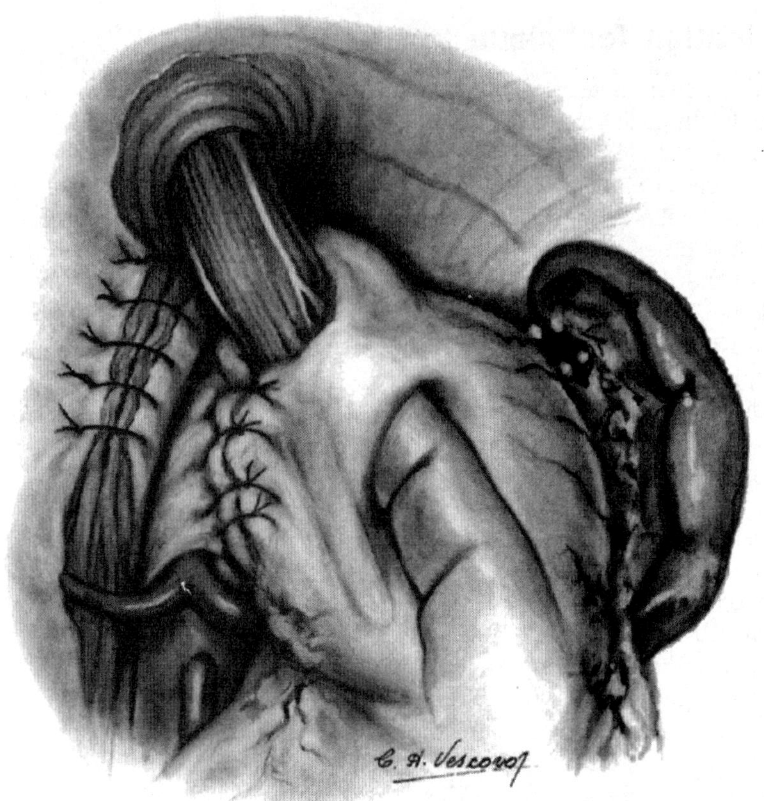

FIGURE 21.13

Nissen Fundoplication Technique

The Nissen fundoplication technique can be carried out by the abdominal or the thoracic approach. However, the thoracic approach has led to many serious postoperative complications, such as esophagopleural or gastropleural fistulas, ulcers in the fundoplication, and so on (18, 60, 80). These and other complications have led to a very rare usage of the thoracic approach. We will only refer to the abdominal route.

The transabdominal Nissen technique consists of carrying out a 360° wrapping around the lower esophagus, using the gastric fundus. The original Nissen technique (64, 65), even though it results in good control of gastroesophageal reflux, can also lead to several postoperative complications. For this reason, it has been modified in order to avoid some of the complications, while conserving its value as an antireflux procedure. The complications that are observed in the classical Nissen procedure include dysphagia, difficulty in burping or vomiting, "gas-bloat syndrome," slippage of the fundoplication downward into the gastric body, giving rise to gastric obstruction, slippage of the fundoplication toward the thorax, dehiscence of the fundoplication, ulcerations of the gastric wrapping, and so on (10, 12, 24, 25, 28, 41, 47).

The Nissen operation does not consist of simply wrapping the stomach around the lower esophagus. It is indispensable to have enough experience to correctly perform this procedure and good criteria for patient selection. With this technique it is important to evaluate the degree of compression that the gastric fundus must exert on the esophagus, the height that the fundic wrapping must have, and to make a very strict selection of the segment of the stomach with which to perform the wrapping of the esophagus. Many of the complications of this procedure are due to utilization of an inadequate technique and poor patient selection. Patients should not undergo the Nissen procedure if they have motor alterations of the esophagus, motor incoordination, weak waves, or aperistalsis, especially those who, for these reasons, present symptoms of dysphagia. Patients with severe esophagitis and stricture or shortening of the esophagus in which it is impossible to bring down a sufficient length of the esophagus into the abdomen, or in which there is residual traction upon the esophagus, should not be subjected to this procedure. Complete study of the patient preoperatively including manometry and 24 hour pH are indispensable to carry out a correct selection of the patients to be submitted to this procedure.

The Nissen procedure is the most frequently performed procedure in the treatment of hiatus hernia with reflux. Technical modifications introduced following the original Nissen technique have considerably diminished the incidence of complications (6, 7, 18–20, 25, 28, 81–83, 92–94). We will now proceed to describe the Nissen technique with the modifications that have been introduced in recent years. Liberation of the lower esophagus and the gastric fundus is exactly the same as that described in the Hill operation.

Nissen Fundoplication Technique

FIGURE 21.14
The drawing shows that the lower esophagus and the esophagogastric junction have been freed. The gastrophrenic ligament has been divided, and three short vessels have been divided and tied off proximally. The patient has a No. 18 F nasogastric tube in place. The esophageal hiatus has been sutured behind the esophagus with five sutures, using nonabsorbable material. Some surgeons believe that it is not necessary to tie off any short vessels in order to perform the Nissen procedure (76). However, the great majority believe that it is indispensable to tie and divide at least three short vessels to permit an adequate mobilization of the gastric fundus, selecting the most appropriate segment of fundus and performing a 360° wrapping without any tension.

Nissen Fundoplication Technique

FIGURE 21.15
Before proceeding with the fundoplasty, it is necessary to be sure that the esophageal hiatus has been closed correctly. This means that between the esophagus, which has an 18 F nasogastric tube within it, and the edge of the hiatus, the tip of the right index finger should be exactly admissible, as shown in the drawing. If the tip of the index finger cannot pass through the hiatus, it means that the hiatus is too narrow and the location of the most proximal suture into the esophagus should be modified. If the remaining space is too ample, it will be necessary to add one or two stitches until only the tip of the index finger will pass. If the space between the esophagus and the edge of the hiatus is too wide, it will facilitate displacement of the fundoplication into the thorax.

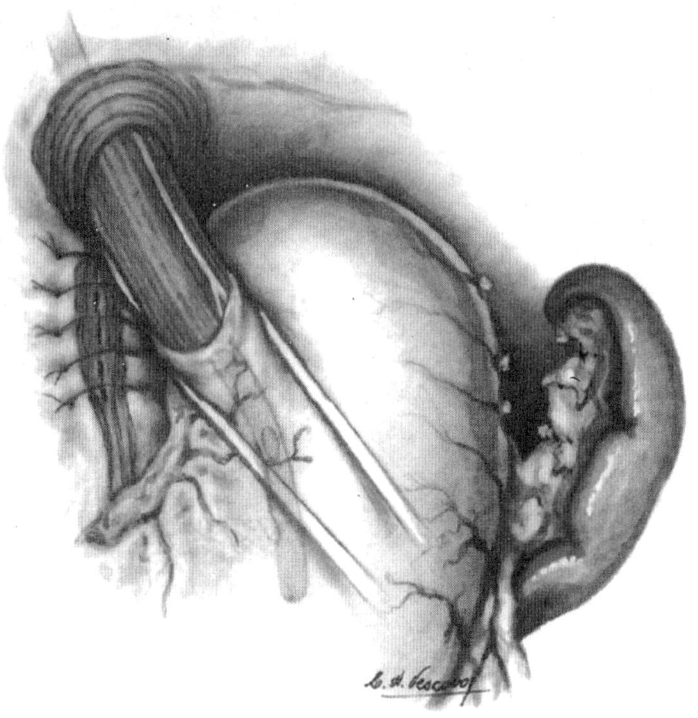

FIGURE 21.14

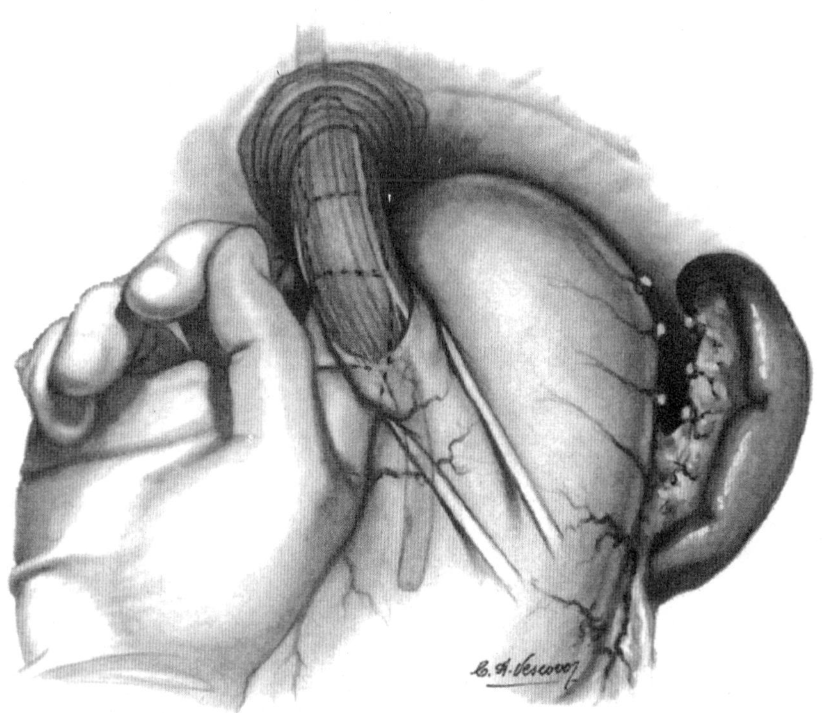

FIGURE 21.15

Nissen Fundoplication Technique

FIGURE 21.16

The drawing shows the moment when the lower esophagus is being wrapped with the gastric fundus. The surgeon performs the wrapping maneuver using the index and middle fingers of the right hand. When the fundus has passed the right edge of the esophagus, it is grasped with a Babcock clamp to complete the wrapping maneuver. As previously mentioned, this maneuver can be performed correctly and without traction if three short vessels in the upper stomach have been divided. The drawing shows that the esophagus has been brought down into the abdomen sufficiently to permit wrapping of the stomach without traction. The abdominal esophagus should be 4 to 7 cm long. The wrapping should be performed using only the gastric fundus. The proximal portion of the gastric body should not be part of the wrapping.

There is an important functional difference between the muscular fibers of the gastric fundus and the gastric body. The muscular fibers of the fundus contract and relax synchronously with the lower esophageal sphincter. When swallowing occurs, if the esophagus is wrapped by the gastric fundus, at the moment in which the lower esophageal sphincter relaxes, the gastric fundus relaxes simultaneously and the bolus of food passes without difficulty into the stomach. If a segment of the proximal portion of the gastric body has been used in performing the wrapping, this segment will not relax to allow passage of the bolus of food and dysphagia will occur postoperatively (6, 25, 28, 55, 56). DeMeester and co-workers (25, 47) have demonstrated that it is easy to make the mistake of using part of the gastric body to wrap around the esophagus. Some patients have one or two or even more short vessels running retroperitoneally, which makes it easy to err.

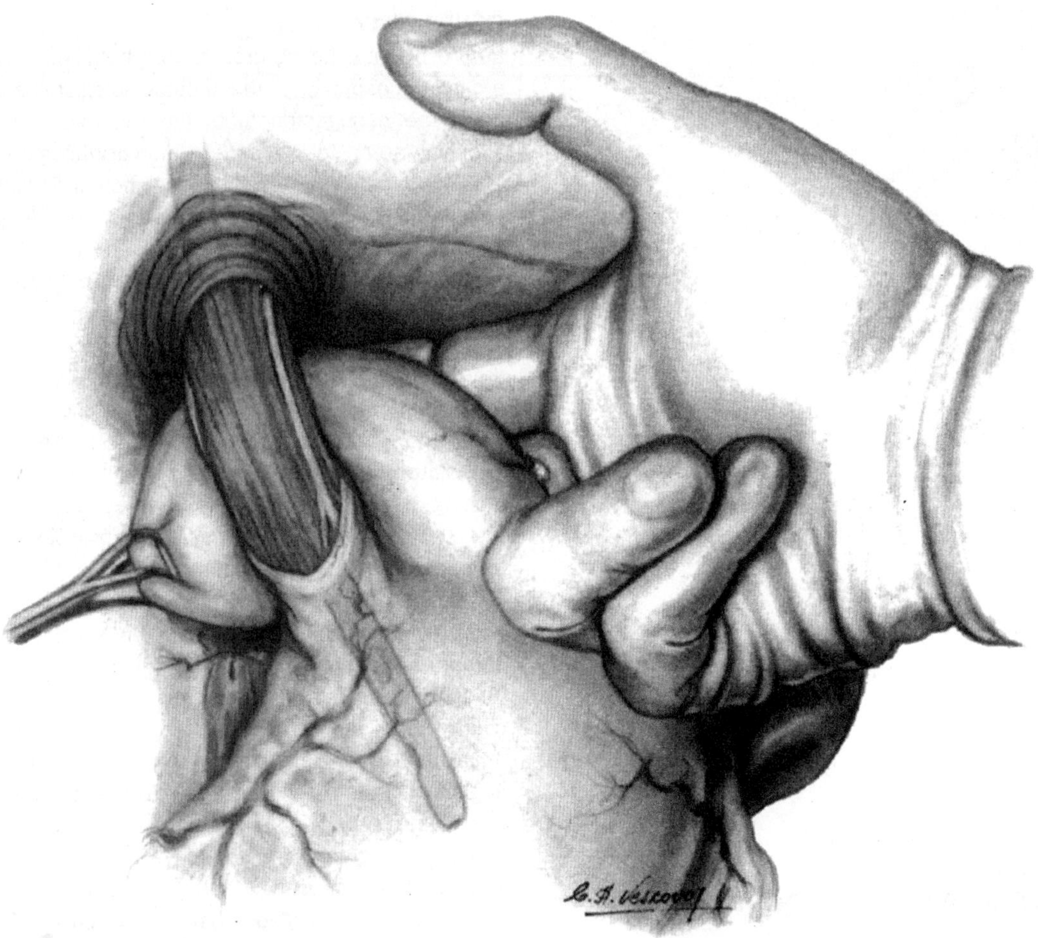

FIGURE 21.16

FIGURE 21.17

Before placing the sutures to join both sides of the fundus around the esophagus, the anesthesiologist is instructed to remove the nasogastric tube into the middle portion of the esophagus and to introduce a mercury bougie of the Hurt or Maloney type, 50 F. This dilating mercury bougie should be passed after the lower esophagus has been wrapped with the gastric fundus. If the bougie is passed before the sutures are tied, it can make the wrapping more difficult. The object of the mercury bougie is to keep the wrapping from compressing the esophagus excessively, leading to dysphagia, "gas-bloat" syndrome, or difficulty in burping or vomiting. It has been shown that it is not necessary to have a tight fundoplication to attain good cardial competence (6, 25, 28, 47). In addition, it should be pointed out that the Nissen technique has another factor leading to compression of the lower esophagus, that is, air in the stomach, which, upon rising, compresses the esophagus through the fold in the fundus (18).

The drawing shows the Hurst 50 F bougie in place. Two Prolene 2-0 sutures have been placed, including, on one side, the serous layer, the muscular layer, and the submucosa of the fundic fold on the left, later passing the esophageal wall, including both muscular layers, and then including the serosa, muscularis, and submucosa of the fundic fold on the right. It is important that the sutures include the submucosa because this is the strongest layer in the gastrointestinal tract. One should take great care not to perforate the mucosa of the stomach or the esophagus to avoid serious postoperative complications. Some surgeons use smaller caliber bougies, 36 to 40 F (7, 81); other surgeons use larger bougies, over 60 F (25, 47). Not all authors pass the sutures through the muscular wall of the esophagus because they believe that it has little value due to the poor consistency of these layers (81–83). Other authors, however, affirm that the sutures in the esophagus favor adhesion of the fundic wrapping to it (5, 18, 25, 47).

Nissen Fundoplication Technique

FIGURE 21.18

The two Prolene 2-0 sutures used in the fundic wrapping have been tied with the Hurst 50 F bougie in place. Under these conditions it should be possible to introduce a finger between the esophagus and the fundic wrapping without any difficulty. If the finger cannot be introduced or fits too snugly, the fundoplication should be corrected. Likewise, if the finger should find great amplitude between the fundic fold and the esophagus, the necessary correction should be performed. The height of the anterior segment of the fundoplication should be between 1.5 and 2 cm. This is the height that is attained using two sutures. A greater height may lead to obstructive symptoms. DeMeester (25, 47) performs a fundic wrapping only 1 cm in height, placing only one mattress suture through Teflon pledgets.

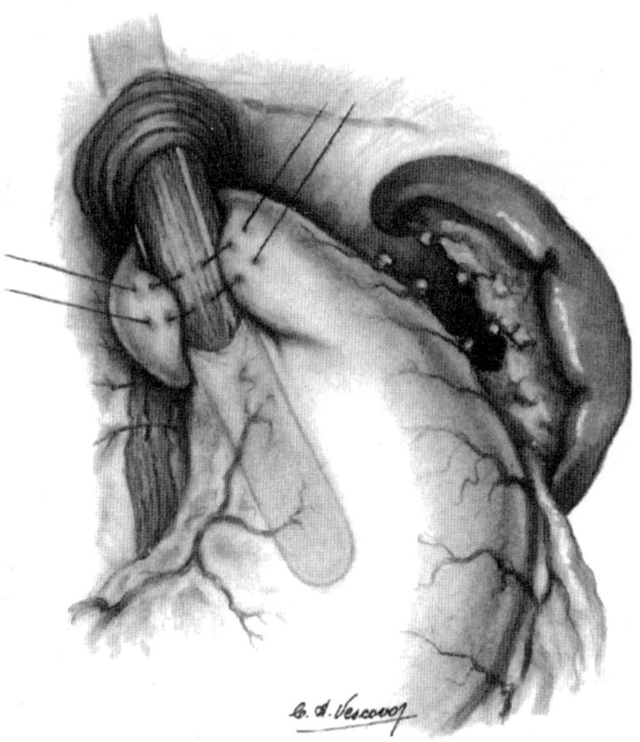

FIGURE 21.17

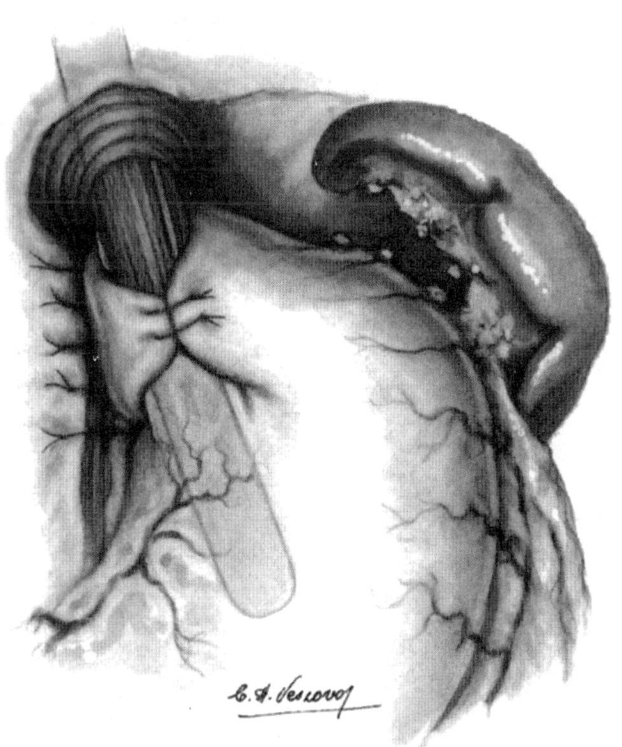

FIGURE 21.18

FIGURE 21.19

Once the fundoplasty has been constructed, the mercury bougie is removed and the nasogastric tube that had been partially removed is reintroduced. The maneuver of introduction of the index finger between the esophagus and the wrapping is again repeated, as shown in the drawing. Without the mercury bougie in place, the index finger should logically enter more easily, and the space may even admit two fingers. With the above described technique, postoperative obstructive complications are few. In some patients, however, even though these precautions are taken, swallowing may present some difficulty postoperatively, lasting 2 to 4 weeks, due to local surgical edema. In some patients swallowing difficulties may be more prolonged. For this reason it is advisable to leave a nasogastric tube in place for at least one week. In order to avoid the discomfort of having a nasogastric tube in place for one week, some surgeons prefer to attain gastric decompression by means of a gastrostomy (6). The gastrostomy, in addition to allowing for a very efficient decompression, contributes to fixing the stomach to the anterior abdominal wall to prevent its possible displacement into the chest. With this in mind, some surgeons have proposed performing the fixing of the gastric wrapping to the right crux of the diaphragm (16). Others have proposed fixing the gastric wrapping to the medial arcuate ligament with several sutures (52). To increase the fixation of the fundic wrapping, Rossetti (81–83) has proposed the placement of two or three sutures including the gastric fold and the anterior wall of the stomach as shown in the insert.

Nissen Fundoplication Technique

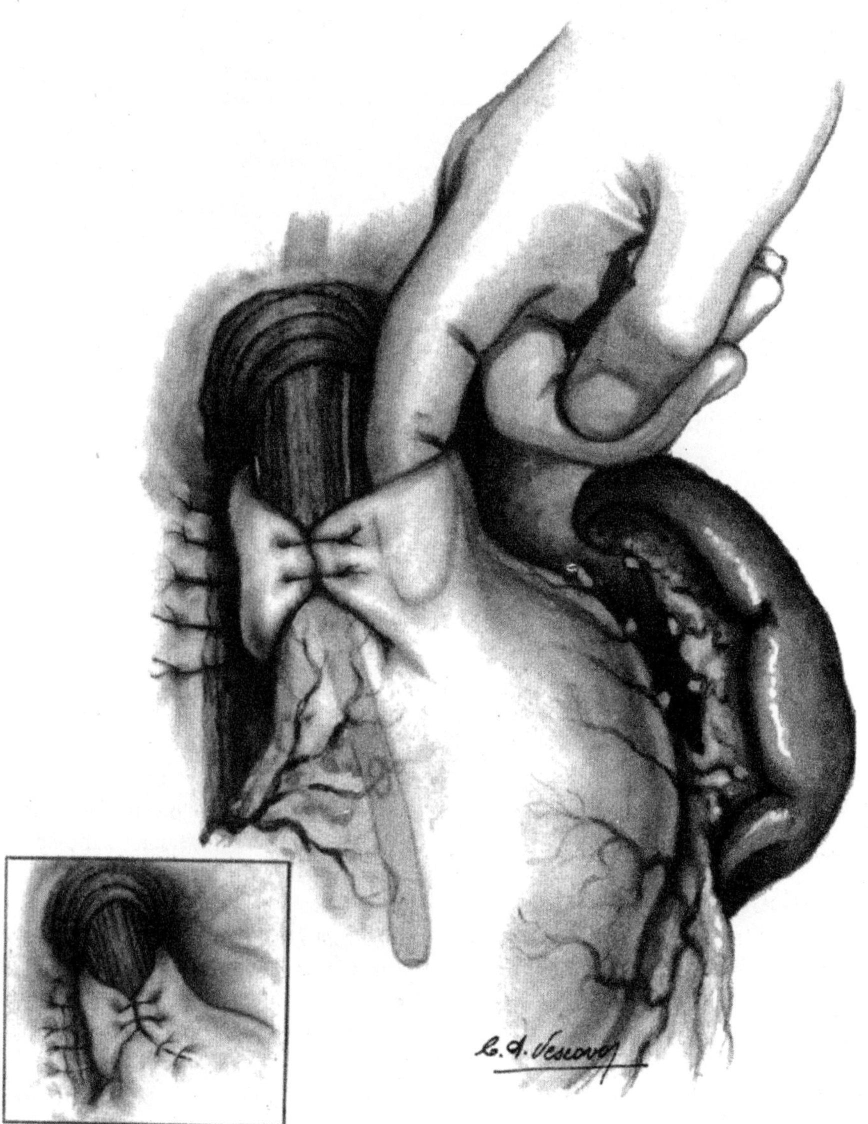

FIGURE 21.19

FIGURE 21.20
This is a schematic section of the lower esophagus and the proximal superior end of the stomach in a patient who has been subjected to a Nissen fundoplication. This drawing graphically illustrates that, besides the compression exerted on the esophagus by the gastric wrapping, there is another compression factor on the lower esophagus, which is generally not taken into account when the Nissen procedure is performed. This factor is composed of the gastric air that rises to the zone of gastric wrapping, exerting pressure on the walls of the lower esophagus through the wrapping. The compression that this gastric air will exert on the lower esophagus should be taken into consideration when the Nissen procedure is performed to prevent obstructive symptoms of the esophagus (18).

Nissen Fundoplication Technique

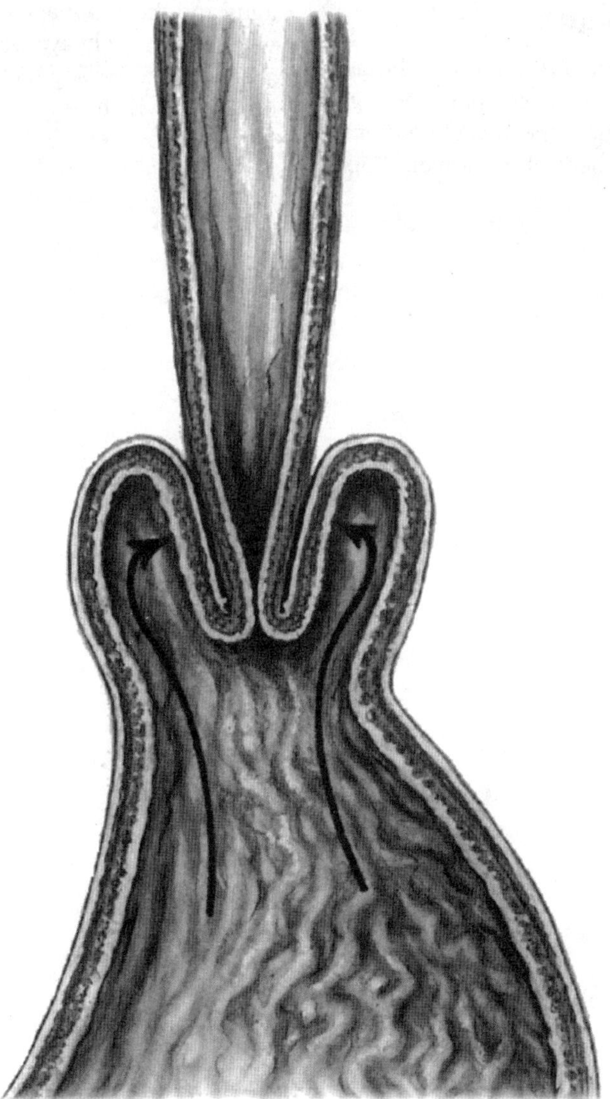

FIGURE 21.20

Belsey Mark IV Technique

The Belsey technique is performed through the thoracic approach. This permits mobilization of the esophagus from the diaphragm to the arch of the aorta, frequently making it possible to bring segment of the lower esophagus and the esophagogastric junction into the abdomen, which cannot always be done through the abdomen. In addition, the Belsey technique includes a fundoplication of 240°, which efficiently contributes to creating an antireflux barrier.

Belsey Mark IV Technique

FIGURE 21.21
The thoracic incision is generally performed through the left sixth intercostal space. In cases in which one expects to have to work in the abdomen in addition to the chest, be it due to a very complicated sliding hernia or due to performing a reoperation of a hiatal hernia with reflux that has recurred one or more times, it is advisable to enter through the seventh intercostal space, which would facilitate a transdiaphragmatic operation and which can also be prolonged into the abdomen, creating a thoracolaparotomy. Once the thoracic incision is completed, the Finochietto retractor is introduced and spread slowly, taking at least 10 minutes, to avoid fracture of the ribs. The inferior pulmonary ligament is divided and tied, and the lung is reflected using moist compresses being retracted by the hands of the second assistant. It is preferable to retract the lungs with the hand instead of using Harrington or other retractors. A dotted line shows the site of the incision in the mediastinal pleura and the fundus of the costal diaphragmatic sac.

Belsey Mark IV Technique

FIGURE 21.22
The mediastinal pleura has been incised and its edges held with traction sutures on both sides. In addition, the pleura over the costodiaphragmatic sac has been incised.

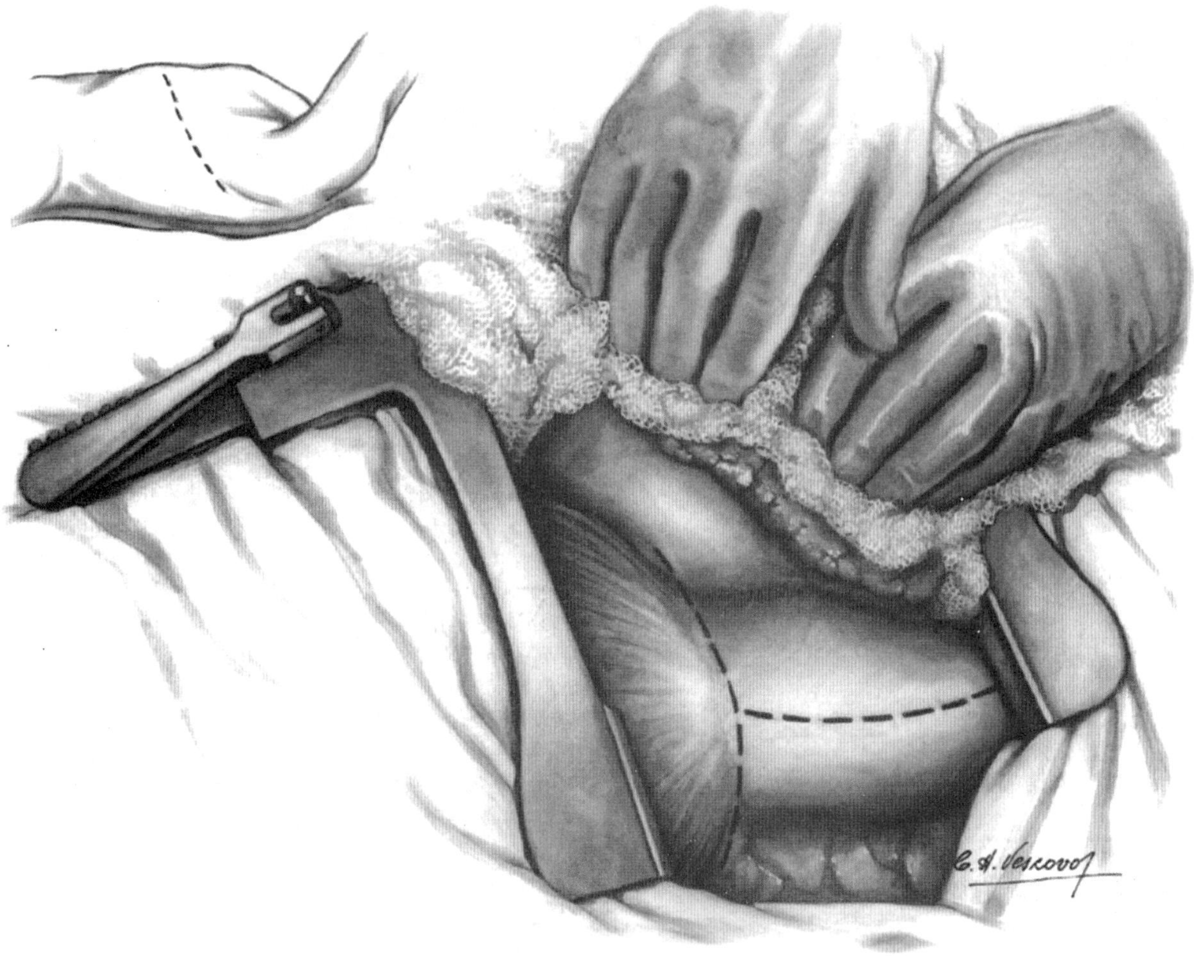

FIGURE 21.21

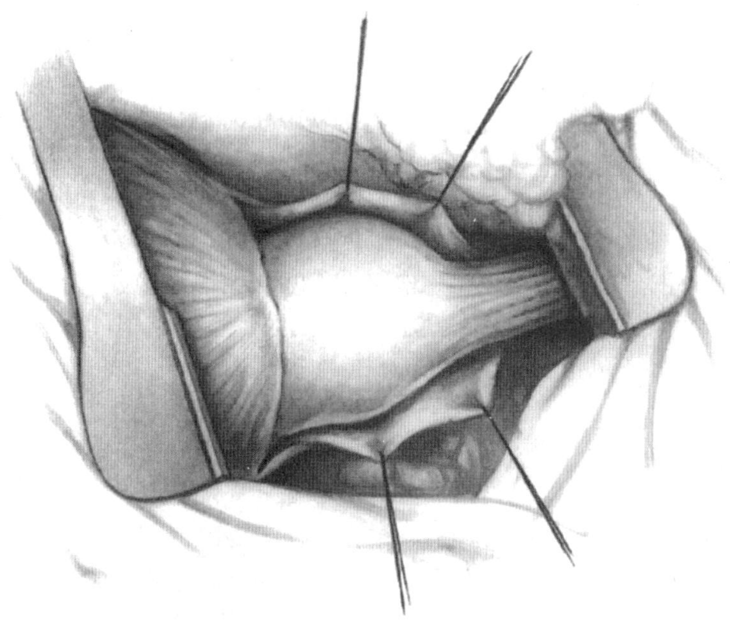

FIGURE 21.22

FIGURE 21.23
The esophagus has been freed above the esophagogastric junction and a rubber tube is being placed around it to facilitate applying traction and further dissection of the esophagus. Dissection of the esophagus in the Belsey technique should be carried out up to the arch of the aorta. In order to obtain an adequate descent of the esophagogastric junction, it is necessary to ligate the superior and inferior left bronchial arteries, which arise in the descending aorta. It is at times necessary to divide two or three small esophageal arteries. These ligations do not affect the intramural circulation of the esophagus (4, 24, 47, 89, 92, 94, 95).

Belsey Mark IV Technique

FIGURE 21.24
The esophagus is held retracted upward. Using a dissecting clamp, a small fold of the phrenoesophageal membrane together with the peritoneum of the hernial sac has been grasped and is being incised to enter the peritoneal cavity.

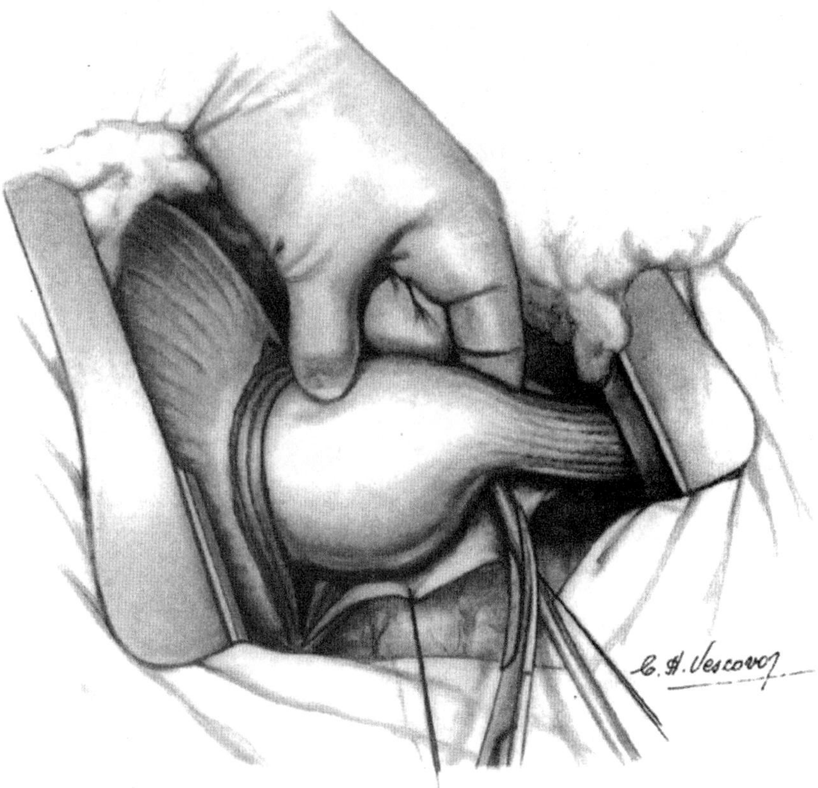

FIGURE 21.23

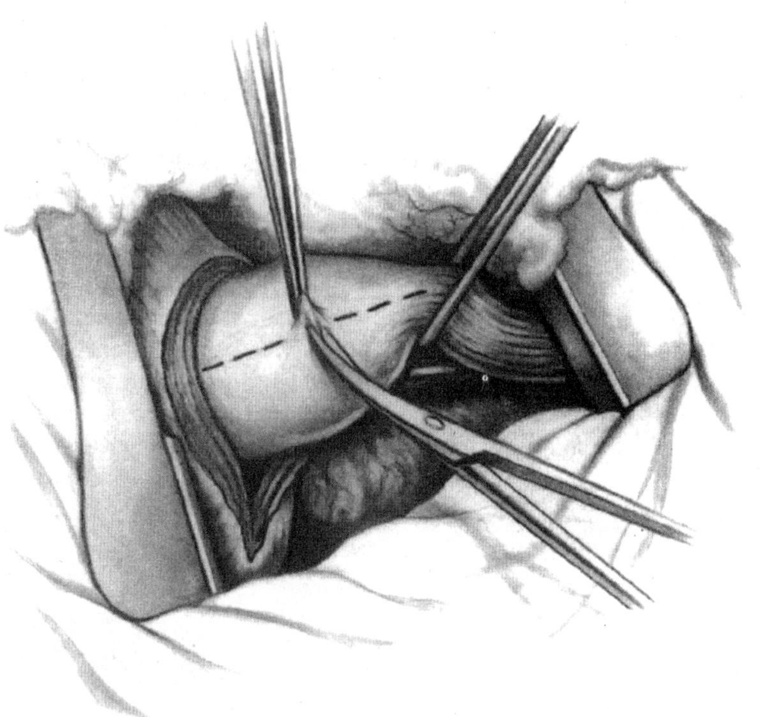

FIGURE 21.24

FIGURE 21.25
After the hernial sac is opened, it is resected using scissors, as shown in the drawing.

Belsey Mark IV Technique

FIGURE 21.26
The entire circumference of the stomach has been freed from the esophageal hiatus. In this liberation it is generally necessary to ligate at least two short vessels and an artery that communicates the left inferior phrenic artery with the ascending branch of the left gastric artery. Ligation of this artery, called the artery of Belsey (89, 92, 93), facilitates liberation of the posterior wall of the stomach without blood loss. If this artery is transected without previously being ligated, it will retract into the abdomen, where it is very difficult to grasp. Once the esophagus and the stomach are freed, the fatty vascular pillow that is always found anterior to the esophagogastric junction is resected, as shown in the drawing. In doing this portion of the operation one should avoid damaging the vagus nerves, which must be carefully retracted posteriorly. Dissection of the above mentioned cushion will facilitate adhesion of the fundoplication to the esophagus without intervening tissue and will permit a better identification of the esophagogastric junction.

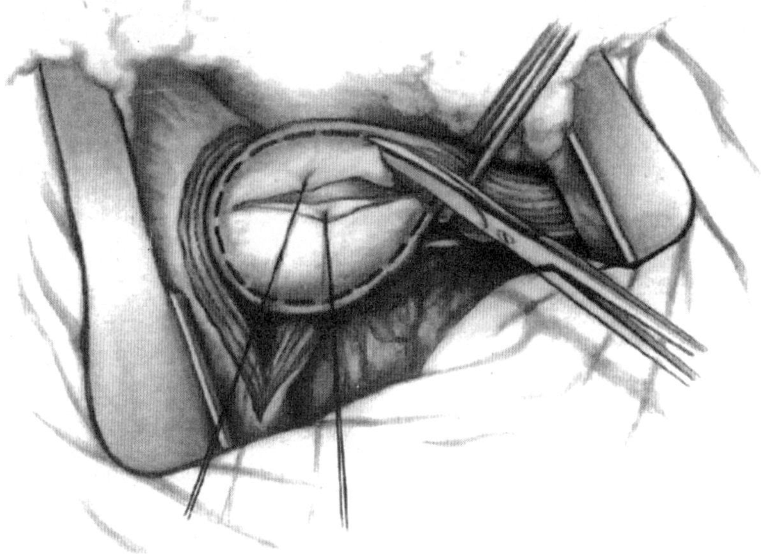

FIGURE 21.25

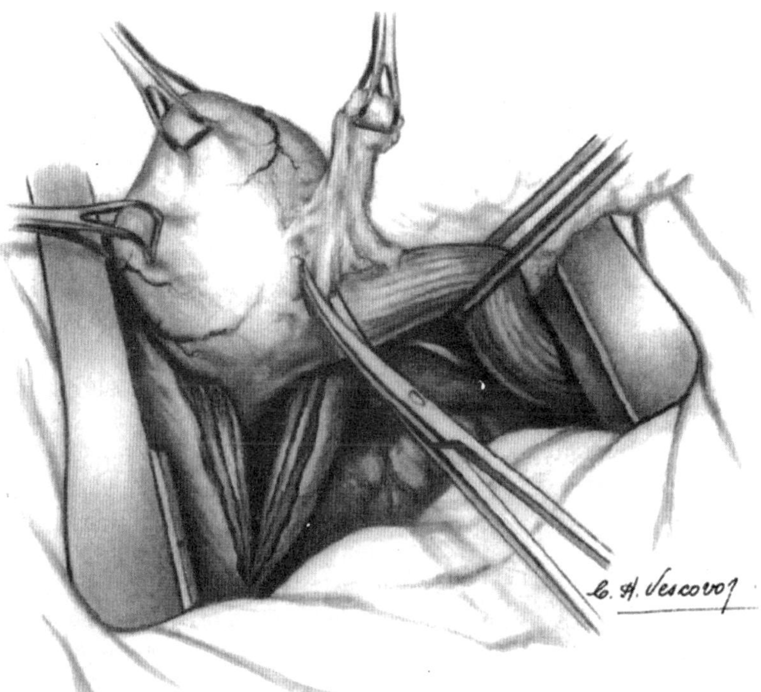

FIGURE 21.26

FIGURE 21.27
Before the fundoplasty is begun, the sutures used to close the esophageal hiatus behind the esophagus are placed. These sutures will be tied after the esophagogastric junction and the stomach have been reduced into the abdomen. Five or six sutures are usually necessary to close the esophageal hiatus. The material used is usually cotton, silk, or nonabsorbable synthetic material. The sutures should include a substantial bite in the edge of the hiatus, including pleura and fascia. Each bite should include about 15 mm, and the sutures should be about 10 mm apart.

Belsey Mark IV Technique

FIGURE 21.28
The Belsey operation includes a partial fundoplication of about 240° around the lower two thirds of the esophagus. To carry out this partial fundoplication, two rows of three mattress sutures each are placed so that some 4 cm of the inferior esophagus will be wrapped by the stomach below the diaphragm. In the drawing one can see that two mattress sutures are in place, one on the left side and the other on the middle portion of the esophagogastric junction. The third mattress suture to be placed in the right side of the esophagogastric junction has not yet been placed because, in order to place this suture in the exact correct position, it is necessary to rotate the esophagus and the stomach to the left, as shown in the following figure. The sutures are performed using 2-0 silk. The mattress sutures are placed in the following manner: The needle is introduced into the seromuscular layer of the stomach some 2 cm from the esophagogastric junction going upward. The needle is removed from the stomach and introduced into the esophagus about 2 cm from the esophagogastric junction, then in the reverse direction from the esophagus to the stomach, as shown in the drawing. This suture is the left one. Later, the mattress suture in the middle is placed as shown. In passing through the wall of the stomach, the needle should include the seromuscular layer and the submucosa, and in passing through the esophagus, the needle should include the muscular layer and the submucosa. One should be careful not to perforate the mucosa of the esophagus or the stomach.

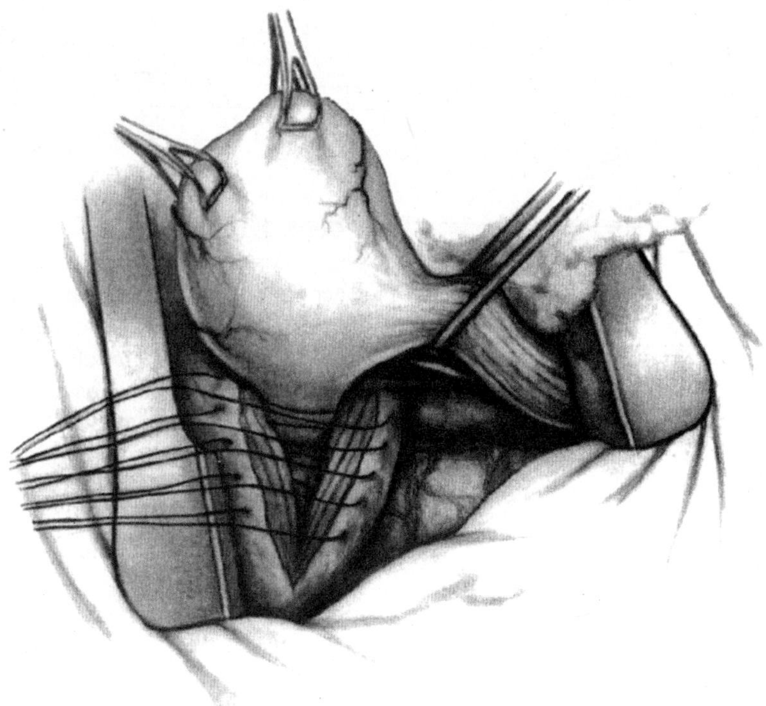

FIGURE 21.27

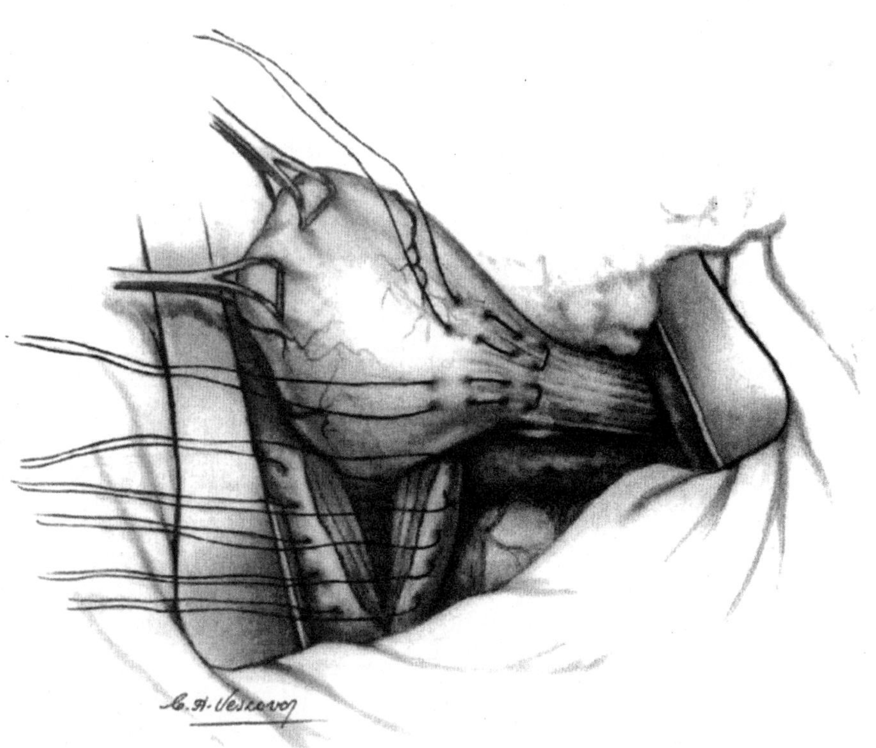

FIGURE 21.28

FIGURE 21.29
The drawing shows that the third or right mattress suture is in place, and this will complete the first row of mattress sutures between the esophagus and the stomach. To place this last suture, it was necessary to rotate the stomach toward the left using two Babcock clamps, as shown in the drawing. The esophagus also had to be rotated to place this third suture. The correct position of this suture over the right side is very important to obtain a fundoplication of 240°. A common mistake is placement of this third suture near the middle suture in the anterior wall and not to the right as shown. This mistake may lead to a less than 240° fundoplication, which will then not create an antireflux barrier and cause the procedure to fail.

Belsey Mark IV Technique

FIGURE 21.30
The mattress sutures in the first row of the fundoplication are being tied. Two sutures have been tied, and a third one is being tied. Tying of the sutures should be done gently so as not to rupture the muscular layer of the esophagus.

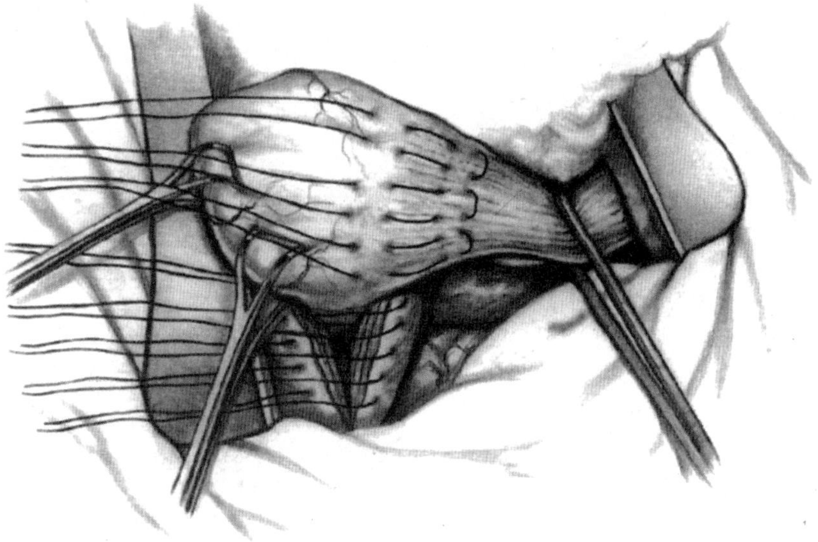

FIGURE 21.29

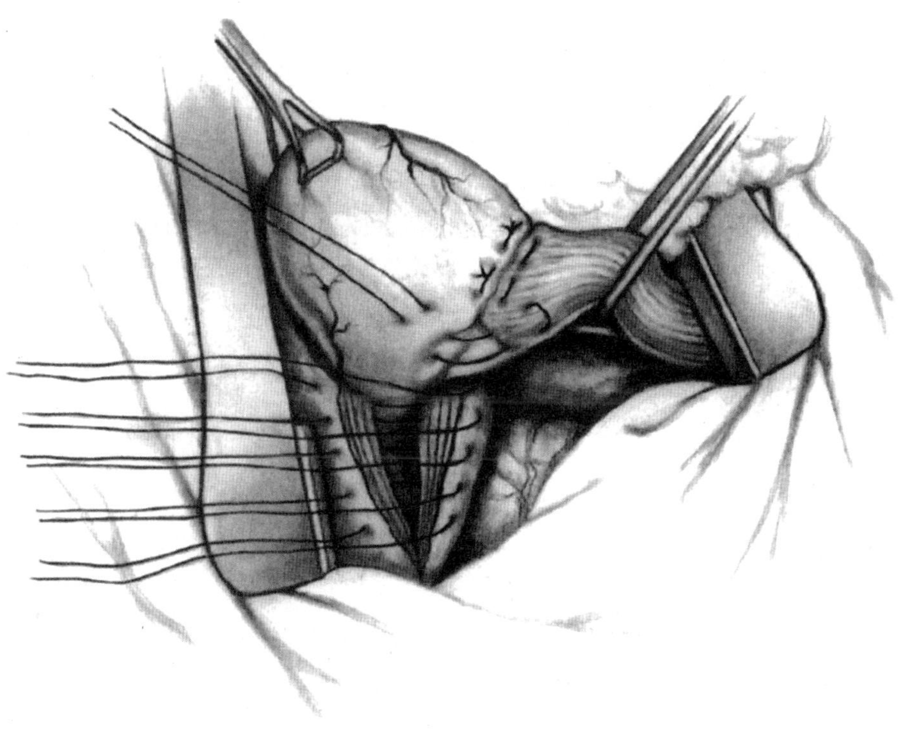

FIGURE 21.30

FIGURE 21.31

The first row of mattress sutures has been tied, and the mattress sutures of the second layer are in place. Different from the first row, the sutures of the second row, in addition to including bites of esophagus and stomach, are placed through the diaphragm.

The second row of sutures are positioned in exactly the same location as those of the first row. The sutures of the second row are placed in the following manner: The needle is first passed through the diaphragm about 2 cm from the edge of the esophageal hiatus from outside in. The needle is then passed through the stomach about 2 cm from the first row of sutures and posteriorly through the esophagus about 2 cm from the first row of sutures. The suture is then turned and the direction of the needle reversed, as shown in the drawing, passing some 2 cm from the edge of the hiatus. In passing the suture through the diaphragm, it is necessary to avoid injuring any abdominal viscera. To avoid injuring an abdominal viscus, it is useful to place a malleable retractor, previously bent, under the diaphragm below the point where the needle will pass, or to use a Belsey spoon retractor.

Belsey Mark IV Technique

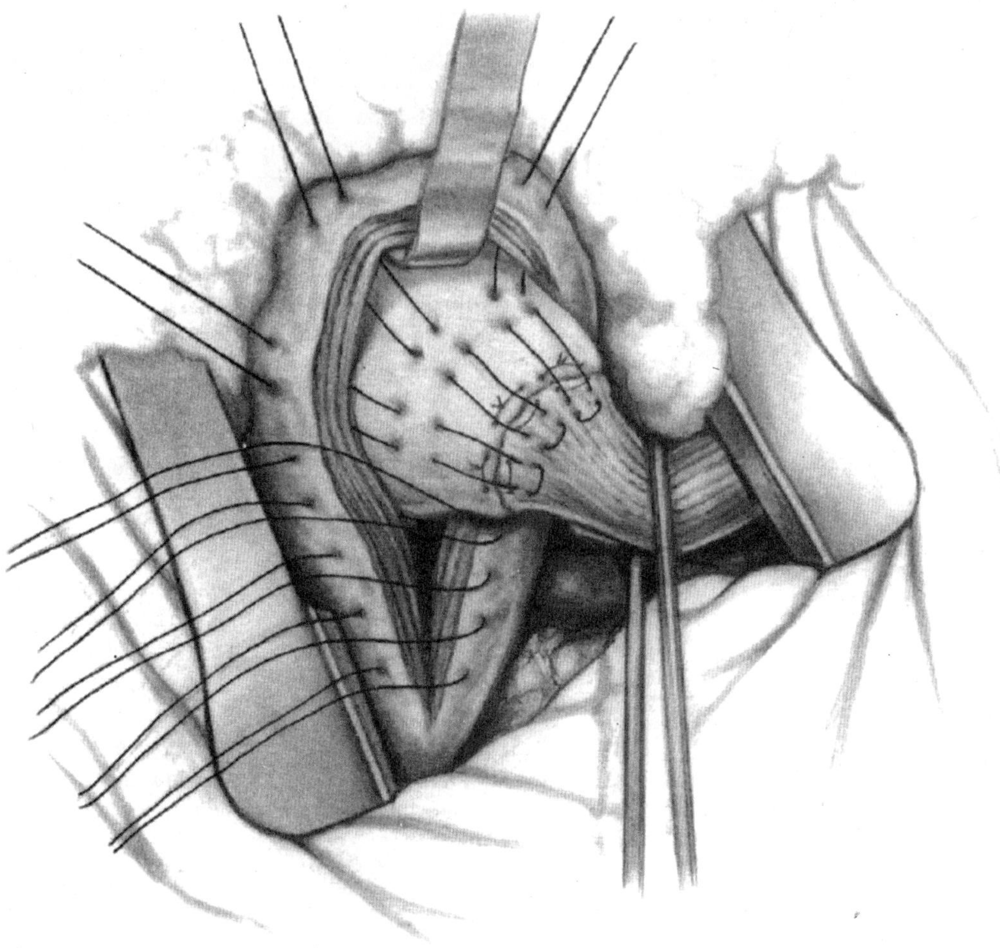

FIGURE 21.31

FIGURE 21.32

The sutures of the second row have been adjusted and tied, having replaced the inferior esophagus and the fundoplication into the abdomen. Introduction of the fundoplasty into the abdomen and tying of the sutures should be done with great caution, without using traction on the sutures in the esophagus, since this may lead to tearing of the muscular wall, which is fragile. The lower esophagus, partially covered by the stomach, is manually replaced under the diaphragm and should remain in that position spontaneously without need for traction. This descent of the esophagogastric junction is obtained when mobilization of the esophagus has been correctly performed. If the esophagogastric junction were to remain in the abdomen under tension it would lead to failure of the operation.

Once the esophagogastric junction has been reduced into the abdomen, the mattress sutures of the second row are tied, as can be seen in the drawing. The previously placed sutures in the esophageal hiatus are then tied. It is considered that the hiatus is correctly closed (figure on the right) when the tip of the right index finger can be passed between the esophagus with a nasogastric tube in it and the edge of the hiatus. Belsey does not use a nasogastric tube to decompress the stomach postoperatively. However, it is felt that it is always necessary to decompress the stomach postoperatively in patients operated on for hiatus hernia in whom a fundoplasty has been performed, be it complete or partial, or in cases in which calibration of the esophagogastric junction has been performed. If the nasogastric tube is not placed during the procedure, it will be very difficult to introduce it postoperatively if gastric decompression becomes necessary.

In patients who are reoperated for reflux esophagitis that has recurred one or more times, dissection of the esophagus and the stomach, as well as identification of the vagus nerves or its branches, is very difficult and dangerous. In these cases, one may involuntarily transect one or both vagus nerves or their branches, which may lead to problems with postoperative gastric function and failure of the procedure. For this reason, it is advisable, in operations for recurrences, to perform a pyloroplasty to facilitate pyloric emptying. This does not become a difficult problem because in reoperations for reflux esophagitis, it is generally necessary to perform a thoracolaparotomy.

With the Belsey operation, one obtains at least 4 cm of the lower esophagus below the diaphragm. Two cm are obtained with the first row of mattress sutures and 2 cm with the second row of mattress sutures.

Belsey Mark IV Technique

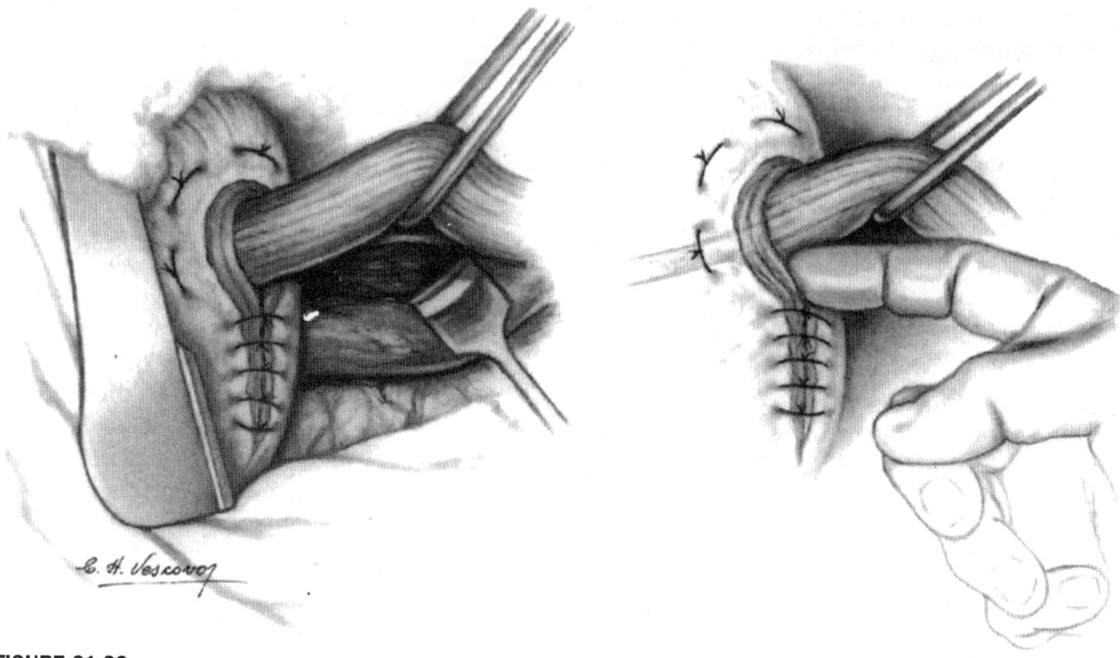

FIGURE 21.32

Shortening and stricture of the esophagus due to gastroesophageal reflux

The treatment of patients with reflux esophagitis complicated by shortening and stricture of the esophagus varies greatly according to the degree of shortening, the degree of stricture, failures of previous operations, the presence of other esophageal lesions, and the age and general condition of the patient. In order to select the most adequate treatment for each patient, it is necessary to identify several situations. Some of them will be analyzed here.

1. There are patients with shortening of the esophagus due to reflux esophagitis in whom, with an extensive mobilization of the esophagus, it is possible to carry the esophagogastric junction into the abdomen without traction and construct a 240° fundoplasty using the Belsey technique (88, 89, 92–94). It is felt that these patients do have shortened esophaguses but that these can be brought into the abdomen.
2. Other patients simultaneously present shortening and fibrous stricture of the esophagus but the stricture is dilatable. In these patients it may also be possible to bring the esophagogastric junction into the abdomen without traction and perform a Belsey fundoplasty. These patients have a shortened esophagus with a dilatable stricture but that can be brought into the abdomen.
3. Some other patients may present shortening of the esophagus but differ from the preceding ones in that, in spite of complete mobilization of the esophagus, it is not possible to carry the esophagogastric junction into the abdomen. These are patients with a short esophagus that cannot be brought into the abdomen. These patients may be treated using the Collis-Nissen technique, which consists in elongating the esophagus at the expense of the lesser curvature of the stomach (14, 15). To this technique one adds a Nissen antireflux procedure (64, 65, 67, 69).
4. There are patients with shortening of the esophagus to the point that it cannot be brought into the abdomen who also have a dilatable fibrous stricture. These patients, too, can be treated with a Collis-Nissen procedure.
5. Other patients may present a fibrous stricture of the esophagus that is dilatable with or without longitudinal shortening but due to the patient's poor general condition it is not possible to perform the complete esophageal mobilization without running a very serious risk. These patients should receive medical treatment with periodic dilations of the esophagus because the peptic stricture recurs readily if reflux has not been suppressed.
6. There are patients with a fibrous stricture of the esophagus that cannot be dilated or who have undergone forced dilation of the esophagus, leading to perforation. The only possible surgical indication for these patients is resection of their affected esophagus and replacement, using a segment of the left colon (4, 7, 18, 35, 61, 104) or a jejunal loop (7, 18, 77), both of which can be brought up in isoperistaltic fashion.
7. Another group is composed of patients who have been operated upon several times for esophagitis due to reflux with poor results (107). These patients have very altered esophagus but one that allows the passage of food or presents a dilatable stricture. These patients cannot undergo a thoracic procedure. They may benefit from the procedure proposed by Payne (71, 72), which consists of an operation performed completely through the abdomen—including hemigastrectomy, bilateral vagotomy and anastomosis of the gastric stump to a jejunal loop brought up in Roux-en-Y fashion, or interposing a jejunal loop longer than 35 cm between the gastric stump and the duodenum. With both procedures the acid secretion of the stomach diminishes and the biliary secretion is diverted. In patients in whom is it not possible to perform a truncal vagotomy by the abdominal route due to the difficulties caused by previous surgery, it is advisable to perform a 70% gastrectomy instead of a hemigastrectomy (18, 71, 72, 84).

Collis-Nissen Technique

In the majority of patients with shortening of the esophagus due to reflux esophagitis, it is possible to bring the esophagogastric junction down into the abdomen without traction if a complete mobilization of the esophagus through the thoracic approach following the Belsey technique is performed (24, 88, 89, 92–94). In patients who present a fibrous stricture of peptic origin that is dilatable in addition to a shortening of the esophagus, it is also frequently possible to bring the esophagogastric junction into the abdomen. However, in other patients with a shortened esophagus and a dilatable stricture or without stricture, it is not possible to bring the esophagogastric junction down into the abdomen even though an extensive mobilization of the esophagus is performed. Extensive mobilization of the esophagus is not complete if the left superior and inferior bronchial arteries and two or three esophageal minor arteries are not divided and tied (88, 92–94). The patients with a shortened esophagus in whom it is not possible to bring the esophagogastric junction down into the abdomen, can be efficaciously treated using the Collis-Nissen procedure (7, 14, 15, 18, 64–67, 69).

The operation originated by Collis (14, 15) consists in producing a lengthening of the esophagus at the expense of the lesser curvature of the stomach. A neoesophagus is constructed using a gastric tube. The neoesophagus is logically without any antireflux mechanism and is therefore exposed to permanent reflux of the contents of the rest of the stomach. To prevent this reflux, the Belsey fundoplication was used with poor results (66). Later, a Nissen type of fundoplasty was used to construct the antireflux barrier with better results (7, 18, 67, 69). This is the technique that will be described in the following. It is necessary to point out that the Collis-Nissen operation cannot be performed in patients presenting a shortening of the esophagus greater than 7 cm nor in patients who have undergone gastrectomy. Patients who suffer from a shortening of the esophagus simultaneous with a fibrous stricture of the esophagus that is not dilatable cannot be treated by this procedure.

FIGURE 21.33

The most frequently used incision for the Collis-Nissen operation is through the left sixth intercostal space. In patients operated on for recurrence of esophagitis with reflux, it is preferable to enter the thorax through the seventh left intercostal space because this permits an easier approach into the abdomen, be it through the diaphragm or by prolonging the incision into the abdomen and transecting the costal margin (thoracoabdominal incision). For a simultaneous approach into the thorax and the abdomen it is necessary to place the patient in the right lateral position with the thorax rotated to the left to give the surgeon standing on the left side of the patient good visualization of both the thoracic and the abdominal fields. Once the thorax is opened, the operative maneuvers previously described in the Belsey procedure are performed. This includes introduction of the self-retaining Finochietto retractor, ligating and dividing the inferior pulmonary ligament, dividing the mediastinum pleura and the pleura of the costodiaphragmatic sinus, and mobilization of the esophagus to the arch of the aorta. One must be careful not to traumatize the esophagus during this mobilization, since it frequently presents very inflamed and fragile walls. One must also avoid damaging the vagus nerves or its branches.

Collis-Nissen Technique

Once mobilization of the esophagus is complete, the fatty cushion some 3 cm in diameter located on the anterior lateral surface of the cardia is resected. The phrenoesophageal ligament is then divided together with the peritoneum over the anterior wall of the hernial sac, allowing entrance into the peritoneal cavity. The phrenoesophageal membrane and the peritoneum of the hernial sac are resected. The right hand is introduced into the peritoneal cavity, and the stomach is freed from the entire circumference of the esophageal hiatus. The proximal segment of the hepatogastric ligament is then divided. All the short vessels in a 15 cm length of the greater curvature of the stomach are divided and tied. Once the proximal half of the stomach is freed, the anesthesiologist is instructed to introduce a dilating mercury Hurst or Maloney bougie 50–60 F through the esophagus into the stomach. If the patient has a stricture of the esophagus that could not be sufficiently dilated preoperatively to permit passage of the bougie, the dilation should be completed during the surgical procedure. In this situation the surgeon, from the chest, will facilitate introduction of the dilating bougies until the necessary diameter is obtained. If, during mobilization of the esophagus, the right pleura is traumatized, the pleural orifice should be covered with one or two gauze compresses to prevent any amount of blood from entering the right pleural cavity.

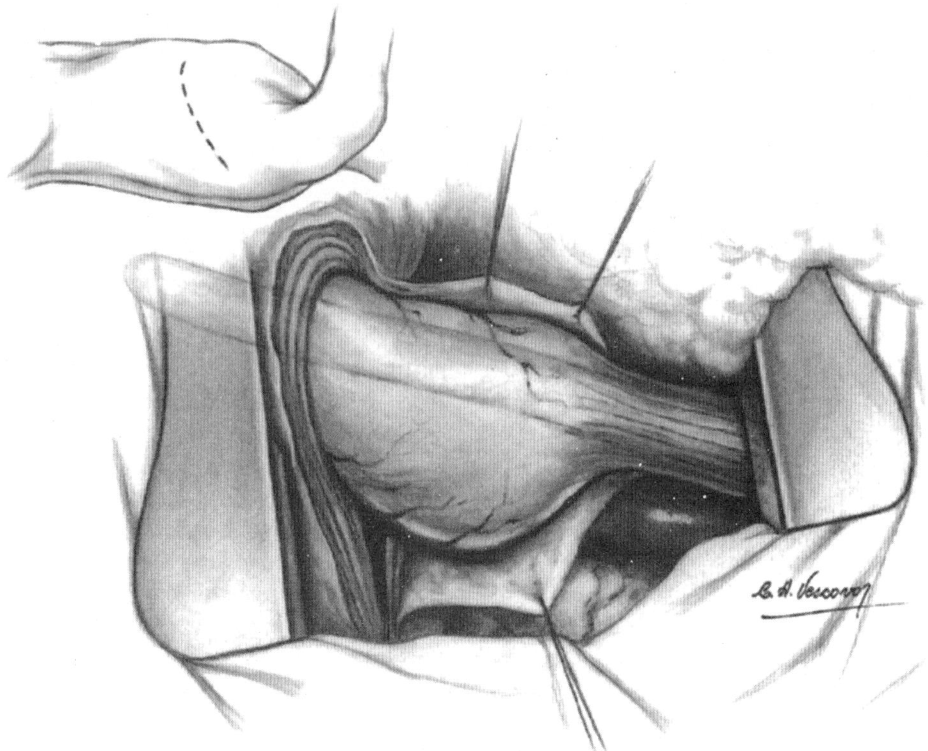

FIGURE 21.33

FIGURE 21.34
The Hurst bougie introduced into the stomach is led along the lesser curvature and held in this position by the first assistant. Using two Babcock clamps placed on the greater curvature, traction is applied in the opposite direction allowing the placement of an 8 cm GIA stapler parallel to and proximal to the mercury bougie. Once the GIA has been correctly placed, it is fired and then removed. The edges where the staples were placed are then inspected to see that they are all correctly positioned and to determine if any leakage exists.

Collis-Nissen Technique

FIGURE 21.35
With firings of the Gia stapler, some 7 to 8 cm of elongation of the esophagus has been obtained.

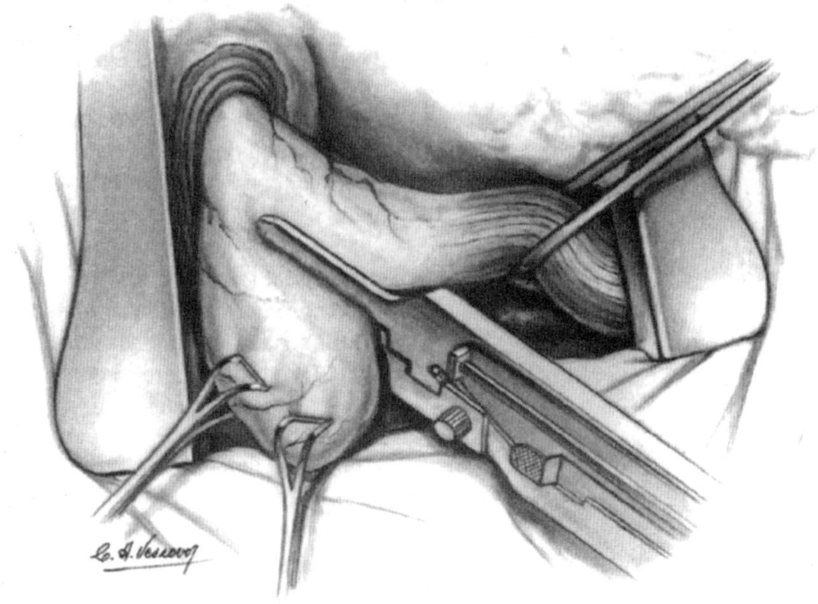

FIGURE 21.34

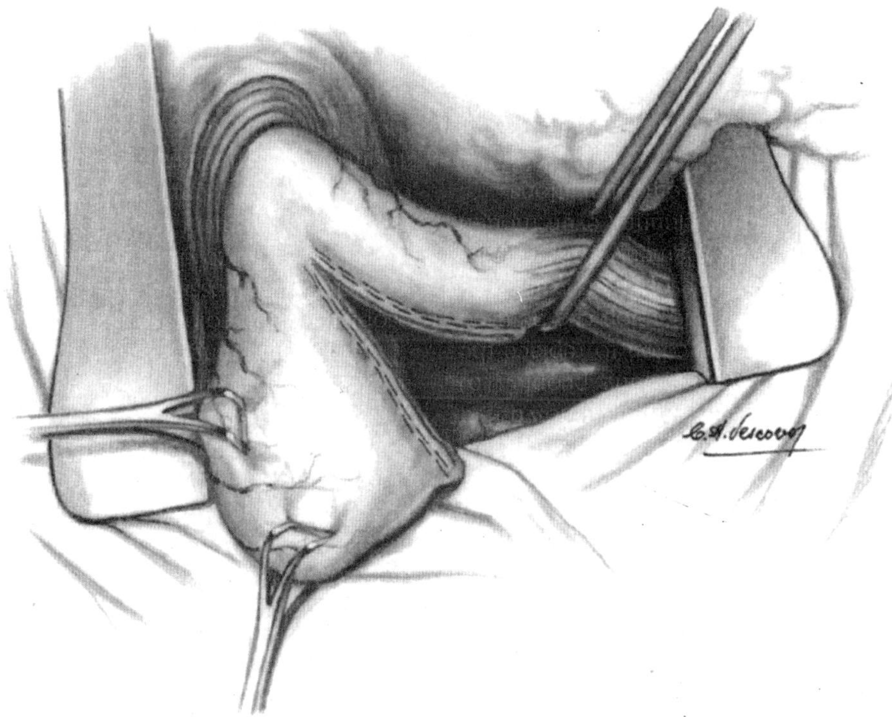

FIGURE 21.35

FIGURE 21.36
Some surgeons trust the suture line performed with the stapler and do not invert the suture line with another layer of sutures. However, it is considered safer to add another suture line to invert the line of staples applied by the GIA instrument. This second layer can be performed with a continuous suture or interrupted sutures. It is preferable to use interrupted sutures, as shown in the drawing, on the neoesophageal tube as well as on the gastric fundus. Interrupted sutures, in addition to affording greater safety, have no tendency to shorten the neoesophagus. The suture material that is used is Prolene 4-0. Up to now we have described the original Collis procedure (14, 15) with the difference that, instead of being constructed with clamps, the neoesophagus has been constructed using the Gia stapler. The only thing that is still missing is adding a Nissen type of fundoplasty as an antireflux barrier to the Collis operation. The fundoplasty that is added to the Collis operation is not a typical Nissen procedure, but only a Nissen type of procedure (18), since what remains of the fundus will not allow a complete fundoplication. In addition, the fundic wrapping is not performed around the abdominal esophagus, a sine qua non of the Nissen procedure. It is done around the neoesophagus, which is a tube constructed from the stomach.

Collis-Nissen Technique

FIGURE 21.37
One can observe in the drawing that the end of the gastric fundus has been grasped with a Babcock clamp to be able to pass it around the neoesophagus and wrap it completely around while the Hurst mercury bougie, 50 F, is still in place.

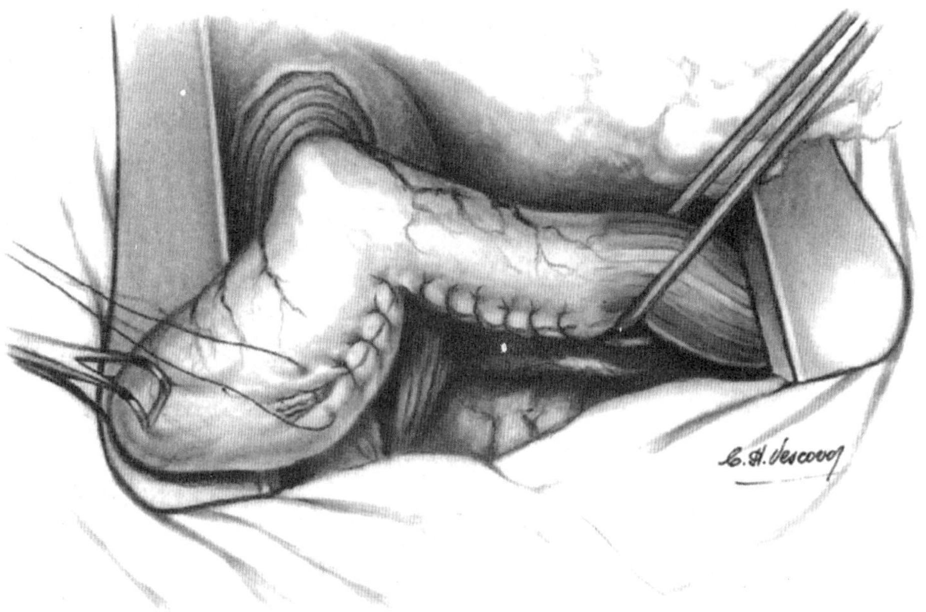

FIGURE 21.36

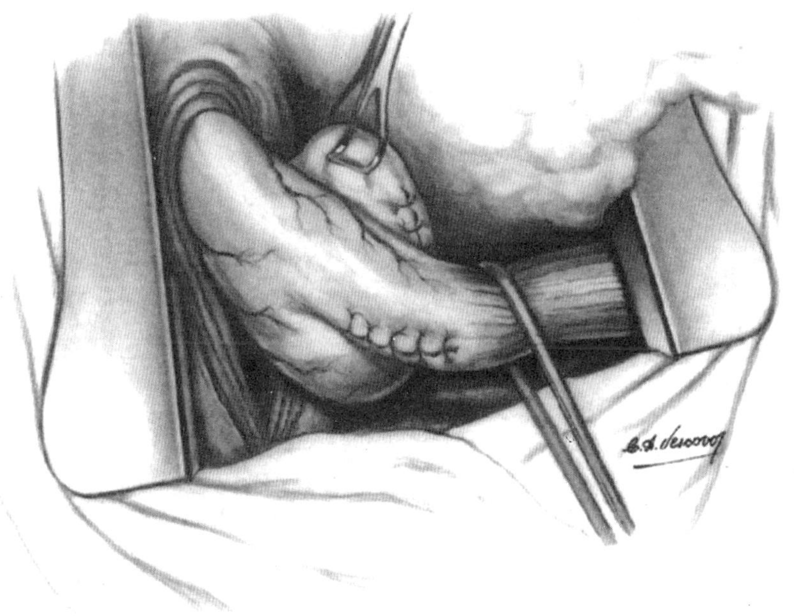

FIGURE 21.37

FIGURE 21.38
The entire circumference of the neoesophagus has been surrounded using the gastric fundus. The end of the gastric fundus is being sutured to the rest of the gastric fundus. Usually, two interrupted Prolene 2-0 sutures are used, leaving a distance of 1 cm between them. The sutures include on one side, the left side of the fundus, then the neoesophagus, and finally the right side of the fundus. The sutures should include the serosa, muscularis, and submucosa of the stomach as well as that of the neoesophagus. Some authors use three or four sutures. It has been shown that the height of the fundic wrapping has great importance in the swallowing movement. The higher and tighter that the fundoplication is performed, the greater difficulty there will be in making the swallowing movement. Once the fundoplasty around the neoesophagus is completed with the mercury bougie still within it, it is possible to introduce a finger comfortably between the neoesophagus and the fundic wrapping. This maneuver shows that the fundic wrapping does not excessively compress the neoesophagus. In this operation, as in the typical Nissen procedure, one should count on the compressive effect that will be exerted by the air in the stomach, postoperatively, on the neoesophagus.

Collis-Nissen Technique

FIGURE 21.39
Once the fundoplication has been completed, the mercury bougie is removed and replaced by a No. 18 F nasogastric tube. One then proceeds to place the sutures, closing the esophageal hiatus behind the neoesophagus. These sutures will not be tied until the neoesophagus surrounded by its fundoplication has been introduced into the abdomen. The drawing shows the maneuver used to perform this. The neoesophagus surrounded by the fundoplication is grasped by the right index finger and thumb and delivered into the abdomen, where it should remain without having to apply any traction.

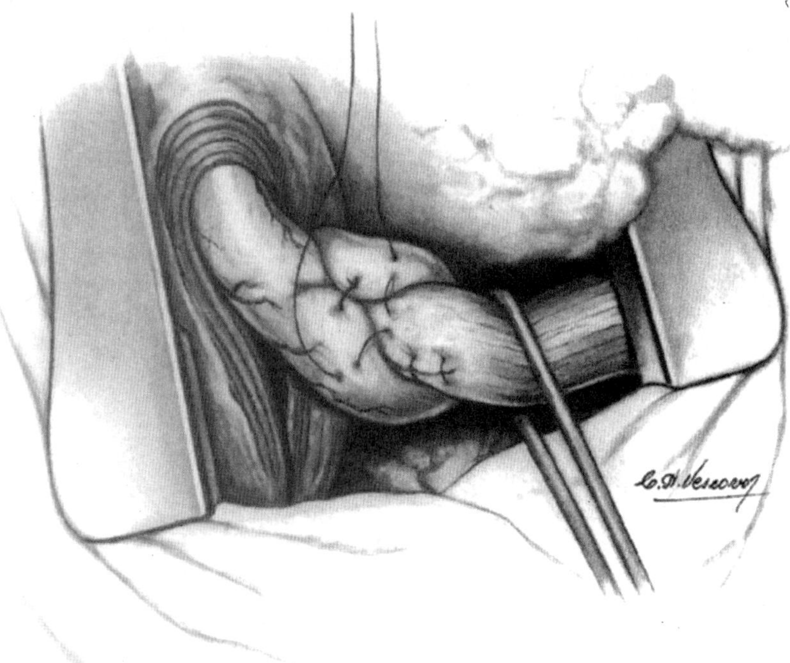

FIGURE 21.38

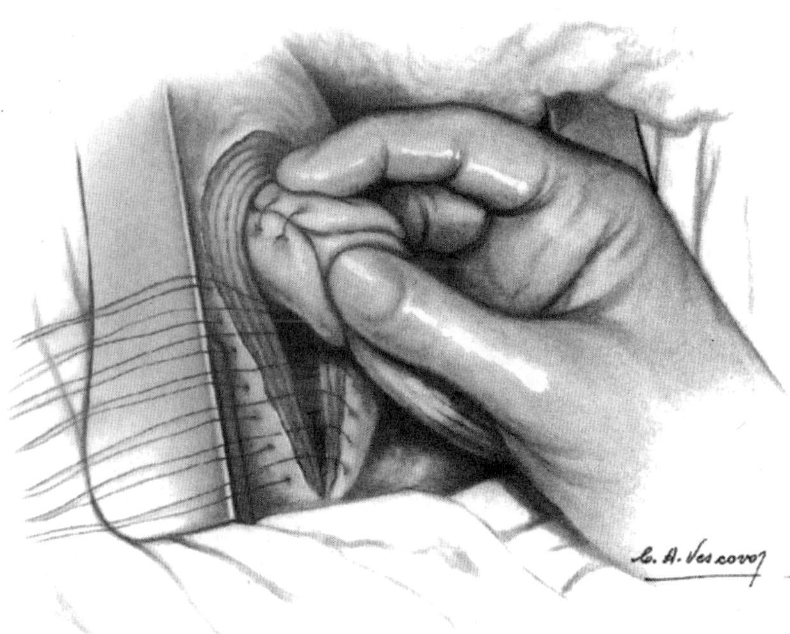

FIGURE 21.39

FIGURE 21.40
The neoesophagus with its fundic wrapping has been introduced into the abdomen. The sutures closing the hiatus will then be tied and adjusted so that the hiatus will be closed.

Collis-Nissen Technique

FIGURE 21.41
The esophageal hiatus has been closed. It is demonstrated that between the esophagus with a nasogastric tube within it and the edge of the hiatus, only the tip of the right index finger can be admitted. The pleural cavity is irrigated with warm saline solution, and the left chest is drained with a No. 38 plastic tube with several perforations.

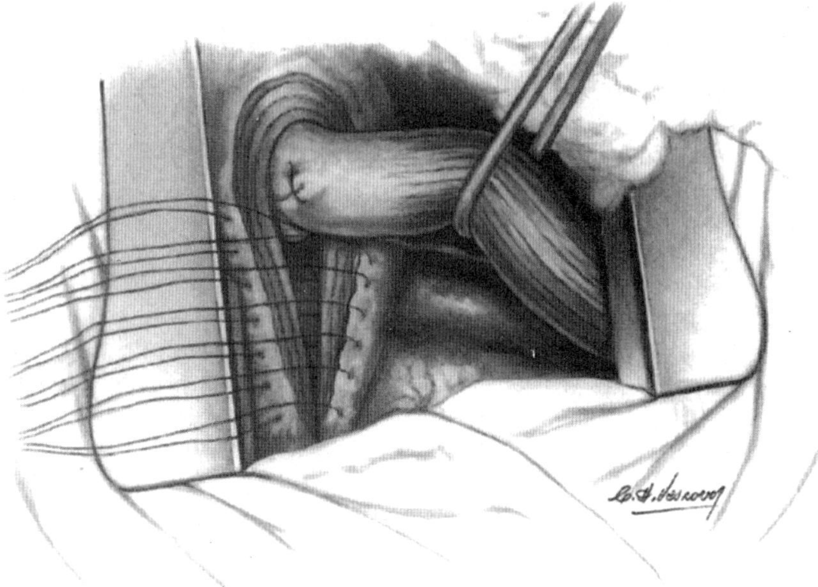

FIGURE 21.40

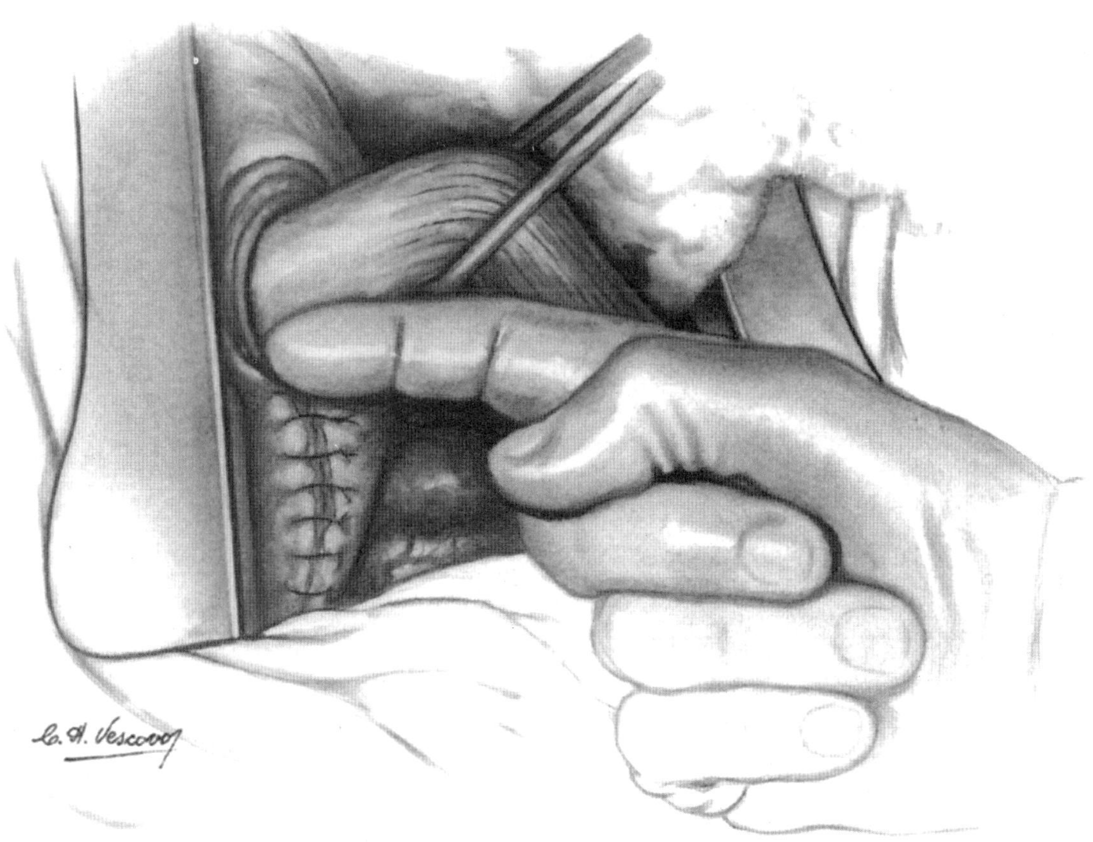

FIGURE 21.41

Esophageal resection with colon interposition

Until recently, strictures of the esophagus of peptic origin were frequently resected. At present, these strictures are very rarely resected. The diminution in the number of resections is due to the success attained with dilations performed by specialized gastroenterologists and to the making of the diagnosis before a nondistensible stricture is established. It should be added that the success of dilation is assured by the performance of an antireflux procedure (4, 7, 17, 18, 35, 62, 92–94).

The colon and the jejunum are the organs most frequently used to replace the esophagus that has been resected because of a peptic stricture. The colon, and in particular the left colon, brought up in isoperistaltic fashion, is the one preferred by the majority of surgeons. The reasons for this are these: (a) The colon has shown that it has good tolerance, especially in young people. (b) The preparation of the segment of colon to replace the esophagus is easy to perform. (c) The colon can be used to replace a short segment of the esophagus (distal lesion) as well as to replace a long segment of the esophagus (midesophageal region). The jejunum, even though it replaces the esophagus well, has some limitations:

1. One limitation is due to the vascular arcades of the jejunum.
2. The maximum viable extension that can be obtained with a segment of jejunum to replace the esophagus varies between 15 and 20 cm.
3. The jejunum is only useful to replace the distal segment of the esophagus.
4. Preparation of the jejunal limb to be interposed is more difficult than preparation of a colonic loop (7, 18, 77).

The segment of the colon generally used to replace the esophagus is the segment irrigated by the left colic artery, the ascending branch of the inferior mesenteric artery. Distal lesions of the esophagus can be replaced with a short segment of colon. The distal esophagus is the most frequent location of strictures of peptic origin. In patients presenting a peptic stricture located more proximally, one should use a long segment of the left colon. Irrigation of the long segment will be supplied, as will that of the short segment, by the left colic artery, but it will be necessary to ligate the midcolic artery to allow a greater displacement of the colon upward (7).

Before planning to use the colon to replace the esophagus, the colon should be studied radiographically to exclude the possible presence of diverticula in the selected area and to discard any other pathologic change. It is also convenient to perform a selective angiography of the colon to eliminate the presence of any vascular anomaly, in particular in the marginal artery, which, even though it is infrequent, can occur. One should also bear in mind the susceptibility of the distal aorta and the inferior mesenteric artery to arteriosclerosis (7). The colon should be prepared in a similar fashion as when it is to be resected.

Esophageal Resection with Colon Interposition

Esophageal Resection with Colon Interposition

FIGURE 21.42
This drawing shows a sliding esophageal hiatus hernia with a fibrous stricture of the distal esophagus. This is the most frequent location of peptic strictures of the esophagus. Distal strictures can be replaced by a short segment of the left colon or a segment of jejunum.

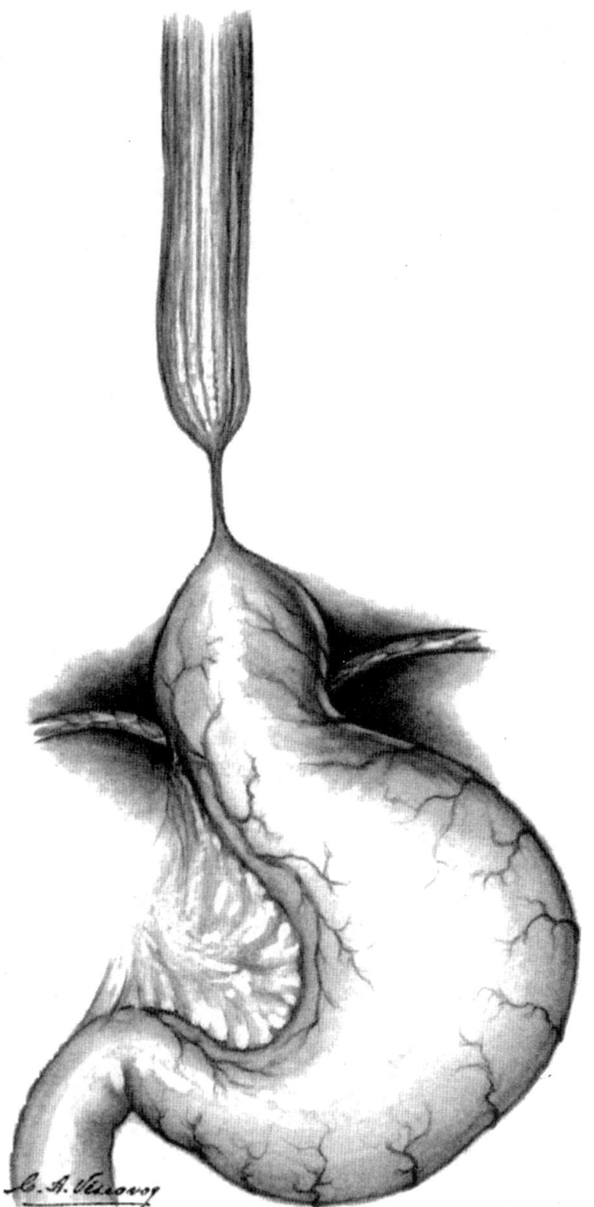

FIGURE 21.42

Esophageal Resection with Colon Interposition

FIGURE 21.43
X-ray of a patient 27 years old with nondistensible stricture of the distal esophagus subjected to a resection of this segment replaced by a segment of the left colon.

FIGURE 21.44
X-ray of a patient 43 years old presenting a fibrous peptic stricture more proximally than the previous patient. She was subjected to several esophageal dilations without success. In the last dilation the esophagus was traumatized. The injured esophagus was resected and replaced by a long segment of the left colon.

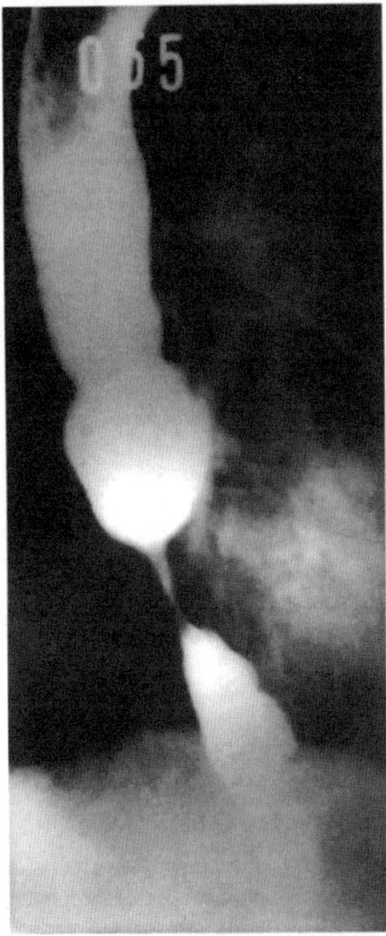

FIGURE 21.43

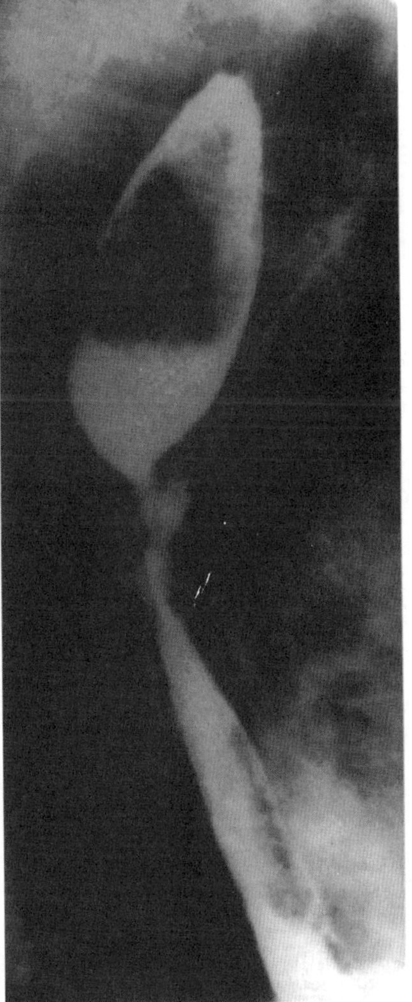

FIGURE 21.44

Esophageal Resection with Colon Interposition

FIGURE 21.45
Schematic drawing of the colon with the arteries that supply it. The portion marked by oblique lines represents a short segment of the left colon. This is the segment that is used to replace the strictured distal esophagus. In these cases it is not necessary to ligate the middle colic artery. However, this artery should be ligated when a long segment of colon is used.

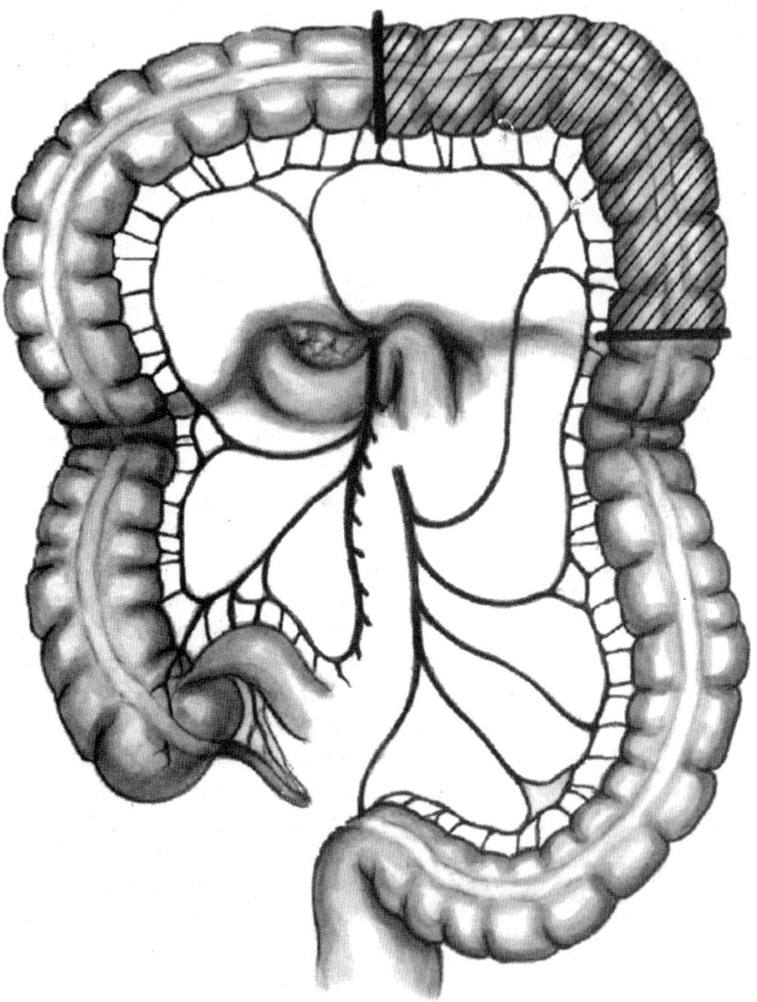

FIGURE 21.45

FIGURE 21.46
This drawing shows the completed operation. A short segment of colon has been placed in isoperistaltic position to replace the resected distal esophagus. The segment of colon has been passed behind the stomach and through the esophageal hiatus. Its upper end has been anastomosed in end-to-end fashion to the transected end of the inferior esophagus. The lower end of the colon has been anastomosed to the anterior wall of the stomach about 8 to 10 cm below the cardia, anteriorly.

Esophageal Resection with Colon Interposition

In patients who have been operated upon several times it is advisable to perform a pyloromyotomy or a pyloroplasty in case the trunks of the vagus nerves or some of its branches have been injured in previous operations. The pyloromyotomy or pyloroplasty is a preventive measure to avoid functional disturbances of the stomach (7, 18). The surgical procedure is terminated by performing a gastrostomy to decompress the stomach postoperatively. Some surgeons decompress the stomach by passing a nasogastric tube through the interposed segment of colon (7). Others perform a feeding jejunostomy to nourish patients postoperatively. This entire procedure is performed through a thoracolaparotomy.

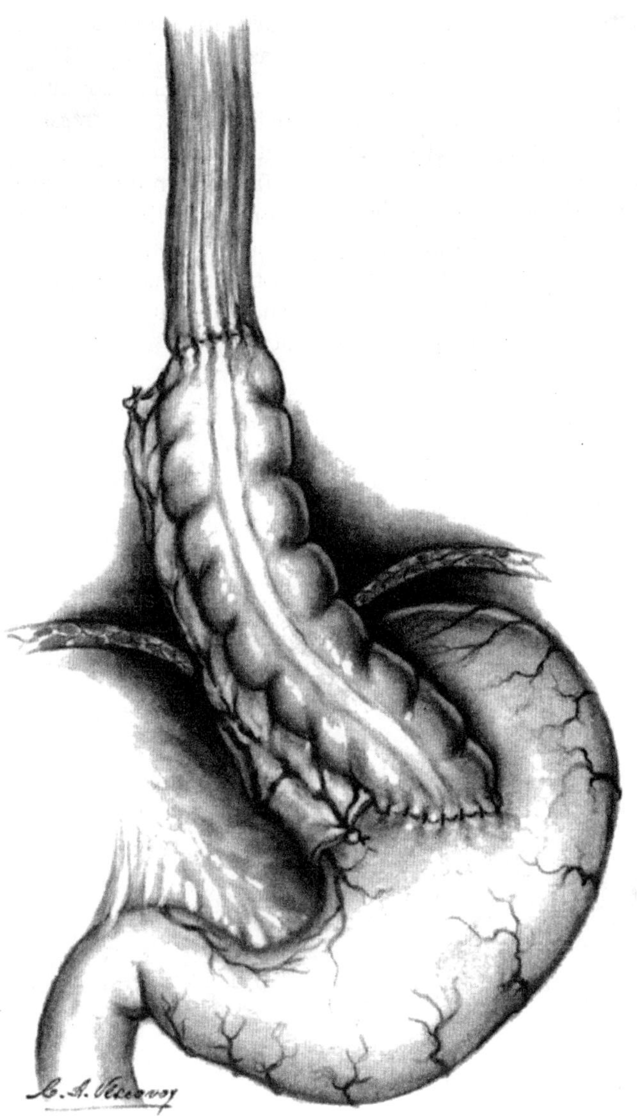

FIGURE 21.46

Esophageal resection with jejunal interposition

Jejunal interposition is a good alternative in the treatment of peptic strictures of the distal esophagus. However, when the esophageal lesion extends above the inferior pulmonary vein, the possibility of using the jejunum should be discarded. The maximum length of jejunal segment that can be transplanted into the thorax varies between 15 and 20 cm. On the other hand, it is necessary to point out that, in order for the segmental jejunum to have any value as an antireflux barrier, it should be at least 15 cm long (77).

The peristaltic contractions of the jejunum are very efficient in the progression of the alimentary bolus. Patients with an interposed segment of jejunum do not notice any difference in the swallowing movement following surgery from what they had when their esophagus was normal, whereas some patients with colonic interposition may notice a certain slowness in the progression of the bolus. The transplanted colon loses a large part of its peristaltic activity (7).

Esophageal Resection with Jejunal Interposition

FIGURE 21.47

This drawing shows the completed operation. A segment of jejunum located in isoperistaltic position replaces the resected distal esophagus. The jejunal segment has been passed through the transverse mesocolon and behind the stomach, through the esophageal hiatus. Its upper end has been anastomosed in end-to-side fashion with the esophagus, and its lower end has been anastomosed to the anterior wall of the stomach near the lesser curvature some 5 or 6 cm below the transected and closed cardia of the stomach. When doing interpositions of either the jejunum or the colon, careful attention should be given not only to the arterial circulation, but the venous circulation as well.

Esophageal Resection with Jejunal Interposition

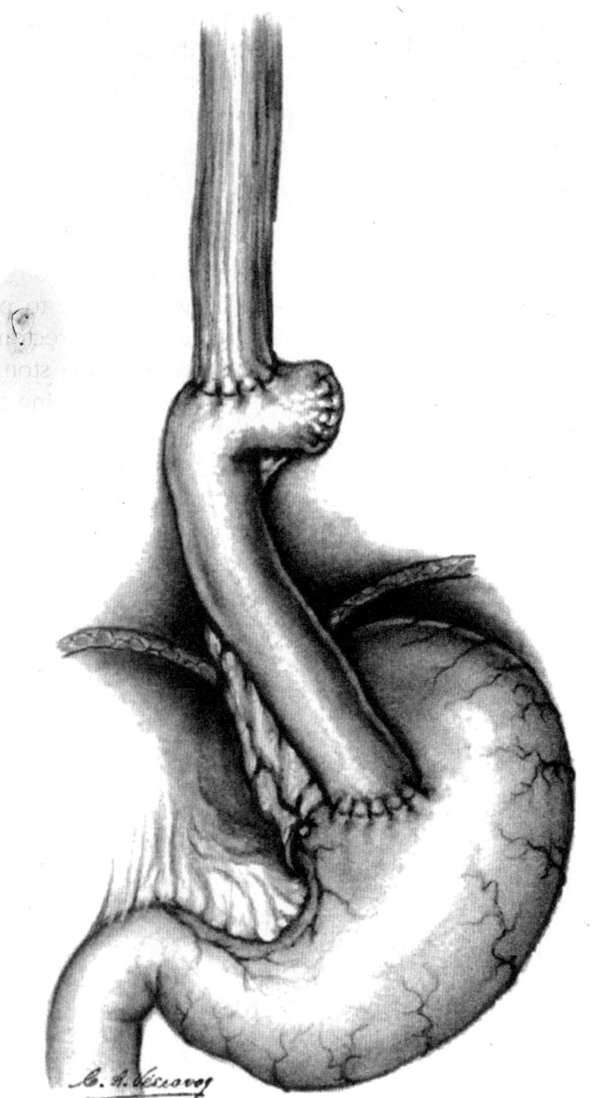

FIGURE 21.47

Hemigastrectomy, vagotomy and drainage with a jejunal loop disposed in Roux-en-Y fashion (Payne)

Patients with esophageal reflux that have been subjected to several operations without success can benefit from the operation proposed by Payne. The operation is performed completely through the abdomen, staying away from the previously invaded areas, be they abdominal or thoracic. The operation consists of a hemigastrectomy, truncal vagotomy and anastomosis of the gastric stump to a Roux-en-Y jejunal loop. The end-to-side jejunojejunal anastomosis of the Roux-en-Y is performed 40 to 50 cm distal to the gastrojejunal anastomosis. With good results, similar to those obtained with the Roux-en-Y anastomosis previously described, Payne has also proposed, instead of the Roux-en-Y anastomosis, the interposition of a segment of jejunum 40 to 50 cm long, in isoperistaltic fashion, between the gastric stump of the hemigastrectomy and the duodenum (71, 72).

In patients who have been operated upon several times and in patients who present a shortening of the esophagus, it is not always possible to perform a bilateral truncal vagotomy through the abdomen. In these patients, it is advisable to perform a 70% gastrectomy instead of a hemigastrectomy to reduce the hydrochloric acid secretion of the stomach. This approach is less aggressive than attempting to perform a truncal vagotomy by the thoracic approach.

Hemigastrectomy, Vagotomy and Drainage with a Jejunal Loop Disposed in Roux-en-Y Fashion (Payne)

Hemigastrectomy, Vagotomy and Drainage with a Jejunal Loop Disposed in Roux-en-Y Fashion (Payne)

FIGURE 21.48

This drawing shows one of the procedures proposed by Payne: Hemigastrectomy, as shown in the insert on the left, and bilateral vagotomy. The duodenal stump, with the performance of an end-to-side jejunojejunal anastomosis some 50 cm beyond the gastrojejunal anastomosis, is closed in two layers and a jejunal limb brought up in Roux-en-Y fashion, whose ascending limb has been anastomosed to the gastric stump in end-to-side fashion some 50 cm from the gastrojejunal anastomosis. This procedure creates a peristaltic barrier preventing reflux of biliary and pancreatic secretions. If there is difficulty in performing a vagotomy, a 70% gastrectomy must be done.

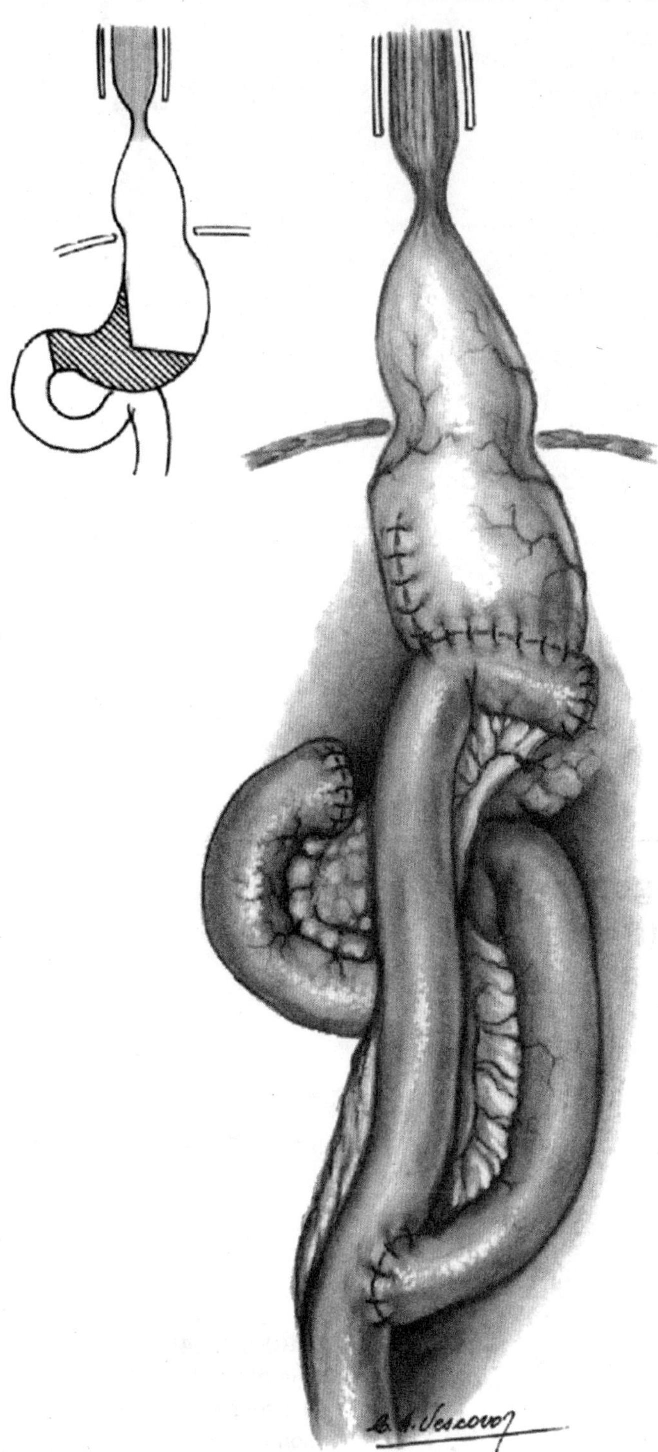

FIGURE 21.48

Hemigastrectomy, Vagotomy and Jejunal Interposition (Payne)

FIGURE 21.49
The drawing shows the other procedure proposed by Payne in the treatment of recurrence of reflux esophagitis. The operation consists of a hemigastrectomy, truncal vagotomy, and interposition of a segment of jejunum 40 to 50 cm long. The interposed jejunal segment also creates a peristaltic barrier, preventing reflux of biliary and pancreatic secretions.

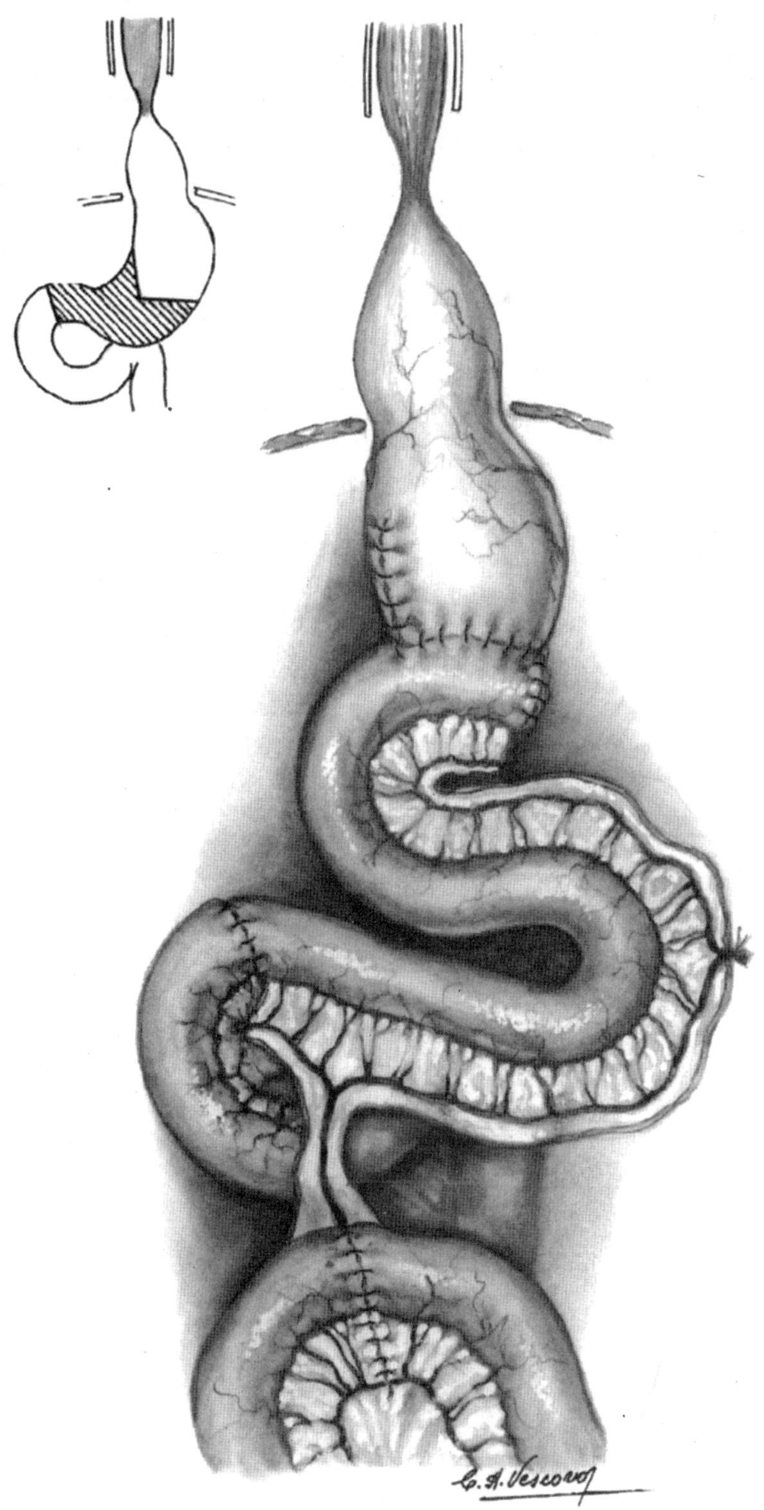

FIGURE 21.49

FIGURE 21.50
The jejunal loop to be interposed is being prepared. Generally, the third or fourth jejunal loop distal to the ligament of Treitz is used. Vascularization of the jejunum must be carefully studied by means of transillumination. The broken line shows where the incision of the mesentery and the ligation of the vascular structures have to be made.

Hemigastrectomy, Vagotomy and Jejunal Interposition (Payne)

FIGURE 21.51
The jejunal loop has been isolated, preserving its venous and arterial circulation. This loop will be disposed in isoperistaltic fashion, performing an anastomosis to the gastric stump in its upper end and to the duodenum in its lower end.

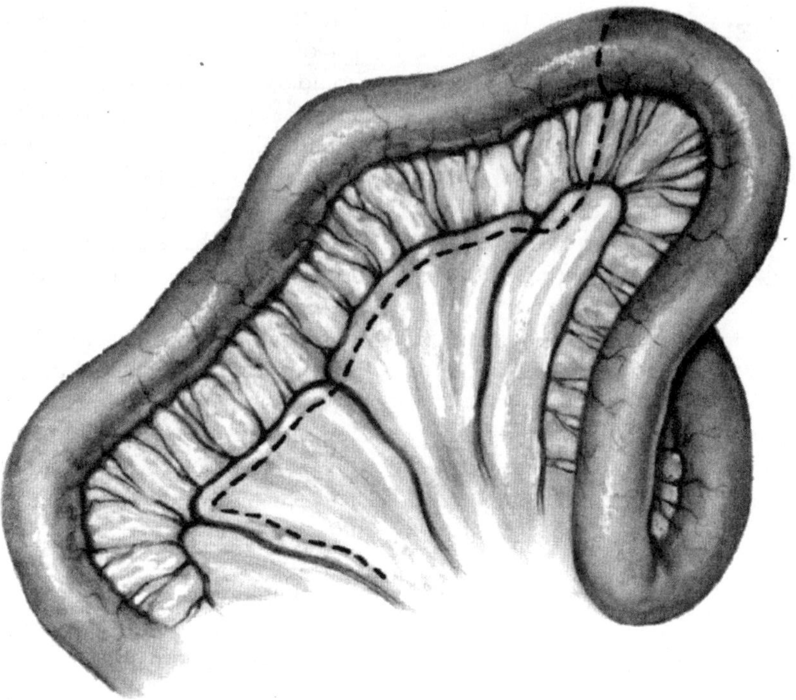

FIGURE 21.50

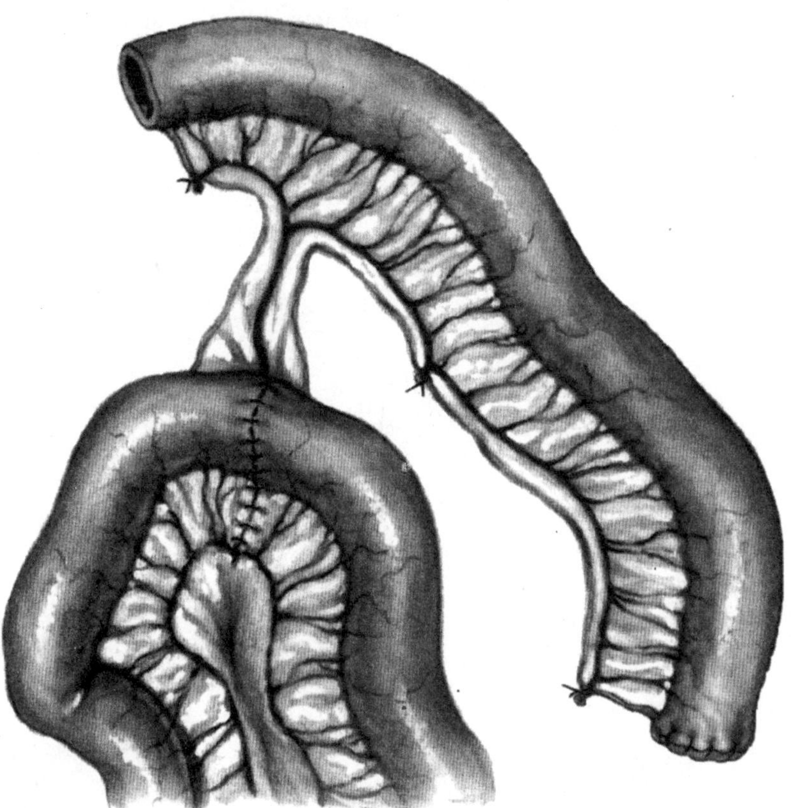

FIGURE 21.51

Paraesophageal Hiatus Hernia

Paraesophageal hiatus hernia is seen less frequently. This variety of hiatus hernia differs from the sliding hiatus hernia because the esophagogastric junction remains below the diaphragm, fixed to the preaortic fascia and the median arcuate ligament. These hernias do not present changes in the mechanism of the competence of the cardia. Paraesophageal hernias have a complete peritoneal sac wrapped around the stomach that has migrated into the thorax. Complications of paraesophageal hernia are exclusively mechanical, sometimes very serious. The stomach progressively ascends into the thorax, first the fundus, and then the greater curvature, which, as it ascends, becomes rotated upward while the lesser curvature remains in its low position. With time the entire stomach may migrate into the thorax wrapped in its parietal peritoneum. In spite of the migration of the entire stomach into the thorax, together with migration of other abdominal organs, the esophagogastric junction stays fixed in its normal infradiaphragmatic position. In a few cases, the esophagogastric junction may also migrate into the thorax, giving place to a mixed hernia that frequently includes incompetence of the cardia.

Complicated paraesophageal hernias have an elevated mortality, making it advisable that patients with paraesophageal hernias be operated on before they become complicated even though they are completely asymptomatic, as long as the patient's general condition will tolerate the procedure. It has been shown that when 60 to 70% of the stomach has migrated to the thorax, patients should be operated upon. Surgery for paraesophageal hiatus hernia is easier to perform than surgery for sliding hernia because, in the great majority of cases, it is not necessary to perform an antireflux procedure. The operation consists simply in reduction of stomach and other viscera if they have migrated into the thorax, resection of the hernial sac, and closure of the esophageal hiatus. If the esophagogastric junction is fixed below the diaphragm, it is necessary to take precautions to keep this fixation from being damaged. Only in mixed hernias should an antireflux procedure be performed. Some authors, however, advise performing an antireflux procedure in all cases of paraesophageal hernia (7). A complete study of patients preoperatively will determine if there is or not an accompanying sliding hernia with reflux. The surgical approach to paraesophageal hernia is not complicated, generally being approached through the abdominal route. Patients with symptoms, which means that the hernia has been complicated by volvulus, incarceration, ischemia, gangrene, or perforation, should be approached through the thoracic or thoracoabdominal route. The author uses the abdominal approach in cases that are not complicated. If it is necessary a thoracotomy can be added in patients in whom the hernial sac is adhered to the mediastinum or the stomach is adherent to the hernial sac. The technique to be described is that proposed by Ellis and colleagues (30, 31).

Paraesophageal Hiatus Hernia

FIGURE 21.52

A midline supraumbilical incision has been performed. If a wider operative field is necessary, the xiphoid process is resected and the incision is extended 5 or 6 cm below the umbilicus. Once the peritoneum is open, a self-retaining large Balfour retractor is inserted. It is very useful to have available an upper-hand retractor to elevate the inferior portion of the sternum and the costal cartridges, making it easier to visualize the esophageal hiatus. The drawing shows that more than 50% of the stomach has migrated into the thorax in an asymptomatic patient. A Harrington retractor holds the left lobe of the liver upward. As has been mentioned previously, it is not always necessary to divide the left triangular ligament of the liver to have good visualization of the esophageal hiatus. In some patients the entire stomach is rotated and has ascended into the chest. Rotation of the stomach may carry with it the greater omentum and transverse colon. In some cases some loops of small intestine also migrate into the thorax.

Paraesophageal Hiatus Hernia

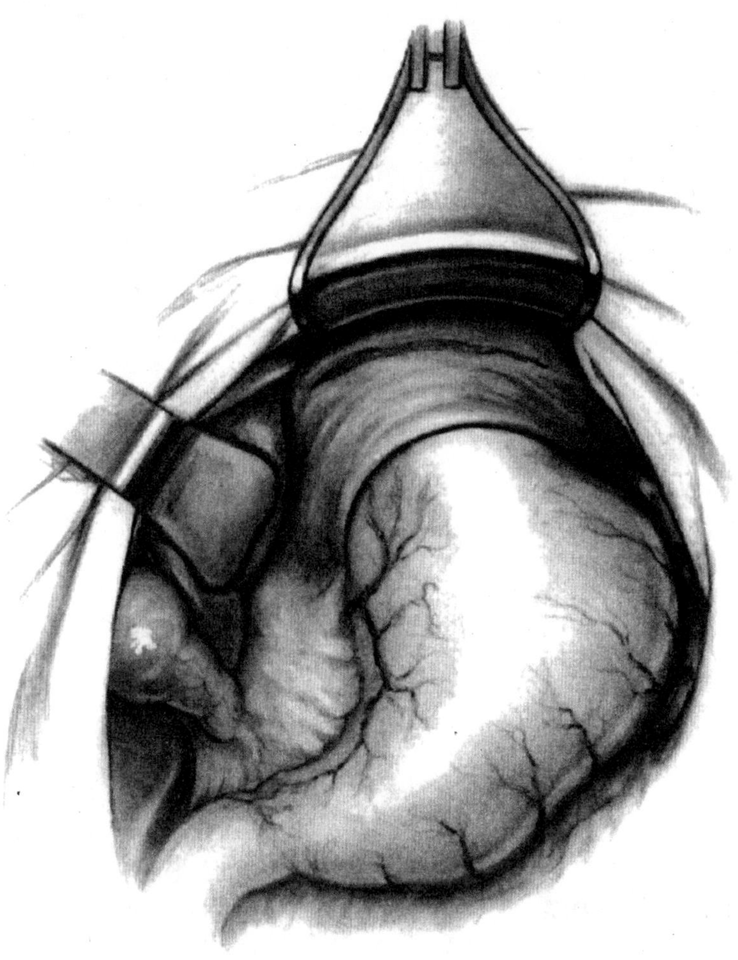

FIGURE 21.52

FIGURE 21.53
Using gentle traction with the right hand, the stomach is reduced into the abdomen. The same technique is used if other viscera have migrated into the thorax. In some patients the stomach is adherent to the hernial sac. The same may occur with other viscera that have migrated. In this situation it may be very difficult to reduce the viscera using the abdominal approach exclusively. In these cases, the incision may be extended into the thorax, or better, the abdominal incision closed, the patient changed in position, and a left thoracotomy performed to treat the paraesophageal hernia through the thoracic approach.

Paraesophageal Hiatus Hernia

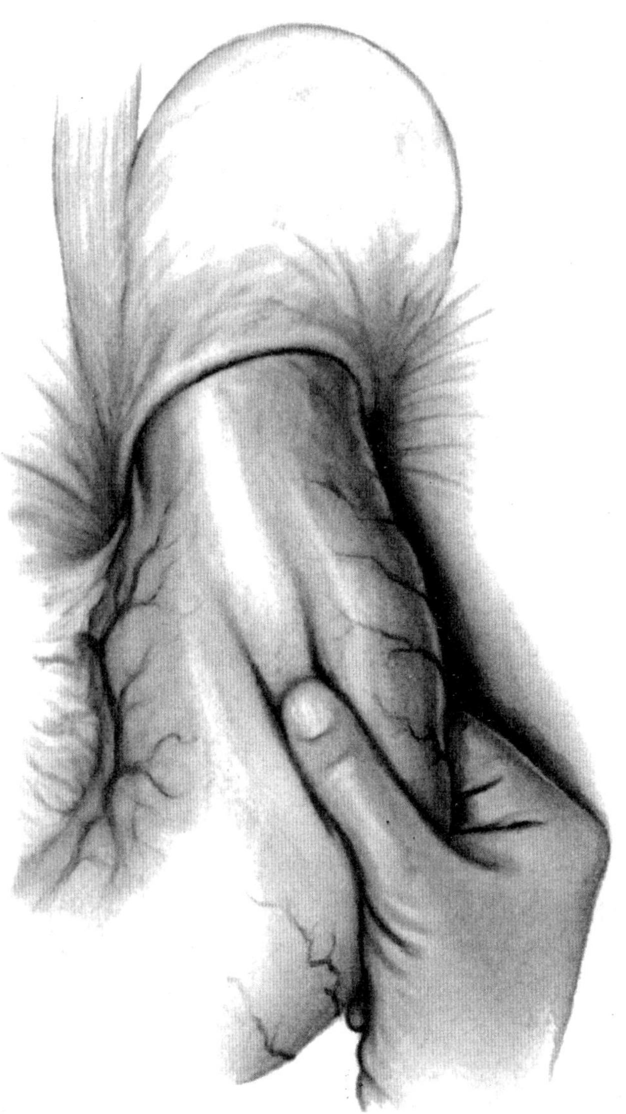

FIGURE 21.53

Paraesophageal Hiatus Hernia

FIGURE 21.54
Once the stomach has been reduced, the hernial sac is resected, applying traction to it toward the abdomen with Allis or Babcock clamps and using blunt dissection. It is necessary to resect the sac in order to prevent a possible recurrence of the hernia.

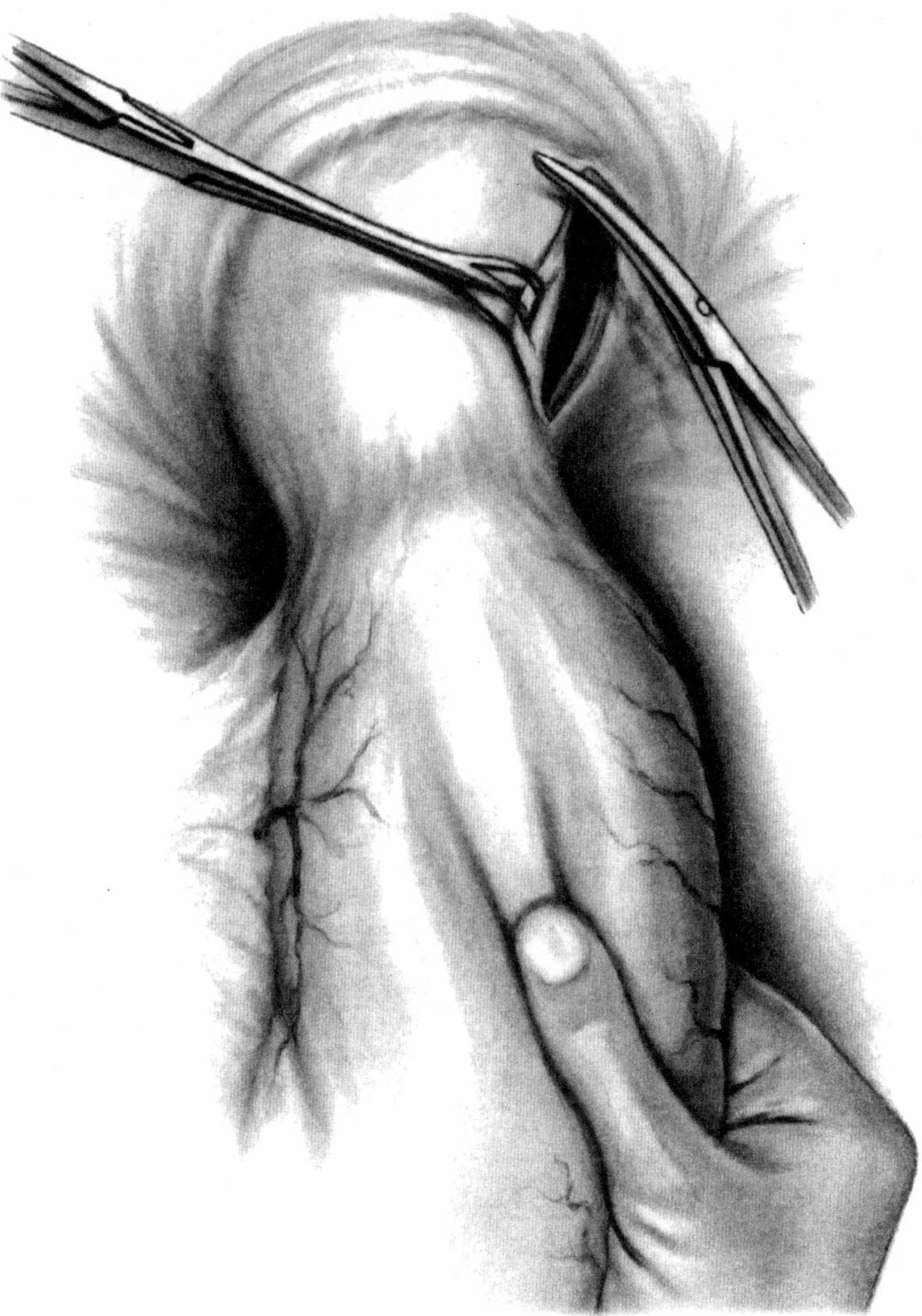

FIGURE 21.54

Paraesophageal Hiatus Hernia

FIGURE 21.55

The stomach has been reduced into the abdomen and the hernial sac resected. The rest of the surgical procedure consists of closure of the hiatus with interrupted silk or cotton sutures, as can be seen in the drawing. The closure is performed in front of the stomach and not behind the stomach as is usually done in sliding hiatal hernia with reflux. The purpose of performing the closure in front of the stomach is not to interfere with the normal fixation of the esophagogastric junction to the preaortic fascia and medial arcuate ligament.

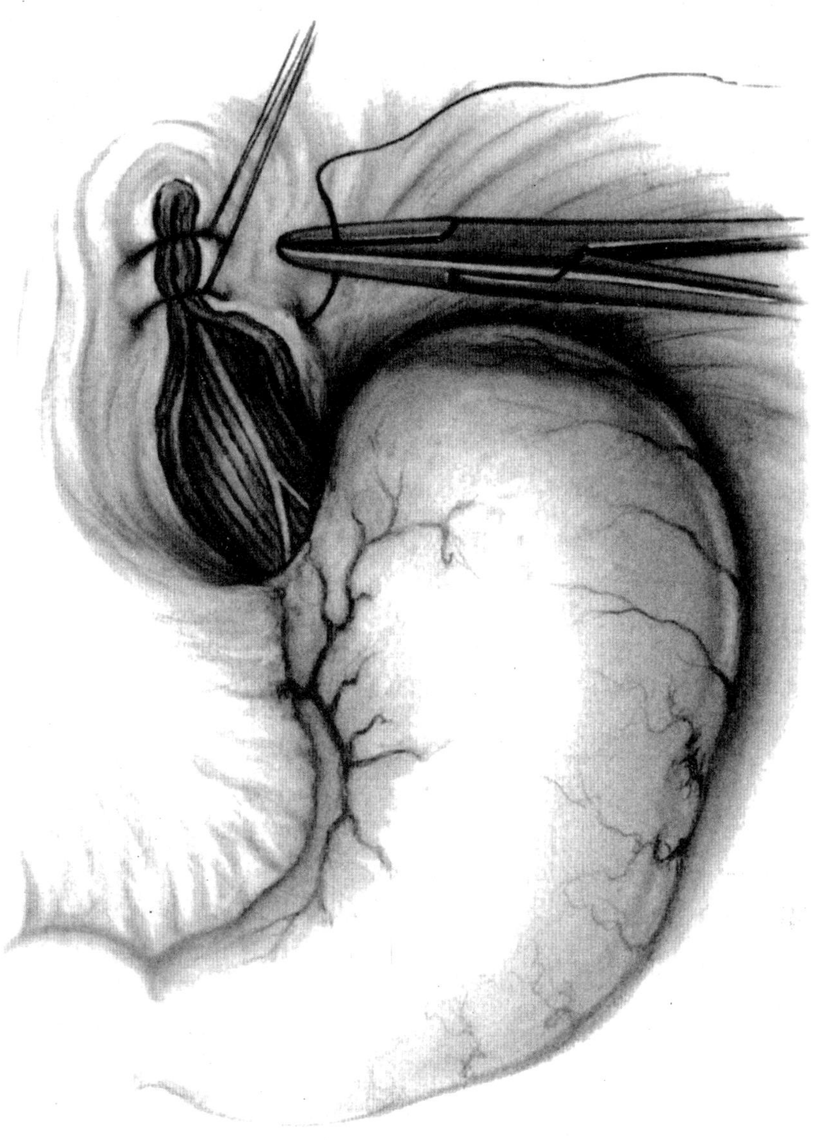

FIGURE 21.55

FIGURE 21.56
The closure of the hiatus in front of the stomach has been completed and the correctness of this closure is being tested. If the tip of the right index finger can pass between the wall of the esophagus with an 18 F nasogastric tube within it and the edge of the hiatus, the closure can be deemed to be correct. In patients in whom a large part of the stomach or all of the stomach has migrated into the chest, as well as other abdominal organs, it is advisable to finish the procedure with a gastrostomy, as shown in the insert. The gastrostomy fixes the stomach to the abdominal wall, making recurrence more difficult by migration of the stomach into the chest.

Paraesophageal Hiatus Hernia

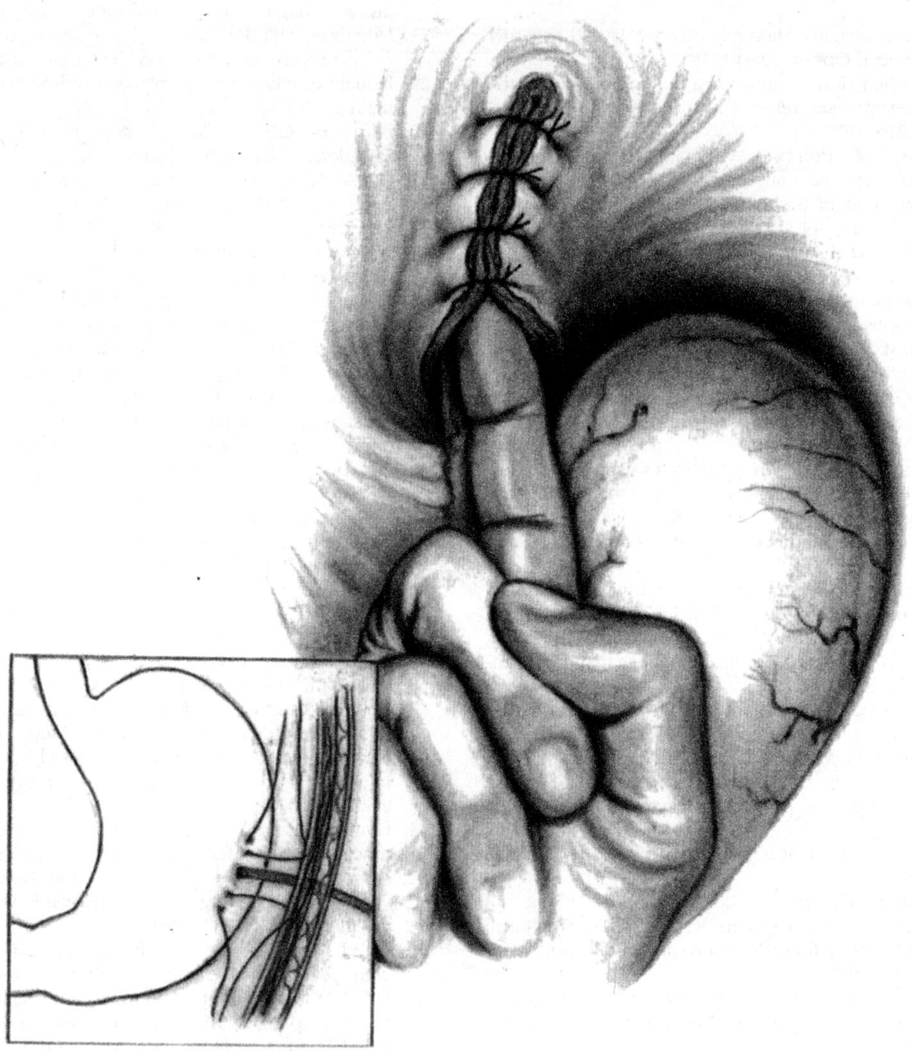

FIGURE 21.56

References

1. Allison, P.R. Reflux esophagitis: Sliding hiatus hernia and anatomy of repair. Surg. Gynecol. Obstet. 92:419, 1951.
2. Angelchick, J.P., Cohen, R.A. A new surgical procedure for the treatment of gastroesophageal reflux and hiatal hernia. Surg. Gynecol. Obstet. 148:246, 1979.
3. Battle, W.S., Nyhus, L.M., Bombeck, C.T. Gastreoesophageal reflux: Diagnosis and treatment. Ann. Surg. 177:560, 1973.
4. Belsey, R. Reconstruction of the esophagus with the left colon. J. Thorac. Cardiovasc. Surg. 49:33, 1965.
5. Bombeck, C.T., Dillard, D.H., Nyhus, L.M. Muscular anatomy of the gastroesophageal junction and role of phrenoesophageal ligament: Autopsy study of the sphincter mechanism. Ann. Surg. 164:643, 1966.
6. Bombeck, C.T. Esophageal hiatal hernia and gastroesophageal reflux. In Nyhus, L.M., Condon, R.E. (Eds.) Hernia. Ed. 3, p. 584. Lippincott, Philadelphia, 1989.
7. Bredenberg, C.E. Gastroesophageal reflux and hiatus hernia. In Fromm, D. (Ed.) Gastrointestinal surgery. Vol. I, p. 163. Churchill Livingstone, New York, 1985.
8. Bremner, C.G., Lynch, V.P., Ellis, F.H. Jr. Barrett's esophagus: Congenital or acquired? An experimental study of esophageal mucosa regeneration in the dog. Surgery 68:209, 1970.
9. Bremner, C.G. The columnar lined (Barrett's) esophagus. Surg. Annu. 9:103, 1977.
10. Bremner, C.G. Gastric ulcer after the Nissen fundoplication. A complication of alkaline reflux. Afr. Med. J. 51:791, 1977.
11. Bremner, C.G., Crookes, P.F., DeMeester, T.R., Peters, J.H., Stein, H.J. Concentration of refluxed acid and esophageal mucosal injury. Am. J. Surg. 164:522, 1992.
12. Bushkin, F.L., Woodward, E.R., O'Learly, J.P. Occurrence of gastric ulcer after Nissen fundoplication. Am. Surg. 42:821, 1976.
13. Caporossi, M., Ginevri, P., Manzo, D., Maffi, C., Arca, R., Moraldi, A., Iascone, C., Stipa, S. Valutazione degli insuccessi della chirurgia del reflusso gastroesofageo ed orientamenti terapeutici. Chirurgie 2:197, 1989.
14. Collis, J.L. An operation for hiatus hernia with short esophagus. Thorax 12:181, 1957.
15. Collis, J.L. Gastroplasty. Thorax 16:197, 1961.
16. Cordiano, C., Róvere, G.Q.D., Agugiaro, S., Mazzilli, G. Technical modification of the Nissen fundoplication procedure. Surg. Gynecol. Obstet. 143:977, 1976.
17. Cougard, P., Bernard, A., Viard, H. Récidive de reflux gastro-oesophagien traité inicialment par voie thoracique. Lyon Chirurgical 88:275, 1992.
18. Chassin, J.L. Operative strategy. In General surgery. Vol. II, p. 255. Springer-Verlag, New York, 1984.
19. DeMeester, T.R., Johnson, L.F., Kent, A.H. Evaluation of current operations for the prevention of gastroesophageal reflux. Ann. Surg. 180:511, 1974.
20. DeMeester, T.R., Johnson, L.F. Evaluation of the Nissen antireflux procedure by esophogeal manometry and twenty-four-hour pH monitoring. Ann. Surg. 129:94, 1975.
21. DeMeester, T.R., Johnson, L.F., Joseph, G.J., Toscano, M.S., Hall, A.W., Skinner, D.B. Patients of gastroesophageal reflux in health and disease. Ann. Surg. 184:459, 1976.
22. DeMeester, T.R., Wang, C.I., Wernly, J.A., Pellegrini, C.A., Little, A.G., Klementschitsch, P., Bermudz, G., Johnson, L.S., Skinner, D.B. Technique, indication and clinical use of 24 hour esophageal pH monitoring. J. Thorac. Cardiovasc. Surg. 79:656, 1980.
23. DeMeester, T.R., Lafontaine, E., Joelsson, B.F. et al. Relationship of hiatal hernia to the function of the body of the esophagus and the gastroesophageal junction. J. Thorac. Cardiovasc. Surg. 82:547, 1981.
24. DeMeester, T.R. Transthoracic antireflux procedures. In Nyhus, L.M., Baker, R.J. (Eds.) Mastery of surgery. Vol. I, p. 381. Little, Brown, Boston, 1984.
25. DeMeester, T.R., Bonavina, L., Albertucci, M. Nissen fundoplication for gastroesophageal reflux disease: Evaluation of primary repair in 100 consecutive patients. Ann. Surg. 204:9, 1986.
26. Dilling, E.W., Peyton, M.D., Cannon, J.P., Kanaly, P.J. et al. Comparison of Nissen fundoplication and Belsey Mark IV in the management of gastroesophageal reflux. Am. J. Surg. 134:730, 1977.
27. Dodds, W.J., Hogan, W.J., Helm, J.F., Dent, J. Pathogenesis of reflux esophagitis. Gastroenterology 81:376, 1981.
28. Donahue, P.E., Bombeck, C.T. The modified Nissen fundoplication, reflux prevention without gas bloat. Chir. Gastroenterol. 11:15, 1977.
29. Donahue, P.E. Gastroesophageal reflux: Some of the mystery remains. Curr. Surg. 36:75, 1979.
30. Ellis, F.H., Olsen, A.M. Achalasia of the esophagus. p. 174. W.B. Saunders, Philadelphia, 1969.
31. Ellis, F.H. Jr. Paraesophageal hiatus hernia: A surgical disease. Surg. Rounds 12:28, 1989.
32. Evander, A., Little, A.G., Riddell Walther, B., Skinner, D.B. Composition of the refluxed material determines the degree of reflux esophagitis in the dog. Gastroenterology 93:28, 1987.
33. Fyke, F.E. Jr., Code, C.F., Schlegel, J.F. The gastroesophageal sphincter in healthy human beings. Gastroenterology 85:135, 1956.
34. Gahagan, T.H. The function of the musculature of the esophagus and stomach in the esophagogastric sphincter mechanism. Surg. Gynecol. Obstet. 114:293, 1962.
35. Glasgow, J.C., Cannon, J.P., Elkin, R.C. Colon interposition for benign esophageal diseases. Am. J. Surg. 137:175, 1979.
36. Goldberg, H.L., Dodds, W.J., Gee, S., Montgomery, C., Zboralske, F.F. Role of acid and pepsin in acute experimental esophagitis. Gastroenterology 56:223, 1969.
37. Goldstein, J.L., Schlessinger, P.K., Moswecz, H.L., Layden, T.J. Esophageal mucosa resistance: A factor in esophagitis. Gastroenterol. Clin. North. Am. 3:365, 1990.
38. Harmon, J.W., Johnson, L.F., Mayodonovich, C.L. Effects of acid and bilis salts on the rabbit esophageal mucosa. Dig. Dis. Sci. 26:72, 1981.
39. Helm, J.F., Dodds, W.J., Pelc, L.R., Palmer, D.W., Hogan, W.J., Teeter, B.C. Effect of esophageal emptying and saliva on clearance of acid from esophagus. N. Engl. J. Med. 310:284, 1984.
40. Henderson, R.D., Mugashe, F.L., Jeejeebhoy, K.N. et al. Synergism of acid and bile salts in the production of experimental esophagitis. Can. J. Surg. 16:12, 1973.
41. Henderson, R.D. Nissen hiatal hernia repair: Problems of recurrence and continued symptoms. Ann. Thorac. Surg. 28:587, 1979.
42. Hetzel, D.J., Dent, J., Reed, W.D. et al. Healing and relapse of severe peptic esophagitis after treatment with Omeprazole. Gastroenterology 95:903, 1988.
43. Hill, L.D., Tobías, J.A. An effective operation for hiatal hernia: An eight-year appraisal. Ann. Surg. 166:681, 1967.
44. Hill, L.D., Gelfand, M., Bauermeïster, D. Simplified management of reflux esophagitis with stricture. Ann. Surg. 172:638, 1970.
45. Hill, L.D. Intraoperative measurement of lower esophageal sphincter pressure. J. Thorac. Cardiovasc. Surg. 75:378, 1978.
46. Hill, L.D., Kozarek, R., McCallum, R., Mercer, C.D. The Esophagus. p. 90. W.B. Saunders, Philadelphia, 1988.
47. Hinder, R.A., DeMeester, T.R. Gastroesophageal reflux diseases and hiatal hernia in adults. In Scott, H.W. Jr., Sawyers, J.L. (Eds.) Surgery of the stomach, duodenum and small intestine. Ed. 2, p. 402. Blackwell, Boston, 1992.
48. Iascone, C., DeMeester, T.R., Little, A.G., Skinner, D.B. Barrett's esophagus: Functional assessment, proposed pathogenesis and surgical therapy. Arch. Surg. 118:543, 1983.
49. Imail-Beigi, F., Pope, C.E. Distribution of histological changes of gastroesophageal reflux in the distal esophagus of man. Gastroenterology 66:1109, 1975.
50. Johnson, L.F., DeMeester, T.R. Twenty-four hour pH monitoring of the distal esophagus: A quantitative measure of gastroesophageal reflux. Am. J. Gastroenterol. 62:325, 1974.
51. Johnson, L.F., Joelsson, B., Floren, C.H. Bile salts in the esophagus of patients with esophagitis. Scand. J. Gastroenterol. 23:712, 1988.
52. Kaminski, D.L., Codd, J.E., Sigmund, C.J. Evaluation of the use of the median arcuate ligament in fundoplication for reflux esophagitis. Am. J. Surg. 134:724, 1977.
53. Kivilaakso, E., Fromm, D., Silent, W. Effect of bile salts and related compounds on isolated esophageal mucosa. Surgery. 87:280, 1980.
54. Lind, J.F., Duthie, H.L., Schlegal, J.R. et al. Motility of the gastric fundus. Am. J. Physiol. 201:197, 1961.
55. Liebermann-Meffert, D. Architecture of the musculature at the gastroesophageal junction and in the fundus. Chir. Gastroenterol. 9:425, 1975.

56. Liebermann-Meffert, D., Allgöwer, M., Schmid, P., Blum, A.L. Muscular equivalent of the lower esophageal sphincter. Gastroenterology 76:31, 1979.
57. Lilliemoe, K.L., Johnson, L.F., Harmon, J.W. Akaline esophagitis: A comparison of the ability of components of gastroduodenal contents to injure the rabbit esophagus. Gastroenterology 85:621, 1985.
58. Siewert, J.R., Hölscher, A.H. eds. Diseases of the esophagus. p. 857. Springer-Verlag, New York, 1988.
59. McCallum, R.W., Berkowitz, D.M., Lerner, E. Gastric emptying in patients with gastroesophageal reflux. Gastroenterology 80:285, 1981.
60. Mansour, K.A., Burton, H.G., Miller, J.I. Jr., Hatcher, C.R. Jr. Complications of intrathoracic Nissen fundoplication. Ann. Thorac. Surg. 32:1973, 1981.
61. Mansour, K.A., Hansen, H.A., Hersh, T., Miller, J.I. Jr. et al. Colon interposition for advanced non malignant esophageal stricture: Experience with 40 patients. Ann. Thorac. Surg. 32:584, 1981.
62. Mercer, C.D., Hill, L.D. Surgical treatment of peptic esophageal stricture. Analysis of 20 year experience. J. Thorac. Cardiovasc. Surg. 91:371, 1986.
63. Merendino, K.A., Dillard, D.H. The concept of sphincter substitution by an interposed jejunal segment for anatomic and physiological abnormalities at the esophagogastric junction. Ann. Surg. 142:486, 1955.
64. Nissen, R. Eine einfache operation zur beein flussung der refluxoesophagitis. Schweitz Med. Wochenschr. 86:590, 1956.
65. Nissen, R. Gastropexy and "fundoplication" in surgical treatment of hiatal hernia. Am. J. Dig. Dis. 6:954, 1961.
66. Orringer, M.B., Sloan, H. Complications and failings of the combined Collis-Belsey operation. J. Thorac. Cardiovasc. Surg. 74:726, 1977.
67. Orringer, M.B., Sloan, H. Combined Collis-Nissen reconstruction of the esophagogastric junction. Ann. Thorac. Surg. 25:16, 1978.
68. Orringer, M.B., Schneider, R., Williams, G.W., Sloan, H. Intraoperative esophageal manometry: Is it valid? Ann. Thorac. Surg. 30:13, 1980.
69. Orringer, M.B., Orringer, J.S. The combined Collis-Nissen operation: Early assessment of reflux control. Ann. Thorac. Surg. 33:534, 1982.
70. O'Sullivan, G.C., DeMeester, T.R., Joelsson, B.E., Smith, R.B., Blough, R.R., Johnson, L.F., Skinner, D.R. Am. J. Surg. 143:40, 1982.
71. Payne, W.S. Surgical treatment of reflux esophagitis and stricture associated with permanent incompetence of the cardia. Mayo Clin. Proc. 45:553, 1970.
72. Payne, W.S., Olsen, A.M. (Eds.). The esophagus. p. 174. Lea & Febiger, Philadelphia, 1974.
73. Pennell, T.C. Supradiaphragmatic correction of esophageal reflux strictures. Ann. Surg. 193:655, 1981.
74. Petterson, G.B., Bombeck, C.T., Nyhus, L.M. The lower esophageal sphincter: Mechanism of opening and closure. Surgery 88:307, 1980.
75. Petterson, G.B., Bombeck, C.T., Nyhus, L.M. The influence of hiatal hernia on lower esophageal sphincter function: An experimental study. Ann. Surg. 193:214, 1981.
76. Polk, H.C. Jr. Fundoplication for reflux esophagitis: Misadventures with the operation of choice. Ann. Surg. 182:645, 1976.
77. Polk, H.C. Jr. Jeyunal interposition for reflux esophagitis and esophageal stricture unresponsive to valvuloplasty. World J. Surg. 4:731, 1980.
78. Pope, C.E. II. Progress in gastroenterology, pathophysiology and diagnosis of reflux esophagitis. Gastroenterology 70:445, 1976.
79. Postlethwait, R.W. Surgery of the esophagus. p. 196. Appleton Century Crofts, New York, 1979.
80. Richardson, J.D., Larson, G.M., Polk, H.C. Jr. Intrathoracic fundoplication for shortened esophagus. Am. J. Surg. 143: 29, 1982.
81. Rossetti, M., Hell, K.T. Sliding hiatus hernia. Fundoplication or Nissen repair. In Nyhus, L.M., Condon, R.E. (Eds.) Hernia. Ed. 2, p. 668. Lippincott, Philadelphia, 1979.
82. Rossetti, M., Hell, K.T., Nissen, R. Antireflux operation. In Nyhus, L.M., Baker, R.J. (Eds.) Mastery of surgery. Vol. I, p. 368. Little, Brown, Boston, 1984.
83. Rossetti, M. Thirty years of Nissen procedure: Development of fundoplication In Siewert, J.R., Hölscher, A.H. (Eds.) Diseases of the esophagus. p. 1239. Springer-Verlag, New York, 1988.
84. Royston, C.M.S., Dowling, B.L., Spencer, J. Antrectomy with Roux-en-Y anastomosis in the treatment of peptic oesophagitis with stricture. Br. J. Surg. 62:605, 1975.
85. Salo, J.A., Kivilaakso, E. The role of bile salts and trypsin in the pathogenesis of experimental alkaline esophagitis. Surgery 93:525, 1983.
86. Salzman, M., Barwick, K., McCallum, R.W. Progression of cimetidine treated reflux esophagitis to a Barrett's stricture. Dig. Dis. Sci. 27:281, 1982.
87. Samelson, S.L., Bombeck, C.T., Nyhus, L.M. et al. A new concept in the surgical treatment of gastroesophageal reflux. Ann. Surg. 197:254, 1983.
88. Skinner, D.B., Belsey, R.H.R. Surgical management of esophageal reflux and hiatus hernia: Long term results with 1030 patients. J. Thorac. Cadiovasc. Surg. 53:33, 1967.
89. Skinner, D.B., Belsey, R.H.R., Hendrix, T.R., Zuidema, G.D. (Eds.) Gastroesophageal reflux and hiatal hernia. Little, Brown, Boston, 1972.
90. Skinner, D.B., DeMeester, T.R. Gastroesophageal reflux. Curr. Probl. Surg. 13:1, 1976.
91. Skinner, D.B. Pathophysiology of gastroesophageal reflux. Ann. Surg. 202:546, 1985.
92. Skinner, D.B., Belsey, R.H.R. Management of esophageal disease. p. 485. W.B. Saunders, Philadelphia, 1988.
93. Skinner, D.B., Belsey, R.H.R. Management of esophageal disease. p. 487. W.B. Saunders, Philadelphia, 1988.
94. Skinner, D.B. Atlas of esophageal surgery. p. 115. Churchill Livingstone, New York, 1991.
95. Skinner, D.B. Hiatal hernia and gastroesophageal reflux. In Sabiston, D.C. Jr. (Ed.) Ed. 14, p. 704. W.B. Saunders, Philadelphia, 1991.
96. Smith, J., Payne, W.S. Surgical technique for management of reflux esophagitis after esophagogastrectomy for malignancy: Further application of the Roux-en-Y principle. Mayo Clin. Proc. 50:588, 1975.
97. Stein, H.J., Bremner, R.M., Jamieson, J., DeMeester, T.R. Effect of Nissen fundoplication on esophageal motor function. Arch. Surg. 127:788, 1982.
98. Stein, H.J., Barlow, A.P., DeMeester, T.R., Hinder, R.A. Complications of gastroesophageal reflux disease. Ann. Surg. 216:35, 1992.
99. Testart, J., Peillon, C. Les complications de l'opération de Collis. Lyon Chir. 88:193, 1992.
100. Vansant, J.H., Baker, J.W., Ross, D.G. Modifications of the Hill technique for repair of hiatal hernia. Surg. Gynecol. Obstet. 143:637, 1976.
101. Vantertoll, D.J., Ellis, H.F., Schlegel, J.F. et al. An experimental study of the role of gastric and esophageal muscle in gastroesophageal competence. Surg. Gynecol. Obstet. 122:575, 1966.
102. Warshaw, A.L. Simplified isolation of the median arcuate ligament for posterior gastropexy. Surg. Gynecol. Obstet. 154:733, 1982.
103. Way, L.W. Current Surgical. Diagnosis and treatment. Ed. 9, p. 400. Appleton Lange, Norwalk, CT, 1991.
104. Wilkins, E.W. Jr. Long segment colon substitution for the esophagus. Ann. Surg. 192:722, 1980.
105. Zaninotto, G., DeMeester, T.R., Schwizer, W., Johansson, K.E., Cheng, S.C. The lower esophageal sphincter in health and disease. Am. J. Surg. 155:104, 1988.
106. Zinner, M.J. Atlas of gastric surgery. In Skinner, D.B. (Ed.) Surgical practice illustrated. p. 103. Churchill Livingstone, New York, 1992.
107. Zucker, K., Peskin, G.W., Saik, R.P. Recurrent hiatal hernia repair: A potential surgical dilemma. Arch. Surg. 117:413, 1982.

[illegible]

Section E

Hiatus Hernia

CHAPTER **22**

Laparoscopic Surgery of Esophageal Hiatus Hernia

The original discussion of open surgery of esophageal hiatus hernia insisted upon the need for a complete examination for an adequate preoperative evaluation in order to correctly select the surgical procedure and the surgical approach to be used, and to adapt the procedure to the functional and organic alterations in each patient.

The development of laparoscopic surgery and its progressive use in different operations—cholecystectomy, appendectomy, various gynecologic operations, hernia surgery, and so on—stimulated the use of this technique in the treatment of gastroesophageal reflux that did not respond to medical therapy (10, 11). The most frequently used procedure in the treatment of hiatal hernia with reflux is a 360° Nissen fundoplication with various modifications introduced after its original description in order to prevent, or at least diminish, postoperative complications (12, 22, 23, 25). Bernard Dallemagne, from Belgium, was the first surgeon to perform a laparoscopic Nissen procedure (10, 11, 32). Partial fundoplications, such as the Toupet technique for partial posterior fundoplication, have been used less frequently (7–9, 31). The Dor partial anterior fundoplication has also been infrequently used (13). The technique proposed by Narbona-Arnau and colleagues, using the ligamentum teres, has also been used (6, 7, 20, 21). Recently Lucius Hill and his group have been performing, by the laparoscopic approach, a posterior gastropexy combined with calibration of the esophagogastric junction proposed by Hill in 1967 (2, 15, 16).

Placement of the Angelchik prosthesis has also been performed by laparoscopy (1, 4, 6, 24).

Laparoscopic surgery has not yet been used in the treatment of esophageal hiatal hernia as frequently as with open surgery. It has only been used in restricted fashion due to the difficulties of applying the laparoscopic procedure and adapting it to the various functional and organic alterations associated with hiatal hernia.

Some published reports of results of the laparoscopic Nissen operation appear promising (3, 7–11). A longer follow-up is necessary, however, in order to evaluate the procedure more adequately.

According to Swanstrom (26, 30), 17.5% of patients with surgical indication due to reflux were turned down due to the results of pH monitoring for 24 hours and manometric studies of esophageal motility.

It has been shown that many of the failures of antireflux surgery are due to a lack of precise preoperative evaluation, which frequently leads to inadequate operative techniques and a poor result (11, 12, 14, 26–28, 30, 32).

The surgeon who has the responsibility of carrying out an antireflux operation should be experienced in esophageal surgery. If a laparoscopic approach is to be used, he or she should also be experienced in this technique.

CONTRAINDICATIONS OF LAPAROSCOPIC SURGERY IN THE TREATMENT OF GASTROESOPHAGEAL REFLUX

Many situations contraindicate the use of laparoscopic surgery for gastroesophageal reflux. Some of these are as follows:

1. Patients in whom the distal esophagus cannot be brought down into the abdomen sufficiently. This is frequently seen in shortened esophagus due to fibrosis, stricture, ulcer, Barrett esophagus, etc.
2. Patients with previous surgery for hiatal hernia with reflux that has recurred. The contraindication holds for previous abdominal as well as thoracic procedures.
3. Gastrectomized patients.
4. Previous splenectomy.
5. Patients with motor alterations of the esophagus, weak peristaltic waves that are not propulsive, motor dysfunction of the lower esophagus, diffuse spasm, etc.

Some of the complications of antireflux surgery, performed laparoscopically, particularly of the Nissen technique, which is the most used, are dysphagia, recurrence of hernia and/or reflux, proximal or distal slipping of the fundic wrap, inability to vomit or regurgitate, "gas-bloat" syndrome, gastrointestinal alterations, early satiety, diarrhea, odinophagia, and so on (30). Additional complications may be caused by the laparoscopy itself.

OPERATIVE TECHNIQUE

A description of the 360° Nissen fundoplication will be made in the following illustrations, since this is the most frequently used technique, either by the open or laparoscopic approach.

Operative Technique

Operative Technique

FIGURE 22.1

The patient should be prepared for both the laparoscopic as well as the open approach in case a change in the approach becomes necessary. The pneumoperitoneum is carried out in the same manner as described for cholecystectomy. The patient is placed in dorsal decubitus with the operating table in reverse Trendelenburg with 20° tilt, so as to better expose the cardioesophageal area. For this procedure five trochars with their respective 10 mm cannulas should be introduced. One trochar should be placed in the midline, about 5 cm above the umbilicus; another trochar is placed about 5 cm below the xiphoid process; one trochar is placed in the left midclavicular line, about 4 to 5 cm from the costal arch; another trochar is placed in the left side at the level of the umbilicus. The last trochar is placed in the midclavicular line, about 5 cm from the costal arch. The laparoscope with the 30 to 45° angle together with the video camera is passed through the supraumbilical cannula. The upper midline cannula and the left subcostal midclavicular cannula are used to introduce instruments for the hiatal dissection and are handled by the surgeon. The right subcostal midclavicular cannula is used to introduce the retractor for the left lobe of the liver. The most commonly used retractor is one that spreads out like a fan and can be fixed in one position during the entire operation. The left lateral cannula is used to introduce instruments held by an assistant to apply downward traction to the stomach.

The trochar used to introduce the laparoscope, and the video camera is introduced first. The four other trochars are then inserted under visual control.

An 18 F nasogastric tube should be in place. Additionally a 50 F Hurst or Maloney mercury bougie should be introduced with its distal end in the lower third of the esophagus so that it can be passed into the stomach when necessary.

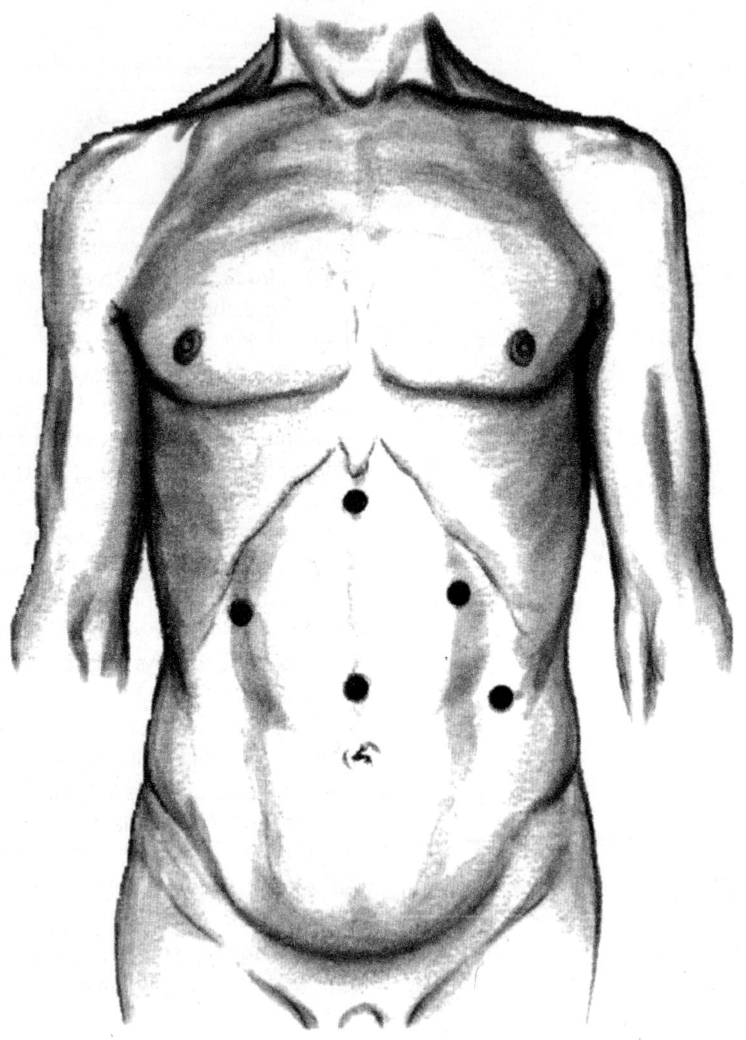

FIGURE 22.1

FIGURE 22.2

With the object of elevating the left lobe of the liver, a retractor is introduced through the right subcostal midclavicular cannula and disposed as a fan. This retractor is fixed in place to avoid having an assistant holding it during the entire procedure. Traction is applied to the upper anterior gastric wall using two atraumatic graspers. Elevation of the left lobe of the liver and downward traction on the stomach exposes the cardioesophageal area. Using a curved scissors or a hook connected to the electrocautery, the peritoneum covering the anterior esophageal wall is divided. In order to liberate the right edge of the esophagus, it is necessary to transect, with the electrocautery, the proximal portion of the gastrohepatic ligament beginning with its pars flaccida. In the dissection of the pars condensa of the gastrohepatic ligament, an aberrant left hepatic artery should be looked for to preserve it and prevent necrosis of the left lobe of the liver. If an aberrant left hepatic artery is identified, it should not be ligated. Once the right edge of the esophagus is freed, the right crus of the diaphragm is exposed. A superelastic dissector with variable curvature (superelastic dissector, U.S. Surgical, Norwalk, CT) is very useful to dissect the posterior esophageal wall. The anterior vagus nerve, which is usually adherent to the anterior esophageal wall, is usually viable, as is the posterior vagus bordering the right pillar of the diaphragm (see drawing).

Operative Technique

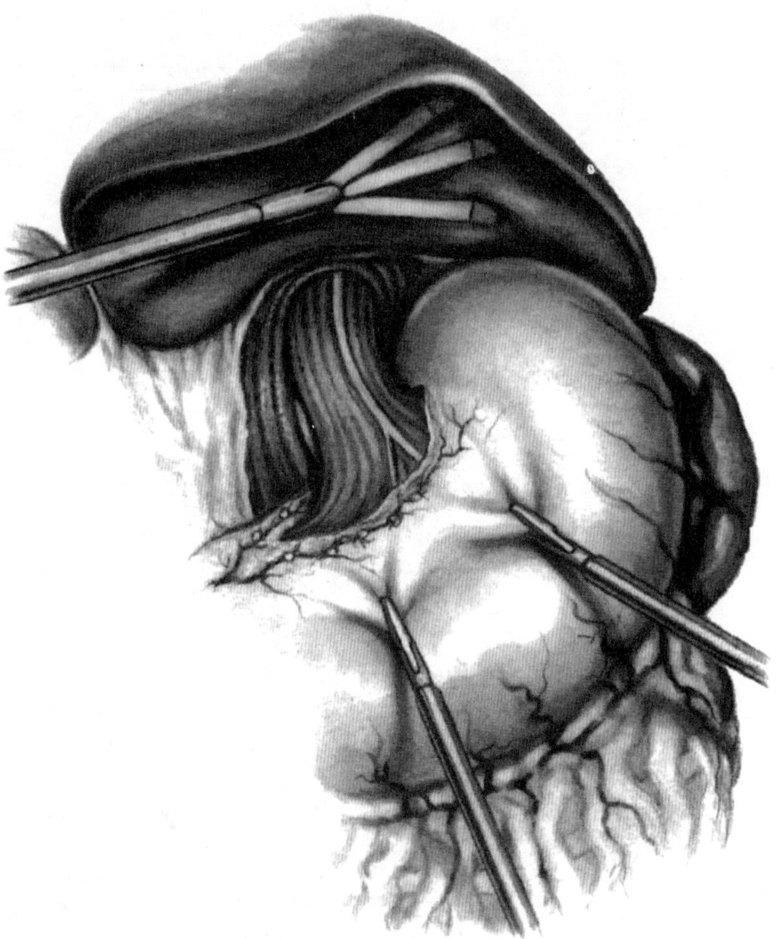

FIGURE 22.2

FIGURE 22.3

Once the distal esophagus is freed, the gastric fundus and the upper portion of the greater curvature of the stomach are liberated so as to prepare the 360° gastric wrapping of the esophagus without traction. The liberation of the gastric fundus is carried out by dividing the gastrophrenic ligament using electrocautery. The anterior gastric wall is then grasped, with an atraumatic grasper, near the greater curvature at the level of the spleen, and moderate traction is applied, to the right, to expose the short gastric vessels. The short vessels are ligated with clips, applying two clips on each side for greater safety, as seen in the drawing. The short vessels should be dissected, ligated, and divided individually. It is usually necessary to ligate the upper three or four short vessels to free at least 15 cm of the fundus and greater curvature of the stomach, from the angle of His. The drawing shows transection of the four most proximal short vessels with two clips on each side.

Operative Technique

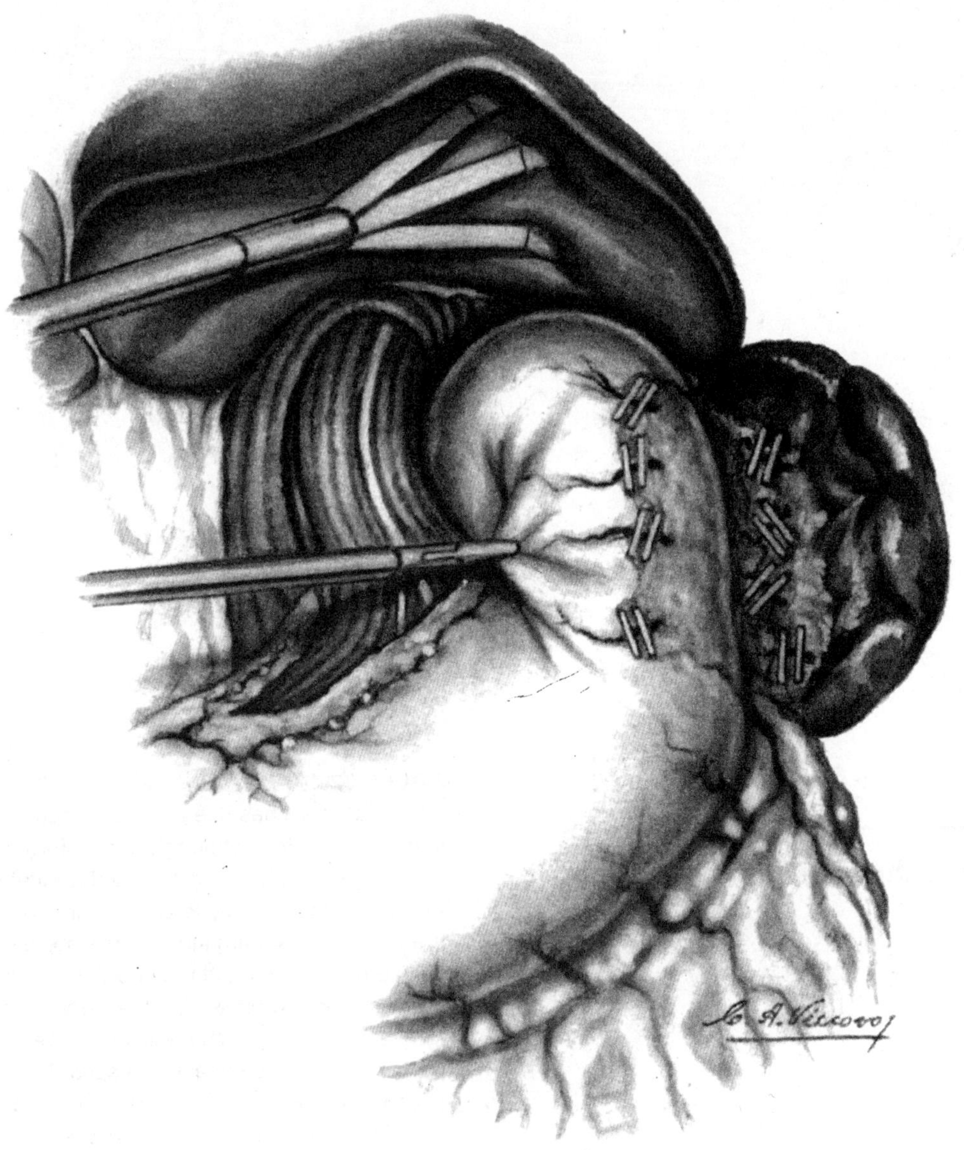

FIGURE 22.3

Operative Technique

FIGURE 22.4

A Penrose drain has been passed around the lower esophagus in order to apply traction to the esophagus to the left so as to expose the esophageal hiatus and facilitate its closure with interrupted, nonabsorbable sutures. In order to be able to pass the Penrose drain around the esophagus, a right-angle clamp should be introduced through a flexible cannula, the need for which should have been foreseen. The clamp is passed behind the esophagus, and the end of the Penrose is grasped and passed around the distal esophagus. Traction is applied to the ends of the Penrose, which are brought to the outside through a small stab wound. The drawing shows the esophagus retracted to the left and the esophageal hiatus being closed with interrupted sutures. The necessary sutures should be placed, leaving a 10 mm space between the esophageal border and the most proximal suture. Closure should be performed with an 18 F nasogastric tube in place.

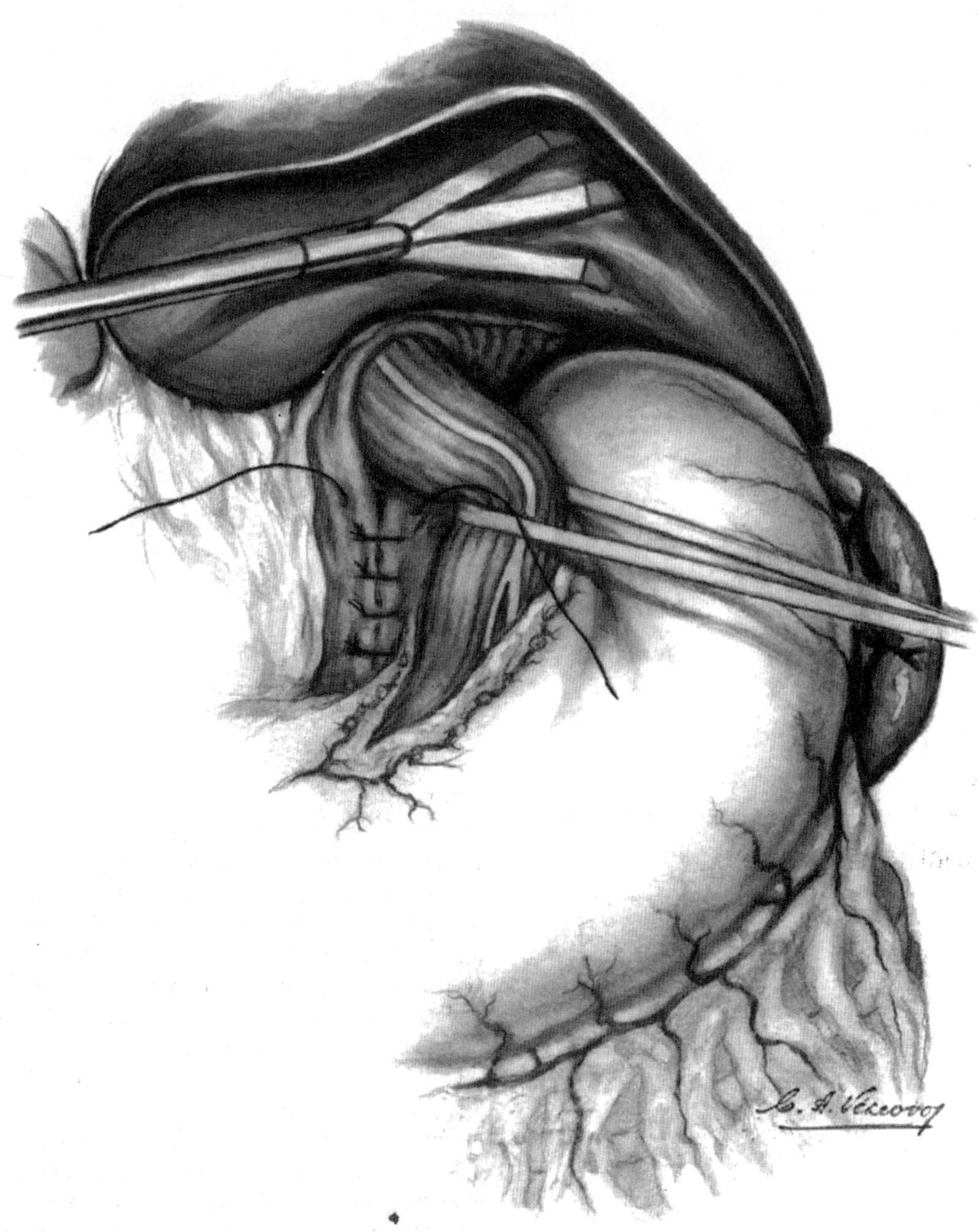

FIGURE 22.4

Operative Technique

FIGURE 22.5

The drawing shows that the gastric fundus has been passed behind the distal esophagus in order to proceed with the Nissen fundoplasty. In order to pass the gastric fundus around the esophagus, a Babcock clamp is passed behind the esophagus from the right. With the help of another Babcock or a Glassman clamp, traction is applied to the gastric fundus, passing it behind the esophagus. The drawing shows traction being applied to the gastric fundus with two Babcock clamps after passing it behind the esophagus. Once the gastric fundus has been passed behind the esophagus, the nasogastric tube is pulled back proximally and the mercury bougie that had been left in the distal third of the esophagus is introduced into the stomach. The mercury bougie should not be introduced into the stomach before passing the gastric fundus to the right of the esophagus to avoid difficulty in fashioning the fundoplasty.

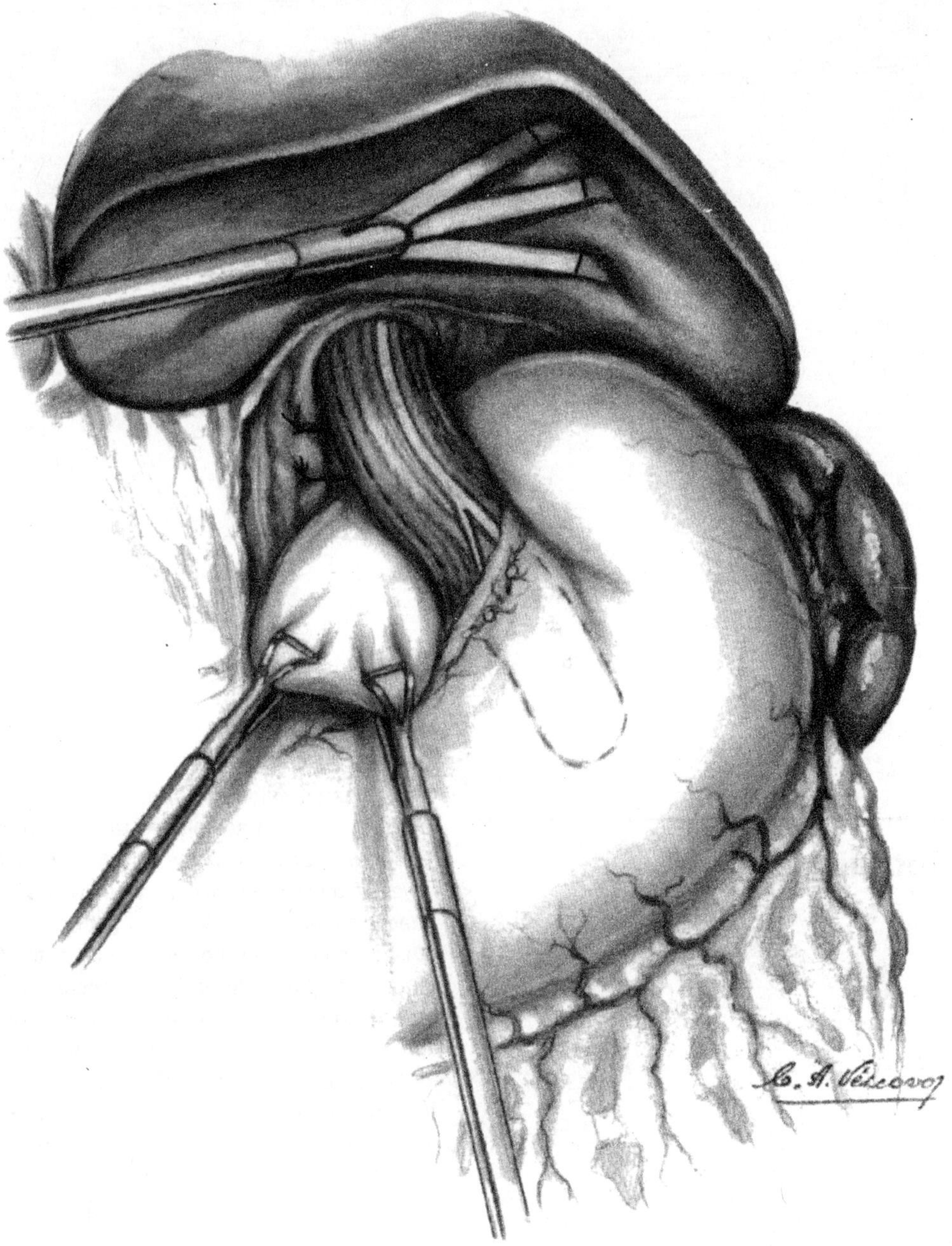

FIGURE 22.5

FIGURE 22.6
Both gastric folds are being sutured. Usually two nonabsorbable sutures are placed that grasp, on the one side, the seromuscular layer of the left gastric fold, then the muscular layer of the esophagus, and finally the seromuscular layer of the right gastric fold. Some surgeons use three or four sutures. It is not convenient, however, to carry the fundoplication higher than 3 cm due to the frequent occurrence of dysphagia. Once the suturing of the stomach has been completed, the mercury bougie is removed and the nasogastric tube is reintroduced. In order to confirm the degree of constriction exerted by the fundoplication on the esophagus, a 5-mm diameter explorer is used. This should easily pass between the esophageal wall and the fundoplication.

Operative Technique

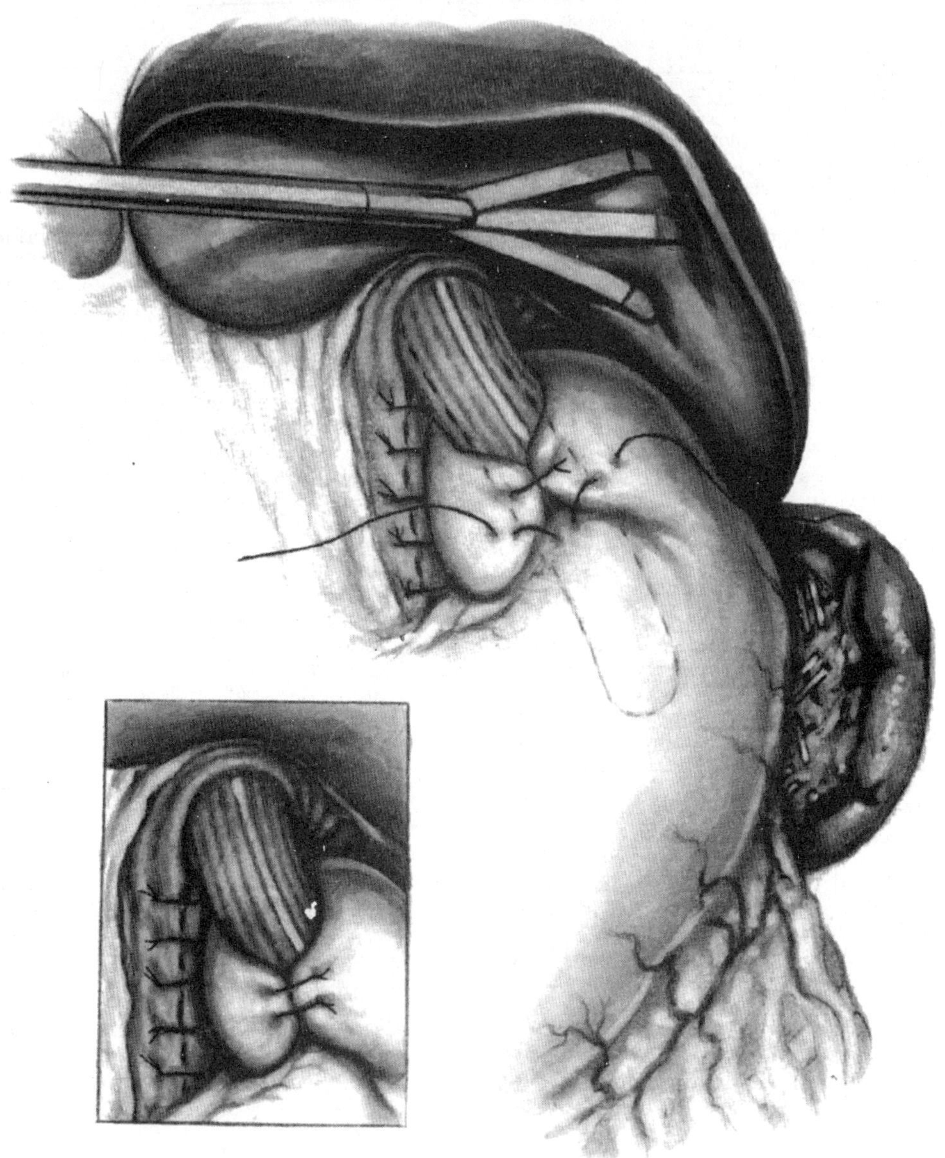

FIGURE 22.6

References

1. Angelchik, J.P., Cohen, R. A new surgical procedure for the treatment of gastroesophageal reflux. Surg. Gynecol. Obstet. 148:246, 1979.
2. Aye, R.W., Hill, L.D., Kraemer, S.J.M., Snopkowski, P. Early results with the laparoscopic Hill repair. Am. J. Surg. 167:542, 1994.
3. Bagnato, V.J. Laparoscopic Nissen fundoplication. Surg. Laparosc. Endosc. 2:188, 1992.
4. Berguer, R., Steigmann, G.V., Yamamoto, M., Kim, J., Mansour, A., Denton, J., Norton, L.W., Angelchik, J.P. Minimal access surgery for gastroesophageal reflux: Laparoscopic placement of the Angelchik prosthesis in the pig. Surg. Endosc. 5:123, 1991.
5. Boutelier, P., Jonsell, G. An alternative fundoplicative maneuver for gastroesophageal reflux. Am. J. Surg. 143:260, 1982.
6. Cuschieri, A.E., Shimi, S., Nathanson, L.K. Laparoscopic reduction, crural repair and fundoplication of large hiatal hernia. Am. J. Surg. 163:425, 1992.
7. Cuschieri, A.E., Nathanson, L.K., Shimi, S. Laparoscopic antireflux surgery. In Cuschieri, A.E., Buess, G., Perissat, J. (Eds.) Operative manual of endoscopic surgery. p. 280. Springer-Verlag, Berlin, 1992.
8. Cuschieri, A.E. Hiatal hernia and reflux esophagitis. In Hunter, J.G., Sachier, J.M. (Eds.) Minimally invasive surgery. p. 87. McGraw-Hill, New York, 1993.
9. Cuschieri, A.E. Laparoscopic antireflux surgery and repair of hiatal hernia. World J. Surg. 17:40, 1993.
10. Dallemagne, B., Weerts, J.M., Jehaes, C., Markiewicz, S., Lombard, R. Laparoscopic Nissen fundoplication: Preliminary report. Surg. Laparosc. Endosc. 1:138, 1991.
11. Dallemagne, B., Weerts, J.M., Jehaes, C., Markiewicz, S., Lombard, R. Laparoscopic management of gastroesophageal reflux. In Zucker, K.A. (Ed.) Surgical laparoscopy update. p. 217. Quality Medical Publishing, St. Louis, 1993.
12. DeMeester, T.R., Bonavina, L., Albertucci, M. Nissen fundoplication for gastroesophageal reflux disease: Evaluation of primary repair in 100 consecutive patients. Ann. Surg. 204:9, 1986.
13. Dor, J., Humbert, P., Dor, V. L'intérêt de la technique de Nissen modifiée dans le prevention du reflux après cardiomiotomie extramuqueuse de Heller. Mem. Acad. Chir. 27:877, 1962.
14. Dunnington, G., DeMeester, T. Outcome effect of adherence to operative principles of Nissen fundoplication by multiple surgeons. Am. J. Surg. 166:654, 1993.
15. Hill, L.D., Chapman, K.W., Morgan, E.H. Objective evaluation of surgery for hiatus hernia and esophagitis. J. Thorac. Cardiovasc. Surg. 41:60, 1961.
16. Hill, L.D. An effective operation for hiatal hernia: An eight year appraisal. Ann. Surg. 166:681, 1967.
17. Hinder, R.A., Filipi, C.J. The technique of laparoscopic Nissen fundoplication. Surg. Laparosc. Endosc. 2:265, 1992.
18. Liebermann-Meffert, D., Allgower, M., Schmid, P., Math, S.D., Blum, A.L. Muscular equivalent of the lower esophageal sphincter. Gastroenterology 76:31, 1978.
19. Linder, H.H. The arcuate ligament of the diaphragm. In Nihus, L.M. (Ed.) Hernia. Ed. 2, p. 708. Lippincott, Philadelphia, 1978.
20. Narbona-Arnau, B., Olavarietta, L., Lloris, J.M., Narbona-Calvo, B. Reflujo gastroesofágico. Hernia Hiatal. Rehabilitación quirúrgica del músculo esofágico, mediante pexia con el ligamento redondo. Resultados (1.143 casos operados en 15 años). Bol. Soc. Val. Digest. 1:21, 1980.
21. Nathanson, L.K., Shimi, S., Cuschieri, A. Laparoscopic ligamentum teres (round ligament) cariopexy. Br. J. Surg. 78:947, 1991.
22. Nissen, R. Eine einfache operation zur beeinflussung der reflex oesophagitis. Schweiz Med. Wochenschr. 86:590, 1956.
23. Nissen, R. Gastropexy and fundoplication in surgical treatment of hiatal hernia. Am. J. Dig. Dis. 6:954, 1961.
24. Postlethwait, R.W. The Angelchik antireflux prosthesis: A critical review. In Simmons, R.U. (Ed.) Debates in clinical surgery. p. 111. C.V. Mosby, St. Louis, 1991.
25. Rosetti, M., Hill, K. Fundoplication for the treatment of gastroesophageal reflux in hiatal hernia. World J. Surg. 1:439, 1977.
26. Sangster, W., Swanstrom, L. Preoperative testing for patients with gastroesophageal reflux disease. Surg. Endosc. 7:118, 1993.
27. Siewert, R., Jennewein, H.M., Waldeck, F., Weiser, H.F. Mechanism of action of fundoplication. J. Abdom. Surg. 18:131, 1976.
28. Siewert, R., Lepsien, G., Weiser, H.F., Schattenmann, G., Peiper, H.J. Das teleskop-phenomen. Eine komplikationsmoglichkeit nach fundoplication. Chirurgia 48:640, 1977.
29. Siewert, R., Hölscher, A.H. (Eds.). Diseases of the esophagus. p. 857. Springer-Verlag, Berlin, 1988.
30. Swanstrom, L., Wayne, R. Spectrum of gastrointestinal symptoms after laparoscopic fundoplication. Am. J. Surg. 167:538, 1994.
31. Toupet, A. Technique d'oesophago-gastroplastie avec phreno gastropexie dans la cure radicale des hernies hiatales et comme complement de l'operation de Heller dans les cardiospasmes. Acad. Chir. 394:399, 1963.
32. Weerts, J., Dallemagne, B., Hamoir, E., Demarche, M. Laparoscopic Nissen fundoplication: Detailed analysis of 132 patients. Surg. Laparosc. Endosc. 3:395, 1993.

Section F

Surgery of the Stomach and Duodenum

CHAPTER 23

Surgical Treatment of Peptic Gastroduodenal Ulcers

One frequently finds in the medical literature the term "gastroduodenal ulcers" used to include both gastric and duodenal ulcers in the belief that these are identical illnesses. Even though some authors (36) share that opinion, the great majority of gastroenterologists recognize etiologic, clinical, and therapeutic differences between both conditions.

We will use the following outline to describe the surgical treatment of peptic gastroduodenal ulcers.

A. Gastric Ulcer
   1. Surgical indications.
   2. Selection of the surgical procedure to be used in gastric ulcers.
   3. Gastric ulcers complicated by hemorrhage, perforation, or obstruction.

B. Duodenal Ulcer
   1. Surgical indications.
   2. Selection of the surgical procedure to be used in duodenal ulcers that are resistant to medical therapy.
   3. Duodenal ulcers complicated by hemorrhage, perforation, or obstruction.

GASTRIC ULCER

In 1963 Daintree Johnson (34), using anatomic and physiologic criteria, proposed the classification of gastric ulcers into three types:

Type I: Ulcers localized on the lesser curvature of the body of the stomach.

Type II: Simultaneous presentation of a gastric ulcer as in Type I and a duodenal ulcer, be it active or healed.

Type III: Ulcers in the prepyloric region of the stomach.

Gastric ulcers of Type I are usually associated with low gastric acidity, and the gastric mucosa is frequently atrophic. Type II patients with simultaneous gastric and duodenal ulcers frequently have gastric hypersecretion or at least a normal level of gastric acidity. Type III, or prepyloric ulcers, are frequently similar to duodenal ulcers and are frequently associated with gastric hyperacidity.

Surgical Indications

Gastric ulcers that appear to be benign should always be treated medically. Surgical therapy should only be contemplated in ulcers that are refractory to medical treatment or when malignancy cannot be excluded.

Medical literature frequently refers to "intractability" of gastric or duodenal ulcers, or to "intractable" ulcers. This is not correct, since an ulcer that cannot be cured with medical treatment can be cured with surgical treatment. This means that the ulcer is not "intractable" but resistant to medical treatment (but curable with surgical treatment). Some 15 to 20% of gastric ulcers are refractory to medical treatment, and about 50% of ulcers that respond to medical care may recur (57), this recurrence manifesting itself by hemorrhage, perforation, or obstruction. If there are frequent recurrences, medical therapy should not be insisted upon due to the possibility of acute complications, which may lead to urgent surgery. If a gastric ulcer is not completely healed with medical care in 12 weeks, the ulcer is refractory to medical care or malignant, even though previously performed biopsies may have been negative.

Today it is relatively easy to distinguish between a benign or malignant gastric ulcer. An adequate radiologic examination performed by an expert is very important, but there is no doubt that an examination with a fiberoptic gastroscope together with 4 to 7 biopsies and brushings of the ulcer for cytologic examination are basic in the differential diagnosis.

It is not always possible to obtain a complete endoscopic view of the gastric lesion due to its location, and at times it is not possible to get adequate biopsies or cytologic brushings of the ulcer. On the other hand, one should keep in mind that a malignant ulcer may disappear with medical treatment and become covered with gastric epithelium of normal appearance. These observations point to the need for strict periodic evaluations for at least 2 years. In case of any doubt, surgical treatment should be advised. Surgery should also be advised when ulcers heal easily, only to recur rapidly, even though histologic studies do not show any sign of malignancy.

Selection of the Surgical Procedure in the Treatment of Gastric Ulcers

The procedure of choice in the surgical treatment of gastric ulcers with surgical indications is gastric resection. Gastric ulcers located in the distal part of the stomach are treated by hemigastrectomy. Gastric ulcers in proximal areas of the stomach are treated by gastric resection with the level of gastric transection at some 3 cm above the edge of the ulcer. Reestablishment of the digestive tract can be carried out by a Billroth I or a Billroth II technique. Either technique can be used in gastric ulcers with the same good results. The same results are not obtained using the Billroth I technique in duodenal ulcers, since this type of procedure leads to recurrent anastomotic ulcers with greater frequency. If a truncal vagotomy is added to the gastrectomy, the probability of recurrence is just as low with the Billroth I as with the Billroth II technique. Some surgeons will add a truncal vagotomy to a hemigastrectomy in cases of pyloric or prepyloric ulcer with gastric acid hypersecretion (6, 52, 53).

Patients with both gastric and duodenal ulcers (Johnson Type II) are also treated by gastric resection. If the resection is a hemigastrectomy it is necessary to add a truncal vagotomy due to the duodenal ulcer. If the resection involves removal of 70% or more of the stomach, it is not necessary to add a vagotomy due to the duodenal ulcer.

Patients with gastric ulcers high on the lesser curvature or near the cardia should undergo an extended gastrectomy with resection of the ulcer using the classical Pauchet technique, which will be described later. There are surgeons who, instead of performing the Pauchet operation, only resect the high-lying ulcer and close the gastric defect in two layers, adding a truncal vagotomy and a pyloroplasty (37). Some surgeons remain loyal to the Kelling-Madlener procedure, which consists of performing a resection only up to below the cardial or subcardial ulcer.

Pauchet's technique is undoubtedly the most adequate and safest in the treatment of these high ulcers, specially if they are associated with hemorrhage.

All the above mentioned techniques can only be used if one is sure the ulcer is benign. If the cardial or subcardial ulcer is proven malignant, the surgery used should respect the oncologic principles that apply to the treatment of an ulcerated cancer of the proximal end of the stomach.

Gastric Ulcers Complicated by Hemorrhage, Perforation, or Obstruction

Hemorrhagic gastric ulcers

Gastric resection is the safest and most adequate procedure for gastric ulcers complicated by hemorrhage that do not respond to medical therapy. The Pauchet technique should be used if the ulcer is located high on the lesser curvature in the cardial area. Some surgeons, however, only carry out hemostasis of the bleeding ulcer by suturing the ulcerated bleeding area (54, 55). Other surgeons resect the ulcer without performing a gastrectomy and close the defect with two layers of sutures (54, 55). To the local resection of the ulcer they usually add a truncal vagotomy and a pyloroplasty (54). Suturing of the bleeding ulcer as well as local resection of the ulcer does not guarantee control of hemorrhage, and bleeding will frequently recur. The addition of a pyloroplasty and a truncal vagotomy does not effectively improve the results. Procedures that do not include gastric resection together with resection of the ulcer should be reserved for patients in very poor general condition, who are unable to tolerate a gastric resection, or cases in which the surgeon is not experienced in gastric resection, especially the Pauchet technique. Some patients are very hard to maintain stable when they lose a lot of blood. In those patients it is useful to immediately stop the loss of blood, temporarily, as soon as the abdomen is opened, to allow the patient to become stable, and then be able to proceed with a gastric resection that includes the ulcer. The procedure is as follows: The ulcer is located and a gastrotomy done. Since the incised gastric walls generally bleed profusely, several large nontraumatic Duval clamps are placed on the borders of the gastric incision, both to control the bleeding and to apply traction to the walls to better see the interior of the stomach. The surgeon, using both hands, then removes the blood clots from within the stomach. The use of suction to remove clots usually fails and frequently injures the gastric mucosa, increasing hemorrhage. The ulcer and its bleeding points are identified, and sutures are placed to attain temporary hemostasis. Once this objective is attained, the gastrotomy is closed with a continuous suture and the gastric resection, including the ulcer area, is carried out.

One should always remember that about 15% of bleeding gastric ulcers are malignant (67).

Some patients with bleeding gastric ulcers can be treated preoperatively with endoscopic temporary control or diminution of the bleeding by means of electrocautery, a heater-probe, or laser ray.

Hemorrhages due to acute gastric erosions

These lesions are frequently called "acute hemorrhagic gastritis," "erosive gastritis," "erosive stress gastritis," or simply "stress gastritis," and are frequently seen postoperatively in very sick or septic patients (43). Actually, the incidence of bleeding due to this cause has diminished significantly due to preventive measures systematically carried out in intensive care units. In cases in which hemorrhage occurs in spite of prophylactic measures, it usually stops under present-day medical measures. If the bleeding does not stop, one can resort to endoscopic treatment, which leads to good results. If nonsurgical measures fail, surgery can be used as a last resort. At present, few patients with stress gastritis need to be subjected to surgery. If surgery becomes necessary, a gastrotomy is performed using the previously mentioned technique and sutures are placed in the more acute ulcers or erosions that are bleeding more severely. If an acceptable hemostasis is attained, the gastrotomy is closed and the operation completed with a truncal vagotomy and a pyloroplasty. This technique is not always successful. If it should fail, one can perform a 75% gastrectomy or a 90% gastrectomy and, exceptionally, a total gastrectomy. When a 75 to 90% gastrectomy is performed, the surgeon should check the residual gastric remnant for bleeding. If there is bleeding, it can be controlled with sutures before reestablishment of digestive continuity. Gastric resection in these patients is a procedure of last resort, since it carries a very elevated mortality rate.

Perforated gastric ulcers

Every patient with a perforation of a gastric ulcer into the peritoneal cavity should be operated upon as an emergency. The exception to this is cases of perforated ulcer that have been sealed by a reaction in adjacent tissues and can be efficiently treated with a more conservative method.

The author believes that the most efficient procedure in the treatment of perforated gastric ulcers is gastric resection. However, some patients are in no condition to tolerate a gastric resection. Others present, at the time of surgery, such severe contamination that resection is very dangerous. In these cases suturing the perforation and adding an omentoplasty can be resorted to. However, it is not always possible to perform a simple closure of the perforation safely, either due to the size of the perforation or due to the inflammatory reaction that is usually present around the perforation. This reaction is at times of such consistency that sutures will not hold, making a safe closure of the perforation very difficult. If the perforated ulcer is small, closure with suturing and omentoplasty is less exposed to failure. Suturing of a perforation of a prepyloric ulcer may lead to gastric emptying problems, and pyloroplasty may be necessary to facilitate gastric emptying. In some patients with a perforated gastric ulcer that is difficult to close, and in patients in very poor general condition, the following procedure may be lifesaving. A rubber catheter is introduced through the perforation and then wrapped with the greater omentum. The anterior gastric wall around the perforation is sutured to the parietal peritoneum, bringing the tube to the outside. This means that the perforation is converted to a gastrostomy to save the situation.

It should be remembered that some perforated gastric ulcers are malignant, which would contraindicate a simple closure of the perforation. In all patients with perforated gastric ulcer a histologic examination of the borders of the perforation should be performed.

Obstruction due to gastric ulcer

Gastric ulcers that can cause obstruction are those that are located in the prepyloric area. Only rarely do more proximally located ulcers produce obstruction. The initial treatment of these ulcers is nasogastric intubation, which involves suction and reestablishment of electrolytic balance. If the obstruction is due to edema, it generally subsides in 3 or 4 days. In these cases medical treatment can be continued as long as histologic studies of the ulcerated lesion do not show signs of malignancy. If the lesion does not improve with medical treatment, surgery should be advised. The most effective treatment for obstructing gastric ulcers is gastrectomy. In cases in which the patient cannot tolerate a resection, a gastroenterostomy can be done, to be followed by the definitive treatment if the condition of the patient permits it.

DUODENAL ULCER

Treatment of duodenal ulcer is essentially medical. Some 95% of uncomplicated duodenal ulcers are cured by medical therapy within three months. Surgical treatment for duodenal ulcers has diminished considerably in recent years, and patients who are referred for surgery frequently have life-threatening complications. This change in therapy is due to the efficient action of H_2 antagonists and to omeprazole, an inhibitor of the proton pump that leads to a great diminution of the secretion of gastric acid.

Surgical Indications

Surgery for duodenal ulcer is now limited to the group of patients who are refractory to medical treatment and to ulcers that are complicated by hemorrhage, perforation, or obstruction.

Surgical treatment of duodenal ulcer should comply with the following requisites: (a) Cure the ulcer. (b) Morbidity and mortality should be low. (c) The incidence of recurrence should be minimal. (d) There should be few side effects due to the surgery (diarrhea, loss of weight, dumping, etc.).

Selection of the Surgical Procedure in the Treatment of Duodenal Ulcers That Are Refractory to Medical Therapy

There are many surgical procedures in the treatment of duodenal ulcers that are refractory to medical therapy. The principal ones are:

1. Seventy percent gastrectomy (68).
2. Hemigastrectomy with truncal vagotomy (6, 9, 12, 24–26, 29, 52, 53, 55).
3. Truncal vagotomy with drainage procedure, pyloroplasty, or gastroenterostomy (8, 65, 66).
4. Selective vagotomy with drainage procedure (16, 32, 54).
5. Proximal gastric vagotomy (6, 7, 19, 21, 25, 30).
6. Proximal gastric vagotomy and sphincteroplasty. Holle (29, 30).

Seventy percent gastrectomy

A 70% gastrectomy has been the procedure of choice in surgical treatment for duodenal ulcer for many years. In this procedure the entire gastric antrum is resected together with a considerable segment of the gastric body and its acid secreting parietal cells. This operation has the advantage of leading to a low incidence of postoperative anastomotic ulcers, if the digestive tract is reestablished by the Billroth II technique (17). If the digestive transit is reestablished by the Billroth I technique, there will be a 15% incidence of anastomotic ulcer (17, 23). However, if a truncal vagotomy is added to the Billroth I procedure, the possibility of an anastomotic ulcer diminishes dramatically, becoming as low as that in 70% gastrectomy with Billroth II anastomosis (17, 23). This confirms the need to always add a truncal vagotomy when the surgeon decides to perform a Billroth I type of anastomosis.

A 70% gastrectomy may cause some postoperative symptoms due to the extent of the gastric resection. Some of these symptoms are weight loss and dumping syndrome. If reconstruction of digestive transit is done using the Billroth I technique and a truncal vagotomy is added to lower the possibility of anastomotic ulcer, other symptoms may occur due to the truncal vagotomy, such as diarrhea, functional alterations of the biliary tract, gallstones, and so on.

In order to perform a gastric resection for duodenal ulcer, the surgeon must be familiar with the techniques for gastrectomy and with the handling of the difficult duodenum.

In a 70% gastrectomy the level of gastric transection is arbitrary, but the gastric arteries can serve as a guide. Division of the stomach on the lesser curvature side is carried out where the left gastric artery comes in contact with the lesser curvature after giving off the cardioesophageal artery. This is about 3 cm distal to the gastroesophageal junction. At the greater curvature the stomach is transected at the level of the first short vessel, or at the point where the left gastroepiploic artery touches the stomach, or level with the lower pole of the spleen, if this is normal (67, 68).

Hemigastrectomy with truncal vagotomy

This is a frequently used operation in the surgical treatment of duodenal ulcer. An extended gastric resection is not necessary if a vagotomy is done. A hemigastrectomy is enough, since, with this technique, the incidence of postoperative anastomotic ulcers comes down to 1% (67, 68), be it with a Billroth I or Billroth II anastomosis. It must be pointed out that a Billroth I anastomosis is not always possible in a large duodenal ulcer penetrating into the pancreas or in postbulbar ulcers, and so on, which make adequate duodenal mobilization to attain an anastomosis to the gastric stump without tension very difficult. In patients who undergo truncal vagotomy operative complications may occur such as esophageal perforation and splenic hemorrhage as well as postoperative complications such as diarrhea and functional alterations or calculi in the biliary system, as previously mentioned. Addition of the truncal vagotomy may lead to a slight, though low, rise in morbidity and mortality if the gastric resection is performed by a surgeon experienced in gastric surgery and the handling of a difficult duodenum.

Hemigastrectomy with truncal vagotomy has replaced the classical 70% gastrectomy in many surgical centers.

The important part of this technique is to resect all the antral mucosa, which extends upward much higher on the lesser curvature than on the greater curvature. The limits of the gastric resection are arbitrary, but, as stated before, it is useful to follow the vascular landmarks. The level of transection of the stomach on the lesser curvature side is usually where the left gastric artery has given off its third collateral branch to irrigate the anterior gastric wall. It is preferable to transect the stomach a little higher to make sure all the antral mucosa has been removed. The level of transection on the greater curvature is at the point where the left gastroepiploic artery joins the right gastroepiploic. This junction is generally manifested by a narrowing of the gastroepiploic arch and at other times by a separation of both arteries. At times it is impossible to determine the site of junction of these arteries. In the latter situation the level of transection can be arbitrarily chosen as 4 cm below the inferior pole of the spleen, at the level at which the left gastroepiploic artery runs up against the stomach. It should be pointed out that some of these landmarks may not coincide with those of other surgeons. Medical literature frequently uses hemigastrectomy and antrectomy as synonymous.

Hemigastrectomy in the treatment of duodenal ulcer should always be accompanied by a truncal vagotomy in order to avoid the frequent incidence of anastomotic ulcers. If a truncal vagotomy cannot be performed, be it because of previous operations, great obesity, or body habitus with a very elevated diaphragm, making the performance of a complete vagotomy without complications very difficult, it is preferable to perform a 70% gastrectomy without a vagotomy or a hemigastrectomy with truncal vagotomy by the thoracic supradiaphragmatic approach, as performed by Dragstedt and Owens in their first two cases (8, 9).

Truncal vagotomy plus a drainage procedure

This technique is easy and can be done rapidly, with very low morbidity and mortality. The biggest problem with this procedure is the very high risk of recurrent ulcers that is associated with it, 24–30% (67, 68). There are also possible surgical complications and postoperative diarrhea due to the vagotomy, which occurs in 15% of patients. Truncal vagotomy should be accompanied by a pyloroplasty. If a pyloroplasty is too difficult, a gastroenterostomy can be done.

Selective vagotomy

This technique consists in sectioning the vagus nerves after the celiac and hepatic branches have been given off. The main object is to avoid functional alterations of the biliary tract, the small bowel, and the proximal colon. This procedure, just as with truncal vagotomy, leads to alterations of gastric motility and has to be accompanied by a drainage procedure. This procedure is more complex than truncal vagotomy and has practically been replaced by proximal gastric vagotomy (7, 15, 18, 19, 22, 36).

Proximal gastric vagotomy

This operation is characterized by transection of the vagal branches that innervate the gastric body, preserving the nerve supply to the antrum and pylorus, and permitting regulation of gastric emptying and the grinding of solid foods. With this procedure it is not necessary to carry out a drainage procedure. At present, proximal gastric vagotomy is performed less frequently due to the high incidence of recurrent ulcers. Some surgeons argue that, if the ulcer recurs after this procedure, a hemigastrectomy can be performed as a second procedure, without inconveniences.

Proximal gastric vagotomy with pyloroplasty

This operation, proposed by Holle (29, 30), adds a pyloroplasty to the proximal vagotomy with the object, according to the author, of insuring gastric emptying. This technique has not improved the result originally obtained with proximal gastric vagotomy without pyloroplasty, the frequency of recurrent ulcers being very similar.

Selection of the best operative technique for each patient should be realized taking into consideration various factors such as age, sex, body habitus, obesity, general condition, cardiovascular status, inadequate weight, gastric secretion, mental attitude, intestinal transit, patients with diarrhea or soft feces, patients who have had hemorrhages, osteoporosis, patients with a difficult duodenum or postbulbar ulcer, and whether or not the surgeon has experience in gastrectomy or in the handling of a difficult duodenum. For example, an obese patient can be subjected to a 70% gastrectomy. On the other hand, this resection is not advisable for thin patients, particularly females, or those who present some mental instability, since it is in these patients that dumping and other vasomotor symptoms are more frequent. A truncal vagotomy should not be advised in patients with diarrhea or soft stools. If the operating surgeon is not experienced in gastrectomy or in the handling of a difficult duodenum, he can perform a proximal gastric vagotomy or a truncal vagotomy with pyloroplasty. Proximal gastric vagotomy is not indicated in duodenal ulcers with hemorrhage, perforation, or obstruction. Truncal vagotomy may be used in elderly patients in poor general health or in patients with several bleeding duodenal ulcers, as long as local control of the bleeding has been possible. In patients with an actively bleeding duodenal ulcer in whom a gastric resection is performed it is advisable to reestablish digestive transit by means of a Billroth II procedure and not by a Billroth I procedure because the former is a safer technique to control hemorrhage. In addition the control of hemorrhage is performed by ligature of arteries outside the duodenum, which is more certain to control bleeding. Also, it is not always possible to perform a Billroth I procedure in duodenal ulcers penetrating into the pancreas, postbulbar ulcers, or severe fibrous retraction of the duodenum.

DUODENAL ULCERS COMPLICATED BY HEMORRHAGE, PERFORATION, OR OBSTRUCTION

Duodenal Ulcers with Hemorrhage

Patients with massive bleeding from duodenal ulcer who have lost more than 2 liters of blood should be treated surgically. Surgery is also indicated in patients without massive blood loss but with recurrent hemorrhage or cardiovascular problems, particularly in older patients or in places where a sufficient amount of blood is not available.

The safest operation in the treatment of duodenal ulcer with hemorrhage is a 70% gastrectomy or a hemigastrectomy with truncal vagotomy.

In elderly patients in poor general condition, or if the surgeon is not experienced in gastric resections or the handling of a difficult duodenum, local hemostasis of the ulcer by means of suture ligatures in the bleeding area can be resorted to. If the hemorrhage arises from one of the arteries of the gastroduodenal arterial complex, three suture ligatures should be placed as shown by Berne and Rosoff. One suture ligature should be placed above the ulcer to occlude the gastroduodenal artery. Another suture ligature should be placed under the ulcer to occlude the gastroduodenal artery and prevent the flow of blood from the right gastroepiploic and pancreatoduodenal arteries. In addition, another suture ligature should be placed to the left of the ulcer to occlude the transverse pancreatic artery. This technique will be described later. More infrequently bleeding is not from the gastroduodenal arterial complex. This makes the bleeding less severe and much easier to control. Local control of a bleeding ulcer is not as sure as control by means of a gastric resection and reestablishment of the digestive tract with a Billroth II procedure. Local hemostasis is prone to frequent recurrences. If the requirements of the Berne and Rosoff technique are complied with, it is very probable that recurrence of hemorrhage will be less frequent. After local control of hemorrhage from the duodenal ulcer, the operation is usually completed with a truncal vagotomy and pyloroplasty, taking into consideration the incision made in the duodenum for local hemostasis.

Perforation of Duodenal Ulcers

The surgeon's mission in a patient with perforated ulcer is first to save the patient's life and then to carry out definitive treatment of the ulcer. In some patients both objectives can be carried out in the same procedure.

The most frequent operation performed to treat a perforated duodenal ulcer is simple closure of the ulcer with an omentoplasty. In about 30 to 50% of patients so treated the ulcer recurs and the patients have to be operated upon a second time for definitive treatment. The rest of the patients are cured and need no further intervention, especially now, with the availability of very efficient medications to treat the ulcer.

If the patient is young and little peritoneal contamination has taken place, a 70% gastrectomy can be done. It is not advisable to perform a hemigastrectomy with truncal vagotomy because of the danger of an infectious mediastinal complication.

In some cases it is possible to excise the ulcer area, which is always anterior, and perform a pyloroplasty. Some surgeons, in addition to simple closure of the ulcer, carry out a proximal gastric vagotomy. For reasons previously mentioned, when faced by an infectious peritoneal process, it is not suitable to expose the patient to a mediastinitis by opening the posterior mediastinum.

Obstruction Due To Duodenal Ulcer

If the clinical picture has not improved with medical treatment, gastric intubation, and reestablishment of electrolytic balance, surgical intervention should be undertaken. Hemigastrectomy with truncal vagotomy is the treatment of choice. It is not advisable to perform a proximal gastric vagotomy due to the presence of obstruction. If the surgeon is not able to perform a gastric resection, he or she can resort to a truncal vagotomy with a pyloroplasty. It should be noted, however, that it is not always possible to perform a conventional pyloroplasty in patients with obstruction. In these cases a gastroenterostomy or a Jaboulay gastroduodenostomy can be carried out.

Truncal Vagotomy: Surgical Technique

FIGURE 23.1
Schematic drawing showing by means of a darker area the level at which a truncal vagotomy is performed. In a truncal vagotomy the vagus nerves are transected at the level of the abdominal esophagus, before the hepatic branch of the anterior vagus and the celiac branch of the posterior vagus are given off. Truncal vagotomy removes the parasympathetic nerve supply to most of the abdominal organs, such as the gallbladder, biliary tract, pancreas, duodenum, small bowel, and proximal colon. It should always be accompanied by a drainage procedure.

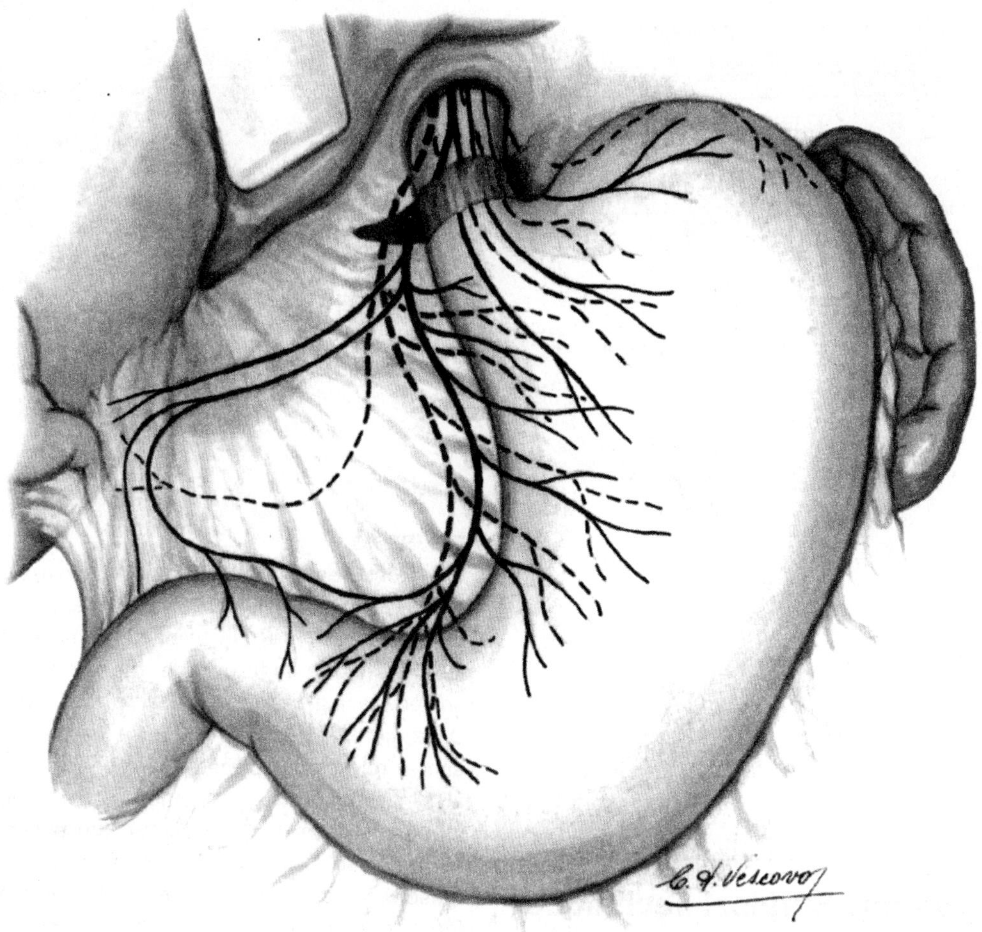

FIGURE 23.1

Truncal Vagotomy: Surgical Technique

FIGURE 23.2

The most frequently used incision for truncal vagotomy is a xiphoumbilical incision. In most patients this incision should be extended 4 to 6 cm below the umbilicus. If the operative field is still not large enough, the xiphoid process can be resected, taking care not to injure the pericardium or pleura. Once the peritoneum is open, a large self-retaining Balfour or similar retractor is placed. An upper-hand type of retractor is also necessary to elevate the anterior inferior portion of the thoracic cage to better visualize the esophagodiaphragmatic area. Before exploring the abdomen for other pathology, the presence of adhesions of the great omentum must be looked for, in order to divide them and avoid traction upon them, which could lead to bleeding from the splenic capsule. Exploration then centers on the stomach and duodenum to identify the duodenal ulcer, its size, its degree of penetration into the pancreas, fibrous duodenal retraction, and the possibility of performing a pyloroplasty. The second assistant grasps the stomach with both hands and applies gentle traction downward and to the left, as seen in the drawing. In order to make this traction stable, it is convenient to displace the Levine nasogastric tube toward the greater curvature so that the assistant can grasp it together with the stomach. The peritoneum over the esophagogastric junction is then incised and the abdominal esophagus freed circumferentially using blunt dissection. The traction applied by the second assistant frequently permits, before the esophagodiaphragmatic peritoneum is divided, visualization of the anterior vagus and its hepatic branch. After the peritoneum is divided, the nerve is not only more evident, it can be palpated.

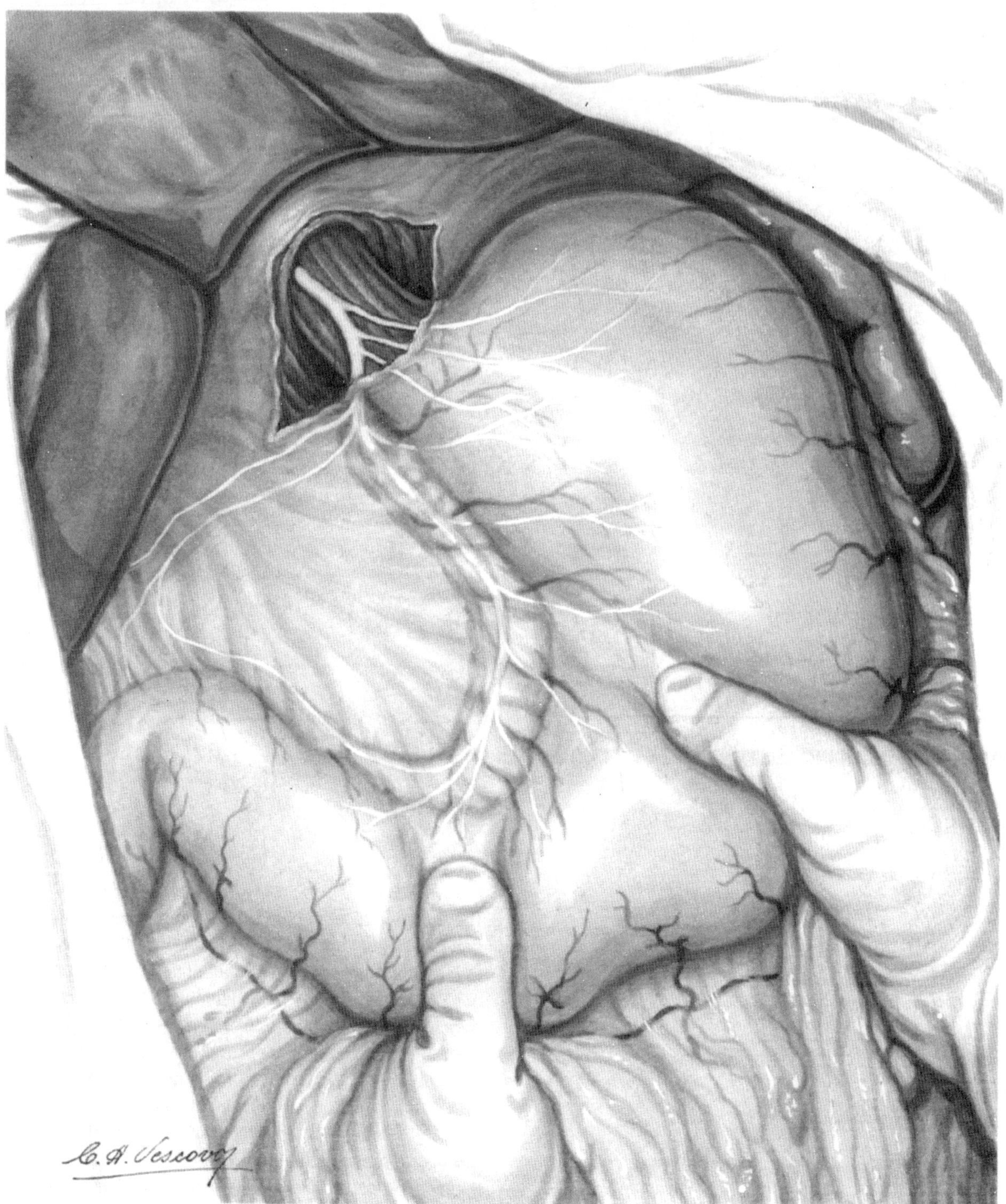

FIGURE 23.2

Truncal Vagotomy: Surgical Technique

FIGURE 23.3

The abdominal esophagus has been freed digitally from its periesophageal areolar tissue, and both the anterior and posterior vagal trunks have been identified by palpation. The anterior trunk has already been identified. The posterior vagus is then identified. The posterior vagus is relatively frequently separated from the esophageal wall, leaning on the right crux of the diaphragm. Localization of this nerve should be performed with great care to avoid missing it, as has happened in some cases. It is said that the degree of certainty of identification of the posterior vagus is directly related to the experience of the surgeon. Once the posterior vagal trunk, which appears like a violin string, of greater thickness than the anterior trunk, has been palpated, it is pushed to the right by the index finger of the surgeon, as seen in the drawing, to be caught with a nerve hook. The anterior vagus may have divisions, and in some cases it may be plexiform in appearance.

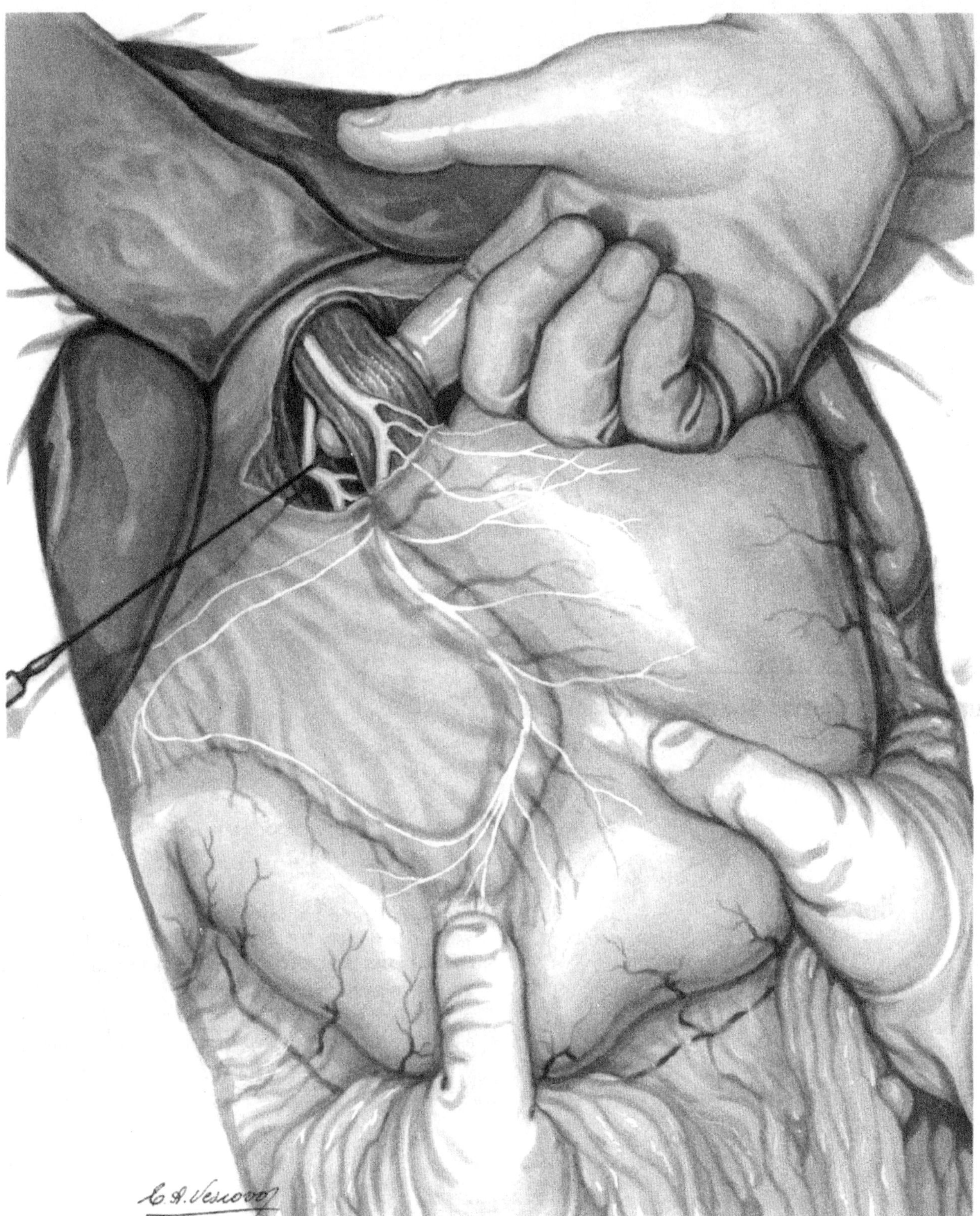

FIGURE 23.3

Truncal Vagotomy: Surgical Technique

FIGURE 23.4
Both vagal trunks are being retracted with nerve hooks, the anterior one to the left and the posterior one to the right, to better expose them. The posterior trunk has been surrounded by two separate sutures, about 3 to 4 cm apart. Some surgeons believe these ligatures are not necessary; however, after the nerves are divided without previously ligating them, bleeding can be observed from blood vessels that accompany them.

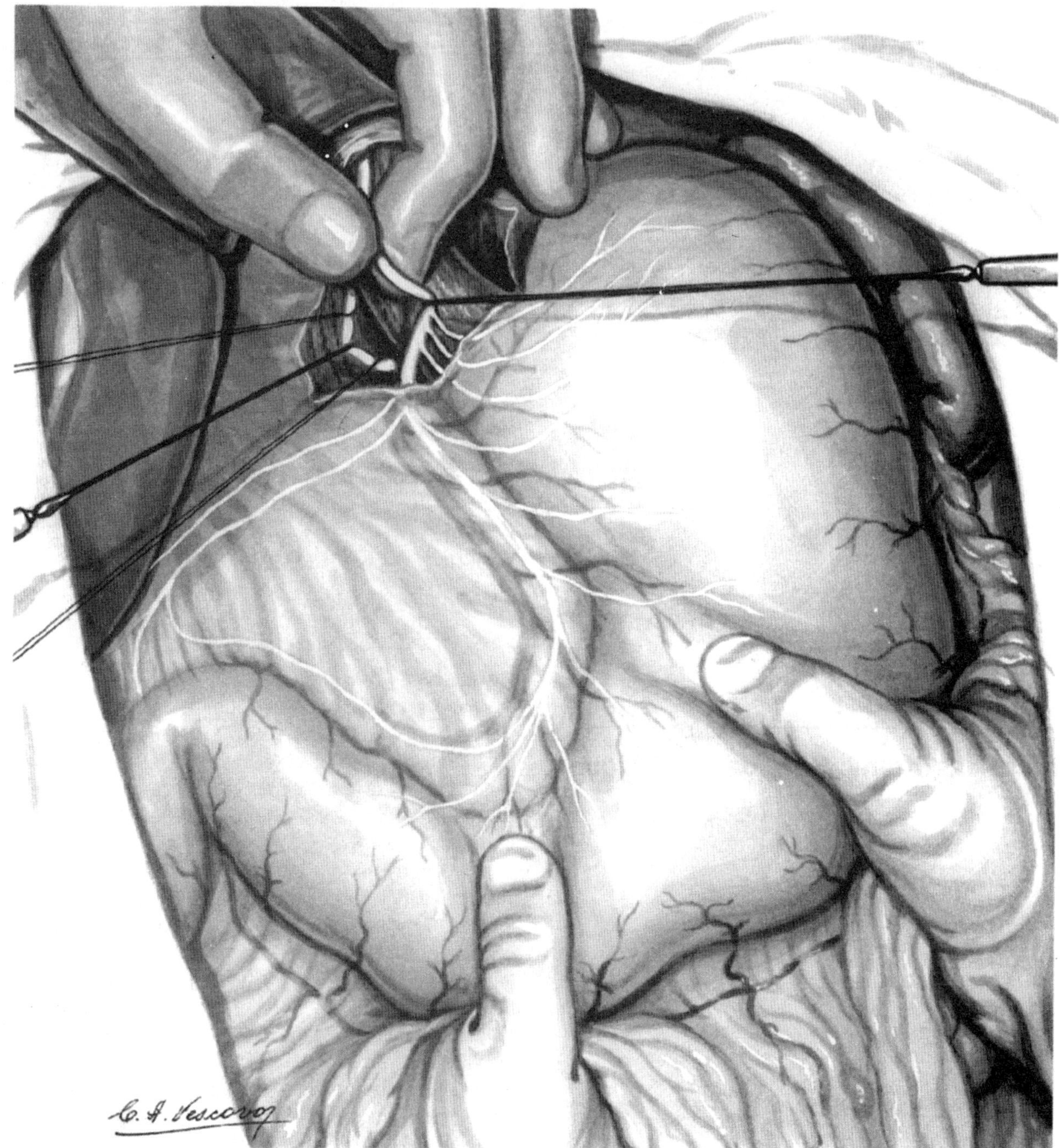

FIGURE 23.4

Truncal Vagotomy: Surgical Technique

FIGURE 23.5

The lower esophagus is pulled down and to the left by a rubber loop. A 3- to 4-cm segment of the posterior vagus, whose retracted stumps cannot be seen, has been resected. A 3- to 4-cm segment of the anterior vagus has also been removed between ligatures, whose ends are visible in the drawing. After the vagal trunks are divided, the presence of branches of the trunks directed toward the stomach should be searched for. These branches may be the cause of an incomplete vagotomy, leading to failure of this operation. A branch of the anterior vagus may innervate the anterior wall of the gastric fundus (anterior criminal nerve of Grassi). Posteriorly another nerve may exist, sometimes two branches of the posterior vagal trunk (posterior criminal nerve of Grassi), which, if they are not identified and divided, may render the truncal vagotomy ineffective. It is also necessary to look for fine vagal branches which may be in contact with the longitudinal muscular layer of the esophagus. These small rami should be identified with delicate nerve hooks so that they can be sectioned, as seen in the drawing.

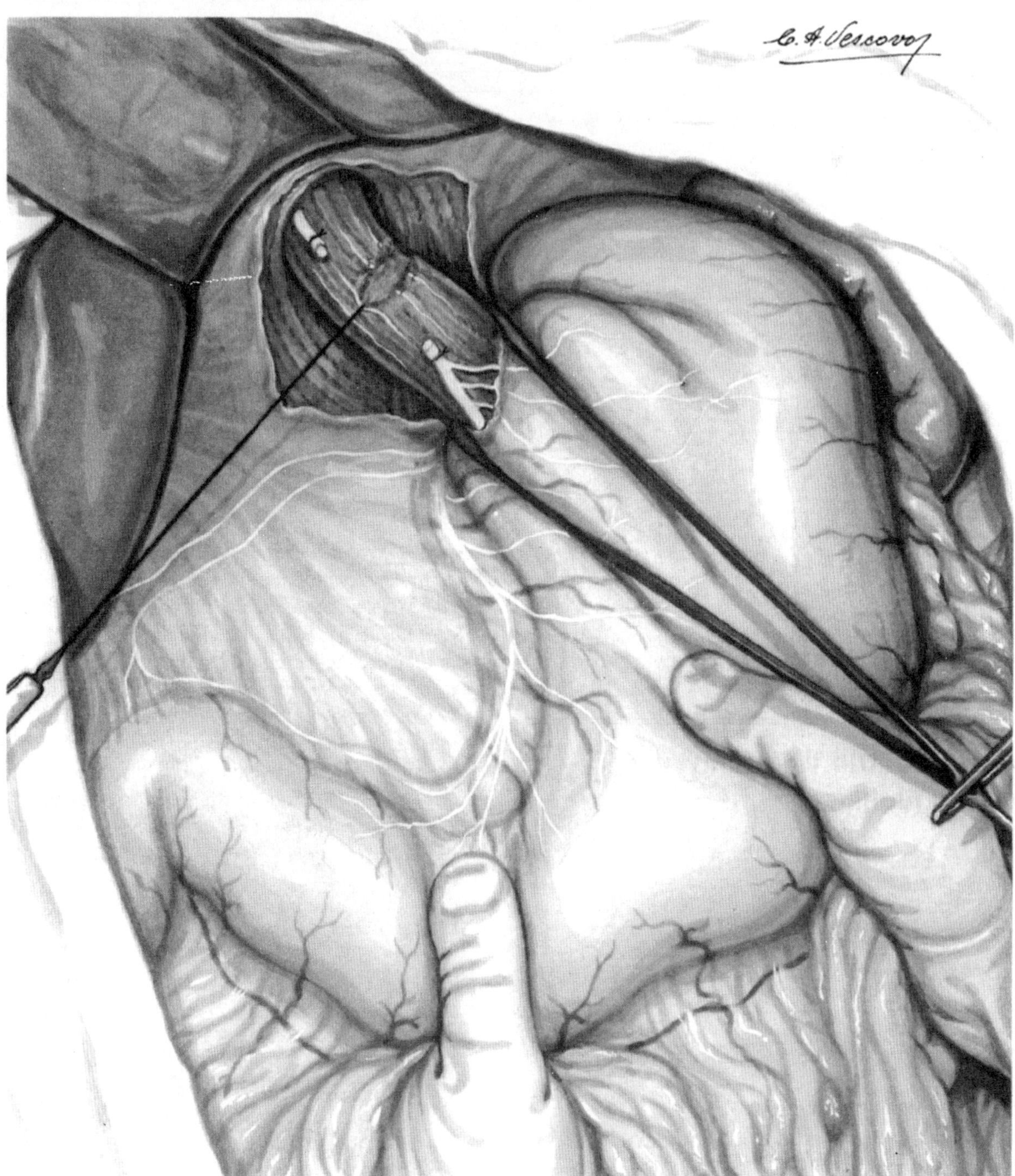

FIGURE 23.5

FIGURE 23.6
Schematic drawing showing, by means of a darker colored band, the level where the division of the vagus nerves is carried out in selective vagotomy. The nerves are divided after the anterior vagus has given off the hepatic branch (sometimes there are two hepatic branches) and the posterior vagus has given off the celiac branch (15, 32). Division of the vagus nerves at this level prevents the development of functional alterations of other abdominal organs with parasympathetic nerve supply and the development of diarrhea, biliary calculi, and so on. On the other hand, selective vagotomy produces severe motor changes of the stomach, making a drainage procedure mandatory.

Selective Gastric Vagotomy: Operative Technique

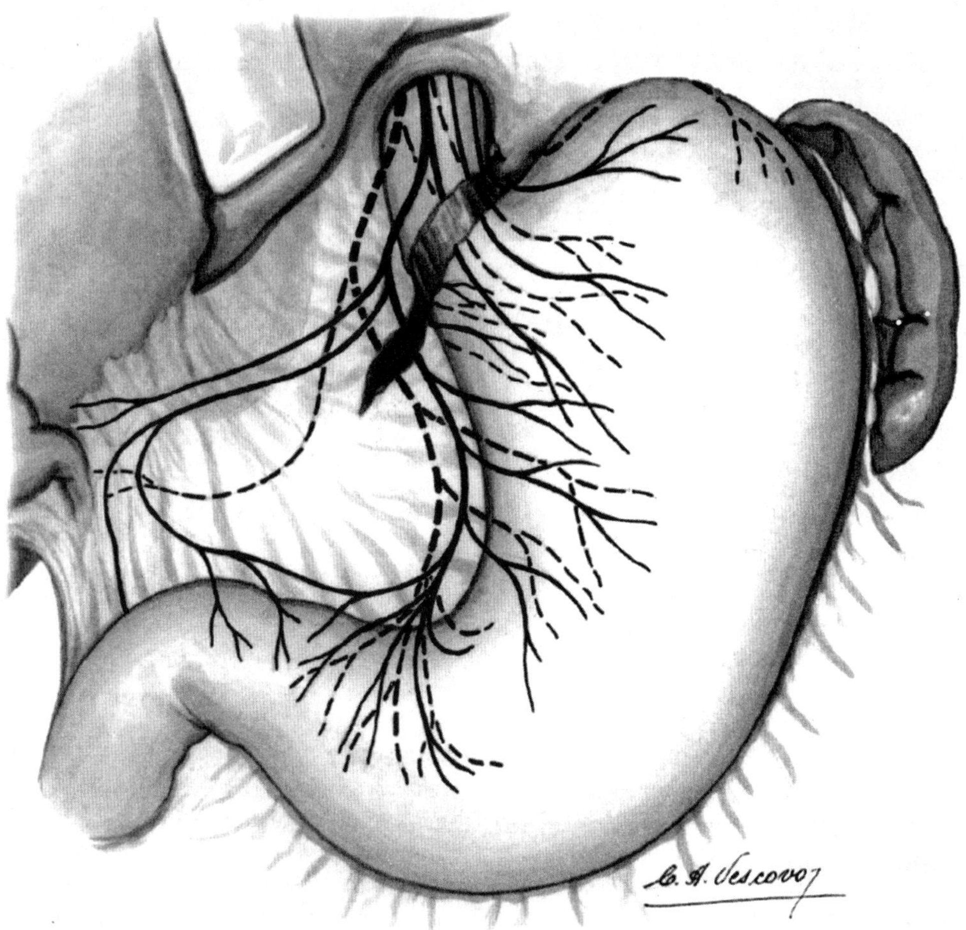

FIGURE 23.6

Selective Gastric Vagotomy: Operative Technique

FIGURE 23.7
In the performance of this technique the same incision is used as in truncal vagotomy, as well as all the precautions pointed out in describing truncal vagotomy. The second assistant applies traction to the stomach downward and to the left, including the Levine tube bordering the inside of the greater curvature. Traction should be applied gently to avoid tearing vessels in the gastrohepatic or gastrosplenic ligaments, especially if the latter is short, which could lead to a tear of the splenic capsule, making splenectomy necessary. Splenectomy should be avoided because ligature of the short vessels would leave the gastric remnant very deficient in its blood supply in case a gastric resection becomes necessary during a second operation for recurrent ulcer. This is particularly true when the inferior diaphragmatic artery arises from the left gastric or coronary artery. The traction applied by the assistant on the stomach may permit visualization of the anterior vagus and its hepatic branch. The esophagodiaphragmatic peritoneum is incised and the anterior vagus grasped with a nerve hook, applying traction to the right as shown in the drawing. The hepatic branch or branches are then identified and traction applied upward with nerve hooks to avoid dividing them.

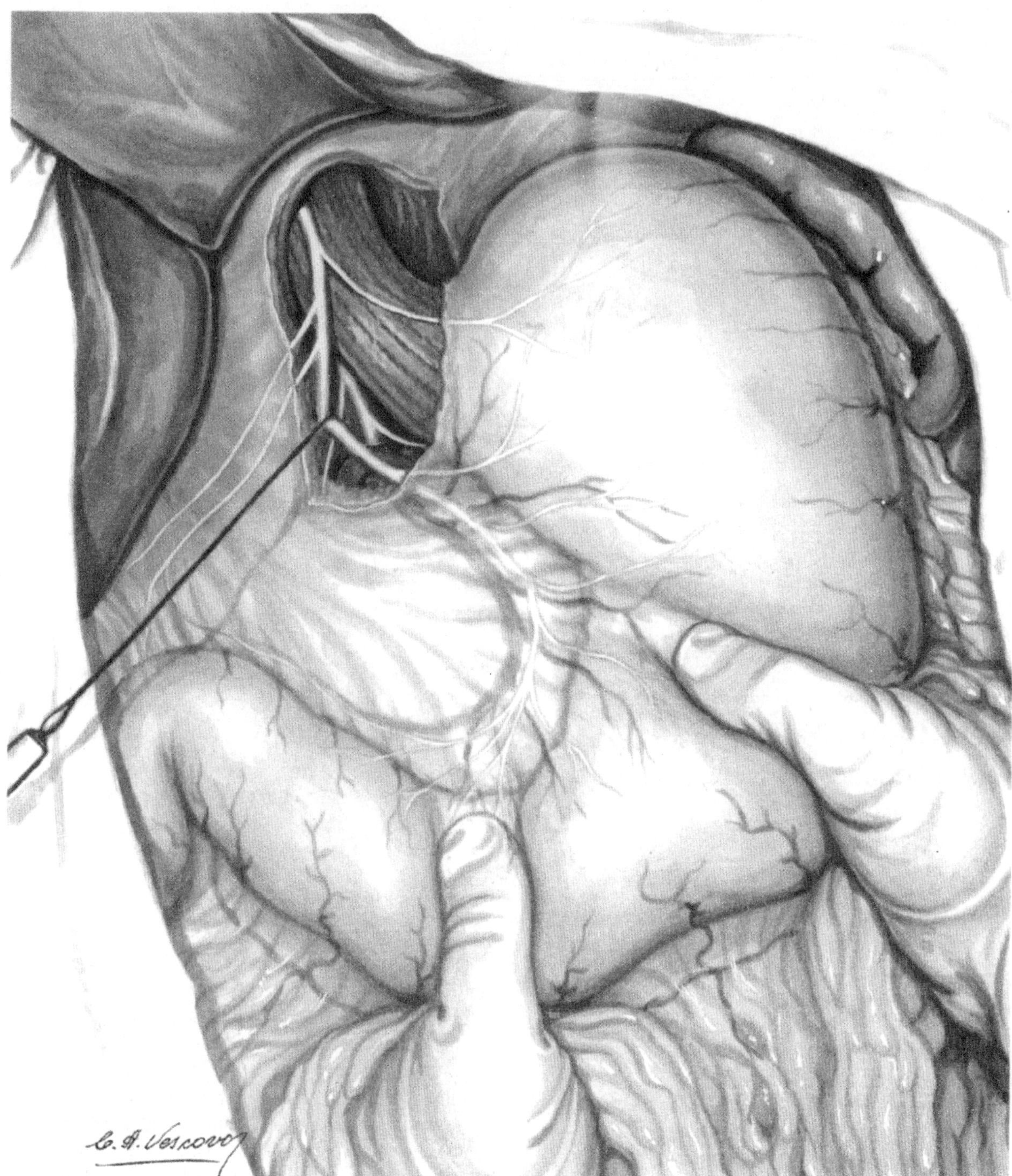

FIGURE 23.7

Selective Gastric Vagotomy: Operative Technique

FIGURE 23.8
A 3- to 4-cm long segment of the anterior vagus has been removed between ligatures from below the hepatic branch. A branch of the anterior vagus entering the anterior wall of the gastric fundus (anterior criminal nerve of Grassi) can also be seen. All tissue located between the anterior vagus and the lesser curvature of the stomach is then transected. The posterior vagus nerve is then identified after giving off its celiac branch. At times the celiac branch can be felt as a guitar or banjo string when traction is applied to the posterior vagus.

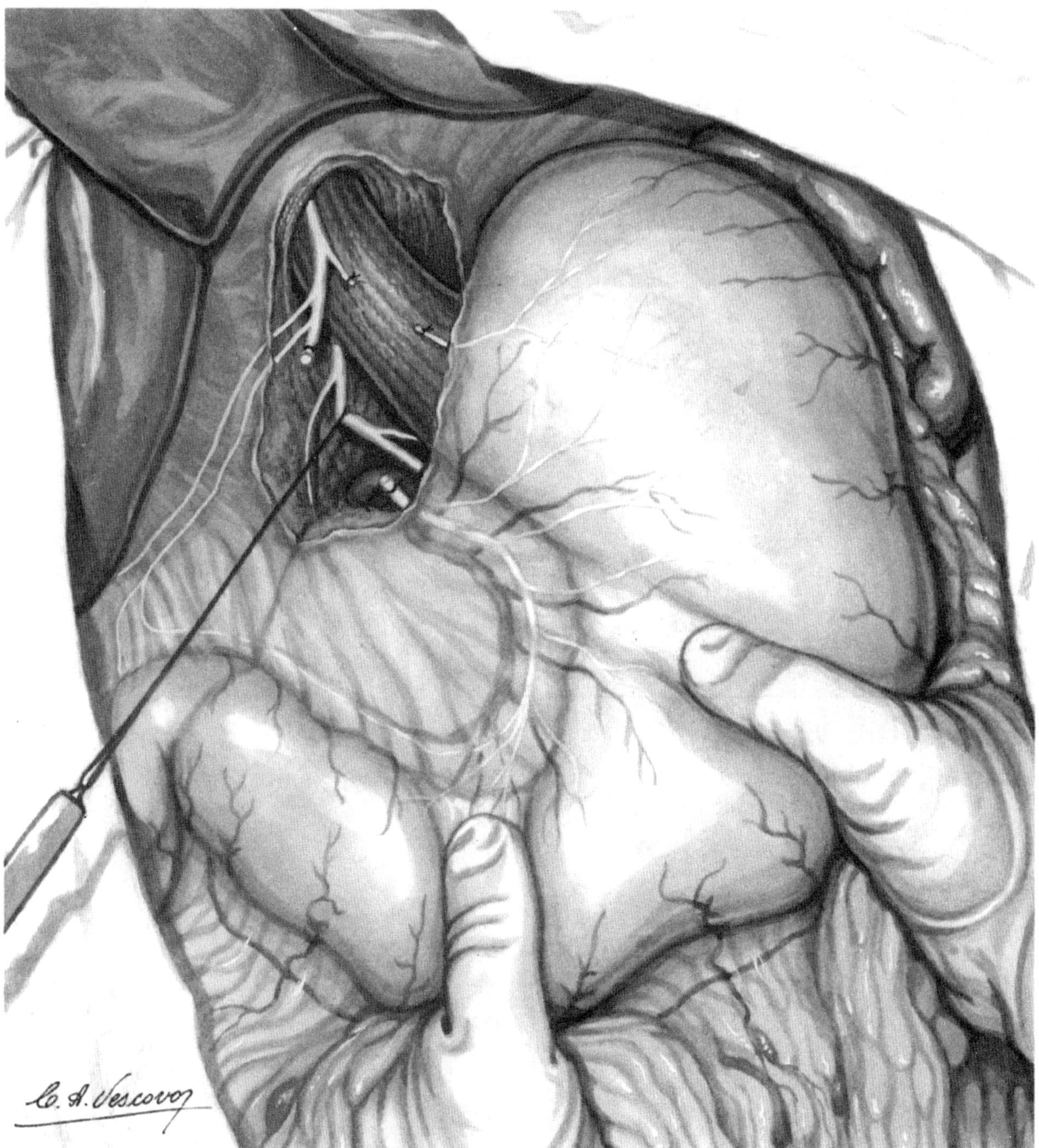

FIGURE 23.8

Selective Gastric Vagotomy: Operative Technique

FIGURE 23.9
The anterior vagus nerve has been transected below the hepatic branches. In order to be able to resect a segment of the posterior vagus nerve below the celiac nerve it is necessary to ligate the left gastric artery at its arch. A 3-cm segment of the posterior vagus is then resected. The posterior criminal nerve of Grassi has been identified by applying traction to it with a nerve hook so that it can be transected.

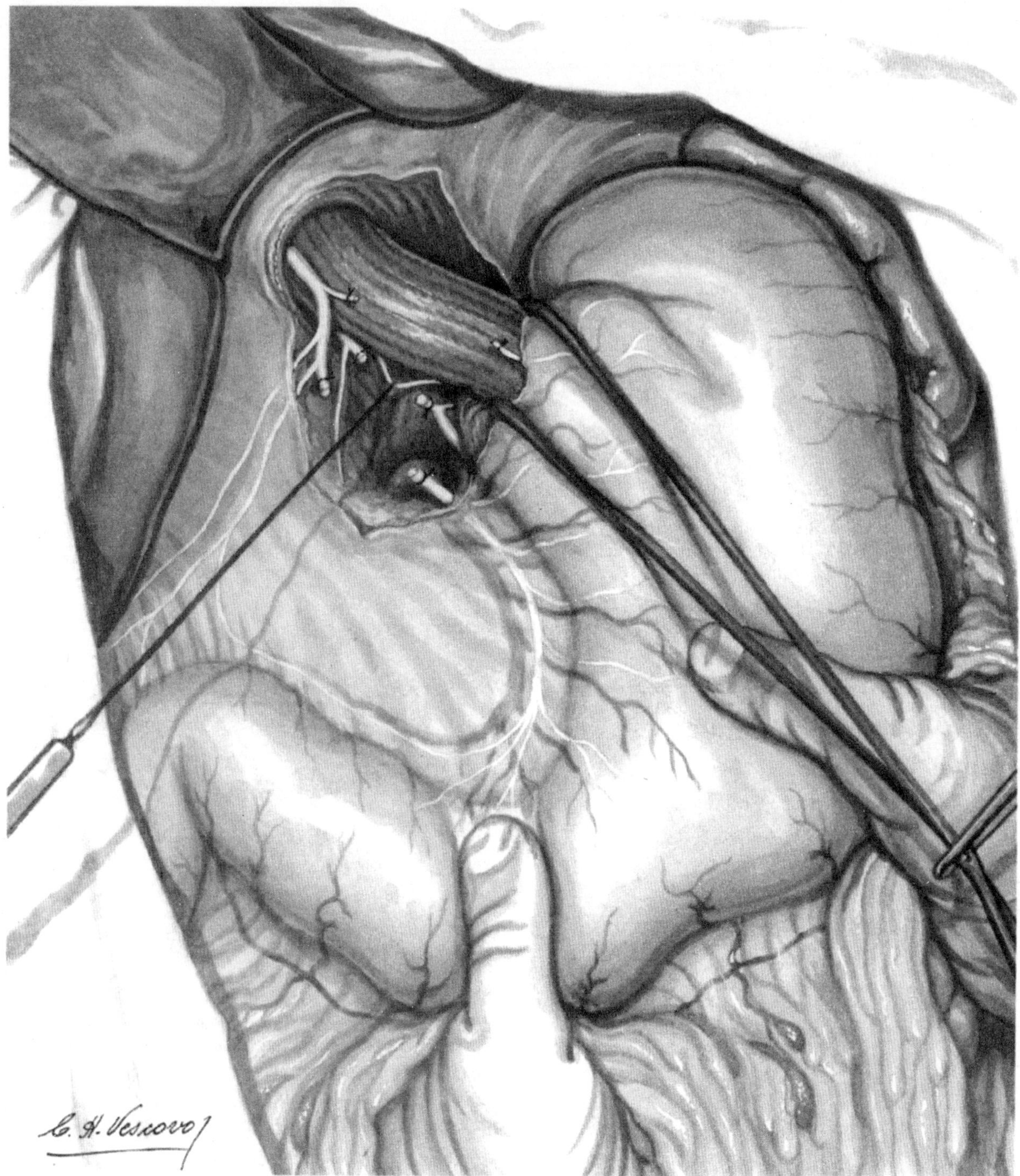

FIGURE 23.9

Selective Gastric Vagotomy: Operative Technique

FIGURE 23.10
After the vagus nerves below the hepatic and celiac branches have been transected and the anterior and posterior criminal nerves have been cut, some 5 or 6 cm of the distal esophagus is freed and a search made for very fine vagal branches, which are at times very adherent to the longitudinal muscular layer of the esophagus. These small nerves are raised with a fine hook so that they can be transected. An electric scalpel should not be used because it may produce necrosis or even perforation of the esophageal wall.

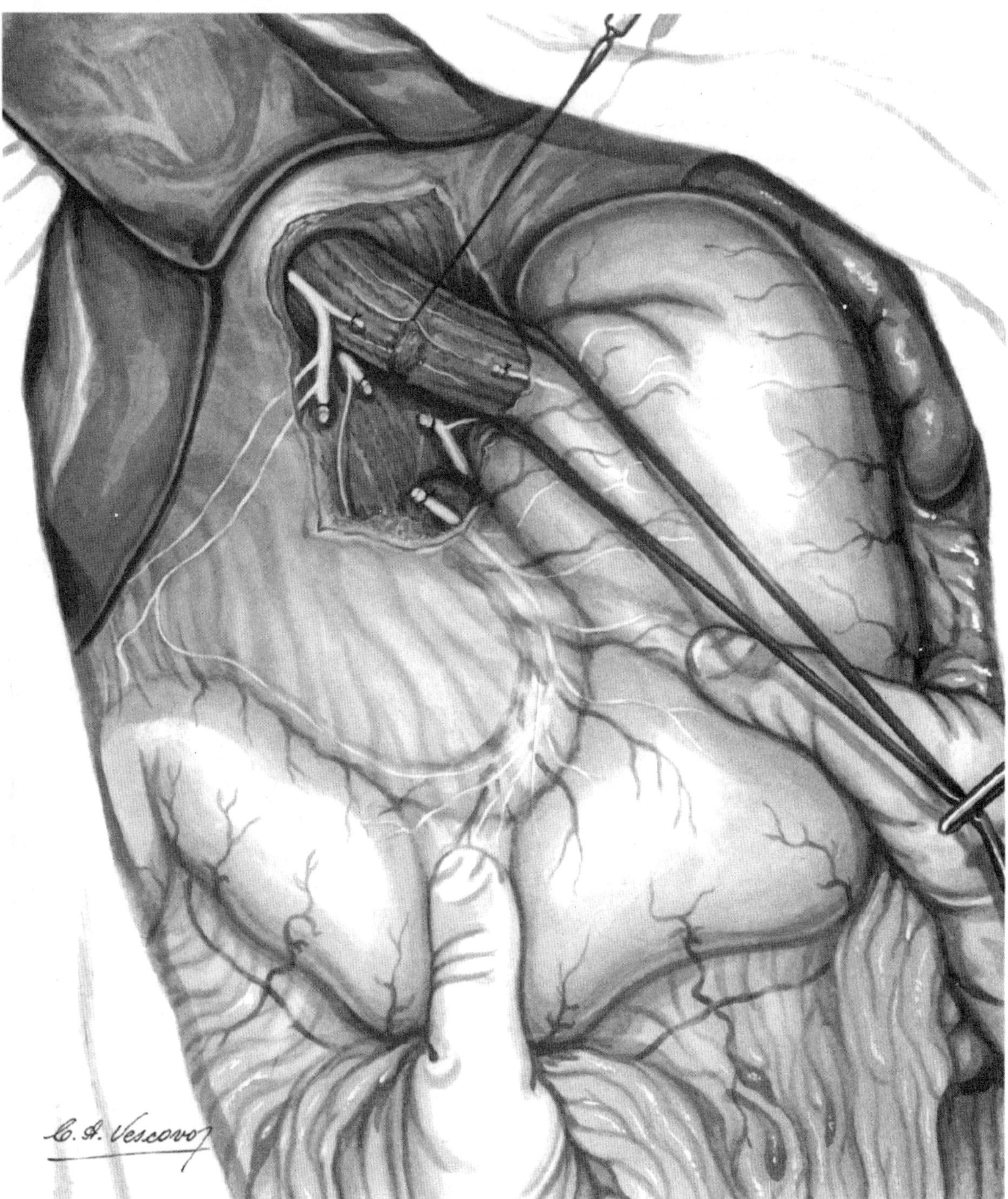

FIGURE 23.10

PROXIMAL GASTRIC VAGOTOMY: SURGICAL TECHNIQUE

Proximal gastric vagotomy has been known by different names such as partial vagotomy (21, 22) superselective vagotomy, highly selective vagotomy, selective proximal vagotomy, and parietal cell vagotomy. To avoid confusion, the present tendency is to designate this operation as proximal gastric vagotomy. The object of this operation is to attain vagal denervation of the gastric fundus and body in order to lower secretory activity of the parietal cell mass; to skeletonize the lower 5 to 6 cm of the esophagus to ensure a complete vagotomy of the parietal cells; to preserve the hepatic branch of the anterior vagus and the celiac branch of the posterior vagus, thereby avoiding functional alterations of the biliary tract, small bowel, and proximal colon; and to preserve the anterior and posterior nerves of Latarjet along their course next to the lesser curvature of the stomach as well as in their terminal branches, the crow's foot, which spread both anteriorly and posteriorly over the gastric antrum. The terminal branches which form the crow's foot are the ones that regulate antropyloric motility, making it unnecessary to perform a drainage procedure if they are preserved.

Griffith and Harkins in 1957 (21, 22) performed this operation experimentally in dogs with good results but did not perform it on humans. In 1967, Holle and Hart (29, 30), performed this operation for the first time on humans, adding a pyloroplasty that Griffith and Harkins did not consider necessary to facilitate gastric emptying. Amdrup and Jensen, of Denmark (2), performed this operation in 1970 on human beings without adding the pyloroplasty that Griffith and Harkins had thought unnecessary. Amdrup designated this procedure as parietal cell vagotomy. Johnston and Wilkinson, in 1970 (35, 36), developed this technique in England designating it "highly selective vagotomy."

Realization of a proximal gastric vagotomy demands that the surgeon have ample knowledge of the anatomy of the distal esophagus and stomach, as well as the need to respect the basic principles of this operation. This procedure is much more complex than truncal vagotomy.

Proximal Gastric Vagotomy: Surgical Technique

FIGURE 23.11
Schematic drawing showing by means of a darker area where the vagal branches have to be transected in performing a proximal gastric vagotomy. The anterior vagus runs along the anterior wall of the lower esophagus and enters the gastrohepatic ligament, where it gives off one or two (sometimes three) hepatic branches. In the drawing it is shown as a continuous line. The anterior vagus nerve then runs along the lesser curvature of the stomach, bordering it on the anterior leaf of the gastrohepatic ligament. In its course along the lesser curvature the anterior vagus gives off numerous collateral vagal branches in right-angle fashion to innervate the anterior wall of the lesser curvature of the stomach. After giving off the hepatic branch, the nerve changes its name to anterior gastric nerve of Latarjet. The nerve of Latarjet ends in three terminal branches (at times four) over the anterior wall of the gastric antrum, where it resembles a crow's foot. The posterior vagus (broken line) descends from the posterior wall of the lower esophagus and introduces itself into the gastrohepatic ligament, where it gives off the celiac nerve and then continues along the lesser curvature of the stomach, bordering it on the posterior leaf of the gastrohepatic ligament. The posterior vagus nerve, after giving off its celiac branch, changes its name to posterior nerve of Latarjet. During its course along the lesser curvature the posterior nerve of Latarjet gives off numerous branches in right angle fashion to innervate the posterior wall of the lesser curvature of the stomach. The posterior nerve of Latarjet ends in the posterior wall of the gastric antrum as three branches, forming the posterior crow's foot. The many collateral branches of both nerves of Latarjet run with the vascular collateral blood vessels of the left gastric or coronary vessels, forming neurovascular bundles. In the drawing both nerves of Latarjet have been placed somewhat away from the lesser curvature so as not to superimpose them and to make the area where the collateral gastric nerves are divided more visible.

Proximal Gastric Vagotomy: Surgical Technique

The abdominal incision is the same as that used in truncal and selective vagotomies.

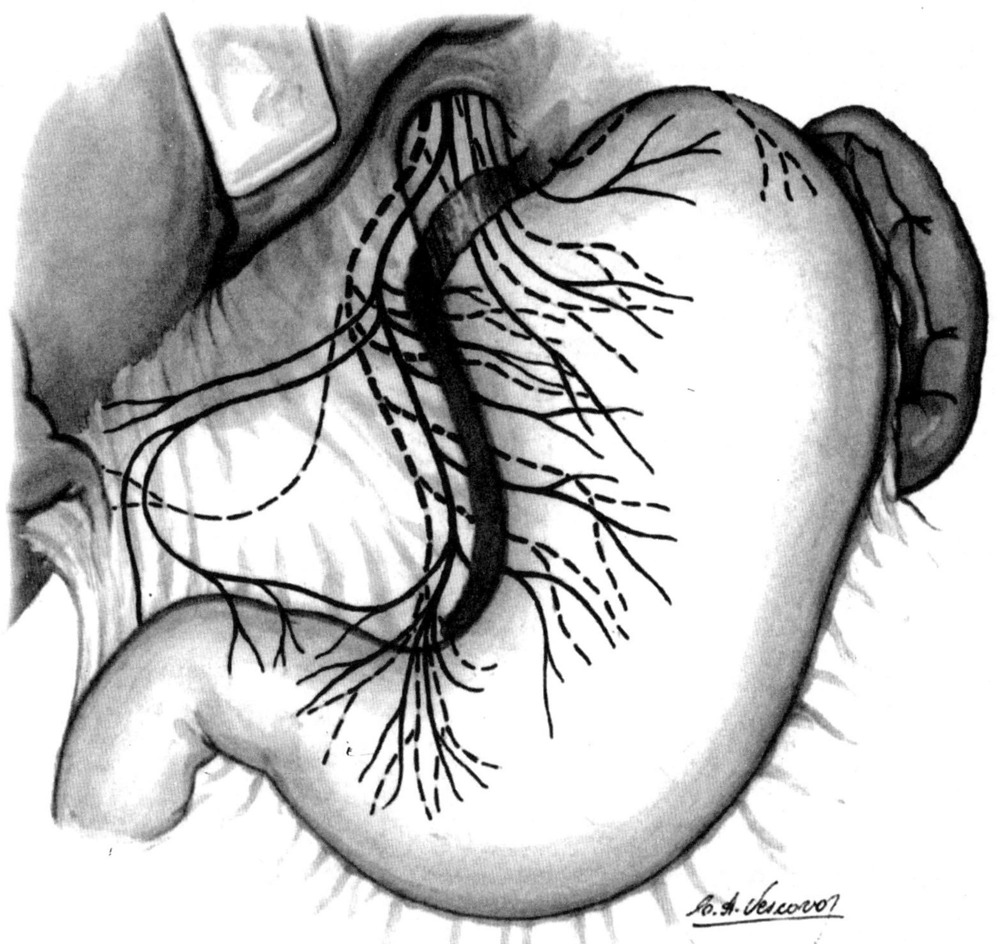

FIGURE 23.11

Proximal Gastric Vagotomy: Surgical Technique

FIGURE 23.12
The second assistant applies traction to the greater curvature of the stomach downward and to the left with both hands. In order for traction to be more effective, it is useful to displace the Levine tube toward the greater curvature so that the tube can be grasped together with the stomach.

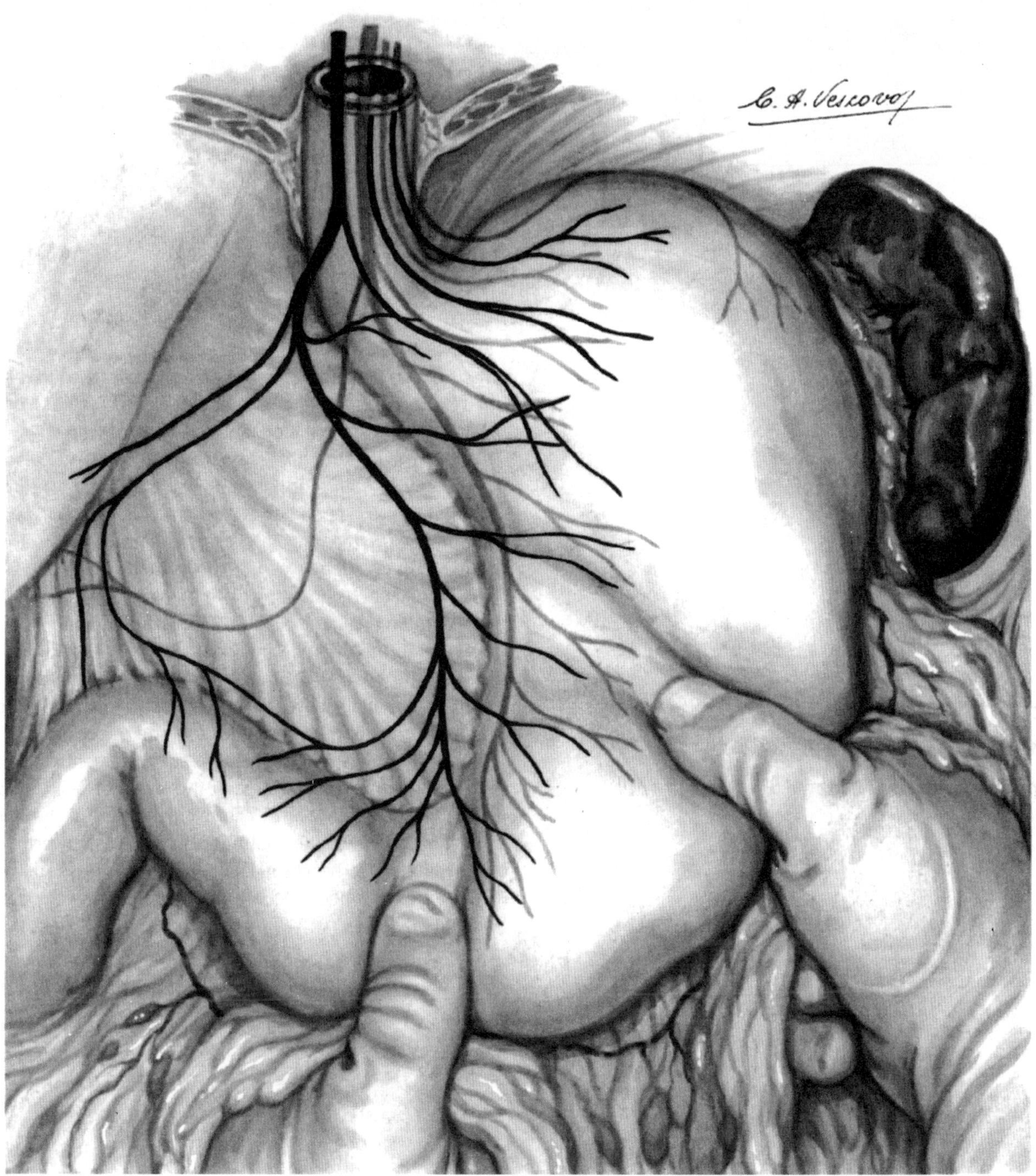

FIGURE 23.12

FIGURE 23.13

The traction applied by the assistant permits the identification, in thin persons, of the anterior nerve of Latarjet as a fine whitish string running along the gastrohepatic ligament next to the lesser curvature of the stomach. At times it is also possible to see the three or four terminal branches of the nerve of Latarjet, which spread over the anterior wall of the gastric antrum below the angular incisure of the lesser curvature, forming what is known as the crow's foot. It is important to visualize a fictitious line running from the esophagogastric angle of His to the angular incisure, which is located some 6 or 7 cm proximal to the pylorus. In obese patients it is very difficult to identify the nerve of Latarjet. The collateral branches of the nerve of Latarjet above the crow's foot should be transected so as not to produce alterations in the motor activity of the antrum and pylorus. The gastrohepatic ligament is cut with a scissors in an avascular area at the level of the incisura in order to introduce the index and middle fingers of the left hand to apply traction on the gastrohepatic ligament toward the right to separate the nerve of Latarjet from the lesser curvature of the stomach and facilitate the transection of the collateral gastric branches.

Proximal Gastric Vagotomy: Surgical Technique

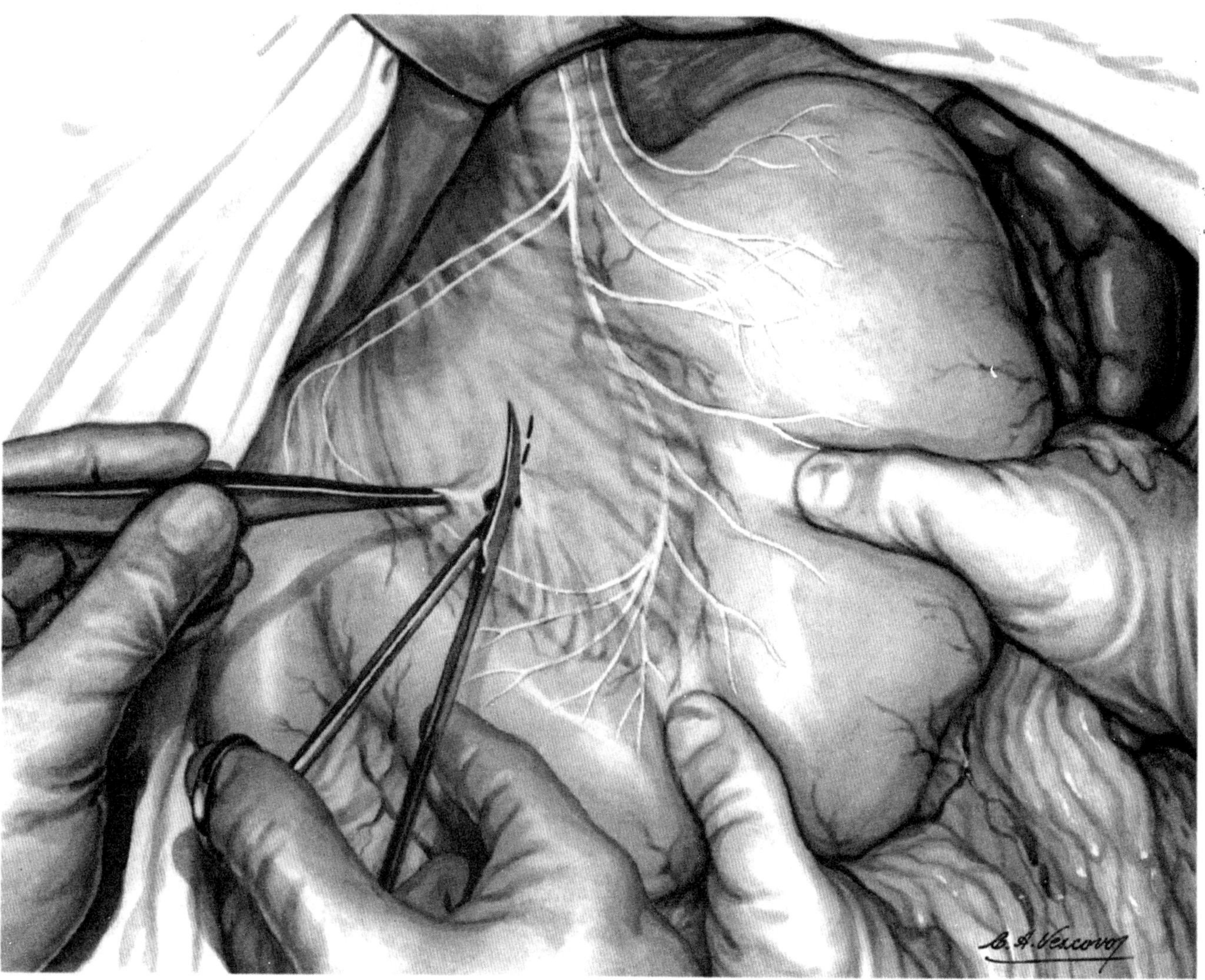

FIGURE 23.13

Proximal Gastric Vagotomy: Surgical Technique

FIGURE 23.14

Instead of applying traction to the right on the gastrohepatic ligament with the index and middle fingers, the following maneuver, which produces good results, can be used. The opening in the gastrohepatic ligament as well as the introduced index and middle fingers can be used. The end of a delicate curved clamp is introduced between the edge of the lesser curvature of the stomach, above the terminal branches of the nerve of Latarjet and, assisted by the left index and middle fingers, into the lesser omental sac.

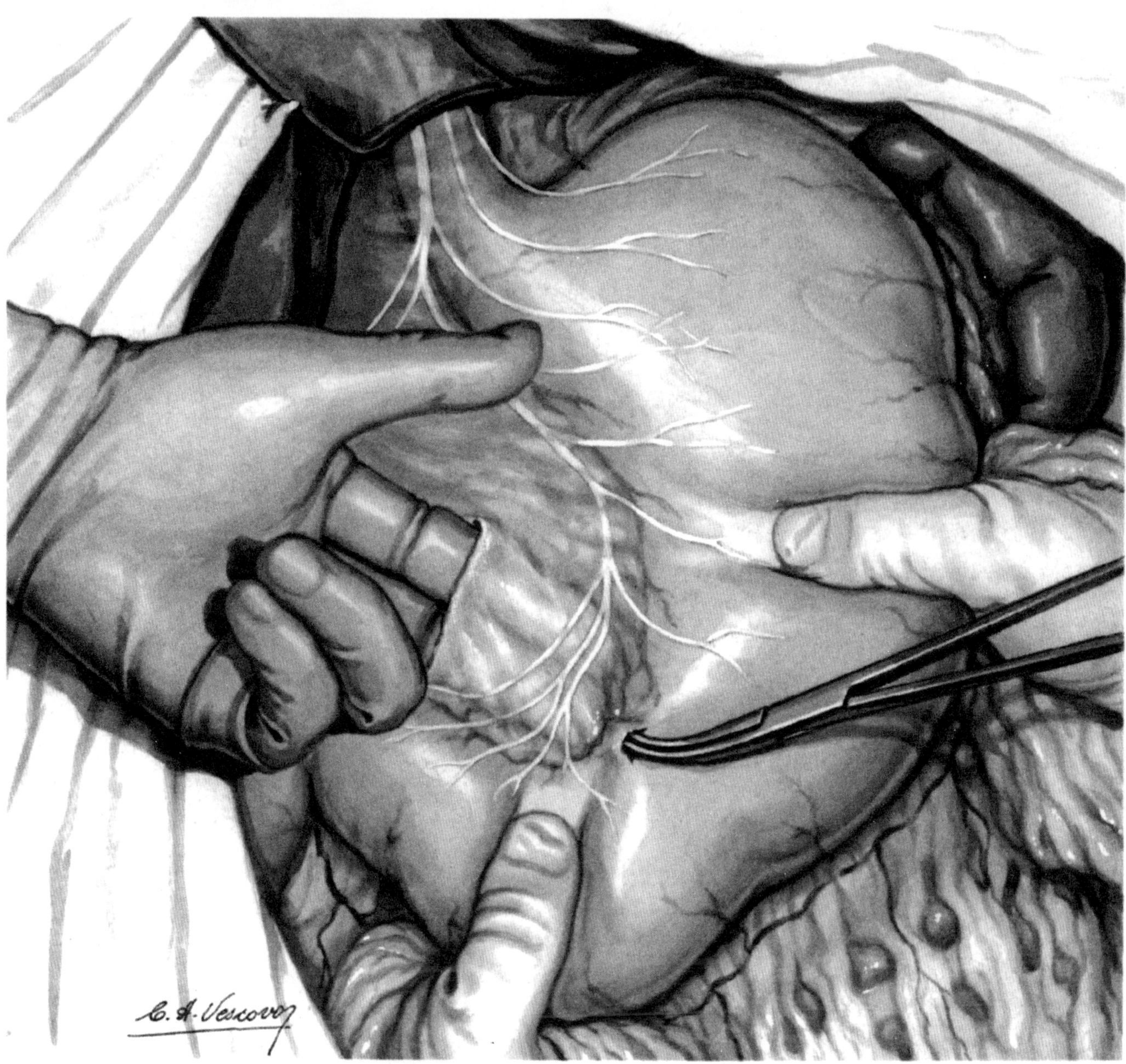

FIGURE 23.14

Proximal Gastric Vagotomy: Surgical Technique

FIGURE 23.15
Once the end of the curved clamp is passed into the lesser omental sac flush with the edge of the lesser curvature, it is advanced through the opening in the gastrohepatic ligament, where a thin rubber tube is grasped and brought back out the small buttonhole on the edge of the lesser curvature.

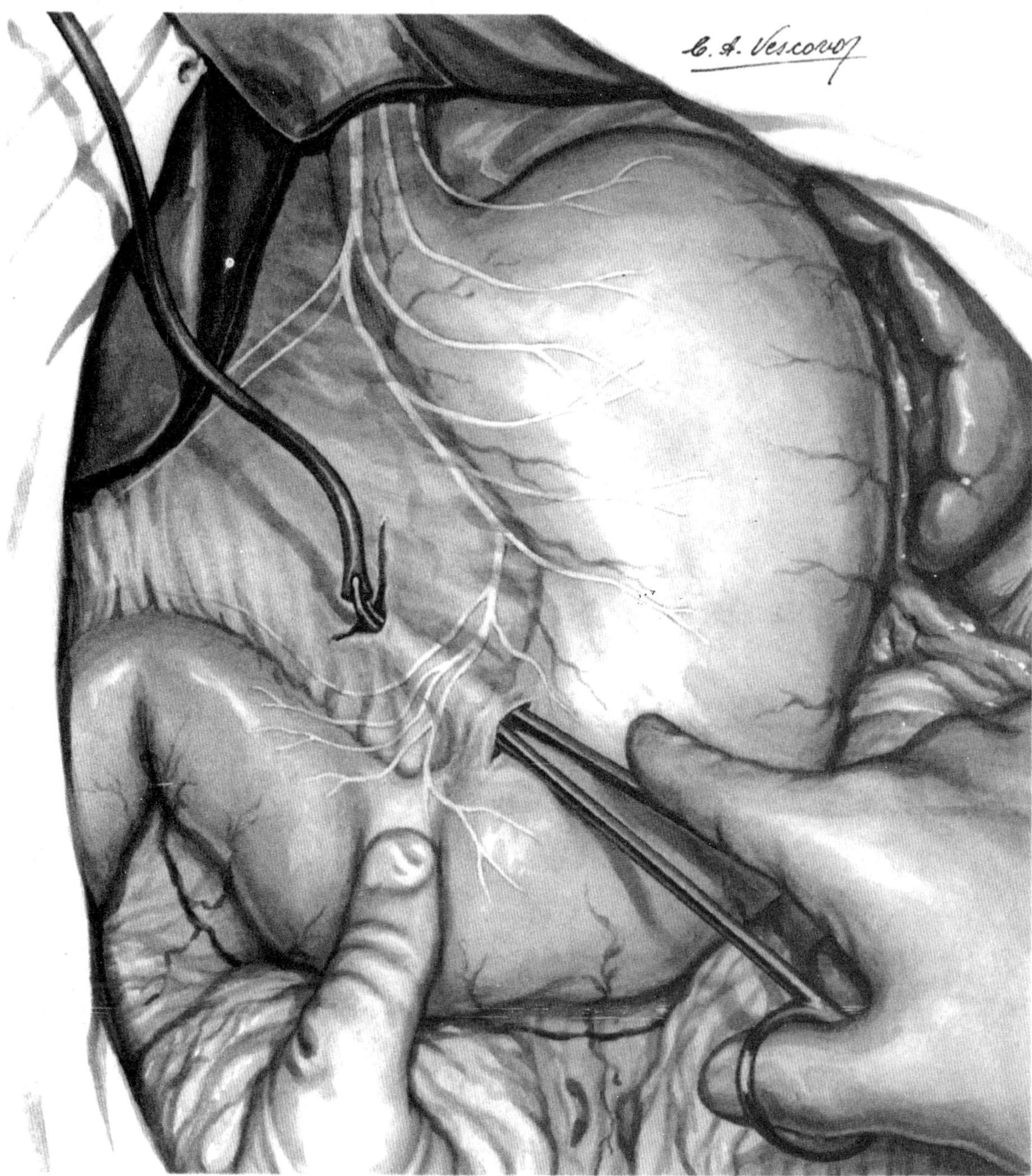

FIGURE 23.15

Proximal Gastric Vagotomy: Surgical Technique

FIGURE 23.16
The ends of the rubber tube are grasped by a clamp, and traction is applied toward the right to separate the nerve of Latarjet from the lesser curvature and to facilitate ligation and division of its collateral gastric branches.

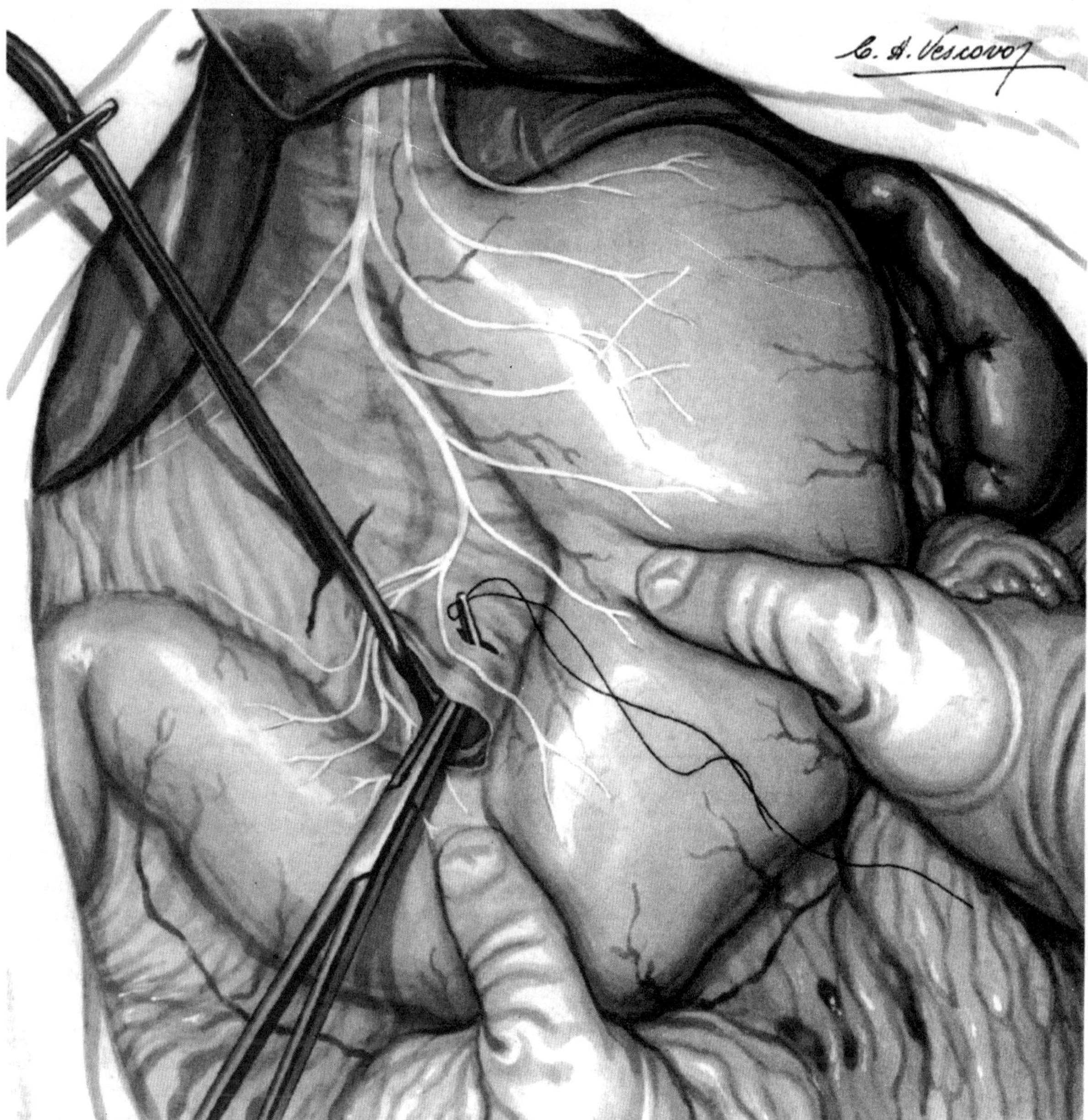

FIGURE 23.16

Proximal Gastric Vagotomy: Surgical Technique

FIGURE 23.17

Traction is applied to the rubber tube toward the right while the assistant pulls the greater curvature down and to the left. Several neurovascular bundles have been ligated and transected, including the collateral branches of the anterior and posterior nerves of Latarjet, as seen in the drawing. The procedure continues by tying off and dividing these bundles from below upward all the way to the esophagogastric junction. If the patient is thin, two or three anterior bundles can be tied and divided, the surgeon proceeding immediately to ligature and division of the posterior bundles, as shown in the drawing. However, if the patient is obese, it is more convenient to ligate and divide all the anterior bundles and then repeat the procedure on the collateral branches of the posterior nerve of Latarjet. Some surgeons tie off and divide the collateral bundles from above downward, but it is simpler and safer to perform the ligature and division of the bundles from below upward, as shown in the drawings. It is not beneficial to include more than one bundle at a time to accelerate the procedure. Even though it is frequently possible to ligate and divide the bundles formed by a collateral branch of the nerve of Latarjet and an arterial and venous branch, at times this is not possible, as can be seen in the drawing, where an isolated collateral nerve branch is about to be tied and divided because the blood vessels are some distance away from it.

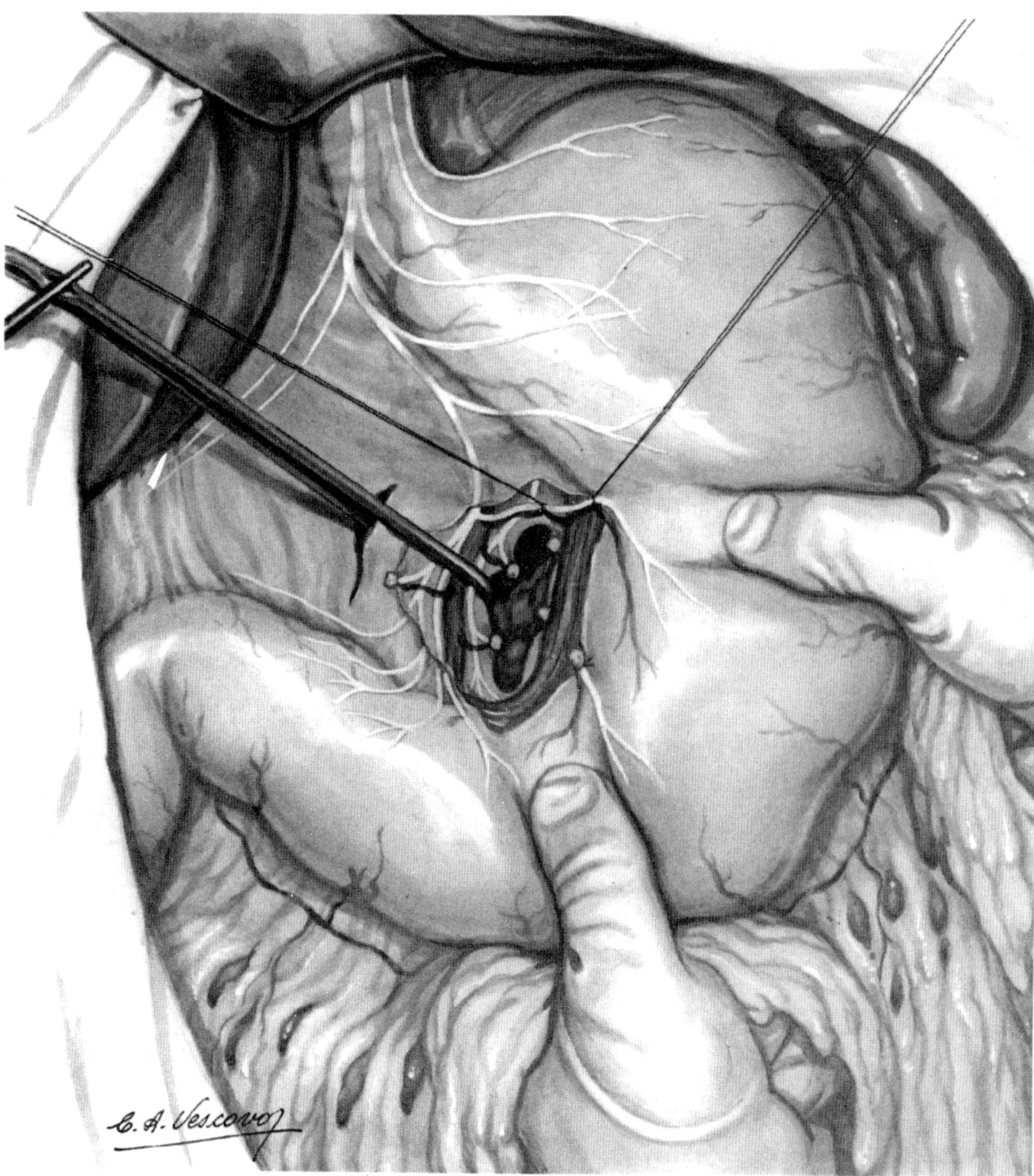

FIGURE 23.17

Proximal Gastric Vagotomy: Surgical Technique

FIGURE 23.18
Several collateral nerve branches have been ligated and divided together with the arteries and veins accompanying them, approaching the esophagogastric junction, where another bundle is being ligated.

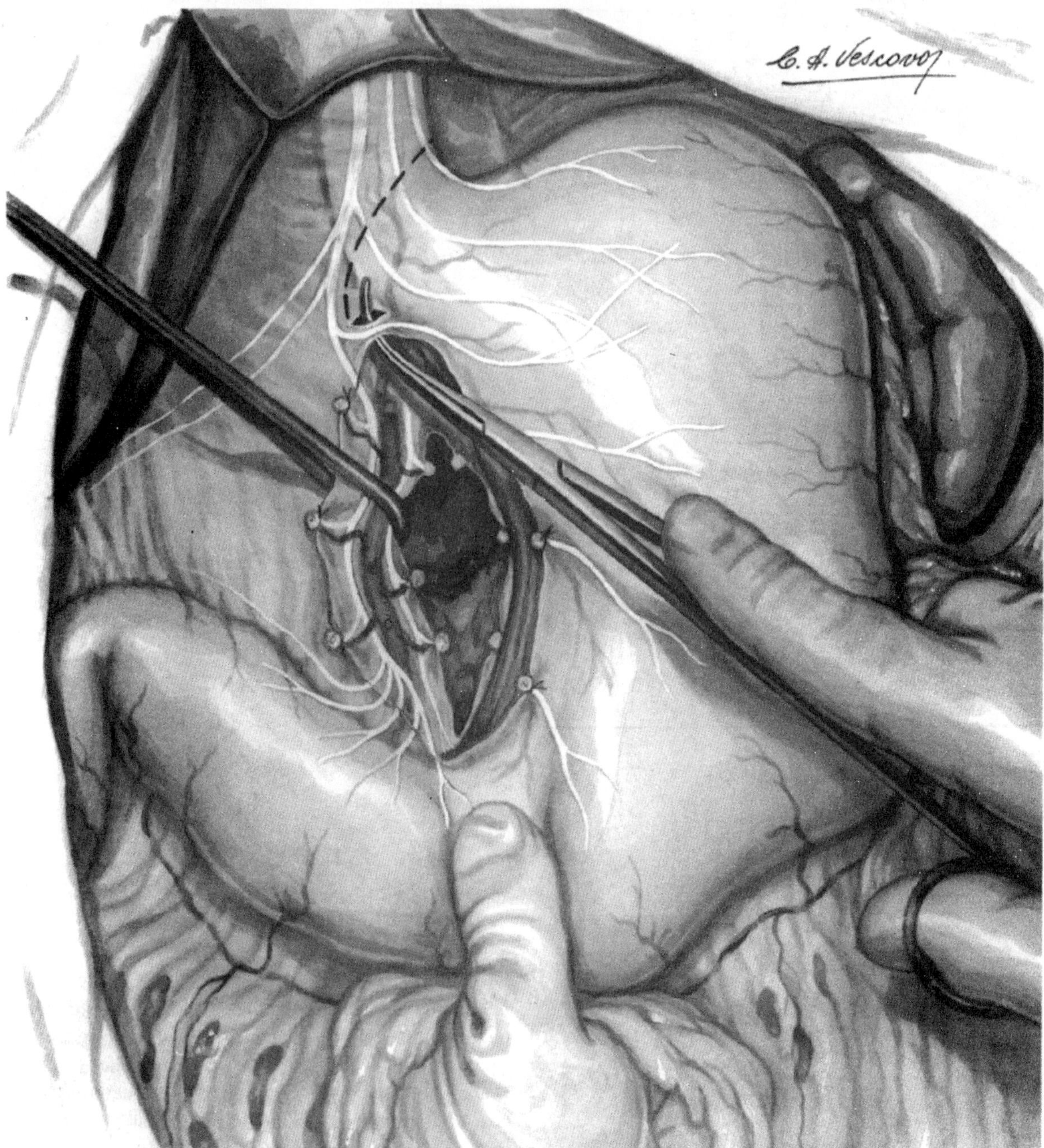

FIGURE 23.18

Proximal Gastric Vagotomy: Surgical Technique

FIGURE 23.19

All the neurovascular bundles have been ligated and transected, from the crow's foot to the esophagogastric junction. Upon arriving at this level, the peritoneum covering the anterior wall of the esophagus is incised in the direction of the angle of His. The anterior and posterior vagal trunks, together with their hepatic and celiac branches, are retracted to the right, and some 5 to 6 cm of the distal esophagus is skeletonized circumferentially, as shown in the drawing.

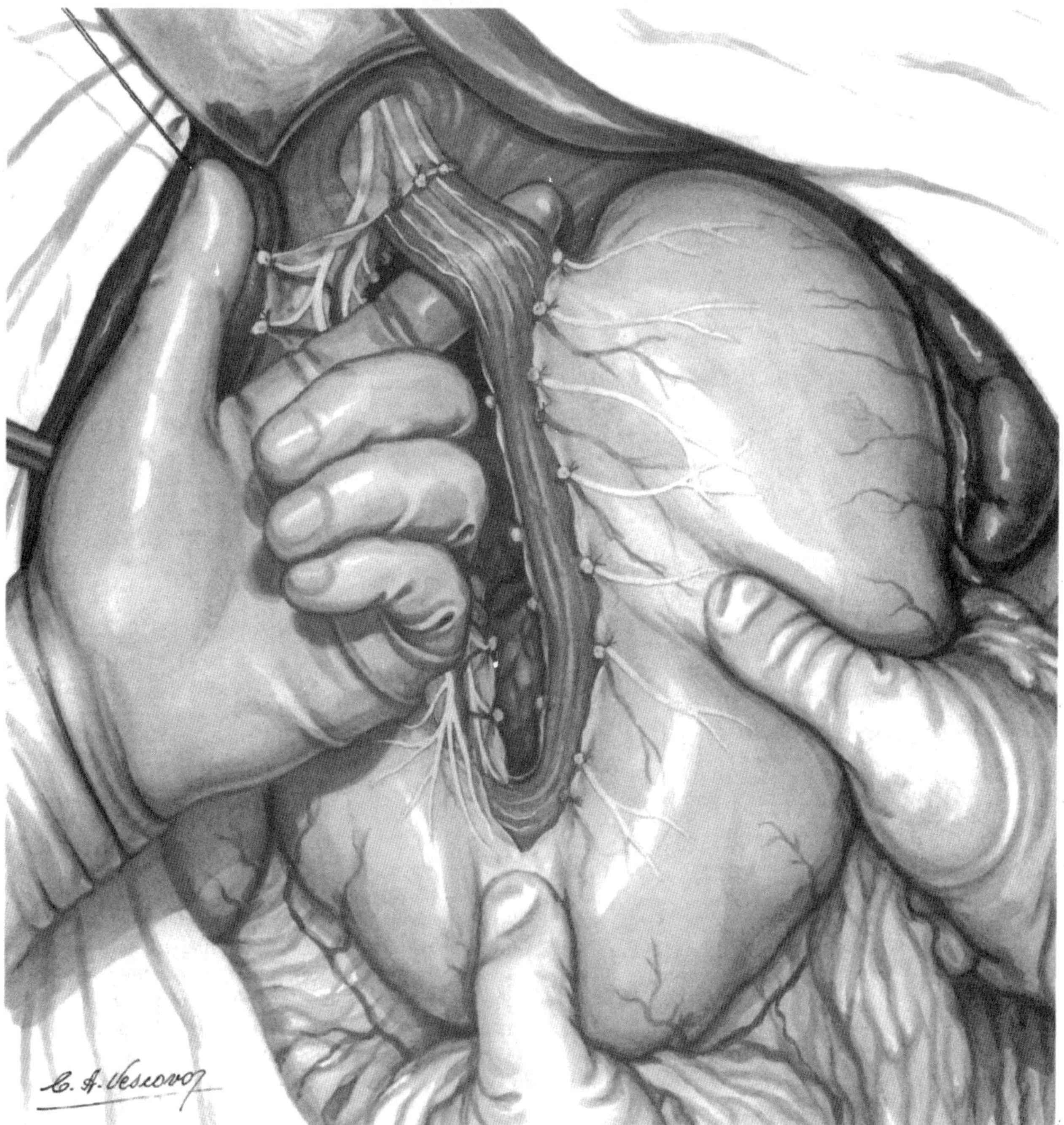

FIGURE 23.19

Proximal Gastric Vagotomy: Surgical Technique

FIGURE 23.20

Two branches of the anterior vagal trunk running toward the proximal portion of the anterior gastric wall have been divided. A branch of the posterior vagus running to the posterior wall of the fundus (posterior criminal nerve of Grassi) has been retracted to the right with a nerve hook. The posterior criminal nerve of Grassi should always be searched for and divided because it can lead to failure of the surgery. A loop has been passed around the esophagus to apply traction to it downward and to the left, to better identify and transect nerve branches that may cause recurrences of ulcers. One can also observe that the terminal branches of the nerve of Latarjet, which form the crow's foot, remain intact, partially retracted to the right by the rubber tube.

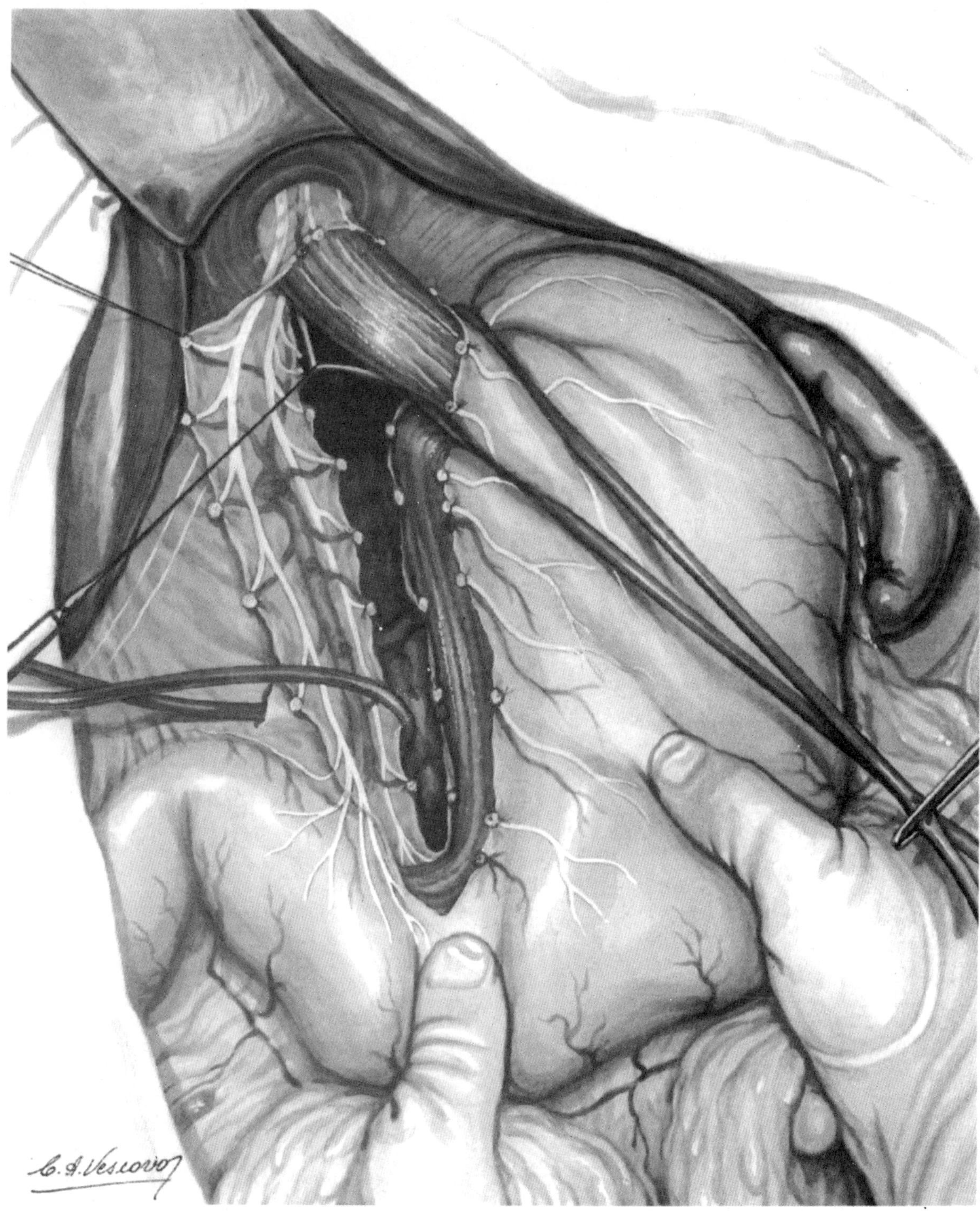

FIGURE 23.20

Proximal Gastric Vagotomy: Surgical Technique

FIGURE 23.21
The transected ends of the posterior criminal nerve of Grassi can be seen. In the esophageal wall some fine vagal fibers can be seen adherent to its longitudinal muscle layer. Using a fine nerve hook, these are identified and transected. At times it is necessary to divide some of the superficial fibers of the longitudinal muscle layer of the esophagus to be able to transect some very thin nerve fibers. It is necessary to skeletonize the distal 5 or 6 cm of the esophagus and divide all the nerve fibers to be sure a complete vagotomy has been performed.

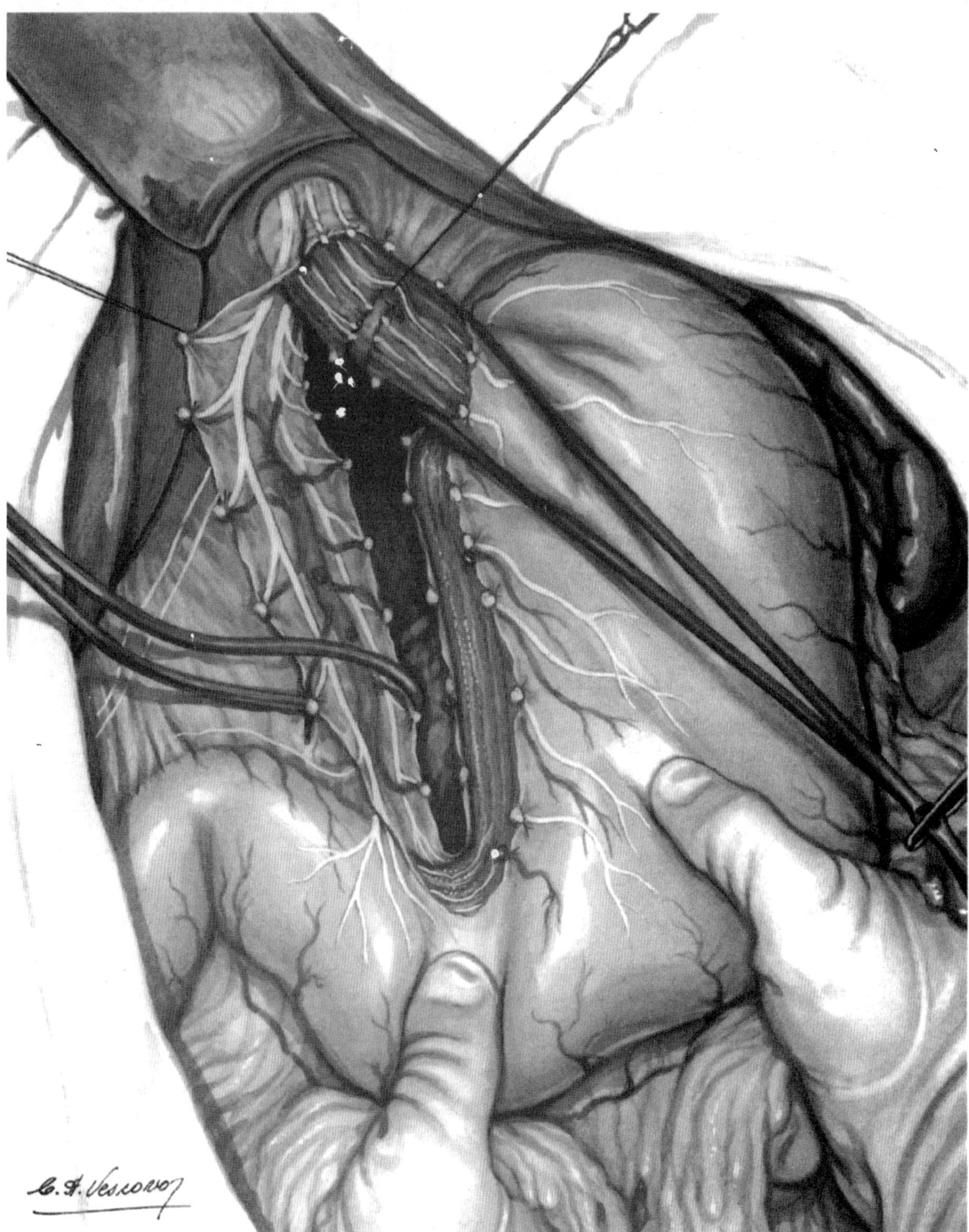

FIGURE 23.21

Proximal Gastric Vagotomy: Surgical Technique

FIGURE 23.22
Several small vagal fibers in the esophageal wall have been identified and divided. Due to their adhesion to the longitudinal muscle layer, it became necessary to perform a superficial transection of some muscle fibers. Some retrograde nerve fibers from the nerves of Latarjet are being divided at the level of the incisura.

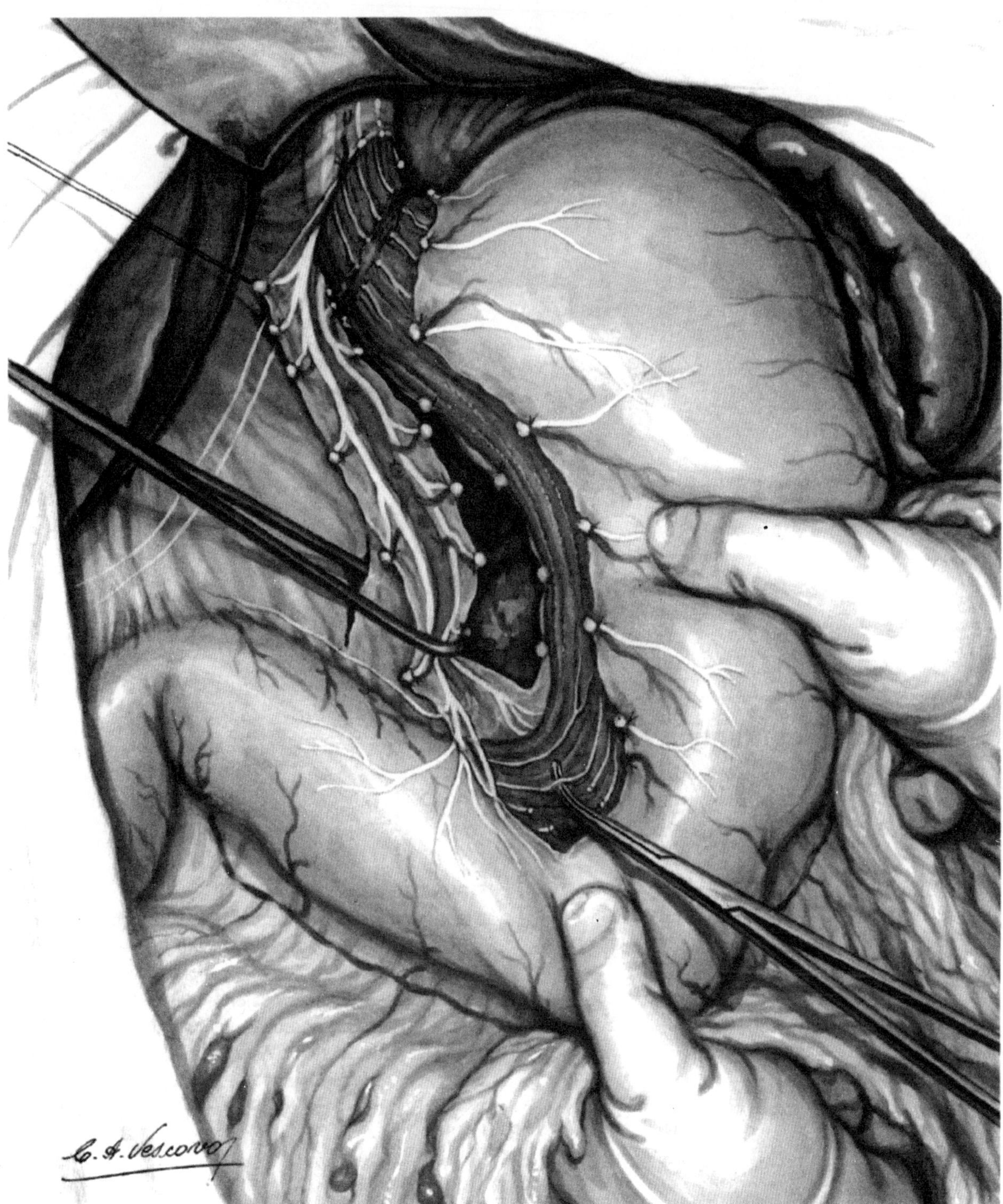

FIGURE 23.22

Proximal Gastric Vagotomy: Surgical Technique

FIGURE 23.23

Using interrupted sutures the lesser curvature of the stomach is being reperitonealized. When the lesser curvature is being dissected to tie off the multiple neurovascular bundles, hematomas and other lesions of the lesser curvature can develop, including necrosis, which can lead to serious postoperative complications. As a protective measure reperitonealization of the lesser curvature is advisable.

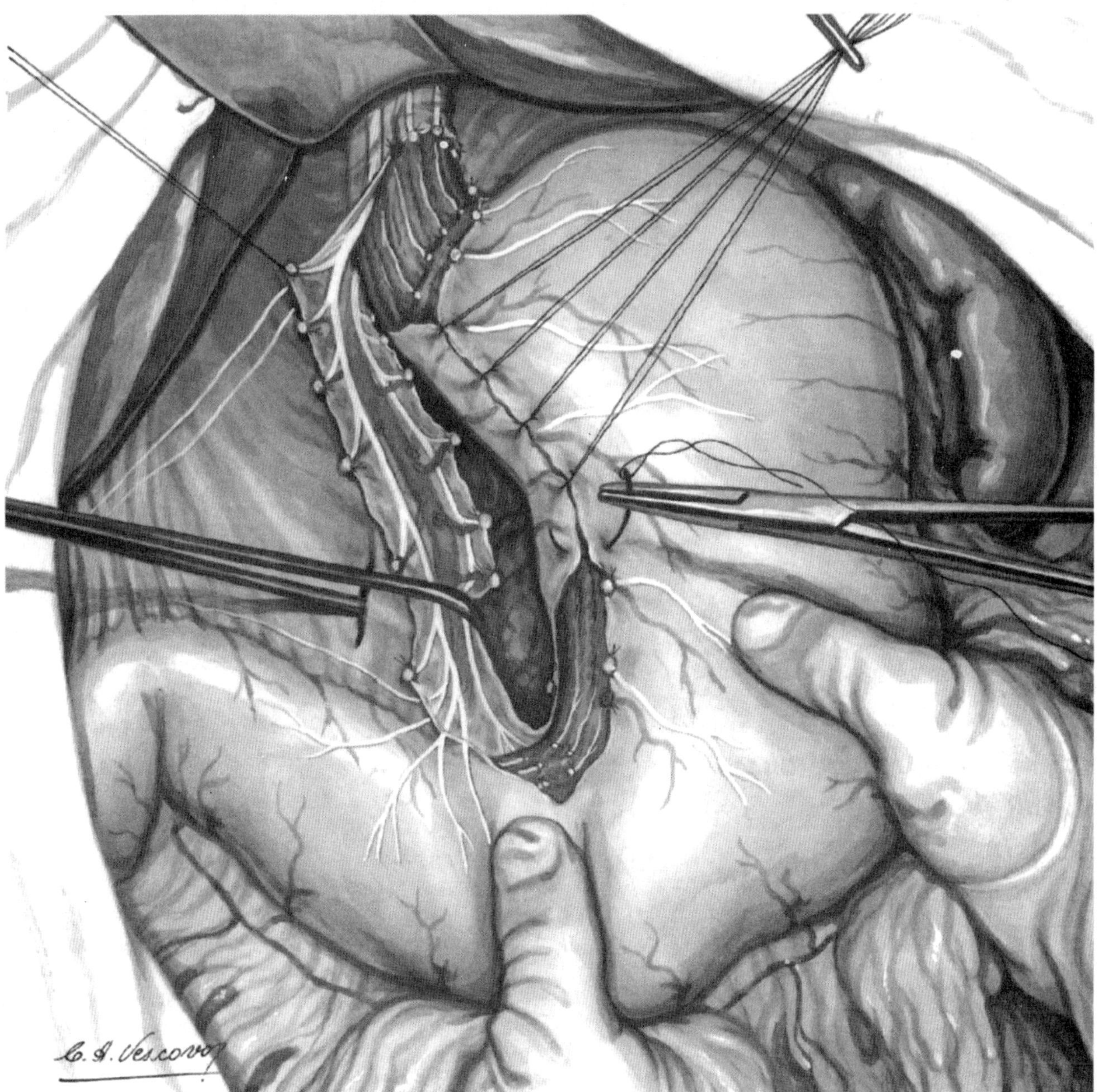

FIGURE 23.23

Proximal Gastric Vagotomy: Surgical Technique

FIGURE 23.24

To avoid leaving a defect between the lesser curvature and the edge of the gastrohepatic ligament, the edge of the ligament is sutured to the lesser curvature of the stomach, being careful not to include the nerves of Latarjet or the branches of the crow's foot in the sutures. The small incision in the avascular area of the gastrohepatic ligament can be closed with two or three sutures.

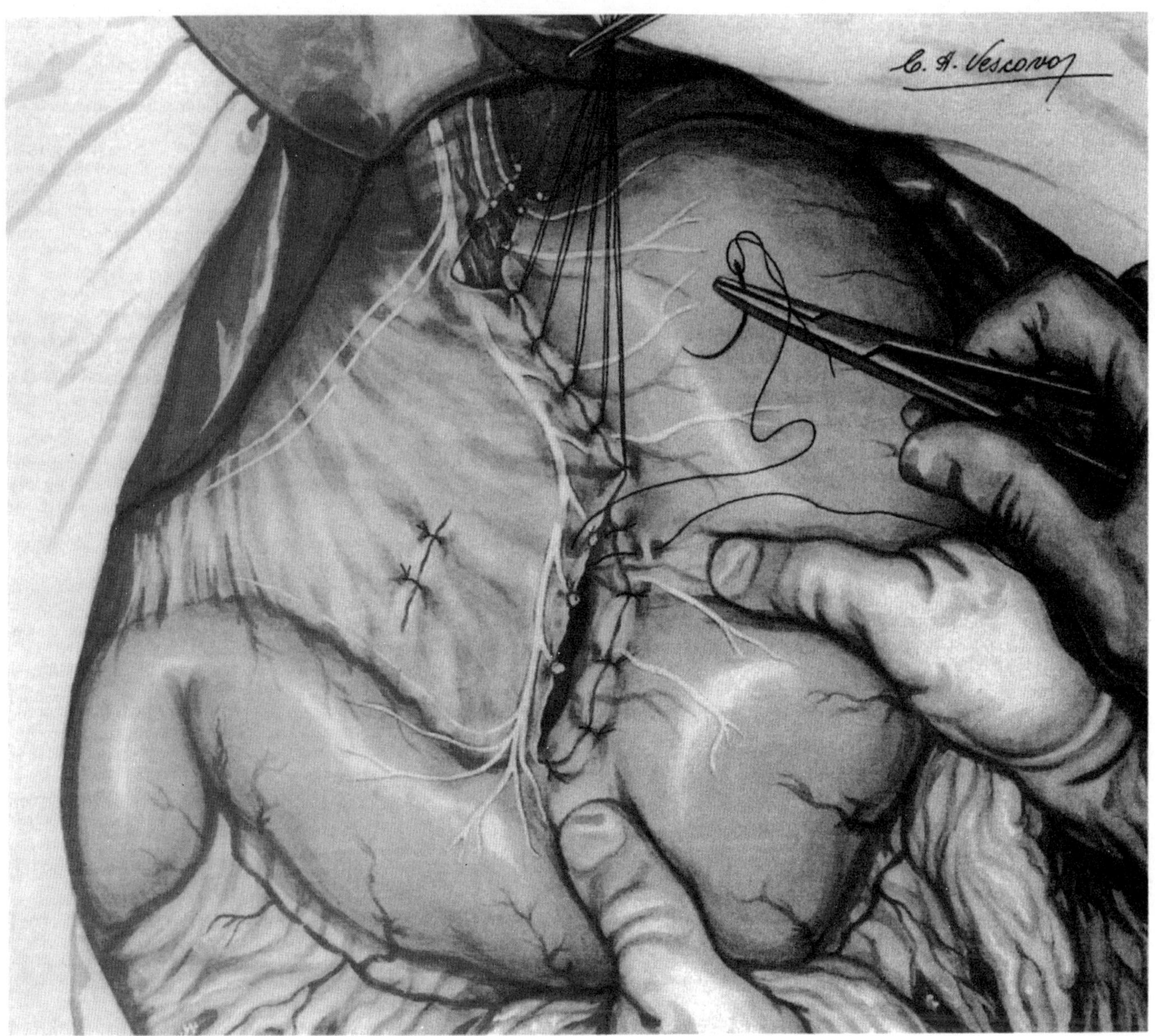

FIGURE 23.24

References

1. Amdrup, B.M., Griffith, C.A. Selective vagotomy of the parietal cell mass: I, with preservation of the innervated antrum and pylorus. Ann. Surg. 170:207, 1969.
2. Amdrup, E., Jensen, H.E. Selective vagotomy of the parietal cell mass preserving innervation of the undrained antrum. Gastroenterology 69:552, 1970.
3. Bircher, E. Die technik der magenchirurgie enke. p. 20. Stuttgart 1925.
4. Burgh, H. Vagotomy in the treatment of peptic ulceration Postgrad. Med. J. 36:2, 1960.
5. Burgh, H. Vagotomy. Edward Arnold, London, 1964.
6. Chassin, J.L. Operative stratgey in general surgery. Vol. I, p. 115. Springer-Verlag, New York, 1980.
7. De Miguel, J. Vagotomía gástrica proximal sin drenaje en el tratamiento de la úlcera duodenal. Rev. Enferm. Apar. Dig. 31:337, 1970.
8. Dragstedt, L.R., Owens, F.M. Supradiaphragmatic section of the vagus nerves in treatment of duodenal ulcer. Proc. Soc. Exp. Biol. Med. 53:152, 1943.
9. Dragstedt, L.R., Owens, F.M. Jr. Supradiaphragmatic section of the vagus nerves in the treatment of duodenal ulcer. Surg. Gynecol. Obstet. 85:461, 1947.
10. Druckerman, L.J., Weinstein, V., Klingenstein, P., Colp, R.A. Comparative study of subtotal gastrectomy with and without infradiaphragmatic vagotomy in the surgical therapy of duodenal ulcer. Ann. Surg. 136:211, 1952.
11. Edwards, L.W., Herrington, J.L. Jr., Cate, W.R. Jr., Scott, H.W. Jr., Carhon, R.I., Phillips, R.J., Stephenson, S.E. Jr. Duodenal ulcer: Treatment by vagotomy and removal of the gastric antrum. Ann. Surg. 145:5, 1957.
12. Etala, E. Gastrectomy for peptic ulcer. Contemp. Surg. 13:21, 1978.
13. Exner, A., Schwartzmann, E. Tabische krisen ulcus ventriculi and vagus. Vienna Klin. Wochenschr. 25:1405, 1912.
14. Finney, J.M.T. A new method of pyloroplasty. Bull. Johns Hopkins Hosp. 13:155, 1902.
15. Franksson, C. Selective abdominal vagotomy. Acta Chir. Scand. 96:409, 1948.
16. Gledhill, T., Clark, C.G. Vagotomy for cimetidine resistant ulcer. Lancet 2:697, 1984.
17. Goligher, J.C., Pulvertaft, C.N., de Dombal, F.T., Conyers, J.H., Duthie, H.L., Feather, D.B., Latchmore, A.J.C., Harrop-Shoesmith, J.H., Smiddy, F.G., Wilson-Petter, J. Five to eight year results of Leeds/York controlled trial of elective surgery for duodenal ulcer. Br. Med. J. 2:781, 1968.
18. Grassi, G. My experience of selective vagotomy in the treatment of ulcer disease. Acta. Chir. Scand. 136:423, 1970.
19. Grassi, G. The technique of proximal selective vagotomy. Chir. Gastroenterol. 5:399, 1971.
20. Grassi, G., Orecchia, C. A comparison of intraoperative tests of completeness of vagal section. Surgery 75:155, 1974.
21. Griffith, C.A. Selective gastric vagotomy. Surg. Clin. North Am. 46:367, 1966.
22. Griffith, C.A. Anatomic consideration in gastroduodenal surgery. In Nyhus, L.M., Baker, R.J. (Eds.) Vol. I, p. 479. Little, Brown, Boston, 1984.
23. Grimson, K.S. Surgical procedures for peptic ulcer: Critique of commitee report. Gastroenterology 24:275, 1953.
24. Harkins, H.N., Lesseph, J.E., Stevenson, J.K., Nyhus, L.M. The combined operation for peptic ulcer. Arch. Surg. 80:743, 1960.
25. Harkins, H.N., Chopman, N.D., Condon, R.E., Nyhus, L.M., Stevenson, J.K., Jesseph, J.E. Combined operation: Vagotomy-antrectomy for gastroduodenal ulcer. Arch. Surg. 85:936, 1962.
26. Herrington, J.L. Jr. The pyloric antrum: The relative extent of distal gastrectomy necessary to insure its complete extirpation. Surgery 44:775, 1958.
27. Herrington, J.L. Jr., Sawyers, J.L. A 25 year experience with vagotomy-antrectomy. Arch. Surg. 106:469, 1973.
28. Herrington, J.L. Discussion of O'Learly, J.P., Woodward, E.R., Hollenbeck, J.I. Vagotomy and drainage procedure for duodenal ulcer: The results of seventeen years' experience. Ann. Surg. 183:613, 1976.
29. Holle, F., Heinrich, G. Die subdiaphragmatische fundektomie. Langenbecks Arch. Klin. Chir. 293:396, 1960.
30. Holle. F., Andresson, A. Vagotomy, latest advances. Springer-Verlag, New York, 1974.
31. Jaboulay, M. La gastroenterostomie, la jejunoduodenostomie, la resection du pylore. Arch. Prov. Chir. 1:1, 1892.
32. Jackson, R.G. Anatomic study of the vagus nerves, with a technique of transabdominal selective gastric vagus resection. Arch. Surg. 57:333, 1948.
33. Jensen, H.E., Kjaergaard, J., Meisner, S. Ulcer recurrence two to twelve years after parietal cellvagotomy for duodenal ulcer. Surgery 94:802, 1983.
34. Johnson, H.D. Gastric ulcer: Classificaion, blood group characteristics, secretion patterns and pathogenesis. Ann. Surg. 162:996, 1963.
35. Johnston, D., Wilkinson, A.R. Selective vagotomy with innervated antrum without a drainage procedure in the treatment of duodenal ulcer. Br. J. Surg. 56:626, 1969.
36. Johnston, D., Wilkinson, A.R. Highly selective vagotomy without a drainage procedure in the treatment of duodenal ulcer. Br. J. Surg. 57:289, 1970.
37. Johnston, D. Division and repair of the sphincteric mechanism at the gastric outlet in emergency operations for bleeding peptic-ulcer: A new technique for use in combination with suture ligation of the bleeding point and highly selective vagotomy. Ann. Surg. 186:723, 1977.
38. Jordan, P.H.J. Duodenal ulcers and their surgical treatment: Where did they come? Am. J. Surg. 149:2, 1985.
39. Klein, E. Left vagus section and partial gastrectomy for duodenal ulcer with hyperaciditv. Ann. Surg. 90:65, 1929.
40. Latarjet, A. Résection des nerfs de l'estomac. Technique opératoire. Résultats cliniques. Bull. Acad. Natl. Med. 87:681, 1922.
41. Latarjet, A., Wortheimer, P. La vagotomie dans l'ulcer duodenal Presse Méd. 31:993, 1923.
42. Littman, A. Veteran Administration cooperative study on gastric ulcer: Healing, recurrence, cancer. Gastroenterology 61:567, 1971.
43. Menguy, R., Gadacz, T., Zajtchuk, R. The surgical management of acute gastric mucosa bleeding. Arch. Surg. 99:198, 1969.
44. McGregor, D.B., Savage, L.E., McVay, C.B. Vagotomy and drainage for elective treatment of peptic ulcers. Surg. Gynecol. Obstet. 146:349, 1978.
45. Nobles, E.R. Jr. Vagotomy and gastroenterostomy Am. Surg. 32:177, 1966.
46. Nyhus, L.M., Donahue, P.E., Krystosek, R.J. et al. Complete vagotomy: The evolution of an effective technique. Arch. Surg. 115:264, 1980.
47. Oberhelman, H.A. Jr. Vagotomy and pyloroplasty or gastrojejunostomy. In Nora, P.F. (Ed.) Operative surgery. Ed. 3, p. 520. W.B. Saunders, Philadelphia, 1990.
48. O'Learly, J.P., Woodward, E.R., Hollenbeck, J.I., Dragstedt, L.R. Vagotomy and drainage procedure for duodenal ulcer: The results of seventeen years' experience. Ann. Surg. 183:613, 1976.
49. Pemberton, J.H., van Heerden, J.A. Vagotomy and pyloroplasty in the treatment of duodenal ulceration: Long-term results. Mayo Clin. Proc. 55:14, 1980.
50. Pi-Figueras, J. Práctica quirúrgica. Ed. 2, vol. II, p. 148. Salvat, Barcelona, 1986.
51. Ruding, R., Hirdes, W.H. Extent of gastric antrum and its significance. Surgery 53:743, 1963.
52. Sawyers, J.L., Edwards, L.W., Herrington, J.L., Scott, H.W. Jr. Vagotomy and antrectomy for duodenal ulcer. 20th Congrès de la Société Internationale de Chirurgie, p. 1022. Imprimérie Médicale et Scientifique, Brussels, 1963.
53. Sawyers, J.L., Herrington, J.L. Jr. Vagotomy and antrectomy. In Nyhus, L.M., Wastell, C. (Eds.) Surgery of the stomach and duodenum. Ed. 3, p. 343. Little, Brown, Boston, 1977.
54. Sawyers, J.L. Selective vagotomy and Pyloroplasty. In Nyhus, L.M., Baker, R.J. (Eds.) Mastery of surgery. Vol. I, p. 522, Little, Brown, Boston, 1984.
55. Sawyers, J.L., Goligher, J.C. Proximal gastric vagotomy. In Scott, H.W. Jr., Sawyers, J.L. (Eds.) Surgery of the stomach, duodenum and small intestine. Ed. 2, p. 510. Blackwell, Boston, 1992.
56. Scott, H.W. Jr., Sawyers, J.L., Gobbel, W.G. Jr., Herrington, J.L. Jr., Edwards, W.H., Edwards, L.W. Vagotomy and antrectomy in surgi-

cal treatment of duodenal ulcer disease. Surg. Clin. North Am. 46:349, 1966.

57. Scott, H.W. Jr., Sawyers, J.L., Gobbel, W.G. Jr., Herrington, J.L. Jr. Definitive surgical treatment in duodenal ulcer disease. Curr. Probl. Surg. October 1968.
58. Schiassi, B.M. The role of the pyloroduodenal nerve supply in the surgery of duodenal ulcer. Di una cosidetta "operazione nuove" Il Policlínico 54:1189, 1937.
59. Schwartz, S.I., Ellis, H., eds. Abdominal operations. Ed. 9, vol. I., p. 647. Appleton Lange, Norwalk, CT, 1990.
60. Smithwick, R.H., Harrower, H.W., Former, D.A. Hemigastrectomy and vagotomy in the treatment of duodenal ulcer. Am. J. Surg. 101:325, 1961.
61. Smithwick, R.H., Former, D.A., Harrower, H.W. Heimgastrectomy and truncal vagotomy in the treatment of duodenal ulcer. Am. J. Surg. 127:631, 1974.
62. Thompson, J.C., Peskin, G.W. Collective review. The gastric antrum in the operative treatment of duodenal ulcer. Surg. Gynecol. Obstet. 112:205, 1961.
63. Thompson, J.C. The stomach and duodenum. In Sabiston, D.C. (Ed.) Textbook of surgery. Ed. 14, p. 756. W.B. Saunders, Philadelphia, 1981.
64. Walters, W., Lynn, T.E. Billroth I and Billroth II operations. Arch. Surg. 74:680, 1957.
65. Weinberg, J.A. Vagotomy with pyloroplasty in the treatment of duodenal ulcer. Am. J. Gastroenterol. 21:296, 1954.
66. Weinberg, J.A. Vagotomy and pyloroplasty in the treatment of duodenal ulcer. Am. J. Surg. 92:202, 1956.
67. Welch, C.E., Rodkey, G.V., von Gryska, P. One thousand operations for peptic ulcer disease. Ann. Surg. 204:454, 1986.
68. Welch, C.E. Gastric resection for duodenal ulcer. In Scott, H.W. Jr., Sawyers, J.L. (Eds.) Gastric resection for duodenal ulcer. Ed. 2, p. 540. Blackwell, Boston, 1992.
69. Woodward, E.R. Truncal vagotomy in the treatment of duodenal ulcer. In Scott, H.W. Jr., Sawyers, J.L. (Eds.) Ed. 2, p. 497. Blackwell, Boston, 1992.

Section F

Surgery of the Stomach and Duodenum

CHAPTER 24

Gastric Drainage and Pyloroplasty

GASTRIC DRAINAGE PROCEDURES AND PYLOROPLASTY

Truncal and selective vagotomy significantly reduce the tonicity and contractility of gastric musculature, leading to a severe disturbance of the mechanism of gastric emptying. To treat this complication, Dragstedt and Owens (4, 5) added a drainage procedure to the truncal vagotomy. This was originally a gastrojejunostomy and was later replaced by a Heineke-Mikulicz pyloroplasty (22). Pyloroplasty was originally proposed in the past century for the treatment of duodenal ulcers by Heineke-Mikulicz. Since this operation was a failure in the treatment of duodenal ulcers, it was forgotten for many years until it was used, not for its original purpose, but as a drainage procedure in patients submitted to a truncal vagotomy for the treatment for duodenal ulcers. The following are some of the advantages of the Heineke-Mikulicz pyloroplasty over a gastrojejunostomy:

1. A correctly performed pyloroplasty ensures ample drainage of the stomach.
2. It is simpler to perform than a gastrojejunostomy.
3. Pyloroplasty does not alter gastroduodenal continuity, allowing the physiologic mixture of duodenal, pancreatic, and biliary secretions with food.
4. In addition, pyloroplasty allows the surgeon to directly inspect the duodenal mucosa and the ulcer, making it possible to determine its extent, the degree of penetration, and the presence of sacciform dilations (false diverticula) due to long-standing duodenal ulcers.
5. In patients with bleeding duodenal ulcers it permits accurate localization of the bleeding and performing local hemostasis by the use of one or more suture ligatures (2, 9, 10, 25, 29).

As will later be seen, besides gastrojejunostomy and the Heineke-Mikulicz pyloroplasty, there are other drainage procedures. The surgeon should select the procedure that is best adapted to the local findings in the patient.

The Heineke-Mikulicz pyloroplasty is considered the procedure of choice, so it is the drainage procedure used most. There are a very few cases in actual surgical practice in which this technique cannot be used because of lack of tissue flexibility, excessive local edema, fibrotic thickening or retraction, and pyloroduodenal hardening. In these cases a gastrojejunostomy or a Jaboulay gastroduodenostomy should be done (15, 20, 24).

The Heineke-Mikulicz technique has its basis on a longitudinal transection following the axis of the stomach, the anterior wall of the proximal portion of the duodenum, the pylorus, and the distal segment of the gastric antrum, followed by a transverse closure of the opening.

Both Heineke and Mikulicz performed the transverse closure in two layers, a mucosal and a seromuscular layer. Suturing in two layers will not lead to stenosis if done correctly. Stenosis is generally due to incorrectly performed closure or a poor selection of a patient for pyloroplasty. Transverse closure of a Heineke-Mikulicz pyloroplasty is no different from anastomoses performed in other segments of the gastrointestinal tract (19). If done correctly by suturing the edge of the gastric mucosa (not a fold) with the edge of the duodenal mucosa, as well as the seromuscular layer of the stomach (not a fold), with the edge of the seromuscular layer of the duodenum, there is no reason for an increased incidence of stricture compared to a one-layer closure.

Another method for transverse closure of a Heineke-Mikulicz pyloroplasty is that proposed by Weinberg (31), who proposed a one-layer transverse closure using interrupted through and through sutures with the object of avoiding excessive inversion of the mucosa, a complication that would lead, according to Weinberg, to a greater probability of stricture if two layers are used.

Some surgeons perform a one-layer transverse closure using the through and through sutures proposed by Gambee (11, 29, 30, 33) for visceral anastomoses of the gastrointestinal tract (11). Gambee proposed the so-called Gambee stitch, to be described later, to prevent excessive inversion of the mucosa, which would be produced by a one-layer closure with through and through sutures. The object of the Gambee stitch is to join the mucosal layer of one side with the mucosal layer of the other side, and the seromuscular layer of one edge to the opposite seromuscular layer. This means that with the Gambee stitch one attempts to attain the same result as in the two-layer closure. Some surgeons perform the closure transversely in one plane, using extramucosal sutures, not through and through sutures.

In the medical literature there are numerous variations of the Heineke-Mikulicz pyloroplasty that are rarely used at present. One of these is the Judd technique (16–18). This technique was used in the treatment of duodenal ulcers of the anterior wall of the first portion of the duodenum. In performing the longitudinal duodenopylorogastric incision, the anterior duodenal ulcer is resected and a transverse closure carried out in classical fashion.

A TA 55 stapler is usually used to close the Heineke-Mikulicz pyloroplasty. However, this technique cannot be used successfully if the tissues are not completely pliable and flexible.

The longitudinal incision of the Heineke-Mikulicz technique must not be too long, because this can lead to tension in the transverse closure. An incision 5 cm long, 2 cm on the duodenal side and 3 cm on the gastric side, is generally long enough to attain an ample pyloroplasty without tension. The incision on the gastric side should always be longer than on the duodenal side because the stomach is more pliable than the duodenum.

Is it necessary to perform a Vautrin-Kocher maneuver to carry out a Heineke-Mikulicz pyloroplasty?

In many cases this maneuver is not necessary, and the majority of surgeons do not perform it. However, partial mobilization of the duodenum facilitates approximation of the duodenum, permitting suturing without tension. Complete mobilization of the duodenum is rarely necessary in the Heineke-Mikulicz pyloroplasty, but, as we will see later, it is indispensable for the Jaboulay gastroduodenostomy (15) and the Finney pyloroplasty (8). Once the transverse closure of the pyloroplasty is completed, the suture line should be covered with a viable segment of greater omentum. The omentoplasty is done to prevent adhesion of the suture line to the lower surface of the liver, to prevent the duodenum from becoming kinked and leading to obstructive symptoms. If an omentoplasty is done the omentum will become adherent and not the duodenal suture line, diminishing the possibility of kinking of the duodenum. Omentoplasty to protect the closure from dehiscence is controversial (3). If an omentoplasty is performed, the omental segment selected should be well vascularized and cover the entire length of the suture line. The sutures holding the omentum in place should not be too tight in order to avoid necrosis.

Should the pyloroplasty be performed before or after the truncal vagotomy?

The pyloroplasty should be performed after the vagotomy to prevent probable contamination of the mediastinum. It is well known that duodenal ulcers are usually associated with hyperchlorhydria, making gastric contents usually sterile. At present, because of the use of H_2 antagonists, the intragastric pH is usually elevated, diminishing its bactericidal power and favoring contamination (10). In patients with massive hemorrhage the order should be inverted (first stopping the bleeding to stabilize the patient), and the pyloroplasty should be performed before the vagotomy. In these patients antibiotics should be used before, during, and after the operation (10).

Due to the Heineke-Mikulicz pyloroplasty, the duodenal folds become distorted, giving a radiologic image simulating the presence of an ulcer. Patients should be advised of this possibility to avoid errors in radiologic interpretation.

SPHINCTEROPLASTY WITH RESECTION OF THE ANTERIOR SEGMENT OF THE PYLORUS: ANTERIOR HEMIPYLORECTOMY

Resection of the anterior half of the pyloric muscle with suturing of the anterior wall of the stomach to the anterior wall of the duodenum has been proposed as a substitute for the Heineke-Mikulicz pyloroplasty. Resection of the anterior segment of the pyloric muscle can be performed submucosally, without entering the gastroduodenal lumen (anterior submucosal hemipylorectomy) (1), or by resecting the entire wall (open anterior hemipylorectomy) (13). Anterior submucosal and open hemipylorectomy are infrequently used in association with truncal vagotomy. These techniques are more frequently used in esophagogastrectomies or in cases in which a proximal gastric vagotomy has been done and there are remaining doubts of pyloric permeability.

The Jaboulay technique (15) is really a gastroduodenostomy and not a pyloroplasty. It is used infrequently, generally in patients in whom the Heineke-Mikulicz sphincteroplasty cannot be performed.

The Finney procedure (8) is also a gastroduodenal anastomosis, with an added transection of the pyloric sphincter. This technique is rarely used at present.

The Ramstedt pyloromyotomy (27) has no indications in conjunction with truncal vagotomy, being used only in congenital hypertrophy of the pylorus.

Pyloroplasty: Heineke-Mikulicz Technique

FIGURE 24.1

The drawing shows a Vautrin-Kocher maneuver being performed. The first assistant grasps the duodenum with two hands and exerts gentle traction upward and to the left. Manual traction is better than that applied with instruments because there is less danger of injuring the duodenal wall. Using scissors, the peritoneum near the external border of the duodenum, which is stretched by the traction, is transected. The extent of this incision varies with the local needs. Once the peritoneum is incised, the dissection is carried deeper, using scissors, dividing the avascular membrane joining the duodenum to the retroperitoneum. Some surgeons use their fingers in this dissection. It is not always necessary to carry out the Vautrin-Kocher maneuver in the Heineke-Mikulicz pyloroplasty, but it can be very useful in some patients.

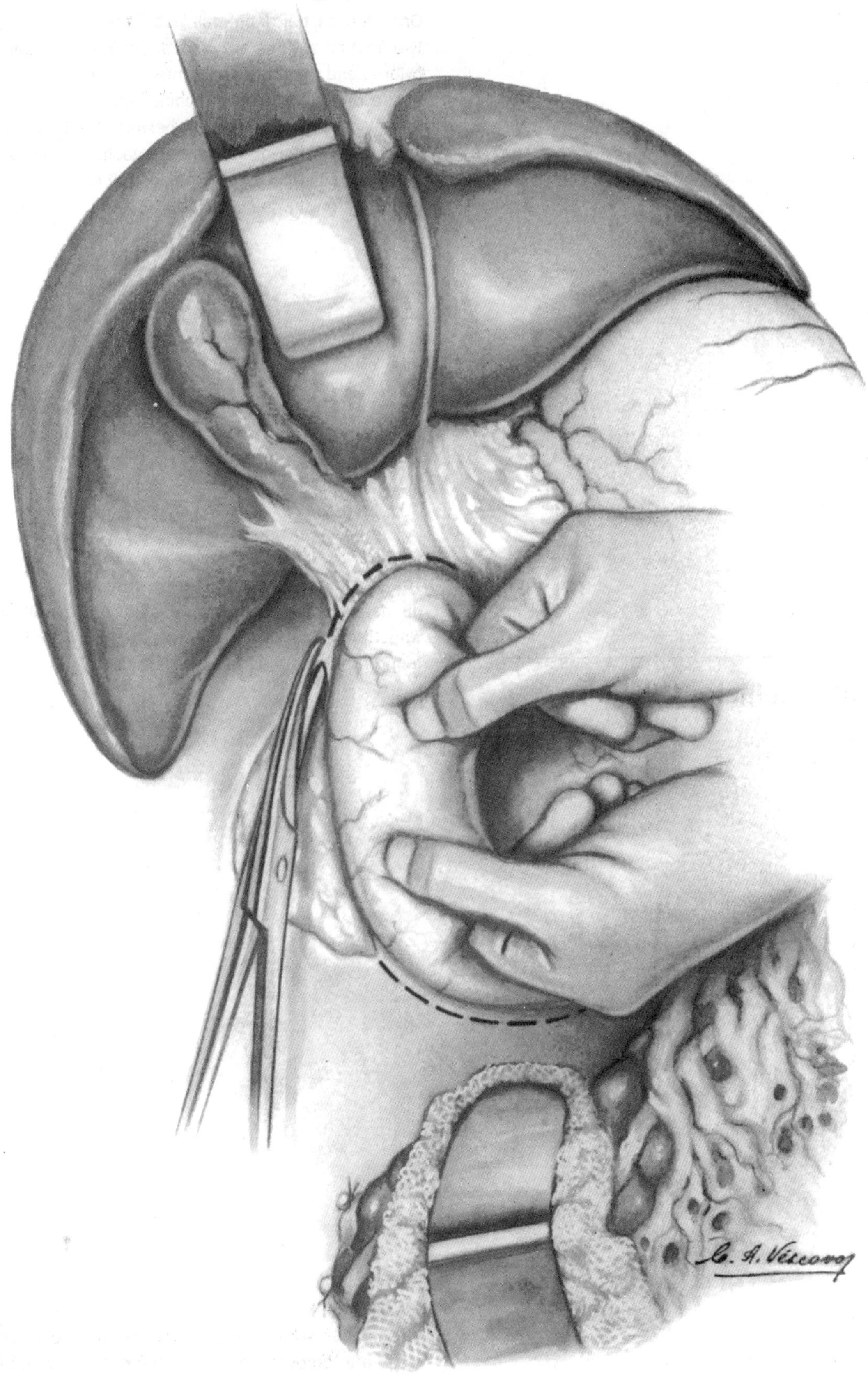

FIGURE 24.1

FIGURE 24.2
Once the partial duodenal mobilization has been carried out, two traction sutures are placed, one on the superior end of the pylorus and the other on its inferior end, to apply traction in opposite directions. The midpoint between the two traction sutures is identified in order to perform the longitudinal incision, which follows the axis of the stomach, as marked in the drawing. The incision is some 5 cm long, 2 cm on the duodenal side and 3 cm on the gastric side.

Pyloroplasty: Heineke-Mikulicz Technique

FIGURE 24.3
The longitudinal incision has been made, entering the gastroduodenal lumen. Bleeding vessels in the wall are controlled with transfixion sutures. The Mayo pyloric vein is commonly found running subserosally in the direction of the pylorus.

FIGURE 24.4
The traction sutures in the superior and inferior ends of the pylorus are removed; to replace them, two sutures are placed in the edges of the pyloric incision to apply traction in the opposite direction, converting the longitudinal incision into a transverse incision, as can be seen in the drawing

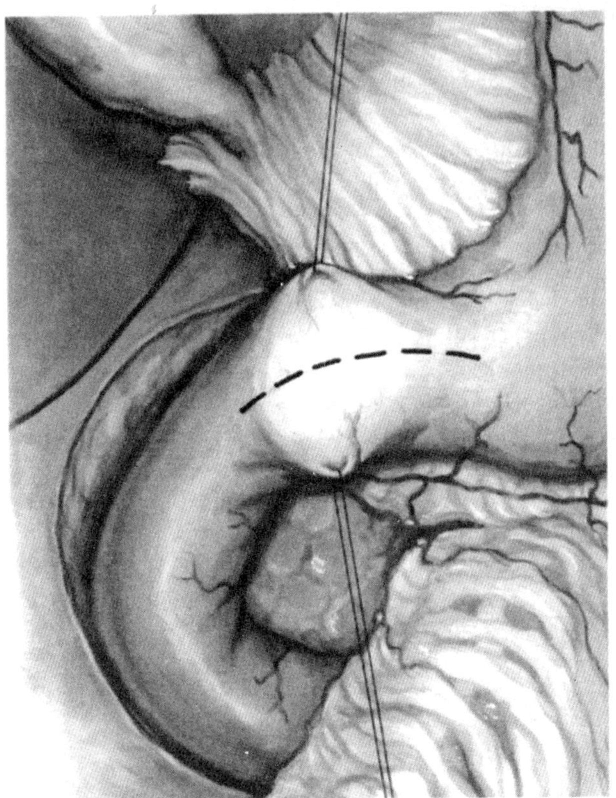

FIGURE 24.2

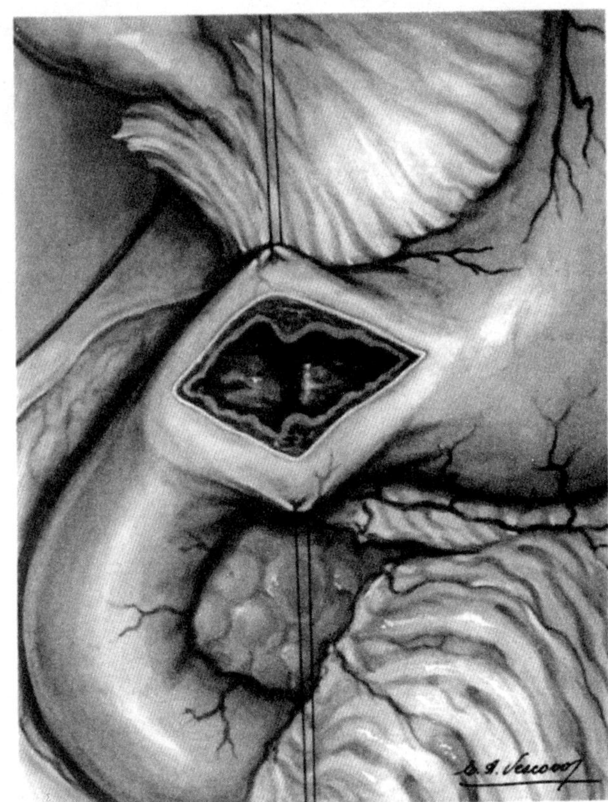

FIGURE 24.3

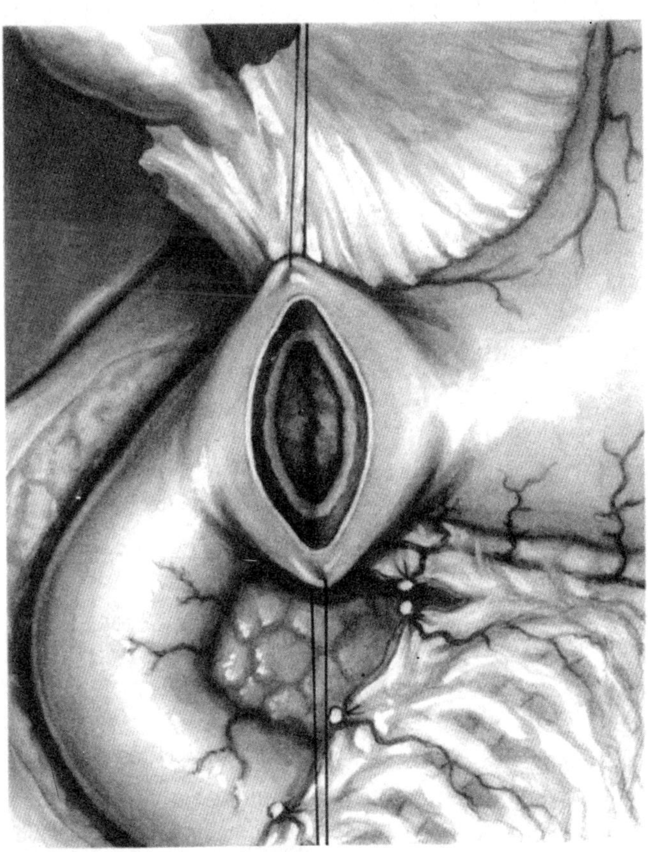

FIGURE 24.4

FIGURE 24.5
The opening into the duodenal lumen is used to inspect the duodenal mucosa and the ulcer. Digital intraluminal exploration of the duodenum distally should be carried out, as shown in the drawing, to determine if there is any duodenal stenosis beyond the 2-cm point in the duodenum that was missed in preoperative examinations. If there is stenosis, the Heineke-Mikulicz pyloroplasty is contraindicated and a gastrojejunostomy or Finney pyloroplasty performed. If the patient has a massively bleeding ulcer, local control of the hemorrhage should be carried out using cotton sutures in U-shaped fashion placed deeply in the ulcer bed. Sometimes more than two U-shaped sutures may be needed. In patients with a bleeding duodenal ulcer in which the bleeding artery belongs to the gastroduodenal artery complex, hemostasis should be carried out by the Berne and Rosoff technique. The hemostatic sutures should be nonabsorbable and adequate in caliber, with a strong enough needle.

Pyloroplasty: Heineke-Mikulicz Technique

FIGURE 24.6
The transverse closure of the pyloroplasty is being carried out in two layers, a mucosal and a seromuscular layer. The mucosal plane is closed with 2-0 chromic catgut. Three guide sutures are placed, in the superior and inferior ends, and in the midpoint of the incision. The remaining sutures are then placed, completing the closure of the mucosal plane.

FIGURE 24.7
The mucosal plane has been closed and the seromuscular plane is being closed using interrupted sutures of cotton, silk, or synthetic nonabsorbable material. Three guide sutures are used in a fashion similar to that used in closing the mucosal layer.

FIGURE 24.8
The maneuver shown in the drawing is performed to confirm the amplitude of the sphincteroplasty.

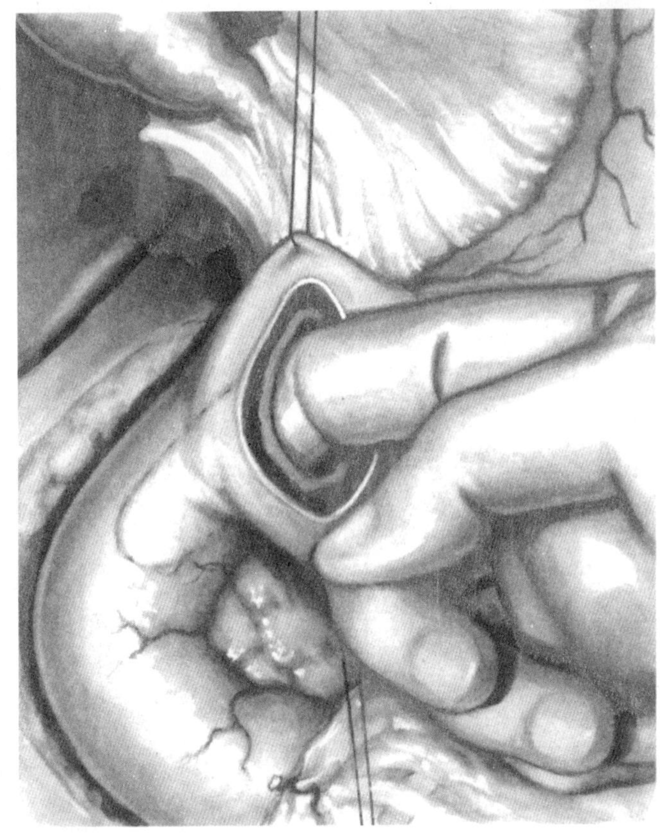

FIGURE 24.5

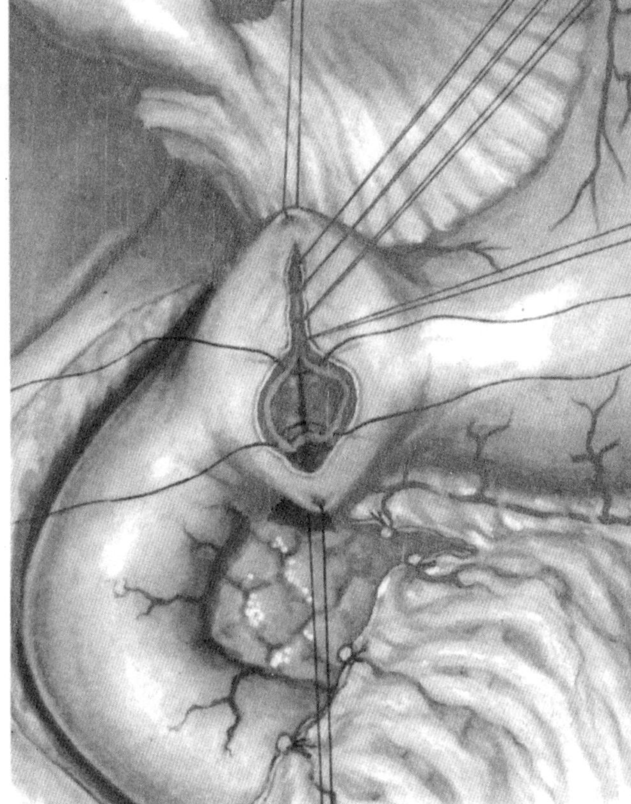

FIGURE 24.6

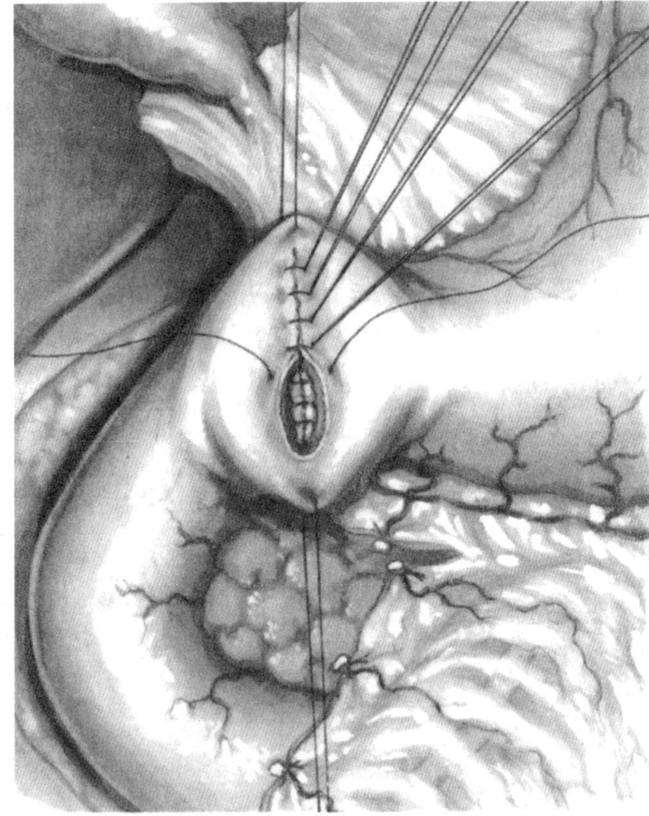

FIGURE 24.7

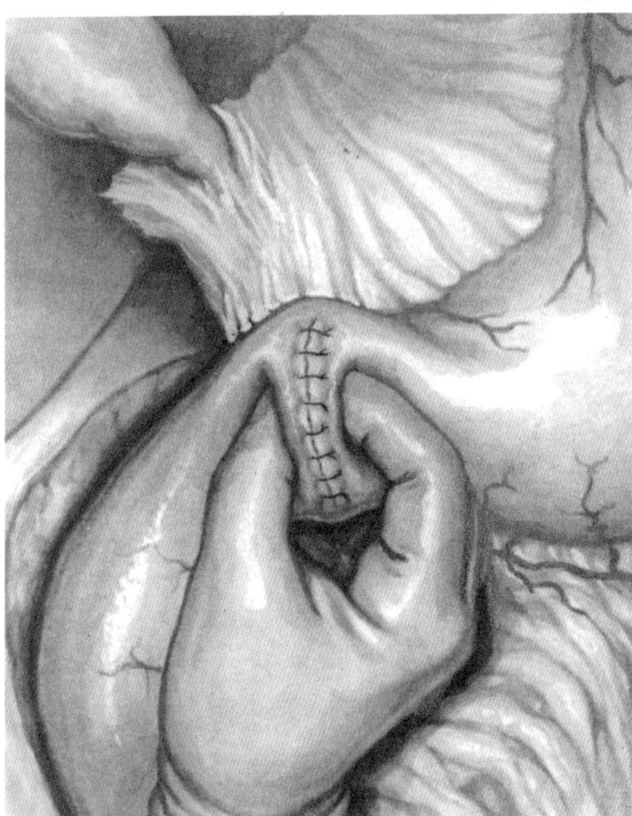

FIGURE 24.8

Pyloroplasty: Heineke-Mikulicz Technique

FIGURE 24.9

It is advisable to cover the suture line with an omentoplasty using a vascularized segment of greater omentum. The sutures fixing the omentum to the gastroduodenal area should not be tied too tightly to avoid producing necrosis. The omentoplasty is a precautionary measure. The closed duodenum has a great tendency to adhere to the undersurface of the liver, leading to kinking and obstructive symptoms in some cases. Covering the suture line with omentum prevents direct adhesion of the duodenum and its possible consequences.

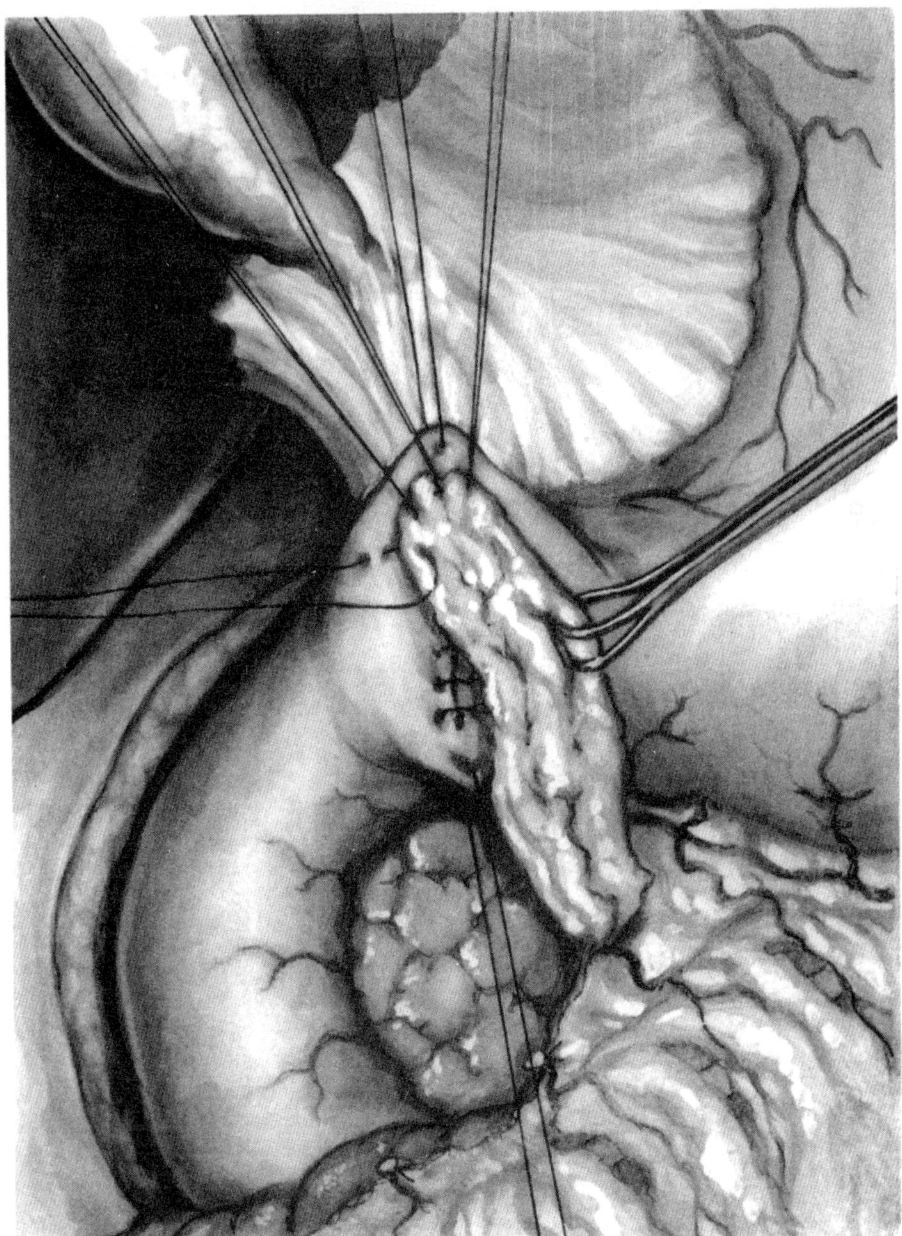

FIGURE 24.9

FIGURE 24.10
Weinberg proposed a one-layer closure with through and through sutures for the Heineke-Mikulicz pyloroplasty. The object of Weinberg's technique is to avoid excessive inversion of gastric and duodenal mucosa and the possibility of producing a stricture. The drawing shows the through and through sutures being placed after the two guide sutures.

Heineke-Mikulicz Pyloroplasty with One-Layer Closure, Gambee Suture and One-Layer Extramucosal Sutures

FIGURE 24.11
Transverse closure of the Heineke-Mikulicz pyloroplasty can be carried out with through and through Gambee sutures. These sutures were proposed by Gambee for one-layer anastomoses of the gastrointestinal tract with the object of approximating the mucosa of one side to the mucosa of the other side as well as approximating the seromuscular layers of both sides. It is easier to understand the Gambee suture by looking at the explanatory insert. The needle, after having gone through the entire gastric wall, is reinserted near the edge to pass only through the mucosa, the muscularis mucosa, and the submucosa. The needle is again extracted and is then passed through the opposite duodenal wall in reverse order, passing first through the submucosa, muscularis mucosa, and the mucosa, and is then reinserted to go through the entire duodenal wall from mucosa to serosa. The sutures are not tied until they are all in place. A suture is placed at each end, another in the middle, and then the rest of the sutures. This technique approximates the gastric and duodenal mucosa as well as both seromuscular layers.

FIGURE 24.12
The drawing shows a closure of a Heineke-Mikulicz pyloroplasty in one layer using extramucosal sutures.

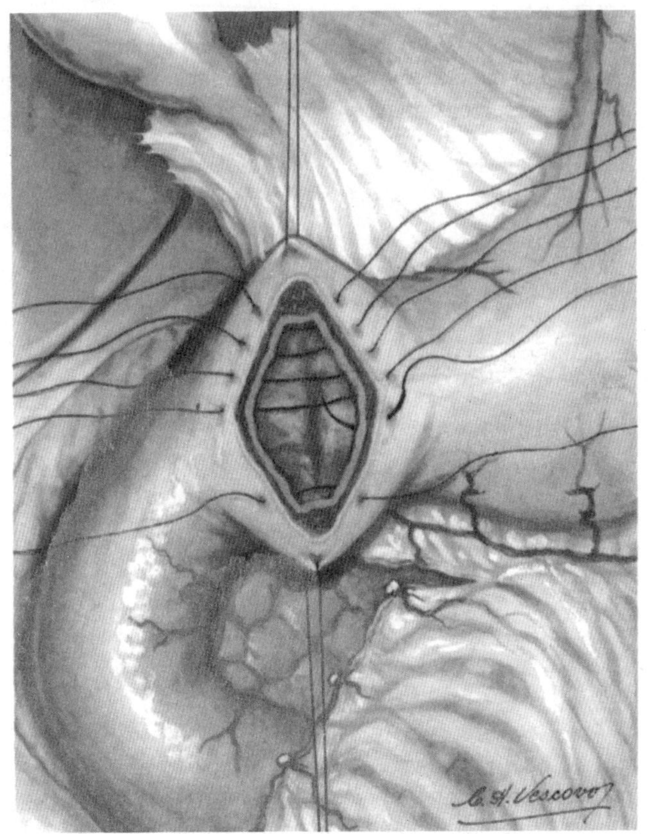

FIGURE 24.10

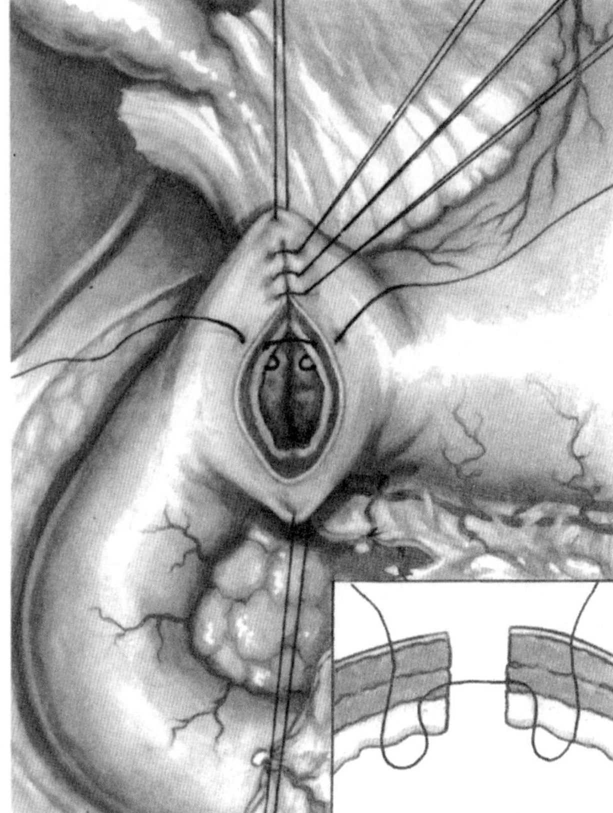

FIGURE 24.11

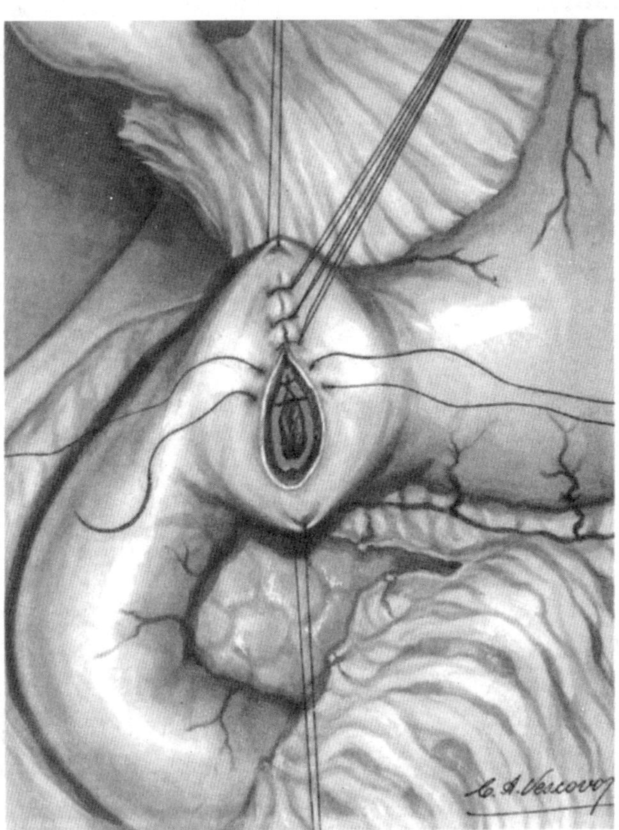

FIGURE 24.12

FIGURE 24.13
One suture is placed at the superior end and another at the inferior end of the pylorus. The broken lines show the oval of tissue to be resected without entering the gastroduodenal lumen.

Anterior Submucosal Hemipylorectomy (Closed Hemipylorectomy)

FIGURE 24.14
The tissue is being resected with a scalpel down to the submucosa. The lower end of the oval segment of tissue is grasped with a Babcock clamp, and traction is applied upward to facilitate dissection of the pyloric muscle in the submucosal plane. If the mucosa is perforated during this dissection, it is closed with silk or cotton sutures.

FIGURE 24.15
Once the anterior half of the pylorus has been resected, careful hemostasis is carried out and suturing of the seromuscular layer is begun with cotton, silk, or synthetic nonabsorbable interrupted sutures. The insert shows the technique schematically.

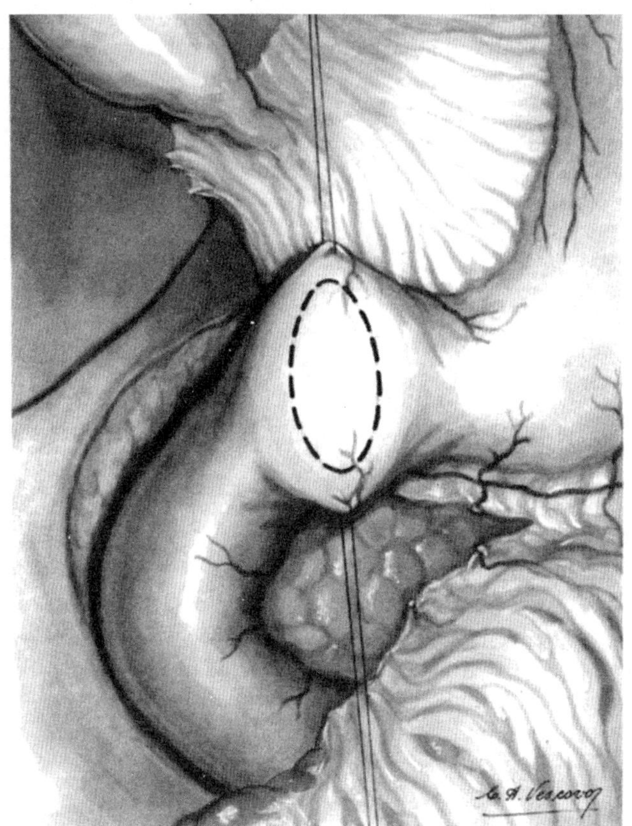

FIGURE 24.13

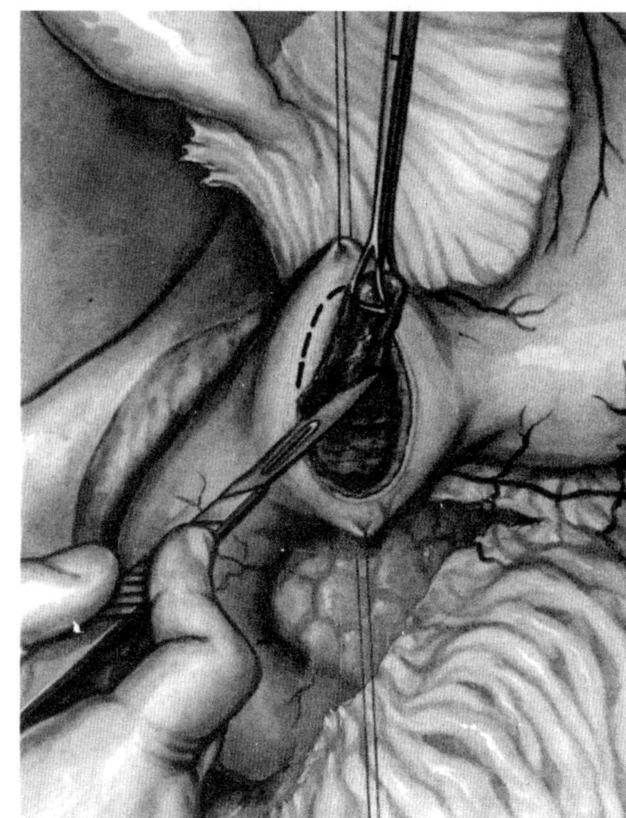

FIGURE 24.14

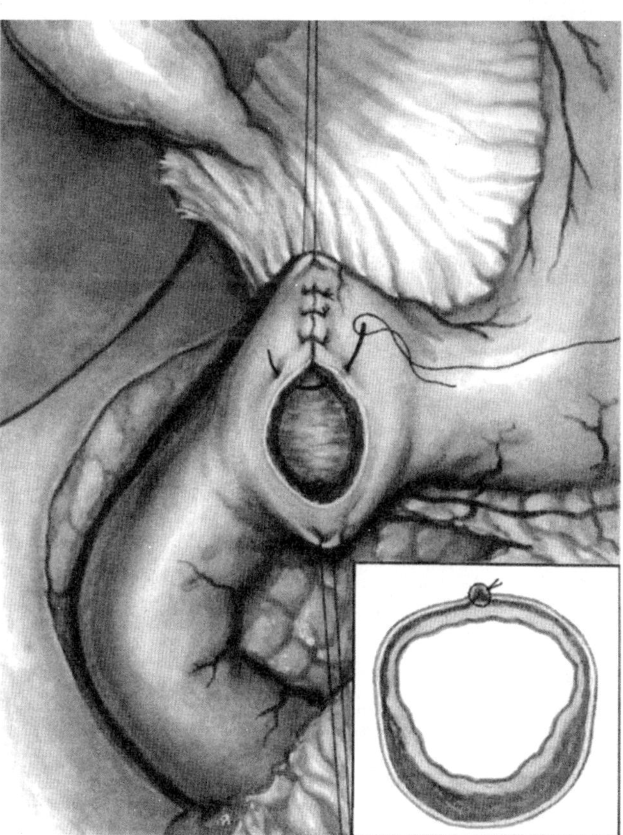

FIGURE 24.15

FIGURE 24.16
Resection of the anterior segment of the pylorus can be carried out entering the gastroduodenal lumen. Sutures are placed at the superior and inferior ends of the pylorus to apply traction in opposite directions. The broken line shows the oval of tissue to be resected.

FIGURE 24.17
Using a scalpel the seromuscular layer has been sectioned along the marked oval. The entire anterior wall has been incised, using a scalpel, until the lumen has been entered. Resection of the entire oval of tissue including the seromuscular layer, the pylorus, and the mucosa is then performed, as shown in the drawing.

Open Anterior Hemipylorectomy

FIGURE 24.18
The gastroduodenal wall is closed in two layers, like the closure of the Heineke-Mikulicz pyloroplasty. The drawing shows the closing of the seromuscular layer after closing the mucosa with 2-0 chromic catgut.

FIGURE 24.19
Once closure is complete, an omentoplasty is carried out by the previously described technique.

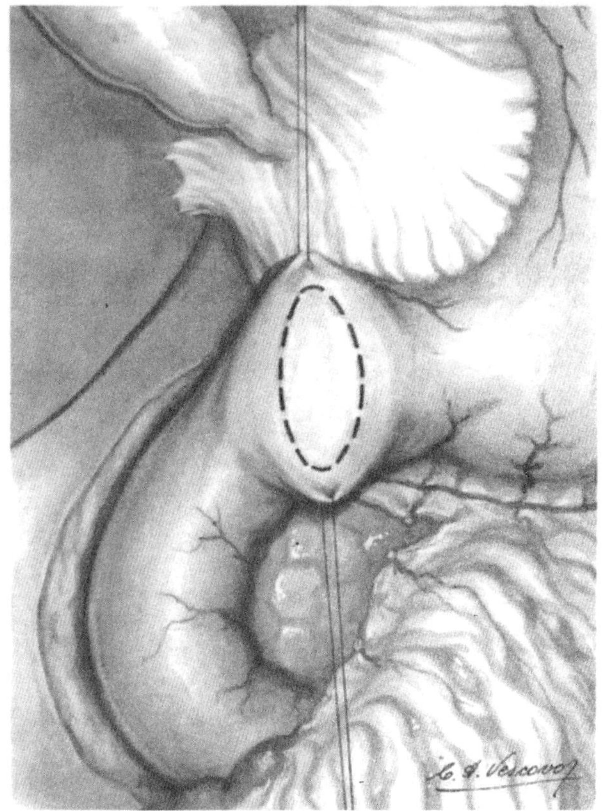

FIGURE 24.16

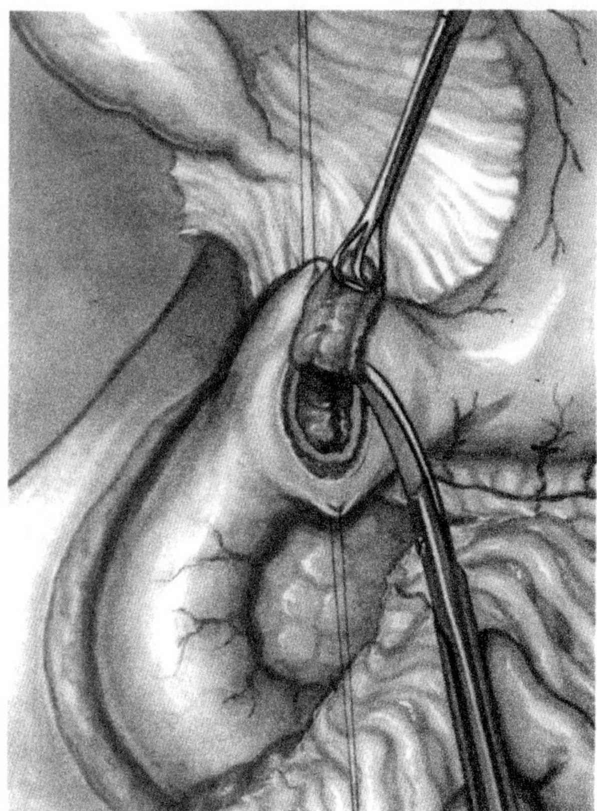

FIGURE 24.17

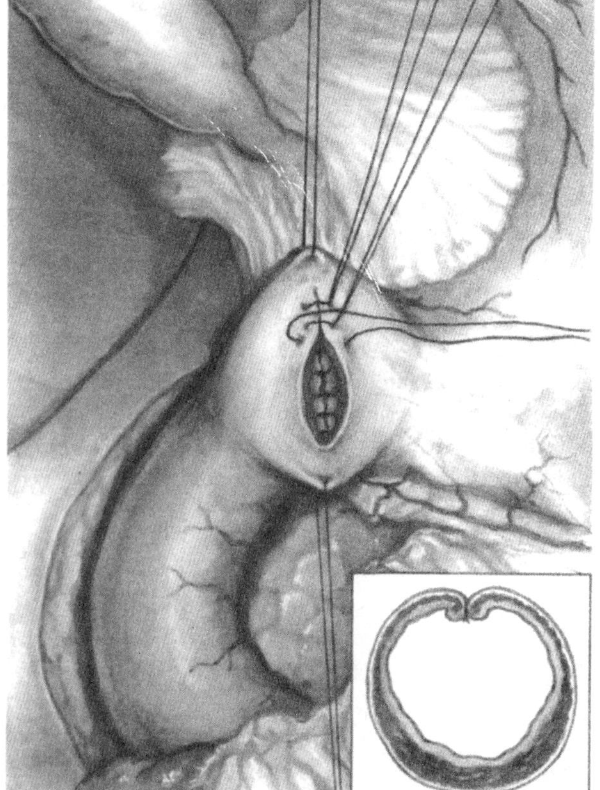

FIGURE 24.18

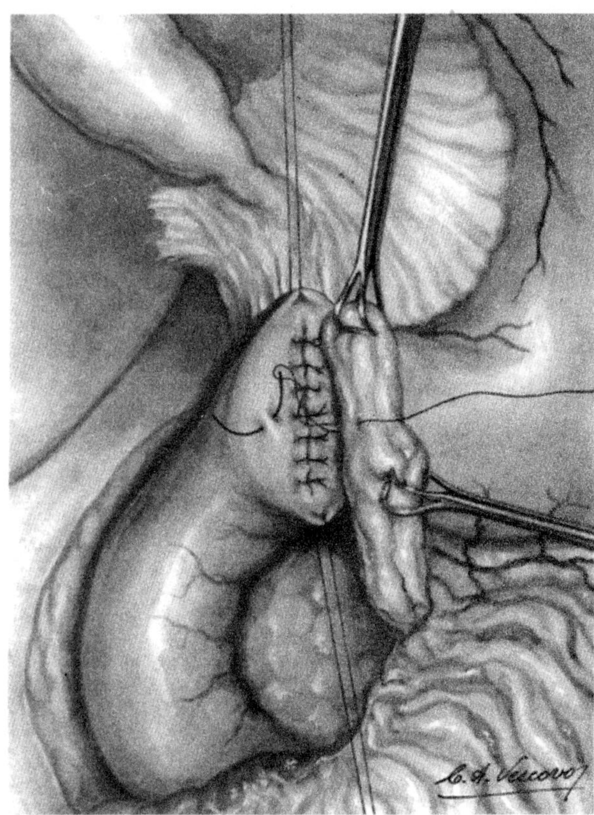

FIGURE 24.19

FIGURE 24.20
To carry out a Finney pyloroplasty, ample pancreatoduodenal mobilization must be attained by the Vautrin-Kocher maneuver. Additionally, ligation and resection of the gastrocolic omentum from the greater curvature of the gastric antrum has to be done. Three traction sutures have been placed, one in the superior end of the pylorus, another in the medial border for the second portion of the duodenum some 6 or 7 cm away from the pylorus, and a third suture near the greater curvature of the gastric antrum some 6 or 7 cm proximal to the pylorus.

Pyloroplasty by the Finney Technique

FIGURE 24.21
Traction is applied upward on the suture in the pylorus and downward on the sutures in the duodenum and antrum. This allows the second portion of the duodenum and the gastric antrum to be brought together in parallel position, touching each other. The posterior seromuscular line of sutures between the second portion of the duodenum and the gastric antrum have been placed, using cotton, silk or synthetic nonabsorbable material, over a 5 to 6 cm length. The sutures are placed near the internal border of the duodenum and near the greater curvature of the gastric antrum. A broken line shows where the inverted U-shaped incision will pass through the duodenum, pylorus, and gastric antrum.

FIGURE 24.22
The duodenum, pylorus, and gastric antrum have been incised. The posterior perforating plane is being closed with interrupted through and through 2-0 chromic catgut sutures. The perforating plane can be closed with a continuous suture.

FIGURE 24.23
The anterior perforating plane is being closed with through and through sutures.

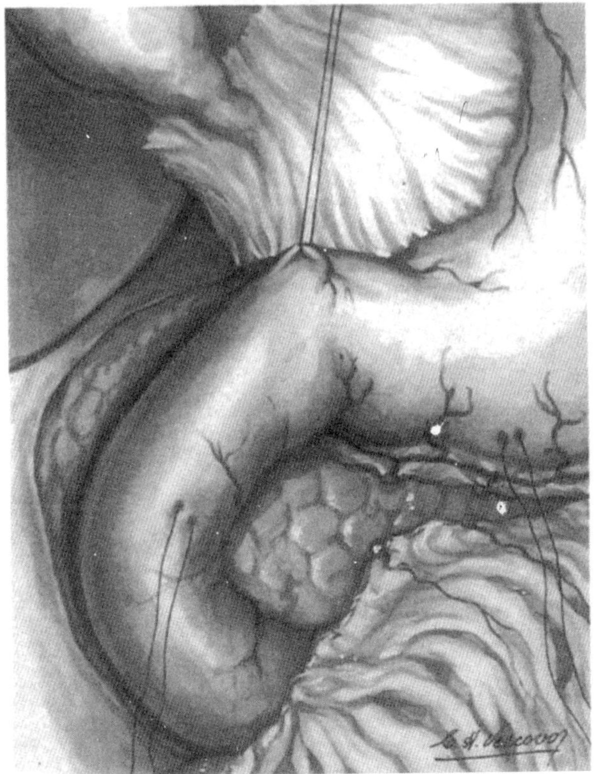
FIGURE 24.20

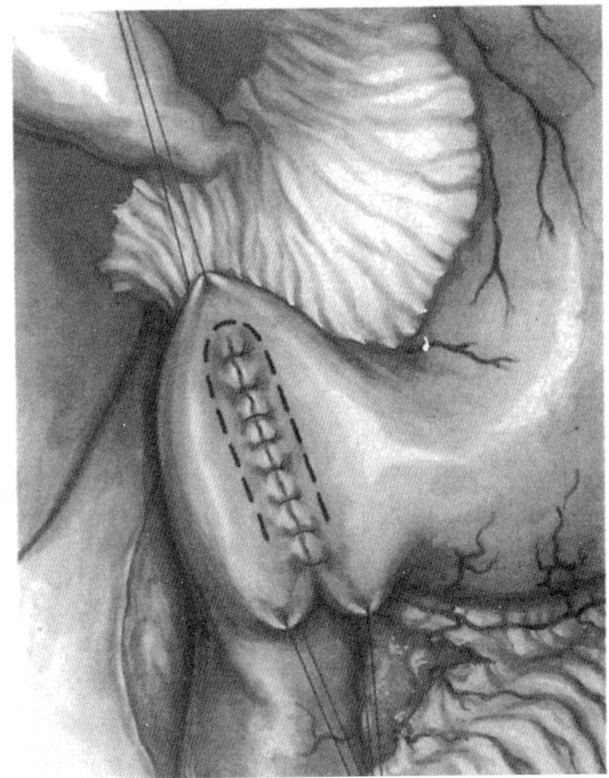
FIGURE 24.21

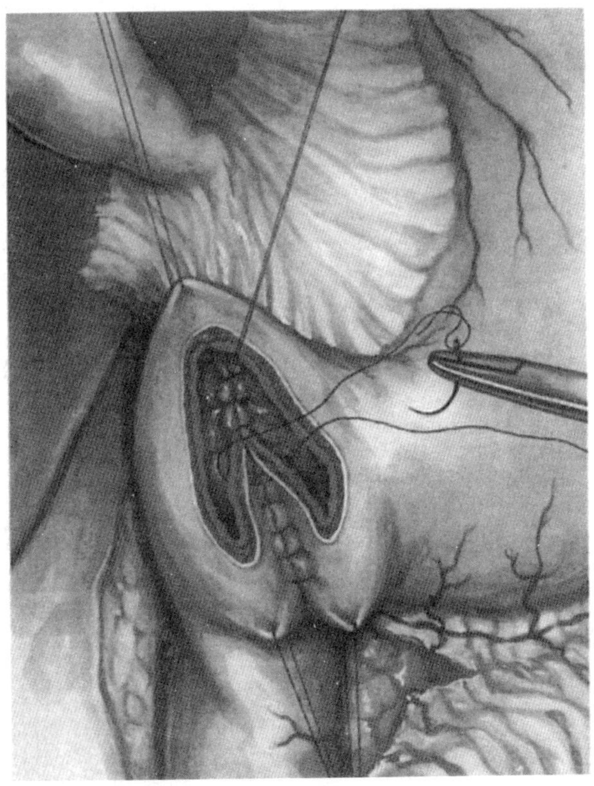
FIGURE 24.22

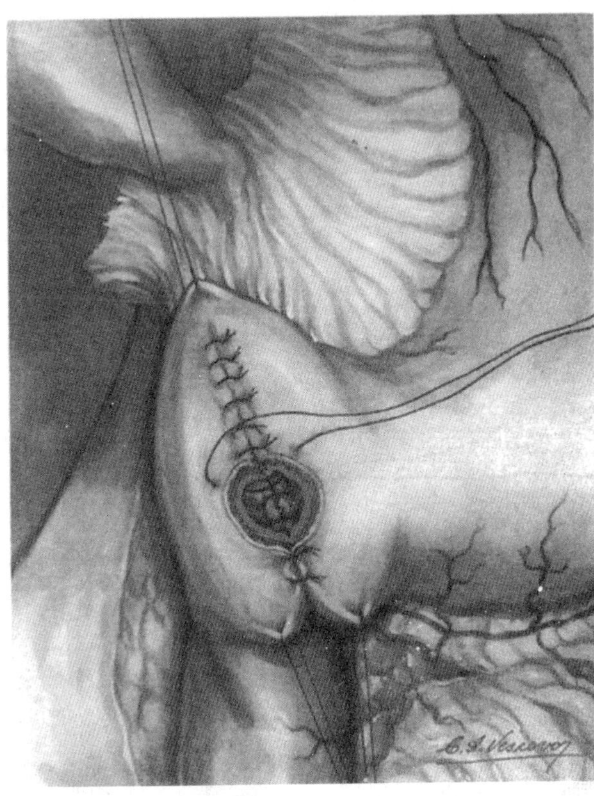
FIGURE 24.23

Pyloroplasty by the Finney Technique

FIGURE 24.24
The anterior seromuscular layer has been closed, completing the Finney pyloroplasty.

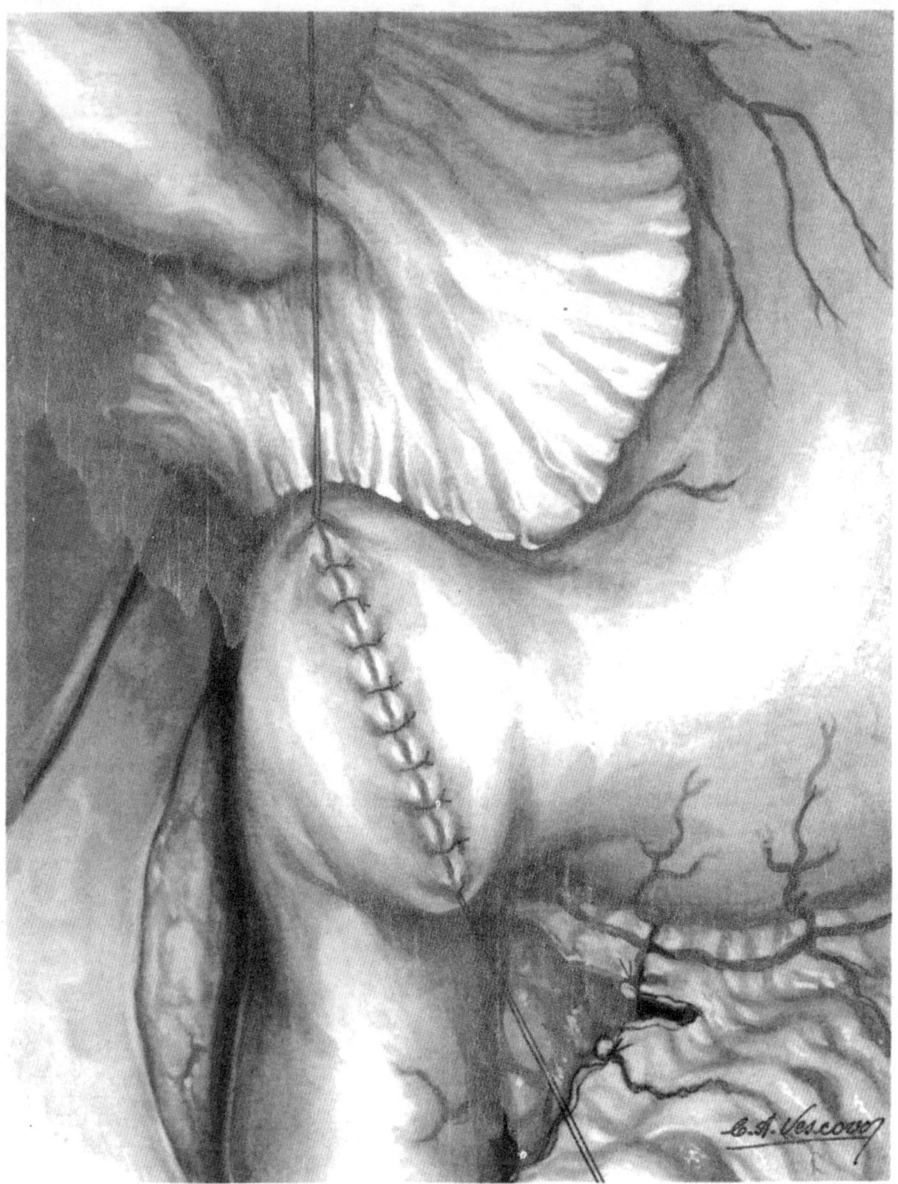

FIGURE 24.24

FIGURE 24.25
A complete Vautrin-Kocher maneuver as well as ligation and resection of the gastrocolic ligament from the greater curvature of the gastric antrum must be carried out in the Jaboulay technique as in the Finney procedure. Traction is being applied to the sutures placed in the superior end of the pylorus, in the internal border of the duodenum some 6 or 7 cm distal to the pylorus, and in the greater curvature of the gastric antrum some 6 or 7 cm proximal to the pylorus. Two broken lines have been drawn to show the site and the length of the incisions to be performed in the duodenum and the gastric antrum. In the Jaboulay technique the pylorus is not transected, this being he only difference from the Finney technique. The operative steps to be described are very similar to the Finney technique.

Gastroduodenostomy (Jaboulay)

FIGURE 24.26
The posterior seromuscular layer has been sutured with interrupted sutures over 6 or 7 cm. Incisions have been made near the internal border of the duodenum and near the greater curvature of the gastric antrum. The incisions are some 5 cm long. The posterior perforating layer is being closed with interrupted sutures. This layer can be closed with a continuous suture.

FIGURE 24.27
The anterior perforating layer is being closed with interrupted through and through sutures.

FIGURE 24.28
The Jaboulay gastroduodenostomy has been completed, establishing an ample communication between the stomach and the duodenum. The Jaboulay technique does not include transection of the pylorus, and therefore may be indicated in some cases in which a pyloroplasty is impractical.

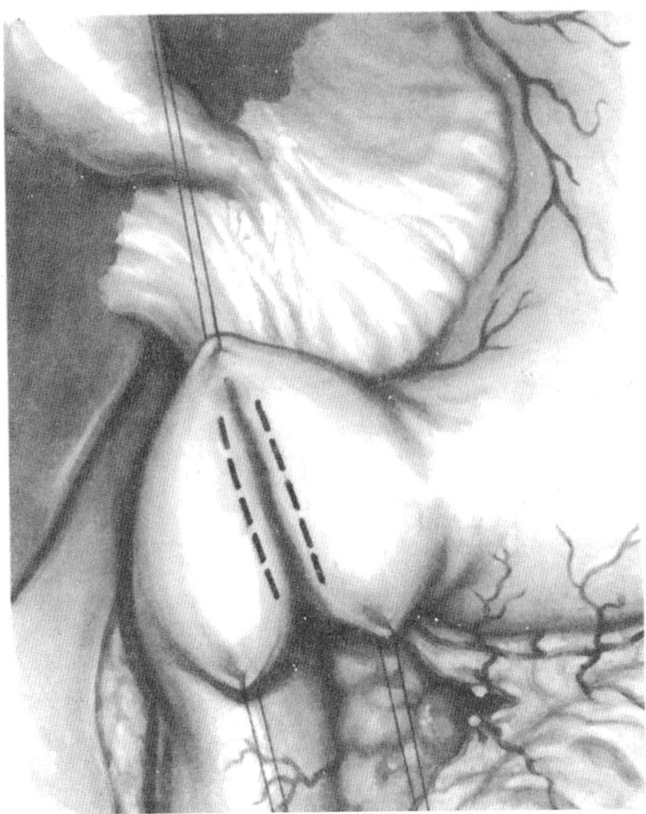

FIGURE 24.25

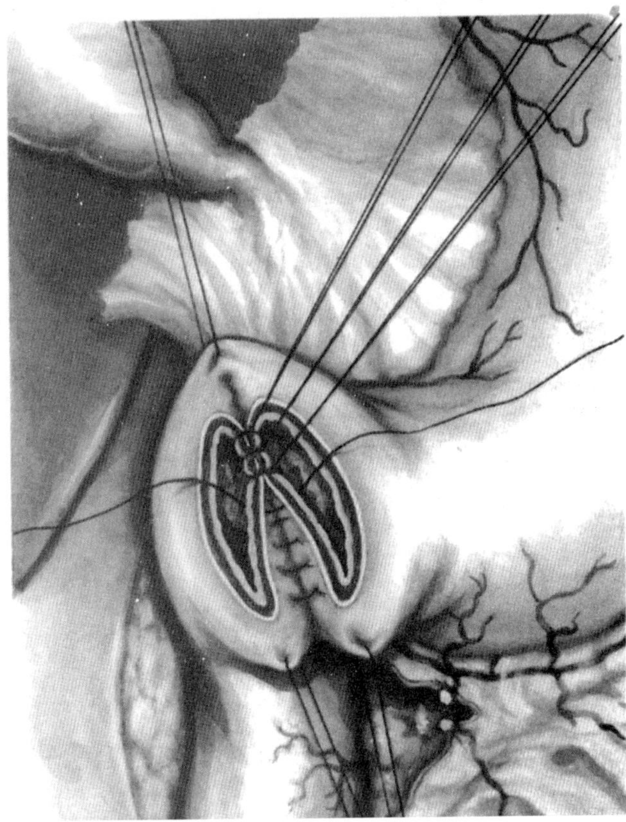

FIGURE 24.26

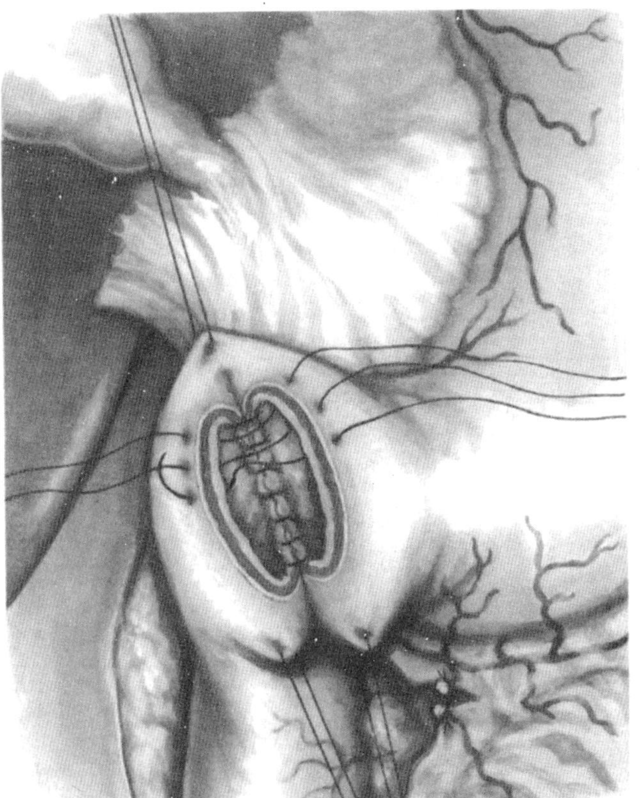

FIGURE 24.27

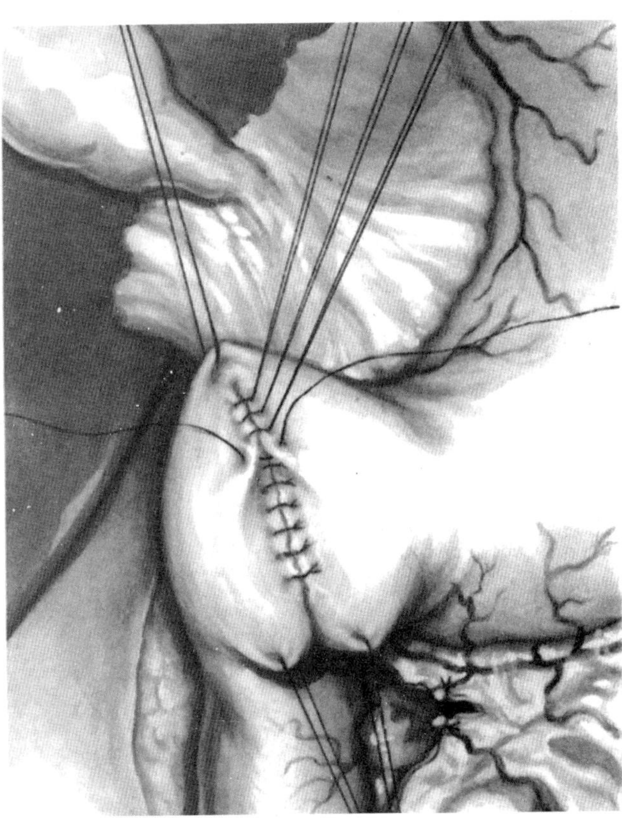

FIGURE 24.28

References

1. Aust, L.B. A new technique for pyloroplasty. Surgery 53:309, 1963.
2. Berne, C.J., Rosoff, L. Peptic ulcer perforation of the gastroduodenal artery complex. Ann. Surg. 169:143, 1969.
3. Chassin, J.L. Operative strategy in general surgery. Vol. I, p. 133. Springer-Verlag, New York, 1980.
4. Dragstedt, L.R., Owens, F.M. Jr. Supradiaphragmatic section of the vagus nerves in the treatment of duodenal ulcer. Proc. Soc. Exp. Biol. Med. 53:152, 1943.
5. Dragstedt, L.R. Vagotomy and gastroenterostomy or pyloroplasty. Present technique. Surg. Clin. North Am. 41:23, 1961.
6. Dragstedt, L.R., Lulu, D.J. Truncal vagotomy and pyloroplasty. Critical evaluation of one hundred cases. Am. J. Surg. 128:344, 1974.
7. Feggetter, G.Y., Pringle, R. The long term results of bilateral vagotomy and gastrojejunostomy for chronic duodenal ulcer. Surg. Gynecol. Obstet. 116:175, 1963.
8. Finney, J.M.T. A new method of pyloroplasty. Bull. Johns Hopkins Hosp. 13:155, 1902.
9. Foster, J.H. Pyloroplasty, vagotomy and suture-ligation for bleeding duodenal ulcer. In Nyhus, L.M., Baker, R.J. (Eds.) Mastery of surgery. Ed. 2, vol. I, p. 696. Little, Brown, Boston, 1992.
10. Fromm, D. Gastrointestinal surgery. Vol. I, p. 254. Churchill Livingstone, New York, 1985.
11. Gambee, L.P. A single layer open intestinal anastomosis applicable to the small as well as the large intestine. West. J. Surg. 59:1, 1951.
12. Hoerr, S.O. Evaluation of vagotomy with gastroenterostomy performed for chronic duodenal ulcer. Report based on five years follow-up of 145 patients. Surgery 38:149, 1955.
13. Holle, F., Anderson, S. Vagotomy, latest advances. P. 198. Springer-Verlag, New York, 1974.
14. Hollender, L.F., Keller, D. Pyloric Drainage. In Becker, H.D., Herfath, C., Lierse, W., Schreiber, H.W. (Eds.) Surgery of the stomach. P. 229. Springer-Verlag, Berlin 1986.
15. Jaboulay, M. La gastro-entérostomie, la jejuno-duodénostomie, la resection du pylore. Arch. Prov. Chir. Paris 1:1, 1892.
16. Judd, E.S. Excision of ulcer of duodenum. Lancet 1:381, 1922.
17. Judd, E.S., Nagel, G.W. Excision of ulcer of duodenum. Surg. Gynecol. Obstet. 45:17, 1927.
18. Judd, E.S., Tanska, K. Technique of pyloroplasty for duodenal ulcer. Ann. Surg. 162:946, 1965.
19. Madden, J.L. Abdominal wall hernias. P. 264. W.B. Saunders, Philadelphia, 1989.
20. Maingot, R. Vagotomy and gastrojejunostomy for duodenal ulcer. Ed. 7, vol. I, p. 341. Appleton Century Crofts, New York, 1980.
21. Misalaret, J. A propos de la pyloroplastie associée a une vagotomie. Mém. Acad. Chir. 90:264, 1964.
22. Mikulicz, J. Zur operativen behandlung des stenosierenden magengeschwüres. Arch. Klin. Chir. 37:79, 1888.
23. Nobles, E.R. Jr. Vagotomy and gastroenterostomy. Am. Surg. 32:177, 1966.
24. Oberhelman, H.A. Jr. Vagotomy and pyloroplasty or gastrojejunostomy. In Nora, P.F. (Ed.) Operative surgery. Ed. 3, p. 520. W.B. Saunders. Philadelphia, 1990.
25. Pi-Figueras, J. Práctica quirúrgica. Ed. 2, vol. II, p. 102. Salvat, Barcelona, 1986.
26. Raymond, J. L'operation de Judd associé a la vagotomie dan le traitement des ulcéres duodénaux. Arch. Mal. Appar. Dig. 51:1250, 1962.
27. Reyes, H.M. Congenital pyloric stenosis and duodenal obstruction. In Nyhus, L.M. Baker, R.J. (Eds.). Mastery of surgery. Ed. 2, vol. I, p. 705. Little, Brown, Boston, 1992.
28. Ruddell, W.S.J., Axon, A.T.R., Findlay, J.M. et al. Effect of cimetidine on the gastric bacterial flora. Lancet 1:672, 1980.
29. Sawyers, J.L. Selective vagotomy and pyloroplasty. In Nyhus, L.M., Baker, R.J. (Ed.) Mastery of surgery. Ed. 2. vol. I, p. 672. Little, Brown, Boston, 1992.
30. Sawyers, J.L. Selective gastric vagotomy. In Scott, H.W. Jr., Sawyers, J.L. (Eds.) Surgery of the stomach, duodenum and small intestine. Ed. 2, p. 503. Blackwell, Boston, 1992.
31. Weinberg, J.A. Vagotomy with pyloroplasty in the treatment of duodenal ulcer, surgical aspects. Am. J. Gastroenterol. 21:296, 1954.
32. Weinberg, J.A. Modified Heineke-Mikulicz pyloroplasty with vagotomy for treatment duodenal ulcer. In Maingot, R. (Ed.). Abdominal operations. Ed. 7. vol. I, p. 325. Appleton Century Crofts, New York, 1980.
33. Zinner, M.J. Atlas of gastric surgery. P. 16. Churchill Livingstone, New York, 1992.

Index

A

D

E

I

R

S

T

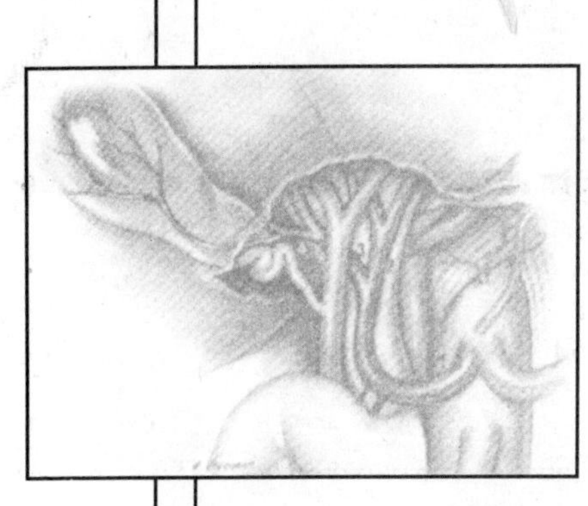

Atlas of Gastrointestinal Surgery

胃肠道外科手术图谱

（下卷）

Volume II

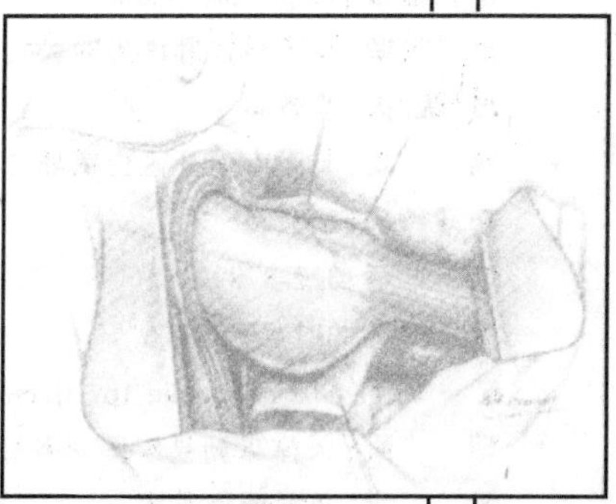

Emilio Etala

Lippincott Williams & Wilkins Inc. 授权
天津科技翻译出版公司出版

著作权合同登记号:图字:02-2002-6

图书在版编目(CIP)数据

胃肠道外科手术图谱/(美)埃泰赖(Etala,E.)编著.—影印版.—天津:天津科技翻译出版公司,2002.6
ISBN 7-5433-1499-1
书名原文:Atlas of Gastrointestinal Surgery

Ⅰ.胃...　Ⅱ.埃...　Ⅲ.胃肠病-外科手术-图谱　Ⅳ.R656-64

中国版本图书馆 CIP 数据核字(2002)第 010729 号

Copyright © 1997 by Lippincott Williams & Wilkins Inc.

All right reserved. This book is protected by copyright. No part of this book may be reproduced in any form or by any means, including photocopying, or utilized by any information storage and retrieval system without written permission from the copyright owner.

Reprint authorized by Lippincott Williams & Wilkins Inc. Reprint is authorized for sale in the People's Republic of China only.

授权单位:Lippincott Williams & Wilkins Inc.
出　　版:天津科技翻译出版公司
出 版 人:邢淑琴
地　　址:天津市南开区白堤路 244 号
邮政编码:300192
电　　话:022-87893561
传　　真:022-87892476
E - mail:tsttbc@public.tpt.tj.cn
印　　刷:天津市蓟县宏图印务有限公司印刷
发　　行:全国新华书店
版本记录:880×1230　16 开本　157.5 印张　3700 千字
2002 年 6 月第 1 版　2002 年 6 月第 1 次印刷
定价:430.00 元(上、下卷)

(如发现印装问题,可与出版社调换)

Atlas of
Gastrointestinal Surgery

Volume II

Editor: Carroll C. Cann
Managing Editor: Susan Hunsberger
Production Coordinator: Peter J. Carley
Copy Editor: Robert Magee
Designer: Nancy Hagan Abbott
Illustration Planner: Danielle Hagan
Cover Designer: Nancy Hagan Abbott
Typesetter: Graphic World, Inc.
Printer: RR Donnelley & Sons Company
Digitized Illustrations: Graphic World, Inc.
Binder: RR Donnelley & Sons Company

Copyright © 1997 Williams & Wilkins

351 West Camden Street
Baltimore, Maryland 21201-2436 USA

Rose Tree Corporate Center
1400 North Providence Road
Building II, Suite 5025
Media, Pennsylvania 19063-2043 USA

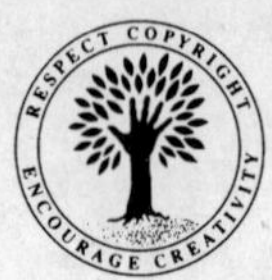

All rights reserved. This book is protected by copyright. No part of this book may be reproduced in any form or by any means, including photocopying, or utilized by any information storage and retrieval system without written permission from the copyright owner.

Accurate indications, adverse reactions and dosage schedules for drugs are provided in this book, but it is possible that they may change. The reader is urged to review the package information data of the manufacturers of the medications mentioned.

Printed in Hong Kong

First Edition.

Library of Congress Cataloging-in-Publication Data

Atlas of gastrointestinal surgery / edited by Emilio Etala :
translated by Alfred Axtmayer.
p. cm.
Includes index.
ISBN 0-683-02837-5
1. Gastrointestinal system—Surgery—Atlases. I. Etala, Emilio, M.D.
[DNLM: 1. Gastrointestinal System—surgery—atlases.
2. Gastrointestinal Diseases—surgery—atlases. WI 17 A8793 1996]
RD540.A845 1996
617.4'3—dc20
DNLM/DLC
for Library of Congress 96-21197
CIP

The publishers have made every effort to trace the copyright holders for borrowed material. If they have inadvertently overlooked any, they will be pleased to make the necessary arrangements at the first opportunity.

To purchase additional copies of this book, call our customer service department at **(800) 638-0672** or fax orders to **(800) 447-8438.** For other book services, including chapter reprints and large quantity sales, ask for the Special Sales department.

Canadian customers should call **(800) 268-4178,** or fax **(905) 470-6780.** For all other calls originating outside of the United States, please call **(410) 528-4223** or fax us at **(410) 528-8550.**

Visit Williams & Wilkins on the Internet: **http://www.wwilkins.com** or contact our customer service department at **custserv@wwilkins.com.** Williams & Wilkins customer service representatives are available from 8:30 am to 6:00 pm. EST. Monday through Friday, for telephone access.

97 98 99
2 3 4 5 6 7 8 9 10

To my wife Celia
To the memory of my parents

Foreword

I first met Dr. Emilio Etala in Ireland at the meeting of the International Society of Surgery in 1961. A true friendship having been established there, it remains to this day.

Dr. Etala has garnered many honors as a surgeon, among them: membership in the Societe Internationale de Chirurgie (1956) and election to the Honorary Fellowship in the American College of Surgeons (1971). It was my honor as Presenter to him of that election to the ACS.

Without reservation, this is an important work, destined to become an integral part of every general surgeon's library. Unique in its single authorship, *Atlas of Surgery of the Gastrointestinal Tract* provides detailed explanations of all techniques performed on all organs of the gastrointestinal tract and a wealth of exquisitely detailed clinical observations not readily available in the existing surgical literature. This can only serve to improve the safety of each operation and to prevent complications. All of these qualities are evident throughout the book, but none are more evident than in the chapters on *Choledochal Cysts* and *Portal Hypertension,* which mandate reading from anyone who is preparing to perform any of these procedures.

Illustrations are critical to the explanation of any surgical procedure and I give this presentation here the highest possible praise. The outstanding art throughout this volume is the work of a single artist who worked closely with Dr. Etala throughout the performance of every operation depicted. Each illustration rendered is from the surgeon's perspective, which provides the reader with a highly accurate view of the operative field and the related surgical anatomy at each step of each operation.

I am pleased to see this wonderful book come to fruition. Dr. Etala is a surgeon *non pareil.* His work here is destined to become a world classic. Shakespeare may best describe Dr. Etala and his work:

I dare do all that becomes a man, who dares do more is none.

John L. Madden, MD

Preface

The completion of the Atlas of Gastrointestinal Surgery would have filled Master Professor of Surgery Pablo L. Mirizzi, whose name is inseparable from operative cholangiography and biliary tract surgery, with satisfaction.

This book describes the surgical procedures used to treat diseases of the gastrointestinal tract. However, the author has always had the conviction that an atlas of surgery should not be limited to a description of surgical techniques, because this means an incomplete vision of reality. So, in addition to the description of the surgical anatomy, the clinical picture, the preoperative and intraoperative diagnosis, and the surgical indications are also presented. It has been proven that the success of an operation does not depend exclusively on surgical technique but is influenced by other factors, such as the stage of the illness, the opportunity of the operation, and the selection of the procedure to be used. All these factors should be carefully contemplated by the surgeon, since they may be decisive in diminishing the number of complications.

For more than 30 years, the author has conducted courses in gastrointestinal surgery for graduate students with surgical sessions transmitted directly. This has allowed the author to understand the most common difficulties that affect graduates with a desire to learn.

The surgical procedures described in this atlas are those that are practiced by the author, and they have produced good results. Alternative techniques are described in separate chapters for when the usual procedures are inappropriate or contraindicated.

Care has been taken to avoid publishing an encyclopedia which could lead to confusion or uncertainty. Afflictions have been detailed that, though rare, can be mortal if not treated adequately and promptly. These illnesses are not usually included in an atlas of surgery. Examples of these illnesses are complicated diverticuli ol the second or third portion of the duodenum, gastric ulcers of the cardia, pancreaticocutaneous fistulas, and duodenal fistulas.

The descriptions of surgical techniques have been written to include both manual suturing and staplers. The most accepted laparoscopic procedures have also been described.

This atlas has been written by a single author. This is not the usual present day practice. However, a book written by a single experienced author offers great uniformity and, at times, is a necessity.

The illustrations are the work of the excellent artist Carlos A. Vescovo. The author and the artist have collaborated very closely to present the most representative and, at the same time, didactic illustrations. The illustrations were made directly in the operating room and later modified to make them more representative and explicit for teaching purposes.

This atlas can be useful for both general surgeons and gastrointestinal surgeons. Colonic surgeons and anorectal surgeons will also find it useful, as well as senior surgeons who may need a concise update of infrequently performed procedures.

The atlas was translated into English by Dr. Alfred L. Axtmayer of Puerto Rico, who has realized the difficult task of interpreting the author's concepts with fidelity. The author would like to express his deepest gratitude.

The author has also been privileged by Dr. John L. Madden of New York, who has written the Foreword. Dr. Madden is one of the world's masters of surgery and the author of an Atlas of Surgery that has spread to all the countries of the world. The author is grateful for Dr. Madden's constant encouragement.

Williams and Wilkins has not limited its efforts in producing an excellent book, for which the author expresses deep gratitude.

Mr. Carroll C. Cann, Executive Editor, has been a great proponent of the book, and the author is grateful for the continuous and extraordinary enthusiasm shown by him in overcoming all difficulties.

The author is also grateful to Ms. Susan Hunsberger for her excellent work in organizing and coordinating the atlas.

To Mr. Peter Carley, Production Coordinator, whose work was a decisive factor in publishing the Atlas, as well as to Mr. Andrew Potter for his brilliant task in correcting manuscripts, the author gives his sincere gratitude.

Emilio Etala, M.D.
Buenos Aires

CONTENTS 目 录

Volume Ⅱ 第Ⅱ卷

Section F

Surgery of the Stomach and Duodenum

CHAPTER 25

Gastrojejunostomy

Gastrojejunostomy is a surgical procedure that used to be performed frequently in the early 20th century in the surgical treatment of duodenal ulcer. With the passage of time the operation was gradually abandoned because anastomotic ulcers frequently developed. In 1943 Dragstedt proposed truncal vagotomy in the treatment of duodenal ulcer with the addition of a gastrojejunostomy at a later stage as a drainage procedure because of the severe motor changes produced by truncal vagotomy. In most cases, gastrojejunostomy was rapidly replaced by the Heineke-Mikulicz pyloroplasty. Gastrojejunostomy has been reserved for some patients in whom pyloroplasty is impracticable. Gastrojejunostomy has additional indications as a palliative drainage procedure in patients with unresectable antropyloric carcinomas, in carcinomas of the pancreas, and in periampullary carcinomas with obstruction or with imminent duodenal obstruction.

The first gastrojejunostomy was performed in Vienna, Austria, in 1881, by Anton Wölfler (13), a disciple of Billroth. Wölfler was operating on a patient with obstructing antropyloric carcinoma and had decided to close the abdomen, considering the case inoperable. At that moment another one of Billroth's disciples, Nicoladoni, suggested Wölfler perform a bypass procedure and he accepted. The procedure Wölfler performed was to bring a long jejunal loop in front of the greater omentum and transverse colon to anastomose it to the anterior gastric wall. This technique is known as an antecolic gastrojejunostomy. It has also been designated as a Wölfler or Wölfler-Nicoladoni gastrojejunostomy (to include the intellectual author of the procedure).

In 1885 Billroth himself (6) proposed another technique for a gastrojejunostomy, bringing a loop of jejunum through the transverse mesocolon and then passing it through the gastrocolic ligament to anastomose it to the anterior gastric wall. This technique is known as an anterior retrocolic gastrojejunostomy.

In the same year, 1885, von Hacker (12), another one of Billroth's disciples, proposed performing the gastrojejunostomy by the shortest route, making the anastomosis with the posterior gastric wall behind the colon, through the transverse mesocolon. The von Hacker procedure is known as posterior retrocolic gastrojejunostomy. These three gastrojejunostomy techniques, proposed in the 19th century, have undergone many modifications and are still performed, but with varying frequency. The posterior retrocolic gastrojejunostomy is undoubtedly the most frequently performed of the techniques. However, it has not been shown to be better than the others if they are well executed. Functional differences have not been demonstrated between posterior, anterior, or marginal anastomoses, or if the anastomotic opening is in a vertical, horizontal, or oblique position (5). It is unanimously accepted, however, that in duodenal ulcers it is advisable to perform the anastomosis near the pylorus, no more than 5 to 7 cm away (2, 3, 8, 14, 15), while in antropyloric carcinomas the anastomosis should be performed as far away as possible from the pylorus and the tumor to avoid early recurrent obstruction (10, 11, 15).

The posterior retrocolic gastrojejunostomy, which is the technique preferred by surgeons (3, 5, 10, 11), can usually be performed except in cases with a very short mesocolon, or in very obese patients, or when the stomach is too high, or when the mesocolon, instead of having the usual blood supply, has numerous blood vessels, which make it very difficult to find an avascular area where the anastomosis can be performed. In some patients the impossibility of carrying out a retrocolic anastomosis is due to the patient having had pancreatitis previously. In these patients the lesser sac may be partially or completely obliterated by fibrosis. In these cases an anterior antecolic gastrojejunostomy should be opted for, since its results are similar.

DIAMETER OF THE ANASTOMOTIC OPENING

It is not necessary that the anastomotic opening be very big, since gastric emptying will be controlled by the diameter of the efferent jejunal loop and not by the diameter of the new opening (3). Many surgeons admit that it is not necessary for the new opening to be more than 4 cm in diameter (2, 4, 14), and many adopt an even smaller diameter (2, 3, 14). It should be remembered, however, that it is common for inflammatory swelling to occur in the new opening, and if the anastomosis is small in diameter, this may lead to emptying problems. To avoid this possible complication, the author prefers a gastrojejunal anastomosis of no less than 6 cm in diameter. Once the anastomosis is complete, the surgeon should evaluate its permeability by introducing two fingers through the new opening.

In patients with duodenal ulcer in which the gastrojejunal anastomosis should be done with the gastric antrum or with the greater curvature, one should remember that frequently the posterior wall of the antrum is adherent to the transverse mesocolon. These adhesions should be carefully divided to avoid vascular injuries and permit a correct anastomosis.

IDENTIFICATION OF THE FIRST JEJUNAL LOOP

The duodenojejunal junction is a fixed point to the left of the second lumbar vertebra. The ligament of Treitz should be carefully identified, as should the distal duodenum. One should always remember that the duodenojejunal junction is situated immediately under the transverse mesocolon. The transverse mesocolon is palpated with the right hand extended with the palm facing upward. The first jejunal loop can be easily pulled gently, confirming its fixation at the ligament of Treitz. In patients with many adhesions due to previous operations, identification of the first jejunal loop must be made taking all precautions to avoid committing the error of grasping a more distal loop of jejunum or a loop of ileum, which could lead to serious postoperative complications.

Once the first jejunal loop has been identified, the ligament of Treitz is divided with the object of shortening the jejunal anastomotic loop but avoiding tension on the anastomosis. It should be remembered that a loop that is too short, besides leading to tension on the anastomosis, may produce kinking or lead to rotation of the anastomosis. In the posterior retrocolic gastrojejunostomy the anastomotic loop should not be more than 10 to 15 cm from the duodenojejunal junction. Some surgeons prefer an even shorter distance of 8 to 10 cm (2, 3, 14).

GASTROJEJUNAL ANASTOMOSIS WITH OR WITHOUT CLAMPS?

Gastrojejunal anastomosis with or without clamps has been the subject of discussion for many years and the controversy continues. Gastrojejunal anastomosis with atraumatic, elastic clamps permits the performance of a clean operation. It has not been proven that atraumatic clamps have altered the viability of the viscera being anastomosed. The author always uses the Finochietto twin clamps to perform a gastrojejunostomy, with excellent results.

ANASTOMOSIS OF THE AFFERENT WITH THE EFFERENT LOOP

In antecolic anastomoses a long jejunal loop should be used. In thin patients with little fat in the greater omentum, the jejunal loop is usually 20 to 25 cm long from the duodenojejunal angle. In obese patients with the greater omentum loaded with fat, the jejunal loop is usually 35 to 40 cm long from the duodenojejunal angle.

When antecolic gastrojejunal anastomoses with a long loop were first carried out, an anastomosis between the afferent and the efferent loop was frequently performed. This was also called a Braun jejunojejunostomy for its original proponent (6). In antecolic gastrojejunostomies for duodenal ulcer the Braun anastomosis would favor the development of anastomotic ulcers. At present this possibility is lowered by the performance of a truncal vagotomy at the same time. However, a Braun anastomosis should be avoided in duodenal ulcers. In patients with antropyloric cancer, carcinoma of the head of the pancreas, or periampullary cancer in whom a palliative gastrojejunostomy is performed, there is no reason to carry out a Braun anastomosis because life expectancy is short and anastomotic ulcers rarely occur, since patients with these diagnoses have little tendency to develop anastomotic ulcers.

GASTRIC ASPIRATION

Patients with pyloroduodenal obstruction should be adequately prepared preoperatively by using a Levine tube to aspirate gastric contents. If patients do not have obstruction, the Levine tube is introduced in the operating room after the patient is anesthetized.

GASTROJEJUNAL SUTURING IN ONE OR TWO LAYERS?

The author always uses two layers of sutures in gastrojejunostomies. One layer joins gastric mucosa to jejunal mucosa; the other joins the seromuscular layers. The mucosal layer is sutured with 2-0 chromic catgut or synthetic reabsorable material. Many surgeons use a one-layer closure with very good results.

The position of the afferent and efferent jejunal loops varies with the type of anastomosis that is performed. In the posterior vertical retrocolic anastomosis the afferent loop should be on the lesser curvature side, with the efferent loop on the greater curvature. In the horizontal anastomosis the afferent loop should be placed on the proximal portion of the stomach (cardia) and the efferent loop on the distal portion (pylorus).

SURGICAL TECHNIQUE

Posterior Retrocolic Gastrojejunostomy

This is the most frequently used technique. The first jejunal loop is anastomosed to the posterior wall of the stomach through an opening in the transverse mesocolon (4, 6, 10–12, 15). The anastomosis can be performed in vertical, horizontal or oblique fashion, near or directly on the greater curvature, either on the body or the antrum of the stomach. In patients with duodenal ulcer it is advisable to perform the gastrojejunal anastomosis near the pylorus.

The incision generally used is the xiphoumbilical incision, since it is adequate to perform a palliative gastrojejunostomy in an inoperable obstructing carcinoma of the stomach or carcinoma of the pancreatic head or periampullary region. In these patients a vagotomy is not necessary due to their short survival period and because anastomotic ulcers are rare in these patients.

In patients with duodenal ulcer, in whom a truncal vagotomy should be done during the same operation, the incision should be longer, extending 4 to 6 cm below the umbilicus. It may occasionally be necessary to resect the xiphoid process to enlarge the operative field.

FIGURE 25.1
A palliative gastrojejunostomy does not have to be performed near the pylorus, but in patients with duodenal ulcer, it is advisable to place the anastomosis about 5 to 7 cm proximal to the pylorus.

Posterior Retrocolic Gastrojejunostomy

Once the peritoneum is open the entire abdominal cavity should be explored, the presence of a duodenal ulcer should be certified, and the pathologic changes that have occurred making it impossible to perform a pyloroplasty, which is the preferred drainage procedure, should be confirmed. The surgeon should also confirm that no impediment for a posterior retrocolic anastomosis exists. In case an impediment does exist, an anterior antecolic anastomosis can be done.

Once these possibilities have been discarded, the transverse mesocolon is pulled upward, exposing its inferior surface and identifying the first jejunal loop, as previously described. The ligament of Treitz is then divided to shorten the trajectory of the afferent jejunal loop. Once the first jejunal loop is identified, it is grasped with a smooth atraumatic Foerster clamp to make it easier to find when the anastomosis with the stomach is performed. The surgeon holds the transverse colon upward with the thumb forward and his remaining four fingers, placed behind the colon, pushing the posterior gastric wall downward to bring it in contact with the transverse mesocolon. With his right hand the surgeon incises the transverse mesocolon with a scalpel in an avascular area between the middle colic vessels and the marginal arcade to grasp the stomach with two Babcock clamps. The incision in the transverse mesocolon should be made more to the right in cases in whom the anastomosis must be carried out only 5 to 7 cm proximal to the pylorus.

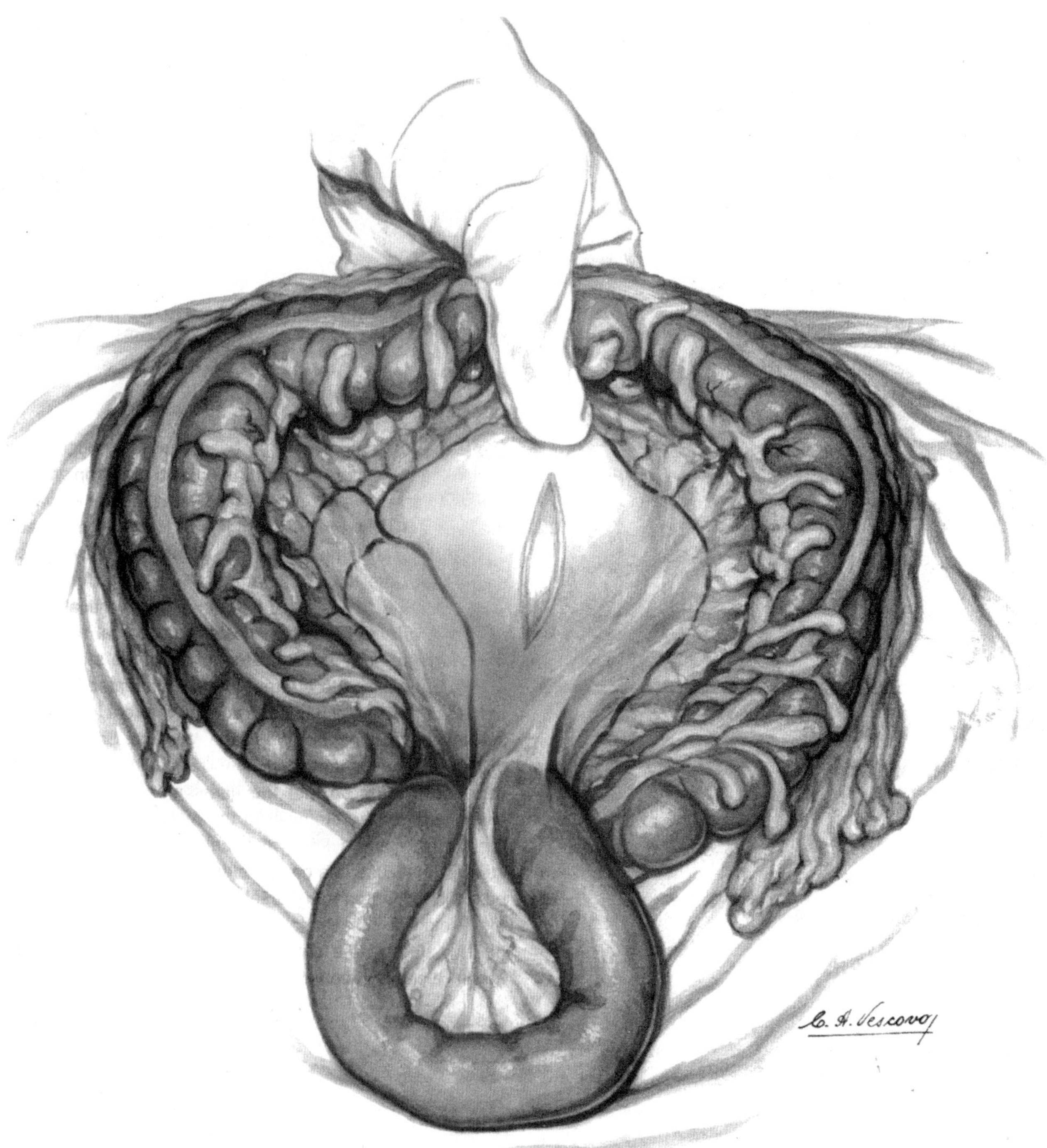

FIGURE 25.1

FIGURE 25.2

The posterior gastric wall has been passed through the incision in the transverse mesocolon. A Babcock clamp grasps the superior part of the stomach, which is the greater curvature of the stomach, where the efferent jejunal loop will be placed. Another Babcock clamp grasps the inferior end, which corresponds with the lesser curvature, where the afferent jejunal loop will enter. If instead of performing a vertical posterior retrocolic von Hacker anastomosis, a horizontal anastomosis is performed, be it in the posterior wall of the stomach or its greater curvature, the afferent loop should enter the proximal portion of the stomach (cardia) and the efferent loop should be in the distal (pyloric) portion of the stomach. Some 4 or 5 cm of the posterior gastric wall should pass through the transverse mesocolon so that the anastomosis with the jejunum and fixation of the stomach to the mesocolon can be carried out. The fixation is performed only on the right side of the stomach because it is on this side that the jejunal wall should be placed, oriented transversely. Fixation of the stomach to the mesocolon is indispensable to prevent intestinal loops from passing through the defect in the mesocolon, leading to obstructive complications.

Posterior Retrocolic Gastrojejunostomy

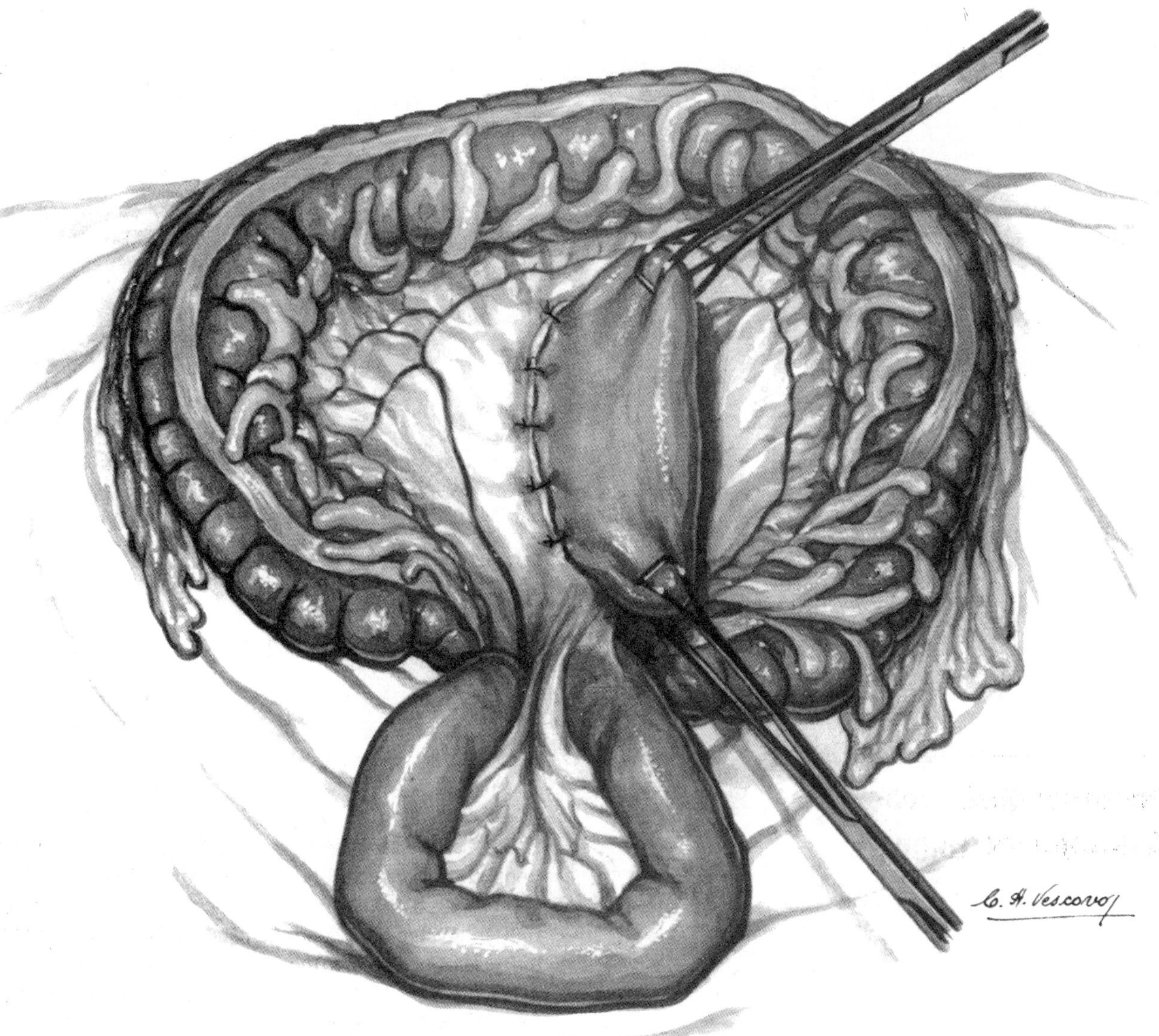

FIGURE 25.2

Posterior Retrocolic Gastrojejunostomy

FIGURE 25.3

Fixation of the stomach to the right edge of the opening in the transverse mesocolon has been completed. The stomach is approximated to the first jejunal loop that had been grasped with a Foerster clamp and the jejunal loop is placed parallel to the stomach to begin the anastomosis. The afferent jejunal loop is in the inferior portion, near the lesser curvature, and the efferent loop is in the superior portion, near the greater curvature. Both ends are held in place by Babcock clamps.

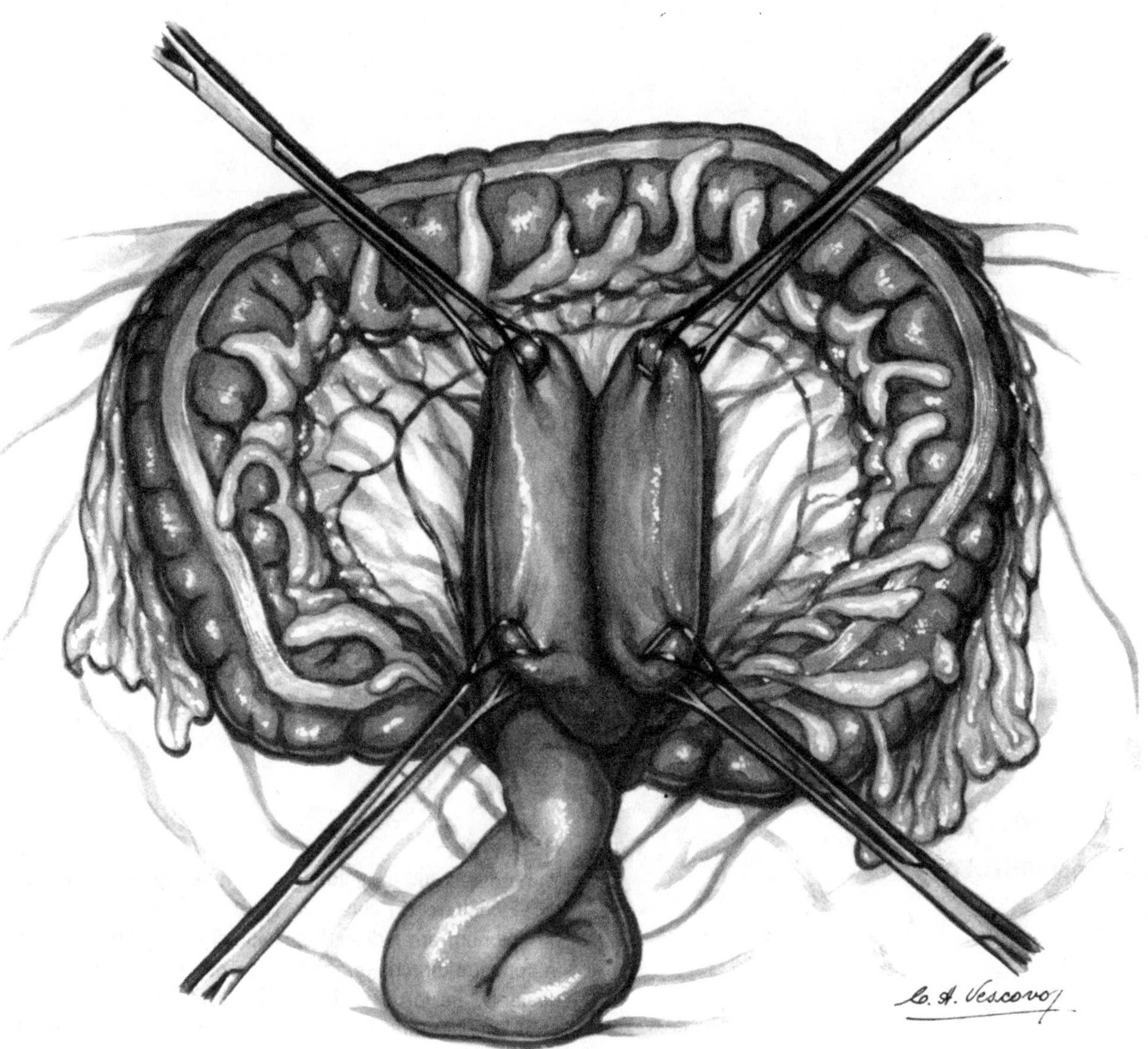

FIGURE 25.3

Posterior Retrocolic Gastrojejunostomy

FIGURE 25.4

The stomach and the jejunum have been grasped by the elastic Finochietto twin clamps. The borders of the stomach and the jejunum are held by Babcock clamps and traction applied in opposite directions, making the posterior gastrojejunal layer easier to perform. Guide sutures have been placed at each end. The posterior seromuscular layer of sutures has been started using interrupted sutures of cotton, silk, or nonabsorbable synthetic material.

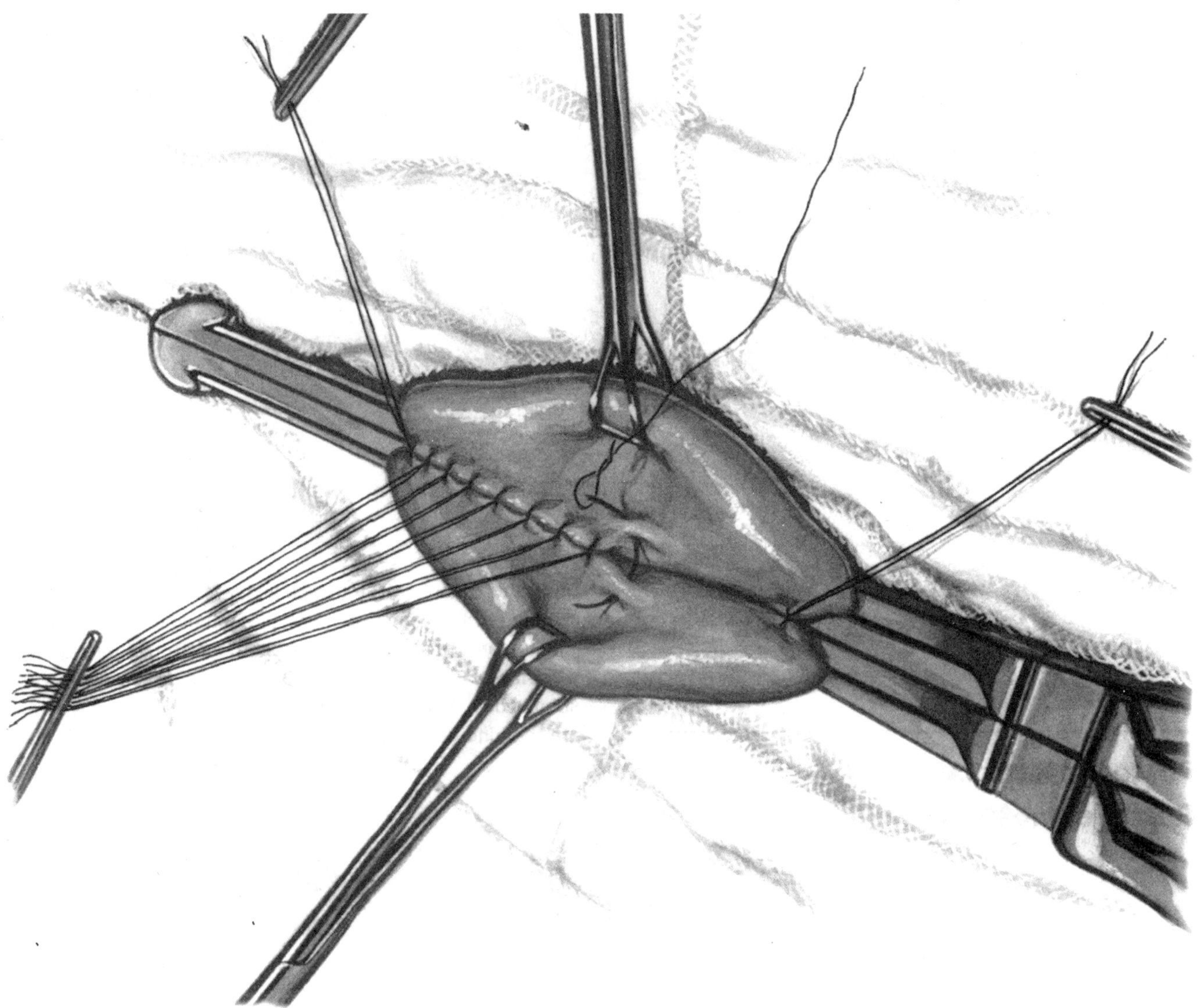

FIGURE 25.4

FIGURE 25.5
Once the posterior seromuscular layer of sutures has been completed, the gastric wall and the antimesenteric wall of the jejunum are incised. It is advisable to incise the gastric wall in two stages. In the first stage the wall is incised down to the submucosa, where numerous blood vessels can be seen that are then individually ligated.

Posterior Retrocolic Gastrojejunostomy

FIGURE 25.6
The incisions in the gastric and jejunal walls have been completed, exposing both mucosas.

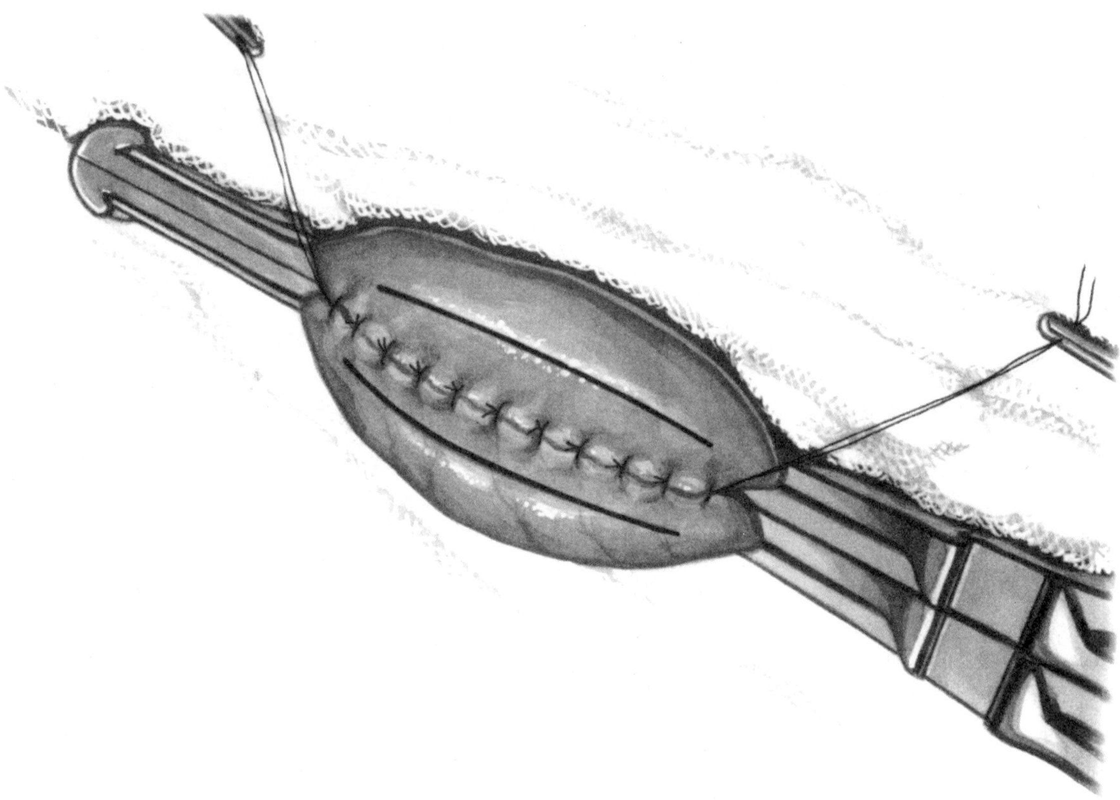

FIGURE 25.5

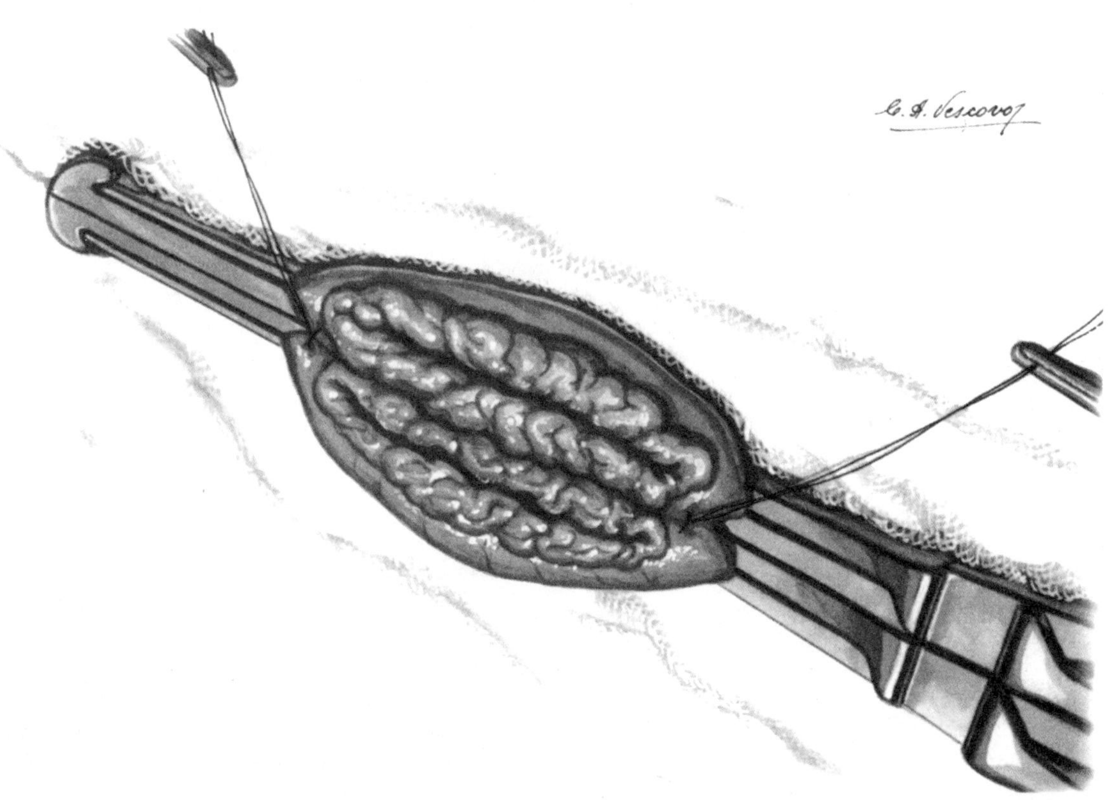

FIGURE 25.7
The posterior perforating incision is being sutured with 2-0 chromic catgut using a continuous reabsorable suture on a straight or curved needle.

Posterior Retrocolic Gastrojejunostomy

FIGURE 25.8
The drawing shows the anterior performing layer being sutured. The author prefers the Schmieden suture in the closure of the anterior perforating layer because it results in very good invagination of the mucosa. As can be seen in the drawing, the Schmieden suture is performed bringing the needle from mucosa to serosa and then going to the opposite side where it enters the mucosa and exits through the serosa, passing again to the other side to enter through the mucosa again.

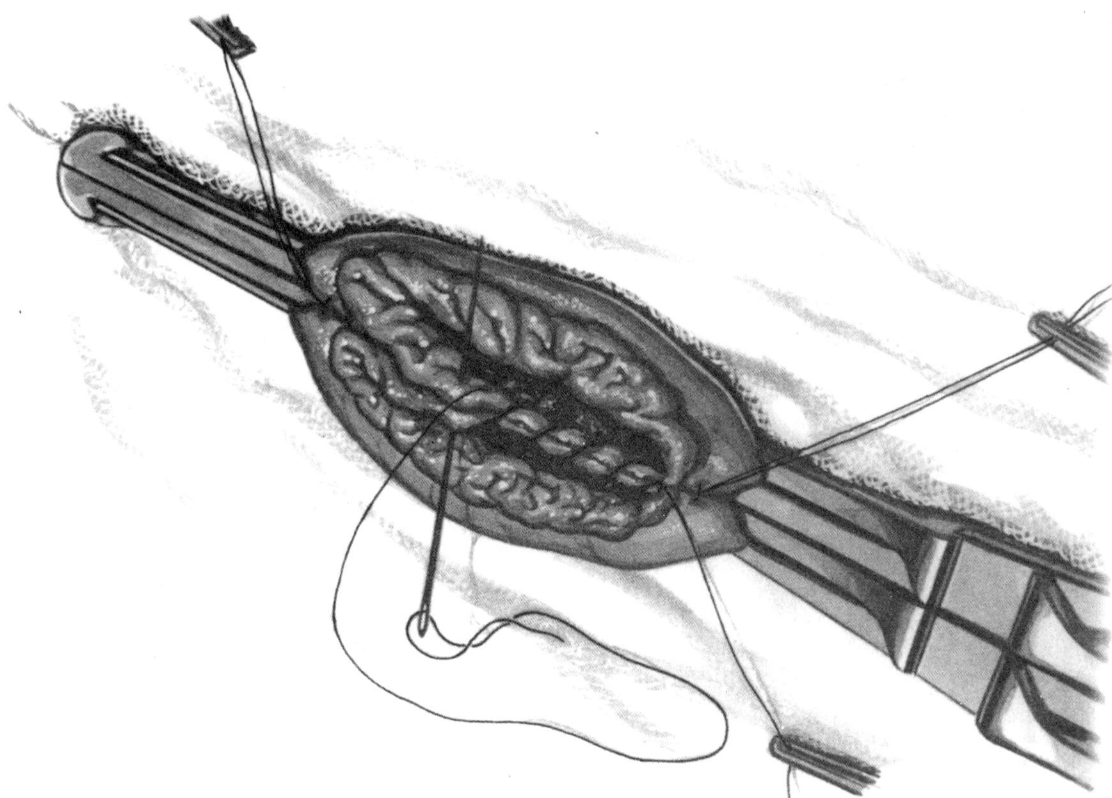

FIGURE 25.7

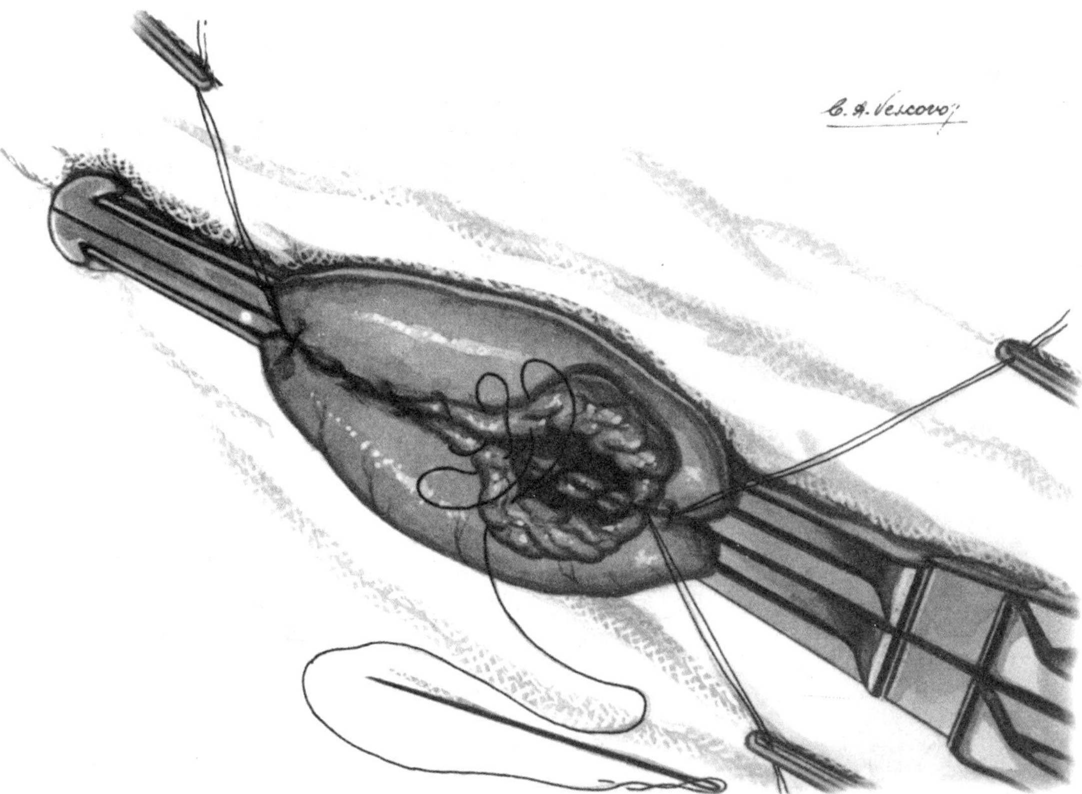

FIGURE 25.8

Posterior Retrocolic Gastrojejunostomy

FIGURE 25.9
Once the anterior perforating layer has been closed, the anterior seromuscular layer is sutured with interrupted cotton, silk, or nonabsorbable synthetic material. The seromuscular layer can be closed with a continuous suture. Some surgeons close the gastrojejunostomy in one layer.

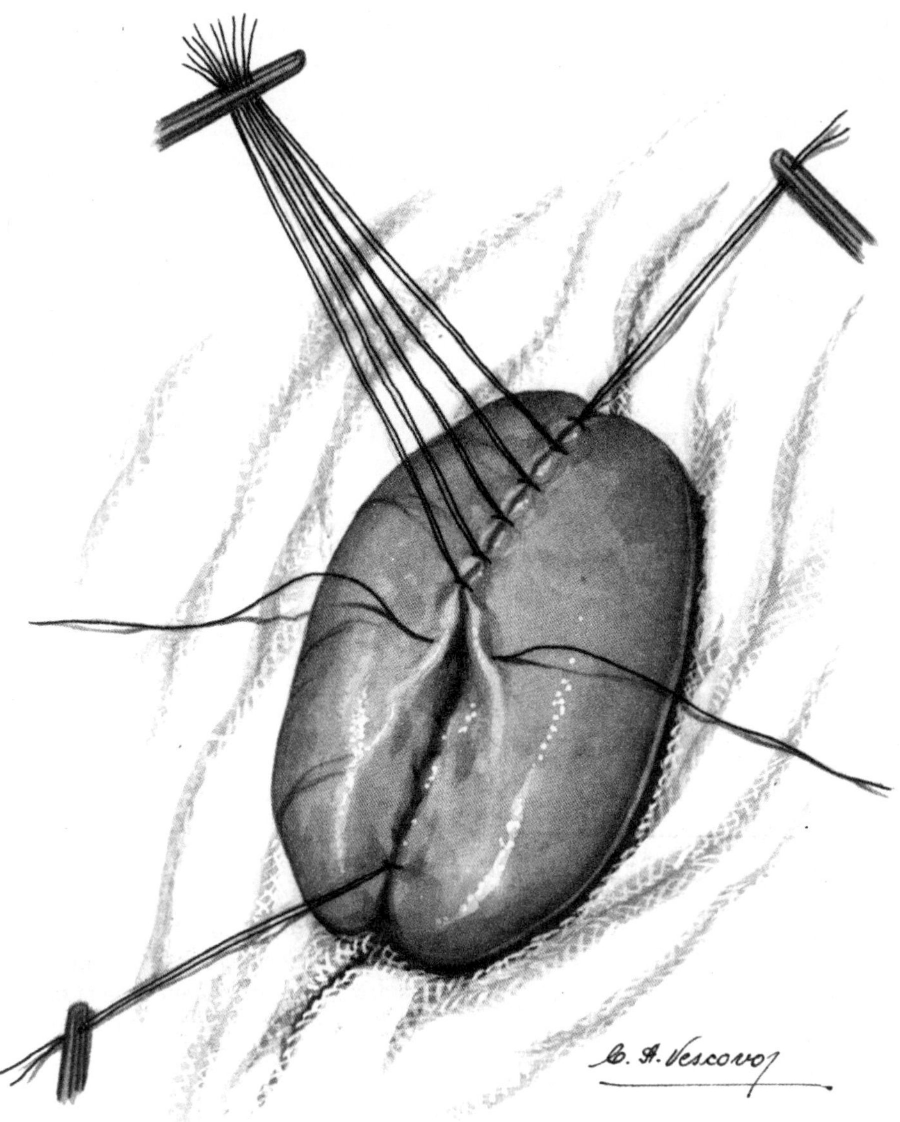

FIGURE 25.9

Posterior Retrocolic Gastrojejunostomy

FIGURE 25.10
Once the anterior seromuscular layer has been completed, the stomach is fixed to the left edge of the transverse mesocolon, using interrupted sutures, thus completing the posterior retrocolic gastrojejunostomy.

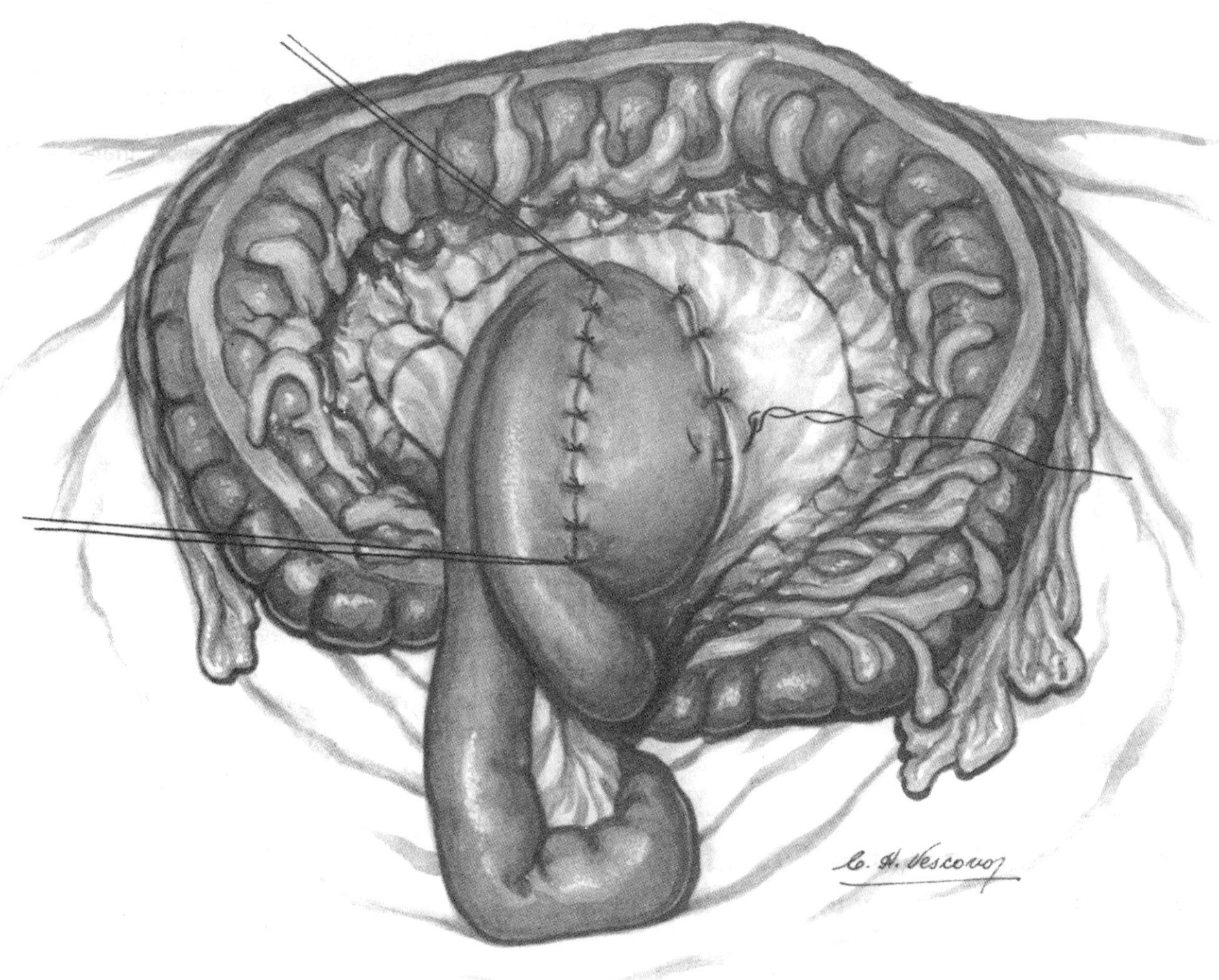

FIGURE 25.10

FIGURE 25.11
In patients with duodenal ulcer in whom it becomes necessary to perform a gastrojejunostomy with truncal vagotomy, the anastomosis should be placed as close as possible to the pylorus, near the greater curvature, with a short afferent loop, as can be seen in the drawing.

FIGURE 25.12
The antecolic gastrojejunostomy is used as a palliative procedure in patients with pyloric obstruction due to carcinoma. In these patients the anastomosis of the jejunum to the anterior wall of the stomach should be performed as far away from the tumor as possible.

Posterior Retrocolic, Antecolic and Anterior Retrocolic Gastrojejunostomy

FIGURE 25.13
The anterior retrocolic gastrojejunostomy is infrequently used. The jejunal loop is brought up through the transverse mesocolon and then through the gastrocolic ligament to be anastomosed to the stomach in the vicinity of the greater curvature.

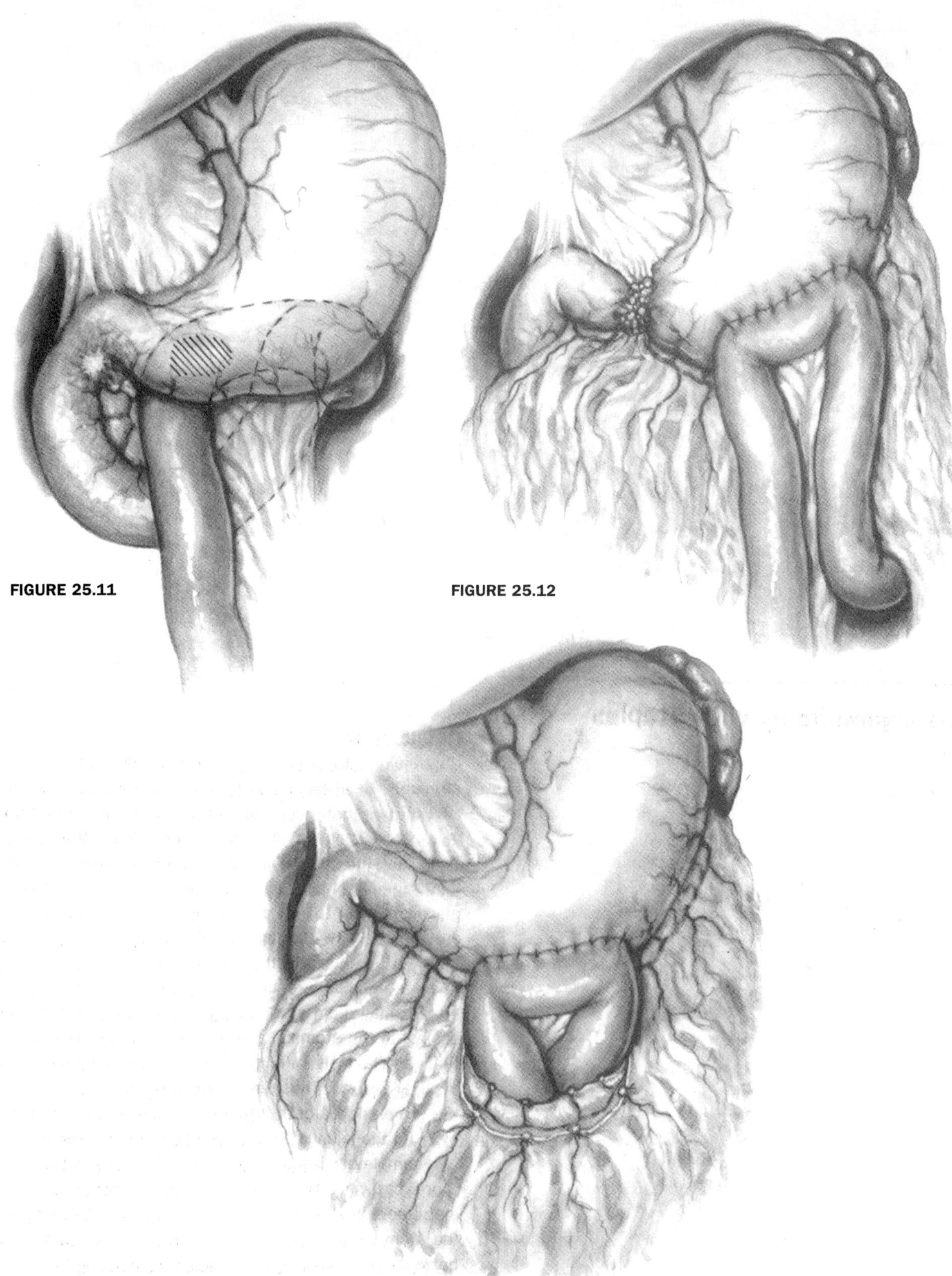

FIGURE 25.11

FIGURE 25.12

FIGURE 25.13

Gastrojejunostomy with Staples

FIGURE 25.14
Gastrojejunostomy can be performed with a stapler. The most frequently used technique for this anastomosis is as follows: Part of the greater curvature of the stomach is freed from the gastrocolic ligament. The first jejunal loop, the ligament of Treitz, and the duodenojejunal junction are identified. The proximal segment of jejunum is brought up in front of the colon and placed parallel to the anterior gastric wall, near the greater curvature, so that the antimesenteric border of the jejunum is in direct contact with the gastric wall. Two seromuscular sutures are placed in each of the ends of the future anastomosis. A small 1-cm stab wound is performed with the electric scalpel in the stomach about 8 cm from the pylorus, and another similar incision is made in the jejunum opposite the gastric stab wound. These incisions serve for the introduction of the two branches of the GIA stapler, one into the stomach and one into the jejunum. The branches of the instrument are usually completely introduced. Some surgeons introduce them 5 or 6 cm. Once the limbs of the GIA stapler are inserted, the instrument is closed and fired. The double row of staples joins the stomach with the jejunum, and the blade cuts the tissue between the double row of staples, completing the anastomosis. The instrument is then removed and the stab wounds in the stomach and jejunum closed with a TA 30 stapler or with two layers of sutures.

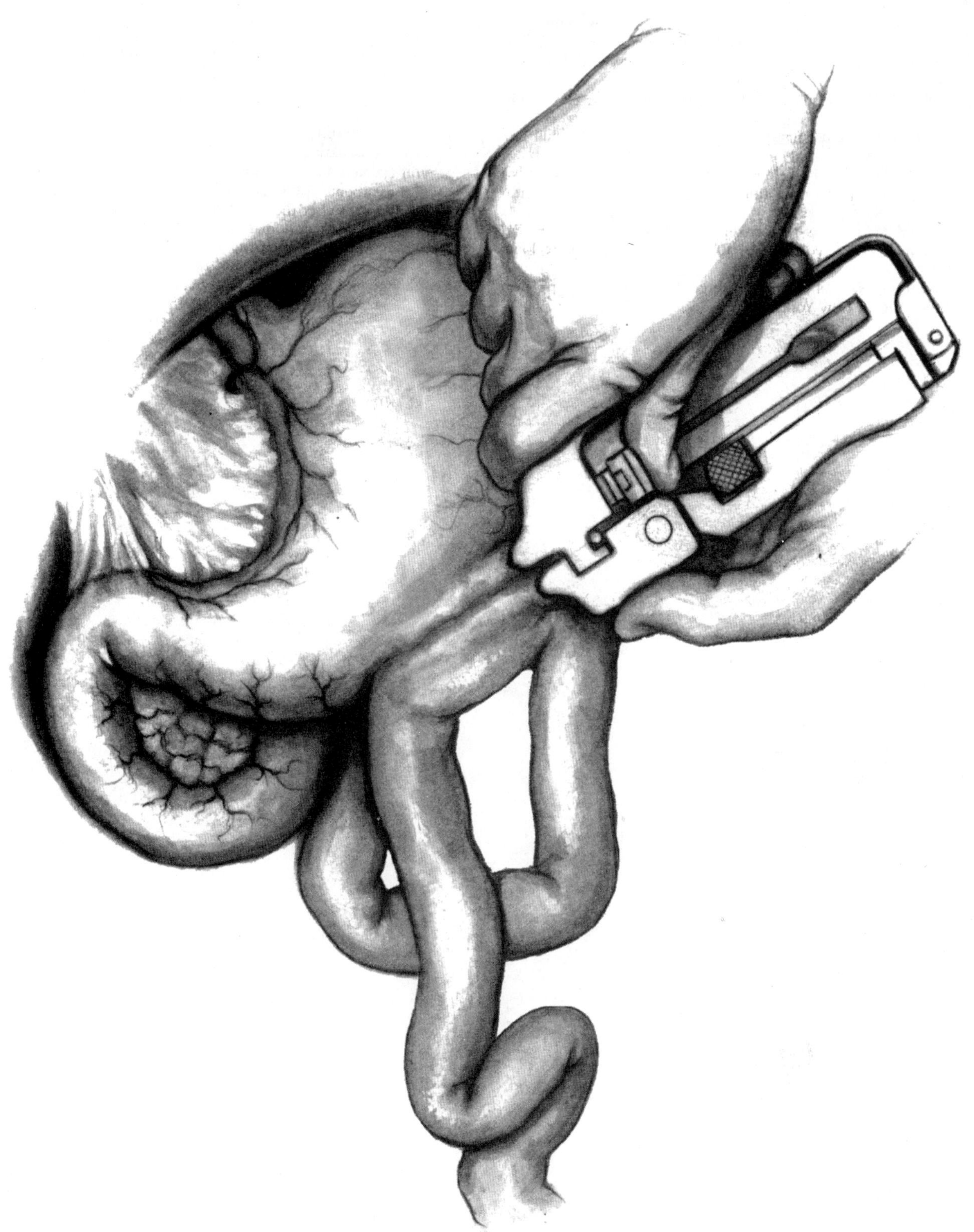

FIGURE 25.14

References

1. Becker, H.D., Herfarth, C., Lierse, W., Schreiber, H.W. Surgery of the stomach. P. 24. Springer-Verlag, Berlin, 1986.
2. Chassin, J.L. Operative strategy in general surgery. Vol. I, p. 142. Springer-Verlag, New York, 1980.
3. Fromm, D. Complications of gastric surgery. Wiley, New York, 1977.
4. Fromm, D. Gastrointestinal surgery. Vol. I, p. 257. Churchill Livingstone, New York, 1985.
5. Kirk, R.M. Drainage Procedures. In Schwartz, S.I., Ellis, H. (Eds.) Maingot's abdominal operations. Ed. 9, vol. I, p. 667. Appleton Lange, Norwalk, CT, 1990.
6. Kirschner, M., Guleke, N., Zenker, R. Operaciones en la cavidad abdominal. Ed. 2, vol. VII, p. 107. Editorial Labor, Barcelona, 1954.
7. Madden, J.L. Atlas of technics in surgery. Ed. 2, p. 224. Appleton Century Crofts. New York, 1964.
8. Oberhelman, H.A. Jr. Vagotomy or pyloroplasty or gastrojejunostomy. In Nora, P.F. (Ed.) Operative surgery. Ed. 3, p. 520. W.B. Saunders, Philadelphia, 1990.
9. Olch, P.D., Harkins, H.N. A historical review of gastric surgery. In Harkins, H.N., Nyhus, L.M. (Eds.) Surgery of the stomach and duodenum. P. 3. Little, Brown, Boston, 1962.
10. Pi-Figueras, J. Práctica quirúrgica. Ed. 2, vol. II, p. 92. Salvat, Madrid, 1986.
11. Valdoni, P. Abdominal surgery. An atlas of operative technqiues. P. 40. W.B. Saunders, Philadelphia, 1976.
12. von Hacker, V. Zur carnistik und statistik der magenresektionen und gastroenterostomien. Arch. Klin. Chir. 32:616, 1885.
13. Wölfler, A. Ueber die von herren Prof. Billroth, ansgeföhrten resektionen des karzinomatösen pylorus. Zentralbl. Chir. 8:359, 1881.
14. Zinner, M.J. Atlas of gastric surgery. P. 18. Churchill Livingstone, New York, 1992.
15. Zollinger, R.M., Zollinger, R.M. Jr. Atlas of surgical operations. Ed. 4, p. 34. Macmillan, New York, 1975.

Section F

Surgery of the Stomach and Duodenum

CHAPTER 26

Gastrostomy

GENERAL CONSIDERATIONS

Gastrostomy is one of the oldest abdominal operations. It is performed to establish a communication between the gastric lumen and the outside of the abdomen, through the abdominal wall.

Gastrostomy is performed to decompress the stomach or for feeding purposes. Decompressive gastrostomies are usually indicated in aged patients with postoperative bronchopulmonary problems, in neurotic patients who do not tolerate nasogastric intubation, or in patients in whom gastric decompression may last several days. It is well known that patients with esophagitis due to reflux do not tolerate intubation well. Cases have been reported of serious esophageal strictures in patients with esophageal reflux who have been intubated. Even though this complication is infrequent, it must be kept in mind (3). There are surgeons who prefer gastrostomy for decompression over postoperative nasogastric intubation (8). Nasogastric intubation should not be replaced by gastrostomy, except in special cases such as those mentioned above.

Feeding gastrostomy may be temporary or permanent. Temporary feeding gastrostomy is performed using the same technique as decompressive gastrostomy, the only variation being the caliber of the catheter, which should be greater in the feeding gastrostomy. An 18 F catheter is used for decompression, whereas in a temporary feeding gastrostomy the caliber of the catheter should be 18 to 22 F.

Permanent feeding gastrostomies are indicated in patients with serious problems in swallowing, in oral, pharyngeal, or esophageal diseases, in neurologic illnesses, and so on.

Permanent feeding gastrostomies are performed by constructing a tube with a flap of the gastric wall. The external surface of the tube remains covered by serosa while the internal surface stays lined by gastric mucosa. The tube is brought out and sutured to the abdominal wall. Patients with this type of permanent feeding gastrostomy do not need to have a catheter continuously, since the catheter is introduced into the stomach through the gastric tube only at the time of feeding. The catheter is removed after each feeding and reinserted at the time of the next feeding. The patients do not have a catheter between feedings.

BRIEF HISTORY OF GASTROSTOMY

Knowledge of the history of the evolution of the technique of gastrostomy from its beginnings to the present time is of great interest to point out the efforts made by surgeons of many countries to lower the mortality and many complications of the original techniques. The bad results obtained at the outset were the result of poor techniques—in particular, opening the stomach directly to the skin of the abdomen. This would make introduction of food easy but at the same time allowed gastric secretions to reflux continuously to the outside, digesting the skin and leading to the formation of ulcers, which caused great suffering to the patient. This serious complication stimulated surgeons to modify surgical technique so as to make introduction of food easy and, at the same time, make it difficult for gastric contents to come out.

Gastrostomy was originally proposed by a Norwegian military surgeon named Egeberg, in 1841 (7), to treat a patient with esophageal stricture. Egeberg, however, never performed the operation. The first surgeon to perform a gastrostomy was Sédillot, a French surgeon from Strasbourg, on November 13, 1849 (2, 28). The patient operated on by Sédillot died a few hours after surgery. The surgeon blamed the patient's death on having performed the operation in only one stage. On January 21, 1853, Sédillot performed another gastrostomy, this time in two stages. In the first stage he fixed the stomach to the anterior abdominal wall to create adhesions and open the stomach in a later second stage. In spite of these precautions, the patient also died. The first gastrostomy with survival was performed by Sydney Jones of St. Thomas Hospital, in London, in 1875 (16). The patient died 40 days later. In 1876, Verneuil, of France (35), using a partial modification of Sédillot's technique, obtained a 1-year, 4-month survival. At the end of the last century and the beginning of the 1900s, many techniques had been proposed showing that the results were less than optimal in all of them (1, 2, 13, 14, 17, 20, 31, 33, 34).

In 1891, Witzel, of Germany (39), proposed a technique that substantially modified the future of gastrostomized patients. The Witzel technique consisted of forming a tunnel of gastric serosa, through which a catheter was passed, preventing gastric secretions from passing directly to the outside. The tunnel created by the Witzel technique ran transversely, the same as the Marwedel technique. This technique was proposed later, and instead of constructing the tunnel with serosa, the tunnel was constructed in the submucosa. Other gastrostomy techniques also created a tunnel, but instead of disposing it transversely as Witzel, and later Marwedel, recommended, they disposed it vertically. Among these last gastrostomies were the Stamm, Senn, Kader, Fontan, and other techniques (2, 17, 33). These and similar techniques were used as temporary decompressive and feeding gastrostomies.

The most frequently used technique for permanent feeding gastrostomy is the Depage-Janeway techniques (5, 12). This technique has been modified to create a valvelike mechanism that will prevent spillage of gastric secretions onto the skin as much as possible (20, 32, 34). These modifications have not convinced many surgeons and, for this reason, are performed infrequently. The Beck-Jianu technique is a variation of the Depage-Janeway procedure. It is also known in medical literature as the Beck-Carrel-Jianu because Beck and Carrel first described it in 1905 (2) and carried out the operation experimentally in dogs. Jianu, however, published it in 1912 (15). Another variation of the Depage-Janeway technique is the Rutkowsky technique (24).

SURGICAL GASTROSTOMY PROCEDURES TO BE DESCRIBED

The gastrostomy procedures to be described are the following:

1. Decompressive and temporary feeding gastrostomy: Stamm technique. Reference will be made to the endoscopic percutaneous gastrostomy.
2. Permanent feeding gastrostomy: The following techniques will be described, which can be adapted to different situations.
   A. Depage-Janeway technique
      i. with manual sutures
      ii. sutured with stapler
   B. Beck-Carrel-Jianu technique: Manual suturing will be described, though the procedure can also be performed with a stapler.
   C. Rutkowsky technique: Suturing with a stapler will be described, though the procedure can also be performed manually.
   D. The Depage-Janeway technique, performed using laparoscopy and a guided stapler, will be mentioned.

Surgical Technique

FIGURE 26.1

The usual incision for this procedure is a midline xiphoumbilical incision some 10 cm long. In patients with the stomach retracted upward, the incision can be extended in that direction as needed. If the gastrostomy is for permanent feeding, it is frequently necessary to make the incision longer, since the procedure is more complex. The gastrostomy catheter should never be brought out through the incision. It should be brought out through a small transverse incision a few centimeters to the left of the midline incision, which generally corresponds to the area of the left rectus muscle and its sheath. A short transverse broken line shows the small incision in the drawing. If a permanent feeding gastrostomy is being performed, the gastric tube should also be brought out through a separate small incision and sutured to the skin, as will be shown later.

Temporary Decompressive and Feeding Gastrostomy: Stamm Technique

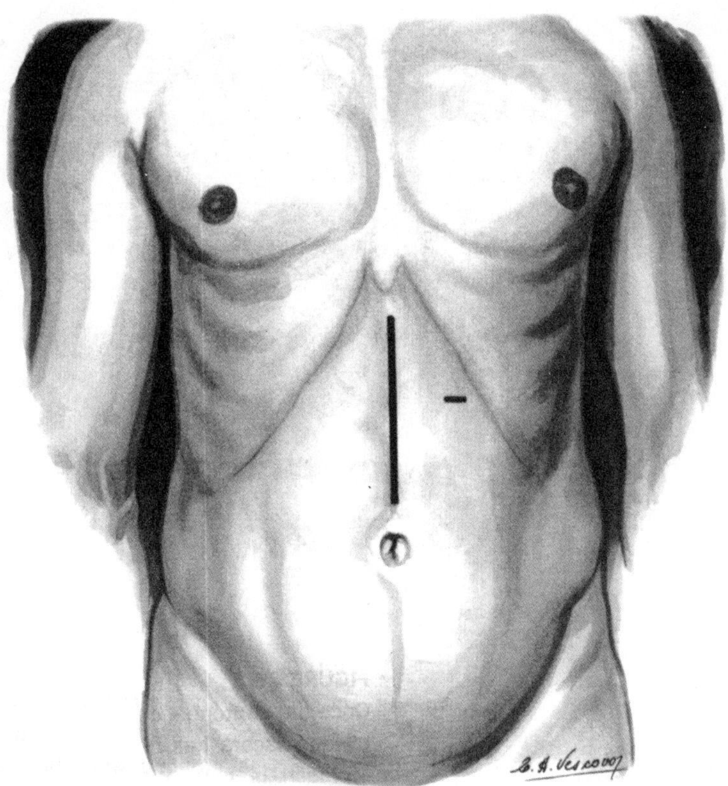

FIGURE 26.1

Temporary Decompressive and Feeding Gastrostomy: Stamm Technique

FIGURE 26.2
Once the peritoneal cavity has been opened and exploration of all the viscera has been performed, the anterior wall of the stomach is grasped with three Babcock clamps near the greater curvature, at its middle third. The author prefers to make a 15 mm incision in the gastric wall, shown by the horizontal line, cutting the seromuscular layer to expose the very vascular submucosa, before placing the purse string sutures that will invaginate the tissue around the catheter.

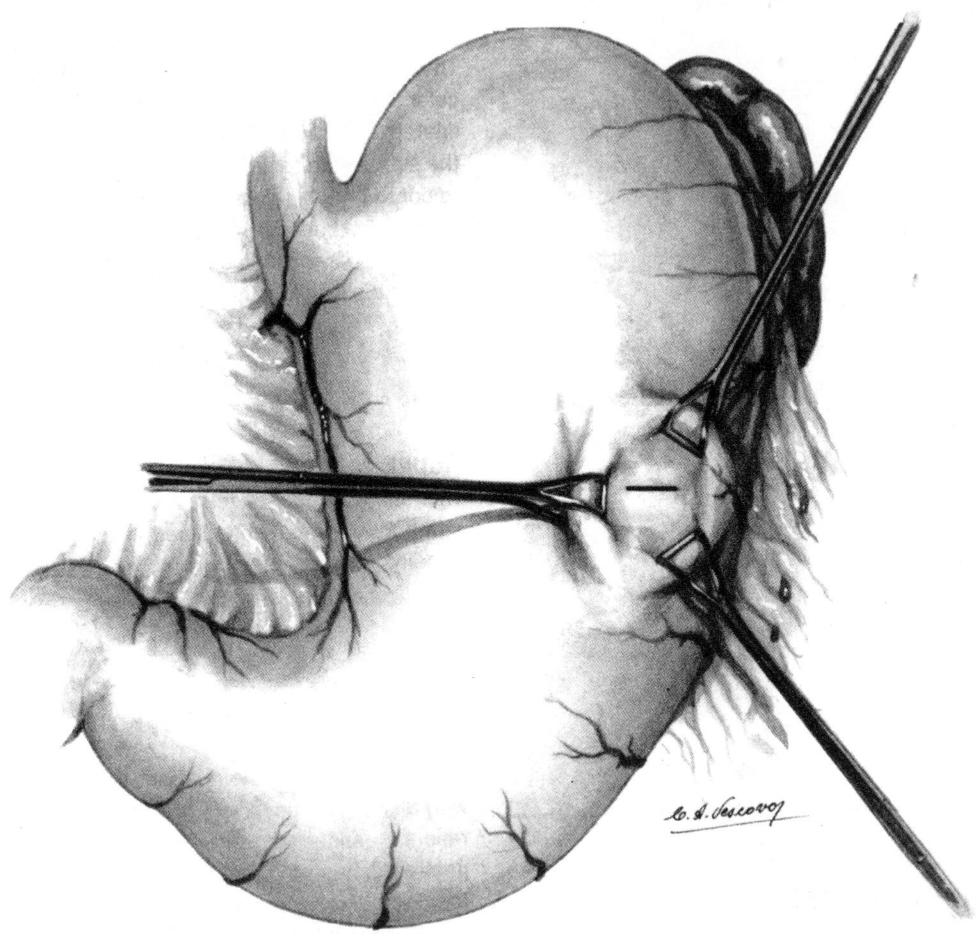

FIGURE 26.2

FIGURE 26.3
The seromuscular layer has been incised, showing the very vascular submucosal layer. The more prominent vessels are suture ligated, as shown. It is known that profuse bleeding occurs when the submucosal arterioles are cut, and it is not always possible to control the bleeding by simply tying the purse string sutures against the catheter. Once the submucosal vessels have been ligated, a purse string suture is placed in the submucosal layer around the incision, using nonabsorbable material.

FIGURE 26.4
The submucosal vessels have been ligated and the purse string suture has been placed in the submucosal layer, which is being incised, as shown.

Temporary Decompressive and Feeding Gastrostomy: Stamm Technique

FIGURE 26.5
The drawing shows the moment an 18 F Pezzer catheter, held with a clamp, is being introduced into the stomach through the recently made opening in the mucosa. In decompressive gastrostomies an 18 F catheter is usually used. In temporary feeding gastrostomies 18 to 22 F catheters are usually employed. A Malecot (mushroom) catheter or a Foley catheter can be used, instead of a Pezzer, with the same good results.

FIGURE 26.6
The Pezzer catheter has been inserted into the stomach, and the purse string suture has been tied. It is desirable to keep the three Babcock clamps in the same place to facilitate further maneuvers.

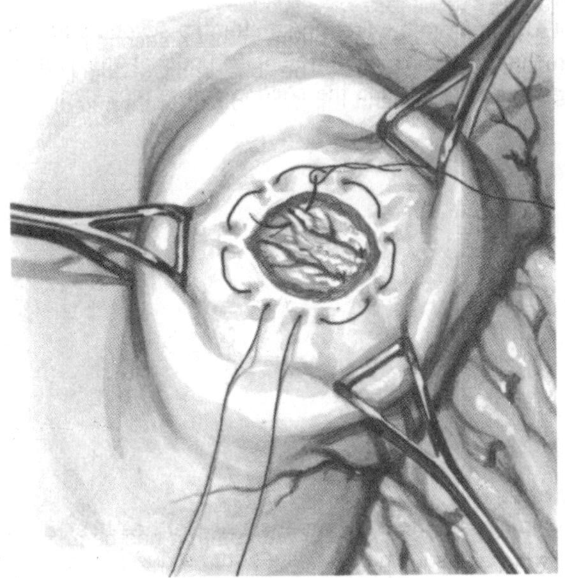

FIGURE 26.3

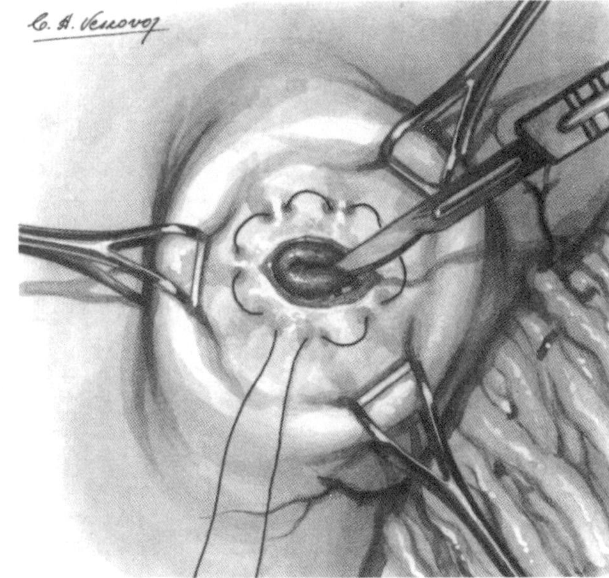

FIGURE 26.4

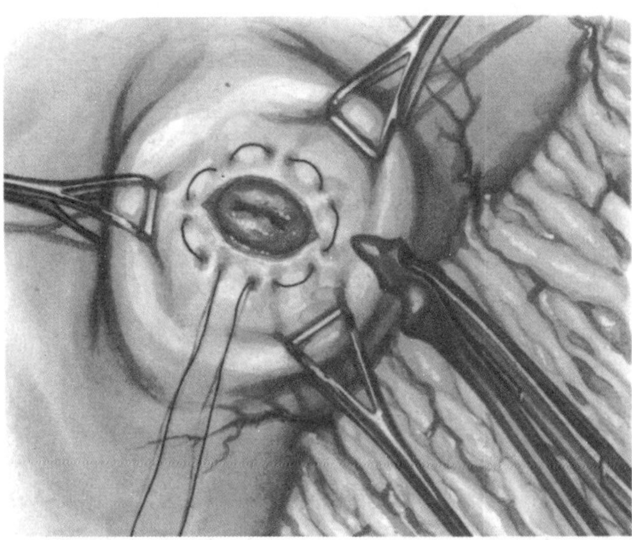

FIGURE 26.5

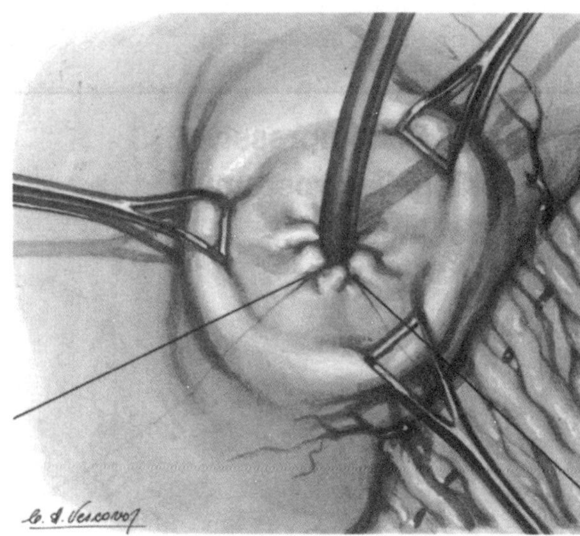

FIGURE 26.6

FIGURE 26.7
About 15 mm from the first purse string, a second purse string suture has been inserted. The long ends of the first purse string suture are cut and the second one is then tied.

FIGURE 26.8
Section of the stomach where the catheter has been inserted and two invaginating purse string sutures are in place. A third purse string will be added about 15 mm from the second. This will invaginate about 45 mm of the anterior gastric wall around the catheter.

Temporary Decompressive and Feeding Gastrostomy: Stamm Technique

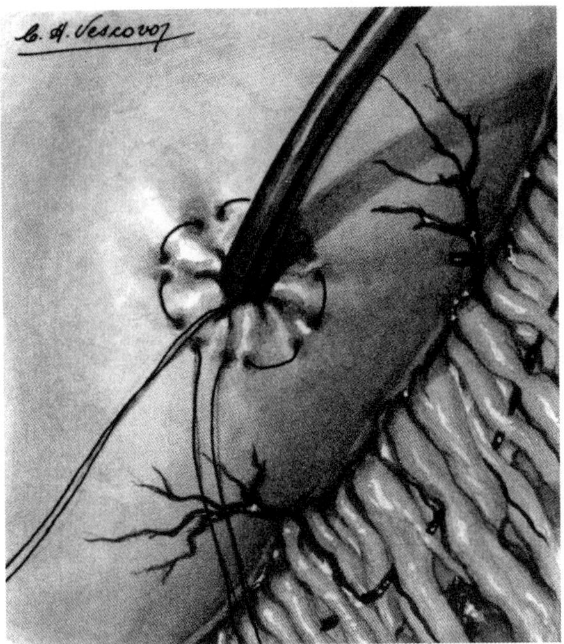

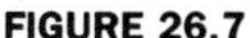
FIGURE 26.7

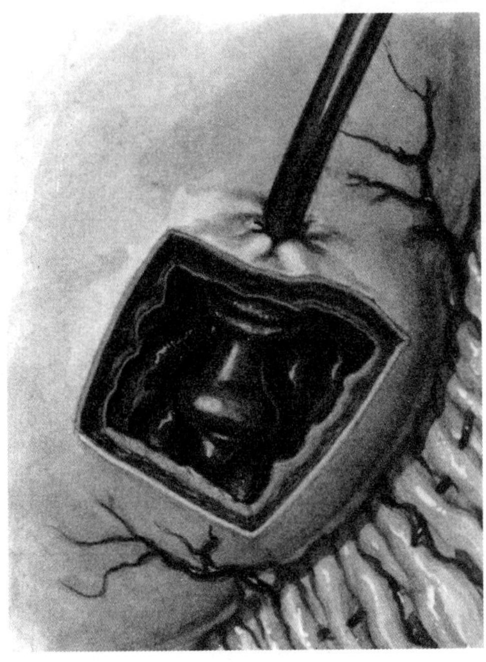

FIGURE 26.8

FIGURE 26.9
Once the three purse string sutures are in place, the ends of the third suture are left long. A 15 mm incision has been made in the skin a few centimeters to the left of the midline and later carried through the left anterior rectus muscle. This stab wound will be used to bring the gastrostomy catheter out. Using Allis clamps the peritoneum and the fascia of the left edge of the midline incision have been grasped in order to apply traction upward and to the left to expose the site where the parietal peritoneum will be incised, avoiding any injury to abdominal viscera.

Temporary Decompressive and Feeding Gastrostomy: Stamm Technique

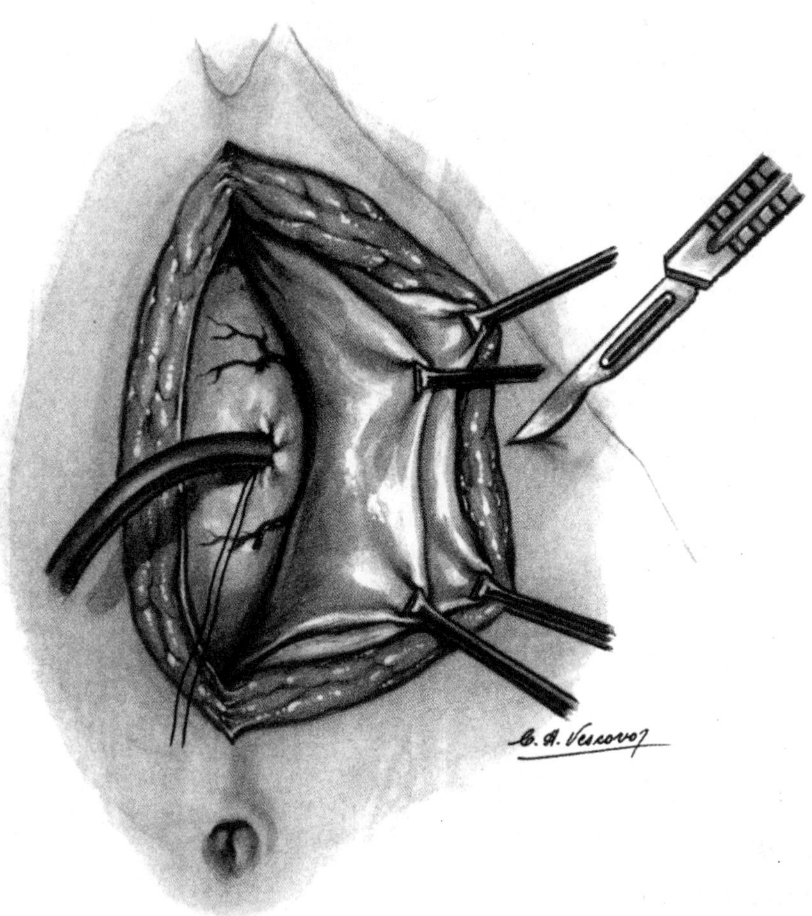

FIGURE 26.9

Temporary Decompressive and Feeding Gastrostomy: Stamm Technique

FIGURE 26.10

The stab wound through which the gastrostomy catheter will be passed has been completed. A large curved clamp has been passed through the stab wound to keep it open to facilitate placement of sutures from the stomach to the parietal peritoneum to protect the exit of the catheter from the rest of the abdominal cavity. This is done by placing three sutures from the seromuscular layer of the stomach to the edge of the peritoneum distal to the catheter and three similar sutures on the proximal side. The drawing shows the sutures from the seromuscular layer of the stomach and the edge of the parietal peritoneum distal to the catheter. The insert shows that the sutures distal to the catheter have been tied.

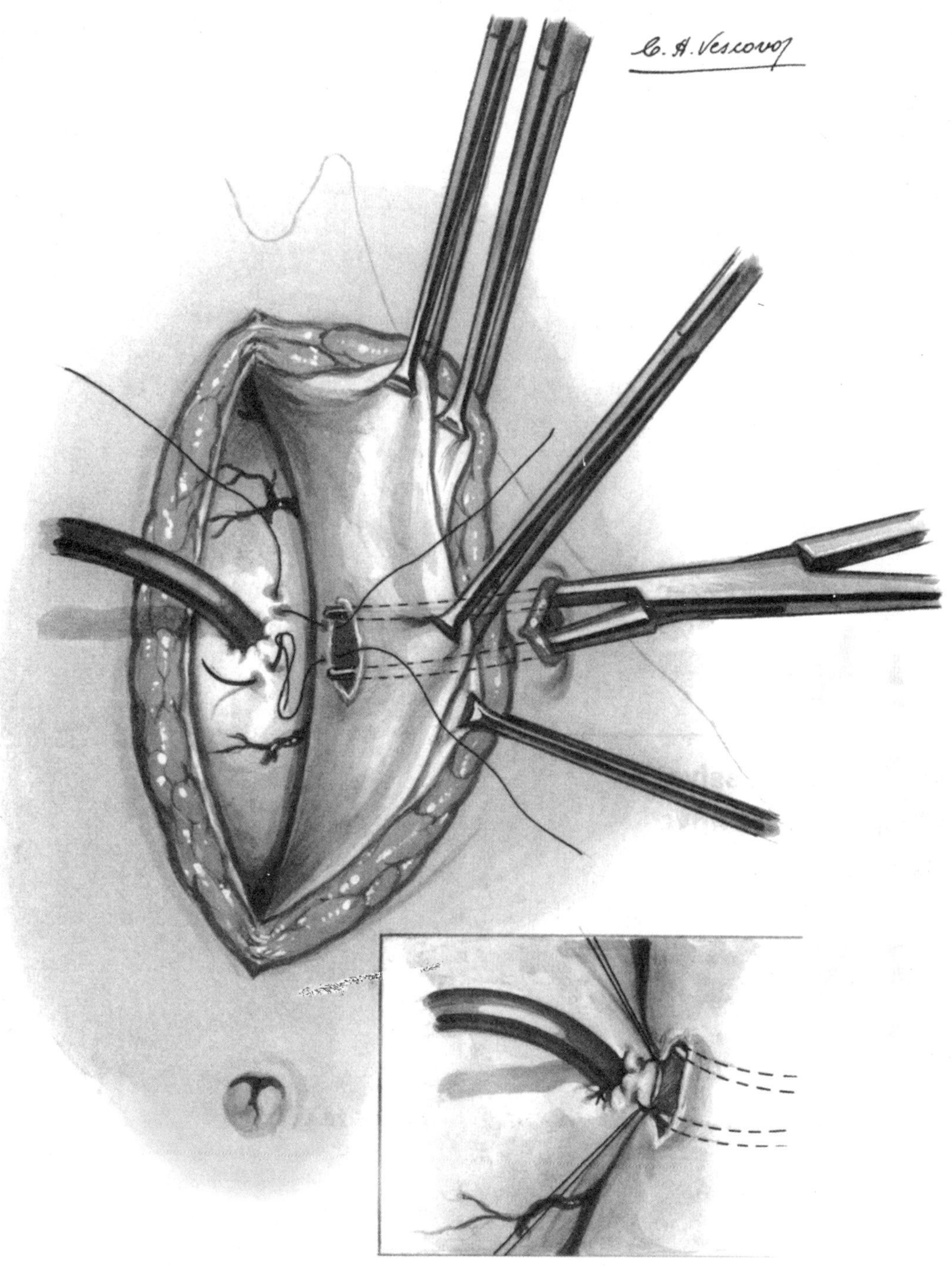

FIGURE 26.10

Temporary Decompressive and Feeding Gastrostomy: Stamm Technique

FIGURE 26.11
Once the distal sutures have been inserted and tied, the catheter is passed through the stab wound. In order to do this, the clamp through the stab wound has been opened to grasp the end of the Pezzer catheter and bring it to the outside.

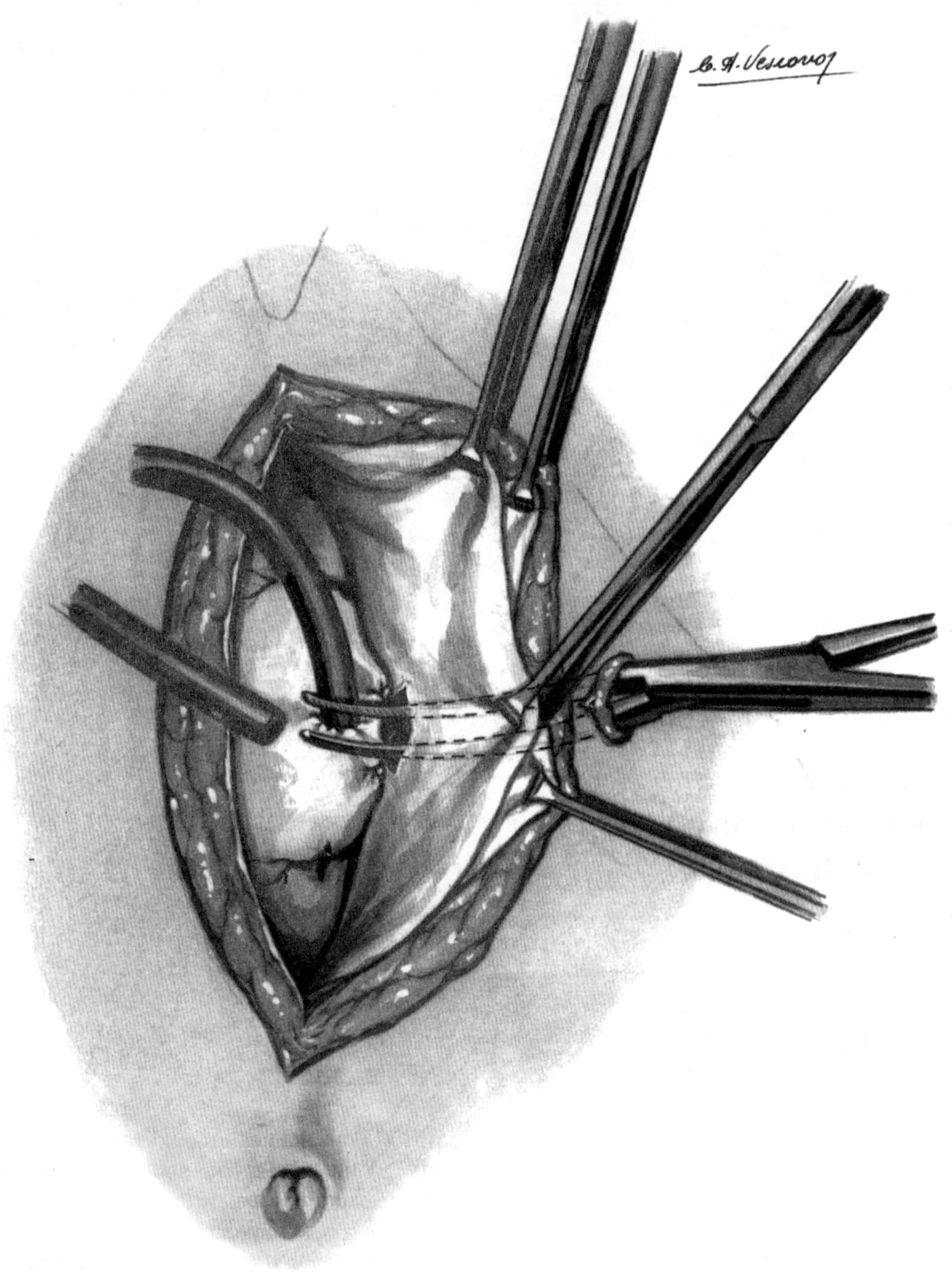

FIGURE 26.11

Temporary Decompressive and Feeding Gastrostomy: Stamm Technique

FIGURE 26.12
The Pezzer catheter has been passed through the stab wound. The proximal sutures from the seromuscular layer of the stomach and the edge of the parietal peritoneum are in place. The upper suture has been tied. The insert shows that the peritoneum around the catheter has been completely blocked off and the catheter has been carefully fixed to the skin of the stab wound to keep it from being accidentally displaced. Blocking off the peritoneum around the gastrostomy orifice is of capital importance to avoid filtration of gastric secretions.

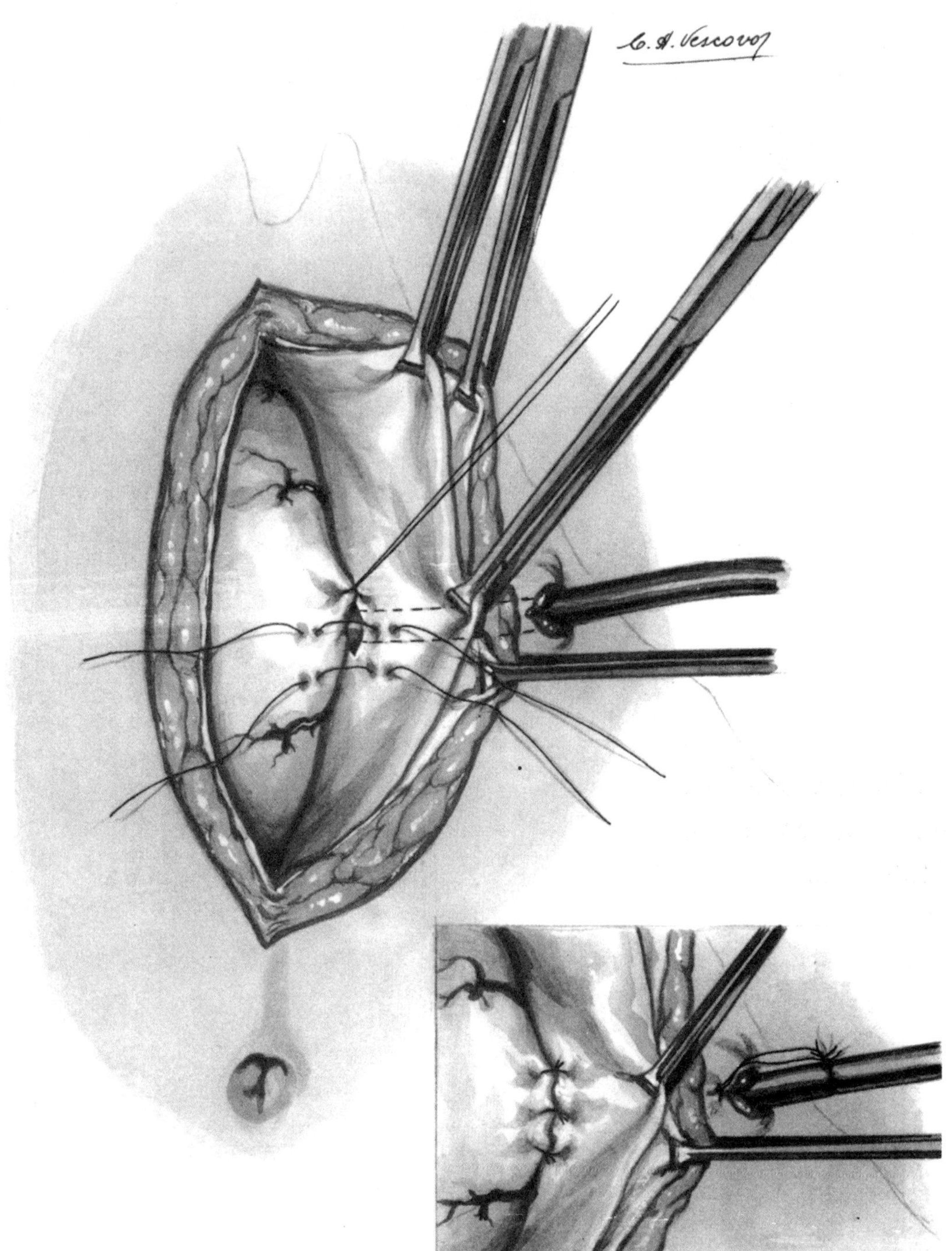

FIGURE 26.12

Temporary Decompressive and Feeding Gastrostomy: Stamm Technique

FIGURE 26.13
The operation is over. The midline incision has been closed in layers. The Pezzer catheter has been connected to a bottle to the left of the patient's bed. Gastric contents will drain by gravity.

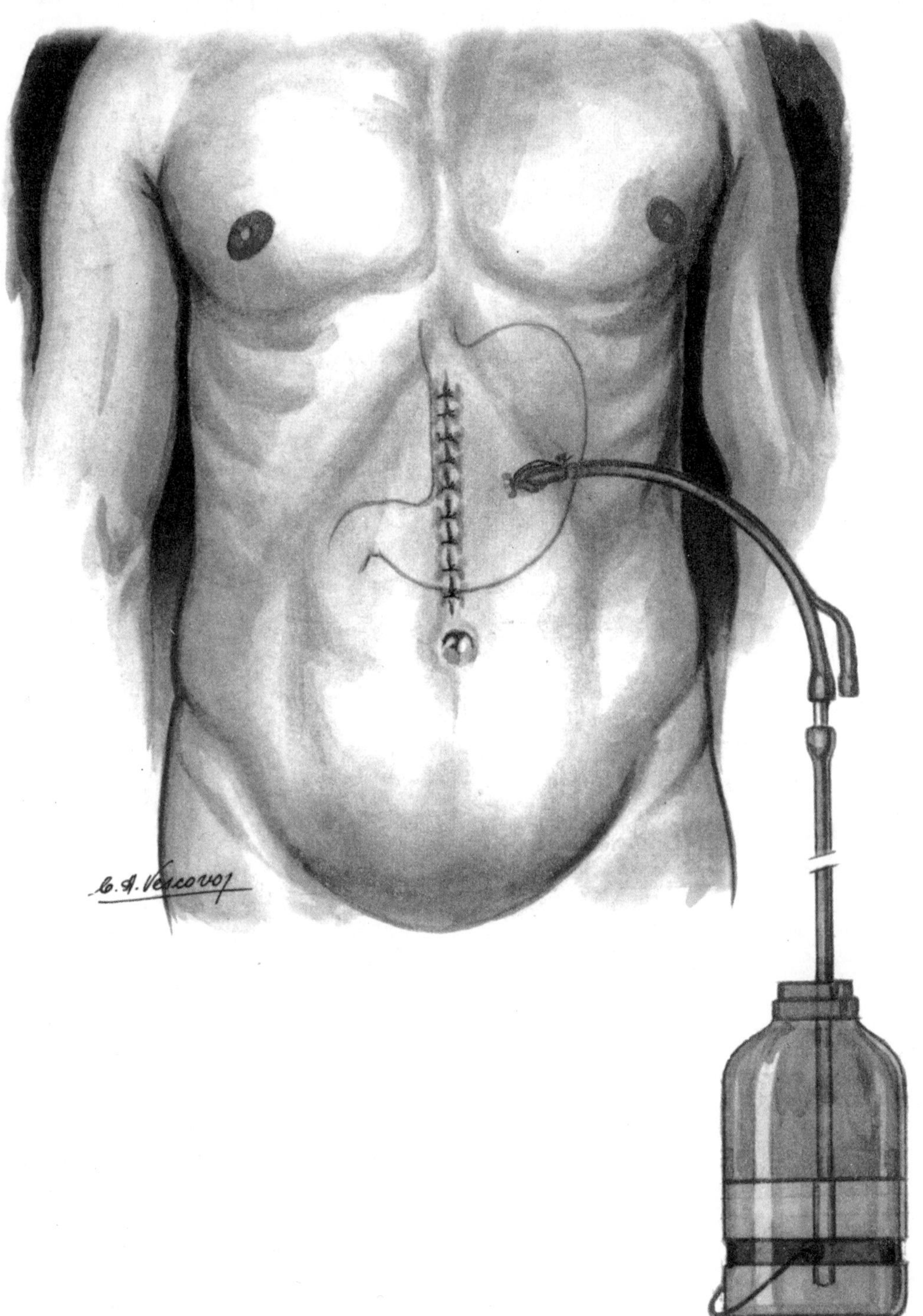

FIGURE 26.13

Temporary Decompressive and Feeding Gastrostomy: Stamm Technique

FIGURE 26.14

If a Foley catheter is to be used instead of a Malecot or a Pezzer, it is advisable to pass the end of the Foley through the stab wound and then insert it into the stomach where submucosal layer hemostasis has been carried out, the seromuscular purse string has been inserted, and the gastric mucosa has been incised. The second purse string is then tied and the balloon inflated in the stomach. If it is considered necessary, a third purse string is inserted and then the peritoneum around the catheter is blocked off in the same way as with the Pezzer catheter.

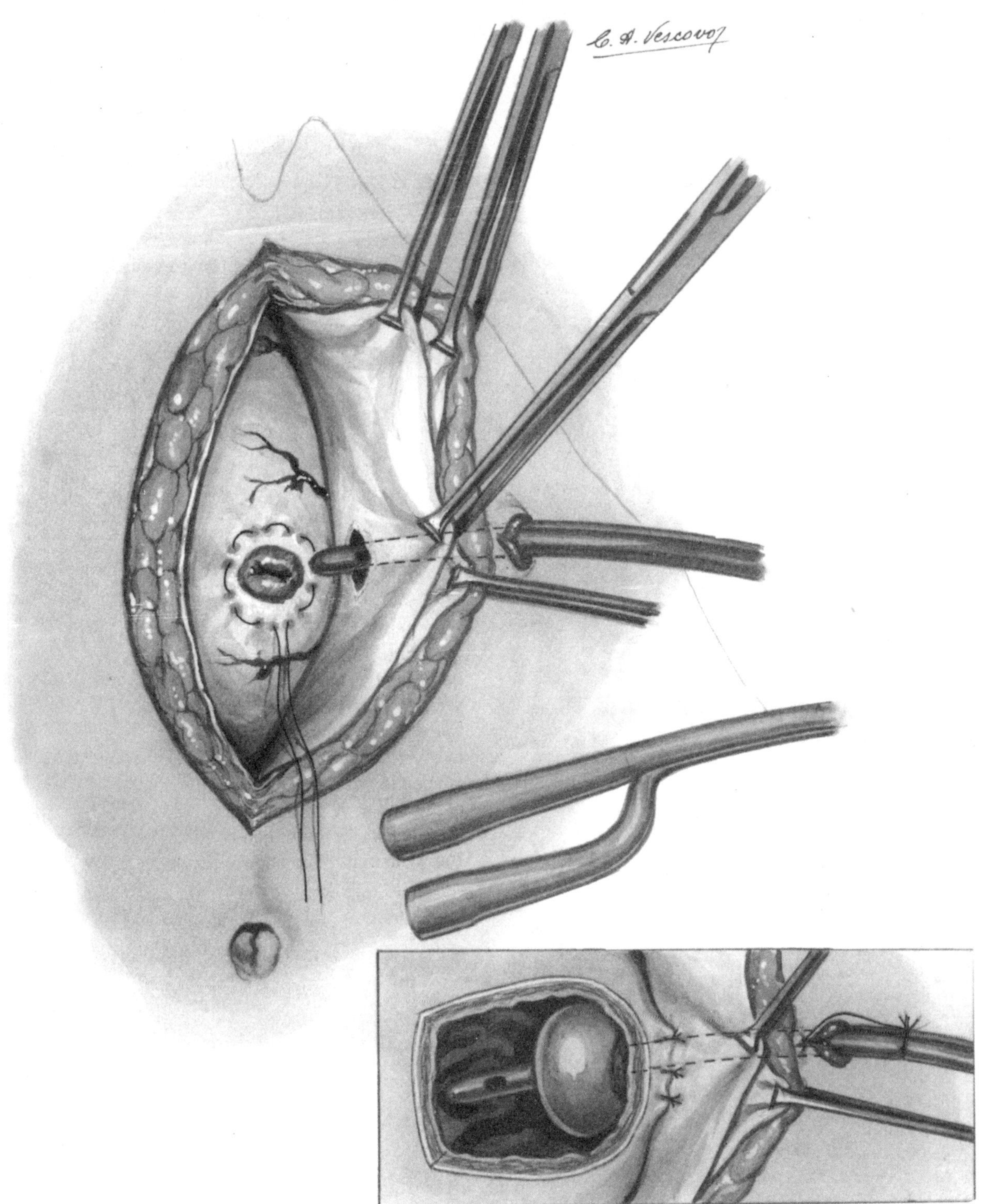

FIGURE 26.14

Depage-Janeway Technique with Manual Sutures

FIGURE 26.15
The drawing shows by means of a broken line a rectangle of the anterior gastric wall. Its superior border is 1.5 cm from the lesser curvature and its base some 2.5 cm from the greater curvature. This broken line shows where the stomach wall will be incised to form a flap with which a gastric tube will be developed to connect the gastric lumen with the outside, through the anterior abdominal wall. The gastric flap should be 8 cm long and must be no less than 4 cm wide, which is the length needed to pass through the anterior abdominal wall. The width of the flap should be carefully calculated to be sure the 18 to 22 F feeding catheter can be easily introduced and removed. The width of the flap should therefore be no less than 5 cm.

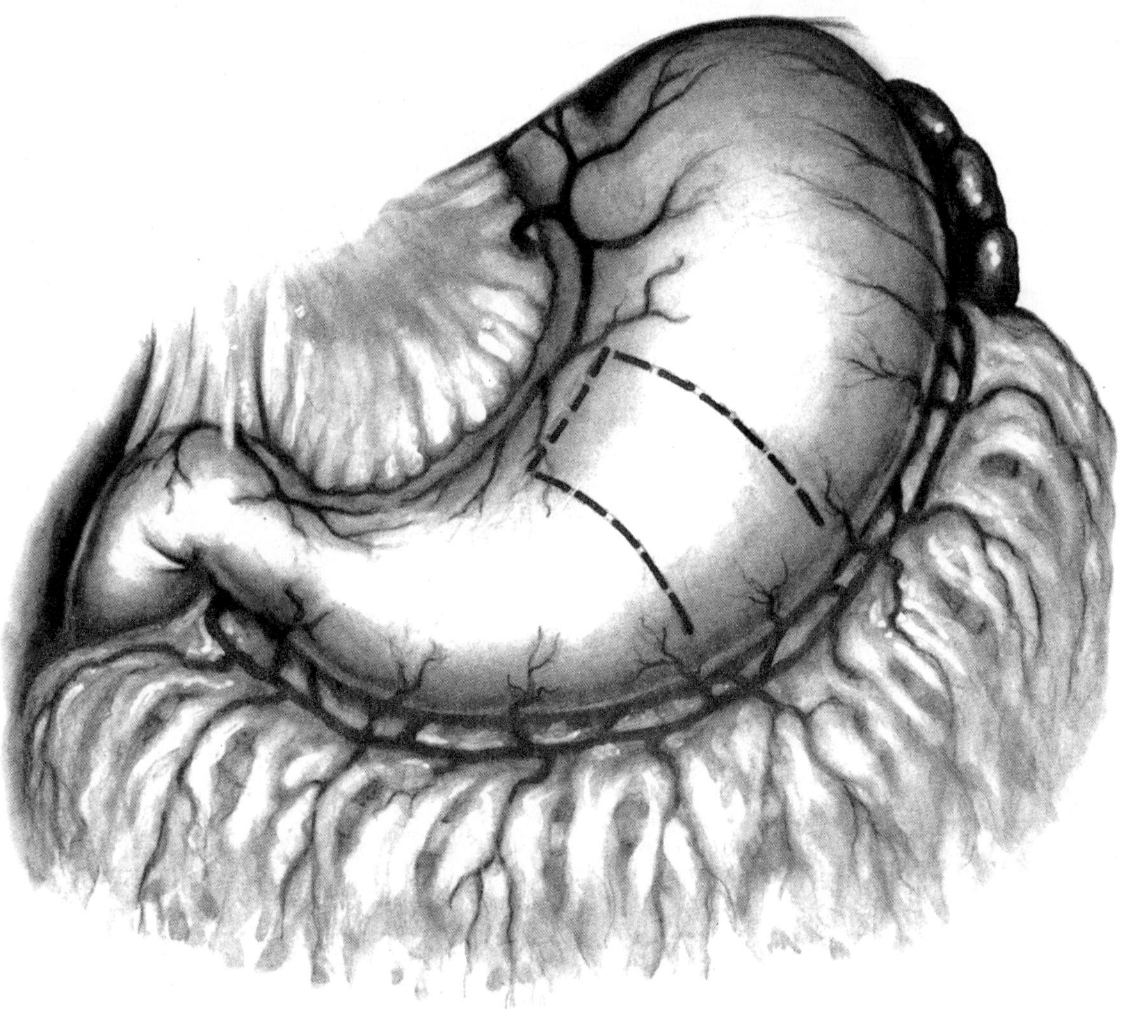

FIGURE 26.15

Depage-Janeway Technique with Manual Sutures

FIGURE 26.16
Once the anterior gastric wall is incised, the tube is constructed. To do this, traction is applied to the lesser curvature by means of an Allis clamp and two other Allis clamps are used to apply traction to the gastric flap. The insert shows the first layer of sutures being placed on the gastric tube. This layer is done as a continuous suture, using 2-0 chromic catgut, with the feeding catheter in place to facilitate the construction of the tube and better calculate its diameter.

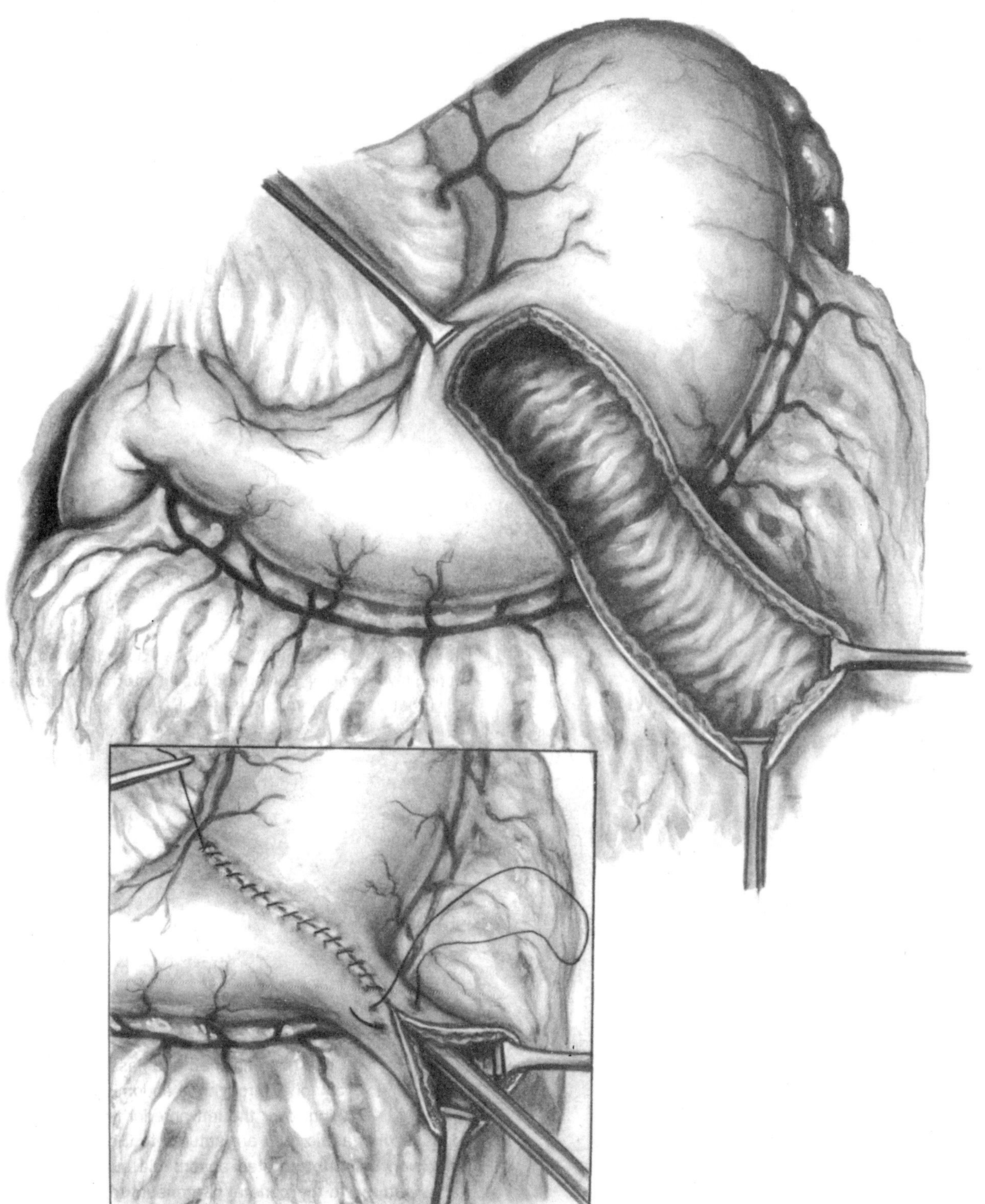

FIGURE 26.16

FIGURE 26.17
The first layer of continuous suture has been finished, and the second layer is being performed, using interrupted cotton, silk, or synthetic nonabsorbable material.

Depage-Janeway Technique with Manual Sutures

FIGURE 26.18
The gastric tube has been finished and passed through a stab wound 1.5 to 2 cm long, through the abdominal wall, to the left of the main incision, over the left anterior rectus muscle. The edges of the gastric tube are sutured to the skin of the counterincision using interrupted absorbable sutures. The gastric wall is sutured to the parietal peritoneum to keep gastric contractions from causing retraction of the gastric tube with possible dehiscence of the suture line and leakage into the peritoneal cavity. The feeding tube should not be removed during the first 10 days postoperatively. This time is necessary for the sutures to heal. After these 10 days the catheter will be introduced for feeding and immediately removed. The insert shows the location of the opening of the gastrostomy over the left anterior rectus muscle, to the left of the midline incision, a few centimeters from the costal margin.

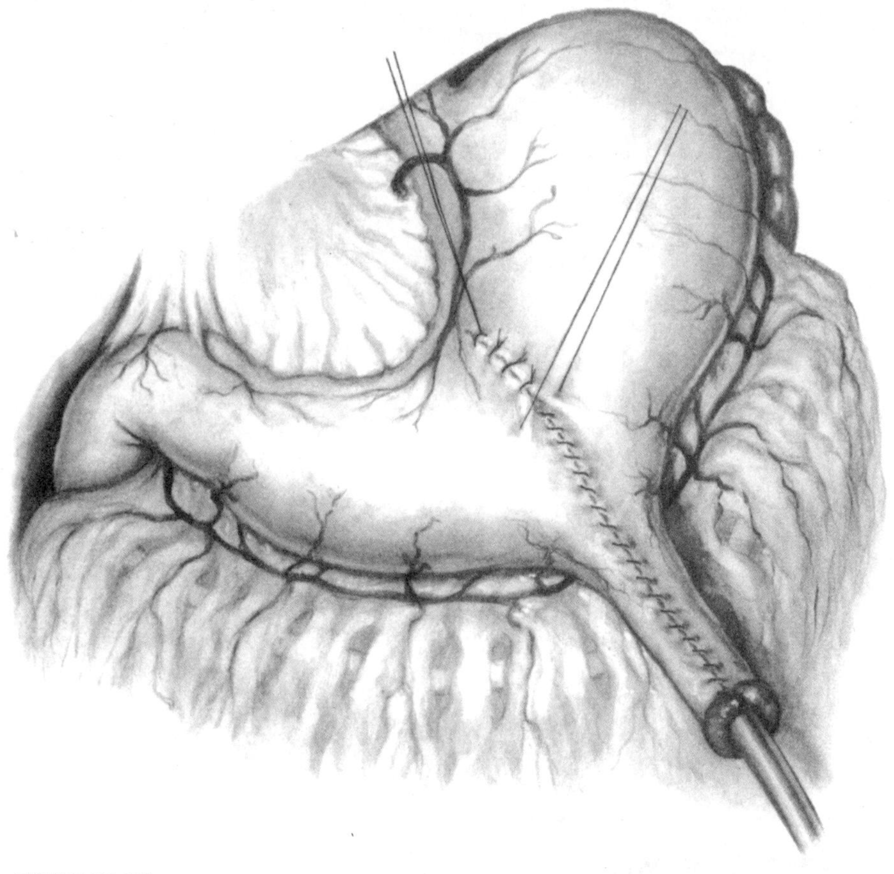

FIGURE 26.17

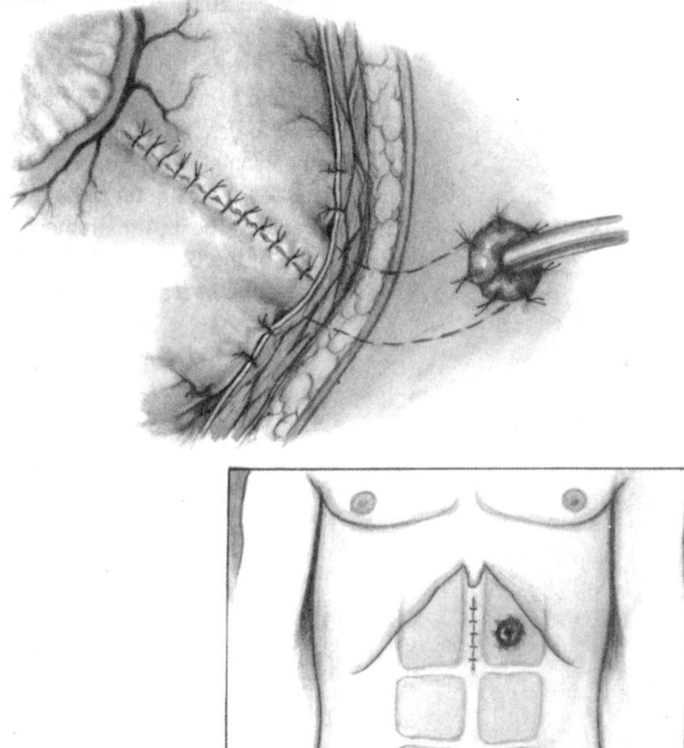

FIGURE 26.18

Depage-Janeway Technique with Stapler

FIGURE 26.19 DEPAGE-JANEWAY TECHNIQUE WITH STAPLER The Depage-Janeway technique can be performed with a stapler, in the following manner. Traction is applied upward by means of two Babcock clamps applied to the anterior gastric wall to construct an 8- to 10-cm-long gastric tube. In addition, the diameter of the tube should be calculated to allow an 18 to 22 F catheter to be introduced and removed to feed the patient. The GIA instrument is placed as shown. The suture line of the GIA instrument should stop about 2.5 cm from the greater curvature.

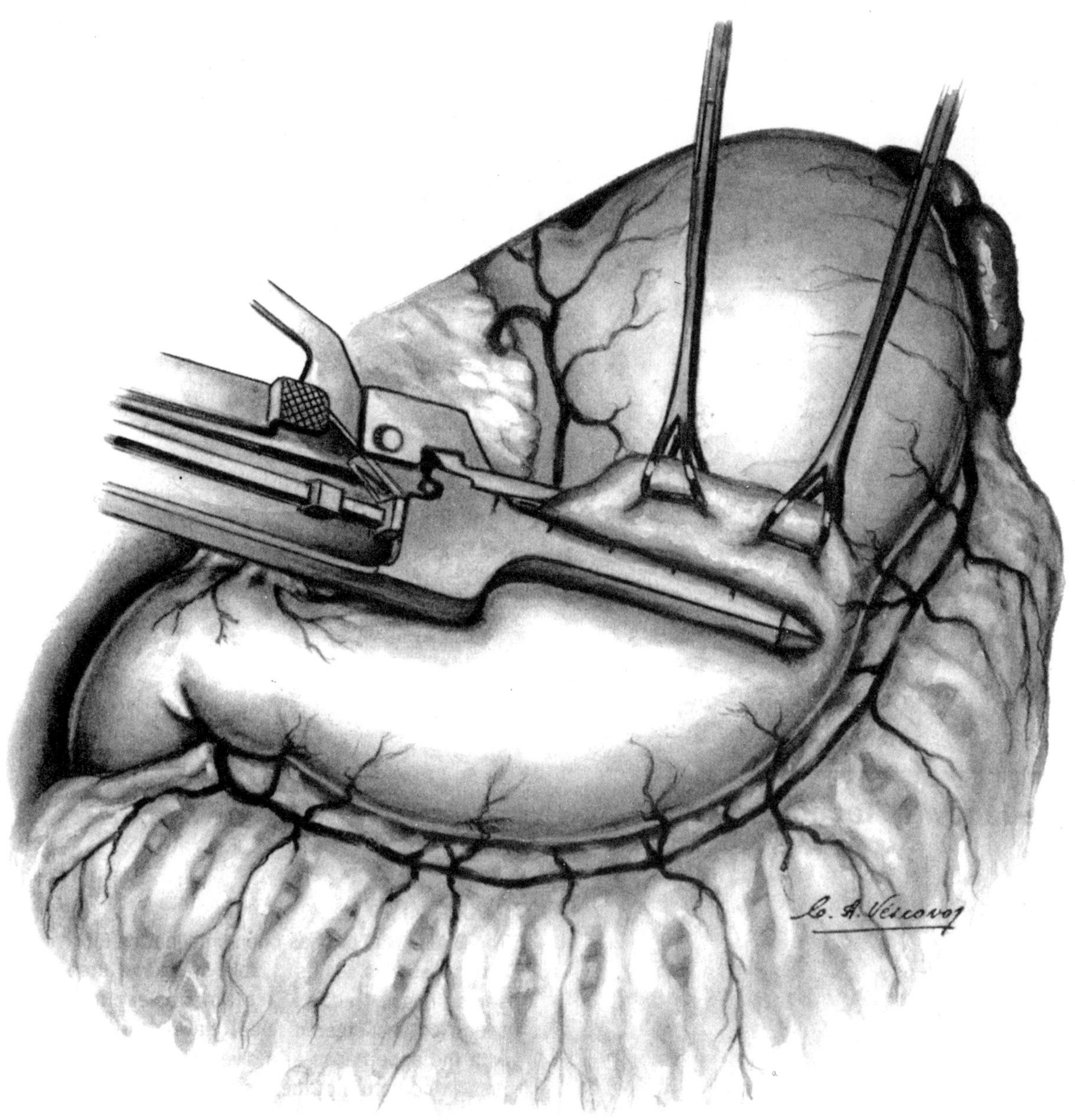

FIGURE 26.19 DEPAGE-JANEWAY TECHNIQUE WITH STAPLER

Depage-Janeway Technique with Stapler

FIGURE 26.20
The GIA instrument has been fired leaving four rows of staples, two on each side, as double staggered staple lines. At the same firing the knife of the GIA stapler cuts the stomach between both staggered lines, leaving the closed gastric tube with the appearance of a diverticulum with the base near the greater curvature of the stomach.

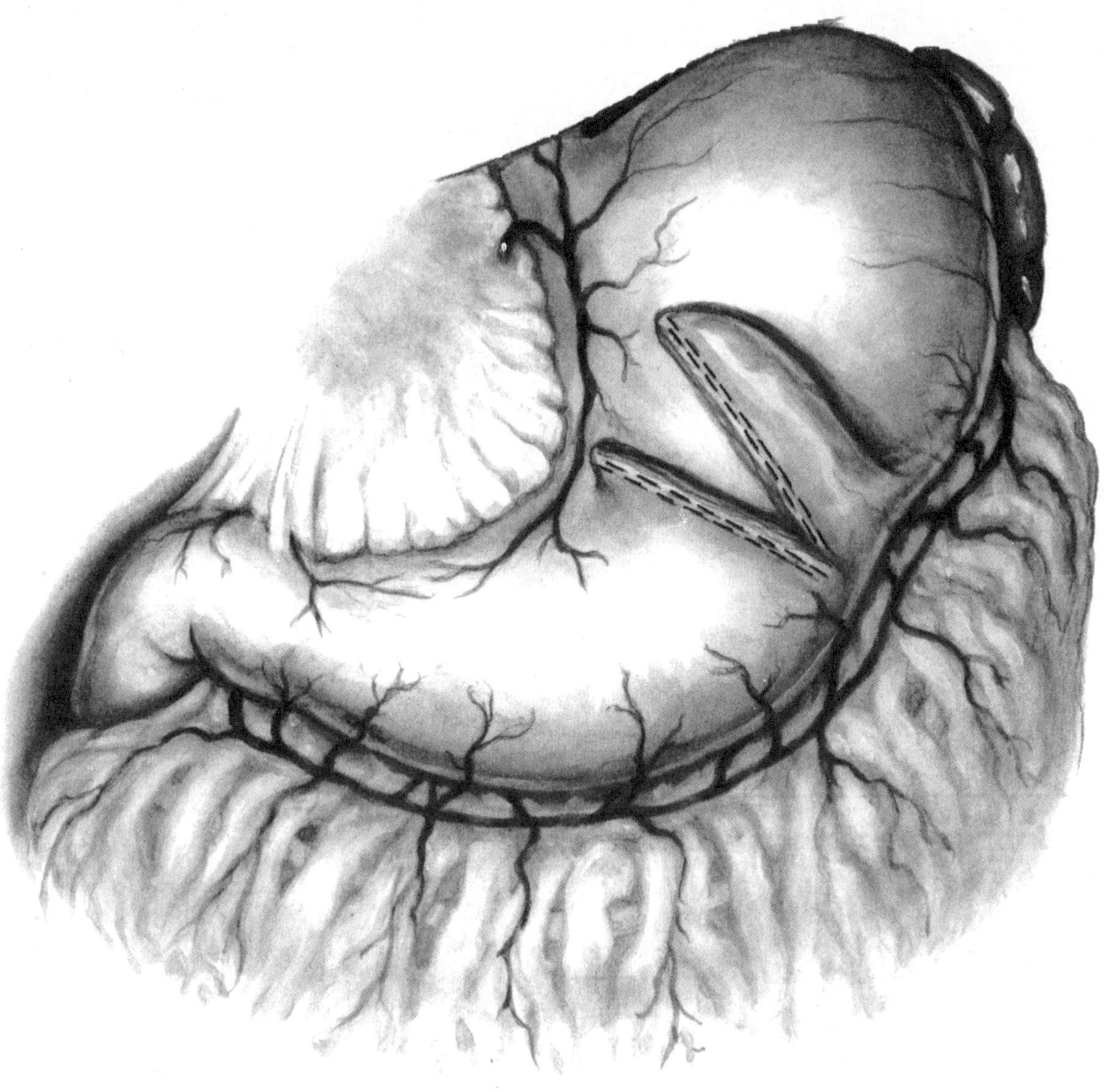

FIGURE 26.20

Depage-Janeway Technique with Stapler

FIGURE 26.21
Using interrupted cotton or silk sutures, the GIA suture line is inverted to make it safer.

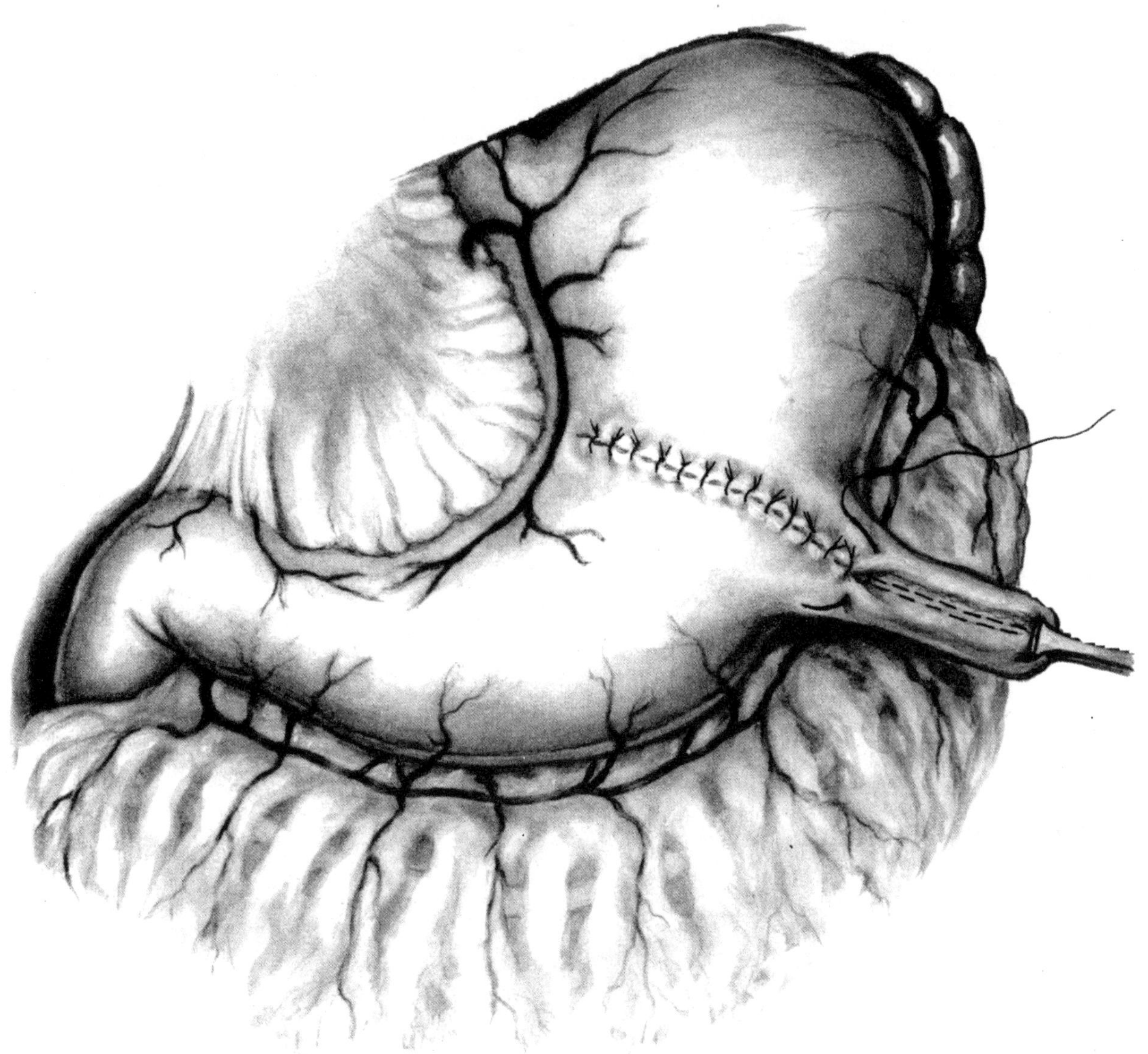

FIGURE 26.21

Depage-Janeway Technique with Stapler

FIGURE 26.22
A stab wound 1.5 to 2 cm long is made to the left of the incision, over the middle of the left anterior rectus muscle. The gastric tube is passed through this stab wound. This is done by passing an Allis clamp through the stab wound, grasping the end of the tube, and bringing it to the outside. The gastric body is fixed with several sutures to the parietal peritoneum to keep the tube from retracting. The end of the constructed gastric diverticulum is incised, bleeding is controlled, and an 18 to 22 F feeding catheter is introduced. This tube will be left in place for one week. The edges of the gastric tube are sutured to the skin with absorbable sutures.

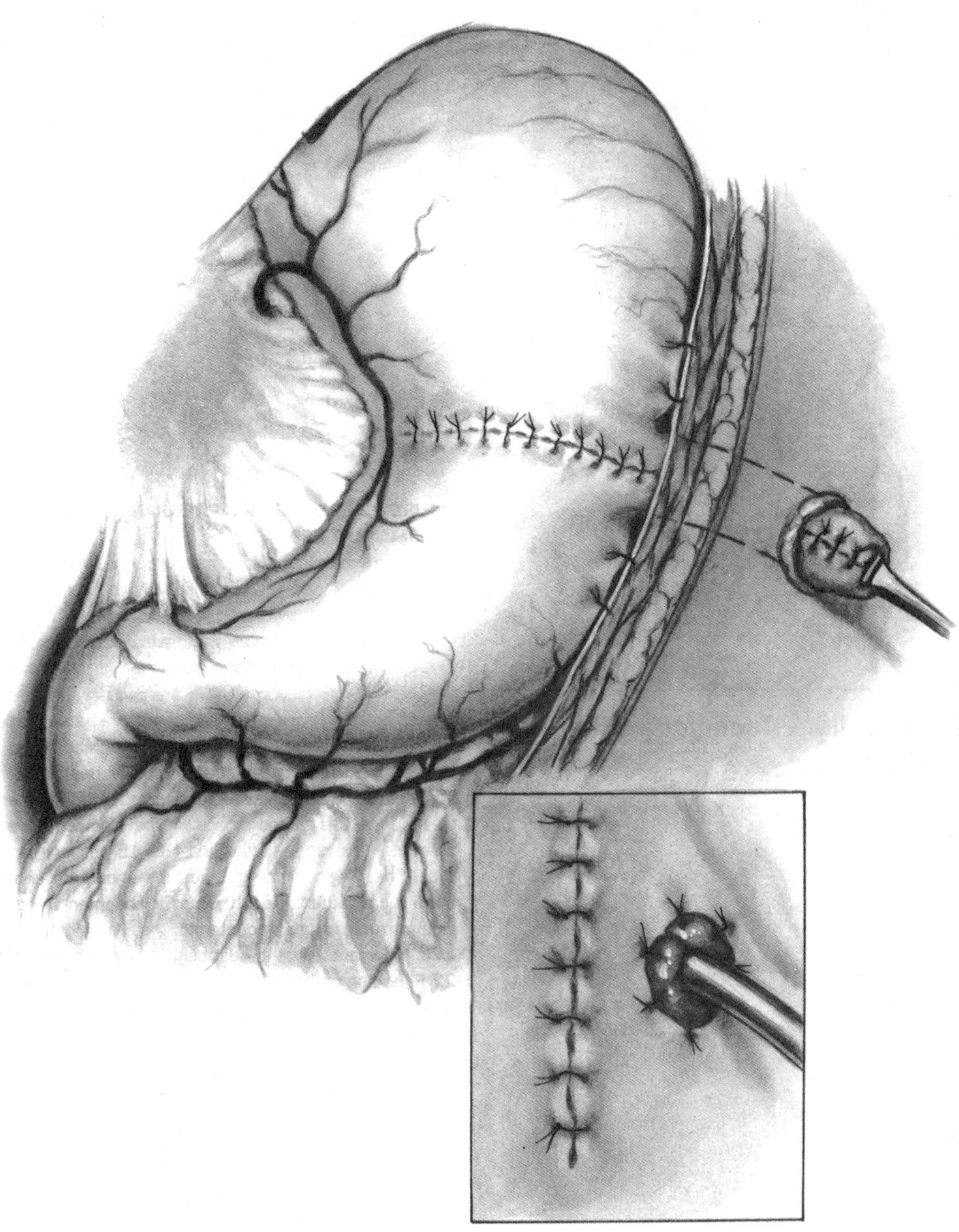

FIGURE 26.22

Beck-Carrel-Jianu Technique with Manual Sutures

FIGURE 26.23 BECK-CARREL-JIANU TECHNIQUE WITH MANUAL SUTURES

This technique consists of constructing a gastric tube at the expense of the greater curvature with its base in the proximal part of the stomach. The operation is begun by dividing the gastrocolic ligament below the gastroepiploic arcade in order to preserve circulation to the greater curvature of the stomach. The right gastroepiploic vessels are divided at the level of the gastric antrum in order to place two curved atraumatic clamps parallel to the longitudinal axis of the stomach. The stomach is then divided between the clamps with straight scissors, strictly following the greater curvature. Traction is then applied to separate the gastric tube from the stomach for a few centimeters. The tube is usually 14 to 15 cm long and 2.5 cm wide. The length of the gastric tube should be enough to be able to carry the tube to the upper abdomen where it will be exteriorized through a counterincision. The width of the tube is also important, since it must permit easy passage of the 18 to 22 F feeding catheter. The gastric tube is supplied by the left gastroepiploic artery.

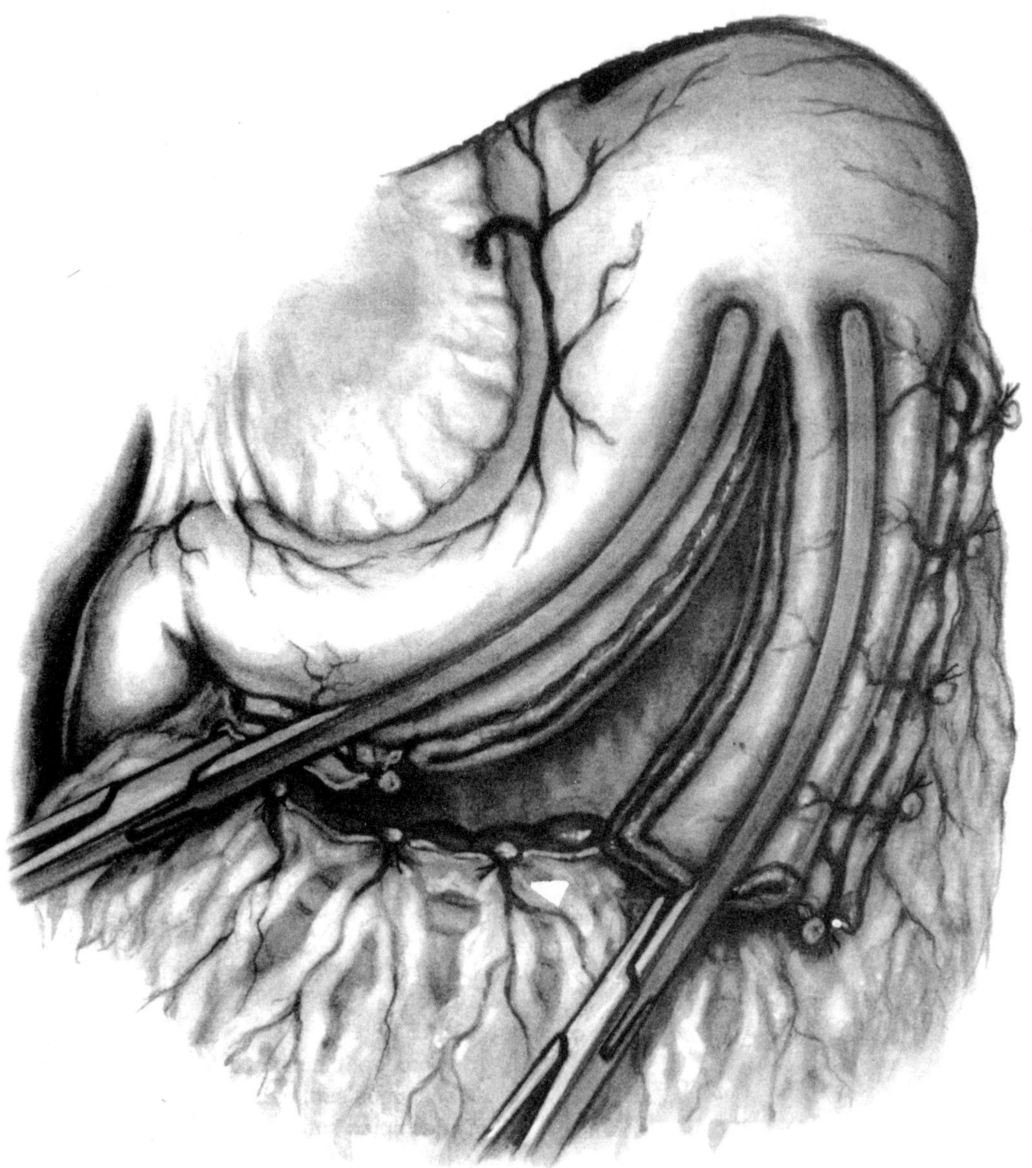

FIGURE 26.23 BECK-CARREL-JIANU TECHNIQUE WITH MANUAL SUTURES

Beck-Carrel-Jianu Technique with Manual Sutures

FIGURE 26.24

The border of the stomach and the gastric tube are closed with a continuous suture using absorbable material. A second layer of interrupted sutures using nonabsorbable material is then inserted. The insert shows the finished operation. The gastric tube is exteriorized through a stab wound high in the abdomen, to the left of the midline, over the left anterior rectus muscle. The edges of the gastric tube are sutured to the skin using interrupted sutures of absorbable material. The insert shows the completed operation, without the feeding tube in place, which as has been said, should be left in place for 10 days following surgery.

Rutkowsky Technique with Stapler: This technique is similar to the Beck-Carrel-Jianu method, with the difference that the tube constructed at the expense of the greater curvature of the stomach is based distally, in the gastric antrum. The blood supply of the gastric tube will come from the right gastroepiploic artery, which has a better blood flow than the left. With this technique the motor activity of the gastric tube will be isoperistaltic and not antiperistaltic, as in the Beck-Carrel-Jianu technique. The Rutkowsky technique can be carried out manually or with a stapler. We will describe the technique using staplers.

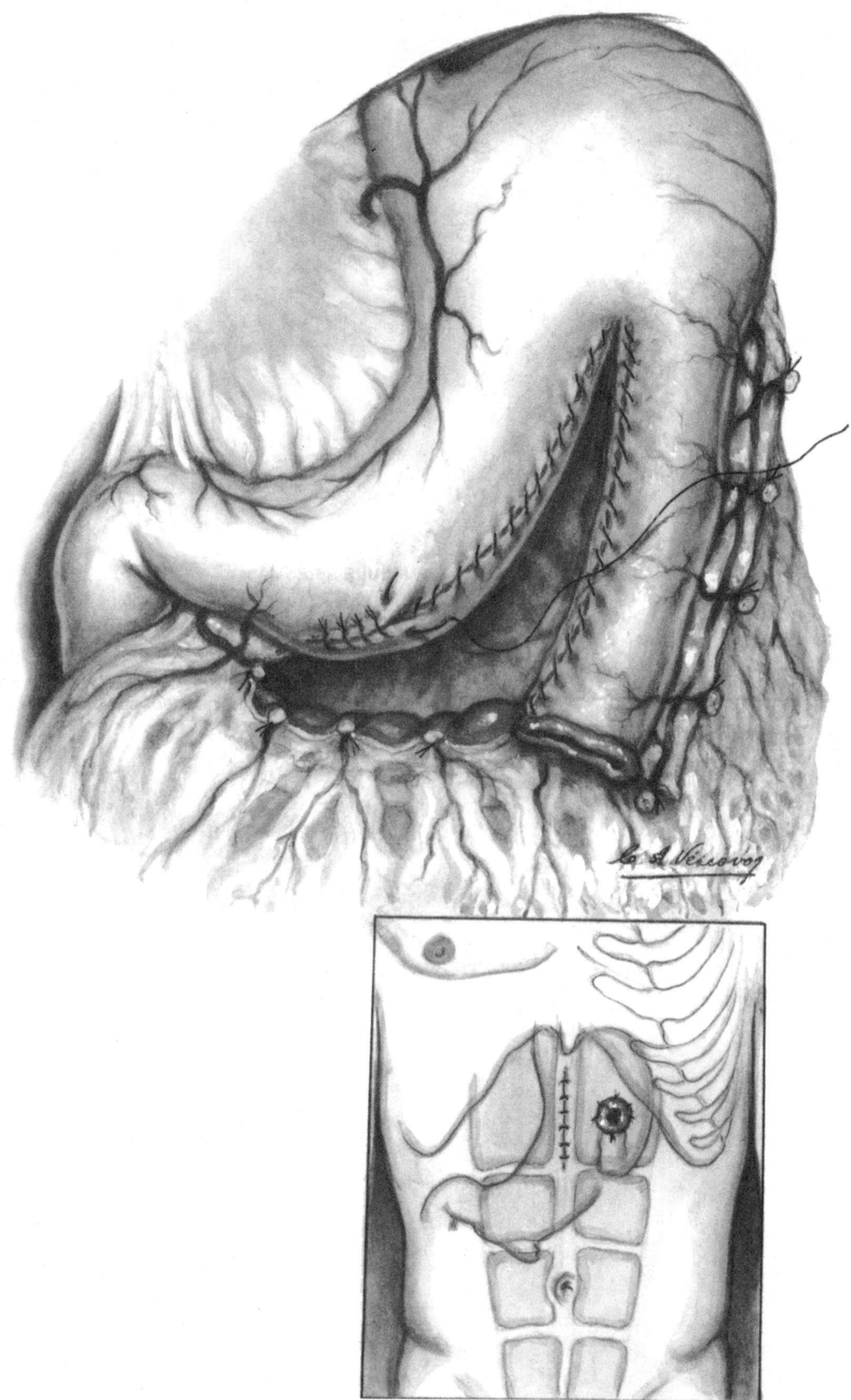

FIGURE 26.24

FIGURE 26.25
The procedure is started by dividing the gastrocolic ligament below the gastroepiploic arcade. The left gastroepiploic vessels are tied and divided to allow insertion of the GIA stapler. Using two Babcock clamps to apply traction to the stomach, the GIA instrument is inserted, pointing distally, as seen.

Rutkowsky Technique with Stapler

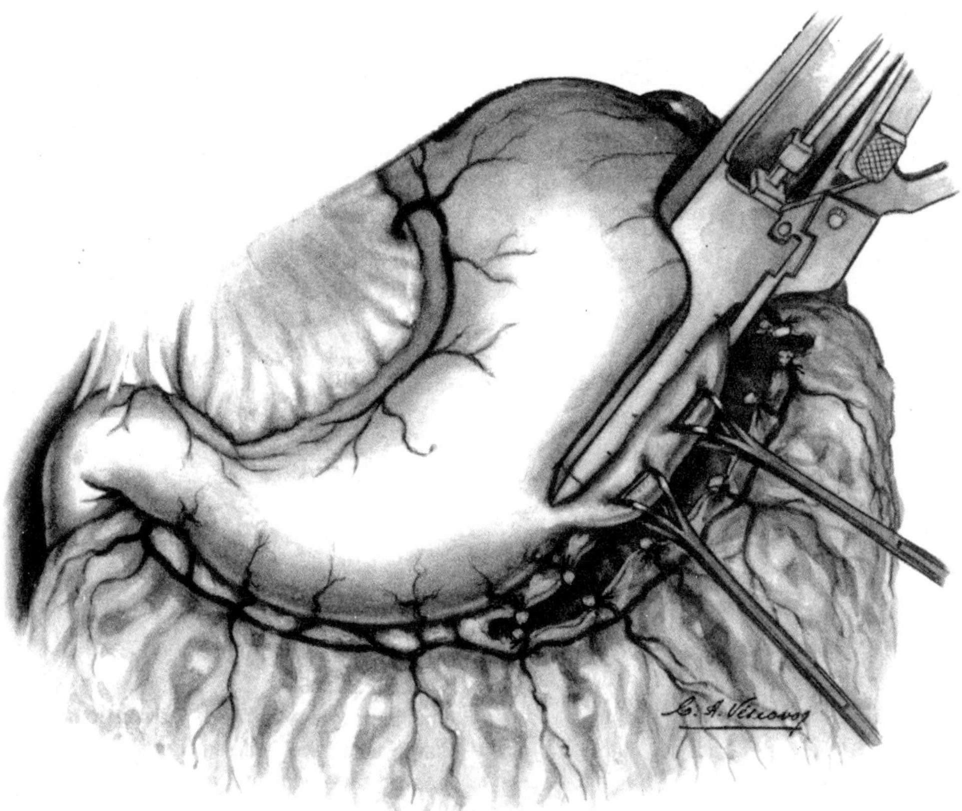

FIGURE 26.25

FIGURE 26.26
The instrument is fired, leaving four rows of staples. At the same time, the knife in the GIA cuts the stomach, creating a gastric tube with two rows of staggered staples and its base near the gastric antrum. The suture lines made with the GIA are inverted with interrupted nonabsorbable sutures to make them more secure.

Rutkowsky Technique with Stapler

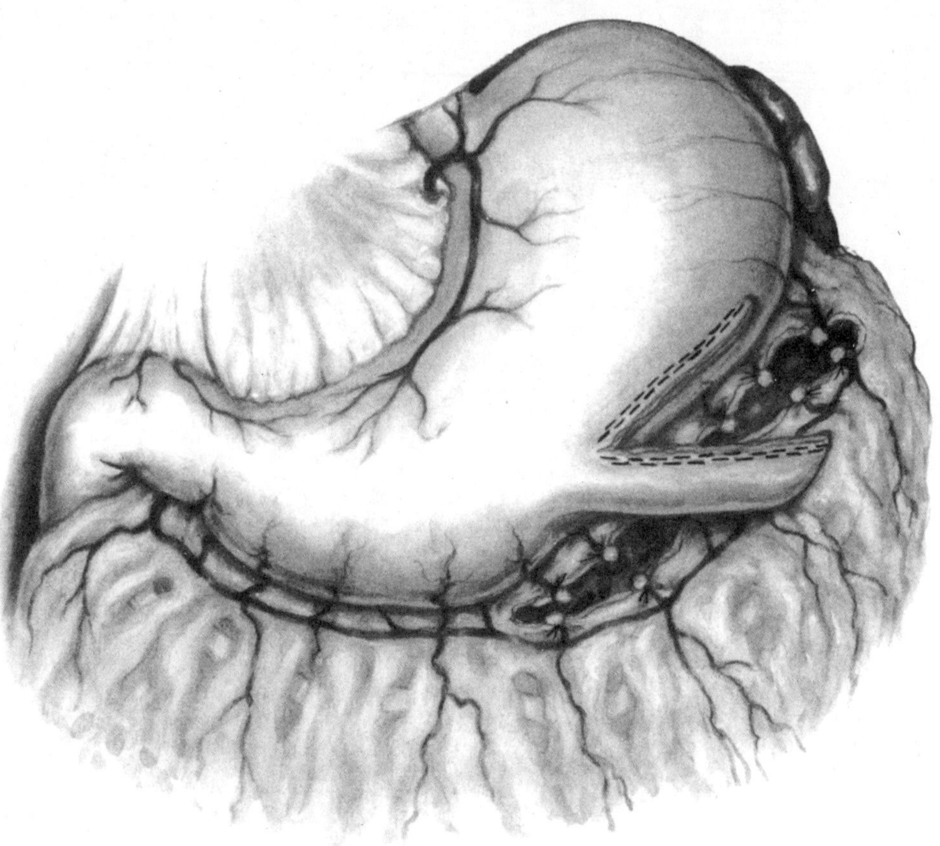

FIGURE 26.26

Rutkowsky Technique with Stapler

FIGURE 26.27
The gastric tube is exteriorized through a stab wound in the anterior abdominal wall. To keep the gastric tube from retracting, the stomach is fixed to the parietal peritoneum with some nonabsorbable sutures. The end of the gastric tube is sutured to the skin with absorbable sutures, leaving the feeding tube in place.

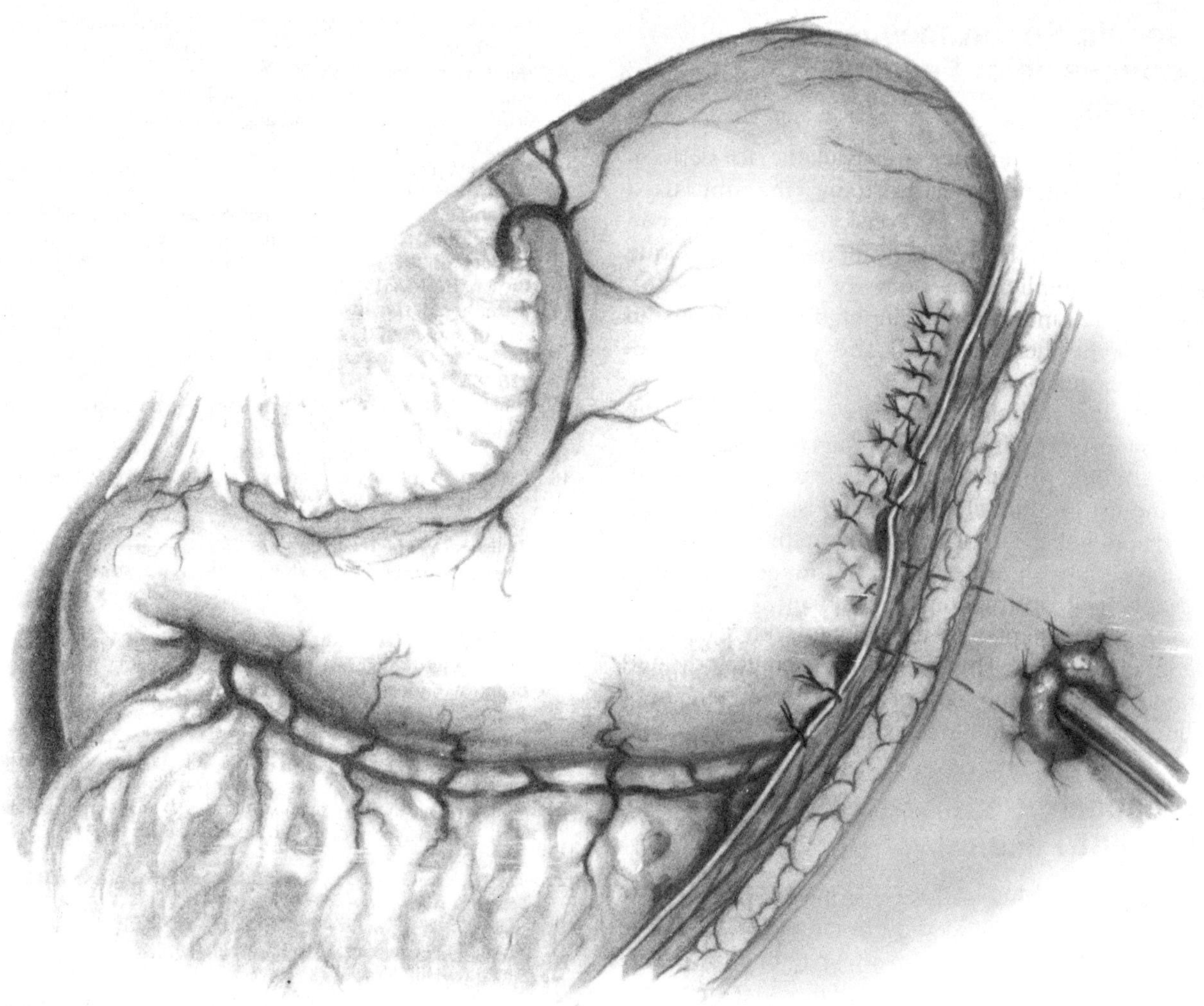

FIGURE 26.27

Endoscopic Percutaneous Decompressive or Feeding Gastrostomy

Although several techniques are available to perform endoscopic percutaneous gastrostomy, the one used most is the one proposed by Ponsky and Gauderer in 1981 (21) with some later modifications. This technique is not free of complications, some of them serious (6). The most exact indication is in high-risk patients in whom local anesthesia is used. This procedure is becoming increasingly popular.

In short, the technique consists in expanding the stomach by insufflation until the stomach wall is in contact with the anterior abdominal wall. With transillumination, and using a Russel kit, the gastrostomy tube is introduced and well secured to the abdominal wall.

This procedure should not be performed in patients with esophageal obstruction or esophageal varices, in gastrectomized patients, or in patients with gastric or duodenal obstruction. This procedure is contraindicated in patients in whom the light of the gastroscope cannot transilluminate the abdominal wall.

Laparoscopic Gastrostomy for Permanent Feeding

The possibility of using stapling instruments through the laparoscope has permitted performing permanent gastrostomies by the Depage-Janeway technique in a very similar way as with the abdomen open.

References

1. Connar, R.G., Sealy, W.C. Gastrostomy and its complications. Ann. Surg. 143:245, 1956.
2. Corachán, M. Cirugía gástrica. Vol. 2, p. 213. Salvat, Barcelona, 1934.
3. Chassin, J.L. Operative strategy in general surgery. Vol. 1, p. 192. Springer-Verlag, New York, 1980.
4. Davis, J.B. Jr., Bowden, T.A., Roves, D.A. Percutaneous endoscopic gastroenterologists get the same results? Am. Surg. 56:47, 1990.
5. Depage, A. Nouveau procédé pour la gastrostomie. J. Chir. Ann. Soc. Belg. Chir. 1:715:1901.
6. Ditesheim, J.A., Richards, W., Sharp, K. Fatal and disastrous complications following percutaneous endoscopic gastrostomy. Am. Surg. 55:92, 1989.
7. Egeberg, quoted by Corachán, M. Cirugía gástrica. Vol. 2, p. 215, Salvat, Barcelona, 1934.
8. Farris, J.M., Smith, G.K. An evaluation of temporary gastrostomy. Ann. Surg. 144:457, 1956.
9. Glassman, J.A. Some modifications on aseptic double valved tube-gastrostomy. Surg. Gynecol. Obstet. 74:843, 1942.
10. Ho, C.S., Yee, A.C.N., McPherson, R. Complications of surgical and percutaneous non endoscopic gastrostomy. Review of 233 patients. Gastroenterology 95:1206, 1988.
11. Hunter, J.G., Laurentano, L., Shellito, P.C. Percutaneous endoscopic gastrostomy in head and neck cancer patients. Ann. Surg. 210:42, 1989.
12. Janeway, H.H. Eine neue gastrostomie-methode. Munch. Med. Wochenschr. 60:1705, 1913.
13. Jesseph, J.E., Csicsko J.F. Miscellaneous techniques for operations on the stomach and duodenum. In Nyhus, L.M., Westell, C. (Eds.). Surgery of the stomach and duodenum. Ed. 3, p. 715. Little, Brown, Boston, 1977.
14. Jesseph, J.M. Gastrostomy. In Nyhus, L.M., Baker, R.J. (Eds.). Mastery of surgery. Ed. 2, vol. 1, p. 633. Little, Brown, Boston, 1992.
15. Jianu, A. Gastrostomie und oesophagoplastik. Dtsch. Z. Chir. 118:383, 1912.
16. Jones, S. Gastrostomy for stricture (cancerous) of esophagus. Lancet 1:678, 1875.
17. Kader, B. Zur technik der gastrostomie. Zentralbl. Chir. 23:665, 1896.
18. Lathrop, J.C., Felix, E.J., Lauber, D. Laparoscopic Janeway gastrostomy using an endoscopic stapling device. J. Laparoendosc. Surg. 1:335, 1991.
19. Ochsner, A. The relative merits of temporary gastrostomy and nasogastric suction of the stomach. Postgrad. Med. 35:358, 1964.
20. Patton, R. A modified valvular gastrostomy. Arch. Surg. 70:859, 1955.
21. Ponsky, J.L., Gauderer, M.W. Percutaneous endoscopic gastrostomy: A nonoperative technique for feeding gastrostomy. Gastrointest. Endosc. 27:9, 1981.
22. Ponsky, J.L. Percutaneous endoscopic stomas. Surg. Clin. North Am. 69:1227, 1989.
23. Reiner, D.S., Leitman, I.M., Ward, R.J. Laparoscopic Stamm Gastrostomy with gastropexy. Surg. Laparosc. Endosc. 1:189, 1991.
24. Rutkowsky, quoted by Christmann, F.E., Ottolenghi, C.E., Raffo, J.M., von Grolman, G. Técnica quirrgica. Ed. 10, p. 732. El Ateneo, Buenos Aires, 1970.
25. Sacks, B.A., Glotzer, D.J. Percutaneous re-establishment of feeding gastrostomies. Surgery 85:575, 1979.
26. Sangster, W., Hunter, J.G. Surgical access for enteral nutrition. In Hunter, J.G., Sackier, J.M. (Eds.) Minimally invasive surgery. P. 113. McGraw-Hill, New York, 1993.
27. Santiago-Delpín, E.A. The use of T-tubes for gastrostomy. Surg. Gynecol. Obstet. 138:765, 1974.
28. Sédillot, C.E. Observation de gastrostomie. Gaz Hôp 26:160, 1853.
29. Senter, K.L. Complications of temporary tube gastrostomy. Arch. Surg. 81:103, 1960.
30. Shellito, P.C., Malt, R.A. Tube gastrostomy: Techniques and complications. Ann. Surg. 2012:180, 1985.
31. Spivack, J.L. Eine neue methode der gastrostomy. Beitr. Klin. Chir. 147:308, 1929.
32. Spivack, J.L. Evolution of gastrostomy. Am. J. Surg. 69:47, 1945.
33. Stamm, M. Gastrostomy: A new method. M. News. 65:324, 1894.
34. Thorek, M. Tubovalvular gastrostomy. History and technique. J. Mich. Med. Soc. 44:3, 1945.
35. Verneuil, M. Observation de gastrostomie pratiqué avec succès pour rétrécissement cicatriciel infranchissable de l'oesophage. Bull. Acad. Med. (Paris) 5:1023, 1876.
36. Welch, C.E. Gastrostomy. Am. J. Surg. 101:279, 1961.
37. Welch, C.E. Surgery of the stomach and duodenum. Ed. 4, p. 80. Year Book, Chicago, 1969.
38. Wilkinson, W.A., Pickleman, J. Feeding gastrostomy: A reappraisal. Am. Surg. 48:273, 1982.
39. Witzel, O. Zür technic der magenstelanlegung. Zentralbl. Chir. 18:601, 1891.

Section F

Surgery of the Stomach and Duodenum

CHAPTER **27**

Gastrectomy

BILLROTH II GASTRECTOMY

Historical Data

The first successful gastrectomy was performed by Christian Albert Theodor Billroth on January 29, 1881, in Vienna, Austria. The patient, Thérèse Heller, 43 years old, had cancer of the pylorus. The operation performed by Billroth was a very limited resection of the stomach, a pylorectomy, with transection of the gastric antrum only 20 mm proximal to the macroscopic edge of the tumor and the duodenum some 15 mm beyond the pylorus (65). Reestablishment of digestive continuity was carried out by anastomosing the transected duodenum to the cut end of the stomach, on its lesser curvature (21, 51, 52, 55, 58, 65). Later, Billroth performed the anastomosis of the duodenum to the greater curvature side of the transected edge of the stomach (65). This type of reconstruction of the gastrointestinal transit was later designated as a gastrectomy with Billroth I anastomosis. The patient died of metastases 4 months after the surgical intervention (48, 65).

Before Billroth's successful operation, this same procedure had been performed experimentally in dogs by a brilliant disciple of Michaelis, named Daniel Carr Theodor Merren, who, in 1809, when he was only 20 years old (48), successfully carried out, at his teacher's request, the first gastric resections using a technique similar to the one that Billroth used later. The first gastric resection in humans was performed by Jules Péan, of Paris (51), in a patient with cancer of the pylorus, in 1879. The technique used by Péan was similar to the one used by Merren and, later, by Billroth. The patient on whom Péan operated died on the fifth postoperative day. Although an autopsy was not authorized, it is supposed, by the patient's course, that death was due to peritonitis caused by dehiscence of the gastroduodenostomy, which was performed entirely with catgut. Some authors do not discard the possibility that death could have been due to the effect of two small blood transfusions given to the patient, one of 50 mL and the other of 80 mL, in an era in which blood types were unknown. Blood types were discovered 40 years later (65). Another surgeon, also before Billroth, Ludwig

Rydygier (55), Polish, performed a pylorectomy for pyloric cancer in 1880, when he was 29 years old (48). Rydygier's patient died 12 hours following the surgical intervention. In addition, Rydygier performed the first successful pylorectomy for benign pyloric ulcer on November 21, 1881. The editor of the journal *Zentralblatt für Chirurgie,* said, in a footnote, "I expect it to be the last one" (48, 65). In both procedures Rydygier performed the anastomosis of the duodenum to the greater curvature of the stomach.

The gastrectomy technique later designated as the Billroth II technique was carried out by him on January 15, 1885, in Vienna (48, 65), with survival of the patient. Billroth had planned to perform the operation in two stages because it was for an obstructing pyloric cancer. In the first stage he planned to perform only an antecolic gastrojejunostomy, anastomosing a jejunal loop to the anterior gastric wall, above the tumor. In the second stage he planned to resect the stomach distal to the anastomosis, together with the tumor. Since the patient tolerated the gastrojejunostomy well, Billroth decided to go ahead with the resection of the distal stomach and the tumor in the same operation (48, 65). In spite of the fact that the Billroth I operation was the first technique used by Billroth, I will first describe the evolution of the Billroth II technique, since it is more frequently used in the majority of the surgical centers of the world.

Evolution of the Billroth II Technique

The Billroth II gastrectomy has undergone innumerable modifications over the course of time, and has now reached a certain degree of standardization. The modifications particularly refer to the extent of the resection and the type of anastomosis.

The most important modifications will be pointed out in the following. The first modification, certainly a very logical one, was introduced by Ulrich Rudolph Kronlein on May 24, 1888. Krönlein proposed anastomosing the jejunum, not to the anterior or posterior gastric wall, as Billroth continued to do, but to the transected end of the stomach (45, 65). This same modification was first performed by Reichel, in Germany, in 1908, and later by Polya, in Hungary, in 1911 (52, 65). The only difference from the Krönlein procedure is that Reichel, as well as Polya, performed a retrocolic instead of the antecolic anastomosis that Kronlein performed. In the scientific world this modification is unjustly known as the Polya technique.

In 1889, Anton Eiselsberg (65) proposed the reduction of the gastrojejunal anastomotic opening, believing it was not necessary to anastomose the jejunum with the entire diameter of the transected stomach. To carry out this objective, Eiselsberg would close the gastric end on the lesser curvature side, anastomosing only the jejunum to the greater curvature side of the stomach opening. Eiselsberg performed an antecolic gastrojejunostomy, the same as Billroth and Krönlein.

In 1905 Franz von Hofmeister in Germany, and later, Hans Finsterer, of Vienna, in 1914, also proposed making the anastomotic opening smaller but by the retrocolic route (48, 65). In addition, these surgeons, after closing the transected end of the stomach on its lesser curvature, sutured the afferent loop of jejunum over the previously closed lesser curvature. This gastric resection technique is known by the Polya-Hofmeister name although Polya had nothing to do with reducing the new stoma and Hofmeister was not the first to perform it.

The retrocolic gastrectomy has the advantage of using a short afferent loop, which can be shortened more by dividing the ligament of Treitz. The antecolic anastomosis is used much more frequently because it is easier to perform and permits a more extensive gastric resection without inconveniences. An extensive gastric resection with a transmesocolic gastrojejunostomy produces marked upward retraction of the transverse mesocolon toward the high portion of the abdomen, which can cause postoperative problems. Experience has shown that in the results there are no important functional differences between retrocolic and antecolic anastomosis.

The position in which the afferent as well as the efferent jejunal loop should be placed has also given rise to controversy. Most surgeons bring the afferent loop to the lesser curvature and the efferent loop to the greater curvature. Other surgeons have similar results doing it in the opposite way.

Advantages and Disadvantages of the Billroth II Gastrectomy

Advantages

a. The Billroth II technique permits an extensive resection of the stomach without producing tension on the gastrojejunal suture line.
b. In patients with duodenal ulcer there are fewer postoperative anastomotic ulcers complicating the patients with Billroth II technique than those with the Billroth I technique.
c. In patients with duodenal ulcer who need a gastric resection but have gross pathologic duodenal changes, it is frequently easier to close the duodenal stump using techniques that will be described later rather than to anastomose it to the stomach (29).
d. The only possible reestablishment of gastrointestinal transit in patients in whom a Finsterer-Bancroft-Plenk exclusion and resection procedure for nonresectable duodenal ulcer has been done is by the Billroth II technique (1, 10, 11).
e. Anastomotic ulcers should be treated by the Billroth II technique (61).

f. Reestablishment of gastrointestinal transit in patients subjected to a gastric resection for carcinoma of the stomach should be by the Billroth II technique (61, 71, 72).

Disadvantages

a. The probability of dumping is somewhat higher with the Billroth II than the Billroth I technique.
b. The Billroth II technique may produce an afferent loop syndrome, though this complication is rare.
c. There is the possibility of other complications such as internal hernias that occur rarely.

Indications for the Billroth II Gastrectomy

As has been said previously, the Billroth II technique has more indications than the Billroth I, since it can also be performed for gastric ulcers in any location—distal, middle, or proximal thirds. The Billroth II technique is more frequently indicated for peptic ulcers than the Billroth I. If a hemigastrectomy is done using the Billroth II technique, it is necessary to add a truncal vagotomy. If the Billroth II procedure includes a 70% gastrectomy, a truncal vagotomy need not be added, except in patients with severe ulcer diathesis. As has been said previously, the Billroth II gastrectomy is indicated in anastomotic ulcers as well as in the exclusion gastrectomy for duodenal ulcer. Finally, the Billroth II technique is indicated in gastric cancer because it permits a more extensive resection of the stomach and its lymph node bearing areas, as well as a greater extension of the duodenal resection than in the Billroth I technique. This fact is of great importance because the pylorus does not constitute a barrier to duodenal invasion by an antropyloric cancer (71, 72). On the other hand, radical gastrectomy for cancer should include resection of periduodenal lymph nodes and some periduodenal blood vessels, which may lead to residual diminished vascularity of the duodenum (61). In addition, local recurrences of gastric neoplasms tend to occur in the vicinity of the localization of the primary tumor, which may lead to obstruction with the Billroth I technique and is much less probable with the Billroth II technique.

BILLROTH I GASTRECTOMY

Historical Data

As was previously mentioned, the first successful gastric resection was performed by Billroth on January 29, 1881, with reestablishment of gastrointestinal transit by anastomosing the duodenum to the lesser curvature of the stomach, though he later did it toward the greater curvature.

Rydygier, on November 21, 1881, performed the first gastrectomy for peptic ulcer of the pylorus with survival of the patient, using the same technique. In 1882, Vincenz von Czerny performed another successful gastrectomy for peptic ulcer (48, 55, 56).

Evolution of the Billroth I Technique

Surgeons of the Billroth I era, including Billroth himself, were very worried about the gastroduodenal suture line because of the frequent incidence of dehiscences. Of the 34 cases of gastric cancer operated upon by Billroth, almost 50% died (48, 65). With the object of reducing the incidence of gastroduodenal dehiscences, in 1891, Theodore Kocher proposed closing the transected end of the stomach and anastomosing the duodenum to the posterior gastric wall. A little later Kocher proposed anastomosing the duodenum to the anterior instead of the posterior gastric wall (48, 65). With the object of attaining a suture line between the duodenum and the posterior gastric wall, Kocher added the mobilization of the duodenum, which he published in 1903. This maneuver became known as the Kocher maneuver, even though Kocher was not the first to perform it. It was first performed experimentally in France, in 1895, by Jourdan, and in humans by Vautrin, who first used it in biliary tract surgery, in 1896. In 1899, in France, Wiart performed this maneuver more completely by adding the lowering of the hepatic flexure to facilitate mobilization of the distal half of the second portion and the lateral segment of the third portion of the duodenum (39). The technique proposed by Kocher, anastomosis of the duodenum to the anterior or posterior gastric wall, was not well accepted by surgeons of that era.

In 1911, Schoemaker, from the Hague (58), proposed resecting the lesser curvature of the stomach with the object of making the gastric stump similar in size to the diameter of the duodenum. Schoemaker's technique was well accepted both in European countries and in the United States, and produced good results. It is used at present in Billroth I gastrectomies and in gastric resections in patients with ulcers located high on the lesser curvature or in the subcardial area, using the Billroth I or Billroth II technique.

In 1922, Hans von Haberer (63, 64) proposed, for gastric resections for peptic ulcer as well as for cancer, closing the duodenum and performing the gastroduodenal anastomosis between the lateral wall of the duodenum and the transected stomach. This same procedure was proposed by Finney, in the United States, in 1923, and for this reason it is usually known as the Haberer-Finney technique. In 1926, Horsley introduced another modification of the Billroth I procedure, which consisted in incising the cut end of the duodenum for a distance of 2 to 3 cm to facilitate the performance of a more ample, and therefore safer, gastroduodenal anastomosis. In 1933, von Haberer introduced another modification to the Billroth I technique, which consisted of making the gastric lumen narrower by placing some sutures so as to gather in the transected end of the stomach, making it smaller, approximating the diameter of the transected duodenum. Hans von Haberer was a great proponent of the Billroth I technique (63, 64).

Advantages and Disadvantages of the Billroth I Technique

Advantages

a. The Billroth I technique does not alter the normal anatomy or function of the gastrointestinal tract, since it anastomoses the gastric stump to the duodenum. This anatomic continuity favors digestion of foods, since these pass from the stomach to the duodenum, where they mix with duodenal, biliary, and pancreatic secretions. In the Billroth II technique, food is mixed with these secretions in the jejunum. The absence of the pylorus in the Billroth I technique, however, allows food to pass rapidly from the stomach into the duodenum and immediately into the jejunum, making the mixture of food and secretions take place, practically, in the jejunum, thereby making any functional differences more theoretical than real. The greater loss of fat through the intestine in patients subjected to the Billroth II technique has no clinical significance.
b. The Billroth I technique is easier than the Billroth II. In addition, the entire procedure is performed in the supramesocolic compartment of the abdomen.
c. Dumping syndrome is less frequent in the Billroth I technique than in the Billroth II.
d. For obvious reasons, the Billroth I technique cannot give rise to afferent loop syndrome or internal hernias.

Disadvantages

a. Anastomotic ulcers occur more frequently with the Billroth I technique, especially in resections for duodenal ulcer.
b. It is not always possible to free the duodenum enough to be able to anastomose it to the stomach without tension on the suture line. This problem usually occurs in duodenal ulcers penetrating into the pancreas with fibrous retraction and narrowing, in the presence of pseudodiverticula in long-standing ulcers, and in ulcers of the proximal stomach.
c. There are surgeons who are very enthusiastic about the Billroth I technique, insisting at times on carrying it out in unfavorable situations with danger of postoperative dehiscence of the suture line. The surgeon should desist from performing a Billroth I procedure when there are difficulties in performing it adequately and safely, opting for a Billroth II.
d. Even though it is said that the Billroth I technique is simpler than the Billroth II, it is necessary that the technique for the procedure be very carefully learned, respecting its indications precisely.
e. In order to carry out a Billroth I procedure without tension on the suture line, it is necessary, in some patients, not only to completely mobilize the duodenum but to also mobilize the gastric stump and the spleen, tying off and dividing the short gastric vessels to diminish the distance between the duodenum and the stomach. This extensive mobilization not only complicates the operation but increases the risk unnecessarily (29).
f. As has been previously stated, the Billroth I technique should not be used to treat gastric cancer.

Indications for the Billroth I Technique

a. The least controversial indication for the Billroth I technique is peptic gastric ulcers. In gastric ulcers both a hemigastrectomy or a 70% gastric resection will give good results without adding a truncal vagotomy, except in prepyloric or pyloric peptic ulcers with gastric acid hypersecretion.
b. Duodenal ulcers treated with hemigastrectomy or a 70% gastrectomy with a Billroth I reconstruction should be accompanied by a truncal vagotomy. If a truncal vagotomy cannot be performed, a 70% Billroth II gastrectomy should be done. If a hemigastrectomy with Billroth II technique is performed, a truncal vagotomy should be added.

BILLROTH I GASTRECTOMY FOR PEPTIC ULCERS

Operative Technique

Before beginning a Billroth I gastrectomy, it is necessary to carefully examine the duodenum and the stomach in order to confirm the diagnosis and determine both the convenience and the feasibility of carrying out this technique. Exploration before performing a Billroth I gastrectomy should be more rigorous than exploration before a Billroth II gastrectomy.

In order to perform a gastroduodenal anastomosis without risk, it is indispensable for the duodenum to have healthy, well vascularized walls. Permeability of the lumen of the second, third, and fourth portions of the duodenum must be assured. If it becomes necessary to ligate the gastroduodenal artery, a Billroth I gastrectomy is not advisable. Some surgeons affirm that a Billroth I gastrectomy is always feasible and resort at times to real surgical acrobatics in their technique, resulting in serious risks for the patients. In order to perform a Billroth I gastrectomy, the extent of resection should not be sacrificed and the gastroduodenostomy should not be under tension. Many of the technical modifications recommended in the past have no indication at present. The anastomosis between the stomach and duodenum should always be an end-to-end anastomosis, using interrupted sutures so that the new stomach remains flexible, elastic, and without stricture.

In all cases in which a Billroth I procedure is performed, a Vautrin-Kocher maneuver should be carried out to facilitate the gastroduodenostomy. Transection of the duodenum should be performed about 3 to 4 cm from the pylorus. It is not advisable to transect the duodenum more than 4 cm from the pylorus because the duodenum may not be long enough for the anastomosis. Transection should not be too close to the pylorus to "save" tissue for the anastomosis.

Mobilization of the stomach is performed by means of a technique similar to the one used in the Billrotb II procedure. In some patients, it is necessary to mobilize the spleen and to ligate and divide the short gastric vessels to be able to perform the gastroduodenostomy without tension. In addition, the gastric stump has to be narrowed down to a diameter similar to that of the duodenum. Resection of the lesser curvature of the stomach by the Shoemaker technique is necessary to attain this. This technique will be described in detail when resection of cardial and subcardial ulcers is described.

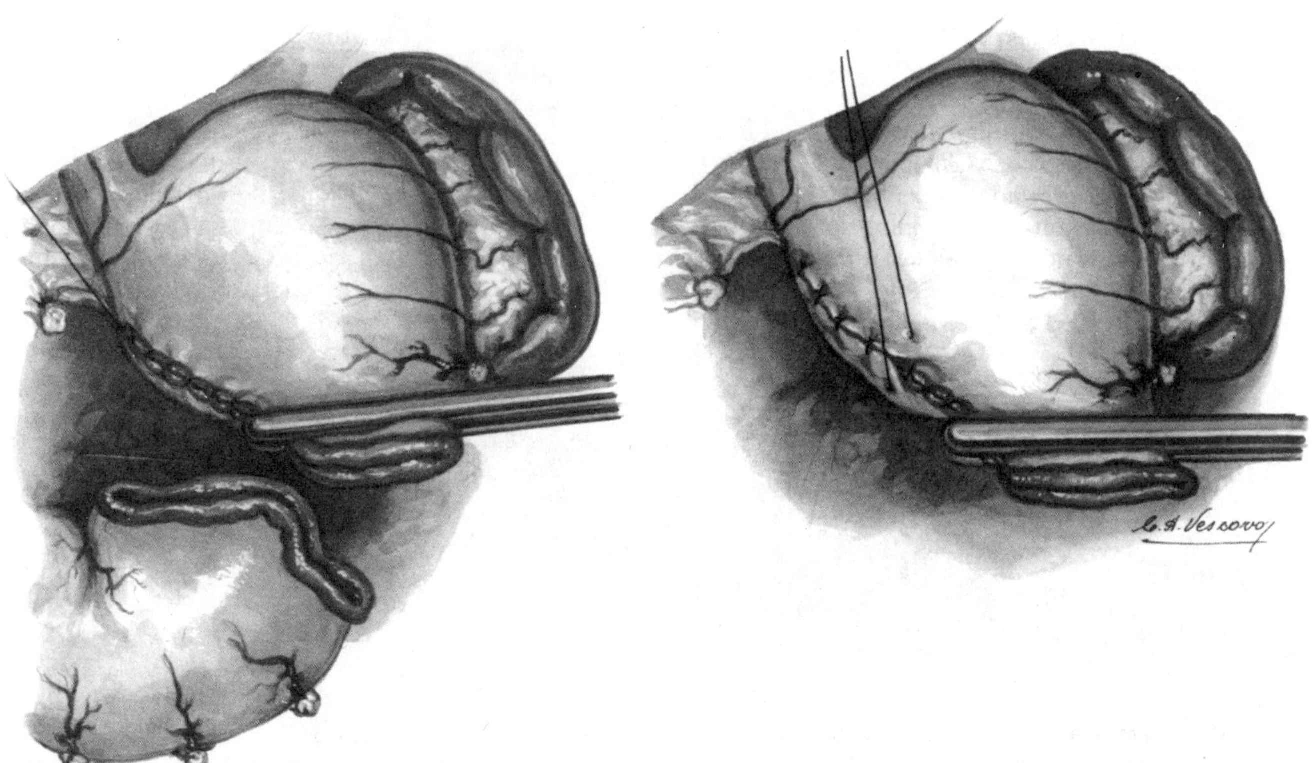

The stomach and duodenum have been freed using the same technique as in the Billroth I gastrectomy. (a) The greater curvature has been freed up to the second short vessel in order to resect an ample portion of the stomach. Part of the lesser curvature has been removed to diminish the diameter of the gastric stump. The mucosa of the lesser curvature has been closed with interrupted 2-0 chromic catgut sutures. The stomach has been grasped with the upper portion of the Finochietto twin clamp. (b) The lesser curvature of the stomach is being peritonealized with interrupted cotton seromuscular sutures.

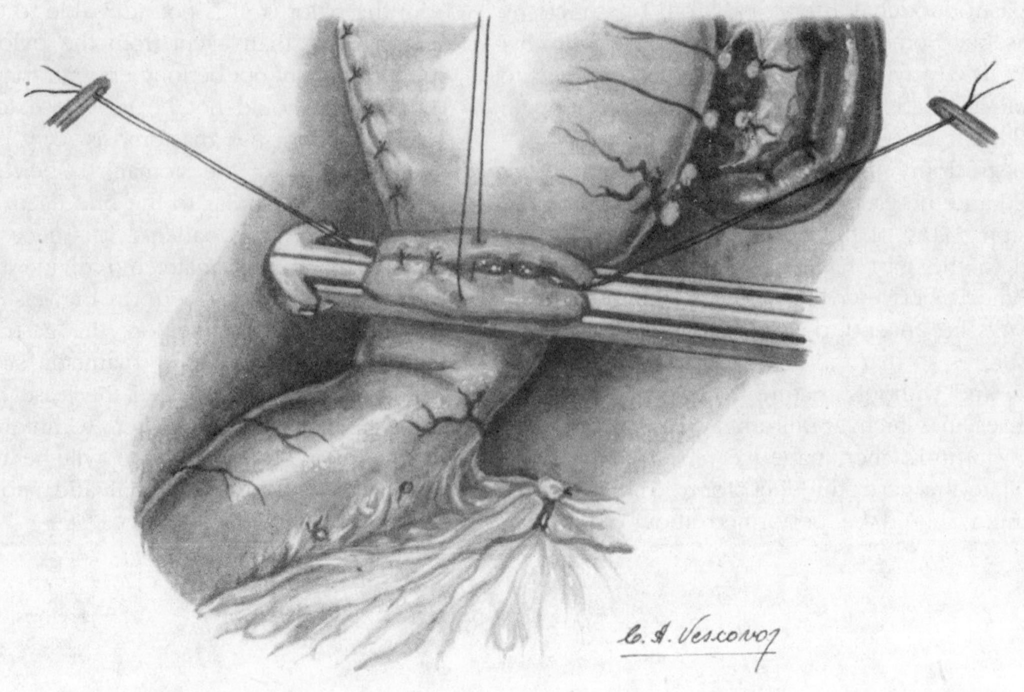

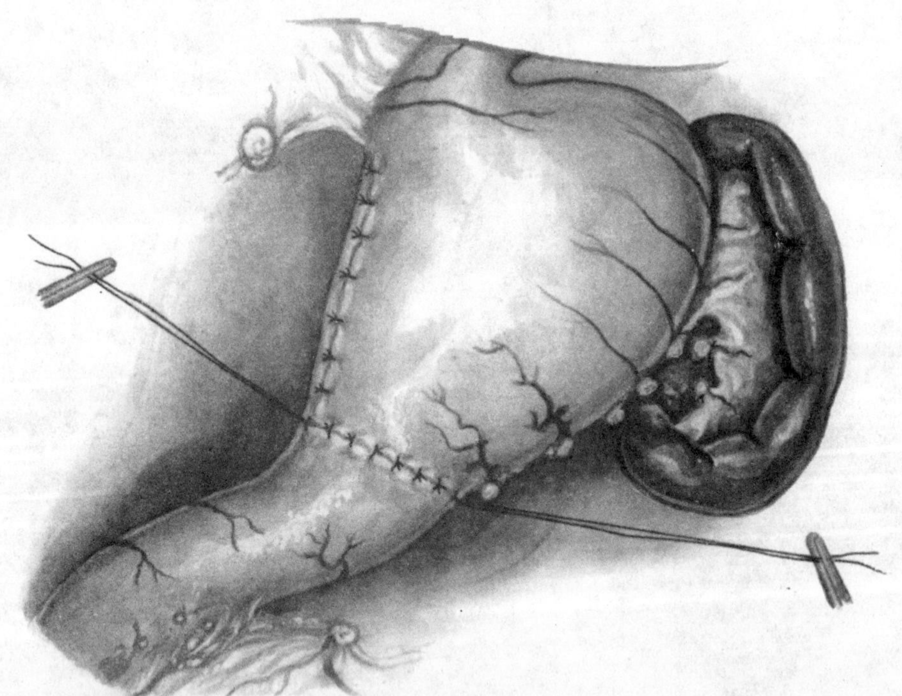

(a) The duodenum has been adequately mobilized by the Vautrin-Kocher maneuver and grasped with the inferior portion of the Finochietto twin clamp. It is being sutured to the gastric stump in two layers of interrupted sutures. The posterior seromuscular layer is the first to be closed with cotton or silk. The posterior and anterior perforating layers are closed in that order, with 2-0 chromic catgut interrupted sutures. Finally the anterior seromuscular layer is closed with silk or cotton. (b) The gastroduodenal anastomosis has been completed without tension.

BILLROTH II GASTRECTOMY FOR PEPTIC ULCER

Surgical Technique: Antecolic Anastomosis

The xiphoumbilical incision is the most frequently used incision in gastrectomy. The possibility of adhesions of the greater omentum to the spleen must be investigated before performing intraabdominal exploration. These adhesions must be divided between clamps before applying traction to the stomach, greater omentum, or transverse colon, to avoid tears of the splenic capsule. The rest of the abdominal organs are then explored, followed by a detailed examination of the stomach and duodenum. The stomach should be completely examined by visualization and palpation, including both the anterior and posterior wall, as well as both curvatures and the cardia and pylorus. To explore the posterior wall, the gastrocolic ligament should be divided below the gastroepiploic arcade, entering the lesser sac, to see and feel the posterior gastric wall. This maneuver allows the surgeon to visualize and feel the anterior surface of the pancreas, where a gastrinoma, chronic pancreatitis, pseudocysts, pancreatic cancer, and so on may be found occasionally. The gastric curvatures and the cardiac and pyloric areas are then explored. The most frequent sites for gastric ulcers are the distal and middle thirds of the lesser curvature; with less frequency peptic ulcers occur in the subcardial region, the anterior and posterior walls, the greater curvature, or the fundus. Peptic ulcers of the stomach may vary from small to giant size. Ulcers may be callous and penetrating into the pancreas, the inferior surface of the liver, or the posterior abdominal wall.

The absence of malignancy in a gastric ulcer is usually determined preoperatively by means of gastroscopic examination with multiple biopsies and brushings. If any doubt about the benign or malignant nature of the gastric ulcer persists, a gastrotomy with several biopsies should be done in order to clarify the diagnosis. With this technique, if the ulcer is malignant, spillage of gastric contents containing neoplastic cells will occur, producing peritoneal seeding. To avoid this possibility the author performs the biopsies in the following manner: A purse string suture is placed in the anterior gastric wall opposite the ulcer and a small incision made in its center through which a lucite scope, illuminated by a cold light, is introduced. The purse string suture is snugged up, the ulcer visualized, and the necessary biopsies taken for histologic examination. This technique prevents spillage of gastric contents with its possible consequences.

In patients being operated on for duodenal ulcer a careful exploration of the duodenum should be carried out, before mobilizing the duodenum, to determine if there is a penetration into the pancreas, a giant duodenal ulcer (over 2 cm in diameter), a postbulbar ulcer, fibrous retraction of the duodenum, or a close connection between the ulcer and the main or accessory pancreatic ducts or the bile duct, or the hepatic artery and/or the portal vein. The possibility of performing a safe duodenal closure or a duodenal closure using the Nissen or Strauss technique has to be investigated. For these techniques the anterolateral duodenal wall must be normal in appearance, pliable, and not thickened or infiltrated with fibrous tissue. If thorough exploration reveals that the duodenal closure is not going to be safe, a truncal vagotomy with drainage procedure or, as preferred by the author, a Finsterer-Bancroft-Plenk exclusion resection, with an added truncal vagotomy, should be performed.

Surgical Technique: Billroth II Gastrectomy Antecolic Anastomosis

FIGURE 27.1

Once the decision has been made to perform a Billroth II gastrectomy, the second assistant grasps the stomach with the right hand and, with the left hand, applies gentle traction on the colon and gastrocolic ligament in the opposite direction to be able to see the greater curvature of the stomach and the gastroepiploic vascular arch with its gastric collateral branches. Liberation of the greater curvatures is begun at its middle third, where there are usually no adhesions between the transverse mesocolon and the gastrocolic ligament. The author frees the greater curvature of the stomach inside the gastroepiploic vascular arcade and not on the outer side of the arcade, as many surgeons do in order to save time. In order to ligate the collateral pedicles of the gastroepiploic arcade, the surgeon passes a curved clamp around the vascular pedicle. The first assistant loads the clamp with the end of a cotton or silk thread. The surgeon grasps the thread with the left hand and applies moderate traction to facilitate passage of another clamp, which is loaded with another thread, which is then passed around the vascular pedicle.

FIGURE 27.2

The surgeon applies traction to the first thread with the left hand. The clamp has again been passed with the surgeon's right hand to grasp another thread. Once both threads have been passed, they are tied around the vascular pedicle. The suture held in the surgeon's left hand is tied by him against the greater curvature of the stomach, and the second thread is tied up against the gastroepiploic vascular arcade by the first assistant. Both ligatures are performed synchronously. The rest of the greater curvature is freed in similar fashion. Liberation of the greater curvature by this method significantly reduces the time it takes, making it unnecessary to perform the ligatures on the outside of the arcade to save time. Although partial or complete necrosis of the omentum rarely occurs with ligation of the branches of the arcade on the outside of the arch, this possibility always exists. The greater curvature is freed proximally. If a 70% gastrectomy is to be performed, the greater curvature is to be transected at the level of the first short vessels. If a hemigastrectomy has been planned, the greater curvature is to be transected where the left gastroepiploic artery joins the right gastroepiploic. If a hemigastrectomy is done for a duodenal ulcer, a truncal vagotomy should be added, and done before beginning liberation of the stomach.

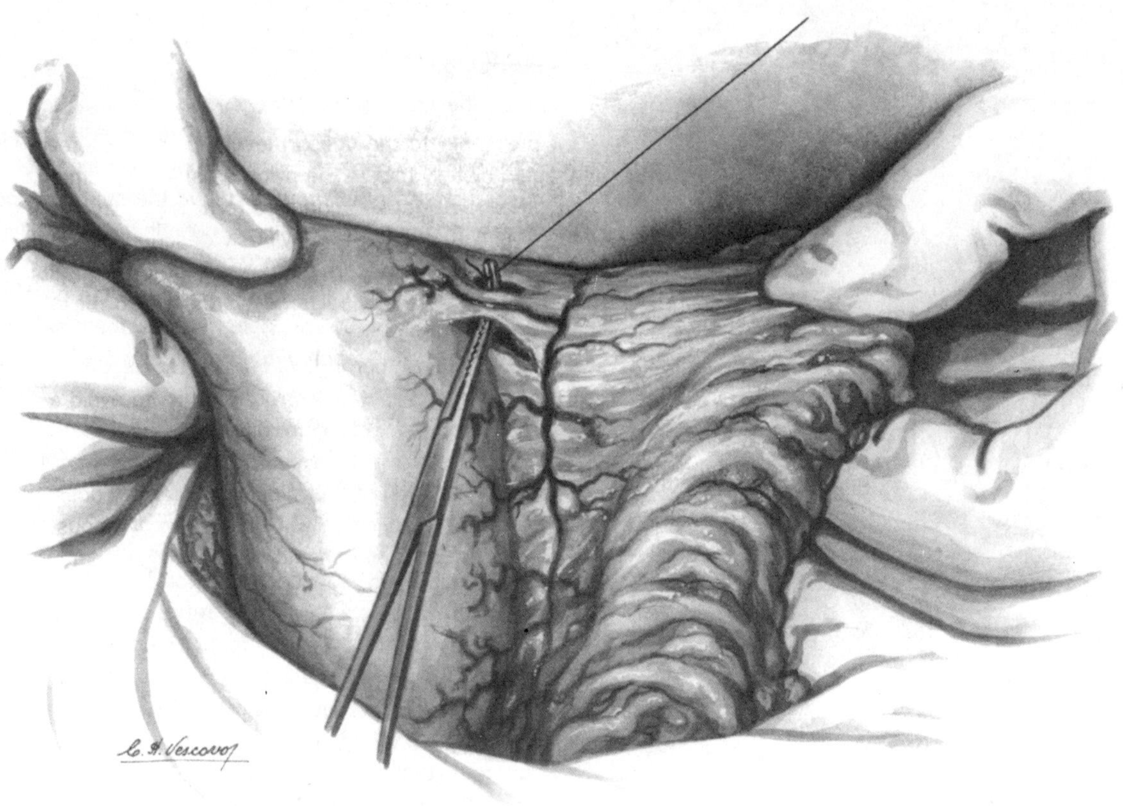

FIGURE 27.1

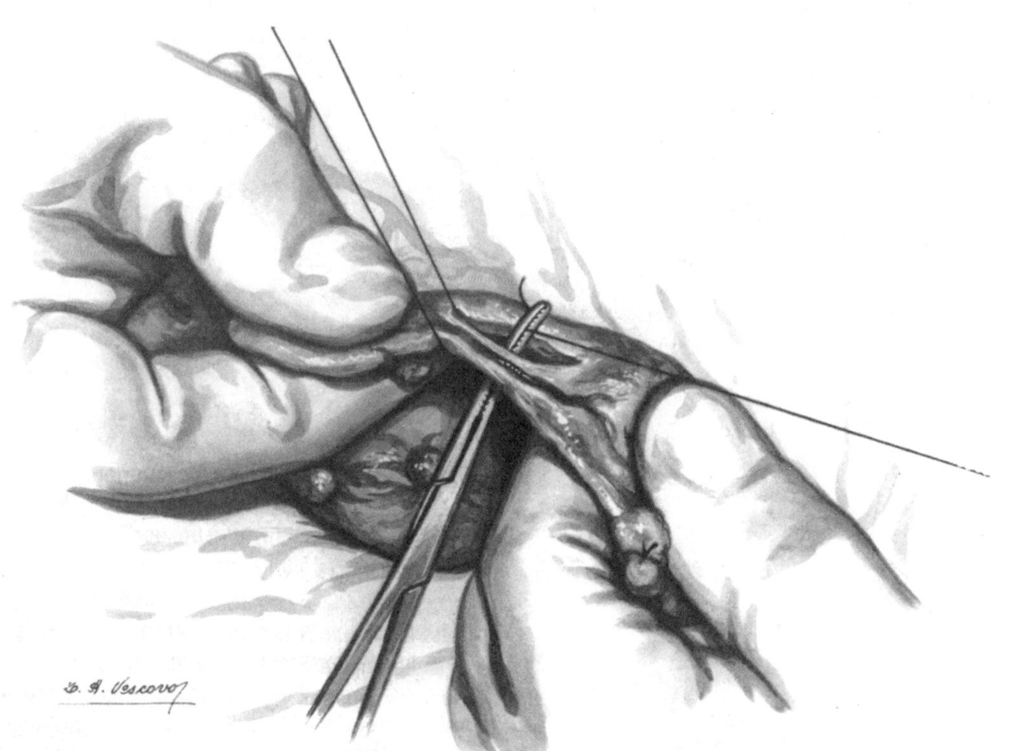

FIGURE 27.2

FIGURE 27.3
Once the greater curvature of the stomach has been freed proximally to the chosen level, liberation is reversed and carried distally toward the pylorus using the same technique. The second assistant continues to hold the stomach and the gastrocolic ligament as previously described. As the liberation of the greater curvature nears the gastric antrum it is frequent to find the gastrocolic ligament adherent to the posterior wall of the antrum and, at times, fused with the transverse mesocolon. During liberation of the greater curvature it is necessary to carefully separate both structures to avoid a possible error that is occasionally committed, namely ligation of the middle colic artery, which is confused with the right gastroepiploic artery. Ligation of the middle colic artery does not mean that the transverse colon will become gangrenous. If this should occur the surgeon should continue the operation and observe the colon. If any changes are noted, the transverse colon should be resected. Liberation of the greater curvature is continued distally, freeing the inferior border of the first portion of the duodenum and ligating the right gastroepiploic artery and vein. Dissection of the posterior wall of the first portion of the duodenum is carried out, revealing several short vessels that run from the gastroduodenal artery to the duodenum, and which should be ligated individually.

Surgical Technique: Billroth II Gastrectomy Antecolic Anastomosis

FIGURE 27.4
The greater curvature of the stomach has been liberated over the necessary extent, as well as the inferior border and the posterior wall of the first portion of the duodenum. The next step will be to ligate the right gastric (pyloric) artery and its accompanying vein. To carry out this step the edge of the gastric antrum is grasped with a Duval triangular clamp, which is pulled upward and to the left by the first assistant, while the surgeon passes his left hand through the flaccid portion of the gastrohepatic ligament to place the segment of this ligament that contains the right gastric vessels under tension.

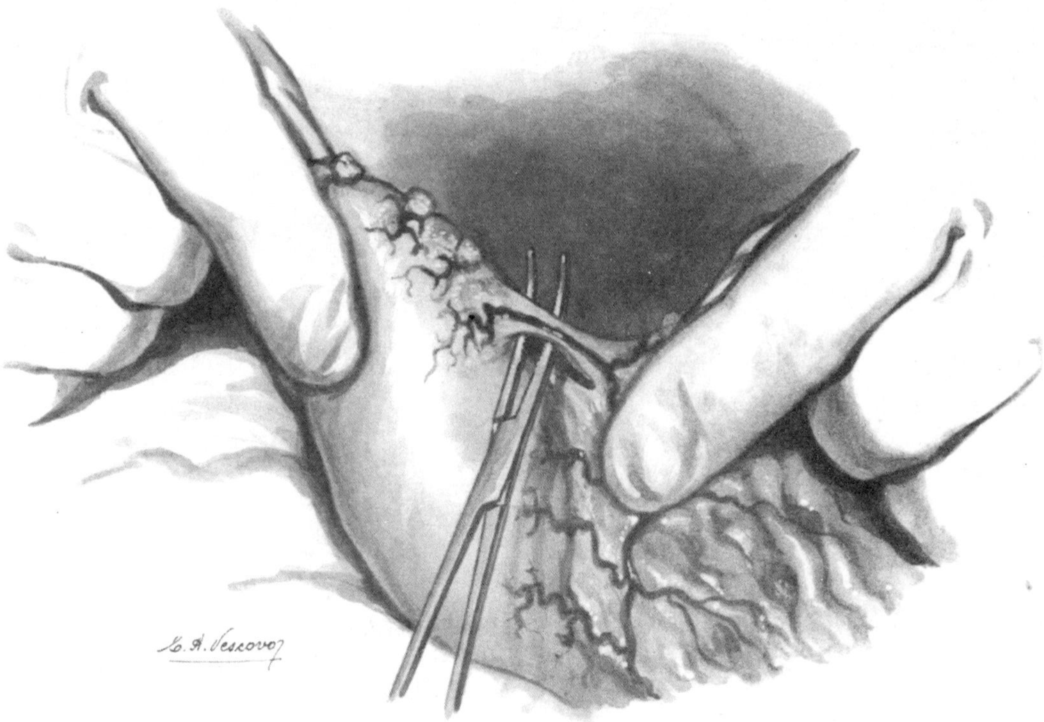

FIGURE 27.3

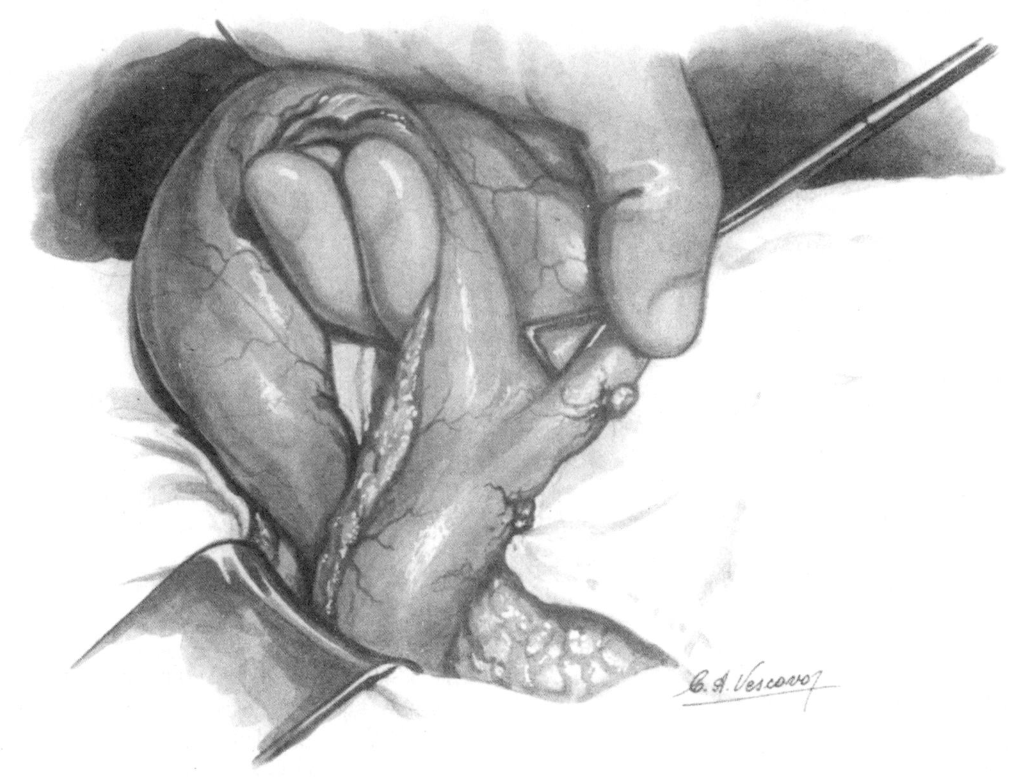

FIGURE 27.4

FIGURE 27.5
The surgeon applies traction to the gastric antrum and the lesser curvature of the stomach upward and to the left, which further demonstrates the right gastric vessels, and proceeds with their ligation by passing a curved clamp, which he handles with his right hand.

Surgical Technique: Billroth II Gastrectomy Antecolic Anastomosis

FIGURE 27.6
A silk or cotton thread has been passed and is held by the first assistant while the surgeon passes another curved clamp, which will be loaded with a similar thread. The assistant then ties both ligatures, leaving enough space for the surgeon to cut the vessels, using a scissors with his right hand, as seen in the insert.

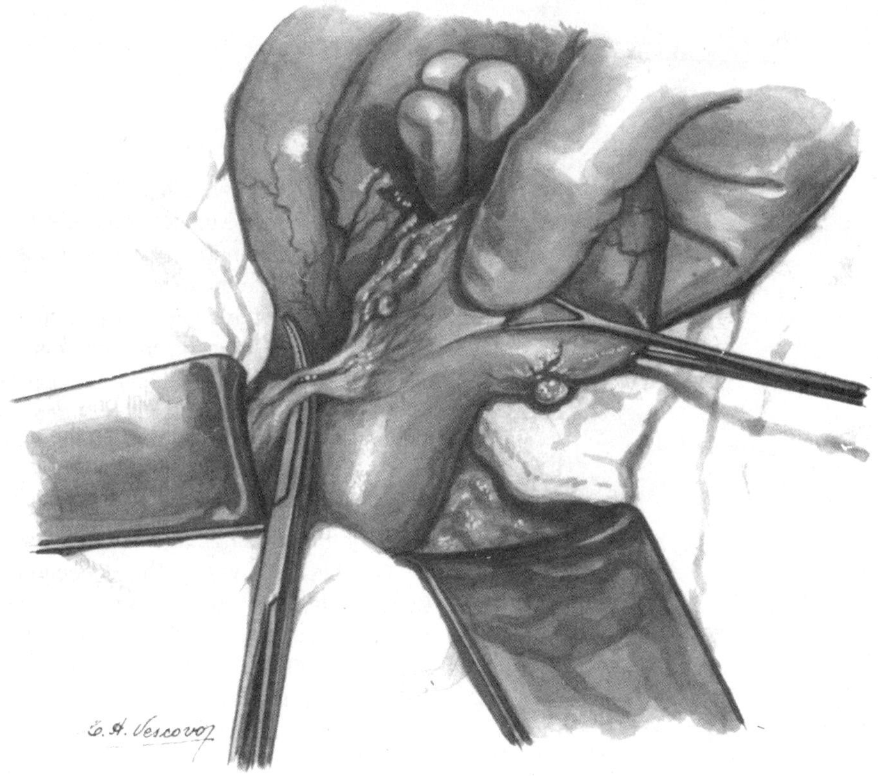

FIGURE 27.5

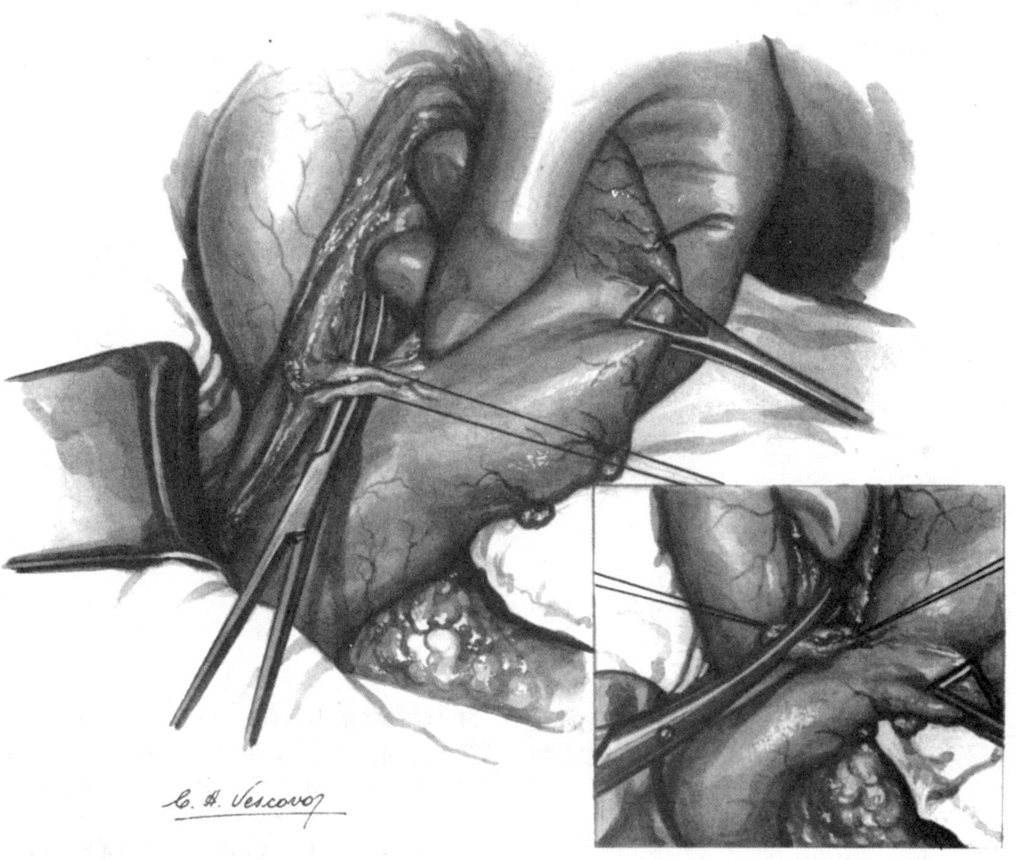

FIGURE 27.6

FIGURE 27.7
Once the greater curvature of the stomach and the first portion of the duodenum have been freed and the right gastric vessels ligated, the duodenum should be transected and closed. In cases in which the duodenum does not present any important pathologic alterations, division and suturing of the duodenum should generally present no problems. There are many techniques for closing the duodenum, which can be used according to the circumstances. We will only describe some of the techniques of duodenal closure when the duodenum does not present severe pathologic alterations. Management and closure of the difficult duodenum will be described later. The technique shown in the drawing has been used by the author, with good results, for many years. The duodenum is grasped with two Babcock clamps. Above the Babcock clamps a clamp designed by the author, which uses the same principle as the Furniss clamp, is applied across the duodenum. A straight needle with silk or cotton is passed through the clamp, as shown. Chronic catgut or a reabsorable synthetic suture can also be used.

Surgical Technique: Billroth II Gastrectomy Antecolic Anastomosis

FIGURE 27.8
The straight needle has been passed through the clamp. The duodenum is transected, with a scalpel, just above the clamp. The proximal transected duodenum is covered with a gauze held in place with a Duval clamp, as shown in the insert.

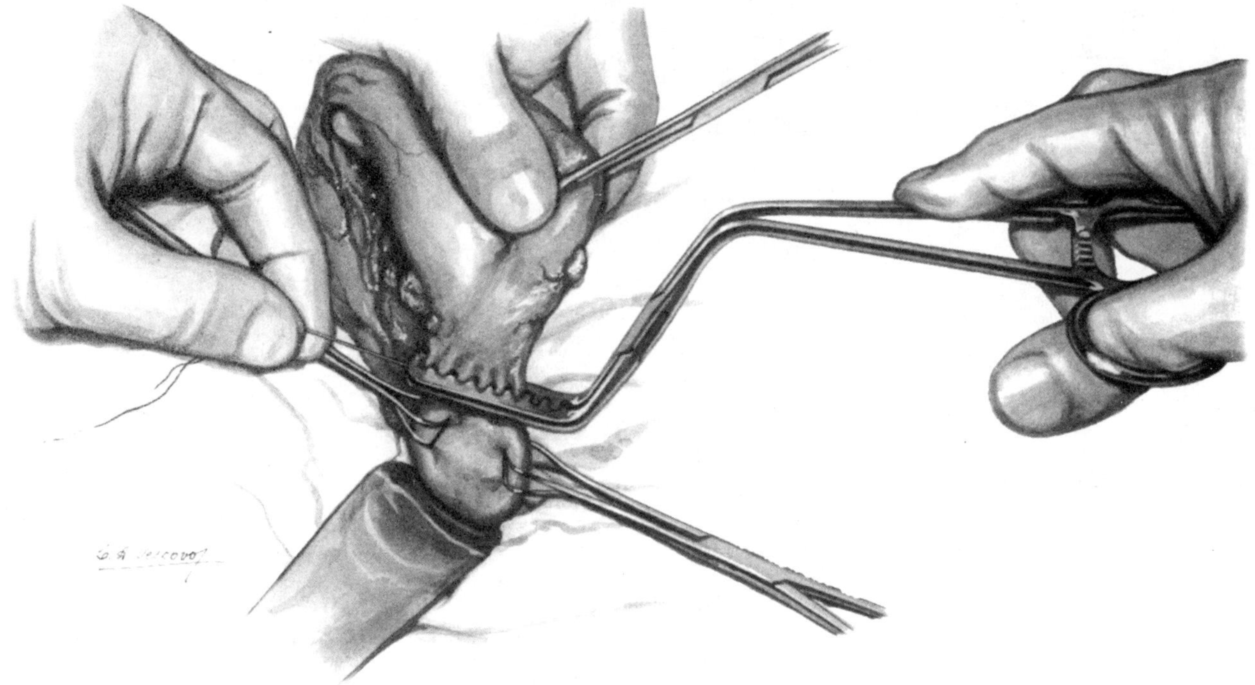

FIGURE 27.7

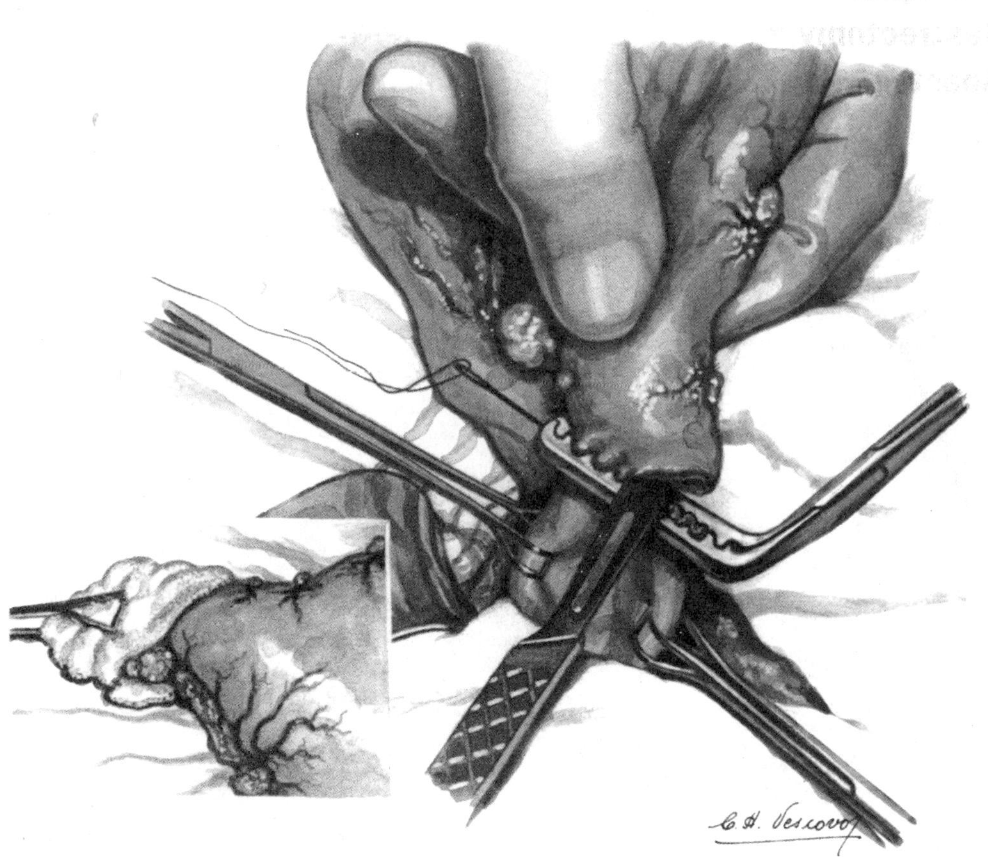

FIGURE 27.8

FIGURE 27.9
The clamp has been removed. Using a Péan clamp, the needle is grasped to remove it from the duodenum.

Surgical Technique: Billroth II Gastrectomy Antecolic Anastomosis

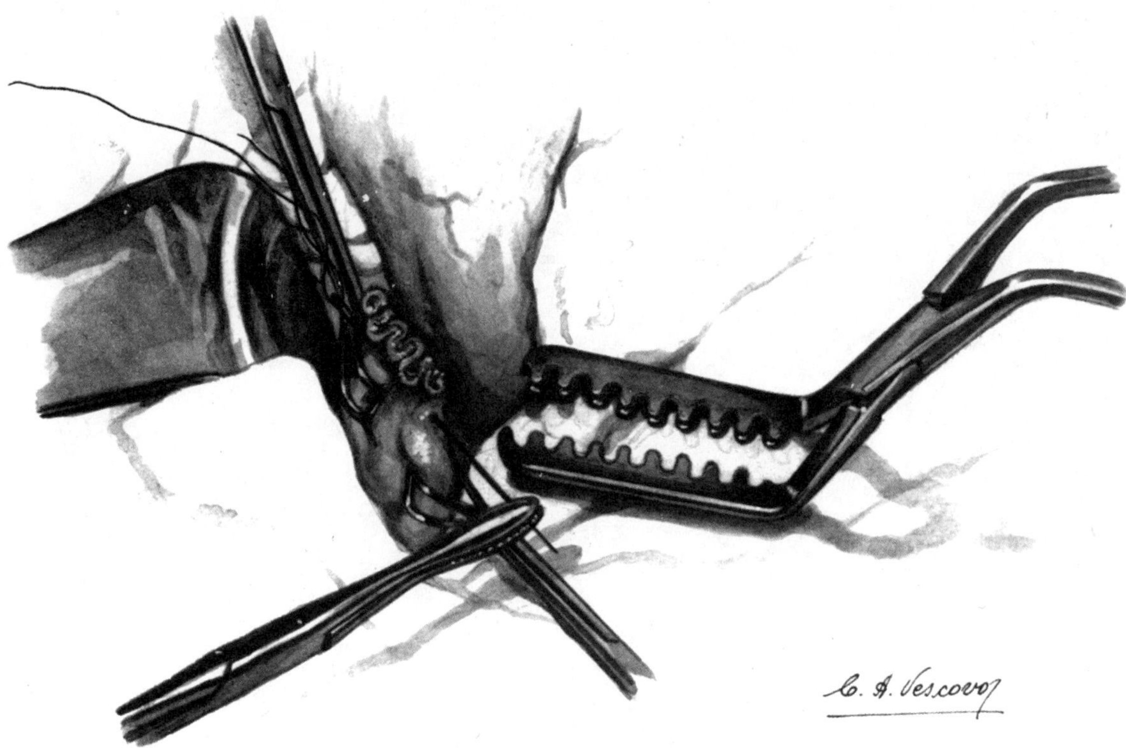

FIGURE 27.9

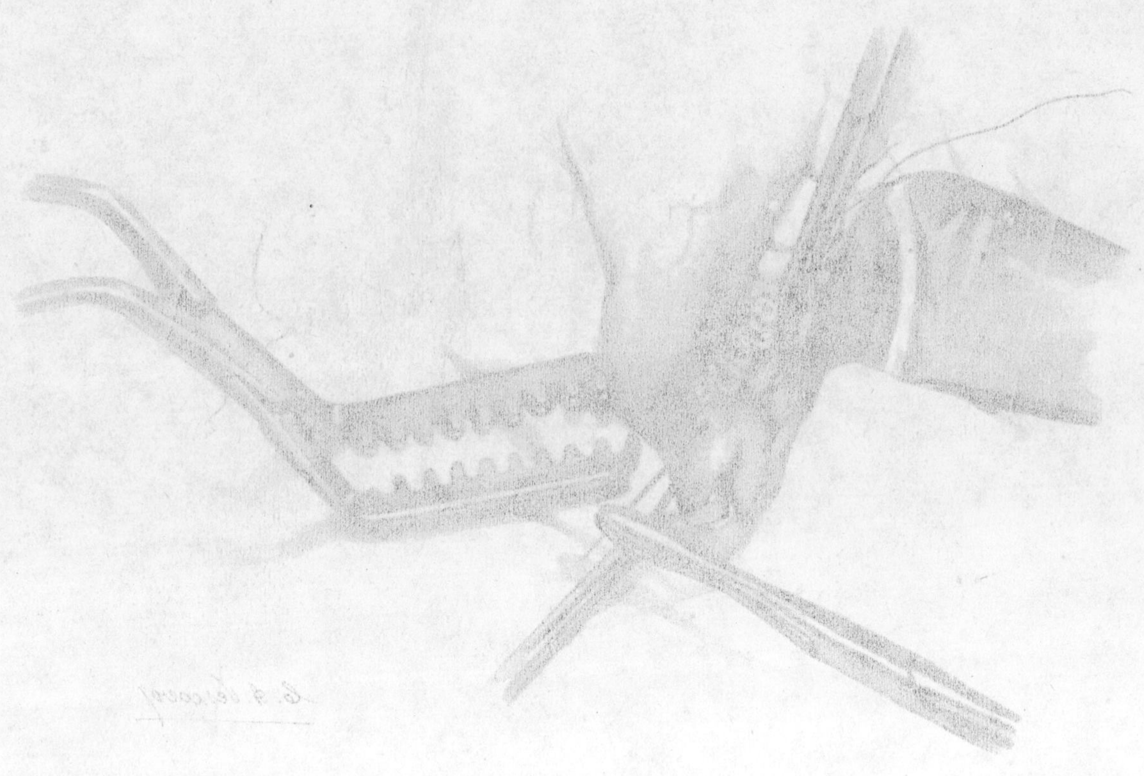

Surgical Technique: Billroth II Gastrectomy Antecolic Anastomosis

FIGURE 27.10

(a) Once the needle is pulled out of the duodenum, it is closed in a manner similar to a purse string suture. The ends of the suture are pulled up and tied. (b) If there is any doubt as to the safety of the suture, 2 or 3 interrupted sutures can be added, as seen in the drawing. (c) A classical purse string suture is used to complete the duodenal closure. (d) The second purse string is being pulled up to invaginate the first purse string.

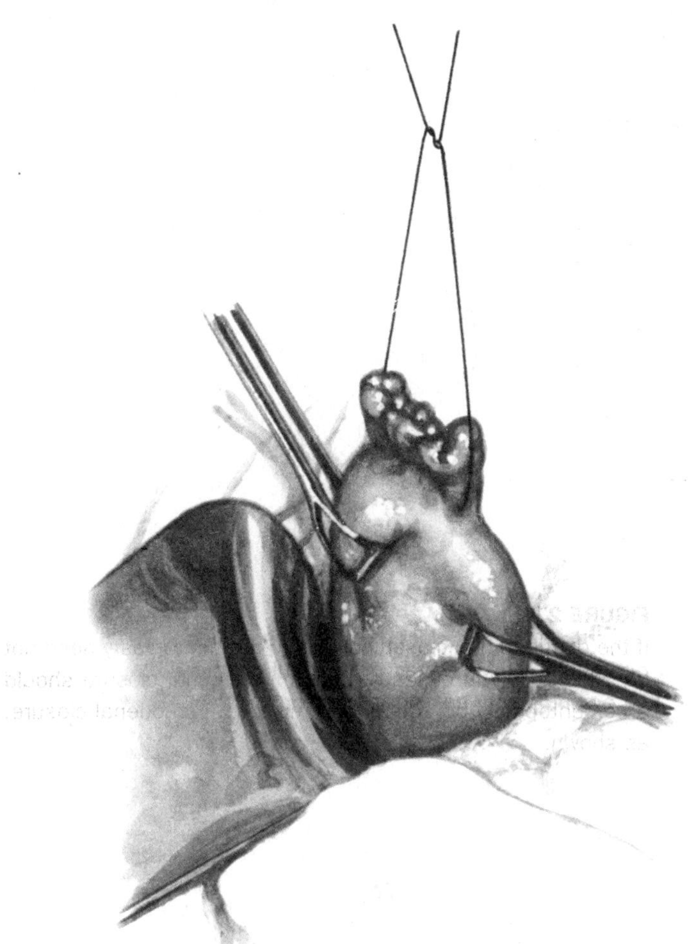

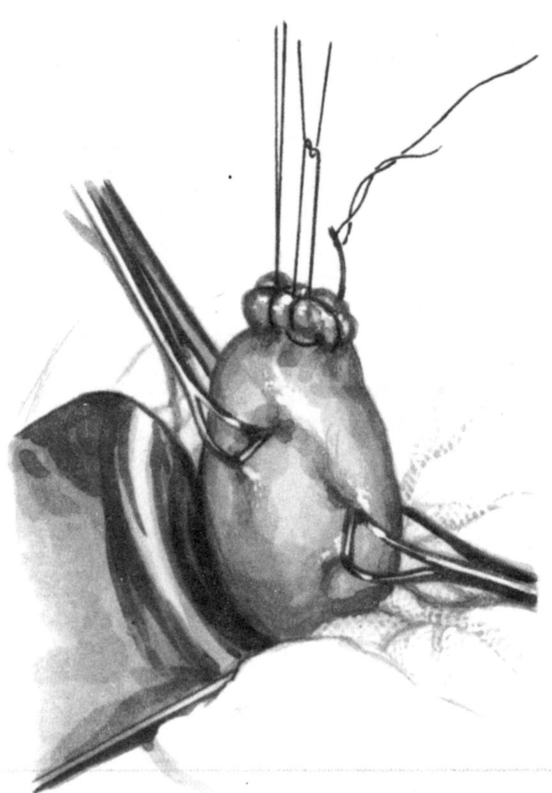

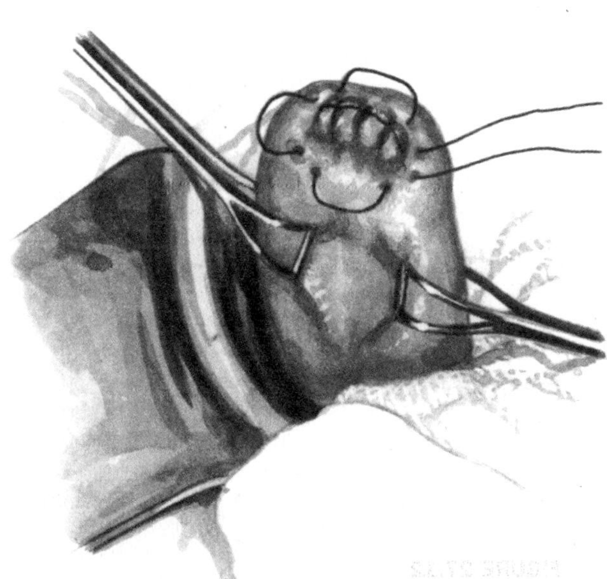

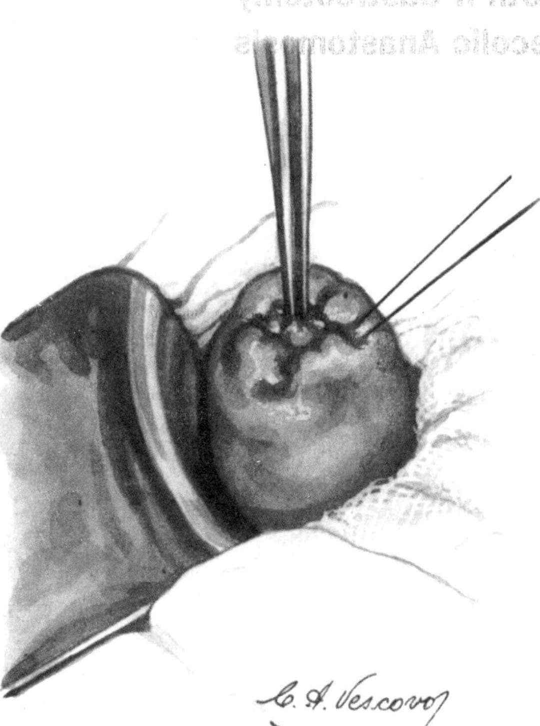

FIGURE 27.10

FIGURE 27.11
If the duodenum is closed correctly, an omentoplasty need not be added. Only in cases of doubtful duodenal closure should an omentoplasty be added to complete the duodenal closure, as shown.

Surgical Technique: Billroth II Gastrectomy Antecolic Anastomosis

FIGURE 27.12
A simple and safe duodenal closure consists of two layers of interrupted silk or cotton sutures. (a) The first layer includes the entire duodenal wall. Some surgeons prefer chromic catgut for this layer. (b) Once the perforating layer is closed, the closure is completed with an invaginating seromuscular layer with silk or linen. (c) The suture line is completed.

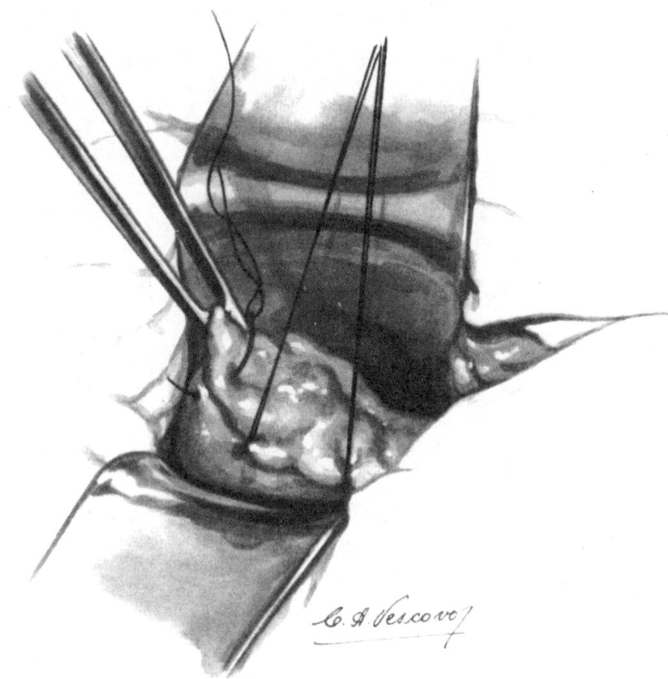

FIGURE 27.11

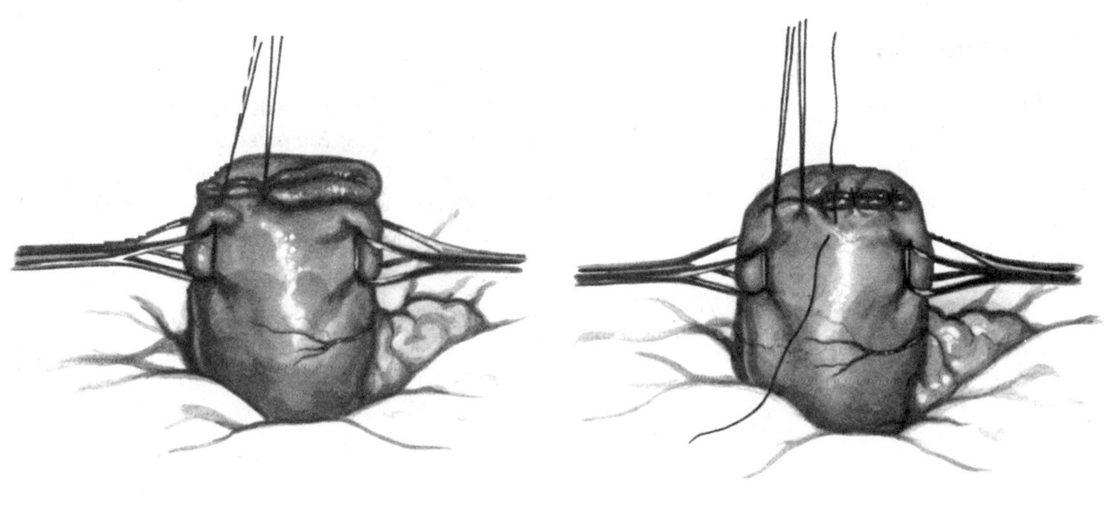

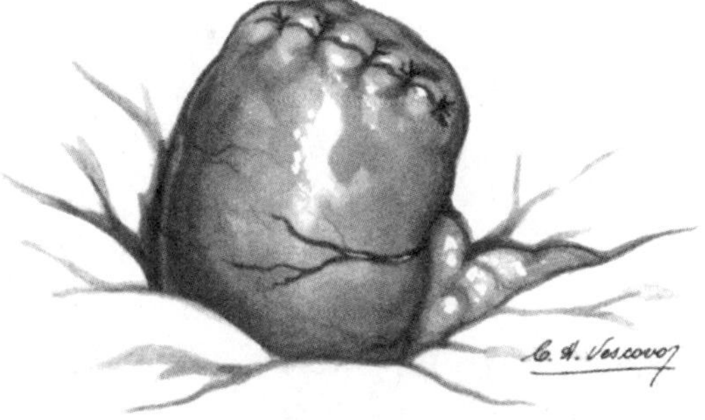

FIGURE 27.12

Surgical Technique: Billroth II Gastrectomy Antecolic Anastomosis

FIGURE 27.13
Some surgeons close the duodenum with a double purse string of silk or cotton. (a) The purse string suture has been inserted. (b) The second purse string is in place, and the first one is being invaginated. (c) The duodenal stump is closed. This technique can only be used if the duodenum is small in diameter.

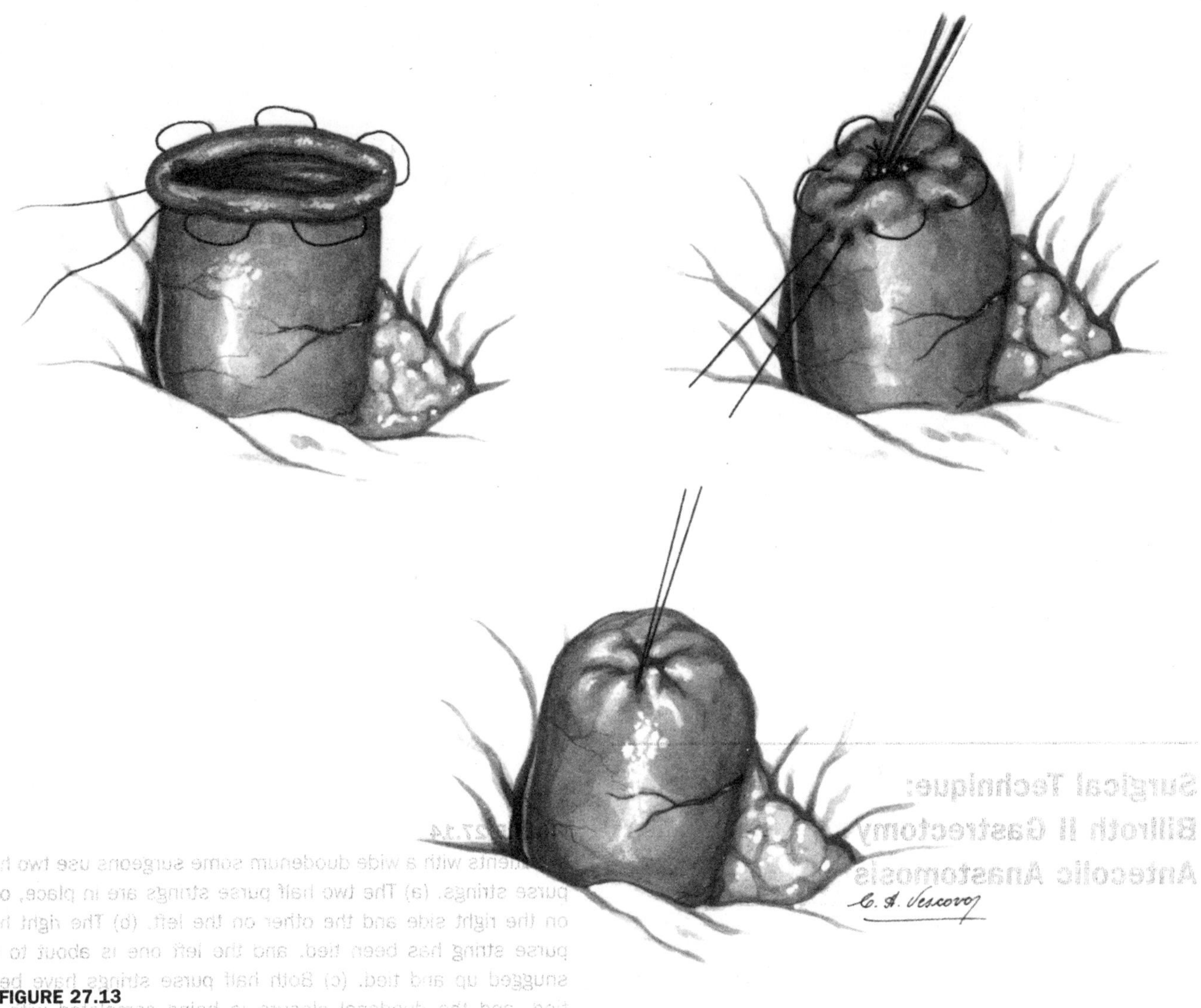

FIGURE 27.13

Surgical Technique: Billroth II Gastrectomy Antecolic Anastomosis

FIGURE 27.14

In patients with a wide duodenum some surgeons use two half purse strings. (a) The two half purse strings are in place, one on the right side and the other on the left. (b) The right half purse string has been tied, and the left one is about to be snugged up and tied. (c) Both half purse strings have been tied, and the duodenal closure is being completed with invaginating seromuscular sutures.

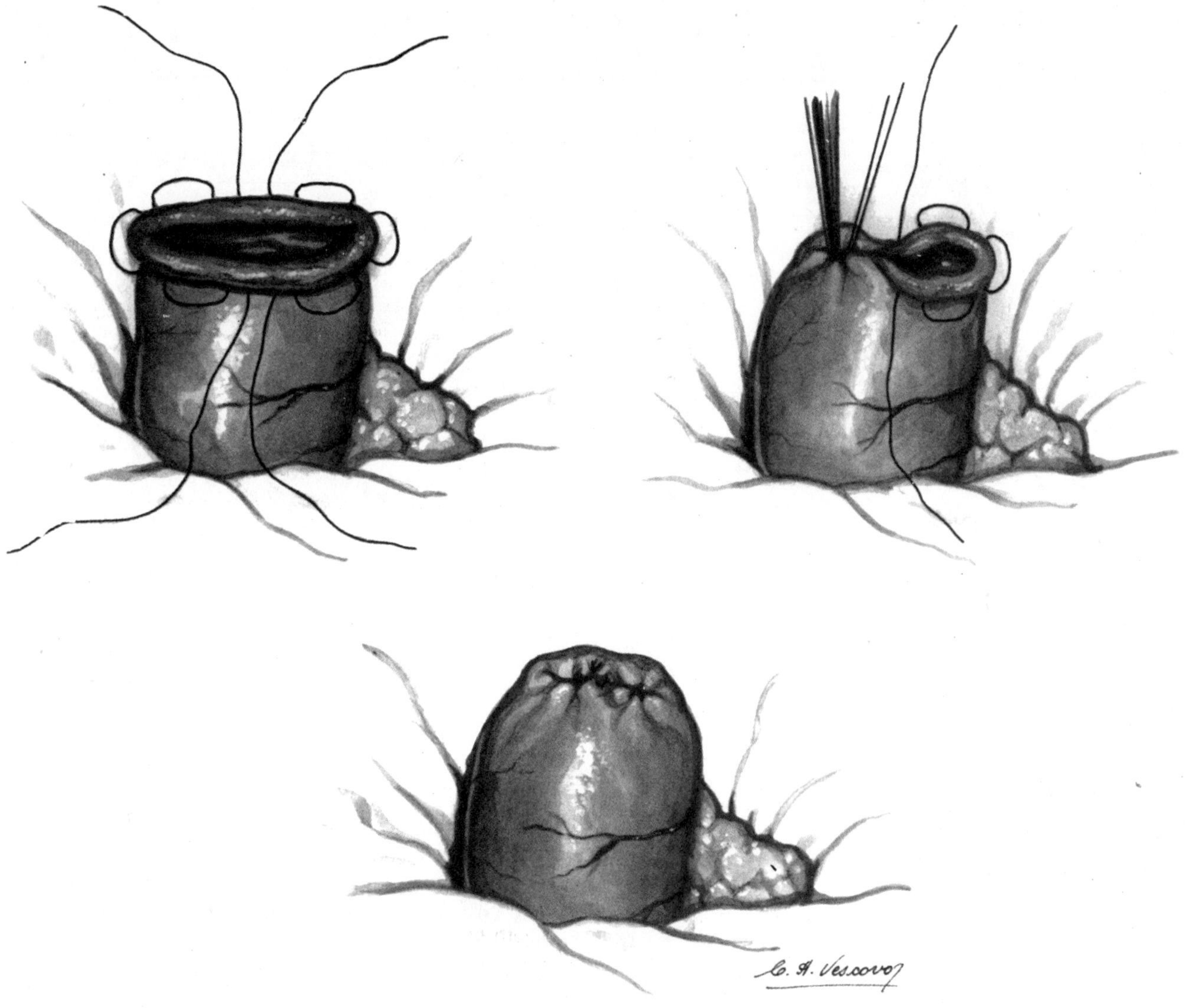

FIGURE 27.14

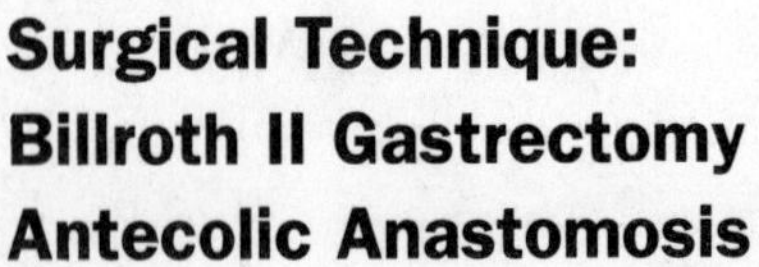

Surgical Technique: Billroth II Gastrectomy Antecolic Anastomosis

FIGURE 27.15
A duodenal closure procedure, frequently used, is the Mayo procedure, shown in this drawing. (a) The duodenum is closed with a Crile clamp and a running suture is applied in through and through fashion, passing the suture over the Crile clamp. (b) The Crile clamp is loosened and removed, applying traction to both ends of the suture, which are then tied. (c) The duodenal closure is completed with invaginating interrupted seromuscular sutures.

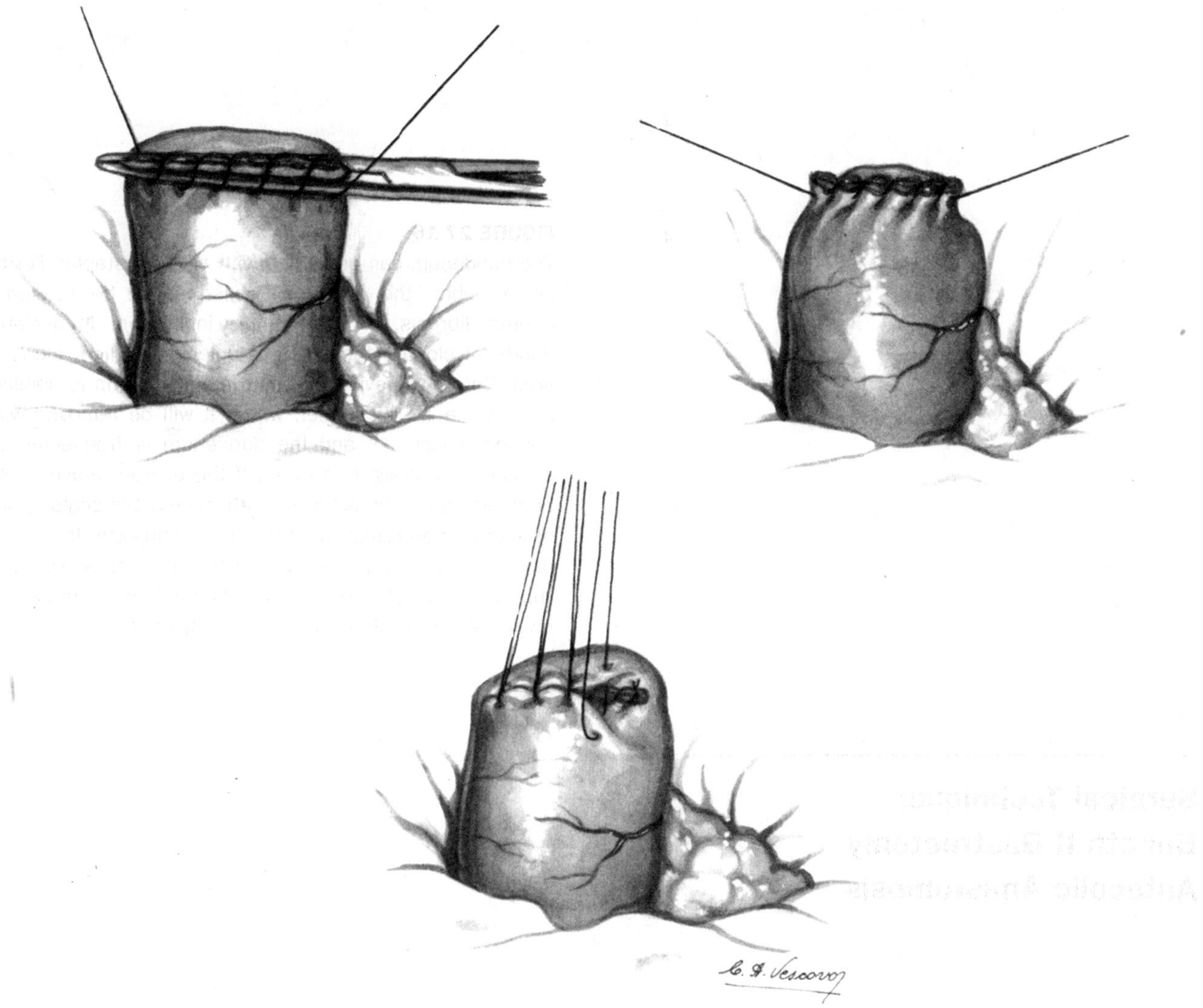

FIGURE 27.15

FIGURE 27.16
The duodenum can be closed with a TA 55 stapler. For this to be possible, the duodenal walls cannot be thickened by edema, fibrosis, or inflammatory infiltration. To perform the duodenal closure the TA 55 stapler is applied, closed, and fired. Before removing the instrument a clamp is applied parallel to the TA 55 stapler, where it will be removed with the surgical specimen, and the duodenum is transected with a scalpel or a straight scissors. If the everted mucosa bleeds, hemostasis can be achieved with the electric scalpel, and the stapler is then removed. Most of the surgeons that close the duodenum with staplers do not use an inverting layer of interrupted sutures for more security. When they do not perform an inverting suture, they add an omentoplasty.

Surgical Technique: Billroth II Gastrectomy Antecolic Anastomosis

FIGURE 27.17
Once the duodenum has been transected and closed, the stomach is reflected upward to complete its liberation for the resection. The next step is the ligation and transection of the left gastric vessels. To carry this out the surgeon introduces his left index finger between the border of the lesser curvature and the left gastric pedicle, separating the vascular pedicle from its bed, as can been seen in the drawing. While holding the left gastric vascular pedicle apart, the surgeon passes a curved clamp, using his or her right hand, which the assistant loads with a cotton or silk thread. This first thread will be used to tie the distal end of the vascular pedicle, which will be removed with the surgical specimen. Two more silk or cotton threads, which will be tied in the proximal part of the pedicle, are then passed. The vascular pedicle will then be divided between the distal suture to be removed with the specimen, and the two proximal sutures, which remain, as shown in the insert.

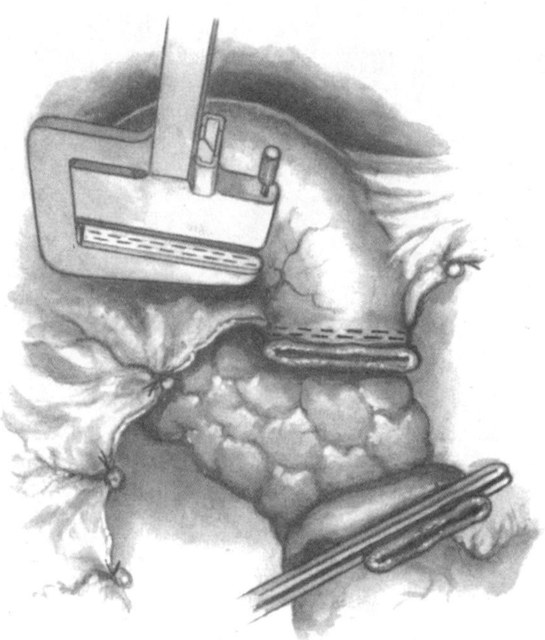

FIGURE 27.16

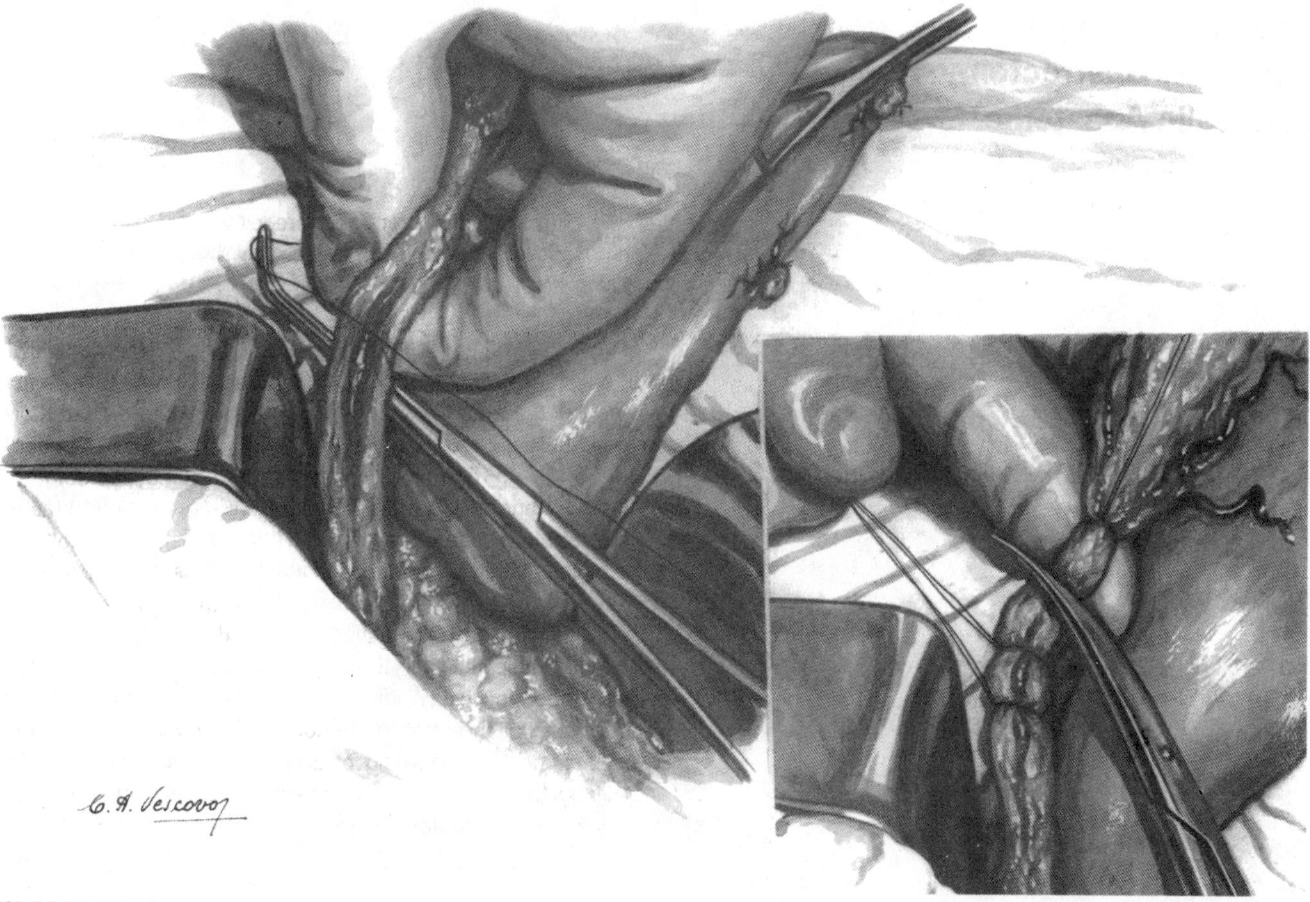

FIGURE 27.17

Surgical Technique: Billroth II Gastrectomy Antecolic Anastomosis

FIGURE 27.18

The lesser curvature of the stomach is generally twisted on itself. This curling effect is more pronounced in cases with chronic callous ulcers in this location. When a gastrectomy is performed, a very useful maneuver consists of untwisting the lesser curvature so that it attains its real length, which will permit the gastric resection to be more exact. In order to untwist the lesser curvature, the surgeon grasps the distal stump of the ligature of the right gastric vessels between the left thumb and index finger exerting moderate traction upward, as seen in the drawing. This maneuver frequently traumatizes some collateral branches of the left coronary vein and, less frequently, collateral branches of the artery. These traumatized collateral branches bleed and must be clamped to attain hemostasis, as seen in the drawing. The proximal stump of the left gastric vessels can be distinguished in the drawing by its location and because the black threads used in the vessels' ligature have been left long. When the maneuver to untwist the lesser curvature of the stomach is complete, a more ample area of the stomach will be void of peritoneum, clearly showing the longitudinal muscle fibers bordering the lesser curvature. This space will be reperitonealized.

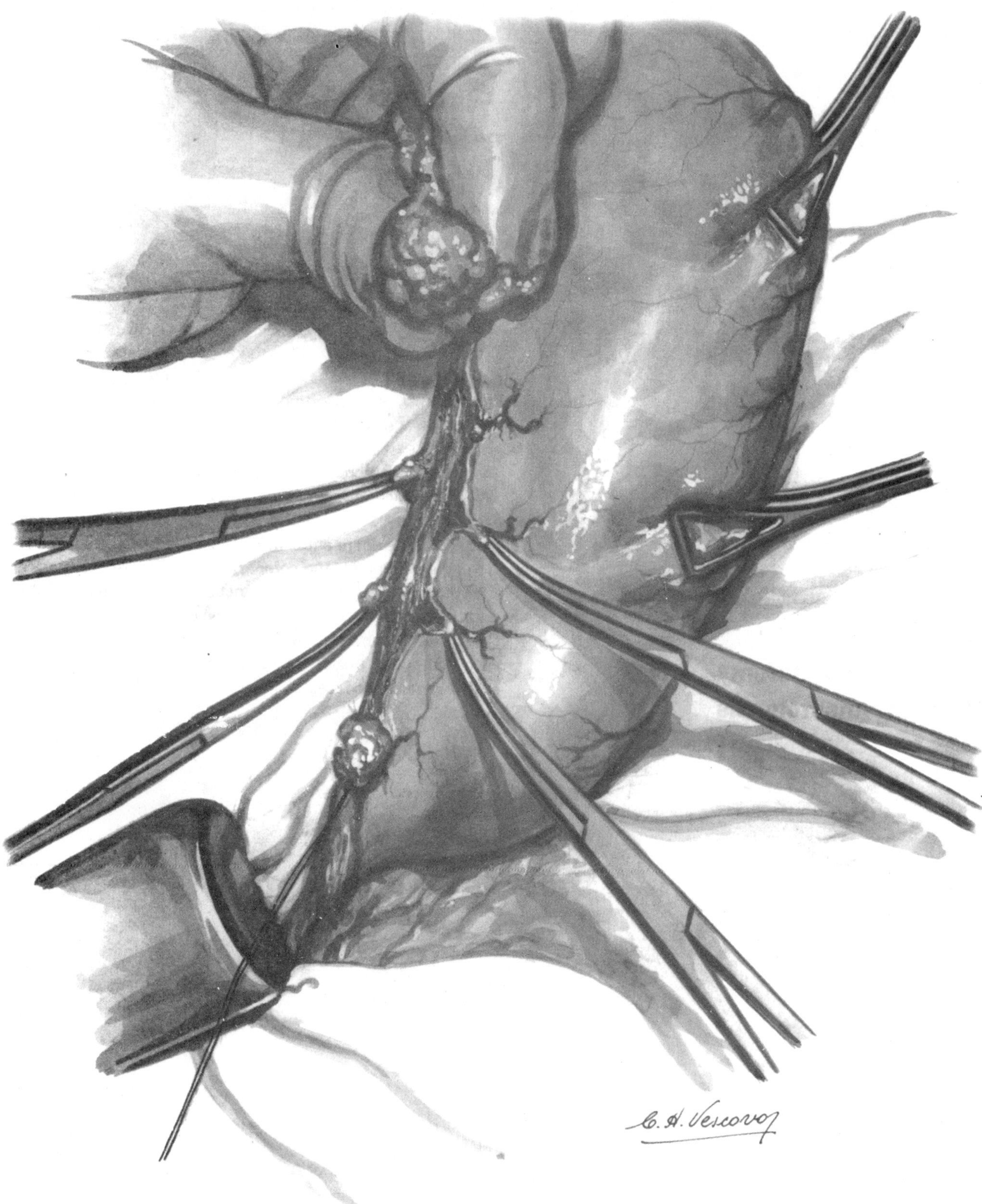

FIGURE 27.18

FIGURE 27.19

The lesser curvature of the stomach has been reperitonealized using interrupted silk or cotton sutures, and the level at which the stomach is to be transected for a hemigastrectomy or a 70% resection is chosen. To carry out a hemigastrectomy the gastric transection should be at the level of the third collateral branch of the coronary or left gastric artery. In patients with duodenal ulcer it is advisable to transect the stomach at the level of the first collateral branch of the coronary artery to be sure that the entire antral mucosa has been resected. The first collateral branch of the coronary artery is located some 3 cm distal to the esophagogastric junction. If the resection is a 70% gastrectomy, the level of transection will be at this point. Once the level of gastric transection has been chosen, the superior portion of the elastic twin Finochietto clamp is placed 2 cm above the chosen level.

Surgical Technique: Billroth II Gastrectomy Antecolic Anastomosis

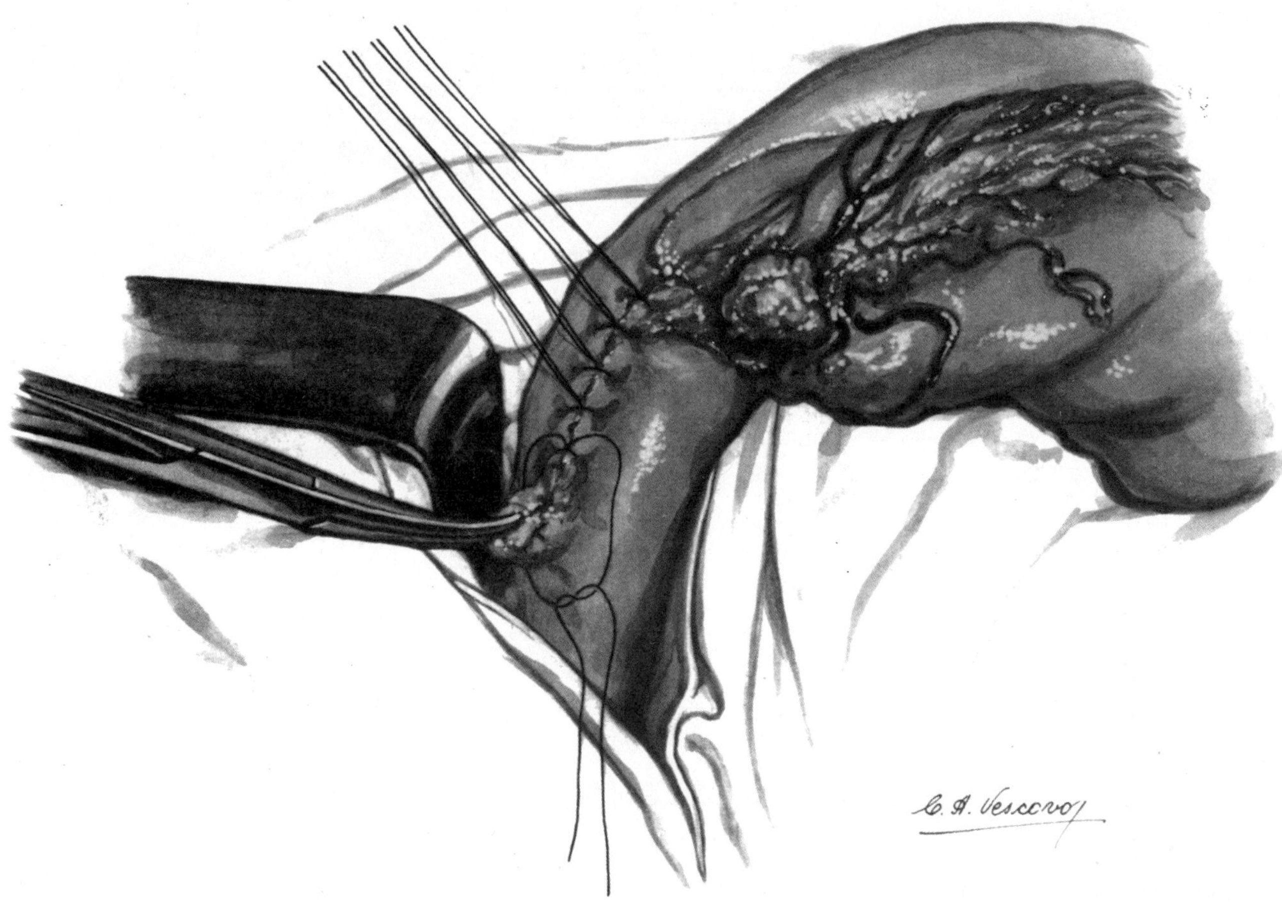

FIGURE 27.19

Surgical Technique: Billroth II Gastrectomy Antecolic Anastomosis

FIGURE 27.20
The superior portion of the Finochietto clamp is in place, the first assistant pulls the colon and transverse mesocolon upward, and the first jejunal loop, the duodenojejunal junction, and the ligament of Treitz are identified. The first jejunal loop has been grasped with a smooth Foerster clamp.

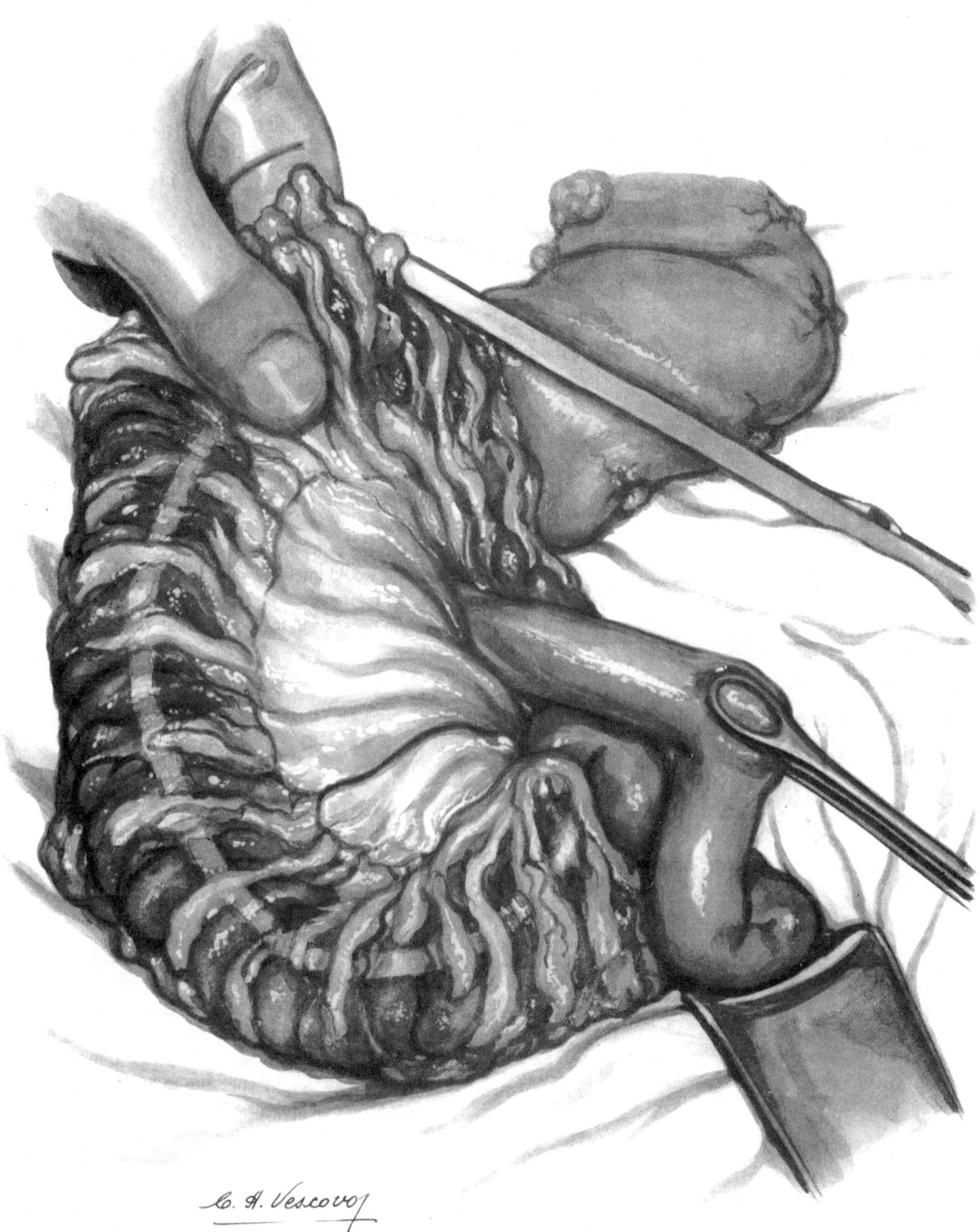

FIGURE 27.20

FIGURE 27.21
The drawing shows the moment at which the surgeon is applying the inferior portion of the Finochietto clamp to the jejunal loop, which is held in place with two Babcock clamps. The insert shows that the clamp has been placed in the correct location. The clamp should not be placed too close to the mesenteric border of the jejunum because that would cause compression of the mesenteric vessels. It should not be placed too close to the antimesenteric border of the jejunum because it would interfere with the performance of the gastrojejunal anastomosis. The superior portion of the Finochietto clamp can be seen in the background, placed on the stomach.

Surgical Technique: Billroth II Gastrectomy Antecolic Anastomosis

FIGURE 27.22
The two parts of the Finochietto twin clamp have been joined. The superior portion grasps the stomach, and the lower portion grasps the jejunum. The jejunum has been brought up in front of the colon with the object of performing an antecolic gastrojejunostomy. An elastic clamp has been placed on the stomach after milking its contents to prevent spillage and contamination of the operative field when the stomach is transected. To perform the gastrojejunal anastomosis, three seromuscular guide sutures from the stomach and the jejunum have been placed. The space between the left and middle guide sutures will determine the length of the gastrojejunal stoma, which is usually 6 cm long. The segment between the middle and right guide sutures points to the portion of the stomach that is to be closed, and therefore will not be part of the anastomosis, according to the Hofmeister-Finsterer technique. A Babcock clamp grasps the border of the jejunum, reclining it downward, to facilitate the placement of the sutures of the posterior seromuscular layer.

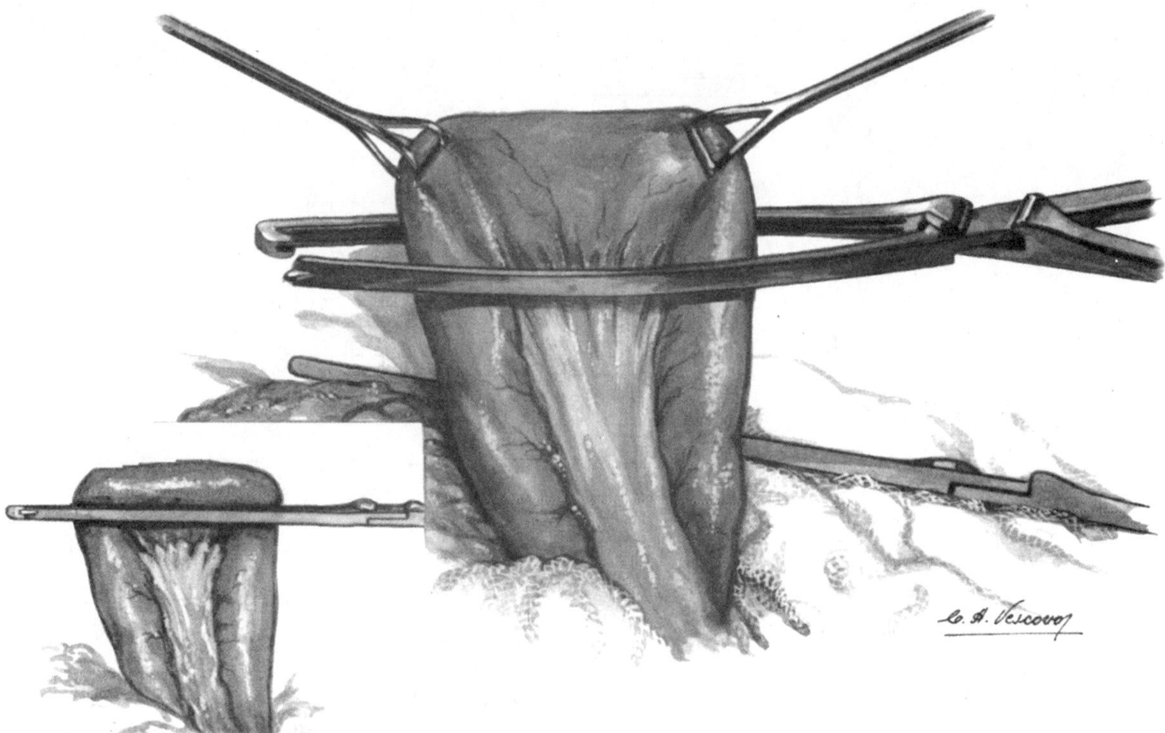

FIGURE 27.21

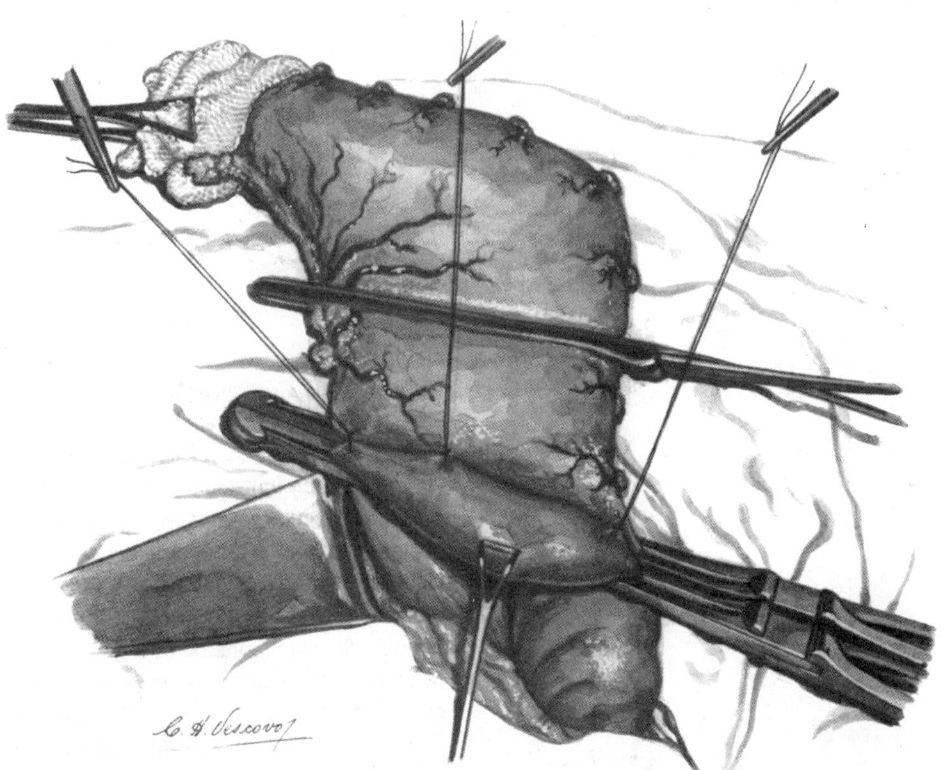

FIGURE 27.22

FIGURE 27.23
The sutures of the posterior seromuscular layer have been placed in the spaces between the three guide sutures and are being cut with straight scissors.

Surgical Technique: Billroth II Gastrectomy Antecolic Anastomosis

FIGURE 27.24
The seromuscular layer of the posterior gastric wall has been incised, with a scalpel, 10 to 12 mm above the twin Finochietto clamp, revealing the submucosal blood vessels. These must be individually ligated near the proximal border of the seromuscular layer. Even though they are small in caliber, the submucosal arterioles bleed profusely when traumatized. Ligation of these arterioles is a preventive measure to avoid bleeding from the gastric wall in the immediate postoperative period. Many surgeons do not ligate the submucosal arterioles believing it to be unnecessary since hemostasis is carried out by the continuous suture of the gastrojejunal anastomosis. The author has seen postgastrectomy bleeding in patients in whom individual ligation of the submucosal arterioles of the stomach has not been carried out.

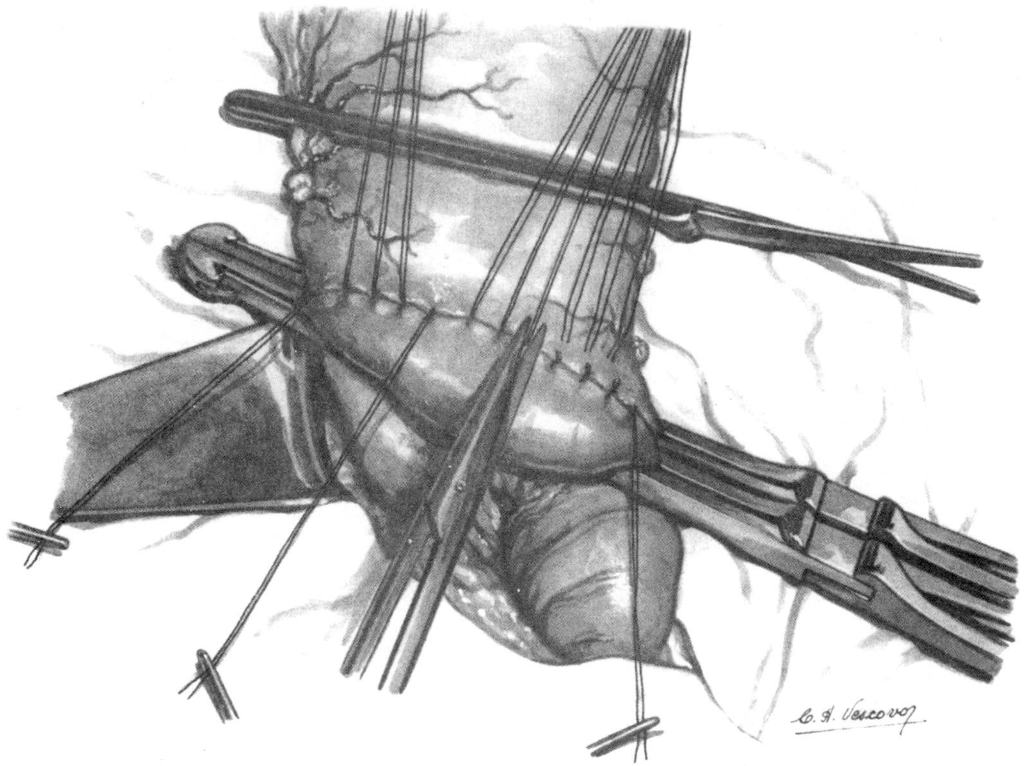

FIGURE 27.23

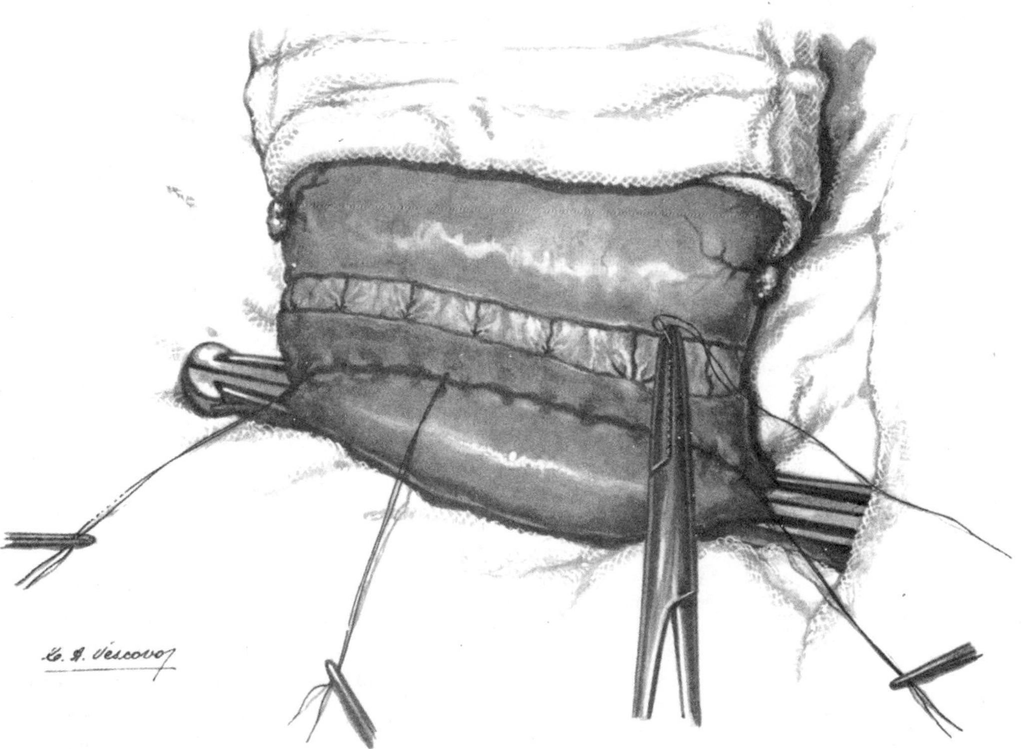

FIGURE 27.24

FIGURE 27.25
The stomach has been turned over to incise the seromuscular layer of the anterior gastric wall and facilitate ligation of the arterioles of the anterior gastric wall, just as the posterior ones were ligated.

Surgical Technique: Billroth II Gastrectomy Antecolic Anastomosis

FIGURE 27.26
Once ligation of the arterioles of the gastric submucosa has been completed, the stomach is divided, using a straight Mayo scissors, following the broken line. The posterior gastric wall is transected first, followed by the anterior wall in its entire extent. A broken line shows the line of incision of the antimesenteric border of the jejunum, extending up to the middle guide suture.

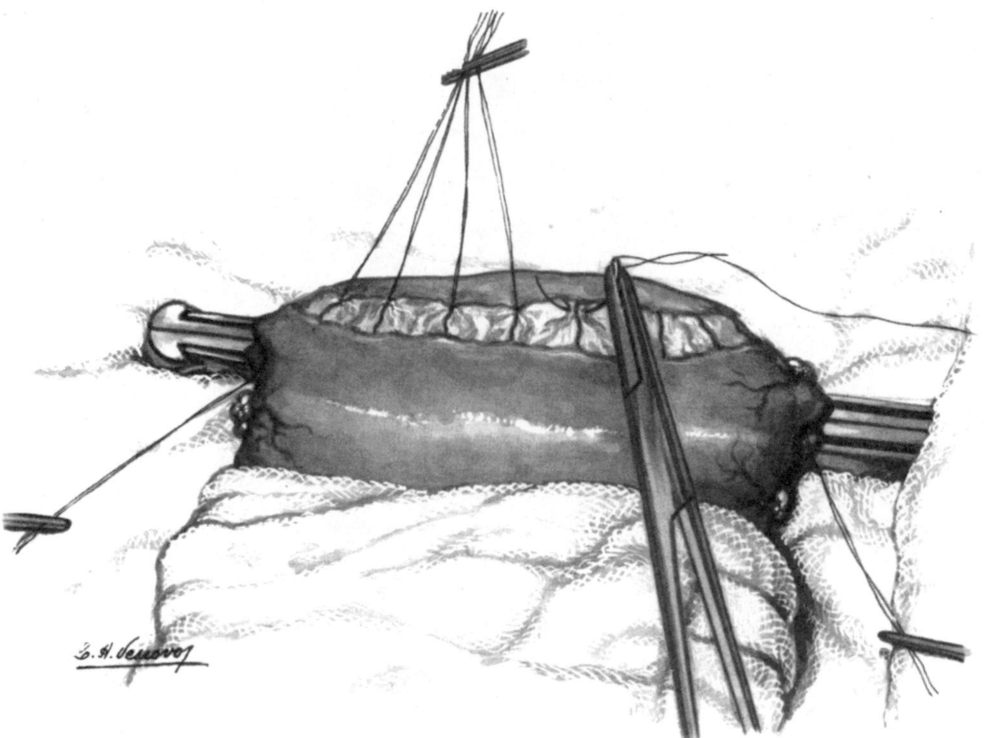

FIGURE 27.25

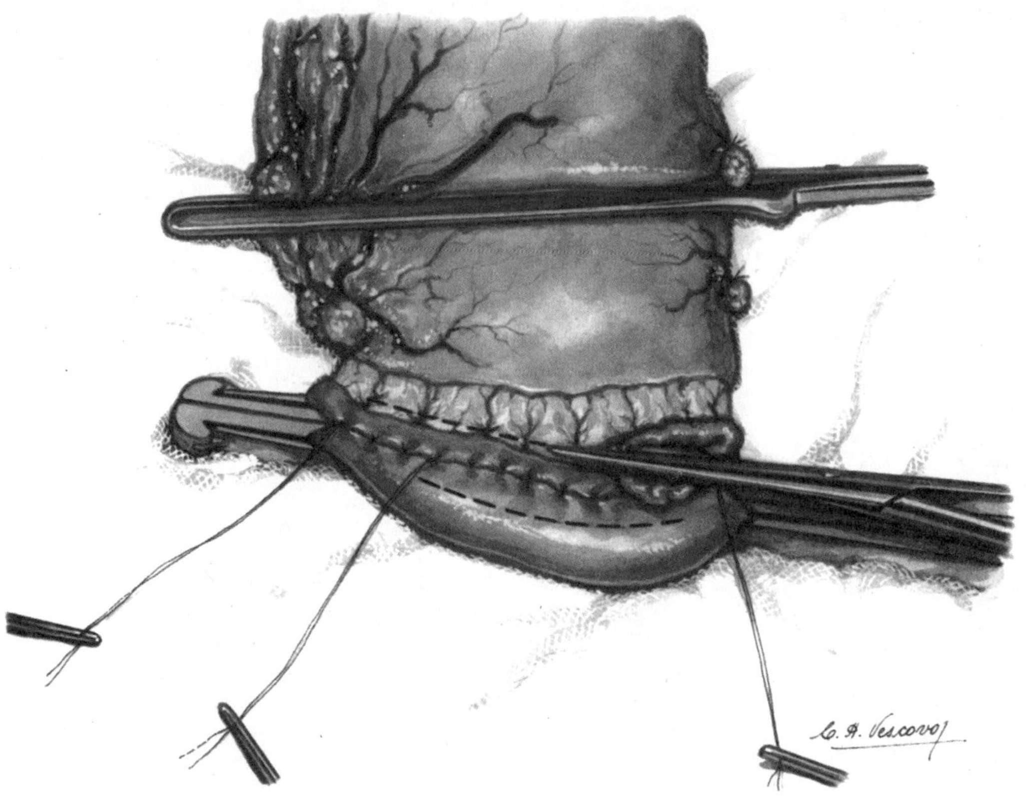

FIGURE 27.26

Surgical Technique: Billroth II Gastrectomy Antecolic Anastomosis

FIGURE 27.27
The stomach has been completely transected and the jejunum has been opened from the middle guide suture to the left guide suture. The posterior complete perforating layer is being closed with a continuous suture using a straight needle. Many surgeons use a curved needle for this continuous suture. Chromic catgut or synthetic reabsorable material is the most frequently used material for the posterior perforating layer. Many surgeons also use silk or cotton for this layer, without any inconveniences.

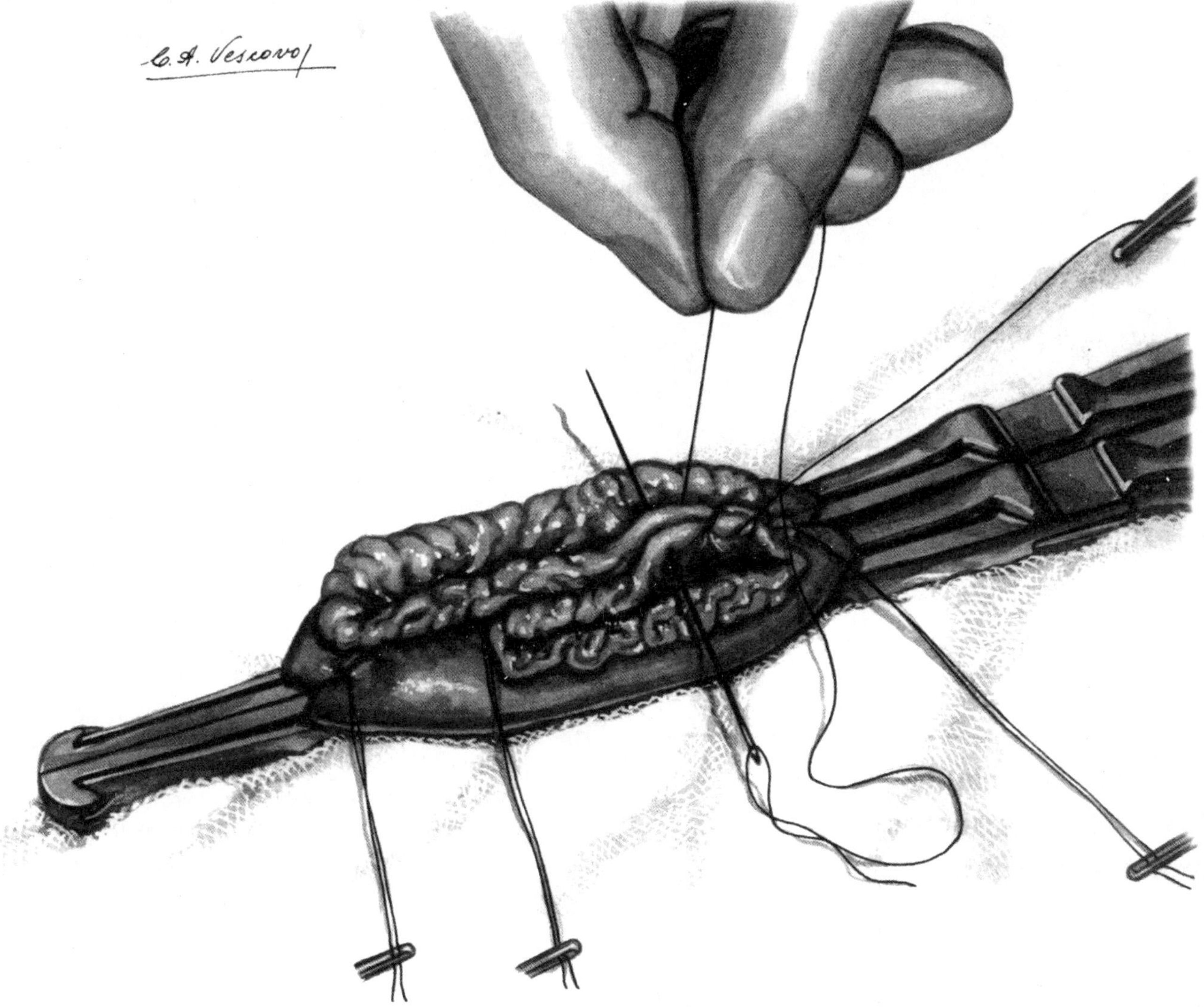

FIGURE 27.27

Surgical Technique: Billroth II Gastrectomy Antecolic Anastomosis

FIGURE 27.28
The continuous perforating suture of the posterior layer between the stomach and jejunum has been completed, and the segment of stomach that will not form part of the new anastomotic stoma is being closed with the same continuous suture.

FIGURE 27.29
Once the continuous suture of the segment of stomach that will not be part of the stoma has been completed toward the lesser curvature, this same segment is oversewn using the same needle and thread making a double through and through closure and continuing with the new gastrojejunal anastomosis.

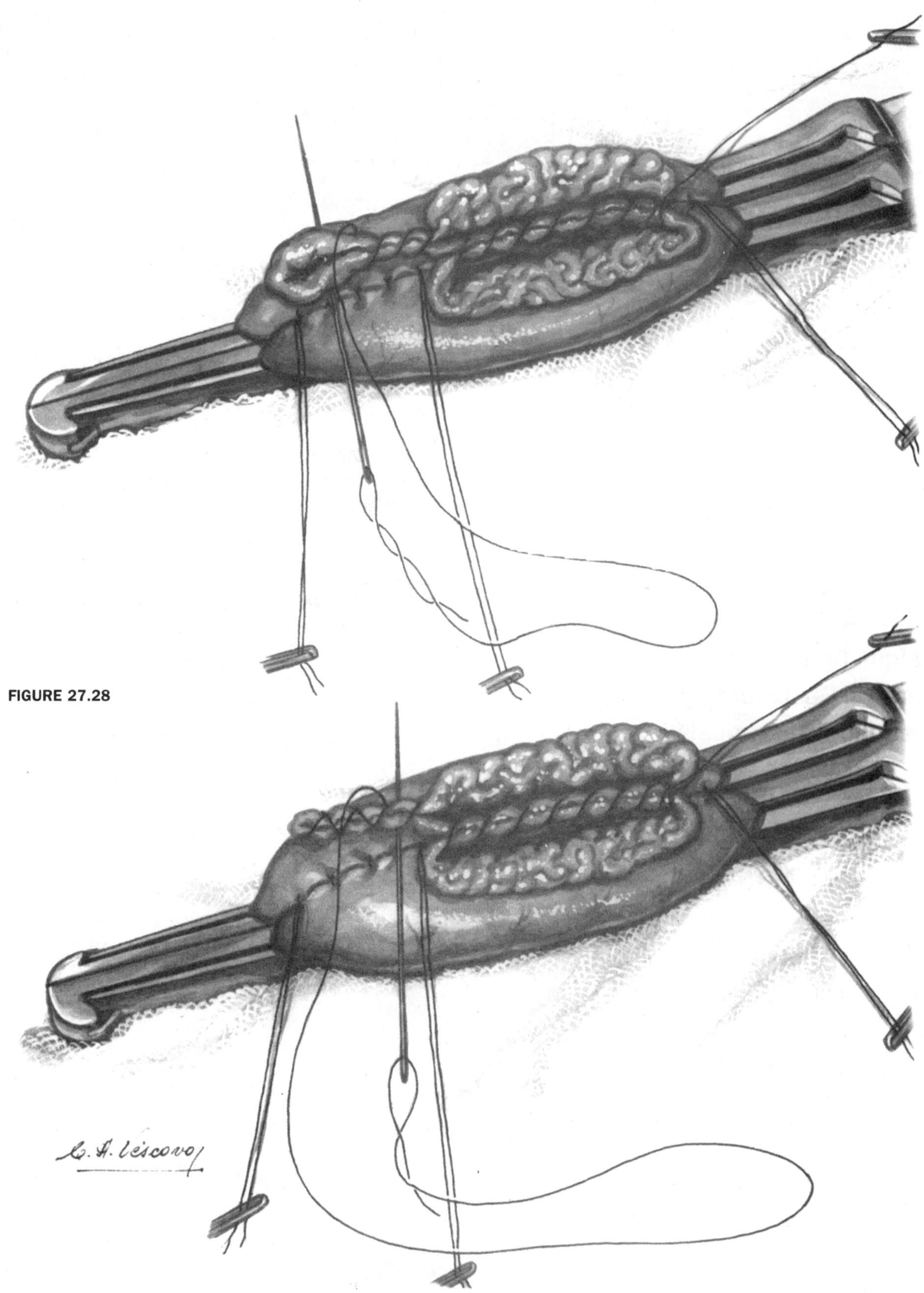

FIGURE 27.28

FIGURE 27.29

FIGURE 27.30
Once the double suture closing the gastric segment has been completed, the gastrojejunostomy is constructed with the same needle and thread using Schmieden sutures, which result in an excellent invagination of the gastric and jejunal mucosa. The Schmieden suture is performed by passing the needle into the mucosa and out the serosa, then over to the other side, entering the mucosa again.

Surgical Technique: Billroth II Gastrectomy Antecolic Anastomosis

FIGURE 27.31
The anterior perforating layer has been completed. The seromuscular layer will be closed with interrupted sutures, after removing the Finochietto clamp.

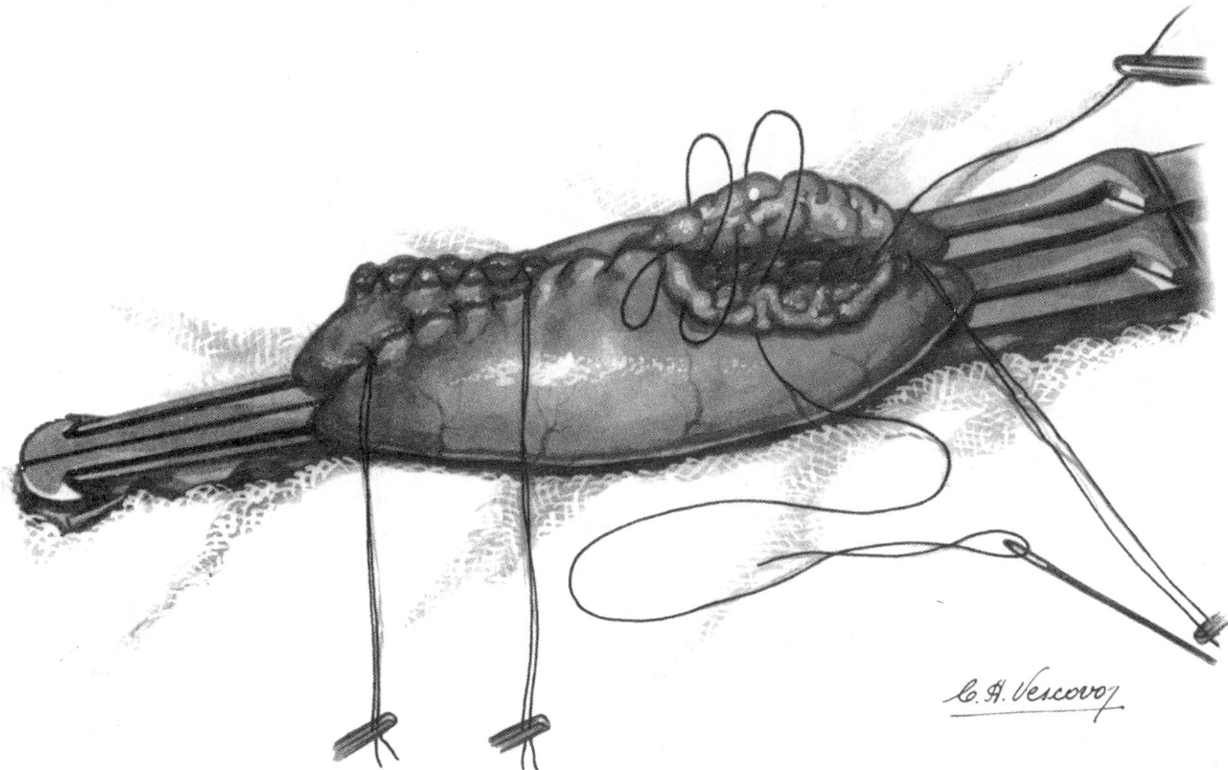

FIGURE 27.30

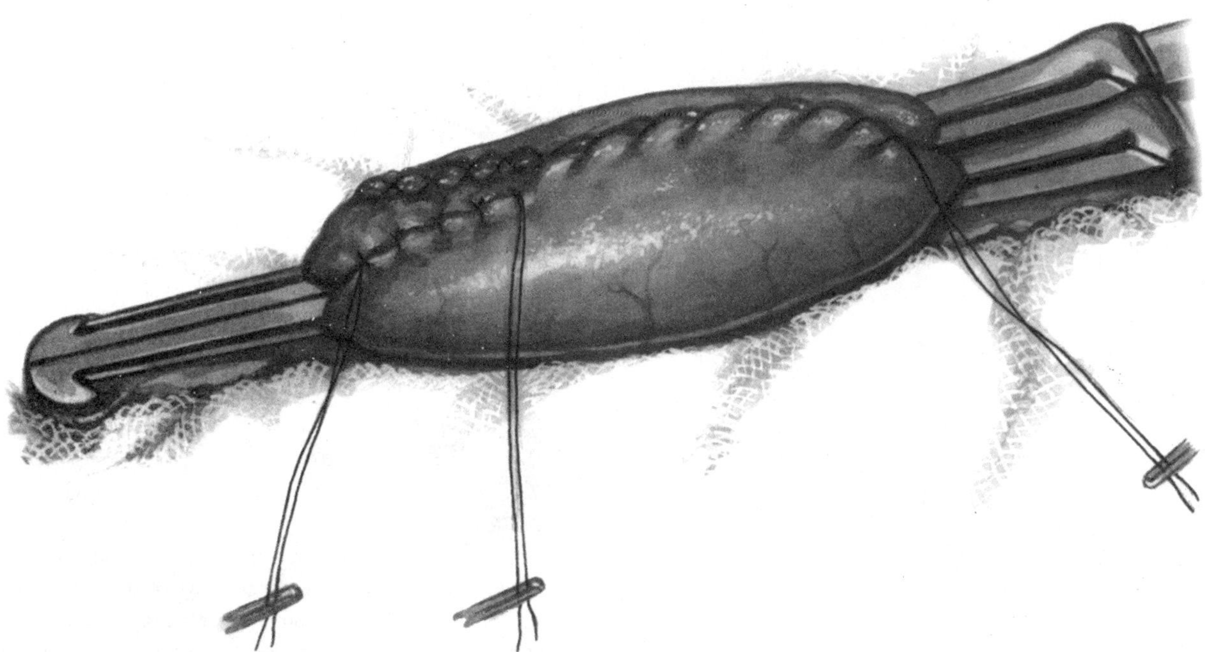

FIGURE 27.31

FIGURE 27.32
The clamp has been loosened so it can be removed. Some surgeons do not use clamps in performing a gastrectomy, believing it is unnecessary. The author always uses a clamp since it permits a cleaner operation. On the other hand, the author has never experienced a complication due to the use of the elastic clamp.

Surgical Technique: Billroth II Gastrectomy Antecolic Anastomosis

FIGURE 27.33
The seromuscular layer has been started beginning with the segment that is not going to be part of the anastomosis. As seen in the drawing, sutures are placed between the gastric seromuscular layer and the jejunal seromuscular layer to cover the perforating gastric suture.

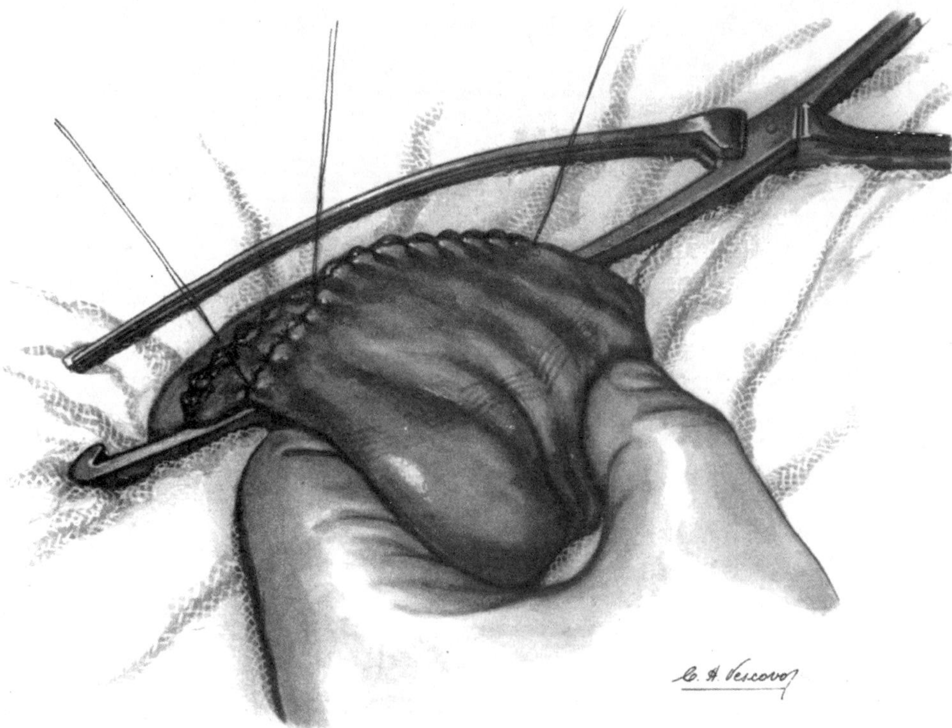

FIGURE 27.32

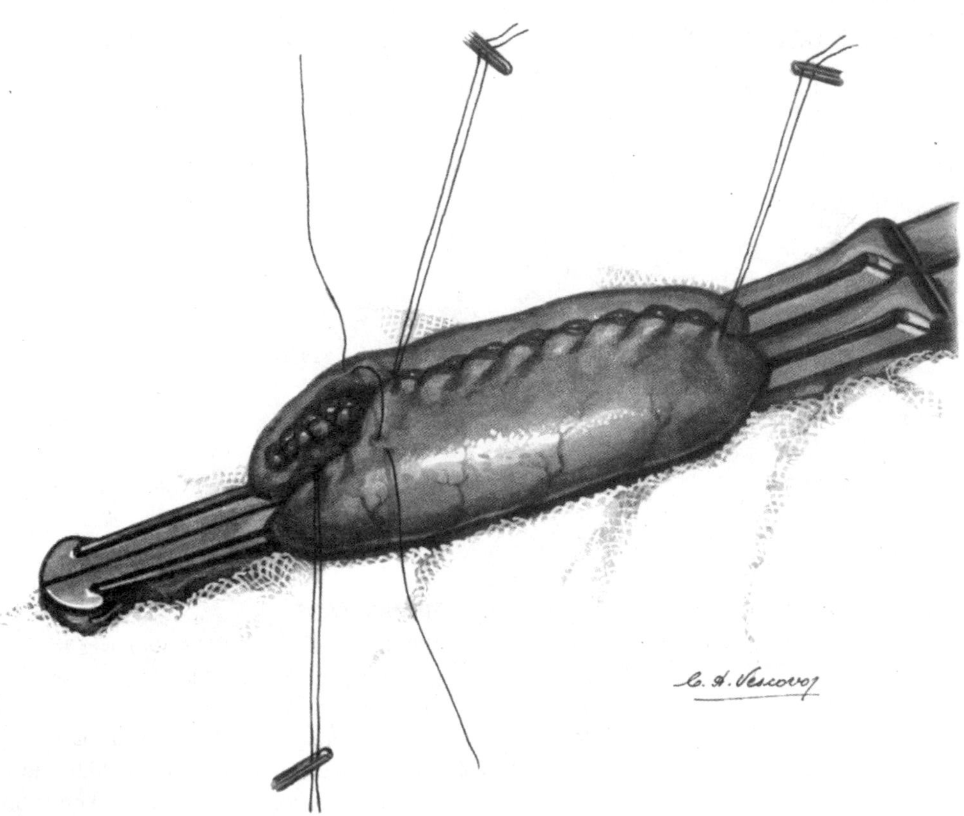

FIGURE 27.33

FIGURE 27.34
The suturing of the gastric angle, which will be completely covered by the seromuscular sutures, is being completed.

Surgical Technique: Billroth II Gastrectomy Antecolic Anastomosis

FIGURE 27.35
The seromuscular sutures of the gastric segment, which will not form part of the anastomosis, have been completed. This segment extends to the middle guide suture, which is being held upward by a clamp. Four gastrojejunal seromuscular sutures have been tied, and a fifth one is about to be tied. The seromuscular suture line will be continued up to the guide suture on the right, which is also being held up by a clamp.

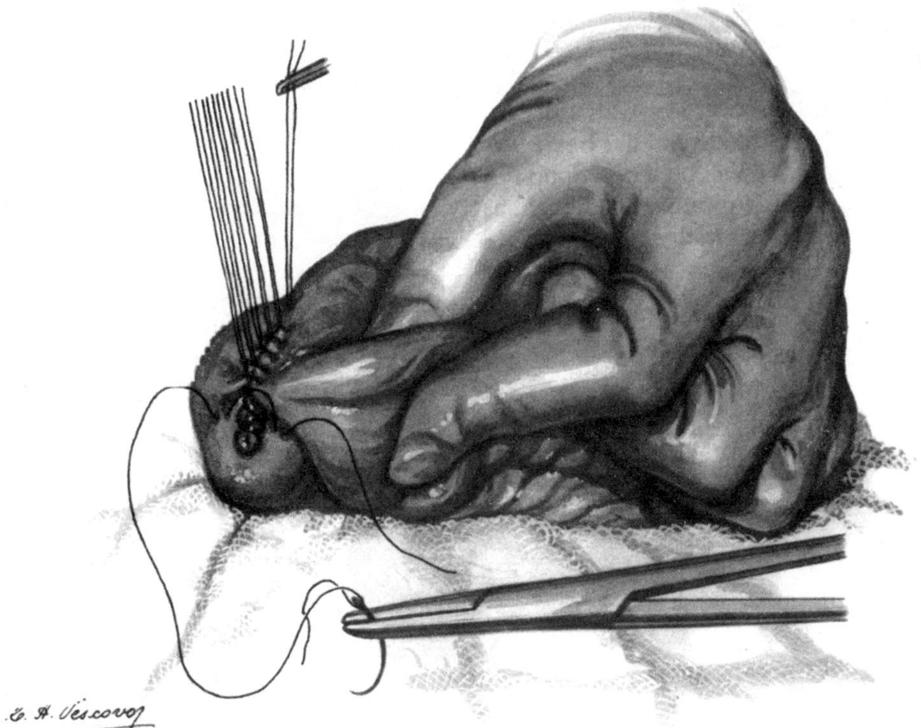

FIGURE 27.34

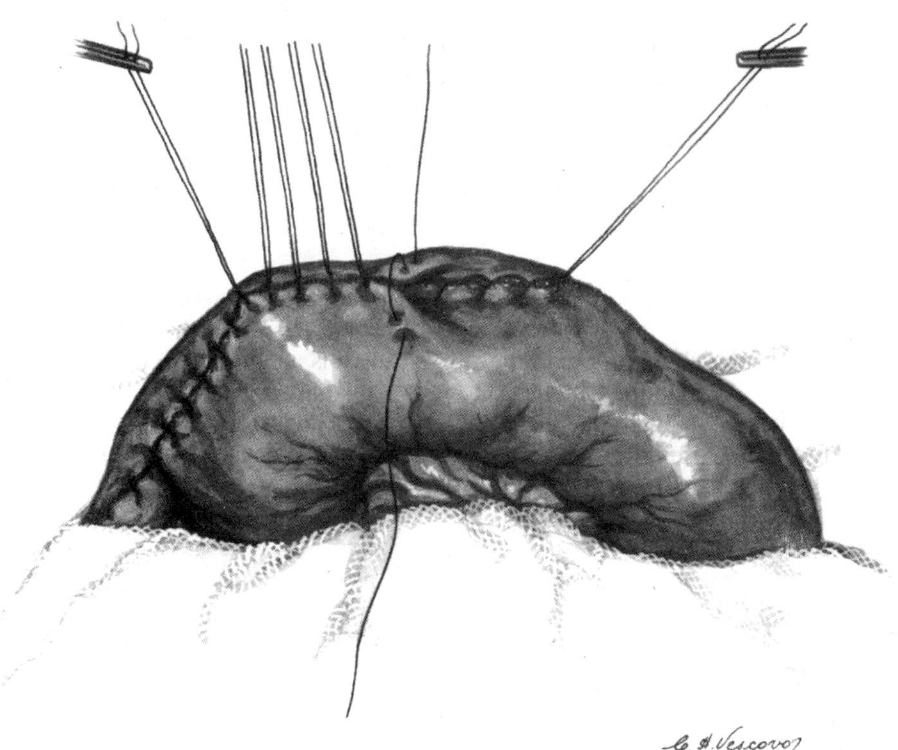

FIGURE 27.35

BILLROTH II GASTRECTOMY WITH STAPLER

Surgeons frequently perform gastrectomies with a stapler. Transection and closure of the duodenum has been previously described. The following will be a description of the technique used to divide and suture the stomach, as well as a gastrojejunal anastomosis with stapler.

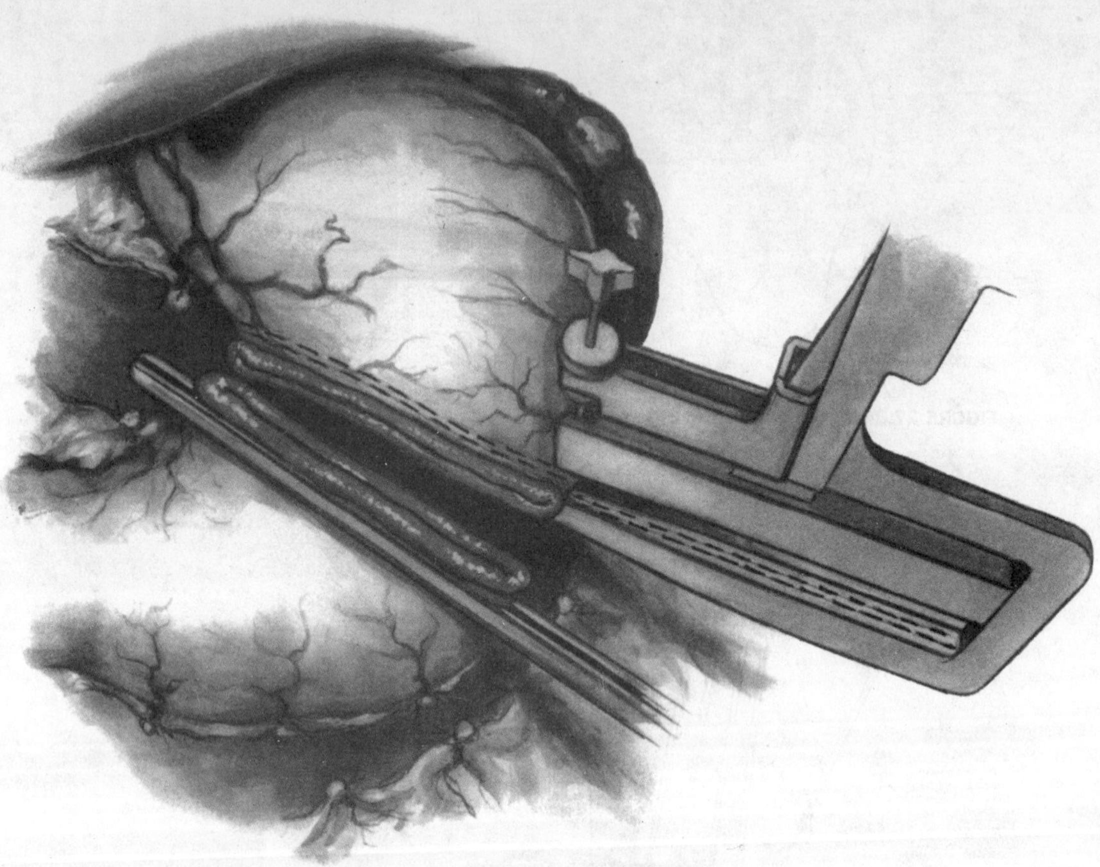

a. To suture and then transect the stomach a TA 90 stapler is placed on it so as to perform the closure with a stapler. The TA 90 stapler should include the entire width of the stomach. Once the stapler is correctly placed at the planned height, the instrument is closed and fired. Before removing the stapler, a clamp is placed below it that also includes the entire width of the stomach. The stomach is then transected below the TA 90 with scalpel or straight Mayo scissors. If the everted mucosa bleeds, hemostasis is attained with electrocautery or with transfixion sutures. Once hemostasis is attained, the TA 90 is removed. At this point, since the duodenum has been transected and both gastric curvatures freed, the surgical specimen can be removed.

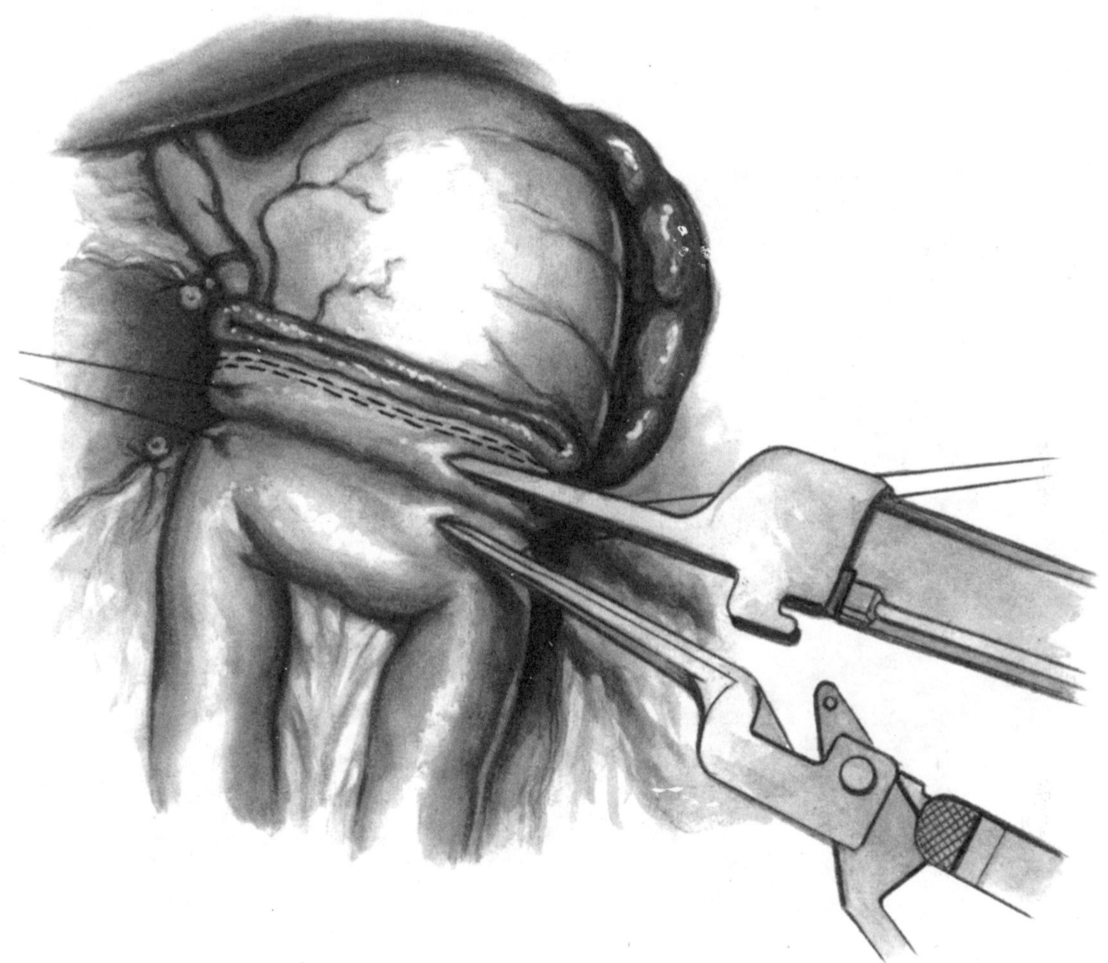

b. The anastomosis of the stomach to the jejunum is then performed. To carry this out, the duodenojejunal junction, the ligament of Treitz, and the first jejunal loop are identified. A segment of the proximal jejunum is brought up in front of the colon and its antimesenteric border placed in contact with the posterior wall of the stomach about 2 or 3 cm from the suture line made with the TA 90. Two small stab wounds, 1 cm each, are made, one in the stomach 1 or 2 cm from the greater curvature and the other in the antimesenteric border of the jejunum, at the same level as the one in the stomach. The stab wounds are made to introduce the arms of the GIA stapler, one in the stomach and the other in the jejunum. In order not to alter the relation of the stomach and the antimesenteric border of the jejunum, seromuscular sutures are placed at both ends including both the stomach and the jejunum. The arms of the GIA are then introduced to their full extent. Some surgeons introduce 5 or 6 cm of the arm, according to the amplitude they wish to give the anastomosis.

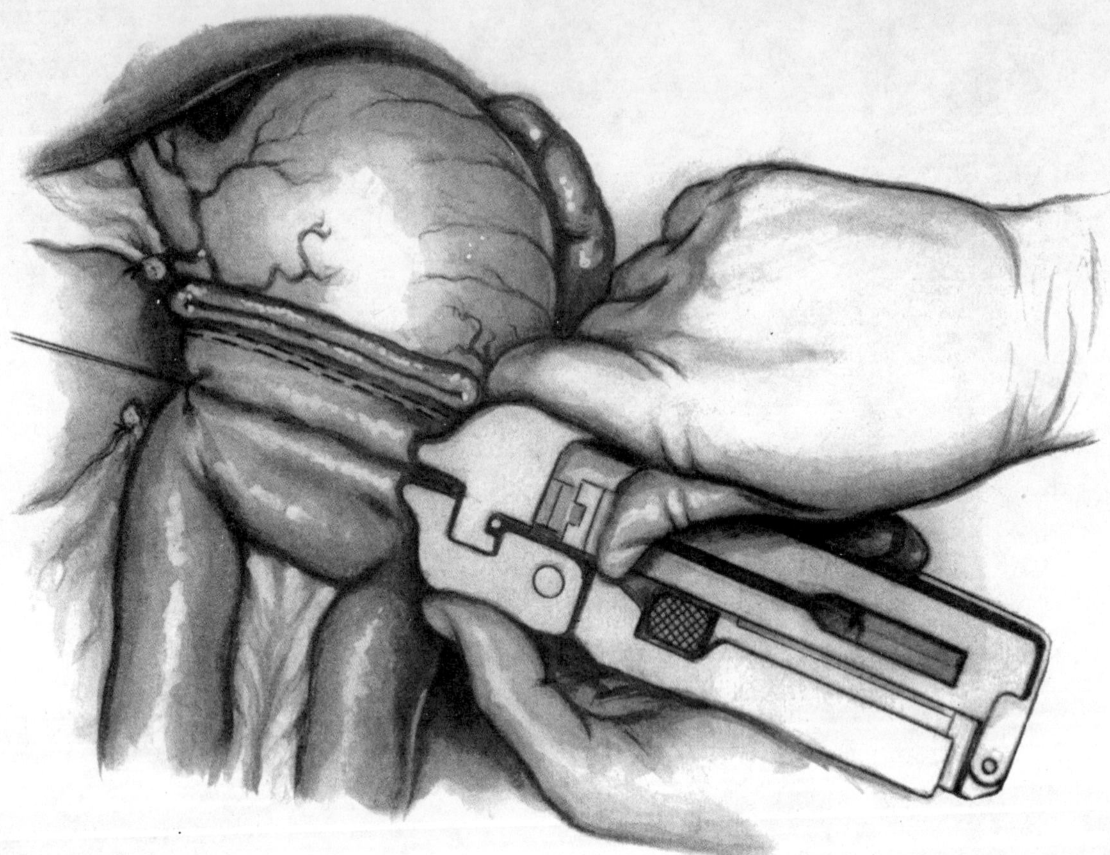

c. The two arms of the GIA stapler have been completely inserted, one in the stomach and the other in the jejunum. At this point the antimesenteric border of the jejunum must be in direct contact with the posterior wall of the stomach. The instrument is then closed and fired. The double row of staples joins both organs, and at the same time the knife blade of the GIA stapler cuts between the double row, creating the anastomosis. The arms of the stapler are removed by performing a small maneuver to separate the arms of the stapler from the bowel tissues. The two stab wounds through which the arms of the GIA stapler were introduced are closed using a TA 30 stapler or a two-layer closure with sutures.

Surgical Technique:
Billroth II Gastrectomy
Transmesocolic Anastomosis

Surgical Technique: Billroth II Gastrectomy Transmesocolic Anastomosis

FIGURE 27.36

The technique in a transmesocolic Billroth II gastrectomy is similar to the antecolic technique. The only difference is that, with the transmesocolic technique, the jejunum is brought up into the upper abdomen through an opening in the mesocolon. The first assistant pulls the transverse colon upward with both hands. The site of the opening in the mesocolon where the opening is to be made is shown by a broken line. This is an avascular zone 8 to 10 cm long.

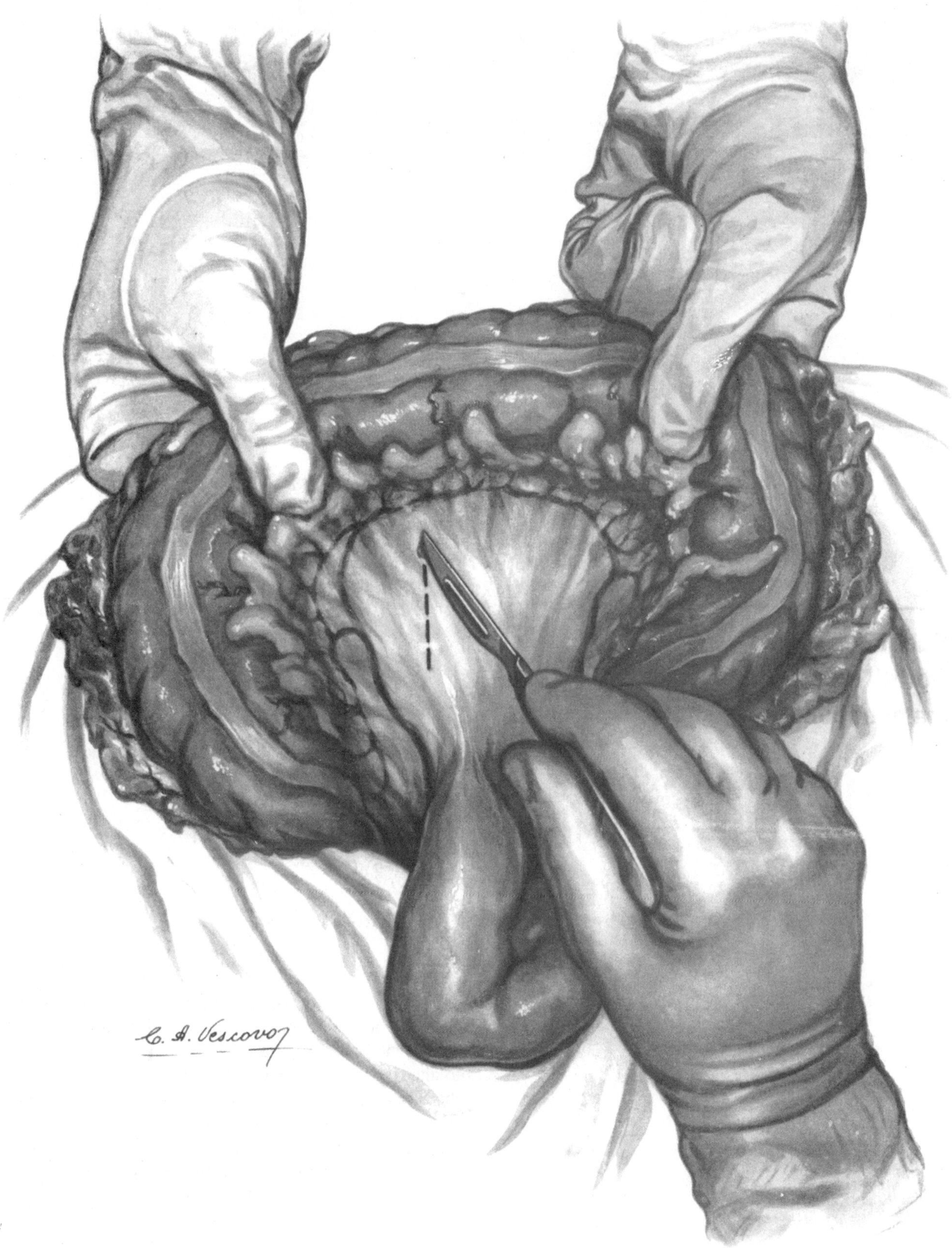

FIGURE 27.36

Surgical Technique: Billroth II Gastrectomy Transmesocolic Anastomosis

FIGURE 27.37
The posterior border of the opening in the mesocolon has been fixed to the stomach with interrupted sutures about 10 to 15 mm from the Finochietto clamp. The jejunum has been brought into the supramesocolic portion of the abdomen with two Babcock clamps. The afferent limb of the jejunal loop is placed at the lesser curvature of the stomach and the efferent limb at the greater curvature. This jejunal loop will be grasped with the lower portion of the twin Finochietto clamp. The gastrojejunal anastomosis is carried out like the previously described anastomosis for the Billroth II gastrectomy.

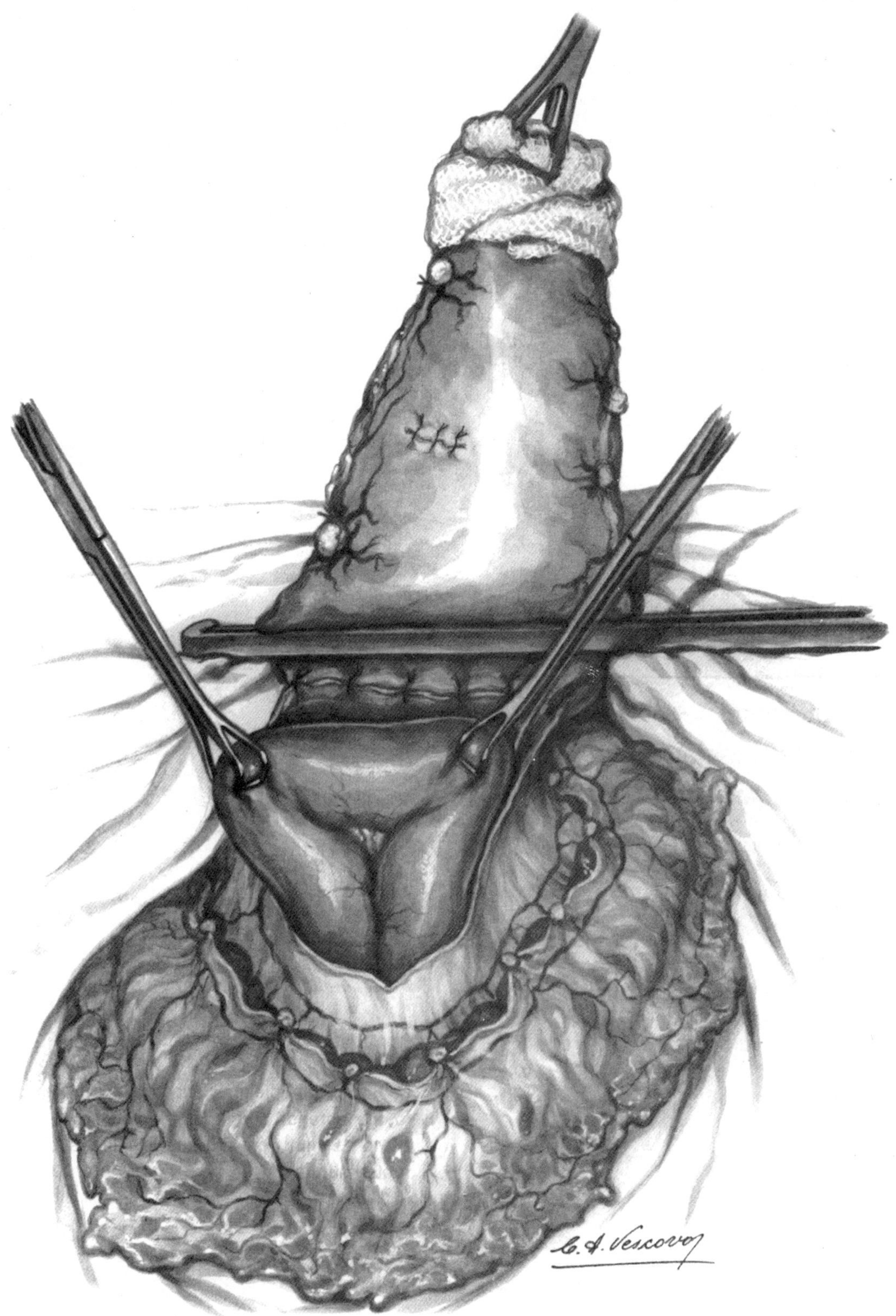

FIGURE 27.37

Surgical Technique: Billroth II Gastrectomy Transmesocolic Anastomosis

FIGURE 27.38
Once the gastrojejunal anastomosis is completed, it is fixed to the anterior border of the mesocolic opening at a point 10 to 15 mm from the gastrojejunal suture line, using interrupted sutures.

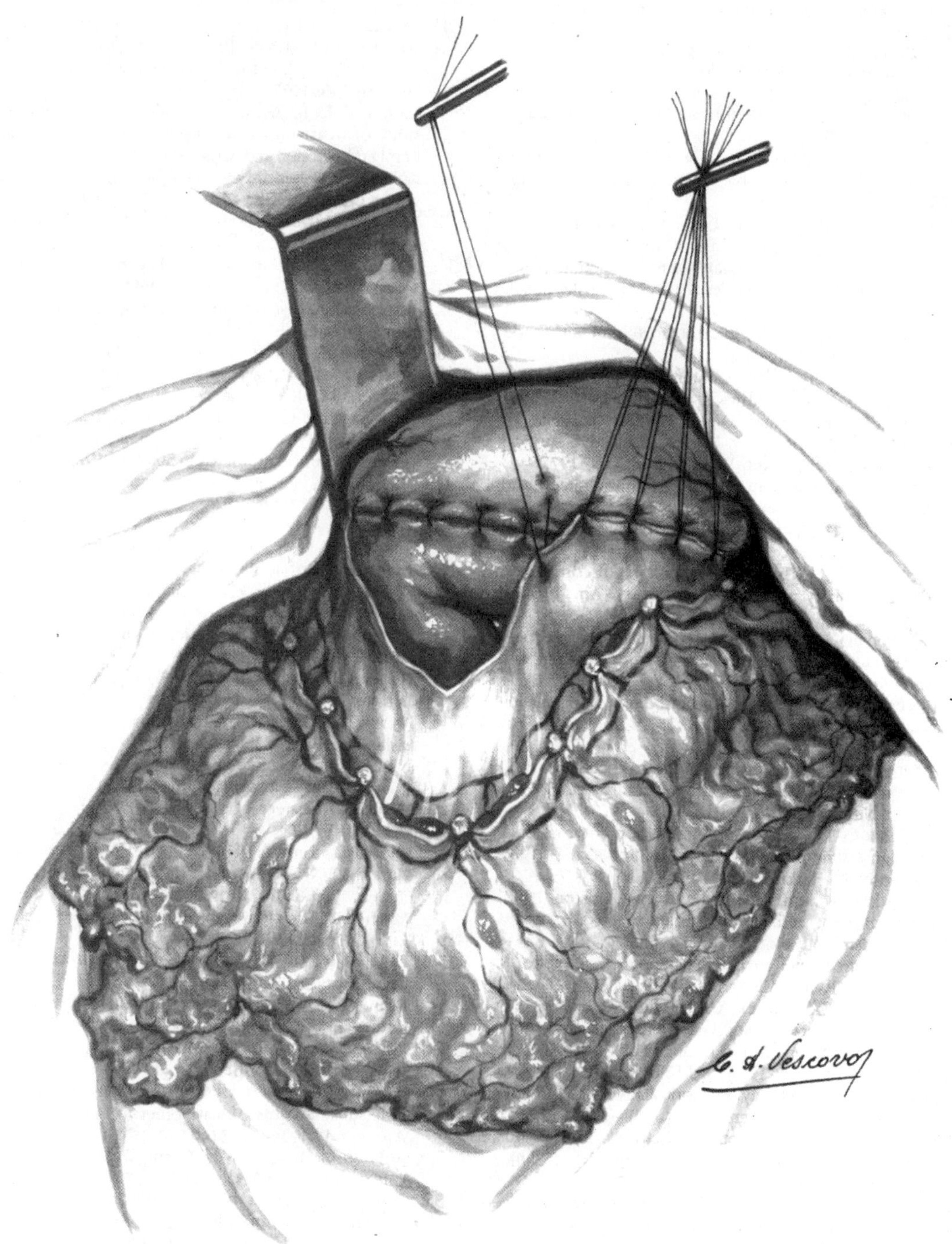

FIGURE 27.38

References

1. Bancroft, F. Pyloric exclusion for duodenal ulcer. Am. J. Surg. 16:223, 1932.
2. Berne, C.J., Rosoff, L. Peptic ulcer perforation of the gastroduodenal artery complex. Ann. Surg. 169:141, 1969.
3. Czendes, A., Lazo, M., Braghetto, I. A surgical technique for high (cardial or juxtacardial) benign chronic gastric ulcer. Am. J. Surg. 135:857, 1978.
4. Devin, R., Lataste, J., Maillet, P. Noveau Traité de technique chirurgicale. Vol. 10, p. 257. Masson et Cie, Paris, 1968.
5. Dragstedt, L.R., Owens, F.M. Jr. Supradiaphragmatic section of the vagus nerves in the treatment of duodenal ulcer. Surg. Gynecol. Obstet. 85:461, 1947.
6. Duval, J. La gastrectomie dans les ulcéres très haut situés de l'estomac. Presse Méd. 61:389, 1953.
7. Etala, E. Gastrectomy for peptic ulcer. Contemp. Surg. 13:21, 1978.
8. Farmer, D.A., Harrower, H.W., Smithwick, R.H. Hemigastrectomy-vagotomy for duodenal ulcer. Am. J. Digest. Dis. 7:195, 1962.
9. Feldman, S.D., Wise, L., Ballinger, N.F. Review of elective surgical treatment of chronic duodenal ulcer. World J. Surg. 1:9, 1977.
10. Finsterer, H. The surgical treatment of ulcer of the stomach and duodenum. Surg. Gynecol. Obstet. 36:454, 1923.
11. Finsterer, H., Chuna, F. The surgical treatment of duodenal ulcer. Surg. Gynecol. Obstet. 52:1099, 1931.
12. Florence, M.G., Hart, M.J., White, T.T. Ampullary disconnection during the course of biliary and duodenal surgery. Am. J. Surg. 142:100, 1981.
13. Frederick, P.L., Osborne, M.P. The development of surgical procedures for the treatment of peptic ulceration of the stomach and duodenum. Surgery 58:884, 1965.
14. Fromm, D. Ulceration of the stomach and duodenum. In Fromm, D. (Ed.) Gastrointestinal surgery. Vol. I, p. 233. Churchill Livingstone, New York, 1985.
15. Graham, R.R. Surgical therapy in lesions of the stomach and duodenum. In Bancroft, F.W. (Ed.) Operative surgery, p. 545 D. Appleton Century, New York, 1941.
16. Greenal, M.J., Lehnert, T. Vagotomy or gastrectomy for elective treatment of benign gastric ulceration? Dig. Dis. Sci. 30:353, 1985.
17. Griffith, C.A. Anatomy. In Harkins, H.N., Nyhus, L.M. (Eds.) Surgery of the stomach and duodenum. P. 21. Little, Brown, Boston, 1962.
18. Grimson, K.S. Surgical procedures for peptic ulcer: Critique of commitee report. Gastroenterology 24:275, 1953.
19. Gueullette, R. La gastrectomie pour exclusion. In Gueullette, R. Chirurgie de l'estomac. P. 117. Masson et Cie, Paris, 1956.
20. Gustavsson, S., Kelly, K.A., Hench, V.S., Melton, L.J. III. Giant gastric and duodenal ulcers: A population-based study with a comparison of nongiant ulcers. World J. Surg. 11:333, 1987.
21. Haeger, K. History of surgery. P. 199. Harold Starke, London, 1990.
22. Hampson, L.G. Partial Gastrectomy. In Nora, P.F. (Ed.) Operative surgery. Ed. 3, p. 497. W.B. Saunders, Philadelphia, 1990.
23. Harkins, H.N. Gastric resection: Billroth I. In Harkins, H.N., Nyhus, L.M. (Eds.) Surgery of the stomach and duodenum. Ed. 2. Little, Brown, Boston, 1969.
24. Herrington, J.L. Jr. The pyloric antrum: The relative extent of distal gastrectomy necessary to ensure its complete extirpation. Surgery 44:775, 1958.
25. Herrington, J.L. Jr., Edwards, L.W., Classen, K.L., Carlson, R.I., Edwards, W.H., Scott, H.W. Jr. Vagotomy and antral resection in treatment of duodenal ulcer. Results in 514 patients. Ann. Surg. 150:499, 1959.
26. Herrington, J.L. Jr., Sawyers, J.L. A 25 year experience with vagotomy-antrectomy. Arch. Surg. 106:469, 1973.
27. Herrington, J.L. Jr., Davidson, J III. Bleeding gastroduodenal ulcers: Choice of operations. World J. Surg. 11:304, 1987.
28. Herrington, J.L. Jr. Historical Aspects of Gastric Surgery. In Scott, H.W. Jr., Sawyers, J.L. (Eds.) Surgery of the stomach, duodenum and small intestine. Ed. 2, p. 1. Blackwell, Boston, 1992.
29. Hoerr, S.O., Steiger, E. Billroth II Gastrectomy. In Nyhus, L.M., Baker, R.J. (Eds.) Mastery of surgery. Ed. 2, vol. I, p. 649. Little, Brown, Boston, 1992.
30. Hunt, P.S. Bleeding gastroduodenal ulcers: Selection of patients for surgery. World J. Surg. 11:289, 1987.
31. Jensen, H.E., Hoffmann, J., Jorgensen, P.W. High gastric ulcer. World J. Surg. 11:325, 1987.
32. Jones, R.C., et al. Difficult closures of the duodenum stump. Arch. Surg. 94:696, 1967.
33. Jordan, G.L. Jr. Acute gastroduodenal perforation: Comparative study of treatment with simple closure, subtotal gastrectomy and hemigastrectomy and vagotomy. Arch. Surg. 92:449, 1966.
34. Kelling, G. Ueber die operative behandlung des chronischen ulcus ventriculi. Arch. Klin. Chir. 109:775, 1918.
35. Kelly, K.A., Malagelada, J.R. Medical and surgical treatment of chronic gastric ulcer. Clin. Gastroenterol. 13:621, 1984.
36. Kirschner, P.A., Garlock, J.H. The rationale of routine omentectomy in subtotal gastrectomy. Surgery 36:884, 1954.
37. Lewisohn, R. The frequency of gastroduodenal ulcers. Surg. Gynecol. Obstet. 40:70, 1925.
38. Lewisohn, R. Changes in surgical treatment of chronic duodenal ulcers during the past 50 years. Arch. Surg. 77:61, 1958.
39. Madden, J.L., Kandalaft, S., Eghran, M. Surgical maneuver incorrectly credited to Kocher. Surgery 63:522, 1968.
40. Madlener, M. Ueber pylorektomie bie pylorus fermen magengeschwar. Zentralbl. Chir. 50:1313, 1923.
41. Madlener, M. Pylorectomy as indirect operation for ulcer. Zentralbl. Chir. 51:1896, 1924.
42. Mayo, W.J. A review of 500 cases of gastroenterostomies, including pyloroplasty, gastroduodenostomy and gastrojejunostomy. Ann. Surg. 42:641, 1905.
43. Moore, F.P., Wyllie, J.H. Ischaemic necrosis of lesser curve after proximal gastric vagotomy. Br. Med. J. 4:328, 1975.
44. Moynihan, B.G.A. On duodenal ulcer and its surgical treatment. Lancet 2:1656, 1901.
45. Nissen, R. Duodenal and jejunal peptic ulcer. W. Heinemann, London, 1952.
46. Nyhus, L.M. Gastric Ulcer. In Harkins, H.N., Nyhus, L.M. (Eds.) Surgery of the stomach and duodenum. P. 159. Little, Brown, Boston 1962.
47. Nyhus, L.M. Selective vagotomy, antrectomy and gastroduodenostomy for the treatment of duodenal ulcer. In Nyhus, L.M., Baker, R.J. (Eds.) Mastery of surgery. Ed. 2, vol. I, p. 662. Little, Brown, Boston, 1992.
48. Olch, P.D., Harkins, H.N. A historical review of gastric surgery. In Harkins, H.N., Nyhus, L.M. (Eds.) Surgery of the stomach and duodenum. P. 3. Little, Brown, Boston, 1962.
49. Pauchet, V. Practique chirurgicale illustrée. Vol. 7. Gastron Doin, Paris, 145:149, 1927.
50. Pauchet, V. Sur la technique de la gastrectomie. Bull. Mem. Soc. Chir. (Paris) 23:243, 1931.
51. Péan, J.E. De l'ablation des tumeurs de l'estomac par la gastrectomie. Gaz. Hôp. 52:473, 1887.
52. Polya, E. Re-establishment of the gastrointestinal passage after gastric resection. Surg. Gynecol. Obstet. 70:270, 1940.
53. Quénu, J., Loygue, J., Perrotin, J., Dubost, C., Moreaux, J. Opérations sur les parois de l'abdomen et sur le tube digestive. P. 453. Masson et Cie, Paris, 1968.
54. Ruding, R., Hirdes, W.H. Extent of gastric antrum and its significance. Surgery 53:743, 1963.
55. Rydygier, L. Ueber magenresektion mit demonstration von präparaten. Arch. Klin. Chir. 26:271, 1881.
56. Siewert, J.R., Hoelscher, A.H. Billroth I gastrectomy. In Nyhus, L.M., Baker, R.J. (Eds.) Mastery of surgery. Ed. 2, vol. I, p. 639. Little, Brown, Boston, 1992.
57. Scott, H.W. Jr., Sawyers, J.L., Gobbel, W.G. Jr., Herrington, J.L. Jr., Edwards, W.H., Edwards, L.W. Vagotomy and antrectomy in surgical treatment of duodenal ulcer disease. Surg. Clin. North Am. 46:349, 1966.
58. Schoemaker, J. Zur technik der magenresektion nach Billroth I. Arch. Klin. Chir. 121:268, 1922.
59. Spencer, F.C. Ischemic necrosis of the remaining stomach following subtotal gastrectomy. Arch. Surg. 73:844, 1956.
60. Stempien, S.J., Lee, E.R., Dagradi, A.E. The role of distal gastrectomy with and without vagotomy in the control of cephalic secretion and peptic ulcer disease. Surgery 71:110, 1972.
61. Tanner, N.C. Billroth II Gastrectomy. In Nyhus, L.M., Wastell, C. (Eds.) Surgery of the stomach and duodenum. Ed. 3. Little, Brown, Boston, 1977.

62. Thompson, N.W. Ischemic necrosis of proximal gastric remnant following subtotal gastrectomy. Surgery 54:434, 1963.
63. von Haberer, H. Meine erfahrungen mit 183 magenresektionen. Arch. Klin. Chir. 106:533, 1915.
64. von Haberer, H. Meine technick der magenresektion. Munchen Wochenschr. 80:915, 1933.
65. Wangensteen, O.H., Wagensteen, S.D. History of gastric surgery: Glimpses into its early and more recent past. In Nyhus, L.M., Wastell, C. (Eds.) Surgery of the stomach and duodenum. Ed. 3, p. 43. Little, Brown, Boston, 1977
66. Wastell, C. Partial and total gastrectomy. In Schwartz, S.I., Ellis, H. (Eds.). Maingot's abdominal operations. Ed. 9, vol. 1 p. 731. Appleton Lange, Norwalk, CT, 1990.
67. Welch, C.E., Rodkey, G.V., von Gryska, P. One thousand operations for peptic ulcer disease. Ann. Surg. 204:454, 1986.
68. Welch, C.E. Gastric resection for duodenal ulcer. In Scott, H.W. Jr., Sawyers, J.L. (Eds.). Surgery of the stomach, duodenum and small intestine. Ed. 2, p. 540. Blackwell, Boston, 1992.
69. Ziegler, H. Billroth erste magenresektion. Krebsarzt 4:49, 1949.
70. Zinner, M.J. Atlas of gastric surgery. P. 30. Churchill Livingstone, New York, 1992.
71. Zinninger, M.M., Collins, W.T. Extension of carcinoma of stomach into duodenum and esophagus. Ann. Surg. 130:557, 1949.
72. Zinninger, M.M. Extension of gastric cancer in the intramural lymphatics and its relation to gastrectomy. Am. Surg. 20:920, 1954.
73. Zollinger, R.M., Zollinger, R.M. Jr. (Eds.) Atlas of surgical operations. Ed. 4, p. 46. Macmillan, New York, 1975.
74. Zollinger, R.M., Zollinger, R.M. Jr. (Eds.) Atlas of surgical operations. Ed. 4, p. 50. Macmillan, New York, 1975.

Section F

Surgery of the Stomach and Duodenum

CHAPTER 28

Dissection and Closure of the Difficult Duodenal Stump

Closure of the duodenum in patients with gastric ulcer or carcinoma is not usually difficult and rarely becomes complicated if it is done correctly. The situation is very different in patients with duodenal ulcer, particularly when the ulcers are big and perforating into the pancreas, and the duodenal walls are edematous and friable, with severe fibrous retraction due to chronic ulceration. This fibrous retraction produces a dangerous proximity of the ulcer to the papilla as well as to the main and accessory pancreatic ducts. Occasionally the inflammatory process surrounding the ulcer can compromise the common bile duct and the common hepatic artery. The fibrosis and retraction can cause severe alterations in the regional anatomy, making it essential to take all possible precautionary measures to prevent complications, which can be very severe.

EVALUATION OF THE DUODENUM

Before opting for a gastrectomy, the surgeon must previously carry out a careful evaluation of the condition of the duodenum to determine its surgical possibilities. In this exploration the surgeon will determine the size and location of the ulcer, whether it is perforating into the pancreas, the distance between the ulcer and the pylorus, the degree of pancreatic reaction, and the proximity of the ulcer to the choledochus and the papilla of Vater. It is also important to determine whether the anterior duodenal wall is healthy, pliable, and normal in extent, because most of the techniques of duodenal stump closure are based on generous utilization of the anterior duodenal wall (8, 10, 11, 16, 24). To make it easier to evaluate the duodenum, it is very useful to mobilize the duodenum by performing a Vautrin-Kocher maneuver, which also brings the duodenum up to a more superficial position. In case there is any doubt about the relation between the ulcer and the common bile duct, it is advisable to perform a transverse choledochostomy long enough to insert a thin biliary probe to determine the course of the common duct and the location of the papilla of Vater.

Some surgeons are afraid to perform a choledochostomy in bile ducts of normal caliber because of the fear of causing a postoperative stricture. Although some cases of postoperative stricture of the common duct have been reported in longitudinal choledochostomies, a stricture has never been proven to have occurred after a transverse choledochostomy. In all patients in whom a choledochostomy is performed it should be completed by inserting a fine T-tube with short transverse limbs. Placement of a T-tube, in addition to being indispensable after a choledochostomy, contributes to healing of the closure of the duodenal stump by diminishing the intraluminal pressure.

Exploration of the duodenum is extremely valuable in orienting the surgeon's decision. However, the conclusions reached at exploration are not always definitive (27, 28).

DUODENAL ULCERS THAT ARE UNRESECTABLE OR OF HIGH RISK TO THE PATIENT

If evaluation of duodenal exploration reveals that the ulcer is unresectable or that its resection carries a high risk, the surgeon should choose an operation in which resection of the pathologic duodenum is unnecessary. In this situation many surgeons resort to a truncal vagotomy with a gastric drainage procedure, either a pyloroplasty or a gastrojejunostomy. Sometimes pyloroplasty cannot be performed due to edema and fibrosis of the pylorus or the duodenum. In these cases a gastrojejunostomy or Jaboulay gastroduodenostomy can be done (7). The author prefers to perform a Finsterer-Bancroft-Plenk exclusion gastrectomy with an added truncal vagotomy in patients with an unresectable or high-risk duodenal ulcer. An exclusion gastrectomy gives good results when technically well carried out. Before deciding for this procedure one must be sure that the gastric antrum is well vascularized and a duodenotomy or pyloroplasty has not been performed.

THE SURGEON'S DECISION

Once duodenal exploration has been completed, the surgeon faces one of these three situations:

1. The surgeon realizes that the duodenal ulcer is unresectable or its resection involves grave risk and decides to carry out a lesser surgical procedure.
2. The surgeon believes that duodenal closure will be difficult but that it will be possible to carry it out using one of the techniques designed to handle the difficult duodenum.
3. The surgeon is sure that closure of the duodenal stump will not present difficulties but during the course of the operation realizes the opposite at a moment at which he or she cannot turn back. The final result will depend on the surgeon's experience and ability to resolve this complex problem.

In some patients the ulcerated duodenum is very retracted and appears to be wrapped in fibrous tissue, giving the impression of a very difficult duodenum to manage surgically. However, by removing the fibrous wrappings it is possible to determine that the apparently difficult case is really an easy duodenum to manage.

We will now describe some of the techniques designed to manage the difficult duodenum.

The Surgeon's Decision

Apparently Difficult Duodenum

FIGURE 28.1
In some patients, like the one shown in the drawing, the duodenum is completely wrapped in layers of fibrous tissue, giving the impression of a duodenum that is very difficult to manage and close. However, after the fibrous membranes covering the duodenum with scissors are divided, it becomes evident that the walls of the duodenum appear healthy in spite of the callous ulcer of the anterior duodenal wall, near the pylorus. In this case the Billroth II gastrectomy and the duodenal closure were performed without any difficulty.

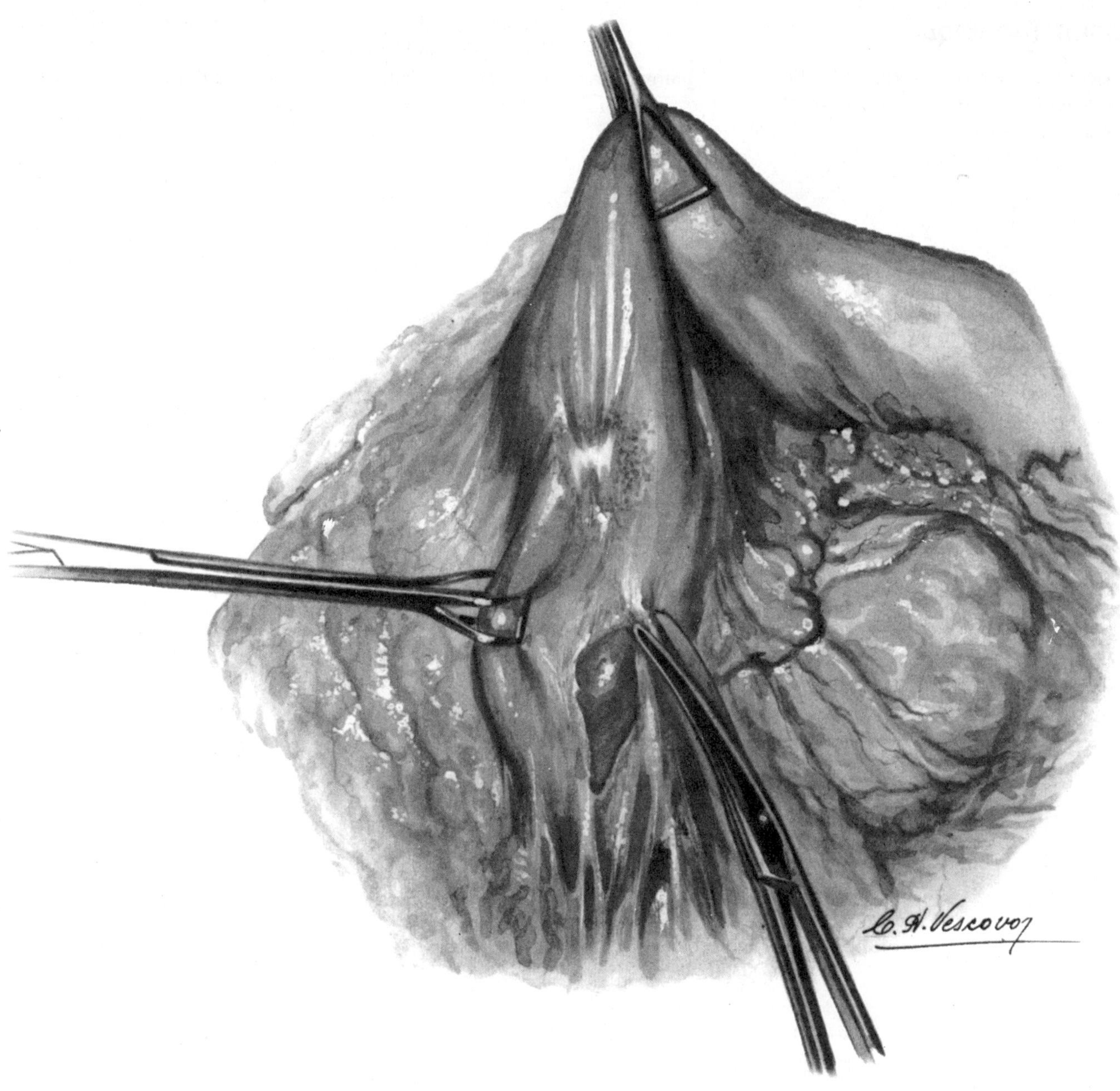

FIGURE 28.1

Nissen Technique

To be able to close a difficult duodenum using the Nissen technique it is indispensable that the anterior duodenal wall appear normal, without edema or fibrosis. The Nissen technique is a simple and efficacious procedure for the treatment of posterior duodenal wall ulcers that penetrate into the pancreas.

Nissen Technique

FIGURE 28.2

A, The drawing shows the ulcer bed in the posterior duodenal wall penetrating into the pancreas. The first suture of the first layer of interrupted sutures has been inserted using silk, cotton, or other nonabsorbable material. As observed in the drawing, the suture includes, on one side, the free duodenal edge (anterior wall) and, on the other side, the inferior edge of the ulcer. **B,** This drawing shows several sutures in place, as described under **A.**

Nissen Technique

FIGURE 28.3

A, The first layer of sutures has been completed between the free duodenal border and the inferior border of the ulcer. **B,** The second layer of sutures, between the anterior duodenal wall and the superior border of the ulcer, is being completed using the same material as in the first layer. **C,** Once the second layer is complete, the third layer is begun between the anterior duodenal wall and the pancreatic capsule, and including a substantial part of the pancreatic parenchyma to make the sutures stronger. An omentoplasty is added when the third layer is completed.

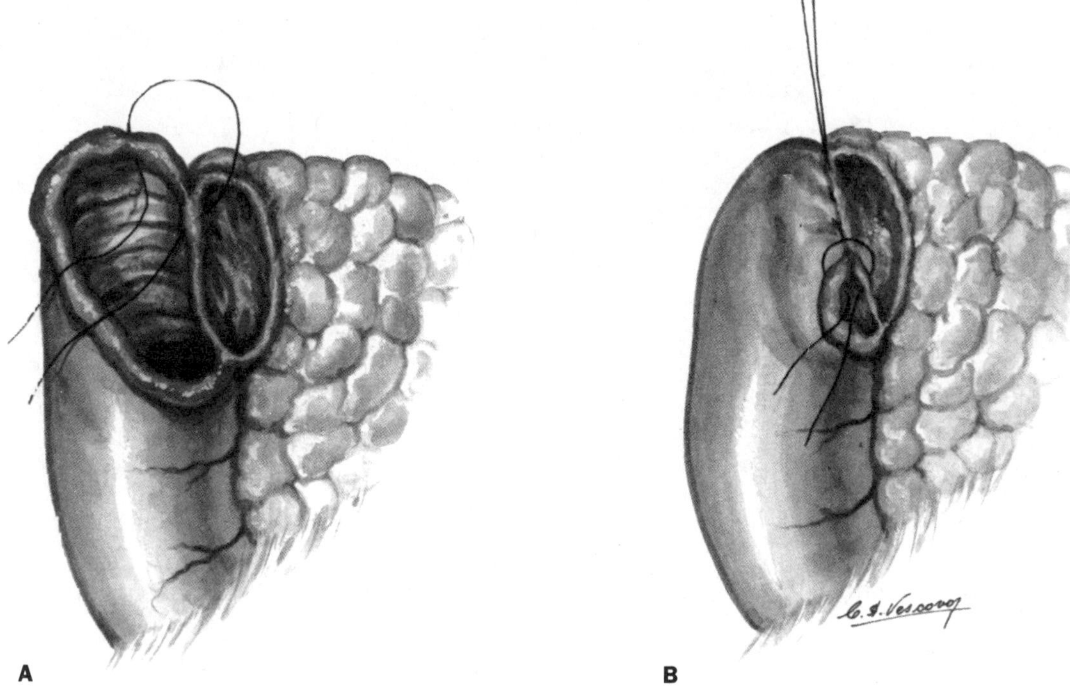

A B

FIGURE 28.2

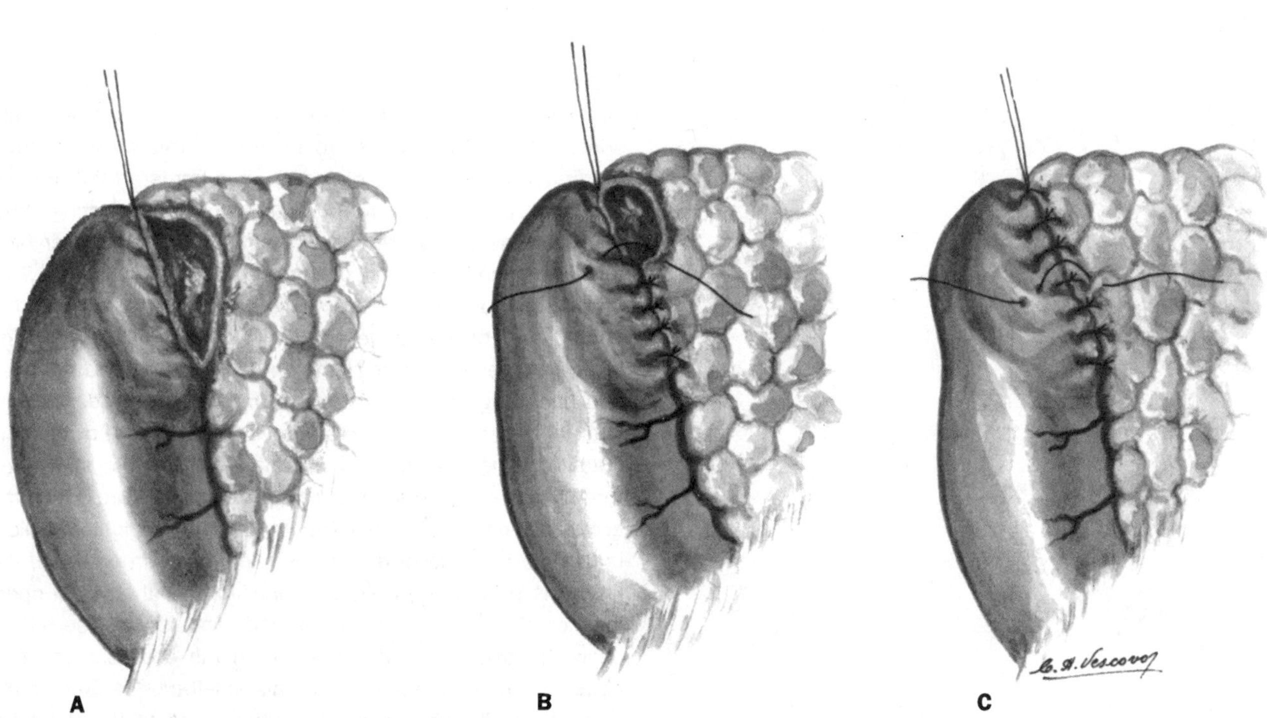

A B C

FIGURE 28.3

Nissen Technique

FIGURE 28.4

Schematic pancreatoduodenal section to better illustrate some details of the Nissen technique. **A,** This drawing shows the first layer of sutures joining the free border of the anterior duodenal wall and the inferior border of the penetrating ulcer. If the accessory pancreatic duct empties into the ulcer bed, this layer should not be performed (see lower figure). This drawing also shows the second layer of sutures between the anterior wall of the duodenum and the superior border of the ulcer, and the first suture of the third layer, which has not been tied, including, on the one hand, the anterior duodenal wall, and, on the other, the pancreatic capsule with part of the pancreatic parenchyma. **B,** This schematic section also shows the three layers of sutures described in the upper figure. Here, the accessory pancreatic duct (Santorini) empties into the ulcer bed and the first layer of sutures cannot be carried out. If the suture is performed, a small rubber tube, with several openings on the side of the ulcer bed, should be inserted to allow the pancreatic secretions from the accessory duct to pass into the duodenal lumen. This small tube is fixed to the duodenal wall with two cotton sutures and to the duodenal mucosa with one or more cotton sutures.

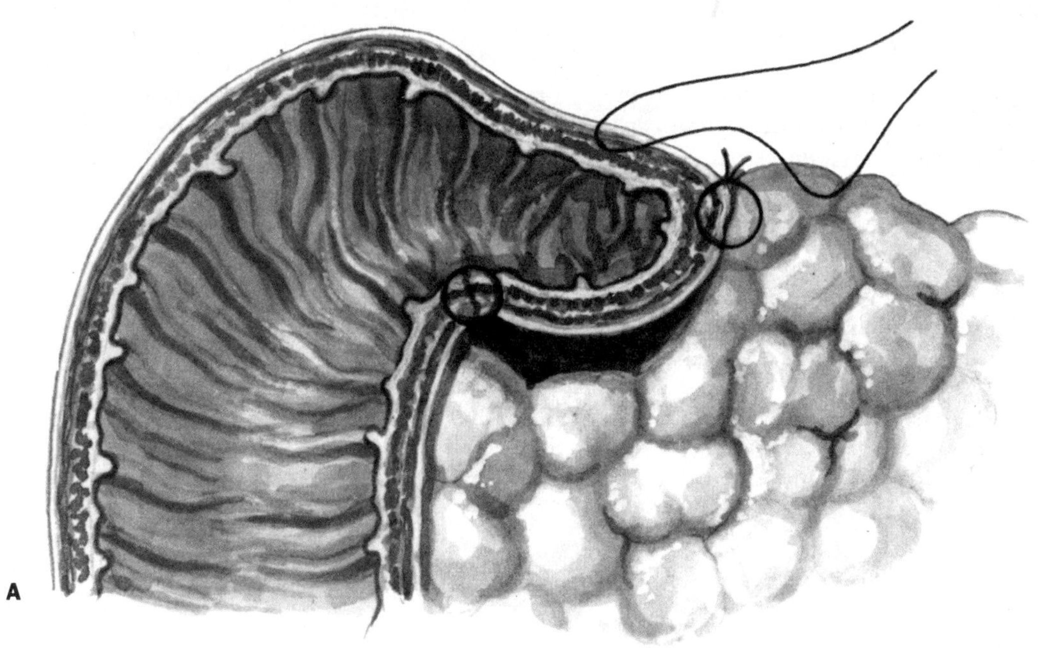

A

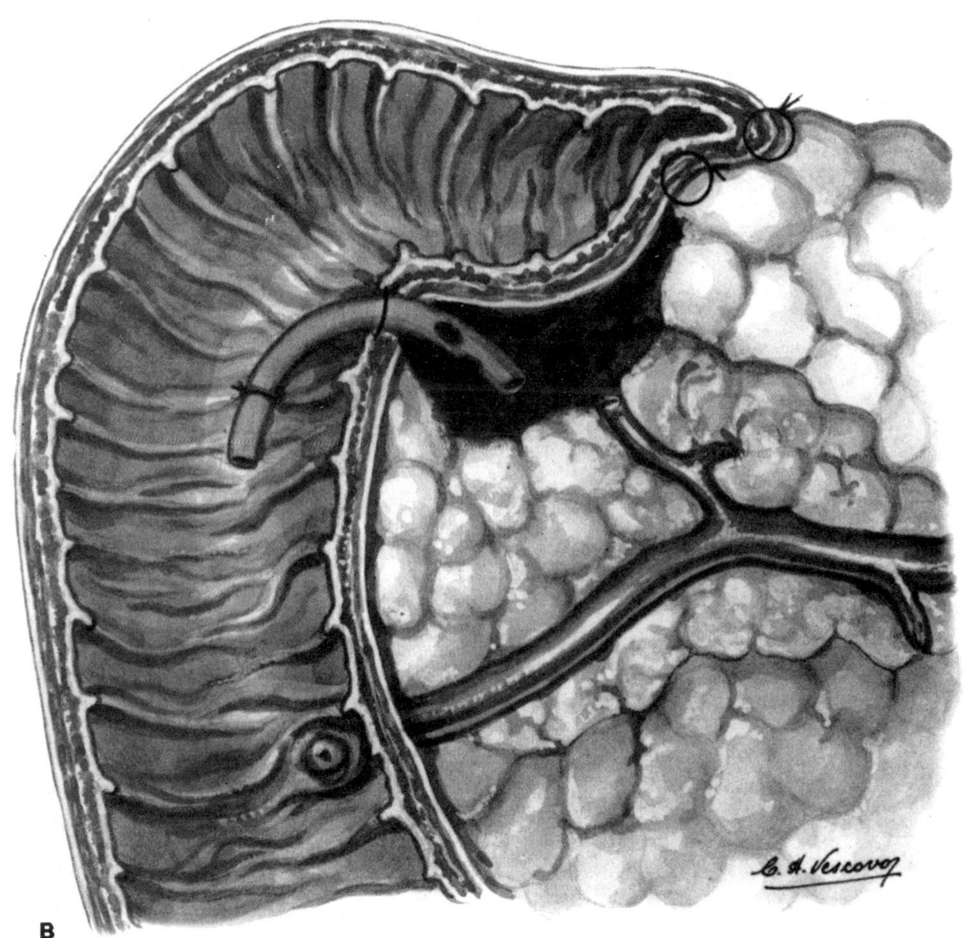

B

FIGURE 28.4

Catheter Duodenostomy

In a difficult to handle duodenum placement of an intraduodenal catheter can prevent a postoperative catastrophe. The main object of an intraduodenal catheter (catheter duodenostomy) is intraduodenal decompres sion. Catheter duodenostomy has been used by numerous surgeons since 1933 and was greatly enhanced by Welch and Rodkey's publication in 1954 (1, 6, 7, 12, 13, 15, 17, 19–21, 23, 25, 28).

Catheter Duodenostomy

FIGURE 28.5
A 16 F rubber catheter has been placed into the duodenal lumen up to the middle third of the second portion of the duodenum. The duodenal stump has been closed with interrupted cotton or silk sutures and the hydraulic test has been performed to test the closure. The catheter will be brought out a small incision and fixed firmly to the skin to avoid its being pulled out by a confused patient.

Catheter Duodenostomy

FIGURE 28.6
A, The duodenal stump can also be closed with a cotton or silk purse string suture. **B,** The catheter and the upper part of the duodenum are being wrapped in the greater omentum to better protect the duodenostomy. **C,** The superior part of the duodenum and the catheter have almost been completely wrapped with omentum. The upper end of the omental wrap has been fixed with several sutures to the parietal peritoneum around the catheter and, below, to the duodenum to keep the omentum from folding and not carrying out its protective function. The catheter is brought out through a small abdominal incision and firmly fixed to the skin. Before the incision is closed, the abdominal cavity is drained with two Penrose drains placed in the subhepatic space and brought out of the abdomen through small separate incisions.

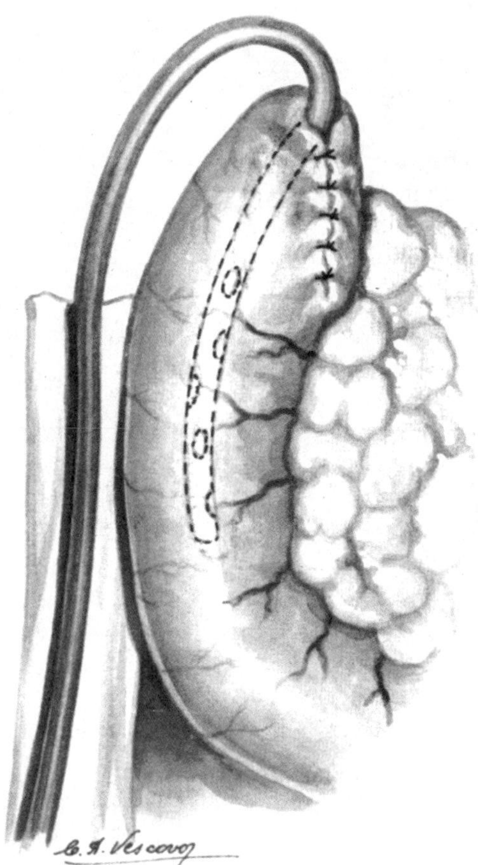

FIGURE 28.5

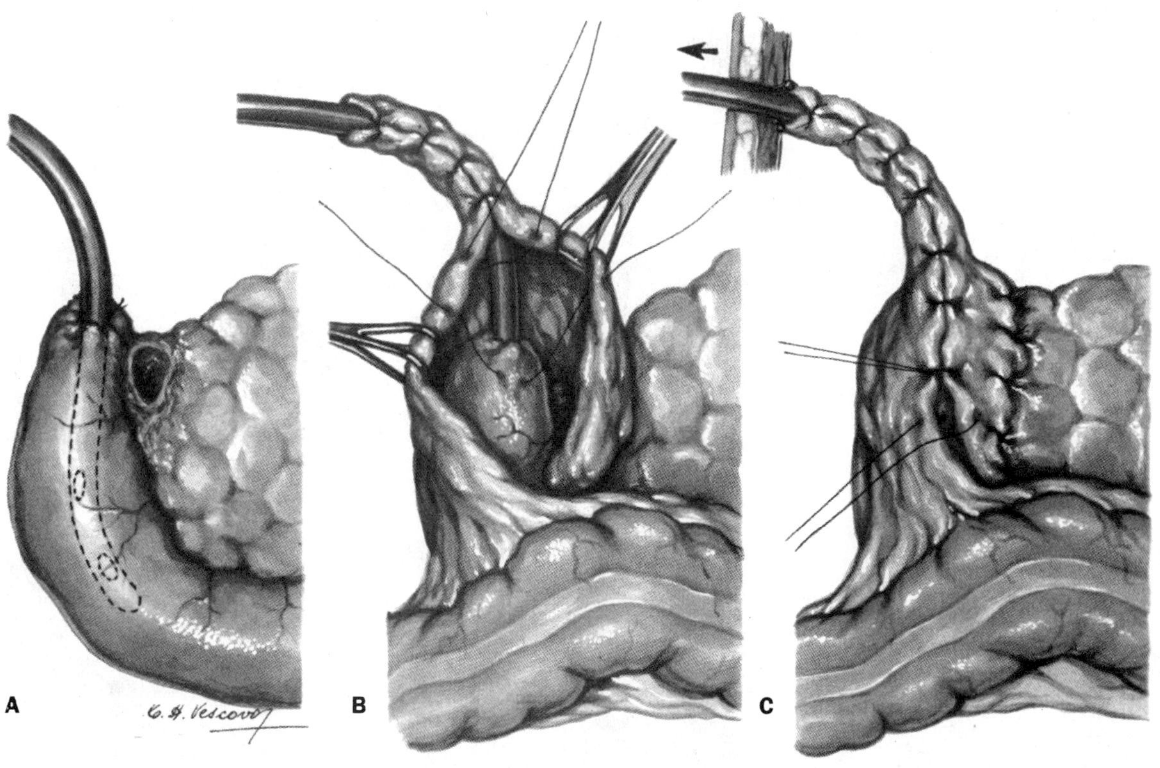

FIGURE 28.6

CLOSURE OF THE DIFFICULT DUODENUM BY THE STRAUSS TECHNIQUE

The Alfred Strauss technique (10, 11) is very effective in the treatment of duodenal ulcers that penetrate into the pancreas, but it must be carried out with precise technique and great care to avoid very serious complications.

Closure of the Difficult Duodenum by the Strauss Technique

Closure of the Difficult Duodenum by the Strauss Technique

FIGURE 28.7

An exploration of the duodenum has been performed and has shown that there is a large duodenal ulcer that penetrates the pancreas. The Strauss technique has been chosen. This technique has the advantage of dissecting the duodenum from right to left, instead of from left to right, which permits conserving a few millimeters of the posterior duodenal wall below the ulcer, which will make it possible to close the duodenum with less difficulty. The duodenum has been mobilized by means of the Vautrin-Kocher maneuver. The papilla of Vater and the course of the common bile duct are identified by doing a transverse choledochostomy to permit passage of a biliary probe, as seen in the drawing. With the probe inside the duct it is possible to determine the relation of the duct to the ulcer.

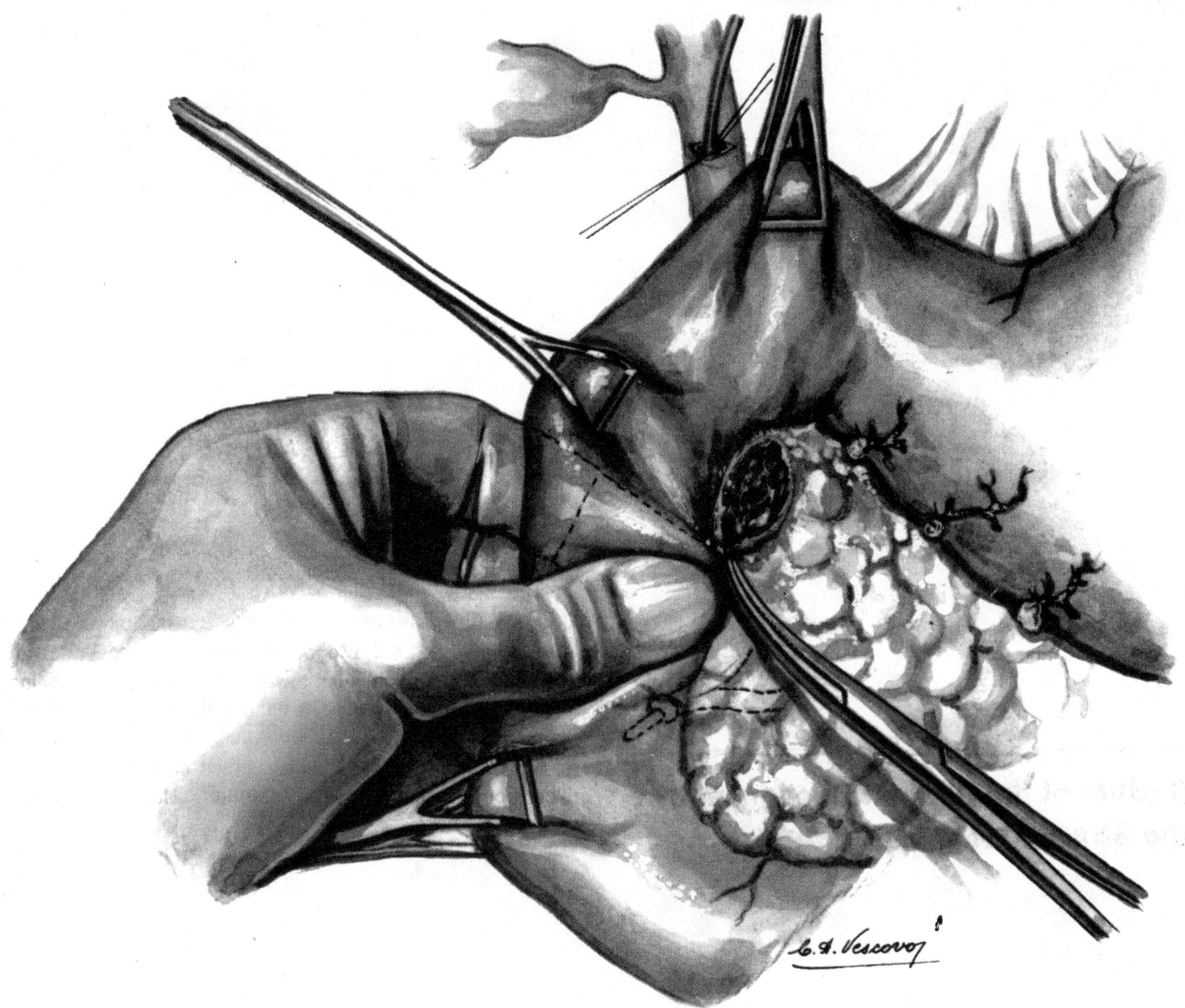

FIGURE 28.7

FIGURE 28.8
Using a Babcock clamp traction is applied upward on the duodenum, and with two other Babcock clamps traction is applied to the duodenum toward the right. With the index and middle fingers of the left hand behind the duodenum and the thumb in front, the surgeon localizes the inferior border of the ulcer and passes a fine curved clamp just below the ulcer from the anterior to the posterior surface as shown.

Closure of the Difficult Duodenum by the Strauss Technique

FIGURE 28.9
A, Traction is applied to the rubber catheter upward. The broken line shows the level where the duodenum is to be transected. This line runs obliquely in order to conserve as much as possible of the anterior duodenal wall. This wall should appear normal in order to be able to suture it to the very short posterior wall. **B,** The duodenal stump has been transected and closed without difficulty using interrupted sutures. Using scissors, the upper segment of the duodenum is being separated from the edges of the ulcer, leaving the perforation into the pancreas intact. Because it is outside the gastric secretions, it will heal rapidly.

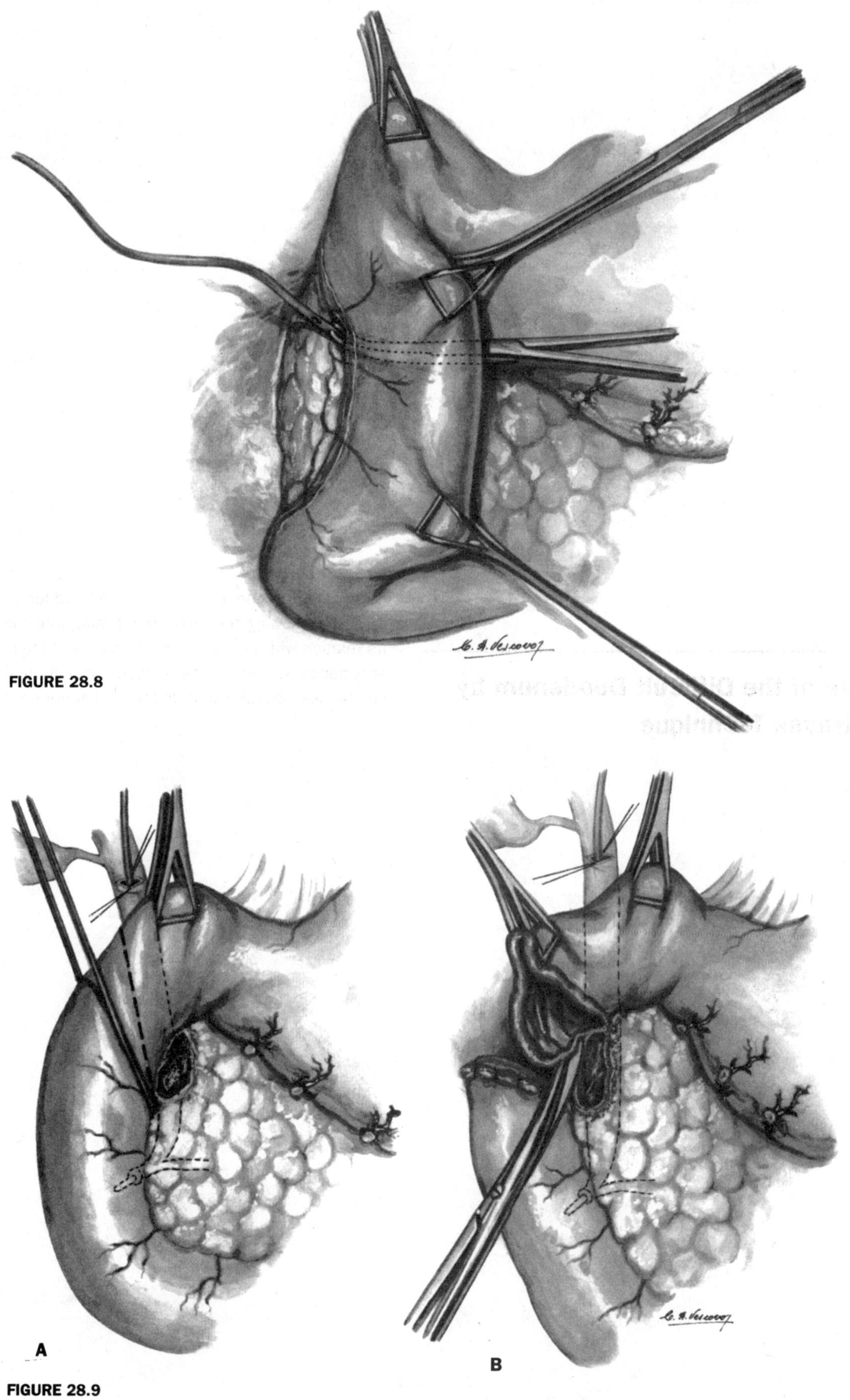

FIGURE 28.8

A

B

FIGURE 28.9

FIGURE 28.10
Schematic section of the pancreatoduodenal area with the object of showing the ulcer penetrating into the pancreas and its relation with the common bile duct and the main and accessory pancreatic ducts. The oblique transection of the duodenum can be seen passing just under the inferior border of the ulcer.

Closure of the Difficult Duodenum by the Strauss Technique

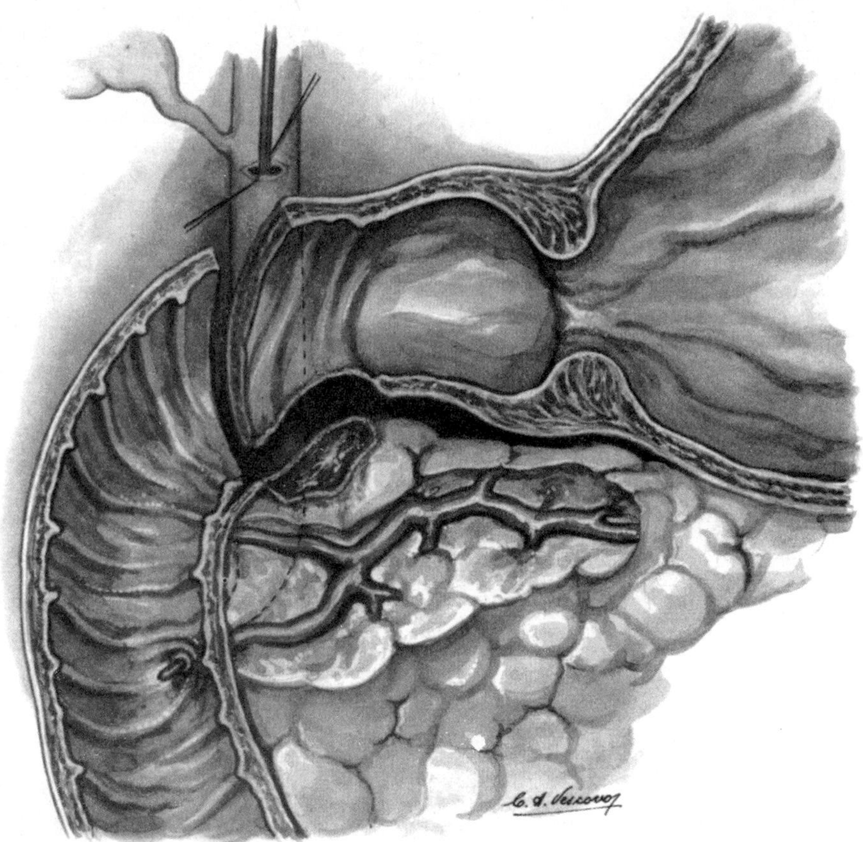

FIGURE 28.10

Closure of the Difficult Duodenum by the Strauss Technique

FIGURE 28.11
The proximal segment of duodenum is covered with a gauze and held with a large triangular Duval clamp to continue the gastrectomy. The biliary probe is replaced by a thin T-tube with short limbs, and the transverse choledochostomy is closed with 3-0 chromic catgut sutures. Closure of a transverse choledochotomy does not lead to common duct stricture.

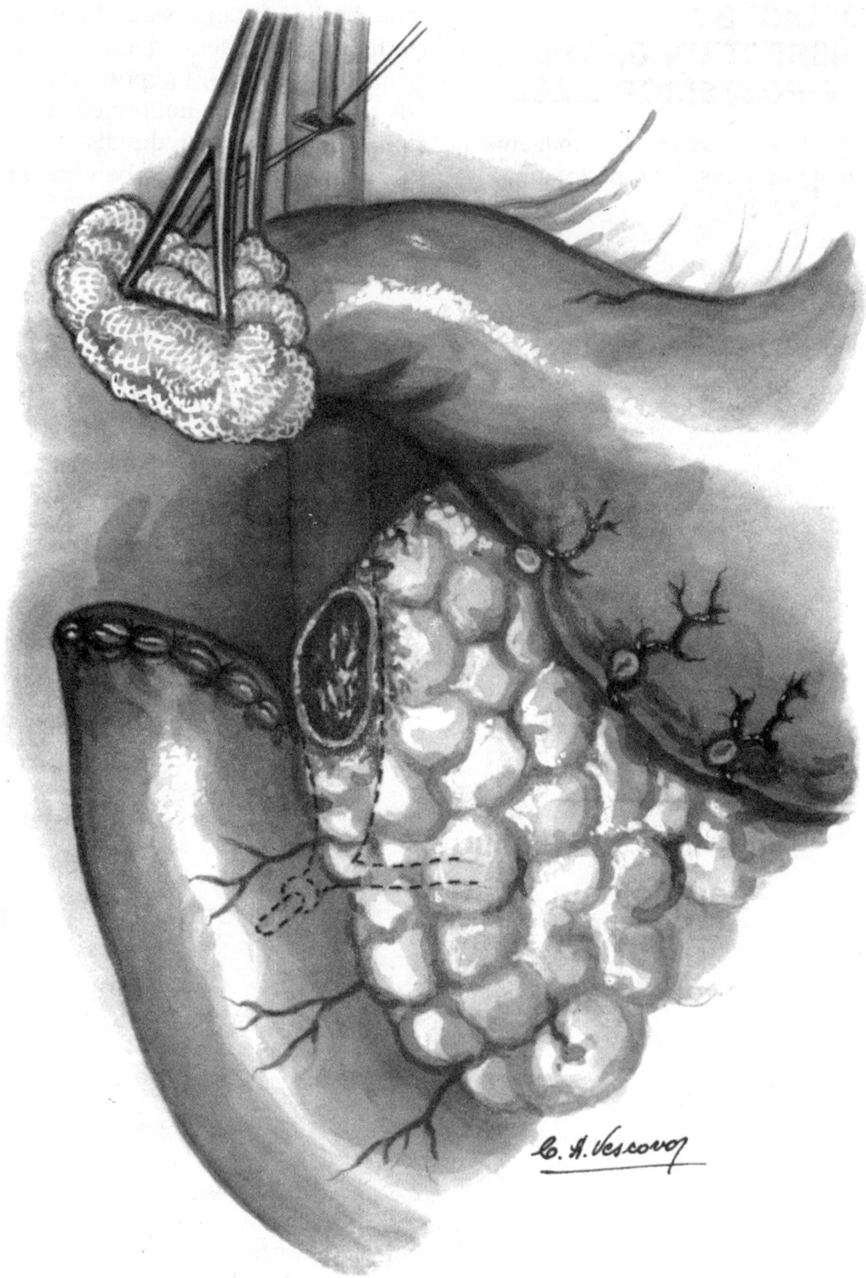

FIGURE 28.11

DUODENAL CLOSURE BY INTRAMURAL DISSECTION OF THE MUCOSA OF THE POSTERIOR WALL

This technique is extremely effective in the management of a difficult duodenal stump caused by perforating ulcers of the posterior wall of the duodenum. which, due to their periduodenal fibrotic and inflammatory process, make dissection of the posterior duodenal wall difficult. If, instead of being performed on the outside of the posterior duodenal wall, the dissection is performed in the submucosal layer, it will be very simplified (4, 22, 23).

Duodenal Closure by Intramural Dissection of the Mucosa of the Posterior Wall

FIGURE 28.12
Liberation of the posterior duodenal wall makes it necessary to individually ligate numerous small vessels coming from the gastroduodenal vessels. One of these small vessels is being ligated in the drawing.

Duodenal Closure by Intramural Dissection of the Mucosa of the Posterior Wall

FIGURE 28.13
If the fibrous periduodenal process caused by the ulcer makes it impossible to continue liberation of the posterior duodenal wall, it is appropriate to transect the seromuscular layer of the duodenum and continue the dissection in the submucosal plane following the broken line shown in **A.** The drawing on the right, **B,** shows the transected seromuscular layer, exposing the intramural submucosal layer, which can be easily dissected.

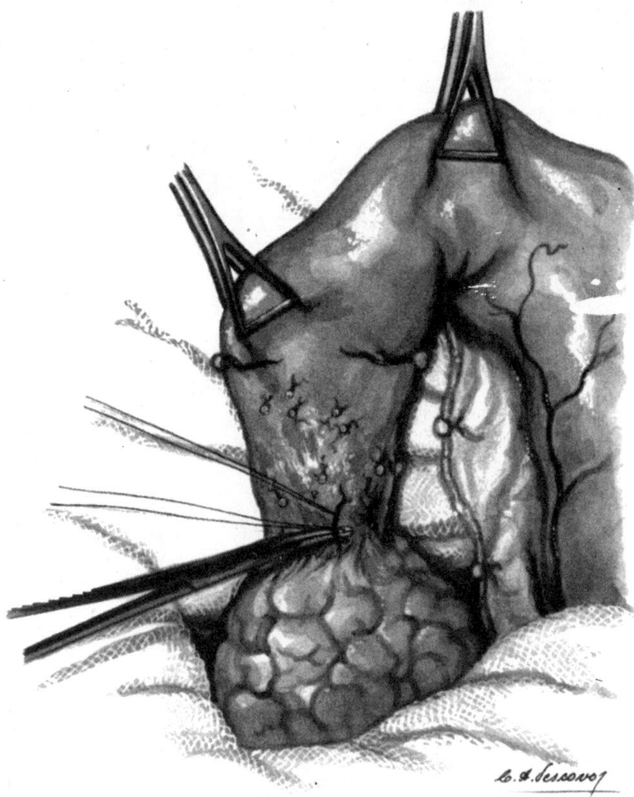

FIGURE 28.12

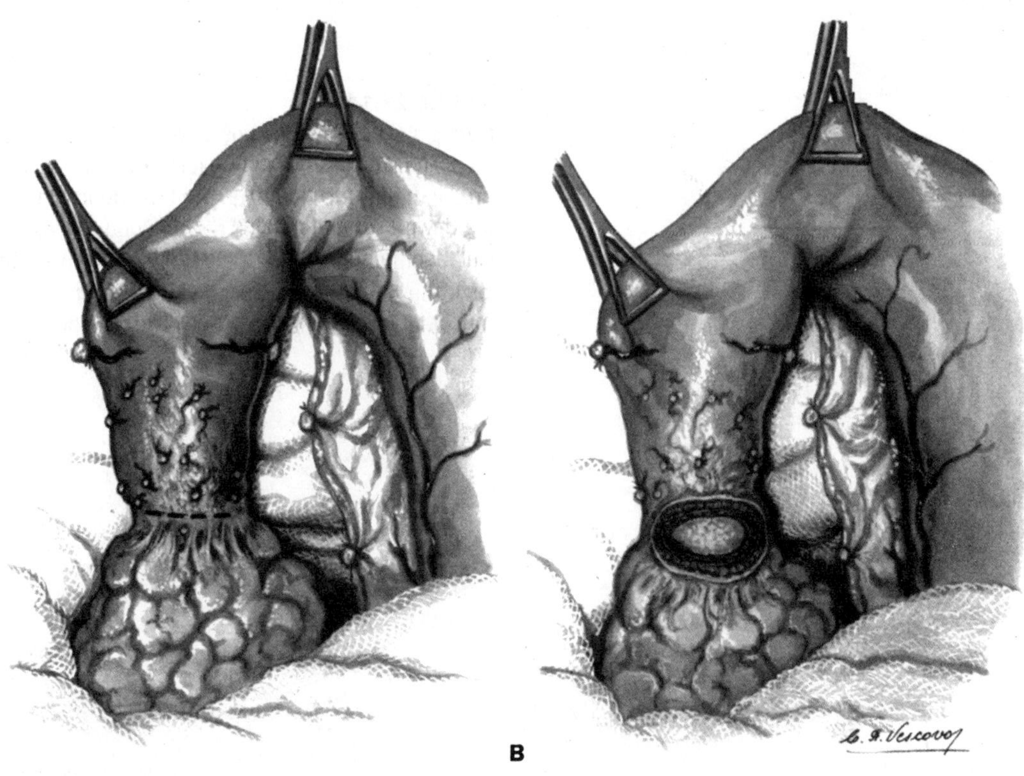

FIGURE 28.13

Duodenal Closure by Intramural Dissection of the Mucosa of the Posterior Wall

FIGURE 28.14
During dissection of the posterior duodenal wall the mucosa may be perforated. If this occurs, it is advisable to suture the inferior end of the perforation to prevent the duodenal tear from extending downward and making a safe duodenal closure impossible. Once some sutures are inserted to close the duodenal perforation, the submucosal dissection is continued cutting the seromuscular layer along the broken line, as shown in the drawing.

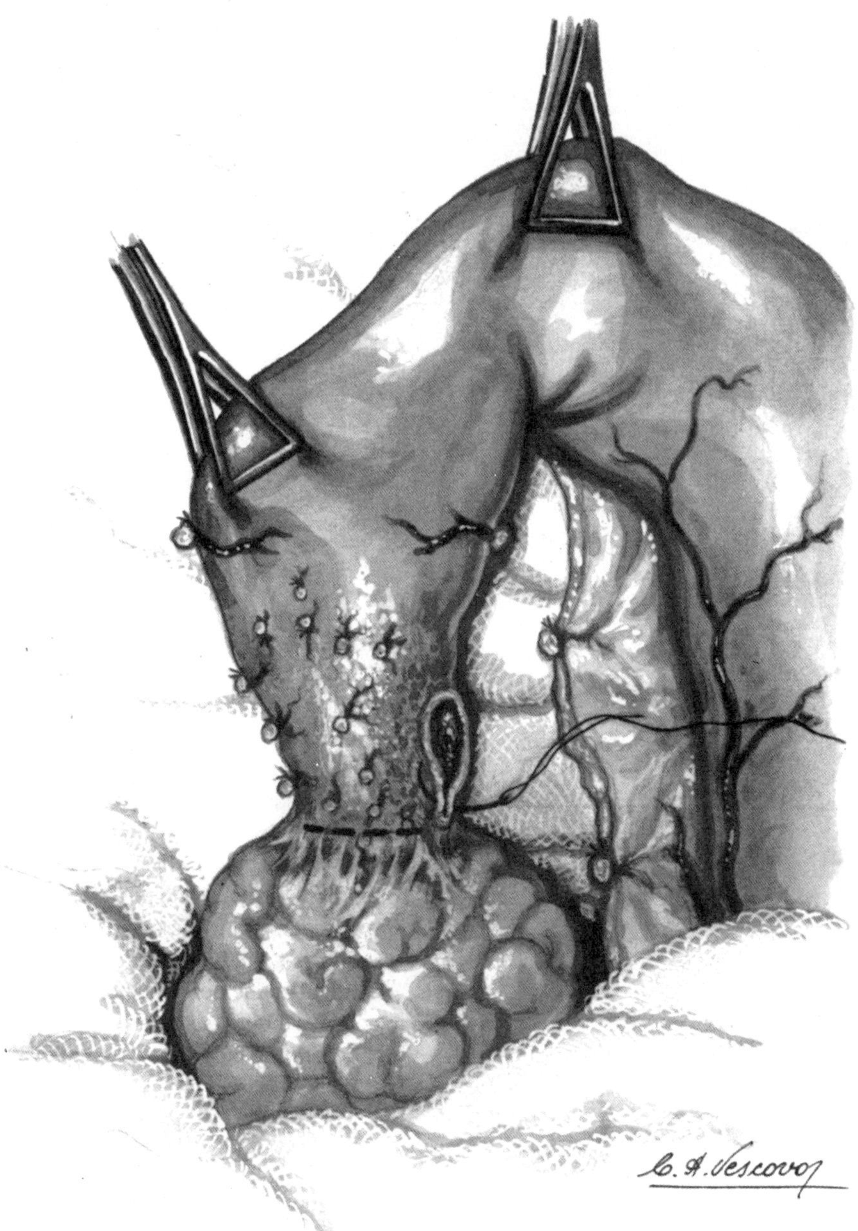

FIGURE 28.14

FIGURE 28.15
A, Schematic section of the duodenum showing the seromuscular layer separated from the mucosa after the submucosal dissection. **B,** A cotton purse string suture has been placed that includes all the layers of the anterior wall and only the posterior mucosal layer. **C,** The purse string suture has been tied. Outside the first purse string is inserted another purse string suture, which includes only the seromuscular wall of both the anterior and posterior duodenal walls. The stump of the first purse string is being invaginated to then tie the second purse string. **D,** The duodenal stump has been satisfactorily closed. It must be remembered that the duodenum is completely covered by visceral peritoneum except at its internal border, where the blood vessels and common bile duct enter it.

Duodenal Closure by Intramural Dissection of the Mucosa of the Posterior Wall

FIGURE 28.16
Schematic section of the duodenal stump, showing in detail the purse string sutures for a safe closure of the duodenum by this technique. **A,** The first purse string has been tied including the entire thickness of the anterior wall of the duodenal stump and only the mucosa of the posterior wall. **B,** Once the first purse string is tied and invaginated, another purse string, which includes only the seromuscular layer, is added.

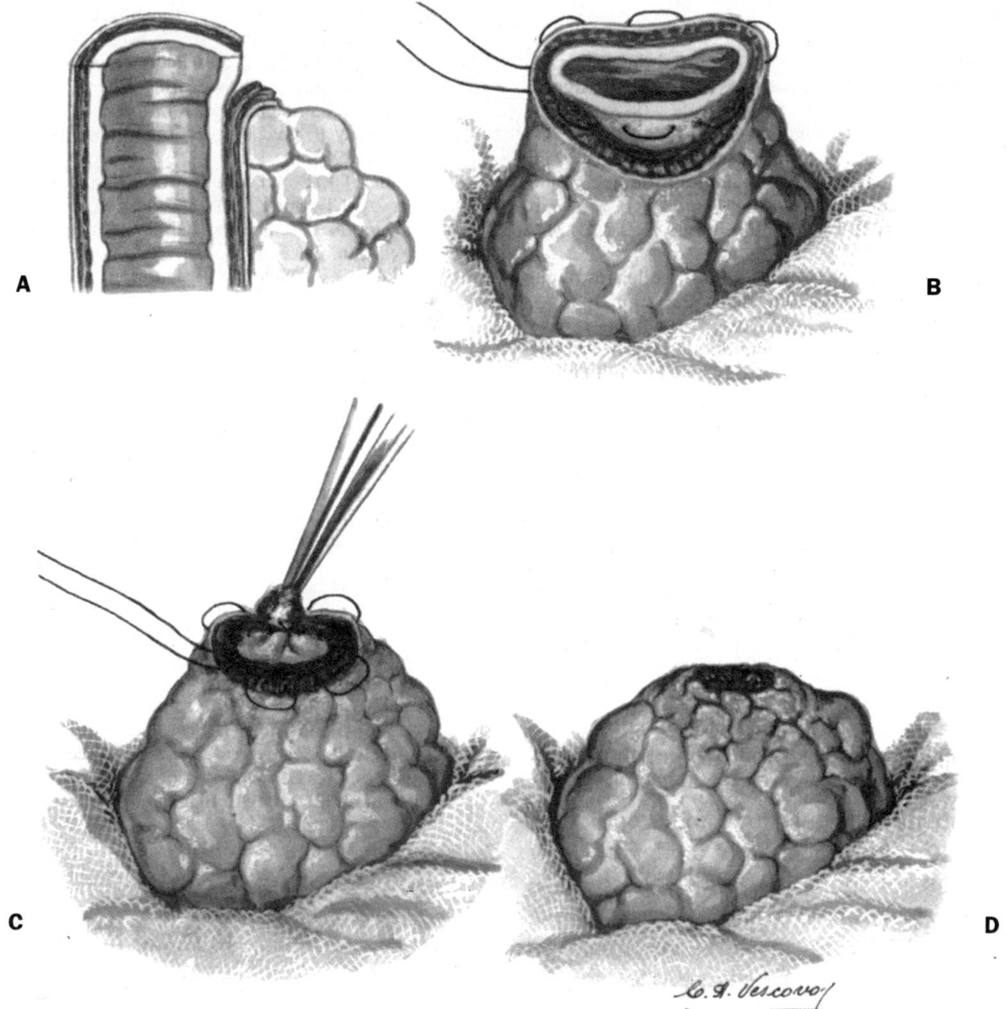

FIGURE 28.15

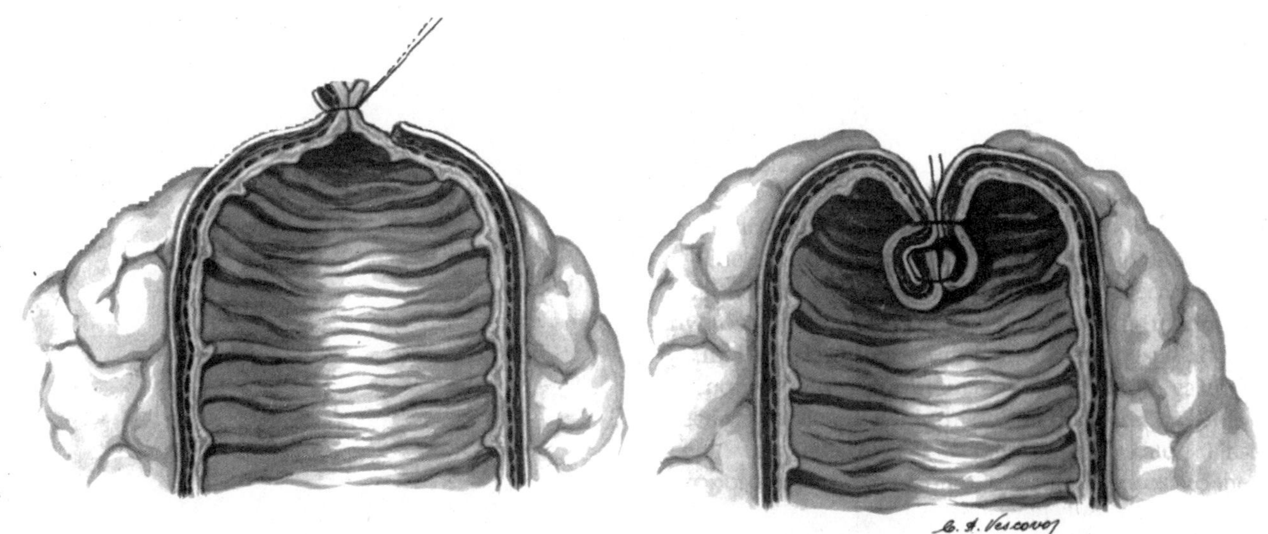

FIGURE 28.16

References

1. Aguirre, C., Halabi, M. Cierre del muñón duodenal dificil por úlcera duodenal penetrante en el páncreas. Prens. Med. Argent. 44:3624, 1957.
2. Bassett, A. Duodenostomie à la Witzel. J. Chir. 41:689, 1933.
3. Corachán, M. Cirugía gástrica. Vol. 2, p. 321. Salvat, Barcelona, 1943.
4. Devin, R., Lataste, J., Maillet, P. Nouveau traité de technique chirurgicale. Vol. 10, p. 342. Masson et Cie, Paris, 1968.
5. Finochietto, E., Finochietto, R. Técnica quirúrgica. Vol. II A, p. 271. Ediar, Buenos Aires, 1962.
6. Friedman, M. Ueber hilfen und sicherung bei gefahrvollen und technisch schwierigen. Magen operationen. Beitr. Klin. Chir. 163:293, 1936.
7. Fromm, D. Ulceration of the stomach and duodenum. In Fromm, D. (ed.) Gastrointestinal surgery. Vol. 1, p. 233. Churchill Livingstone, New York, 1985.
8. Ginsburg, L. Management of the difficult duodenum stump. Surg. Clin. North Am. 34:473, 1954.
9. Graham, R. Technical surgical procedures for gastric and duodenal ulcer. Surg. Gynecol. Obstet. 66:209, 1936.
10. Harkins, H.N., Nyhus, L.M. Strauss maneuver for division of the duodenum. In Harkness, H.N., Nyhus, L.M. (Eds.) Surgery of the stomach and duodenum. P. 684. Little, Brown, Boston, 1962.
11. Harkins, H.N., Nyhus, L.M. Operative technique for surgical treatment of duodenal ulcer. In Harkins, H.N., Nyhus, L.M. (Eds.) Surgery of the stomach and duodenum. P. 684. Little, Brown, Boston, 1969.
12. Hoerr, S.O., Perryman, R.G. Catheter duodenostomy: A safeguard in gastric resection. Cleve. Clin. Q. 19:49, 1952.
13. Lippert, K.M., Coleman, H.V. Duodenostomy in gastric resection for duodenal ulcer. Am. J. Surg. 95:781, 1958.
14. Maingot, R. Difficult or irremovable duodenal ulcers. In Maingot, R. (Ed.) Abdominal operations. Ed. 7, vol. 1, p. 412. Appleton Century Crofts, New York, 1980.
15. Mayfield, R.C., Abramson, P.D. The use of catheter duodenostomy in subtotal gastrectomy. Am. J. Surg. 90:998, 1955.
16. Nissen, R. Duodenal and jejunal peptic ulcer technique. P. 50 Grune and Stratton, New York, 1943.
17. Pearson, S.C., MacKenzie, R.J., Ross, T. The use of catheter duodenostomy in gastric resection for duodenal ulcer. Am. J. Surg. 106:194, 1963.
18. Priestley, J.T., Butler, D.B. Duodenostomy. Am. J. Surg. 82:163, 1951.
19. Priestley, J.T., Butler, D.B. Duodenostomy: A method of managing the duodenal stump in certain cases of partial gastrectomy. Proc. Mayo. Clin. 26:65, 1951.
20. Rodkey, G.V., Welch, C.E. Duodenal decompression in gastrectomy: Further experiences with duodenostomy. N. Engl. J. Med 262:498, 1960.
21. Sesin, M., Halabi, M., Ciffoniello, A., Aguirre, C. Técnica de Welch en el cierre del muñón duodenal difícil. Pren. Med. Argent. 62:276, 1975.
22. Slattery, L. Intramural dissection and staggered closure of the duodenal stump. Surg. Gynecol. Obstet. 110:252, 1060.
23. Vadra, J.E., Mungiello, R.R. Atlas del cierre del muñón duodenal. Artes gráficas, Buenos Aires, 1973.
24. Wastell, C. Partial and total gastrectomy. In Schwartz, S., Ellis, H. (Eds.) Maingot's abdominal operations. Ed. 9, vol. 1, p. 731. Appleton Lange, Norwalk, CT, 1990.
25. Welch, C.E., Rodkey, G.V. A method after gastrectomy. Surg. Gynecol. Obstet. 98:376, 1954.
26. Welch, C.E. Internal and external gastric, duodenal and biliary fistulas. In Manigot, R. (Ed.) Abdominal operations. Ed. 7, vol. 1, p. 157. Appleton Century Crofts, New York, 1980.
27. Welch, C.E., Rodkey, G.V., von Gryska, P. One thousand operations for peptic ulcer disease. Ann. Surg. 204:454, 1986.
28. Welch, C.E. Gastric resection for duodenal ulcer. In Scott, H.W., Sawyers, J.L. (Eds.) Surgery of the stomach, duodenum and small intestine. Ed. 2, p. 540. Blackwell, Boston, 1992.

Section F

Surgery of the Stomach and Duodenum

CHAPTER 29

Finsterer-Bancroft-Plenk Exclusion Gastrectomy

HISTORIC DATA

In 1895, Anton von Eiselsberg of Austria (4) proposed a palliative operation from unresectable pyloroduodenal tumors, which consisted of transection of the stomach above the tumor, closing the distal gastric segment, and anastomosing the proximal stomach to the jejunum. Among the 18 cases in which von Eiselsberg used this technique were two patients with duodenal ulcer that were thought to have tumors (12, 16). In 1910 von Eiselsberg extended the indications for this technique to patients with unresectable or very risky duodenal ulcers, introducing the concept of antral exclusion. In 1925, Devine of Australia (3) proposed an antral exclusion technique similar to von Eiselsberg's. Shortly thereafter, it was proven that this antral exclusion technique, including gastric transection, was complicated by anastomotic ulcers with alarming frequency.

With the object of avoiding this serious complication, a few surgeons performed the gastric transection with antral exclusion in two stages in some cases presenting with duodenal ulcers that were very difficult to handle. In the first stage they performed the exclusion to allow regression of the inflammatory process and then, in a second stage, within 45 days carried out the antral and duodenal resection, thereby preventing the frequent complication of anastomotic ulcer.

The experiences of Edkins from 1905 to 1908 revealed the importance of the effect of hormonal antral secretions on the hydrochloric acid and peptic secretions of the fundus.

In 1918 Hans Finsterer of Austria proposed adding resection of part of the stomach to the simple gastric transection to decrease chlorhydropeptic secrĕtion. This concept was thus firmly established (5). Later, Finsterer proposed adding excision of the antral mucosa to the gastric resection (6, 12), thereby establishing the presently accepted concept of gastrectomy with exclusion and not of gastric transection with exclusion, as proposed by von Eiselsberg and Devine. In addition, Finsterer advocated resection of the antral mucosa, which is the stimulus for chlorhydropeptic secretion and the cause of anastomotic ulcers (6). In 1932, Bancroft, from the United States (1), proposed a modification of the Devine and von Eiselsberg operation, very similar to the Finsterer operation, in which he added some very interesting technical details in carrying out removal of the antral mucosa. Plenk, from Germany, in 1936 (13) also introduced some technical modifications to carry out a safer closure of the seromuscular antral stump.

The Finsterer exclusion gastrectomy is also known as the Finsterer-Bancroft-Plenk exclusion gastrectomy because of the modifications introduced by the latter two surgeons. In some publications this procedure is known as a Bancroft or Bancroft-Plenk exclusion gastrectomy, without mentioning Finsterer and thereby altering the historic truth (2, 5, 6, 8, 12, 15, 16). Finsterer visited the United States in 1930, having been invited to dictate conferences on gastric surgery and perform several demonstrations of gastric surgery at several American centers. With his experience of more than 5000 gastric resections, he, together with Eugene Polya of Hungary, gave great impetus to the performance of gastrectomy in the United States.

INDICATIONS FOR EXCLUSION GASTRECTOMY

There are few indications for exclusion gastrectomy, but it is important to know the technique because it may be lifesaving in very active duodenal ulcers that penetrate the pancreas, surrounded by dense adhesions, and with a very difficult to handle, very friable duodenum. There is no doubt that as the surgeon gains experience in the handling of the duodenum, the number of unresectable or difficult ulcers is reduced. It has been proven that an exclusion gastrectomy leads to better results than truncal vagotomy with pyloroplasty or gastrojejunostomy and proximal gastric vagotomy (11).

It is important to make the decision to perform an exclusion procedure before mobilizing the gastric antrum because the blood supply of this segment should be kept intact. On the other hand, before deciding to perform an exclusion gastrectomy, the surgeon must be sure that a duodenostomy has not been done to explore the duodenum or to carry out hemostasis in a bleeding ulcer. A pylorotomy should not be done. Exclusion gastrectomies are contraindicated in duodenal ulcers with obstruction or active bleeding.

COMPLICATIONS

The complications that are usually mentioned as disadvantages of this procedure are really due to poor technique. Frequent dehiscence of the antral stump has been attributed to this procedure, being blamed on poor capacity of the muscular layer of the antrum to heal and produce a firm scar. The muscular walls of the antrum will heal very well if they are correctly apposed with adequately placed sutures, without leaving residual dead spaces. It is also important to carry out an adequate hemostasis to prevent the formation of hematomas in the antral walls. The exclusion gastrectomy is also blamed for the occurrence of anastomotic ulcers due to having left remnants of gastric mucosa. This complication is also due to an error in technique, because the antral mucosa should be completely removed up to the pylorus, which can always be done. If a small remnant of pyloric mucosa remains, it is neutralized by the truncal vagotomy, which should be performed in all cases of exclusion gastrectomy before the resection is begun. Exclusion gastrectomy, correctly performed, does not lead to more complications than the classic gastrectomy for duodenal ulcer. Makkas and Marangos, in 1949 (11), reported 2.1% mortality and 95% good results in 415 cases submitted to exclusion gastrectomy.

Operative Technique

FIGURE 29.1
If exploration has confirmed that the duodenal ulcer is unresectable or resection may be too risky for the patient, the surgeon may choose to do an exclusion gastrectomy using the Finsterer-Bancroft-Plenk technique. Once the decision has been made, a truncal vagotomy should be carried out first. A duodenostomy or pylorotomy should be avoided. Since the natural circulation must be preserved, liberation of the greater curvature, if performed inside the gastroepiploic arcade, has to stop some 5 cm from the pylorus. On the lesser curvature side the vascular arcade formed by the right and left gastric vessels is divided about 5 cm from the pylorus. The drawing shows the presence of a large duodenal ulcer, penetrating into the pancreas, with deep alteration of its walls, giving rise to great deformity of the first and second portions of the duodenum. Using Babcock clamps, traction is applied upward on the lesser curvature and downward on the greater curvature. A broken line shows the site where the entire circumference of the seromuscular layer of the antrum will be incised. This line is located some 5 cm from the pylorus.

Operative Technique

FIGURE 29.2
An elastic clamp is placed above this line and the seromuscular layer is incised, as seen in the drawing. The elastic clamp is used to prevent spillage of gastric contents when the mucosa is incised.

FIGURE 29.3
The seromuscular layer is held with one or more Babcock clamps to apply traction and, using scissors and gauze pledgets, the mucosa is dissected following the submucosal plane. This dissection usually presents no difficulty.

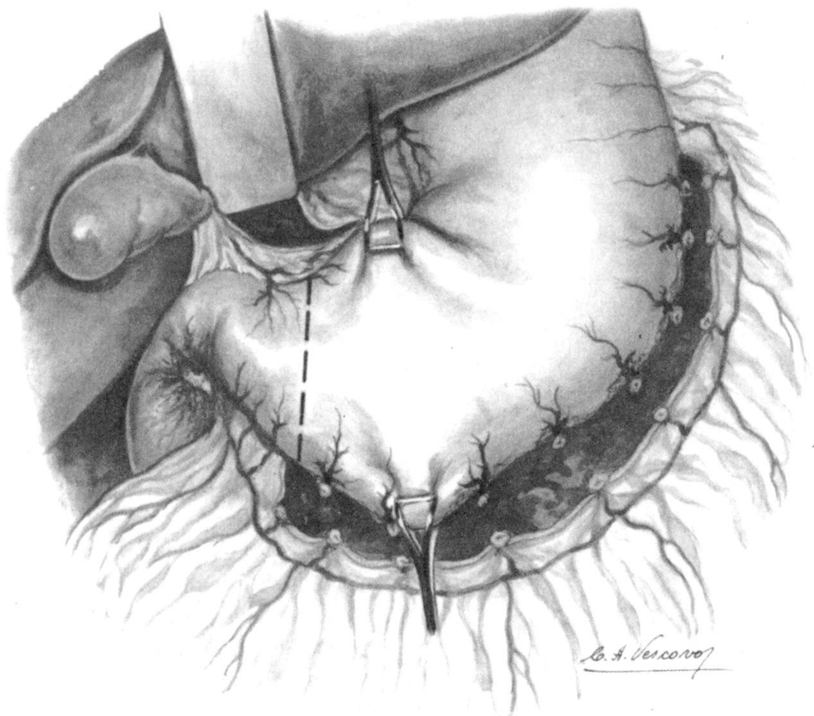

FIGURE 29.1

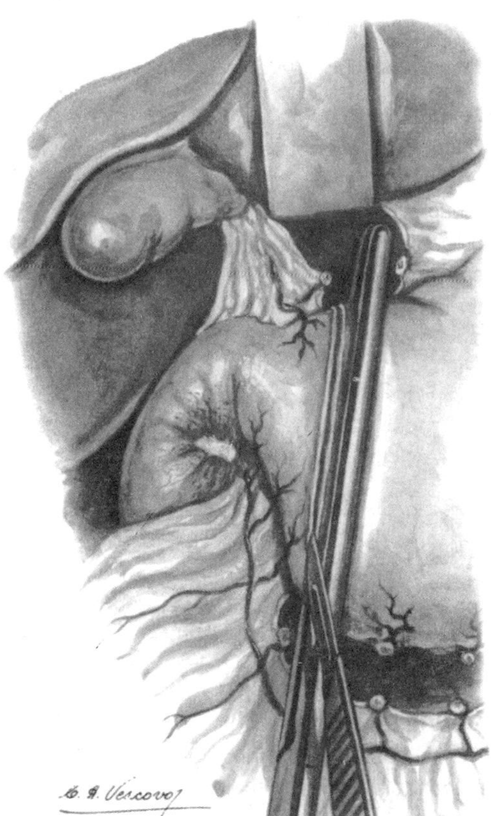

FIGURE 29.2

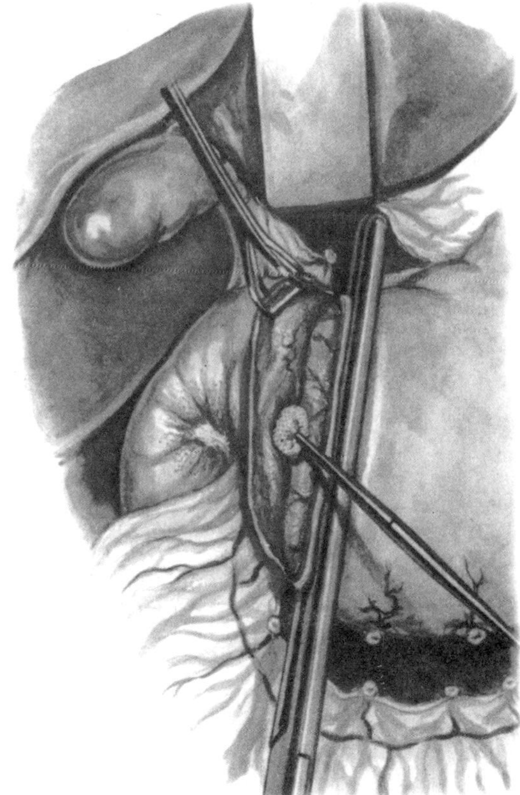

FIGURE 29.3

FIGURE 29.4
Dissection of the antral mucosa should be extended to the pylorus and if, possible, a few millimeters beyond it. As the dissection is carried closer to the pylorus, the submucosal layer can be seen to be thinner, making separation of the seromuscular from the mucosal layer more difficult. Upon reaching the pylorus, the antral mucosa, which has become progressively thinner, is found to be adherent to the pyloric muscle layer, making its dissection more difficult.

FIGURE 29.5
Dissection of the anterior wall and part of the posterior wall of the gastric antrum has been completed. The antral mucosa of both walls is divided with straight Mayo scissors in order to be able to continue dissection of the posterior wall to the pylorus. Dissection of the seromuscular layer should be done delicately to avoid perforating it, specially near the pylorus. Careful hemostasis of bleeding vessels during this dissection is very important. Correct hemostasis will prevent hematoma formation, which may lead to complications.

Operative Technique

FIGURE 29.6
Once dissection has been carried out to the pylorus, an attempt is made to separate the mucosa from the pyloric muscle for a few more millimeters. A purse string suture is placed in the submucosal plane, using a fine needle with fine cotton, avoiding perforation of the mucosa. Mucosal dissection should extend to the pylorus and a little further, if possible, in order to leave as little pyloric mucosa as possible.

FIGURE 29.7
The mucosal purse string suture has been tied down and the mucosa is being transected just above it. This should be done as close to the purse string suture as possible without compromising it.

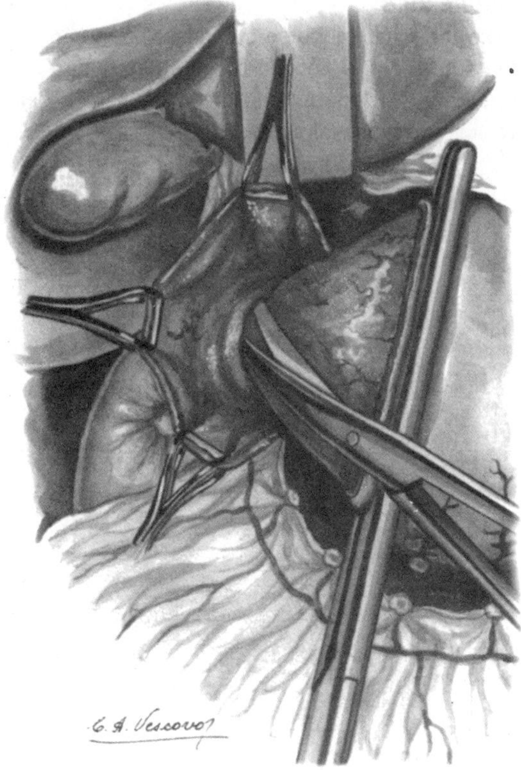

FIGURE 29.4

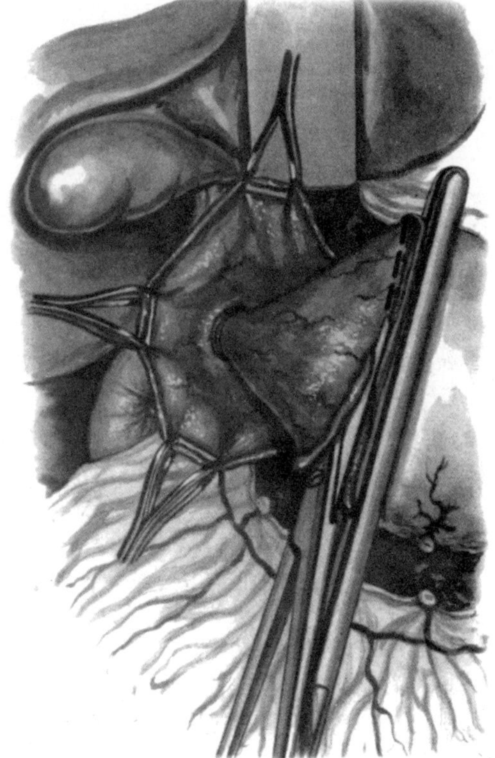

FIGURE 29.5

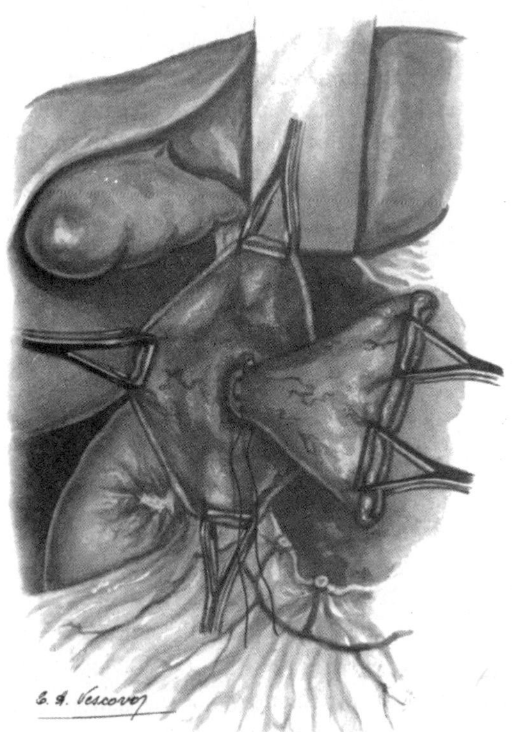

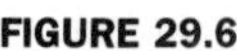

FIGURE 29.6

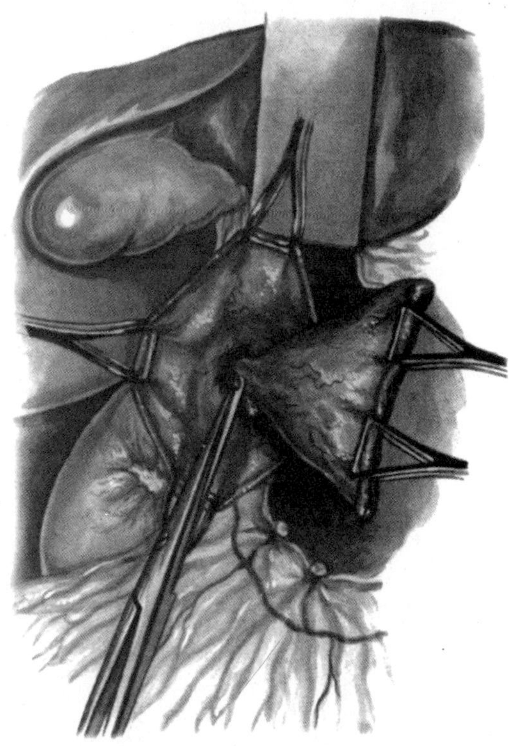

FIGURE 29.7

FIGURE 29.8
Once the mucosal purse string has been tied and the ends of the suture cut, a second purse string suture is placed in the pyloric muscle, permitting the pylorus to be closed after inverting the mucosal stump.

FIGURE 29.9
The mucosal stump has been inverted and the purse string of the pyloric muscle is being closed.

Operative Technique

FIGURE 29.10
The seromuscular layer is then trimmed back, leaving only 2 cm from the pylorus. Conservation of more of the antral seromuscular layer favors formation of dead spaces, which lead to infectious complications and development of fistula. The drawing shows that the circulation of the small antral residual segment has been preserved.

FIGURE 29.11
The residual muscular layer of the antrum is being sutured with interrupted cotton or silk sutures so as to have good apposition, avoiding dead spaces, as seen in the drawing.

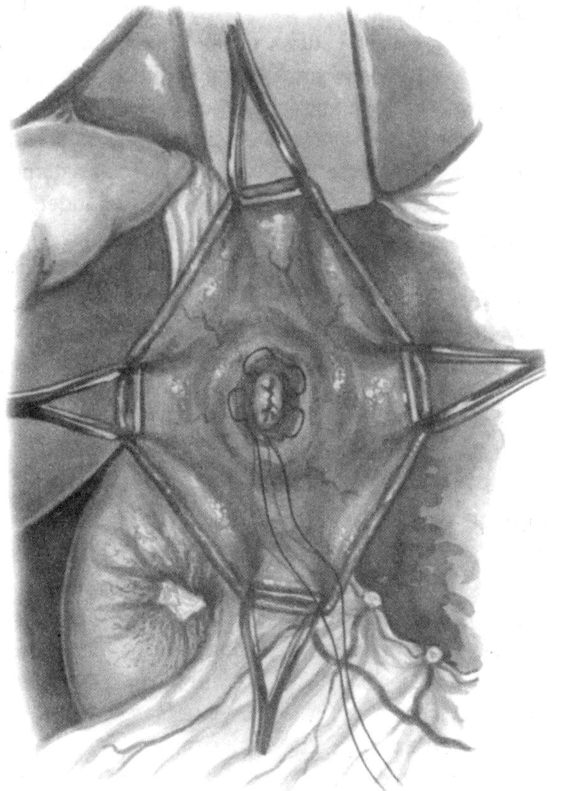

FIGURE 29.8

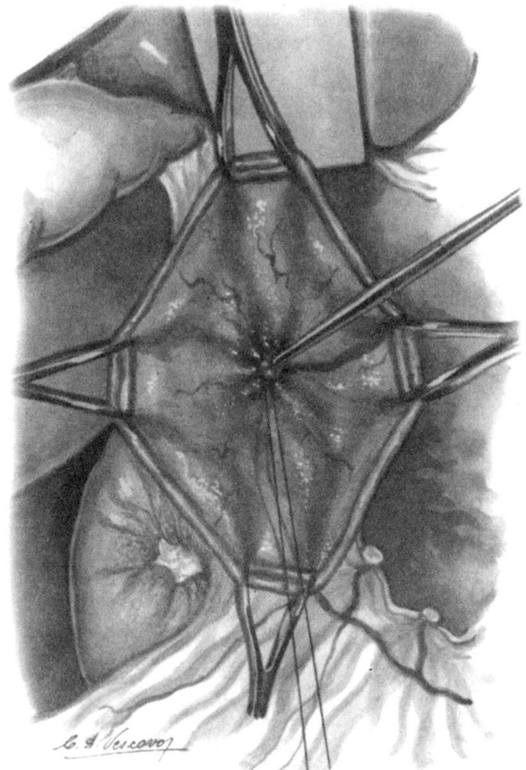

FIGURE 29.9

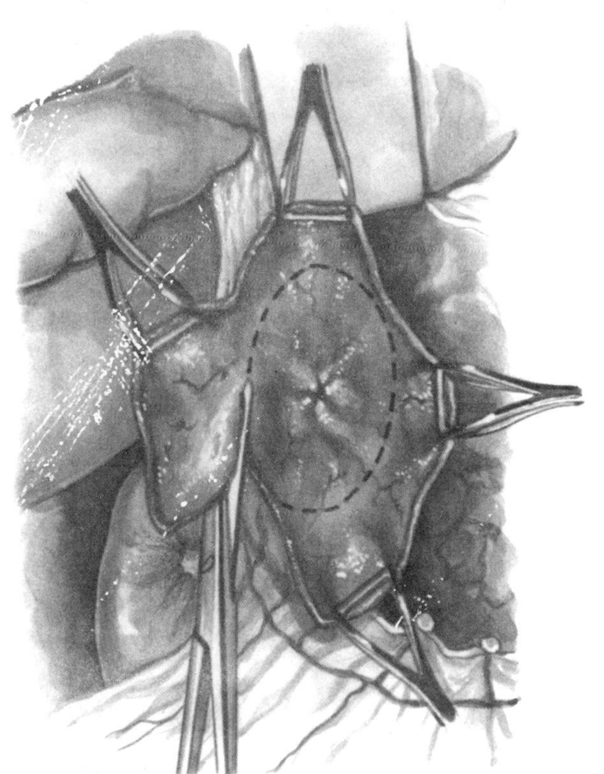
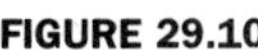

FIGURE 29.10

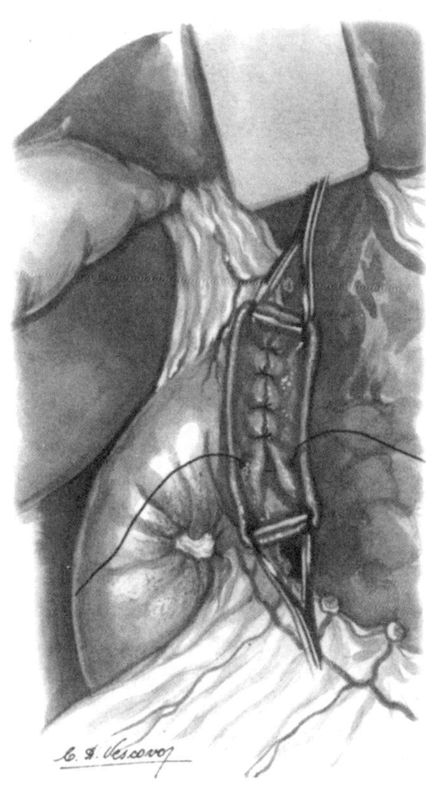

FIGURE 29.11

FIGURE 29.12

Once the apposed sutures of the antral mucosal layer are in place, closure of the small antral seromuscular stump is completed with through and through cotton or linen sutures, which include the entire wall at its edge. The pylorus is marked by an oval dotted line. Once the small seromuscular stump of antrum is satisfactorily closed, an omentoplasty is added using a well vascularized segment of omentum.

The residual antral segment maintains its normal blood supply, as shown in the drawing, through the right gastric and right gastroepiploic arteries. Maintaining good blood supply to the antral segment is an important part of this operation.

FIGURE 29.13

Schematic section showing the duodenum at the end of the operation with the ulceration that led to the indication for and the choice of the exclusion gastrectomy. From left to right one can see the large duodenal ulcer perforating into the pancreas, the stump of the pyloric mucosa closed with a purse string suture and invaginated into the duodenal lumen, the pyloric muscle closed with a purse string suture, the muscular layer of the anterior wall of the antrum, sutured and apposed to the posterior wall, the edge of the seromuscular layer closed with through and through sutures, and finally the omentoplasty. This operation offers good early and later results in the relatively few cases in which it is indicated, if the above mentioned technical details are followed.

Operative Technique

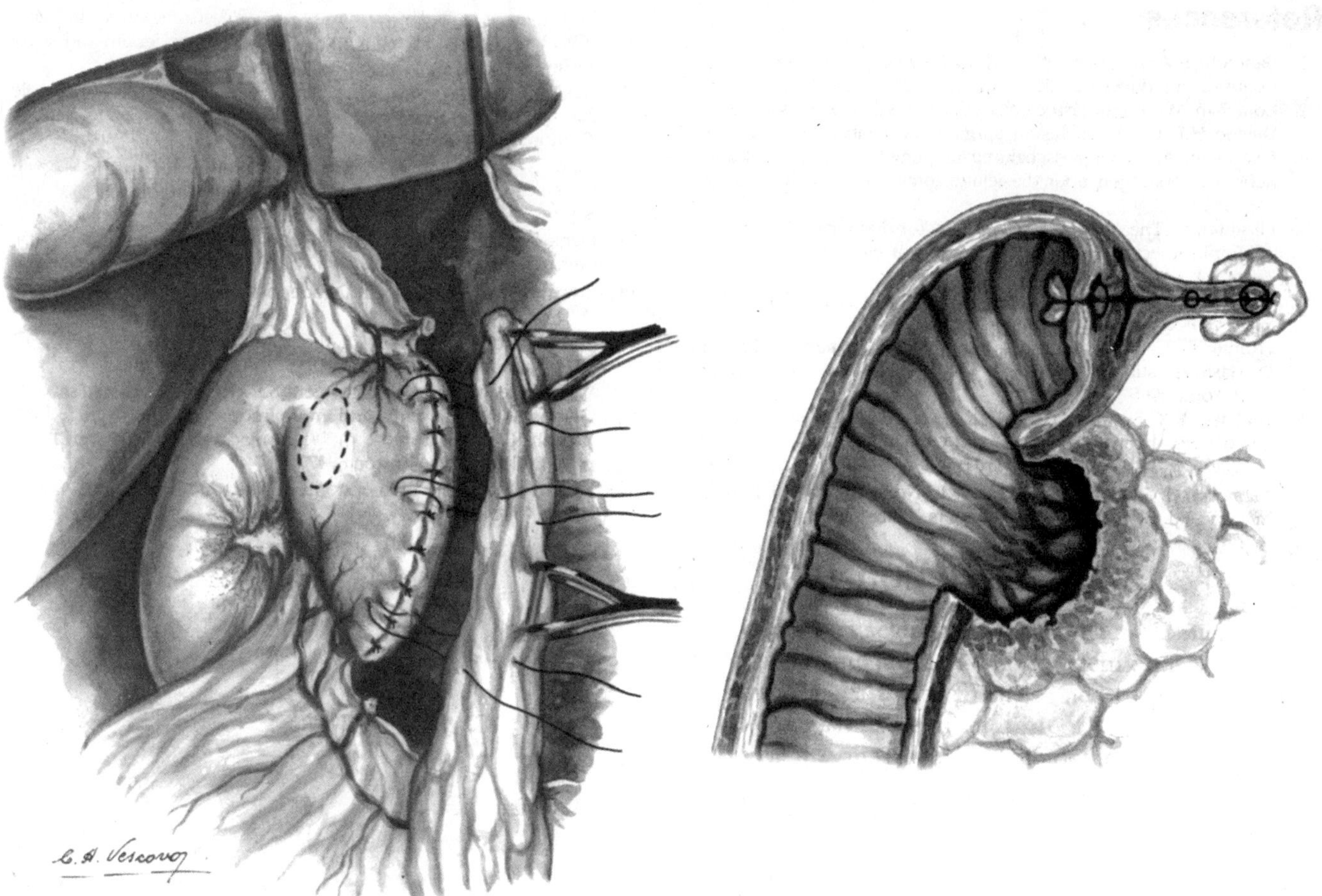

FIGURE 29.12

FIGURE 29.13

References

1. Bancroft, F.W. A modification of the Devine operation of pyloric exclusion for duodenal ulcer. Am. J. Surg. 16:223, 1932.
2. Corachán, M. Cirugía gástrica. Vol. 2, p. 358. Salvat, Barcelona, 1943.
3. Devine, H.B. Gastric exclusion. Surg. Gynecol. Obstet. 47:239, 1928.
4. Eiselsberg, A. Ueber ausschaltung inoperabler pylorus strikturen nebst bemerkungen uber die jejunostomie. Arch. Klin. Chir. 50: 919, 1895.
5. Finsterer, H. The extended gastrectomy for duodenal ulcer instead of simple resection of the duodenum or of the pyloric exclusion. Zentralbl. Chir. 26:434, 1918.
6. Finsterer, H., Chuna, F. The surgical treatment of duodenal ulcer. Surg. Gynecol. Obstet. 52:1099, 1931.
7. Fromm, D. Ulceration of the stomach and duodenum. In Fromm, D. Gastrointestinal surgery. Vol. 1, p. 233. Churchill Livingstone, New York, 1985.
8. Graham, R.R. Surgical Therapy in Lesions of the Stomach and Duodenum. In Bancroft, F.W. (Ed.) Operative surgery. P. 545. Appleton Century, New York, 1941.
9. Hampson, L.G. Partial gastrectomy. In Nora, P.F. (Ed.) Operative surgery. Ed. 3, p. 497. W.B. Saunders, Philadelphia, 1990.
10. Herrington, J.L. Jr. Historical aspects of gastric surgery. In Scott, H.W. Jr., Sawyers, J.L. (Eds.) Surgery of the duodenum and small intestine. Ed. 2, p. 1. Blackwell, Oxford, 1992.
11. Makkas, M., Marangos, G. Surgical treatment of non-resectable duodenal ulcer; antral exclusion (operation Bancroft-Plenk modification). Br. J. Surg. 37:206, 1949.
12. Olch, P.D., Harkins, H.N. A historical review of gastric surgery. In Harkins, H.N., Nyhus, L.M. Surgery of the stomach and duodenum. P. 3. Little, Brown, Boston, 1962.
13. Plenk, V.A. Zur technik der resektion zur ausschaltung. Zentralbl. Chir. 63:3019, 1936.
14. Priestly, J.T., Butler, D.T. Duodenostomy. Am. J. Surg. 82:163, 1951.
15. Shackleford, R.T. Surgery of the alimentary tract. Vol. 1, p. 447. W.B. Saunders, Philadelphia, 1955.
16. Wangensteen, O.H., Wangensteen, S.D. History of gastric surgery: Glimpses into its early and more recent past. In Nyhus, L.M., Wastell, C. (Eds.) Surgery of the stomach and duodenum. Ed. 3, p. 3. Little, Brown, Boston, 1977.
17. Welch, C. Surgery of the stomach and duodenum. Ed. 4. Year Book, Chicago, 1973.

Section F

Surgery of the Stomach and Duodenum

CHAPTER **30**

High-Lying Gastric Ulcers; Cardiac or Subcardiac

GENERAL CONSIDERATIONS

The cardia is a segment of the stomach surrounding the esophagogastric junction whose extension is some 15 to 40 mm. This gastric segment is lined by a mucosa with a different structure from that of the gastric fundus, body, or antrum. The epithelium of the cardia is made up exclusively of mucus secreting cells. The term "cardia" is frequently used to designate the external as well as the internal line of junction of the esophagus and stomach, which is not exactly correct. The junction of the esophageal and gastric mucosa forms an irregular, festooned line, called the ora serrata or Z line, that results from the union of the epidermoid esophageal lining and the cylindrical gastric epithelium. The external esophagogastric junction does not correspond to the internal limit. The external limit can be determined by a horizontal line through the vertex of the angle of His. In tracking this horizontal line one should remember that the line of junction of esophageal and gastric mucosa is a few millimeters above it and, in some individuals, considerably higher (7).

High ulcers of the lesser curvature of the stomach can originate in the cardia itself or below this area. These are known as ulcers of the cardia and subcardia, a name that is more correct than jutxacardiac ulcers. In general, ulcers located within 6 cm from the external esophagogastric junction are considered to be ulcers of the cardia and subcardia. These ulcers constitute 5 to 9% of all gastric ulcers (1, 20–22).

Because these ulcers are usually perforating and frequently callous, they produce a retraction of the lesser curvature of the stomach. Ulcers near the esophagus may compromise the integrity of its walls, be it due to the ulcer itself or to inflammatory reaction around it. Involvement of the esophageal wall is not as frequent as is thought. It is frequently possible, in patients with ulcers of the cardia or subcardia, to obtain sufficient space between the superior border of the ulcer and the esophagus to make it possible to transect the stomach, including the ulcer in the gastrectomy, and still be able to attain a secure gastric closure. If it is impossible to resect the ulcer without severe injury to the esophagus, a different procedure should be carried out (5, 8, 10–13).

The great majority of these high-lying ulcers are on the lesser curvature of the stomach. At times, however, these ulcers are found on the anterior or posterior gastric wall as well as on the greater curvature. Ulcers in these locations present the same or greater surgical problems than ulcers on the lesser curvature.

As was previously pointed out, ulcers of the cardia and subcardia are usually chronic and callous, penetrating into the posterior abdominal wall, frequently into the diaphragmatic crura. Acute ulcers are seen in this area. They frequently bleed massively and should be treated surgically when hemostasis by other therapeutic measures has failed (8, 10).

Ulcers of the cardia and subcardia seen in patients with sliding hiatus hernias are associated with treatment of the hiatal hernias.

SURGICAL INDICATIONS

The indications for surgery in these ulcers are as follows:

1. Ulcers that do not respond to correct medical therapy.
2. Ulcers that recur frequently after healing under medical therapy.
3. Ulcers complicated by massive hemorrhage or recurrent less severe bleeding.
4. Ulcers with acute perforation.
5. Cases in which it is impossible to determine preoperatively whether the ulcers are benign or malignant.
6. Acute ulcers with massive hemorrhage that could no be controlled by other therapeutic means.

SURGICAL PROCEDURES

The most efficient surgical procedure in the treatment of ulcers of the cardia and subcardia is gastric resection including the ulcer (3–5, 15, 16, 21). The author uses the modified Pauchet technique, which will be described later (15, 16). The Kelling-Madlener technique (11, 13) can be used in cases in which gastric resection, including the ulcer, is not possible. Even though the Kelling-Madlener technique is classified as an exclusion procedure, the ulcer is not really excluded from digestive transit, as occurs in the Finsterer-Bancroft-Plenk exclusion gastrectomy, which is used in the surgical treatment of some duodenal ulcers that are unresectable or very risky to resect.

Patients with these ulcers complicated by massive bleeding should also be treated by the modified Pauchet technique, including the bleeding ulcer. Patients in very poor general condition should undergo hemostasis with suture ligatures of the ulcer bed, adding a gastrectomy below the ulcer (Kelling-Madlener technique). In case of massive hemorrhage, some surgeons carry out local resection of the ulcer, later closing the defect in two layers. This technique is not recommended because the bleeding vessels are generally outside the resected tissue and still have to be suture-ligated to obtain hemostasis. Resection of the ulcer is also very difficult because limiting the excision strictly to the affected tissue may give rise to difficulties with the closure and frequently leads to esophageal compromise.

In patients with massive hemorrhage complicating these high ulcers, suture ligation should be carried out, followed by gastric resection in patients in whom suture ligation of the ulcer does not control the bleeding.

Surgical Procedures

FIGURE 30.1
Schematic drawing representing a gastric ulcer with superimposed lines. The drawing shows the relation between the peptic ulcer and the left gastric artery, the celiac trunk, and the ascending esophageal or cardioesophageal artery. This relation changes considerably in patients with ulcers of the cardia or subcardia because these ulcers are chronic, they are perforating, and they cause retraction of the lesser curvature due to surrounding sclerosis and edema. The surgeon should always remember the possibility of an aberrant left hepatic artery arising from the left gastric artery, usually before this artery comes in contact with the lesser curvature. One should avoid ligating this aberrant left hepatic artery to prevent partial or complete necrosis of the left lobe of the liver.

Surgical Procedures

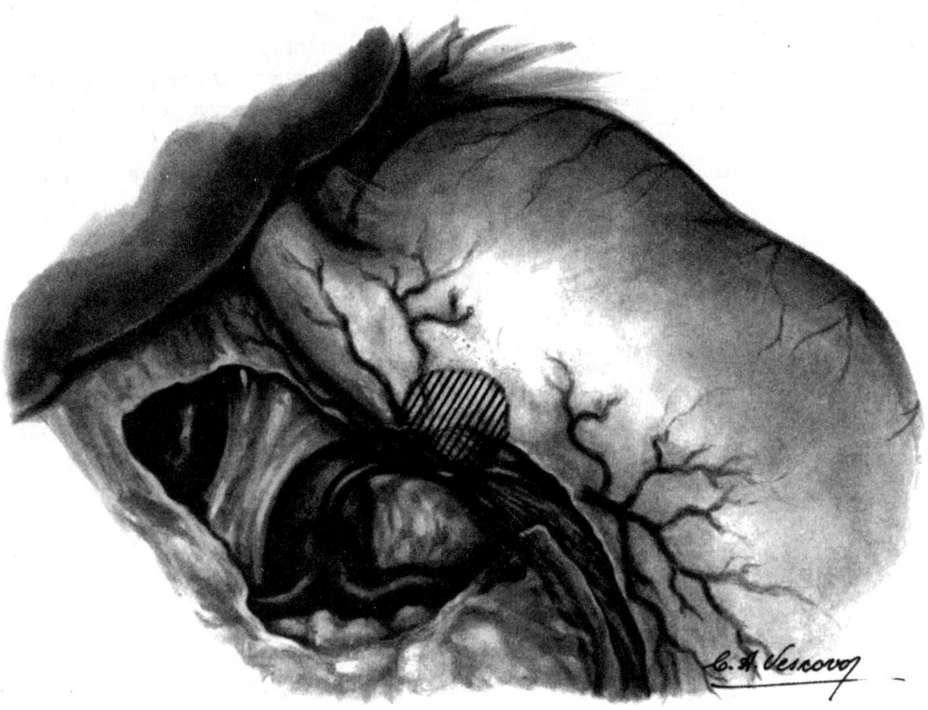

FIGURE 30.1

FIGURE 30.2

It is important to carry out a complete exploration of all the abdominal viscera before performing a gastric resection and then give our full attention to gastric exploration. The surgeon should establish the size of the ulcer, how deeply and into what organ it is penetrating, the relation of the ulcer to the esophagus, and the degree of surrounding inflammation and retraction of the lesser curvature of the stomach. In addition, the celiac trunk and the origin of the left gastric artery from it should be established, as well as the possible concomitant presence of another gastric or duodenal ulcer. In some patients a gastrotomy is necessary to determine if there is enough room between the esophagus and the superior border of the ulcer, so that the surgeon can decide if a gastrectomy with inclusion of the ulcer can be performed, or if this should be avoided because of the danger involved.

In some patients the macroscopic appearance of the ulcer may lead to suspicion of ulcerated carcinoma in spite of negative preoperative biopsies. In this case four or more biopsies should be performed from the edges of the ulcer. Better yet, the biopsies can be done through a lucite anoscope, as previously described, to avoid seeding the operative field with malignant cells. If the ulcer were proven malignant, the surgical procedure should be completely different from the one to be described here.

Once the exploration has been completed and the diagnosis of a peptic ulcer confirmed, the gastrectomy with inclusion of the ulcer is performed using the modified Pauchet technique.

Surgical Procedures

The first maneuver to be performed is ligation and section of the left triangular ligament of the liver to obtain good visualization of the esophagogastric zone. It is not always necessary to divide the left triangular ligament of the liver to obtain good visualization of this area. Most surgeons divide the left triangular ligament without previously ligating it, considering it unnecessary. However, there are patients in whom this ligament may have blood vessels or small aberrant bile ducts, which may cause hemorrhage or spillage of bile, if not ligated (7).

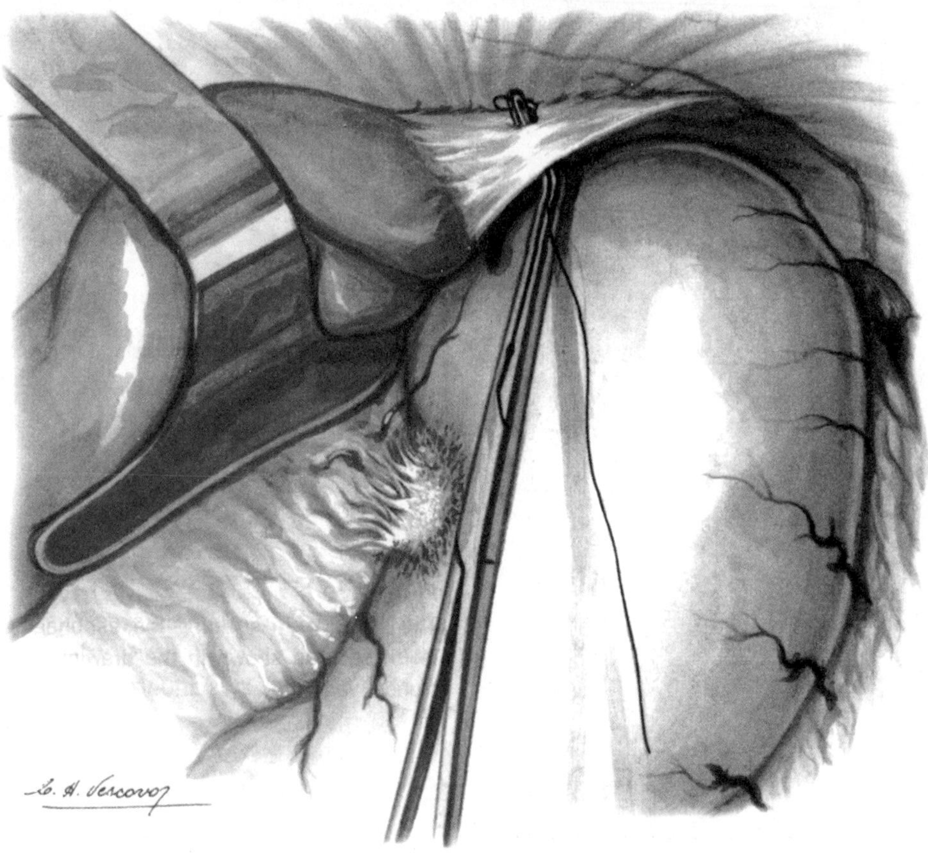

FIGURE 30.2

FIGURE 30.3
The peritoneum covering the esophagus and the diaphragm is incised, as shown in the drawing, in order to carry out a truncal vagotomy.

Surgical Procedures

FIGURE 30.4
With his right index finger the surgeon dissects the periesophageal areolar tissue and identifies the two vagus nerves. Dissection of the esophagus and division of the vagus nerves allows the esophagus to descend and facilitates the necessary maneuvers for the gastrectomy.

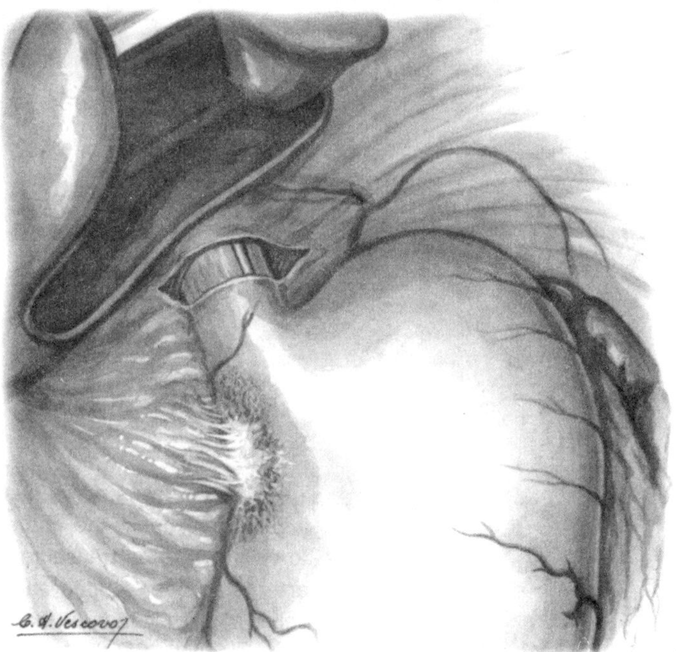

FIGURE 30.3

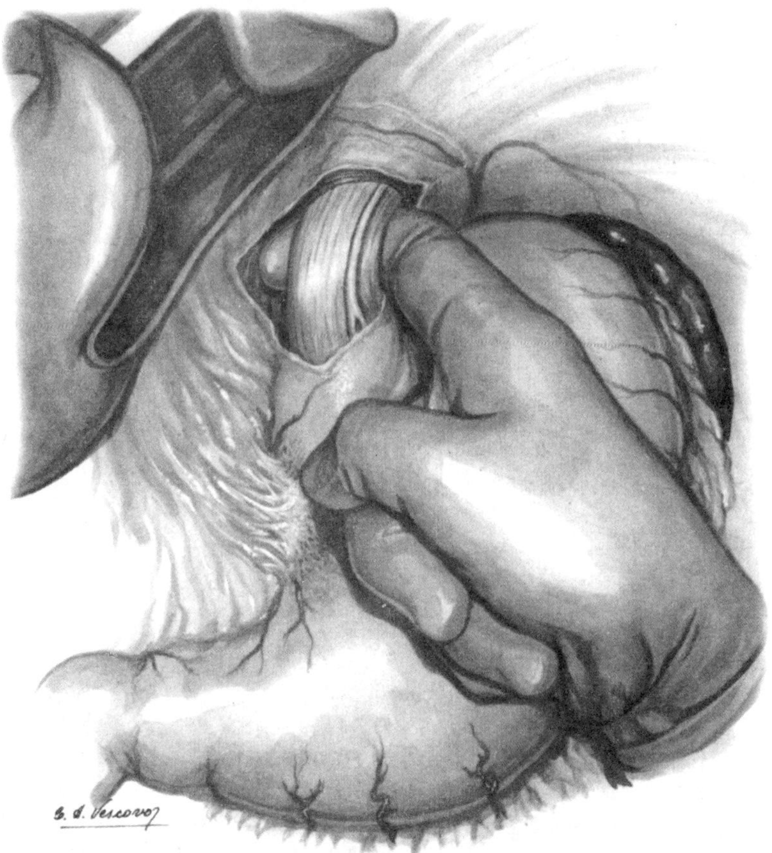

FIGURE 30.4

FIGURE 30.5
The anterior vagus nerve has been identified and divided. Using a nerve hook, the posterior vagus nerve is being pulled to the right, to be transected later. In addition, the left gastric artery has been ligated and transected at its origin from the celiac trunk. Ligation of the coronary artery at this level facilitates dissection of the tissues around the ulcer. If an aberrant left hepatic artery is found, the left gastric artery should not be ligated at this level. A Levine tube has been passed into the stomach for better control of the esophageal walls and their relation to the ulcer. In patients with ulcers that are very close to the esophagus it is better to use a Hurst mercury bougie or a Maloney 50 F tube to calibrate the esophagus and prevent a possible stricture.

Surgical Procedures

FIGURE 30.6
The distal esophagus has been lowered considerably as a result of the truncal vagotomy, the esophageal dissection, and the ligation of the left gastric artery at its origin from the celiac trunk. Lowering the esophagus makes it easier to dissect the ulcer and separate it from the esophagus.

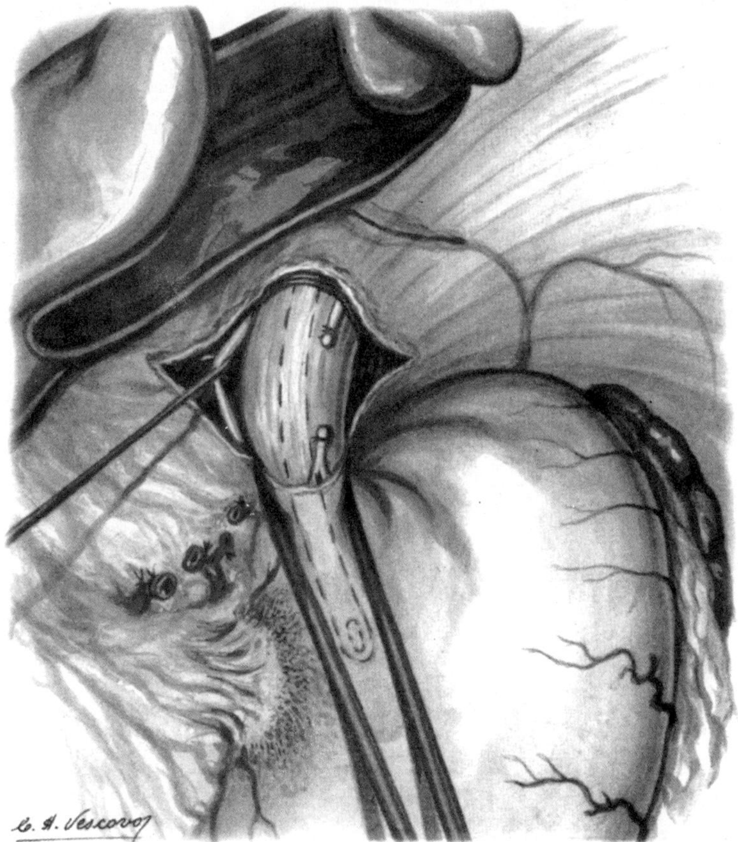

FIGURE 30.5

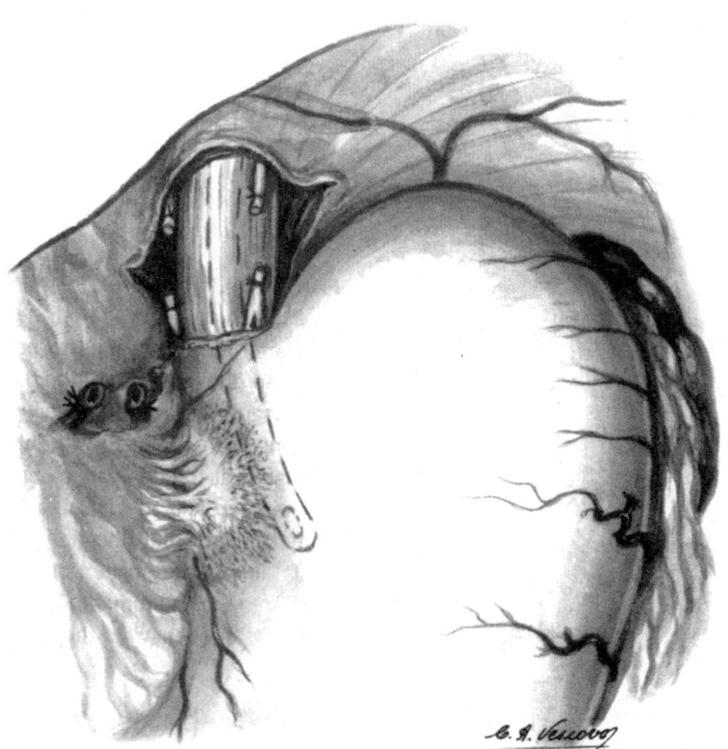

FIGURE 30.6

Surgical Procedures

FIGURE 30.7
It has been determined that there is enough room between the ulcer and the esophagus to be able to transect the stomach between the ulcer and the esophagus without injuring the esophagus. An incision 2 cm long is made in the stomach. This opening is then closed with interrupted sutures, leaving them long so that traction can be applied to them. Another 2 cm of stomach is incised and also closed. This is continued in the same manner until the horizontal line is arrived at. The horizontal line is the portion of the stomach that is to be anastomosed to the jejunum, if a Billroth II Gastrectomy is to be done, or to the duodenum in the case of a Billroth I Gastrectomy.

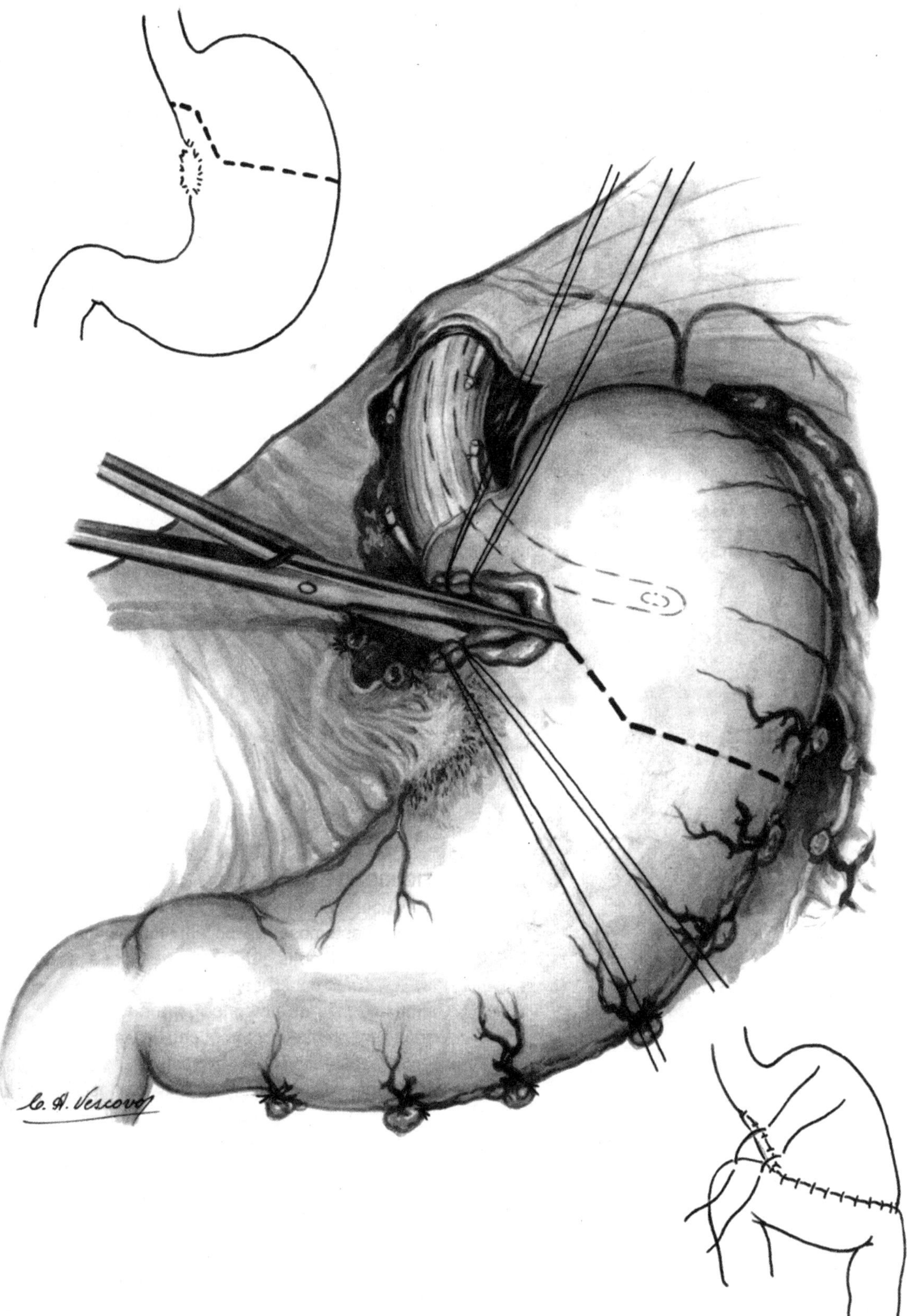

FIGURE 30.7

FIGURE 30.8
Once the oblique line is closed, using through and through interrupted sutures, transection of the stomach is continued along the horizontal line. This segment will be anastomosed to the jejunum. The upper part of the Finochietto clamp is in place. The inferior portion of the clamp will grasp the jejunal loop. The figure shows the previously closed lesser curvature being covered with interrupted seromuscular sutures.

Surgical Procedures

FIGURE 30.9
The operation has been completed. The gastric stump has been anastomosed to an antecolic jejunal loop. The afferent limb of the loop is sutured to the closed portion of the gastric stump. This closed segment will not form part of the anastomotic opening (Hofmeister-Finsterer technique), as is seen in the figure on the left. In patients in whom the ulcer involves the esophageal wall, it is advisable to pass a Hurst or Maloney 50 F mercury bougie to stretch the esophagus and prevent stricturing when the transected stomach is closed. In patients in whom the esophageal closure is not completely satisfactory, it is advisable to carry the afferent limb of the jejunal loop all the way up to the esophagus, where it is sutured to the esophageal wall for greater protection. This maneuver is shown on the left. It should be pointed out that this protection cannot be carried out in the Billroth I Gastrectomy for high-lying gastric ulcers. In order to better protect the esophagus in doubtful cases, Czendes and his colleagues (2) have proposed a Roux-en-Y gastrojejunostomy, as shown on the right, in which the ascending limb of the Roux-en-Y is sutured over the nonfunctioning portion of the anastomosis and the doubtful zone of the esophagus as a protective measure.

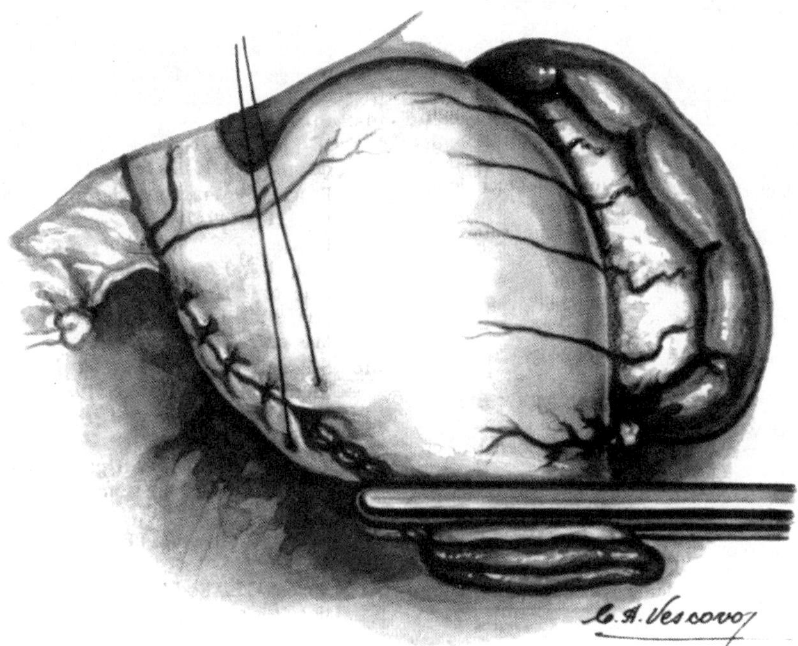

FIGURE 30.8

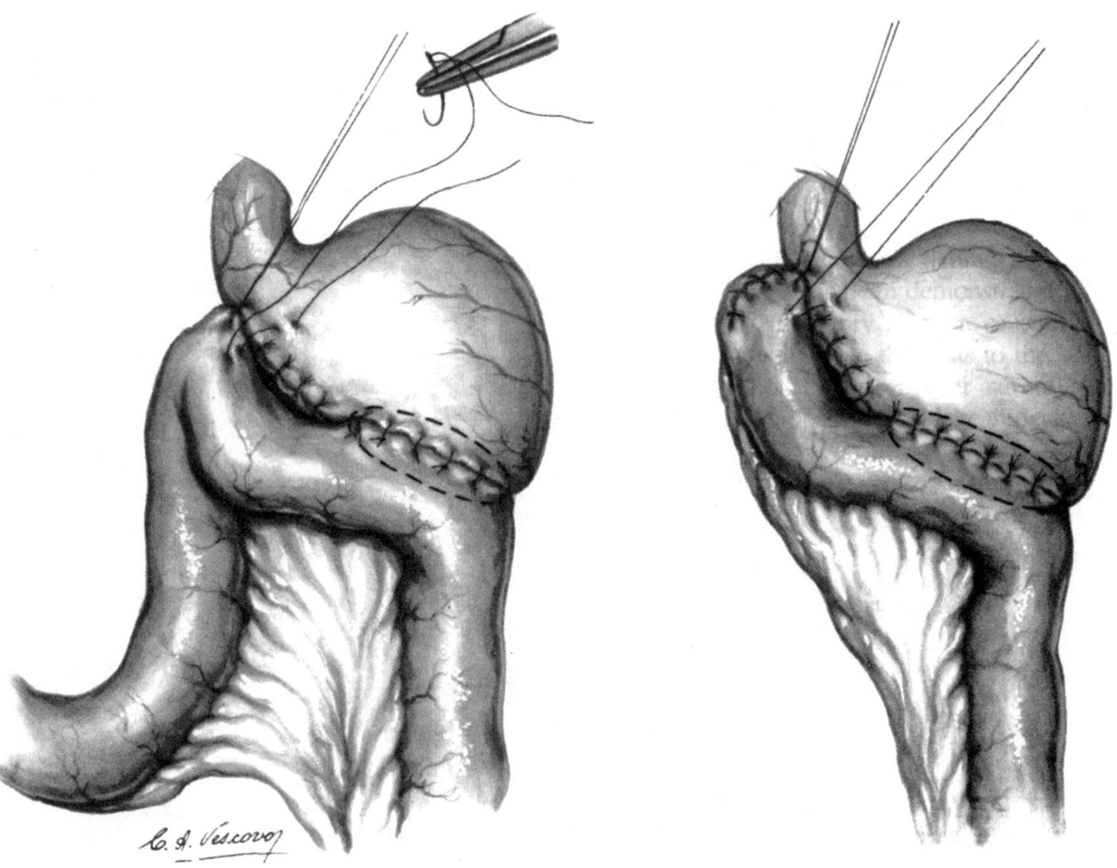

FIGURE 30.9

References

1. Braasch, J.W., Cain, J.C., Priestley, J.T. Juxta-esophageal gastric ulcer. Surg. Gynecol. Obstet. 101:280, 1955.
2. Czendes, A., Lazo, M., Braghetto, J. A surgical technique for high (cardial or juxtacardial) benign chronic gastric ulcer. Am. J. Surg. 135:857, 1978.
3. Devin, R., Lataste, J., Maillet, P. Nouveau traité de technique chirurgicale. Vol 10, p. 257. Masson et Cie, Paris, 1968.
4. Duval, J. La gastrectomie dans les ulcères très haut situés de l'estomac. Presse Méd. 61:389, 1953.
5. Fromm, D. Ulceration of the stomach and duodenum. In Fromm, D. (ed.) Gastrointestinal surgery. Vol. 1, p. 233. Churchill Livingstone, New York, 1985.
6. Gilchrist, R.K., Surgical treatment of high-lying gastric ulcer. J.A.M.A. 162:1039, 1956.
7. Gray, S.W., Skandalakis, J.E. Atlas of surgical anatomy for general surgeons. P. 79. Williams & Wilkins, Baltimore, 1985.
8. Herrington, J.L. Jr. The surgical management of duodenal ulcer and benign gastric ulcer. Int. Surg. 68:299, 1983.
9. Jensen, H.E., Hoffman, J., Jorgensen, P.W. High gastric ulcer. World J. Surg. 11:325, 1987.
10. Jordan, P.H. Gastric ulcer. In Scott, H.W. Jr., Sawyers, J.L. (Eds.) Ed. 2, p. 309. Blackwell, Oxford, 1992.
11. Kelling, G. Ueber die operative behandlung des chronischen ulcus ventriculi. Arch. Klin. Chir. 109:775, 1918.
12. Madlener, M. Ueber pylorektomie bie pylorus fermen magengeschwar. Zentralbl. Chir. 50:1313, 1923.
13. Madlener, M. Pylorectomy as indirect operation for ulcer. Zentralbl. Chir. 51:1896, 1924.
14. Olch, P.O., Harkins, H.N. A historic review of gastric surgery. In Harkins, H.N., Nyhus, L.M. (Eds.) Surgery of the stomach and duodenum. P. 3. Little, Brown, Boston, 1962.
15. Pauchet, V. Practique chirurgicale illustrée. Vol. 7. Gastron Doin, Paris, 145:149, 1927.
16. Pauchet, V. Sur la technique de la gastrectomie. Bull. Mem. Soc. Chir. (Paris) 23:243, 1931.
17. Quénu, J., Loygue, J., Perrotin, J., Dubost, C., Moreaux, I. Opérations sur les parois de l'abdomen et sur le tube digestive. P. 453. Masson et Cie, Paris, 1968.
18. Schoemaker, I. Zur technik der magenresektion nach Billroth I. Arch. Klin. Chir. 121:268, 1922.
19. Tanner, N.C. Surgery of peptic ulceration and its complications. Postgrad. Med. J. 30:448, 1954.
20. Tanner, N.C. Billroth II gastrectomy. In Nyhus, L.M., Wastell, C. (Eds.) Surgery of the stomach and duodenum. Ed. 3. Little, Brown, Boston, 1977.
21. Welch, C.E., Burke, J.F. Gastric ulcer reappraised. Surgery 65:708, 1969.
22. Welch, C.E., Rodkey, G.V., von Gryska, P. One thousand operations for peptic ulcer disease. Ann. Surg. 204:454, 1986.

Section F

Surgery of the Stomach and Duodenum

CHAPTER 31

Gastric Ulcers Penetrating the Pancreas and Inferior Surface of the Liver

PEPTIC GASTRIC ULCERS PENETRATING THE PANCREAS

Peptic gastric ulcers that penetrate into the pancreas and are refractory to medical therapy are very infrequent, due to the efficacy of modern therapeutic measures. At some time or other, however, the surgeon will encounter one of these cases. It is extremely important to remember that the pancreatic ulcer bed should not be treated aggressively, either by resection or by electrocoagulation. Even though the great majority of gastric ulcers that perforate into pancreas are benign in nature, there are cases in which malignancy has been demonstrated in spite of the presence of inflammatory reaction caused by peptic action. If there is still some doubt as to the benign or malignant nature of the ulcer after several preoperative biopsies, these biopsies should be repeated during the operation.

The technique for gastric resection in peptic gastric ulcers that perforate into the pancreas is described, as follows:

FIGURE 31.1
This patient has a great callous peptic ulcer in the lesser curvature of the posterior wall of the gastric body, perforating into the body of the pancreas. The perforation is surrounded by an intense fibrous inflammatory process. The greater curvature of the stomach has been freed and grasped by two Duval triangular clamps, and gentle traction is being applied upward. The duodenum will then be liberated and divided to gain ample access to the posterior gastric wall and the anterior surface of the pancreas.

Peptic Gastric Ulcers Penetrating the Pancreas

FIGURE 31.2
The duodenum has been divided and its distal end closed while its proximal end is wrapped in gauze and held with a Duval clamp. Traction applied upward on the three clamps exposes the perforation into the pancreas and the surrounding fibrotic reaction. Fibrous adhesive bands around the perforation are being divided.

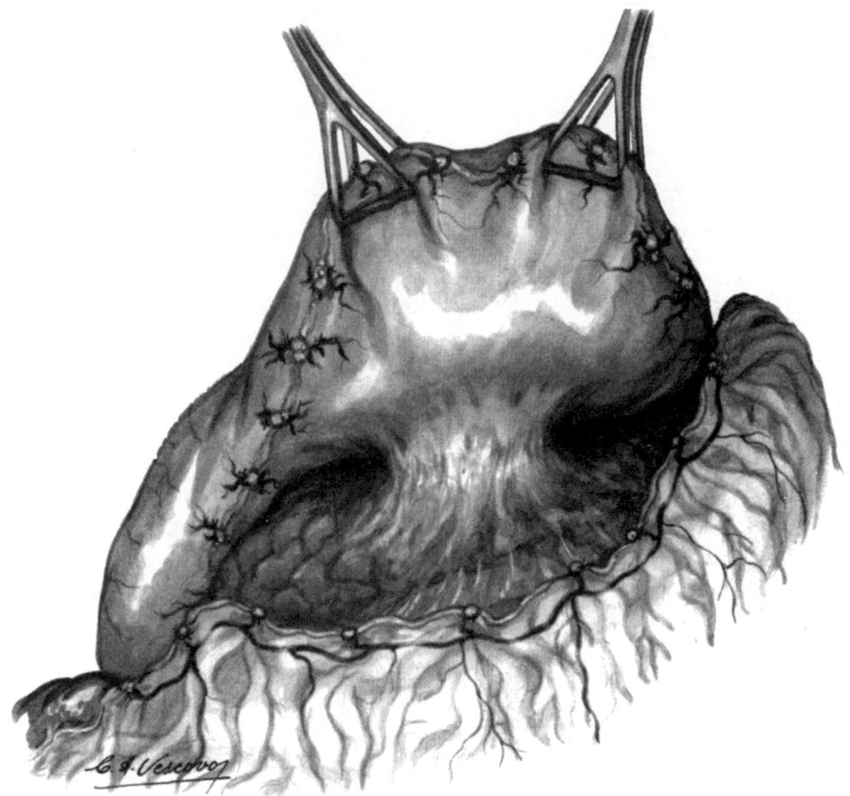

FIGURE 31.1

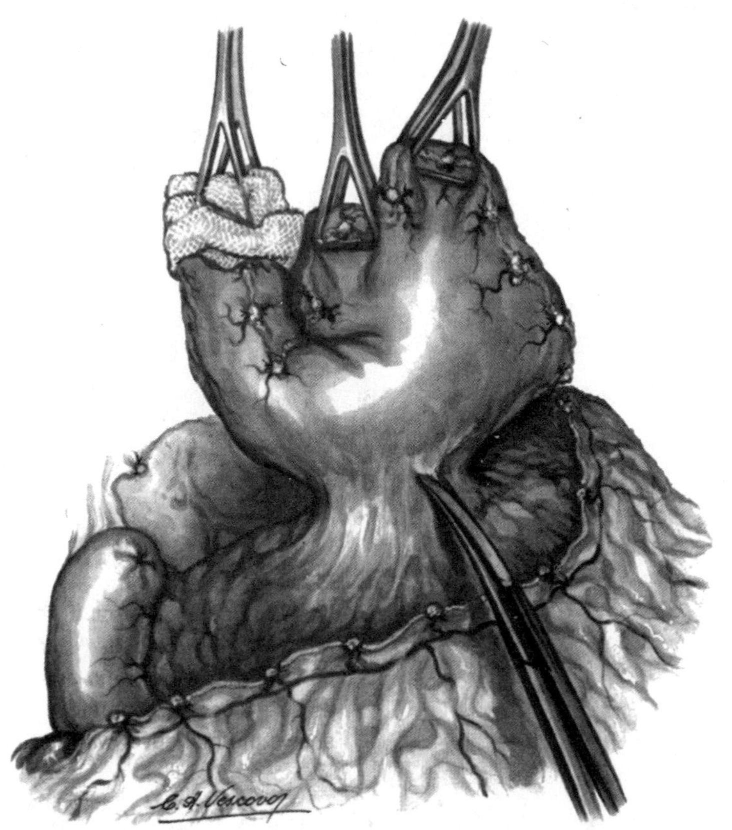

FIGURE 31.2

Peptic Gastric Ulcers Penetrating the Pancreas

FIGURE 31.3
The fibrous bands around the perforation are divided, the perforation is surrounded with the index finger of the right hand to be sure that there is no adherent viscus that could be injured as the ulcer is separated from the pancreas. The drawing shows the maneuver with the rıght index finger.

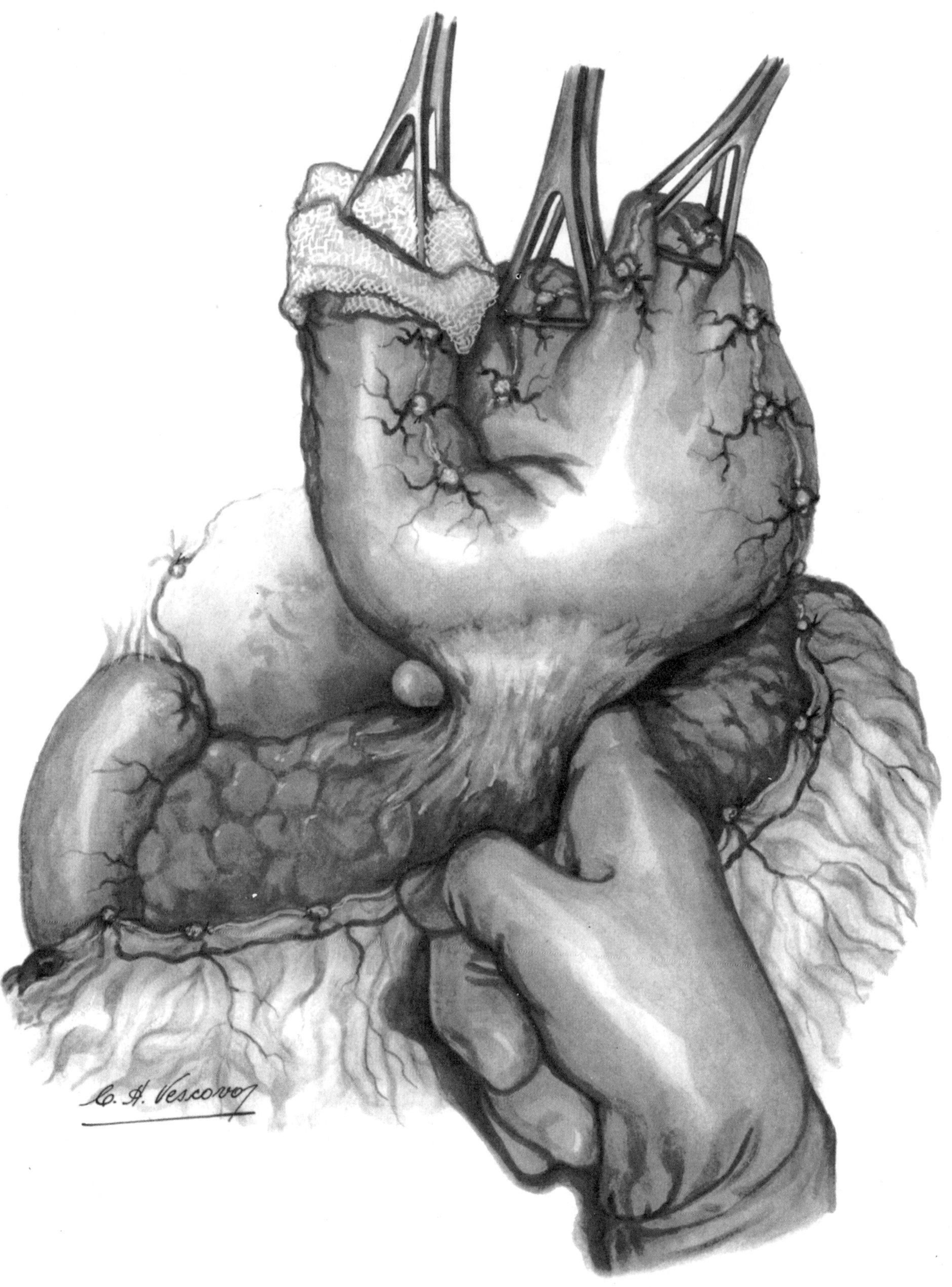

FIGURE 31.3

Peptic Gastric Ulcers Penetrating the Pancreas

FIGURE 31.4
The index finger surrounding the perforation has been replaced with a loop or rubber tube to apply some traction, allowing the edge of the ulcer to be incised with an electric scalpel.

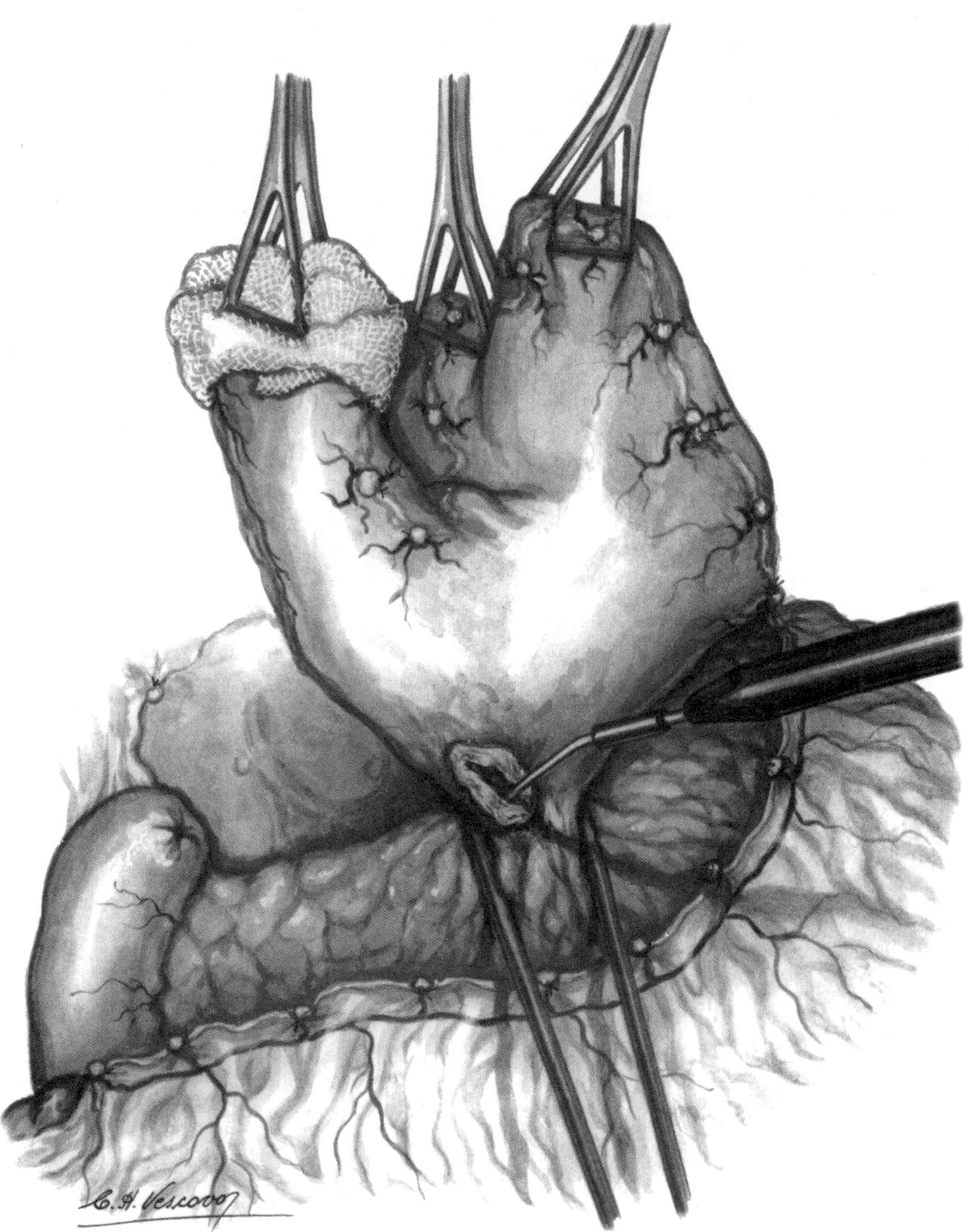

FIGURE 31.4

Peptic Gastric Ulcers Penetrating the Pancreas

FIGURE 31.5
The division of the ulcer edge penetrating into the pancreas is being completed with an electric scalpel.

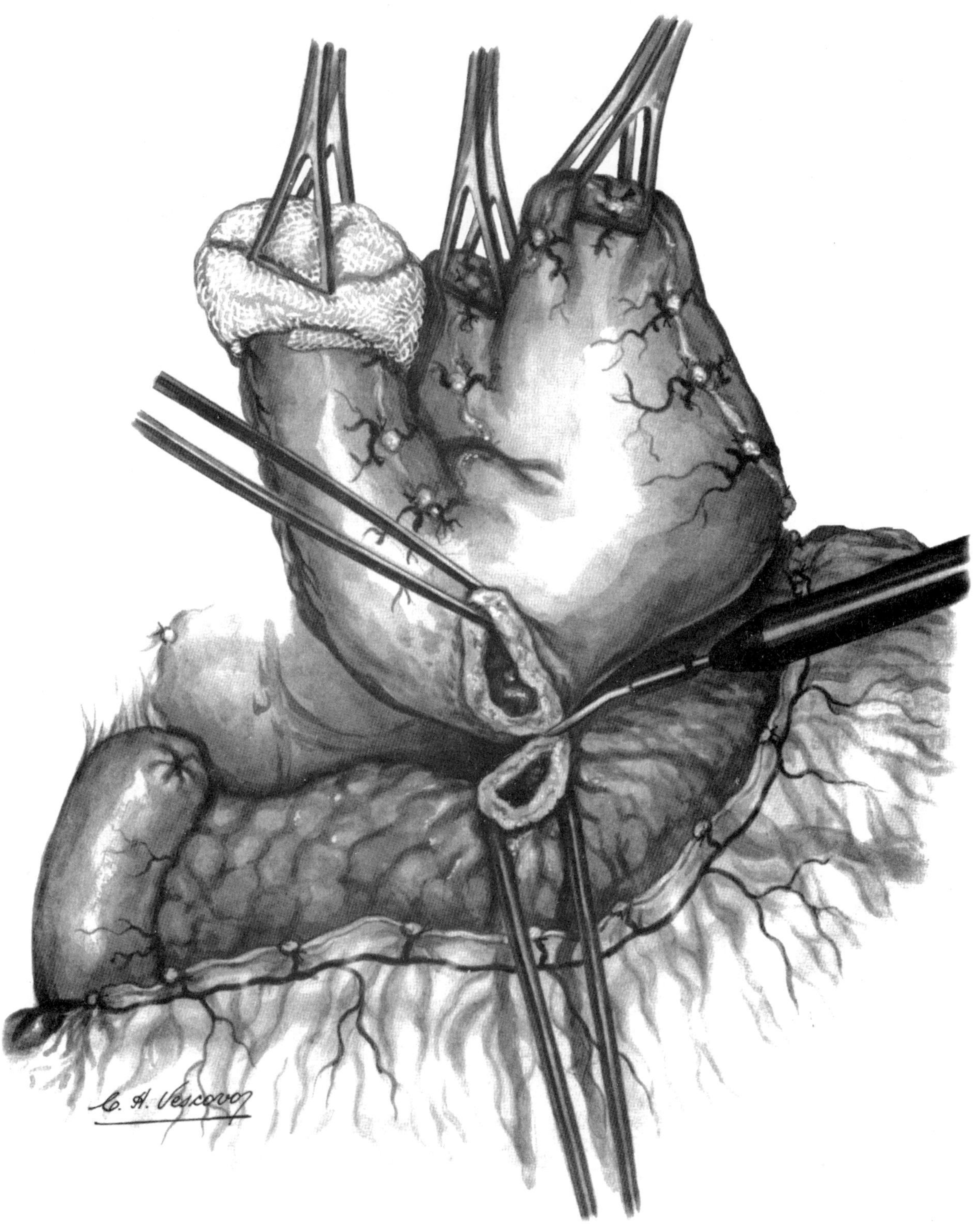

FIGURE 31.5

Peptic Gastric Ulcers Penetrating the Pancreas

FIGURE 31.6

Once the stomach is separated from the pancreas, the gastric perforation is closed to prevent further spillage of gastric contents. The ulcer bed should not be treated aggressively. Some surgeons cover the ulcer bed with some greater omentum to keep small bowel loops from adhering to it.

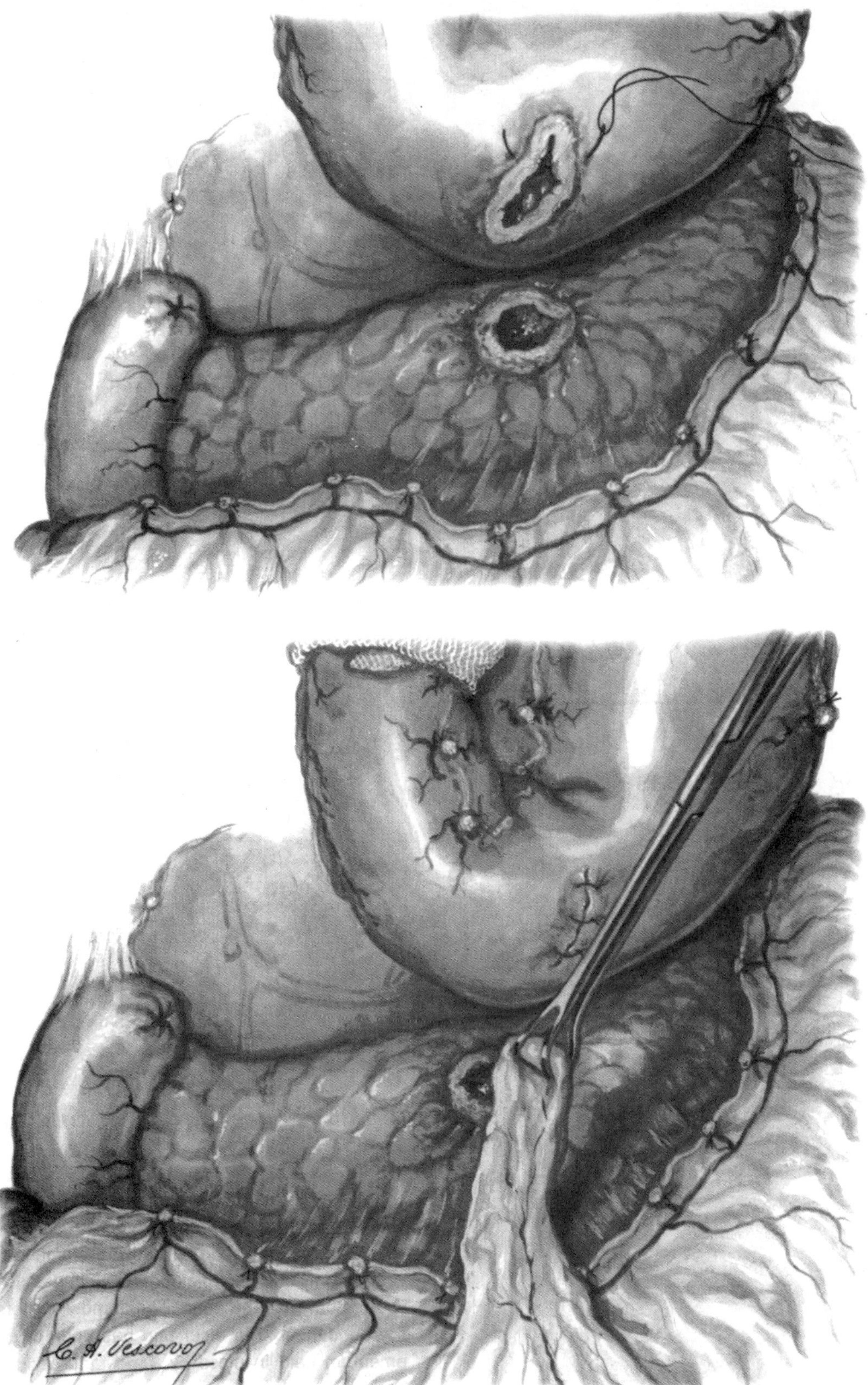

FIGURE 31.6

Peptic Gastric Ulcers Penetrating the Pancreas

FIGURE 31.7
The gastric perforation has been closed with three interrupted sutures, and the upper part of the atraumatic Finochietto twin clamp has been placed across the stomach for the Billroth II gastrectomy and gastrojejunostomy. In gastric ulcer a Billroth I gastrectomy may be used, anastomosing the gastric stump to the duodenum. The ulcer bed has been covered with greater omentum held in place by three sutures into the pancreatic capsule.

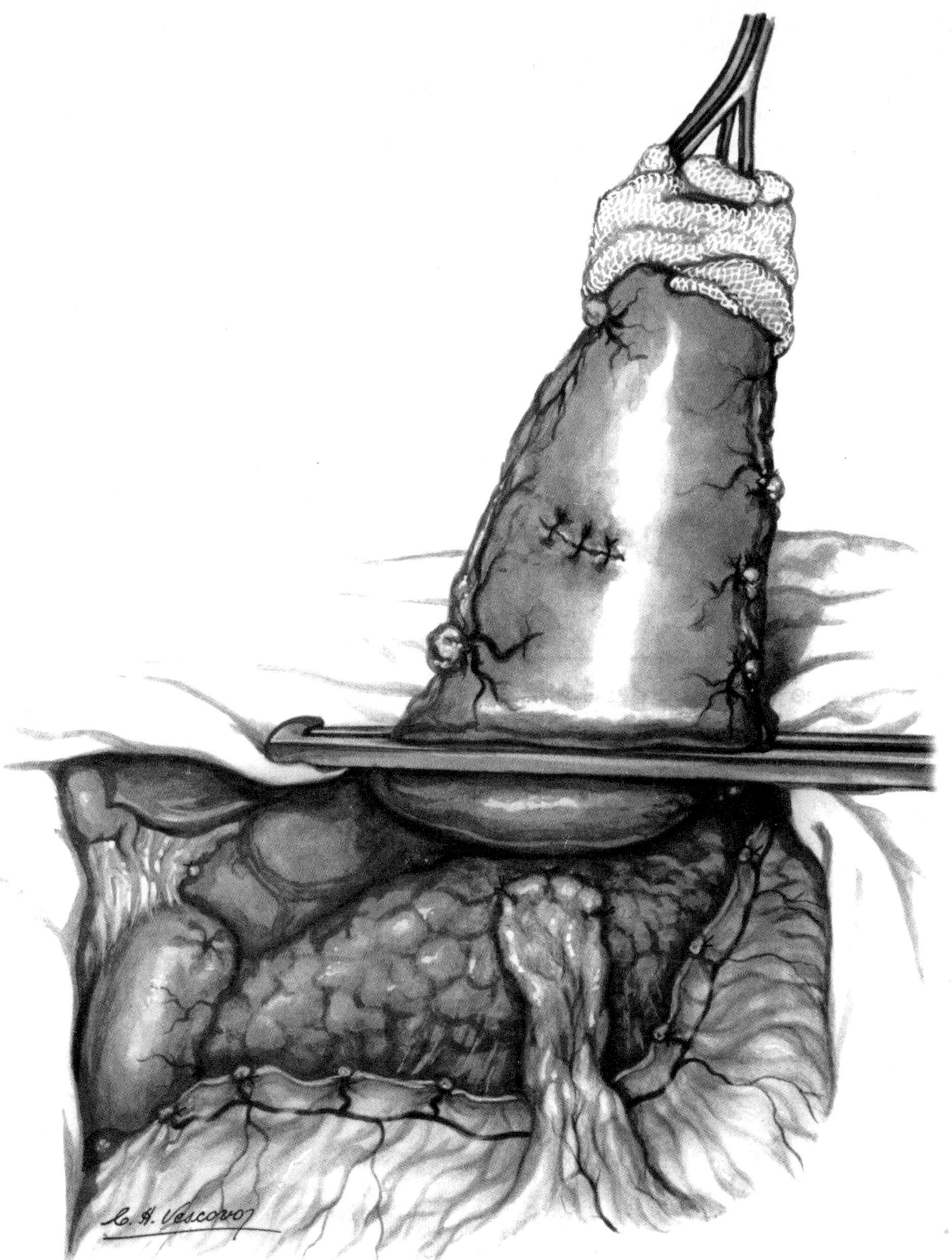

FIGURE 31.7

PEPTIC GASTRIC ULCERS PERFORATING THE INFERIOR SURFACE OF THE LIVER

Peptic ulcers located on the lesser curvature or the anterior wall of the stomach can sometimes perforate into the inferior surface of the liver. Even though this complication is rare, it can give rise to difficulties with the gastric resection due to anatomic alterations and compromise of vital organs.

Peptic Gastric Ulcers Perforating the Inferior Surface of the Liver

FIGURE 31.8
Patient with a chronic callous ulcer of the anterior wall of the lesser curvature of the gastric antrum perforating into the inferior surface of the liver. A part of the greater omentum has become displaced toward the inflammatory area, passing over the anterior wall of the antrum and causing gastric obstruction.

Peptic Gastric Ulcers Perforating the Inferior Surface of the Liver

FIGURE 31.9
A, The callous antral ulcer, which is penetrating into the liver, is surrounded with a ribbon or a rubber tube to exert traction and allow the ulcer edge to be separated from the liver with an electric scalpel. **B,** Once the stomacn has been separated from the liver surface, the gastric opening is sutured to prevent contamination of the peritoneum by gastric contents. The adherent omentum is then divided and ligated. The curved clamp shows where sutures will be passed to ligate the adherent omentum and then proceed with liberation of the stomach to carry out the gastrectomy.

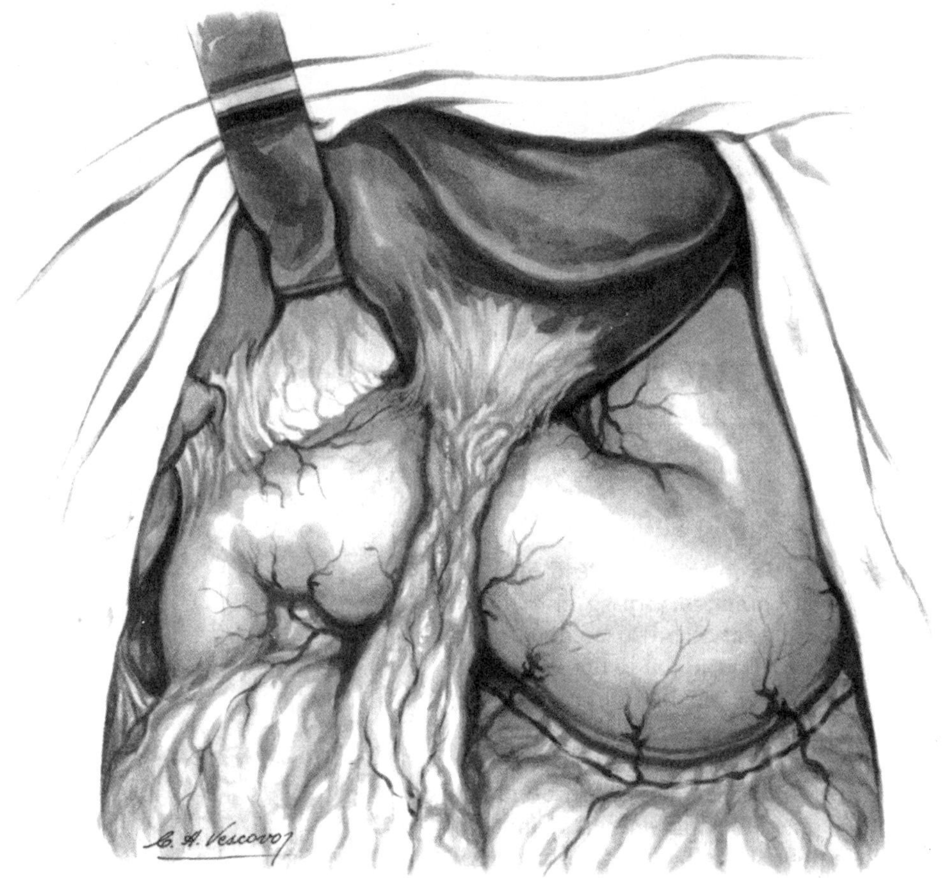

FIGURE 31.8

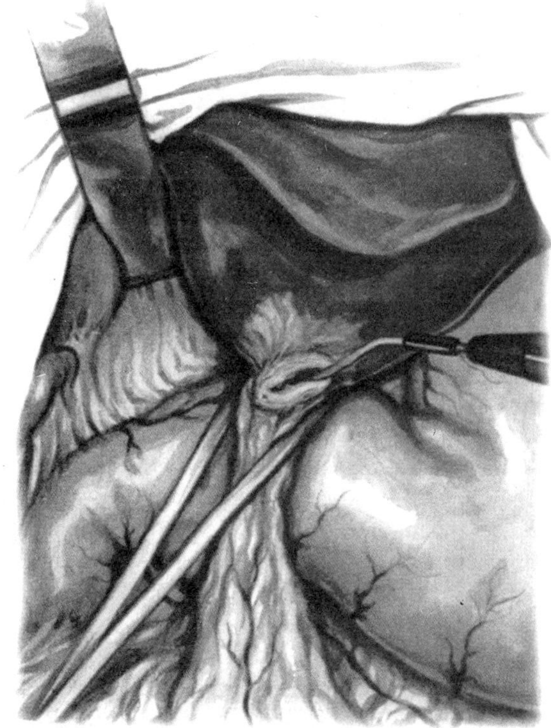

A

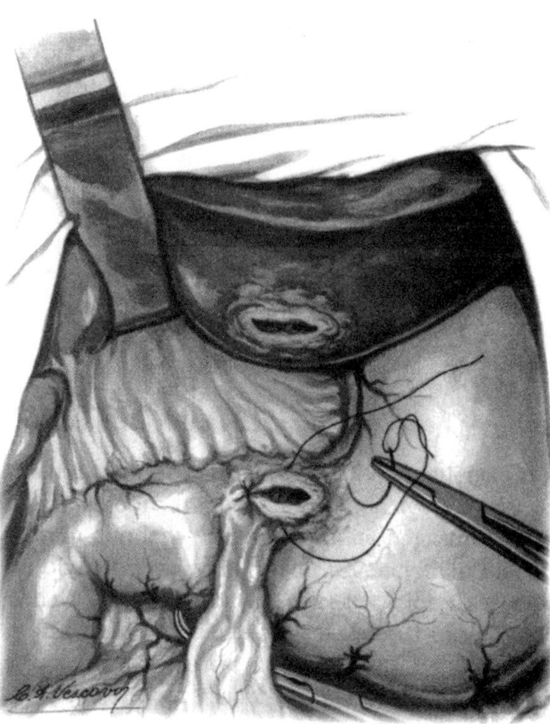

B

FIGURE 31.9

Section F

Surgery of the Stomach and Duodenum

CHAPTER **32**

Surgical Treatment of Bleeding Gastric and Duodenal Ulcers

The best treatment of bleeding gastric and duodenal ulcers is gastric resection. This procedure offers greater guarantee of hemostasis and less recurrence of hemorrhage and of the ulcer. However, gastrectomy may not be tolerated in patients with unstable cardiovascular conditions or in poor general condition due to advanced age and the presence of other simultaneous illnesses. In these cases it is advisable to carry out local hemostasis, which, though far from being the ideal treatment because it can frequently become complicated by recurrent hemorrhage, can save a very difficult situation. The decision to operate on these patients should be made before they become too deteriorated. Several factors may be of help to the surgeon in making the decision:

1. If the hemorrhage produced a state of shock.
2. If the patients bled continuously.
3. If the hemorrhage represented a loss of 30% of the blood volume or the patient had to be transfused 1500 mL of blood every 24 hours.
4. If the patient rebled and had to be transfused under medical therapy during the same hospital stay.
5. If the patient bleeds and has to be transfused after a good response to medical treatment.
6. If an actively bleeding vessel is seen in the ulcer bed during gastroduodenoscopy.

GASTRIC ULCER

Gastric ulcers bleed in 10 to 20% of patients (15). Bleeding is a more frequent indication for surgery in gastric than in duodenal ulcers. In addition, gastric ulcers should be operated on with greater urgency than bleeding duodenal ulcers (15) because gastric ulcers are more common in older patients than duodenal ulcers and hemorrhage from a gastric ulcer is more likely to recur. The great majority of gastric ulcers are localized on the lesser curvature and coexist with a duodenal ulcer in 15% of patients (3, 14, 15). In 10 to 15% of cases gastric ulcers are malignant (15). The probability of malignancy should always be in the surgeon's mind (7).

SURGICAL EXPLORATION OF THE STOMACH IN GASTRIC HEMORRHAGES

Bleeding gastric ulcers can present two situations:

1. The bleeding gastric ulcer can be localized from outside the stomach.
2. The bleeding gastric ulcer cannot be localized from outside the stomach.

In the first case, local hemostasis can be carried out through a longitudinal gastrotomy in the anterior gastric wall, near the ulcer, to facilitate placement of the hemostatic suture ligatures. In the second case a longitudinal gastrotomy is made in the midline of the anterior gastric wall over the extent of the gastric body. Once the gastric wall has been incised, the edges of the gastric wall are grasped with large atraumatic Duval clamps. This nas two objectives:

1. It stops bleeding from the gastric wall, which is very vascular, without having to carry out multiple ligatures of the wall, which will lead to considerable blood loss in addition to the hemorrhage.
2. It allows. by opposite traction on the Duval clamps, opening the stomach widely to explore its interior. The function of the Duval clamps can be complemented by other retractors to explore the stomach, especially its upper portion, the esophagogastric junction, the cardia, and the fundus. Intragastric clots can be removed manually. Suction should not be used to remove clots because this will not work and frequent suction will injure the gastric mucosa and increase the blood loss. The suction cannula can be used directly where the blood is being lost to facilitate vision and correct placement of the hemostatic sutures. If the hemorrhagic ulcer is located high in the area of the cardia or subcardia, placement of the hemostatic sutures can be very difficult. Good illumination is essential. It is very helpful to pass a 50 F Hurst bougie through the esophagus up to but without going beyond the esophagogastric junction so as not to impede the surgeon's vision in placing the sutures into the base of the ulcer without causing narrowing of the esophagus. This procedure is preferable to local excision of the ulcer, as proposed by some surgeons (5) in cases where the condition of the patient does not permit gastrectomy with resection of the ulcer by the Pauchet technique, which is the treatment of choice.

In patients with bleeding ulcers located high near the greater curvature of the stomach (a very infrequent site of peptic ulcer), invagination of the greater curvature with the right hand of the surgeon can be resorted to, to bring the ulcer to a position where it is easier to place the hemostatic sutures. If the bleeding has stopped at the moment of exploration, the sutures should still be placed.

In some patients, instead of carrying out the hemostasis by suturing the ulcer base, resection of a wedge of stomach including the entire ulcer, with later reconstruction of the stomach, can be done (12). Wedge resection is a lesser procedure than gastrectomy but can only be done in limited areas of the stomach. Ulcers of the lesser curvature located above the incisura angularis can be removed by wedge resection without inconvenience. If the ulcer is below the incisura, wedge resection is contraindicated because it will damage the nerve of Latarjet (7).

DUODENAL ULCER

The best procedure for the treatment of bleeding duodenal ulcers is gastric resection, be it a hemigastrectomy with truncal vagotomy or a 70% gastrectomy. Local hemostasis can be resorted to in patients in such precarious condition as to preclude a gastrectomy. However, local hemostasis does not prevent recurrence of bleeding, which happens frequently. To carry out local hemostasis of bleeding duodenal ulcer, a longitudinal duodenotomy 3 cm long can be carried out on the anterior duodenal wall, starting 15 mm below the pylorus, or a 5-cm duodenopyloroantral incision can be carried out with 2 cm of it over the duodenum and some 3 cm over the antral portion. This is the same incision used in the Heineke-Mikulicz pyloroplasty. Massive bleeding of duodenal ulcers is generally due to ulcers of the posterior duodenal wall that penetrate into the pancreas, making hemostasis no easy task. In the majority of cases massive bleeding of a duodenal ulcer is due to erosion of the duodenal arterial complex described by Berne and Rosoff in 1969 (1). Less frequently, bleeding from a duodenal ulcer has no relation to this arterial complex. If the hemorrhage is related to the arterial complex, it is necessary to ligate the gastroduodenal artery above, below, and lateral to the erosion (1). If the ligature of the gastroduodenal artery is done only above the bleeding site, hemorrhage will continue because blood will reach the site through the right gastroepiploic and the superior and anterior pancreatoduodenal branches of the gastroduodenal artery. Suture ligatures of the gastroduodenal artery above and below the eroded area may not be enough in cases in which the transverse pancreatic artery arises medially from the gastroduodenal artery. To carry out hemostasis with less risk of recurrence of bleeding, a triple suture ligature has to be done, as advised by Berne and Rosoff (1, 7). If the hemorrhage is not produced by an artery of the gastroduodenal arterial complex, the suture ligatures should be placed as described for gastric ulcers.

In patients with bleeding from duodenal ulcers localized in the postbulbar region or in the second portion, local hemostasis becomes very important to avoid a very risky resection due to the proximity of the ulcer to the papilla of Vater and the common bile duct.

Once local hemostasis is attained, some surgeons complete the operation with a proximal gastric vagotomy or with a truncal vagotomy and pyloroplasty (4, 7, 11, 14). If it is not possible to perform a safe pyloroplasty because of the previous exploratory duodenal incision, one can opt for a gastrojejunostomy, a Finney pyloroplasty, or a Jaboulay gastroduodenostomy (7).

ANASTOMOTIC ULCERS

In patients with hemorrhage from an anastomotic ulcer the best treatment, if the patient's condition permits it, is gastrectomy. If the patient has had a previous gastrectomy, a regastrectomy should be done. If the patient has had a vagotomy, a revision vagotomy should be done, preferably by the supradiaphragmatic approach. If the patient's condition is very poor, local hemostasis should be resorted to. However, local hemostasis can create technical difficulties for the surgeon if the anastomotic ulcer occurs in a patient with an ample gastrectomy and a retrocolic anastomosis. In some of these patients local hemostasis can only be attained through an abdominothoracic approach. This incision should be used to perform a supradiaphragmatic vagotomy (7).

Surgical Technique

FIGURE 32.1
A midline incision has been made in the anterior gastric wall in order to explore the inside of the stomach to localize the site of the hemorrhage and carry out local hemostasis, if indicated.

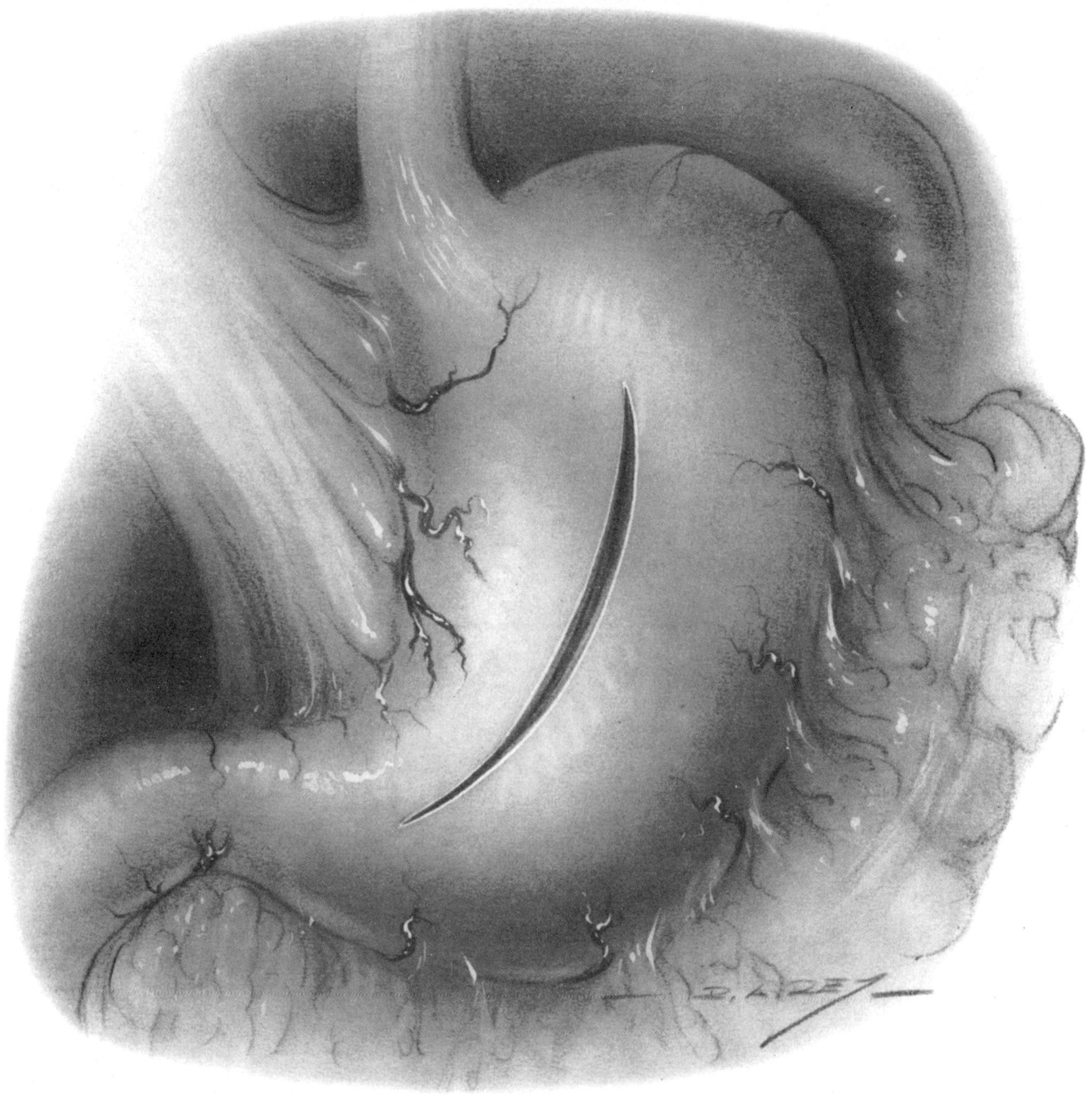

FIGURE 32.1

Surgical Technique

FIGURE 32.2
The anterior gastric wall has been incised and the edges of the stomach grasped with large Duval clamps. This will provide temporary control of bleeding from the numerous vessels in the gastric wall. Traction is applied to the clamps to open the stomach widely for the exploration. Any clots within the stomach should be removed manually.

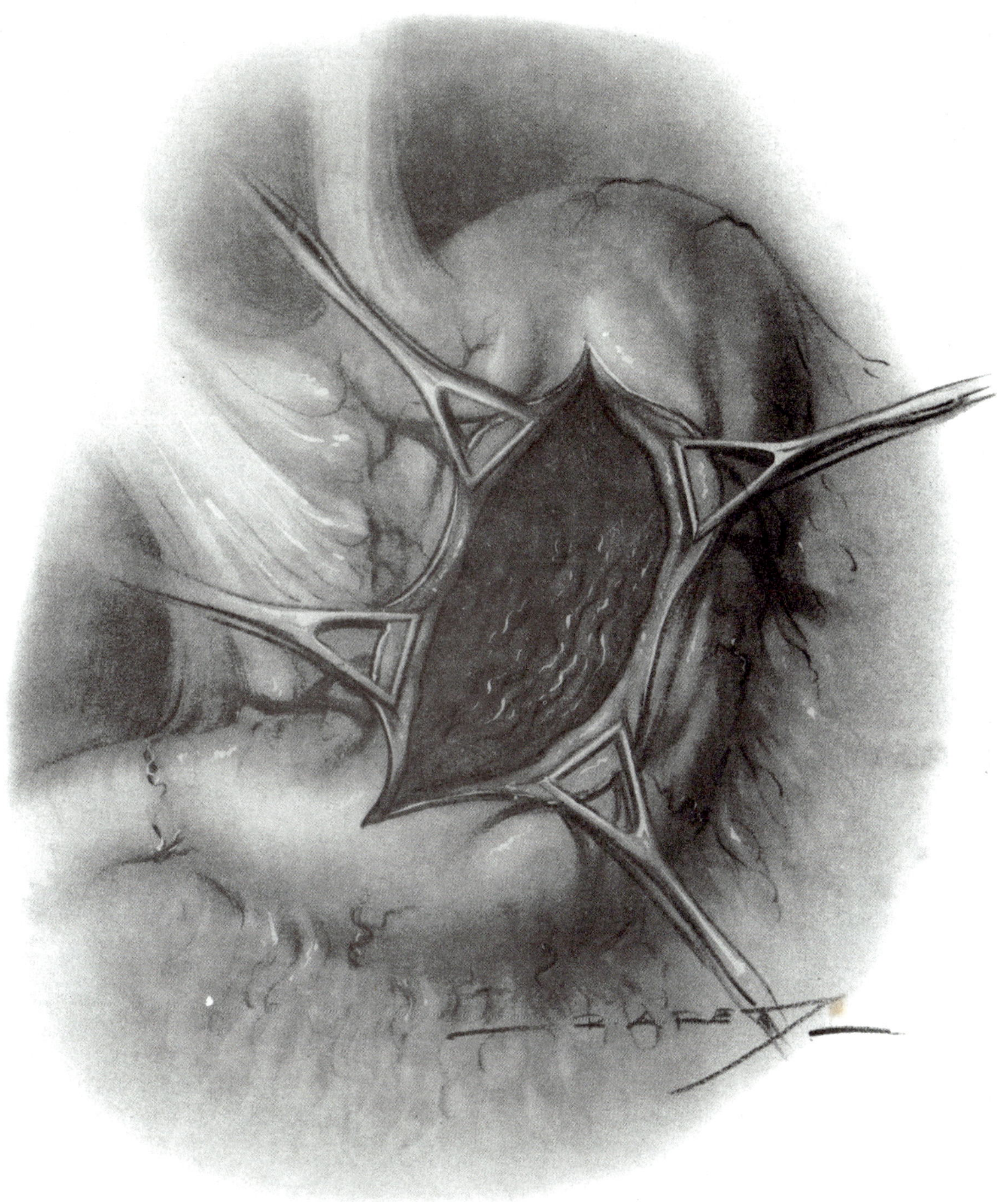

FIGURE 32.2

Surgical Technique

FIGURE 32.3
Gastric exploration can be improved by the use of retractors to explore the upper part of the stomach. Insert **A** shows severe erosive gastritis with several acute ulcers bleeding massively. Insert **B** shows that the bleeding is due to a rupture of the gastric mucosa near the esophagogastric junction (Mallory-Weiss Syndrome). Insert **C** shows a gastric leiomyoma near the cardia as the cause of the hemorrhage.

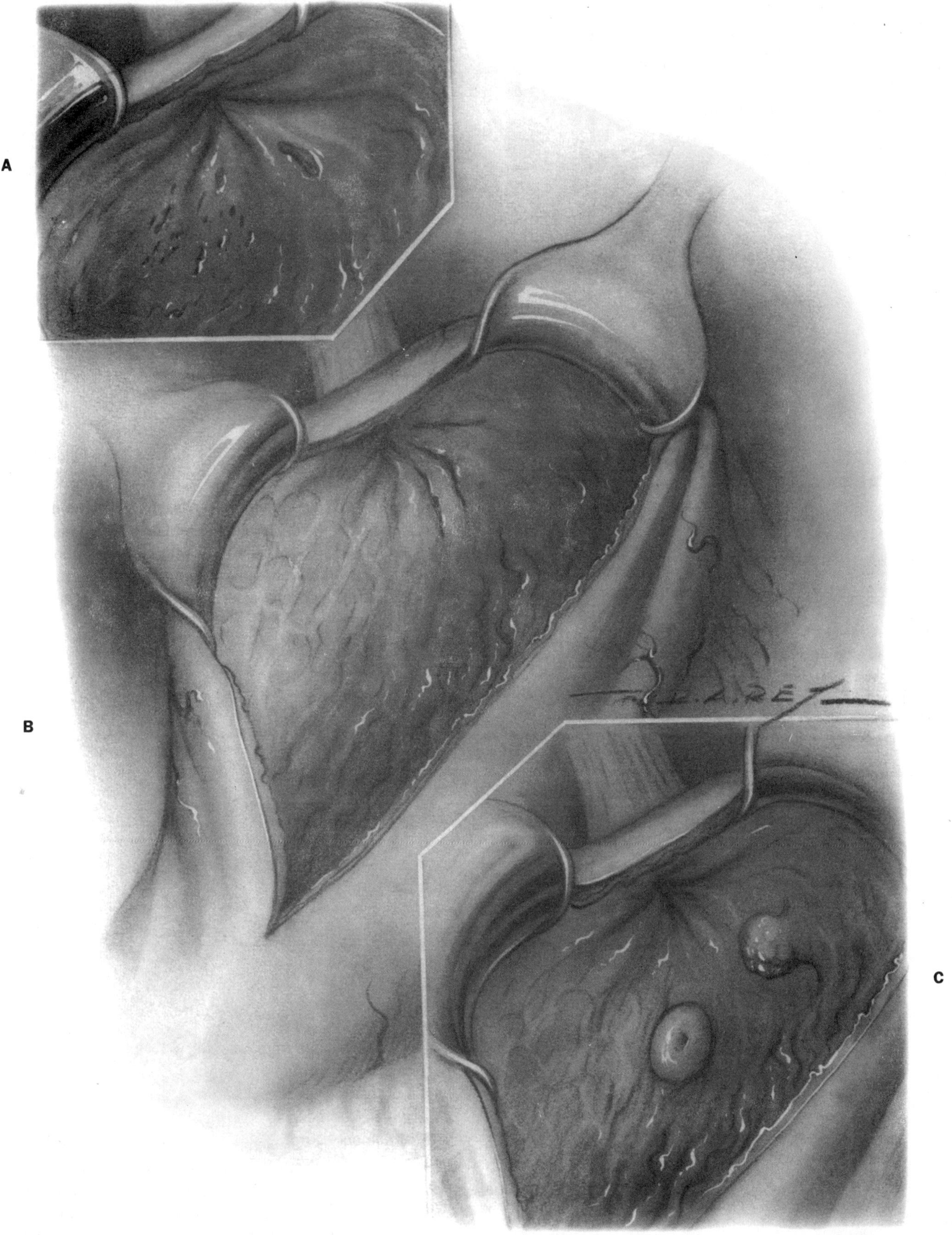

FIGURE 32.3

FIGURE 32.4
A massively bleeding gastric ulcer is shown, located on the posterior wall of the lesser curvature. Local hemostasis is being carried out by closing the ulcer with suture ligatures using nonabsorbable suture material. The number of sutures will be related to the size of the ulcer and their efficiency in controlling the hemorrhage.

Surgical Technique

FIGURE 32.5
Massive hemorrhage from a gastric ulcer located in the upper part of the posterior wall, near the greater curvature. The location of the ulcer is shown by a broken-line oval. The anterior gastric wall has been opened, and its edges are being held with atraumatic Duval clamps. The location of the ulcer impedes adequate local hemostasis. To facilitate placement of the hemostatic sutures, the gastrocolic ligament is divided and ligated for a distance long enough to allow the greater curvature to be invaginated so as to place the ulcer where it is more accessible for local hemostasis.

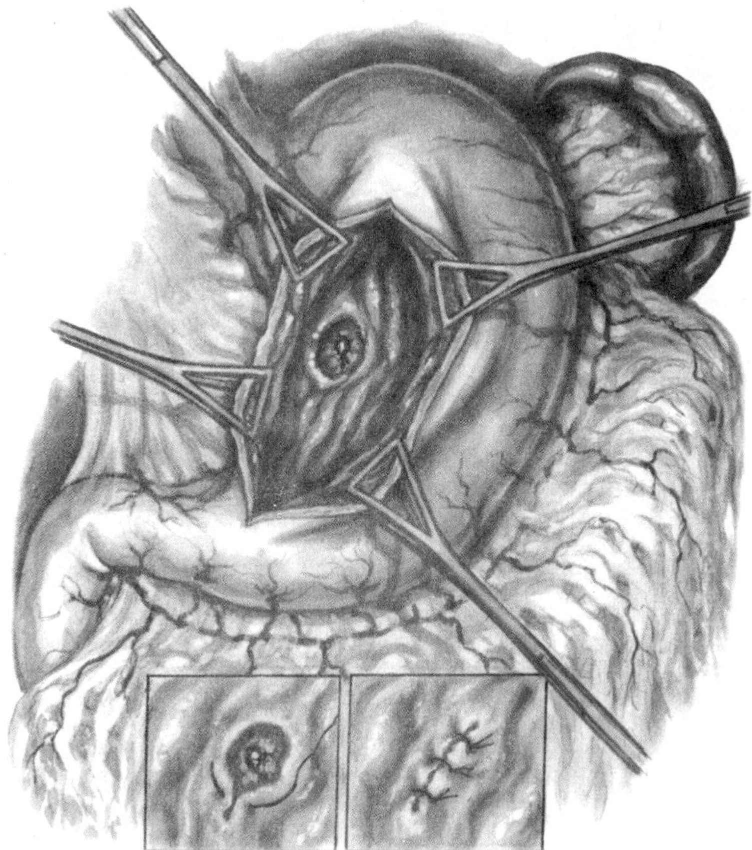

FIGURE 32.4

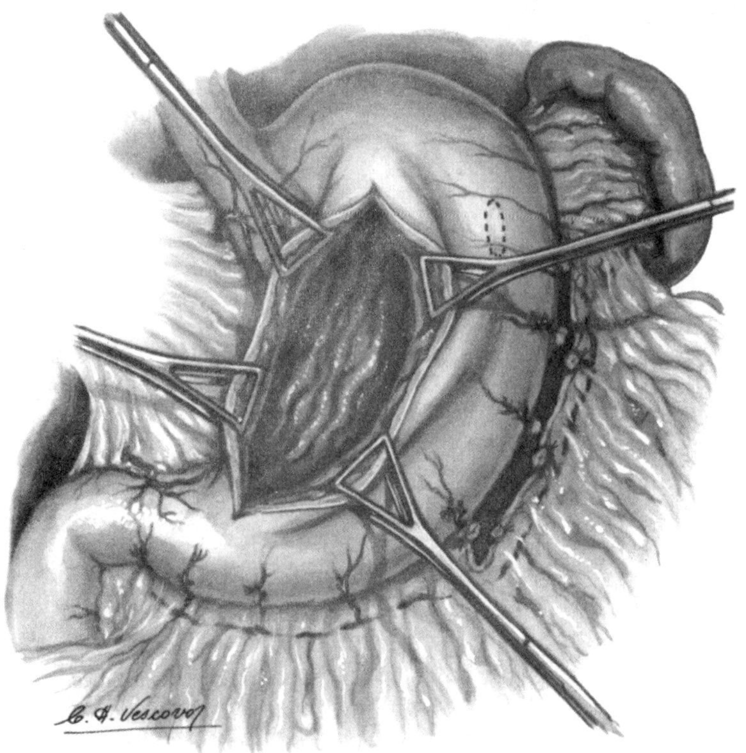

FIGURE 32.5

Surgical Technique

FIGURE 32.6
Manual invagination of the greater curvature has been carried out, placing the ulcer where it is accessible for the hemostatic sutures.

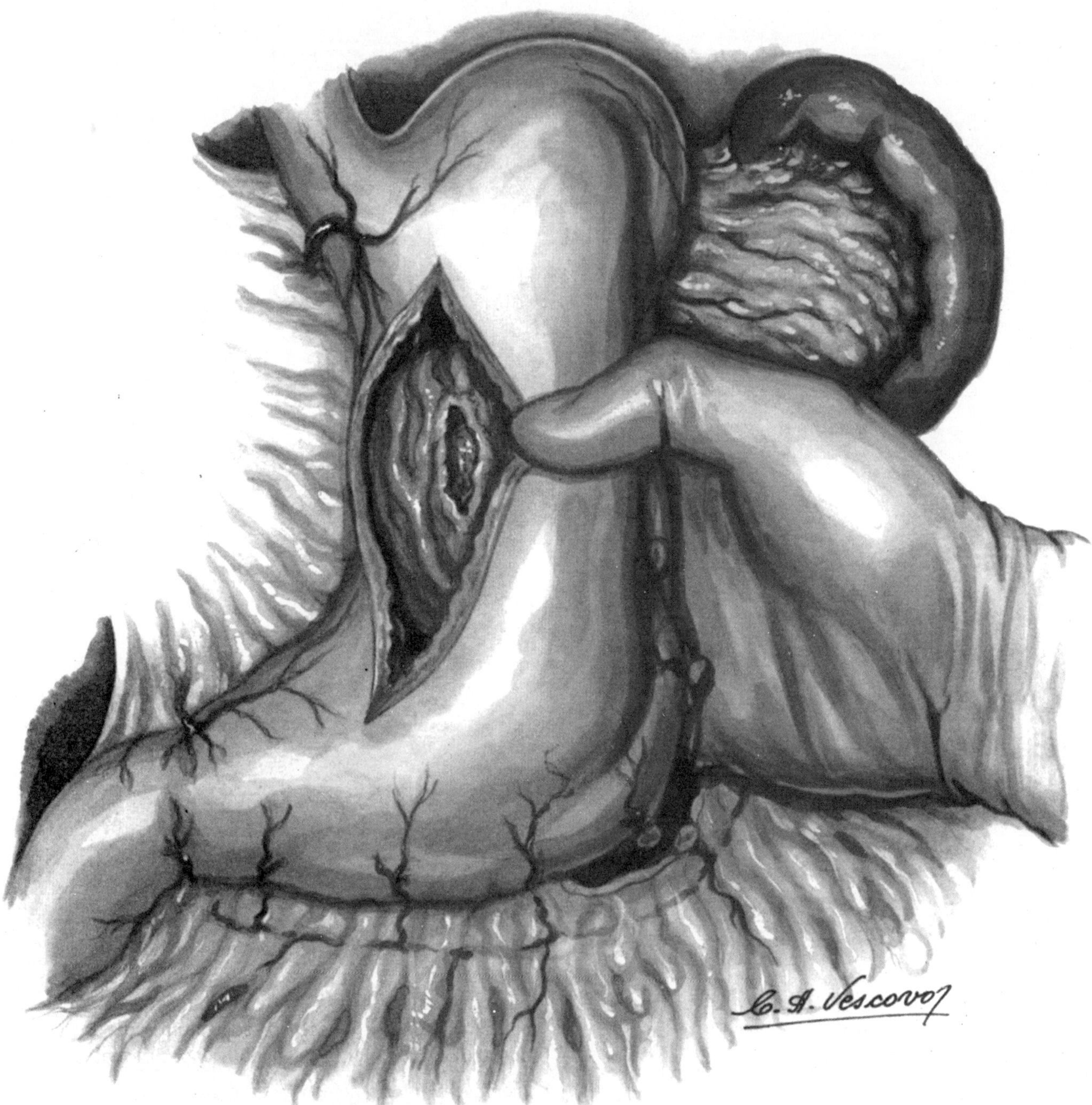

FIGURE 32.6

Surgical Technique

FIGURE 32.7
In some patients, massive hemorrhage from acute gastric ulcers cannot be prevented in spite of the very efficacious preventive treatment that is available at present. Surgery has to be performed when massive bleeding from acute gastric ulcer does not respond to medical and endoscopic therapy. Due to the severity of the hemorrhage, in some patients, gastric resection may be indicated. Acute gastric ulcers are usually not palpable and cannot be located from the outside of the stomach. In order to be sure to resect the highest bleeding ulcer it is useful to place a clip or a suture to mark the site and resect it with the gastrectomy, as shown in the drawing.

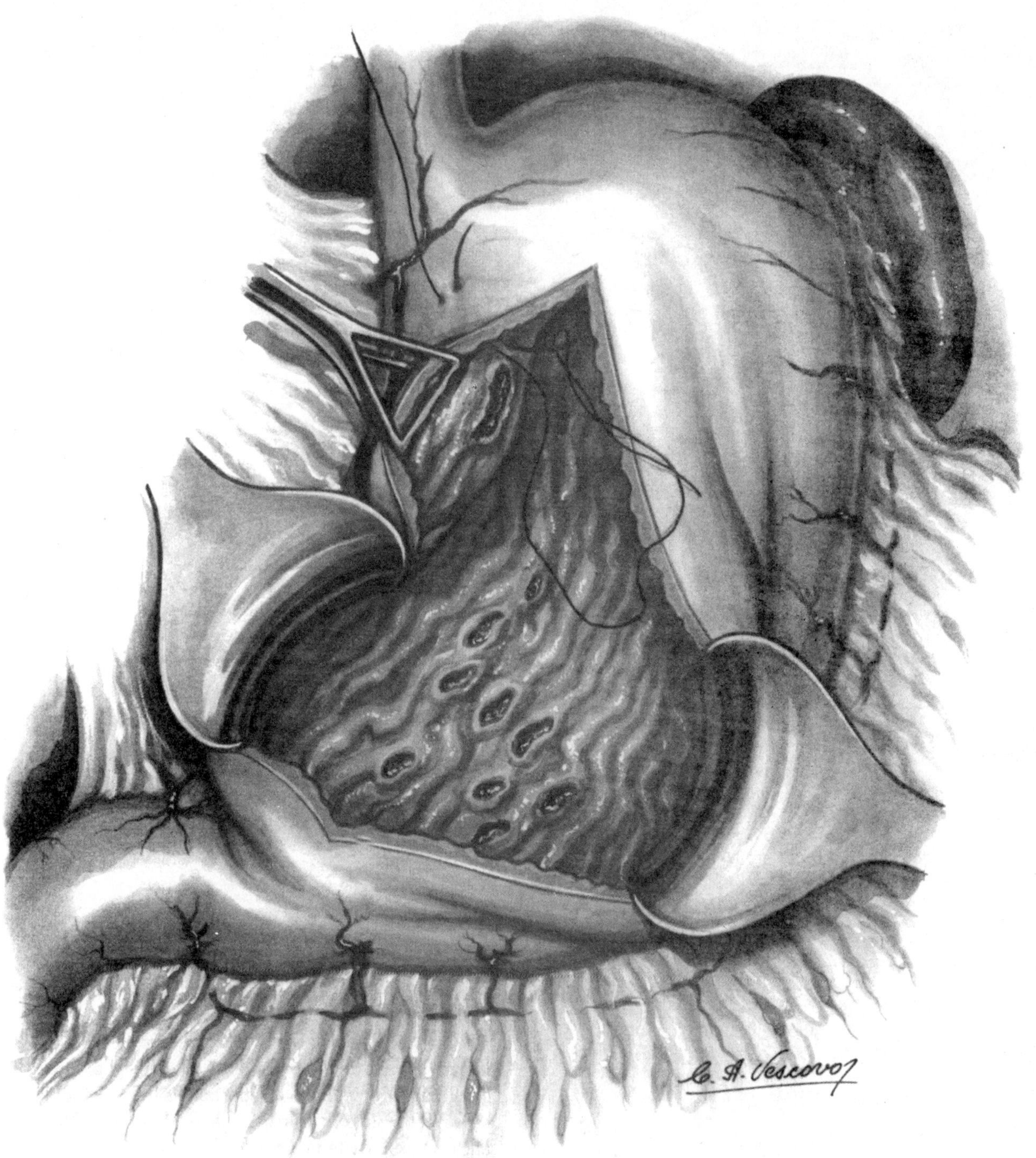

FIGURE 32.7

Surgical Technique

FIGURE 32.8
The highest bleeding acute ulcer has been marked with a suture. The gastrotomy is closed with a running suture and the gastrectomy immediately undertaken. The superior limit of the resection is shown with a broken line. The highest ulcer is shown with a dotted oval line.

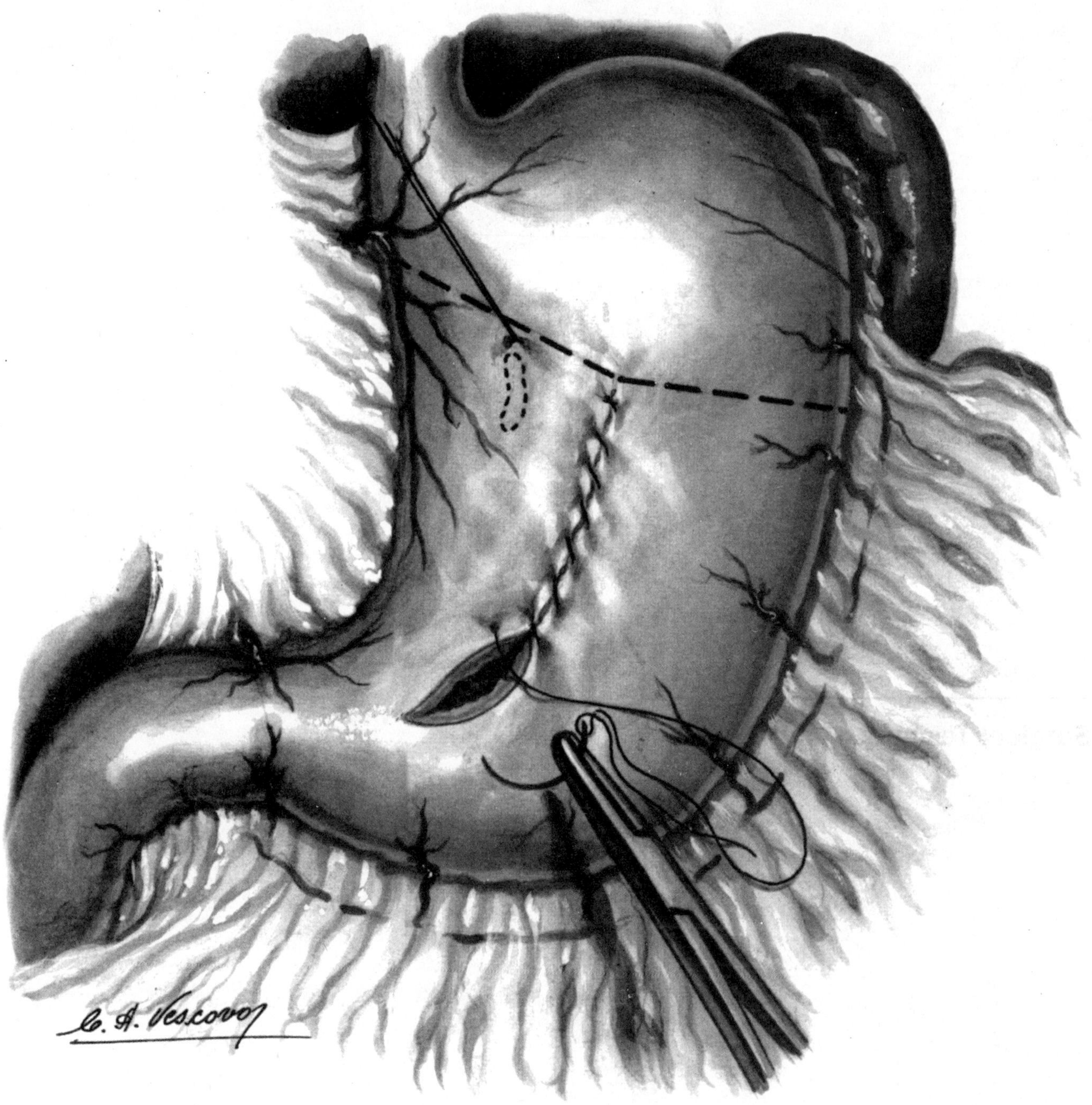

FIGURE 32.8

Surgical Technique

FIGURE 32.9 MALLORY-WEISS SYNDROME
Generally the Mallory-Weiss Syndrome, produced by tears of the gastric mucosa near the esophagogastric junction, responds to medical and endoscopic therapy. In some patients it is necessary to intervene surgically and carry out hemostasis, as seen in the insert, by suturing the lacerated mucosa.

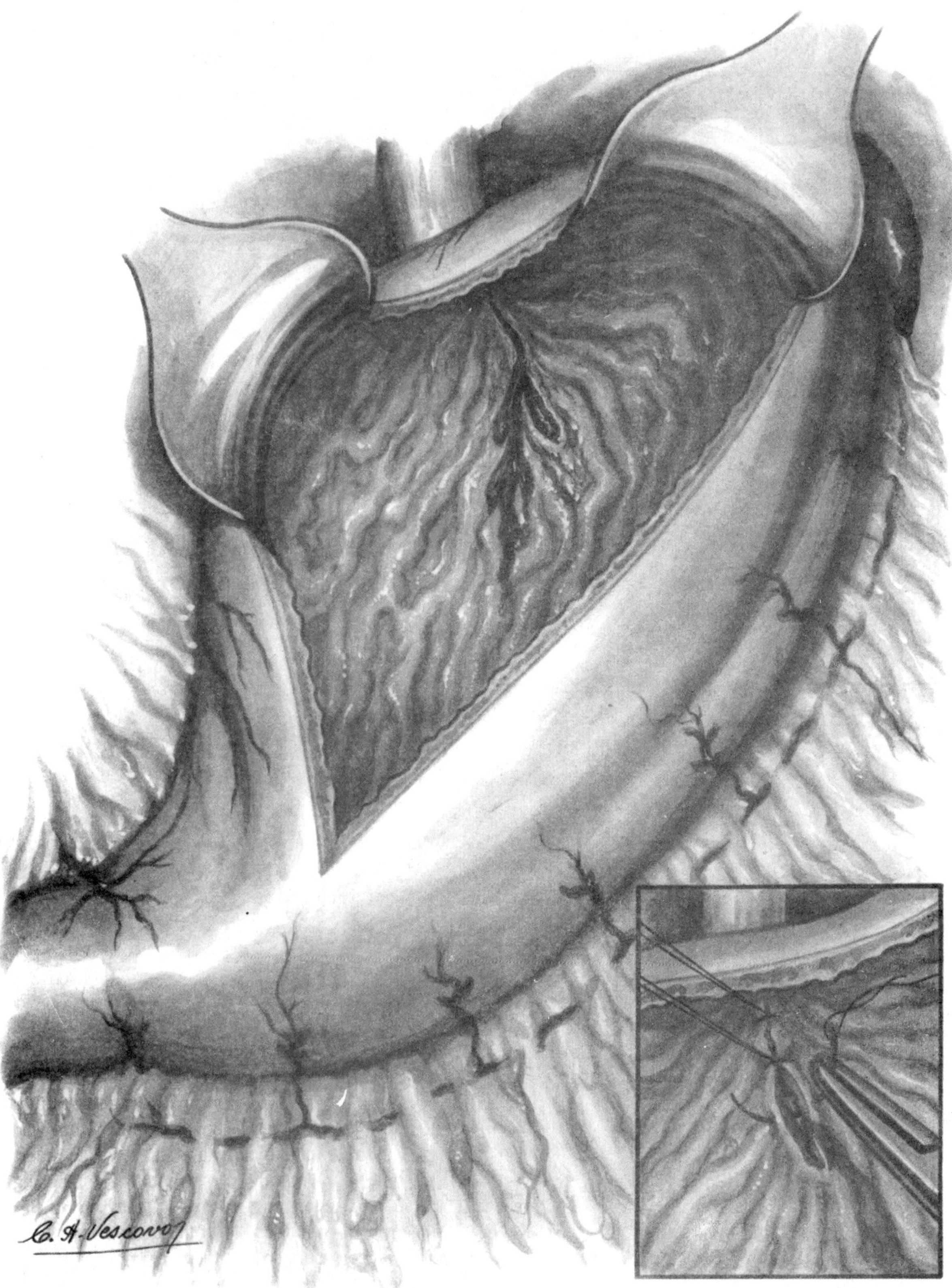

FIGURE 32.9

Surgical Technique

FIGURE 32.10
In some patients with surgical indications to operate for bleeding gastric ulcer, hemostasis can be attained by wedge resection of the area of the ulceration (12). Wedge resection, however, has very limited indications. If the bleeding ulcer is located on the lesser curvature, slightly above the incisura, wedge resection is feasible. If the ulcer is located more proximally, wedge resection is difficult or impossible to perform. If the ulcer is located below the incisura, wedge resection is contraindicated because this technique would transect the nerves of Latarjet. Once the wedge is resected the defect is sutured, as shown in the drawing.

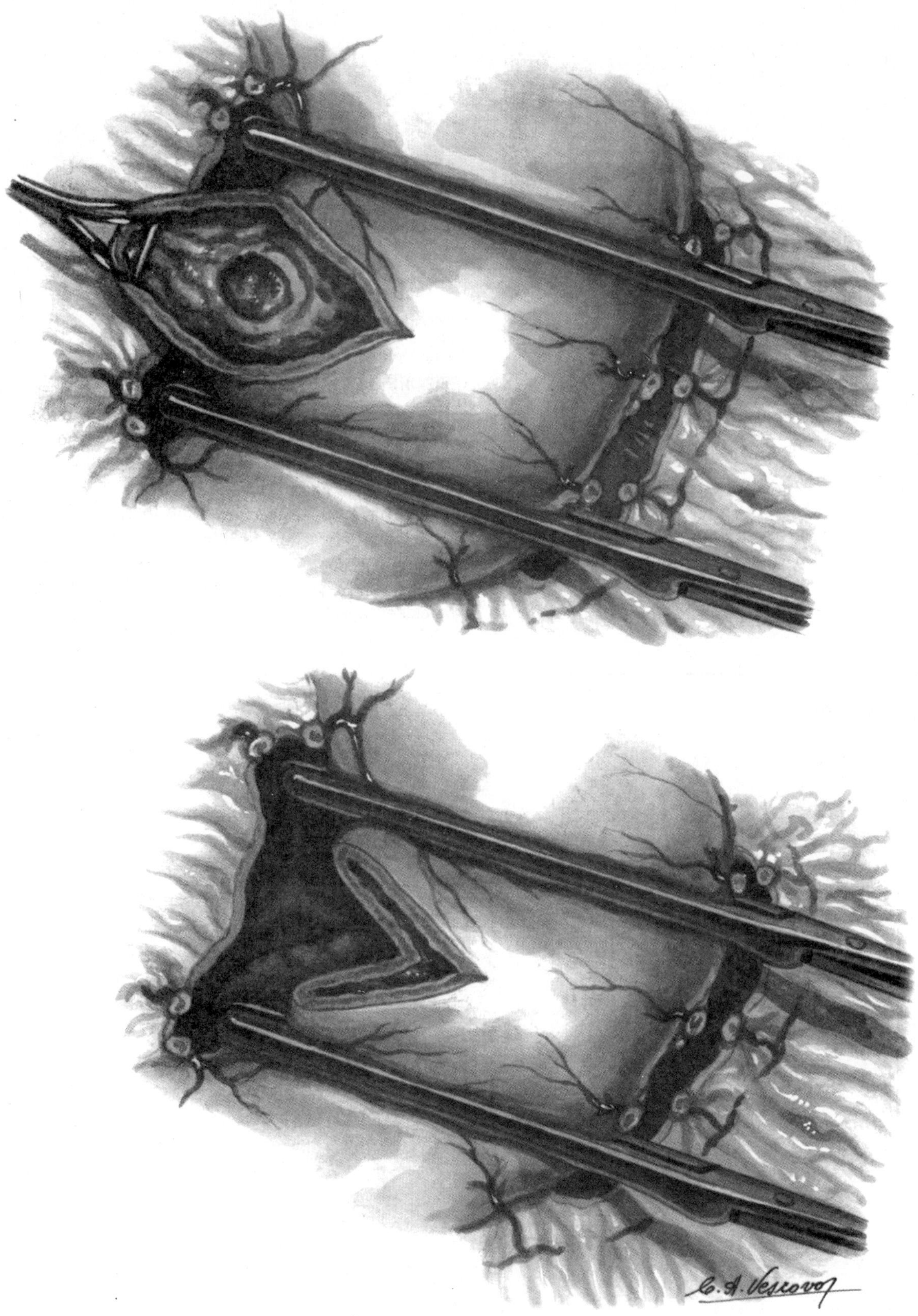

FIGURE 32.10

FIGURE 32.11
Hemorrhagic duodenal ulcer. Bleeding from duodenal ulcers penetrating into the pancreas is frequently associated with the gastroduodenal arterial complex, as described by Berne and Rosoff (1). To carry out hemostasis, a suture has been placed in the base of the ulcer to ligate the gastroduodenal artery above the perforation, another one below the arterial perforation, and a third suture laterally to ligate the transverse pancreatic artery. Once hemostasis is attained, the duodenotomy is closed with two layers of interrupted sutures.

Surgical Technique

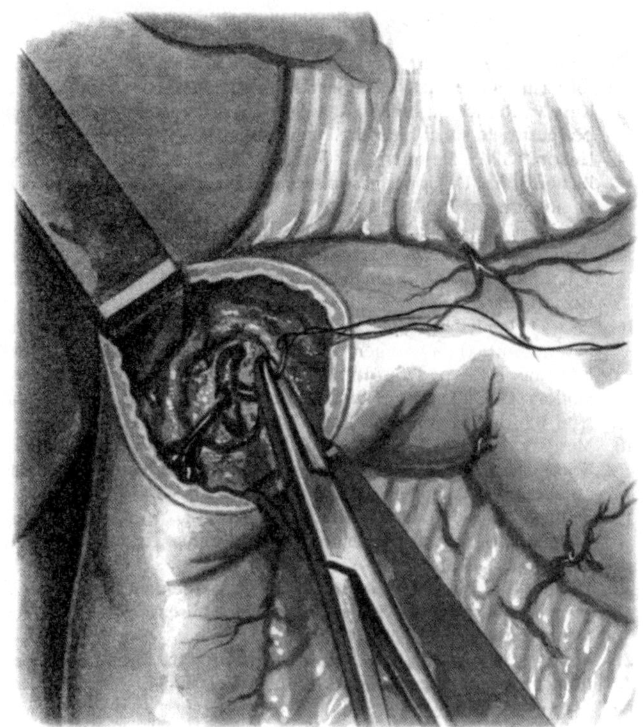

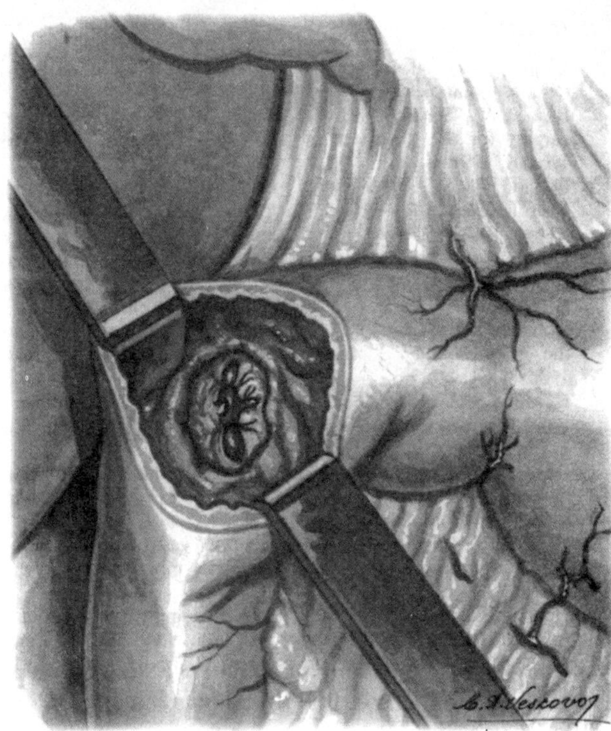

FIGURE 32.11

References

1. Berne, C.J., Rosoff, L. Peptic ulcer perforation of the gastroduodenal artery complex. Ann. Surg. 169:141, 1969.
2. Bliss, D.W., Stabile, B.E. The impact of ulcerogenic drugs on surgery for the treatment of peptic ulcer disease. Arch. Surg. 126:609, 1991.
3. Borland, J.L. Sr., Handcock, W., Borland, J.L. Jr. Recurrent upper gastrointestinal hemorrhage in peptic ulcer. Gastroenterology 52:631, 1967.
4. Donahue, P.E., Nyhus, L.M. Massive upper gastrointestinal hemorrhage. In Nyhus, L.M., Wastell, M.S. (Eds.) Surgery of the stomach and duodenum. Ed. 3, p. 405. Little, Brown, Boston, 1977.
5. Donahue, P.E., Nyhus, L.M. Surgical excision of gastric ulcer near the gastroesophageal junction. Surg. Gynecol. Obstet. 155:85, 1982.
6. Elerding, S.C., Moore, E.E., Wolz, J.R., Norton. I.W. Outcome of operations for upper gastrointestinal tract bleeding. Arch. Surg. 115:1473, 1980.
7. Fromm, D. Ulceration of the stomach and duodenum. In Fromm, D. (Ed.) Gastrointestinal surgery. Vol. I, p. 233. Churchill Livingstone, New York, 1985.
8. Himal, H.S., Perrault, C., Mzabi, R. Upper gastrointestinal hemorrhage. Aggressive management decreases mortality. Surgery 84: 448, 1978.
9. Hunt, P.S., Hansky, J., Korman, M.G. Bleeding carcinomatous ulcer of the stomach—a current review. Ann. Surg. 201:741, 1985.
10. Jones, F.A. Hematemesis and melena. Gastroenterology 30:166, 1956.
11. Jordan, P.H. Jr. Surgery for peptic ulcer disease. Curr. Probl. Surg. 28:267, 1991.
12. Jorgensen, S.J., Halse, C., Poulsen, P.E. Segmental gastric resection for gastric ulcer. Acta Chir. Scand. 140:635, 1974.
13. Kim, V., Rudick, J., Aufses, A.H. Surgical management of acute upper gastrointestinal bleeding. Ann. Surg. 199:44, 1984.
14. Larson, G.M., Schmidt, T., Gott, J., Bond, S., O'Connor, C.A., Richardson, J.D. Upper gastrointestinal bleeding predictors of outcome. Surgery 100:765, 1986.
15. Larson, G.M., Polk, H.C. Massive upper gastrointestinal hemorrhage. In Scott, H.W. Jr., Sawyers, J.L. (Eds.) Surgery of the stomach, duodenum and small intestine. Ed. 2, p. 552. Blackwell. Boston, 1992.
16. Law, D.H., McCarthy, D. Chronic duodenal ulcer. In Scott, H.W. Jr., Sawyers, J.L. (Eds.) Surgery of the stomach, duodenum and small intestine. Ed 2, p. 476. Blackwell, Boston, 1992.
17. Mallory, G.K., Weiss, S. Hemorrhage from the cardiac orifice of the stomach due to vomiting. Am. J. Med. Sci. 178:506, 1929.
18. Menguy, R., Gadacz, T., Zajtchuk, R. The surgical management of acute gastric mucosal bleeding, stress ulcer, acute erosive gastritis and acute hemorrhagic gastritis. Arch. Surg. 99:198, 1969.
19. Schiller, K.F.R., Traelove, S.C., Williams, G.D. Hematemesis and melena with special reference to factors influencing outcome. Br. Med. J. 2:7, 1970.
20. Sloane, R., Cohen, H. Common-sense management of *Helicobacter pylori* associated with gastroduodenal disease. Gastroenterol. Clin. North Am. 22:199, 1993.
21. Welch, C.E., Rodkey, G.V., von Gryska, P. One thousand operations for peptic ulcer disease. Ann. Surg. 204:454, 1986.

Section F

Surgery of the Stomach and Duodenum

CHAPTER 33

Perforated Gastroduodenal Ulcers

The first objective of the surgeon who treats a perforated gastroduodenal ulcer surgically is to save the patient's life. The second objective is to attain a definitive cure of the ulcer. If the general condition of the patient allows it, the surgeon can attain both objectives in one surgical act. Otherwise, definitive treatment of the ulcer will be performed in a second surgical procedure. The treatment of the perforation and definitive treatment of the ulcer can generally be carried out in relatively young patients with recent perforation, in which the peritonitis is more chemical than bacterial in nature. Patients with gastroduodenal perforated ulcer have a positive peritoneal bacterial culture in one-third of cases, even within 12 to 24 hours of perforation (2). In about 10% of cases septic postoperative complications will develop (4, 8). In making a decision the surgeon must consider, in addition to the past history, the patient's general stability, the degree of peritoneal contamination, the time since perforation, and the amount of fluid that has spilled into the peritoneal cavity. Mortality will depend more on the patient's condition than on the technique that is used.

The diagnosis of perforated gastric or duodenal ulcer is easy to make in 80% of cases because of the symptoms, the physical examination, and especially because of the finding of air below the right or both domes of the diaphragm in chest or abdominal X-rays. In the remaining 20% of cases, however, there is no subdiaphragmatic pneumoperitoneum and the diagnosis is made late (4, 5).

SURGICAL EXPLORATION

A nasogastric tube should be passed before transporting the patient to the operating room to aspirate all the gastric contents. The stomach should be completely empty when anesthesia is administered (3).

The best incision to treat perforation of gastric or duodenal ulcers is a xiphoumbilical incision. When the peritoneum is opened, fluid will rise to the surgical incision. The fluid is aspirated and samples taken for culture and sensitivity studies. Exploration is begun by separating the liver upward with a Harrington retractor, which allows visualization of the lesser curvature of the stomach and the duodenum. The perforated ulcer is usually easily seen, and frequently gastric fluid is seen coming out the perforation. The liquid coming out of a perforated duodenal ulcer is bile stained. In some patients the perforation is covered by other viscera and the opening in the perforated ulcer can only be seen after a detailed exploration separating the viscera over the ulcer. Treatment of the perforation is then carried out. The surgical procedures used to close perforated gastric or duodenal ulcers will be described later. Once the perforation is treated, all the accumulated fluid between the superior surface of the liver and the diaphragm, in the subhepatic space, between small bowel loops, in both left and right paracolic gutter spaces, behind the spleen, and in the pouch of Douglas is aspirated. Gauze compresses should not be used to remove fluid from the peritoneal surface because the peritoneum is injured by the gauze (3). Once all the fluid is aspirated, the peritoneal cavity is thoroughly irrigated with warm physiologic solution. It is not usually necessary to drain the abdominal cavity, except in case of purulent contents. The most efficient drainage is a Silastic tube in the bottom of the pouch of Douglas, brought out through a small suprapubic incision. If the peritoneal infection is massive, a subhepatic drainage tube is left in place and brought out through a small incision in the right upper quadrant. Once the operation is complete the abdominal wall is closed in layers. In highly contaminated cases it is not appropriate to close the subcutaneous layers and the skin in the same operative procedure, and close the skin 6 to 8 days later.

SURGICAL PROCEDURES

Treatment of perforated gastric or duodenal ulcers is essentially surgical. Nonsurgical treatment, proposed by Hermon Taylor (10), has very limited indications. The use of this therapy is in patients in very serious condition in which the surgical risk is very high. If this procedure is to be used, one should be sure that the perforation is sealed. This can be confirmed by instilling aqueous radiopaque material through the nasogastric tube. The perforation will be considered to be sealed if the radiopaque substance remains in the stomach without spilling into the peritoneum (1, 4).

PERFORATED GASTRIC ULCERS

The safest and most correct treatment of perforated gastric ulcer is gastric resection. One should not hesitate in performing this operation in patients in good general condition with minor or moderate contamination (1, 3, 4, 11). Gastrectomy is performed more frequently for gastric ulcers than for duodenal ulcers. In patients in poor general condition or with great peritoneal contamination, it is advisable to suture the perforation, adding an omentoplasty, once a frozen section examination of the ulcer proves it to be benign. Not all patients with perforated peptic ulcer can be subjected to simple closure of the perforation, be it because the perforation is large or because the tissue around the perforation is unable to hold the tension on the sutures, due to its fatlike consistency. This would make it impossible to close the perforation safely. In some patients who are not in condition to tolerate a gastric resection or suturing of the perforation, an extreme, possibly lifesaving procedure can be performed. It was proposed by Neumann (4, 7), and consists of placing a 16 F tube into the stomach through the perforation in the ulcer and bringing the tube out of the abdomen. Later, both the tube and the gastric opening are wrapped in greater omentum. The gastric wall around the perforation is sutured to the parietal peritoneum with interrupted sutures that are placed just outside of the omental wrapping. This means converting the opening of the perforation into a gastrostomy. If histologic examination of the ulcer done by frozen section on a biopsy proves the ulcer is malignant (6–15% of perforated gastric ulcers), a gastrectomy should be undertaken even though there will be greater contamination and even though the patient's condition is poor. If such a perforation is sutured, reperforation will frequently develop postoperatively. Even in cases in which frozen section evaluation of the biopsy of the ulcer has been reported negative and the ulcer simply closed, the patient should be carefully evaluated periodically by means of gastroscopy and biopsy due to the possibility that the frozen section study had given a false negative result.

PERFORATED DUODENAL ULCERS

The most efficient operation in the treatment of perforated duodenal ulcer is gastric resection. If this operation cannot be performed due to the poor general condition of the patient or because of severe contamination of the peritoneal cavity, the operation of choice should be closure of the perforation with omentoplasty. It has been shown that in 30 to 50% of patients treated this way the ulcer recurs, and that in some cases, the perforation recurs. It should be remembered, however, that 50 to 70% of patients treated by suturing of the perforation plus omentoplasty are definitively cured. At present, the percentage of cured patients should be higher due to the efficient action of existing antiulcer medications. Some surgeons add a truncal vagotomy or a proximal gastric vagotomy to the closure of the perforation and omentoplasty (4, 8, 9). In the former case a pyloroplasty, if possible, or a gastrojejunostomy is necessary. With a contaminated peritoneum there is danger of producing mediastinitis if a vagotomy is performed. For this reason, in cases in which a gastrectomy is indicated, the author prefers a 70% Billroth II gastrectomy over a hemigastrectomy with truncal vagotomy, to prevent possible mediastinal contamination. Gastrectomy for perforated duodenal ulcer is usually easy to perform because duodenal ulcers are usually located on the anterior wall.

PERFORATED ANASTOMOTIC ULCERS

Perforated anastomotic ulcers should be treated by simple closure of the perforation. Definitive surgical treatment should be carried out in a second stage if medical therapy fails.

Surgical Technique

FIGURE 33.1
Perforated gastric ulcer of the middle third of the lesser curvature. Frozen section biopsy proved it to be benign. Closure of the perforation with omentoplasty is chosen as the procedure of choice because of the poor general condition of the patient. Cotton, silk, or nonabsorbable synthetic suture material can be used.

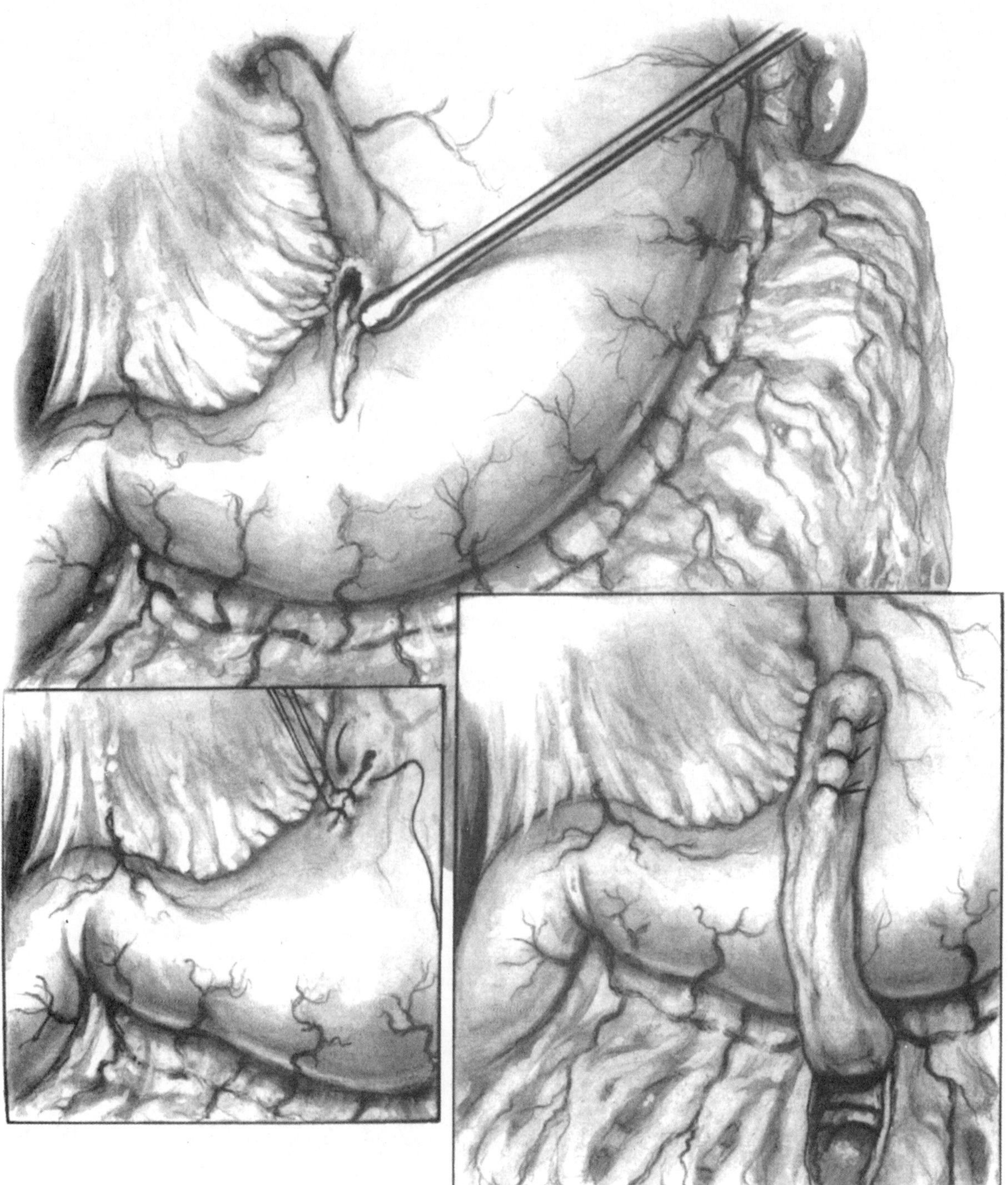

FIGURE 33.1

FIGURE 33.2
Perforated duodenal ulcer. The perforation is closed and an omentoplasty done with nonabsorbable sutures, as seen in the drawing.

Surgical Technique

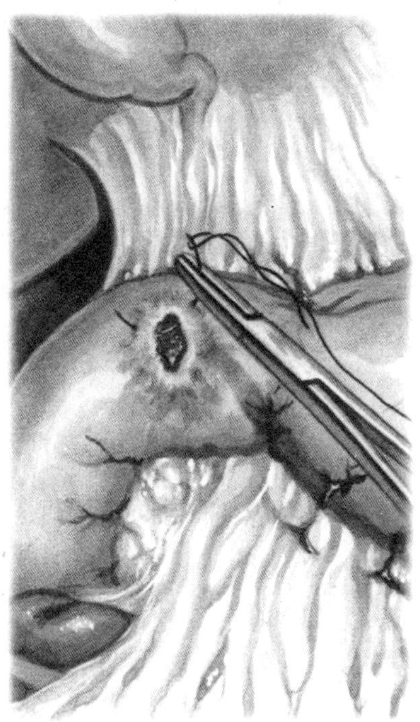
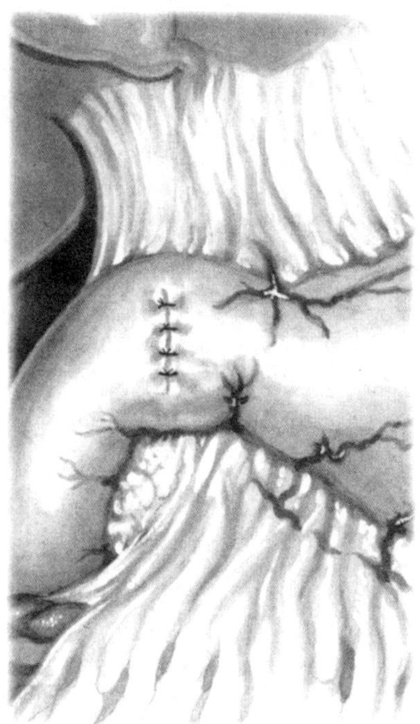
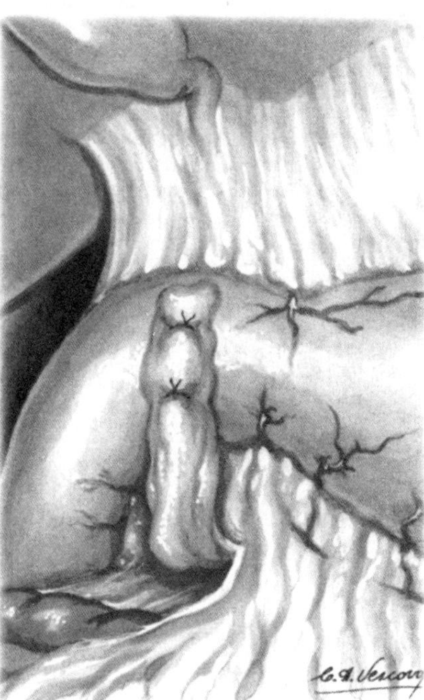

FIGURE 33.2

References

1. Berne, C.J., Rosoff, L. Acute perforation of peptic ulcer. In Nyhus, L.M., Wastell, C. (Eds.) Surgery of the stomach and duodenum. Ed. 3, p. 449. Little, Brown, Boston, 1977.
2. Boey, J., Wong, J., Ong, G.B. Bacteria and septic complications in patients with perforated duodenal ulcers. Am. J. Surg. 143:635, 1982.
3. Chalstry, J. Acute perforated peptic ulcers. In Maingot, R. (Ed.) Abdominal operations. Ed. 7, vol. 1, p. 431. Appleton Century Crofts, New York, 1980.
4. Fromm, D. Ulceration of the stomach and duodenum. In Fromm, D. (Ed.) Gastrointestinal surgery. Vol. 1, p. 233. Churchill Livingstone, New York, 1985.
5. Griffin, G.E., Organ, C.H., Jr. The natural history of the perforated duodenal ulcer treated by suture plication. Ann. Surg. 183:382, 1976.
6. Judd, E.S., Nagel, G.W. Excisions of ulcer of the duodenum. Surg. Gynecol. Obstet. 45:17, 1927.
7. Kirschner, M., Guleke, N., Zenker, R. Allgemeine und spezielle chirurgische operationslehre. Ed. 2, p. 320. Springer-Verlag, Berlin, 1954.
8. Playforth, M.J., McMahon, M.J. The indication for simple closure of perforated duodenal ulcer. Br. J. Surg. 65:699, 1978.
9. Sawyers, J.L., Harrington, J.L. Jr. Perforated duodenal ulcer managed by proximal gastric vagotomy and suture plication. Ann. Surg. 185:656, 1977.
10. Taylor, H. The non surgical treatment of perforated peptic ulcer. Gastroenterology 33:353, 1957.
11. Welch, C.E., Rodkey, G.V., von Gryska, P. One thousand operations for peptic ulcer disease. Ann. Surg. 204:454, 1986.

Section F

Surgery of the Stomach and Duodenum

CHAPTER 34

Complications of Gastric Surgery

ANASTOMOTIC AND RECURRENT PEPTIC ULCERS

Anastomotic peptic ulcers are a complication of gastrointestinal anastomoses. The basic cause of this complication is duodenal ulcer and its operation. It is rare that a gastric peptic ulcer or neoplasm is complicated by an anastomotic ulcer. This complication is more serious and more dangerous than the duodenal ulcer that originated it. The morbidity and mortality that repair of this complication carries has to be added to the risk. No operation for duodenal ulcer that involves a gastrointestinal anastomosis is free of this complication, except total gastrectomy.

Medical literature contains a variety of names, which are considered synonymous, to designate ulcers that occur as a consequence of gastric operations. Some of these are jejunal ulcers, marginal ulcers, anastomotic ulcers, secondary peptic ulcers, postoperative ulcers, recurring or recurrent ulcers, stomal ulcers, gastrojejunal ulcers, etc (19, 20, 22, 24, 27, 29, 32, 40, 44). This variety of names undoubtedly gives rise to confusion, and it is necessary to point out that anastomotic ulcers cannot be considered to be the same as recurrent or recurring ulcers. Anastomotic ulcers are, as their name indicates, a complication of a gastrointestinal anastomosis. The term denotes a new ulcer, one that did not exist before surgery. Therefore, these ulcers cannot be designated as recurrent ulcers. Recurrent ulcers are generally duodenal ulcers that were not resected, only treated with truncal vagotomy and pyloroplasty or by proximal gastric vagotomy. A duodenal ulcer can heal after surgery and, after a variable period of time, become active again. It is then logical to refer to it as a recurrent ulcer.

To make the nomenclature simpler, it is convenient to divide these ulcers into two groups:

1. Peptic anastomotic ulcers that develop as a consequence of a gastrojejunal or gastroduodenal anastomosis or in an interposed segment of jejunum as in

the Henley operation or in an interposition of a segment of colon as in the Moroney operation (32).

2. Recurrent peptic ulcers in cases in which a duodenal ulcer becomes active again, after having healed, in spite of the previously performed truncal vagotomy or proximal gastric vagotomy.

Some authors (29) use the term "postoperative recurrent ulcers," meaning that what recurs is the ulcerative illness, an assertion that is inexact.

In the evolution of the surgical treatment of duodenal ulcers, one can appreciate the great preoccupation that surgeons have shown in trying to prevent anastomotic ulcers and, in recent years, trying to prevent recurrent duodenal ulcers by increasing the use of vagotomy (32).

Gastrojejunostomy was used for many years in surgical treatment of duodenal ulcer. As time passed, it was shown that this operation resulted in a high incidence of anastomotic ulcers, some 35 to 50% of cases (4, 14, 19, 22, 23, 44). It was later shown that gastric resection was more efficacious in the treatment of ulcers, both duodenal and gastric, since it led to a much lower incidence of postoperative anastomotic ulcers. Resections of 65 to 75% of the stomach led to the lowest incidence of anastomotic ulcers, and lesser resections for duodenal ulcer were associated with higher incidence of anastomotic ulcers. This fact stimulated surgeons to use extensive gastric resections to prevent anastomotic ulcers. It was later proven that the Billroth I gastrectomy for duodenal ulcers led to a greater incidence of anastomotic ulcers than the Billroth II (6, 11, 15, 39, 40, 43), which led to the tendency to perform Billroth II anastomoses with a 70% gastrectomy for duodenal ulcers. It was later shown that, if a truncal vagotomy was done, it was not necessary to resect 70% of the stomach, and that a 50% resection of the distal stomach was sufficient to diminish the incidence of postoperative anastomotic ulcers. This technique, known as antrectomy or by its synonym, hemigastrectomy, is based on resection of the entire antral mucosa and part of the fundic glands with an added truncal vagotomy (7, 8, 14, 15, 17, 19, 35, 37, 42, 44).

Hemigastrectomy with vagotomy for duodenal ulcer reduces the frequency of anastomotic ulcers to a minimum, 1 to 2%, if the gastrointestinal transit is reestablished by either a Billroth II or a Billroth I technique. If a Billroth I procedure is performed, the possibility of an incomplete vagotomy has to be kept in mind, since it may favor development of anastomotic ulcers. For this reason, in duodenal ulcer, it is advisable to complement a hemigastrectomy and vagotomy with a Billroth II reconstruction and not a Billroth I (15, 42, 43).

As a result of Dragstedt's studies (7), duodenal ulcers began to be treated with truncal vagotomy with a drainage procedure. Originally the stomach was drained by means of a gastrojejunostomy, but later pyloroplasty was used to drain the stomach (41). Follow-up of these patients revealed frequent complication of the gastrojejunostomy by an anastomotic ulcer, but less frequently than without vagotomy. It was also shown that vagotomy with pyloroplasty frequently produced recurrence of the duodenal ulcer. Selective vagotomy (13) was proposed, and shortly thereafter it was replaced by proximal gastric vagotomy (14, 16, 19, 32, 43). As time passed, recurrent duodenal ulcer became more frequent leading to the conclusion that the best operation for duodenal ulcer is 70% gastrectomy with a Billroth II anastomosis and occasionally a Billroth I or a hemigastrectomy with truncal vagotomy (8, 12, 14, 15, 18, 19, 37).

In patients subjected to an exclusion resection using the Finsterer-Bancroft-Plenk technique (3, 9, 10, 33) for an unresectable or very risky duodenal ulcer, the entire antral mucosa should be removed and a truncal vagotomy added, to prevent anastomotic ulcer as much as possible.

A Braun jejunojejunostomy should not be performed because it favors the development of anastomotic ulcers by keeping the biliopancreatic secretions from bathing the gastrojejunal anastomosis (32). For the same reason a Roux-en-Y is not advisable.

In gastrectomies for duodenal ulcer, particularly if digestive transit is reconstructed by the Billroth I technique, the first portion of the duodenum should also be resected.

It has been said that a long afferent jejunal loop favors formation of anastomotic ulcers. Gastrectomy with an antecolic gastrojejunostomy, which is done relatively frequently, has not confirmed this presumption, however, if the gastrectomy is done correctly and with the necessary extent. In hemigastrectomy the truncal vagotomy should be as complete as possible.

LOCATION OF ANASTOMOTIC PEPTIC ULCERS

Anastomotic ulcers are preferentially located in the efferent jejunal loop up to several centimeters distal to the gastrojejunal anastomosis. Less frequently they are located on the anastomotic line with a preference for the jejunal side and still less frequently on the gastric side. Localization of anastomotic ulcers in the afferent loop is very infrequent because this segment is always bathed by alkaline biliopancreatic secretion. Anastomotic ulcers secondary to a gastric resection with a Billroth I anastomosis more frequently tend to occur on the gastric side of the gastroduodenal anastomosis. Less frequently, they are localized right on the anastomotic line, the duodenal side, or the duodenum itself (15, 29).

SURGICAL PROCEDURES IN THE TREATMENT OF ANASTOMOTIC PEPTIC ULCERS AND RECURRENT DUODENAL ULCERS

Surgical treatment of anastomotic ulcers and recurrent ulcers depends on the previous surgery, since a gastrojejunostomy is not the same as a proximal gastric vagotomy or a 70% gastrectomy. On the other hand, medical therapy should be used before advising surgical treatment because, with the use of H_2 blockers and proton pump inhibitors, it is sometimes possible to attain notable improvement in symptoms, and in some cases even a cure. It should be admitted, however, that recurrence is frequent, with the possibility of hemorrhage, perforation, obstruction or gastrojejunocolic fistula, if it is in a gastrojejunostomy. The best treatment for anastomotic peptic ulcers is surgical, even though reoperations are technically difficult and one can never be sure that another ulcer will not appear postoperatively. If at all possible, the surgeon must avoid the appearance of another ulcer. If an anastomotic ulcer develops in a gastrojejunostomy, it is better to perform a 70% gastrectomy with truncal vagotomy than a hemigastrectomy. Additionally, digestive transit should be reestablished using a Billroth II technique rather than a Billroth I.

TYPES OF OPERATIONS

The operation to be used to treat an anastomotic ulcer depends on the previously performed procedure.

Gastrojejunostomy Without Vagotomy

Surgical treatment will consist of truncal vagotomy that is as complete as possible, and a 70% gastrectomy with resection of the ulcerated anastomotic segment. Resection of 70% of the stomach is preferable over a hemigastrectomy, and reconstruction with a Billroth II procedure is preferred over the Billroth I.

Gastrojejunostomy with Vagotomy

The same procedure should be carried out as in the previous case with revision of the truncal vagotomy.

Vagotomy with Pyloroplasty

A 70% gastrectomy is preferred over a hemigastrectomy. A revision of the truncal vagotomy should be added to the Billroth II reconstruction.

Patients with Proximal Gastric Vagotomy With or Without Pyloroplasty

Surgery should consist of a 70% gastrectomy with Billroth II anastomosis plus a subphrenic truncal vagotomy. If there are many esophagocardiac adhesions due to the previous vagotomy that prevent an adequate truncal vagotomy from being carried out subdiaphragmatically, a supradiaphragmatic approach should be used to perform the truncal vagotomy.

Gastrectomy of Insufficient Extent or Incorrect Technique

In these cases a more extensive gastrectomy with resection of the pathologic segment of jejunum and an added truncal vagotomy should be done. If a Billroth I technique has been used, it should be changed to a Billroth II.

Patient with a Correctly Performed 70% Gastrectomy with Billroth II Anastomosis and Truncal Vagotomy That Has Developed an Anastomotic Ulcer

In this case a supradiaphragmatic truncal vagotomy should be done.

Patient with a Gastrectomy and a Retained Excluded Antrum

The antrum should be resected with a more extensive gastrectomy, resection of the pathologic jejunal segment and a truncal vagotomy.

Pancreatic Gastrinoma with Anastomotic Ulcer (Zollinger-Ellison Syndrome)

A total gastrectomy with esophagojejunal reconstruction of the digestive tract and, if possible. a removal of the gastrinoma, should be carried out.

Gastrojejunocolic Fistula

This is a serious complication of anastomotic ulcer. During its evolution, the anastomotic ulcer perforates into the colon, producing a communication between the stomach, the jejunum, and the colon. Gastrojejunocolic fistulas develop mostly in patients with a posterior transmesocolic gastrojejunal anastomosis for duodenal ulcer.

A few years ago gastrojejunostomy without vagotomy was frequently performed to treat duodenal ulcers. Later, gastrectomy replaced gastrojejunostomy in the treatment of duodenal ulcers. This led to a much lower incidence of this complication, even though it occurs in gastrectomy with transmesocolic gastrojejunostomy. These fistulas rarely occur less than 2 years after gastrojejunal anastomosis, but can appear 20 to 30 years after surgery. These patients are seen by the surgeon in very debilitated condition due to their diarrhea, fecaloid smelling eructation, fecal vomiting, and severe electrolytic imbalance.

Deviation of the fecal stream by means of a proximal colostomy leads to improvement in the patient's condition. In 1939, Pfeiffer and Kent proposed diversion of the fecal stream at the level of the ascending colon prior to surgical resection (30). The ascending colostomy was later replaced by a transverse colostomy because the latter is easier to do and tolerated better. Lahey (20), in 1936, and later Marshall (25), in 1945, proposed deviation of the fecal stream by anastomosing the ileum to the descending colon before resection. In 1936, Pi-Figueras (31), proposed anastomosing the right colon to the left colon with the same objective in mind.

At present, gastrojejunocolic fistula is treated in one stage because patients are better prepared and there is better anesthesia and postoperative care, better preparation of the colon due to the action of antibiotics, and total parenteral nutrition.

Surgery for gastrojejunocolic fistula should include a truncal vagotomy or a revision vagotomy if one had been done during previous surgery. This should be carried out before the gastrojejunostomy is taken down, since the fistula creates a very septic atmosphere that could cause mediastinal contamination. Once the vagotomy has been done, a triple resection should be performed, as follows:

1. 70–80% gastrectomy,
2. resection of the affected jejunal segment, and
3. resection of the transverse colon and the affected mesocolon.

Gastrointestinal transit should then be reestablished by means of an antecolic gastrojejunal anastomosis, a jejunojejunostomy, and a colocolostomy (1, 2, 29, 34, 38).

OPERATIVE TECHNIQUE: ANASTOMOTIC PEPTIC ULCER IN A POSTERIOR TRANSMESOCOLIC GASTROJEJUNOSTOMY

The abdominal cavity is usually entered through the same incision used to perform the gastrojejunostomy, excising the scar. It is advisable to enter the abdomen by incising peritoneum in the lowest portion of the scar because there is less danger of injuring the abdominal viscera, which are frequently adherent to one another or to the parietal peritoneum. Once adhesions are freed, the stomach, the duodenum, and the gastrojejunal anastomosis are explored. Exploration of the duodenum will reveal if the duodenal ulcer for which the patient was subjected to a gastrojejunostomy is healed or active. If the latter is the case, its size, location, and degree of penetration into the pancreas must be determined to plan from the start the most appropriate technique to be used in the handling and closure of the duodenum. The gastrojejunostomy, which is generally a posterior transmesocolic one with a short jejunal loop, is then investigated, as is the anastomotic ulcer. To carry out this exploration, the transverse colon is raised upward with its mesocolon, revealing a tumoral swelling with fibrous tissue and surrounding swelling of the adjacent tissues. Also seen will be the swelling affecting the efferent jejunal loop, the gastrojejunal anastomosis, the stomach, the transverse mesocolon, and a great portion of the greater omentum, which is generally adherent to the inflammatory process. At this moment, the surgeon, if he did not have this information prior to surgery, must determine if a truncal vagotomy had been done in the original procedure to decide if he should perform a vagotomy or a revision vagotomy.

Once this detailed exploration is finalized, the gastrojejunostomy is taken down to carry out the resection of the stomach and the affected jejunal segment.

Operative Technique: Anastomotic Peptic Ulcer in a Posterior Transmesocolic Gastrojejunostomy

FIGURE 34.1
Schematic drawing of a posterior transmesocolic gastrojejunal anastomosis showing, in dark, the extent of the gastric resection. Also shown in dark is the extent of the jejunal segment to be removed, as well as the truncal vagotomy that must always be done with this operation (or a revision vagotomy if the vagotomy was done in the original operation).

Operative Technique: Anastomotic Peptic Ulcer in a Posterior Transmesocolic Gastrojejunostomy

FIGURE 34.2
The resection of the mesocolon has been started, using scissors to liberate the stomach as well as the jejunal loop and the anastomotic ulcer. To carry out this maneuver, the transverse colon and its mesocolon have been raised, exposing the anastomotic loop and the ulcer. The mesocolon is divided in an avascular zone around the gastrojejunal anastomosis. Special care must be taken during this stage of the operation not to injure the marginal arcade or the middle colic artery. If these vessels are not clearly seen, it is advisable to perform the incision of the mesocolon from left to right and very close to the anastomosis.

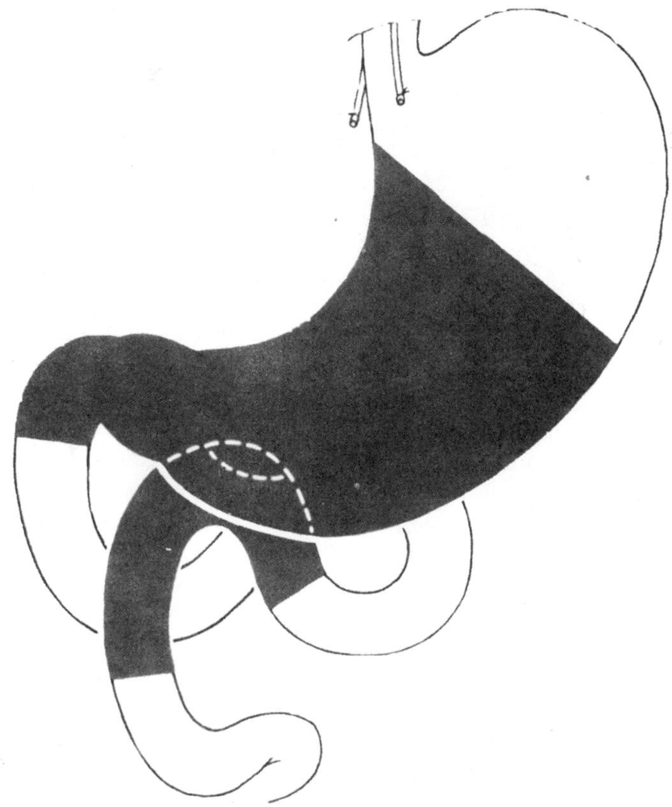

FIGURE 34.1

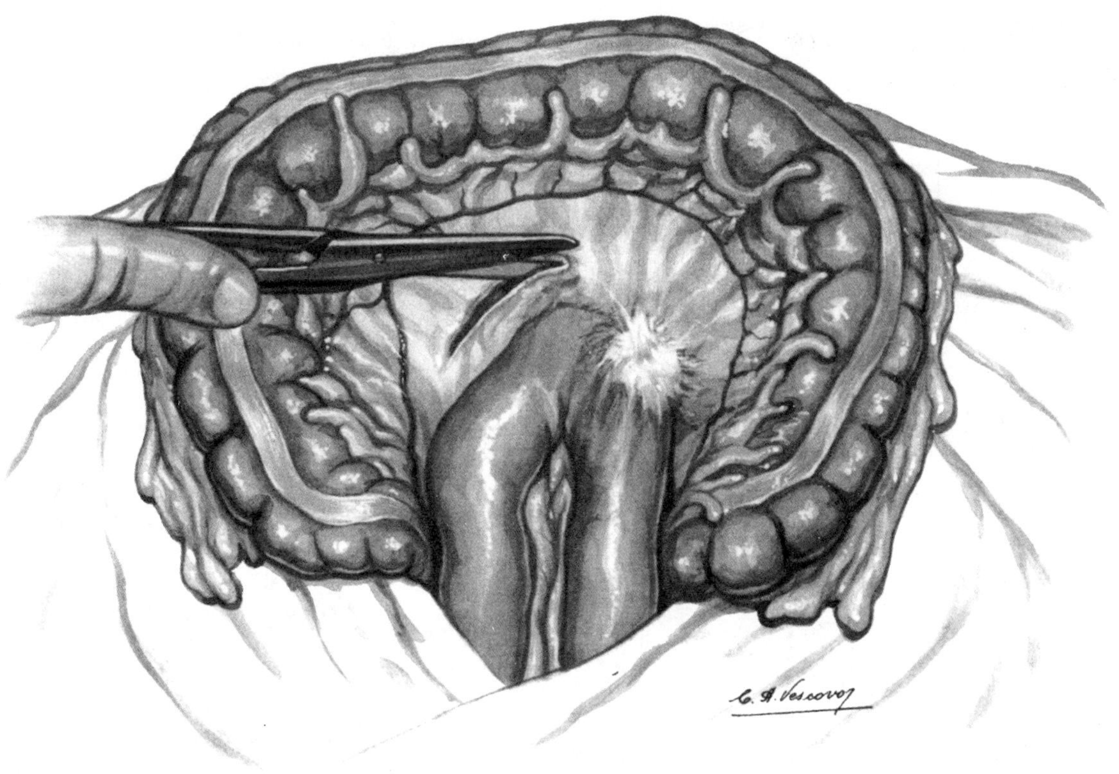

FIGURE 34.2

FIGURE 34.3
Once the mesocolon has been divided, one or two fingers are passed around the anastomosis to be sure it has been completely liberated.

Operative Technique: Anastomotic Peptic Ulcer in a Posterior Transmesocolic Gastrojejunostomy

FIGURE 34.4
Once the gastrojejunal anastomosis has been separated from the mesocolon, traction is applied to the stomach and the jejunal loop with Babcock clamps, to deliver the anastomosis into the supramesocolic compartment of the abdomen. The size of the anastomotic ulcer as well as the inflammatory reaction around it can be observed.

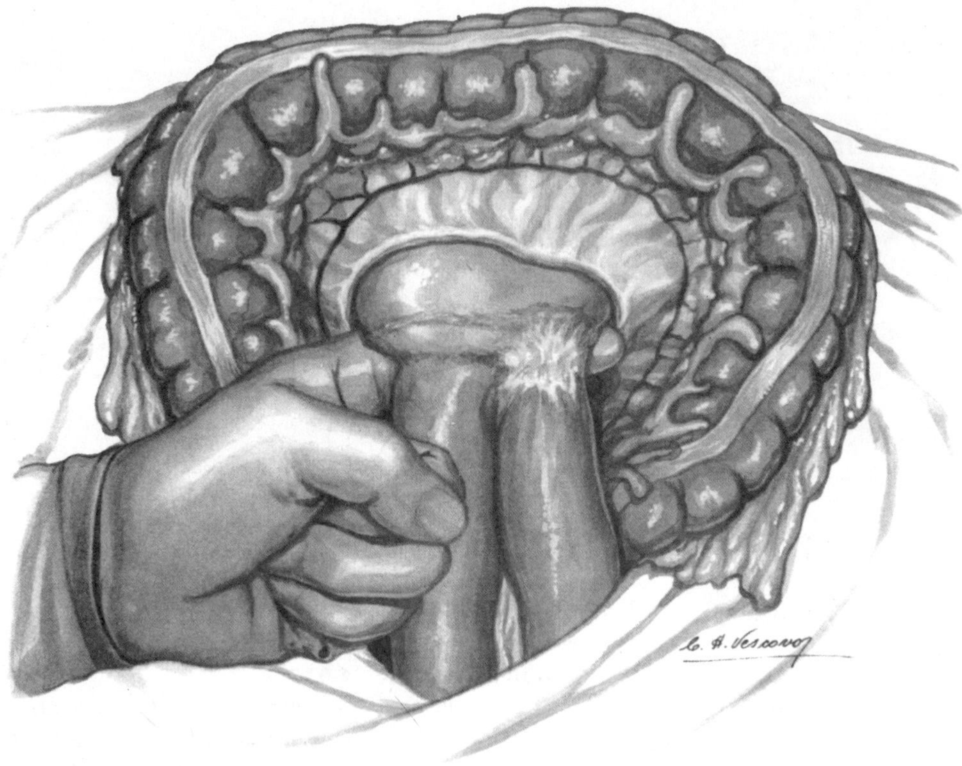

FIGURE 34.3

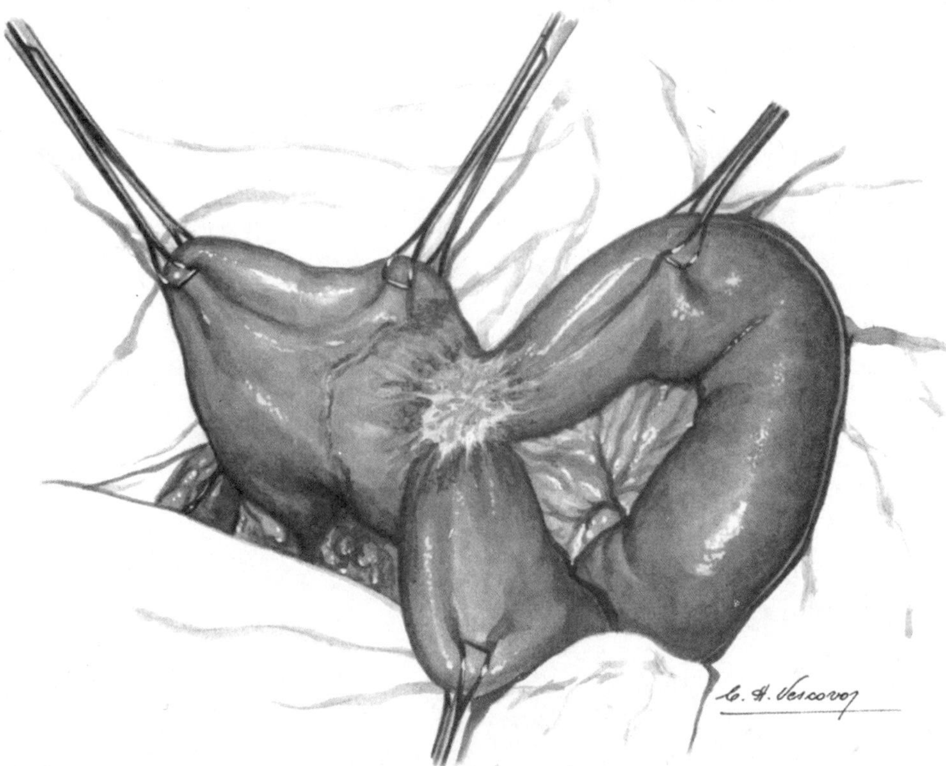

FIGURE 34.4

FIGURE 34.5
In order to facilitate later surgical maneuvers, the stomach and the anastomotic jejunal loop will be transected. One elastic clamp is placed across the stomach, and another is placed grasping both the afferent and the efferent jejunal limbs, to avoid spillage of gastrojejunal contents when the transections are carried out.

Operative Technique: Anastomotic Peptic Ulcer in a Posterior Transmesocolic Gastrojejunostomy

FIGURE 34.6
The stomach is being transected using straight Mayo scissors.

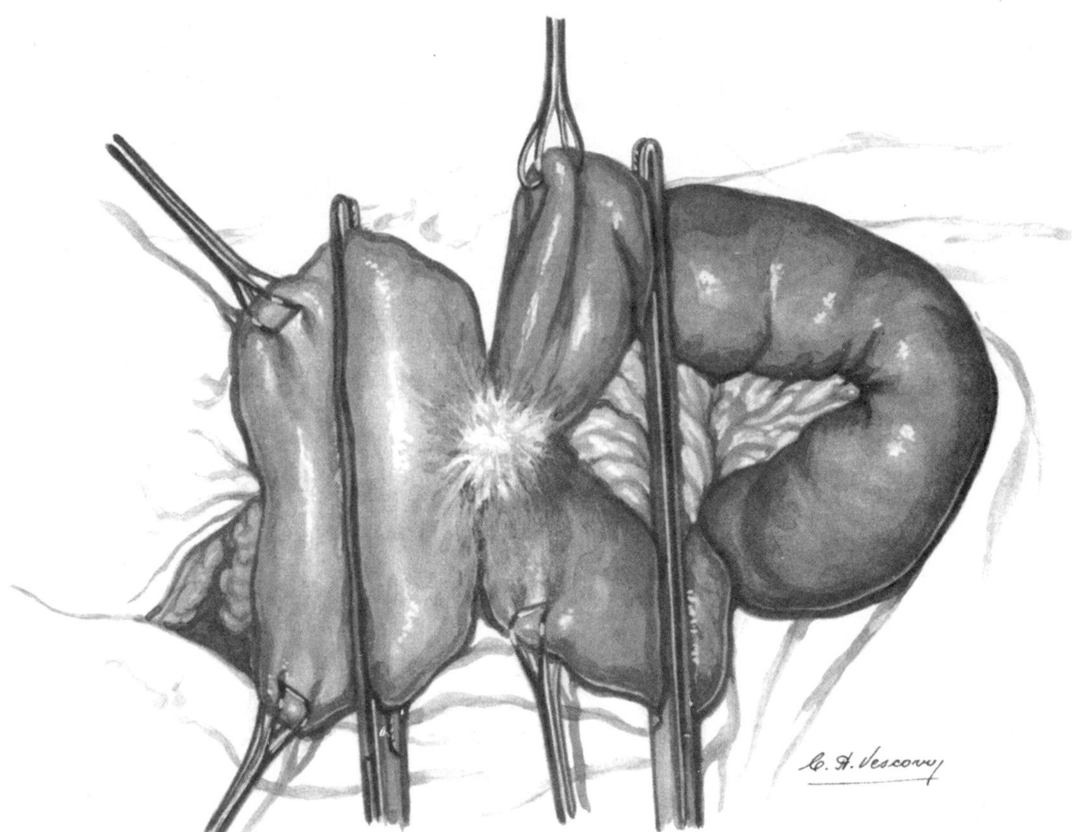

FIGURE 34.5

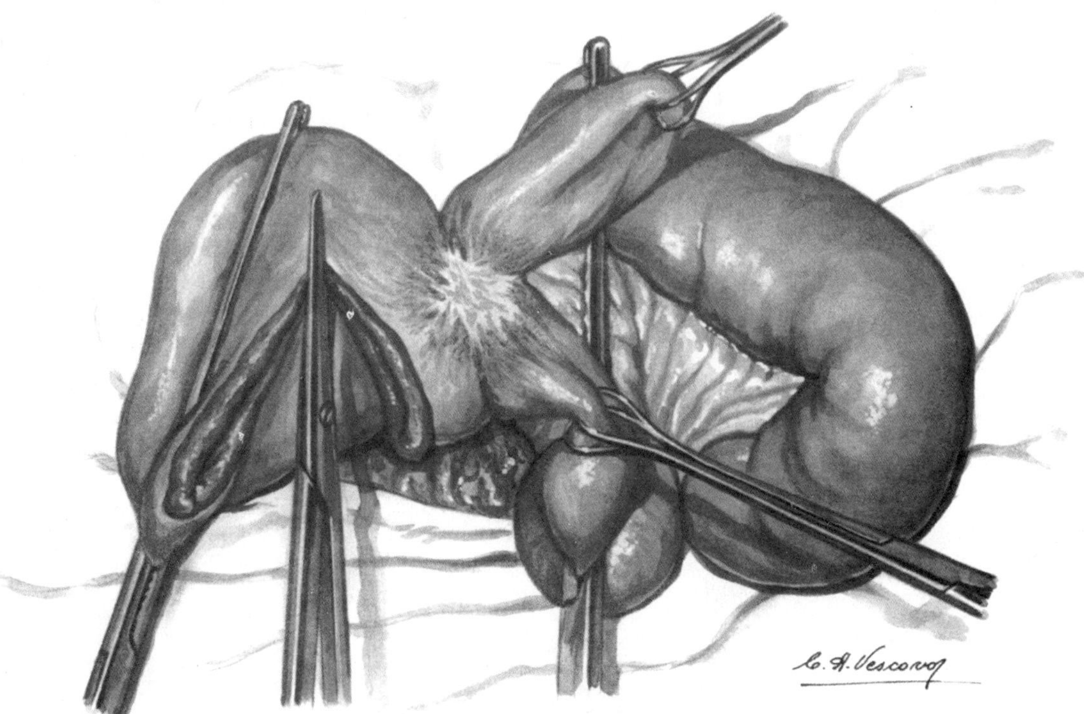

FIGURE 34.6

Operative Technique: Anastomotic Peptic Ulcer in a Posterior Transmesocolic Gastrojejunostomy

FIGURE 34.7
The transected stomach is being held upward with two Babcock clamps, and the afferent loop of jejunum is being transected. A broken line shows where the mesentery and the efferent loop will be transected. The transection of both jejunal loops should be through healthy tissues in order to be able to carry out a safe anastomosis of both ends of the jejunum. The line of transection of both the afferent and efferent limbs of the jejunum is some 6 to 8 cm from the gastrojejunal anastomosis. It should be remembered that if the afferent limb of the posterior gastrojejunostomy is too short it may lead to traction on the jejunojejunostomy, which could cause serious complications. To avoid this, it may be necessary to free the duodenojejunal angle and divide the ligament of Treitz to perform a safe anastomosis, without traction. This problem does not exist in patients with an antecolic gastrojejunostomy.

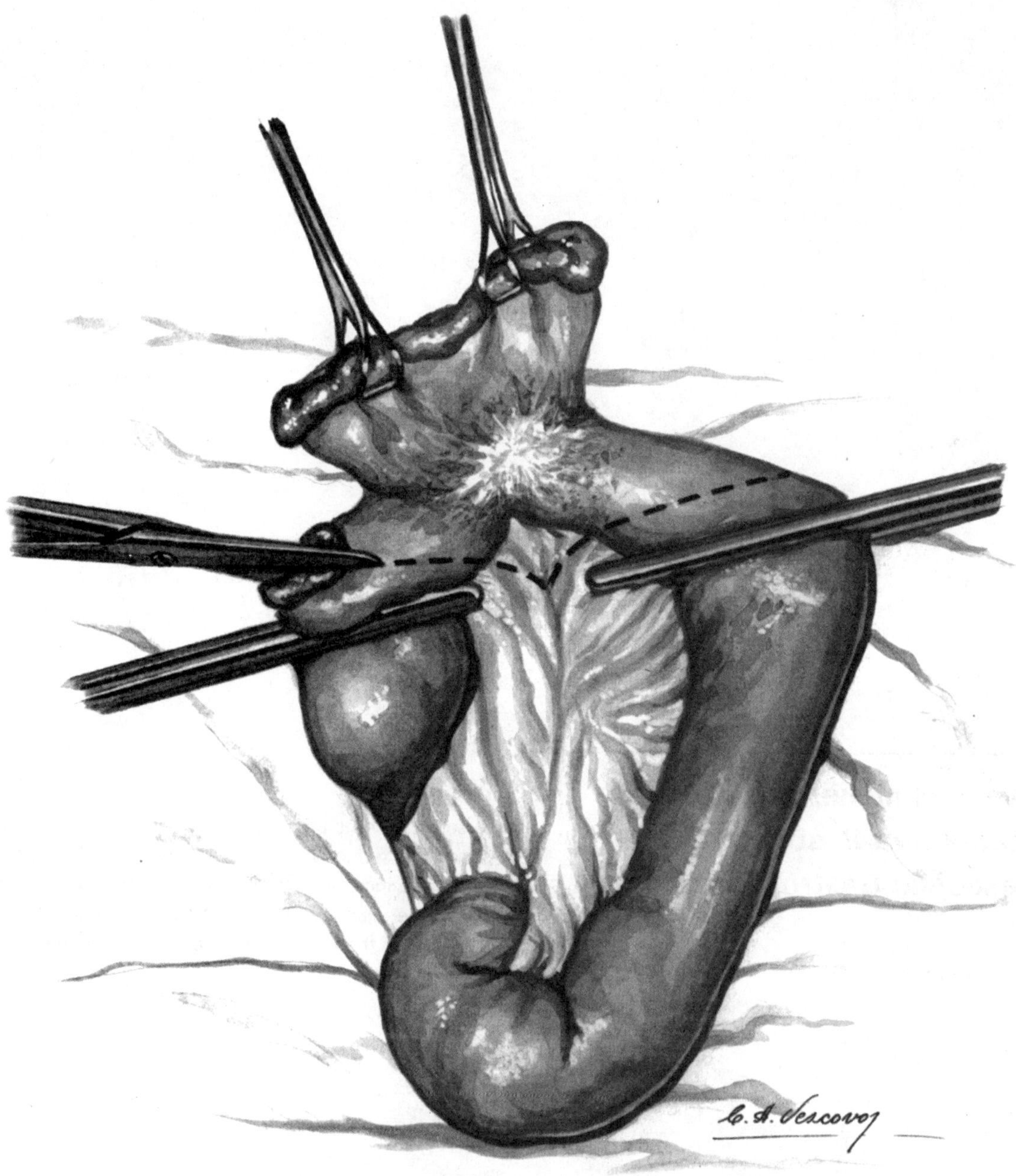

FIGURE 34.7

Operative Technique: Anastomotic Peptic Ulcer in a Posterior Transmesocolic Gastrojejunostomy

FIGURE 34.8

In some patients the caliber of the efferent jejunal loop may be somewhat reduced. In this situation it is advisable to carry out a Cheatle incision about 2 cm long at the antimesenteric border of the jejunum, cutting off the "dog ears" to increase the diameter of the jejunum and carry out an adequate anastomosis, as seen in the drawing.

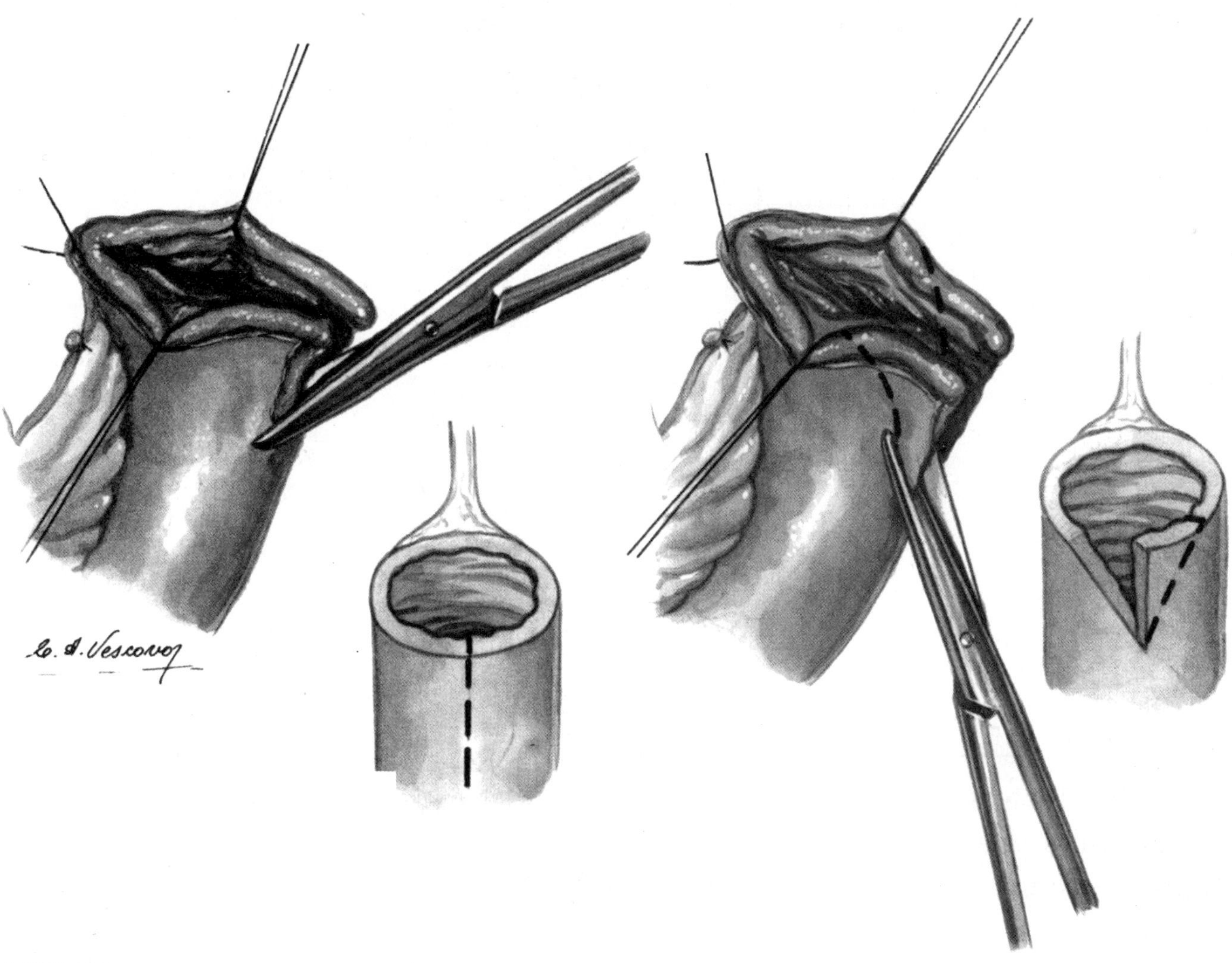

FIGURE 34.8

Operative Technique: Anastomotic Peptic Ulcer in a Posterior Transmesocolic Gastrojejunostomy

FIGURE 34.9

Both jejunal limbs are ready to be anastomosed in two layers of interrupted sutures. The mucosal layer is done with 2-0 chromic catgut and the seromuscular layer with cotton, silk, or other nonabsorbable synthetic suture. The jejunojejunostomy can be performed according to the surgeon's preference, in one or two layers of continuous sutures or with a stapler.

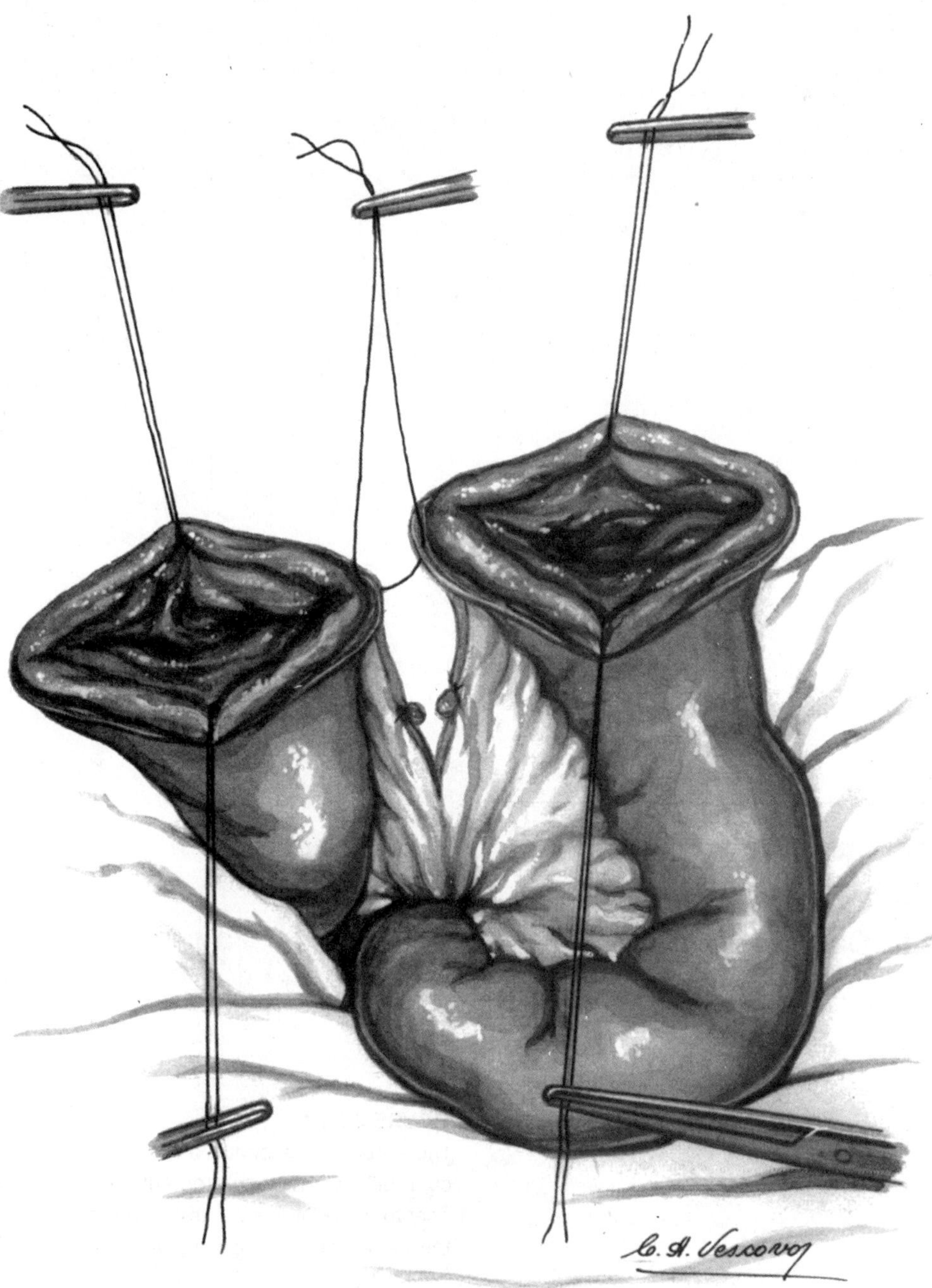

FIGURE 34.9

Operative Technique: Anastomotic Peptic Ulcer in a Posterior Transmesocolic Gastrojejunostomy

FIGURE 34.10
The surgeon has begun anastomosing the posterior seromuscular layer with interrupted sutures. It is advisable to start the anastomosis at the posterior or mesenteric side, since this is the more difficult and risky area.

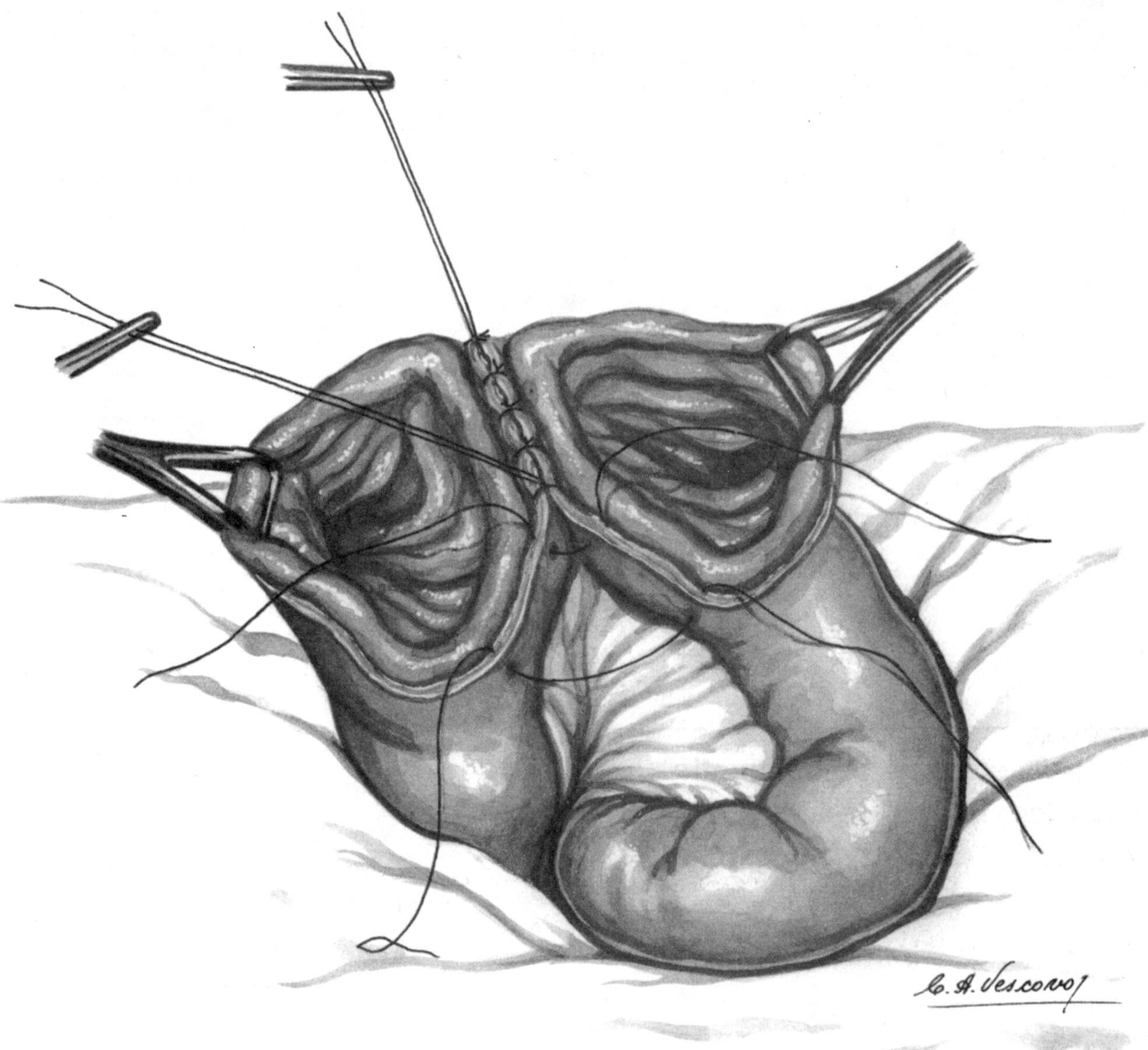

FIGURE 34.10

Operative Technique: Anastomotic Peptic Ulcer in a Posterior Transmesocolic Gastrojejunostomy

FIGURE 34.11
The posterior or mesenteric side has been completed, and the posterior mucosal plane is being sutured.

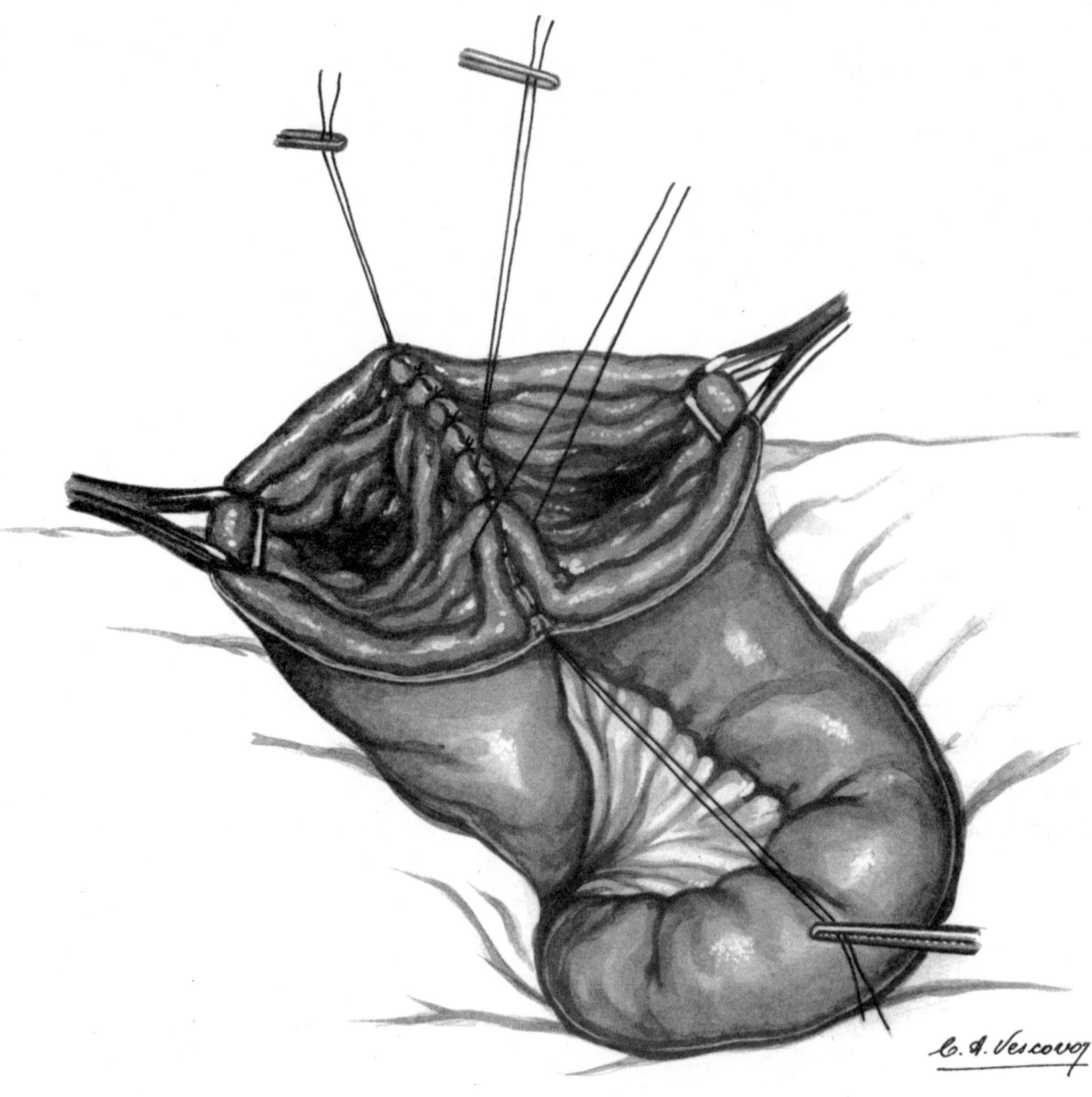

FIGURE 34.11

Operative Technique: Anastomotic Peptic Ulcer in a Posterior Transmesocolic Gastrojejunostomy

FIGURE 34.12
The anterior mucosal plane is being sutured with the knots inside the intestinal lumen.

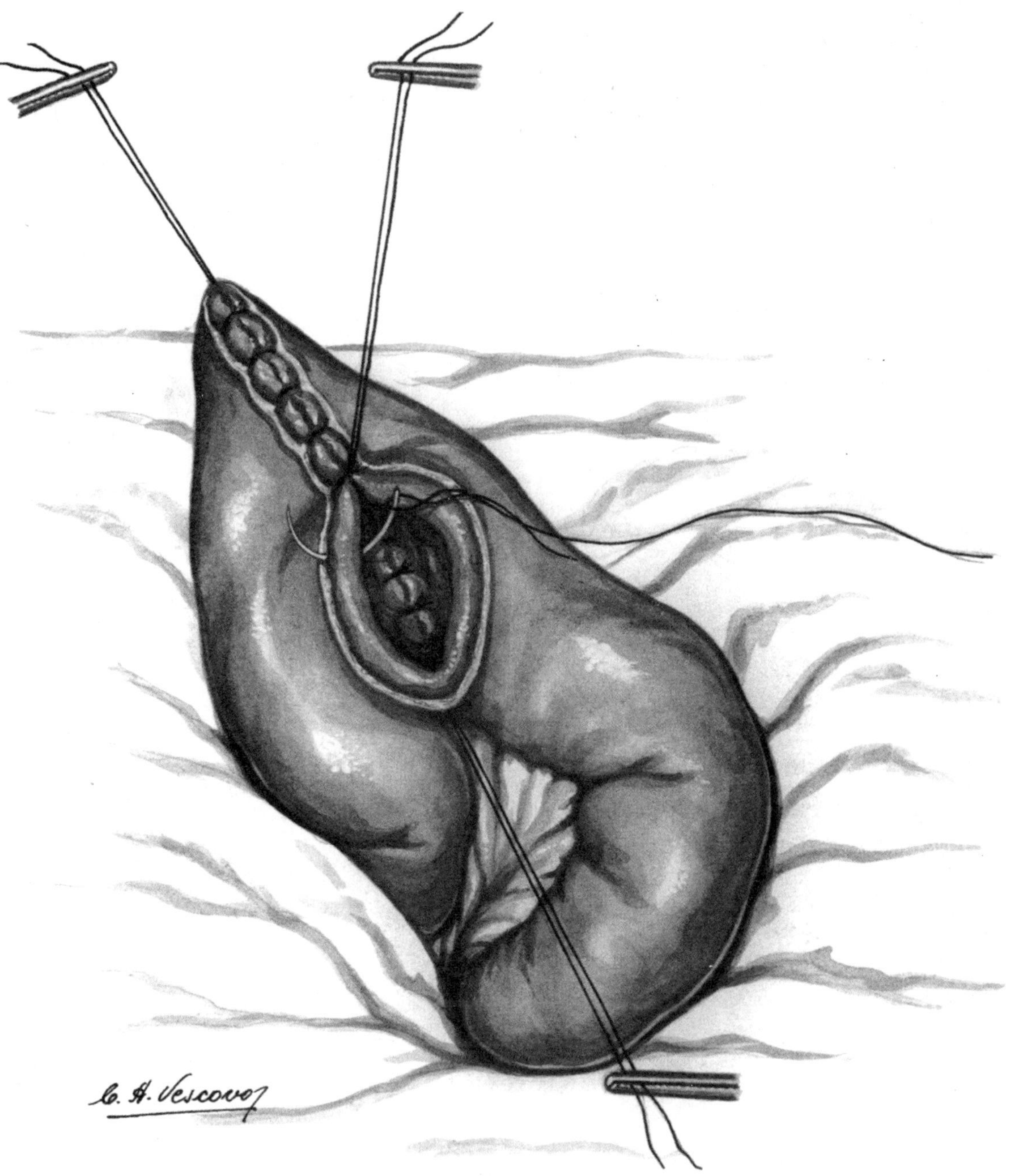

FIGURE 34.12

Operative Technique: Anastomotic Peptic Ulcer in a Posterior Transmesocolic Gastrojejunostomy

FIGURE 34.13
The jejunojejunal anastomosis is complete, with a safe and ample anastomosis.

FIGURE 34.14
The mesenteric defect is being closed with interrupted sutures. In closing the defect care must be taken to avoid damaging the blood supply to the sutured jejunal ends.

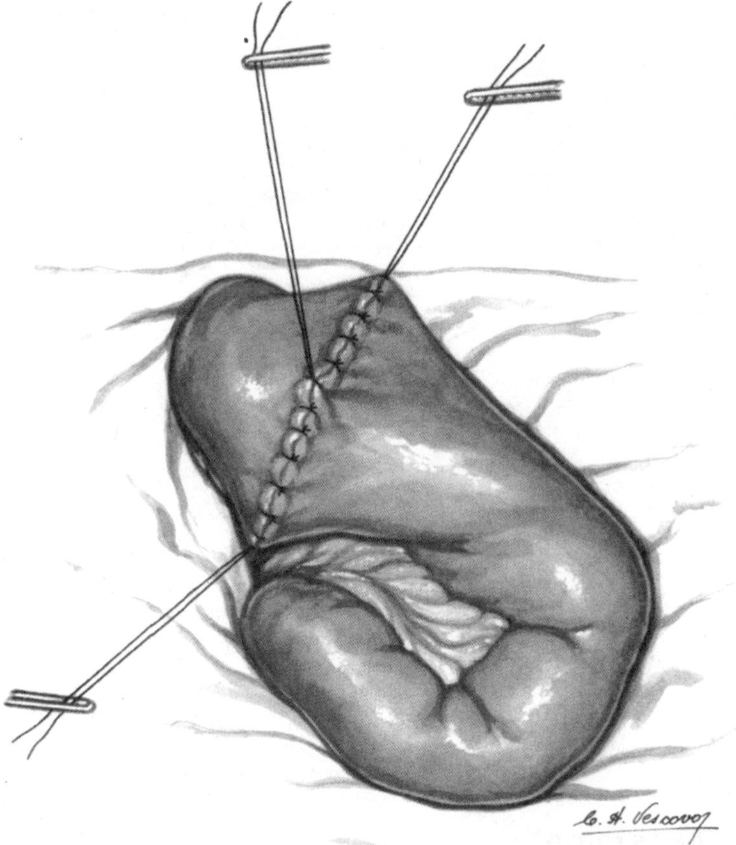

FIGURE 34.13

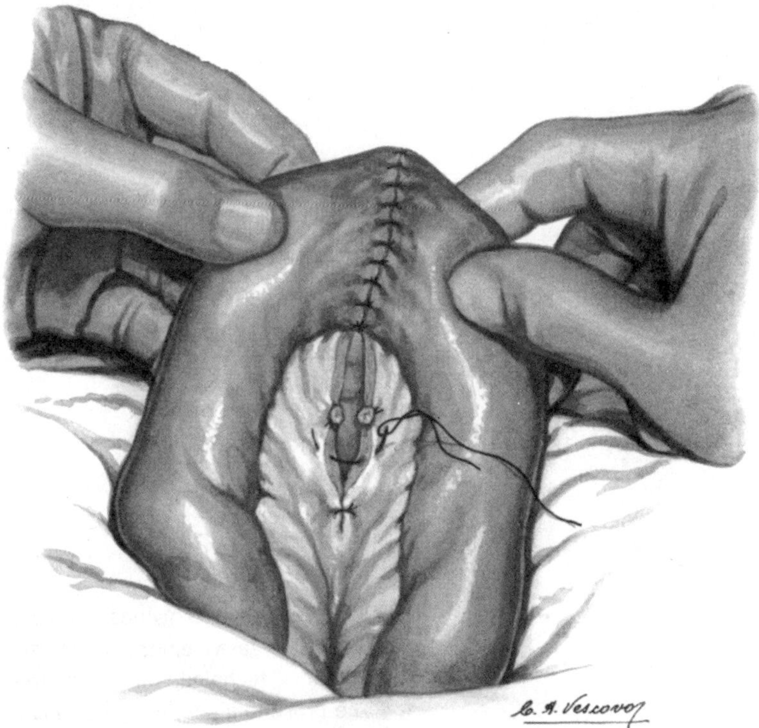

FIGURE 34.14

FIGURE 34.15
Once the jejunojejunostomy is completed, the colon and mesocolon are raised upward to close the defect in the mesocolon with interrupted sutures, as seen in the drawing. The techniques for the gastric resection and the gastrojejunostomy have been previously described.

Operative Technique: Anastomotic Peptic Ulcer in a Posterior Transmesocolic Gastrojejunostomy

FIGURE 34.16
The 70% gastrectomy has been completed with a truncal vagotomy. The gastrojejunostomy has been constructed using the Billroth II technique with a Hofmeister-Finsterer modification. The broken line outlines the functional portion of the gastrojejunostomy. The previously performed jejunojejunal sutures can be seen in the afferent loop. To the left, the duodenal stump can be seen, closed with two layers of sutures.

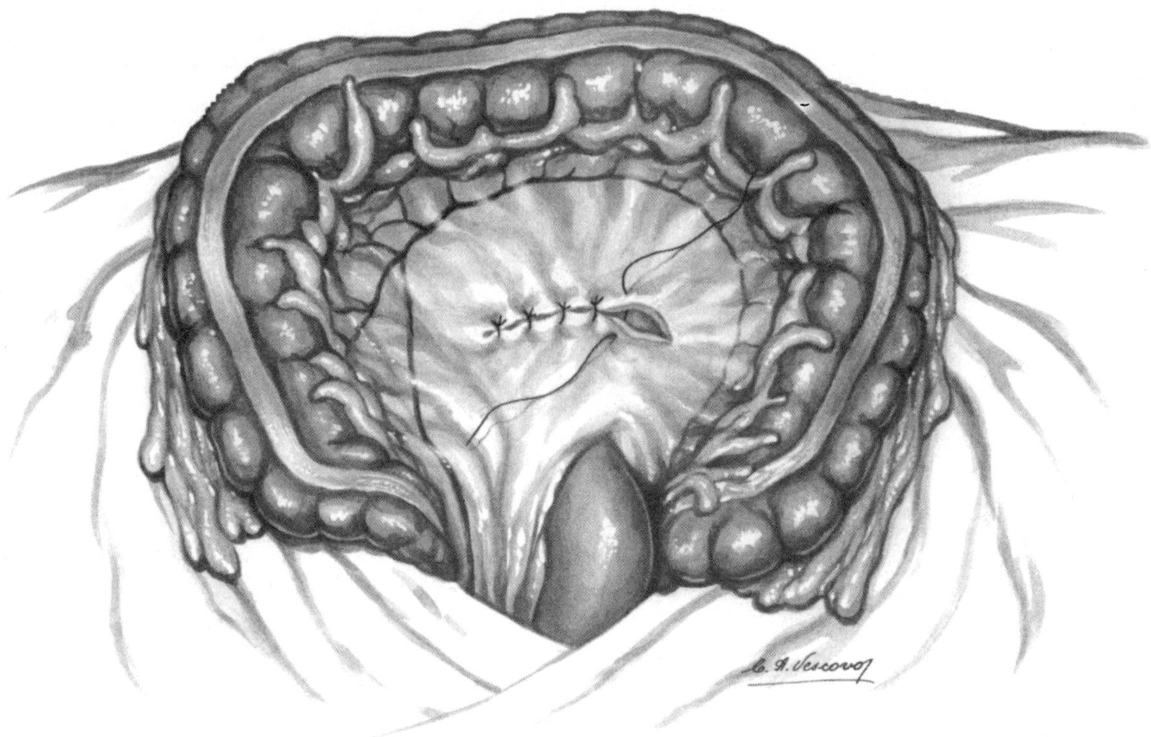

FIGURE 34.15

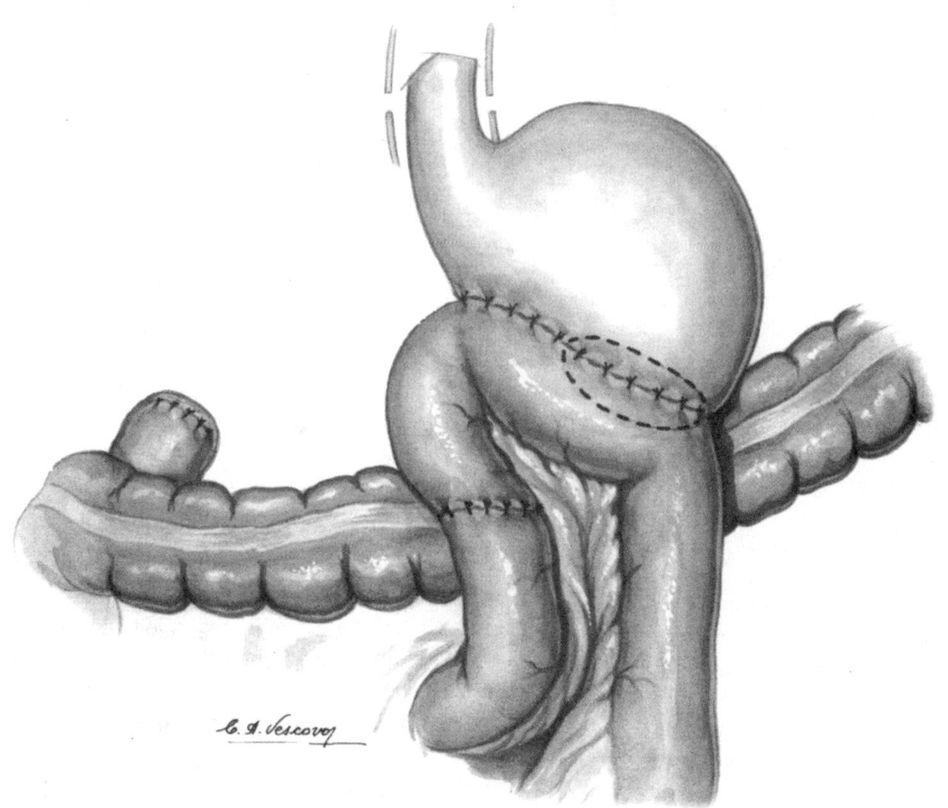

FIGURE 34.16

Gastrojejunocolic Fistula

FIGURE 34.17

The drawing shows a case of gastrojejunocolic fistula as a consequence of a postgastrojejunal anastomosis peptic ulcer. The transverse colon can be seen, densely adherent to the stomach and the efferent loop of jejunum. The fistula has produced deep retraction of the transverse mesocolon. The insert shows a schematic drawing of the communication between the stomach, jejunum, and colon produced by the anastomotic ulcer.

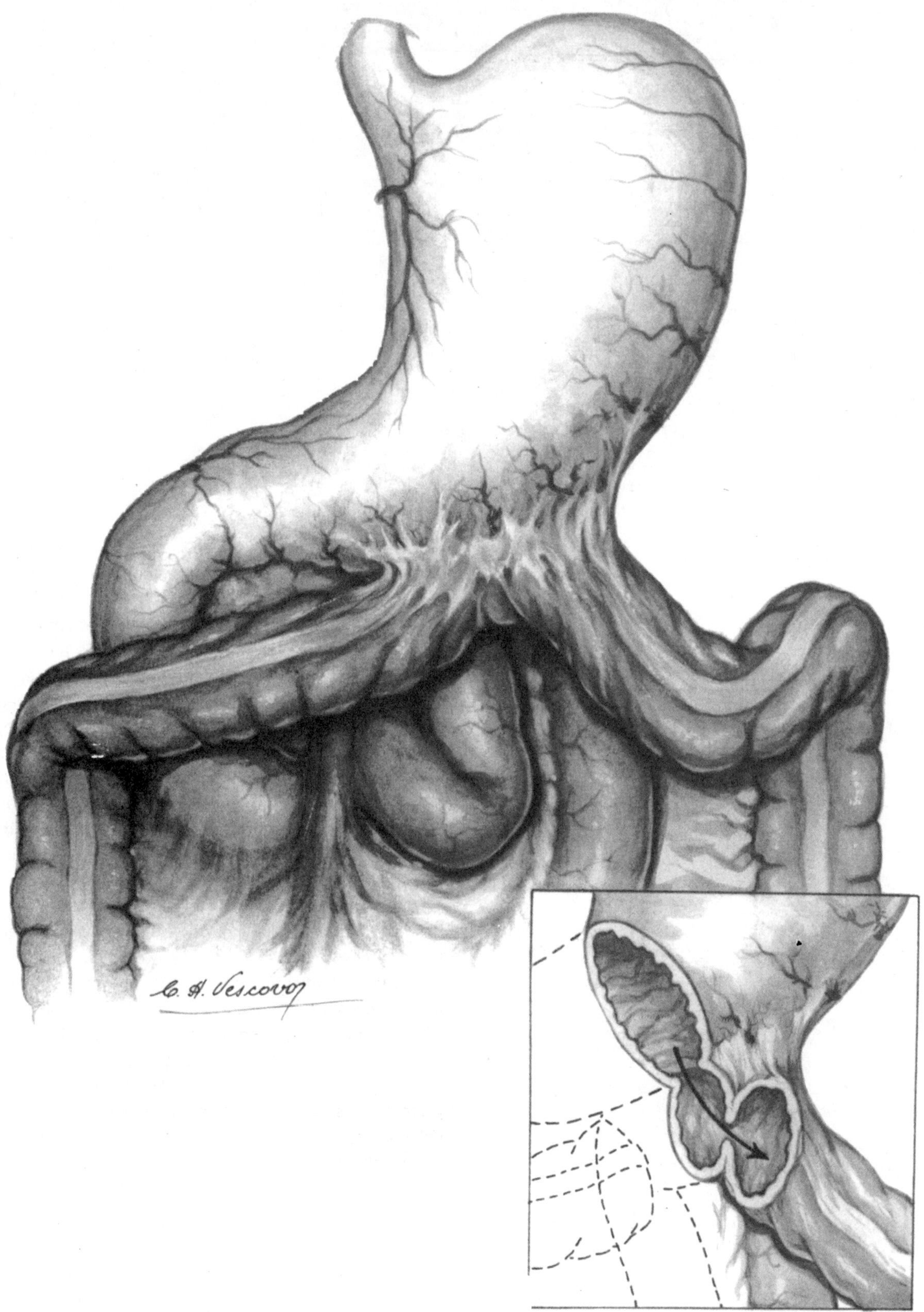

FIGURE 34.17

Gastrojejunocolic Fistula

FIGURE 34.18
Once the diagnosis of a gastrojejunocolic fistula has been made and the surgical treatment planned, the first maneuver to be performed is incision of the esophagodiaphragmatic peritoneal reflection to identify the vagus nerves and do a truncal vagotomy. The vagotomy should be done before beginning the contaminated portion of the operation during repair of the colon and jejunum from the stomach. This avoids septic contamination of the mediastinum. Once the vagotomy has been performed, the transverse colon is separated from the jejunum, to which it is communicated through the fistula. A line illustrates where the stomach and duodenum should be transected to carry out an 80% gastrectomy. A broken line shows where the stomach should be transected if a 70% gastrectomy is to be done. The extent of the jejunal segment to be resected is shown with two solid lines. The segment of transverse colon to be removed is also shown by two lines. In some patients with a limited inflammatory process due to the fistula, it may not be necessary to resect a segment of jejunum or colon because it may be sufficient to remove the affected area and suture the perforation transversely so as not to produce stricturing of the jejunum or the transverse colon (14). It is usually preferable to resect a segment of jejunum and transverse colon in order to be able to carry out a safe reconstruction using healthy tissue.

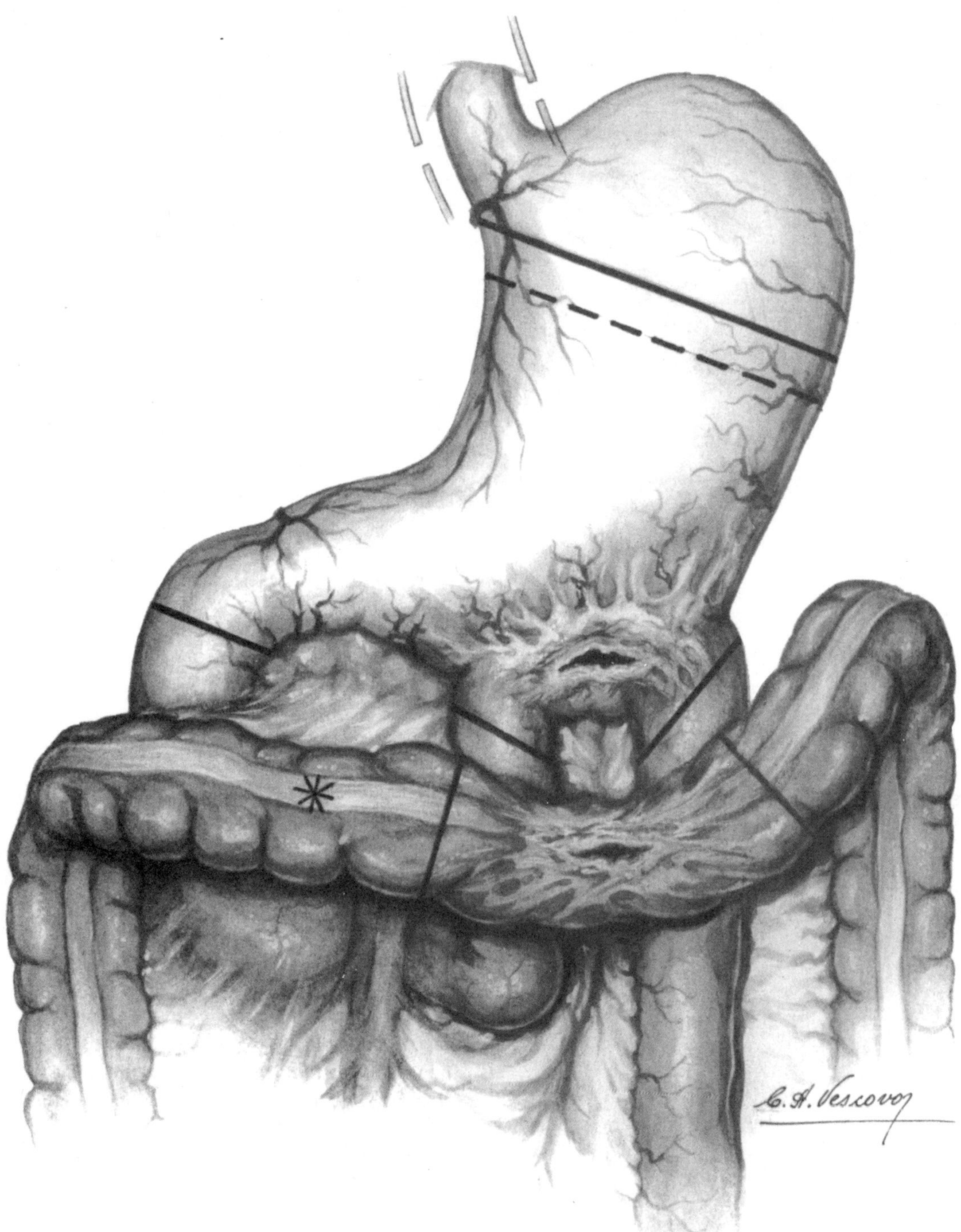

FIGURE 34.18

Gastrojejunocolic Fistula

FIGURE 34.19
What is usually known as a triple resection has been performed on the stomach, a segment of jejunum, and another segment of the transverse colon. Gastrointestinal transit is reestablished by anastomosing the gastric stump to the jejunum in front of the transverse colon (70–80% gastrectomy with Billroth II anastomosis using the Hofmeister-Finsterer modification). The jejunal ends have been anastomosed to each other, as noted in the drawing of the afferent jejunal loop. The colonic ends have also been anastomosed, as seen in the drawing immediately to the right of the afferent jejunal loop. The duodenal stump has been closed with two purse string sutures. The vagal trunks have been transected. This complex surgical procedure, which used to be done in two or three stages several years ago, is now carried out in one procedure.

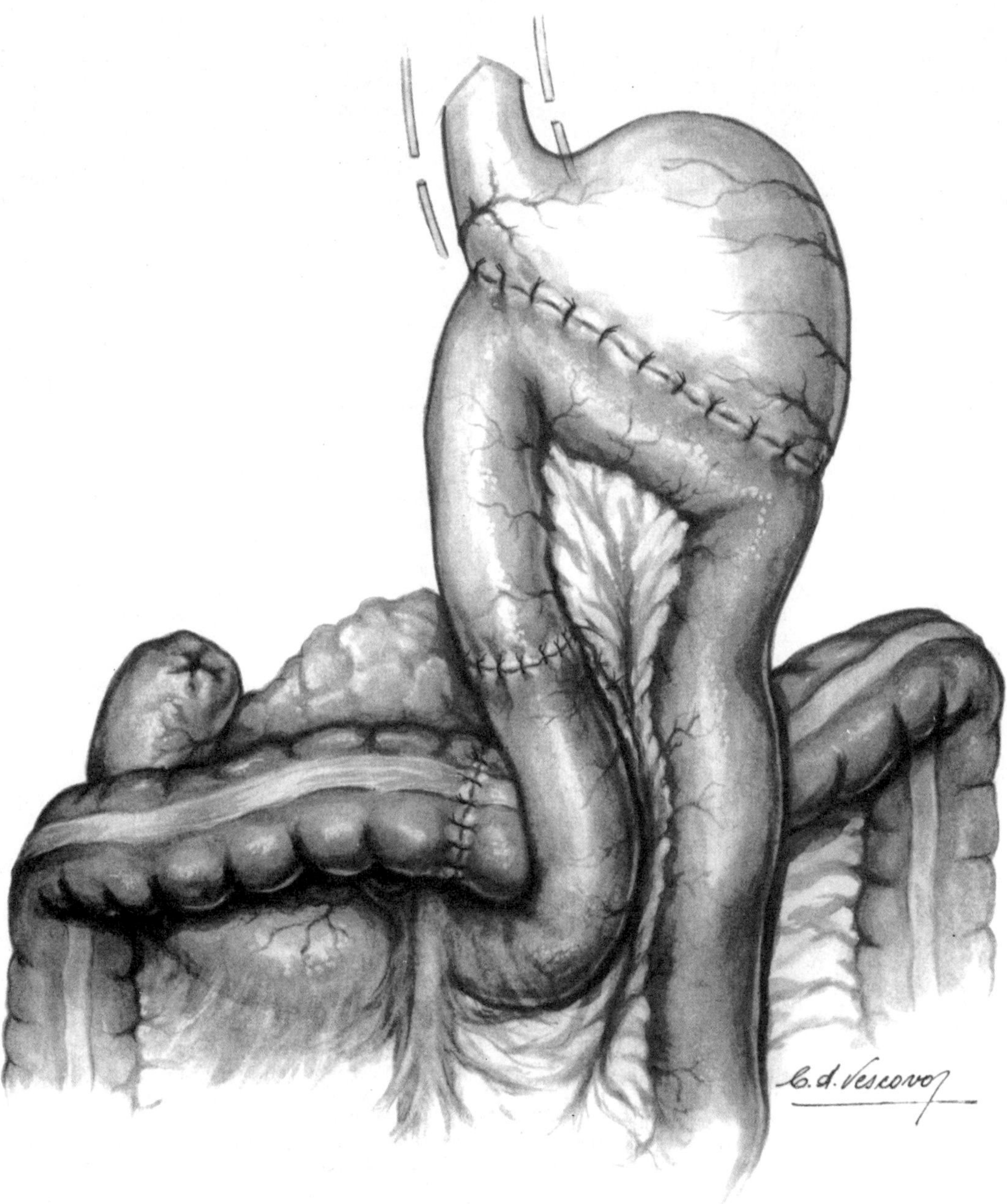

FIGURE 34.19

References

1. Barber, K.W. Jr., Waugh, J.M., Priestley, J.T. Operation in one stage for gastrojejunocolic fistula. Surg. Clin. North Am. 42:1443, 1962.
2. Barber, K.W. Jr., Waugh, J.M., Priestley, J.T. Operation in one stage for gastrojejunocolic fistula. Report of 12 cases and review of the literature. Ann. Surg. 181:376, 1975.
3. Bancroft, F.W. Modification of Devine operation of pyloric exclusion for duodenal ulcer. Am. J. Surg. 16:223, 1932.
4. Baron, J.H. Clinical tests of gastric secretin. Oxford University Press, New York, 1979.
5. Callum, K.G., Talbot, J.E. The surgical treatment of peptic ulcer: A 15 year review. Br. J. Surg. 60:511, 1973.
6. Dinbar, A., Avigad, I., Shafir, R., Tulcinsky, D.B. Long-term results of subtotal gastrectomy for duodenal ulcer. World J. Surg. 4:625, 1980.
7. Dragstedt, L.R., Owen, F.M. Jr. Supra-diaphragmatic section of the vagus nerves in treatment of duodenal ulcer. Proc. Soc. Exp. Biol. Med. 53:152, 1943.
8. Farmer, D.A., Smithwick, R.H. Hemigastrectomy combined with resection of vagus nerves. N. Engl. J. Med. 247:1017, 1952.
9. Finsterer, H. The extended gastrectomy for duodenal ulcer instead of simple resection of the duodenum or of the pyloric exclusion. Zentralbl. Chir. 26:434, 1918.
10. Finsterer, H., Chuna, F. The surgical treatment of duodenal ulcer. Surg. Gynecol. Obstet. 52:1099, 1931.
11. Fischer, P.B., Jordan. G.L. Jr. The Billroth I Gastrectomy for the treatment of duodenal ulcer. Am. Surg. 24:922, 1958.
12. Fischer, P.B. Twenty five years after Billroth II Gastrectomy for duodenal ulcer. World J. Surg. 8:293, 1984.
13. Franksson, C. Selective abdominal vagotomy. Acta Chir. Scand. 96:409, 1948.
14. Fromm, D. Complications of gastric surgery. Wiley, New York, 1977.
15. Goligher, J.C., Moir, P.J., Wrigley, J.H. The Billroth I and Polya operations for duodenal ulcer: A comparison. Lancet 1:220, 1956.
16. Harkins, H.N., Stavney, L.S., Griffth, C.A., Savage, L.E., Kato, T., Nyhus, L.M. Selective gastric vagotomy. Ann. Surg. 158:448, 1963.
17. Herrington, J.L. Jr. Current operation for duodenal ulcer. Curr. Probl. Surg. 1:61, 1972.
18. Herrington, J.L. Jr., Sawyers, J.L., Scott, H.W. Jr. A 25 year experience with vagotomy-antrectomy. Arch. Surg. 106:469, 1973.
19. Jordan, G.L. Jr. Recurrent Ulcer. In Scott, H.W. Jr., Sawyers J.L. (Ed.) Surgery of the stomach, duodenum and small intestine. Ed. 2, p. 593. Blackwell, Boston 1992.
20. Lahey, F.H. Experiences with postoperative jejunal ulcer gastrojejunocolic fistula. Am. J. Dig. Dis. 2:675, 1936.
21. Lewisohn, R. The frequency of gastroduodenal ulcers. Surg. Gynecol. Obstet. 40:70, 1925.
22. Lewisohn, R. Frequency of gastrojejunal ulcers following gastroenterostomy for duodenal ulcers. J.A.M.A. 154:1301, 1954.
23. Lewisohn, R. Changes in surgical treatment of chronic duodenal ulcers during the past 50 years. Arch. Surg. 77:61, 1958.
24. Lindenauer, S.M., Dent, T.L. Management of recurrent ulcer. Arch. Surg. 110:531, 1975.
25. Marshall, S.F. Plan for surgical management of gastrojejunocolic fistula. Ann. Surg. 121:620, 1945.
26. Mathewson, C. Preliminary colostomy for gastrocolic and gastrojejunocolic fistulae. Ann. Surg. 114:1004, 1941.
27. Mouchet, A., Marquant, J., Guivare, H., Maisel, A. A propos de 36 cas d'ulcères peptiques post-opératoires. J. Chir. 94:129, 1967.
28. Nobles, E.R. Jr. Vagotomy and gastroenterostomy. Am. J. Surg. 32:177, 1962.
29. Nyhus, L.M. Stomal Ulcer. In Harkins, H.N., Nyhus, L.M. (Eds.) Surgery of the stomach and duodenum. P. 196. Little, Brown, Boston, 1962.
30. Pfeiffer, D.B., Kent, E.M. The value of preliminary colostomy in the correction of gastrojejunocolic fistula. Ann. Surg. 110:659, 1939.
31. Pi-Figueras Badía, J. Sobre el tratamiento de la fistula gastroyeyunocólica con una nueva técnica de derivación. Rev. Esp. Ap. Dig. Nutr. 25:979, 1966.
32. Pi-Figueras, J. Ulcera péptica anastomótica. In Pi-Figueras, J. (ed) Práctica quirúrgica. Ed. 2, vol. 1, p. 194. Salvat, Barcelona, 1986.
33. Plenk, A. Zur technik der resektion zur ausschaltung. Zentralbl. 63:3019, 1936.
34. Quénu, J., Loygue, J., Perrotin, J., Dubost, C., Moreaux, J. Opérations sur les parois de l'abdomen et sur le tube digestif. P. 576. Masson et Cie, Paris, 1968.
35. Ruding, R., Hirdes, W.H. Extent of the gastric antrum and its significance. Surgery 53:743, 1963.
36. Strauss, A.A., Bloch, L., Friedman, J.G. Gastrojejunal ulcer, medical and surgical considerations. J.A.M.A. 90:181, 1928.
37. Smithwick, R.H. Conservative gastric resection combined with vagotomy. Surgery 41:144, 1957.
38. Walters, W., Clagett, O.T. Gastrojejunocolic ulcer and fistula. Am. J. Surg. 46:94, 1939.
39. Walters, W., Lynn, T.E. Results of 237 Billroth I gastric resections for peptic ulcer: A 6 to 15 year follow-up. Ann. Surg. 144:464, 1956.
40. Walters, W., Lynn, T.E. The Billroth I and Billroth II operations: Comparison of the results six to ten years after operations for gastric, duodenal and gastrojejunal ulcers. Arch. Surg. 74:680, 1957.
41. Weinberg, J.A. Pyloroplasty and vagotomy for duodenal ulcer. Curr. Probl. Surg. 3:36, 1964.
42. Welch, C.E., Rodkey, G.V. Partial gastrectomy for duodenal ulcer. Am. J. Surg. 105:338, 1963.
43. Welch, C.E., Rodkey, G.V., von Griska, P. One thousand operations for peptic ulcer disease. Ann. Surg. 204:454, 1986.
44. Wychulis, A.R., Priestley, J.T., Foulk, W.T. A study of 360 patients with gastrojejunal ulceration. Surg. Gynecol. Obstet. 122:89, 1966.
45. Zollinger, R.M., Ellison, E.C. Primary peptic ulcerations of the jejunum associated with islet cell tumors of the pancreas. Ann. Surg. 142:709, 1955.

Section F

Surgery of the Stomach and Duodenum

CHAPTER 35

Uncommon Complications of Gastric Surgery

In addition to anastomotic ulcers, gastric surgery can give rise to other, less frequent complications, which must be understood to be able to treat them adequately. Some of these infrequent complications will be described here.

AFFERENT LOOP SYNDROME

This is an infrequent complication of the Billroth II gastrectomy. It is usually due to excess accumulation of biliopancreatic secretions in the afferent loop. This complication is usually the result of defective technique in the gastrojejunal anastomosis. In very rare cases the syndrome is caused by adhesive bands that cause kinking of the afferent loop and interfere with emptying of the loop. In some patients part of the liquids that are ingested can run into the afferent loop and considerably increase its contents (11, 12, 14, 16).

Patients usually complain of abdominal distension and epigastric pain followed by bilious vomiting and momentary relief. Vomiting can become repetitive and may contain food particles (18, 19). The afferent loop syndrome may become manifest a few days after surgery or late after surgery.

This syndrome was first described by Mimpris and Birt in 1948 (26) and later by Wells and Welbourn (39). According to Alexander-Williams, this syndrome is not due to accumulation of biliary and pancreatic secretions in the afferent loop but to an alkaline gastritis in patients with a susceptible gastric mucosa. Both Jordan (21, 22) and Herrington (17–19) have affirmed that the afferent loop syndrome should be differentiated from alkaline gastritis. DuPlessis (9), Lawson (23), Bushkin (4), Dahlgren (7) and others have reached the same conclusion.

The clinical picture of the afferent loop syndrome is not serious, but in cases where the intensity and frequency of symptoms increase, surgical intervention may be necessary.

Several surgical procedures have been proposed to correct this complication. Among these is the interposition of a jejunal loop between the gastric stump and the duodenum using the Henley technique, to which a truncal vagotomy should always be added. Conversion of a Billroth II anastomosis to a gastrectomy with a Roux-en-Y anastomosis or conversion of a Billroth II to a Billroth I have also been proposed. This latter procedure is probably the preferred procedure. One of these techniques will be described later.

In cases in which the patient is in poor general condition because of frequent pain and vomiting, some surgeons have resorted to a simple anastomosis between the afferent and the efferent loops (Braun jejunojejunostomy). Even though this is not an optimal procedure, it can be done as an emergency. The Braun anastomosis favors the development of anastomic ulcers, since the alkaline pancreatic and biliary secretions will not bathe the gastrojejunostomy by bypassing it through the Braun anastomosis.

HEMORRHAGE FROM THE GASTROJEJUNAL ANASTOMOSIS

Postoperative hemorrhage from the gastrojejunal suture line is an infrequent complication that occurs when the suture is not correctly performed.

This complication usually occurs in the immediate postoperative period and arises in the gastric submucosal arterioles. These arterioles bleed freely when transected. Even one of these vessels that is not ligated can lead to the patient's death. Because of this particularity of the submucosal arterioles, it is advisable to ligate each one individually before transecting the stomach, as pointed out in the gastrectomy technique.

During the first postoperative day one should observe that a serosanguinous fluid comes out through the Levine tube, which later changes to stained bile. If blood continues to come out of the Levine tube instead of a serosanguinous fluid, it means that the hemorrhage persists. In this situation the stomach should be irrigated with chilled water through the Levine tube. If blood loss continues and it becomes necessary to transfuse the patient with one or more units of blood, H_2 blockers (ranitidine) or proton pump inhibitors (omeprazole) should be ordered and attempts made to control bleeding endoscopically using electrocoagulation, laser, or heater probe. If bleeding cannot be controlled endoscopically, surgery should be carried out for control. In most cases hemostasis can be attained without taking down the gastrojejunal anastomosis by opening the anterior wall of the stomach, parallel to the anastomosis, 3 to 4 cm above it. Once the stomach is opened, retained blood clots are removed manually and the interior of the stomach is explored for possible bleeding from an overlooked superficial gastric ulcer. The suture line is then explored and hemostasis carried out using the technique described by Nissen (29) and used successfully by various surgeons (3, 15, 16, 30, 32). This technique will now be described.

Hemorrhage from the Gastrojejunal Anastomosis

Hemorrhage from the Gastrojejunal Anastomosis

FIGURE 35.1 HEMORRHAGE FROM THE GASTROJEJUNAL SUTURE LINE: REOPERATION

Once the peritoneum is open, the abdominal cavity is protected with pads to avoid contamination. A transverse incision is made in the anterior gastric wall some 3 or 4 cm above the gastrojejunal suture line. Using both hands, the blood clots are removed. It is not advisable to aspirate the gastric contents with a metallic cannula because these can produce diffuse bleeding from the gastric mucosa. Using two or three Babcock or Duval clamps, the superior edge of the gastric wall is clamped. This has two objectives: achieving hemostasis and improving the visualization of the gastric interior by pulling the clamps upward. The inferior border of the gastric wall is then grasped with one or more Babcock or Duval clamps to exert downward traction. With the fingers of the left hand the surgeon retracts the inferior border of the gastric wall at the same time as he or she pushes the posterior gastrojejunal suture line forward, to expose the entire gastrojejunostomy. If the hemorrhage is confined to a small area, hemostasis is easily attained by using a couple of suture ligatures. In the rare case in which the bleeding is diffuse, a continuous suture is performed with nonabsorbable material placed over the previous gastrojejunal suture line, as seen in the drawing. Once hemostasis is assured, the gastrotomy is closed in two layers and the end of the Levine tube is placed so that gastric contents can be aspirated efficiently.

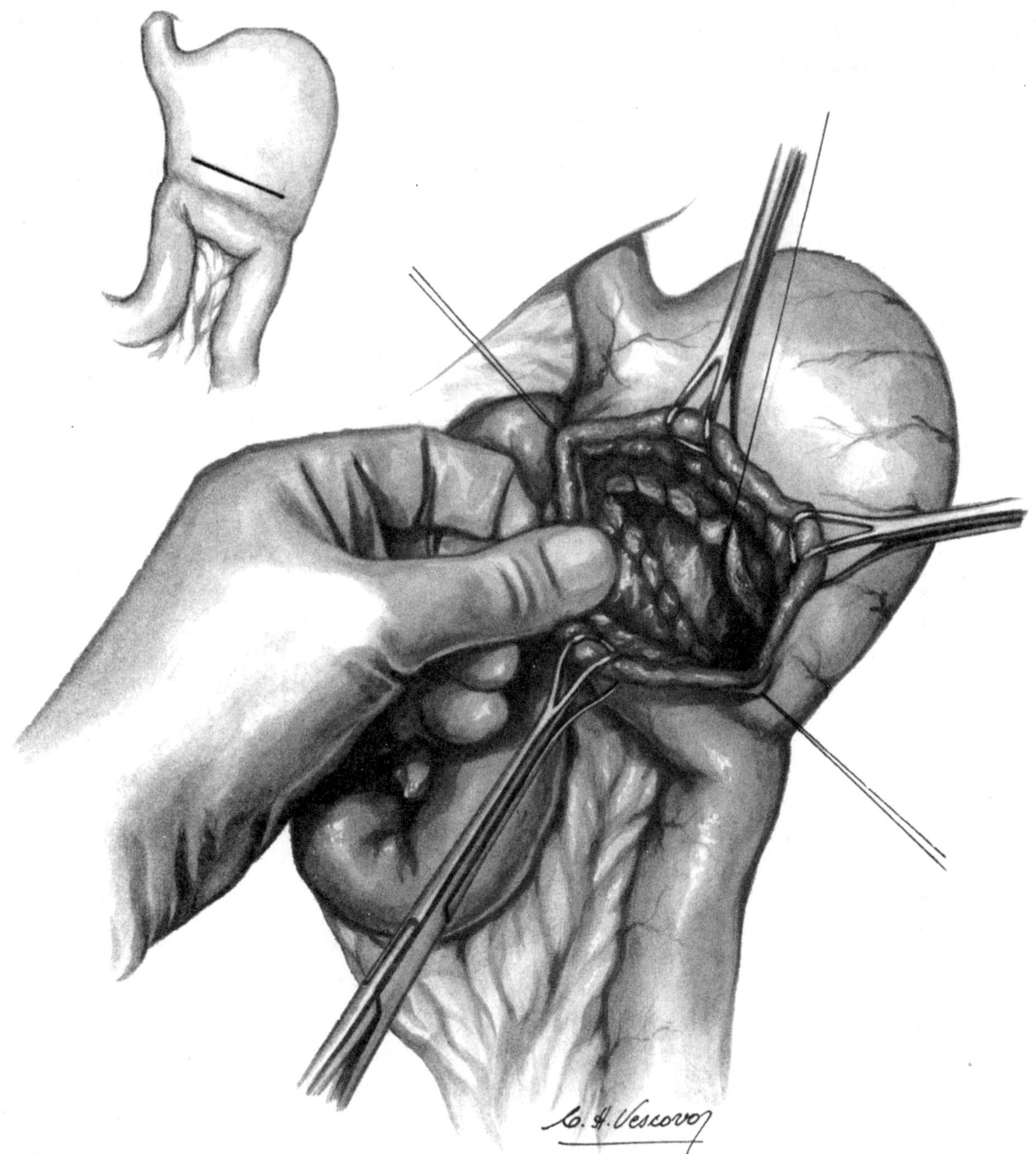

FIGURE 35.1 HEMORRHAGE FROM THE GASTROJEJUNAL SUTURE LINE: REOPERATION

SMALL BOWEL HERNIATION THROUGH THE TRANSVERSE MESOCOLON

This rare complication can occur in retrocolic gastrectomies or gastrojejunostomies in which the gastric stump has not been correctly fixed to the transverse mesocolon. In the opening that has been left between the gastric walls and the transverse mesocolon a loop of small bowel can be introduced. In some patients this small bowel hernia can be completely asymptomatic; in others it can produce moderate intermittent pain, nausea, and vomiting; and in still other patients it can cause severe small bowel obstruction with urgent indications for surgery. Treatment will vary according to the condition of the circulation of the herniated bowel. If the circulation of the intestinal wall is not compromised, treatment will consist of reduction of the herniated bowel into the inframesocolic compartment and closing the defect in the mesocolon. If the intestinal wall is affected, it becomes necessary to resect the gangrenous segment, reestablishing bowel continuity with a two-layer anastomosis between the healthy bowel ends and closing the mesocolic defect to prevent recurrences.

Just as sometimes the mistake is made of not suturing the stomach to the transverse mesocolon correctly, leading to the complication described earlier, the mistake can also be made of fixing the anastomotic jejunal limb to the transverse mesocolon instead of the stomach. If this error is made, the patients will usually present postoperative obstructive symptoms due to the tendency of the mesocolon to produce diminution of the jejunal lumen, since the wall of the jejunum is more easily compressed than that of the stomach.

Small Bowel Herniation Through the Transverse Mesocolon

Small Bowel Herniation Through the Transverse Mesocolon

FIGURE 35.2
The drawing shows herniation of the small bowel through a space between the gastric stump and the transverse mesocolon. An arrow shown in the insert illustrates the route of the herniated small bowel. In this case the herniated loop showed no circulatory compromise and treatment simply consisted of reducing the herniated loop back into the inframesocolic space and closing the defect between the gastric stump and the transverse mesocolon.

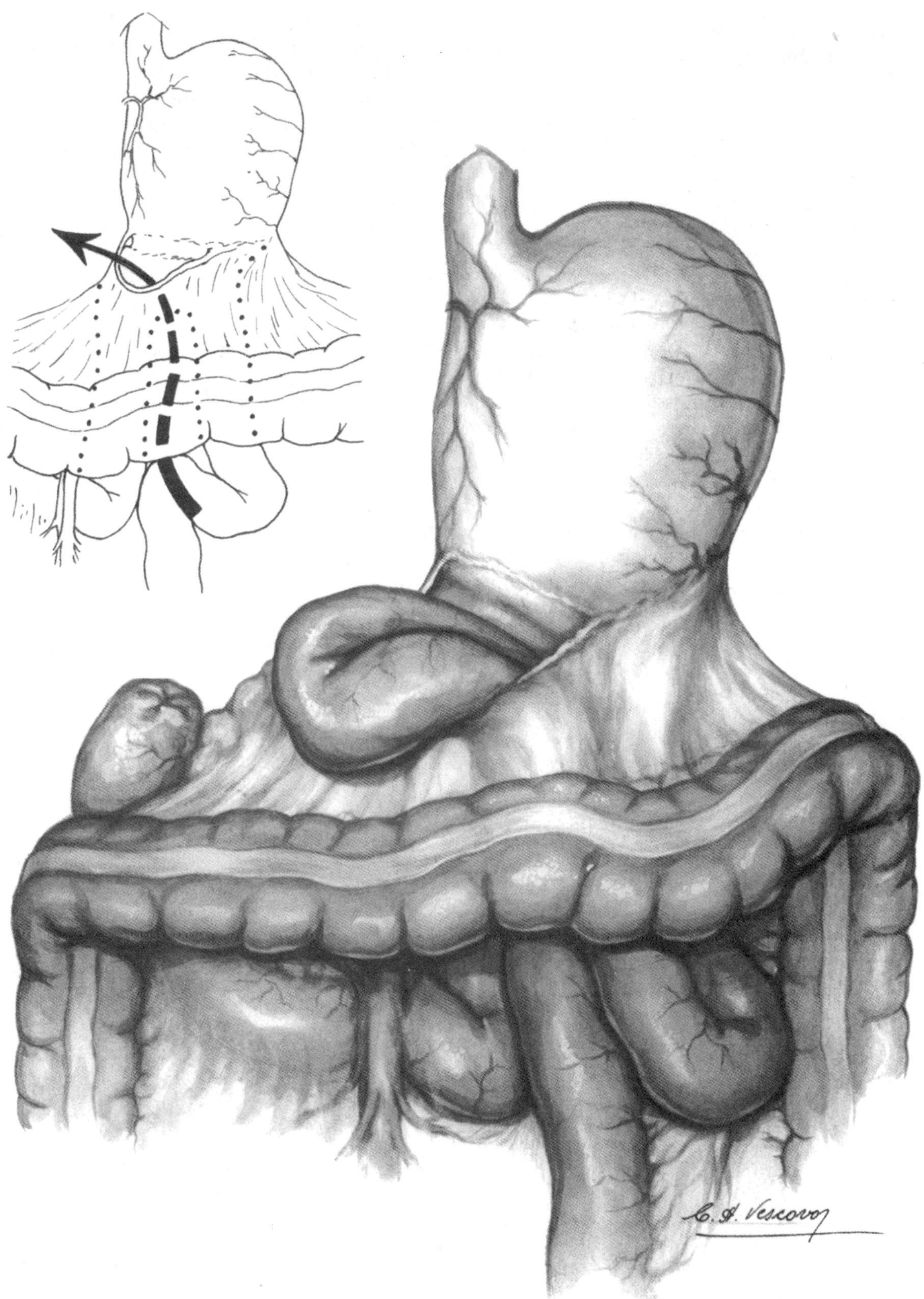

FIGURE 35.2

RETROANASTOMOTIC INTERNAL HERNIAS

Internal postgastrectomy hernias are rare, occurring in antecolic as well as retrocolic Billroth II procedures, although much less frequently in the latter. On rare occasions these hernias can occur in gastrojejunal anastomoses. Retroanastomotic internal hernias may appear immediately after surgery or in the late postoperative period. Half of these hernias manifest themselves within the first postoperative month (11, 12). The herniated segment can be the efferent loop, the afferent loop, or both simultaneously. The efferent loop becomes herniated more frequently. The afferent loop is herniated less frequently, and very rarely both loops are herniated simultaneously.

Symptomatology in retroanastomotic hernias varies a lot from one patient to another. Some of these hernias are completely asymptomatic; others present moderate intermittent symptoms with epigastric pain, distension, nausea, and vomiting. In other patients the clinical picture is one of serious bowel obstruction, making urgent surgery mandatory. In these cases the small bowel may be gangrenous. According to Stammers (38) the symptoms of patients with retroanastomotic hernias begin 3 to 6 days after surgery. If the hernia involves the afferent loop, the vomitus will not usually be bilious, because this loop is obstructed (11, 12). The majority of these hernias are from right to left and not from left to right. To prevent these hernias it is necessary to close the space behind the gastrojejunostomy with interrupted sutures.

This complication was originally described by Petersen in 1900 and is known as a Petersen hernia in his honor. Gray (13), in 1904, proposed the closure of the posterior gastrojejunal space in all gastrectomies to prevent these hernias. Morton, Alrich, and Hill (28), in 1955, again insisted on the need to close this space. It is exceptional, however, for surgeons to carry this out to prevent this complication.

Surgical treatment of retroanastomotic hernias consists of reducing the herniated bowel and closing the posterior gastrojejunal space. If the circulation of the herniated bowel loop has been compromised, the hernia should be resected. If the herniated loop cannot be reduced, the gastrojejunostomy should be taken down, the herniated bowel reduced, and the gastrojejunal anastomosis reconstructed (25, 34, 38).

Retroanastomotic Internal Hernias

Retroanastomotic Internal Hernias

FIGURE 35.3 INTERNAL RETROANASTOMOTIC POSTGASTRECTOMY HERNIA
The herniated efferent loop is not compromised in its circulation. The loop is reduced and the retroanastomotic space closed with several sutures to prevent recurrences.

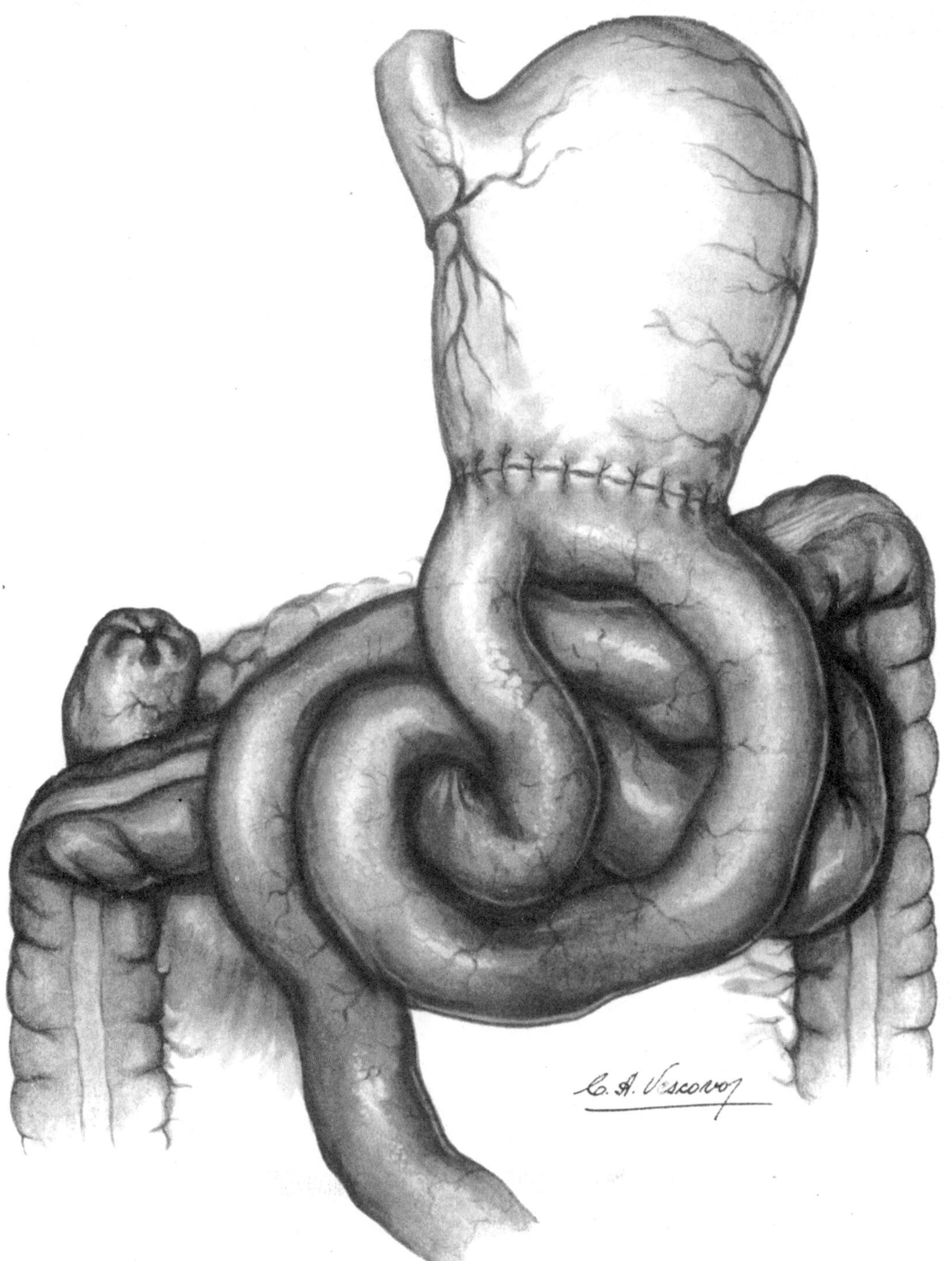

FIGURE 35.3 INTERNAL RETROANASTOMOTIC POSTGASTRECTOMY HERNIA

DUMPING SYNDROME

In patients with gastric surgery the dumping syndrome may appear due to loss of the regulatory action of the pylorus in controlling gastric emptying. Loss of this pyloric regulatory action can be caused by the following:

1. Pyloric transection (pyloroplasty).
2. Pyloric bypass (gastrojejunostomy).
3. Pyloric resection (Billroth I or Billroth II gastrectomy).

The term "dumping" was originally used by Mix, in 1922 (27), meaning that the stomach emptied very rapidly.

Dumping syndrome is characterized by vasomotor and gastrointestinal symptoms. Vasomotor symptoms are due to stimulation of the adrenergic system and consist of tachycardia, flushing, restlessness, weakness, anxiety, respiratory distress, and so on. The most frequent gastrointestinal symptoms are abdominal distension, nausea, vomiting, abdominal cramps, and diarrhea. Ingested hypertonic solutions reproduce symptoms of dumping when they enter the jejunum. On the other hand, the rapid gastric emptying together with accelerated intestinal transit and distension of the efferent loop give rise to diminution of plasma volume. Dumping syndrome also produces other neurohumoral alterations such as increase in vasoactive intestinal peptides, neurotensin, pancreatic polypeptides, insulin, and glucagon. It has been shown that analogous somatostatin (octeotride) inhibits the secretion of the above mentioned hormones, thereby preventing symptoms of dumping, for which reason it is used in treating dumping.

The symptoms of dumping appear during ingestion of food or up to 45 minutes later. For this reason the symptoms that appear during or a few minutes after eating are designated as precocious dumping syndrome, to differentiate this from other episodes of dumping that may appear one or more hours after eating, which is known as late dumping. These symptoms vary a lot from one individual to another but, taken together, are similar to the clinical picture of hypoglycemia because, in reality, dumping is due to a decrease in the blood sugar level. For this reason, this syndrome is frequently designated as reactive hypoglycemic syndrome, which causes a reaction of the adrenal medulla and an increase in epinephrine production. Late dumping syndrome can be prevented or neutralized by injecting analogous somatostatin.

Dumping syndrome is usually tolerable and gradually disappears spontaneously. There are few patients with serious symptoms or who are incapacitated by dumping syndrome.

Dumping syndrome appears in patients operated on for duodenal peptic ulcer and rarely occurs in patients operated on for gastric ulcer or cancer. Patients with duodenal ulcer frequently have psychosomatic alterations that favor the appearance of dumping syndrome. This fact makes it important to adapt the selection of the surgical procedure to be performed not only to the pathologic alterations of the ulcer but also to the psychosomatic condition of the patient. The treatment of dumping syndrome, either early or late, is medical in nature. Surgery for dumping syndrome is only rarely indicated and has very controversial results.

Early dumping syndrome usually improves greatly when the patient takes several small meals daily. The meals should be mainly protein and fat with very little carbohydrate content. Patients should not take liquids with their meals: Liquids should be taken between meals. The use of sedatives and antihistaminics is important. It is also important that, early after surgery, the patients eat while lying down, especially on their left side. This position considerably diminishes the symptoms of precocious dumping.

Somatostatin is very efficient in preventing or making the symptoms of precocious dumping disappear, as well as those of late dumping.

This hormone is frequently used as long acting analogous somatostatin (octeotride), which is injected subcutaneously 20 minutes before meals.

Many surgical procedures have been proposed to treat precocious dumping syndrome, especially in incapacitated cases. It can be affirmed that none of these procedures has proven to be efficacious.

Some of these procedures are as follows (18, 19):

1. Interposition of a segment of jejunum 20 to 25 cm long placed in isoperistaltic fashion between the gastric stump and the duodenum with an added truncal vagotomy to prevent the development of an anastomotic ulcer.
2. Interposition of a double jejunal segment 10 to 12 cm long, one in isoperistaltic fashion and the other in antiperistaltic fashion, both joined by a jejunojejunal anastomosis.
3. Interposition of an antiperistaltic segment of jejunum 10 cm long between the stomach and the duodenal stump.
4. Roux-en-Y gastrojejunostomy together with antrectomy and truncal vagotomy to prevent anastomotic ulceration.
5. Conversion of a Billroth II gastrectomy to a Billroth I.

NECROSIS OF THE GASTRIC STUMP

Necrosis of the gastrectomy stump is a very rare complication of gastric surgery. The great majority of cases have occurred in extensive subtotal gastrectomies for carcinoma and only a few in gastrectomies for gastroduodenal ulcers (10–12, 33, 35, 37). In 1959, Casebolt (5) asserted that the circulation of the gastric remnant depends on the presence of the ascending branch of the left gastric or coronary artery, on the presence of the short gastric vessels, and on the presence of the right inferior phrenic artery. In order to avoid necrosis of the gastric stump, at least one of the above vessels must be preserved. In patients in whom the left gastric artery is ligated at its origin from the celiac trunk and the spleen is removed, which means the short vessels are ligated, the only residual circulation to the gastric stump is through the right inferior phrenic artery. It should be kept in mind that the right inferior phrenic artery or both inferior phrenic arteries may arise from the left gastric artery in 2.6% of patients. This means that, if the left gastric artery is ligated near the celiac trunk and the spleen has been removed, the gastric remnant will lose its arterial supply and will inevitably become necrotic.

Cate and Dawson (6), in an experimental study on dogs, were able to prove that necrosis of the gastric stump was more frequent with larger gastric stumps. If the gastric stump was small, the possibility of necrosis was less. Jackson (20) was able to prove that necrosis of the stump (due to arteriosclerosis of the vessels) can occur even if the short gastric vessels are preserved. In a personal communication, Henry N. Harkins (1960) stated that he had observed two cases of necrosis of the stump in 500 gastrectomies which he called Blue Stomach Syndrome. In those two cases Harkins had ligated the left gastric artery and the short vessels. He also suggested that truncal vagotomy in extensive gastrectomies can cause gastric stump necrosis due to possible injury of the inferior phrenic arteries during dissection of the vagus nerves.

The prognosis in patients with necrosis of the gastric stump remnant is very serious and frequently mortal. The indicated surgical procedure is resection of the necrotic stump (total gastrectomy) and anastomosis of the esophagus to the jejunum.

JEJUNOGASTRIC INTUSSUSCEPTION

Retrograde jejunogastric intussusception is a very rare complication, both in gastrojejunostomies and in the Billroth II gastrectomy, either antecolic or retrocolic. For obvious reasons, the Billroth I gastrectomy is not exposed to this complication.

Jejunogastric intussusception generally occurs late postoperatively, although in some patients this complication occurs 3 or 4 days after surgery (11, 12). Diagnosis is very difficult when the complication occurs early.

The most frequent intussusception that occurs in both gastrectomies as well as gastrojejunostomy is that of the efferent loop. In gastrojejunostomies the afferent loop becomes intussuscepted much more frequently, although at times both loops (afferent and efferent) can be affected. In gastrectomies the afferent loop becomes intussuscepted more rarely.

Retrograde jejunogastric intussusception is manifested by epigastric pain and vomiting, and at times by a palpable epigastric mass if a large loop becomes intussuscepted. Diagnosis of the complication is made clinically, by radiologic study, or by endoscopy. In some patients symptoms are moderate and intermittent. Surgery is indicated in these cases if the clinical picture recurs frequently and leads to nutritional problems and inability to work.

If patients present an acute abdominal problem due to this complication, they should be operated upon urgently. If surgery reveals no vascular compromise of the intussuscepted jejunal loop, the loop can be reduced. If there is vascular compromise of the loop, it should be resected.

In gastrectomized patients with frequent symptoms of jejunogastric intussusception, as well as in patients with acute intussusception, it is advisable to convert the Billroth II gastrectomy to a Billroth I. In patients with gastrojejunostomies the simplest procedure is taking down the gastrojejunostomy and performing a pyloroplasty with truncal vagotomy (11, 12, 16, 18, 19).

CONVERSION OF A BILLROTH II GASTRECTOMY TO BILLROTH I

It is very rarely necessary to convert a Billroth II gastrectomy to a Billroth I. It has been mentioned that this conversion may be necessary in some cases of afferent loop syndrome or retrograde jejunogastric intussusception. Some surgeons have recommended conversion in patients with dumping syndrome. Conversion of a Billroth II gastrectomy to a Billroth I in the treatment of dumping syndrome, as has been stated before, does not have a scientific basis, since patients with a Billroth I gastrectomy are also prone to suffer from dumping syndrome. One of the techniques used to carry out the conversion is that of Soupault and Bucaille described in Paris in 1955 (36).

The Soupault-Boucaille technique will be described as follows:

Conversion of a Billroth II Gastrectomy to Billroth I

FIGURE 35.4A

Incision through the old scar. Intraperitoneal adhesions are freed. The colon and transverse mesocolon is elevated upward dividing the mesocolon around the gastric stump, being especially careful to avoid injuring the middle colic or marginal arteries. The afferent loop, the duodenojejunal junction, and the efferent loop are identified. The broken line illustrates where the afferent loop (next to the stomach), the efferent loop (15 cm below the gastrojejunal anastomosis), and the mesentery will be divided in order to preserve the circulation of the jejunal loop to be transposed. If a truncal vagotomy has not been previously performed, it should be carried out before dividing the bowel.

FIGURE 35.4B

The afferent loop has been divided flush on the lesser curvature of the gastric stump and closed in two layers. The proximal end of the afferent loop is grasped with a Babcock clamp, as shown in the drawing. The efferent loop is transected about 15 cm from the gastrojejunal anastomosis and both transected ends are held with Babcock clamps. Observe that the jejunal loop to be transposed is well vascularized by arterial mesenteric branches. The afferent loop will be anastomosed to the distal end of the efferent loop to reestablish intestinal continuity while the proximal segment of the efferent loop will be anastomosed to the duodenum.

FIGURE 35.4C

The anastomosis of the proximal end of the afferent jejunal loop to the distal end of the efferent loop has been performed. The proximal end of the efferent jejunal loop is grasped with a Babcock clamp, brought into the supramesocolic region, and anastomosed to the anterior wall of duodenum. The anterior duodenal wall has been incised to receive the end of the jejunum.

FIGURE 35.4D

The proximal portion of the efferent jejunal segment has beer transposed to the supramesocolic region and anastomosed terminolaterally to the anterior wall of the duodenum. During this transposition strict attention must be given to avoid traction or excessive rotation on the transposed segment so as to avoid endangering its circulation. The mesentery of the transposed segment is fixed to the mesocolon with several sutures to avoid possible internal hernias. When the Billroth II gastrectomy is antecolic, conversion is much easier.

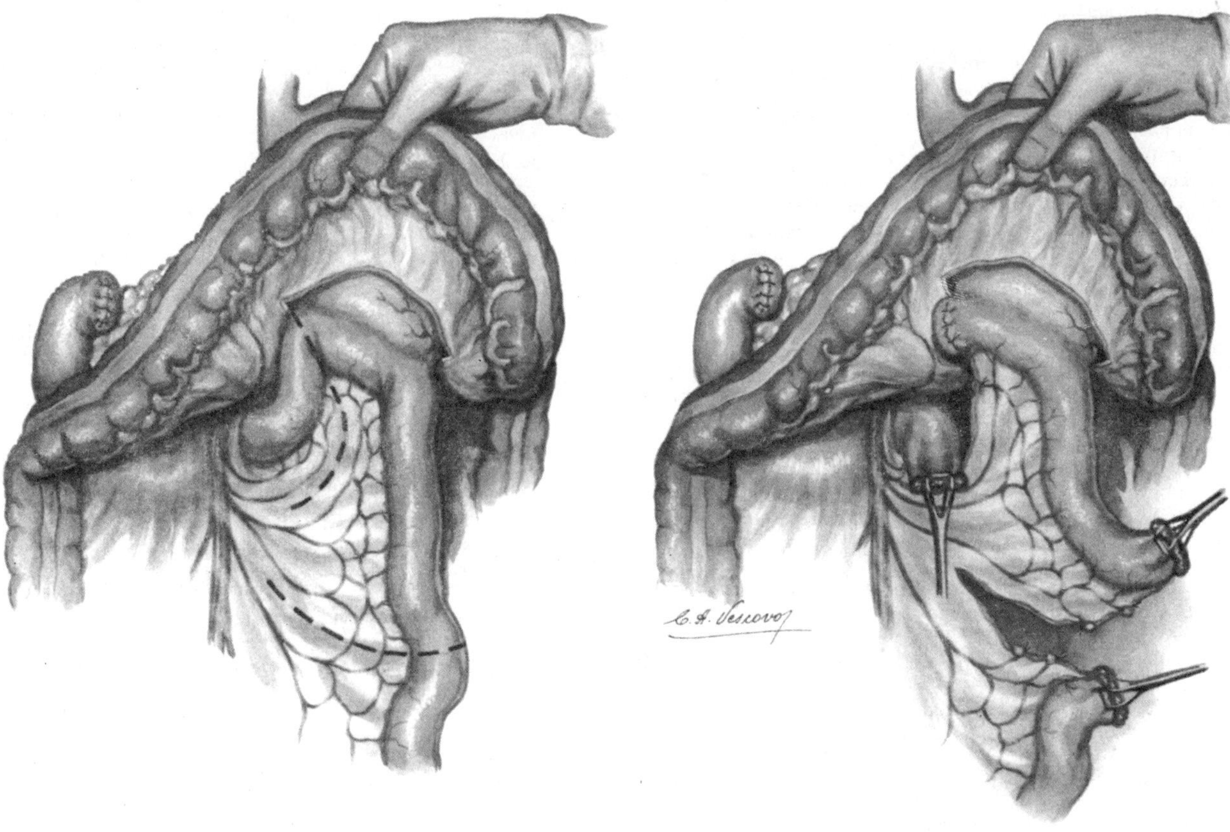

FIGURE 35.4A

FIGURE 35.4B

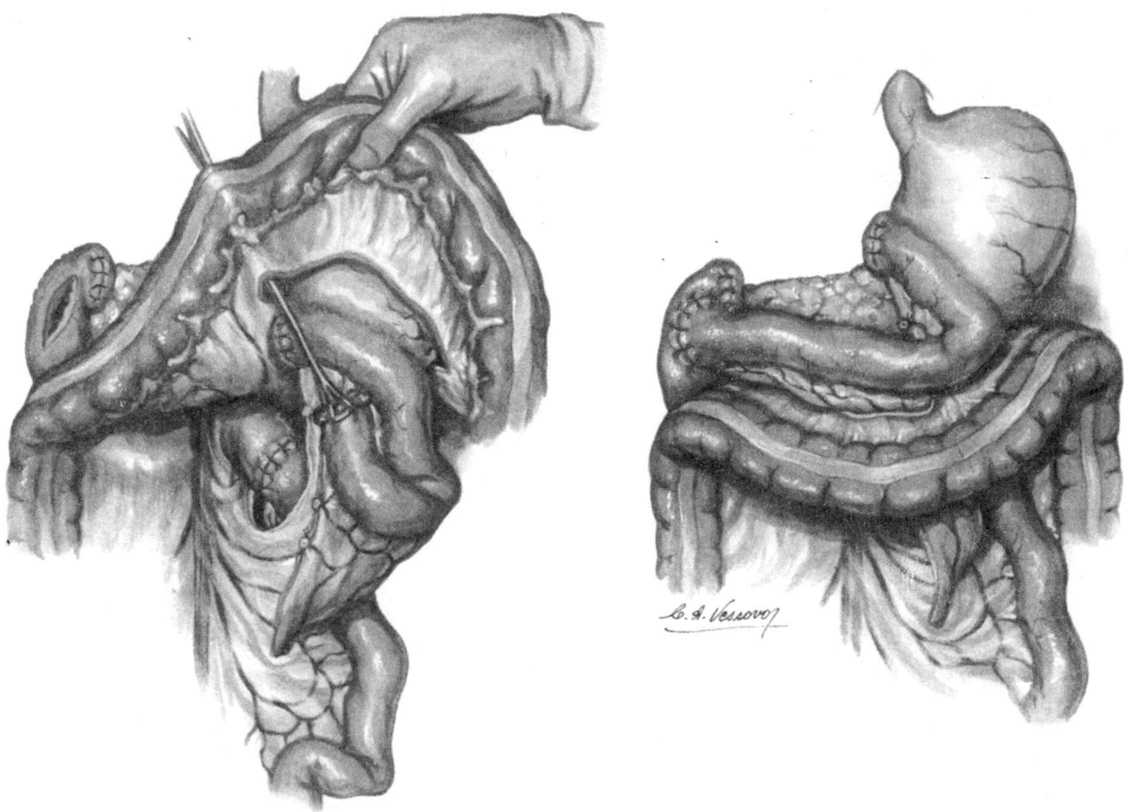

FIGURE 35.4C

FIGURE 35.4D

References

1. Alexander-Williams, J. Gastric reconstructive surgery. Ann. R. Coll. Surg. Engl. 52:1, 1972.
2. Anfres, P., Pi-Figueras Badía, J. Complicaciones post-operatorias. In Pi-Figueras, J. (ed) Práctica quirúrgica. Ed. 2, Vol. 2, p. 267. Salvat, Barcelona, 1986.
3. Becker, H.D., Herfarth, C., Lierse, W., Schreiber, H.W. Surgery of the stomach. P. 330. Springer-Verlag, Berlin, 1988.
4. Bushkin, F.L., Wickbom, G., DeFord, J.M., Woodward, E.R. Postoperative alkaline reflux gastritis. Surg. Gynecol. Obstet. 138:933, 1974.
5. Casebolt, B.T. Ischemic anastomotic break-down and gangrene of the gastric remnant following subtotal gastrectomy. J. Int. Coll. Surg. 31:269, 1959.
6. Cate, W.R. Jr., Dawson, R.E. The viability of proximal gastric remnants following radical subtotal gastrectomy and gastroduodenostomy. Surgery 41:401, 1957.
7. Dahlgren, S. The afferent loop syndrome. Acta Chir. Scand. 327:1, 1964.
8. Dunphy, J.E. A method of handling jejunal loop and gastrectomy with posterior anastomosis. Surg. Gynecol. Obstet. 110:109, 1960.
9. DuPlessis, D.J. Gastric mucosa changes after operations on the stomach. S. Afr. Med. J. 36:471, 1962.
10. Fell, S.C., Seindenberg, B., Hurwitt, E.S. Ischemic necrosis of the gastric remnant: An uncommon complication of radical subtotal gastrectomy. Surgery 43:490, 1958.
11. Fromm, D. Complications of gastric surgery. Wiley, New York, 1977.
12. Fromm, D. Ulceration of the stomach and duodenum. In Fromm, D. Gastrointestinal surgery. P. 233. Churchill Livingstone, New York, 1985.
13. Gray, H.M.W. A cause of intestinal obstruction after gastroenterostomy. Lancet 2:526, 1904.
14. Griffith, C.A. Anatomy. In Nyhus, L.M., Wastell, C. (Eds.) Surgery of the stomach and duodenum. Ed. 3, p. 41. Little, Brown, Boston, 1977.
15. Hardy, J.D. Problems associated with gastric surgery: A review of 604 consecutive patients with annotation.
16. Hardy, J.D. Complications of gastric surgery. In Artz, C.P., Hardy, J.D. (eds.) Management of surgical complications, Ed. 3, p. 445. W.B. Saunders, Philadelphia, 1975.
17. Herrington, J.L. Jr. Experiences with the surgical management of the afferent loop syndrome. Ann. Surg. 164:797, 1966.
18. Herrington, J.L. Jr., Sawyers, J.L. Remedial operations. In Nyhus, L.M., Wastell, C. (Eds.) Surgery of the stomach and duodenum. Ed. 3, p. 537. Little, Brown, Boston, 1977.
19. Herrington, J.L. Jr., Sawyers, J.L. Complications following gastric operations. In Schwartz, S.I., Ellis, H. (Eds.) Maingot's abdominal operations. Ed. 9, vol. I, p. 701. Appleton Lange, Norwalk, CT, 1990.
20. Jackson, P.P. Ischemic necrosis of the proximal gastric remnant following sub-total gastrectomy. Ann. Surg. 150:1071, 1959.
21. Jordan, G.L. Jr. The afferent loop syndrome. Surgery 38:1027, 1955.
22. Iordan, G.L. Jr. The post-gastrectomy syndromes. J.A.M.A. 163: 1485, 1957.
23. Lawson, H.H. Effect of duodenal contents on the gastric mucosa under experimental conditions. Lancet 1:469, 1964.
24. Lygidakis, N.J. The value of revisional surgery for the treatment of post-operative alkaline reflux gastritis. World J. Surg. 6:226, 1982.
25. Markowitz, A.M. Internal hernia after gastrojejunostomy. Surgery 49:185, 1961.
26. Mimpris, T.W., Birt, S.J.N.C. Results of partial gastrectomy for peptic ulcer. Br. Med. J. 2:1095, 1948.
27. Mix, C.L. Dumping stomach following gastrojejunostomy. Surg. Clin. North Am. 2:617, 1922.
28. Morton, C.B., Alrich, E.M., Hill, L.D. Internal hernia after gastrectomy. Ann. Surg. 141:759, 1955.
29. Nissen, R. Die resektion die tiefsintzenden duodenal geschwürs. Zentralbl. Chir. 60:483, 1933.
30. Pearse, C.W., Jordan, G.L. Jr., De Bakey, M.E. Intra-abdominal complications following distal subtotal gastrectomy for benign gastroduodenal ulceration. Surgery 42:447, 1957.
31. Phillips, R.B., Child, W.A. Post-gastrectomy hemorrhage. Ann. Surg. 95:411; 1958.
32. Robb, H.J., Nickel, W.O. Surgery in post-gastrectomy bleeding. Surgery 42:474, 1957.
33. Rodgers, J.B. Infarction of the gastric remnant following subtotal gastrectomy. Arch. Surg. 92:917, 1966.
34. Rutledge, R.H. Retroanastomotic hernia after gastrojejunal anastomosis. Ann. Surg. 177:547, 1971.
35. Rutter, A.G. Ischemic necrosis of the stomach following subtotal gastrectomy. Lancet 2:1021, 1953.
36. Soupault, R., Bucaille, M. La transplantation au duodénum de l'anse efférente. Operation corrective de certains troubles des gastrectomies subtotales. Presse Méd. 63:27, 1955
37. Spencer, F.C. Ischemic necrosis of remaining stomach following subtotal gastrectomy. Arch. Surg. 73:844, 1956.
38. Stammers, F.A.R. Remarks on fifteen cases of small-bowel obstruction following antecolic partial gastrectomy and one case following retrocolic partial gastrectomy. Br. J. Surg. 42:34, 1954.
39. Wells, C.A., Welbourn, R.B. Post-gastrectomy syndromes: A study in applied physiology. Br. Med. J. 1:546, 1951

Section F

Surgery of the Stomach and Duodenum

CHAPTER 36

Surgical Treatment of Gastric Diverticula

Gastric diverticula are infrequently seen. It is quite probable that the thickness of the muscular part of the gastric wall is a barrier in their development (5, 7, 8). Even though gastric diverticula are really infrequent, improved radiologic and endoscopic means of examination allow the diagnosis of diverticula to be made with greater frequency. From the structural point of view gastric diverticula are made up of all layers of the gastric wall and are therefore true diverticula (10, 11). The great majority of gastric diverticula are asymptomatic, and surgery is rarely necessary except for acute diverticulitis or for bleeding (9, 11). Most diverticula are located high in the posterior gastric wall, near the cardia, with the diverticulum emptying more frequently near the greater than the lesser curvature (1, 4, 7, 8, 10).

The surgical procedure to be carried out for gastric diverticula must be adapted to their localization.

The most frequently used surgical procedure for gastric diverticula is resection of the diverticulum with immediate two-layer closure of the residual opening. Some surgeons prefer to invaginate the diverticulum into the gastric lumen, closing the defect in the gastric wall in two layers (10).

In the few cases in which the diverticulum is located in the pyloric region, gastric resection should be done, especially if the diverticulum is complicated by a stenosis of the pylorus or coexists with a gastric or duodenal ulcer (2, 4, 10, 12).

The surgical procedure to be described in the following corresponds to a complicated diverticulum localized in the upper part of the posterior wall of the stomach, which is its most frequent location.

Surgical Technique

FIGURE 36.1

A midline xiphoumbilical incision is made. In patients with diverticula located high in the posterior gastric wall, it is useful to remove the xiphoid process to be able to extend the incision upward so as to attain deeper exposure. The entire abdominal cavity should be explored first, to exclude the possibility of some other cause for the symptoms that have been attributed to the diverticulum. The next step is identification of the diverticulum. Since most diverticula are located high in the posterior wall of the stomach, as in this case, identification of the diverticulum can be done by palpation. If the diverticulum cannot be identified by palpation, the stomach should be compressed, with both hands, to fill it with air and fluid, making it palpable (10). If this maneuver is not successful, air can be injected through a nasogastric Levine tube after an atraumatic clamp is placed across the gastric antrum. If the diverticulum is still not demonstrable, physiologic saline solution can be injected through the Levine tube to fill the diverticulum.

Once identified, the diverticulum has to be exposed so that it can be resected. For this purpose the left half of the gastroepiploic ligament is divided outside the gastroepiploic arcade together with all the gastrosplenic ligament and short gastric vessels. To make the posterior wall of the gastric fundus more accessible, it is convenient to divide the gastrophrenic ligament. The greater curvature is grasped with two Duval clamps and traction applied to the right, exposing the posterior wall of the stomach, where a 7-cm-long diverticulum is seen. It is 4 cm wide transversely near its fundus and 2.5 cm wide at its neck. There are extensive peridiverticular adhesions to the gastric wall due to peridiverticular inflammation. The insert shows the location and direction of the diverticulum with its fundus directed downward and its ostium directed upward near the cardia.

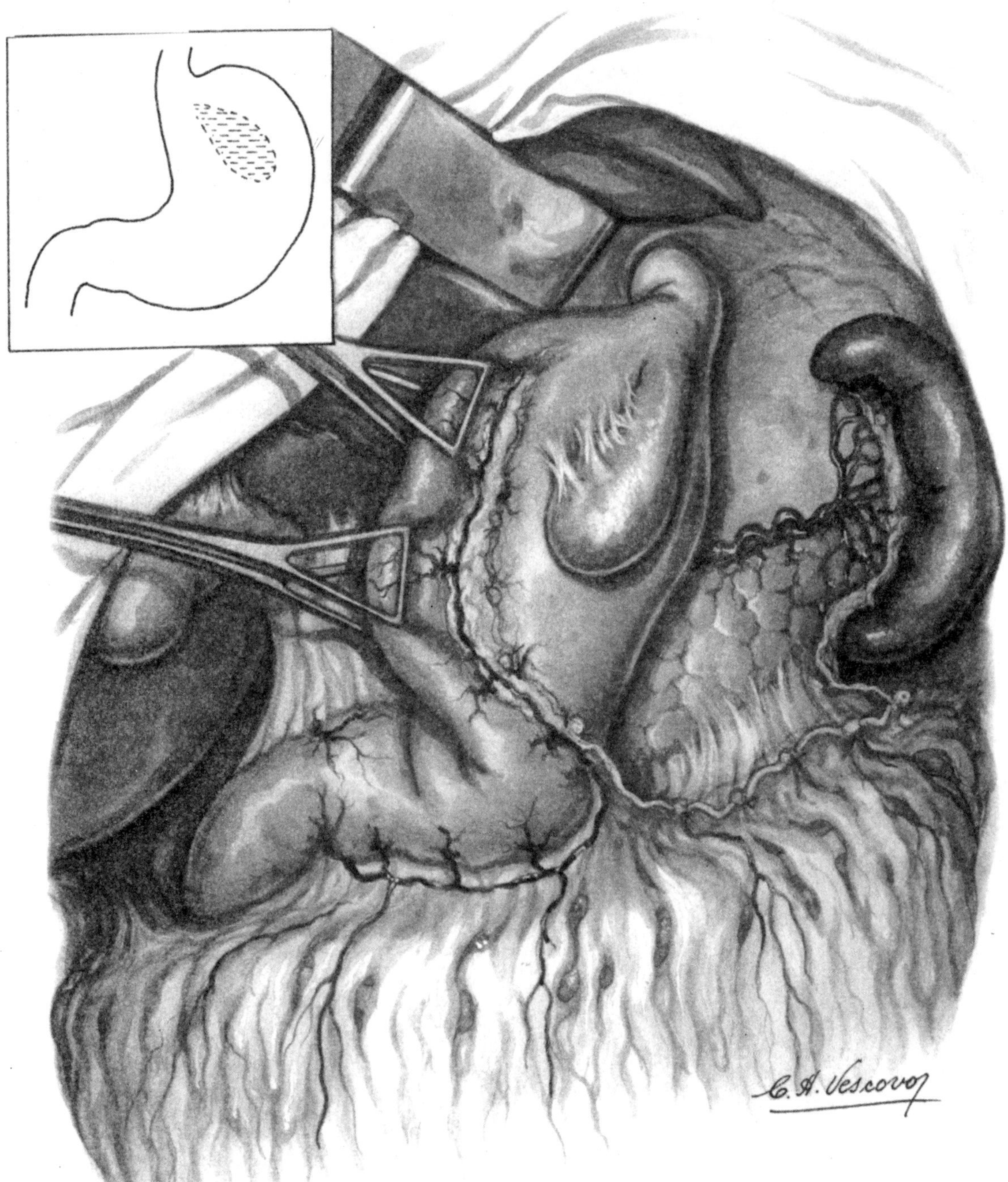

FIGURE 36.1

Surgical Technique

FIGURE 36.2
Using straight Mayo scissors the diverticulum is being resected while it is being held up with a Babcock clamp, the adhesions binding it to the stomach having been divided. To facilitate resection of the diverticulum, two seromuscular sutures have been placed near the posterior gastric wall and traction has been applied to them in opposite directions. A small segment of the gastric wall surrounding the diverticulum should be resected with it to make closure of the gastric wall easier.

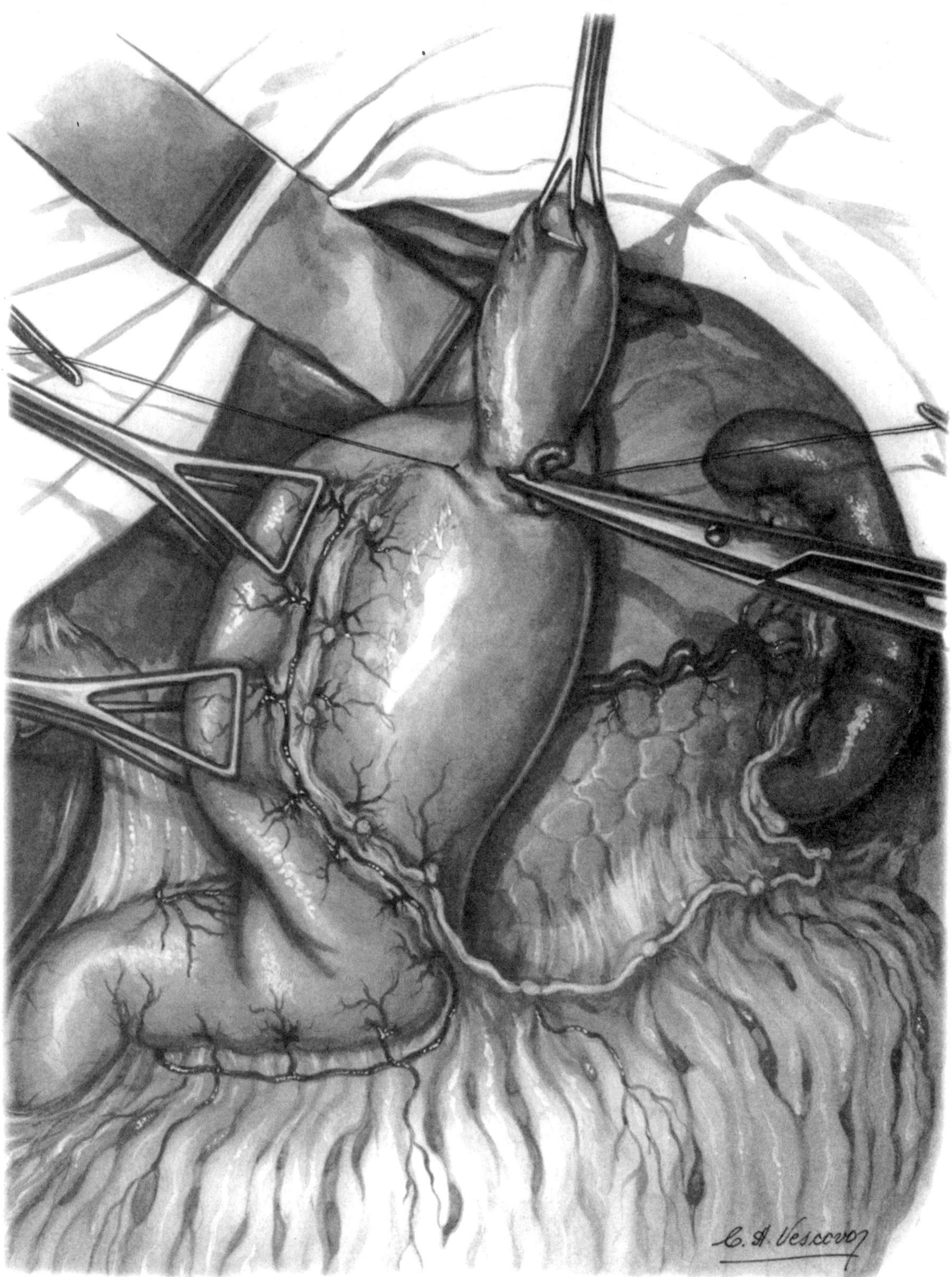

FIGURE 36.2

FIGURE 36.3
The diverticulum has been resected and the gastric mucosa is being closed with interrupted 2-0 chromic catgut sutures.

Surgical Technique

FIGURE 36.4
Once the mucosal layer is closed, the seromuscular layer is closed with interrupted cotton, silk, or nonabsorbable synthetic interrupted sutures.

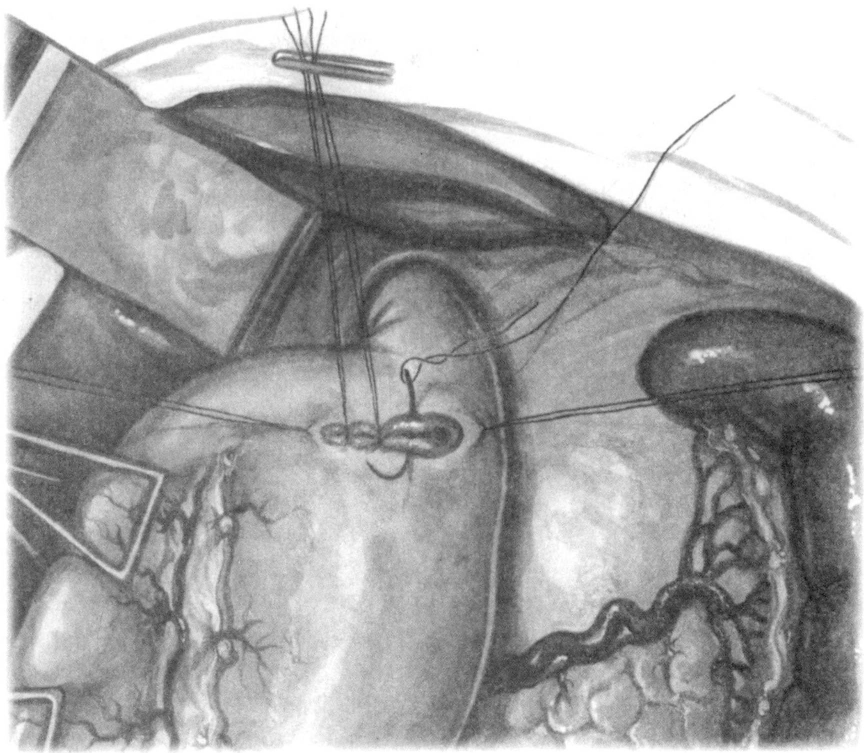

FIGURE 36.3

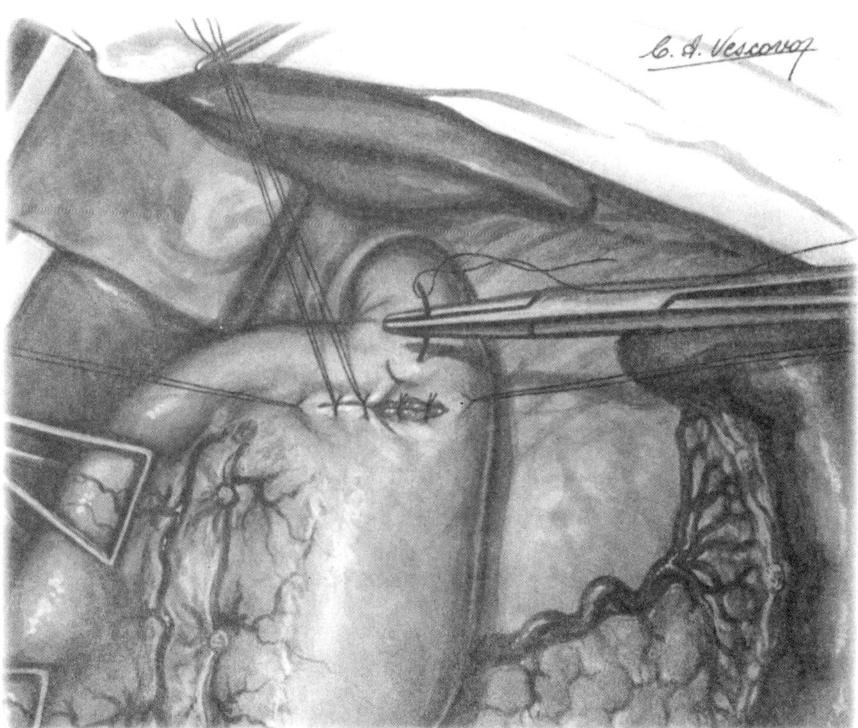

FIGURE 36.4

References

1. Big, R.L., Judd, E.S. Gastric diverticula. Am. J. Surg. 105:239, 1963.
2. Cosman, B., Kellum, J., Kingsbury, H. Gastric diverticula and massive gastrointestinal hemorrhage. Am. J. Surg. 94:144, 1957.
3. Dragomiresco, L., Freschin, D., Paun, C., Bandila, T.R. Deux cas de diverticule gastric invaginé dans l'esophage. J. Chir. 86:192, 1963.
4. Ellis, H. Diverticula of the stomach and duodenum. In Schwartz, S.I., Ellis, H. (eds) Maingot's abdominal operations. Ed. 9, vol. 1, p. 575. Appleton Lange, Norwalk, CT, 1990.
5. Finochietto, R. Divertículos gástricos. Pren. Med. Argent. 47:1860, 1960.
6. Heijboer, M.P., Nieuwenhuizen, L.N. Gastric diverticula. Neth. J. Surg. 32:16, 1980.
7. Mallet-Guy, P., Marion, P. Le traitement chirurgical des diverticles sous cardiaques de l'estomac. J. Chir. 57:466, 1947.
8. Meeroff, M., Gollan, J.R.M. Gastric diverticulum. Am. J. Gastroenterol. 47:189, 1967.
9. Palmer, E.D. Gastric diverticula. A collective review. Surg. Gynecol. Obstet. 92:417, 1951.
10. Puig-Massana, M. Divertículos gástricos. In Pi-Figueras, J. (Ed.) Práctica quirúrgica. Ed. 2, vol. 2, p. 68. Salvat, Barcelona, 1986.
11. Rivers, A. B., Stevens, G.A., Kirklin, B.R. Diverticula of stomach. Surg. Gynecol. Obstet. 60:106, 1935.
12. Young, H.B. Juxta-oesophageal diverticula of the stomach. Br. J. Surg. 50:150, 1962.

Section F

Surgery of the Stomach and Duodenum

CHAPTER **37**

Surgery for Benign Gastric Tumors

Benign gastric tumors are not very frequent, comprising slightly less than 2% of all gastric neoplasms (1, 8, 10, 11, 18, 25). The majority of benign tumors are asymptomatic and are discovered in double contrast radiographic or endoscopic examinations for some other condition. Polyps are sometimes found during surgical exploration of the stomach for some other pathologic process (7, 10, 13). In some cases they are found when the stomach is opened after resection for carcinoma in another part of the stomach or near the carcinoma (8, 13, 18). Gastric polyps can also be findings of carefully performed autopsies (1, 8, 10, 11, 13, 18, 20, 25). Benign gastric tumors become symptomatic when they develop complications, such as ulceration and hemorrhage from the mucosa on the surface of the polyp, or in cases of obstruction due to a pedunculated antral polyp prolapsing through the pylorus into the duodenum. Prolapse can also occur in cases of sessile polyps carried by peristaltic contractions. In recent years more benign gastric tumors have been diagnosed because of improvement in radiographic techniques and increase in frequency and precision of gastroscopic studies (1, 6, 8).

MEANING OF THE TERM POLYP

Polyp comes from the Greek *polypus*, which means "many feet." This name and that of polypoid tumors are used to designate any tumor formation that protrudes into the gastric lumen with a tendency to form a pedicle. The term "polyp" does not distinguish between benign or malignant tumors, or of epithelial, mesenchymal, or hamartomatous origin, referring only to the macroscopic appearance of the tumor and not to its pathology. We will only refer here to tumors strictly of epithelial origin (8, 10, 11).

CLASSIFICATION OF BENIGN GASTRIC TUMORS

As previously stated, benign tumors are not frequent, but exact knowledge about them is of great importance because there are significant differences in their behavior due to varying malignant potential.

Surgeons or gastroenterologists must always be aware of the different pathologic and evolutionary characteristics of benign gastric tumors so that they can recommend the most appropriate treatment in each case. One of the most frequently used classification of benign tumors establishes two groups of benign tumors according to their origin: (a) benign epithelial tumors and (b) benign nonepithelial tumors. Benign tumors of nonepithelial origin are designated by some authors (6, 8, 11) as intramural tumors, the great majority of which are localized in the submucosa. Tumors of nonepithelial origin are also frequently designated as mesenchymatous, which is not exactly correct. Tumors of mesenchymatous origin include leiomyomas, which are undoubtedly the most frequent, fibromas, neurogenic tumors, lipomas, and vascular tumors. Nonepithelial or intramural tumors also include a heterogenous group:

1. Heterotopic pancreas.
2. Inflammatory tumors, which are really pseudotumors.
3. Peutz-Jeghers tumors.
4. Hamartomas.

Benign Tumors of Epithelial Origin

Two different types of tumors should be distinguished within this group. They have similar macroscopic appearance but different histology and malignant potential: hyperplastic polyps and adenomatous polyps.

Hyperplastic polyps, also called regenerative, inflammatory polyps (6, 11, 17, 20), represent 75% of polyps of epithelial origin, constituting the most frequent group of polyps of epithelial origin (6, 7, 20). Hyperplastic polyps are benign and have no malignant potential. These tumors are usually less than 2 cm in size and are just as common in the antrum as in the body of the stomach. Most of them are sessile, and less frequently they have a pedicle. Because they are sessile, it is more difficult to remove them endoscopically. Hyperplastic polyps are single or multiple. Even though they are benign and have no malignant potential, they can coexist with gastric carcinoma, located in some other portion of the gastric mucosa, in 29% of cases (8, 17, 25).

From the microscopic point of view, hyperplastic polyps are the result of glandular proliferation with cystic formations. The polyp is generally covered by epithelium similar to the epithelium of the mucosa surrounding the polyp.

Hyperplastic gastric polyps can appear in patients with familiar polyposis of the colon. In these cases the polyps are limited to the gastric body (11, 20). Familiar colonic polyposis can also be accompanied by lymphoid gastric polyps or even adenomatous gastric polyps. These polyps are usually localized in the antrum and duodenum, in contrast with hyperplastic polyps, which are generally localized in the gastric body. It is exceptional that these polyps, which coexist with familiar colonic polyposis, be they hyperplastic, lymphoid, or adenomatous, end in cancer (11).

Diffuse gastric polyposis can be due to either hyperplastic or adenomatous polyps. Hyperplastic polyposis will not degenerate in malignancy, diffuse hyperplasia is one of the forms of Menetrier's disease. Adenomatous polyposis can degenerate in cancer (10, 11, 17, 25).

Adenomatous polyps are much less frequent than hyperplastic polyps and usually larger. They can be sessile or pedunculated, with a tendency to be more frequent in the antrum than in other parts of the stomach. They are more commonly single than multiple. Adenomatous polyps, in contrast with hyperplastic polyps, coexist with gastric carcinoma in another part of the stomach in 59% of cases (11, 25).

Adenomatous polyps are premalignant lesions, especially when they are over 2 cm in size. Malignant change is more frequent in sessile polyps than in the pedunculated polyps.

Small pedunculated polyps are frequently benign. When adenomatous polyps are over 2 cm in size, the presence of malignant degeneration should be suspected. It should be pointed out, however, that this does not mean that all adenomatous polyps larger than 2 cm are malignant, since many of them are benign in spite of their size. According to Tomasulo (25), 24% of adenomatous polyps 2 cm or more in size show malignant degeneration whereas adenomatous polyps smaller than 2 cm are malignant in only 4% of cases. On the other hand, adenomatous polyps over 2 cm in size show dysplasia, carcinoma in situ, or invasive carcinoma more frequently (23).

Achlorhydria is present in 85% of patients with gastric polyps. At the same time achlorhydric patients have a greater tendency to have polyps. Polyps are more frequent in patients with atrophic gastritis, pernicious anemia, and gastric cancer.

Microscopically, adenomatous polyps are made up of basophilic cells, arranged in tubules, secreting very little or no mucus, and with small nuclei in the base of the cell.

Surgical Treatment of Gastric Polyps of Epithelial Origin

All polyps should be biopsied endoscopically. The entire stomach should be explored in search of a gastric carcinoma, which, as was stated previously, can coexist with adenomatous or hyperplastic polyps (although in different ratios) in another part of the stomach. The polyp should be removed entirely endoscopically and immediately examined microscopically to apply the best treatment. If the polyp is hyperplastic, treatment is complete with endoscopic excision. If the polyp is a benign adenomatous polyp, excision completes the treatment. If the polyp shows carcinoma in situ, meaning no invasion of the muscularis mucosa, many gastroenterologists or surgeons will periodically reexamine the patient radiologically and endoscopically to detect possible recurrences. The author prefers to carry out a gastrectomy to offer more security to the patient. With more reason, the author adopts the same attitude when the resected adenomatous polyp shows invasive carcinoma (surpassing the muscularis mucosa). Surgical intervention should be carried out in cases in which endoscopy has been unable to determine whether the polyp is benign or malignant, as well as when the polyp cannot be resected completely. Surgical resection should also be performed in sessile polyps 2 cm or larger in size, as well as in polyps that are not accessible for endoscopic resection.

Surgical resection of gastric polyps is done through a gastrotomy. Gastrotomy, which has been previously described, is done through a longitudinal incision in the anterior wall of the stomach. Gastrotomy should be avoided in the greater curvature, at the junction of the proximal and middle thirds, since the gastric pacemaker is located there (11, 14). If the polyp is localized in the gastric fundus, where exploration and resection may be difficult, the surgeon can invert the fundus, using his right hand to make the polyp more accessible and easier to resect. This maneuver must be done with care to avoid injuring the splenic capsule or a short vessel. If necessary, the short vessels can be divided and ligated to facilitate the maneuver.

Once the stomach has been completely explored, the polyp is completely resected with a safe margin of mucosa round it. Frozen section examination of the polyp will determine its nature and the presence or absence of malignant degeneration so the correct treatment can be carried out. Patients with multiple polyps, not with diffuse polyposis, localized in the distal half of the stomach should be treated by a distal gastrectomy of 50 to 75%. If some polyps were to still remain proximally, they should be removed and examined microscopically. Definitive treatment should be adapted to the results of this examination.

Symptomatic gastric polyps, complicated by hemorrhage or obstruction, can be resected endoscopically, if possible, and subjected to pathologic examination to determine their nature. In case of profuse bleeding it is more convenient to resect them surgically. The same is true in antral polyps that have prolapsed into the duodenum.

Benign Tumors of Nonepithelial Origin

The most common nonepithelial benign tumor is the leiomyoma, whose size varies from millimeters to various centimeters in diameter. Its most common location is in the gastric antrum, although it may be found in any area of the stomach. Leiomyomas develop more frequently toward the gastric mucosa, which they frequently ulcerate, possibly leading to hemorrhage. Less frequently they develop toward the serosa or remain localized in the muscular layer itself.

Endoscopic biopsy of leiomyomas, and of all submucosal tumors in general, is unsure and difficult, even with perfect technique. It has been shown that there is only a 40 to 50% chance of a positive biopsy in leiomyomas with ulcerated gastric mucosa (11).

Treatment of leiomyomas can be performed endoscopically if the tumor grows toward the mucosa and is not large. Careful examination of the resected specimen will help determine if the tumor has been removed completely. Treatment of leiomyomas is safer when done surgically by gastrectomy or a local gastric resection. Enucleation of leiomyomas is not advisable, except in some circumstances, since these tumors do not have a capsule. Enucleation can be indicated in leiomyomas of the fundus or cardia with the object of avoiding a very complex and risky operation. On the other hand, some leiomyomas can appear benign grossly but histologic examination may reveal many mitoses, making at least a local resection advisable (11).

In leiomyomas localized on the lesser curvature of the stomach that must be resected, care should be taken not to divide the nerve of Latarjet so that the antral innervation will remain intact.

If the tumor is large and located in the distal half of the stomach, gastrectomy is the indicated procedure.

Operative Technique

FIGURE 37.1 SURGICAL REMOVAL OF A PEDUNCULATED GASTRIC POLYP

A longitudinal gastrotomy has been made in the anterior gastric wall. Exploration of the interior of the stomach has been negative for other lesion. The 18-mm pedunculated polyp is pulled upward with a Babcock clamp. A circle around the pedicle marks the extent of gastric mucosa that is to be removed for a greater margin of security. The resected polyp and surrounding mucosa are delivered to the pathologist for frozen section examination. The mucosa is closed with interrupted reabsorbable synthetic sutures while the specimen is evaluated. The pathologist has reported the polyp as completely benign, so the gastrotomy is closed in two layers.

Exploratory gastrotomy should be avoided in cases where the polyps are suspicious for malignancy. If this exploration is necessary, because of lack of sure data, the operative field should be carefully walled off to prevent implantation of cells from the malignant polyp. If the endoscopic biopsy proves the polyp malignant preoperatively, a gastric resection should be done without a gastrotomy for exploration.

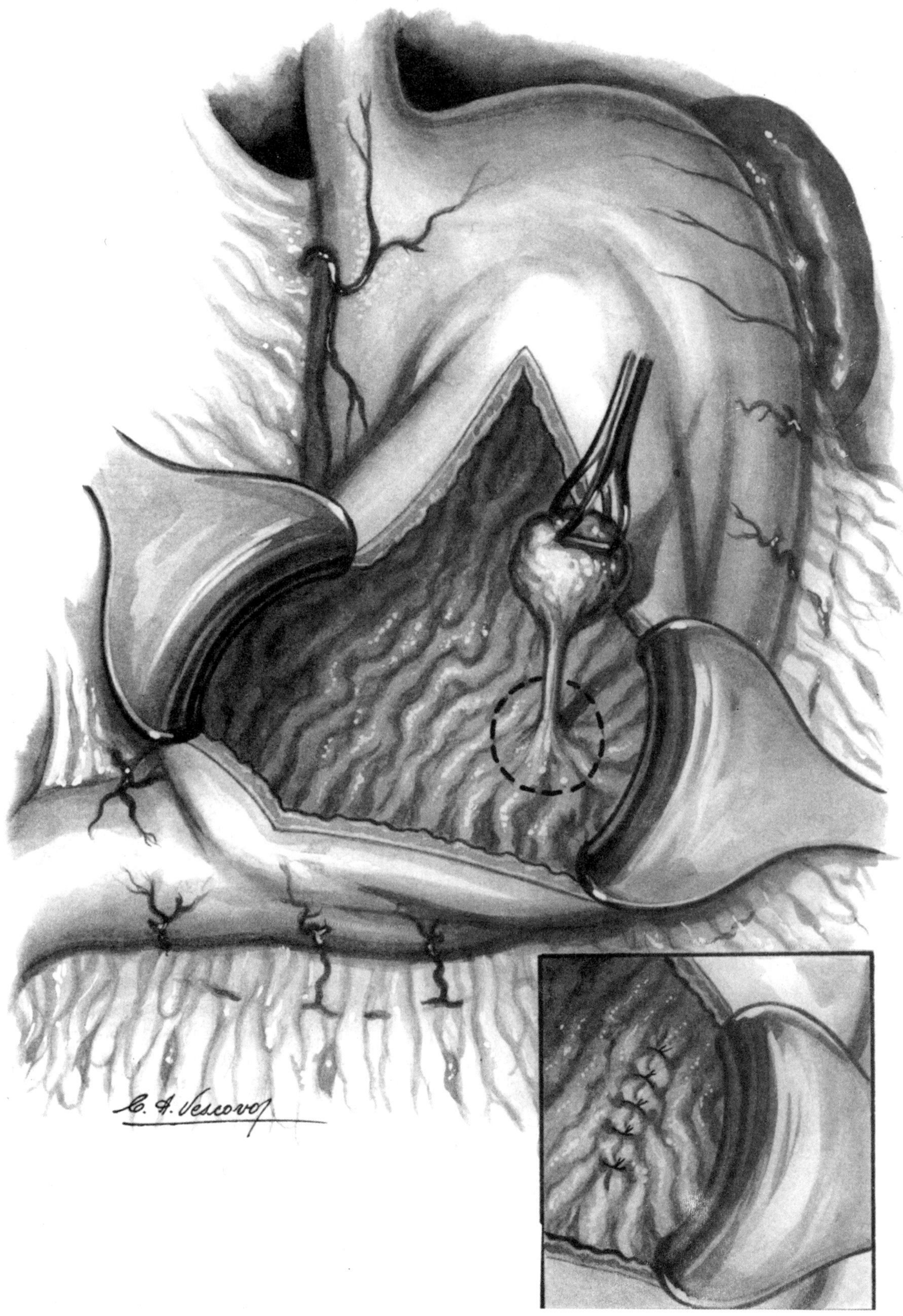

FIGURE 37.1 SURGICAL REMOVAL OF A PEDUNCULATED GASTRIC POLYP

Operative Technique

FIGURE 37.2
Local gastric resection for a sessile polyp in the proximal third of the stomach. A longitudinal gastrotomy has been made, showing the presence of a sessile polyp 15 mm in diameter located high in the posterior wall of the gastric body. The appearance of the polyp suggested malignancy, so the operation was discontinued and the gastrotomy closed with two layers of sutures.

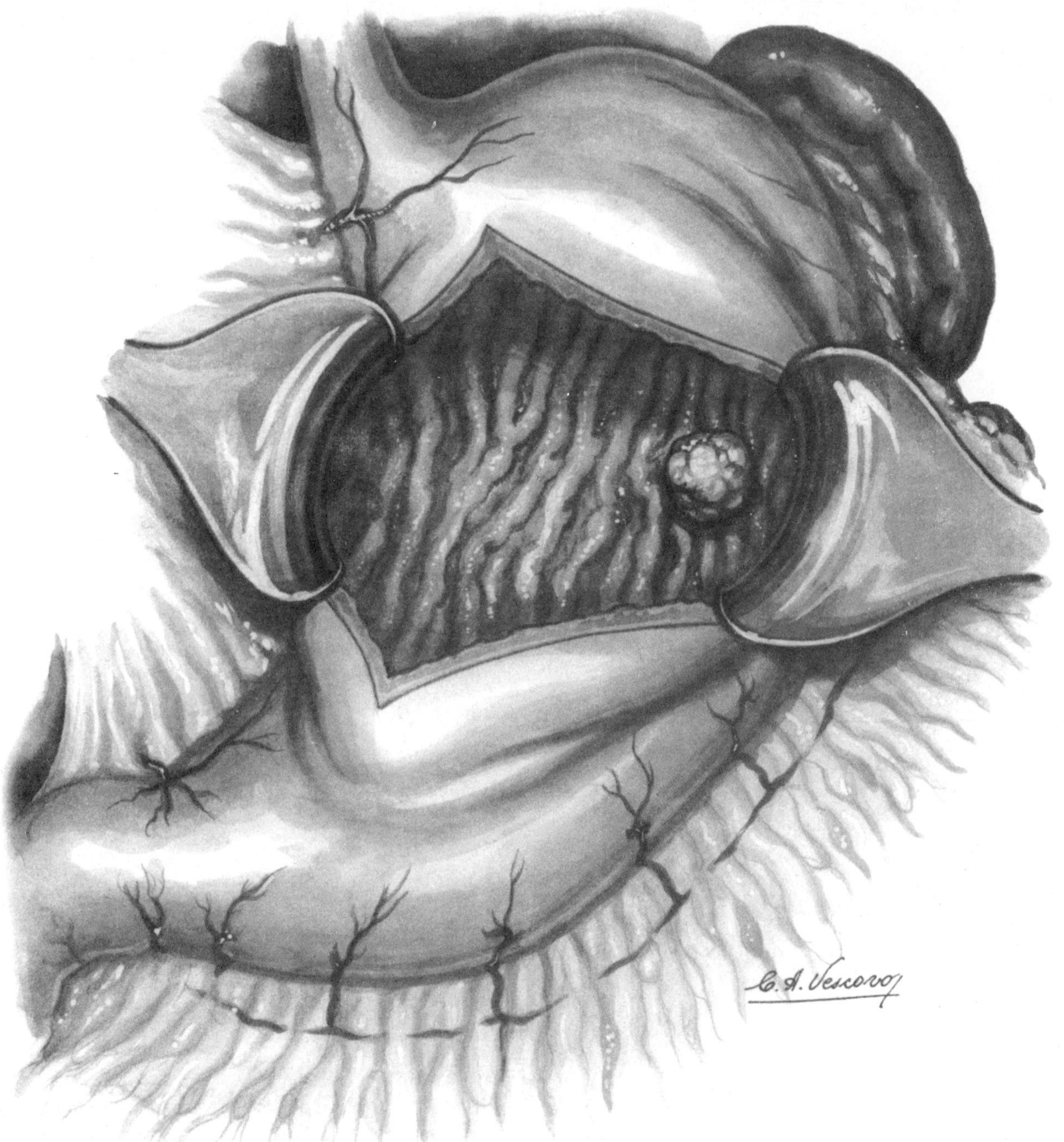

FIGURE 37.2

Operative Technique

FIGURE 37.3
The gastrotomy has been closed and the greater curvature of the stomach has been freed in the area where the polyp is located so that two atraumatic clamps can be placed, as shown, and so that a local gastric resection, including the sessile polyp, can be performed, to submit the polyp to frozen section study.

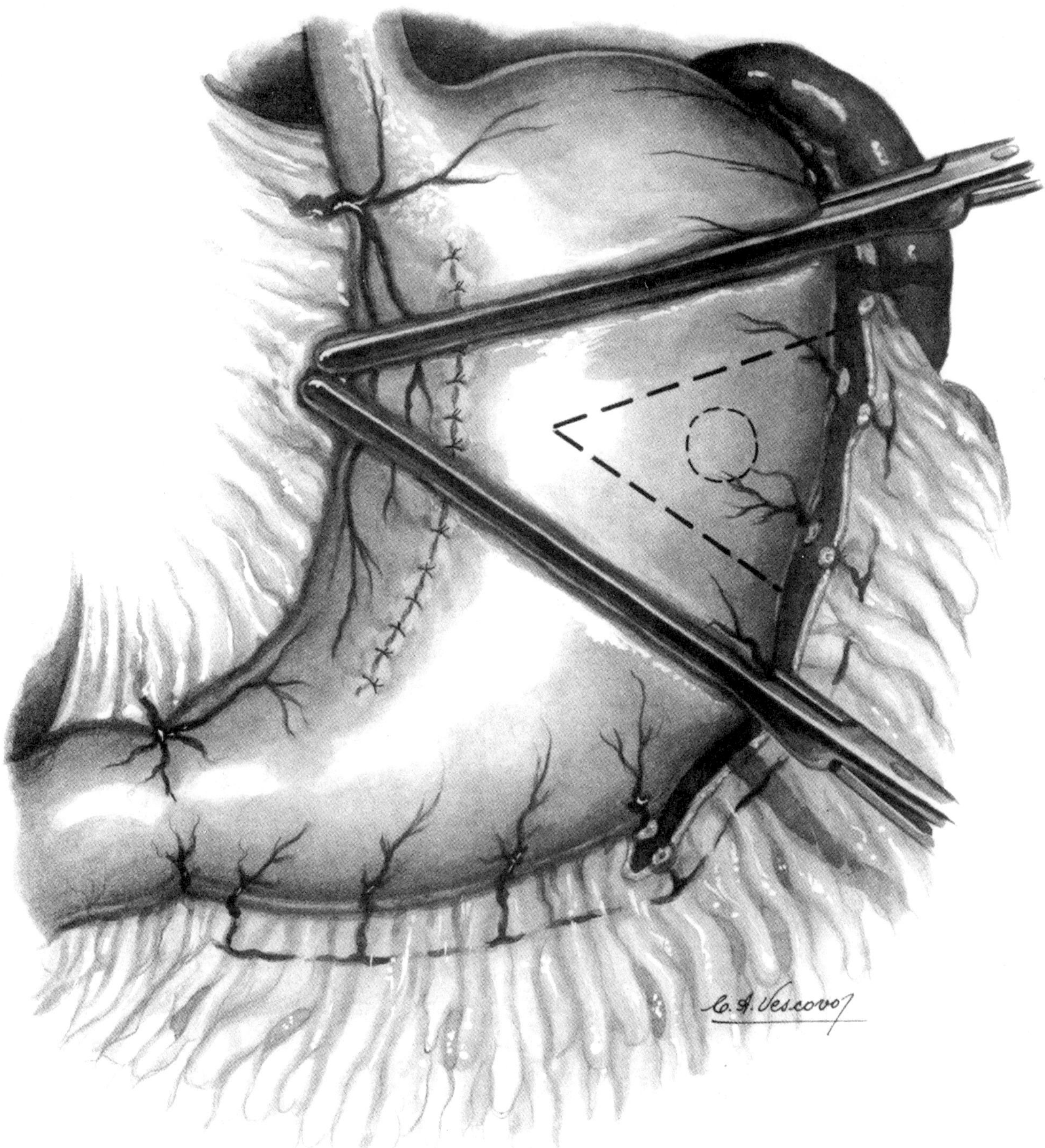

FIGURE 37.3

Operative Technique

FIGURE 37.4
The microscopic examination revealed that the polyp was hyperplastic, so the stomach was closed in two layers of sutures.

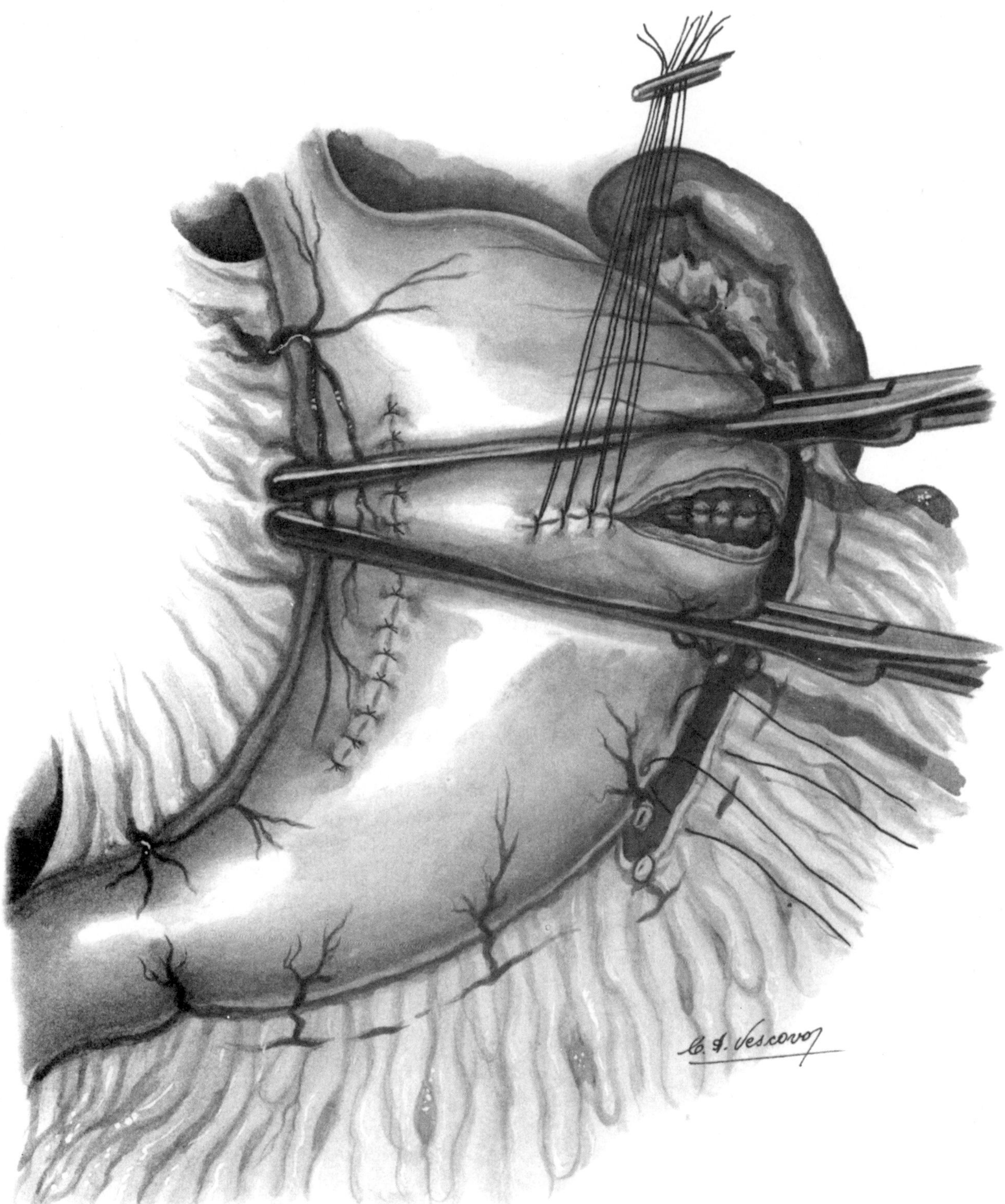

FIGURE 37.4

Operative Technique

FIGURE 37.5
Local gastric resection to remove a subserous gastric leiomyoma. A, The broken line shows where the gastric walls will be transected to remove the leiomyoma. B and C show the gastric closure after resection confirmed the lesion to be a leiomyoma.

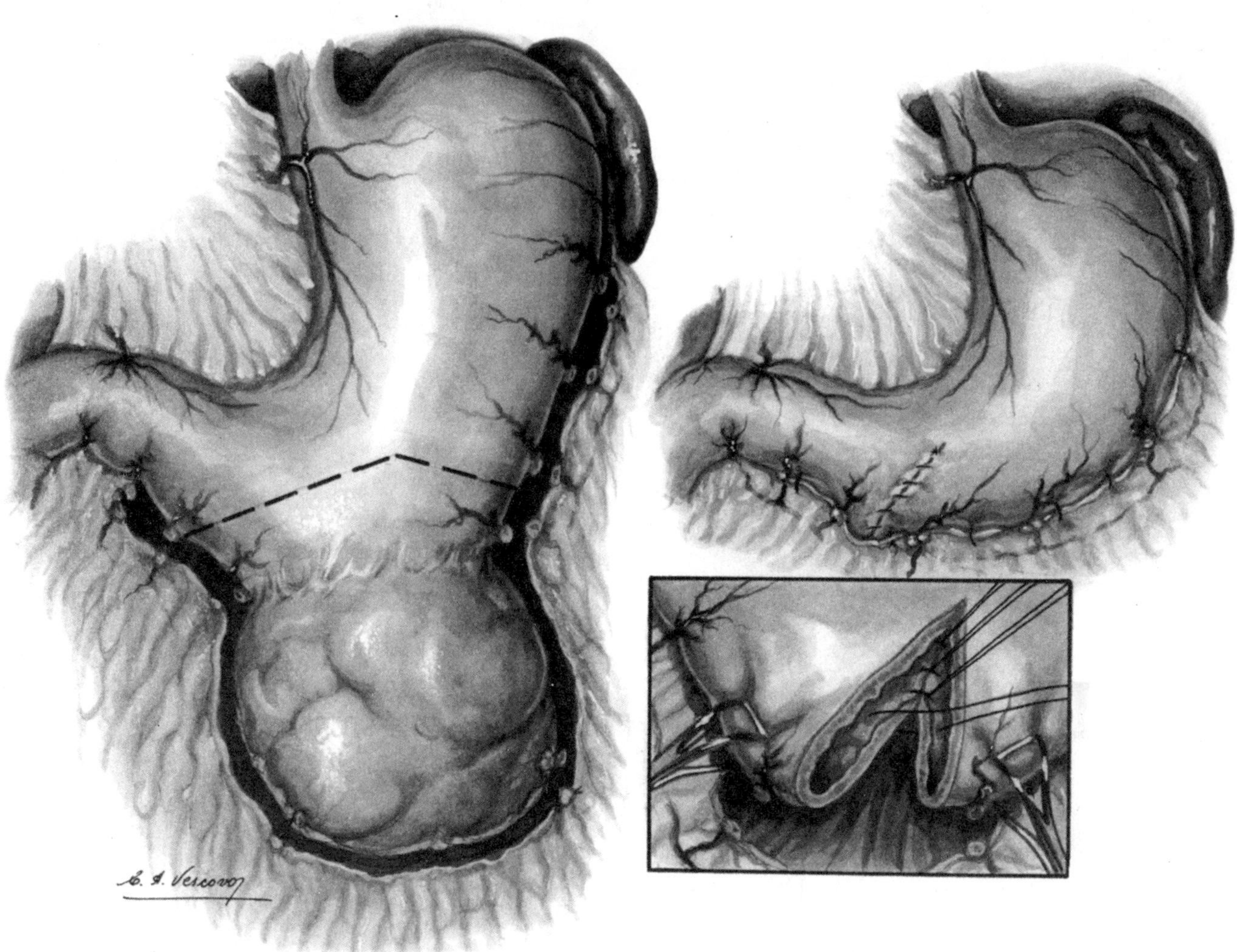

FIGURE 37.5

Operative Technique

FIGURE 37.6
Enucleation of an actively bleeding 2-cm leiomyoma on the posterior wall of the fundus. The best surgical treatment of leiomyomas is gastric resection. In cases where the leiomyoma is small and located in the fundus or near the cardia an enucleation can be performed to avoid a complex and risky procedure. **A,** The location of the ulcerated bleeding leiomyoma. The line of incision of the gastric mucosa is shown by the broken line. **B,** The leiomyoma is being dissected out with scissors. Resection by enucleation can be laborious because leiomyomas do not have a capsule. **C,** Once the tumor is removed, its bed is sutured and the gastrotomy closed in two layers.

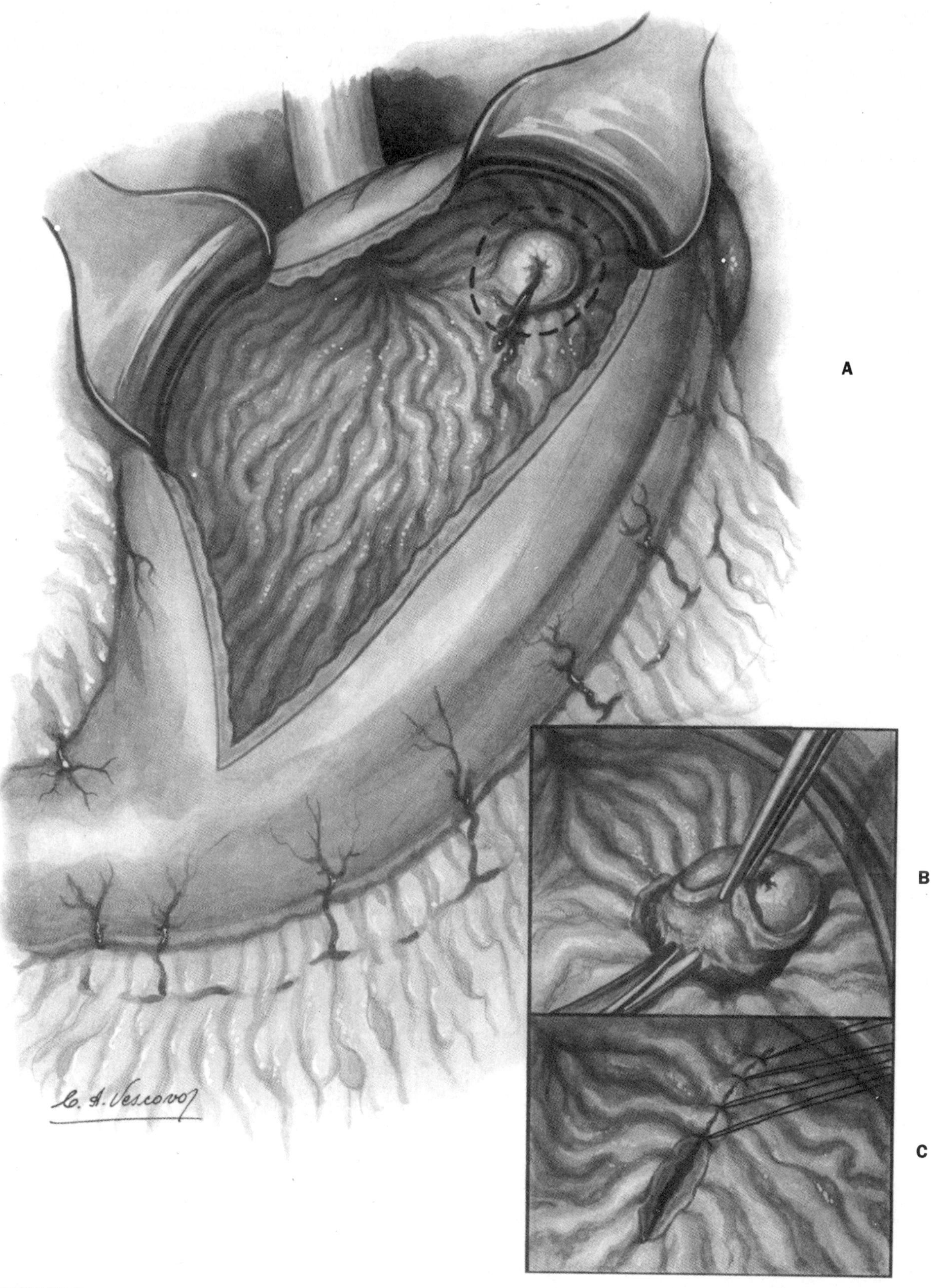

FIGURE 37.6

References

1. Akwari, O.E. Benign tumors of the stomach. In Sabiston, D.C. Jr. (Ed.) Ed. 14, p. 787. W.B. Saunders, Philadelphia, 1991.
2. Berg, J.W. Histological aspects of the relation between gastric adenomatous polyps and gastric cancer. Cancer 11:149, 1958.
3. Carey, J.B., Hay, L. Gastric polyps. Symposium. Gastroenterology 14:280, 1950.
4. Carlson, E., Ward, J.G. Surgical consideration in gastric polyps, gastric polyposis and giant hypertrophic gastritis in 74 cases. Surg. Gynecol. Obstet. 107:727, 1958.
5. Classen, M., Demling, L. Operative Gastroskopie fiberendoskische polypenabtragung im magen. Dtsch. Med. Wschr. 96:1466, 1971.
6. Debray, C., Veyne, S. Les tumeurs bénignes gastriques. Clinique, Radiology, Endoscopie. Actual. Hôtel Dieu 2:36, 1966.
7. Deppisch, L.M., Rona, V.T. Gastric epithelial polyps: A 10-years study. J. Clin. Gastroenterol. 11:110, 1989.
8. Edis, A.J. Benign tumors of the stomach. In Maingot, R. (Ed.) Abdominal operations. Ed. 7, vol. 1, p. 582. Appleton Century Crofts, New York, 1980.
9. Eliason, E.L., Wright, V.W.M. Benign tumors of the stomach. Surg. Gynecol. Obstet. 41:461, 1925.
10. Eklöff, O., Eriksson, E., Sahlin, O. Benign epithelial tumors of the stomach and duodenum. Acta Chir. Scand. 255:1, 1960.
11. Fromm, D. Benign Tumors. In Fromm, D. Gastrointestinal surgery Vol. I, p. 366. Churchill Livingstone, New York, 1985.
12. Hay, L.J. Polyps and adenomas of the stomach. Surgery 33:446, 1953.
13. Huppler, E.G., Priestley, J.T., Marlock, C.G., et al. Diagnosis and results of treatment in gastric polyps. Surg. Gynecol. Obstet. 110:309, 1960.
14. Kelly, K.A., Code, C.F. Canine gastric pacemaker. Am. J. Physiol. 220:112, 1971.
15. Kleinhaus, V., Weich, L.Y., Maoz, S. Gastroduodenal intussusception secondary to prolapsing gastric tumors. Gastrointest. Radiol 11:229, 1986.
16. Marshall, S.F. Gastric tumors other than carcinoma. Surg. Clin. America 35:693, 1955.
17. Ming, S.C., Goldman, H. Gastric polyps: Histogenetic classification and its relation to carcinoma. Cancer 18:721, 1965.
18. Monaco, A.P., Roth, S.I., Castleman, B., Welch, C. Adenomatous polyps of the stomach. Cancer 15:456, 1962.
19. Morgan, B.K., Compton, C., Talbert, M., Gallagher, W.J., Wood, W.C. Benign smooth muscle tumors of the gastrointestinal tract. Ann. Surg. 211:63, 1990.
20. Morson, B.C. Gastric polyps composed of intestinal epithelium. Br. J. Cancer 9:550, 1959.
21. Palmer, E.D. Benign intramural tumors of the stomach. Medicine 30:81, 1951.
22. Rosin, R.D. Tumours of the stomach. In Schwartz, S.I., Ellis, H. (Eds.) Maingot's abdominal operations. Ed. 9, vol. 1, p. 679. Appleton Lange, Norwalk, CT, 1990.
23. Seifert, E., Gail, K., Weismuller, J. Gastric polypectomy. Endoscopy 15:8, 1985.
24. Stout, A.P. Bizarre smooth muscle tumors of the stomach. Cancer 15:400, 1962.
25. Tomasulo, J. Gastric polyps: Histologic types and their relationship to gastric carcinoma. Cancer 27:346, 1971.

Section F
Surgery of the Stomach and Duodenum

CHAPTER 38
Surgical Treatment of Cancer of the Stomach

Up to 1940 cancer of the stomach was the most frequent malignant disease in the United States, as shown by statistics (23, 33, 40, 77, 126). Since then, the incidence of this disease has progressively decreased, and no adequate explanation of this phenomenon has yet been given. In 1930 the mortality for cancer of the stomach in the United States was 30 per 100,000 (40, 102), but by 1989 (40) the number of deaths per 100,000 had fallen to 6.6 for men and 3.4 in women. This progressive decrease continued until 1960, after which it became less significant. At present the mortality of cancer of the stomach is stable. It is evident that this decrease in mortality is not due to greater efficiency of surgical treatment, at least not in the Western countries (31, 32).

The diminution in the frequency of cancer of the stomach has been manifested not only in the United States, but also in other countries of Europe and America with the exception of some countries in which the mortality of gastric cancer has remained elevated such as Finland, Iceland, some countries in Eastern Europe, and some in Central and South America such as Costa Rica, Colombia, and Chile. Japan is a country where the incidence of gastric cancer is very frequent and continued to rise annually up to 1960. Since that time a moderate diminution of mortality from gastric cancer has occurred (40, 112). This mortality was 58.8 per 100,000 males and 27.5 in females. This moderate decrease in mortality is probably due to a compulsory mass screening program carried out in Japan among every person over 45 years of age. This had yielded an increase in the early diagnosis of gastric carcinoma, which in Japan is over 30% of the gastric cancers subjected to gastric resection (29, 39, 60, 61, 93). The screening program carried out in Japan cannot be carried out in Western countries, one of the reasons being their low incidence of gastric cancer.

In addition to a decrease in gastric carcinoma in Western countries, there has also been a variation in the site of the disease within the stomach. In 1927, Rehfuss (102) pointed out that 60.8% of gastric cancers occurred in the antropyloric area and only 8% were located in the proximal third of the stomach. In a recent study by the American College of Surgeons, Wanebo et al. (126) reported the incidence, in 19,000 cases, of the following locations: 30.5% in the proximal third of the stomach, 13.9% in the middle third, and 26% in the distal third. The increased occurrence of gastric cancer in its proximal third has led to diminution of the possibility of cure. Because treatment of cancer of the proximal stomach is more complex, postoperative complications are more frequent and lymphatic spread is more extensive.

PATHOLOGY OF GASTRIC CANCER AND ITS RELATION TO SURGICAL TREATMENT

Gastric carcinoma starts in the neck of the mucosal glands. From there it extends to the surface as well as to the depths of the mucosal layer. After invading the mucosa, the carcinoma passes through the muscularis mucosa and penetrates the submucosa. While it is limited to the mucosa, only rarely does it produce lymphatic or hematogenous metastases. However, these have been observed (60, 61). If the carcinoma has invaded the submucosa, the incidence of lymphatic metastases rises from 4 to 20% (39, 60, 61, 93). Lymphatic metastases are generally localized in the N_1 lymphatic barrier but can also invade the N_2 barrier (60).

In some cases invasion of the mucosa is much more extensive than invasion of the submucosa. In other cases there are areas of submucosal invasion with intervening areas that are not infiltrated by tumor. The extent of submucosal invasion is related to the lymphatic invasion (60, 61).

Dissemination of neoplastic infiltration through the submucosa occurs very easily and can extend several centimeters beyond the visible or palpable macroscopic limit of the primary tumor (132, 133). Submucosal spread of the carcinoma occurs distally as well as proximally. In general, proximal spread is more extensive than distal spread (133). Proximal transection of the stomach in gastrectomy for cancer should be carried out at least 6 cm from the macroscopic limit of the primary tumor to avoid tissue that has been invaded by the tumor (31, 36).

Antropyloric carcinomas can infiltrate the proximal duodenum in 30% of cases (137). For this reason, in gastrectomies the duodenum should be transected at least 3 cm from the pylorus, even though submucosal and subserosal infiltration of the duodenal walls has been observed up to 8 cm beyond the pylorus. Because microscopic invasion of the duodenum is not apparent grossly or by radiologic examinations, it was thought for many years that the pylorus was a barrier to the invasion of cancer (137, 138). The frequent invasion of the duodenum in antropyloric cancers is a very important indication for the use of the Billroth II technique and not the Billroth I technique.

Macroscopic invasion of the submucosa is more extensive in diffusely infiltrating carcinomas than in the expansive intestinal type of tumors described by Lauren and Ming (70, 88). Therefore, in the diffuse infiltrating type of cancer, proximal transection of the stomach should be carried out at least 8 cm away from the tumor. In patients with an intestinal expansive type of tumor (Group I or II of the Borrmann classification) proximal transection of the stomach can be carried out 4 cm from the primary tumor. In order to be sure that the transection of the stomach as well as the duodenum has been carried out through healthy tissue, a microscopic frozen section examination of the transected gastric borders should be done in every case.

Gastric carcinoma, after invading the submucosa, penetrates the muscular wall of the stomach, proceeding into the subserosa and later into the serosa, with the possibility of invading neighboring viscera such as the pancreas, mesocolon, transverse colon, left lobe of the liver, and so on. When the carcinoma has invaded the serosa, neoplastic cells can become detached and fall into the peritoneal cavity, becoming implanted in the visceral peritoneum of the intestine, the parietal peritoneum, and the pouch of Douglas, where they can give rise to solid tumors that are palpable by rectal or vaginal examination (Blumer's shelf), or on the surface of the ovaries, where they can give rise to a Krukenberg tumor.

Gastric cancer cells can enter the lymphatics and invade the regional lymph nodes of the stomach by embolization or by lymphatic permeation (132, 133). During surgery, the surgeon should try to establish the extent of lymphatic invasion by frozen section study of biopsies, studying several sections of each node, especially those of the N_3 group. The greater the penetration of the tumor into the gastric wall, the greater will be its lymphatic dissemination. On the other hand, tumors of the diffuse infiltrative type lead to more lymphatic spread than do the intestinal expansive types.

Invasion of lymph nodes of the stomach differs from invasion of nodes in colon cancer. In the stomach lymphatic spread does not occur in orderly stages following a certain order as in the colon. In the stomach, invasion of groups of nodes can occur in distant nodes (N_3), leaving nodes near the tumor free (N_0). Patients subjected to gastric resection for cancer have metastases to nodes in 50 to 70% of cases. It has been shown in the Western world that the 5 year survival in patients with positive nodes decreases from 50% to 20%. In Japan, the 5 year survival rate is higher (90, 10, 60, 117). The 5 year survival rates are not only related to the presence of positive nodes, but also to their number and location.

Cells of gastric cancer can enter the bloodstream and lead to secondary tumors in the liver, lungs, and bones, as well as in other organs. The presence of distant metastases in cases of gastric cancer is a contraindication for surgery, except under special conditions or complications such as hemorrhage, perforation, or obstruction of the primary tumor.

Frequently the surgeon, after performing a gastric resection for cancer of the stomach, with hopes for a cure, affirms that he or she has performed a radical operation, a very common and accepted term used by surgeons. This affirmation, however, is only theoretical and conditional, since it is impossible to be sure that no nodules or groups of neoplastic cells have been left behind. It is only possible to be sure the operation has been radical if the later result confirms it.

MACROSCOPIC CLASSIFICATION OF GASTRIC CANCER

In 1926, Borrmann (12) proposed a macroscopic classification of gastric cancer that, because of its practicality, is still used, not only by pathologists, but also by radiologists, gastroenterologists, and surgeons. The Borrmann classification is the following:

I. Polypoid cancer.
II. Ulcerated cancer with raised borders.
III. Ulcerated cancer with partial or complete infiltration of its borders.
IV. Partial or complete infiltrating cancer (linitis plastica).

Japanese writers consider the Borrmann classification as a classification of advanced gastric cancer. In recent years a fifth group has been added to the Borrmann classification, that of early carcinoma.

It is possible to infer in a general way that groups I and II of the Borrmann classification correspond to the Lauren microscopic intestinal type and the Ming expansive type. At the same time groups III and IV correspond to the Lauren diffuse type and the Ming infiltrative type.

MICROSCOPIC CLASSIFICATION OF GASTRIC CANCER

As will be seen later, even though the histologic characteristics of gastric cancer are important in determining prognosis, it does not form part of the TNM classification. In 1965, Lauren (70) proposed a histologic classification with the object of showing the biologic behavior of gastric cancer. Lauren divided gastric cancer in two types: (a) intestinal and (b) diffuse. The intestinal type forms glandular structures as seen in the intestine, resembling carcinoma of the colon and usually coexisting with metaplasia of the gastric mucosa of the intestinal type. Tumors of the intestinal type have a better prognosis than those of the diffuse type. and are more frequently seen in countries where there is a high incidence of gastric cancer such as Japan, Chile, Costa Rica, and Colombia. In the countries where gastric cancer has diminished in frequency in recent years such as the United States and some European countries, the microscopic type that is diminishing is the intestinal type. The diffuse type of the Lauren classification is made up of isolated cells or small groups of cells with slight inflammatory reaction without forming glandular structures. The diffuse type of carcinoma is more malignant, may affect the entire stomach, as in linitis plastica, and infiltrates the gastric lymph nodes more frequently than the intestinal type.

In 1977, Ming (88) also proposed a histologic classification of gastric cancer with some similarities with the Lauren classification. Ming classified gastric tumors into two types: (a) expansive and (b) infiltrative. The expansive carcinomas are made up of cellular groups that maintain their affiliation and give rise to nodules that displace the normal structures. The infiltrative type is characterized by the presence of cellular infiltrates which retain their individuality. The Lauren intestinal type is similar to the Ming (88) expansive type, and both types have a better prognosis than diffuse or infiltrative carcinomas. The intestinal and expansive types generally produce polypoid tumors, ulcerated or not (Groups I and II of the Borrmann macroscopic classification), while the diffuse or infiltrative types penetrate into the gastric wall, giving rise to partial or total infiltrative lesions, which correspond with Groups III and IV of the Borrmann macroscopic classification (12).

EARLY GASTRIC CARCINOMA

In 1962, the Japanese Society of Endoscopic Gastroenterology defined and proposed a macroscopic classification of early gastric carcinoma, considering it necessary to diagnose gastric cancer at an early stage of its evolution in order to carry out a more effective surgical treatment of gastric cancer.

The society defined as early gastric cancer those carcinomas limited to the mucosa and submucosa, without considering their extension or the presence of invasion of regional lymphatic nodes. In Japan, early gastric carcinoma is found in 30 to 40% of all gastric carcinomas. In Western countries, early carcinoma of the stomach is found in 10% or fewer cases. In a recent publication by Wanebo et al. (126), in which more than 19,000 cases of gastric cancer from various centers were studied, early cancer was found in 17% of cases, an unusually high frequency for Europe and the United States.

In Japan there is an 80 to 90% 5 year survival of patients operated for early carcinoma (29, 39, 60, 61, 93). In Europe and in the United States 5 year survival is 50 to 60%. In Japan the rate of incidence of positive lymph nodes in early gastric cancer varies from 5 to 20%. The involved lymph nodes are usually those of the N_1 group, although invasion of Group N_2 nodes is also observable (31, 32, 39, 60, 61, 92, 134).

Early carcinoma of the stomach is usually asymptomatic. When it does produce symptoms, these are mild and unspecific except in ulcerated carcinomas, which can produce discrete pains or hemorrhages. Some authors (77) maintain that the designation of early carcinoma is not correct and that it is more adequate to call these tumors superficial carcinoma. René Gutmann, Bertrand, and Peristiany, in their 1939 book, *Le Cancer de L'estomac au Debut* (48), were already using the term "superficial carcinoma" when, at that time, all that was available was the radiologic examination. Stout of the United States also used the term "superficial carcinoma" in describing this type of cancer (121).

Macroscopic Classification of Early Carcinoma of the Stomach

The Japanese Society of Endoscopic Gastroenterology classified early carcinomas of the stomach into three types: Type I, early protruded type; Type II, early superficial carcinoma; Type III, early excavated carcinoma. Type II has been subdivided into three varieties: A, elevated; B, flat; and C, depressed. The diagnosis of early gastric carcinoma is made by double contrast radiologic examination and gastroscopy with biopsy.

TNM Classification of Gastric Cancer

It is important to establish a classification of gastric cancer and determine its stage of evolution. This will allow selection of the most adequate treatment for patients and the evaluation of the results of different surgical treatments in order to compare statistics of different surgical centers. The TNM classification was proposed by the American Joint Committee for Cancer Staging and Results Reporting of Cancer in 1970 and modified in 1977 (2, 3, 8, 63). The letter T represents the primary tumor:

- T_1: The carcinoma is limited to the mucosa or submucosa without limits to its localization or extent.
- T_2: The carcinoma has penetrated the muscularis without passing through the serosa.
- T_3: The carcinoma has penetrated the serosa without invading contiguous viscera.
- T_4: The carcinoma has penetrated through the serosa and has invaded contiguous viscera.

The letter N represents the presence or absence of metastases in the regional lymph nodes:

- N_0: Without regional lymph node metastases.
- N_1: Invasion of lymphatic nodes within 3 cm of the carcinoma that can be resected with the gastrectomy.
- N_2: Invasion of lymph nodes more than 3 cm away from the primary tumor that are also resected with the gastrectomy, including the nodes along the left gastric artery, the splenic artery, the celiac trunk, and the common hepatic artery.

The letter R means residual tumor:

- R_0: The gastric resection has been performed without apparently leaving residual tumor behind.
- R_1: The gastrectomy has been performed leaving microscopic residual tumor behind.
- R_2: The gastrectomy has been performed leaving macroscopic residual tumor.

The letter M represents the presents or absence of distant metastases:

- M_0: No known distant metastases.
- M_1: Presence of distant metastases.

LYMPHATIC AREAS OF THE STOMACH

The lymphatics of the stomach were described in Chapter 20. There are numerous studies of the lymph nodes of the stomach, many of them by the Japanese, who have contributed to our knowledge of the lymphatic spread of carcinoma of the stomach (5, 11, 18, 25, 34, 65, 118).

Three lymphatic barriers are recognized in the stomach:

The first lymphatic barrier is composed of the following groups of lymph nodes: 1, right cardiac nodes; 2, lymph nodes of the lesser curvature of the stomach, that is the left gastric (coronary) artery and the right gastric (pyloric) artery; 3, lymph nodes of the greater curvature, that is, the left gastroepiploic artery; 4, infrapyloric nodes; 5, suprapyloric nodes; and 6, retropyloric nodes. All these nodes are removed with the gastric resection.

The second lymphatic barrier is made up of the following groups of lymph nodes: 7, anterior, superior anterior, and inferior pancreatoduodenal nodes; 8, inferior phrenic nodes; 9, celiac nodes; 10, common hepatic artery nodes; 11, cystic lymph nodes; 12, splenic hilar nodes; and 13, superior pancreatic nodes.

The third lymphatic barrier is made up of the following groups of lymph nodes: 14, inferior pancreatic lymph nodes; 15, superior mesenteric lymph nodes; 16, lateral aortic lymph nodes; 17, preaortic lymph nodes; and 18, precaval lymph nodes.

In describing and performing the histologic examination of the different groups of nodes, these should be designated by their localization and not by a number, as some authors do, because the surgeon then has to remember the number assigned to the different locations of the lymphatic groups, which is more complex than remembering the localization. In the TNM classification

N_0 means that the lymph nodes are not invaded.
N_1 means the first lymphatic barrier is invaded.
N_2 means the second lymphatic barrier is invaded.
N_3 means the third lymphatic barrier is invaded.

In gastric resections for cancer, performed in the Western world, the lymph nodes of the N_1 and N_2 barrier are resected, occasionally with some groups of nodes of the N_3 barrier. Surgical resection of the three gastric lymphatic barriers is a difficult task with elevated morbidity and mortality, in spite of opposite opinions (65, 67, 68, 79, 117, 118). Extensive lymphadenectomy is only used in selected cases, since it has not been proven to improve survival (26, 31, 39, 58, 77, 85, 95, 98, 116, 126).

EXTENT OF GASTRIC RESECTION

Total gastrectomy, as a principle, has not been shown to improve the 5 year survival of patients with gastric cancer. Total gastrectomy was very popular in the 1940s and 1950s. At present, in the great majority of surgical centers, subtotal gastrectomy is preferred, reserving total gastrectomy for cases in which a lesser operation would not permit removal of all the neoplastic tissue. In subtotal gastrectomy, transection of the stomach should be at least 6 cm above the tumor, in order not to cut gastric tissue at a level where it could be infiltrated by the carcinoma. In cases in which the carcinoma is of the diffuse infiltrative histologic type (Lauren, Ming), it is preferable to transect the stomach 8 cm above the tumor.

Total gastrectomy is generally indicated in patients with infiltrative carcinoma affecting the entire stomach (linitis plastica), or involving the middle third of the stomach, in very large polypoid tumors of the middle third, in tumors of the proximal third, in patients with gastric cancer and polyposis or gastric cancer and atrophic gastritis, in patients with cancer of the gastric stump after gastrectomy for peptic ulcer, and so on.

In total gastrectomy the level of transection of the esophagus should be at least 5 cm above the esophagogastric junction. It should be remembered that carcinomas of the upper third of the stomach can infiltrate the esophagus up to 10 cm above the esophagogastric junction. For this reason, frozen section study of the transected esophagus is indispensable to determine if there is tumor infiltration. If it is difficult to perform the esophagojejunal anastomosis, due to inability to bring the esophagus down, the Savinyj maneuver, published in 1957 (109), can be very useful, This involves dividing the diaphragm in the midline, from the esophagus forward, for as long as is necessary to improve the operative field. Even though the mortality and morbidity of total gastrectomy have improved in recent years, they continue to be higher than for subtotal gastrectomy. In order to keep the mortality of total gastrectomy below 10%, it should be performed by a team with experience in this procedure. On the other hand, total gastrectomy should not be used palliatively, except in very special circumstances.

In years past, when total gastrectomy was carried out in order to amplify the extent of the lymphadenectomy, the operation was extended by splenectomy to remove the nodes in the hilus of the spleen. In addition, some surgeons resected the tail or the body and tail of the pancreas in order to remove the suprapancreatic lymph nodes. It was soon determined that this extensive operation increased mortality without improving 5 year survival. Splenectomy and resection of the body and tail of the pancreas is not indicated to remove more lymph nodes, but is indicated when the pancreas is invaded by the tumor. At present, in most Western surgical centers, total gastrectomy is performed in 15 to 20% of cases, while subtotal gastrectomy is used in 80 to 85% of cases.

The level of transection on the lesser curvature in gastric cancer is performed very close to the esophagogastric junction. Transection of the greater curvature is performed at the level of the most distal short vessel.

With the object of avoiding a total gastrectomy, some surgeons resort to a greater resection of the stomach, leaving a small stump designated as a high subtotal gastrectomy or a "quasi-total" gastrectomy (14, 30). The anastomosis of this small gastric stump to the jejunum is safer than anastomosis to the esophagus. In this ample gastrectomy the blood supply of the gastric stump should be controlled so that it does not become ischemic due to ligation of the left gastric artery at its origin from the celiac trunk. In addition, in order to perform a quasi-total gastrectomy it is necessary to ligate 2, 3, or more distal short vessels. It should not be forgotten that the number of short vessels varies from 2 to 10, and their actual number in the patient must be determined before proceeding with their ligation.

Transection of the duodenum in gastrectomy for carcinoma of the distal third should be done at least 3 cm from the pylorus as a minimum, since these tumors may infiltrate the proximal duodenum (137, 138). This makes it mandatory to always carry out a frozen section study of the transected duodenal border.

Gastrectomy for cancer, be it subtotal or total, is carried out en bloc, removing the gastrohepatic and gastrocolic ligaments as well as the greater omentum and the lymph nodes with the stomach.

The technique of these procedures will be described later.

PREOPERATIVE STAGING OF GASTRIC CANCER

Gastric cancer should be staged preoperatively. Physical examination of patients with gastric cancer will only reveal signs of advanced cancer. Some of these signs are hepatomegaly with or without metastases; palpable gastric tumor, movable or fixed; presence of a hard fixed mass in Douglas' pouch, palpable on rectal or vaginal examination (Blumer's shelf); in women there can also be a Krukenberg tumor by implantation on the ovarian surface of malignant cells detached from the gastric serosa invaded by the cancer, and a palpable or visible left supraclavicular lymph node described by Virchow in 1848. This lymph node was described by Troisier 38 years later, in 1886 (90) and, at present, it is frequently referred to as the Virchow-Troisier supraclavicular node.

In some cases, an increase in the size of the umbilicus is observed, caused by neoplastic infiltration of the round ligament, which occasionally forms an umbilical mass that has been compared to an iceberg. This neoplastic infiltration of the umbilicus is usually known in the English literature as the Sister Mary Joseph node.

Once the clinical examination is complete, the study of the patient is completed with a double contrast X-ray study of the stomach, a gastroscopy with multiple biopsies, endoscopic ultrasonography, abdominal ultrasonography, computed axial tomography, and so on. All these studies will allow us to approximate the extent of the gastric tumor, in some cases the degree of nodal involvement, and the presence of hepatic pulmonary or bone metastases, and so on.

If these examinations do not reveal the presence of signs of inoperability or of distant metastases, surgical exploration is indicated.

OPERATIVE STAGING OF GASTRIC CANCER

Once the abdomen is opened, a complete visual and palpatory examination of the entire abdominal cavity is carried out, with biopsy of any suspicious lesions. One should first search for distant metastases in the liver, the visceral or parietal peritoneum, the Douglas' pouch, and the ovaries, as well as the presence of ascitic fluid, and so forth. Exploration is then centered on the whole stomach. This is begun by inspection and palpation of the anterior wall of the stomach, then the posterior wall after opening the lesser sac, and then the lesser and greater curvatures. The localization, extension, and mobility of the tumor should be determined, together with the type of tumor, polypoid or infiltrating, as well as the distance from the upper border of the tumor to the esophagogastric junction and the number of short vessels.

The groups of gastric lymph nodes should be explored visually as well as by palpation, always remembering that neither their size nor their consistency can indicate with certainty if they are invaded by tumor. Only frozen section biopsy of the different groups of nodes, with several sections of each node, can confirm the presence of the neoplasm. It is important to carry out resection of one or more of the nodes of the N_3 barrier zone. If one of these nodes is invaded by tumor, the gastrectomy will only be palliative.

It is not advisable to perform a gastrotomy to remove tissue for biopsy to determine if the tumor is of the expansive intestinal or diffuse infiltrative type. Histologic examination of the tumor should be done preoperatively, by obtaining several biopsies during gastroscopy. Biopsy of the tumor by gastrotomy may produce seeding of neoplastic cells in the peritoneal cavity or in the abdominal incision. During the dissection of groups of nodes, transection of the nodes should be avoided because, if the node is invaded by tumor, this may lead to implantation of tumor in the abdomen.

Staging is completed when microscopic study of the operative specimen and each of the resected nodes is finalized. The lymph node groups should be identified by the surgeon and placed in separate jars containing formalin. In cases in which a subtotal gastrectomy is performed, it should be determined if the transected gastric border is or is not infiltrated by the tumor. In patients with a total gastrectomy this determination should be made on the esophageal border. The histologic examination should be completed by studying the border of the transected duodenum for tumor invasion.

Radical Subtotal Gastrectomy and Extended Radical Subtotal Gastrectomy

Radical Subtotal Gastrectomy

FIGURE 38.1
The most frequently used incision is the midline xiphoumbilical incision. This incision can be extended upward, removing the xiphoid process. In these cases the incision is extended to the base of the xiphoid as shown by the dotted line. If necessary, the incision can be extended downward to a point 4 to 6 cm below the umbilicus.

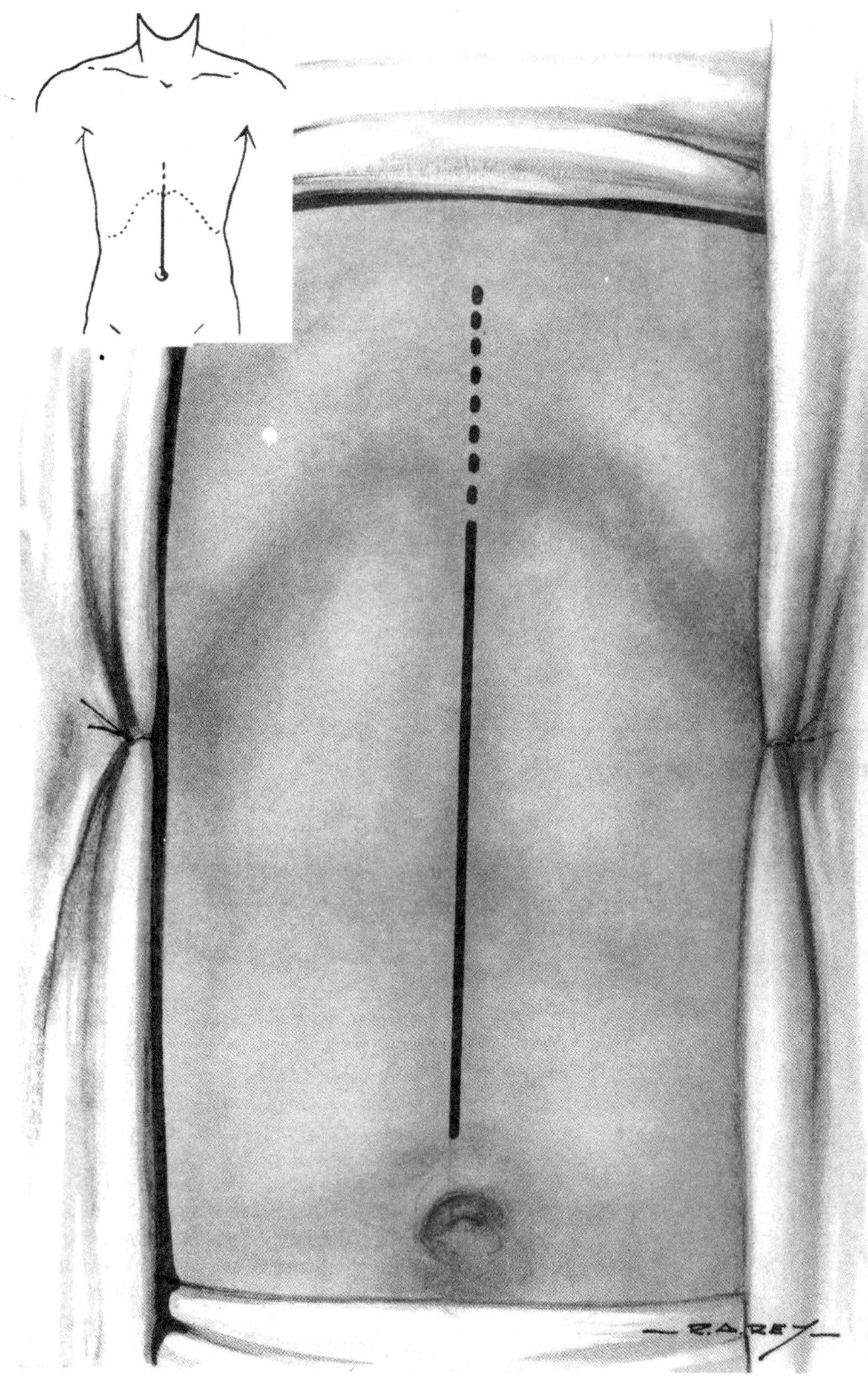

Radical Subtotal Gastrectomy

FIGURE 38.2
The skin, the subcutaneous tissue, and the midline aponeurosis have been incised. **A,** Using a scalpel, a small incision is being made in the peritoneum, at a point halfway from the xiphoid to the umbilicus. For this purpose, the peritoneum has been grasped by two Allis clamps. Before dividing the peritoneum, the surgeon, using the index finger and the thumb, must be sure that an abdominal viscus has not been grasped by the Allis clamps. **B,** The Allis clamps are replaced by hemostatic clamps with which upward traction is applied to the peritoneum, proceeding with division of the peritoneum toward the xiphoid process using scissors. **C,** Again, using the scalpel, the peritoneum is divided downward, protecting the abdominal viscera with the fingers of the left hand.

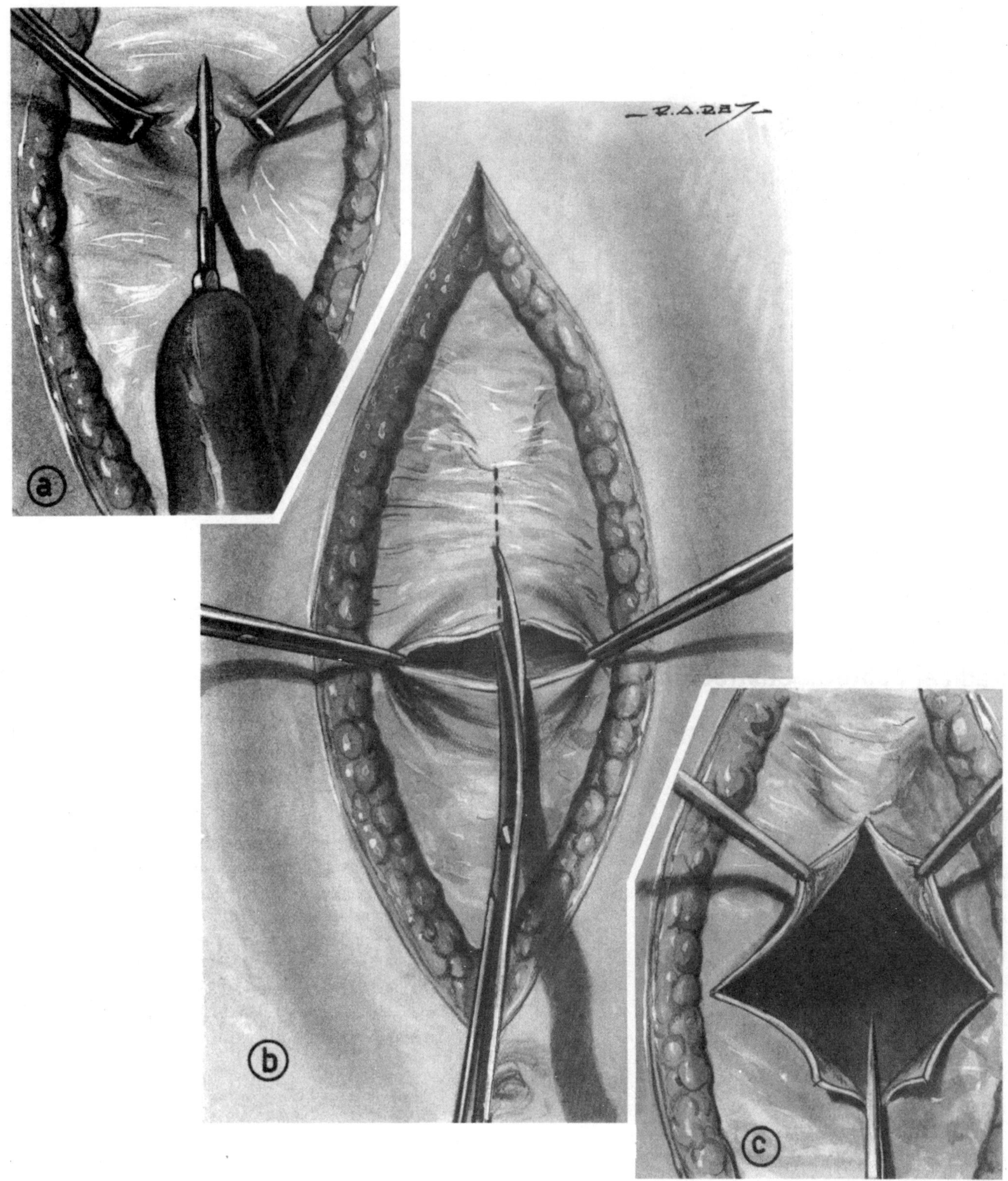

FIGURE 38.2

Radical Subtotal Gastrectomy

FIGURE 38.3

Once the abdominal cavity is open, exploration of the abdomen is carried out as completely as possible, later concentrating on the stomach. A large Balfour or similar retractor is placed to obtain an ample operative field. The xiphoid process has been removed and a blood vessel is being electrocoagulated for hemostasis. In order to obtain good visualization of the esophagodiaphragmatic area, an "upper hand" retractor is used to apply upward traction to the lower portion of the sternum and the costal cartilages.

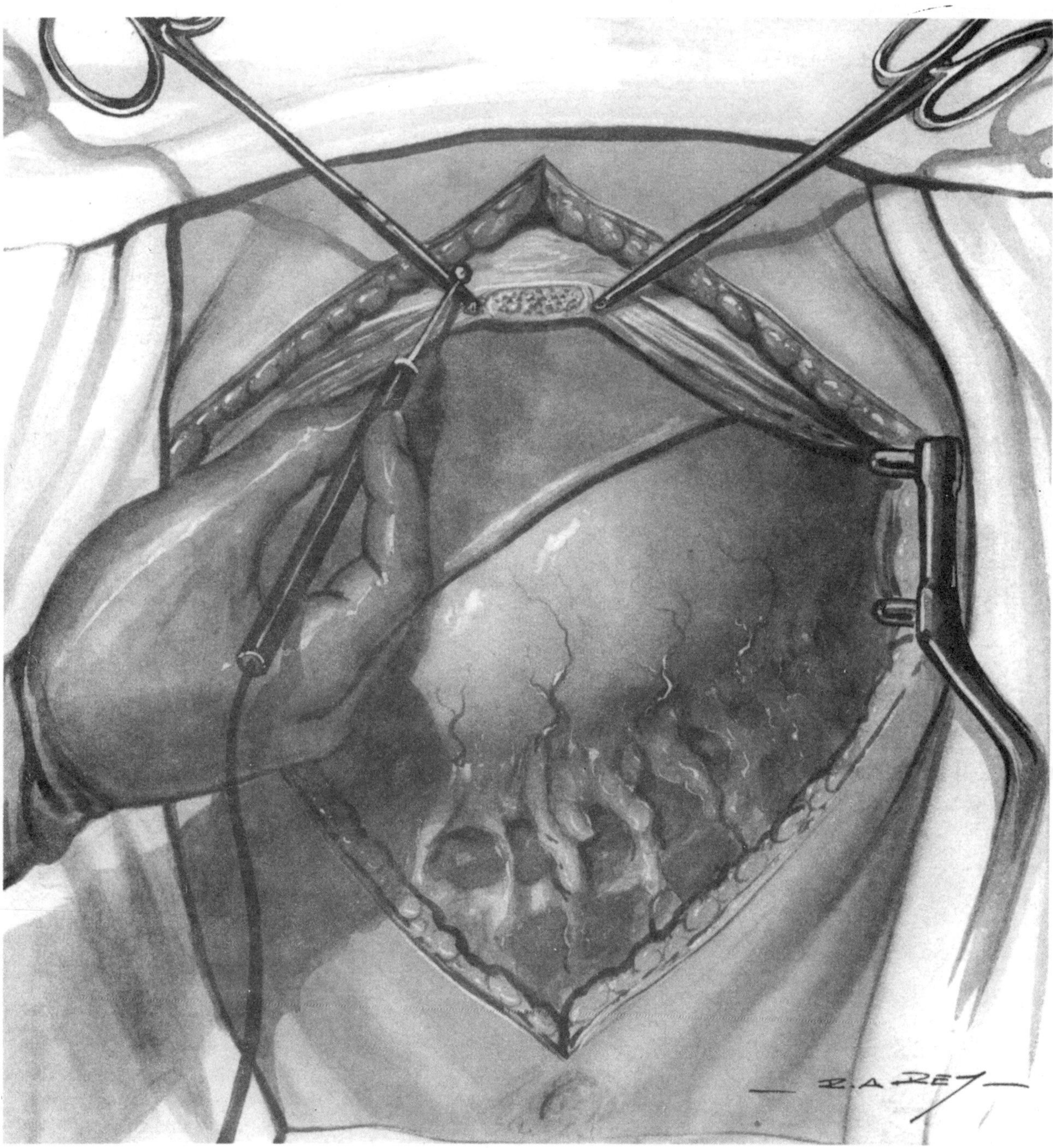

FIGURE 38.3

Radical Subtotal Gastrectomy

FIGURE 38.4
The drawing shows, using broken lines, the limits of the subtotal gastrectomy in cases of carcinoma of the distal third of the stomach or in cases of noninfiltrating carcinomas of the middle third. The extent of the subtotal gastrectomy can vary depending on the following factors: localization, macroscopic type, histologic structure, and so on. The gastrectomy can extend to 70 to 90%, and in some cases, can be a quasi-total resection (30). Gastrectomy for cancer includes en bloc removal of the stomach and the gastrohepatic and gastrocolic ligaments, as well as the greater omentum together with the gastric lymph node bearing area.

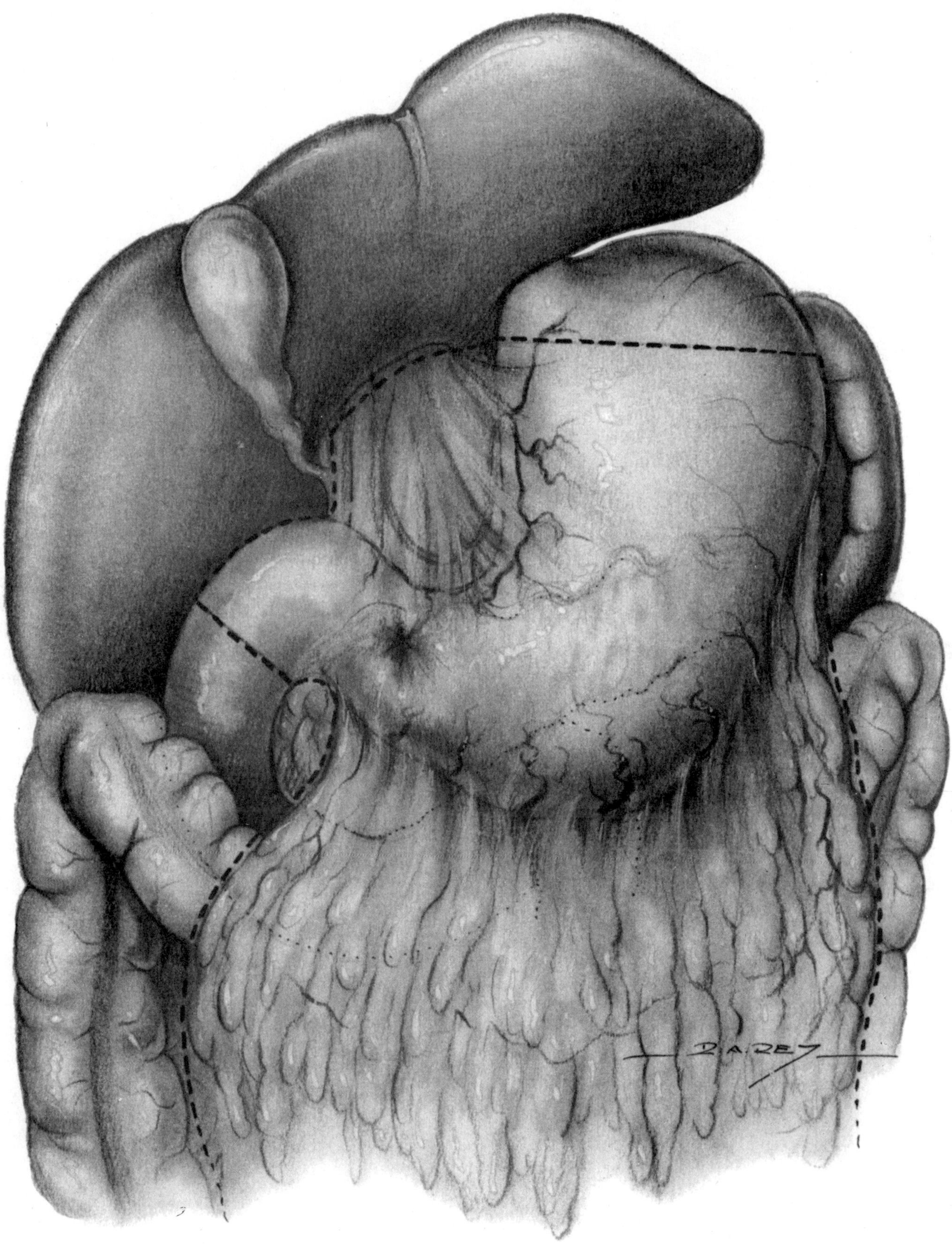

FIGURE 38.4

Radical Subtotal Gastrectomy

FIGURE 38.5
The first step of a radical subtotal gastrectomy consists of separation of the greater omentum from the transverse colon. This maneuver can be realized without blood loss as follows: the first assistant holds the transverse colon with both hands and applies downward traction while the second assistant applies upward traction with two hands to the greater omentum. Using curved scissors, the surgeon then separates the omentum from the transverse colon.

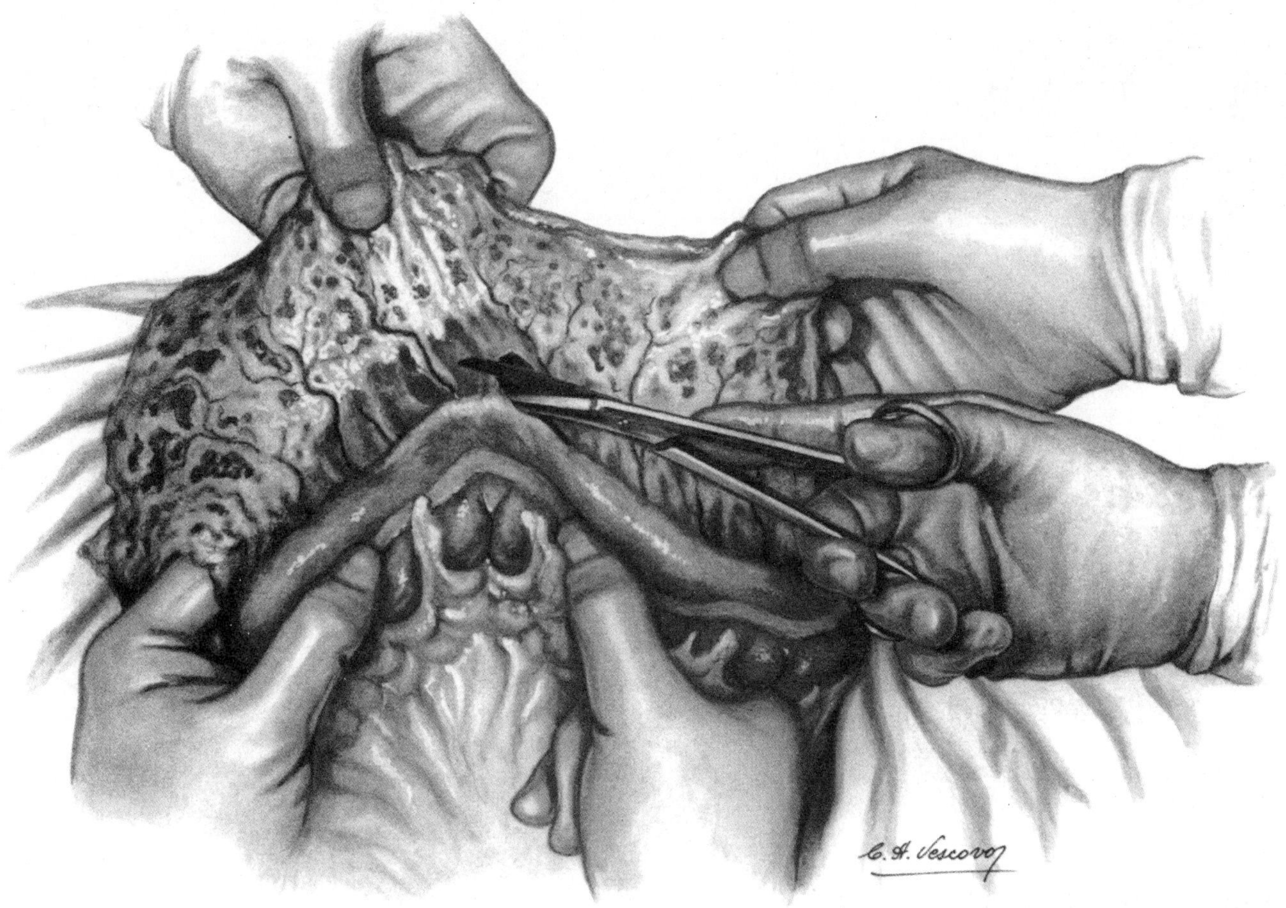

FIGURE 38.5

Radical Subtotal Gastrectomy

FIGURE 38.6
Once the greater omentum is separated from the transverse colon, the superior leaf of the transverse mesocolon is resected, as shown. While carrying out the dissection near the pyloroduodenal area, the gastroepiploic vein and artery are ligated separately, and the anterior pancreatoduodenal and infrapyloric nodes are dissected.

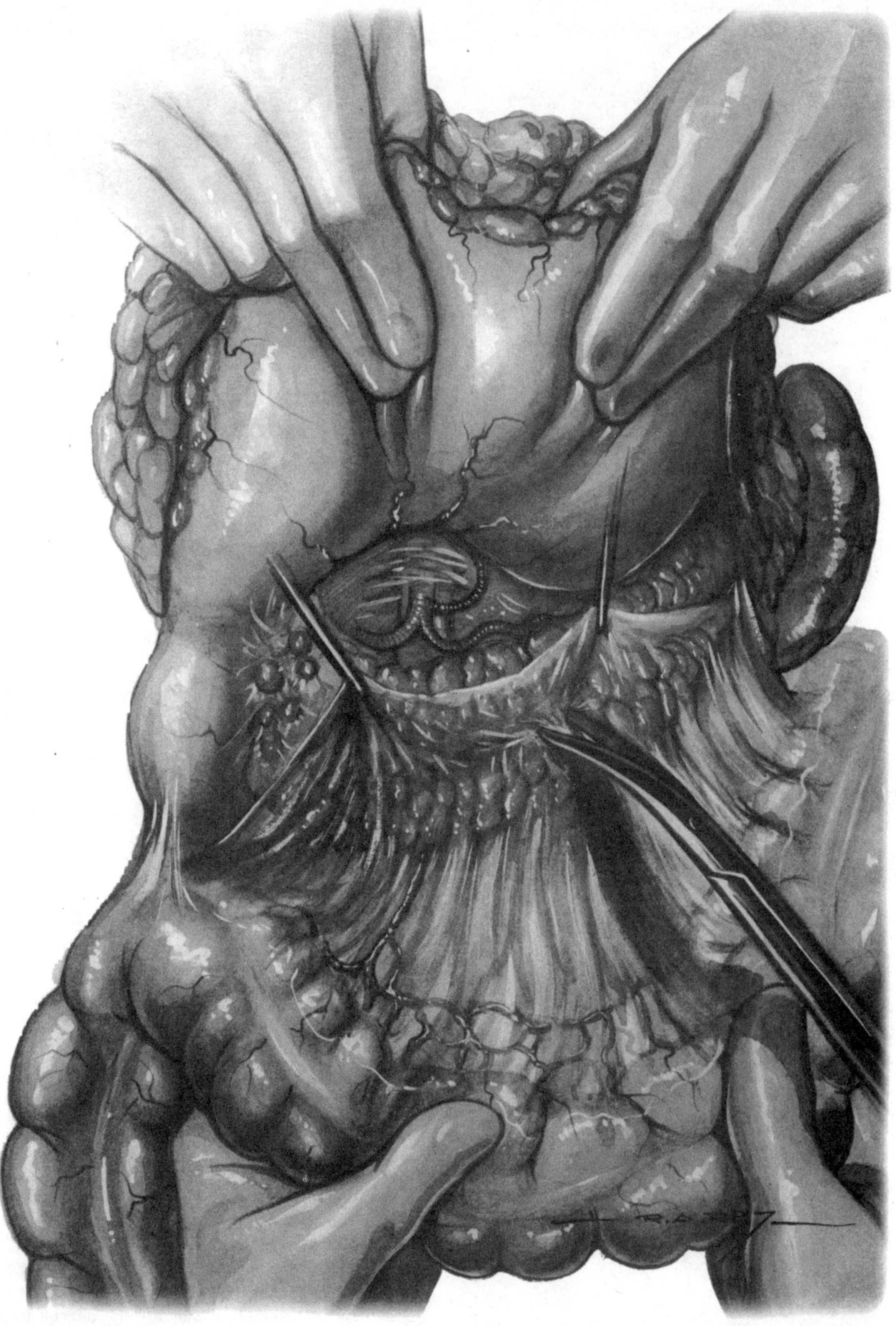

FIGURE 38.6

Radical Subtotal Gastrectomy

FIGURE 38.7
The dissection of the anterior pancreatoduodenal and infra-pyloric nodes is being performed.

FIGURE 38.8
If the retroduodenopancreatic lymph nodes (N_3) are invaded, the possibility of curing the patient is very low or nil. These nodes may be resected, if they are not difficult to resect, in order to carry out more complete staging.

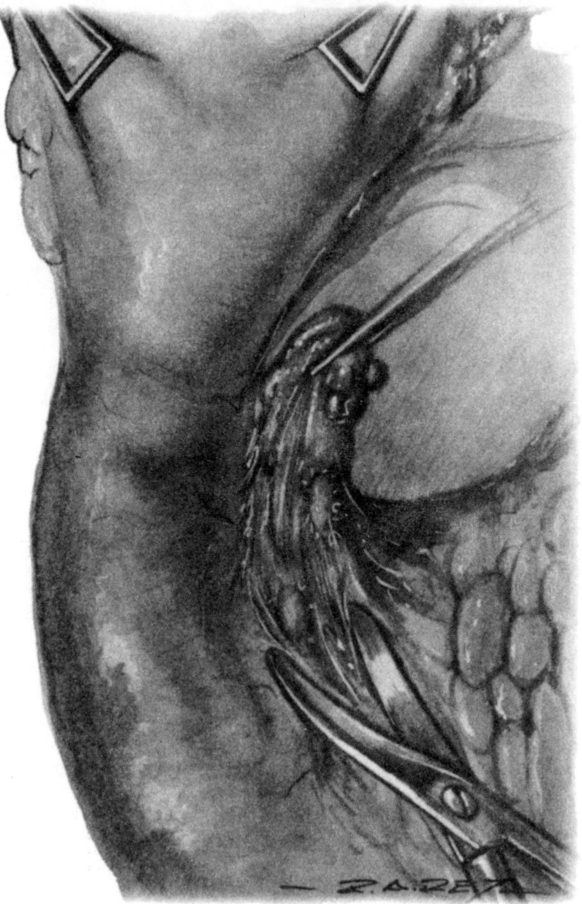

FIGURE 38.7

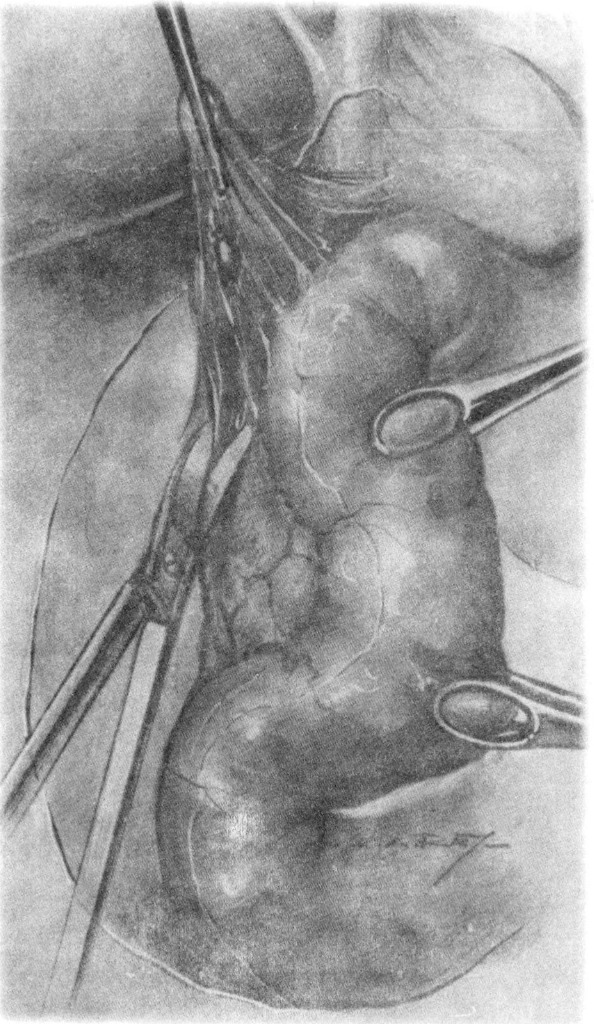

FIGURE 38.8

Radical Subtotal Gastrectomy

FIGURE 38.9

The resection of the nodes of the inferior portion of the hepatoduodenal ligament is being carried out. These nodes are also resected if it is not too difficult in order to have better staging.

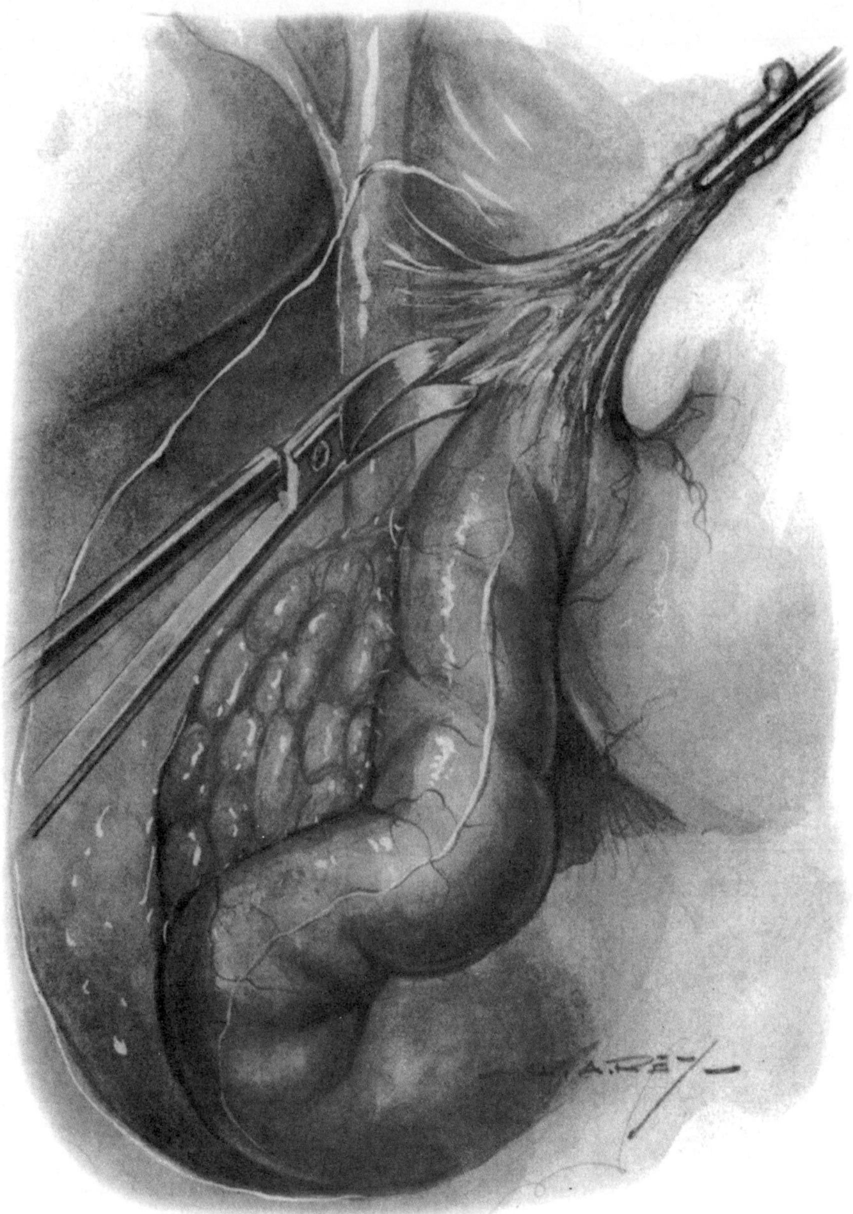

FIGURE 38.9

FIGURE 38.10
The right gastric artery has been ligated and the duodenum has been transected about 3 cm from the pylorus and has been closed. The stomach is being pulled upward and to the left. The posterior parietal peritoneum covering the common hepatic artery has been divided in order to resect two or three nodes usually present at that level (11). The nodes of the vertical portion of the hepatic artery are usually not dissected. Once the nodes of the horizontal portion of the hepatic artery are dissected, the dissection is continued proximally in order to remove the nodes of the celiac trunk en bloc.

Radical Subtotal Gastrectomy

FIGURE 38.11
The dissection of the celiac trunk has been completed, resecting the lymph nodes and the tissue surrounding it after dividing the posterior peritoneum. The cellular tissue, including the nodes, is pulled upward and to the left using a Duval clamp, exposing the celiac trunk and its branches; the hepatic artery, which runs to the right, above the edge of the pancreas; the splenic artery, which runs to the left over the edge or more frequently on the posterior surface of the pancreas; and the left gastric or coronary artery, which runs away from the celiac trunk running to the lesser curvature of the stomach with which it comes into contact about 3 cm distal to the esophagogastric junction. In performing a dissection of the celiac trunk, the surgeon should identify the three arteries that arise from it to avoid the mistake of ligating an artery that is not the left gastric artery.

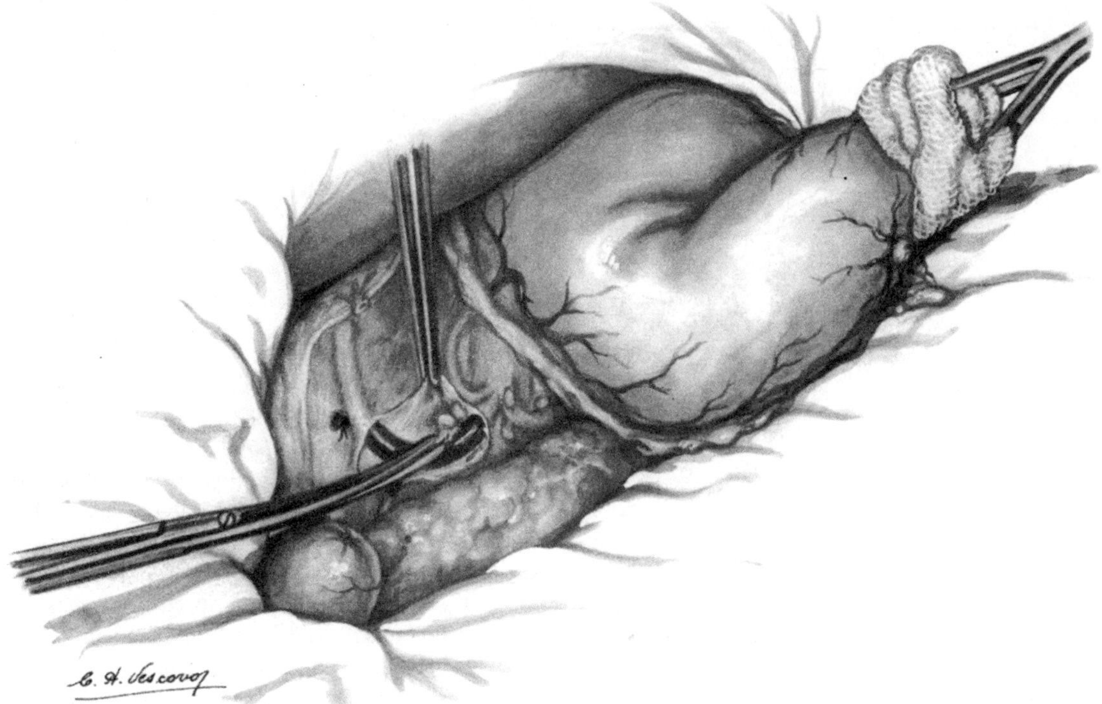

FIGURE 38.10

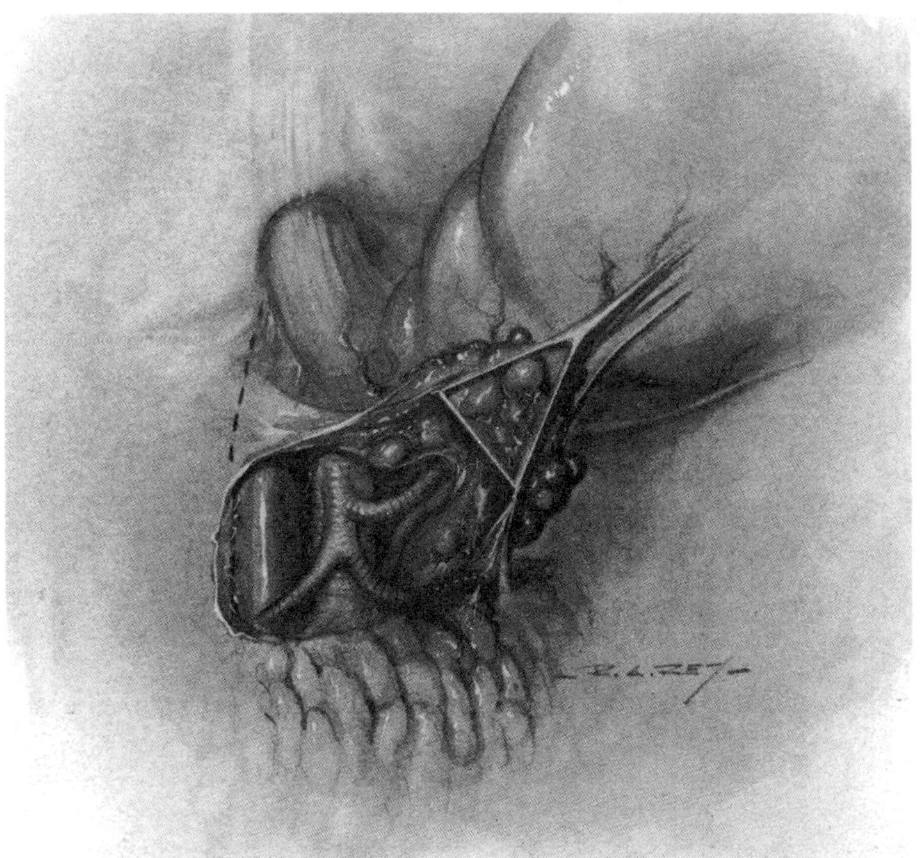

FIGURE 38.11

FIGURE 38.12

The left gastric artery has been ligated at its origin in the celiac trunk. Dissection is continued up to the lesser curvature of the stomach, where the right paracardial zone is dissected in order to remove one or two nodes that are usually found in this site. The left and posterior paracardial nodes cannot be resected by means of a radical subtotal gastrectomy. Usually the left gastric or coronary vein is ligated before the artery is ligated. The level at which the stomach is to be transected in a high subtotal gastrectomy is shown by a broken line. In ample gastrectomies, such as this one, it is necessary to ligate at least 2 or 3 of the distal gastric vessels. Once these are ligated the surgeon must be sure that the gastric remnant has not lost all its blood supply. Before ligating the short vessels it is necessary to note how many of these short vessels are present in the patient. This number should be between 2 and 10.

Radical Subtotal Gastrectomy

FIGURE 38.13

The drawing shows that the dissection of the right paracardial region has been carried out and the dissection is being continued distally.

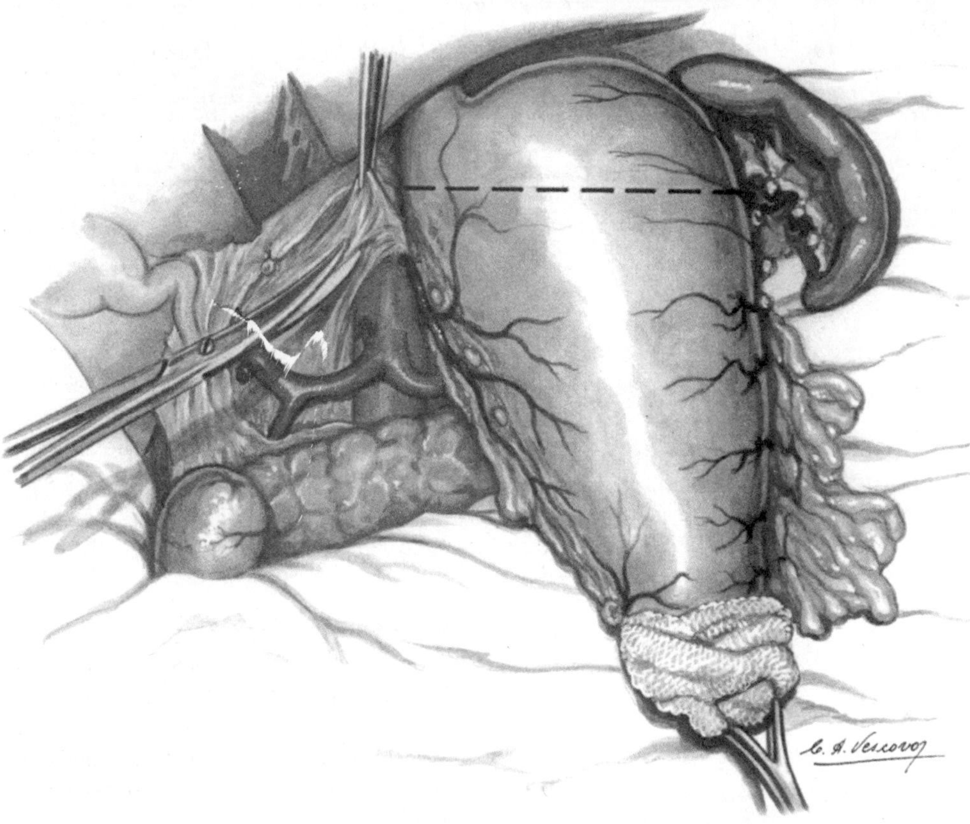

FIGURE 38.12

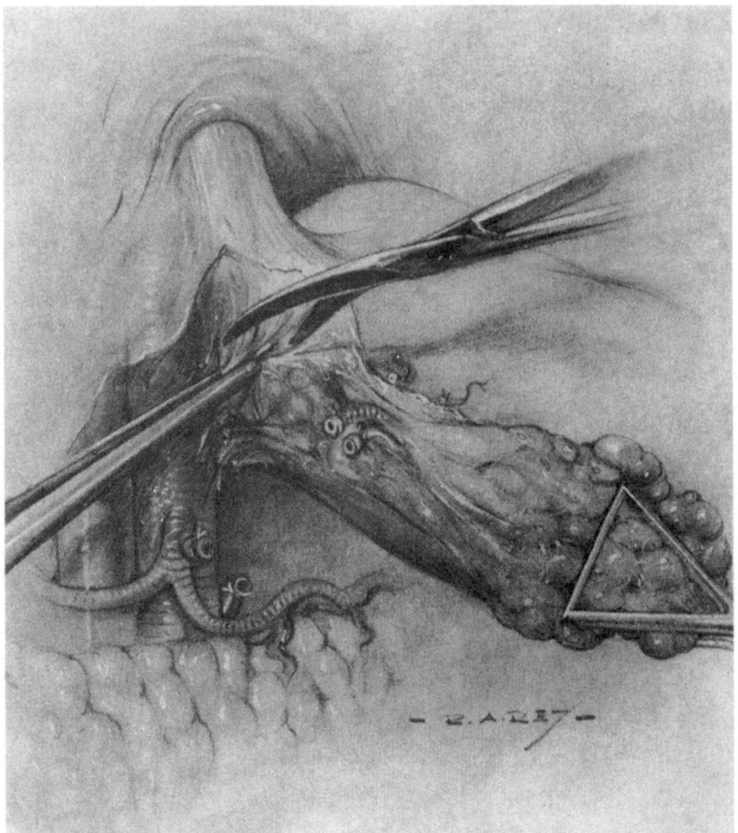

FIGURE 38.13

FIGURE 38.14
The upper portion of the lesser curvature is now free of any cellular or lymph node–bearing tissue. In performing this dissection the lesser curvature is left devoid of peritoneum, and it is advisable to reconstruct the peritoneum of the lesser curvature in order to be able to perform safer gastrojejunal suturing later.

Radical Subtotal Gastrectomy

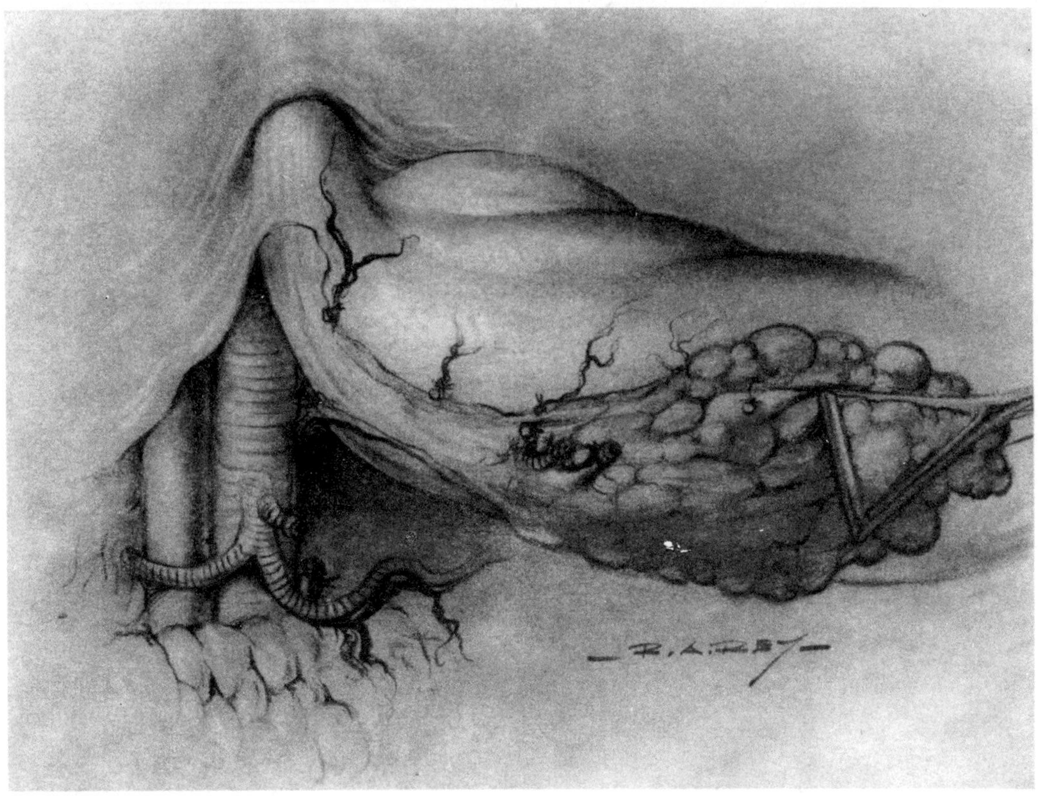

FIGURE 38.14

Radical Subtotal Gastrectomy

FIGURE 38.15

The peritoneum of the lesser curvature of the stomach has been repaired using interrupted cotton sutures. The extent of this reperitonealization of the lesser curvature will vary with the extent of the gastrectomy to be performed.

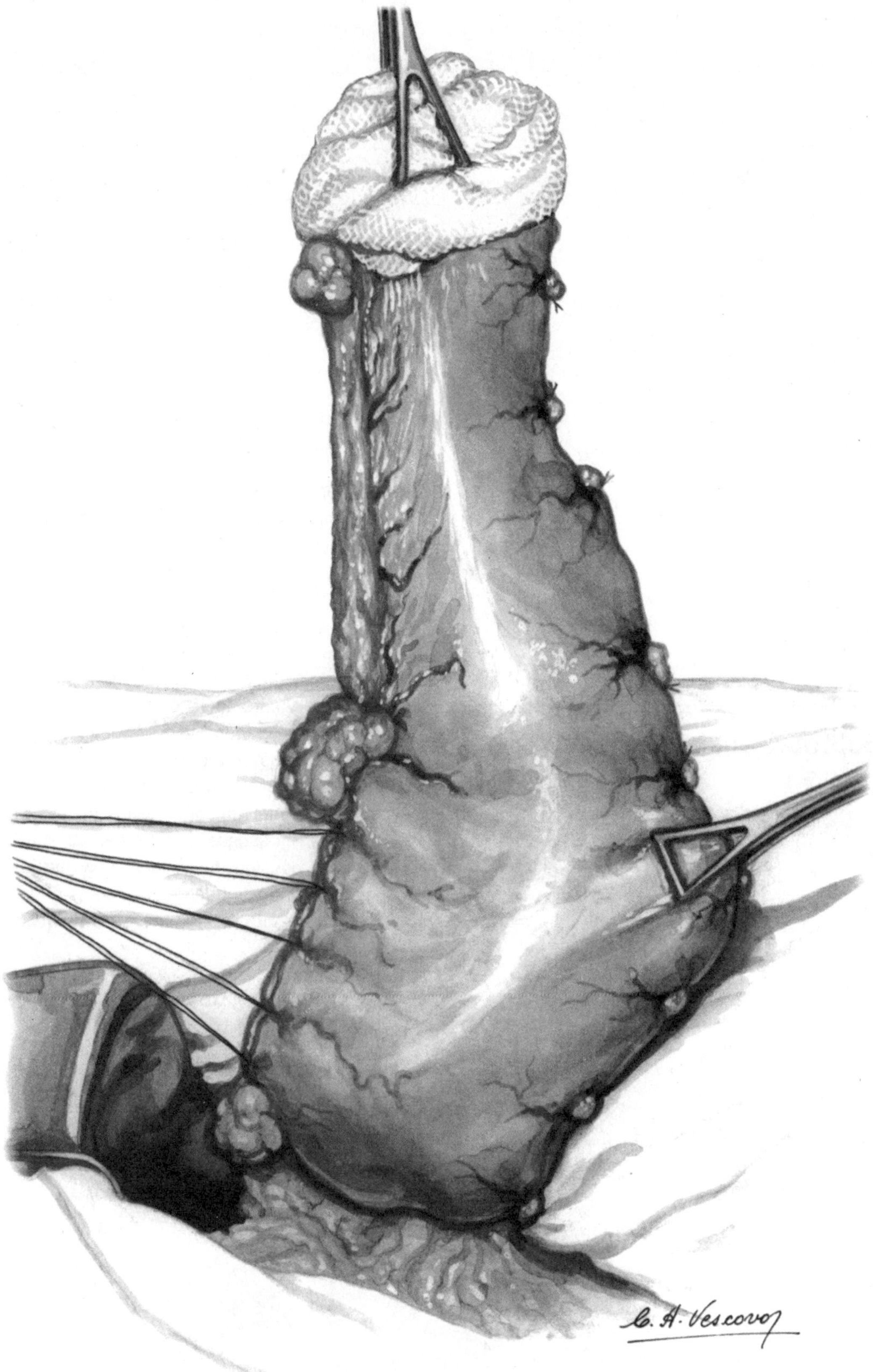

FIGURE 38.15

Radical Subtotal Gastrectomy

FIGURE 38.16

If the gastric resection to be performed is a 70 to 80% resection, it is possible to place atraumatic clamps on the stomach and the jejunum when the anastomosis is performed. In these cases the author uses a twin atraumatic Finochietto clamp. If the gastric resection is more extensive (high subtotal or quasi-total gastrectomy) it is difficult to carry out the gastrojejunal anastomosis using clamps. The author prefers to perform the gastrojejunal anastomosis using clamps whenever possible, because this is cleaner and more precise than the anastomosis without clamps. In the drawing it can be observed that the superior branch of the atraumatic twin Finochietto clamp has been placed (resection of 70% of the stomach). Above the clamp a Levine nasogastric tube can be seen. In the inferior drawing it is possible to observe how the distal arm of the Finochietto clamp has been placed so as to prevent spillage of gastric contents into the abdominal cavity when the stomach is transected.

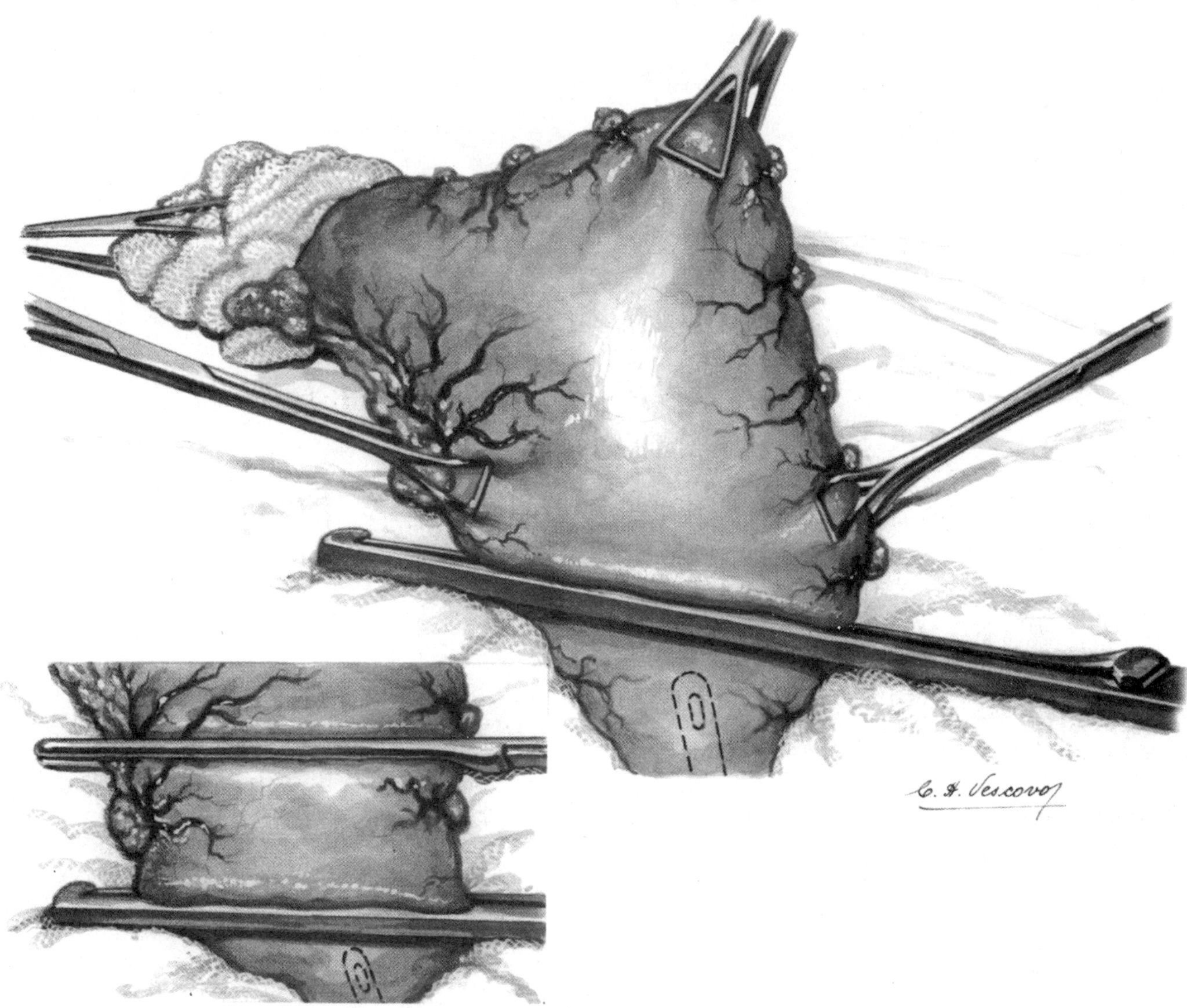

FIGURE 38.16

Radical Subtotal Gastrectomy

FIGURE 38.17

The superior arm of Finochietto twin clamp has been applied to the proximal portion of the stomach. The inferior branch of the clamp is in place on the anastomotic jejunal limb. Later both arms of the clamp will be joined to carry out a two-layer anastomosis in a manner similar to that described in the Billroth II gastrectomy for peptic ulcer.

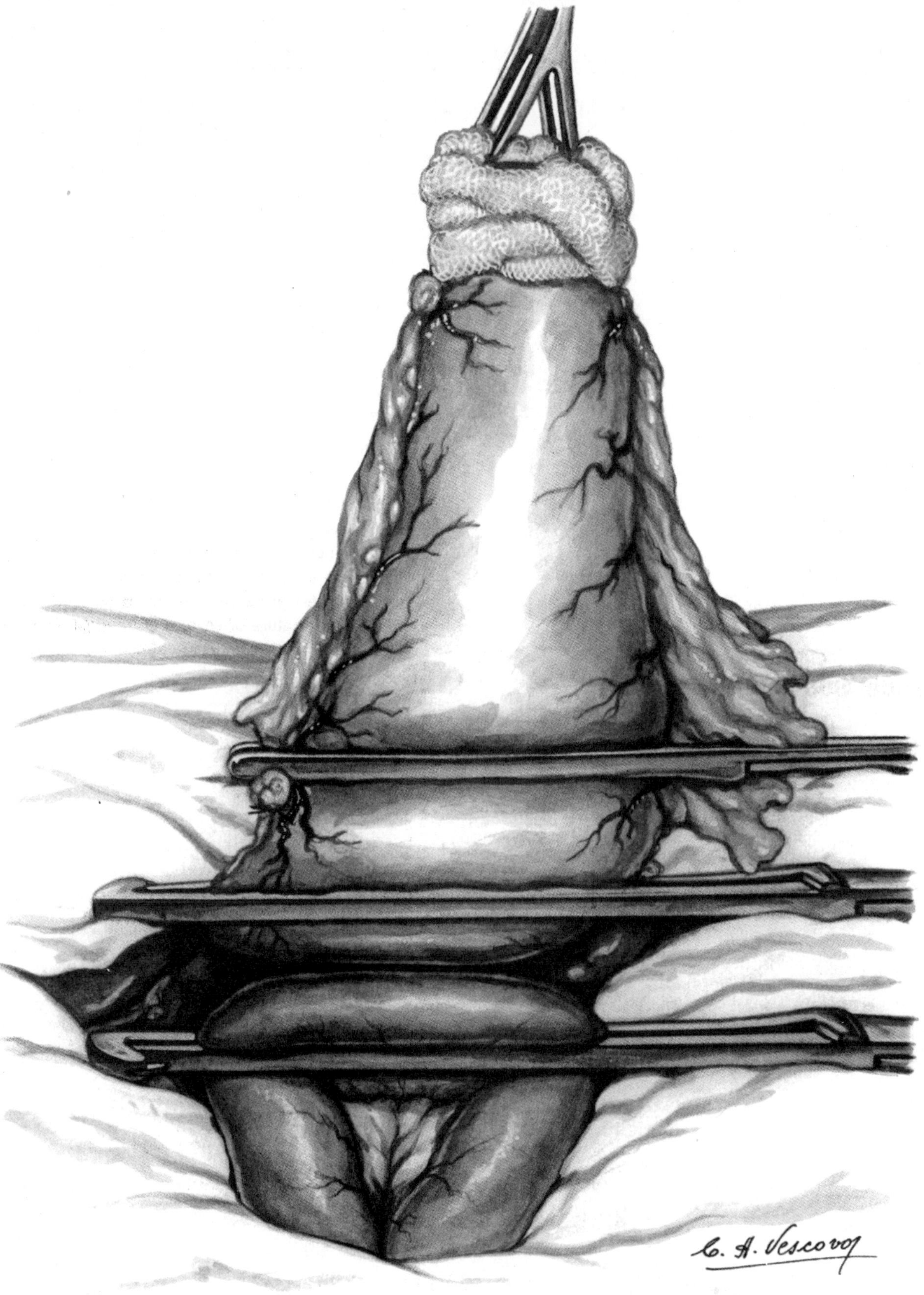

FIGURE 38.17

FIGURE 38.18
The radical subtotal gastrectomy for carcinoma of the distal portion of the stomach is almost complete. The ligature of the left gastric artery at its origin in the celiac trunk can be seen as well as the ligature of several of the short gastric vessels to allow the upper portion of the stomach to be transected.

Radical Subtotal Gastrectomy

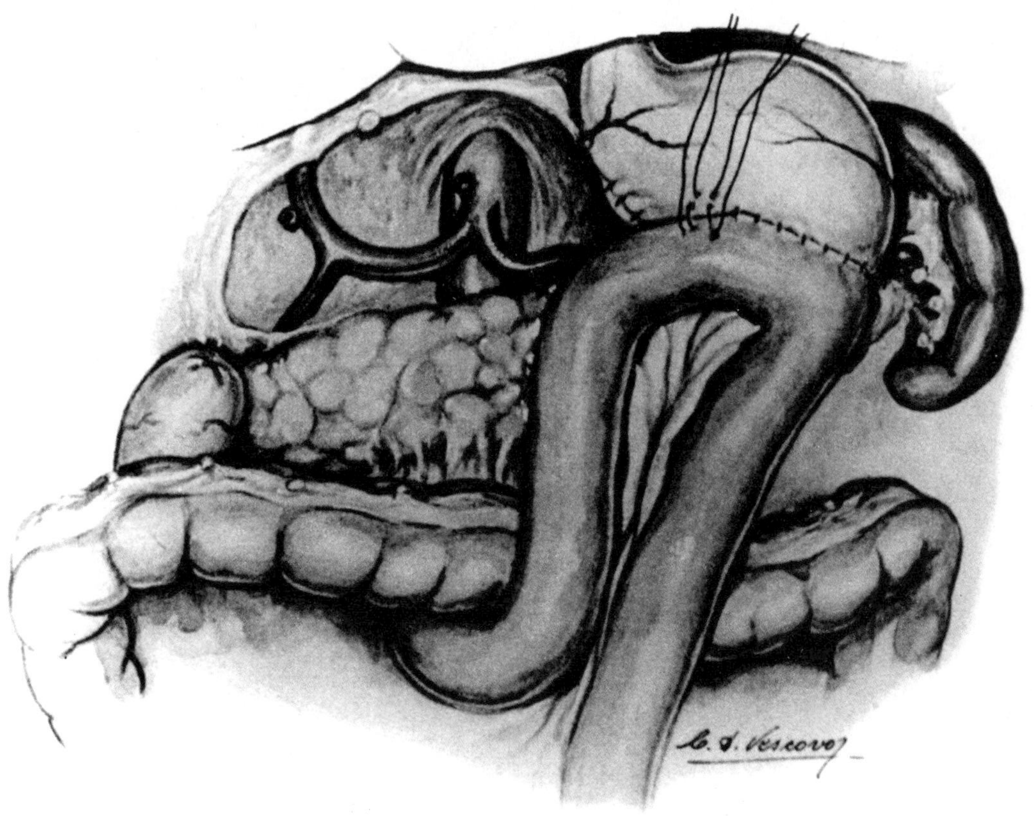

FIGURE 38.18

Extended Radical Subtotal Gastrectomy

FIGURE 38.19
In this case the gastric carcinoma infiltrates an avascular portion of the transverse mesocolon to the left of the middle colic vessels (space of Riolano). In this situation, resection of the mesocolon and the transverse colon, to the extent shown in the drawing, should be added. For this reason it is advisable to prepare the colon for surgery when confronted with a gastric cancer, in case it may become necessary to resect and anastomose a segment of the transverse colon in the same operative procedure.

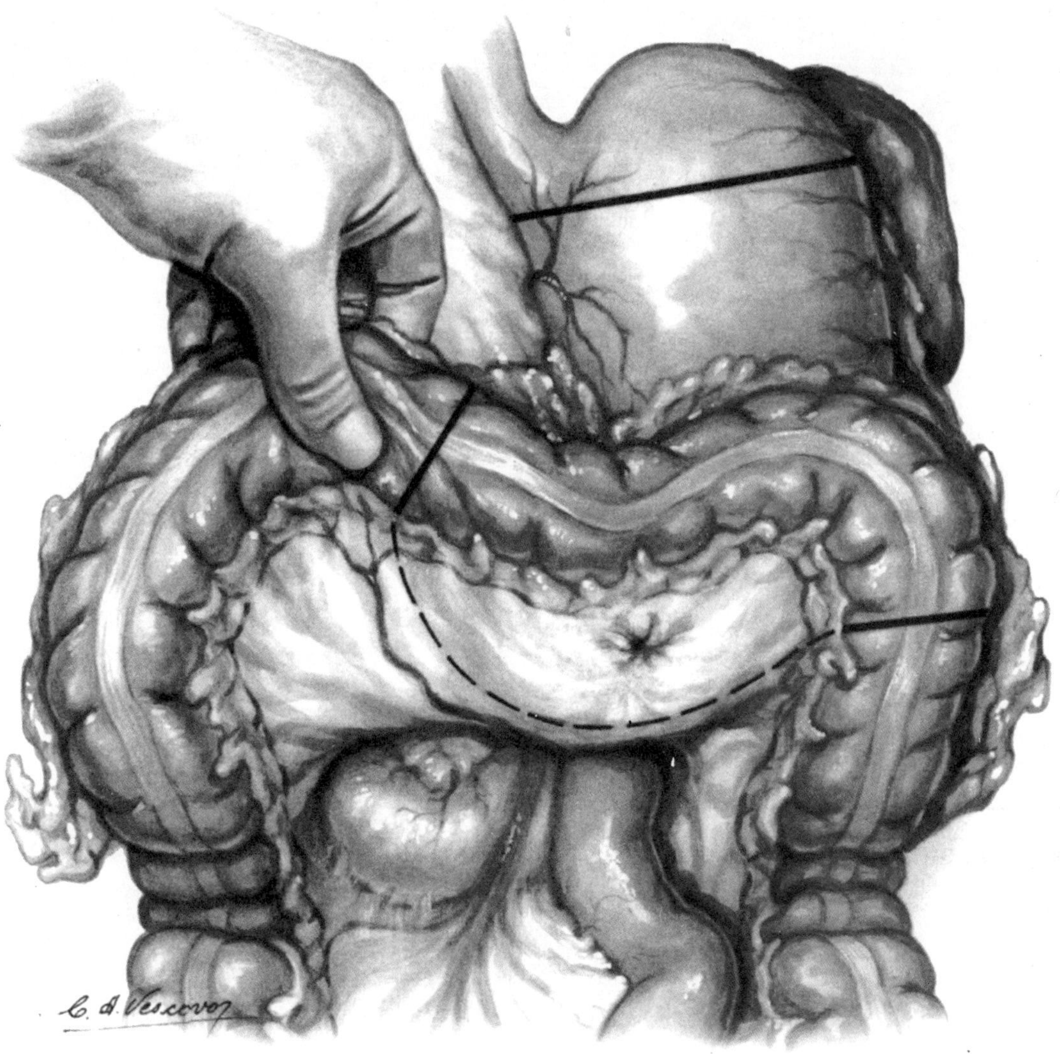

FIGURE 38.19

FIGURE 38.20
The drawing shows a carcinoma of the anterior gastric wall that is infiltrating the transverse colon. To the radical subtotal gastrectomy, a resection of the entire transverse colon, including its mesocolon, should be added. The limits of this resection are shown in the drawing.

Extended Radical Subtotal Gastrectomy

FIGURE 38.21
This drawing shows the limits of an en bloc resection of 80% of the distal stomach together with the transverse mesocolon. The ligature and transection of the middle colic artery can be observed. The ends of the colon are held by atraumatic clamps, ready to be anastomosed.

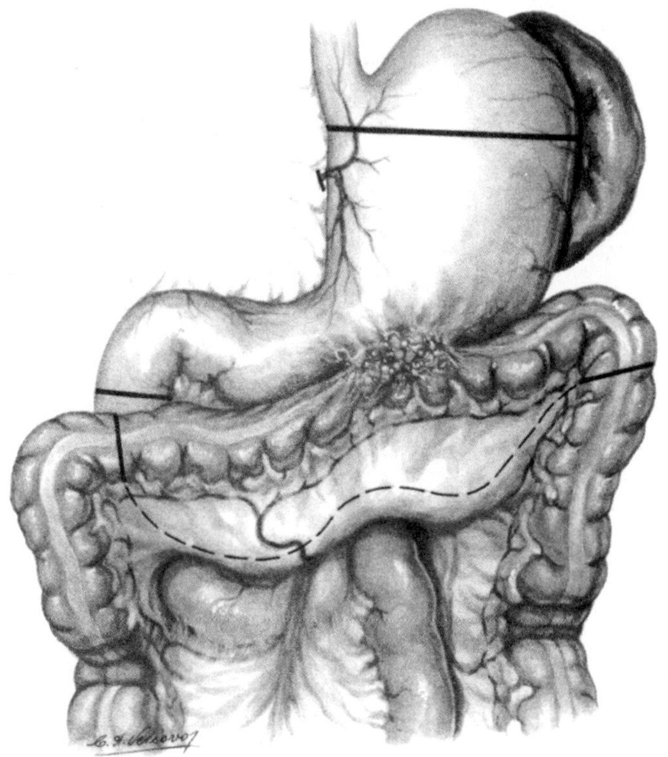

FIGURE 38.20

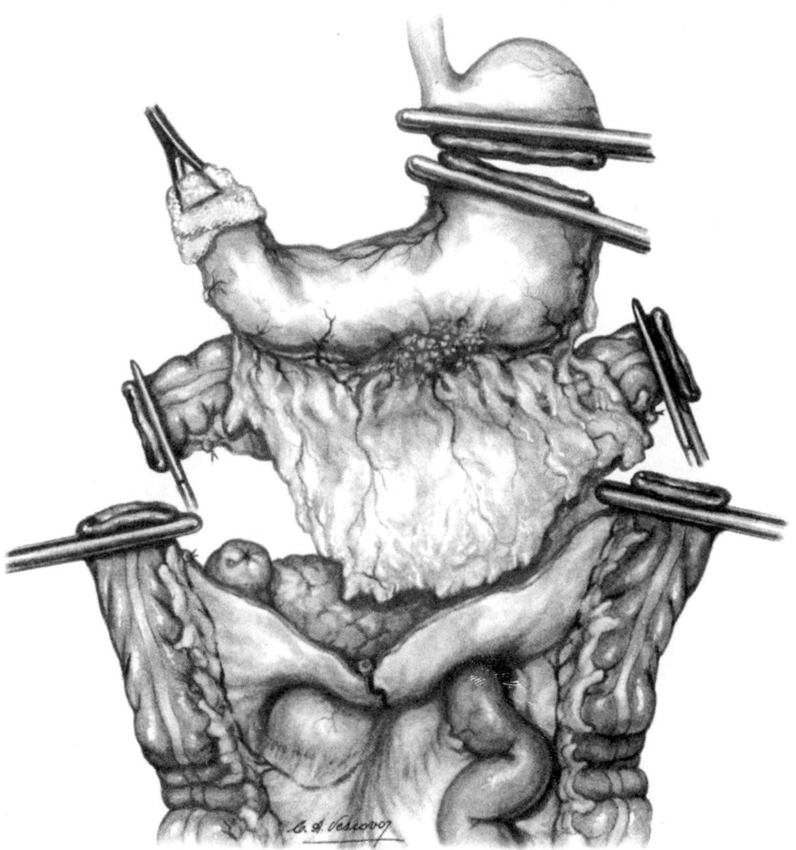

FIGURE 38.21

Extended Radical Subtotal Gastrectomy

FIGURE 38.22
The ends of the transected colon will be anastomosed in end-to-end fashion, using two layers of interrupted sutures: 3-0 chromic catgut on the mucosal layer, and cotton, silk, or some other nonabsorbable synthetic material in the seromuscular plane.

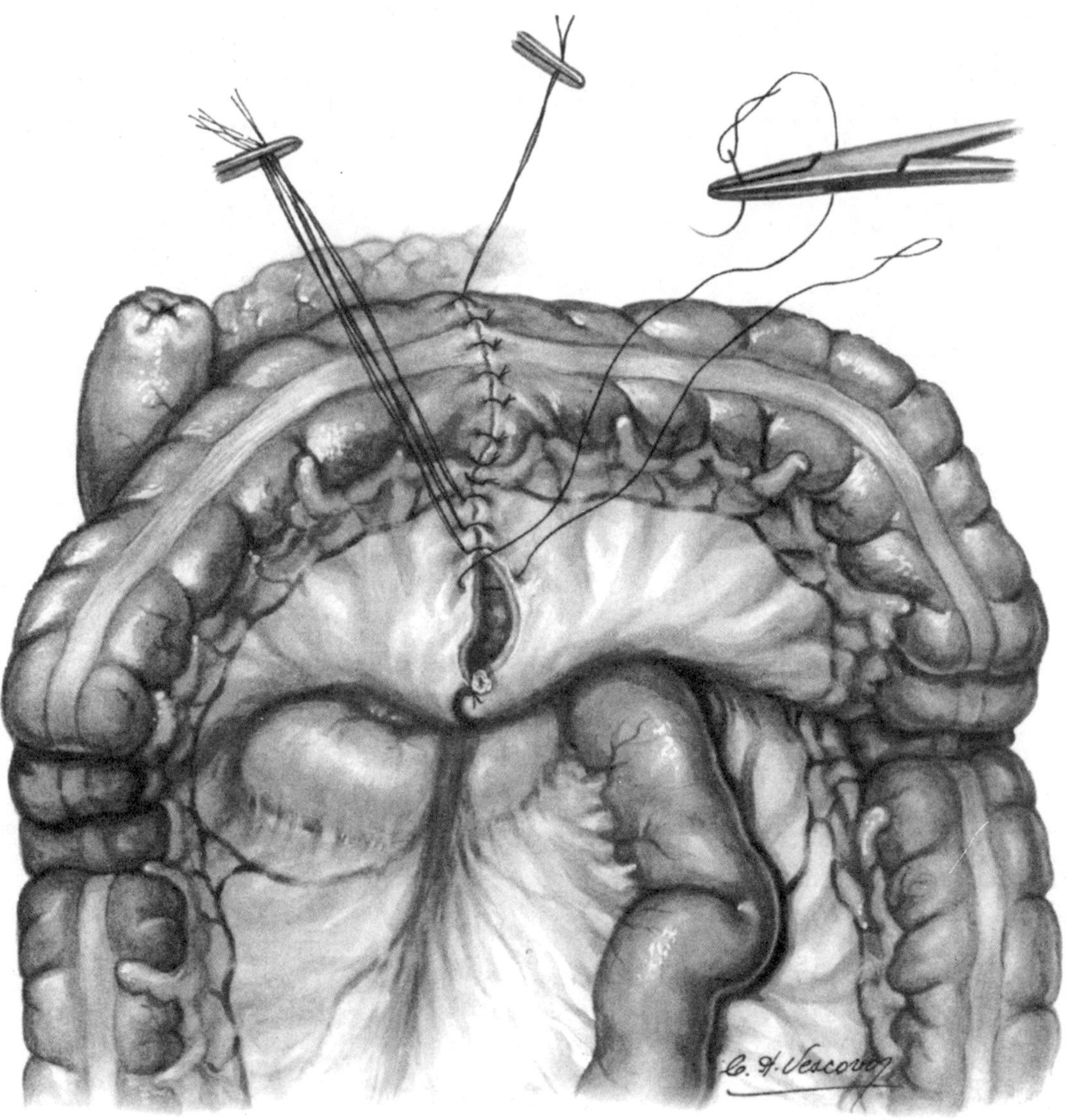

FIGURE 38.22

FIGURE 38.23
This is a case of polypoid carcinoma of the stomach located in the upper portion of the middle third of the stomach, partially infiltrating the left lobe of the liver. The patient was subjected to a quasi-total radical gastrectomy with resection of the invaded segment of the liver. The extent of resection of the left lobe of the liver is shown by the broken line.

Extended Radical Subtotal Gastrectomy

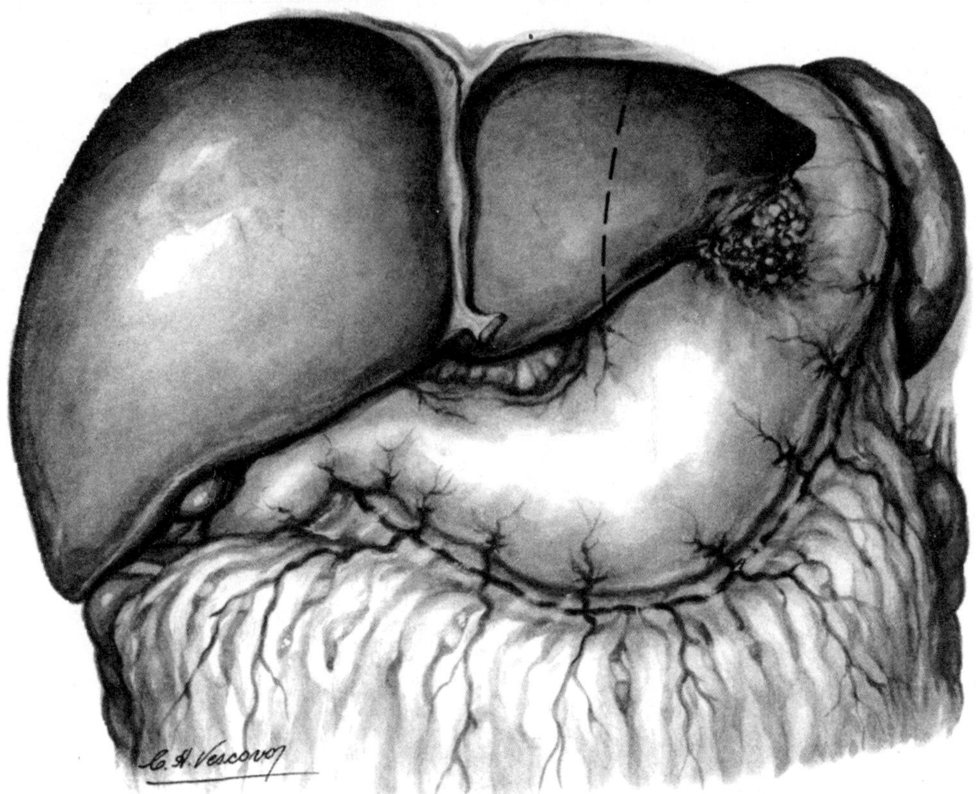

FIGURE 38.23

FIGURE 38.24
Before proceeding to transect the hepatic parenchyma, it must be shown that the index finger of the surgeon can surround the portion of liver invaded by the tumor. The drawing shows this maneuver.

Extended Radical Subtotal Gastrectomy

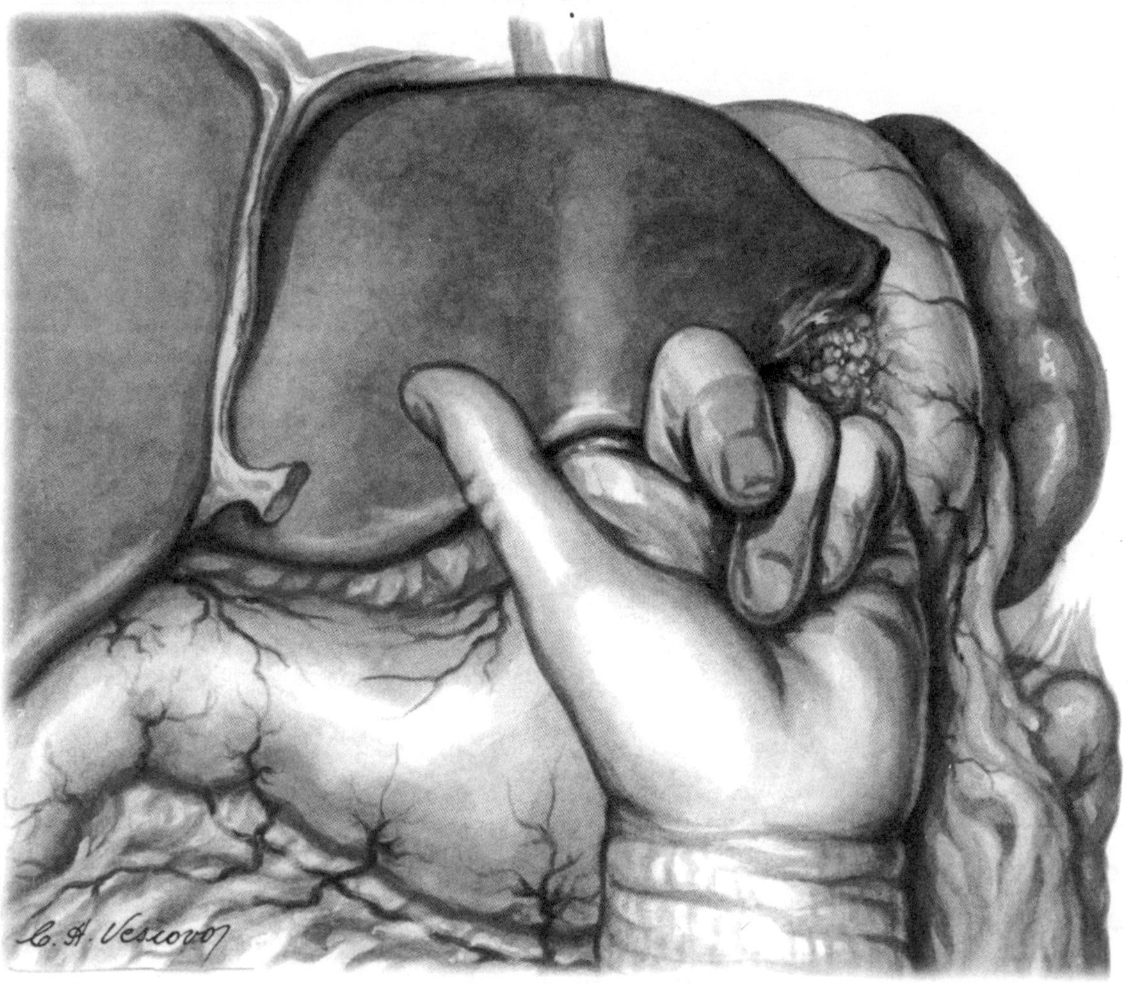

FIGURE 38.24

FIGURE 38.25
Glisson's capsule is incised using the electrocautery. Following this, compression of the hepatic parenchyma is carried out using the index finger and the thumb (digitoclasia or finger fracture). This technique is continued until resistance is encountered, be it due to the presence of a blood vessel, a branch of the hepatic artery, a branch of the portal vein, or an intrahepatic biliary duct. These elements should be isolated, ligated, and divided. Some surgeons use clips to occlude these structures instead of ligating them. Hemostasis in resection of hepatic parenchyma should be exact. In addition, the surgeon should be sure of having ligated all the intrahepatic biliary ducts, because during the operation there may be no visible spillage of bile, but bile may leak postoperatively. Some surgeons do not divide the hepatic parenchyma with the fingers, but use the handle of the scalpel.

Extended Radical Subtotal Gastrectomy

FIGURE 38.26
A blood vessel has been grasped with two hemostatic clamps prior to its division and ligation.

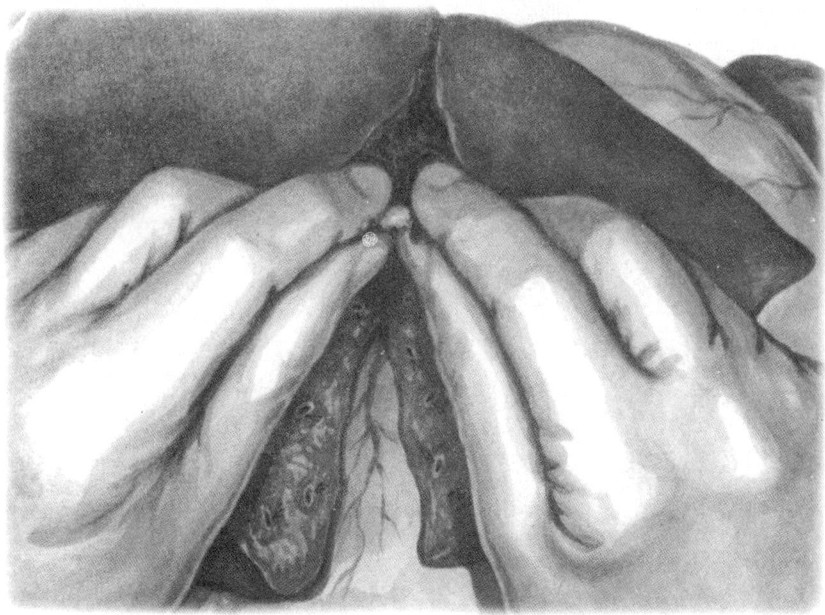

FIGURE 38.25

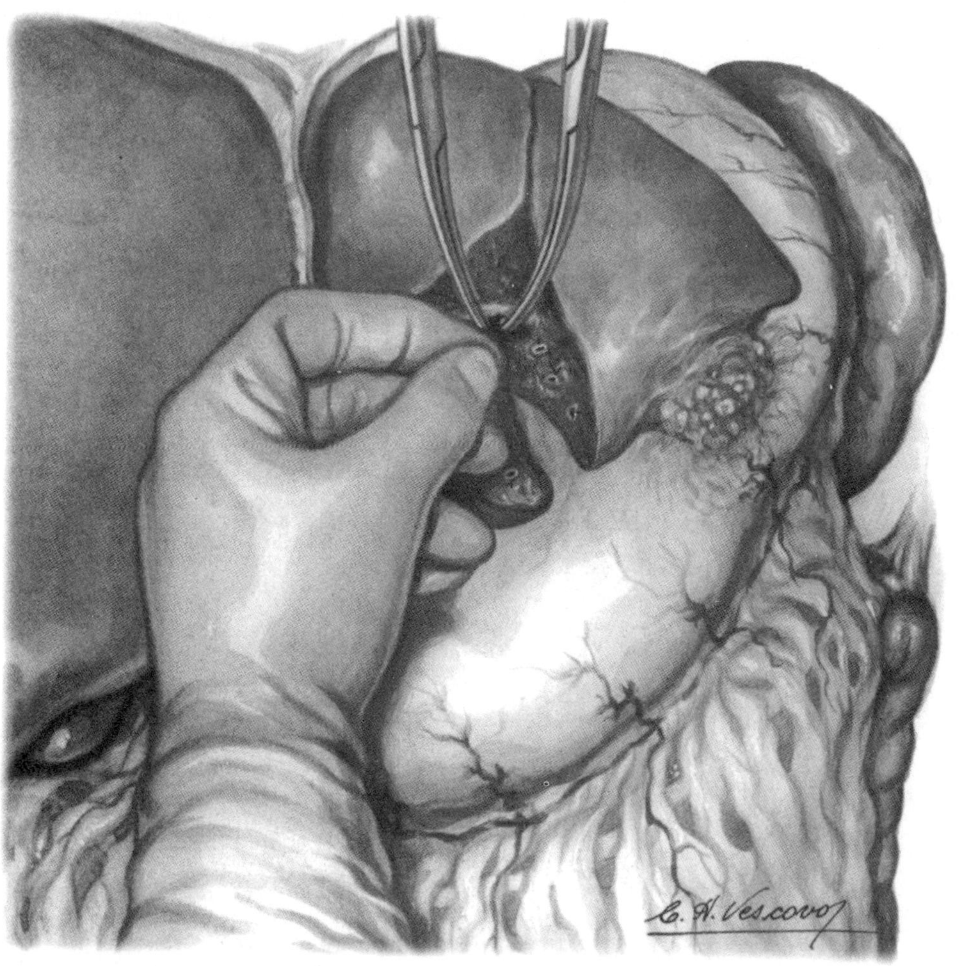

FIGURE 38.26

FIGURE 38.27
If necessary, hemostasis of the hepatic parenchyma may be completed using some hemostatic materials such as surgicel or Gelfoam soaked in thrombin or with Avitene. In some cases, it may be necessary to resort to sutures using heavy catgut. These U sutures are also known as mattress sutures and are placed near the line of transection of the hepatic parenchyma, as seen in the drawing.

Extended Radical Subtotal Gastrectomy

FIGURE 38.28
This figure shows that the greater omentum has been separated from the transverse colon and the duodenum has been divided and its distal side sutured. The left gastric artery has also been ligated and transected at its exit from the celiac trunk. Transection of the stomach will be performed 4 cm above the tumor, since it is polypoid in type. The border of the stomach is not infiltrated microscopically by the carcinoma, a fact that must be confirmed by examining the operative specimen. Histologically this was a case of Lauren intestinal carcinoma.

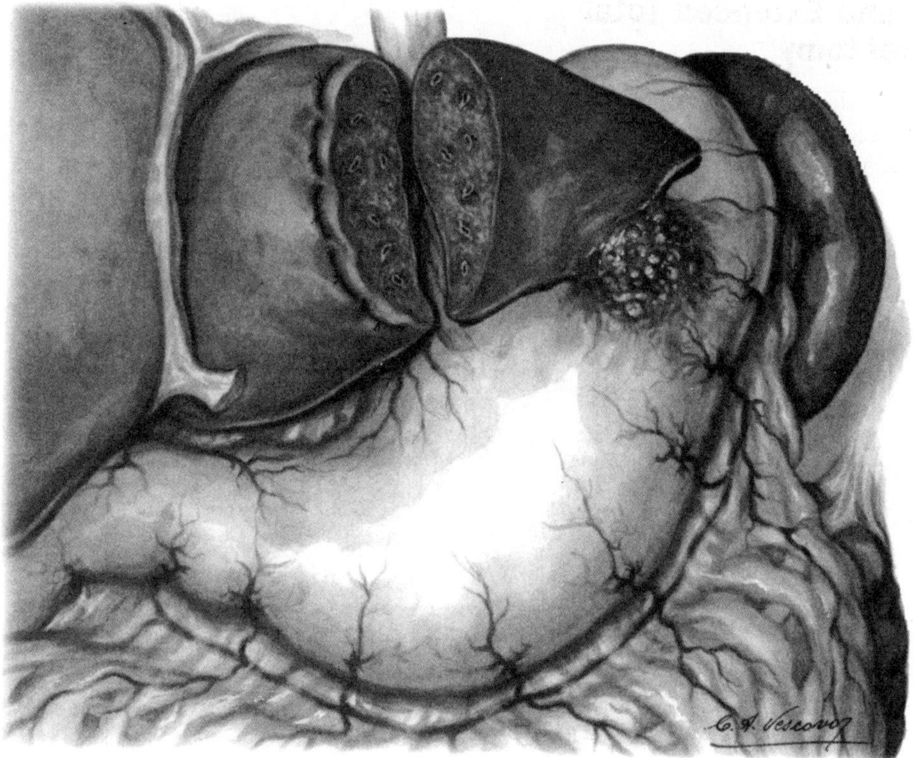

FIGURE 38.27

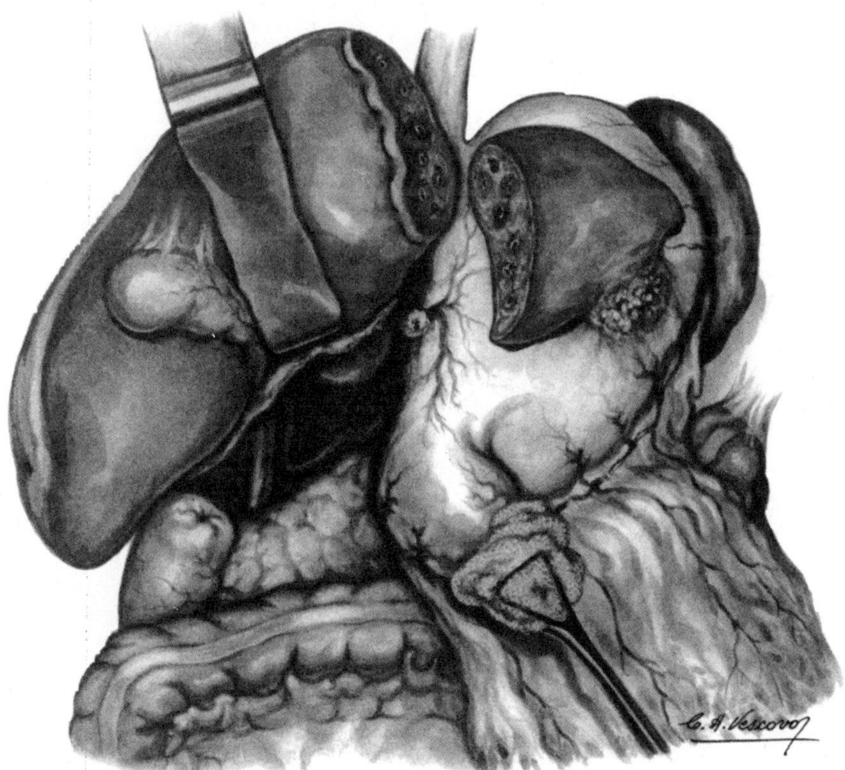

FIGURE 38.28

Total Radical and Extended Total Radical Gastrectomy

The following will be a description of the operative steps of total radical gastrectomy that were not shown in the description of radical subtotal gastrectomy.

Total Radical and Extended Total Radical Gastrectomy

Total Radical and Extended Total Radical Gastrectomy

FIGURE 38.29

The drawing shows a carcinoma of the anterior gastric wall infiltrating the lesser curvature. The distal two thirds of the stomach have been freed, and only the proximal third of the stomach and the distal portion of the esophagus are still to be freed. The left gastric artery has been ligated and divided at its origin in the celiac trunk. The right gastric artery has also been ligated and divided. The duodenal stump has been transected and sutured. Several distal short vessels have been ligated, and the left triangular ligament of the liver is being divided in order to be able to reflect the left lobe of the liver upward. Some authors advise ligating the triangular ligament before dividing it since cases of hemorrhaging after its transection and cases of leakage of bile due to aberrant biliary ducts have been observed.

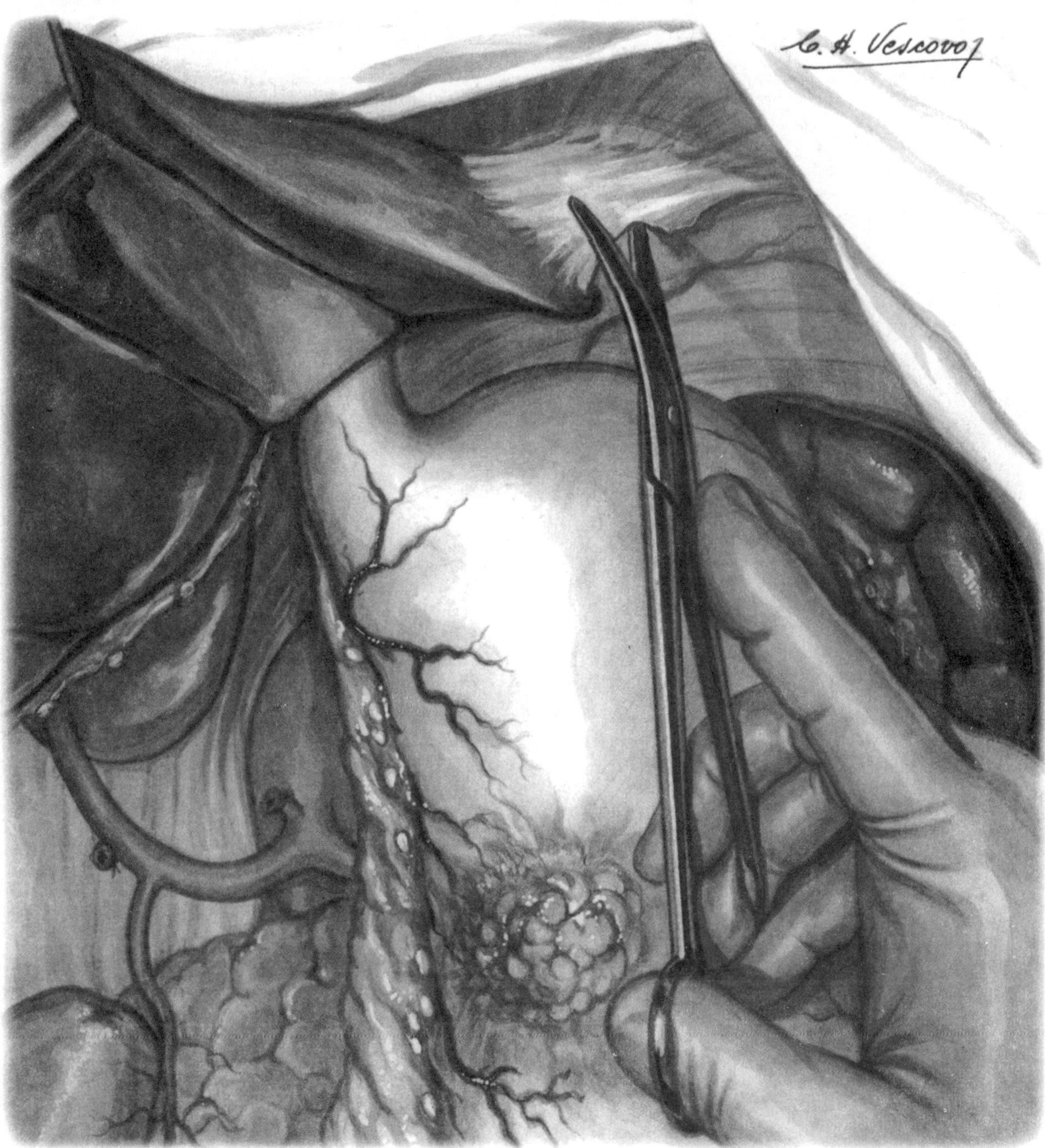

FIGURE 38.29

Total Radical and Extended Total Radical Gastrectomy

FIGURE 38.30
All the short vessels have been divided and ligated, and the gastrophrenic ligament, situated between the first short vessel and the angle of His, is about to be tied and divided. The gastrophrenic ligament is made up of fibrous tissue and can be divided without previous ligation. However, there have been cases in which this ligament has blood vessels in it and its transection was followed by hemorrhage. The author prefers to ligate this ligament before dividing it.

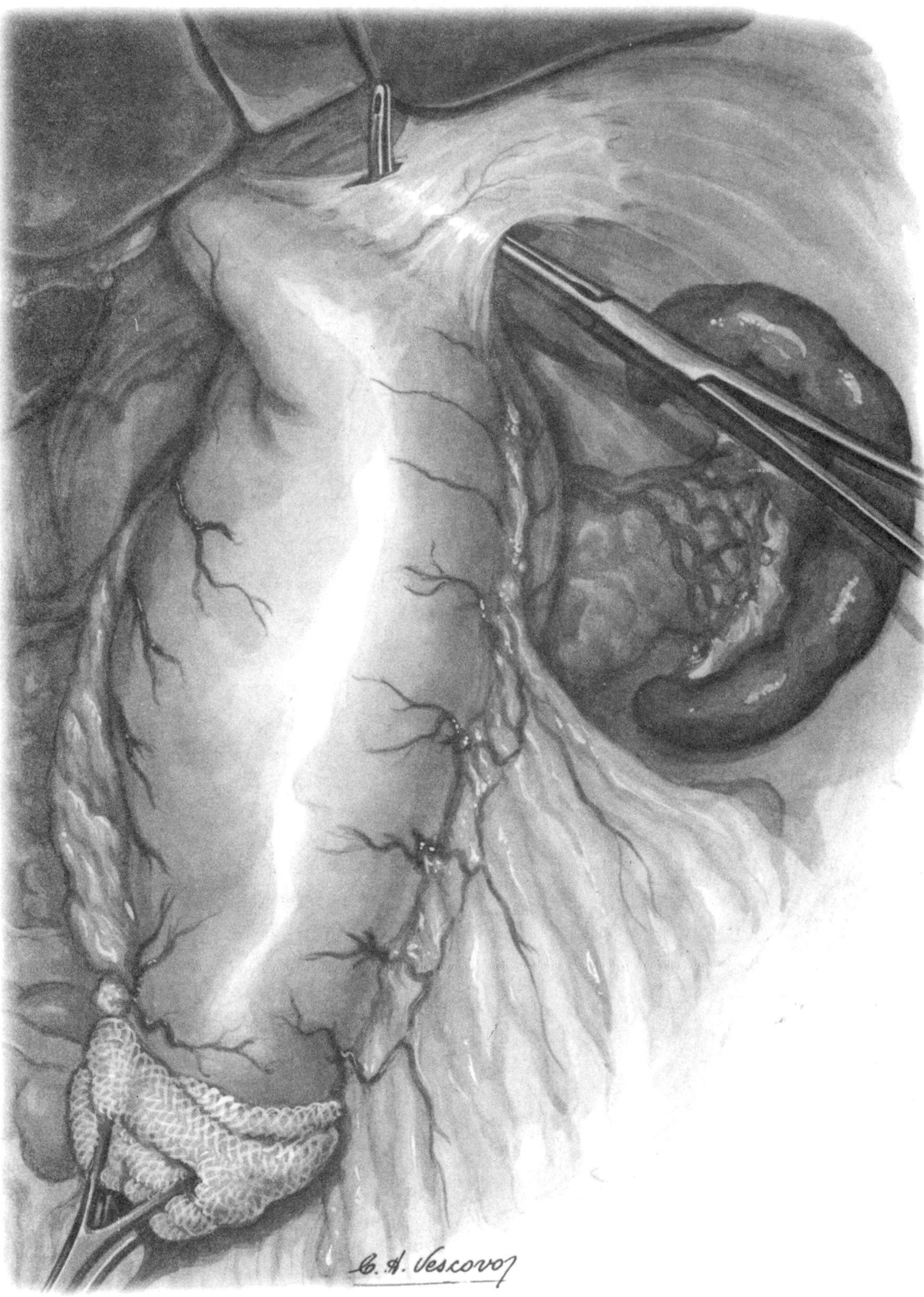

FIGURE 38.30

Total Radical and Extended Total Radical Gastrectomy

FIGURE 38.31
The peritoneum of the esophagodiaphragmatic area is being divided. The right border of the esophagus will then be freed. In order to carry this out it is necessary to divide the upper portion of the gastrohepatic ligament (pars condensa). Before dividing the pars condensa of the gastrohepatic ligament, it is necessary to investigate the possible existence of an aberrant left hepatic artery arising from the left gastric artery, since division of this artery may lead to partial or complete necrosis of the left lobe of the liver.

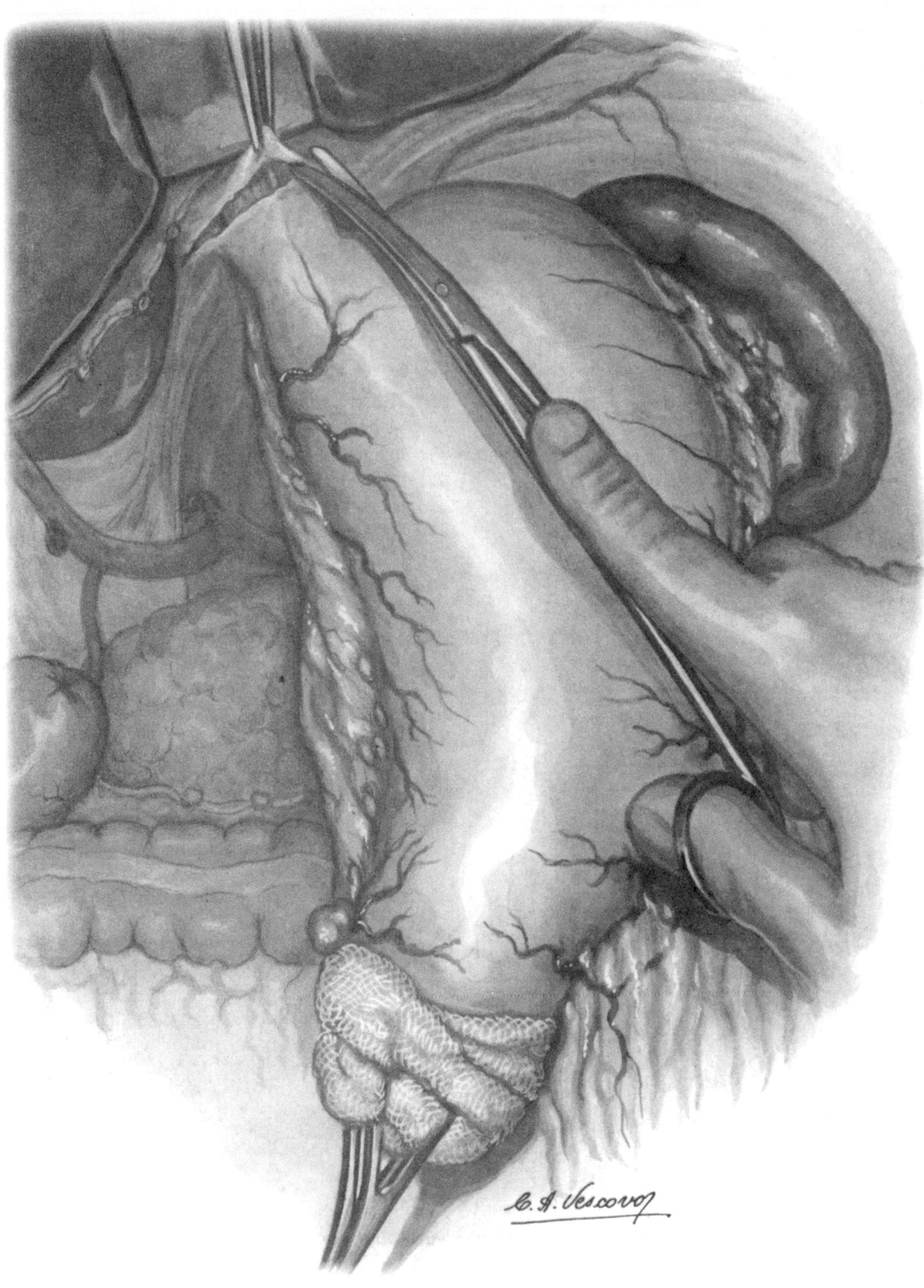

FIGURE 38.31

FIGURE 38.32
Both vagus nerves have been identified and transected, facilitating digital dissection and lowering of the distal esophagus. This descent of the distal esophagus, in addition to making the anastomosis to the jejunum easier, allows division of the esophagus where it is not infiltrated by tumor. For this reason it is indispensable to carry out a frozen section biopsy. In patients in whom there is difficulty in bringing the esophagus down as much as necessary, the surgeon can resort to the Savinyj maneuver, cited previously (109). This consists of dividing the diaphragm from the anterior wall of the esophagus forward as much as necessary, making all maneuvers easier in the lower esophagus. The divided diaphragm does not have to be sutured.

Total Radical and Extended Total Radical Gastrectomy

FIGURE 38.33
A rubber catheter has been passed around the distal esophagus, and traction is being applied to it downward and to the left. Tumors of the middle or proximal third of the stomach may invade several centimeters of the distal esophagus microscopically. This makes it indispensable to perform a frozen section biopsy of the level of transection of the esophagus. The esophagus should be transected at least 5 cm from the esophagogastric junction.

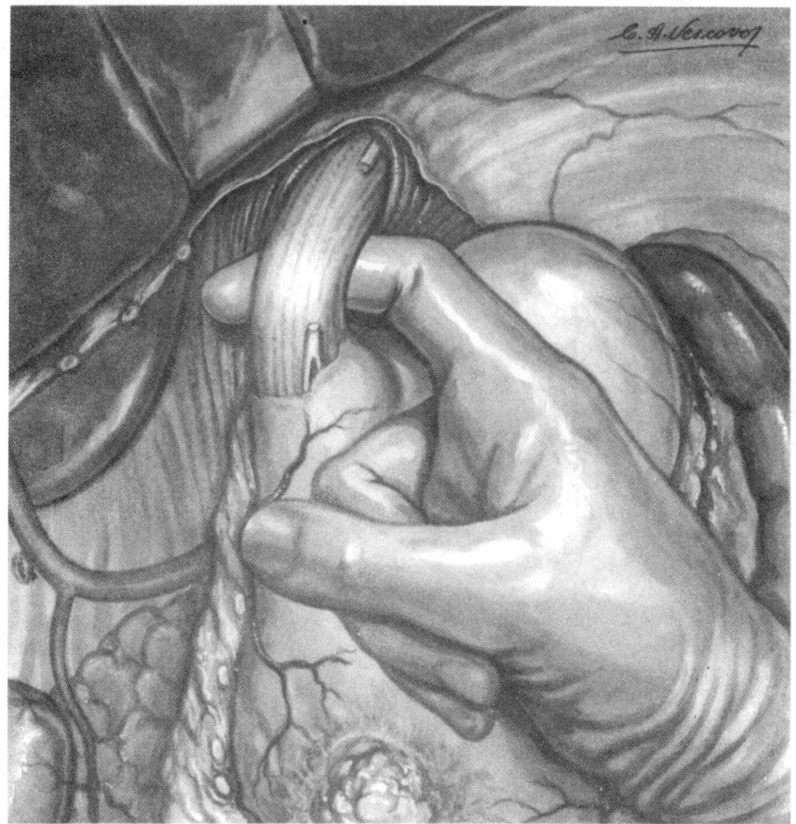

FIGURE 38.32

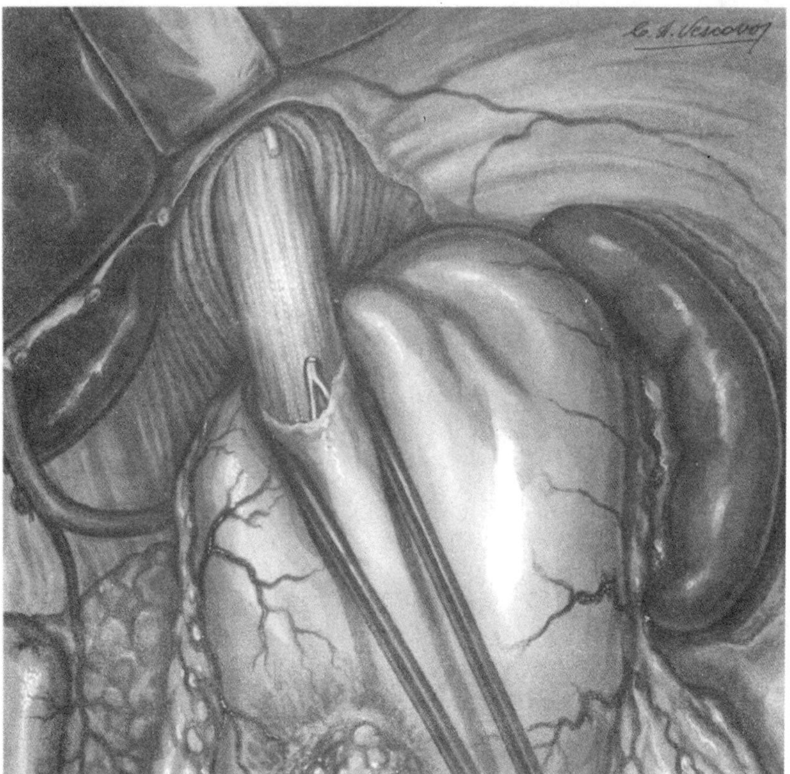

FIGURE 38.33

Total Radical and Extended Total Radical Gastrectomy

FIGURE 38.34 TOTAL RADICAL EXTENDED GASTRECTOMY
Total radical gastrectomy with resection of the tail or the body and the tail of the pancreas, with splenectomy, is indicated in cases in which the gastric carcinoma infiltrates the body or the body and tail of the pancreas. Resection of the body and tail of the pancreas that is added to total gastrectomy is carried out by necessity and not to remove the superior pancreatic nodes or the nodes of the splenic hilus (34). The drawing shows the usual extent of this resection.

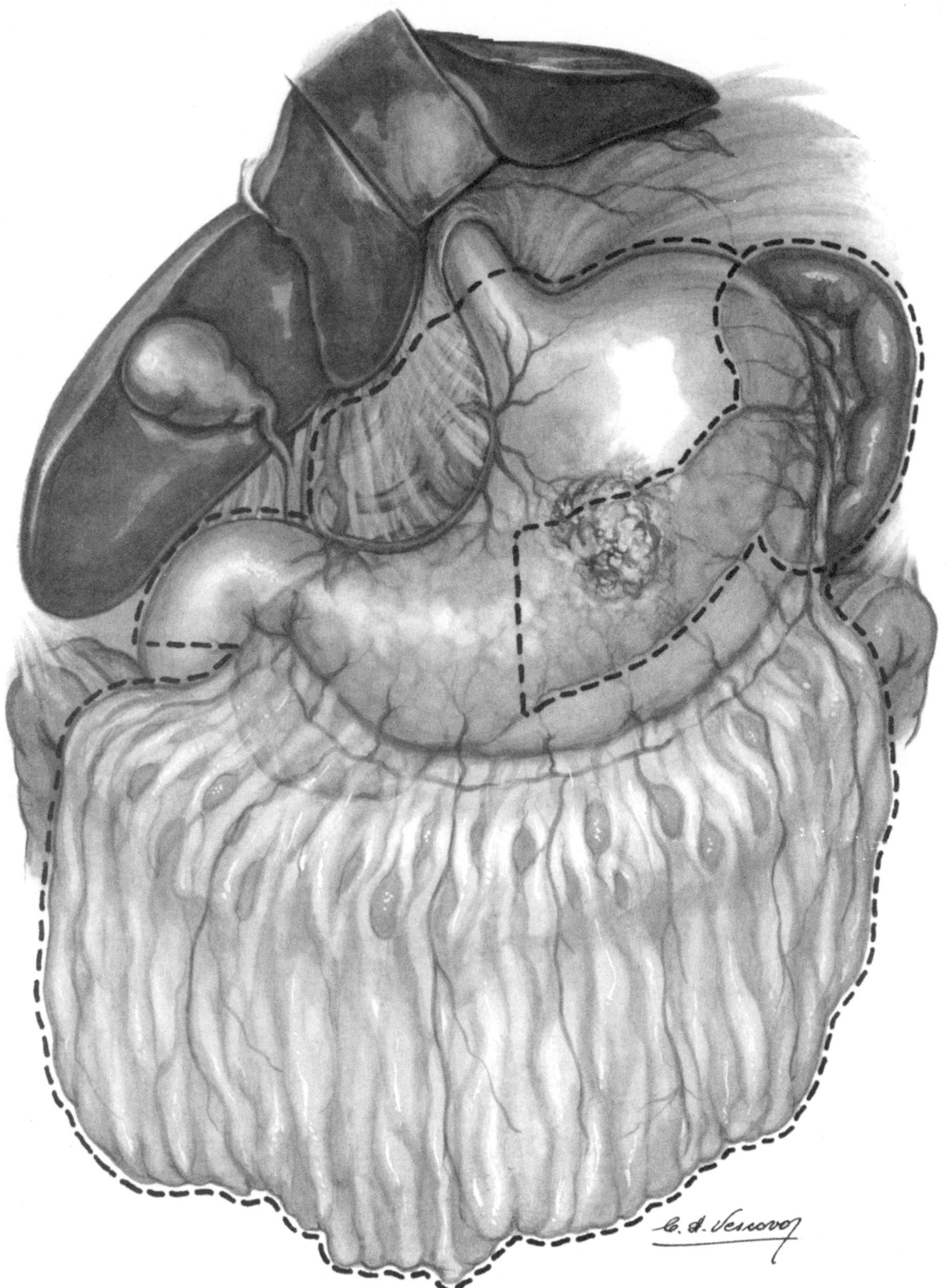

FIGURE 38.34 TOTAL RADICAL EXTENDED GASTRECTOMY

FIGURE 38.35
This drawing shows the surgical steps in resection of the body and tail of the pancreas with splenectomy: **A,** The splenic artery and vein have been ligated at the level where the pancreas is to be transected. Using a scalpel, the body of the pancreas is divided obliquely. **B,** The pancreatic duct has been sutured using two ligatures of nonabsorbable material and the transected edge of the body of the pancreas is being sutured using interrupted sutures of nonabsorbable material. Division of the pancreas obliquely makes this layer of sutures easier to realize. **C,** Suturing of the pancreatic stump has been completed. **D,** The sutured pancreatic stump is covered with a segment of peritoneum fixed over the stump with some sutures.

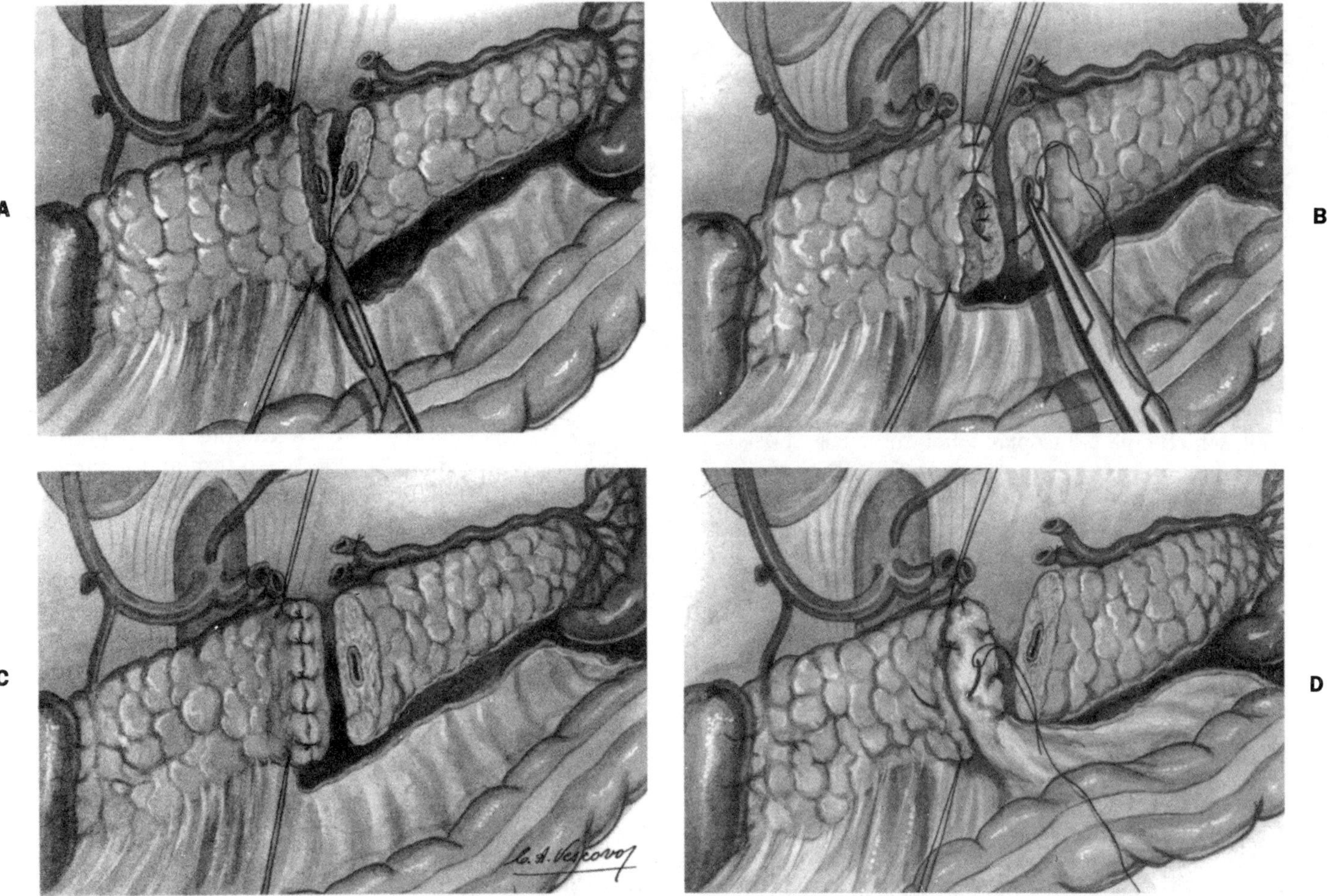

FIGURE 38.35

RECONSTRUCTION OF DIGESTIVE CONTINUITY AFTER TOTAL GASTRECTOMY

Numerous surgical procedures have been proposed to reconstruct the digestive tract after a total gastrectomy. A great variety of reservoirs constructed at the expense of the jejunum to replace the stomach have been designed. None of the proposed procedures has demonstrated to be better than anastomosis of the esophagus with a jejunal loop disposed as a Roux-en-Y in an isoperistaltic fashion.

It is undoubtedly true that total gastrectomy presents greater technical difficulties than subtotal gastrectomy. This is principally due to the fragility of the esophageal wall, which enters into play when the anastomosis with the jejunum is being performed. The esophagojejunal anastomosis is not only difficult, but risky, due to the possibility of disruption of the suture line, which is the most frequent cause of mortality and morbidity.

Gastrectomy and the reestablishment of the digestive transit should be practiced respecting basic principles, some of which will be shown as follows (100):

1. Esophagojejunal suturing should be performed in the most correct fashion possible, always keeping in mind the fragility of the esophageal tissues.
2. When the esophagus is transected it is frequently apparent that the esophageal mucosa has great tendency to retract. This may lead to an incorrect suture line because one or more of the sutures may not include the retracted mucosa, favoring disruption of the suture line. To avoid this inconvenience, some authors (140), before performing the anastomosis, place some 3-0 chromic catgut sutures between the mucosa and the muscularis, preventing retraction of the mucosa. Other authors (100) transect the esophagus in two stages, the first stage including transection of the muscular layer and the second transection of the mucosa a few mm distal to the muscular layer so that if retraction should occur, the mucosa would still be at the same level as the muscular layer.
3. It is important that the esophagojejunal sutures be placed at regular intervals, avoiding superimposition of sutures, so as not to devitalize the esophageal wall (100).
4. If a surgeon has been obtaining good results with a given surgical technique, he or she should continue to use it because this will provide more security than changing the procedure frequently.
5. The reconstruction procedure selected by the surgeon in restoring esophageal transit should lead to minor postoperative functional alterations.
6. The procedure to reconstruct digestive transit should allow the patient to receive enough nutrients to avoid malnutrition.
7. The surgical procedure that is used should not lead to reflux of biliopancreatic secretions into the esophagus.
8. It is advisable that the esophagojejunal anastomosis be constructed so that the terminal end of the esophagus enters the lateral wall of the jejunum. This is because the blood supply of the end of the jejunum is somewhat deficient when compared with the blood supply of the lateral border of the jejunum.
9. Total gastrectomy and reestablishment of digestive transit should be carried out by an experienced team in order to obtain the best functional results and maintain mortality under 10%.

The most commonly used surgical procedures at present are reconstruction of digestive transit after total gastrectomy by the following techniques:

a. Esophagojejunostomy (Roux-en-Y) using manual sutures.
b. Esophagojejunal anastomosis (Roux-en-Y) using mechanical sutures.
c. Anastomosis of the terminal end of the esophagus with a jejunal loop adding a jejunojejunal anastomosis below it.
d. Interposition of a segment of jejunum between the esophagus and the duodenum.

ESOPHAGOJEJUNOSTOMY USING A ROUX-EN-Y JEJUNAL LOOP WITH MANUAL SUTURES

At present this is the most commonly used procedure to reestablish digestive transit after total gastrectomy. Results of this procedure have not been improved by other more complex procedures. If the jejunojejunostomy is performed some 60 cm from the esophagojejunostomy, it is very unusual that biliopancreatic reflux into the esophagus will occur. Best results are obtained when the jejunal limb is carefully selected and long enough so that the esophagojejunal sutures are not under traction and do not interfere with the blood supply. Transillumination can be very helpful in selecting the most adequate jejunal loop. Anastomosis of the esophagus to the jejunum can be carried out in end-to-end fashion or, more adequately, using the end of the esophagus anastomosed to the lateral wall of the jejunum. The jejunal loop can be brought up either behind or in front of the transverse colon. The esophagojejunal anastomosis can be performed manually or using the EEA instrument. We will now describe the terminolateral esophagojejunostomy using manual sutures; later we will describe the same procedure using mechanical sutures.

Esophagojejunostomy Using a Roux-En-Y Jejunal Loop with Manual Sutures

Esophagojejunostomy Using a Roux-En-Y Jejunal Loop with Manual Sutures

FIGURE 38.36
The drawing shows that the most adequate jejunal loop has been selected. This usually corresponds with the third vascular arcade (124). The broken line shows where the incision is to be made. A short broken line has been drawn in an avascular zone of the transverse mesocolon, through which the jejunal loop to be anastomosed to the esophagus will pass (124).

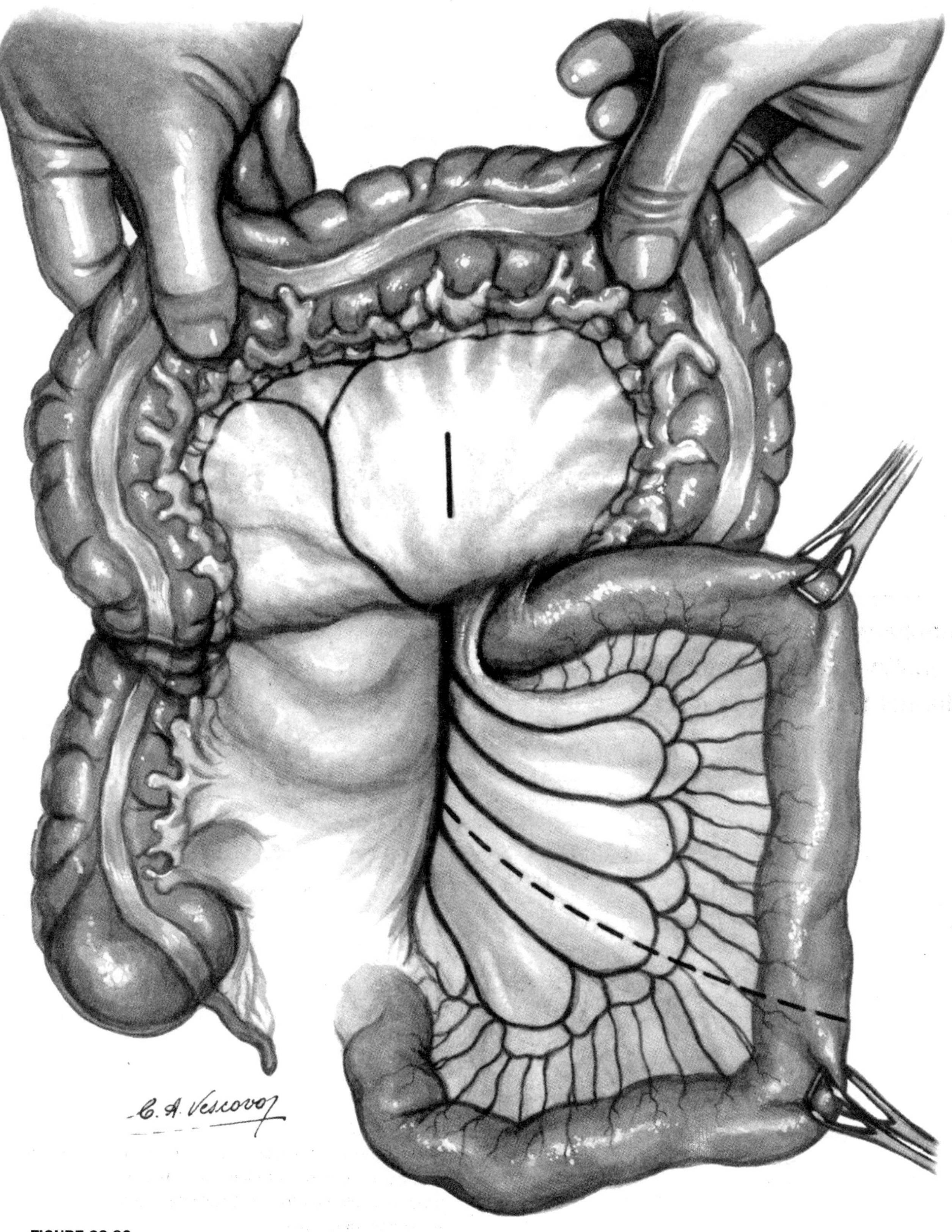

FIGURE 38.36

Esophagojejunostomy Using a Roux-En-Y Jejunal Loop with Manual Sutures

FIGURE 38.37
As shown in the previous figure the jejunum and its mesentery have been divided. Both jejunal ends have been grasped with atraumatic clamps to avoid spillage of intestinal contents into the abdominal cavity.

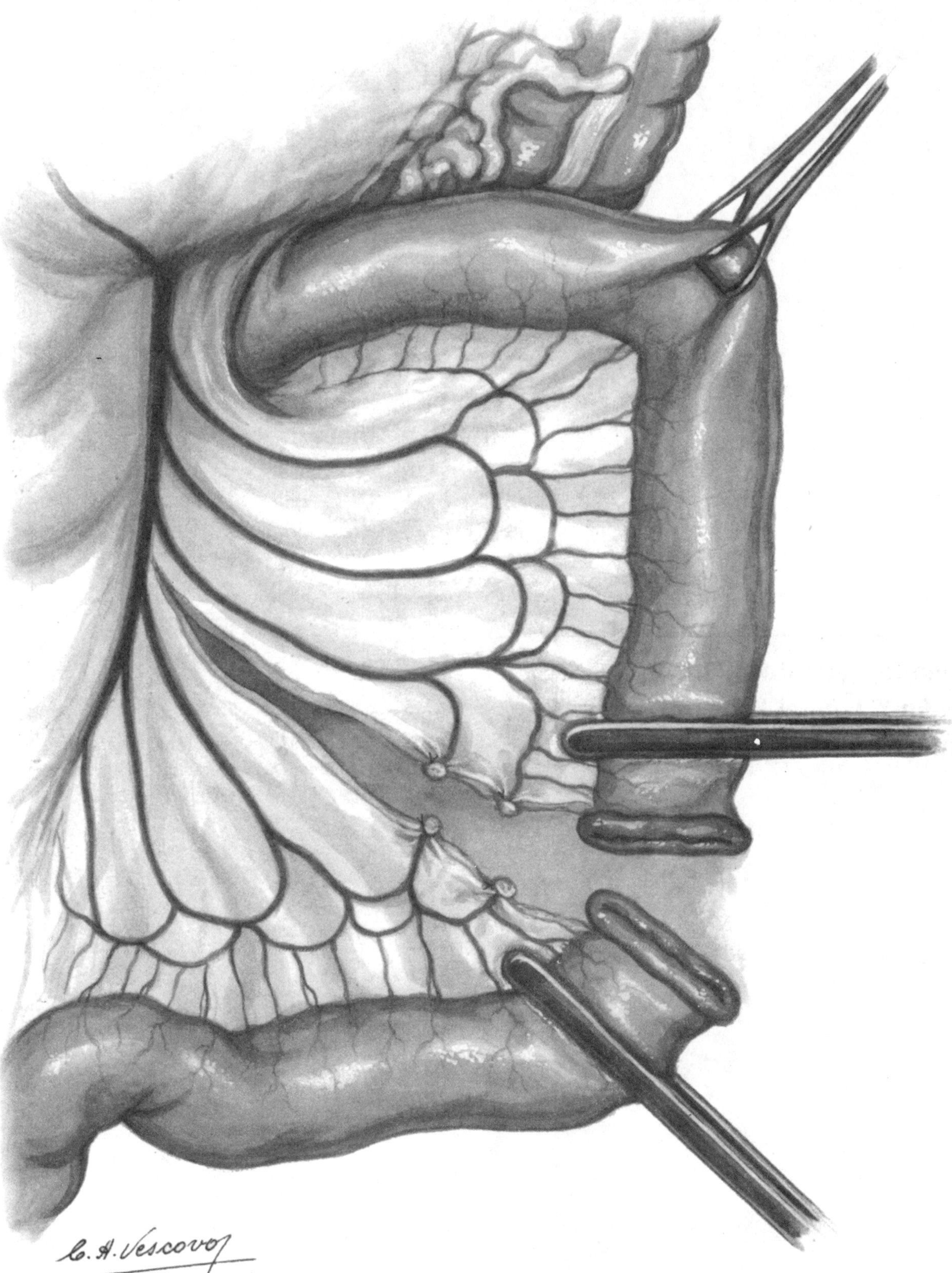

FIGURE 38.37

Esophagojejunostomy Using a Roux-En-Y Jejunal Loop with Manual Sutures

FIGURE 38.38
The distal jejunal end is closed in two layers of sutures using interrupted sutures: **A,** perforating plane; **B,** seromuscular level. **C,** The sutures have been completed.

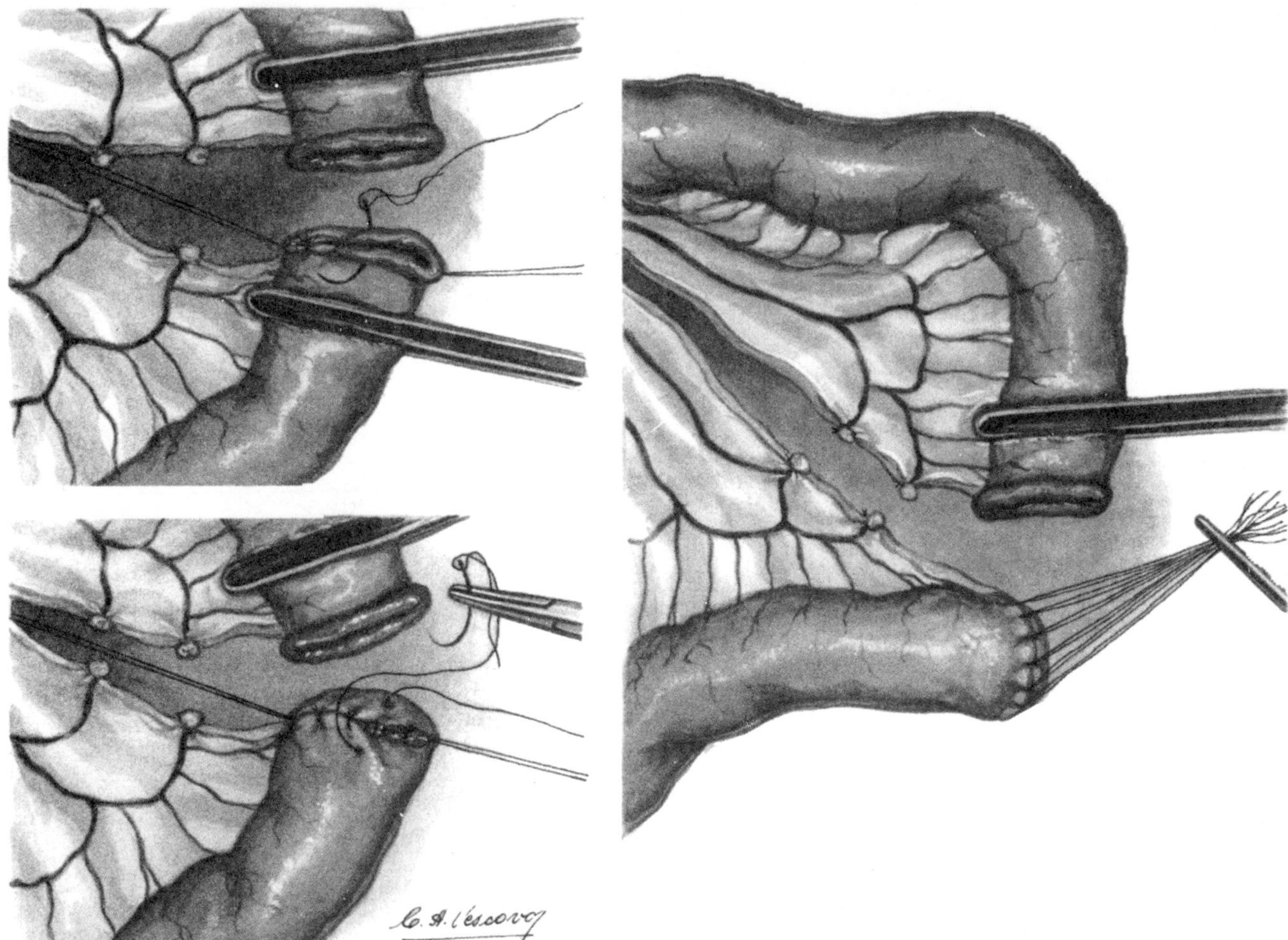

Esophagojejunostomy Using a Roux-En-Y Jejunal Loop with Manual Sutures

FIGURE 38.39
The sutured distal jejunal end has been passed through the transverse mesocolon where it was shown in the previous figure, and brought up to the esophagus, held in place by an atraumatic triangular Duval clamp. The jejunal loop has been marked with a line in its inframesocolic portion where the end of the jejunal loop will be sutured to the distal limb in end-to-side fashion.

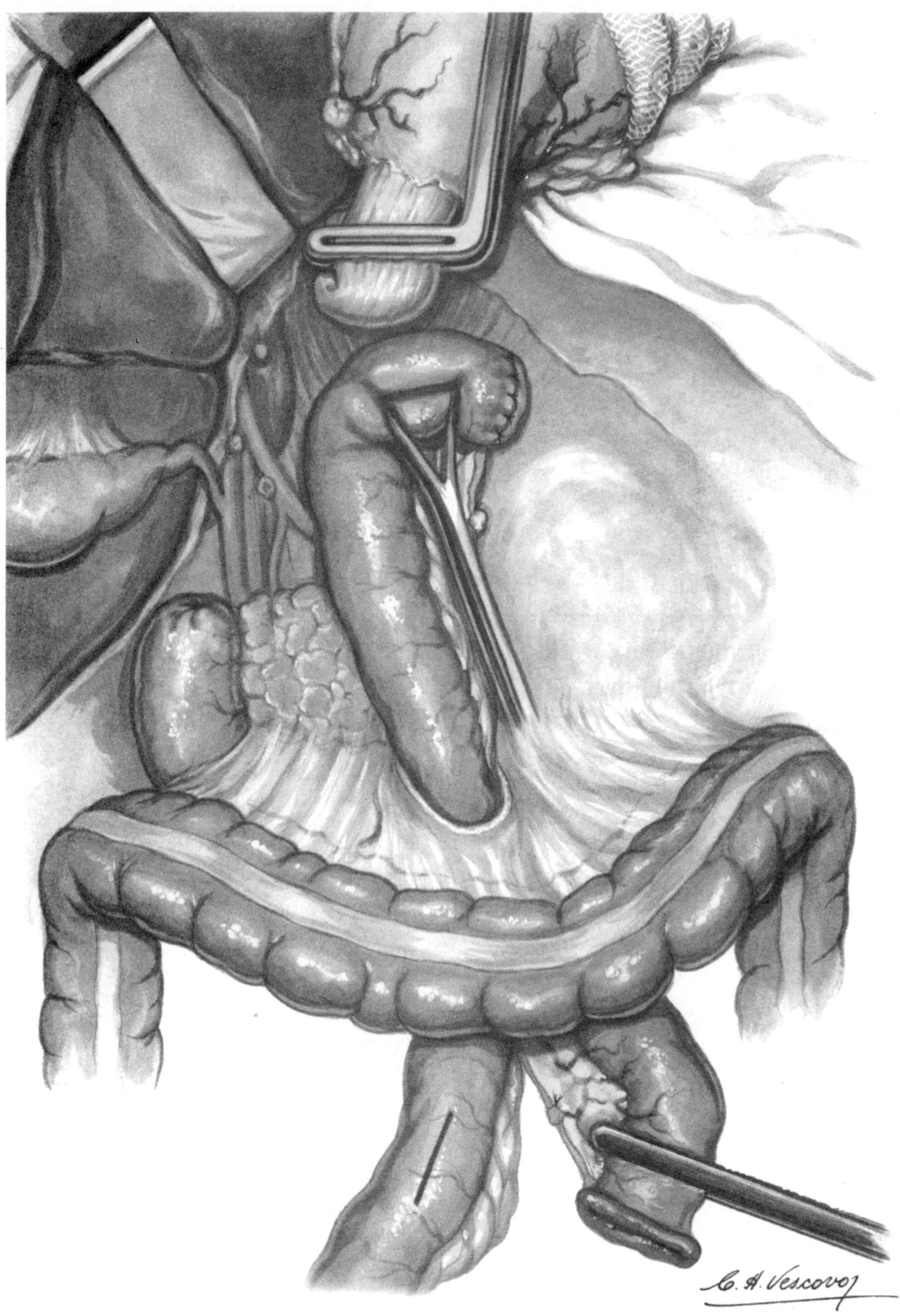

FIGURE 38.39

FIGURE 38.40

A, The distal jejunal limb, held by an atraumatic Duval clamp, is fixed with 3 or 4 sutures using nonabsorbable material to the muscular layer of the diaphragm to prevent traction on the intestine. **B,** The suturing of the muscular layer of the esophagus to the seromuscular layer of the jejunum has begun, using nonabsorbable material.

Esophagojejunostomy Using a Roux-En-Y Jejunal Loop with Manual Sutures

FIGURE 38.41

A, The posterior wall of the esophagus has been incised, and the perforating posterior sutures have begun to be applied between the posterior esophageal wall and the jejunal wall using nonabsorbable material. **B,** Once the posterior layer has been completed, the anterior perforating layer is then realized, after transecting the anterior layer of the esophagus. Suturing of the anterior perforating layer is carried out with the same material, leaving the knot on the inside of the esophagojejunal lumen. The Levine nasogastric tube that had been passed at the beginning of the operation and whose end was left in the middle third of the esophagus is passed under visual control into the jejunal limb.

A

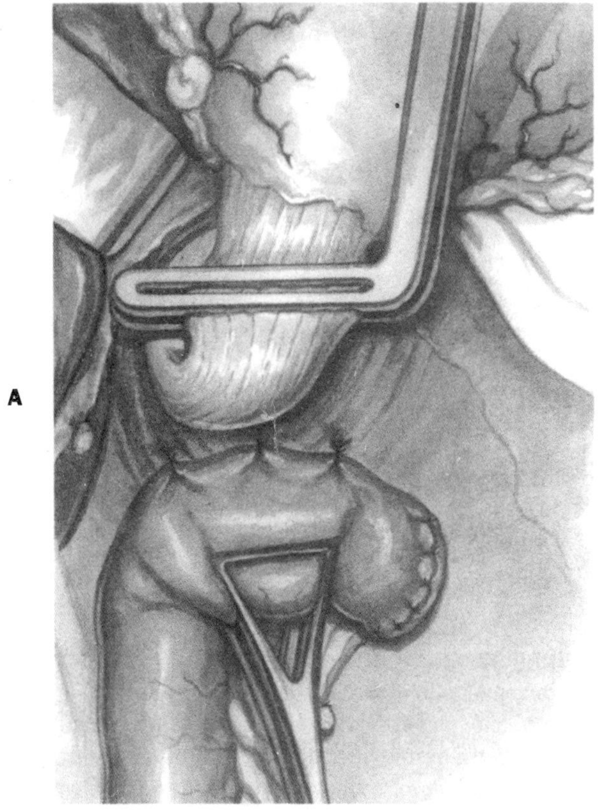

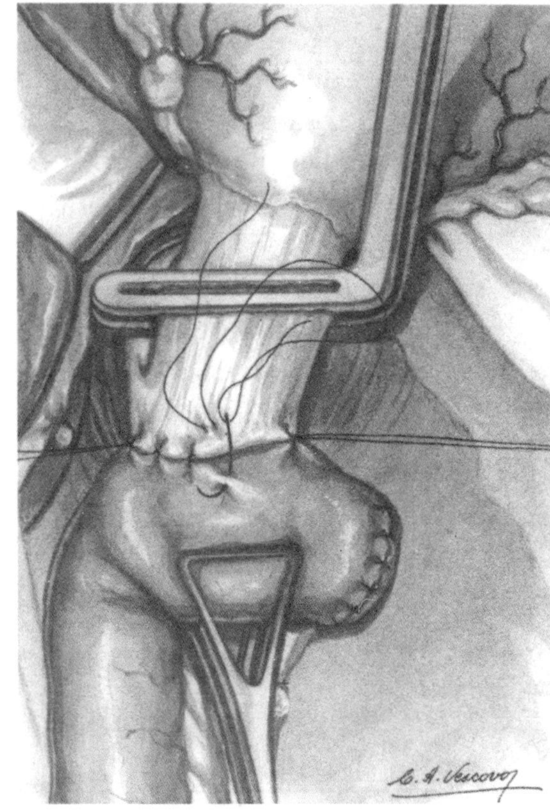

B

FIGURE 38.40

A

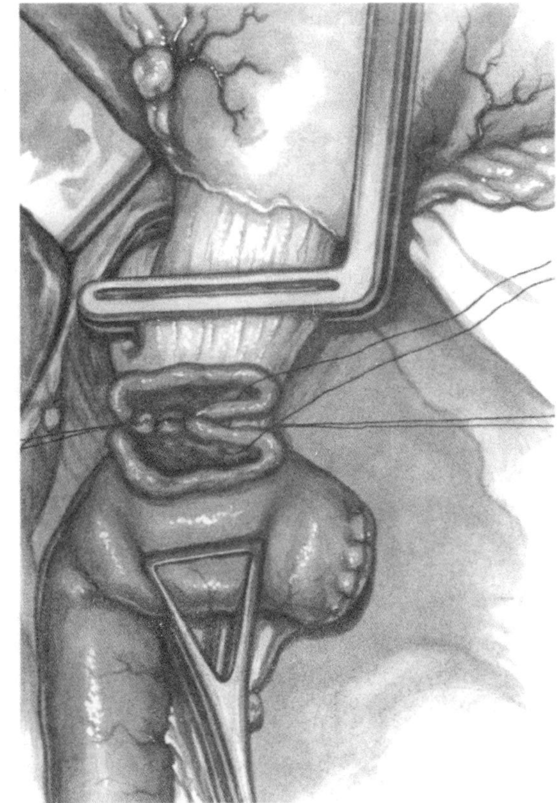

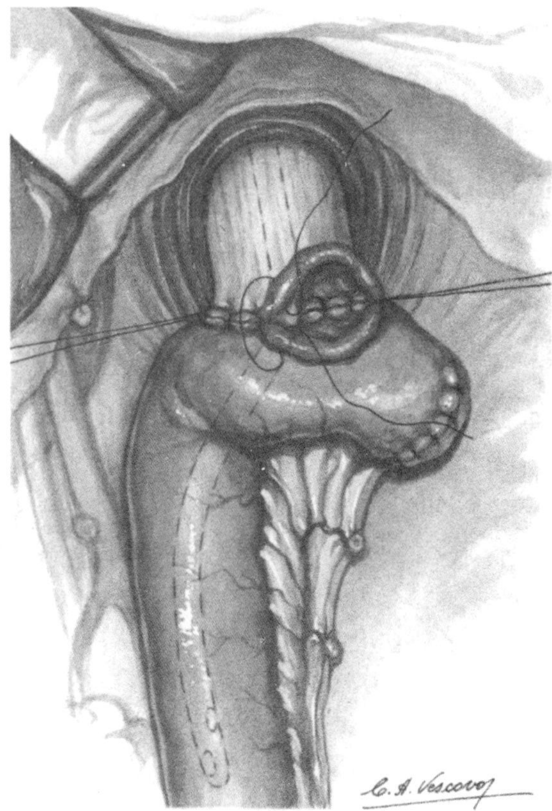

B

FIGURE 38.41

FIGURE 38.42

A, Once the anterior perforating layer of sutures has been completed, the nonperforating sutures of the anterior layer are placed between the muscular layer of the esophagus and the seromuscular layer of the jejunum. **B,** To avoid traction on the esophagojejunal sutures, several interrupted sutures of nonabsorbable material are placed between the esophagodiaphragmatic peritoneum and the seromuscular layer of the jejunal anastomotic limb.

Esophagojejunostomy Using a Roux-En-Y Jejunal Loop with Manual Sutures

FIGURE 38.43

A, Once the esophagojejunal sutures are all in place, the anastomosis between the proximal jejunal limb and the distal jejunal limb is carried out in end-to-side fashion. The posterior seromuscular layer is anastomosed first, followed by the perforating posterior layer and the perforating anterior layer. **B,** The suturing of the anterior seromuscular layer is being carried out.

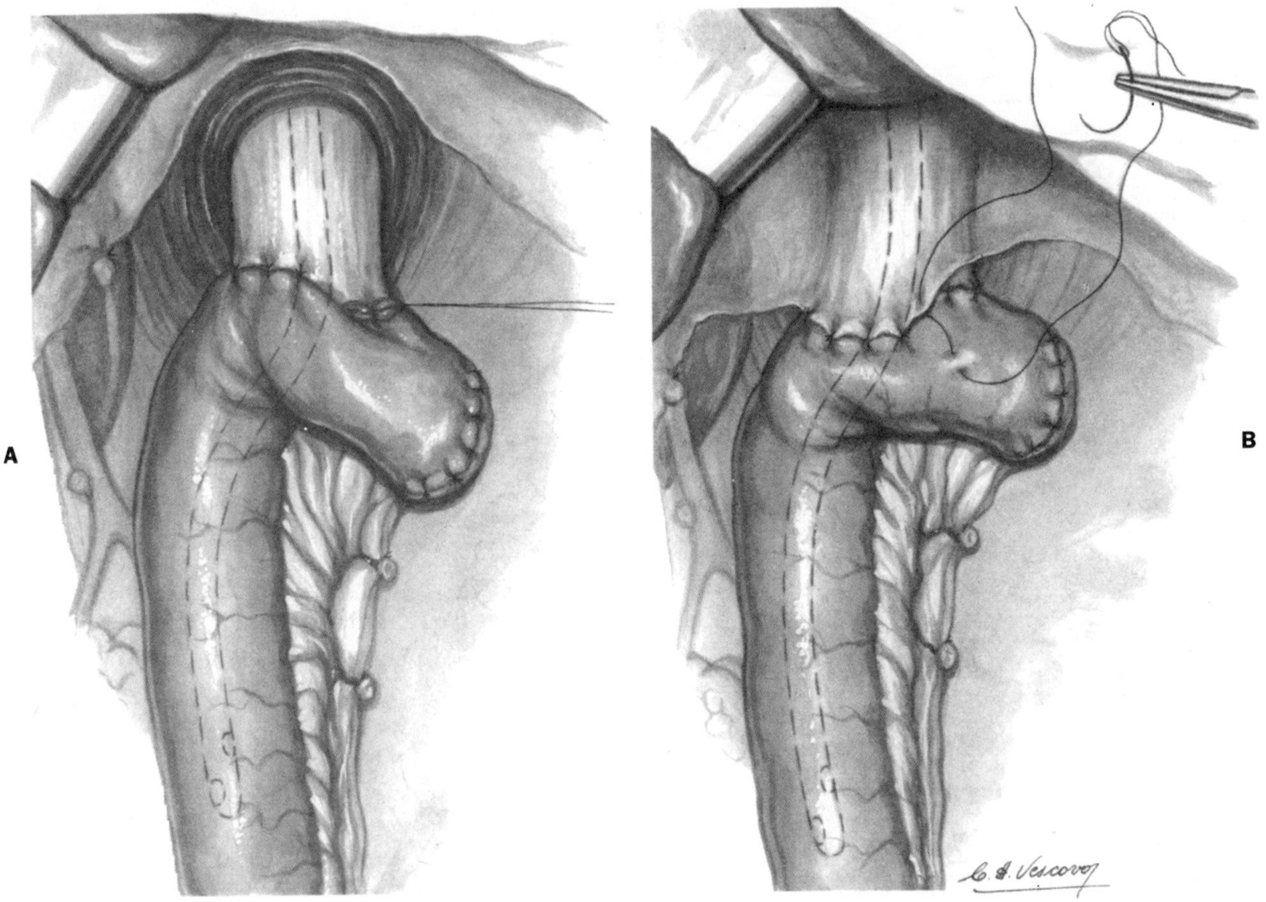

A

B

FIGURE 38.42

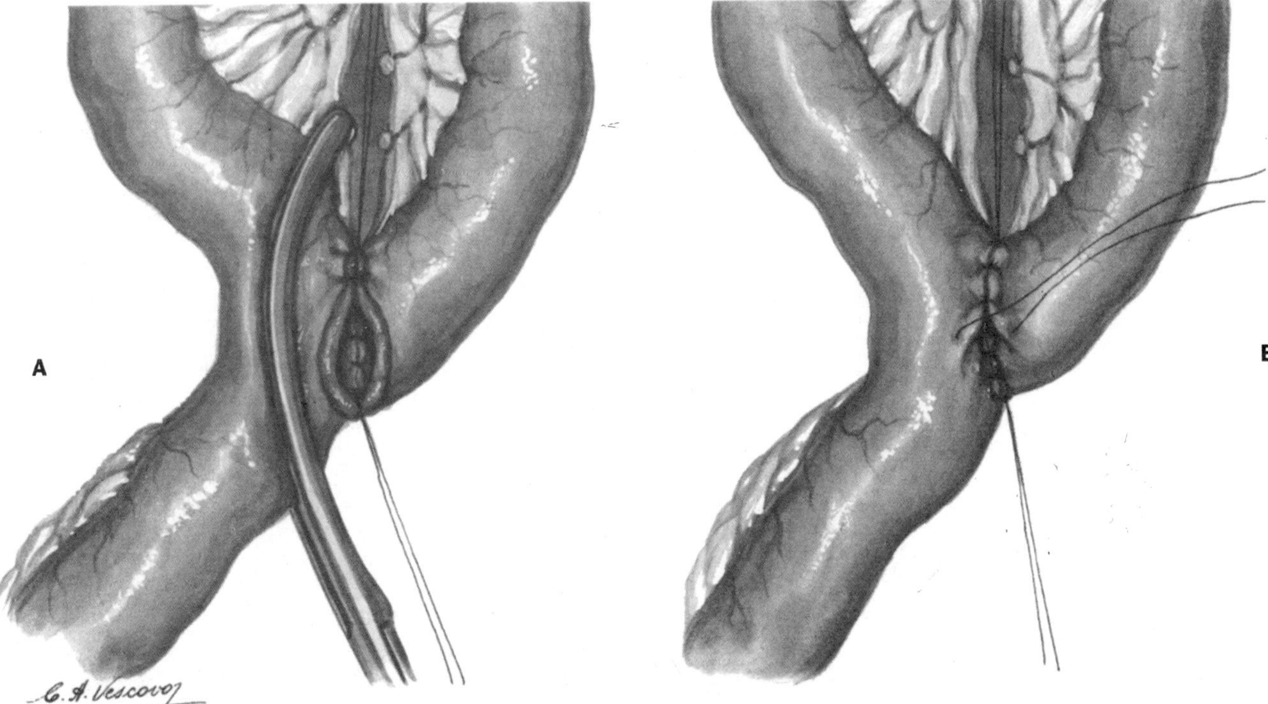

FIGURE 38.43

Esophagojejunostomy Using a Roux-En-Y Jejunal Loop with Manual Sutures

FIGURE 38.44
The defect in the mesentery of the jejunum is being repaired with interrupted sutures.

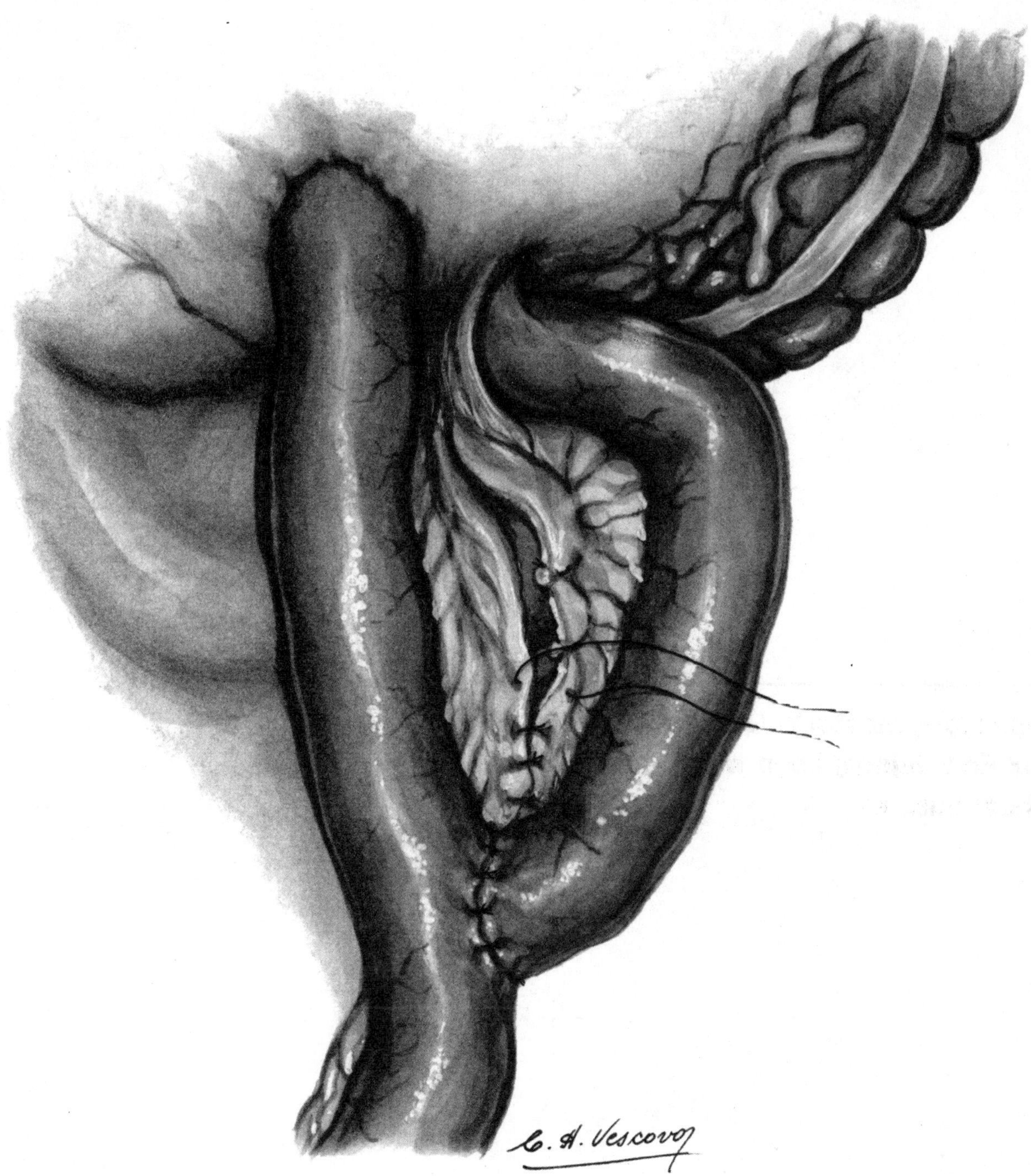

FIGURE 38.44

Esophagojejunostomy Using a Roux-En-Y Jejunal Loop with Manual Sutures

FIGURE 38.45
The establishment of digestive transit after total gastrectomy has been completed with the jejunal loop disposed in Roux-en-Y fashion. The jejunojejunal anastomosis has been completed in end-to-side fashion some 60 cm from the esophagojejunostomy. The anastomotic jejunal limb is fixed with several sutures to the transverse mesocolon to close the space and prevent internal hernia.

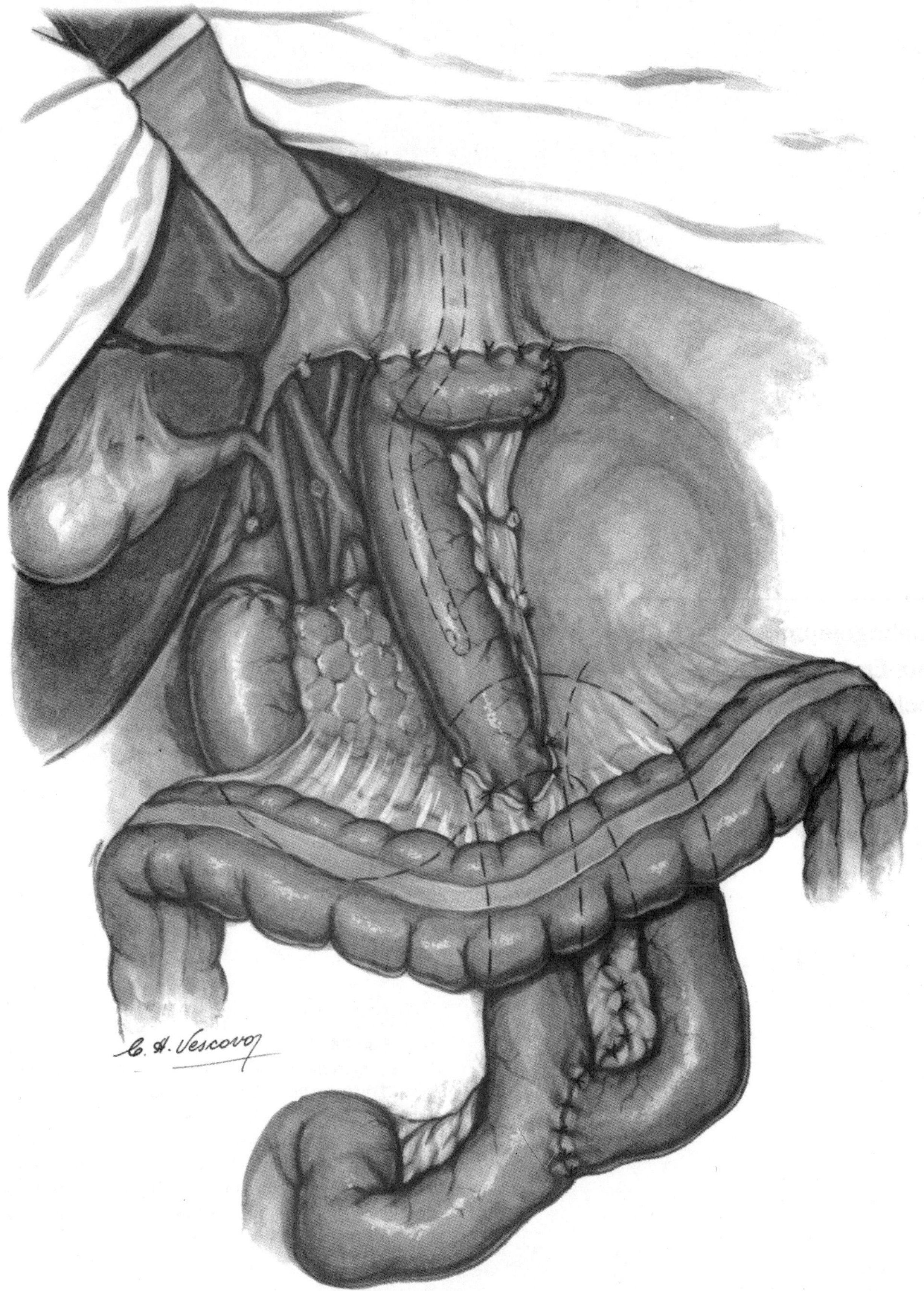

FIGURE 38.45

Esophagojejunostomy with a Roux-En-Y Limb Using Mechanical Sutures

FIGURE 38.46

The EEA instrument (United States Surgical Corporation, Norwalk, CT) without the anvil has been passed through the lumen of the jejunal end. A purse string suture has been placed in the lower end of the esophagus using the purse string instrument or manually. On either side of the lower esophageal end a suture has been placed to apply traction. In this case the jejunal limb has been brought down in front of the transverse colon to anastomose it to the esophagus.

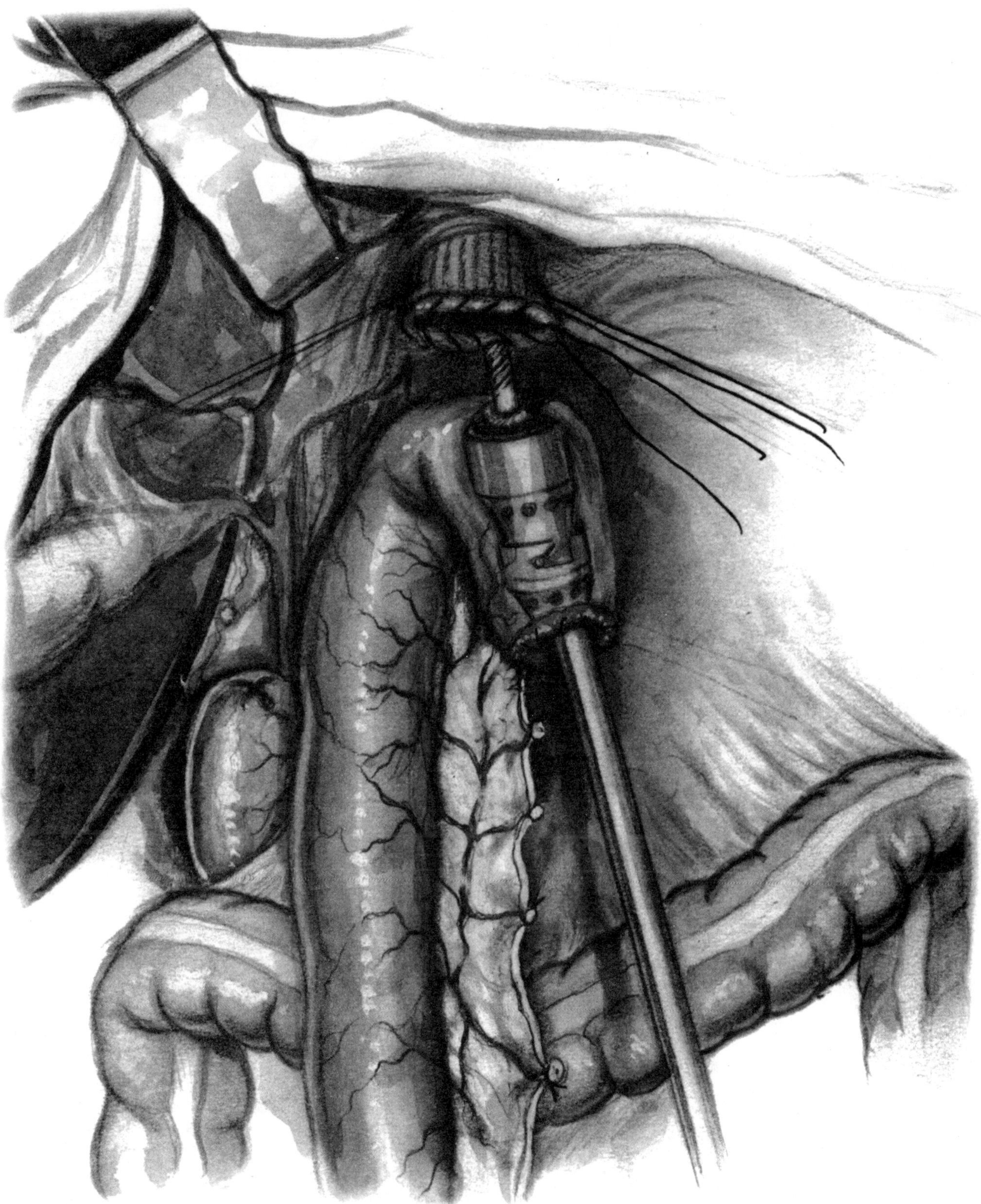

FIGURE 38.46

Esophagojejunostomy with a Roux-En-Y Limb Using Mechanical Sutures

FIGURE 38.47
The rod of the EEA instrument without the anvil has been passed through the antimesenteric wall of the jejunum about 6 to 8 cm from the transected end of the jejunum. If the opening of the antimesenteric border of the jejunum through which the rod of the EEA instrument is passed is too wide, it will be necessary to place a suture to make it smaller. In the lumen of the lower end of the esophagus the anvil of the EEA instrument has been introduced and is held in place by a purse string suture. The anvil will then be united to the rest of the EEA instrument.

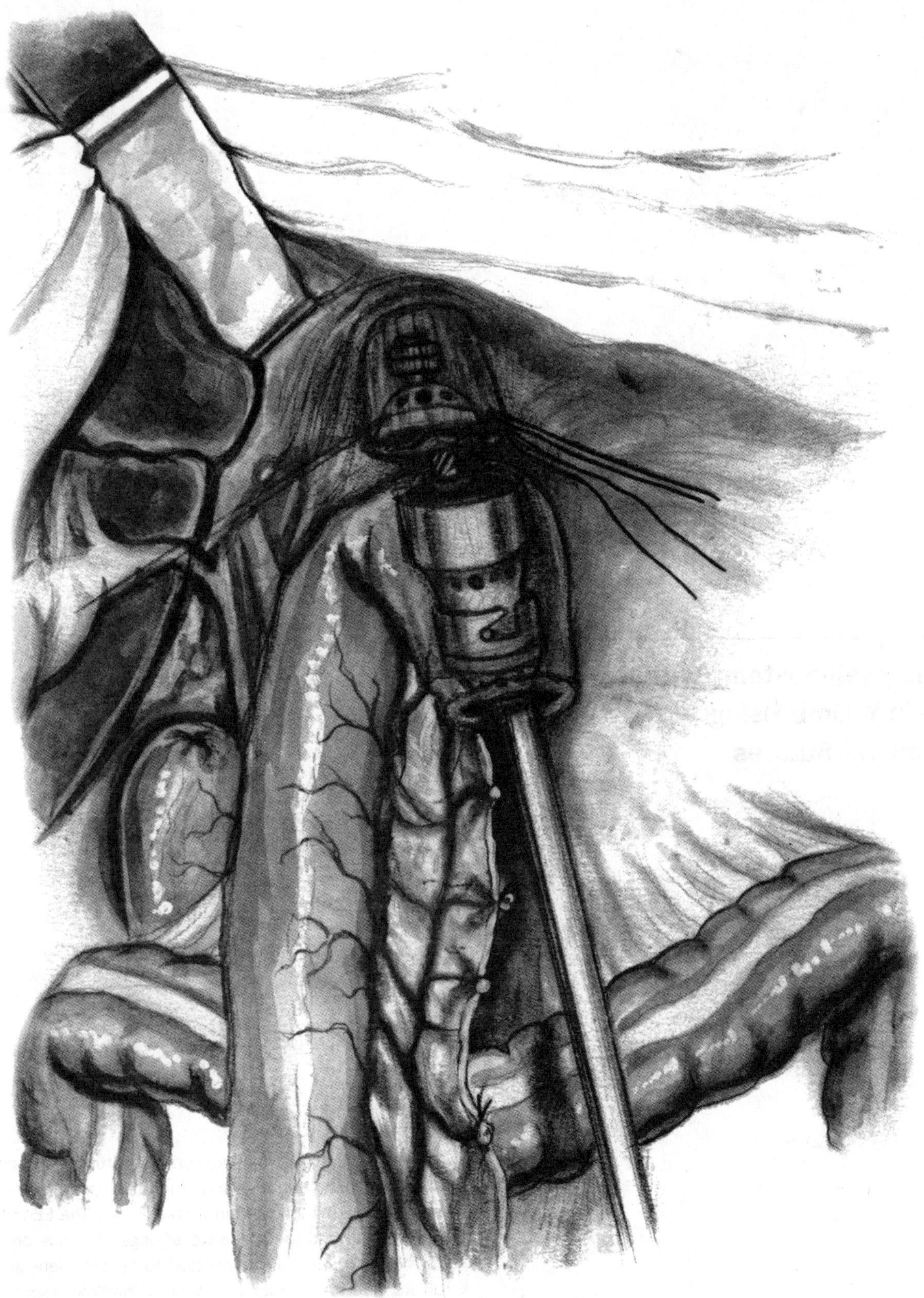

FIGURE 38.47

Esopnagojejunostomy with a Roux-En-Y Limb Using Mechanical Sutures

FIGURE 38.48
In performing the esophagojejunal anastomosis, a double row of staples has been inserted. The instrument is fired, and the staples become inserted in a double row. The EEA instrument is removed, and the presence of rings of tissue on each end of the instrument are confirmed to be complete and include all its layers. In order to be sure that the esophagojejunal suturing (35) is satisfactorily performed, 50 mL of indigo carmine are injected.

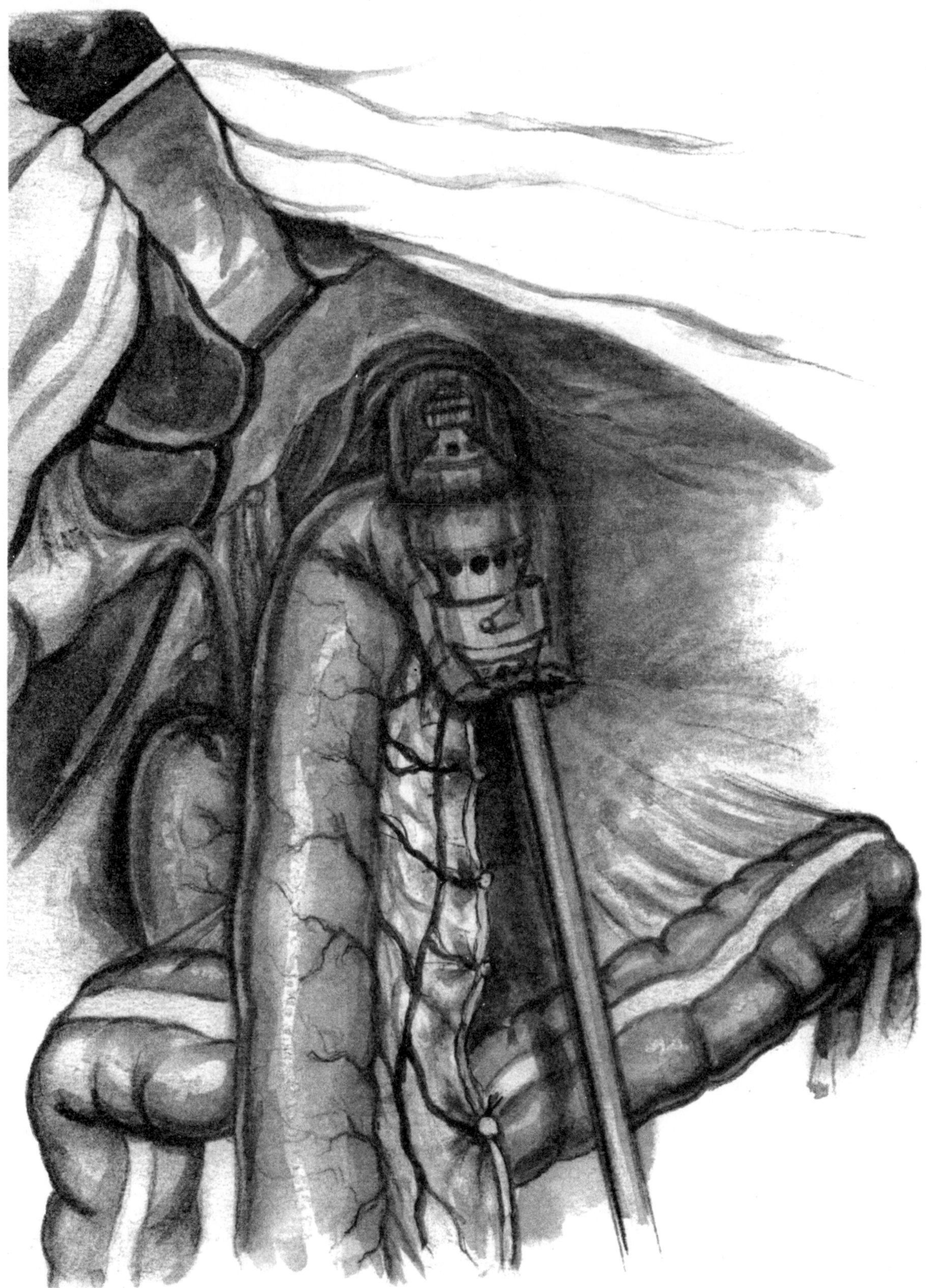

FIGURE 38.48

Esophagojejunostomy with a Roux-En-Y Limb Using Mechanical Sutures

FIGURE 38.49
Once the esophagojejunal suture is found to be impermeable, the end of the jejunum is closed manually or using a TA instrument, as can be seen in the drawing. The mesenteric border of the anastomotic jejunal limb, which has been brought up in front of the transverse colon, is fixed to the transverse mesocolon and the posterior abdominal wall with severa' sutures to prevent rotation.

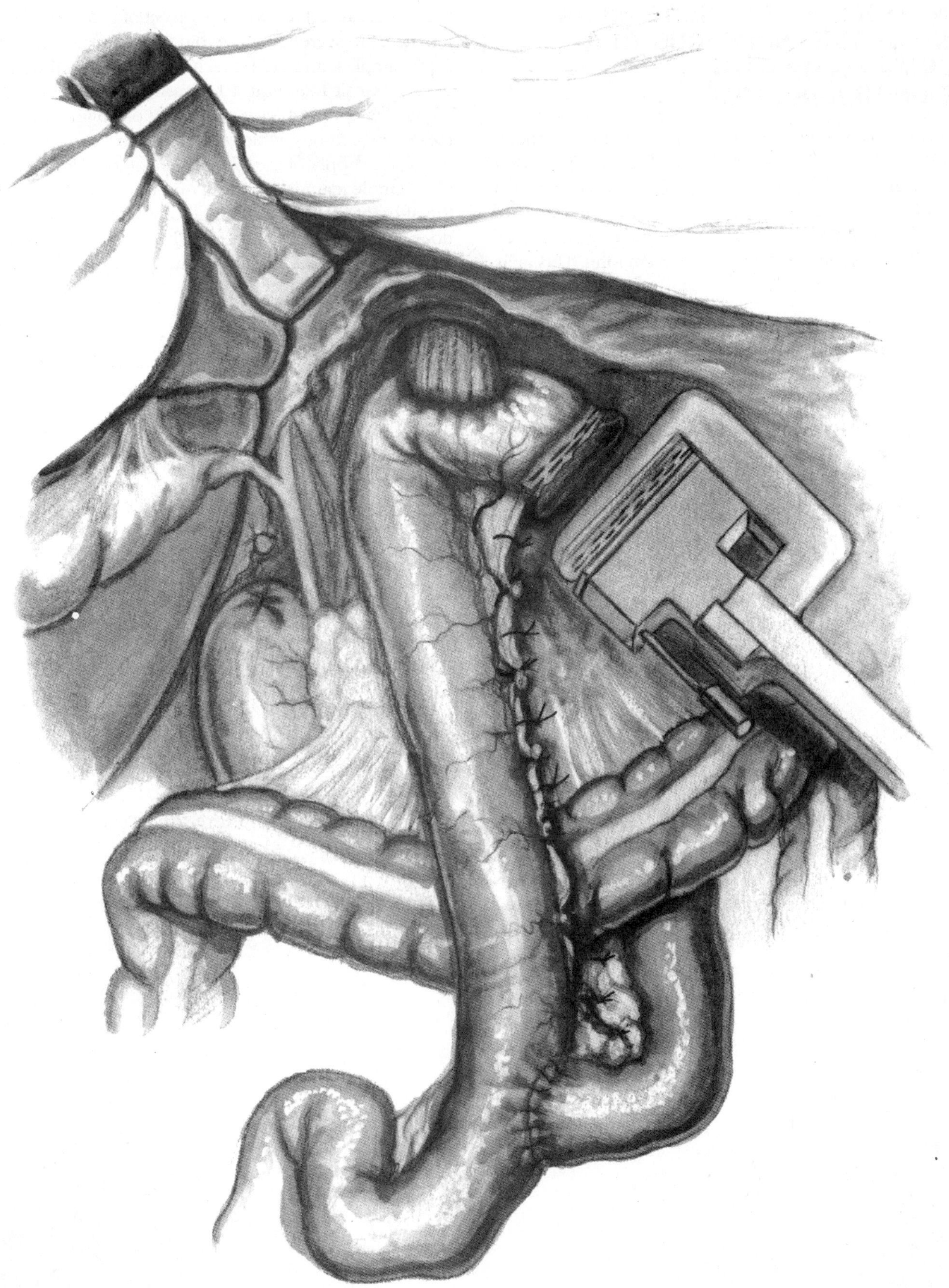

FIGURE 38.49

ANASTOMOSIS OF THE TERMINAL END OF THE ESOPHAGUS TO A JEJUNAL LOOP WITH JEJUNOJEJUNOSTOMY

This procedure is used as an alternative to the esophagojejunostomy using the Roux-en-Y technique. The esophagus is anastomosed in end-to-side fashion with a jejunal loop (Omega anastomosis). About 60 cm from this anastomosis the efferent jejunal loop is joined to the afferent jejunal loop in an anastomosis 6 to 8 cm long. This anastomosis is carried out with the object of detouring the biliopancreatic secretions to avoid esophageal reflux. This is the simplest and fastest technique in reestablishing digestive transit following total gastrectomy. In this technique it is not necessary to identify or divide any of the mesenteric arteries, which could lead to a compromise of the blood supply of the jejunal anastomotic limb. In spite of an ample jejunojejunostomy between the efferent and the afferent limbs at a distance of 60 cm, this procedure does not completely prevent reflux of alkaline secretion into the esophagus and its resulting esophagitis.

Anastomosis of the Terminal End of the Esophagus to a Jejunal Loop with Jejunojejunostomy

Anastomosis of the Terminal End of the Esophagus to a Jejunal Loop with Jejunojejunostomy

FIGURE 38.50

The distal esophagus is freed for about 5 to 8 cm to bring it down and transect it in an area that is not infiltrated by the gastric carcinoma. By bringing down the inferior esophagus its anastomosis to the jejunum is facilitated. The author prefers not to completely transect the esophagus with a later anastomosis with the jejunum. Suturing between the esophagus and the jejunum is facilitated if the stomach is kept joined at the esophagus and held by a Harrington clamp oriented upward. The stomach serves to apply traction to the esophagus.

A jejunal limb of sufficient length to be sutured to the esophagus is selected. The jejunal limb is passed through an avascular area in the transverse mesocolon. It can also be passed in front of the transverse mesocolon. Using a triangular atraumatic Duval clamp the jejunal limb is held next to the esophagus. Before carrying out the anastomosis between the jejunal limb and the esophagus it is important to place 3 or 4 sutures of nonabsorbable material including on one side the seromuscular portion of the posterior side of the jejunal limb and on the other side the diaphragmatic muscle. These sutures serve to hold the jejunal limb so that traction is not exerted on the esophagojejunal anastomosis. Placement of these sutures as well as the esophagojejunal sutures of the posterior plane is facilitated if the jejunal limb continues to be held by the Duval clamp.

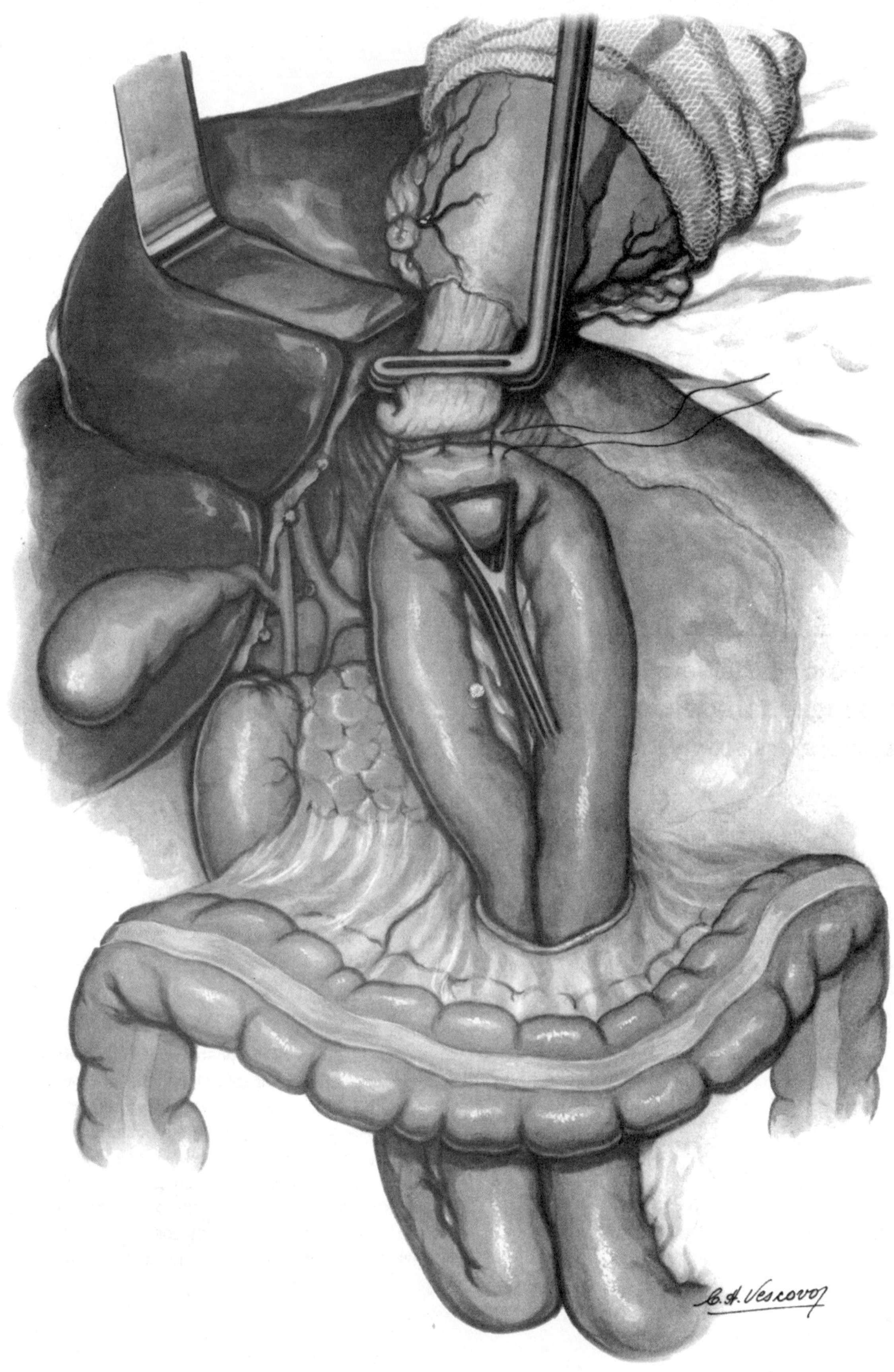

FIGURE 38.50

Anastomosis of the Terminal End of the Esophagus to a Jejunal Loop with Jejunojejunostomy

FIGURE 38.51
Once the jejunal limb has been fixed to the diaphragmatic muscle, suturing of the posterior plane is carried out between the muscular esophageal wall and the seromuscular wall of the jejunum using interrupted sutures of nonabsorbable material. The broken line shows where the posterior wall of the esophagus and the jejunum are to be incised. As was noted previously, transection of the esophageal walls should be done in two stages: In the first one the muscular layer is transected, and in the second one the mucosal layer is transected, a few millimeters distal to the transection of the muscular layer.

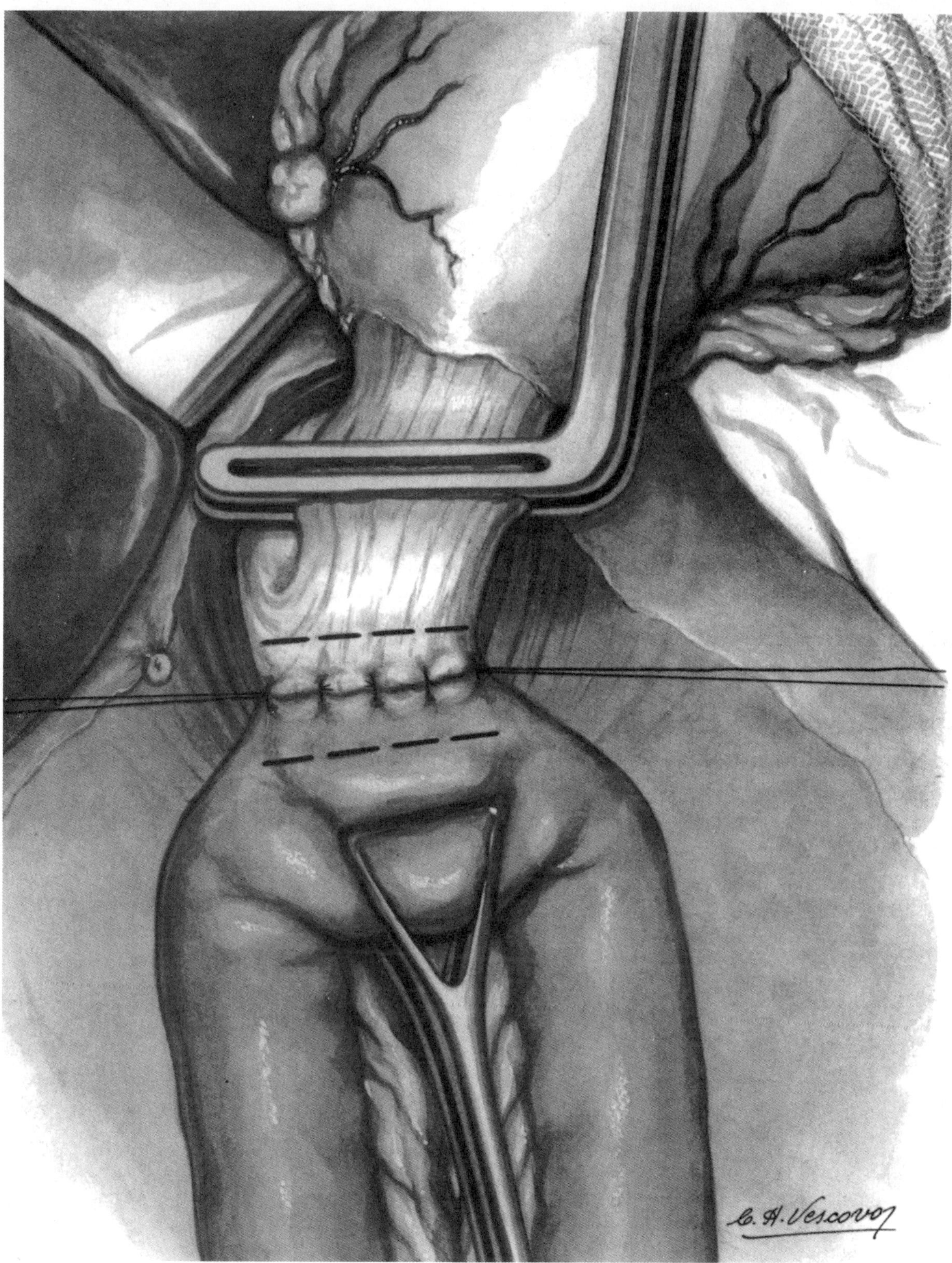

FIGURE 38.51

FIGURE 38.52
A, The posterior wall of the esophagus and the jejunum have been incised, continuing with the suturing of the posterior perforative layer using interrupted sutures of nonabsorbable material. **B,** The posterior layer of perforating sutures is being completed.

Anastomosis of the Terminal End of the Esophagus to a Jejunal Loop with Jejunojejunostomy

FIGURE 38.53
A, The posterior layer of perforating esophagojejunal sutures has been completed. **B,** Using a Sweet right angle scissors the esophagus is being transected, allowing removal of the operative specimen.

A 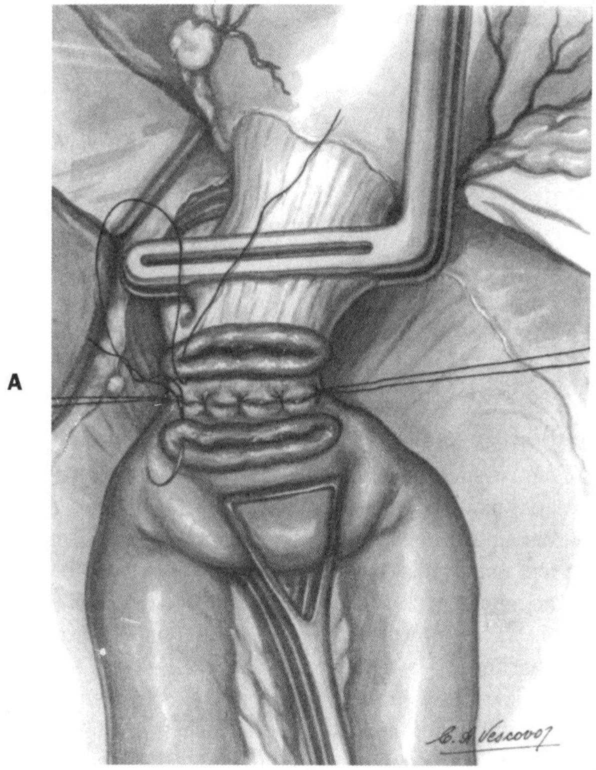

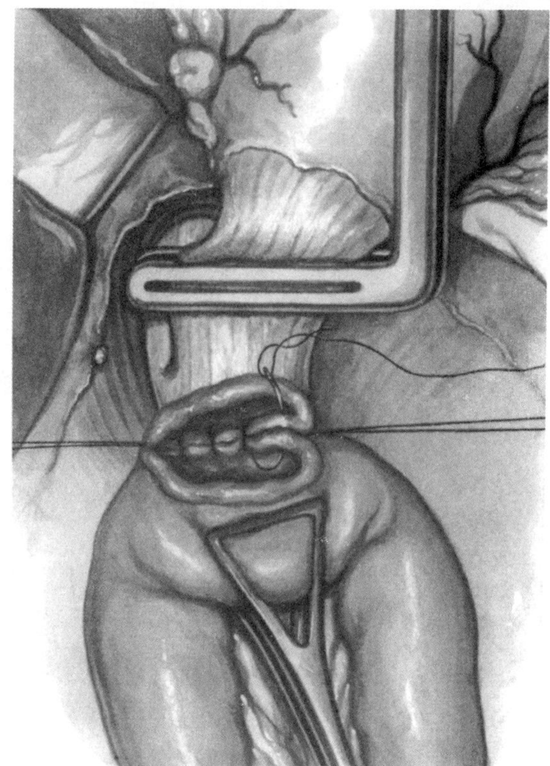 B

FIGURE 38.52

A 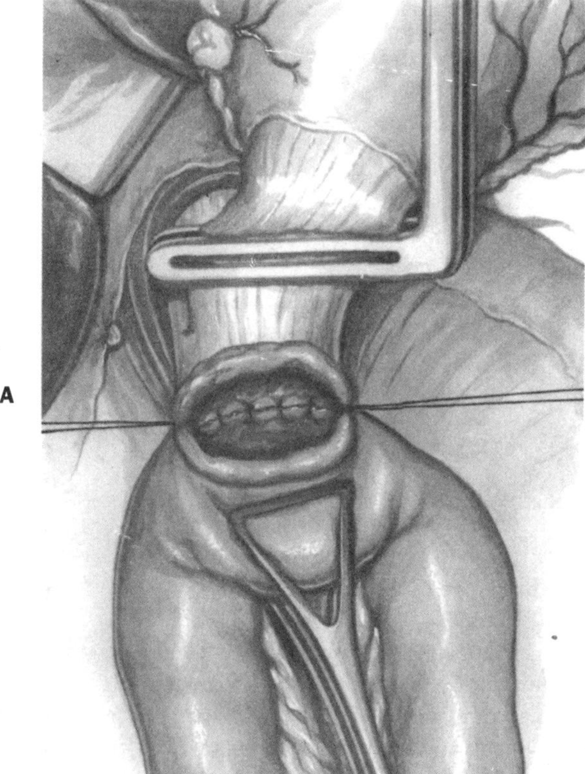

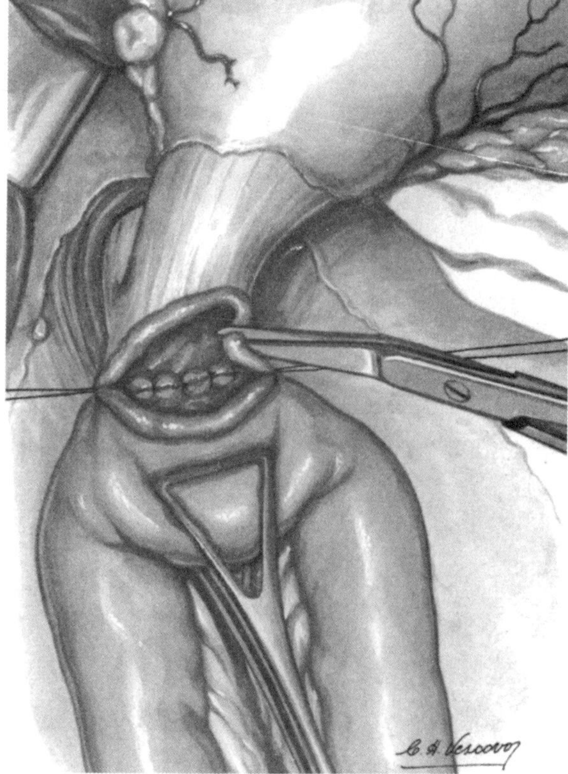 B

FIGURE 38.53

FIGURE 38.54

A, The anterior perforating layer is being sutured, between the wall of the esophagus and the wall of the jejunum, using interrupted sutures with the knot directed inward. The nasogastric Levine tube, whose lower end had been left in the middle third of the esophagus, is passed under visual control a distance of some 15 cm into the efferent jejunal limb. **B,** Once the anterior perforating layer has been sutured, the nonperforating anterior layer is sutured, including the muscular esophageal wall and the seromuscular jejunal wall. The insert shows the transected anastomosis with the end of the esophagus invaginated into the jejunum. Once the anastomosis is completed, 50 mL of indigo carmine are injected to confirm that the esophagojejunostomy is impermeable.

Anastomosis of the Terminal End of the Esophagus to a Jejunal Loop with Jejunojejunostomy

FIGURE 38.55

After the esophagojejunostomy has been completed, several sutures are placed between the anterior border of the esophagodiaphragmatic peritoneum and the anterior wall of the jejunum, as can be seen in the drawing. These sutures are used to hold the jejunum in place so that there will be no traction on the esophagojejunum suture line.

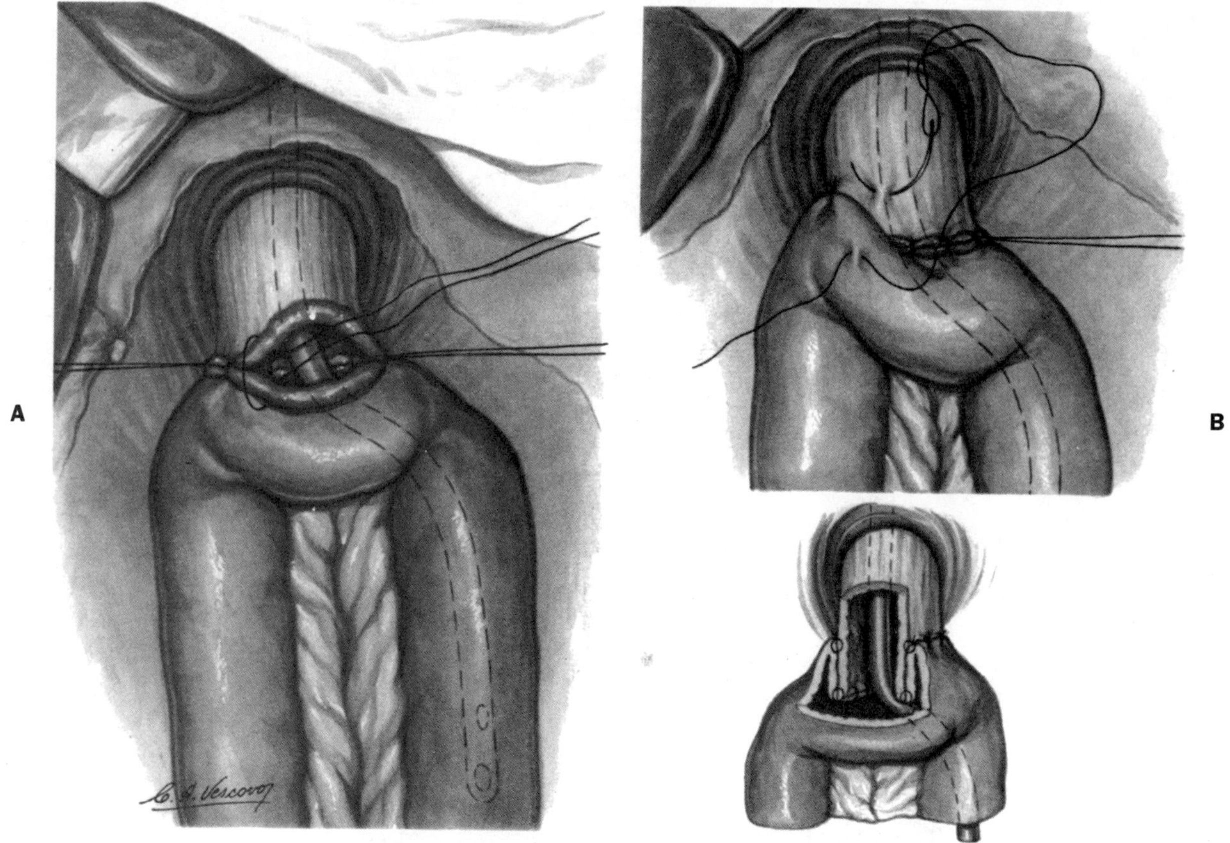

FIGURE 38.54

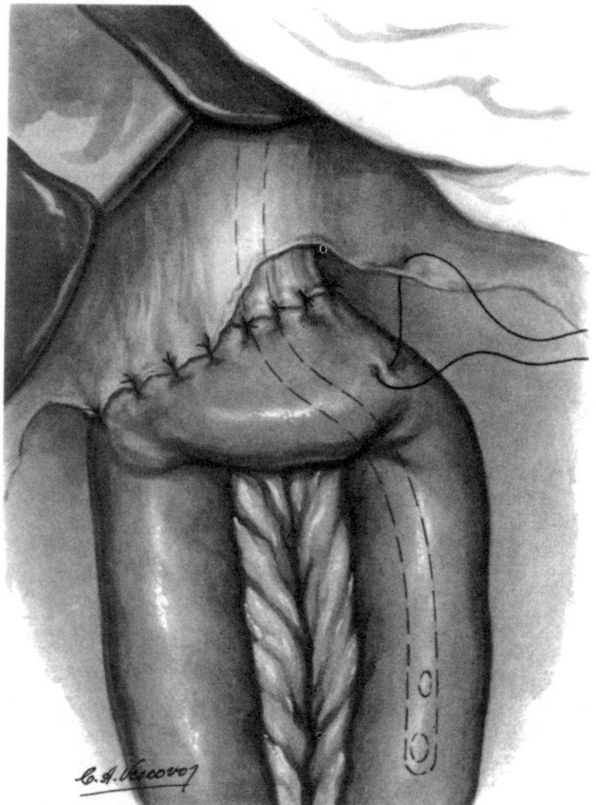

FIGURE 38.55

Anastomosis of the Terminal End of the Esophagus to a Jejunal Loop with Jejunojejunostomy

FIGURE 38.56

Once the esophagojejunostomy has been completed and the jejunal limb suspended posteriorly from the diaphragmatic muscle and anteriorly from the esophagodiaphragmatic peritoneum, the walls of the jejunum are fixed to the transverse mesocolon as it runs into the upper abdomen. These sutures not only fix the jejunum but prevent rotation as well as the production of internal hernias. Below the transverse mesocolon, some 60 cm from the esophagojejunostomy, the afferent jejunal loop is anastomosed to the efferent jejunal loop for a distance of 6 to 8 cm (Braun jejunojejunal anastomosis).

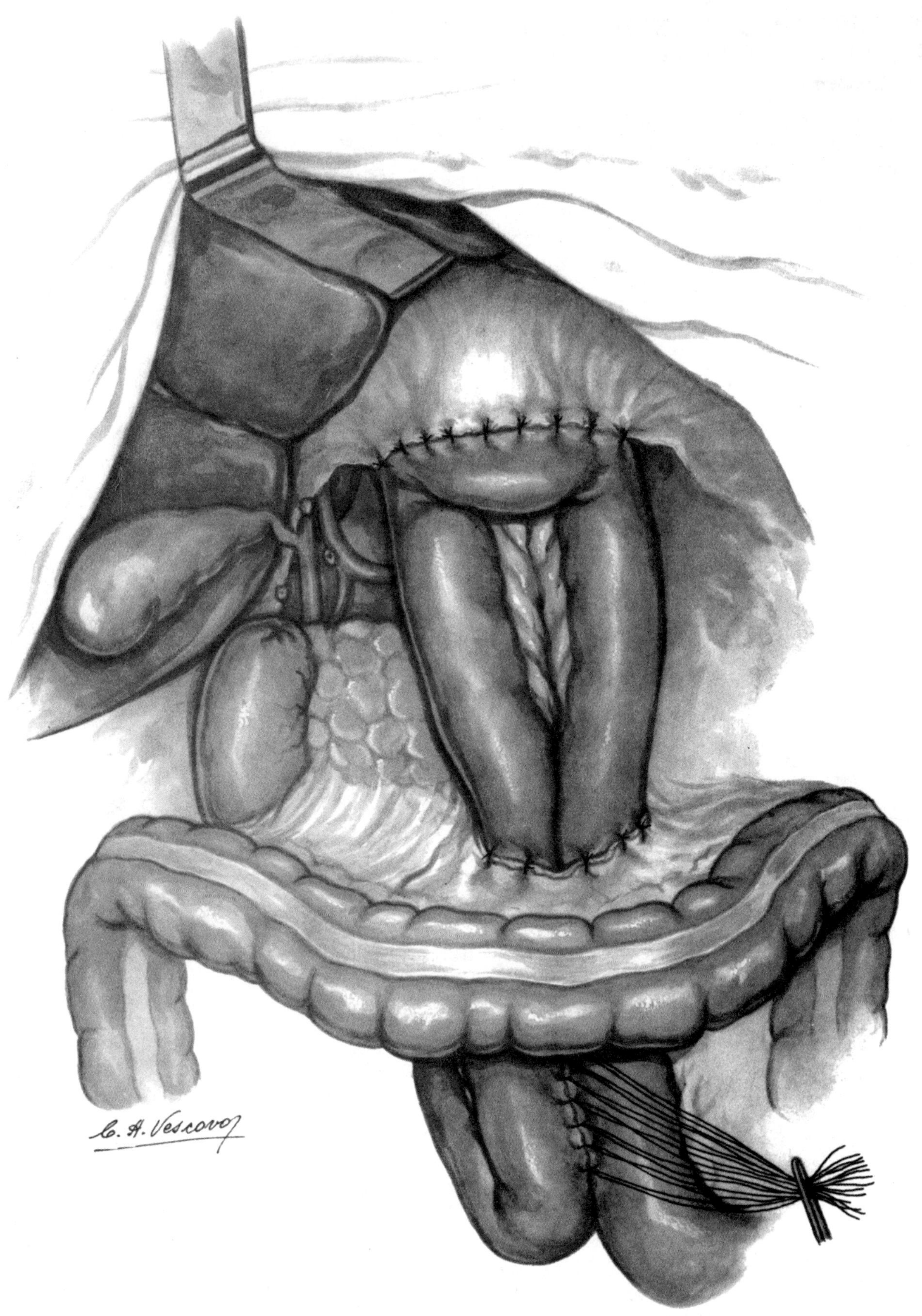

FIGURE 38.56

INTERPOSITION OF A JEJUNAL LOOP BETWEEN THE ESOPHAGUS AND THE DUODENUM

This technique was proposed by Henley, Longmire, and Beal (75–77). A description will be made of the Valdoni technique (124), which is the one used by the author.

Interposition of a Jejunal Loop Between the Esophagus and the Duodenum

Interposition of a Jejunal Loop Between the Esophagus and the Duodenum

FIGURE 38.57
Traction is applied upward to the transverse colon by the second assistant, exposing the proximal jejunal limbs. The broken lines show where the mesentery of the jejunum will be divided. The upper incision passes through the third vascular arch and the lower incision through the fourth vascular arch. The jejunal segment should be at least 35 cm long. An avascular area of the transverse mesocolon has been shown, using a line as the site where the jejunal limb to be interposed will be passed.

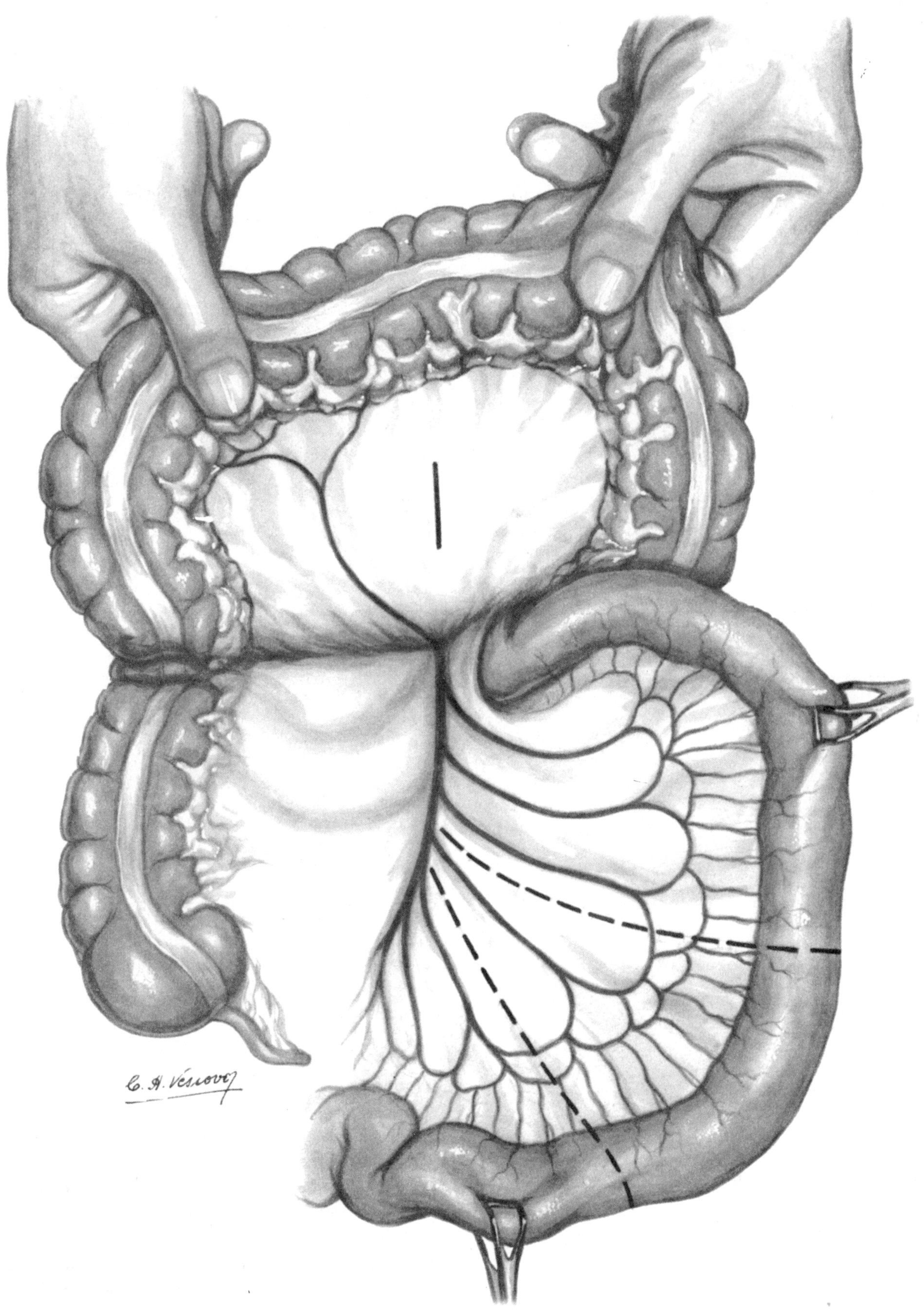

FIGURE 38.57

Interposition of a Jejunal Loop Between the Esophagus and the Duodenum

FIGURE 38.58
The jejunal limb to be interposed has been brought to the upper abdomen through the incision in the avascular area of the transverse mesocolon. The proximal end of the jejunal segment to be interposed has been closed using two layers of interrupted sutures and is held in place by an atraumatic triangular Duval clamp, at a point near the esophagus. The distal end of the jejunal segment to be interposed is grasped with an atraumatic clamp and will be anastomosed to the duodenum in end-to-end fashion using two layers of interrupted sutures.

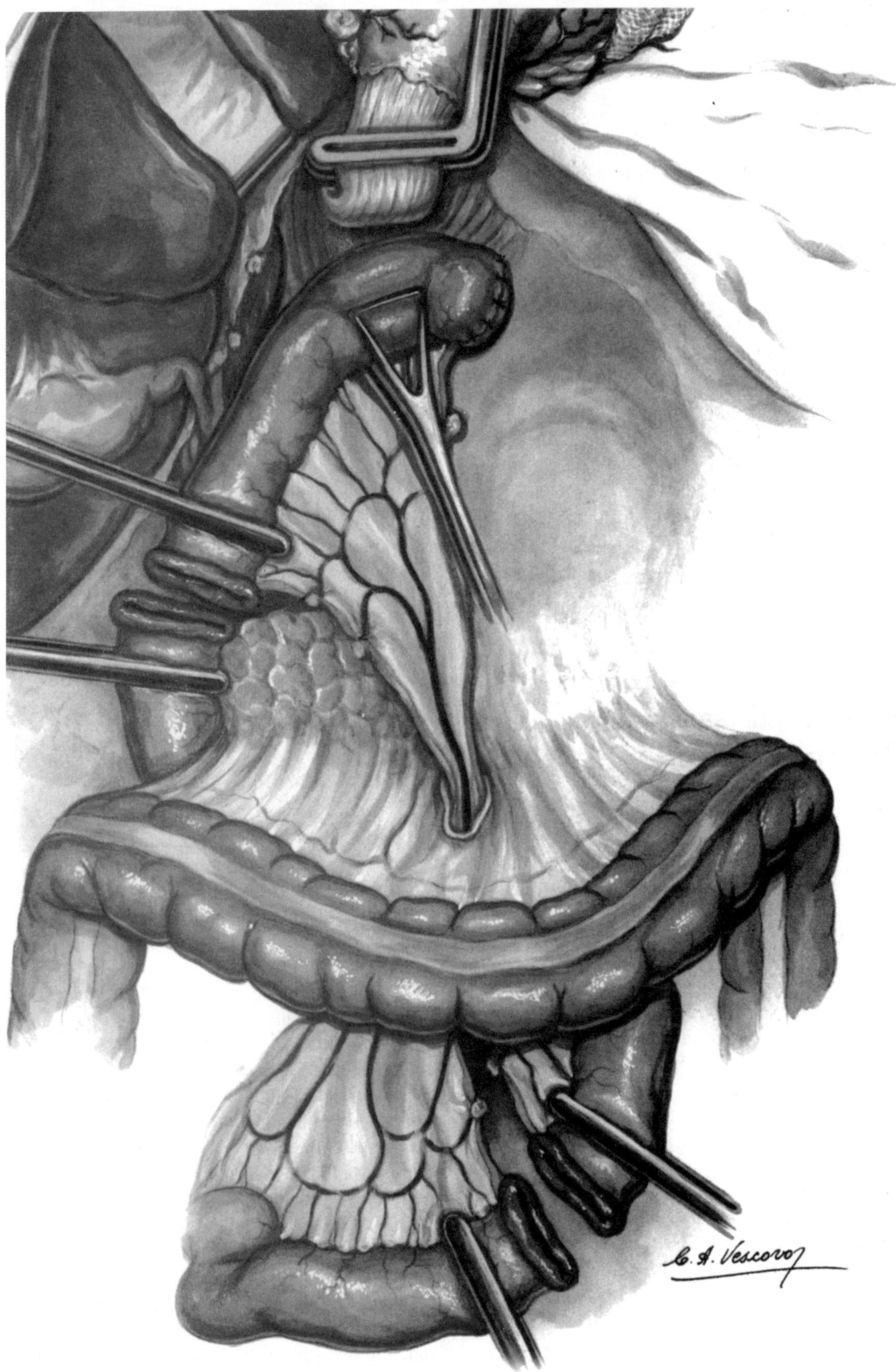

FIGURE 38.58

Interposition of a Jejunal Loop Between the Esophagus and the Duodenum

FIGURE 38.59
The inferior end of the esophagus has been sutured to the jejunum in end-to-side fashion using two layers of sutures. As shown in previous descriptions, it is important to place 3 or 4 sutures to hold the jejunum to the diaphragm to avoid traction on the esophagojejunal suture line. The distal end of the jejunum has been anastomosed to the duodenum in end-to-end fashion using two layers of sutures. The mesentery of the interposed limb of the jejunum has been sutured to the opening in the transverse mesocolon to prevent rotation and internal hernia. The segment of jejunum used for interposition between the esophagus and the duodenum should be held in position to prevent changes in its blood supply. The mesentery of the interposed jejunal limb should be fixed with several sutures to the posterior abdominal wall to prevent rotation or retraction. The ends of the jejunum have been grasped with atraumatic clamps to be anastomosed in end-to-end fashion using two layers of interrupted sutures.

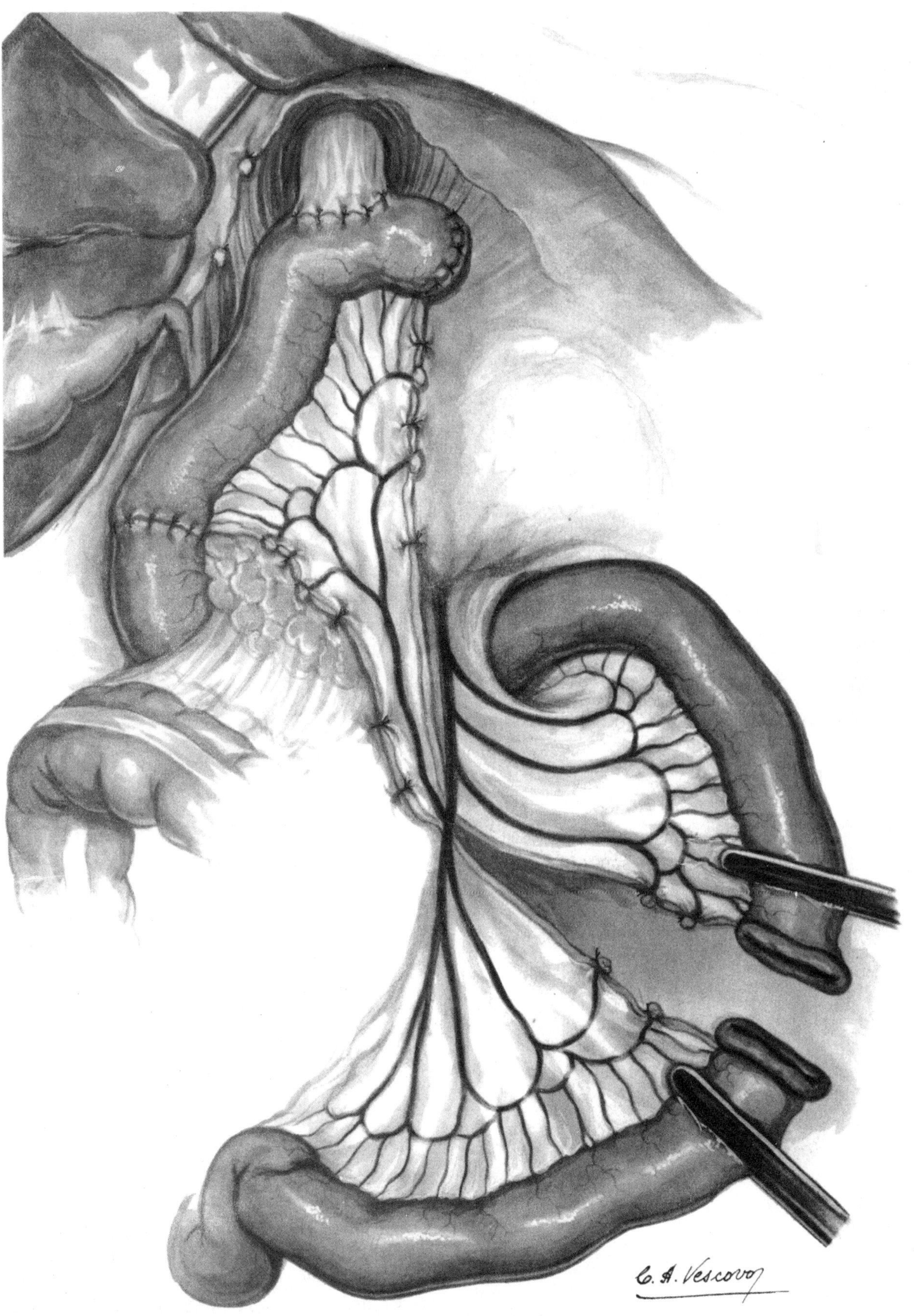

FIGURE 38.59

Interposition of a Jejunal Loop Between the Esophagus and the Duodenum

FIGURE 38.60
Panoramic view of the finished operation. It can be observed that the interposed jejunal limb has been fixed with interrupted sutures to the esophagodiaphragmatic peritoneum, to prevent traction on the esophagojejunal suture. The edges of the jejunal mesentery have been sutured using nonabsorbable material

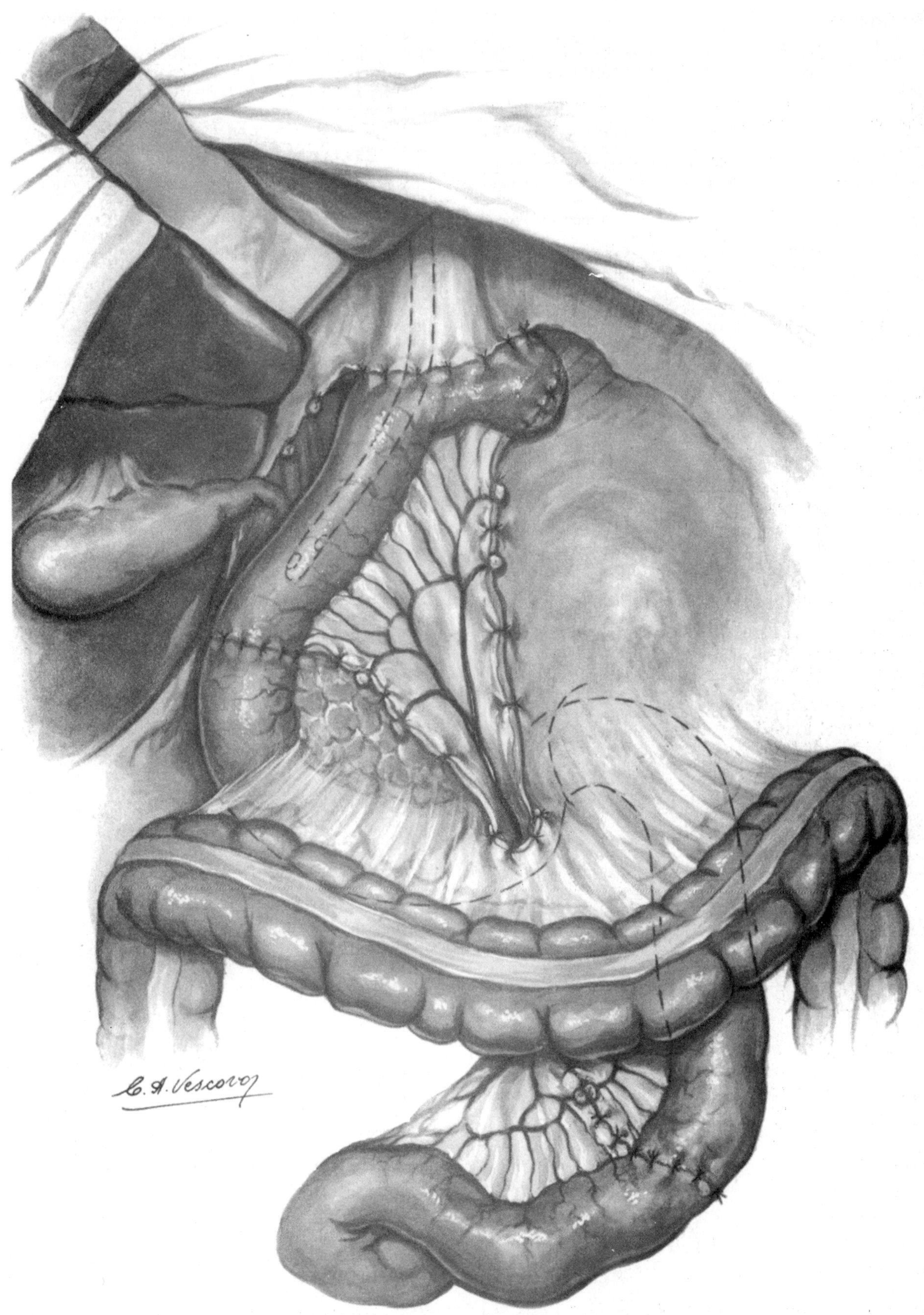

FIGURE 38.60

References

1. Adam, Y.G., Efron, G. Trends and controversies in the management of carcinoma of the stomach. Surg. Gynecol. Obstet. 169:371, 1989.
2. A.J.C. (American Joint Committee for Cancer Staging and Results Reporting). Manual for staging of cancer. The Committee, Chicago, 1972.
3. A.J.C. (American Joint Committee for Cancer Staging and Results Reporting). Manual for staging of cancer. The Committee, Chicago, 1977.
4. Antonioli, D.A., Goldman, H. Changes in the location and type of gastric adenocarcinoma. Cancer 50:775, 1982.
5. Arhelger, S.W., Lober, P.H., Wangensteen, O.H. Dissection of the hepatic pedicle and retropancreaticoduodenal areas for cancer of the stomach. Surgery 38:675, 1955.
6. Armstrong, C.P., Dent, D.M. Factors influencing prognosis in carcinoma of the stomach. Surg. Gynecol. Obstet. 162:343, 1986.
7. Baba, H., Korenaga, D., Okamura, T., Saito, A., Sugimachi, K. Prognostic factors in gastric cancer with serosal invasion: Univariate and multivariate analyses. Arch. Surg. 124:1061, 1989.
8. Beahrs, O.H., Myers, M.H. Manual of staging of cancer. Lippincott, Philadelphia, 1988.
9. Behrns, K.E., Dalton, R.R., Van Heerden, J.A., Sarr, M.G. Extended lymph node dissection for gastric cancer. Surg. Clin. North Am. 72:433, 1992.
10. Becker, H.D., Herfarth, Ch., Lierse, W., Schreiber, H.W. Surgery of the stomach. P. 86. Springer-Verlag, Berlin, 1986.
11. Brenier, J.L. Du problème ganglionnaire dans la gastrectomie pour cancer. Les curages de l'espace rétro-duodénopancréatique et du pédicule hépatique. J. Chir. 80:361, 1960.
12. Borrmann, R., Henke, F., Lubarsch, O. Handbuch der spieziellen pathologischen anatomie und histologie. Vol. 4, p. 865. J. Springer, Berlin, 1926.
13. Bozzetti, F., Bonfanti, L., Boffi, P., Boracchi, P., Marubini, E. Studio policentrico randomizzato sul confronto tra gastrectomia totale e subtotale nei tumori della metá distale dello stomaco. Chirurgia 6:428, 1993.
14. Bozzetti, F., Bonfanti, G., Bufalino, R., Menotti, V., Lersano, S., Andreola, S., Doci, R., Gennari, L. Adequacy of margins of resection in gastrectomy for cancer.
15. Buchholtz, T.W., Welch, C.E., Malt, R.A., Clinical correlates of resectability and survival in gastric carcinoma.
16. Cady, B., Rossi, R.L., Silverman, L.M., et al. Gastric adenocarcinoma: A disease in transition. Arch. Surg. 124:303, 1989.
17. Cassel, P., Robinson, J.O. Cancer of the stomach: A review of 854 patients. Br. J. Surg. 63:603, 1976.
18. Coller, F.A., Kay, E.B., McIntyre, R.S. Regional lymphatic metastases of carcinoma of the stomach. Arch. Surg. 43:748, 1941.
19. Connor, J., Wise, L. Management of gastric lymphoma. Am. J. Surg. 127:102, 1974.
20. Correa, P. A human model of gastric carcinogenesis. Cancer Res. 48:3554, 1988.
21. Czendes, A., Medina, E. Sobrevida de pacientes con cáncer gástrico III: Sobrevida según tipo de resección. Rev. Méd. Chile, 103:244, 1975.
22. Czendes, A., Strauszer, T.F. Cáncer gástrico. P. 143. Editorial Andrés Bello, Sgo. de Chile, 1984.
23. Davis, G.R. Neoplasms of the Stomach. In Sleisenger, M.H., Fordtran, J.S. (Eds.) Gastrointestinal disease. Ed. 3, vol. I, p. 578. W.B. Saunders, Philadelphia, 1983.
24. Day, D.W. Histopathology of gastric cancer. In Fielding, J.E., Newman, C.E., Ford, C.H.J., Jones, B.G. (Eds.) Gastric cancer. P. 95. Pergamon Press, Oxford, 1981.
25. Delamère, G., Poirier, P., Cunéo, B. The lymphatics. Constable, London, 1913.
26. Dent, D.M., Madden, M.V., Price, S.K. Randomized comparison of R1 and R2 gastrectomy for gastric carcinoma. Br. J. Surg. 75:110, 1988.
27. Dupont, B., Cohn, I. Gastric adenocarcinoma. Curr. Probl. Cancer 4:1, 1980.
28. Eberlein, T.J., Lorenzo, F.V., Webster, M.W. Gastric carcinoma following operation for peptic ulcer. Ann. Surg. 187:251, 1978.
29. Farley, D.R., Donahue, J.H. Early gastric cancer. Surg. Clin. North Am. 72:401, 1992.
30. Farquharson, E.L. Textbook of operative surgery. Ed. 3, p. 553. E. and S. Livingstone, Edinburgh and London, 1966.
31. Fielding, J.W.L., Ellis, D.J., et al. Natural history of early gastric cancer. Results of a 10 year regional survey. Br. Med. J. 281:965, 1980.
32. Fielding, J.W.L. Gastric cancer: Different diseases. Br. J. Surg. 76:1227, 1989.
33. Fink, A.S., Longmire, W.P. Jr. Carcinoma of the stomach. In Sabiston, D.C. Jr. (Ed.) Textbook of surgery. Ed. 14, p. 814. W.B. Saunders, Philadelphia, 1991.
34. Fly, O.A. Jr., Waugh, J.M., Dockerty, M.B. Splenic hilar nodal involvement in carcinoma of the distal part of the stomach. Cancer 9:459, 1956.
35. Fujimoto, S., Takahashi, M., Endoh, F., Takai, M., et al. Stapled or manual suturing in esophagojejunostomy after total gastrectomy: A comparison of outcome in 379 patients. Am. J. Surg. 162:256, 1991.
36. Gall, F.P., Hermanek, P. New aspect in the surgical treatment of gastric carcinoma. A comparative study of 1636 patients operated on between 1969 and 1982. Eur. J. Surg. Oncol. 3:219, 1985.
37. Gardner, B. Extended subtotal gastrectomy for cancer. In Nyhus, L.M., Baker, R. (Eds.) Mastery of surgery. Ed. 2, vol. I, p. 713. Little, Brown, Boston, 1992.
38. Gazzola, L.M., Saegesser, F. Cancer of the gastric stump following operations for benign gastric and duodenal ulcers. J. Surg. Oncol. 7:293, 1975.
39. Gentsch, H.H., Groitl, H., Giald, J. Results of surgical treatment of early gastric cancer in 113 patients. World J. Surg. 5:103, 1981.
40. Gilbertsen, V.A. Results of treatment of stomach cancer. An appraisal of efforts for more extensive surgery and a report of 1983 cases. Cancer 23:1305, 1969.
41. Golden, R., Stout, A.P. Superficial spreading carcinoma of the stomach. Am. J. Roentgenol. 59:157, 1948.
42. Goñi Moreno, I. Técnicas para la gastrectomía total. Pren. Méd. Argent. 37:75, 1950.
43. Gouzi, J.L., Huguier, M., Fagniez, P.L., Launois, B., Flamant, Y., Lacaine, F., Paquet, J.C., Hay, J.C. Total versus subtotal gastrectomy for adenocarcinoma of the gastric antrum. A French prospective controlled study. Ann. Surg. 209: 162, 1989.
44. Grabiec, J., Owen, D.A. Carcinoma of the stomach in young persons. Cancer 56:388, 1985.
45. Green, P.H.R., O'Toole, K.M., Weinberg, L.M., Goldfarb, J.P. Early gastric cancer. Gastroenterology 81:247, 1981.
46. Grimes, O., Visalli, J. The embriologic approach to the surgical management of carcinoma of the upper stomach. Surg. Clin. North Am. 44:1227, 1964.
47. Gueullette, R. Chirurgie de l'estomac. P. 347. Masson et Cie., Paris, 1956.
48. Gutmann, R.A., Bertrand, I., Peristiany, T.J. Le cancer de l'estomac au debut. G. Doin and Company, Paris, 1939.
49. Heberer, G., Teichmann, R.K., Kraemling, H.J., Guenter, B. Results of resection for carcinoma of the stomach: The European experience. World J. Surg. 12:374, 1988.
50. Harrington, J.L. Jr. Historical aspects of gastric surgery. In Scott, H.W. Jr., Sawyers, J.L. (Eds.) Surgery of the stomach, duodenum and small intestine. Ed. 2, p. 1. Blackwell, Boston, 1992.
51. Hertzer, N.R., Hoerr, S.O. An interpretative review of lymphoma of the stomach. Surg. Gynecol. Obstet. 143:113, 1976.
52. Hirayama, T. Changing patterns in the incidence of gastric cancer. In Fielding, J.W.L., Newman, C.E., Ford, C.H.J., Jones, B.C. (Eds.) Gastric cancer. P. 1–15. Pergamon Press, Oxford, 1981.
53. Hoerr, S.O. Prognosis for carcinoma of the stomach. Surg. Gynecol. Obstet. 137:205, 1973.
54. Hoerr, S.O. Carcinoma of the stomach. In Nyhus, L.M., Wastell, C. (Eds.). Surgery of the stomach and duodenum. Ed. 3, p. 649. Little, Brown, Boston, 1977.
55. Hoerr, S.O., Hazard, J.B., Bailey, D. Prognosis in carcinoma of the stomach in relation to the microscopic type. Surg. Gynecol. Obstet. 122:485, 1966.
56. Hoerr, S.O., McCormack, L.J., Hertzer, N.R. Prognosis in gastric lymphoma. Arch. Surg. 107:115, 1973.

57. Jaehne, J., Meyer, H., Maschek, H., Gaerling, H., Bruns, E., Pichmagr, R. Lymphadenectomy in gastric carcinoma. Arch. Surg. 127:290, 1992.
58. Jewkes, A., Taylor, E.W., Fielding, J.W.L., Alexander-Williams, J. Radical total gastrectomy for carcinoma. In Nyhus, L.M., Baker, R.S. (Eds.) Mastery of surgery. Ed. 2, vol. I, p. 721. Little, Brown, Boston, 1992.
59. Jordan, G.L. Decreasing incidence of carcinoma of the stomach. Am. J. Surg. 116:407, 1968.
60. Kajitani, T. Early gastric carcinoma from a surgical point of view. Jpn. J. Cancer Clin. 11:787, 1965.
61. Kajitani, T., Fukami, A. Gastric cancer. J. Exp. Med. 51:63, 1974.
62. Kawai, K., Kizu, M., Miyaoka, T. Epidemiology and pathogenesis of gastric cancer. Front. Gastrointest. Res. 6:71, 1980.
63. Kennedy, B.J. T N M Classification for stomach cancer. Cancer. 26:971, 1970.
64. Konjetzni, G.E. Der Magenkrebs. Ferdinant Enke, Stuttgart, 1938.
65. Kodama, Y., Sugimachi, K., Soejima, K., et al. Evaluation of extensive lymph node dissection for carcinoma of the stomach. World J. Surg. 5:241, 1981.
66. Kock, N.G., Lewin, E., Patterson, S. Partial or total gastrectomy for adenocarcinoma of the cardia. Acta Chir. Scand. 135:340, 1969.
67. Koga, S., Nishimura, O. Clinical evaluation of long-term survival after total gastrectomy. Jpn. J. Surg. 8:508, 1978.
68. Koga, S., Kaibara, N. Prognostic significance of combined splenectomy or pancreatosplenectomy in total and proximal gastrectomy for gastric cancer. Am. J. Surg. 142:546, 1981.
69. Lahey, F.H. Total gastrectomy for all patients with operable cancer of the stomach. Surg. Gynecol. Obstet. 90:246, 1950.
70. Lauren, P.T. The two histological main types of gastric carcinoma: Diffuse and so-called intestinal type carcinoma. Acta Pathol. Microbiol. Scand. 64:31, 1965.
71. Laurence, W.J., McNeer, G. An analysis of the role of radical surgery for gastric cancer. Surg. Gynecol. Obstet. 111:691, 1960.
72. Lawrence, W.T., Lawrence, W. Jr. Gastric cancer: The surgeon's viewpoint. Semin. Oncol. 7:400, 1980.
73. Lawrence, W. Jr. Radical gastrectomy. In Nora, P.F. (Ed.) Operative surgery. Ed. 3, p. 544. W.B. Saunders, Philadelphia, 1990.
74. Longmire, W.P. Jr. Total gastrectomy for cancer of the stomach. Surg. Gynecol. Obstet. 84:21, 1947.
75. Longmire, W.P., Beal, J.M. Construction of a substitute gastric reservoir following total gastrectomy. Ann. Surg. 135:637, 1952.
76. Longmire, W.P. Gastric carcinoma: Is radical gastrectomy worthwhile? Ann. R. Coll. Surg. Engl. 62:25, 1980.
77. Longmire, W.P. A current view of gastric cancer [Editorial]. Ann. Surg. 218:579, 1993.
78. Marshall, S.F. Total versus radical partial resection for cancer of the stomach. Surg. Gynecol. Obstet. 104:497, 1957.
79. Maruyana, K., Okabayashi, K., Kinochita, T. Progress in gastric cancer surgery in Japan and its limits of radicality. World J. Surg. 11:418, 1987.
80. Mattingly, S.S., Cibull, M.L., Ram, M.D., et al. Pseudolymphoma of the stomach. Arch. Surg. 116:25, 1981.
81. McNeer, G., Lawrence, W., Ortega, I.G., Sunderland, D.A. Early results of extended total gastrectomy for cancer. Cancer 9:1153, 1956.
82. McNeer, G., Lawrence, W., Ashley, M.P., Pack, G.T. End results in the treatment of gastric cancer. Surgery 43:879, 1958.
83. McNeer, G., Bowden, L., Bocher, R.J., McPeak, C.I. Elective total gastrectomy for cancer of the stomach, end results. Ann. Surg. 180:252, 1974.
84. Menguy, R.B. Surgical treatment of gastric adenocarcinoma. J.A.M.A. 228:1286, 1974.
85. Menguy, R.B. Gastric cancer. In Schwartz, S. (Ed.) Principles of surgery. Ed. 3, vol. II, p. 1158. McGraw-Hill, New York, 1979.
86. Meyers, W.C., Damiano, R.J. Jr., Rotolo, F.S., Postlethwait, R.W. Adenocarcinoma of the stomach: Changing patterns over the last four decades. Ann. Surg. 205:1, 1987.
87. Mine, M., Najima, S., Harada, M., et al. End results of gastrectomy for gastric cancer, effect of extensive lymph node dissection. Surgery 68:753, 1970.
88. Ming, S.C. Gastric carcinoma. A pathobiological classification. Cancer 39:2475, 1977.
89. Mishima, Y., Hirayama, R. The role of lymph node surgery in gastric cancer. World J. Surg. 11:406, 1987.
90. Morgenstern, L. The Virchow-Troisier node: A historical note. Am. J. Surg. 138:703, 1979.
91. Moss, A.A., Schnyder, P., Marks, W., Margulisis, A.R. Gastric adenocarcinoma: A comparison of the accuracy and economics of staging by computed tomography and surgery. Gastroenterology 80:45, 1981.
92. Murakami, T. Surgical treatment of gastric cancer. In Bockus, A.L. (Ed.) Gastroenterology. Ed. 3, vol. I, p. 983. W.B. Saunders, Philadelphia, 1974.
93. Murakami, T. Early cancer of the stomach. World J. Surg. 3:685, 1979.
94. Nagata, T., Ikeda, M., Nakayama, F. Changing perspective of gastric cancer in Japan. Histologic perspective of the past 76 years. Am. J. Surg. 145:226, 1983.
95. Najima, S., Etani, S., Fuyita, I., Tabahashi, T. Evaluation of extended lymph node dissection for gastric cancer. Jpn. J. Surg. 2:1, 1972.
96. Papachristou, D.N., Fortner, J.G. Adenocarcinoma of the gastric cardia: The choice of gastrectomy. Ann. Surg. 192:58, 1980.
97. Park, H.G.M., Chung, S.C., McGuire, L., Li, A.K.C., Croft, T. Intraoperative assessment of lymph node involvement in gastric carcinoma. Ann. R. Coll. Surg. Engl. 1:324, 1989.
98. Patterson, I.M., Easton, D.F., et al. Changing distribution of adenocarcinoma of the stomach. Br. J. Surg. 74:481, 1987.
99. Paulino, F., Roselli, A. Carcinoma of the stomach with special reference to total gastrectomy. In Ravitch, M. (Ed.). Current problems in surgery. Year Book, Chicago, 1973.
100. Preece, P.E., Cuschieri, A., Wellwood, J.M. Cancer of the stomach. P. 209. Grune and Stratton, London, 1986.
101. Quénu, J., Loygue, J., Perrotin, J., Dubost, C., Moreaux, J. Operations sur les parois de l'abdomen et sur le tube digestif. p. 590. Masson et Cie., Paris, 1968.
102. Rehfuss, M.E. Diseases of the stomach. P. 117. W.B. Saunders, Philadelphia, 1927.
103. ReMine, W.H., Priestley, J.T. Trends in prognosis and surgical treatment of cancer of the stomach. J. Surg. 117:177, 1969.
104. ReMine, W.H. Indications and contraindications for surgery in gastric carcinoma. World J. Surg. 3:709, 1979.
105. ReMine, W.H., Spencer Payne, W., van Heerden, J.A. Manual of upper gastrointestinal surgery. P. 99. Springer-Verlag, New York, 1985.
106. Rosin, R.D. Tumors of the stomach. In Schwartz, S., Ellis, H. (Eds.) Maingot's abdominal operations. Ed. 9, vol. I, p. 679. Appleton Lange, Norwalk, CT, 1990.
107. Rouvière, H. Anatomy of the human lymphatic system. Edwards Brothers, Ann Arbor, Michigan, 1938.
108. Salmela, H. Lymphosarcoma of the stomach. Acta Chir. Scand. 134:567, 1968.
109. Savinyj, A.G. Surgical treatment of cancer of the cardia. XXVII Congrès. Soc. Inter. Chir. México City, Oct. 20–27, 1957, p 479. Imprimerie Médicale et Scientifique, Brussels, 1957.
110. Scott, H.W., Adkins, R.B., Sawyers, J.L. Results of an aggressive surgical approach to gastric carcinoma during a twenty-three year period. Surgery 97:55, 1985.
111. Scott, H.W., Longmire, W.P., Gray, G.F. Jr. Carcinoma of the stomach. In Scott, H.W. Jr., Sawyers, J.L. (Eds.) Surgery of the stomach, duodenum and small intestine. Ed. 2 p. 333. Blackwell, Boston, 1992.
112. Schafer, P.W. Stomach: Carcinoma of the stomach. In Schafer, P.W. (Ed.) Pathology in general surgery. Vol. 311, p. 323. University of Chicago Press, Chicago, 1950.
113. Schlatter, C. A unique case of complete removal of the stomach: Successful esophago-enterostomy. Med. Rec. 62:909, 1897.
114. Schrock, T.R., Way, L.W. Total gastrectomy. Am. J. Surg. 135:348, 1978.
115. Sherman, R.S., Wilner, D. Superficial spreading gastric carcinoma; is it detectable roentgenographically? Am. J. Roentgenol. 79:781, 1958.
116. Smith, J.W., Shiu, M.H., Kelsey, I., et al. Morbidity of radical lymphadenectomy in the curative resection of gastric carcinoma. Arch. Surg. 126:1469, 1991.

117. Soga, J., Kobayashi, K., Saito, J., Fujimaki, M., Muto, T. The role of lymphadenectomy in curative surgery for gastric cancer. World J. Surg. 3:701, 1979.
118. Soga, J., Ohyama, S., Miyashita, K., Suzuki, T., Nashimota, A., Tanaka, O., Muto, T. A statistical evaluation of advancement in gastric cancer surgery with special reference to the significance of lymphadenectomy for cure. World J. Surg. 12:398, 1988.
119. Spencer, F.C. Ischemic necrosis of the remaining stomach following subtotal gastrectomy. Arch. Surg. 73:844, 1956.
120. Stout, A.P. Bizarre smooth muscle tumors of the stomach. Cancer 15:400, 1962.
121. Stout, A.P. Pathology of carcinoma of the stomach. Arch. Surg. 46:807, 1985.
122. Terranova, V., Garavello, A., Antonellis, D., Tozzi, M. Cancro gastrico. Analisi stadistiche e valutazioni prognostiche. Chirurgia 6:773, 1993.
123. Thompson, N.W. Ischemic necrosis of proximal gastric remnant following subtotal gastrectomy. Surgery 54:434, 1963.
124. Valdoni, P. Abdominal surgery. P. 61. W.B. Saunders, Philadelphia, 1976.
125. Visalli, J.A., Grimes, O.R. An embryologic and anatomic approach to the treatment of gastric cancer. Surg. Gynecol. Obstet. 103:401, 1956.
126. Wanebo, H.J., Kennedy, B.J., Chmid, J., Steele, G. Jr., Winchester, D., Osteen, R. Cancer of the stomach. A patient care study by the American College of Surgeons. Ann. Surg. 218:583, 1993.
127. Wangensteen, O.H. The problem of gastric cancer. J.A.M.A. 134:1161, 1947.
128. Wangensteen, O.H. The surgeon and problem of gastric cancer. Cancer 7:170, 1957.
129. Wangensteen, O.H., Wangensteen, S.D. History of gastric surgery: Glimpses into its early and more recent past. In Nyhus, L.M., Wastell, C. (Eds.) Surgery of the stomach and duodenum. Ed. 3, p. 3. Little, Brown, Boston, 1977.
130. Way, L.W. Stomach and duodenum. In Way, L.W. (Ed.) Current surgical diagnosis and treatment. Ed. 9, p. 460. Appleton Lange, Norwalk, CT, 1991.
131. Weinberg, J., Greaney, F.M. Identification of regional lymph nodes by means of vital staining dye during surgery of gastric cancer. Surg. Gynecol. Obstet. 90:561, 1950.
132. Willis, R.A. The spread of tumours in the human body. Ed. 2, p. 216. Butterworth, London, 1952.
133. Willis, R.A. Pathology of tumours. Ed. 2, p. 391. Butterworth, London, 1953.
134. Yamada, E., Miyaishi, S., Nakasato, H., Kato, K., Kito, T., Takagi, H., Yasue, M., Kat, T., Morimoto, T., Yamaguchi, M. The surgical treatment of cancer of the stomach. Int. Surg. 65:387, 1980.
135. Zacho, A., Fischermann, K. Total gastrectomy in carcinoma of the stomach. Acta Chir. Scand. 117:278, 1959.
136. Zacho, A., Fischermann, K. The results of surgical treatment of cancer of the stomach. Surg. Gynecol. Obstet. 123:73, 1966.
137. Zinner, M.J. Atlas of gastric surgery. P. 140. Churchill Livingstone, New York, 1992.
138. Zinninger, M.M., Collis, W.T. Extension of carcinoma of the stomach into the duodenum and esophagus. Ann. Surg. 130:557, 1949.
139. Zinninger, M.M. Extension of gastric cancer in the intramural lymphatics and its relation to gastrectomy. Am. Surg. 20:920, 1954.
140. Zollinger, R.M., Zollinger, R.M. Jr. Atlas of surgical operations. Ed. 4, p. 50. Macmillan, New York, 1975.

Section F

Surgery of the Stomach and Duodenum

CHAPTER 39

Jejunal Patch for Duodenal Injury or Fistula

SEROSAL PATCH FOR THE TREATMENT OF TRAUMATIC LESIONS OR DUODENAL FISTULAS

Kubold and Thal, in 1963 (9), experimentally demonstrated the efficacy of serosal patches in the treatment of defects of the duodenal wall using jejunal wall. In 1964, Jones and Steedman (7) proved that the serosa of the jejunal wall used to close the duodenal defect becomes covered with mucosa (2). The serosal patch can be constructed with a simple jejunal loop (12) or with a Roux-en-Y jejunal loop. The jejunal serosa should not be sutured to the edge of the duodenal defect, but to the duodenal serosa about 6 or 7 mm from the edge of the defect (6, 9).

It is necessary to choose the right jejunal loop so that it reaches the injured jejunum easily, without having to exert any traction. It has been shown that some patients in whom a jejunal patch was used developed fistulas (8). This shows the importance of using the highest jejunal loops, to avoid the error of using an ileal loop for the patch. The efficacy of this procedure has been confirmed (2) but has not been widely accepted in surgical circles, probably due to fear of dehiscence of the suture line or the possibility of a fistula developing between the duodenum and the jejunum (2).

The serosal patch is especially indicated in patients who have suffered an abdominal injury that has produced an important defect in the duodenal wall, the closure of which is impossible without compromising the duodenal lumen. The serosal patch is also indicated in lateral duodenal fistulas due to perforated peptic ulcers, in perforated duodenal diverticula, and in dehiscence of a duodenectomy used in various operations. The most frequent indication for jejunal patches is in accidental or iatrogenic injury to the duodenum, such as in right nephrectomy or colectomy, if the surgeon notices it during the surgical procedure.

In patients with lateral duodenal fistulas, it is advisable to add diverticulization of the duodenum to the serosal patch by means of a Billroth II gastrectomy to bypass the flow of food directly toward the jejunum. Diverticulization of the duodenum by closure of the duodenum and a gastrojejunostomy has not always been efficacious (2, 4, 8, 10).

Surgical Technique

FIGURE 39.1
Traumatic defect of the duodenal wall. Suturing of this defect is impossible without producing important changes in the duodenal lumen, for which reason a serosal patch is chosen. To carry this out a high jejunal loop is brought up to the duodenal defect. The jejunal serosa is sutured to the duodenal serosa about 6 or 7 mm from the left border of the duodenal defect, as can be seen in the drawing. Interrupted nonabsorbable sutures are used.

Surgical Technique

FIGURE 39.2
Once the suturing near the left edge of the duodenal defect is completed, the suturing is completed on the right side. A feeding jejunostomy is performed after the serosal patch has been constructed.

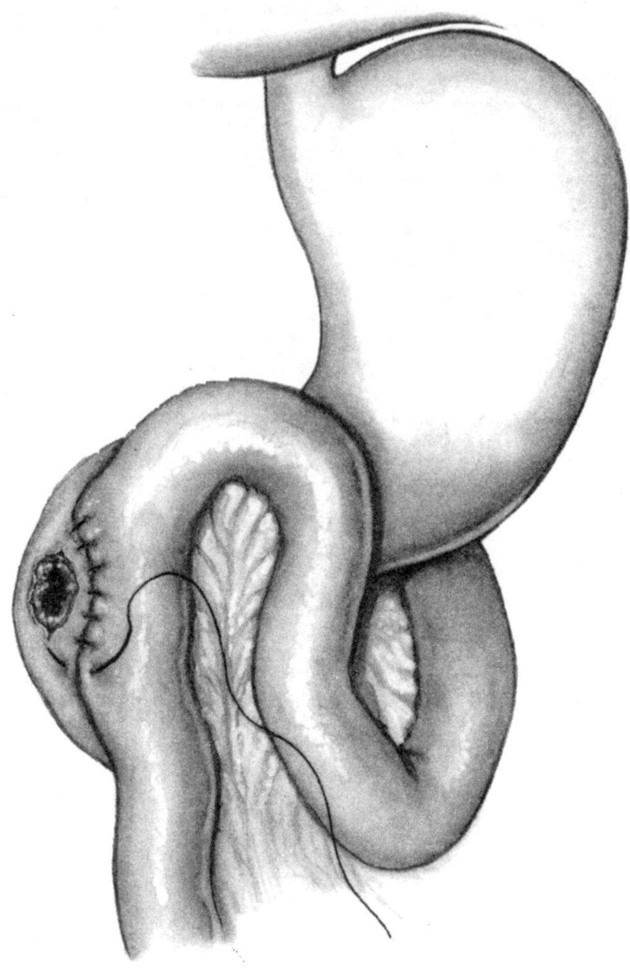

FIGURE 39.1

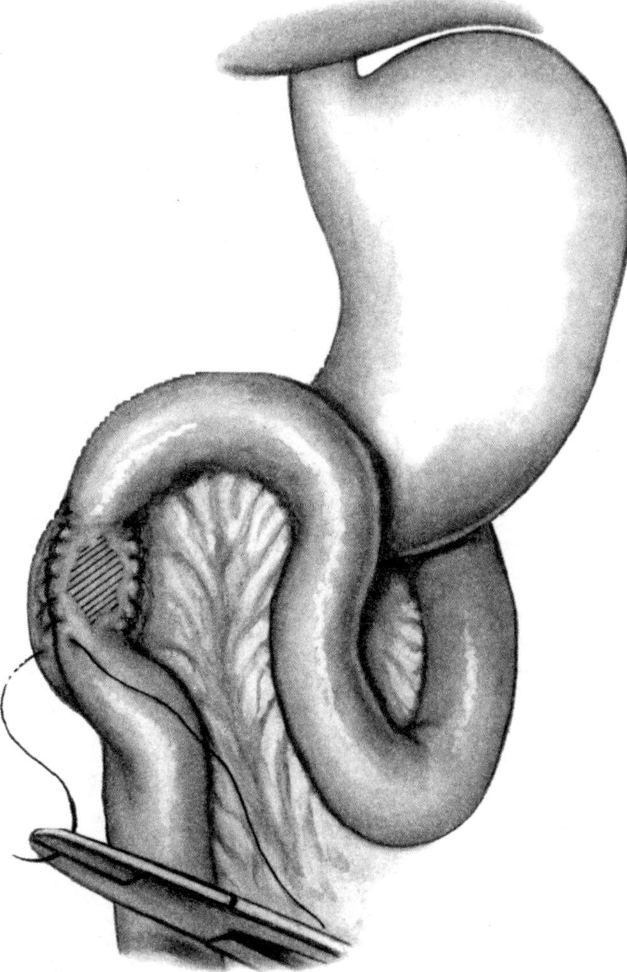

FIGURE 39.2

References

1. Donohue, J.H., Crass, R.S., Trunkey, D. The management of duodenal and other small intestinal traumas. World J. Surg. 9:904, 1985.
2. Ellis, H., Irving, M. Serosal patch technique. In Schwartz, S.I., Ellis, H. (Eds.) Maingot's abdominal operations. Ed. 9, vol. 1, p. 329. Appleton Lange Norwalk, CT, 1990.
3. Etala, E. Nueva técnica de anastomosis biliodigestiva en resecciones pancreatoduodenales con vías biliares de calibre normal. Pren. Méd. Argent. 79:169, 1992.
4. Fromm, D. Lateral duodenal fistula. In Fromm, D. (Ed.) Gastrointestinal surgery. Vol. I, p. 113. Churchill Livingstone. New York, 1985.
5. Jones, S.A., Joergenson, E.J. Closure of duodenal wall defects. Surgery 53:438, 1962.
6. Jones, S.A., Gregory, G., et al. Surgical management of the difficult and perforated duodenal stump. Am. J. Surg. 108:257, 1964.
7. Jones, S.A., Steedman, R. Management of chronic infected intestinal perforation by serosal patch technique. Am. J. Surg. 117:731, 1969.
8. Kellum, J.M., Boucher, J.K., Ballinger, W.F. Serosal patch repair for benign duodenocolic fistula secondary to duodenal diverticulum. Am. J. Surg. 131:607, 1976.
9. Kubold, E.E., Thal, A.P. A simple method for management of experimental wounds of the duodenum. Surg. Gynecol. Obstet. 116:340, 1963.
10. Lowe, R.J. Duodenal trauma. In Nyhus, L.M., Wastell, C. (Eds.) Surgery of the stomach and duodenum. Ed. 3, p. 615. Little, Brown, Boston, 1977.
11. Morton, J., Jordan, G.L. Traumatic duodenal injuries. J. Trauma 8:127, 1968.
12. Schirmer, B., Scott Jones, R. Small Intestine. In Nora, P.F. (Ed.) Operative surgery. Ed. 3, p. 562. W.B. Saunders, Philadelphia, 1990.
13. Ujiki, G.T., Shields, T.W. Roux-en-Y operation in the management of postoperative fistula. Arch. Surg. 116:614, 1981.

Section F

Surgery of the Stomach and Duodenum

CHAPTER **40**

Superior Mesenteric Artery Syndrome

The superior mesenteric artery syndrome is characterized by a clinical picture of obstruction of the third portion of the duodenum due to compression of the bowel by the superior mesenteric artery against the aorta and the vertebral column at the level of the third lumbar vertebra. This syndrome was frequently diagnosed from 1920 to 1935. A duodenojejunostomy, as proposed by Stavely in 1910, was frequently used in treating this syndrome (6, 14). This technique was popularized by Wilkie (14), who, in England in 1921, presented a very complete study of this syndrome. For this reason, some authors even now call this syndrome the Wilkie syndrome (6). Duodenojejunostomy was proposed in the United States by Kellog, Pool, and others (1, 6, 13) and in France by Pierre Duval (6). Some authors later affirmed that the diagnosis of this syndrome was greatly exaggerated, and some even doubted the presence of this syndrome (4, 11, 12, 17). We have concluded that it can be assured that this syndrome exists, but it is now diagnosed much less frequently than from 1920–1935.

SYNONYMS

This syndrome has been designated in many ways. We will point out the most commonly used names to avoid confusion: syndrome of the superior mesenteric artery, vascular compression of the duodenum, aortomesenteric compression of the duodenum, duodenal compression due to the aortomesenteric relation, duodenal stasis, duodenal ileus, chronic vascular compression of the duodenum, Wilkie syndrome.

ANATOMIC DATA

Normally, the superior mesenteric artery arises from the aorta, forming an angle of 50 to 60° (20). The duodenum passes through the space between the aorta and the superior mesenteric artery. This space is 10 to 20 mm wide (6, 20). In general, patients who are affected by the superior mesenteric artery syndrome present a more acute aortomesenteric angle and the space between the aorta and the superior mesenteric artery is less than 10 to 20 mm. The suspensory ligament of Treitz may arise from a high fixation and exert traction upon the jejunal flexure, and even may be fixed to the fourth or third portions of the duodenum. This favors elevation of the third portion of the duodenum, bringing it up into the vertex of the aortomesenteric angle. Seventy percent of the ligaments of Treitz that have been studied histologically have been shown to contain muscular fibers. This may increase the traction exerted on the duodenum (6). Normally, the superior mesenteric artery surrounds the duodenum smoothly without compressing it against the aorta, because of the existence of a fat pad and lymphatic tissue separating the superior mesenteric artery from the duodenum. In patients who lose a lot of weight over a short period of time, this fat pad may disappear and the artery may then compress the duodenum.

FACTORS PRODUCING THE SYNDROME

The superior mesenteric artery syndrome can occur in persons who have lost many kilograms of weight over a short period of time, in patients who remain immobilized in bed in the dorsal position for a long time, and in patients immobilized in hyperextension because of lesions of the vertebral column. In some patients, however, it is not possible to determine what factors cause or precipitate the clinical picture. The symptoms that are usually presented by these patients are distension of the upper abdomen and cramplike pains that are relieved by vomiting. Obstructive symptoms disappear if the patient passes from the upright or dorsal decubitus position to the ventral decubitus or left lateral decubitus. Obstruction is usually intermittent and rarely complete.

Diagnosis is made by the clinical picture, by direct radiologic examination of the upper abdomen showing a great dilation of the duodenum. Gastroduodenal X-ray series with radiopaque substance confirms the dilation of the duodenum with a sudden stoppage of the radiopaque substance at the middle third or distal third of the third portion of the duodenum. Dilation affects the duodenum, and much less frequently, there is dilation of the stomach. If the radiographic examination is performed during an obstructive crisis, it is important to change the patient's position to see if the radiopaque substance passes more easily in the ventral decubitus position. Hypotonic duodenography is also a means that is frequently used in the diagnosis of this syndrome (1, 2, 6). In some selective cases, angiographic studies can be done to show that the aortomesenteric angle is less than 25°. It should be pointed out that some patients may present a stoppage of the radiopaque substance at the level of the third portion of the duodenum without presenting any symptoms.

The initial treatment of this syndrome should be medical, and surgery should only be resorted to if the obstruction persists and the weight loss is accentuated and progressive. The surgical treatment most frequently used to treat this syndrome is laterolateral duodenojejunal bypass. Gregoire, in France (14), in 1920, proposed a duodenojejunal anastomosis in Roux-en-Y fashion, a technique that was used very infrequently in those times but was much more accepted later. This was because the laterolateral duodenojejunal anastomosis sometimes led to a blind loop syndrome with increase in bacteria and changes in the biliary salts with the appearance of malabsorption phenomena. In 1959, Strong (6) proposed treating this syndrome by dividing the suspensory ligament of Treitz and allowing the duodenum to descend within the aortomesenteric angle. Once the ligament of Treitz is divided, it is usually possible for the surgeon to introduce two fingers between the superior border of the third portion of the duodenum and the aortomesenteric arterial angle. This means that the result of division of the ligament will be beneficial. On the other hand, if the duodenum does not descend after dividing the ligament, it will be necessary to add a duodenojejunal anastomosis.

In dividing the suspensory ligament, care must be taken not to injure the inferior mesenteric vein, which is to the left of the duodenojejunal junction. In addition, all the fibers of the suspensory ligament should be divided, those that hold the flexure in place as well as those that sustain the third of fourth portions of the duodenum.

Operative Technique

Operative Technique

FIGURE 40.1
The drawing shows pronounced dilation of the duodenum, produced by compression exerted by the superior mesenteric artery against the aorta and the vertebral column. Duodenal distension stops abruptly at the level of the superior mesenteric vessels.

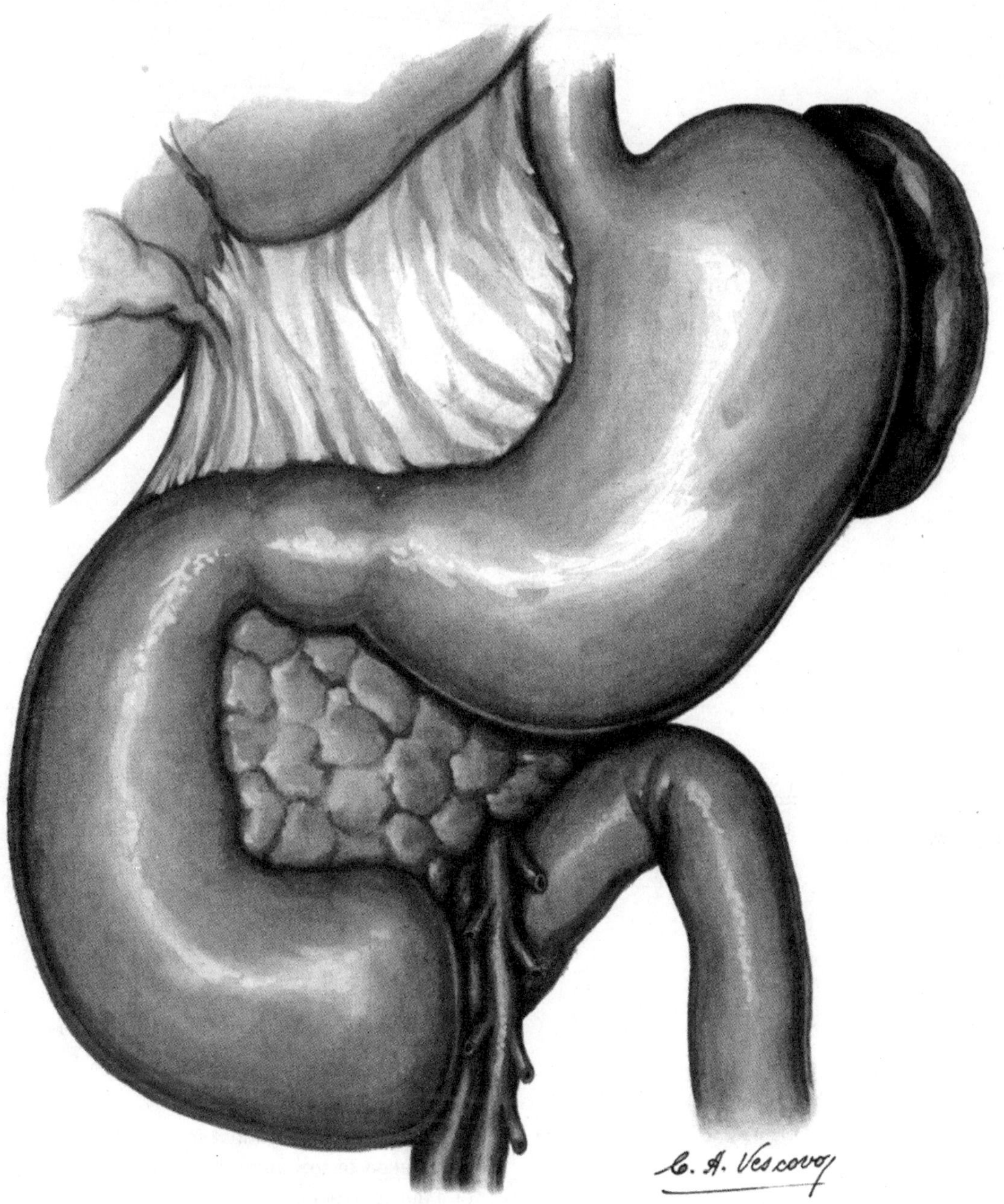

FIGURE 40.1

Operative Technique

FIGURE 40.2

The operation that is most frequently performed to overcome obstruction of the third portion of the duodenum is laterolateral duodenojejunal anastomosis. To carry out this procedure, the transverse colon and its mesocolon are retracted upward, exposing the middle colic vessels and the third portion of the duodenum, which is very dilated and displaces the transverse mesocolon downward. The broken line shows the extent of the incision that is to be performed on the transverse mesocolon to expose the third portion of the duodenum at the site where it joins the second portion.

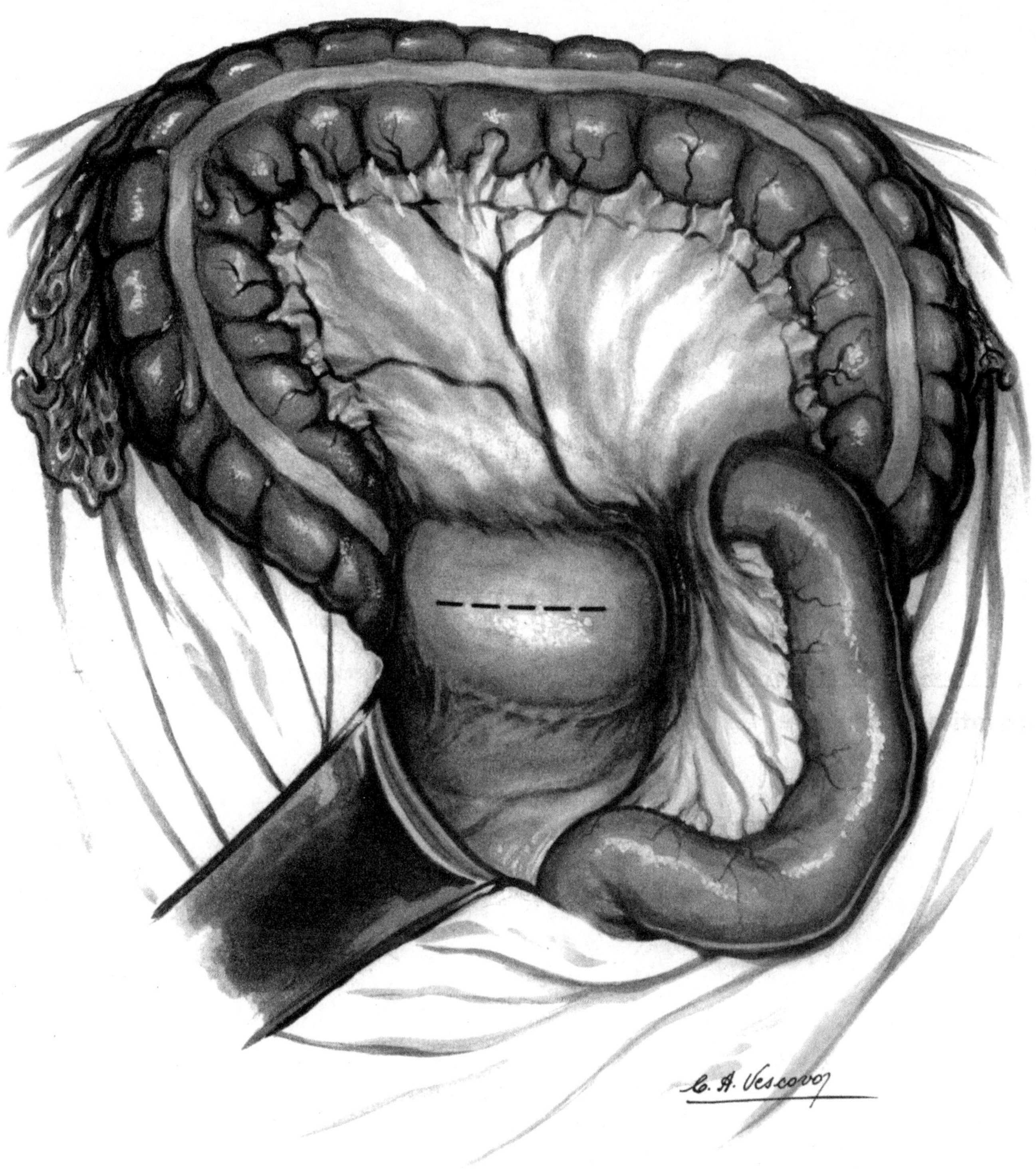

FIGURE 40.2

FIGURE 40.3
Both leaves of the transverse mesocolon have been incised and, using Babcock clamps, the duodenum is brought downward in its second portion, where it joins the third portion. For this purpose, a smooth Foerster clamp should be used.

Operative Technique

FIGURE 40.4
The duodenum has been brought partially down and held with two smooth Foerster clamps. The posterior wall of the duodenum is being fixed to the posterior edge of the transverse mesocolon using interrupted nonabsorbable sutures. The jejunal loop selected to be anastomosed to the duodenum has been grasped with two Babcock clamps. Anastomosis of the jejunal loop to the duodenum is carried out at about 12 to 15 cm from the duodenojejunal flexure.

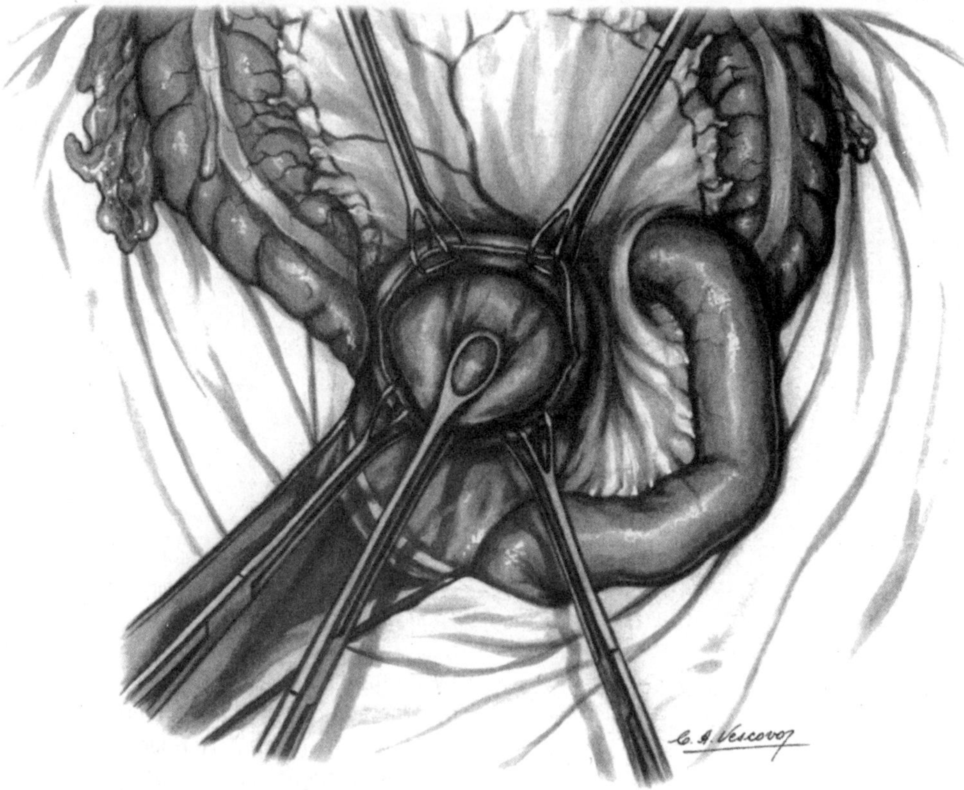

FIGURE 40.3

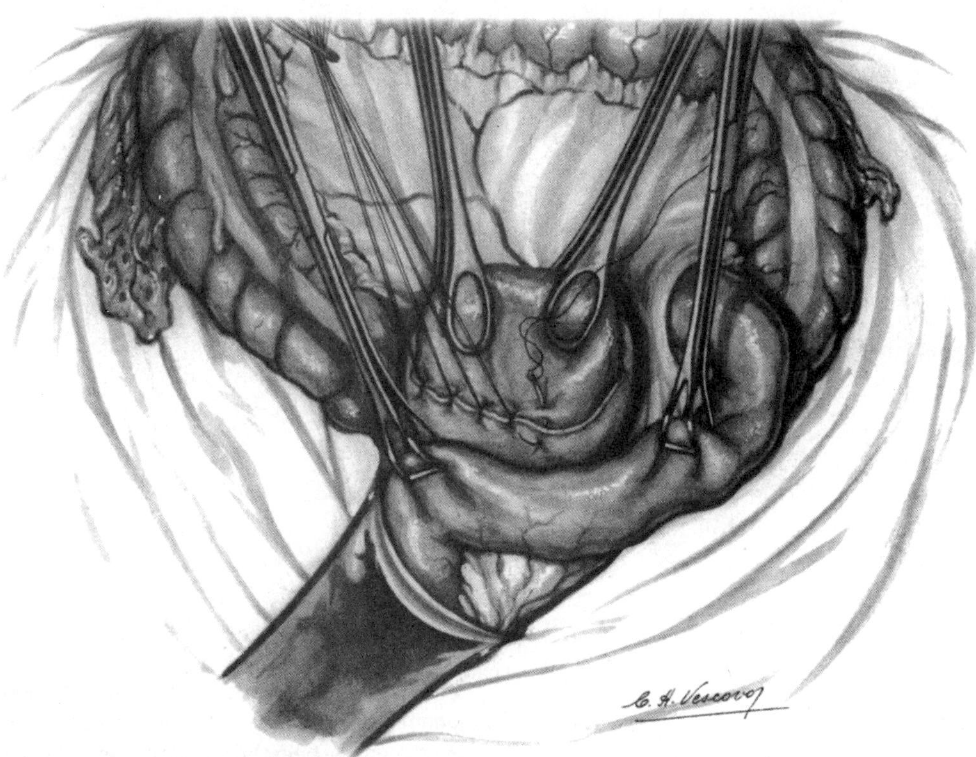

FIGURE 40.4

FIGURE 40.5
To carry out the duodenojejunal anastomosis as cleanly as possible, the atraumatic twin Finochietto clamp is used. A good anastomosis can also be performed without the help of this clamp. Suturing of the posterior seromuscular layer between the duodenum and jejunum has been performed using interrupted nonabsorbable sutures, and suturing of the perforating layer is being performed with interrupted reabsorbable sutures. Duodenojejunal anastomosis can be carried out using continuous sutures with the same good results.

Operative Technique

FIGURE 40.6
The suturing of the anterior layer of the duodenum and the jejunum has been completed and the seromuscular layer of the duodenum is being fixed to the anterior border of the transverse mesocolon, which completes the procedure.

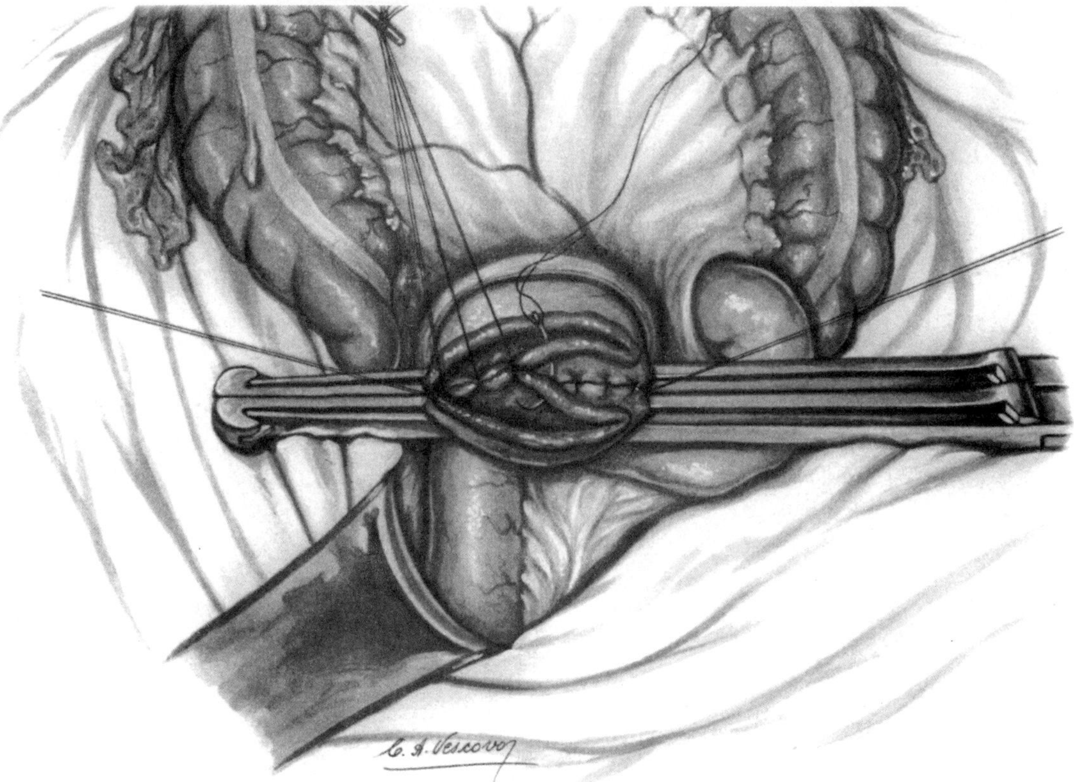

FIGURE 40.5

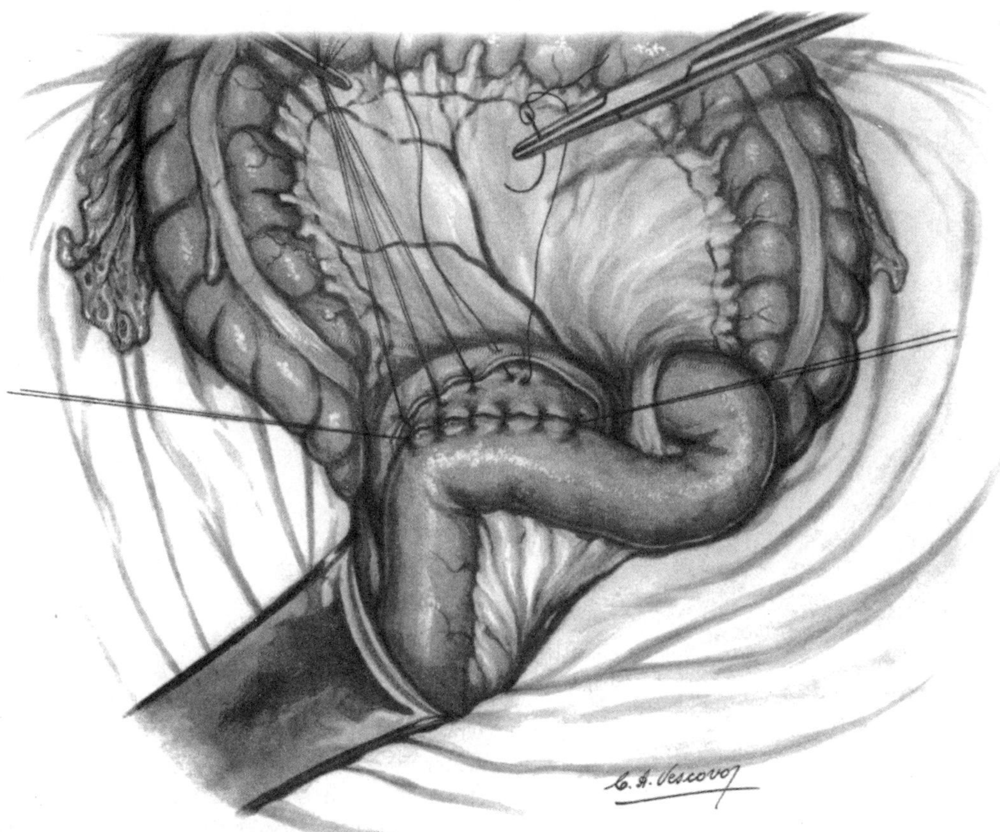

FIGURE 40.6

Operative Technique

FIGURE 40.7
As said previously, some surgeons prefer to perform the duodenojejunal anastomosis using a Roux-en-Y jejunal limb as shown in the drawing to prevent possible development of a blind loop syndrome (5). The distal jejunal limb is anastomosed in end-to-side fashion to the duodenum at the junction of the second and third portions. The proximal jejunal limb is anastomosed in end-to-side fashion to the distal jejunal limb.

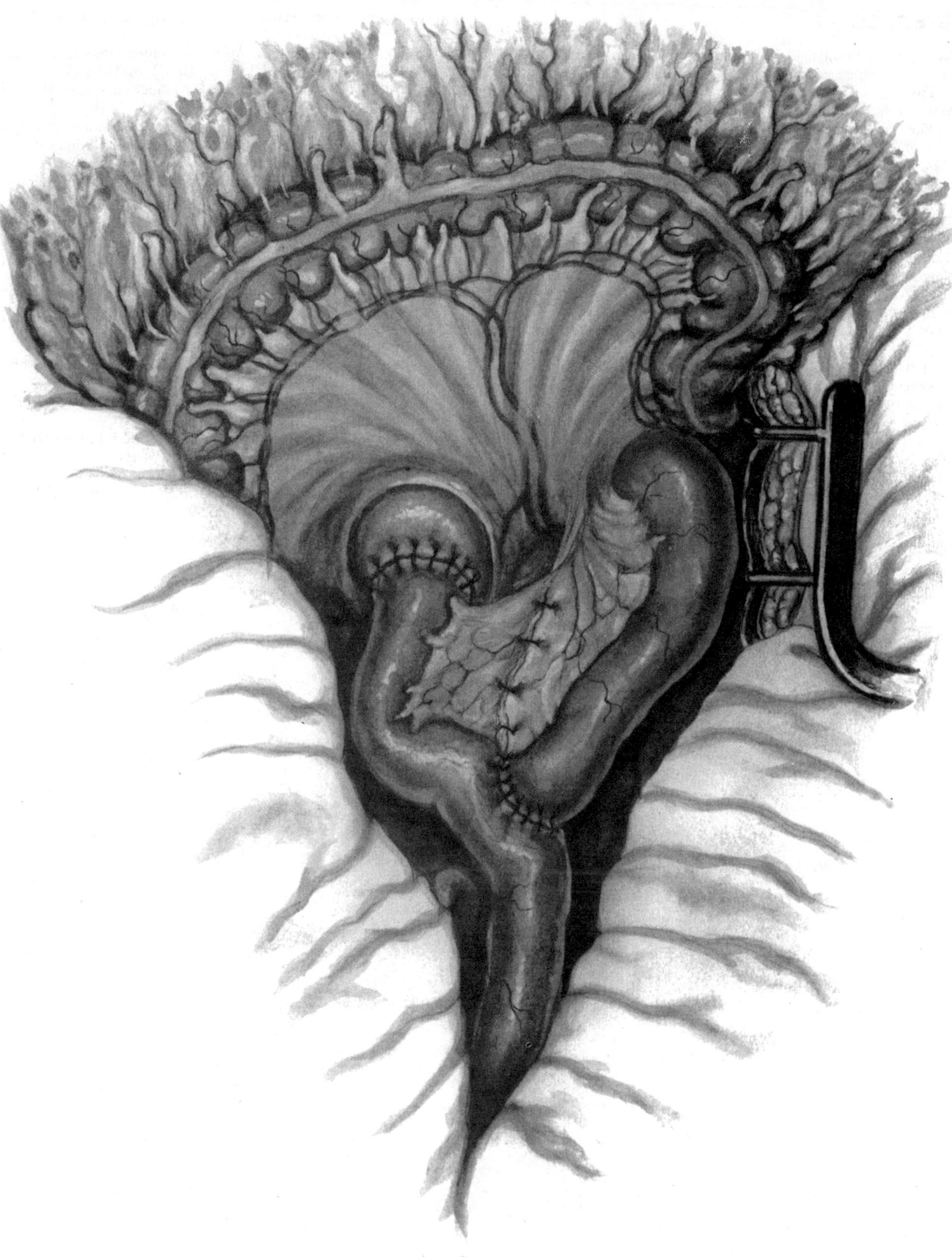

FIGURE 40.7

References

1. Akin, J.T. Jr., Skandalakis, J.E., Gray, S.W. The anatomic basis of vascular compression of the duodenum. Surg. Clin. North Am. 54:1361, 1974.
2. Akin, J.T. Jr., Gray, S.W., Skandalakis, J.E. Vascular compression of the duodenum. Surgery 79:515, 1976.
3. Ellis, H. Superior mesenteric artery syndrome. In Schwartz, S.I., Ellis, H. (Eds.) Maingot's abdominal operations. Ed. 9, vol. I, p. 587. Appleton Lange. Norwalk, CT, 1990.
4. Fischer, H.W. The big duodenum. Am. J. Roentgenol. 83:861, 1960.
5. Fromm, D. Superior mesenteric artery syndrome. In Fromm, D. (Ed.) Gastrointestinal surgery. Vol. I, p. 387. Churchill Livingstone, New York, 1985.
6. Gray, S.W., Skandalakis, J.E. Embryology for surgeons. P. 178. W.B. Saunders, Philadelphia, 1972.
7. Gray, S.W., Skandalakis, J.E. Atlas of surgical anatomy for general surgeons. P. 156. Williams & Wilkins, Baltimore, 1985.
8. Gustaffson, L., Falk, A., Lukes, P.J., Gamklou, R. Diagnosis and treatment of superior mesenteric artery syndrome. Br. J. Surg. 71:499, 1984.
9. Hines, J.R., Gore, R.M., Ballantyne, G.H. Superior mesenteric artery syndrome:Diagnostic criteria and therapeutic approaches. Am. J. Surg. 148:630, 1984.
10. Jones, A.S., Carter, R., Smith, L.L., Jorgensen, E.J. Arteriomesenteric duodenal compression. Am. J. Surg. 100:262, 1960.
11. Kaiser, G.C., Mckain, J.M., Shumacker, H.B. Jr. The superior mesenteric artery syndrome. Surg. Gynecol. Obstet. 110:133, 1960.
12. Lontok, R.M., Taber, K.W. Arterio-mesenteric duodenal occlusion (report of 8 proven cases). Penn. Med. J. 62:1529, 1959.
13. Pool, E.H., Niles, W.L., Martin, K.A. Duodenal stasis: Duodeno-jejunostomy. Ann. Surg. 98:587, 1933.
14. Quenú, J., Joygue, J., Perrotin, J., Dubost, C., Moreaux, J. Opérations sur les parois de l'abdomen et sur le tube digestif. P. 657. Masson et Cie., Paris, 1960.
15. Schirmer, B., Scott Jones, R. Superior mesenteric artery syndrome. In Nora, P.F. (Ed.) Operative surgery. Ed. 3, p. 583. W.B. Saunders, Philadelphia, 1990.
16. Schirmer, B. Vascular compression of the duodenum. In Sabiston, D.C. Jr. (Ed.) Textbook of surgery. Ed. 14, p. 807. W.B. Saunders, Philadelphia, 1991.
17. Thieme, E.T., Postmus, R. Superior mesenteric artery syndrome. Ann. Surg. 154:139, 1961.
18. Thompson, V.W., Stanley, J.C. Vascular compression of the duodenum and peptic ulcer disease. Arch. Surg. 108:674, 1974.
19. Valdoni, P. Abdominal surgery, P. 141. W.B. Saunders, Philadelphia, 1976.
20. Way, L.W. Current surgical diagnosis and treatment. Ed. 9, p. 494. Appleton Lange. Norwalk, CT, 1991.
21. Wilson-Storey, D., Mackinlay, G.A. The superior mesenteric artery syndrome. J. R. Coll. Surg. Edinb. 31:175, 1986.
22. Ylinen, P., Kinnunen, J., Hockerstedt, K. Superior mesenteric artery syndrome: A follow-up study of 16 operated patients. J. Clin. Gastroenterol. 11:386, 1989.

Section F

Surgery of the Stomach and Duodenum

CHAPTER **41**

Duodenal Diverticula—Extraluminal Diverticula

It is generally said that duodenal diverticula are infrequent. It has been shown, however, that the frequency of duodenal diverticula is directly related to the methods of diagnosis and to the interest the examiner takes in finding them. According to McSherry and Glenn (49) the frequency of duodenal diverticula according to writings by anatomists, radiologists, and surgeons is 22% but much more infrequent are the complications of the diverticula and the production of symptoms which make it necessary to treat them surgically. According to Neil and Thompson (54) only 10% of diverticula presents symptoms and only 1% may need surgical treatment.

CLASSIFICATION OF DUODENAL DIVERTICULA

Duodenal diverticula are usually described as a uniform pathologic change, the treatment of which seems to be similar in almost all cases. This opinion, in addition to not being correct, leads to confusion, especially among young surgeons. For this reason the author has found it very necessary to establish, from the beginning, a classification of duodenal diverticula according to their origin, anatomic structure, and location. Surgical treatment will not only differ according to the above mentioned factors, but also according to the clinical picture they may present: acute or chronic, if the surgical procedure was preplanned, an unexpected surgical finding, an iatrogenic complication, and so on.

Duodenal diverticula can be divided into three groups:

Group A: Extraluminal Diverticula. These are the diverticula that are most frequently observed. They are produced by a protrusion of the mucosa, the submucosa, and the muscularis mucosa through a weak point in the duodenal wall. The great majority of these diverticula are located in the internal or pancreatic border of the duodenum, which is the only part of the duodenum without peritoneum.

Group B: Duodenal Diverticula into Which Empty the Common Bile Duct and Pancreatic Ducts. These are diverticula of the second portion of the duodenum and rarely the third portion, which receive the opening of the common bile duct and pancreatic ducts. Surgical treatment of diverticula of this group, when indicated, differs completely from that of group A (3, 4, 13, 24, 64, 66).

Group C: Intraluminal Diverticula. These diverticula develop completely within the duodenal lumen. Their external surface, as well as their internal surface, is covered by duodenal mucosa. This group of diverticula is congenital in origin, and treatment differs from that of groups A and B (1, 7, 21, 25, 29, 34, 35, 41, 44, 52, 53, 60, 67).

In the following we will describe separately the general characteristics of each group of diverticula as well as the different surgical procedures used in treating these groups and subgroups.

Group A: Extraluminal Duodenal Diverticula

Seventy-five percent of extraluminal duodenal diverticula are located in the second portion of the duodenum, 20% in the third portion, and 5% in the fourth portion (22, 38, 54). About 90% of extraluminal diverticula originate in the internal border of the duodenum, and more than 70% are located within 2 cm of the papilla (22, 54). The diverticular sac, as previously stated, is made up of mucosa, submucosa, and muscularis mucosa. The size of the diverticulum varies greatly, from millimeters to several centimeters. These diverticula may grow retropancreatically and, in other cases, may penetrate the pancreatic parenchyma or develop in front of the pancreas. Because of their growth, these diverticula may compress the common bile duct, the pancreatic duct, or both ducts simultaneously. Diverticula located near the papilla of Vater (peripapillary) are the ones that lead to the greatest number of complications. Since the extraluminal diverticula lack a muscular layer, they do not have the capacity to eliminate any food that may accumulate in their interior, which may lead to decubitus ulcerations, infections, compression, and so on. Diverticula with a long neck and extending inferiorly are more prone to complications than those with a wide neck and extending upward (11, 31).

Symptoms

The great majority of extraluminal diverticula are asymptomatic and may be incidental radiographic or endoscopic findings. Symptoms that may be produced by extraluminal diverticula are due to obstruction of the common bile duct or the pancreatic duct, inflammation of the pancreatic parenchyma, acute pancreatitis, recurrent pancreatitis, duodenal obstruction due to the distortion that the weight and traction of a voluminous diverticulum produces, hemorrhages due to ulceration of the diverticulum, acute perforated diverticulitis, and so on. Intermittent obstruction of the biliary tract may lead to the formation of biliary calculi, due to deconjugation of biliary salts (38, 49). In patients with extraluminal duodenal diverticula, an increase in the number of microbial colonies has been shown, and it has also been shown that the calculi that form in these cases are usually pigment calculi (22).

Diagnosis

Diagnosis of extraluminal duodenal diverticula is made by means of conventional gastroduodenal radiographic examinations and by means of double contrast, hypotonic duodenography and duodenal endoscopy. Radiographic examination determines the location of the diverticulum, its size, shape, ascending or descending direction, mobility, relation to the pancreas, and relation to the papilla of Vater, the time that radiopaque substances remain in the interior of the diverticulum, and its sensibility to palpation. Endoscopic duodenal examination complements radiographic examination and determines with greater precision the location of the diverticulum and its proximity to the papilla, the presence of blood emerging from the diverticular opening, and so on. Clinical examination of the patient, ultrasonographic examination, computerized axial tomography, and endoscopic examination of other viscera will help in determining the possible existence of some other pathologic process (biliary lithiasis, gastroduodenal ulcer, irritable colon, etc.) that could explain the symptoms presented by the patient, which had been attributed to the presence of a diverticulum.

When the emergency abdominal clinical findings are due to an acute perforated diverticulitis, the problem is very serious, not only because of its elevated mortality and morbidity, but because it is very difficult to establish the diagnosis before the operation. Mortality of surgical treatment of this complication is nearly 50% (49).

Acute duodenal diverticulitis is frequently confused with acute pancreatitis because of the similarity of the pain and an increase in the serum amylase. Direct abdominal radiographic examination has diagnostic value, since it usually shows an accumulation of air in the right upper quadrant of the abdomen. This examination should be complemented by the ingestion of Hypaque, which will show the duodenal perforation, usually blocked off retroperitoneally. The image of the blocked off perforation coincides topographically with the site of accumulation of air in the retroperitoneum, which was seen in the direct X-ray of the upper abdomen. Examination of the patient is completed by laboratory tests and computed axial tomography.

It is necessary to point out that the diagnosis of perforated duodenal diverticulitis may not be made, even with the abdomen open, if the surgeon is not well informed. The medical literature has many descriptions of cases of acute perforated duodenal diverticulitis in which the diagnosis was not made in spite of the patient having undergone laparotomy (11, 17, 18, 20, 39, 68). To confirm the diagnosis of acute perforated diverticulitis of the duodenum during the surgical procedure, it is indispensable to carry out an ample Vautrin-Kocher maneuver because the perforated diverticular process is generally blocked off retroperitoneally and can only be demonstrated after the Vautrin-Kocher maneuver, which permits observation of the presence of a phlegmon or bile-stained fluid in an abscess (8, 10, 11, 17, 18, 24, 31, 39, 57, 63, 68).

Factors that influence the elevated morbidity and mortality in surgery for extraluminal duodenal diverticula

The morbidity and mortality of surgery for extraluminal duodenal diverticula is elevated. Some of the causative factors are as follows:

1. *Location of the Diverticula.* Seventy percent of extraluminal duodenal diverticula are located within 2 cm from the papilla (peripapillary diverticula), which is a very difficult zone and carries high risk, since the more frequent complications are lateral duodenal fistulas and injuries to the papilla.
2. An important factor of morbidity and mortality is, not having established the diagnosis and the relation between the minor papilla and the common bile duct, before surgery. The common bile duct should be catheterized and the relation between the diverticulum and the papilla established before beginning dissection of the diverticulum. Dissection of a peripapillary duodenal diverticulum may lead to irreparable injury without the surgeon being able to repair the defect, since the structure of extraluminal duodenal diverticula is very fragile.
3. Surgical treatment of extraluminal duodenal diverticula is infrequent, so surgeons cannot have enough experience with the existing surgical procedures.
4. There are not many details in the surgical techniques that should be used in the treatment of extraluminal diverticula in surgical atlases. Surgical technique varies according to location, clinical picture (acute or chronic), iatrogenic perforation of the diverticulum, and so on. This prevents inexperienced surgeons from being able to learn the existing techniques and be prepared when the moment arises in which they have to apply these techniques in urgent cases.

Surgical Procedures for the Resection of Extraluminal Duodenal Diverticula

These surgical procedures vary according to the location of the diverticulum, its relation to the papilla, if it presents an acute or chronic clinical picture, and so on. To avoid confusion in the description of surgical procedures used in the treatment of extraluminal duodenal diverticula, the following order will be followed:

a. Technique for resection for extraluminal duodenal diverticula of the second portion, peripapillary, with chronic clinical picture, performed from the outside of the duodenal lumen.
b. Technique for resection of duodenal diverticula of the second portion, peripapillary, with chronic clinical picture, performed from within the duodenal lumen.
c. Surgical treatment for extraluminal diverticula of the second portion with an acute clinical picture (acute perforated diverticulitis).
d. Surgical technique in cases of iatrogenic perforation of peripapillary diverticula during instrumental exploration of the common bile duct for biliary tract lithiasis.
e. Surgical technique for the resection of extraluminal diverticula of the third portion of the duodenum with a chronic clinical picture.
f. Surgical technique for the treatment of extraluminal diverticula of the third portion of the duodenum with an acute clinical picture (acute perforated diverticulitis).

FIGURE 41.1
Extraluminal diverticula of the second portion of the duodenum may develop behind the pancreas, as seen in the drawing.

Extraluminal Diverticula of the Second Portion of the Duodenum with Chronic Clinical Picture: Resection from the Outside of the Duodenum

FIGURE 41.2
Less frequently extraluminal diverticula of the second portion of the duodenum may develop in front of the pancreas, as seen in the drawing.

FIGURE 41.3
In some cases extraluminal duodenal diverticula may develop into the pancreatic parenchyma, as shown in the drawing. No matter what direction the diverticula take during their development, they can produce compression of the common bile duct or the pancreatic duct, leading to complications such as jaundice, pancreatitis, infection, and so on.

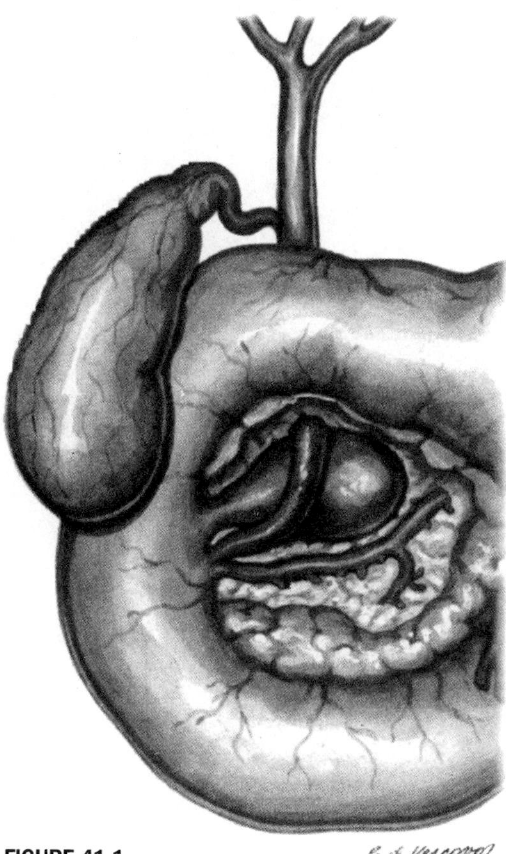

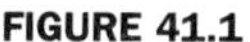

FIGURE 41.1

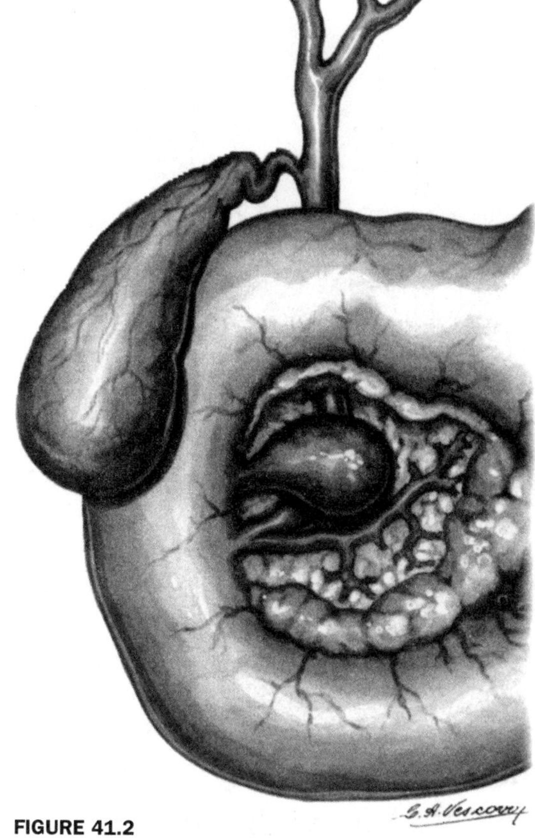

FIGURE 41.2

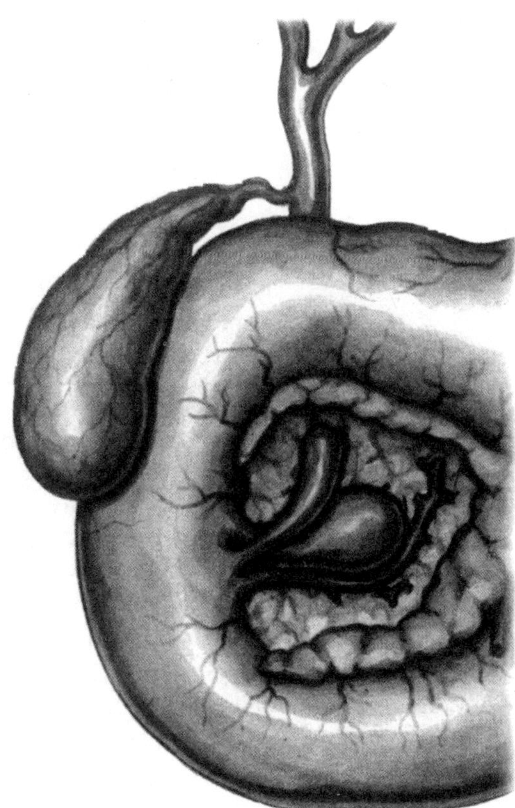

FIGURE 41.3

Extraluminal Diverticula of the Second Portion of the Duodenum with Chronic Clinical Picture: Resection from the Outside of the Duodenum

FIGURE 41.4
Before proceeding with dissection of the diverticulum, it is necessary to determine its exact location and its relation to the papilla of Vater. These precise determinations can be obtained during preoperative study and then completed during the operation. It is very useful to practice operative cholecystocholangiography by puncturing the gallbladder. An ample Vautrin-Kocher maneuver is then carried out to mobilize the duodenum and the head of the pancreas. The Vautrin-Kocher maneuver should be very ample, and the peritoneum over the external border of the duodenum should be incised, not only in the second portion, but also in the first portion and the external segment of the third portion, to the right of the superior mesenteric vessels, as seen in the drawing. A small transverse incision is then made into the common bile duct and a rubber explorer with an olive shaped end introduced.

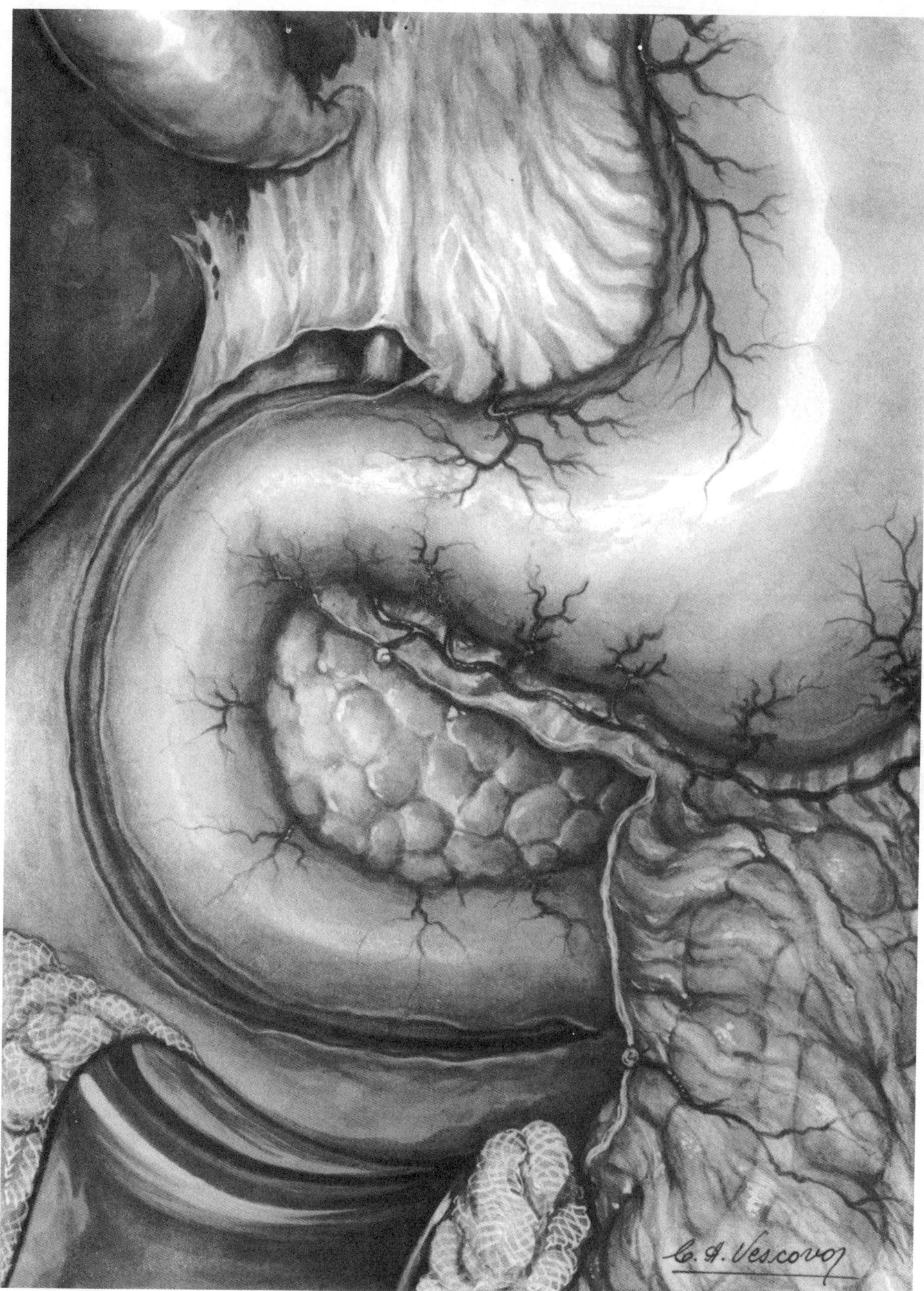

FIGURE 41.4

Extraluminal Diverticula of the Second Portion of the Duodenum with Chronic Clinical Picture: Resection from the Outside of the Duodenum

FIGURE 41.5
Dissection of the diverticulum has begun. The second assistant applies traction to the second portion of the duodenum toward the left with both hands or by means of two Babcock clamps. Dissection of the diverticulum is begun at the internal border of the duodenum at the level of the papilla of Vater. Some diverticula may be very retracted and covered with fibrous tissue, making their identification difficult. It may be useful to use the Mahorner procedure (47, 48). To carry out this maneuver, the Levine nasogastric tube is passed into the duodenum and an atraumatic clamp placed, compressing the third portion of the duodenum. Air is then injected through the Levine tube. The air will fill the diverticulum, facilitating its identification.

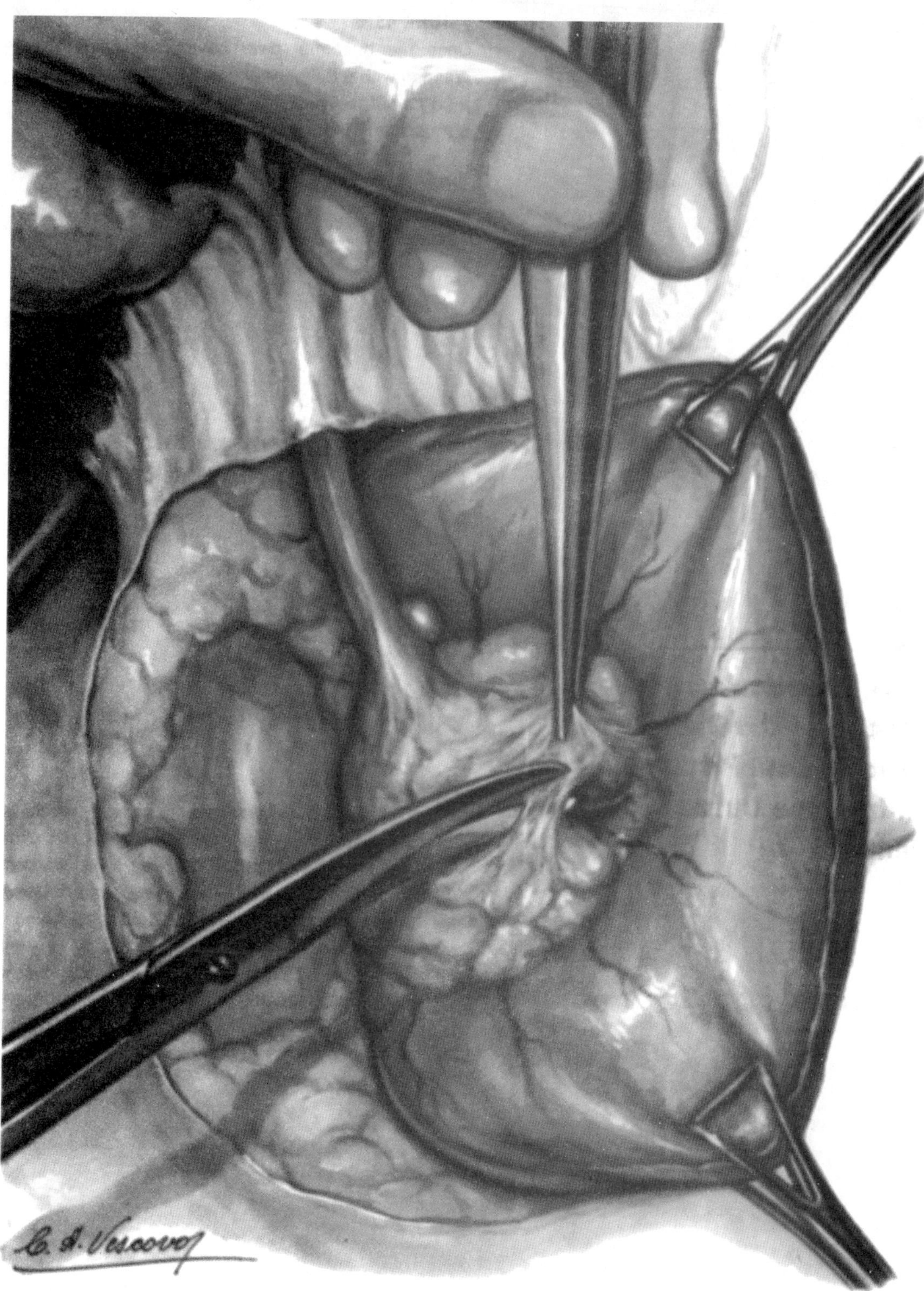

FIGURE 41.5

FIGURE 41.6
Once the duodenal diverticulum has been identified, it is grasped with a Babcock clamp and gentle traction is applied to it so as not to injure it, since its walls are very fragile, lacking a muscularis propria layer.

FIGURE 41.7
Dissection of the diverticulum has been continued, showing that its size is much larger than it seemed to be when dissection was started.

Extraluminal Diverticula of the Second Portion of the Duodenum with Chronic Clinical Picture: Resection from the Outside of the Duodenum

FIGURE 41.8
The diverticulum has been freed to its neck, where two sutures have been applied to place traction in opposite directions and keep the mucosa of the neck of the diverticulum from introducing itself into the inside of the duodenum. Using scissors, the fundus and body of the diverticulum is incised. By means of this maneuver, the diverticulum will be divided into two halves. The mucosa of the neck of the diverticulum will then be sectioned after the catheterized papilla is identified. Section of the diverticulum into two halves is done with object of identifying the papilla and its relation to the diverticulum.

FIGURE 41.9
Once the papilla has been identified, the neck of the diverticulum is transected with scissors. Traction continues to be exerted on the mucosa of the neck of the diverticulum to keep it from extending into the duodenal lumen, which would lead to incomplete suture of the edges of the diverticular opening and the possible postoperative development of a lateral duodenal fistula.

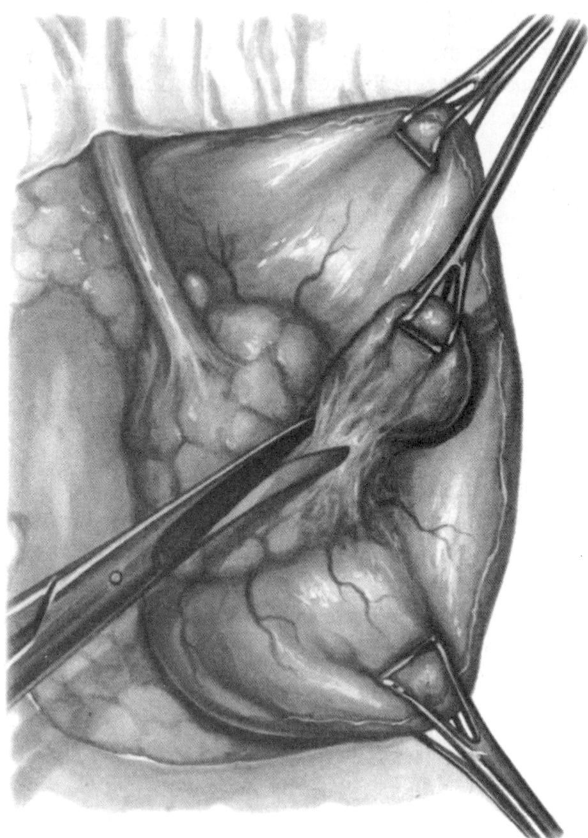

FIGURE 41.6

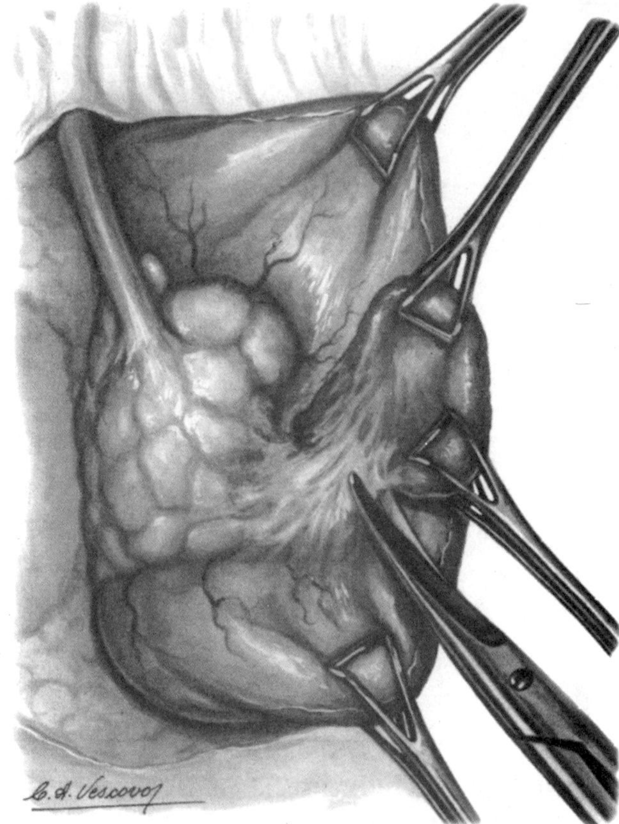

FIGURE 41.7

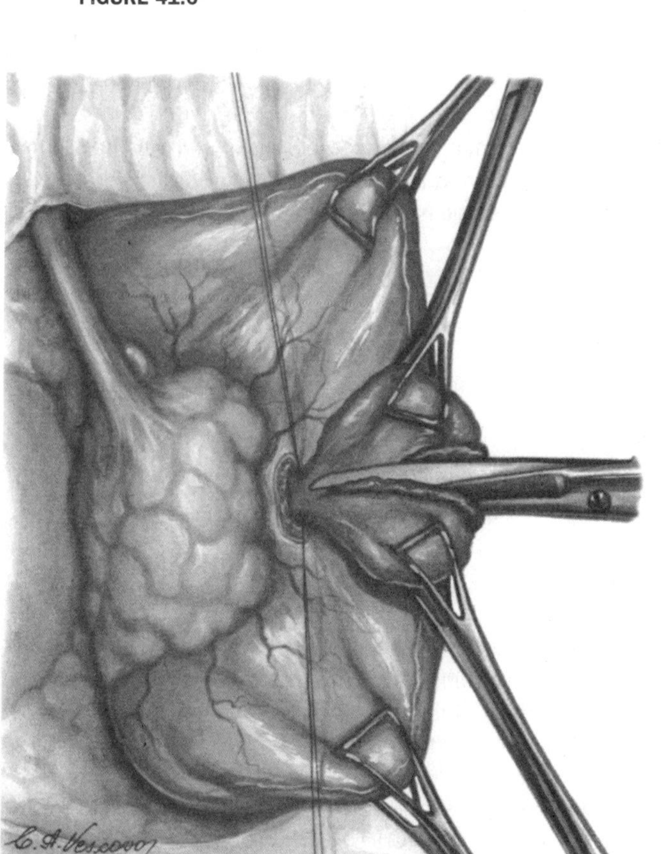

FIGURE 41.8

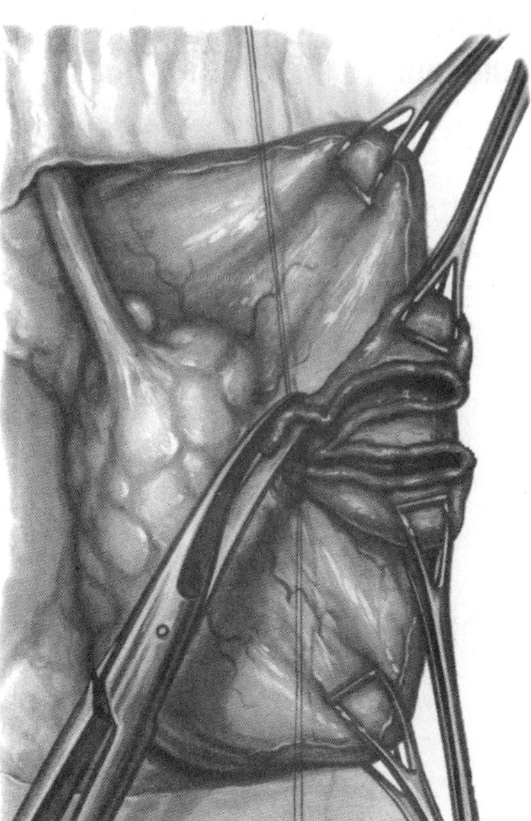

FIGURE 41.9

FIGURE 41.10
Traction on the sutures placed in the mucosa of the neck of the diverticulum permits adequate vision of the catheterized papilla.

FIGURE 41.11
Before proceeding with closure of the duodenal mucosa, it is convenient to remove the inferior and superior traction sutures, leaving only the lateral sutures, to facilitate transverse closure of the duodenal mucosa with interrupted absorbable sutures.

Extraluminal Diverticula of the Second Portion of the Duodenum with Chronic Clinical Picture: Resection from the Outside of the Duodenum

FIGURE 41.12
The mucosa of the duodenum is being sutured with interrupted absorbable sutures, leaving the knots on the inside. Correct closure of the mucosa and submucosa of the duodenum is very important.

FIGURE 41.13
Once the mucosal layer has been sutured, the seromuscular layer is sutured with interrupted nonabsorbable sutures. A fine T-tube is inserted into the common bile duct in order to partially drain bile to the outside. The transverse choledochotomy, if it is closed transversely and a fine T-tube is left in place, in bile ducts of normal caliber will only exceptionally become complicated with a postoperative stricture. If the duodenal diverticulum is far away from the papilla, its resection is simpler and less dangerous.

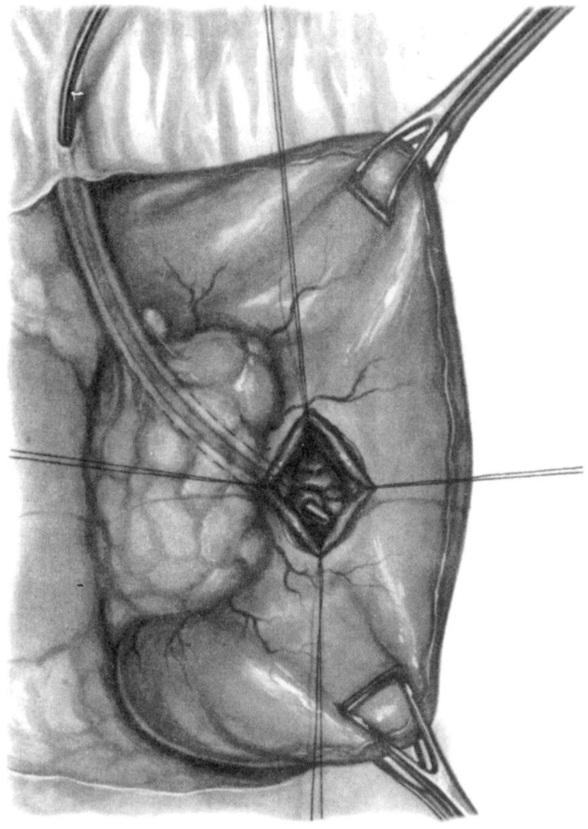
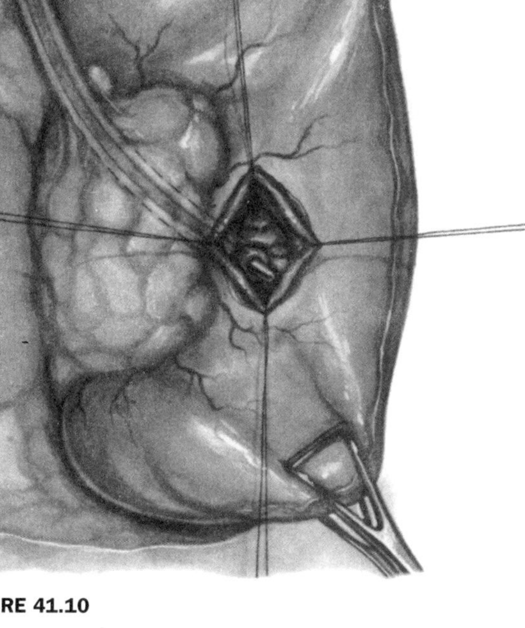

FIGURE 41.10

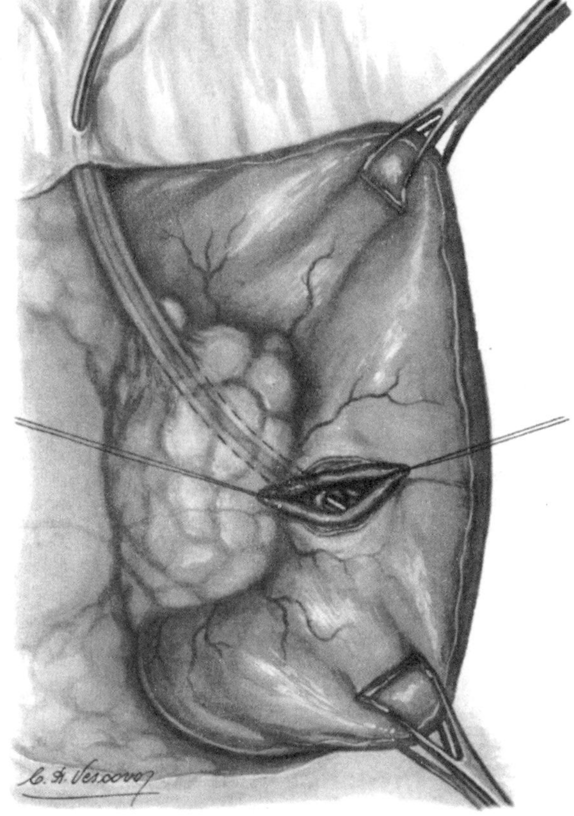

FIGURE 41.11

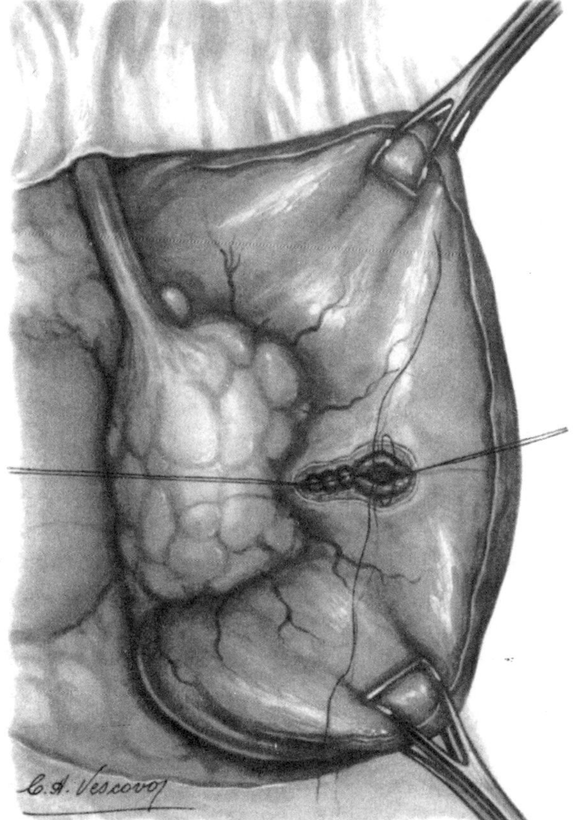
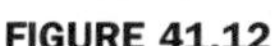

FIGURE 41.12

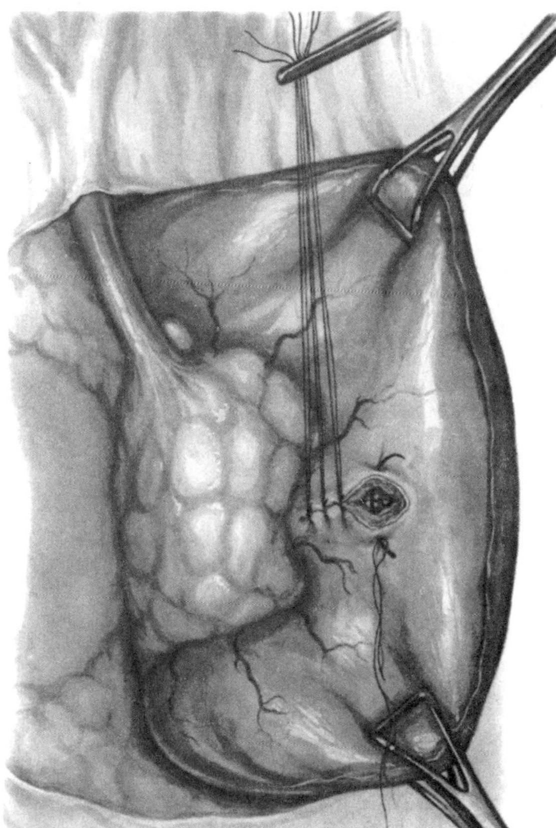

FIGURE 41.13

Extraluminal Diverticula of the Second Portion of the Duodenum with Chronic Clinical Picture: Resection from the Inside of the Duodenum

FIGURE 41.14
The Vautrin-Kocher maneuver has been carried out, and the silhouette of the extraluminal diverticulum is demonstrated with lines including its extraluminal body and fundus, which are projected on the pancreas. The location of the papilla of Vater below the neck of the diverticulum has been pointed out. By means of a broken longitudinal line the incision to be made in the duodenum has been traced. Before dissection of the diverticulum is begun, the common bile duct should be catheterized through a small transverse incision to identify the papilla and its relation with the diverticulum.

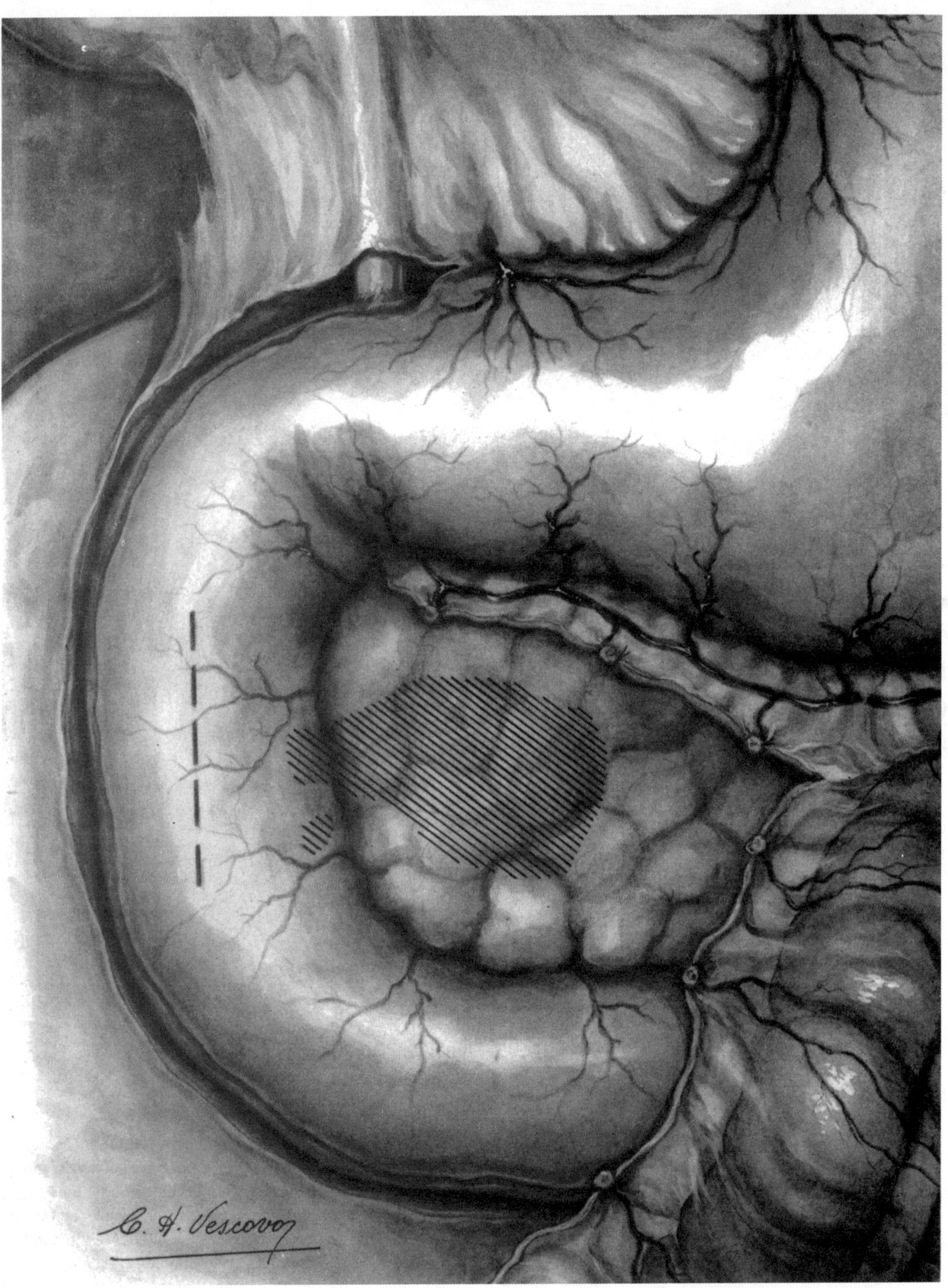
C. H. Vescovo

Extraluminal Diverticula of the Second Portion of the Duodenum with Chronic Clinical Picture: Resection from the Inside of the Duodenum

FIGURE 41.15
The second portion of the duodenum has been opened. The edges of the duodenal wall have been grasped with triangular atraumatic Duval clamps, which, at the same time as they control bleeding temporarily from the duodenal wall, can be used to apply traction and better visualize the interior of the duodenum. The common bile duct has been catheterized. Just above and very near the papilla the entrance of the diverticulum is noted.

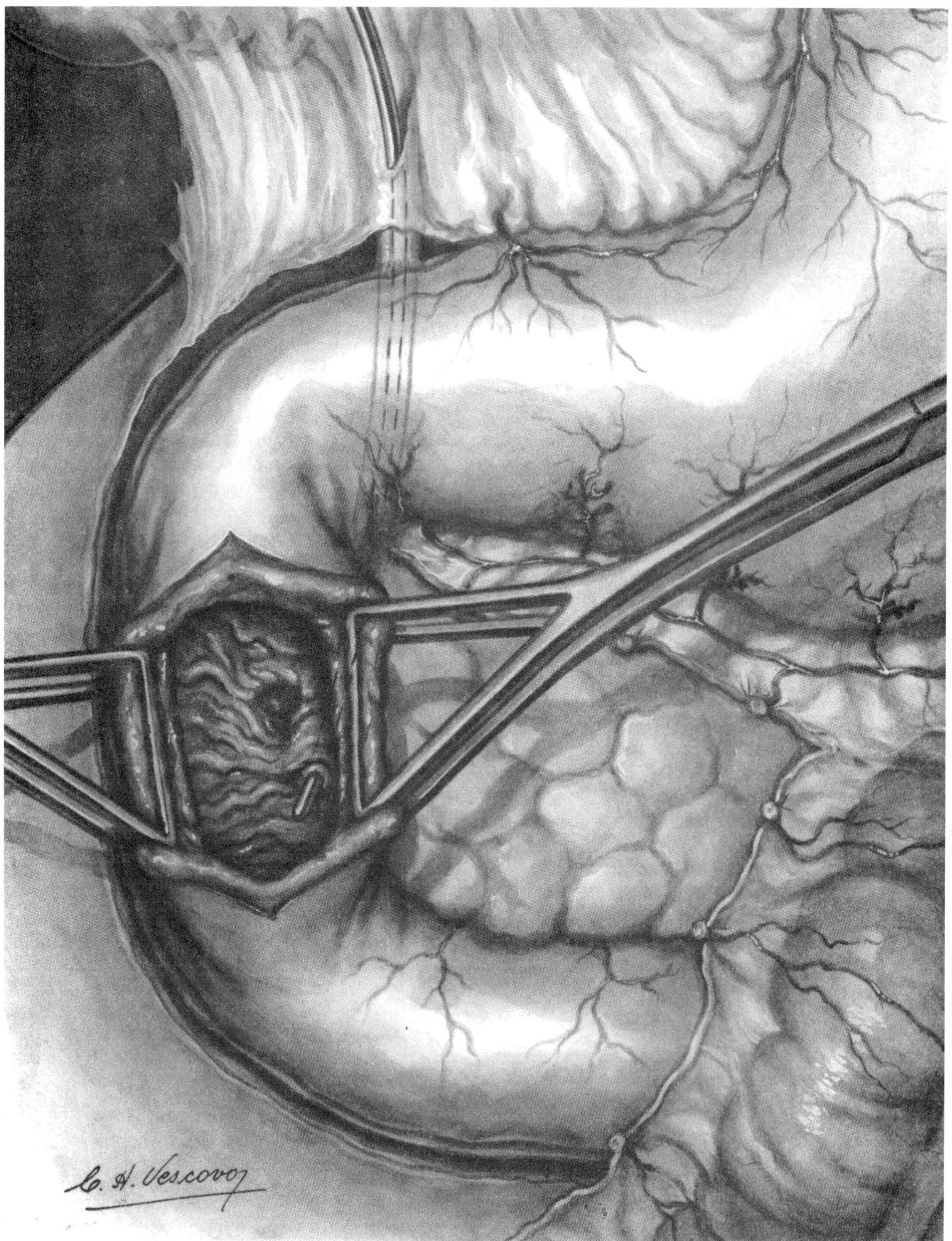

FIGURE 41.15

FIGURE 41.16
An Allis or Babcock clamp is introduced into the entrance of the diverticulum, and the fundus of the diverticulum is grasped. It is made up of mucosa and submucosa, and by applying traction on it, it is partially exposed.

Extraluminal Diverticula of the Second Portion of the Duodenum with Chronic Clinical Picture: Resection from the Inside of the Duodenum

FIGURE 41.17
The diverticulum has been completely exteriorized. The close relation between the neck of the diverticulum and the papilla of Vater can be seen.

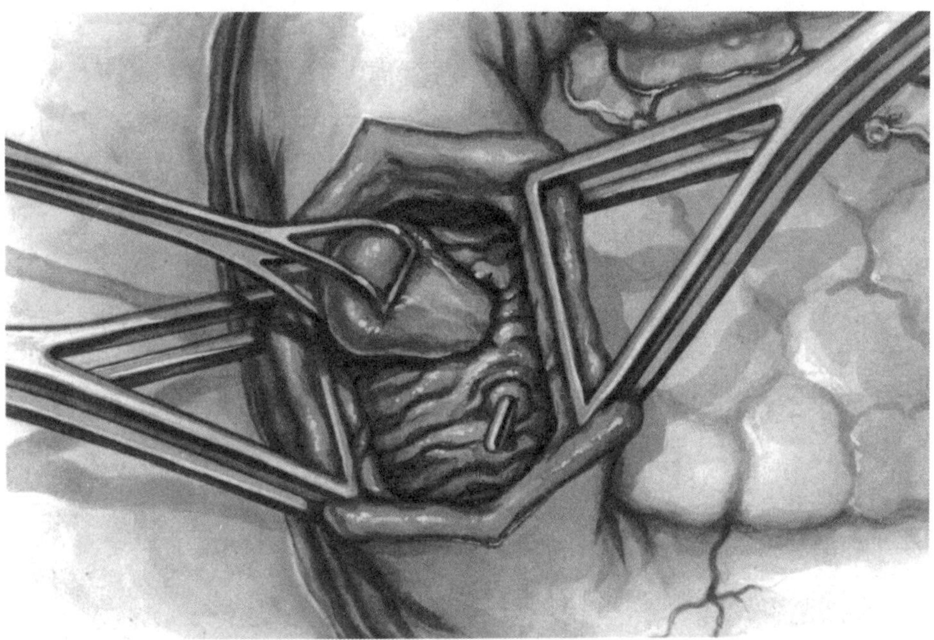

FIGURE 41.16

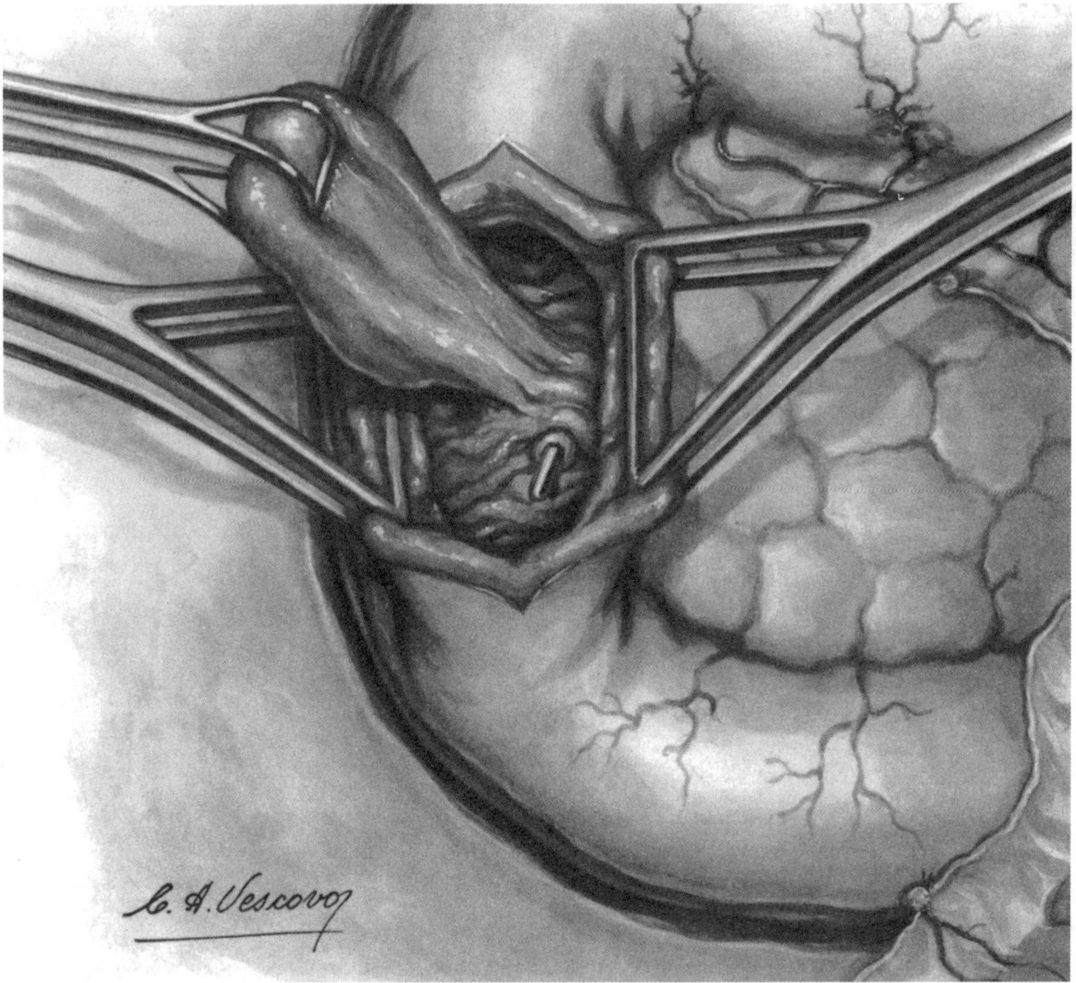

FIGURE 41.17

Extraluminal Diverticula of the Second Portion of the Duodenum with Chronic Clinical Picture: Resection from the Inside of the Duodenum

FIGURE 41.18

Two traction sutures have been placed in the mucosa of the neck of the diverticulum. Above these sutures, transection of the diverticulum has begun, using scissors.

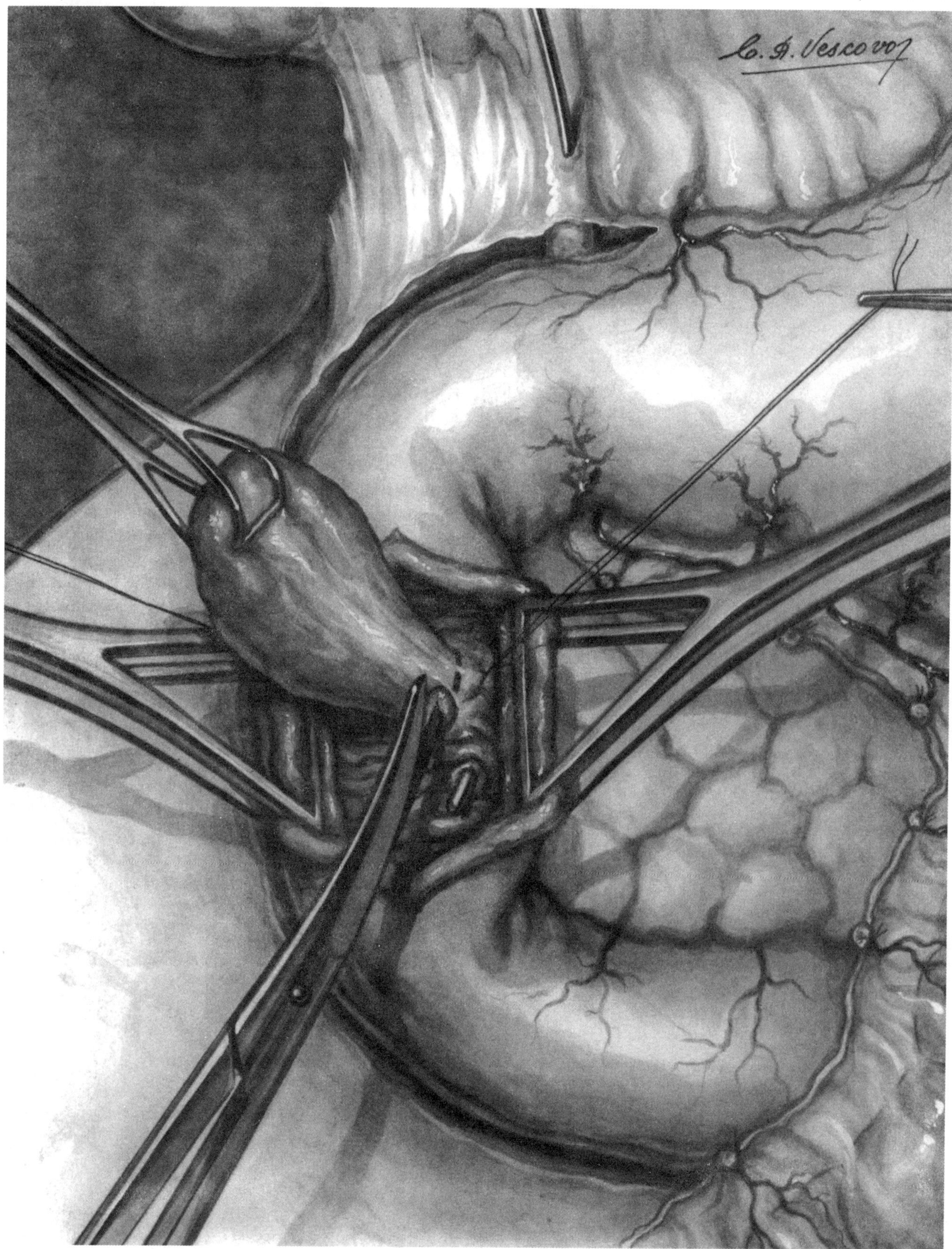

FIGURE 41.18

FIGURE 41.19
A, The diverticulum has been resected. The mucosa at the level of the neck of the diverticulum is pulled in opposite directions using the two sutures. **B,** The needle is being passed in the placement of the first seromuscular suture using nonabsorbable material. **C,** The seromuscular layer has been completely closed. **D,** Once the suture of the seromuscular layer has been completed, the mucosal layer is sutured using absorbable material. Once the opening of the diverticulum has been closed, the incision in the duodenum is closed in two layers using interrupted sutures. The mucosa and submucosal layers are sutured with absorbable material and the seromuscular layer with nonabsorbable material. Once the duodenal closure is completed, a fine T-tube is placed in the common bile duct and secured with two 3-0 chromic catgut sutures.

Extraluminal Diverticula of the Second Portion of the Duodenum with Chronic Clinical Picture: Resection from the Inside of the Duodenum

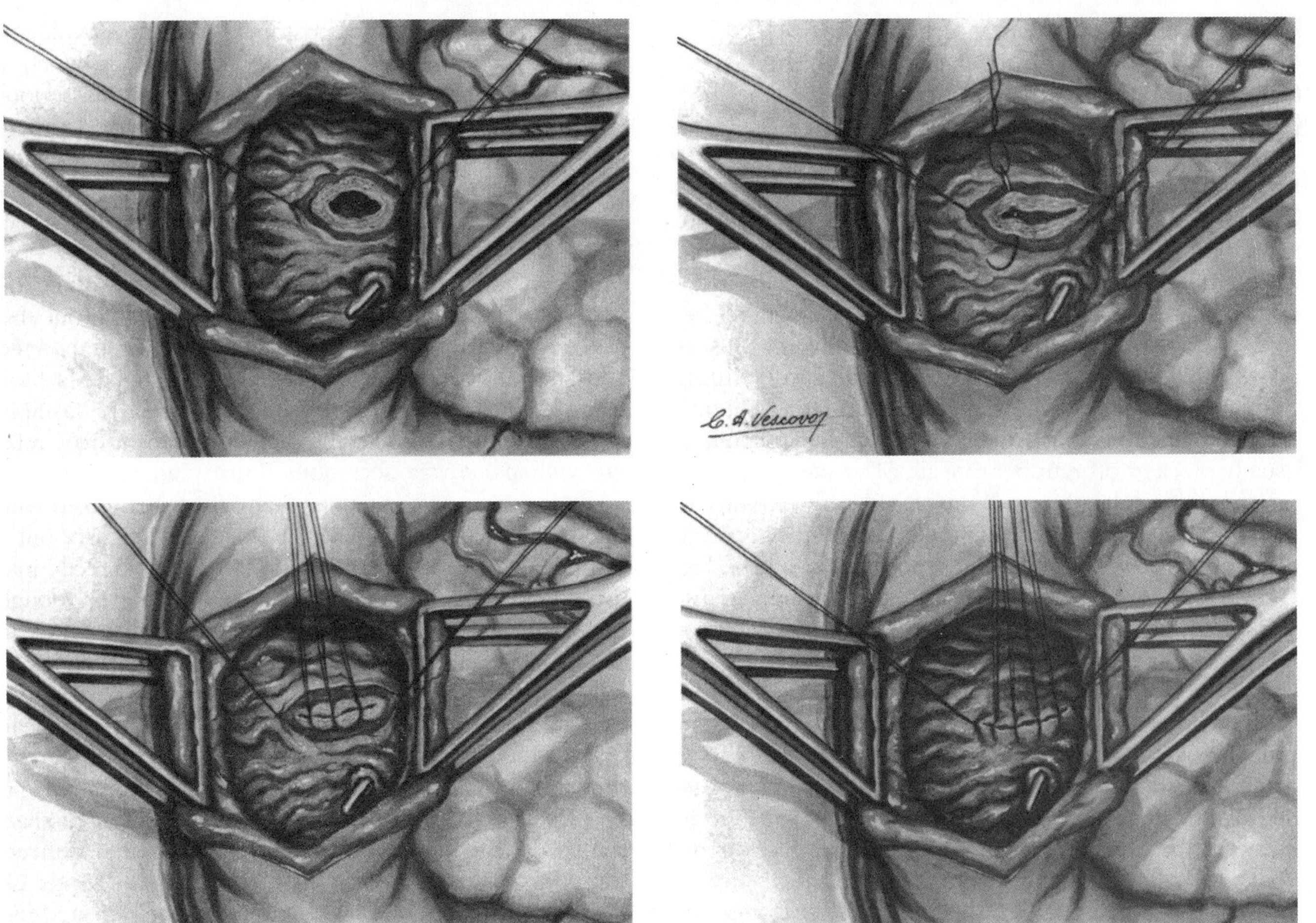

FIGURE 41.19

Treatment of extraluminal duodenal diverticula of the second portion of the duodenum with acute clinical picture (acute perforated diverticulitis)

Diverticula of the duodenum can become infected and give rise to an acute diverticulitis. The diverticula that are more prone to become complicated with an acute clinical picture are those of the second portion of the duodenum, located near the papilla. As has been stated before, preoperative diagnosis of acute diverticulitis is usually difficult. In order to make this diagnosis during the operation, it is necessary to perform the Vautrin-Kocher maneuver, since the perforated diverticulum is usually blocked off retroperitoneally. The site of the perforated diverticulitis has to be explored very carefully to determine the degree of infiltration and edema of the walls of the duodenum, the presence of pus, and so on. Once this exploration has been carried out, a small transverse choledochotomy is performed through which a rubber explorer is passed to establish the relation between the papilla and the perforated diverticulum.

If the perforation is very recent, which is not very probable, since in the majority of cases the diagnosis is made late, some surgeons will opt to close the orifice of the diverticulum directly, using two layers of sutures, by means of the same technique used in the treatment of diverticula of the duodenum with chronic clinical picture (11). However, closure of a diverticulum that is very infiltrated by inflammatory tissue, edema, or suppuration, is very difficult and will most probably be complicated by a lateral duodenal fistula postoperatively, the evolution of which is very serious and the treatment of which is very difficult. The surgeon should prevent this serious complication by using, during the same surgical procedure, a Billroth II gastrectomy to prevent the formation of a lateral duodenal fistula and leave a terminal duodenal fistula, which is easier to treat and has greater possibilities of closing.

A bypass of bile directly to the intestine should be added to the Billroth II gastrectomy. To carry out this procedure, the common bile duct should be transected and anastomosed to a jejunal limb in end-to-side fashion using the jejunal limb disposed in Roux-en-Y fashion. Drainage of the bile into the jejunum keeps it from mixing with pancreatic secretions. Pure pancreatic juice is less aggressive on the tissues than when it is mixed with bile (11, 20, 31, 49, 51, 68). The decision to carry out a Billroth II gastrectomy and to drain the bile directly into the jejunum should be made by the surgeon even though they appear to be excessive measures because they can save the life of the patient. If the patient still has his or her gallbladder and this appears normal, the author prefers to use it to bypass bile into the jejunum instead of anastomosing a normal caliber common bile duct to the jejunum, because this anastomosis, in some cases, is prone to stricture postoperatively. The technique of anastomosis of the gallbladder to the jejunum, after destruction of its valves of Heister, was described in Chapter 24. Some of the stages of this technique will be repeated further on. Before closing the abdominal cavity, a feeding jejunostomy should be performed.

Treatment of Extraluminal Duodenal Diverticula of the Second Portion of the Duodenum with Acute Clinical Picture (Acute Perforated Diverticulitis)

Treatment of Extraluminal Duodenal Diverticula of the Second Portion of the Duodenum with Acute Clinical Picture (Acute Perforated Diverticulitis)

FIGURE 41.20
Peripapillary diverticulum of the second portion of the duodenum with acute diverticulitis and retroperitoneal perforation. The diverticular orifice is sutured, if possible. If this is not possible, it is left open and the Billroth II gastrectomy is carried out to transform the lateral duodenal fistula into a terminal duodenal fistula. The upper drawing shows the line of transection of the duodenum to carry out the Billroth II gastrectomy. The lower drawing shows the transected closed duodenum and the stomach being freed to perform the Billroth II gastrectomy.

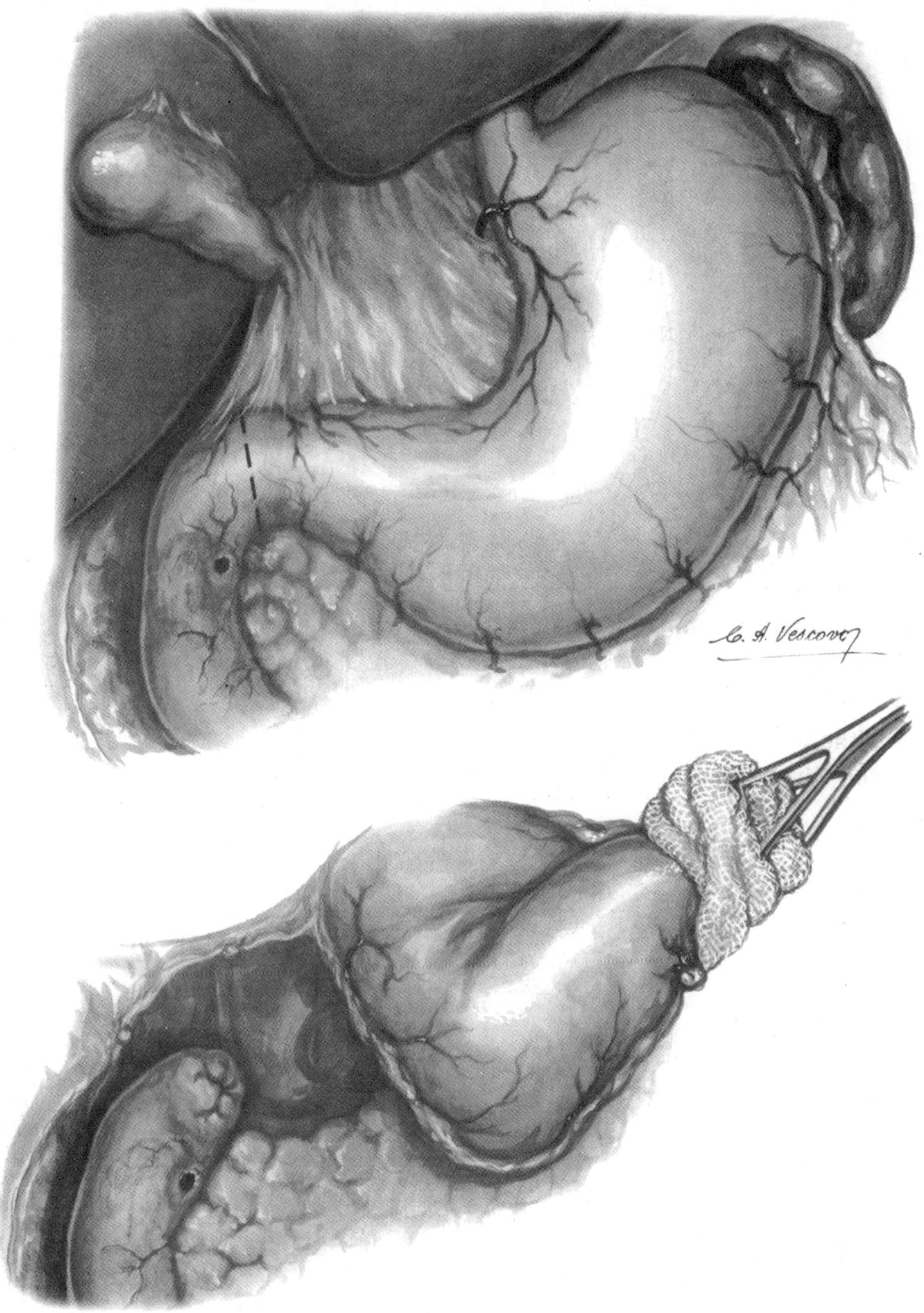

FIGURE 41.20

Treatment of Extraluminal Duodenal Diverticula of the Second Portion of the Duodenum with Acute Clinical Picture (Acute Perforated Diverticulitis)

FIGURE 41.21
The Billroth II gastrectomy has been completed, transforming the lateral duodenal fistula into a terminal duodenal fistula. The subhepatic space is drained by means of a rubber tube. The Billroth II gastrectomy is not sufficient, and it is necessary to drain the bile into the jejunum, as will be shown in Figure 41.22.

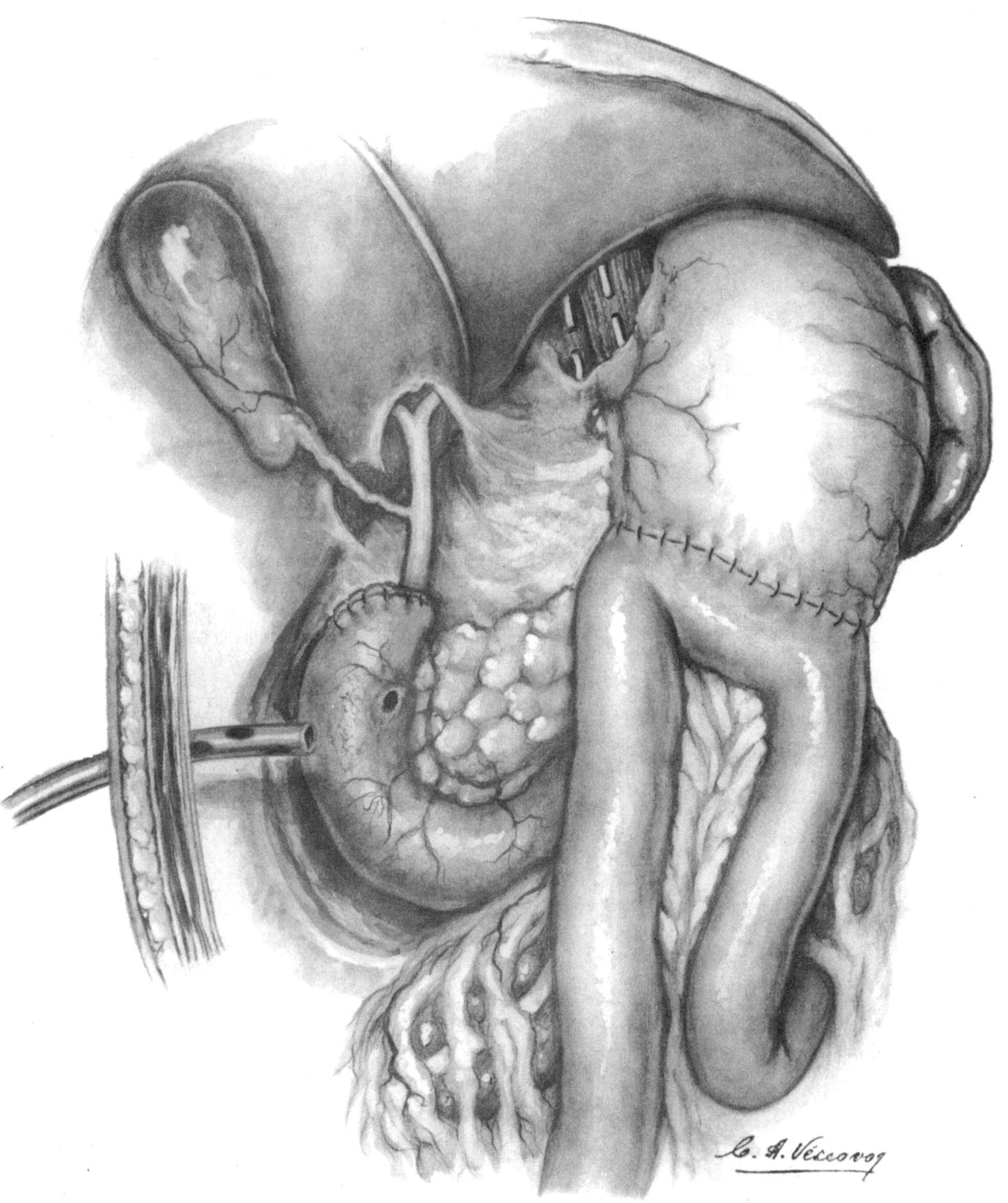

FIGURE 41.21

FIGURE 41.22
The Billroth II gastrectomy should be completed with removal of the gallbladder, as shown in the drawing, later dividing the common bile duct and anastomosing it in end-to-side fashion to a jejunal loop using one layer of nonabsorbable sutures. The details of the choledochojejunal anastomosis can be seen in the insert.

Treatment of Extraluminal Duodenal Diverticula of the Second Portion of the Duodenum with Acute Clinical Picture (Acute Perforated Diverticulitis)

FIGURE 41.23
In patients with a thin common bile duct there exists the possibility that the terminal choledochojejunal anastomosis may become strictured postoperatively. In these cases, the author prefers to destroy the valves of Heister in the cystic duct, transforming the cystic duct into a smooth duct, which will allow bile to pass easily the same way it passes through the hepatic or common bile ducts. The small stump of the common bile duct is closed and the gallbladder sutured to a jejunal loop in end-to-side fashion using two layers of sutures. This anastomosis functions very well. For more details see Chapter 24.

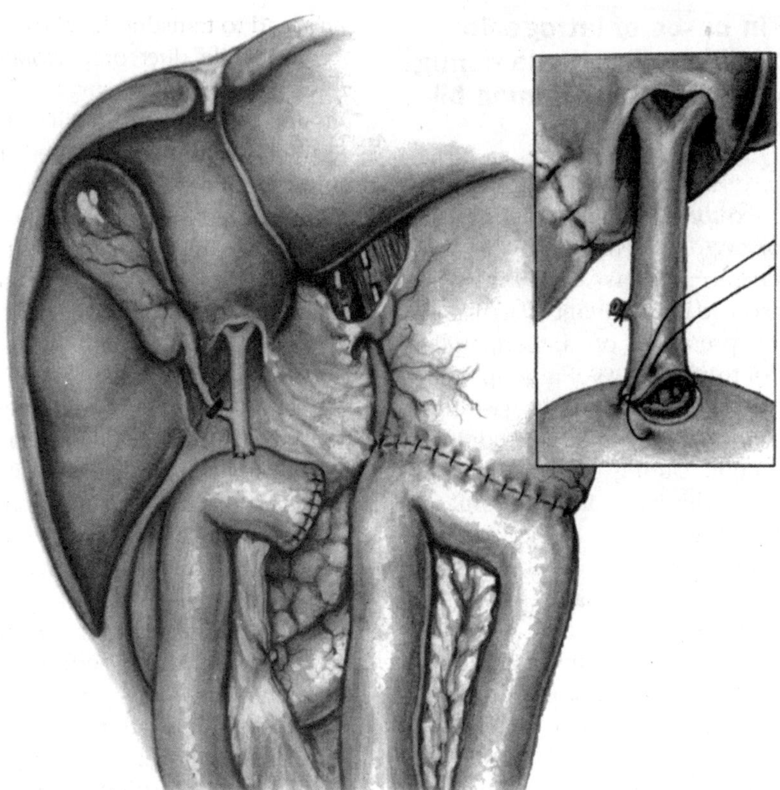

FIGURE 41.22

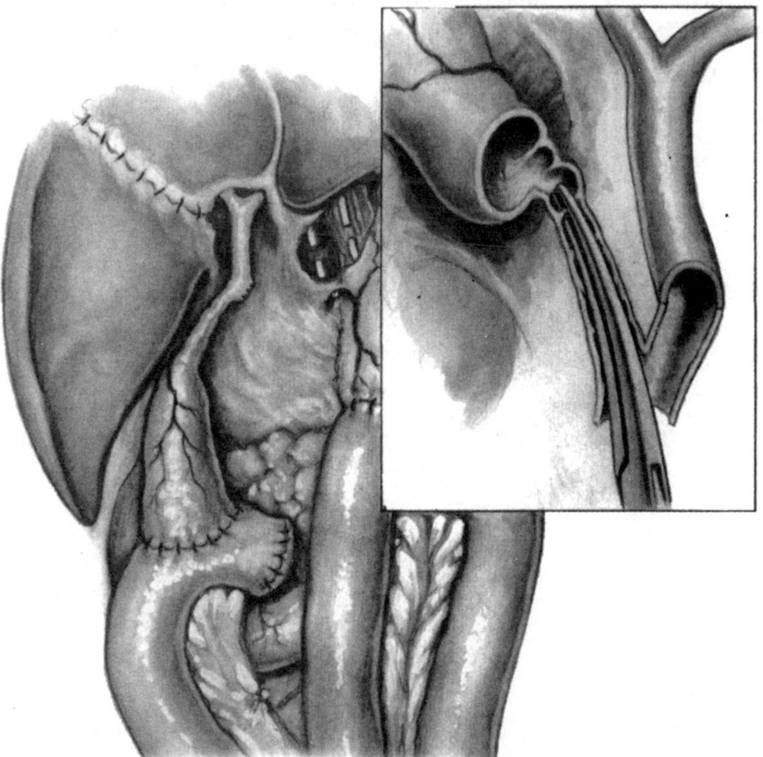

FIGURE 41.23

Surgical technique in cases of iatrogenic perforation of peripapillary diverticula during instrumental exploration of the common bile duct for biliary tract calculi

Instrumental exploration of the common bile duct, particularly when metallic explorers are used, may cause perforation of a peripapillary diverticulum. This is sometimes ignored by the surgeon and has very serious consequences. For this reason it is important that the surgeon know about the presence of a peripapillary diverticulum. Diagnosis of the presence of a peripapillary diverticulum can be made preoperatively by gastroduodenal radiographic examination and by endoscopic examination of the duodenum. During the surgical intervention one should not hesitate in carrying out transcystic operative cholangiography. If the operative cholangiography shows that the bile duct is normal in caliber, that the papilla functions normally, that the radiopaque substance passes easily into the duodenum, and there are no images of calculi or other pathology, it is not necessary to perform a choledochotomy and an instrumental examination of the common bile duct and the papilla.

If it is necessary to perform an instrumental examination of the common bile duct, soft explorers should be used, such as semirigid rubber or silk explorers with an olive shaped end. It is not advisable to use rigid metallic explorers. If the surgeon is accustomed to using metallic explorers, he or she should avoid forcing their passage into the duodenum, which may be of no use at all and may lead to transduodenal (intramural) perforation of the common bile duct or perforation of a peripapillary diverticulum, with the surgeon believing that he or she is passing through the papilla of Vater. A peripapillary diverticulum can be perforated during instrumental exploration. This perforation could have been noticed by the surgeon or the surgeon could have had a sensation of something unusual happening. If the surgeon feels that something rare has happened and stops the introduction of the explorer, he or she could have perforated a periampullary diverticulum without injuring the pancreas. However, if the surgeon believes that the obstacle is the papilla and insists on going through it, the explorer may penetrate the pancreatic parenchyma, giving rise to a serious lesion. If the surgeon simply perforated the diverticulum, the situation can be taken care of by suturing the duodenal mucosa of the diverticular orifice and then suturing the seromuscular layer of the diverticular orifice. The operation is finished leaving a T-tube in the common bile duct and drainage in the subhepatic space. However, if in addition to the perforation of the diverticulum, the surgeon injured the pancreas, the duodenal diverticular orifice should be sutured and the common bile duct then should be transected and anastomosed to a Roux-en-Y jejunal limb. In order to make a diagnosis of injury to the pancreatic parenchyma, the posterior surface of the pancreas, which is usually marked with streaky signs of bleeding, should be observed. If there is still any doubt, operative cholangiography should be carried out, which will show passage of the radiopaque substance through the pancreatic parenchyma.

Surgical Technique for the Resection of Extraluminal Diverticula of the Third Portion of the Duodenum with Chronic Clinical Picture

FIGURE 41.24
Diverticula of the third portion of the duodenum may be approached through a horizontal incision of the posterior parietal peritoneum. This incision may be made to the right or to the left of the superior mesenteric vessels, depending on the location of the diverticulum. The drawing shows the location of the diverticulum in the third portion of the duodenum to the right of the superior mesenteric vessels with the fundus directed toward the pancreas. The broken line shows the course of the incision. A better and more ample approach to the third and fourth portions of the duodenum is attained by means of the Cattell and Braasch maneuver (9).

Surgical Technique for the Resection of Extraluminal Diverticula of the Third Portion of the Duodenum with Chronic Clinical Picture

FIGURE 41.25 CATTELL AND BRAASCH MANEUVER
The broken line includes the cecum, the ascending colon, the terminal ileum and part of the mesentery. This entire area has to be mobilized to obtain access to the third and fourth portions of the duodenum.

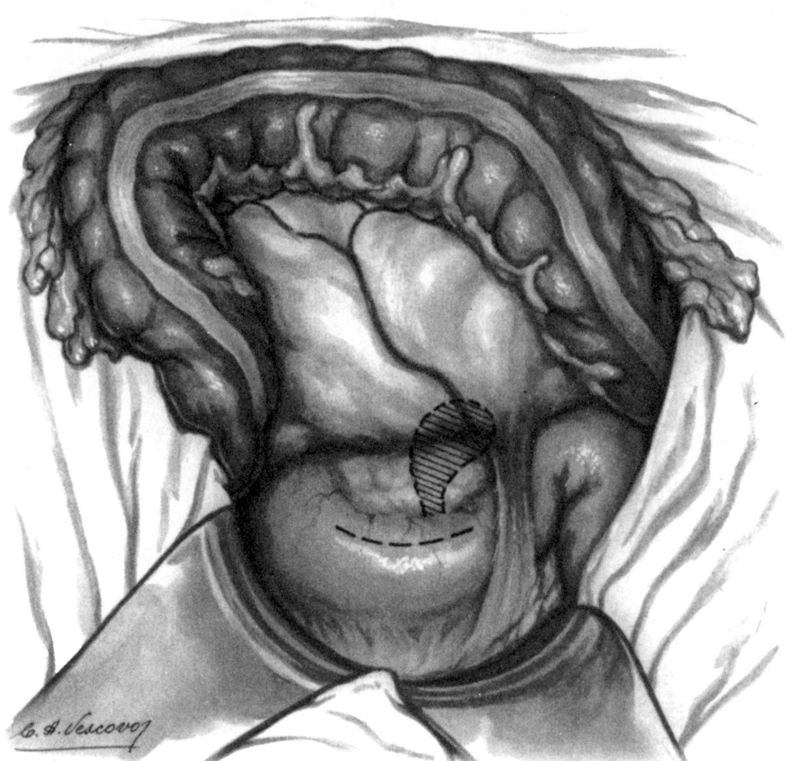

FIGURE 41.24

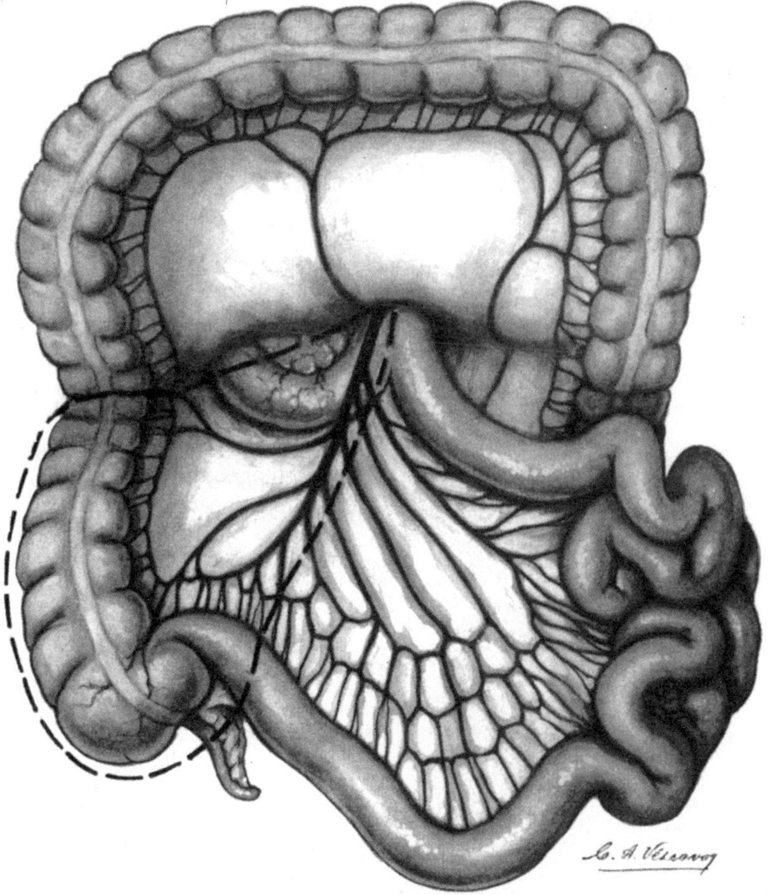

FIGURE 41.25 CATTELL AND BRAASCH MANEUVER

Surgical Technique for the Resection of Extraluminal Diverticula of the Third Portion of the Duodenum with Chronic Clinical Picture

FIGURE 41.26 CATTELL-BRAASCH MANEUVER
The peritoneum bordering the cecum has been incised, and the peritoneum bordering the ascending colon is being divided.

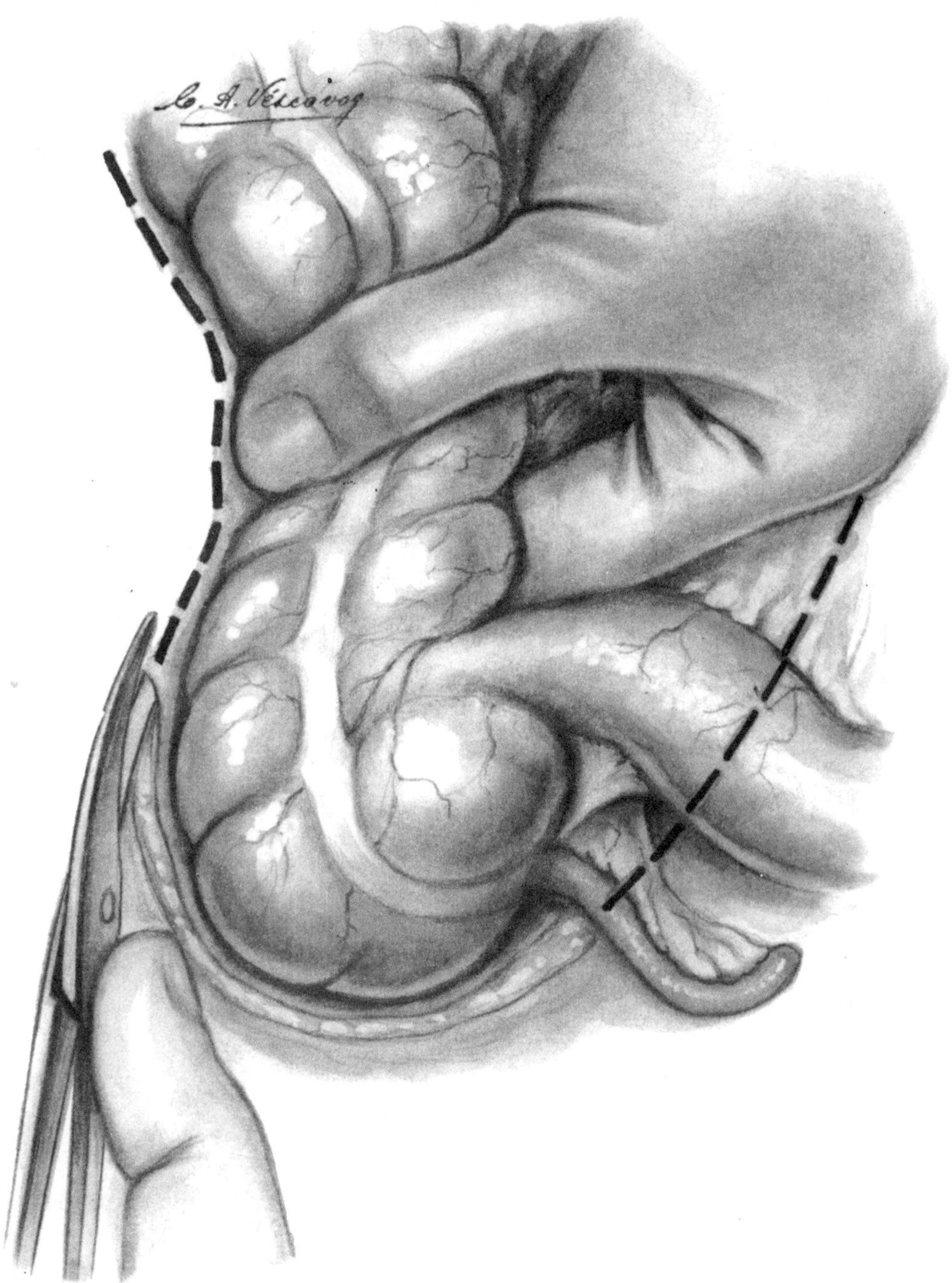

FIGURE 41.26 CATTELL-BRAASCH MANEUVER

Surgical Technique for the Resection of Extraluminal Diverticula of the Third Portion of the Duodenum with Chronic Clinical Picture

FIGURE 41.27 CATTELL-BRAASCH MANEUVER

The cecum has been mobilized, 3, the right colon and the terminal ileum, 4, and the mesentery have also been mobilized through the avascular area exposing the third and fourth portions of the duodenum, 1, as well as the duodenojejunal flexure, 2.

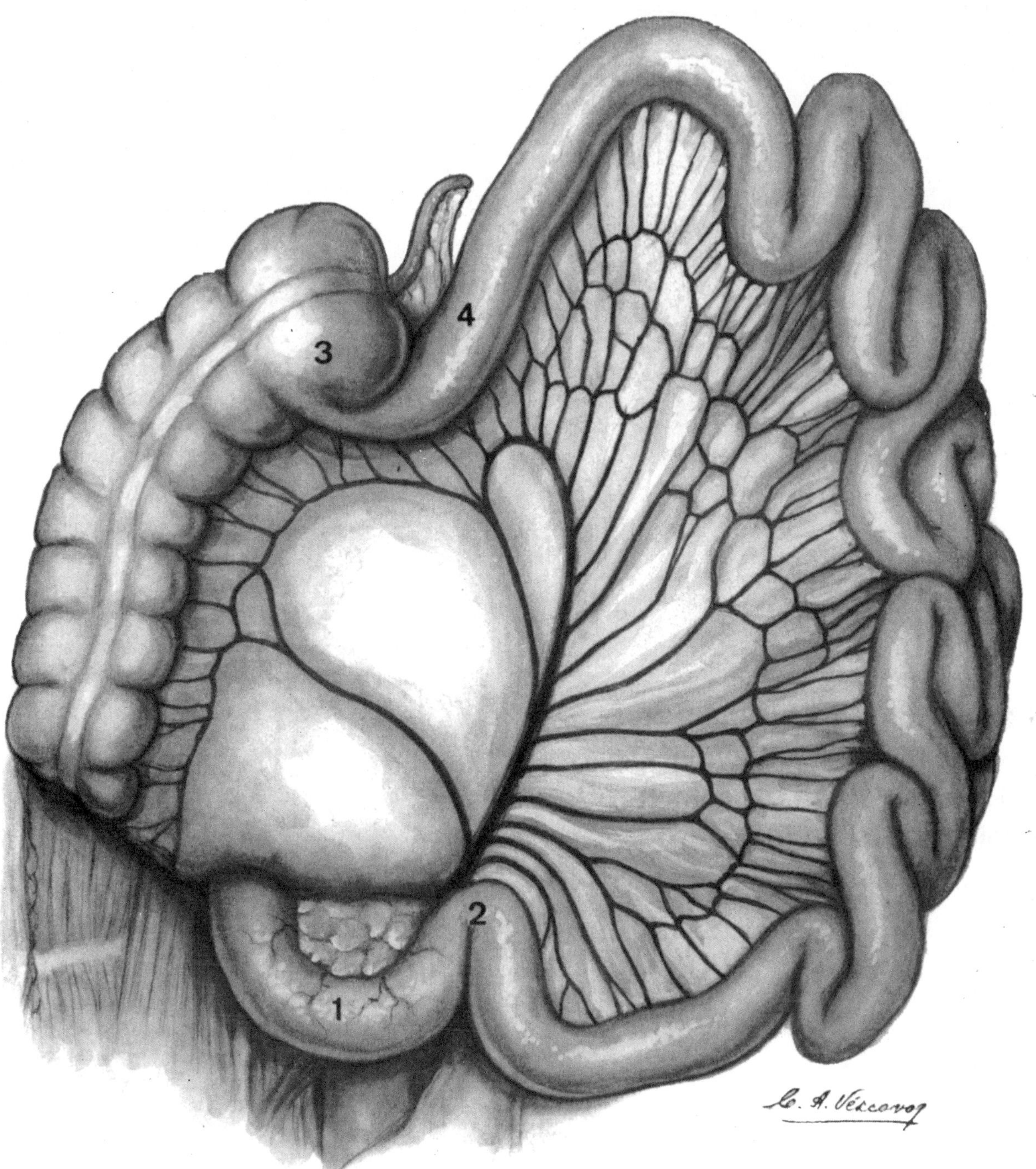

FIGURE 41.27 CATTELL-BRAASCH MANEUVER

Surgical Technique for the Resection of Extraluminal Diverticula of the Third Portion of the Duodenum with Chronic Clinical Picture

FIGURE 41.28
Using a Foerster clamp, traction is applied downward and the third portion of the duodenum and the superior border of this portion of the duodenum is being freed. The neck of the diverticulum can be seen.

FIGURE 41.29
Dissection of the neck of the diverticulum has been completed. Traction is applied to the body of the diverticulum downward using a Babcock clamp, while, by means of a curved scissors, the diverticulum is gently dissected, avoiding injuring it. If the diverticulum is not very inflamed, it is possible to free it from the pancreas with relative ease. In cases in which the diverticulum is very inflamed, be it chronically or acutely, its dissection becomes very difficult.

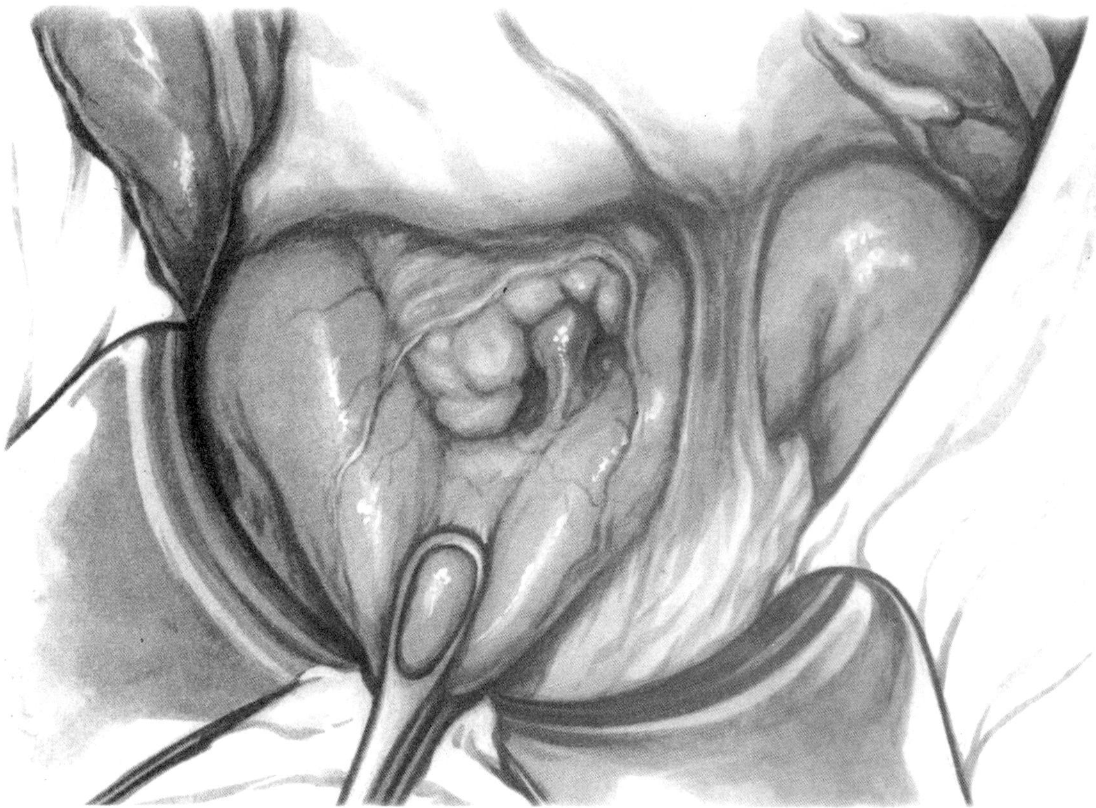

FIGURE 41.28

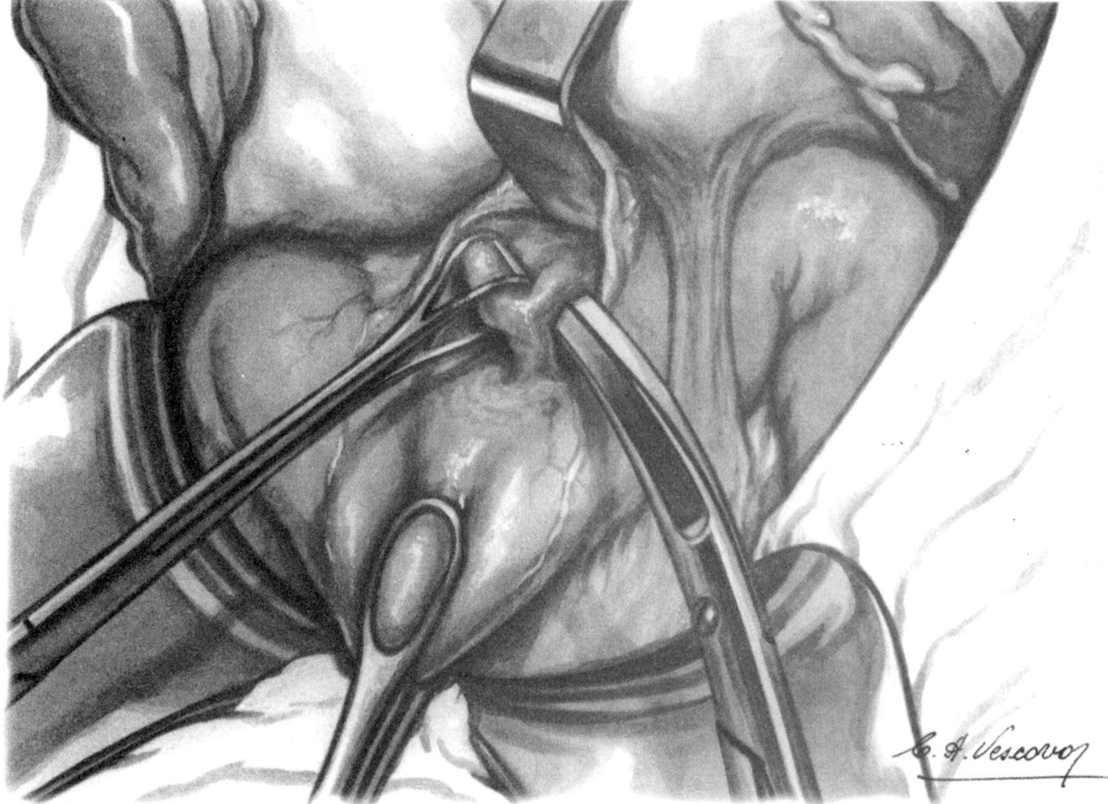

FIGURE 41.29

FIGURE 41.30
The diverticulum has been completely exteriorized and is held by a Babcock clamp. Sutures have been placed in the vicinity of the neck of the diverticulum to apply traction.

Surgical Technique for the Resection of Extraluminal Diverticula of the Third Portion of the Duodenum with Chronic Clinical Picture

FIGURE 41.31
The neck of the diverticulum is being transected with scissors.

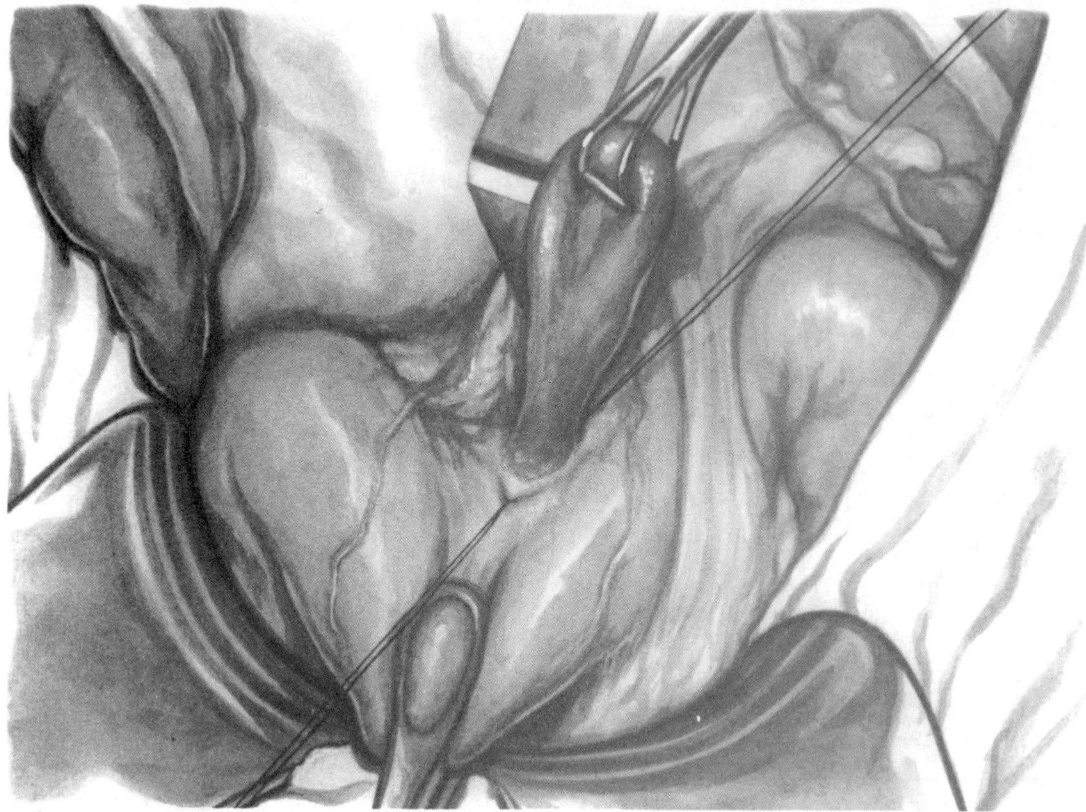

FIGURE 41.30

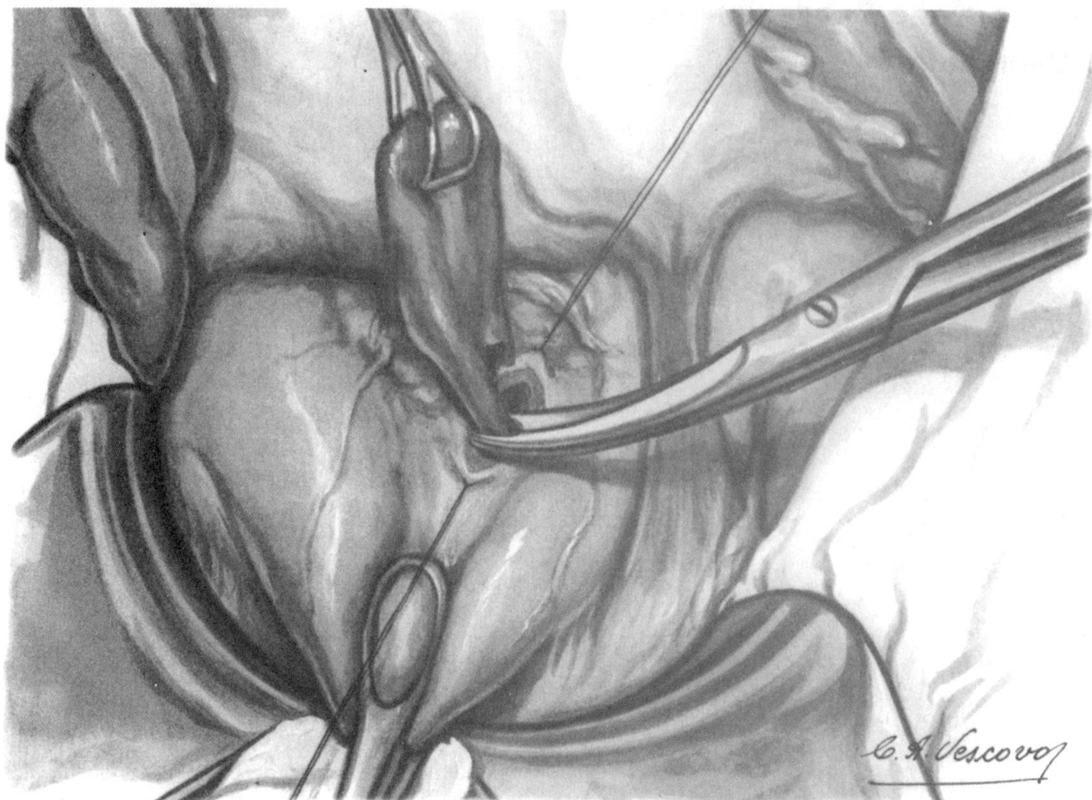

FIGURE 41.31

FIGURE 41.32
The mucosa of the orifice of the diverticulum has been sutured with reabsorbable interrupted sutures, and the seromuscular layer is being sutured with interrupted sutures of nonabsorbable suture material.

Surgical Technique for the Resection of Extraluminal Diverticula of the Third Portion of the Duodenum with Chronic Clinical Picture

FIGURE 41.33
Once the orifice of the diverticulum of the third portion of the duodenum has been closed, the bed of the third portion of the duodenum is reperitonealized using nonabsorbable sutures applied to the peritoneum covering the pancreas and joining it with the peritoneum covering the duodenum.

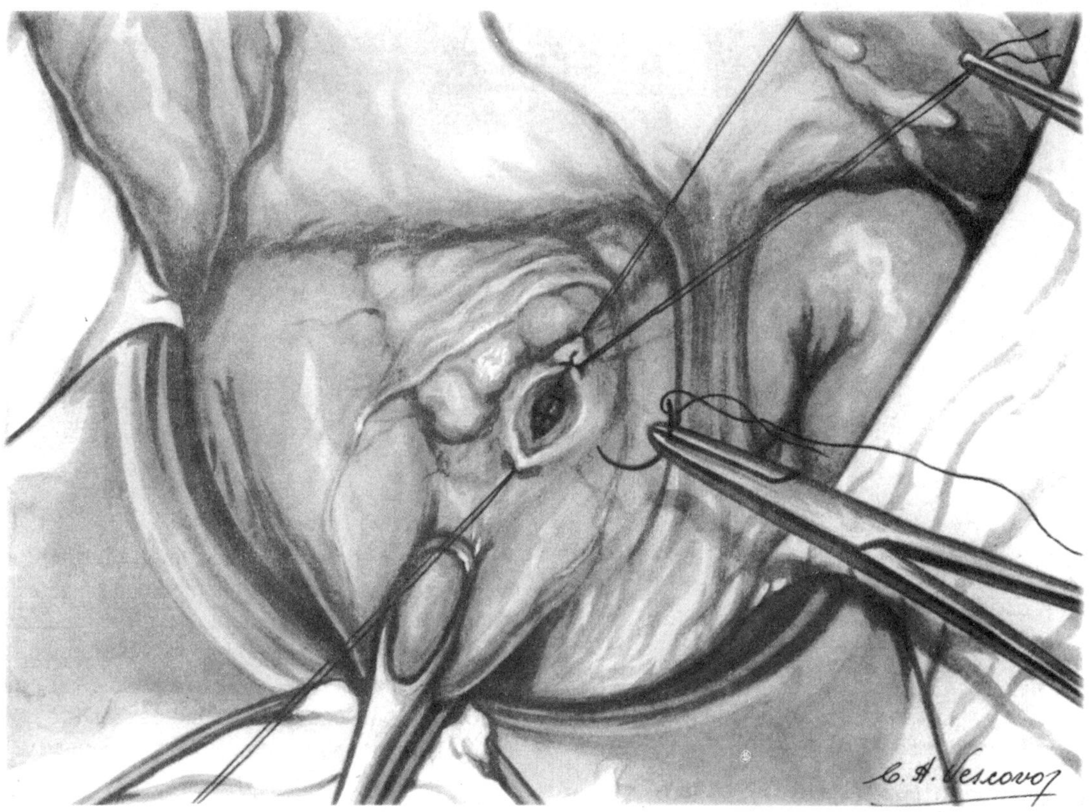

FIGURE 41.32

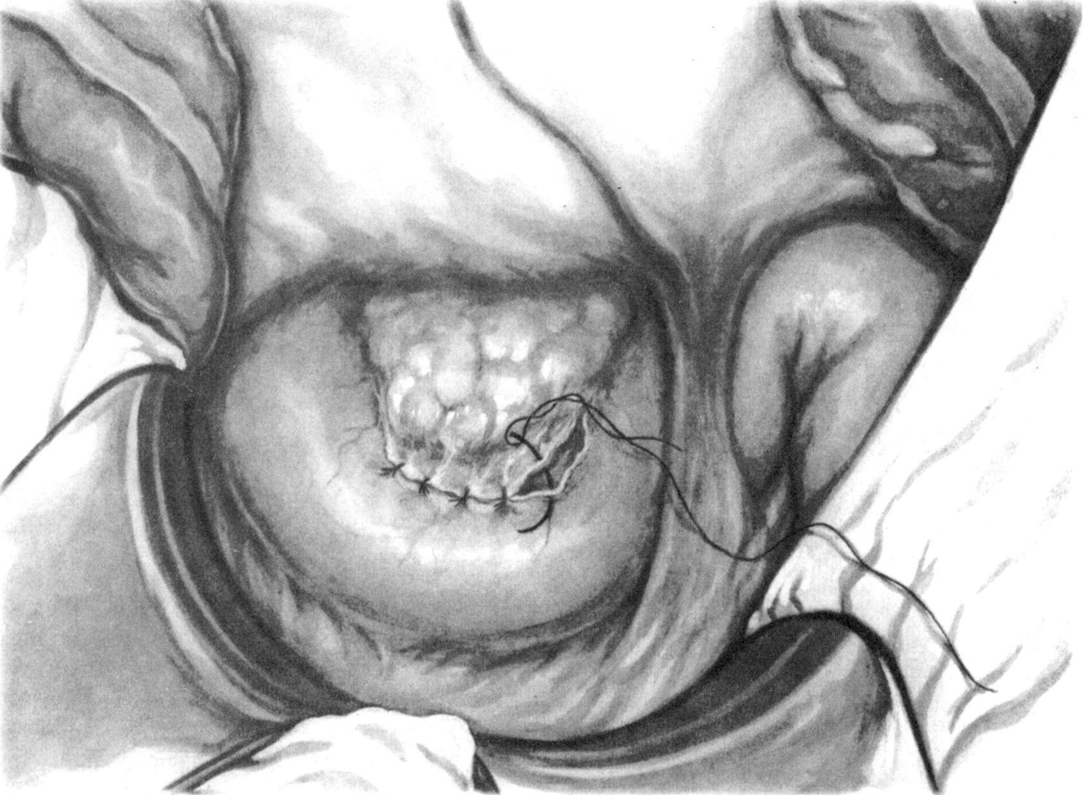

FIGURE 41.33

FIGURE 41.34
The drawing shows a diverticulum in the third portion of the duodenum that is acutely inflamed and perforated. Resection of the diverticulum and suture of the diverticular orifice is generally impossible to perform. If it is performed, the usual result is that dehiscence of the suture line will occur, with very grave consequences because the tissues are highly inflamed. In this situation the surgeon can resort to the procedure shown in Figure 41.35 (31).

Surgical Technique of the Treatment of Extraluminal Diverticula of the Third Portion of the Duodenum with Acute Clinical Picture (Acute Perforated Diverticulitis)

FIGURE 41.35
The duodenum has been transected at the junction of its second and third portion. The distal end of the transected duodenum is closed using two layers of interrupted sutures, while the proximal layer is sutured in end-to-end fashion to a jejunal loop (31). The proximal limb of the jejunum is anastomosed in end-to-side fashion to the jejunal loop that is anastomosed to the duodenum in Roux-en-Y fashion. This procedure may save the life of the patient. Diverticula of the fourth portion of the duodenum are treated in similar fashion.

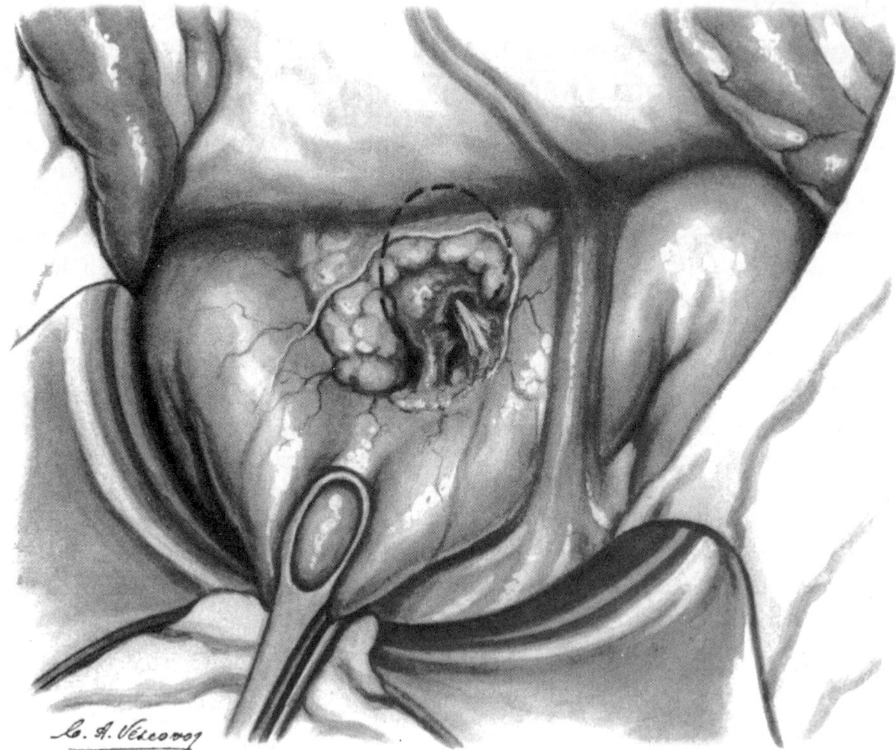

FIGURE 41.34

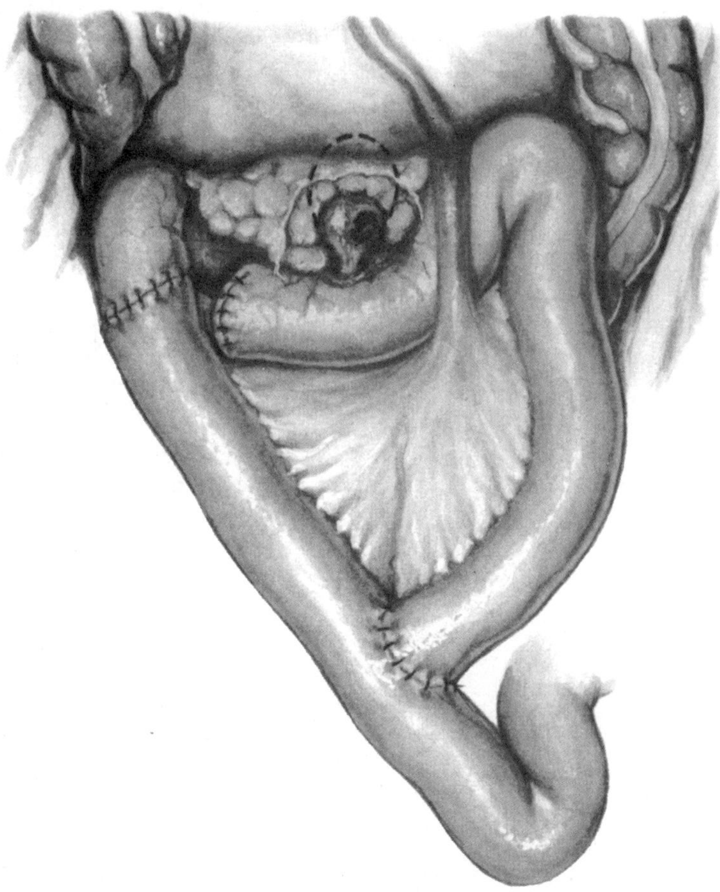

FIGURE 41.35

Group B: Duodenal Diverticula That Have the Common Duct and Pancreatic Duct Emptying into Them

Emptying of the common and pancreatic ducts into a duodenal diverticulum is not very rare, as shown by numerous publications that have appeared in recent years (3, 4, 13, 16, 24, 49, 64, 66). Progress in radiographic technique and more frequent use of operative cholangiography and postoperative cholangiography as well as transparietal hepatic cholangiography and retrograde endoscopic cholangiopancreatography have confirmed this increase. Willox and Costopoulos (64) published 18 cases in a period of 8 years of which 8 had been previously operated upon, undergoing biliary surgery.

Diverticula of the duodenum, into which empty the common bile duct and pancreatic ducts, can lead to stasis and biliary infection and, as a consequence, production of biliary or pancreatic problems. This pathologic change can go undetected if biliary or pancreatic complications that would lead to cholangiographic examination do not occur. This examination should be carried out in a precise fashion if it is dealing with a duodenal diverticulum that receives the opening of the pancreatic or common bile ducts, or if it is simply a superimposed image of the lower common bile duct over the image of the peripapillary duodenal diverticulum. In order to differentiate and clear up this problem, it is necessary to rotate the patient adequately so that the images may be separated clearly. In confronting a duodenal diverticulum into which the common bile duct and pancreatic ducts empty, several situations may be encountered.

1. During a surgical intervention for biliary calculi, operative cholangiography shows a duodenal diverticulum receiving the common bile duct and pancreatic ducts without calculi either in the common bile duct or in the diverticulum and with good passage of radiopaque substance into the duodenum. In this case it is not necessary to carry out any other surgical procedure but finishing the operation.
2. Patient with biliary lithiasis in which operative cholangiography shows the presence of calculi in the common bile duct. In this case, a choledochotomy should be performed, removing the calculi and finishing with a control cholangiography. If the latter shows that all the calculi have been removed and that the radiopaque substance passes readily into the duodenum, it is not necessary to add any other surgical procedure except leaving a T-tube in place in the common bile duct.
3. Patient with biliary lithiasis and calculi in the common bile duct with calculi also within the diverticulum. If the diverticular calculi can be removed through the choledochotomy, it is not necessary to carry out any other surgical procedure.
4. Patient with biliary calculi including calculi in the duodenal diverticulum that cannot be removed through a choledochotomy. In this situation it is necessary to perform a duodenotomy, section of the diverticulum, and removal of the calculi with suturing to the diverticulum at the duodenal wall. The operation is completed by leaving a T-tube in the common bile duct.

Some authors recommend resection of the duodenal diverticulum with implantation of the papilla of Vater into the duodenal wall. The author believes that this procedure, in addition to being unnecessary, is difficult to carry out and has great risk of serious complications with elevated morbidity and mortality.

It is necessary to establish a clear differentiation between diverticula of the duodenum that receive the opening of the common bile duct and pancreatic ducts, and diverticular dilations of the distal end of the common bile duct. Diverticular dilations of the distal common bile duct are caused by impaction of calculi in the prepapillary area of the common bile duct. The impacted calculi within the diverticular dilation of the common bile duct generally lead to protrusion within the internal duodenal wall. These calculi are very difficult to remove through a sphincterotomy of the sphincter of Oddi, and generally incision of the wall of the dilated common duct where it protrudes into the duodenal lumen with removal of the calculi and resuturing of the wall of the dilated common bile duct to the internal wall of the duodenal is necessary.

Group B: Duodenal Diverticula That Have the Common Duct and Pancreatic Duct Emptying into Them

FIGURE 41.36
The drawing shows the usual arrangement presented by patients in whom a duodenal diverticulum receives the opening of the common bile duct and pancreatic ducts through the papilla of Vater.

Group B: Duodenal Diverticula That Have the Common Duct and Pancreatic Duct Emptying into Them

FIGURE 41.37
Operative cholangiography in a patient submitted to surgery for biliary calculi. The operative cholangiography shows a dilated common bile duct with two elongated calculi inside it. The common bile duct empties into a diverticulum of the second portion of the duodenum.

FIGURE 41.38
The visible calculi seen in the previous figure 41.37 have been removed through a supraduodenal choledochotomy. Control cholangiography shows a dilated common bile duct, without calculi, emptying into the duodenal diverticulum. The radiopaque substance passes into the duodenum freely, for which reason it was not necessary to carry out any other surgical procedure.

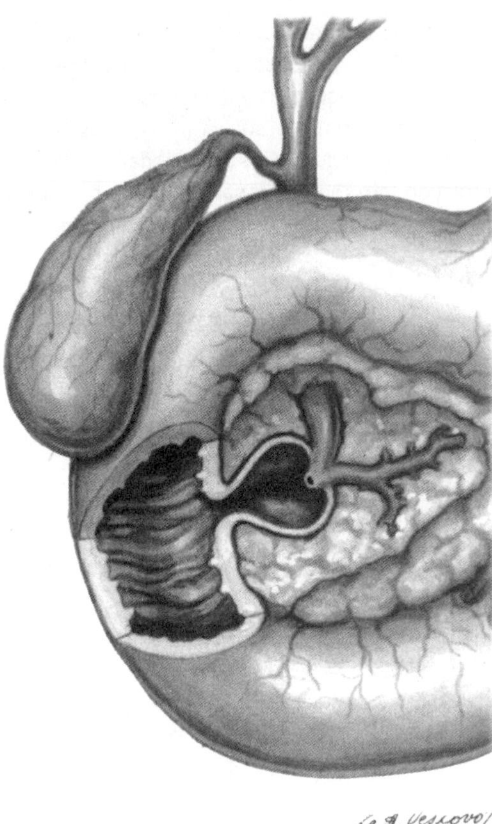

FIGURE 41.36

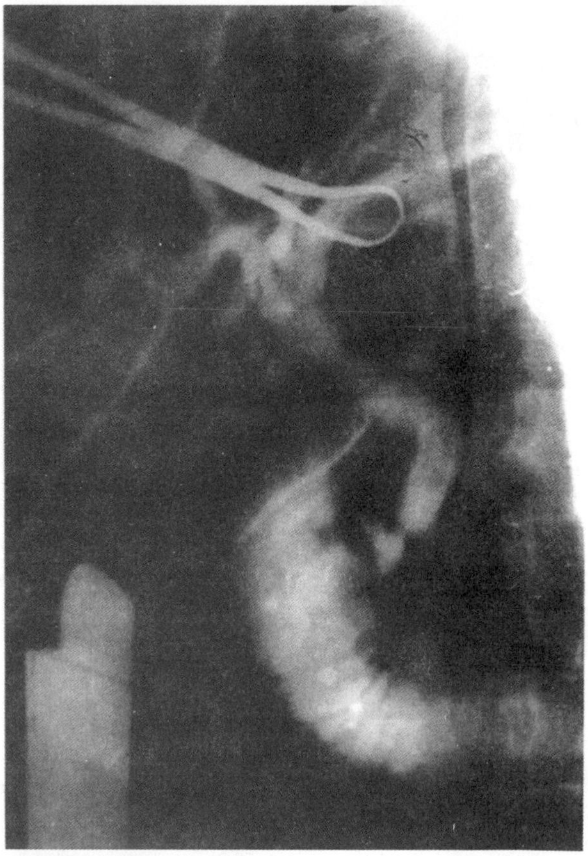

FIGURE 41.37

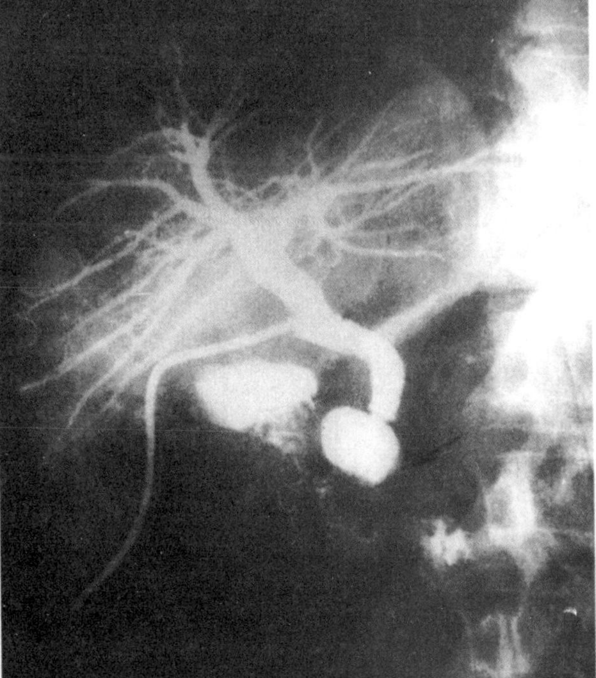

FIGURE 41.38

FIGURE 41.39
If calculi from the common bile duct have passed into the diverticulum and it is not possible to remove them through a supraduodenal choledochotomy, a duodenotomy has to be performed to remove them, as shown in the drawing. Communication of the diverticulum with the duodenum is too narrow. Calculi protrude into the duodenal lumen. To remove them the duodenal wall and the diverticular wall are incised, as shown in the insert.

FIGURE 41.40
Once the duodenal and the diverticular walls have been incised, three calculi can be seen, which will be removed using a Desjardins stone clamp.

Group B: Duodenal Diverticula That Have the Common Duct and Pancreatic Duct Emptying into Them

FIGURE 41.41
The calculi are being removed from the diverticulum with the Desjardins clamp.

FIGURE 41.42
The three calculi that were lodged in the diverticulum have been removed, and the wall of the diverticulum is being sutured to the duodenal wall using nonabsorbable interrupted surgical material. In the bottom of the diverticulum the opening of the papilla can be seen, which functioned normally in the control operative cholangiography. Resection of the diverticulum with anastomosis of the papilla to the duodenum, as proposed by several authors, would have constituted an unnecessary and dangerous surgical excess.

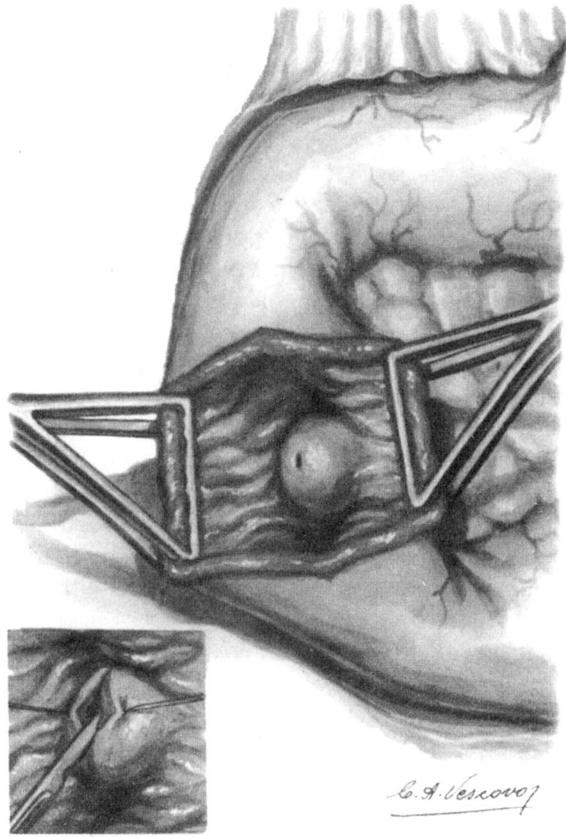

FIGURE 41.39

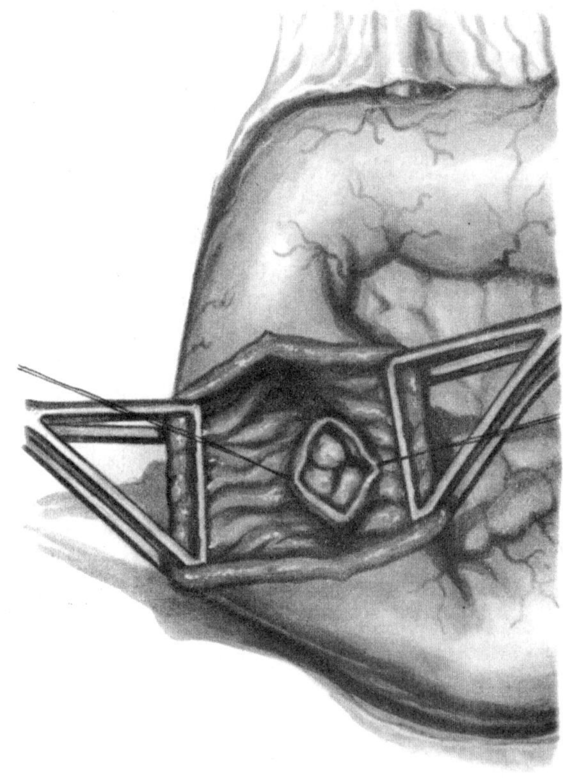

FIGURE 41.40

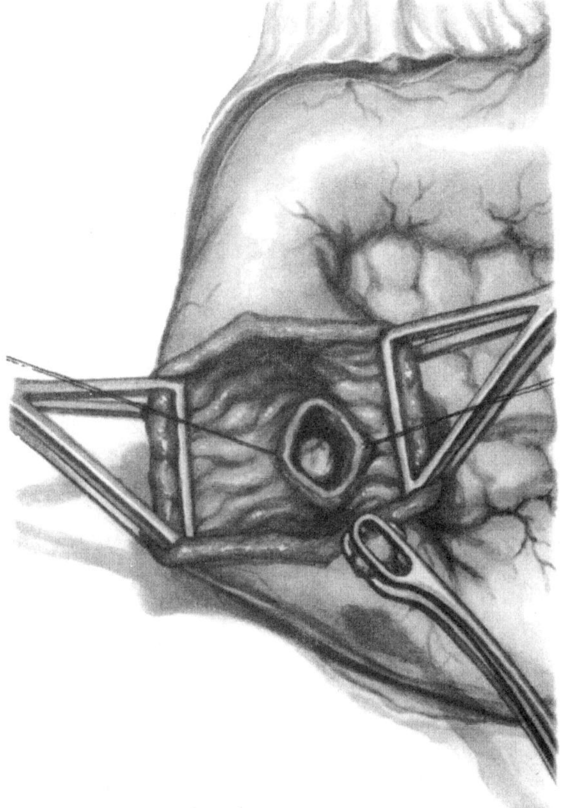

FIGURE 41.41

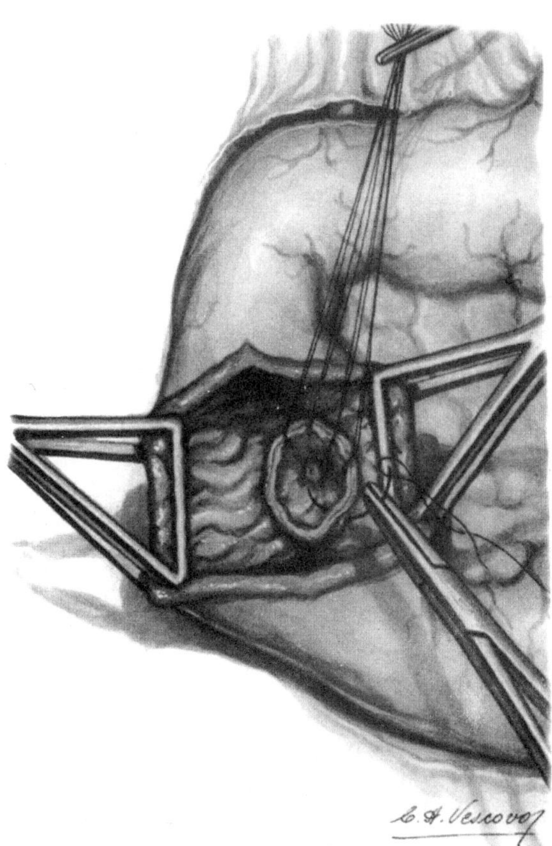

FIGURE 41.42

Group C: Intraluminal Duodenal Diverticula

Intraluminal duodenal diverticula are seen infrequently. Although they are congenital in origin, they are generally not diagnosed until the adult age. Intraluminal diverticula arise near the papilla of Vater and develop distally around the duodenum in irregular shape. Some occupy only the distal portion of the second part of the duodenum, while others occupy the third and fourth portions of the duodenum and some even go beyond the duodenojejunal junction. The exact origin of these diverticula is not known, but it is believed that they are a consequence of persistence of an incomplete congenital diaphragm, which, due to propulsive action of the bolus of food and duodenal peristalsis, develops further. Intraluminal diverticula are covered, on both their internal and external sides, by duodenal mucosa. These diverticula are differentiated from choledochoceles because the latter have their internal surface covered by biliary epithelium and only their external surface is covered by duodenal mucosa.

Patients with intraluminal duodenal diverticula frequently present anomalies of the biliary ducts and the pancreatic ducts. Intraluminal duodenal diverticula may be completely asymptomatic or may lead to partial obstructive symptoms that are intermittent and, in some cases, lead to complete duodenal obstruction produced by the entrance into the inside of the diverticulum of ingested foods. Some patients, in addition to suffering from obstruction of the duodenum, may present pancreatic complications such as acute pancreatitis due to the obstruction of the pancreatic duct by food retained in the diverticulum. When a diagnosis of intraluminal duodenal diverticulum is made, the location of the papilla of Vater, which may present several variations, should be identified. One possibility is that the common bile duct may empty separately from the pancreatic duct into the diverticulum itself. This shows the importance of identifying the papilla and any other anomalies of the intraluminal diverticula when surgery for them is contemplated (1, 21, 25, 29, 33–35, 37, 41, 44).

Diagnosis of intraluminal duodenal diverticula is fundamentally carried out by means of gastroduodenal radiographic examination, which renders a very characteristic image. The diverticulum fills with radiopaque material and is surrounded by a radiolucent halo, which separates it from the duodenal wall. This radiolucent halo is due to the thickness of the wall of the diverticulum. Endoscopic examination is very useful, not only to diagnose the intraluminal diverticulum, but to locate the papilla or any other anomalies. Endoscopic examination, however, has its dangers, because the lumen of the diverticulum may be confused with the lumen of the duodenum. Identification of the papilla and other anomalies, on the other hand, is not always possible. Treatment for these diverticula has been proposed, using endoscopy and electrocautery (34). However, since anomalies are so frequent in these cases, it is very dangerous to treat them by the endoscopic route. Undoubtedly the safest treatment is surgical treatment, the details of which will now be described (1, 21, 34, 37, 41, 67).

Group C: Intraluminal Duodenal Diverticula

FIGURE 41.43
Gastroduodenal radiographic study in which the characteristic image of an intraluminal duodenal diverticulum is seen. The diverticulum occupies the second and third portions of the duodenum, with the fundus extending to the duodenojejunal junction. The diverticulum is surrounded by a clear, smooth, parallel halo. This corresponds to the wall of the diverticulum. Between the clear halo produced by the wall of the diverticulum and the wall of the duodenum there exists a place where a small amount of radiopaque substance passes. The foods that the patient ingested entered the diverticulum in their greatest proportion, and very little reached the jejunum, explaining the clinical picture of duodenal obstruction that the patient presented.

Group C: Intraluminal Duodenal Diverticula

FIGURE 41.44
Schematic drawing of the radiographic study in Figure 41.43. This shows the diverticulum full of radiopaque substance and very little radiopaque substance passing into the jejunum. The fundus of the diverticulum, which has been distended with air, extends to the duodenal jejunal junction. The halo surrounding the diverticulum and produced by the thickness of its wall is very visible.

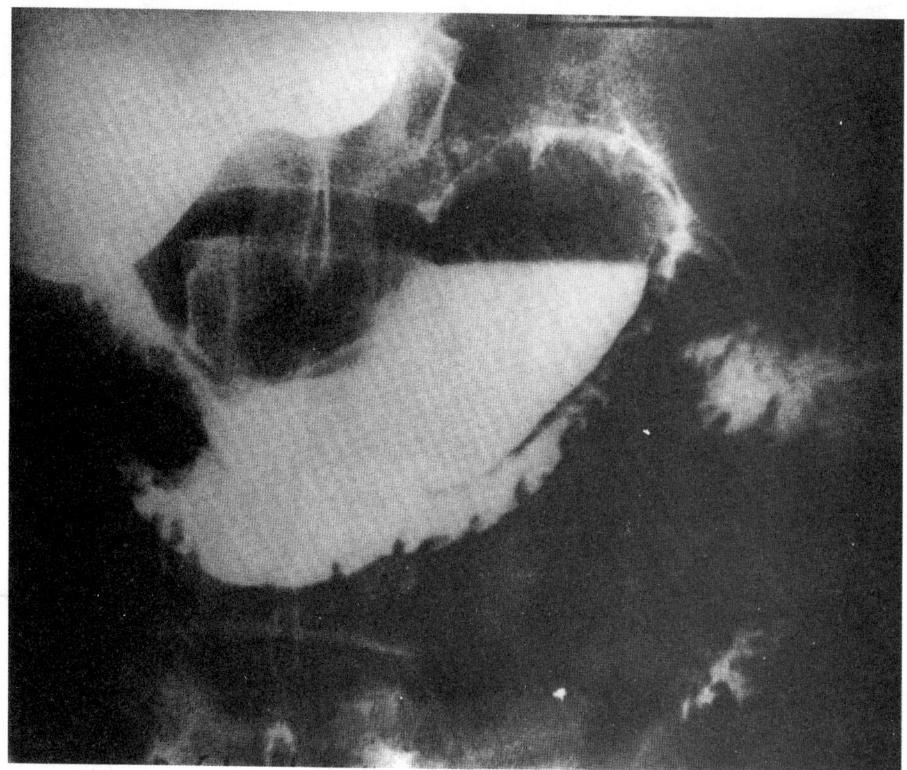

FIGURE 41.43

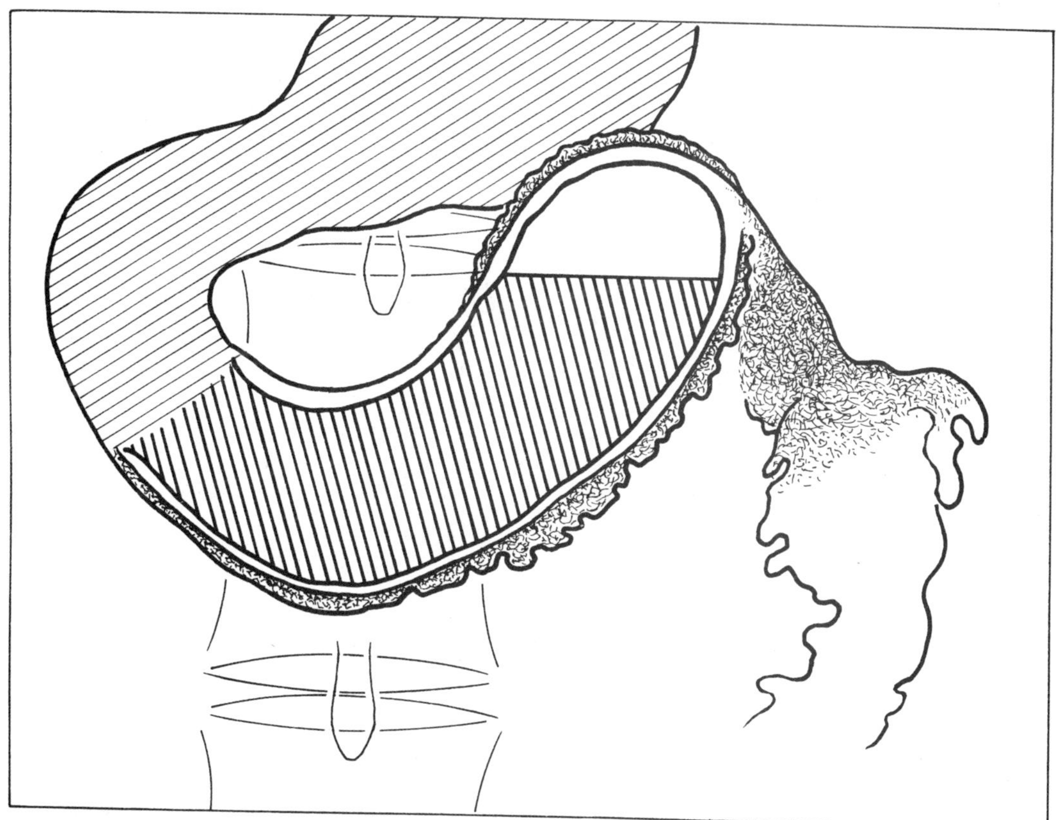

FIGURE 41.44

FIGURE 41.45
Radiographic study of the same patient as in Figure 41.43. The duodenal diverticulum has been filled, not by ingested radiopaque substance, but by injecting it using the lumen of the nasogastric tube that was introduced into the diverticulum. This radiographic examination permits clear observation of the extension of the diverticulum, its diameter, and its end.

Group C: Intraluminal Duodenal Diverticula

FIGURE 41.46
This drawing clears up the image in Figure 41.45, obtained by direct filling of the diverticulum with radiopaque substance by means of the nasogastric tube.

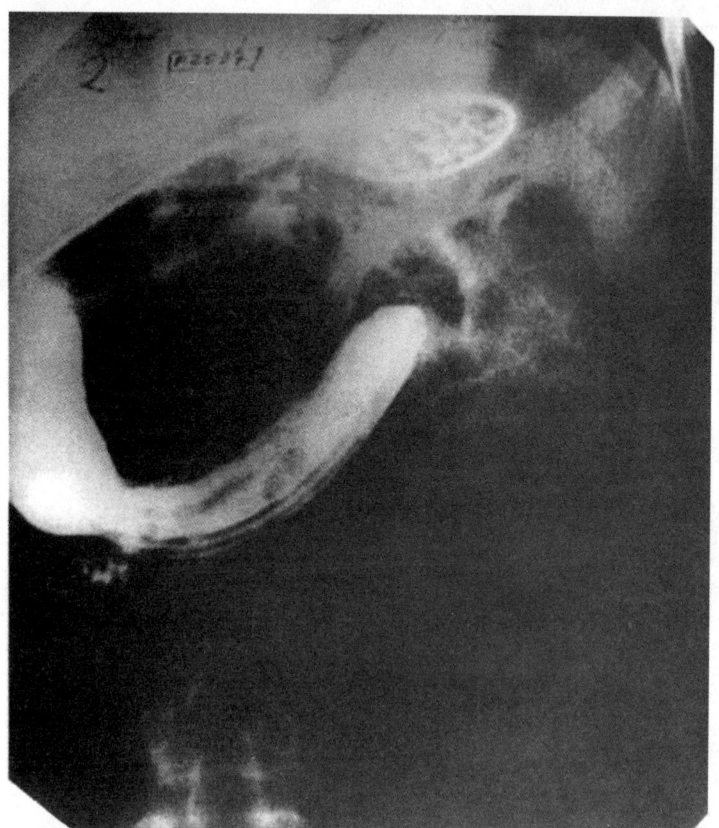

FIGURE 41.45

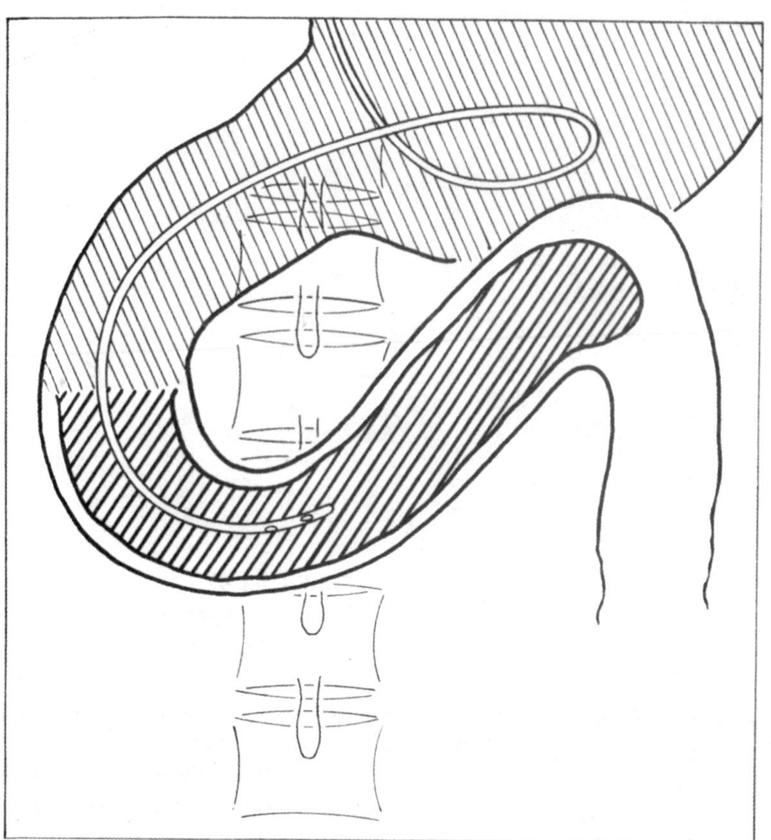

Group C: Intraluminal Duodenal Diverticula

FIGURE 41.47
This drawing shows the probable origin of intraluminal diverticula of the duodenum: **A,** Duodenal diaphragm producing partial partition of the duodenal lumen. This diaphragm is located right near the papilla of Vater. **B** and **C,** Passage of food and duodenal peristalsis will contribute to the formation of a blind sac which will develop progressively until forming an intraluminal diverticulum as shown in **D.** The entrance of the diverticulum can be seen, very near the papilla of Vater.

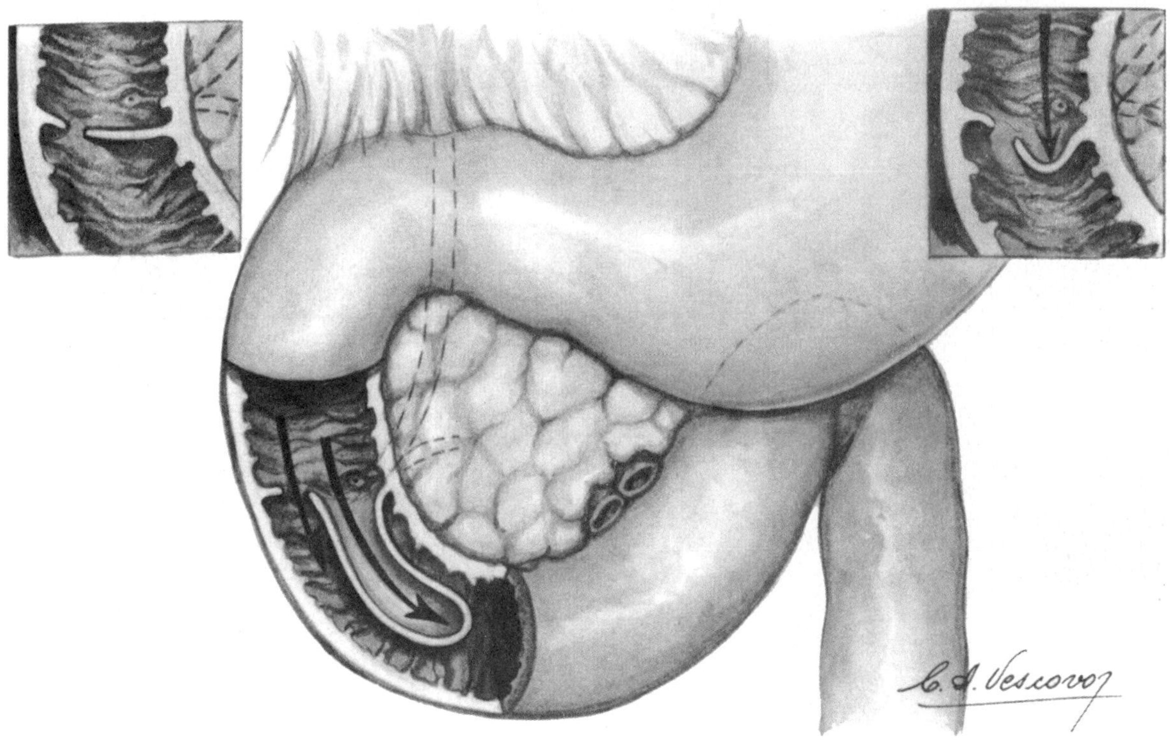

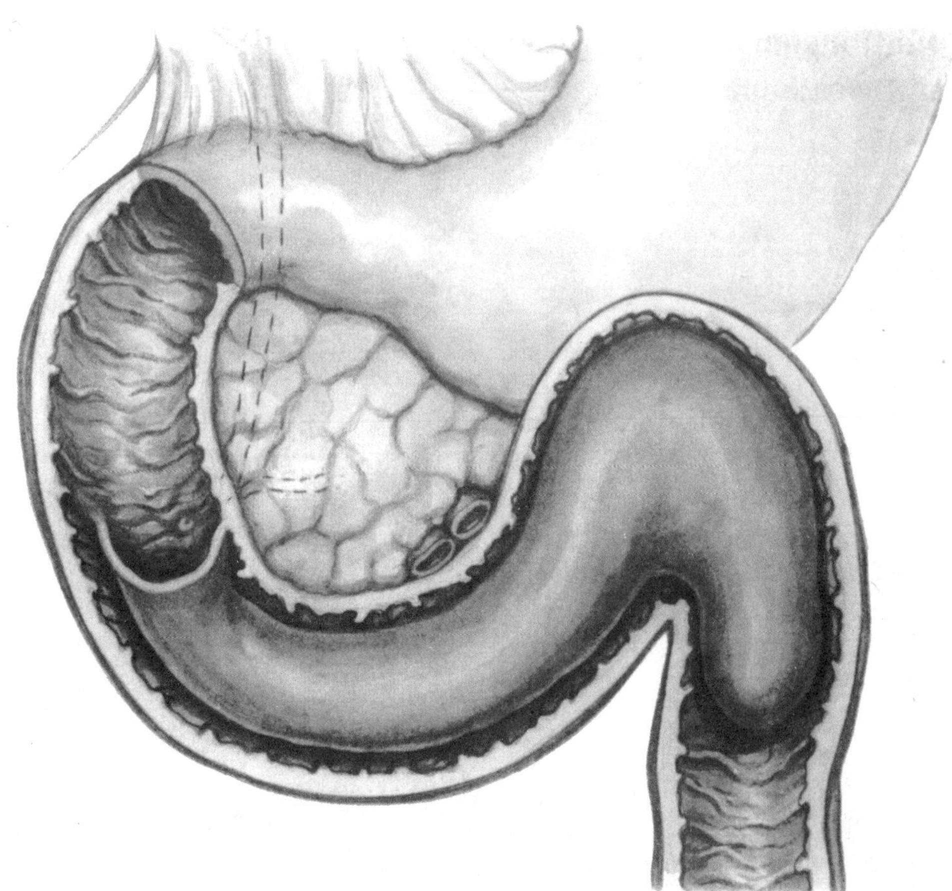

FIGURE 41.47

Group C: Intraluminal Duodenal Diverticula

FIGURE 41.48

The safest and most efficacious treatment of intraluminal duodenal diverticula is by surgical extirpation. Treatment with endoscopic electrocautery is very unsafe and dangerous (1, 34, 37). To carry out resection of these diverticula, a longitudinal duodenotomy has to be made with its center situated in the middle third of the second portion of the duodenum, and measuring about 6 cm. Before carrying out the duodenotomy, as seen in the drawing, an ample Vautrin-Kocher maneuver has to be performed.

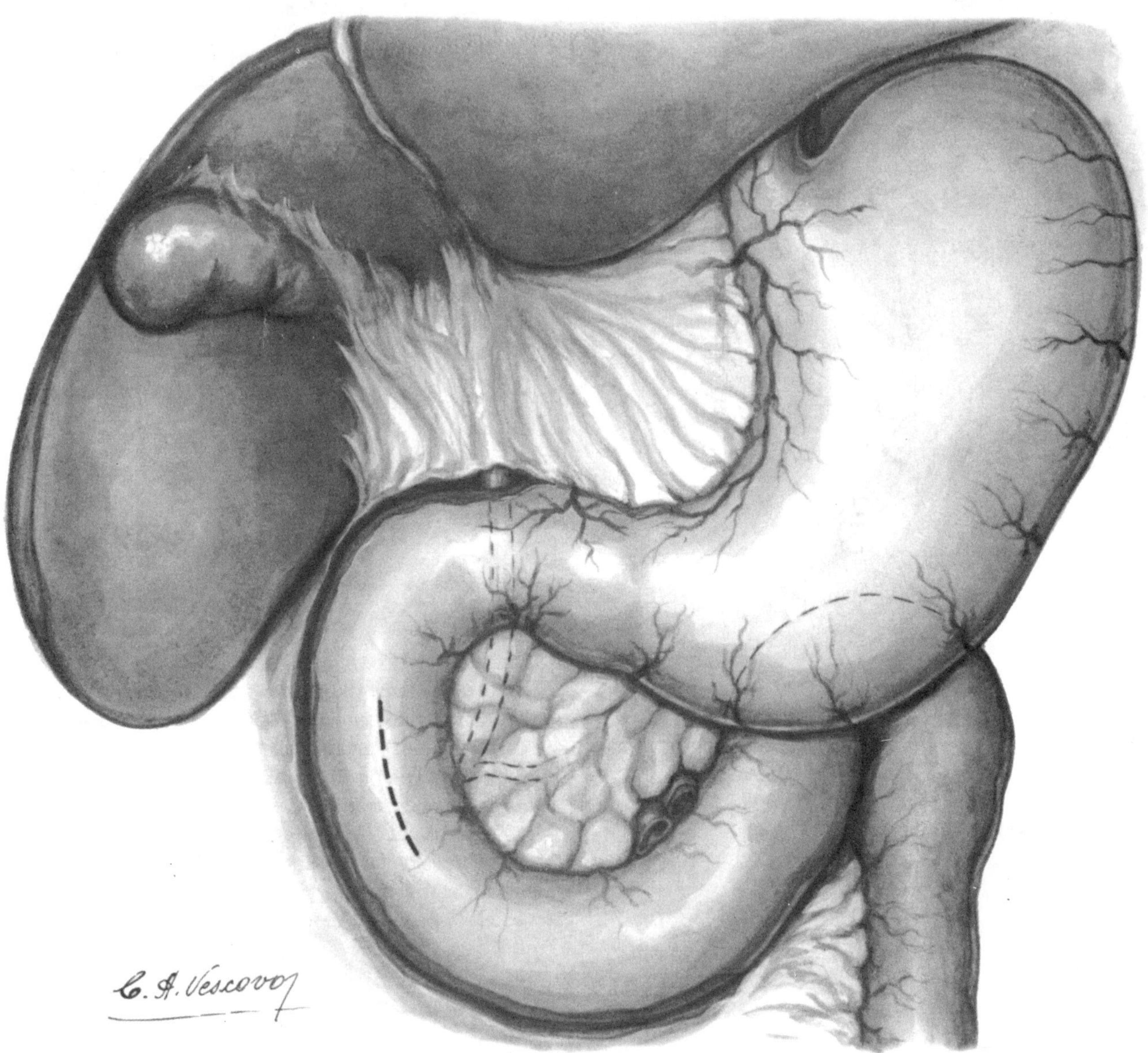

FIGURE 41.48

FIGURE 41.49

Once the duodenotomy has been made, the interior of the duodenum is explored, identifying the entrance to the diverticulum, the papilla of Vater, and the possible presence of anomalies, which are observed in 30 to 40% of cases (1). The diverticulum is palpated to determine is flexibility and mobility, as well as the possibility of exteriorizing it. To bring the diverticulum out of the duodenum, a Babcock clamp is introduced and grasps the wall of the diverticulum, applying gentle traction until the diverticulum is exteriorized.

Group C: Intraluminal Duodenal Diverticula

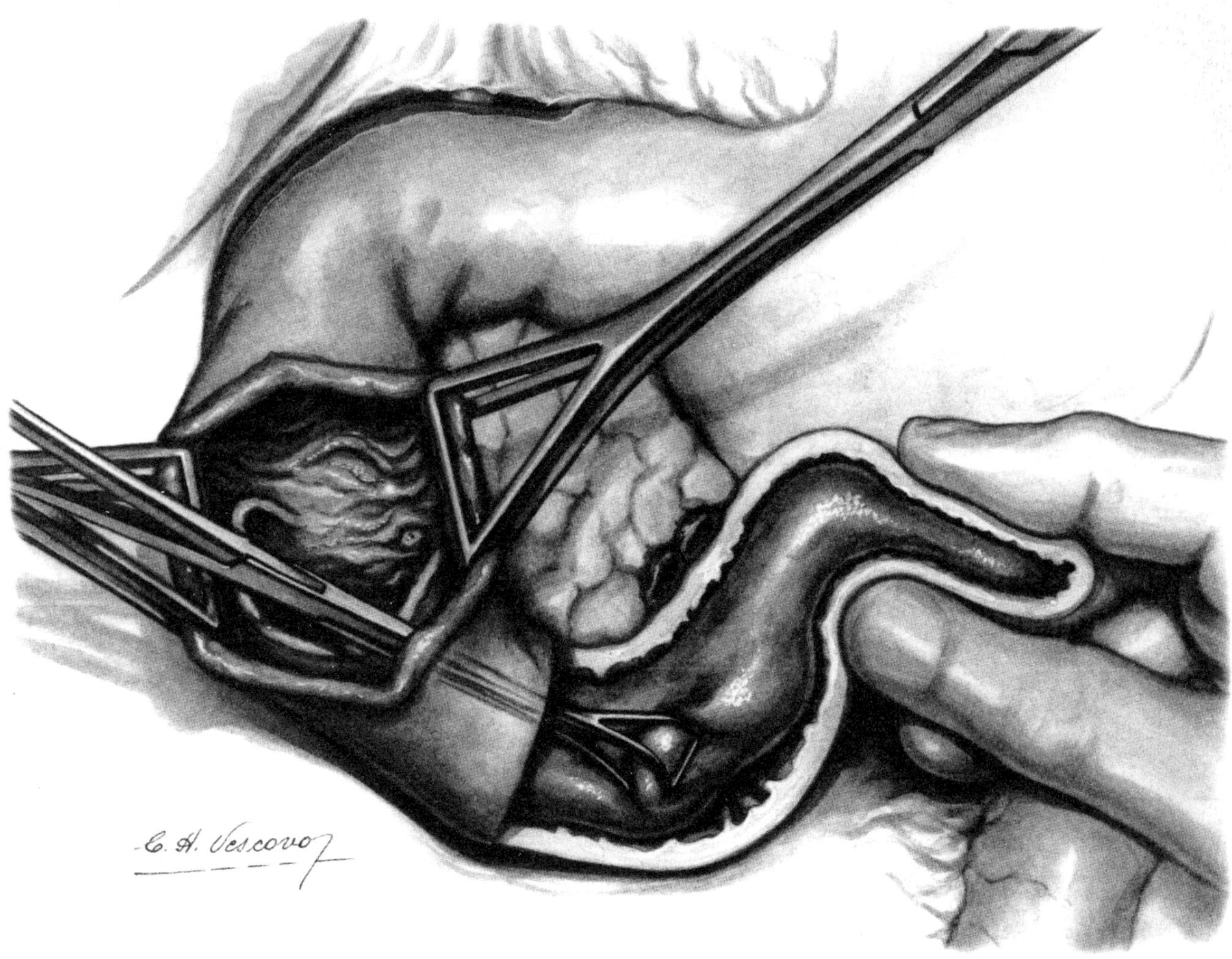

FIGURE 41.49

Group C: Intraluminal Duodenal Diverticula

FIGURE 41.50
The intraluminal duodenal diverticulum has been completely exteriorized. The left index finger has been introduced into it, giving us an approximate idea of its amplitude. One can see that the papilla of Vater is very close to the opening of the diverticulum.

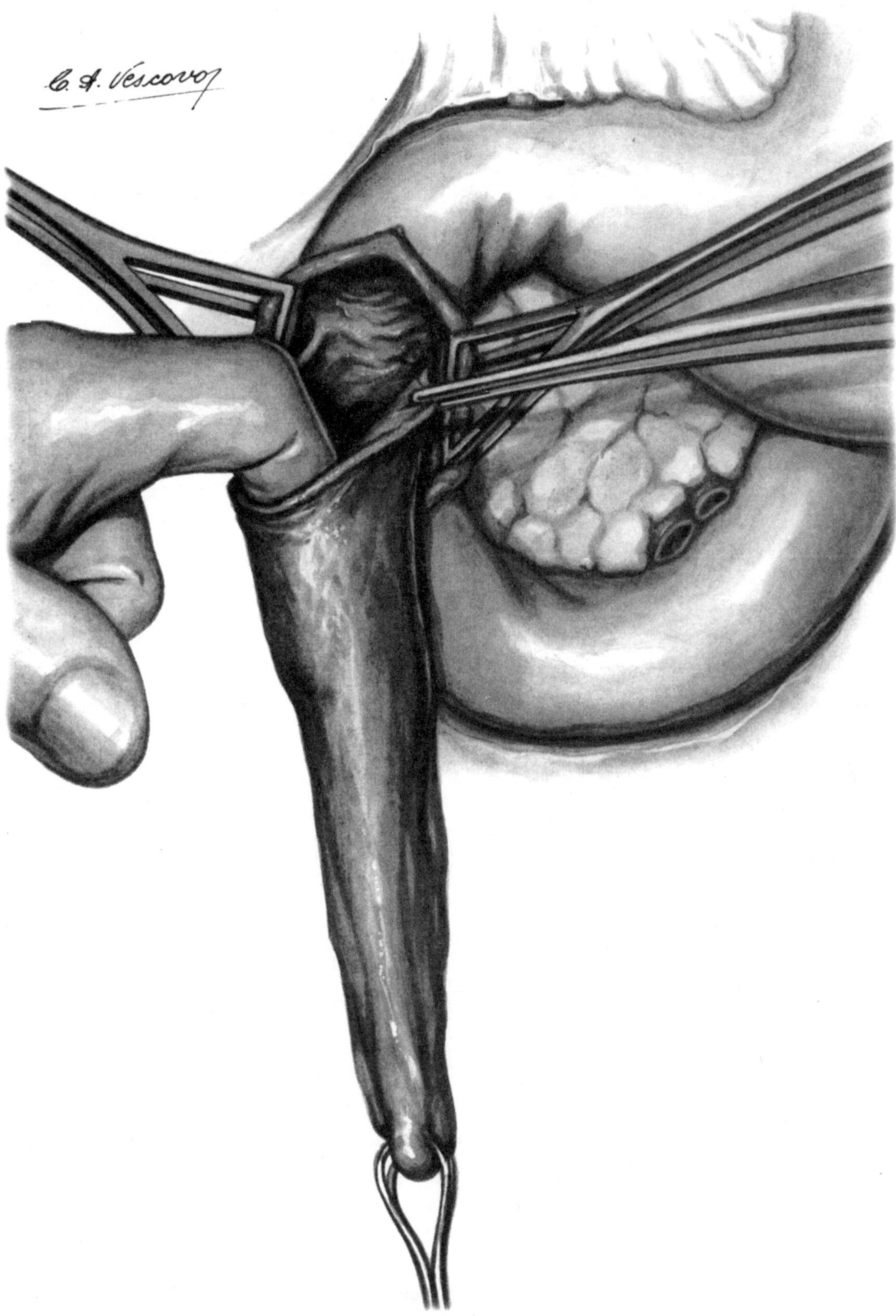

FIGURE 41.50

Group C: Intraluminal Duodenal Diverticula

FIGURE 41.51
Photograph of an intraluminal diverticulum of the duodenum completely exteriorized with the surgeon's index finger introduced inside it, in a patient who presented a clinical picture of duodenal obstruction.

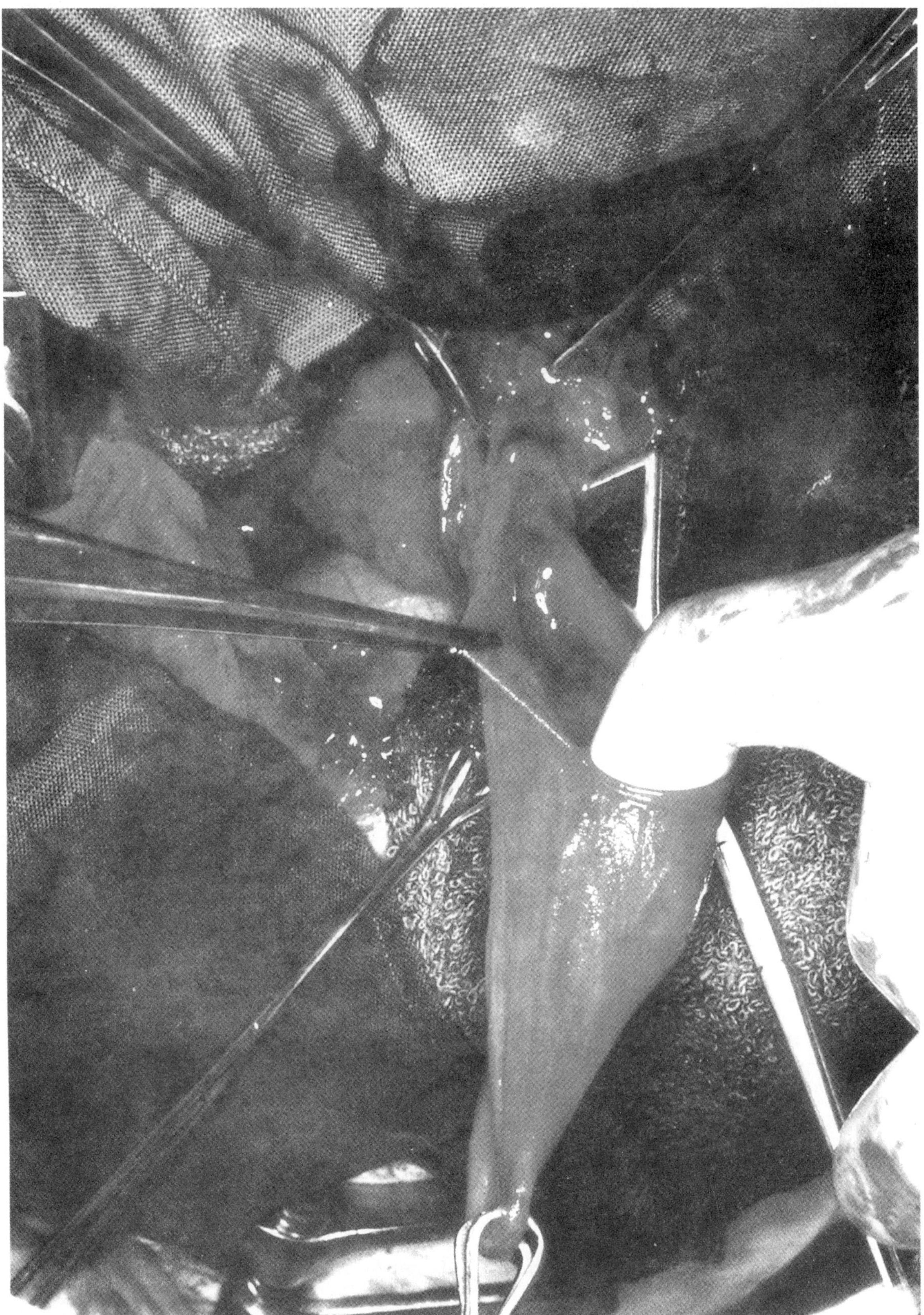

FIGURE 41.51

Group C: Intraluminal Duodenal Diverticula

FIGURE 41.52
The intraluminal duodenal diverticulum has been reflected upward to show its posterior wall and its continuity with the duodenal mucosa.

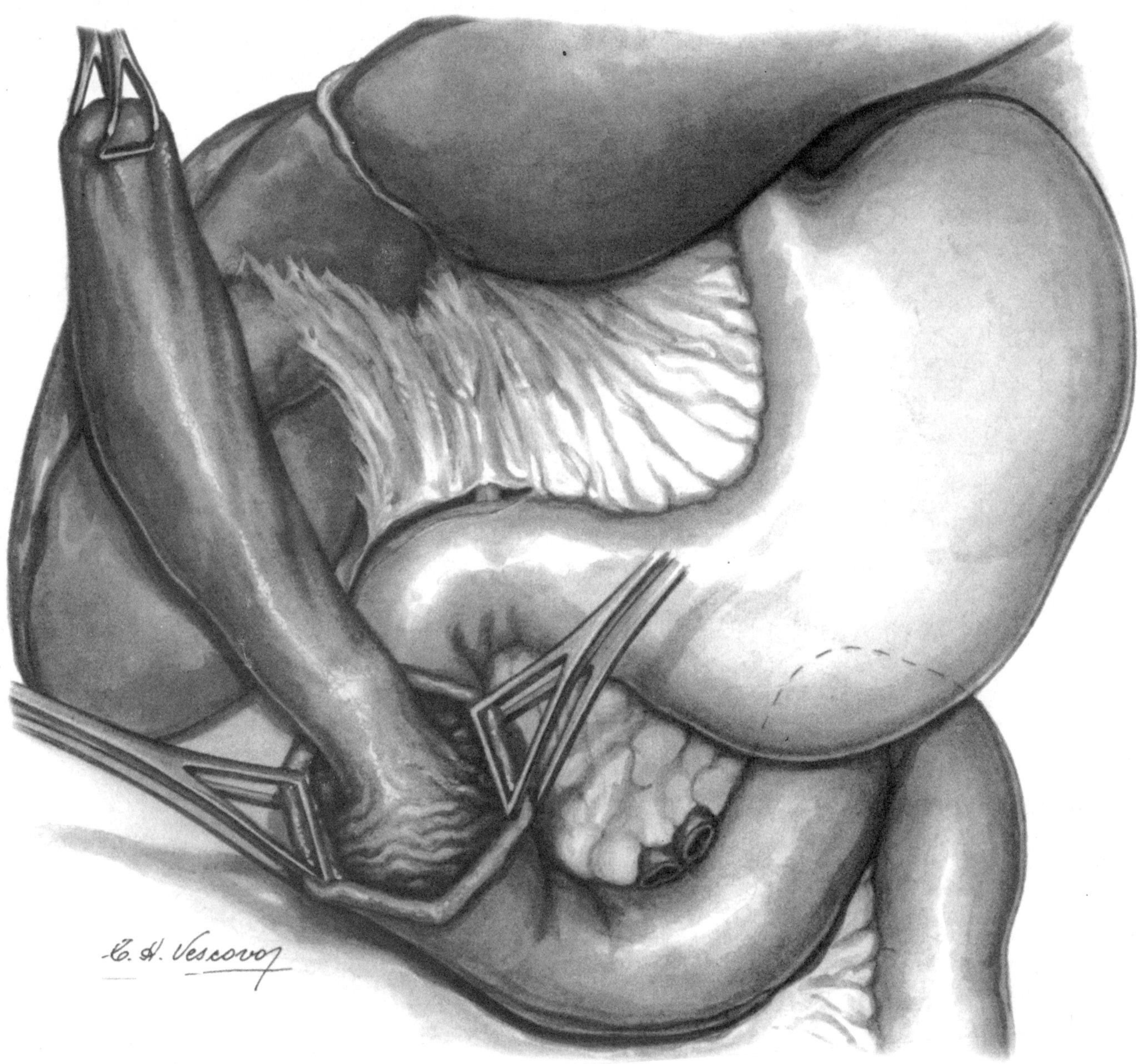

FIGURE 41.52

Group C: Intraluminal Duodenal Diverticula

FIGURE 41.53
Surgical photograph of the same case as that in Figure 41.51, with the diverticulum reflected upward, to show its posterior wall and its continuity with the duodenal mucosa.

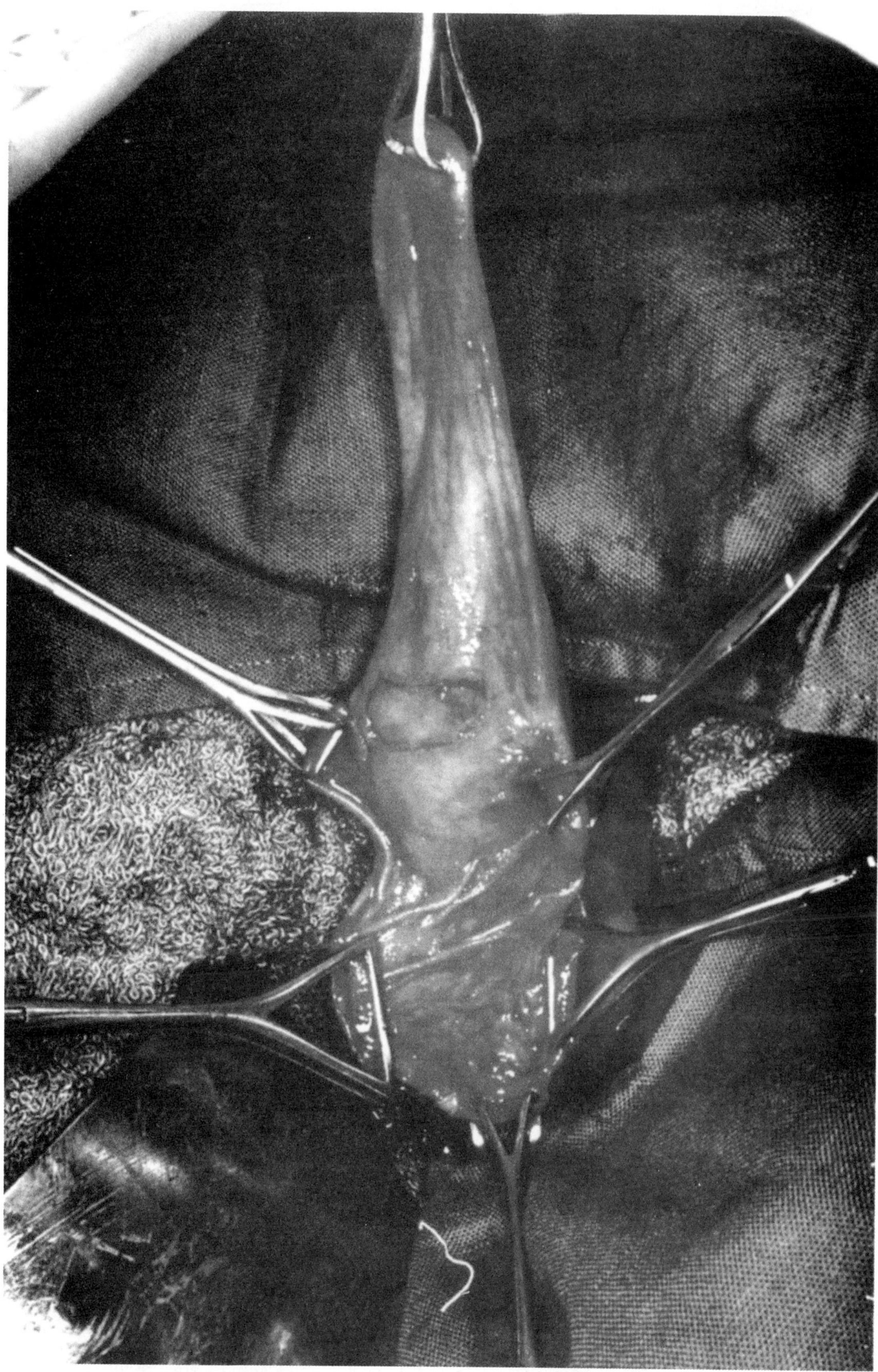

FIGURE 41.53

Group C: Intraluminal Duodenal Diverticula

FIGURE 41.54
Resection of the diverticulum has begun, beginning at its base in the posterior wall of the duodenum. As the wall of the diverticulum is divided, sutures are placed between the edge of the diverticulum and tne duodenal mucosa.

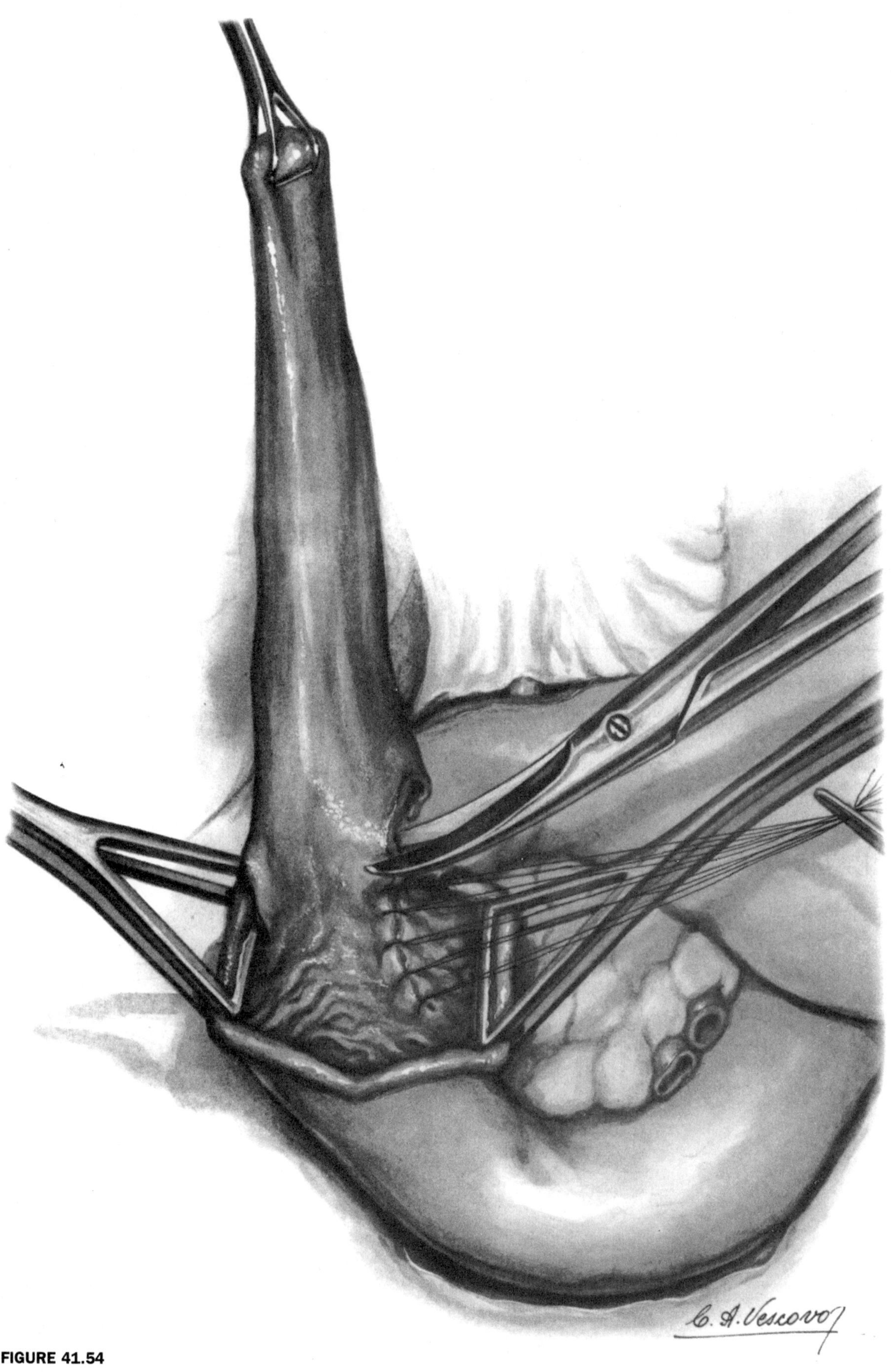

FIGURE 41.54

Group C: Intraluminal Duodenal Diverticula

FIGURE 41.55
Both the left base and the right base of the diverticulum have been divided and sutured, leaving only a small segment left to complete the resection of the diverticulum.

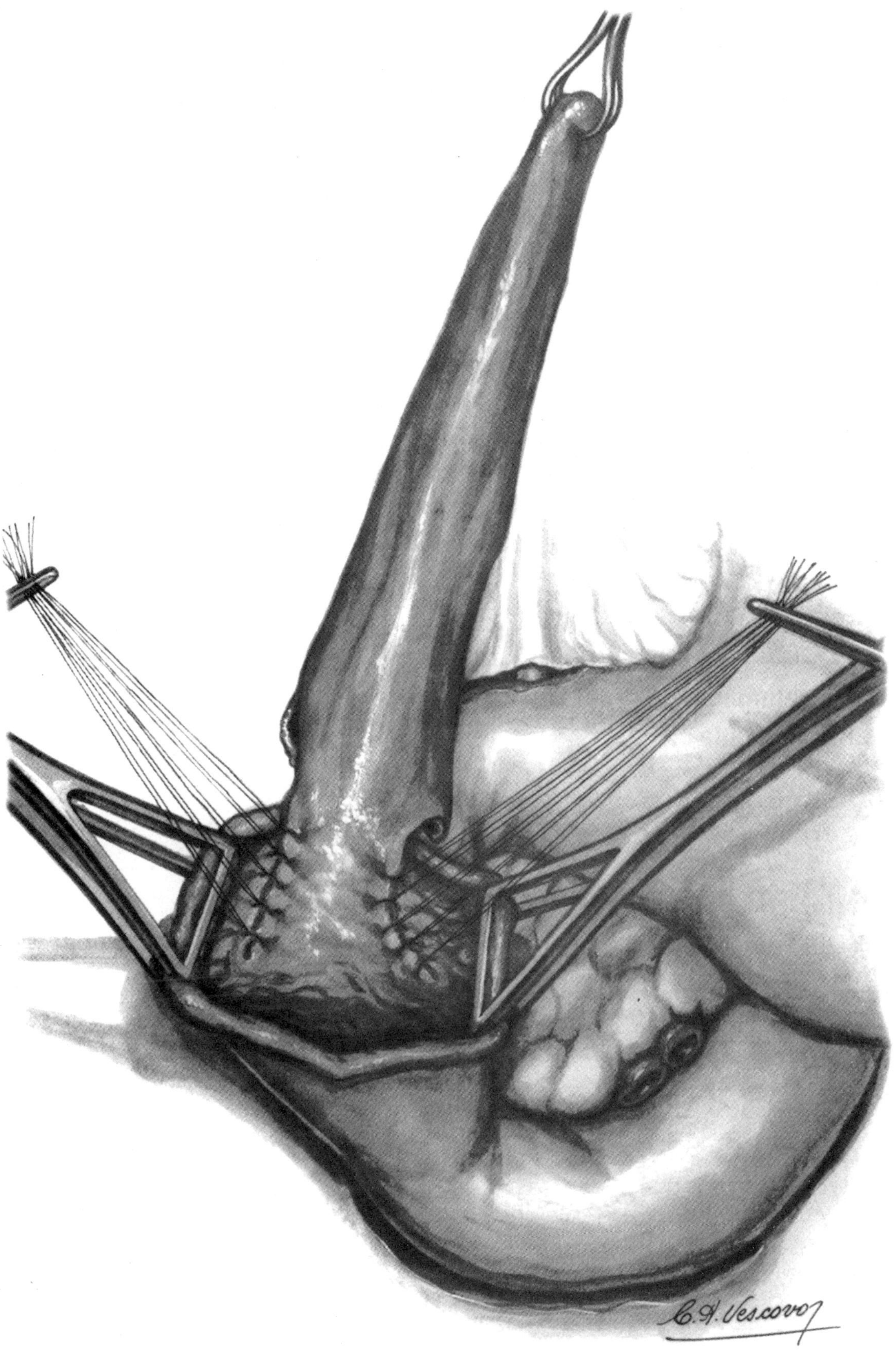

FIGURE 41.55

Group C: Intraluminal Duodenal Diverticula

FIGURE 41.56
To complete the resection of the diverticulum, it is useful to apply traction to the diverticulum downward so that the surgeon can clearly see the site where the diverticulum is to be sectioned using scissors, as shown by the broken line. During resection of an intraluminal diverticulum, precautions should be extreme to determine very precisely the location of the papilla and the course of the common bile duct, because in these patients other anomalies frequently exist.

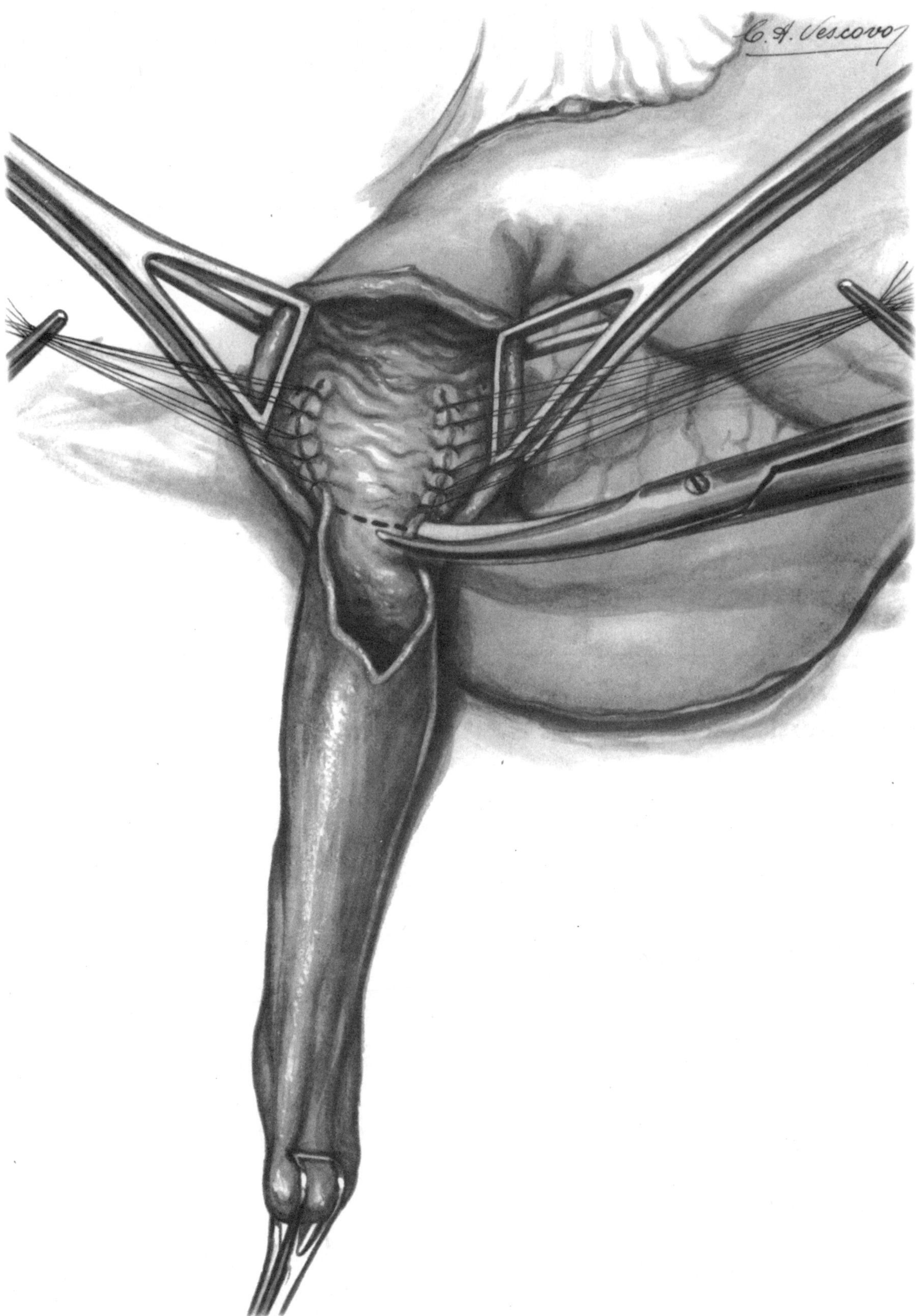

FIGURE 41.56

FIGURE 41.57

The suturing between the mucosa of the base of the diverticulum and the duodenal mucosa has been completed. The drawing shows the location of the papilla, very near to the suture line.

FIGURE 41.58

The longitudinal incision of the duodenum is closed in two separate layers of interrupted sutures. The mucosal layer is closed with absorbable sutures and the seromuscular layer with nonabsorbable sutures.

Group C: Intraluminal Duodenal Diverticula

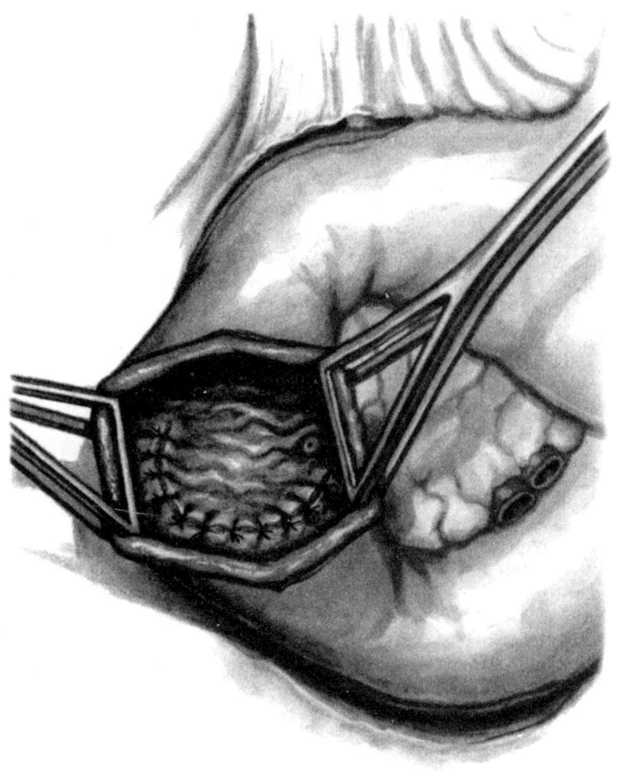

FIGURE 41.57

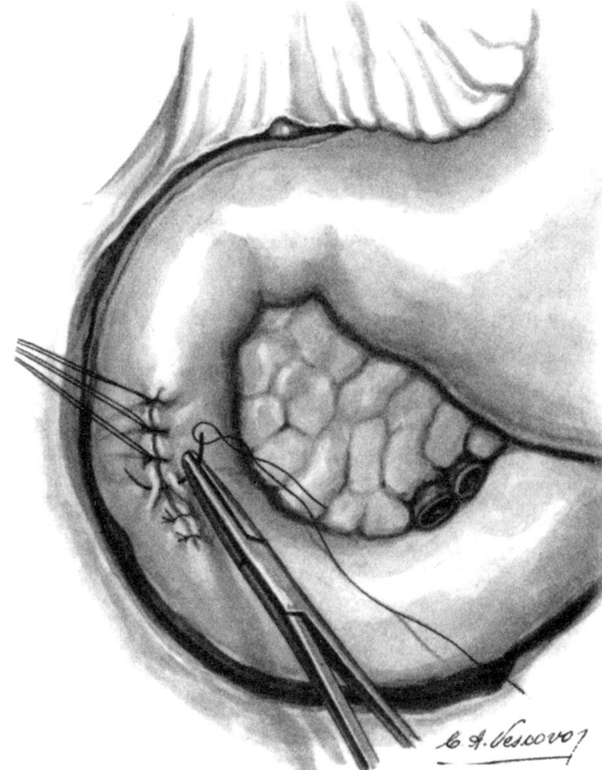

FIGURE 41.58

References

1. Adams, D.B. Management of the intraluminal duodenal diverticulum: Endoscopy or duodenotomy? Am. J. Surg. 151:524, 1986.
2. Ackerman, W. Diverticula and variations of the duodenum. Ann. Surg. 117:403, 1943.
3. Blegen, H.M., Swanberg, A.V., Cox, W.B. Entrance of common bile duct into duodenal diverticulum: Report of a case corrected by surgery. J.A.M.A. 148:195, 1952.
4. Benninghoven, C., Michael, P. Common bile duct emptying into a duodenal diverticulum. A case report. Radiology. 17:579, 1931.
5. Boyd, W. Textbook of pathology. Ed. 4, p. 255. W.B. Saunders, Philadelphia, 1947.
6. Bradham, G.B., Martin, J.B. Massive bleeding from a polyp in a duodenal diverticulum. Ann. Surg. 156:81, 1962.
7. Brompart, M. Atlas of radiologic clinique du tube digestive. Vol. I, p. 32. Masson et Cie., Paris, 1964.
8. Byerly, W.L. Duodenal diverticulitis with perforation: Report of case. Surgery 25:441, 1949.
9. Cattell, R.B., Mudge, T.J. The surgical significance of duodenal diverticula. N. Engl. J. Med. 246:317, 1952.
10. Cavanagh, J.E. Jr. Enteroliths and perforation of duodenal diverticula. Arch. Surg. 100:614, 1970.
11. Chassin, J.L. Operative strategy in general surgery. Ed. 2, p. 571. Springer-Verlag, New York, 1994.
12. Chitamber, A. Duodenal diverticula. Surgery 33:768, 1953.
13. Collett, H.S., Tirman, W.S., Caylor, H.D. Roentgen demonstration of the common duct entering a duodenal diverticulum. Radiology 55:72, 1950.
14. Coors, G.A., Mitchum, W.R. Intraluminal duodenal diverticulum. Am. J. Surg. 103:400, 1962.
15. Critchlow, J.F., Shapiro, M.E., Silen, W. Duodenojejunostomy for the pancreaticobiliary complications of duodenal diverticulum. Ann. Surg. 202:56, 1985.
16. Culver, G.L., Pierson, H.S. The roentgenographic finding, in three cases of termination of the common bile duct in duodenal diverticula. Am. J. Roentgenol. 96:370, 1966.
17. Curtis, L.E., O'Grady, T.J. Duodenal diverticulitis with spontaneous perforation. J.A.M.A. 195:582, 1966.
18. Desmund, A.M. Heald, R.J. Perforated diverticulum of the duodenum and its treatment. Br. J. Surg. 55:396, 1968.
19. Donald, J.W. Major complications of small bowel diverticula. Ann. Surg. 190:183, 1979.
20. Duarte, B., Nagy, K.K., Cintion, J. Perforated duodenal diverticulum. Br. J. Surg. 79:877, 1992.
21. Economides, N.G., McBurney, R.P., Hamilton, F.H. Intraluminal duodenal diverticulum in adult. Ann. Surg. 185:147, 1977.
22. Eggert, A., Teichmann, W., Wittman, D.H. The pathologic implication of duodenal diverticula. Surg. Gynecol. Obstet. 154:62, 1982.
23. Ellis, H. Diverticula of the stomach and duodenum. In Schwartz, S.I., Ellis, H. (Eds.) Maingot's abdominal operations. Ed. 9, vol. I, p. 575. Appleton Lange. Norwalk, CT, 1990.
24. Etala, E., Buroni, J.R. Desembocadura del colédoco y del conducto de Wirsung en divertículo duodenal. Pren. Méd. Argent. 64:386, 1977.
25. Etala, E., Volpacchio, E., Buroni, J.R. Divertículos intraluminales del duodeno. Pren. Méd. Argent. 65:76, 1978.
26. Etala, E. Nueva técnica de anastomosis biliodigestiva en resecciones pancreatoduodenales con vías biliares de calibre normal. Pren. Méd. Argent. 79:169, 1992.
27. Feldman, M. The association of duodenal diverticula with pancreatic disease. Am. J. Gastroenterol. 28:615, 1957.
28. Ferguson, L.K., Cameron, C.S. Jr. Diverticula of the stomach and duodenum. Treatment by invagination and suture. Surg. Gyneol. Obstet. 84:292, 1947.
29. Fleming, C.R., Newcomer, A.D., Stephen, D.H., Carlson, H.C. Intraluminal duodenal diverticulum. Mayo Clin. Proc. 50:244, 1975.
30. Forrest, A.D. Incidence of bleeding in duodenal diverticula. Gastroenterology 33:800, 1957.
31. Fromm, D. Duodenal diverticulum. In Fromm, D. Gastrointestinal surgery. Vol. I, p. 391. Churchill Livingstone, New York, 1985.
32. Griffen, W.O. Diverticula of the duodenum, jejunum, and ileum. In Scott, H.W. Jr., Sawyers, J.L. Surgery of the stomach, duodenum and small intestine. Ed. 2, p. 789. Blackwell, Boston, 1992.
33. Griffin, M., Carey, W.D., Hermann, R., Buonocore, E. Recurrent acute pancreatitis and intussusception complicating an intraluminal dudenal diverticulum. Gastroenterology 81:345, 1981.
34. Hajiro, K., Yamamoto, H., Matsui, H., Yamamoto, T. Endoscopic diagnosis and excision of intraluminal duodenal diverticulum. Gastrointest. Endosc. 25:151, 1979.
35. Heilbrum, N., Boyden, E.A. Intraluminal duodenal diverticulum. Radiology 82:887, 1964.
36. Herrington, J.L. Jr. Massive hemorrhage resulting from benign ulceration in primary duodenal diverticulum. Surgery 43:340, 1958.
37. Howard, J.M., Wynn, B., Lenhart, F.M., Chandnani, P.C. Intraluminal diverticulum: An unusual cause of acute pancreatitis. Am. J. Surg. 151:505, 1986.
38. Jones, T.W., Merendino, K.A. The perplexing duodenal diverticulum. Surgery 48:1068, 1960.
39. Juler, G.L., List, J.W., Stemmer, E.A., et al. Perforating duodenal diverticulitis. Arch. Surg. 99:572, 1969.
40. Kirk, A.P., Summerfield, J.A. Significance of periampullary duodenal diverticula at E R.C P. Gut 19:433, 1978.
41. Knight, M.J., Mousley, J.S., Mitchell, R.C. Endoscopic diagnosis of intraluminal duodenal diverticulum. Gastrointest. Endosc. 24:34, 1977.
42. Landor, J.H., Fulkerson, C.C. Duodenal diverticula. Relations to biliary tract diseases. Arch. Surg. 93:182, 1966.
43. Langman, M.J.S. Duodenal diverticula and hemorrhage. Gut. 4:30, 1963.
44. Lawson, T.L. Intraluminal duodenal diverticulum: A rare cause of acute pancreatitis. Am. J. Dig. Dis. 19:673, 1974.
45. Lida, F. Transduodenal diverticulectomy for periampullar diverticula. World J. Surg. 3:103, 1979.
46. Madden, J.L. Atlas of technics in surgery. Ed. 2, vol. I, p. 320. Appleton Century Crofts, New York, 1964.
47. Mahorner, H., Kisner, W. Diverticula of the duodenum and jejunum. With report of a new technical procedure to facilitate their removal and discussion of surgical significance. Surg. Gynecol. Obstet. 85:607, 1947.
48. Mahorner, H. Diverticula of the duodenum: A report of eight surgical cases. Ann. Surg. 133:697, 1951.
49. McSherry, C.K., Glenn, F. Biliary tract obstruction and duodenal diverticula. Surg. Gynecol. Obstet. 130:829, 1970.
50. Morton, J.J. The surgical treatment of primary duodenal diverticula. Surgery 8:265, 1940.
51. Munnell, E.R., Preston, W.J. Complications of duodenal diverticula. Arch. Surg. 92:152, 1966.
52. Nance, F.C., Cochiara, J., Kinder, K. Acute pancreatitis associated with an intraluminal duodenal diverticulum. Gastroenterology 52:544, 1967.
53. Nance, F.C. Intraluminal duodenal diverticulum. Surg. Gynecol. Obstet. 124:613, 1967.
54. Neil, S.A., Thompson, N.W. The complications of duodenal diverticula and their management. Surg. Gynecol. Obstet. 120:1251, 1965.
55. Newman, A., Nathan, M.H. Intraluminal diverticulum of the duodenum in a child. Am. J. Roentgenol. 103:326, 1968.
56. Nicholson, W.M. Jaundice caused by a duodenal diverticulum. Bull. Johns Hopkins Hosp. 56:305, 1935.
57. Ogilvie, R.F. Duodenal diverticula and their complications with particular reference to acute pancreatic necrosis. Br. J. Surg. 28:362, 1941.
58. Rowlands, B.C., King, P.A. Duodenal diverticula perforating into abdominal aorta causing fatal hemorrhage. Br. J. Surg. 41:415, 1954.
59. Svartz, N., Sjöberg, S.G. Duodenal diverticula as a cause of chronic pancreatitis. Gastroenterology 80:203, 1953.
60. Tandon, V.M., Oesau, H.T. Rassa, R. Intraluminal diverticulum of the duodenum. Ann. Surg. 178:787, 1982.
61. Weig, C.G. Benign ulceration within a duodenal diverticulum. Report of a case. Radiology. 48:143, 1947.
62. Wilbur, B.C., Reimer, G.W., Cresman, R.D. Duodenal diverticula in common duct disease. Am. J. Surg. 92:318, 1956.
63. Wilkinson, G., Greaney, E.M. Jr. Perforated perivaterian duodenal diverticulitis. Am. J. Surg. 111:351, 1966.

64. Willox, G.L., Costopoulos, L.B. Entry of common bile duct and pancreatic ducts into a duodenal diverticulum. Arch. Surg. 98:447, 1969.
65. Whitcomb, J.C. Duodenal diverticulum. Arch. Surg. 88:275, 1964.
66. Wolfson, N.S., Miller, F.B. Anatomic relationship of insertion of the common bile duct and primary duodenal diverticula. Surg. Gynecol. Obstet. 146:628, 1978.
67. Yang, T.S., Greespan, A., Farber, M., Richter, R.M., Bryk, O., Levowitz, B.S. Intraluminal duodenal diverticulum. Arch. Surg. 109:113, 1974.
68. Zeifer, H.D., Goersch, H. Duodenal diverticulitis with perforation. Arch. Surg. 82:746, 1961.
69. Zinninger, M.M. Diverticula of the duodenum: Indications for and technique of surgical treatment. Arch. Surg. 66:836, 1953.

Section F

Surgery of the Stomach and Duodenum

CHAPTER 42

Serosal Patch and Billroth II Gastrectomy in the Treatment of Traumatic Lesions or Fistulas of the Duodenum

Duodenal diverticulization by means of a Billroth II gastrectomy is the most efficient procedure in the treatment of lateral duodenal fistulas that do not respond to well-managed medical therapy (4). The Billroth II gastrectomy can be completed using a serosal patch and a jejunal loop brought up in Roux-en-Y fashion. It is also valuable by deviating biliary flow toward the jejunum, for which reason the common bile duct is divided and anastomosed to the jejunal limb in end-to-side fashion as a Roux-en-Y loop. Details of the biliary bypass were described in the treatment of perforated periampullary duodenal diverticula (6). The serosal patch is used with the object of obtaining an earlier recovery of the patient, since lateral duodenal fistulas are very difficult and complex to treat due to their elevated content of enzymes and their close proximity to the biliary tract and the pancreas.

As mentioned previously, suture of the jejunal serosa should be carried out about 6 to 7 mm from the duodenal defect. In case the duodenal wall shows signs of inflammation or fibrosis, it is advisable to perform the suture further away from the duodenal defect so that healthy duodenal serosa is used.

Serosal Patch and Billroth II Gastrectomy in the Treatment of Traumatic Leions or Fistulas of the Duodenum

FIGURE 42.1
Lateral duodenal fistula treated by a Billroth II gastrectomy with a serosal patch from a jejunal loop brought up in Roux-en-Y fashion. This operation is even more effective if bile is bypassed to the jejunal Roux-en-Y loop, anastomosing the transected common bile duct to the jejunal loop in end-to-side fashion. This biliary bypass should be accompanied at all times by resection of the gallbladder. If the common bile duct is very narrow in diameter, it is useful to use the technique described in the treatment of perforated periampullary diverticula (5).

FIGURE 42.2
This drawing has the object of showing the details of the suturing of the jejunal serosa to the duodenal serosa while the serosal patch operation is performed, using a Roux-en-Y jejunal limb after the Billroth II gastrectomy is performed. In this case the sutures on the duodenal serosa have been placed a little farther away from the defect in the duodenum where the serosa appears healthier and is not involved in the inflammatory process of the duodenal wall.

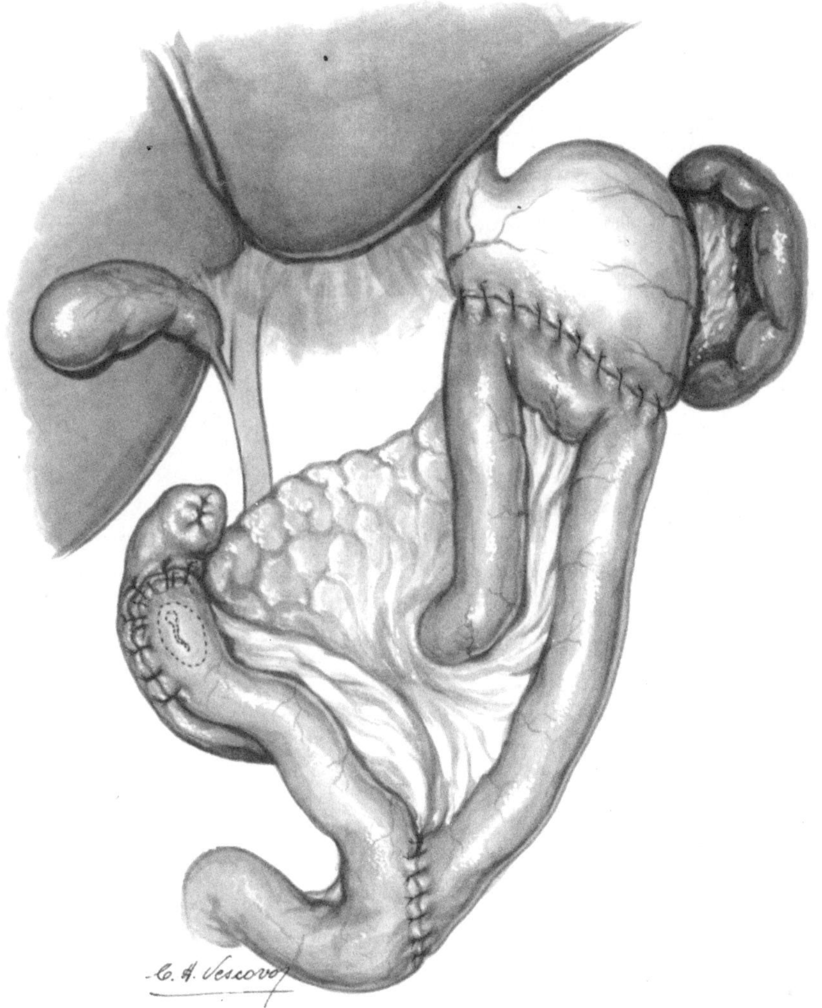

FIGURE 42.1

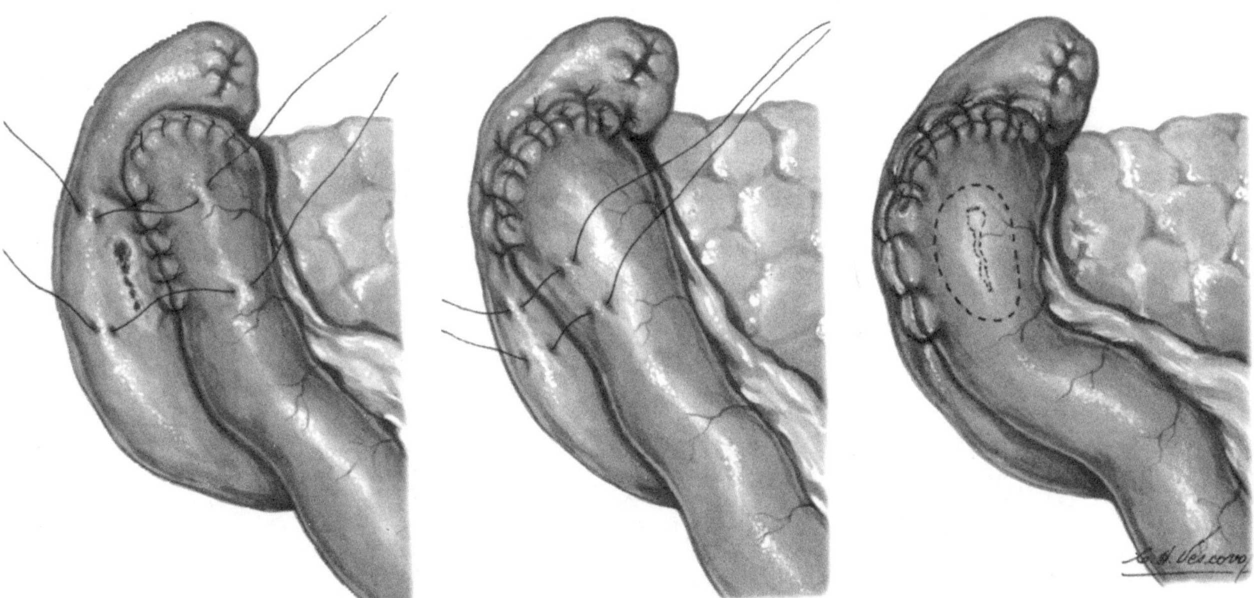

FIGURE 42.2

References

1. Berne, C.J., Donovan, A.J., White, E.J., Yellin, A.E. Duodenal "diverticulization" for duodenal and pancreatic injury. Am. J. Surg. 127:503, 1974.
2. Chassin, J.L. Operative strategy in general surgery. Ed. 2, p. 571. Springer-Verlag, New York, 1994.
3. Duarte, B., Nagy, K.K., Cintron, J. Perforated duodenal diverticulum. Br. J. Surg. 79:877, 1992.
4. Ellis, H., Irving, M. External duodenal fistulae. In Schwartz, S.I., Ellis, H. (Eds.). Maingot's operations. Ed. 9, vol. 1, p. 328. Appleton Lange, Norwalk, CT, 1990.
5. Etala, E. Nueva técnica de anastomosis biliodigestiva en resecciones pancreatoduodenales con vías biliares de calibre normal. Pren. Méd. Argent. 79:169, 1992.
6. Fromm, D. Lateral Duodenal Fistula. In Fromm, D. (Ed.) Gastrointestinal surgery. Vol. 1, p. 113. Churchill Livingstone, New York, 1985.
7. Lowe, R.J. Duodenal trauma. In Nyhus, L.M., Wastell, C. (Eds) Surgery of the stomach and duodenum. Ed. 3, p. 615. Little, Brown, Boston, 1977.
8. Morton, J., Jordan, G.L. Traumatic duodenal injuries. J. Trauma 8:127, 1968.
9. Neil, S.A., Thompson, N.W. The complications of duodenal diverticula and their management. Surg. Gynecol. Obstet. 120:1251, 1965.
10. Sandler, J.T., Deitel, M. Management of duodenal fistulas. Can. J. Surg. 24:124, 1981.
11. Ujiki, G.T., Shields, T.W. Roux-en-Y. Operation in the management of postoperative fistula. Arch. Surg. 116:614, 1981.

PART III

Surgery of the Small Intestine, Colon, Rectum, and Anus

Section G
Small Intestine

CHAPTER 43
Surgery of the Small Intestine

The small intestine extends from the pylorus to the ileocecal junction. From the anatomic as well as the functional point of view, the small intestine should be divided into two separate parts, the duodenum, which is the segment of small intestine that is fixed retroperitoneally and measures about 25 cm, and the jejunoileum or mesenteric portion of the small intestine, made up of free and mobile intestinal loops that occupy a large portion of the abdominal cavity. The jejunoileum extends from the duodenojejunal junction, which is located to the left of the first or second lumbar vertebral body, under the transverse mesocolon, and ends in the ileocecal valve. The usual length of the small intestine varies between 4 and 7 meters.

The surgical anatomy of the duodenum was previously described, for which reason only the surgical anatomy of the jejunoileum will be described, including techniques of resection and anastomosis of the same.

SURGICAL ANATOMY OF THE JEJUNOILEUM

The jejunoileum occupies an ample space in the abdomen, with its superior limit being the transverse mesocolon and the inferior limit constituted partially by the mesosigmoid and the pelvic floor. The greater omentum covers, either completely or partially, the front of the jejunoileal mass, separating it from the parietal peritoneum (16, 28). From its origin in the duodenojejunal angle up to its ileocecal junction, the jejunoileum forms a series of convolutions that form the intestinal loops. The jejunoileum is fixed to the posterior wall of the abdomen by a peritoneal reflection called the mesentery (28). The mesentery is constituted of two peritoneal leaves. In the space between these two leaves blood vessels, nerves, and lymphatic ganglia pass through.

The site where the peritoneal leaves insert into the posterior wall of the abdomen constitutes what is known as the root of the mesentery (4, 28). The mesentery has an intestinal border, which is continuous with the serous covering of the jejunoileum. The intestinal border of the mesentery corresponds to the mesenteric border of the jejunoileum. The mesentery extends from the left side of the second lumbar vertebra all the way to the right iliac fossa at the level of the sacroiliac joint (2). In this oblique course it passes over the front of the third portion of the duodenum, the aorta, the inferior vena cava, the psoas muscle, the ureter, and the right spermatic or ovarian vessels. The mesentery presents two surfaces, one directed upward and to the right, and the other directed downward and to the left. The height of the mesentery is from 10 to 15 cm but, in its proximal as well as its distal ends, the mesentery is not elevated. The median length of the mesentery is about 15 cm (28).

The length of the jejunoileum varies from about 3 to 11 meters (15, 20, 25, 28). The resected jejunoileum of adult persons has a medium length of 6 to 7 meters (4, 13–15). Measurement of the length of the jejunoileum should be carried out during surgical exploration, following the antimesenteric border of the bowel. Measurement of the length of the jejunoileum carried out before resection yields a shorter length than after resection due to the tone of the muscular fibers and periodic tonic contractions of the loops (14). The measurement of the length of the jejunoileum taken before resection should be recorded in the clinical history (14).

The jejunum is wider in diameter than the ileum. The jejunum is 25 to 30 mm in diameter. The diameter of the jejunoileum diminishes distally. The ileum has a diameter of 25 mm, which in its terminal segment is reduced to 20 mm (4, 7, 14, 28). The jejunoileum is very movable, a condition that is widely used in surgery to carry out anastomoses to the esophagus or the stomach, or in the construction of Roux-en-Y anastomotic loops, and so on (2, 4).

The difference in length between the mesentery and the jejunoileum to which it is fixed explains the existence of numerous folds and loops. The jejunum is disposed in transverse loops, while the ileum is disposed in vertical loops. The jejunoileum, due to its location, caliber, mobility, and good blood supply, the good structure of its walls, and the minimal bacterial contamination of its contents, offers good possibilities in surgery (4).

There is no exact limit of demarcation between the jejunum and the ileum, admitting that two fifths of the length of the small bowel belongs to the jejunum and the remaining three fifths correspond to the ileum.

The great majority of jejunal loops are located on the left side of the abdomen, while the ileal loops are located on the right side.

BLOOD SUPPLY OF THE JEJUNOILEUM

The blood that supplies the jejunoileum comes from the superior mesenteric artery, which arises in the aortic wall about 10 mm distal to the origin of the celiac trunk. From its origin, the superior mesenteric artery runs behind the pancreas, passing over the uncinate process and in front of the third portion of the duodenum. After giving off the middle colic artery and two or three small branches to the jejunum, the superior mesenteric artery enters between the peritoneal leaves of the root of the mesentery, giving off 15 to 20 collateral branches destined to irrigate the jejunum and the ileum (4, 16, 28). Within the mesentery, each of the collateral branches of this artery divides in two branches, one superior and one inferior. The superior branches anastomose with the inferior branch of the collateral artery, which is above, and the inferior branch anastomoses with the superior branch of the collateral artery, which is below.

Due to these numerous anastomoses, a series of arterial arches are formed. The first arterial arches are designated primary arches. From these primary arches arise other branches, which bifurcate and anastomose with neighboring arteries, giving rise to another series of arterial arches, which are smaller than the previous ones and are designated as secondary arterial arches. In the ileum, tertiary and even smaller arches are frequently seen, especially in its distal segment. From these arterial arches, be they primary, secondary, tertiary, or other, the straight vessels arise (vasa recta or arteriae rectae). When there is only one arch, the straight arteries are longer and arise further away from the bowel. On the other hand, if the arterial arches are multiple, the straight arteries are shorter and arise closer to the intestine.

The jejunum usually presents one or two arches, and the straight arteries measure 4 to 5 cm. The ileum usually presents 3 or 4 arterial arches, with the straight vessels being shorter and smaller in caliber than the jejunal straight vessels. On the other hand, these straight vessels are more numerous (16, 28). The circulation of the mesenteric side of the jejunoileum is richer than the circulation of the antimesenteric side (14).

LYMPHATIC GANGLIA OF THE JEJUNOILEUM

The mucosa of the jejunoileum presents a great number of lymphatic follicles. These are more frequent in the ileum and particularly in the distal ileum, where, in addition, Peyer's patches are located on its antimesenteric border. Lymph from the jejunoileum enters into the lymphatic ganglia of the mesentery, whose number varies from 100 to 200 ganglia. Three groups of ganglia are discernible in the mesentery. The first group is made up of ganglia located in the vicinity of the arches closest to the jejunoileum (2), the second group is located at the level of the secondary vascular arches, and the third group is located in the root of the mesentery (2).

RESECTION AND ANASTOMOSIS OF THE JEJUNOILEUM

As has been stated before, the excellent structure of the jejunoileum and its good blood supply permit resections and anastomoses to be performed safely. The serosa of the jejunoileum, the well-developed muscular layer, and its well-constituted submucosa permit very trustworthy suturing to be carried out. Jejunoileal surgery should fulfill certain requirements to obtain the best surgical results. Some of these are as follows: (4, 6, 7)

1. The jejunoileal loops should be handled gently.
2. Spillage of intestinal contents into the peritoneal cavity should be avoided as much as possible, particularly in patients with obstruction.
3. The blood supply of the intestinal ends to be anastomosed should be studied in every detail and its pulsating circulation observed.
4. An end-to-end anastomosis should be performed whenever possible, which, in addition to being more physiologic, diminishes the number of sutures needed.
5. The peritoneal cavity should be protected with abdominal pads to avoid contamination as much as possible during the resection and anastomosis.
6. Before applying the atraumatic clamps to the bowel, adequate milking of the intestinal contents should be carried out.
7. Hematomas should be avoided in the mesentery to prevent alterations in the blood supply to the bowel.
8. Interposition of foreign elements in the suture line should be avoided.
9. Sutures should not be under tension. Since the jejunoileum is very mobile, it is difficult to carry out an anastomosis under tension. However, this may occur in suturing proximal to the angle of Treitz and in suturing areas near the ileocecal junction.
10. If interrupted sutures are used, these should be placed 5 mm from each other.
11. Ligature of the blood vessels and division of the mesentery should be carried out before transecting the bowel.
12. Correct suturing is very important, no matter if it is done in two layers, one layer, or using mechanical sutures (6, 12).

Indications for Jejunoileal Resection

Indications for the resection of the jejunoileum are numerous, among which we can point out:

1. Abdominal trauma with lesions of the jejunoileum.
2. Jejunoileal infarction due to arterial or venous thrombosis.
3. Lesions that alter the survival of intestinal loops: volvulus, acute obstruction due to adhesions, intestinal intussusception, strangulated hernia, and so on.
4. Inflammatory lesions of the Jejunoileum: Crohn's disease, some cases of tuberculosis, refractory to medical treatment, and so on.
5. Neoplastic lesions. Benign neoplasms do not offer any difficulty in their resection. Malignant tumors, when they are resectable, do not offer difficulty in carrying out the resection as far as the length of the bowel is concerned, but they do offer difficulty in carrying out the resection deep enough so that it is a radical resection, because it is difficult or impossible to perform a dissection of the lymph nodes in the root of the mesentery.

Extent of Resection of the Jejunoileum

The extent of resection of the jejunoileum is directly related to the nature of the lesion, its location, and its size. In trauma to the abdomen, a small lesion of the wall of the jejunoileum can be produced, which can be repaired with one suture, without having the need to resect a segment of the bowel. In these cases, the edges of the wound should be freshened to be able to carry out a safe suture. For this purpose, the contused edges of the intestinal wound should be trimmed with a scissors. Suturing of the intestinal wound without carrying out a debridement of its edges in order to use healthy tissue can be complicated by a postoperative fistula. Suturing can be carried out transversely or longitudinally, according to the form and extent of the intestinal wound. In some cases a longitudinal suture may lead to stenosis, and this should be kept in mind. If the intestinal lesion is large in size and it is not possible to carry out an adequate repair, resection of a limited segment of the small bowel should be carried out. In these cases it is not necessary to perform a triangular resection of the mesentery, which should be reserved for resections of larger intestinal segments. It is sufficient to ligate and divide the straight vessels near the edge of the bowel as shown in Figure 43.3.

In wide resections of the small bowel due to trauma, gangrene, Crohn's disease, or tumors, resection of the mesentery should always be wide and triangular in shape, as shown in Figure 43.5. Resection of the mesentery in triangular shape has the advantage of reducing the number of vessels that have to be ligated and removing tissue that would be an obstacle to the performance of the intestinal anastomosis. Before carrying out the vascular ligatures, a careful study of the blood supply of the intestines should be performed, be it by palpation, transillumination, or transparency. Some of these mesenteries will offer difficulty in the identification of the blood vessels.

To carry out a resection of an ample segment of small bowel, adequate milking of the intestinal contents should first be performed by squeezing the intestine between the index and the thumb of both hands until at least 10 cm beyond the area to be resected, on each side, can be replaced by atraumatic clamps including only the diameter of the small bowel. Atraumatic clamps are placed at 10 cm from the edges of the involved area of bowel to facilitate maneuverability. Where the intestine is to be transected, traumatic clamps are placed, which will be removed with the resected specimen. Ligature of the mesenteric vessels is then begun, starting with the most important vessels in the apex of the triangle. In order to carry out these ligatures, a delicate curved clamp is passed around the vessel and a nonabsorbable suture is grasped to carry out ligature of the vessel. Some 15 mm from this ligature another similar ligature, which will be removed with the operative specimen, is carried out.

Once the mesenteric vessels related to the segment to be resected have been ligated, the intestine is transected outside the traumatic clamps, removing the operative specimen with both clamps. The intestinal ends are then approximated, being held in place by the atraumatic clamps, and the circulation of the intestinal ends is controlled so that the suturing can be carried out between ends of the intestine, using two layers of interrupted sutures. This is the technique practiced by the author and will be described later (4, 6, 7).

In cases in which the diameter of the intestine is normal, transection of the bowel is carried out transversely. If the diameter of the bowel is somewhat diminished, it is advisable to carry out the division of the bowel in an oblique fashion, with the antimesenteric border shorter than the mesenteric end. In cases in which only one of the intestinal ends is reduced in diameter, this diameter is easily increased using the Cheatle technique, as can be observed in Figures 43.6 and 43.7. In some cases, it may be necessary to use a terminolateral or laterolateral anastomosis.

Technical Variations Due to the Topography of the Lesion

In lesions of the jejunoileum proximal to the angle of Treitz or in the ileocecal area, it may be necessary to resort to some modifications of the above described techniques. In lesions that are very close to the duodenojejunal angle, it may be necessary to mobilize the duodenojejunal flexure and the fourth portion of the duodenum to make possible the anastomosis to the left of the mesenteric vessels. In some patients, it may become necessary to mobilize the duodenum, move it in front of the mesenteric vessels, and carry out the duodenojejunal anastomosis to the right of the mesenteric vessels. In lesions near the ileocecal junction, if it is possible to maintain a segment of distal ileum with good circulation, an end-to-end anastomosis can be performed. If it is not possible to preserve the circulation in the distal ileal segment, some surgeons prefer to anastomose the ileum to the anterior wall of the cecum on the anterior tenia. This is what some authors call "ileocecal implantation" (4, 5, 22, 24).

If the previously mentioned techniques are not practical, a right hemicolectomy should be carried out, which is the technique performed by the majority of surgeons when there is doubt as to the viability of the distal segment of the ileum (4, 5, 12).

Operative Technique

FIGURE 43.1 Drawing of a segment of jejunum showing its vascularization: one or two vascular arches with long, straight vessels.

Operative Technique

FIGURE 43.2 Drawing showing a segment of ileum in which its vascularization can be appreciated: primary, secondary, and tertiary vascular arches. In a segment of the more distal ileum than the one shown in the drawing, the presence of more than three vascular arches is frequent. In the third or fourth vascular arches, the straight vessels arise, being shorter and more numerous than those in the jejunum.

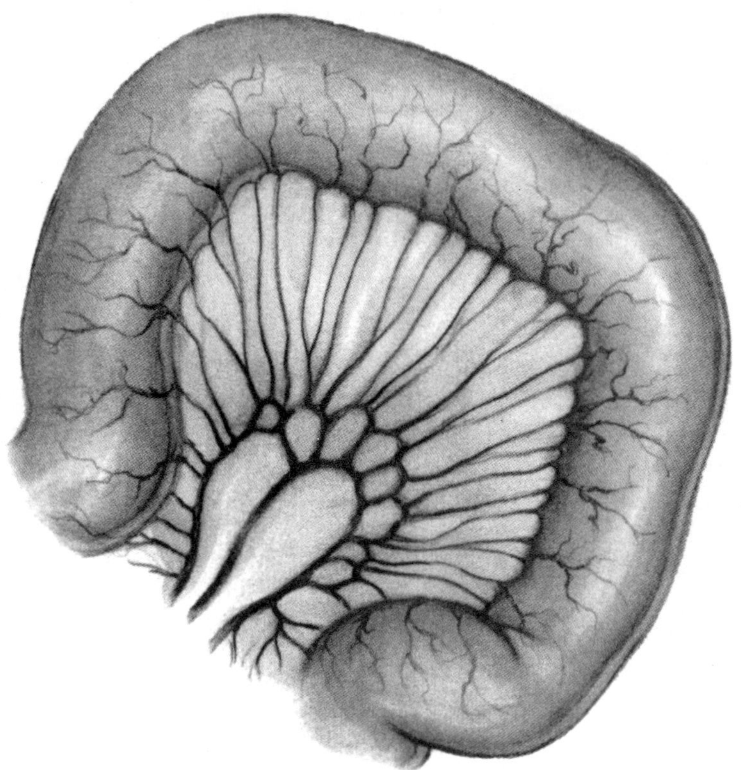

FIGURE 43.1

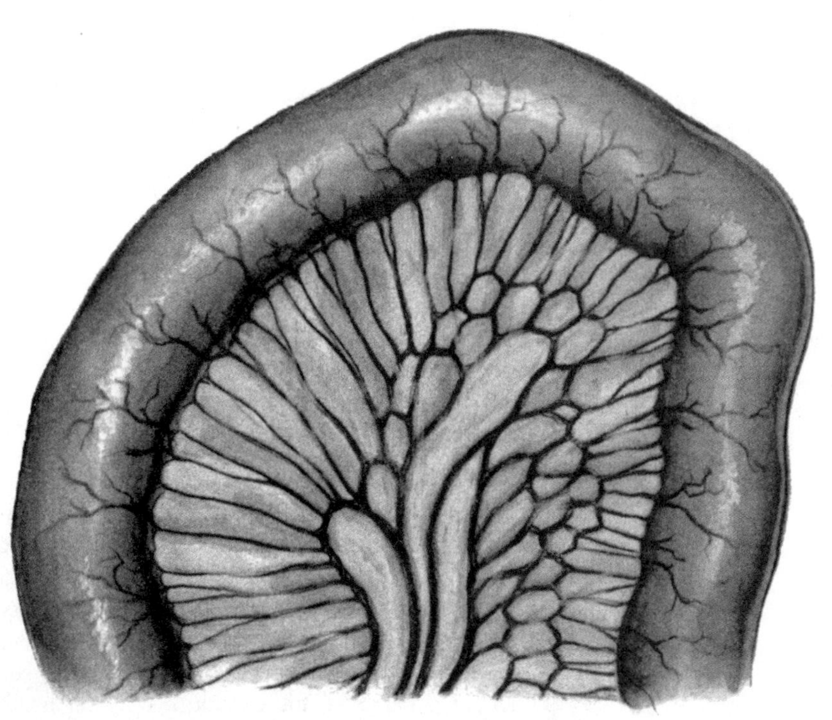

FIGURE 43.3
In traumatic lesions of the jejunum, as shown in this case, or of the ileum, ligature of the straight vessels and transection of the mesentery before the intestinal resection can be carried out in transverse fashion, as shown in the drawing. In lesions limited to the jejunoileum, ligature and transection of the straight vessels does not make suturing of the mesentery more difficult following limited resection of the bowel. The lines on both sides of the intestine show the lines of transection of the bowel.

Operative Technique

FIGURE 43.4
Once the limited resection of the small bowel is carried out, a two-layer anastomosis is being performed between both ends of the bowel. The posterior seromuscular layer has been completed, as well as the posterior mucosal layer and the anterior mucosal layer. Suturing of the anterior seromuscular layer is being completed. All layers are sutured with interrupted sutures, the seromuscular layer using nonabsorbable material, while the mucosal layer is sutured with 3-0 chromic catgut.

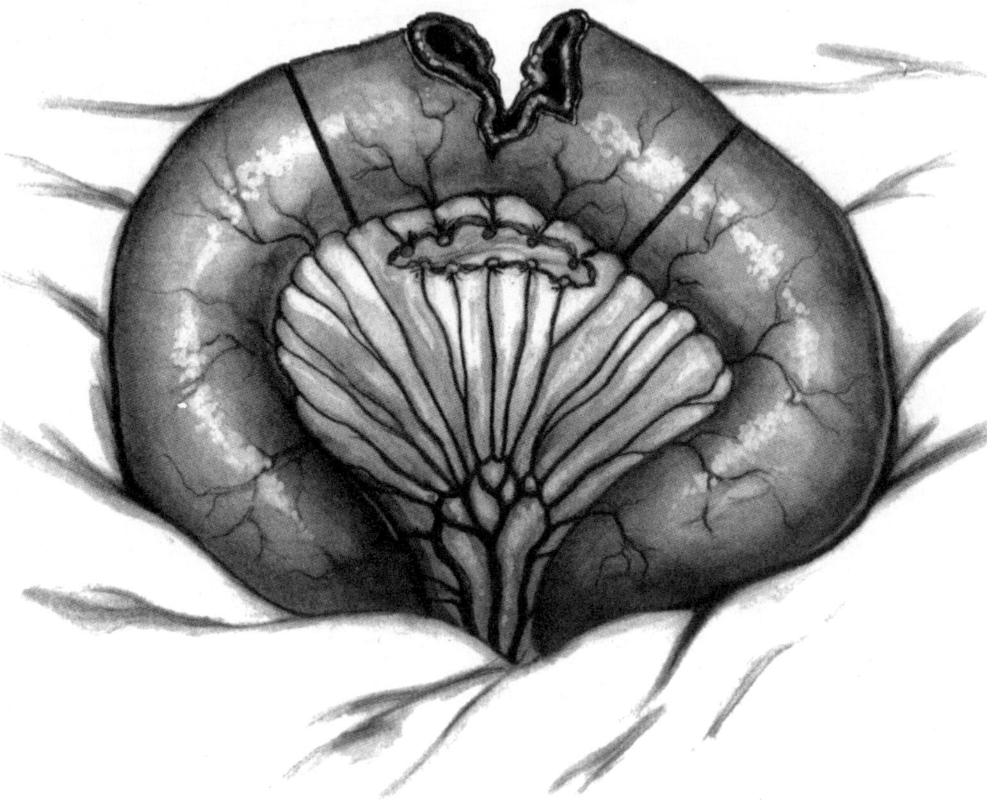

FIGURE 43.3

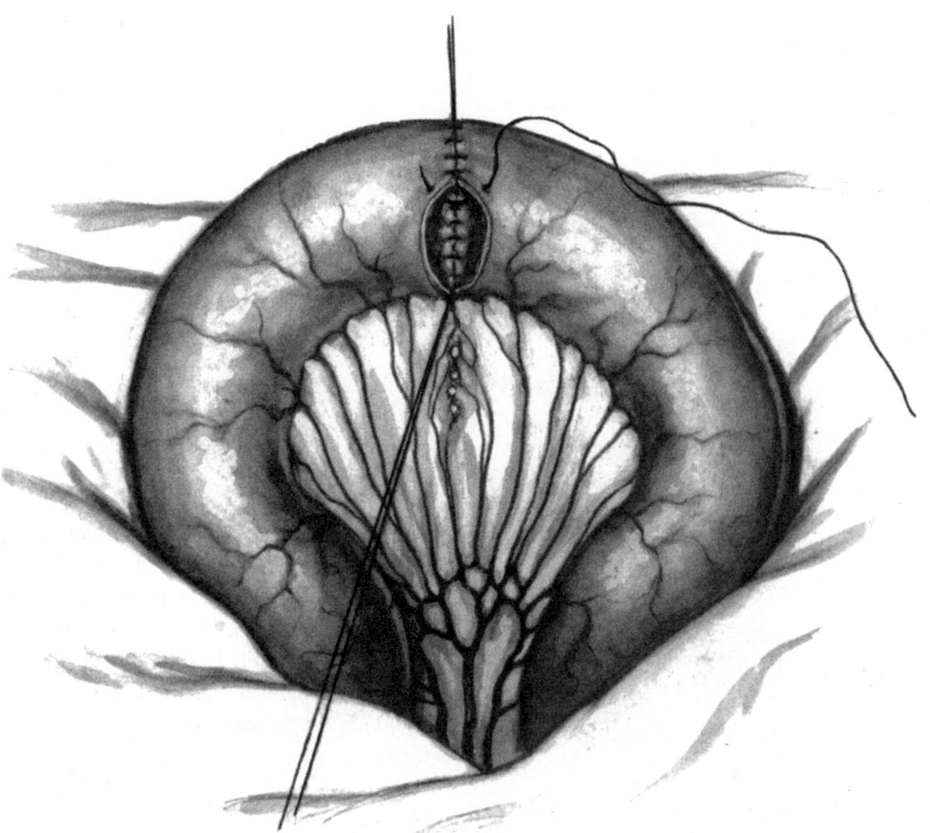

FIGURE 43.4

Operative Technique

FIGURE 43.5

Resection of the jejunum for carcinoma. The bowel proximal to the lesion is dilated. The limits of the resection of the jejunum and its mesentery are shown by a broken line. As shown in the drawing, resection of mesentery is in the form of a triangle with the apex at the site where the more important vessels are to be ligated and the base constituted by the segment of jejunum to be resected.

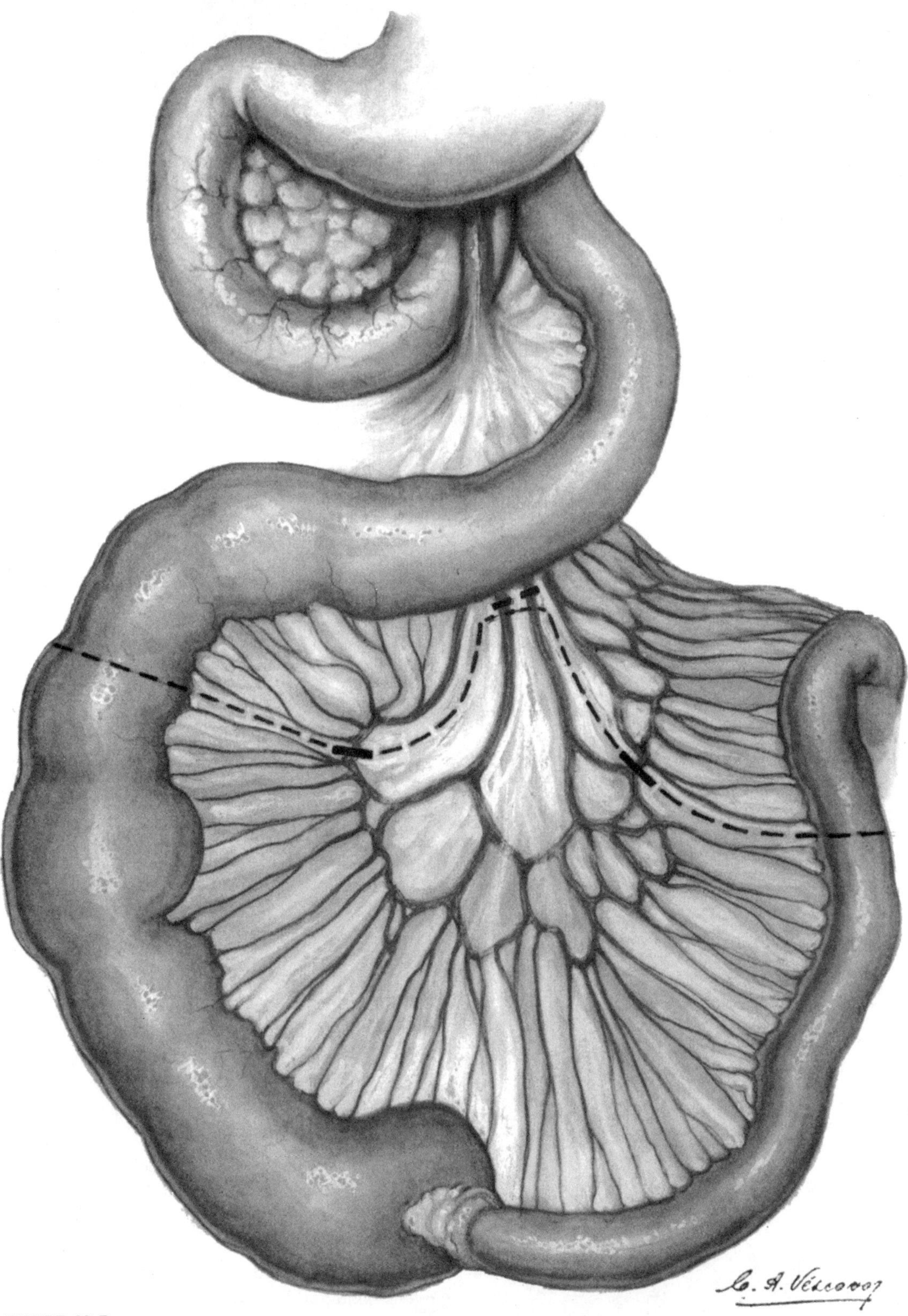

FIGURE 43.5

Operative Technique

FIGURE 43.6

A, B, The difference in caliber that exists between the segment above the anastomosis and the segment below the anastomosis determines the need to increase the diameter of the infrastenotic jejunum in order to carry out an end-to-end anastomosis in correct fashion. In order to do this, a longitudinal incision is made in the antimesenteric edge of the infrastenotic jejunal segment measuring some 2.5 cm in length and the corners of this incision are resected (Cheatle procedure). **C,** The anastomosis of both ends of the small bowel is being carried out after making the diameters similar. Suturing is commenced in the posterior seromuscular layer, placing two traction sutures at the ends and one in the middle. The intermediate sutures are then placed, as shown in **D.** The material used in this layer is not absorbable. **E,** Suturing of the posterior seromuscular layer has been completed, and the posterior mucosal layer is being sutured with 3.0 chromic catgut. **F,** The anterior mucosal layer is being sutured.

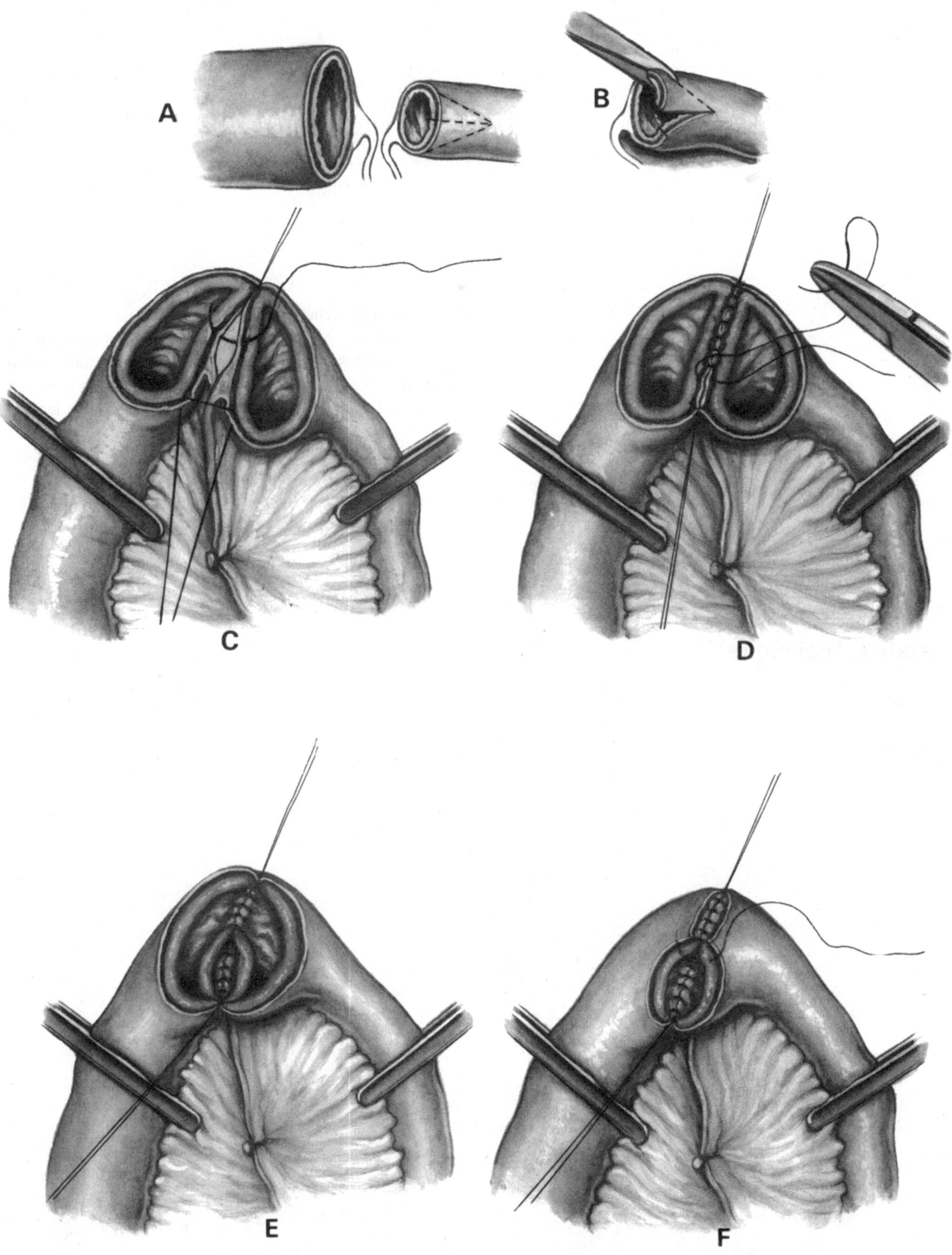

FIGURE 43.6

FIGURE 43.6 CONTINUED
G, The anterior seromuscular layer is being completed. **H,** Once the intestinal anastomosis has been completed, the mesenteric defect is closed. Since it is triangular, it does not offer any difficulty in its closure. The sutures should include only one leaf of the mesentery to avoid injury of a blood vessel. To reinforce the suture line of one of the leaves of the mesentery, the same technique is carried out on the leaf on the opposite side of the mesentery. Suturing both leaves of the mesentery produces more adequate peritonealization.

Operative Technique

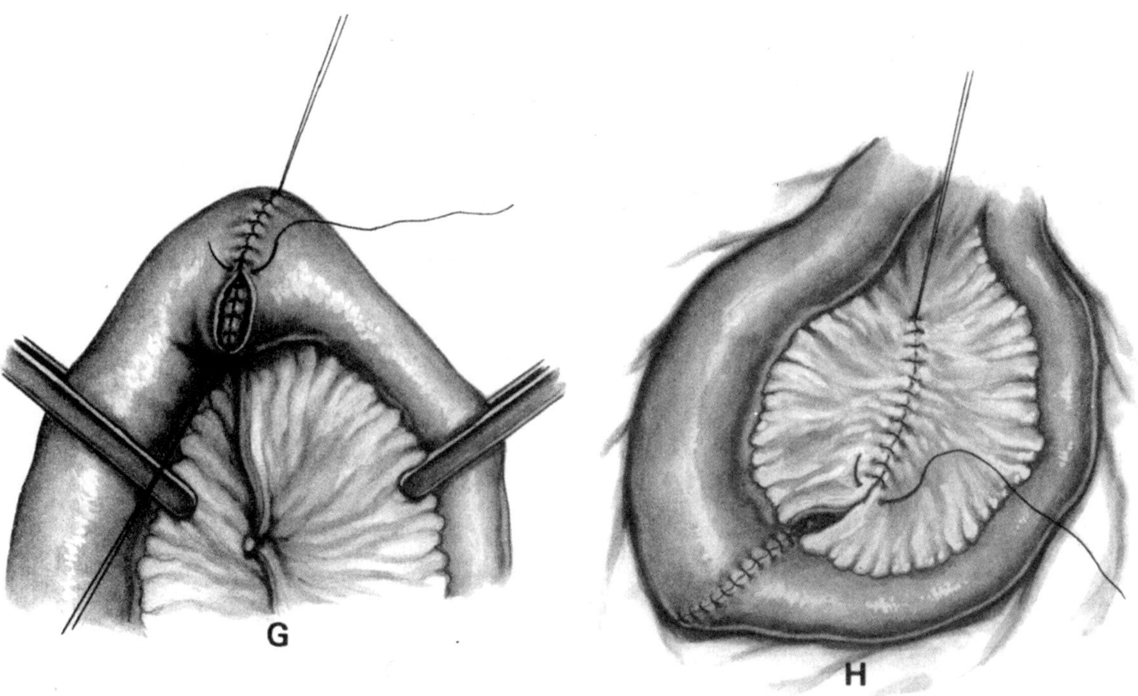

FIGURE 43.6

References

1. Alexander-Williams, J., Haynes, I.G. Conservative operations for Crohn's disease of the small bowel. World J. Surg. 9:945, 1985.
2. Anfres Torrás, P., Nogueras, F.M. Cirugía del intestino delgado. In Pi-Figueras, J. (Ed.) Práctica quirúrgica. Ed 2, p. 317. Salvat, Barcelona, 1986.
3. Asbun, H., Pempinello, C., Halaz, N.A. Small bowel obstruction and its management. Intern. Surg. 74:23, 1989.
4. Bricot, R. Chirurgie de l'intestin grêle. In Lami, J., Louis, R., Michotey, G., Bricot, R., Sarles, J.C. (Eds.) Nouveau traité de technique chirurgicale. Vol. II, p. 3. Masson et Cie., Paris, 1969.
5. Couinaud, C., Pérès, C. La résection de la dernière anse grêle, est-elle une intervention dangeureuse? Faut-il la rejeter au profit de l'hémicolectomie droite? Reflexions sur 5 cas. J. Chir. 73:461, 1957.
6. Chassin, J.L. Operative strategy in general surgery. Ed. 2, p. 267. Springer-Verlag, New York, 1994.
7. Christmann, F.E., Ottolenghi, C.E., Raffo, J.M., von Grolman, G. Técnica quirúrgica. Ed. 10, p. 788. El Ateneo, Buenos Aires, 1970.
8. Dauterive, A.H., Flancbaum, L., Cox, E.F. Blunt intestinal trauma, a modern day review. Ann. Surg. 201:198, 1985.
9. Davis, J.J., Cohn, I. Jr., Nance, F.C. Diagnosis and management of blunt abdominal trauma. Ann. Surg. 183:672, 1976.
10. Farmer, R.G., Whelan, G., Fazio, V.W. Longterm follow-up of patients with Crohn's disease. Gastroenterology 88:1818, 1985.
11. Frileux, C., Thomeret, G., Pillot, P. Pronostic de la résection étendue de l'intestin grêle. A propos de 5 observations. Arch. Mal. App. Dig. 48:1400, 1959.
12. Fromm, D. Small Intestine. In Fromm, D. (Ed.) Gastrointestinal surgery. Vol. I. p. 371. Churchill Livingstone, New York, 1985.
13. Giuliano, A. Clínica y terapéutica quirúrgica. Ed. 3, p. 594. El Ateneo, Buenos Aires, 1976.
14. Gray, S.W., Skandalakis, J.E. Atlas of surgical anatomy for general surgeons. p. 214. Williams & Wilkins, Baltimore, 1985.
15. Hirsch, J.E., Arhens, E.H. Jr., Blankenhorn, D.H. Measurement of the human intestinal length in vivo and some causes of variations. Gastroenterology 31:274, 1956.
16. Hollinshead, W.H. Anatomy for Surgeons. Vol. 2, p. 469. Hoeber-Harper, New York, 1956.
17. Lafargue, P., Lafargue, J. Contribution à la chirurgie de l'angle duodéno-jéjunal. Presse Méd. 62:549, 1954.
18. Lee, E.C.G., Papaioannou, N. Recurrences following surgery for Crohn's disease. Clin. Gastroenterol. 9:419, 1980.
19. Millet, L.D., Mackie, J.A., Rhoads, J.E. The pathophysiology and management of intestinal obstruction. Surg. Clin. North Am. 42:1285, 1962.
20. Monks, G.H. Intestinal localization: review of certain studies (on cadaver) in surgical anatomy of small intestine and its mesentery. Surg. Gynecol. Obstet. 49:213, 1929.
21. Morson, B.C., Dawson, I.M.P. Gastrointestinal pathology. p. 183. Blackwell, Oxford, 1972.
22. Noer, R.J., Deer, J.W., Johnson, C.G. Circulation of the small intestine; evaluation of its revascularizing potential. Ann. Surg. 130:608, 1949.
23. Orlott, M.J., Charters, A.C. Injuries of the small bowel and mesentery and retroperitoneal hematoma. Surg. Clin. North Am. 52:729, 1972.
24. Peycelon, R., Replumaz, J. Duodéno-jéjunectomie segmentaire pour tumeur de l'angle duodéno-jéjunal. J. Chir. 71:125, 1955.
25. Reifferscheid, M. Cirugía del intestino. p. 100. Labor, Barcelona, 1965.
26. Schirmer, B., Scott, Jones, R. Small intestine. In Nora, P.F. (Ed.) Operative surgery. Ed. 3, p. 562. W.B. Saunders, 1990.
27. Schwartz, S.I. Intestinal resection and anastomosis. In Schwartz, S.I., Ellis, H. (Eds.) Maingot's abdominal operations. Ed. 9, vol. 1, p. 933. Appleton Lange. Norwalk, CT, 1990.
28. Testus, L. Tratado de anatomía humana. Ed. 7, vol. 2, p. 255. Salvat, Barcelona, 1912.
29. Valdoni, P. Abdominal surgery. p. 163. W.B. Saunders, Philadelphia, 1976.
30. Wangensteen, O.H. Intestinal obstructions. Ed. 3, p. 128. Charles C Thomas, Springfield, IL, 1955.
31. Zollinger, R.M., Zollinger, R.M. Jr. Atlas of surgical operations. Ed. 4, p. 84. Macmillan, New York, 1975.

Section G

Small Intestine

CHAPTER **44**

Recurring Intestinal Obstruction Due to Postoperative Adhesions

Adhesions are the most frequent cause of intestinal obstructions as a result of surgical abdominal operations. Less frequently, bowel obstructions are due to acute inflammatory processes of the abdomen, such as acute appendicitis, acute diverticulitis, and so on. Generally, adhesions are more frequent and extensive after major operations than after minor ones. Sometimes, however, the opposite occurs and multiple diffuse adhesions are due to more minor operations, such as appendectomy or hernioplasty, while scant adhesions occur after major abdominal operations such as pancreatoduodenectomy or total ileoproctocolectomy (13–15, 26). This means that there probably is an individual predisposition to develop adhesions. On the other hand, there is an obvious disparity in the symptoms presented by different patients, since some patients with few adhesions present severe obstructive symptoms, while other patients with multiple diffuse adhesions remain completely asymptomatic (13, 14, 18, 26). The great majority of patients with postoperative adhesions remain completely asymptomatic. Only those symptomatic patients who do not respond to medical therapy or intubation should be operated on.

In general, acute intestinal obstructions that have to be operated upon urgently are caused by one adhesion. Obstruction is less frequently due to more than one adhesion, while recurring postoperative obstructions are generally due to multiple, diffuse adhesions, which join bowel to bowel, to the abdominal wall, and to the greater omentum. These recurring postoperative adhesions may give rise to serious problems that force the surgeon to carry out repetitive, complex operations.

In spite of numerous investigations carried out to prevent postoperative adhesions, up to the present time they have all failed (10, 13, 14). Prevention of adhesions is an unsolved problem. However, some recommendations can be made, with the object of reducing the incidence of adhesions (7, 25, 26). Some of these are as follows:

1. Strict asepsis.
2. Delicate handling of the tissue during surgical maneuvers.
3. All raw surfaces within the abdomen should be peritonealized.
4. Do not carry out mass ligatures, leaving large vascular stumps.
5. Do not leave any clots.
6. Do not leave accumulations of fibrin.
7. If the greater omentum has been preserved, it should be interposed between the intestinal loops and the abdominal wall.

At present, the majority of surgeons do not give much importance to peritonealization of raw areas within the abdomen. The author, however, has had to carry out urgent surgery in three cases of acute obstruction of the small bowel due to adhesion of the bowel to the gallbladder bed, which had not been peritonealized.

ENTEROLYSIS AND ENTEROPEXY

Treatment of bowel obstruction due to adhesions consists of performing a complete enterolysis of the small bowel. This means liberating all the bowel loops, from the ligament of Treitz to the ileocecal junction. Since it is impossible to prevent the formation of new adhesions, plication and fixation of the bowel loops should be performed carrying out an orderly rearrangement without altering their physiology, so that the new adhesions will not lead to bowel obstruction. The orderly fixation of the bowel was proposed by Wichmann in 1933 (36) and by Noble in 1937 (21–23).

Enterolysis

Reoperation of patients with a clinical picture of obstruction due to adhesions should generally be carried out through the scar of the previous operation, frequently performed 8 to 10 days before. This incision should extend above or below the limits of the previous incision, with the object of being able to enter the abdomen in an area where the bowel is not adherent. Once the peritoneum is opened, the edges of the incision are grasped with several Allis clamps and traction applied upward to allow separation of the bowel loops from the scar and the rest of the anterior abdominal wall. As the intestinal loops that are adherent to the scar are freed, the incision is extended to make it easier to free the bowel loops adherent to each other and to the omentum. The mesenteries of the bowel loops, which are frequently adherent, should also be separated. If the adhesions are laminar in form, they should be freed digitally, and with scissors or scalpel, if they are thick and firm. It is convenient to separate the bowel loops that are easier to separate first and then continue with the more complex adhesions. Great care must be taken in freeing the loops, following a cleavage plane. This is no easy task in a thickened edematous bowel with friable walls. In some cases it is preferable to leave the bowel adherent to the parietal peritoneum or the posterior rectus sheath, avoiding injuring the bowel (18). In normal persons the content of the small bowel is practically sterile, but in patients with bowel obstruction, the intestinal content is not only septic but also toxic (13). Spillage of intestinal contents into the peritoneal cavity should be avoided, and if it occurs, it should be considered catastrophic due to its consequences, which are usually grave (18, 26).

Special attention should be paid to the bowel loops that are adherent to the pelvic floor, since their liberation can cause serious problems. If the serosa of a segment of bowel is injured during enterolysis, most surgeons will ignore it, while others will suture it so that the bowel wall is well peritonealized. If the muscle layer is injured and the mucosa is observed to protrude through it, the seromuscular layer should be immediately sutured. This repair should not be left to the end of this long and laborious operation lest it be forgotten. If the injury of the seromuscular layer cannot be adequately sutured, a patch of jejunal serosa can be applied or a side-to-side anastomosis carried out. A resection of the injured bowel should be performed if the injury is severe or there are doubts as to its viability.

In cases where contamination of the peritoneal cavity has occurred, even though it is only slight, the abdomen should be thoroughly irrigated with warm saline solution before it is closed. In addition, the skin and subcutaneous tissue should not be sutured.

If the intestinal loops are too distended by gas, it is very effective to aspirate them to make enterolysis easier and diminish the danger of contamination of the abdominal cavity by the possible rupture of an intestinal loop during the dissection. This aspiration is performed by using a long, fine needle connected to a closed suction system (16, 18). The needle is inserted almost parallel to the bowel wall, through a subserosal tract, then through a tract in the muscular layer, and finally through a submucosal tract, perforating the mucosa and penetrating the bowel lumen. The entire intramural needle tract is 2.5 to 3.0 cm. This technique prevents leakage of intestinal contents through the orifice left by the needle. It should be recognized that with this technique only 50 to 60 cm of bowel can be decompressed. If it is necessary to decompress another segment of bowel, the needle should be changed for a new sterile one. This technique can be repeated in various segments of bowel.

Enteropexy

Enteropexy means fixation of the bowel. This fixation should be carried out in a predetermined order, so that the bowel physiology is not altered, avoiding recurrence of bowel obstruction by the adhesions that cannot be prevented. Enteropexy is prophylaxis for bowel obstruction. This procedure was proposed by Wichmann, of Finland, in 1933 (36) and by Noble, of the United States, in 1937 (22). The Noble procedure consists of pleating loops of bowel 15 to 20 cm in length to each other, with a continuous catgut suture joining both antimesenteric borders beginning 15 to 20 cm from the angle of Treitz and ending about the same distance from the ileocecal junction. In 1950, Noble had operated upon 260 cases using this technique, with good results and only two deaths. Poth and colleagues (27) had operated on 47 cases with good results, up to 1953. In 1955, Barron and Fallis (4) had operated on 40 cases with good results. All their patients had been operated on at least three times previously, and one of their patients had been operated on 22 times (4, 26). On the other hand, other authors (8, 20, 26, 28, 32, 37) have reported many complications of the Noble operation. This procedure underwent several modifications with the passage of time. One of them was changing the suture material of the plication for nonabsorbable material, and another was the use of interrupted sutures. Reymond (29) proposed plicating only the affected loops. It was later shown (4) that the free loops became obstructed by adhesions, while the previously plicated loops remained in position. The Noble technique will be described later.

Due to the complications of the Noble operation and the prolonged time the procedure takes, Childs and Phillips, in 1965 (11), proposed transmesenteric plication of the small intestine, preserving the Noble principle. These authors place three U-shaped mattress sutures through the mesentery, one in the center and two laterally, using special long needles. This technique does shorten the operating time but leads to many complications, as described by several authors (5, 6, 8, 17, 19). In 1975, McCarthy modified the Childs and Phillips technique. He proposed replacing the catgut transmesenteric sutures with nonabsorbable material. He also changed the point where the sutures pass through the mesentery from 0.3 cm from the bowel, to 3 to 4 cm. McCarthy also proposed joining the three U-shaped transmesenteric sutures. The Childs and Phillips technique, as modified by McCarthy, will be described later.

The Childs and Phillips technique proved that intestinal plication can be done without suturing the intestinal wall, which is usually thickened, edematous, and friable, exposing the patient to fistulous complications. Barron and Fallis (4) confirmed this fact.

The author uses a simplified enteropexy that avoids suturing the bowel with all its inconveniences and the risks of transmesenteric enteropexy. This technique will be described later. The author has operated on 21 patients using this technique, with good early and late results. All the patients had been operated on from 4 to 9 times. Follow-up was from 6 to 21 years.

In 1968, Joel Wilson Baker, an American surgeon, proposed a very interesting technique, consisting of producing plication and fixation of the bowel loops in cases of recurrent obstruction due to adhesions (1–3). This technique is carried out with the Baker (stitchless plication) tube, which, once introduced into the small bowel, produces fixation and plication of the intestinal loops without the need of using sutures in the bowel wall or its mesentery. The Baker tube acts as an intraluminal stent. This tube is 270 cm long, 18 F., with a double lumen and a 5 cm balloon at its end. The tube is usually introduced through a Stamm gastrostomy, though it can also be introduced through the nose, through a jejunostomy, and, in some special cases, in retrograde fashion, through a cecostomy. The Baker tube is left in place from 14 to 21 days. This procedure can also lead to complications, such as fistulas, recurrent obstructions, difficulty in removing the tube, intussusception of the bowel as the tube is removed, and so on (6, 8, 12, 19, 34, 35). The technique for introducing the Baker tube will be described later.

Operative Technique

FIGURE 44.1

This drawing shows multiple, diffuse adhesions kinking and obstructing the small intestine. Liberation of the small bowel loops should be carried out from the ligament of Treitz to the ileocecal valve (total enterolysis). Division of the adhesions between the bowel loops is performed differently according to the type of adhesion, digitally in thin, laminar adhesions, and with scissors or scalpel if the adhesions are thick, as in the drawing.

FIGURE 44.2

During the enterolysis loops of small bowel can be observed to be distended with gas. In these cases it is safer to aspirate the gaseous contents so that the dissection is easier and there is less possibility of rupture. The puncture is carried out with a long 18 F needle, which is introduced parallel to the bowel wall through a subserous tract. The intramural tract made by the needle before entering the lumen is 2.5 to 3 cm long.

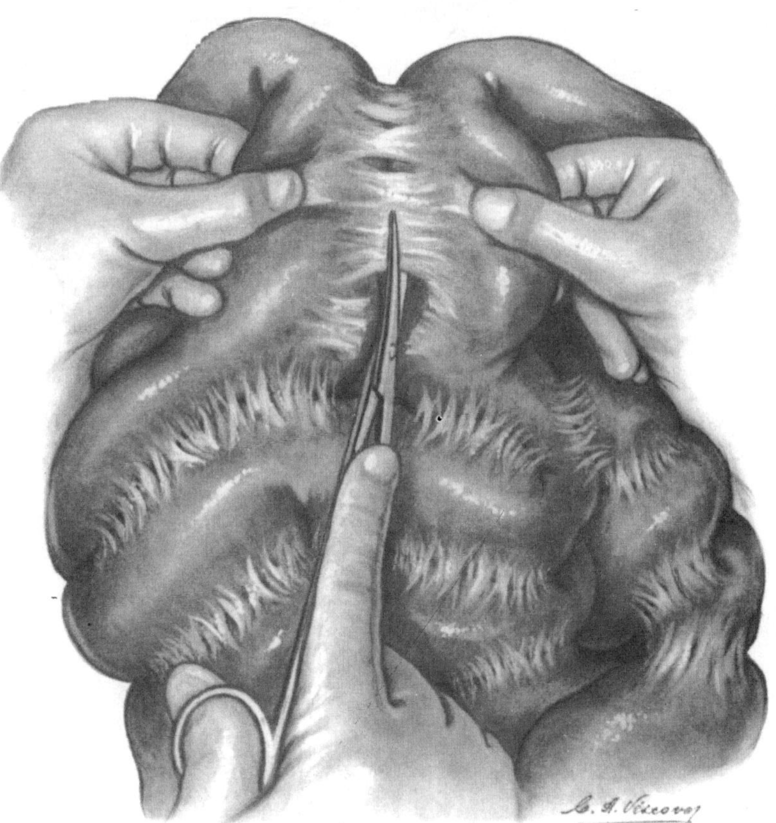

FIGURE 44.1

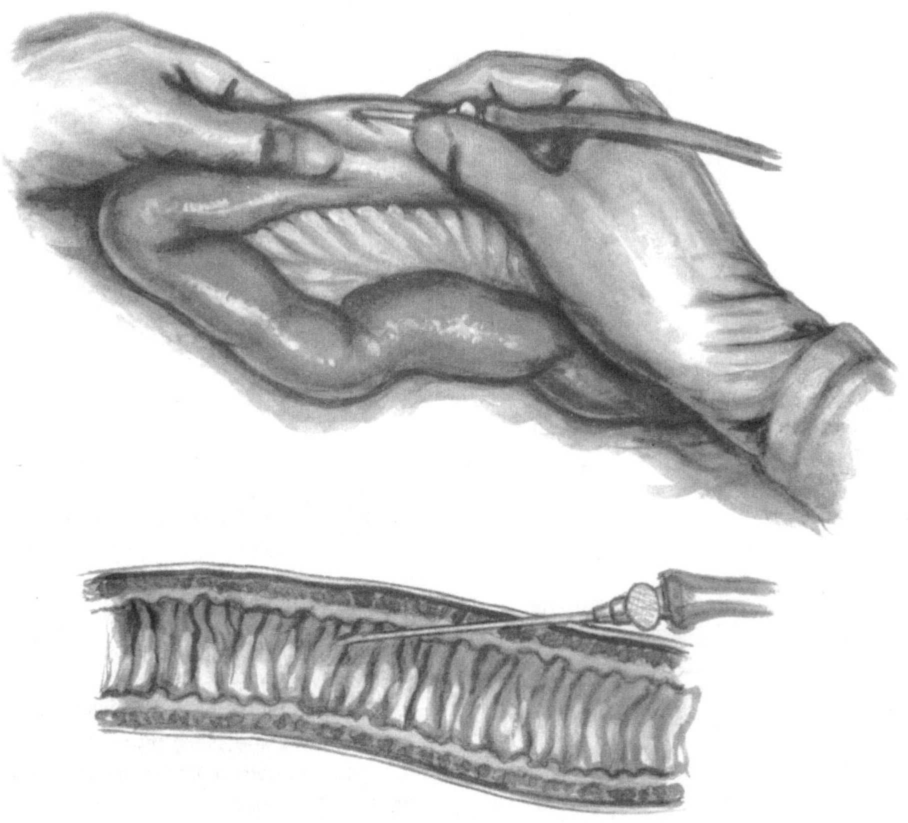

FIGURE 44.2

Operative Technique

FIGURE 44.3 ENTEROPEXY—NOBLE PROCEDURE

After the complete enterolysis is performed, plication of the bowel loops is carried out, joining the loops in stepladder fashion, as seen in the drawing. The antimesenteric borders of the loops are joined by a continuous suture, which includes the seromuscular layer of each loop. The bowel loops are arranged in segments of 15 to 20 cm with gentle curves and avoiding acute angles. The plication should begin about 15 to 20 cm from the ligament of Treitz and end about 15 to 20 cm from the ileocecal valve.

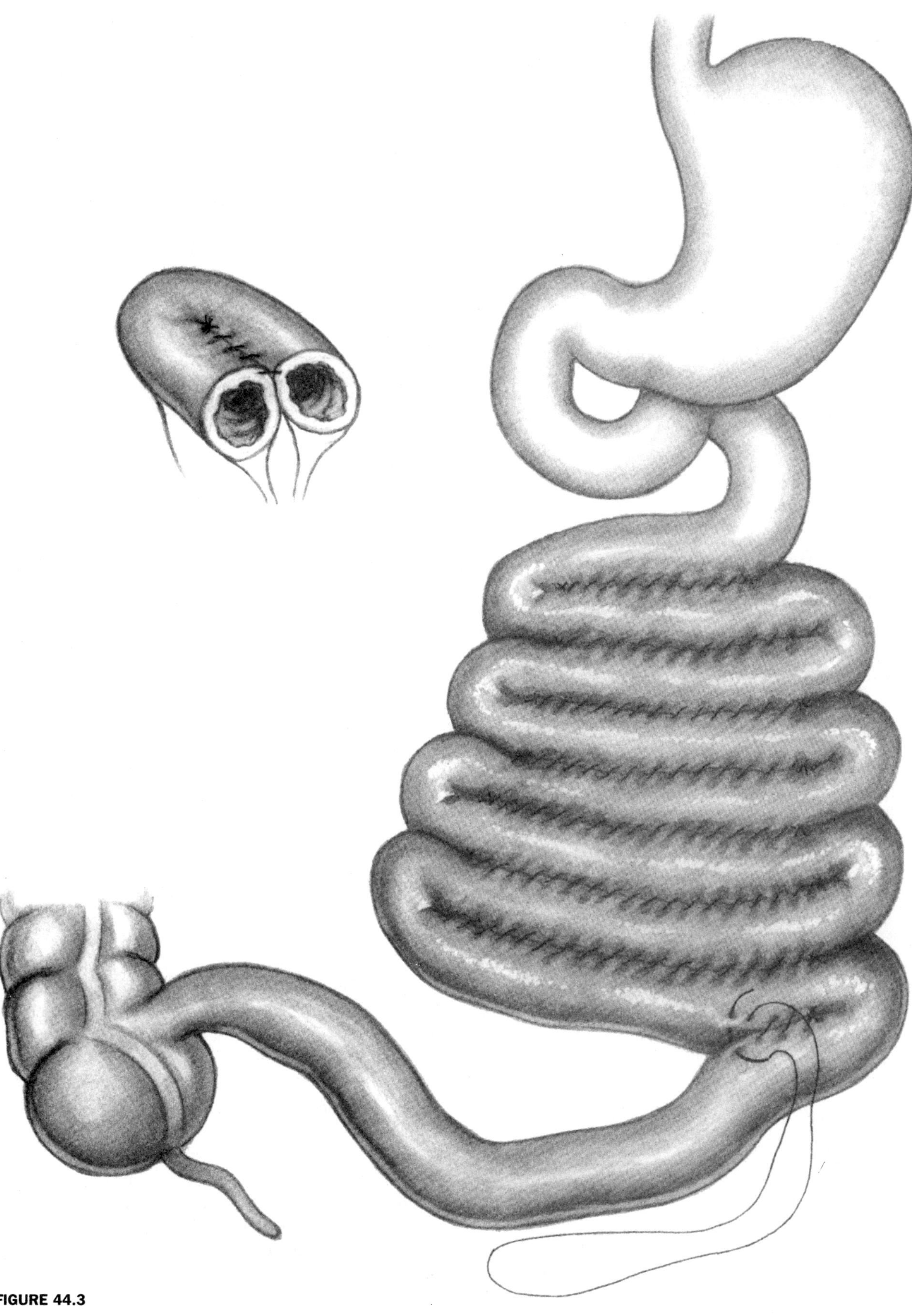

FIGURE 44.3

Operative Technique

FIGURE 44.4 McCARTHY MODIFICATION OF THE CHILDS-PHILLIPS ENTEROPEXY

In this technique the small bowel plication is not held in place by suturing the bowel wall, as in the Noble procedure, but by joining the mesenteries of the bowel loops with the three U-shaped mattress sutures passing through the mesentery. For this purpose the loops of bowel are plicated, as shown, making each segment from 15 to 20 cm long. The U-shaped sutures are inserted with special, long needles, as shown, which perforate the mesentery about 3 to 4 cm from the mesenteric border of the bowel. It is important to study the vessels in the mesentery by transillumination to avoid injuring an important vessel. One U-shaped suture is placed in the middle and the other two in either side. The sutures are adjusted, and their ends joined above and below, as shown.

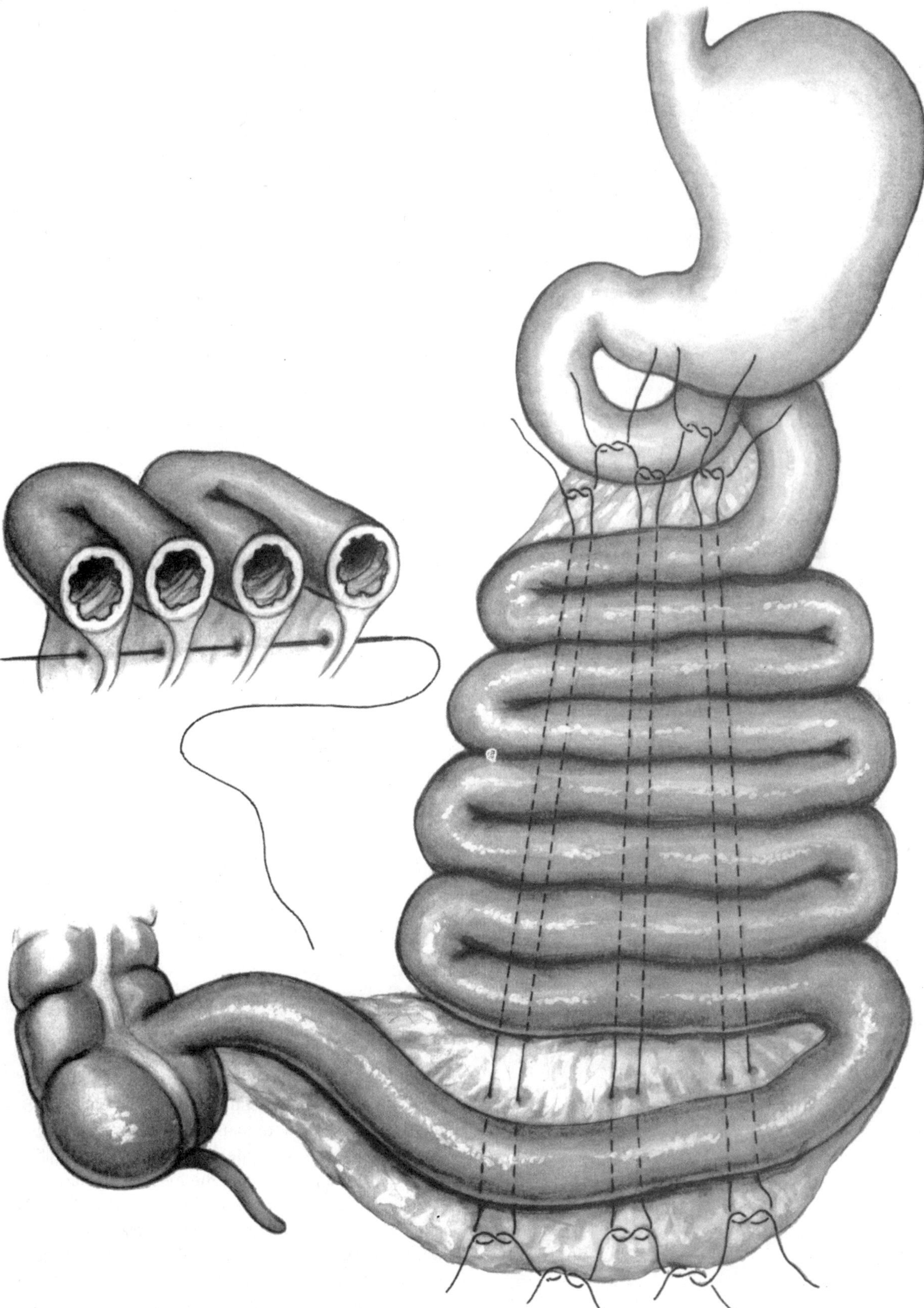

FIGURE 44.4

Operative Technique

FIGURE 44.5 SIMPLIFIED ENTEROPEXY (4, 11)
This is the technique used by the author since 1969. After the enterolysis is complete and the bowel loops arranged as in the above techniques, the enteropexy is done in simplified fashion, using 3 or 4 sutures to join the mesenteric border of one loop with the mesenteric border of the opposite loop. The suture should include a substantial portion of the mesenteric border without including any blood vessel. The site of the placement of the sutures can be clearly seen in the drawing. This technique prevents suturing the intestinal wall, with its possible dangers.

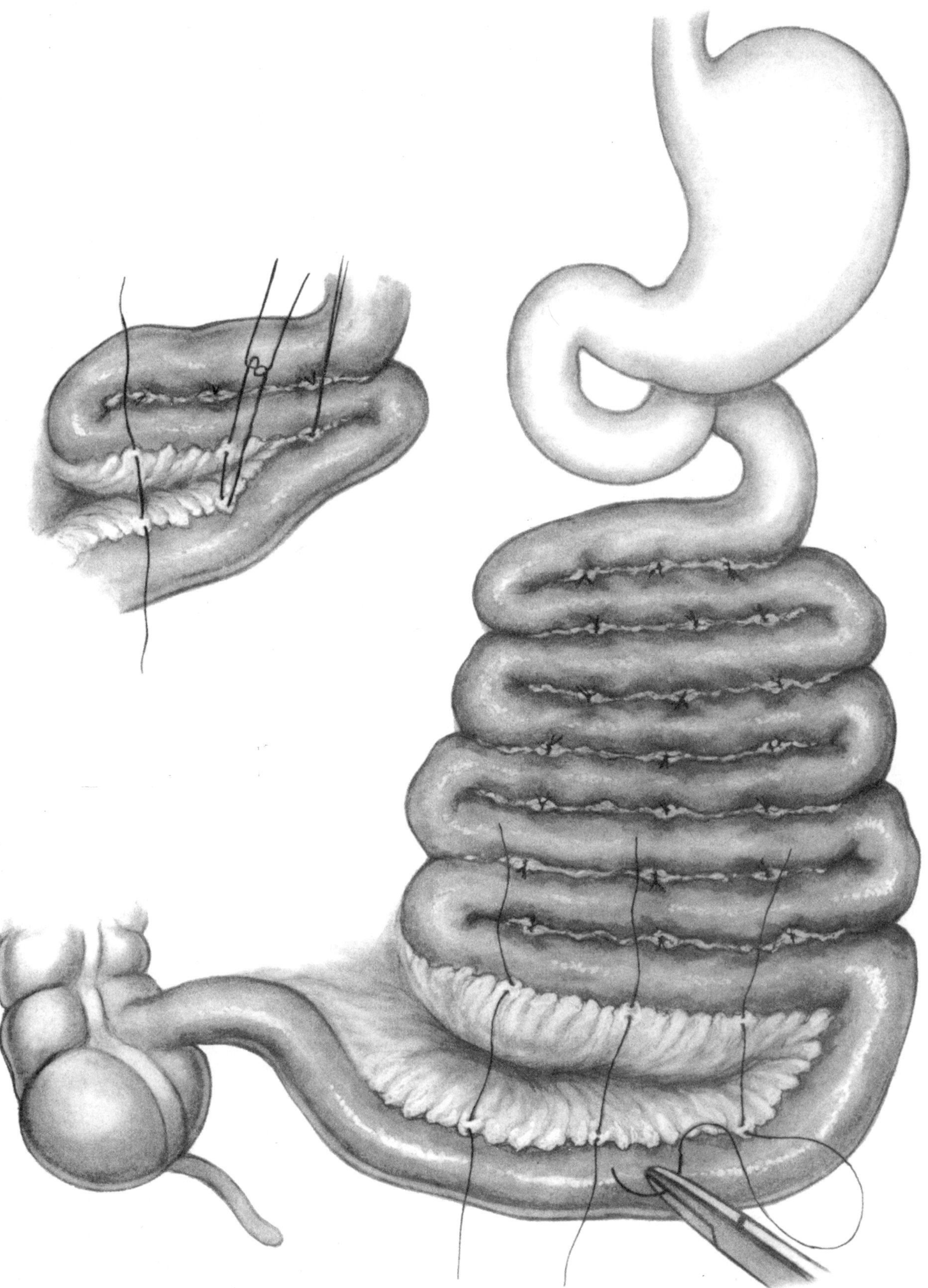

FIGURE 44.5

FIGURE 44.6
Patient, age 18, operated on for acute appendicitis, not perforated. Eight days later he was reoperated on for bowel obstruction due to multiple, diffuse adhesions. The surgeon simply divided the more important adhesions and closed the abdomen. This clinical picture recurred twice, and the surgeon proceeded in the same manner, without success, having to operate again 5 days after the last operation. The photograph shows severe distension of the small bowel with edematous, congested walls and the bowel obstructed and distorted by multiple, diffuse adhesions.

Operative Technique

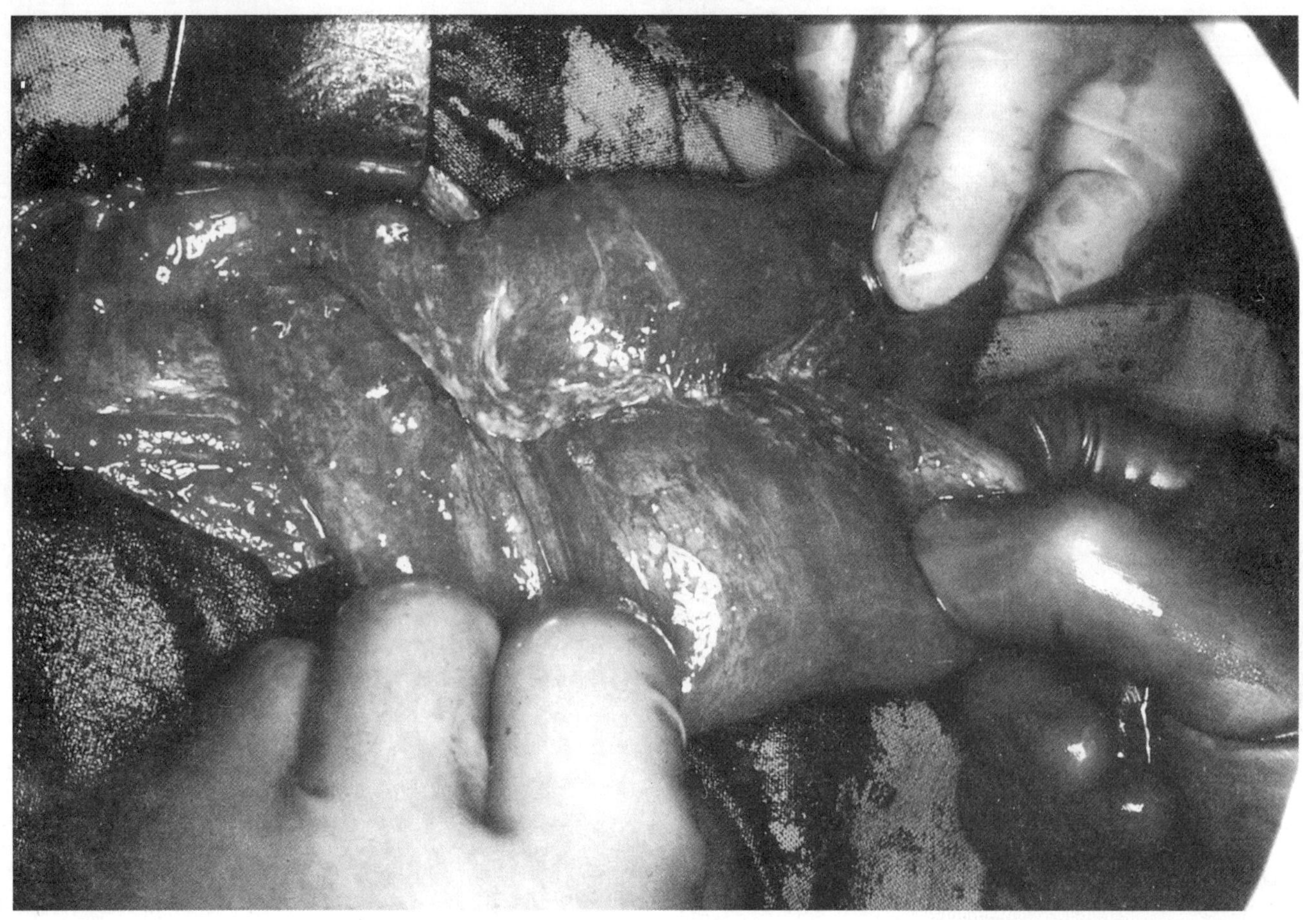

FIGURE 44.6

Operative Technique

FIGURE 44.7
The same patient as in Figure 44.6, after complete enterolysis, from the ligament of Treitz to the ileocecal valve. The previously described enteropexy will be carried out immediately.

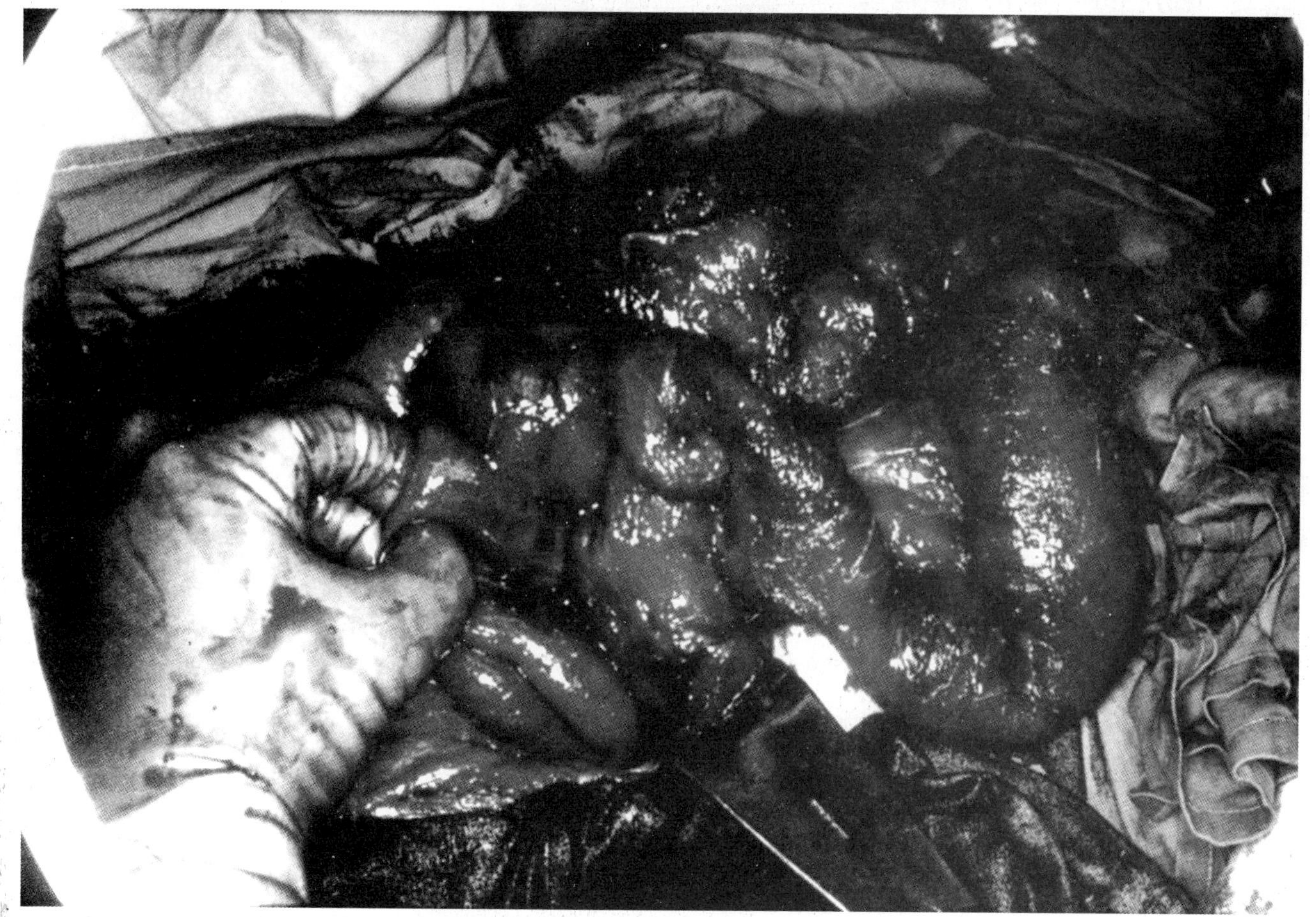

FIGURE 44.7

Operative Technique

FIGURE 44.8
Radiographic examination of the same patient as in Figures 44.6 and 44.7, to study intestinal transit 8 years later. The radiopaque substance can be seen to pass normally through the small bowel.

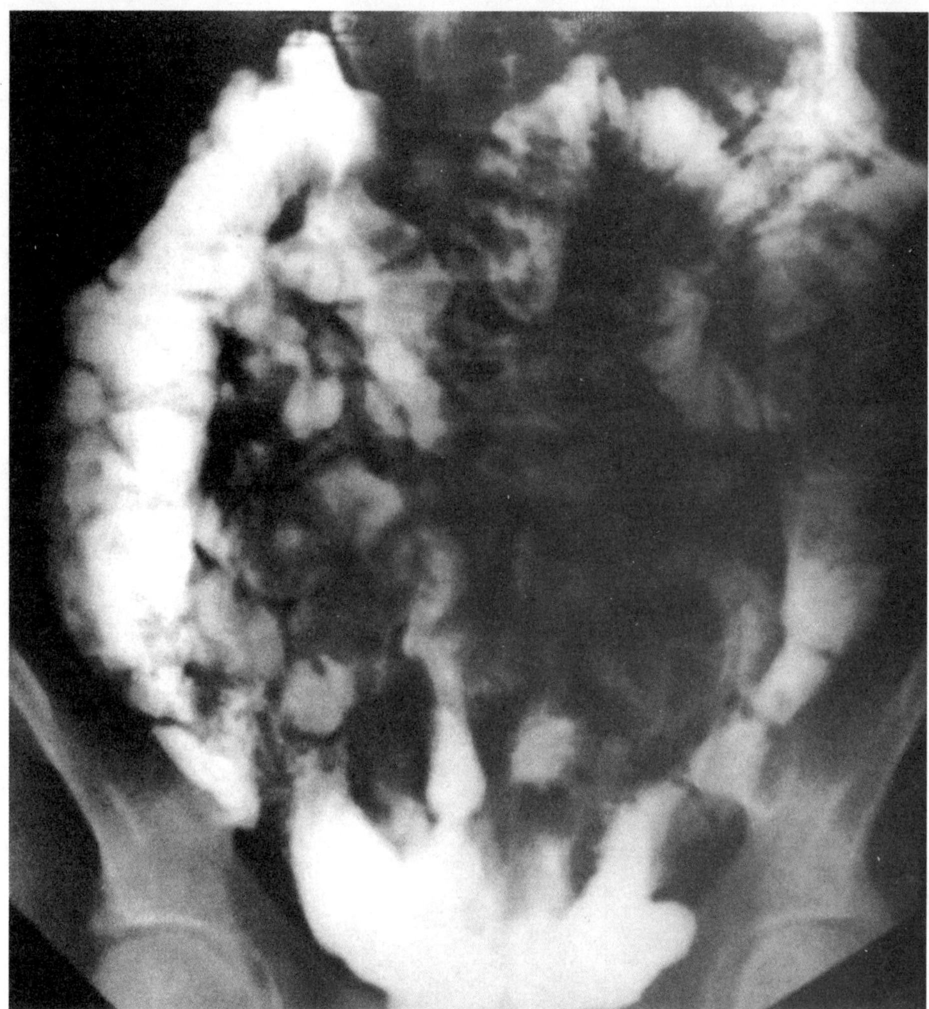

FIGURE 44.8

Operative Technique

FIGURE 44.9
Intestinal decompression and enteropexy with the Baker tube (stitchless plication tube). The most frequent route that is used to introduce a Baker tube at the present time is through a Stamm gastrostomy. The tube is introduced into the stomach with an empty balloon, passing it through the pylorus and the angle of Treitz. The balloon is then partially inflated and passed through the jejunum and ileum manually. When the balloon is near the ileocecal valve, it is emptied completely and passed into the cecum. The balloon is then reinflated and left in that position.

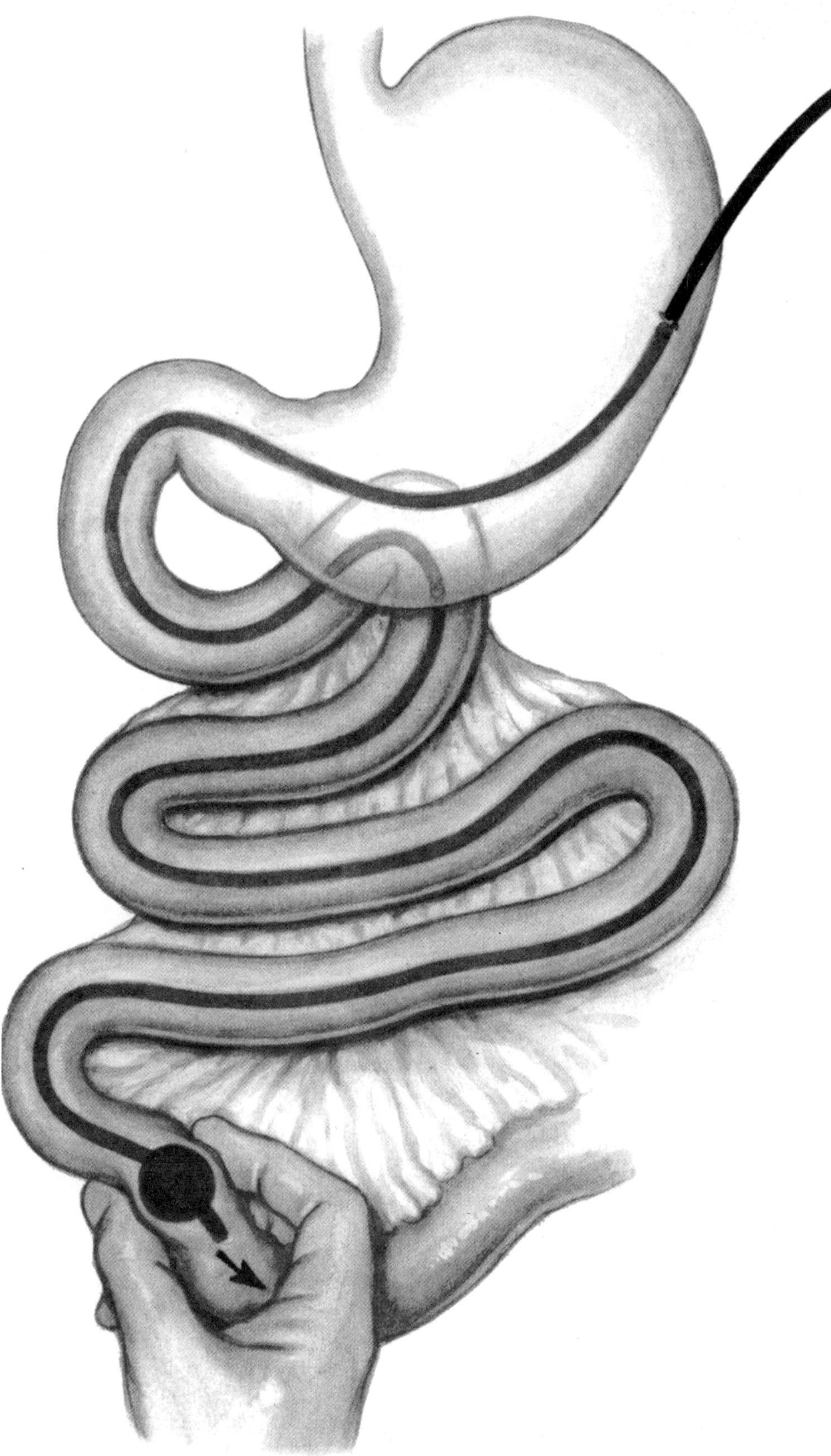

FIGURE 44.9

Operative Technique

FIGURE 44.10
The inflated Baker tube balloon is located in the cecum. The intestinal loops have been plicated in similar fashion as in previous techniques, the Baker tube acting as a stent. About 24 hours later the balloon in the cecum should be emptied to avoid producing an intestinal obstruction. During this period of time the small bowel loops have become adherent to each other, without using any sutures. A Levine nasogastric tube should be left in place to decompress the stomach.

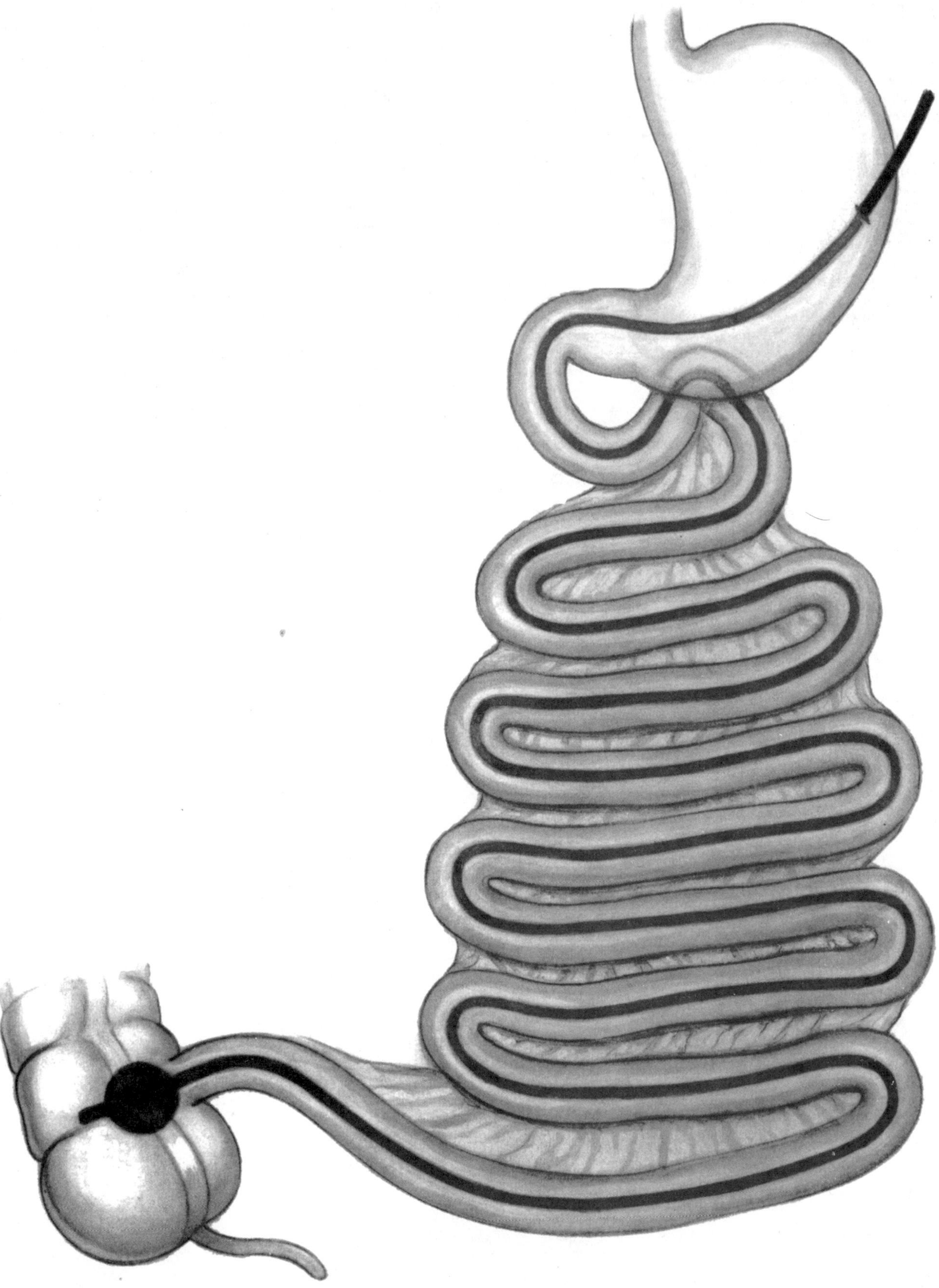

FIGURE 44.10

References

1. Baker, J.W. A long jejunostomy tube for decompressing intestinal obstruction. Surg. Gynecol. Obstet. 109:519, 1959.
2. Baker, J.W. Stitchless plication for recurring obstruction of the small bowel. Am. J. Surg. 116:316, 1968.
3. Baker, J.W. Selective usage of the original and modified Baker intestinal tube. Surg. Gynecol. Obstet. 149:577, 1979.
4. Barron, J., Fallis, L.S. The Noble plication operation for chronic recurring intestinal obstruction. Arch. Surg. 71:518, 1955.
5. Boulvin, R. La plicature mésentérique du grêle ou operation de Childs and Phillips. Ann. Chir. 112:505, 1977.
6. Brightwel, N.L., McFee, A.S., Aust, J.B. Bowel obstruction and the long tube stent. Arch. Surg. 112:505, 1977.
7. Boys, F. The prophylaxis of peritoneal adhesions. A review of the literature. Surgery 11:118, 1942.
8. Close, M.B., Christensen, N.M. Transmesenteric small bowel plication or intraluminal tube stenting. Am. J. Surg. 138:89, 1979.
9. Coletti, L., Bossart, P.A. Intestinal obstruction during the early postoperative period. Arch. Surg. 8:774, 1964.
10. Chassin, J.L. Operative strategy in general surgery. Ed. 2, p. 273. Springer-Verlag, New York, 1994.
11. Childs, W.A., Phillips, R.B. Experience with intestinal plication and a proposed modification. Ann. Surg. 152:258, 1960.
12. Chilimindris, C.P., Stonesifer, G.L. Complications associated with the Baker tube jejunostomy. Am. Surg. 44:707, 1978.
13. Ellis, H. Intestinal Obstruction. Appleton Century Crofts, New York, 1982.
14. Ellis, H. The causes and prevention of intestinal adhesions. Br. J. Surg. 69:241, 1982.
15. Ellis, H. Special forms of intestinal obstruction. In Schwartz, S.I., Ellis, H. (Eds.) Maingot's abdominal operations. Ed. 9, vol. I, p. 905. Appleton Lange, Norwalk, CT, 1990.
16. Farquharson, E.L. Textbook of operative surgery. Ed. 3, p. 640. E. and S. Livingstone, Edinburgh and London, 1966.
17. Ferguson, A.T., Reihmer, V.A., Gaspar, M.R. Transmesenteric plication for small intestinal obstruction. Am. J. Surg. 114:203, 1967.
18. From, D. Small intestine. Obstruction, adhesions. In Fromm, D. (Ed.) Gastrointestinal surgery. Vol. I, p. 371. Churchill Livingstone, New York, 1985.
19. Hollender, L.F., Otten, F., et al. La plicature mésentérique selon Child et Phillips. Lyon Chir. 67:24, 1971.
20. Lamy, J., Louis, R., Michotey, G., Bricot, R., Sarles, J.C. Nouveau traité de technique chirurgicale. Vol. XI, p. 57. Masson et Cie., Paris, 1969.
21. McCarthy, J.D. Further experience with Childs-Phillips plication operation. Am. J. Surg. 130:15, 1975.
22. Noble, T.B. Plication of small intestine as prophylaxis against adhesions. Am. J. Surg. 35:41, 1937.
23. Noble, T.B. Jr. Plication of small intestine. Am. J. Surg. 45:574, 1939.
24. Noble, T.B. Jr. Place of plication in treatment of peritonitis. J. Int. Coll. Surg. 5:513, 1942.
25. Perry, J.F., Smith, G.A., et al. Intestinal obstruction caused by adhesions: A review of 388 cases. Ann. Surg. 142:810, 1955.
26. Pi-Figueras, J. Problema de las adherencias intestinales. In Pi-Figueras, J. (Ed.) Práctica quirúrgica. Ed. 2, vol. II, p. 398. Salvat, Barcelona.
27. Poth, E.J., Lewis, S.R., Wolma, F.J. Treatment of recurrent intestinal obstruction by the plication procedure. Am. Surg. 19:24, 1954.
28. Quenu, J., Thomeret, G. L'opération de Noble. Mém. Acad. Chir. Paris. 77:80, 1951.
29. Reymond, J.C. La plicature segmentaire de l'intestin avec accolement partiel des anses. Sur une façon de réaliser l'operation de Noble. Presse Med. 74:2691, 1966.
30. Richard C.A. La plicature mésentérique. Nouveau traitment des occlusions récidivantes du grêle. Mém. Acad. Chir. 87:256, 1961.
31. Schirmer, B., Scott Jones, R. Small intestine. In Nora, P.F. (Ed.) Operative surgery. Ed. 3, p. 562. W.B. Saunders, Philadelphia, 1990.
32. Sivula, A., Asp, K. Wichmann's plication in the treatment of recurrent intestinal obstruction due to adhesions. Acta Chir. Scand. 131:99, 1966.
33. Vayre, P., Chatelin, C., Grosdidiers Lagache, D., Maillet, P., Pellerin, D. Resultats éloignés de l'operation de Noble et des mésentéricoplicatures. 79 Congr. Franc. Chir. p. 325. Paris, 1977.
34. Weigelt, J.A., Snyder, W.H., Norman, J.L. Complications and results of 160 Baker tube plications. Am. J. Surg. 44:707, 1978.
35. Weigelt, J.A., Snyder, W.H., Norman, J.L. Complications and results of 160 Baker tube plications. Am. J. Surg. 140:810, 1980.
36. Wichmann, S.E. Uber die peritonisierung von wundflachen am dunndarm. Lagenbecks Arch. Chir. 179:589, 1934.
37. Wilson, N.D. Complications of the Noble procedure. Am. J. Surg. 108:264, 1964.

Section G

Small Intestine

CHAPTER **45**

Jejunostomy

Feeding by jejunostomy is an efficacious method in the treatment of patients who are unable to receive nourishment by the normal route. The most frequent indications are in cases of illnesses or surgical interventions of the esophagus, especially esophagogastrectomy, total gastrectomy, gastrectomies that are complicated by gastroduodenal or gastrojejunal fistula, and in the preoperative preparation of malnourished patients who cannot be fed by gastrostomy. By means of a jejunostomy it is possible to provide an adequate amount of elementary nutrition. It is important that the feeding mixtures be given continuously day and night by drops with a stable flow by means of a perfusion pump, under aseptic conditions.

Instead of by means of a jejunal route, feedings can be given by the parenteral route: total parenteral nutrition (TPN), which is frequently used. Some authors (12), however, affirm that jejunal feeding is cheaper than total parenteral nutrition, and if the patient is to continue feedings at home, it is more difficult to do it by the parenteral route than by the jejunal route.

A feeding jejunostomy should have the following conditions fulfilled in order to be efficient:

1. It should be an easy procedure.
2. It should be carried out in the highest possible jejunal segment, in order not to exclude an important part of the small bowel.
3. The jejunostomy should be continent. This means that the feedings that are given should not reflux, neither to the outside nor toward the duodenum.
4. The jejunostomy should not obstruct the transit of biliopancreatic secretions which come from the duodenum.
5. The incision to carry out this procedure should not be placed near the costal border (1, 5–7, 9, 10, 13, 14).

At present, jejunostomy can also be performed by the endoscopic percutaneous route, guided by laparoscopy (3, 4, 11, 12).

Operative Technique

FIGURE 45.1

A midline supraumbilical incision, about 10 cm long, is performed. Once the peritoneum has been opened, the surgeon introduces the right hand into the abdomen to identify the duodenojejunal angle of Treitz, which is located under the transverse mesocolon to the left of the spinal column against the posterior wall of the abdomen. The first jejunal loop is grasped by the surgeon with the right hand and brought out the surgical incision. The rubber jejunostomy tube is to be introduced into the bowel about 30 to 40 cm from the ligament of Treitz. This tube should be 14 F in diameter. The tube should not be placed at a distance of less than 30 cm from the ligament of Treitz, to avoid reflux of feeding into the duodenum. The exteriorized jejunal loop is squeezed between the fingers of both hands to empty it of any contents. The fingers are replaced by two atraumatic clamps, as shown in the drawing, to keep the segment of the jejunum empty of contents. About 35 to 40 cm from the angle of Treitz, in the antimesenteric border of the jejunum, a purse string suture is carried out using 3-0 cotton or silk. Some surgeons perform two concentric purse string sutures to give better support to the tube (14). The surgeon, using the right hand, holds the rubber jejunostomy tube, in which multiple perforations have been made to facilitate the introduction of the feeding solution and diminish the possibility of the tube becoming obstructed. The center point of the purse string is perforated with a fine scalpel or with electrocautery, and, using an atraumatic fine clamp, the opening is held open to facilitate the introduction of the jejunostomy catheter.

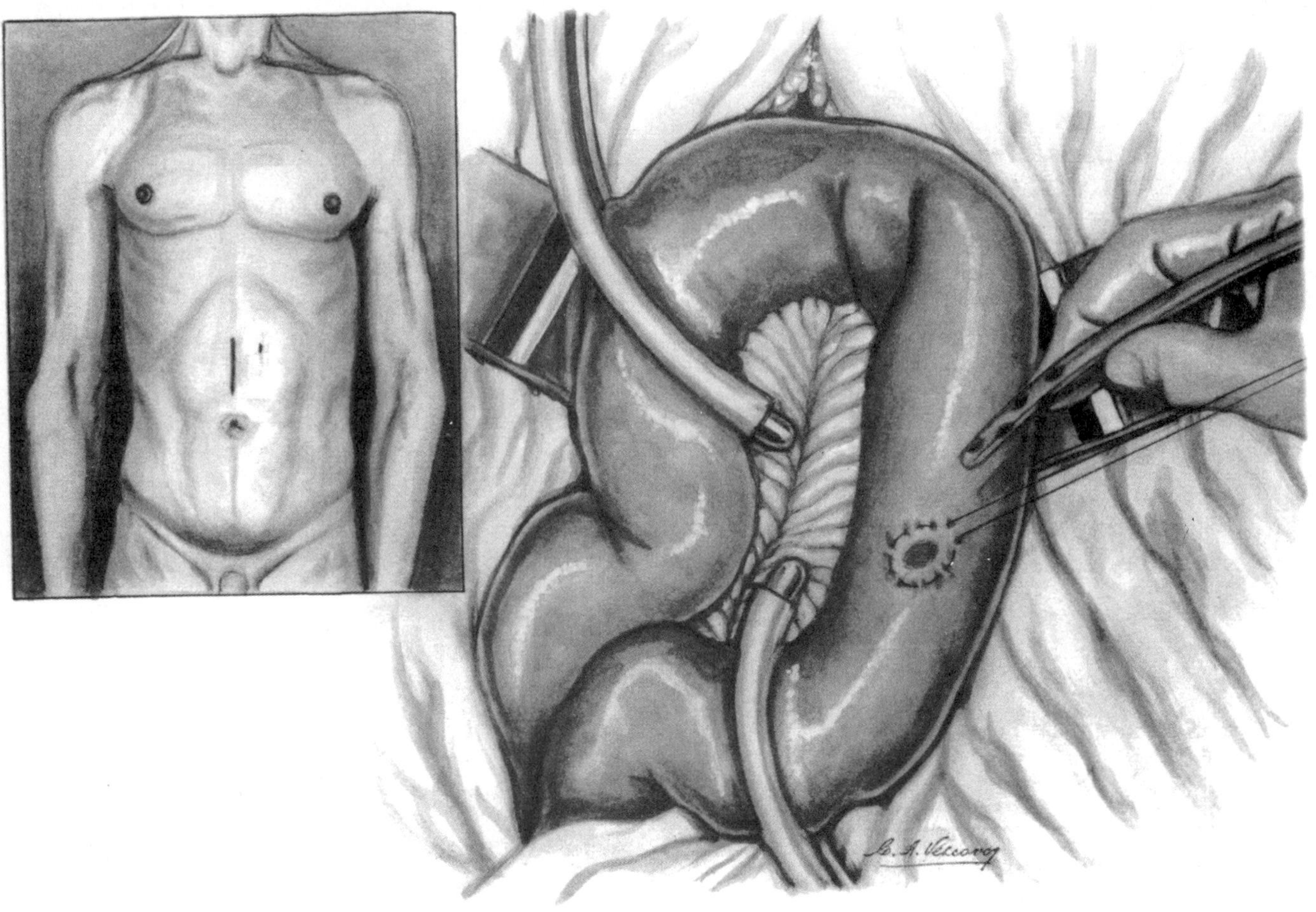

FIGURE 45.1

Operative Technique

FIGURE 45.2
The rubber catheter has been introduced 8 to 10 cm in the same direction as peristalsis. Later the purse string suture is adjusted over the jejunostomy tube.

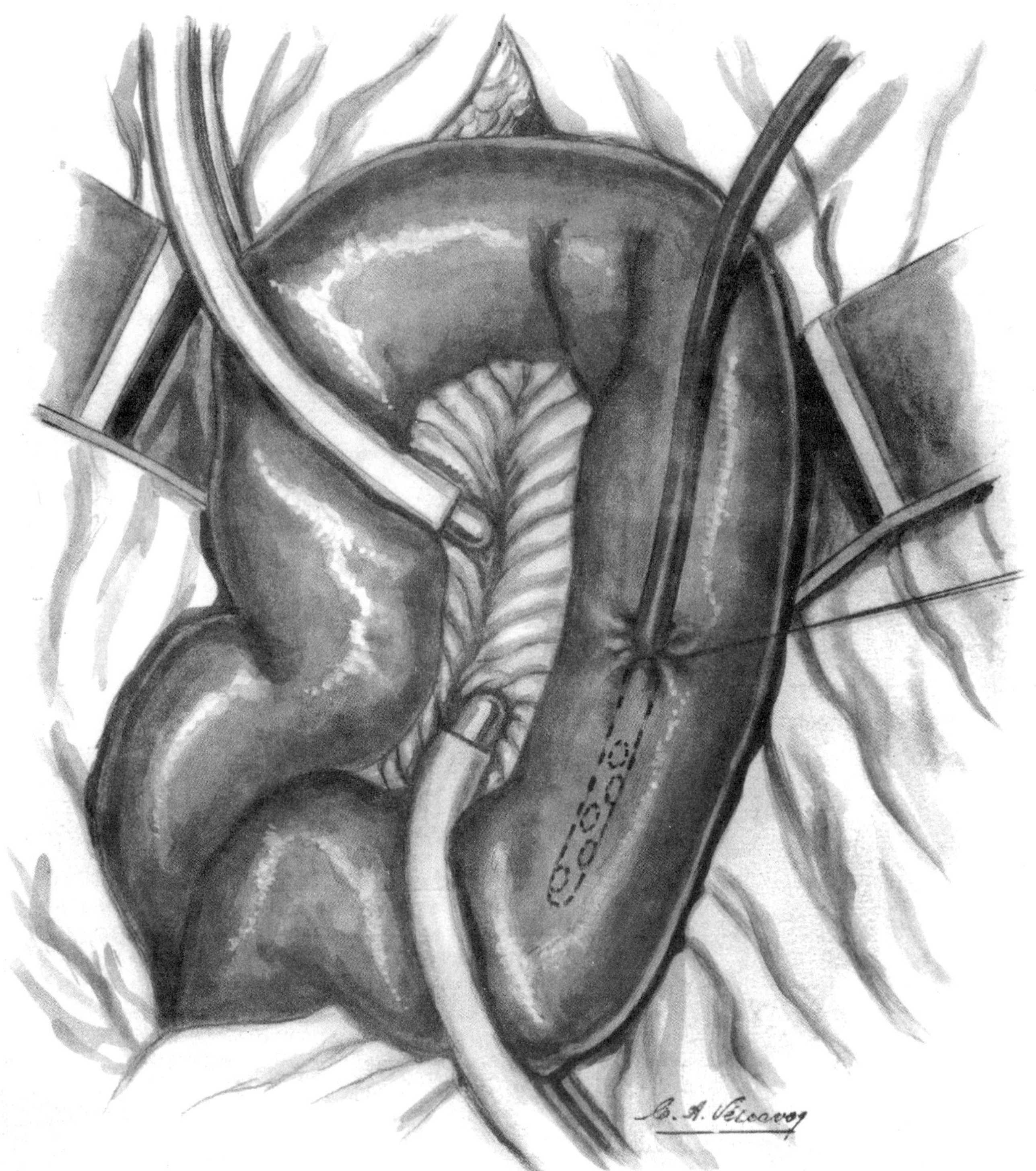

FIGURE 45.2

Operative Technique

FIGURE 45.3
The jejunostomy catheter has been inserted and fixed to the jejunal wall. An extraluminal tunnel will now be constructed using seromuscular sutures according to the Witzel technique. This tunnel should be 8 cm long and carried out using nonabsorbable sutures. A small incision has been made in the upper left quadrant of the anterior abdominal wall in order to allow the jejunostomy catheter to be brought to the outside. A curved long atraumatic clamp has been passed through this cutaneous opening in order to grasp the catheter and bring it out through the abdominal wall.

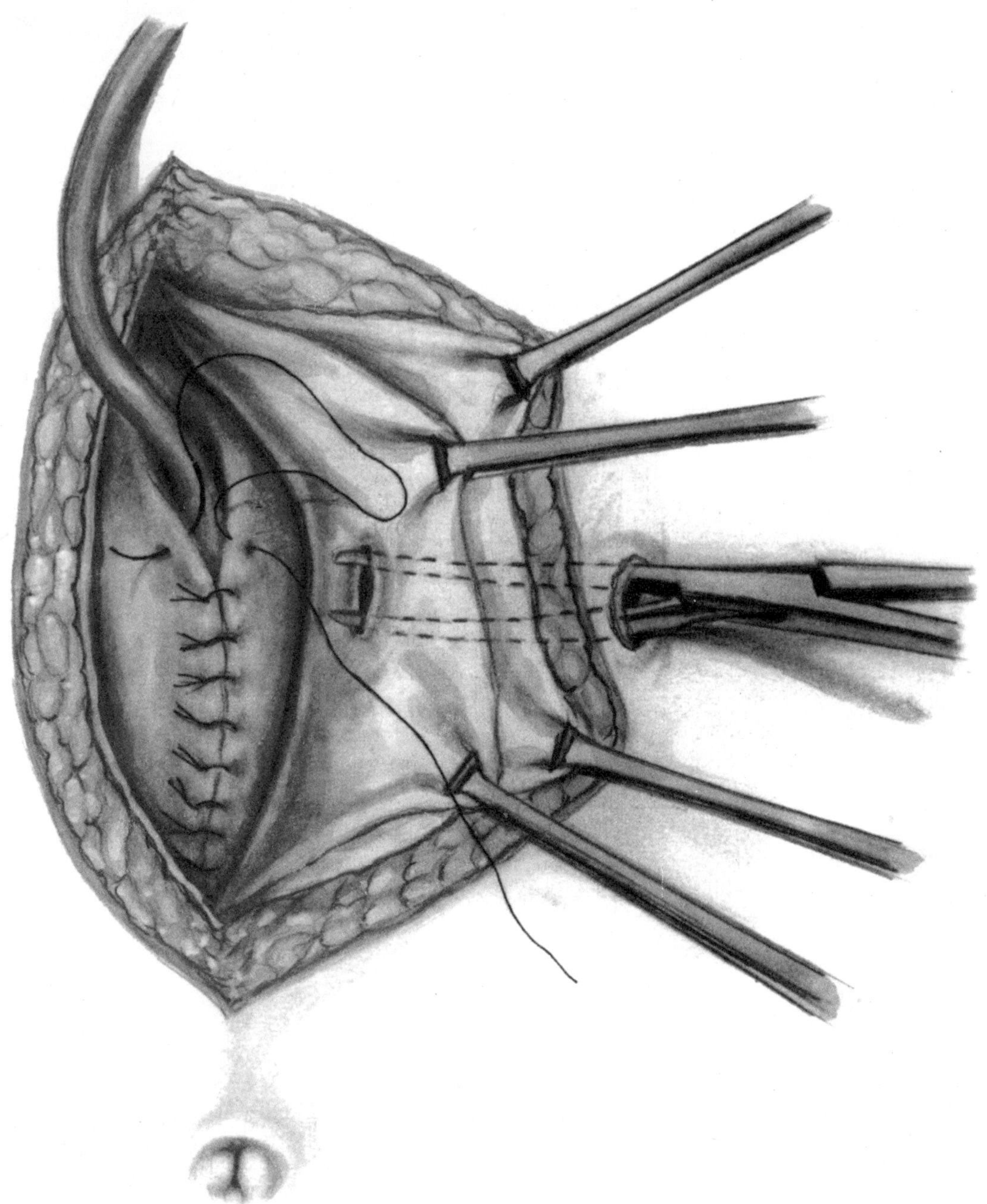

FIGURE 45.3

Operative Technique

FIGURE 45.4
The jejunostomy catheter has been brought out through the abdominal wall, and the jejunal loop is being fixed to the parietal peritoneum and fascia behind the anterior rectus muscle near the exit of the jejunostomy catheter. The jejunum should be fixed to the peritoneum using 3 or 4 sutures. One single suture should not be used because it may lead to a volvulus of the small bowel around the fixed point (14).

The insert shows that the jejunal loop with the tube has been fixed to the parietal peritoneum. The tube has been brought out the small incision in the abdominal wall and is then solidly fixed to the skin with one or more sutures, using nonabsorbable material.

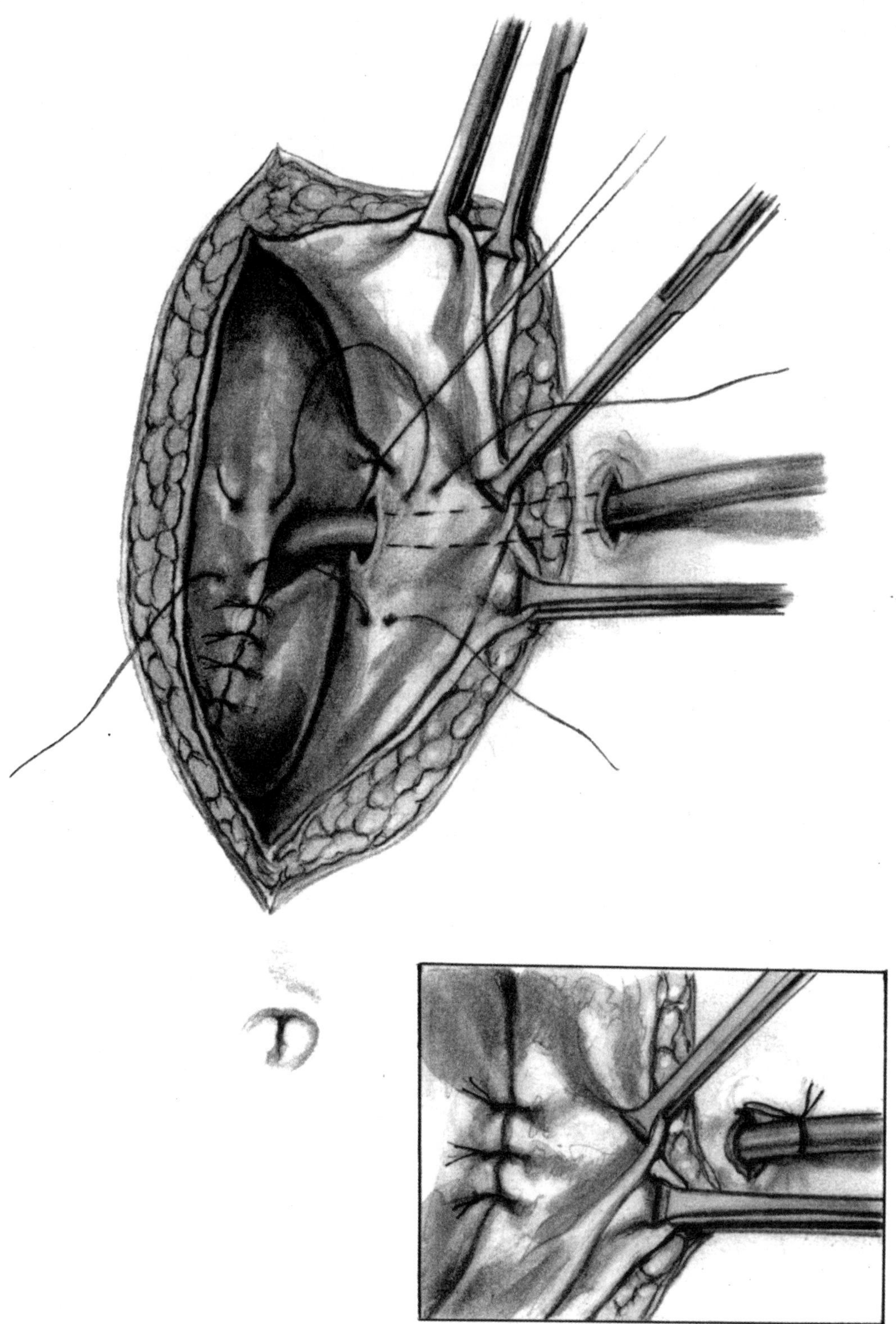

FIGURE 45.4

References

1. Barron, J. Tube feeding of postoperative patients. Surg. Clin. North Am. 39:1481, 1959.
2. Colcock, B.P., Braasch, J.W. Surgery of the small intestine in the adult. p. 178. W.B. Saunders, Philadelphia, 1968.
3. Delany, H.M., Carnevale, N.J., Garvey, J.W. Jejunostomy by a needle catheter technique. Surgery 73:786, 1973.
4. DiSario, J.A., Foutch, P.G., Sanowski, R.A. Poor results with percutaneous endoscopic jejunostomy. Gastrointest. Endosc. 36:257, 1990.
5. Giuliano, A. Clínica y terapéutica quirúrgica. Ed. 3, p. 594. El Ateneo, Buenos Aires, 1976.
6. Herlst, C.A. Continent feeding jejunostomy. Surg. Gynecol. Obstet. 151:555, 1980.
7. Hoover, H.C., Ryan, J.A., Anderson, E.J., Fisher, J.E. Nutritional benefits of immediate postoperative jejunal feeding of an elemental diet. Am. J. Surg. 139:153, 1980.
8. Kirschner, M., Guleke, N., Zenker, R. Allgemeine und spezielle. chirurgische operationslehre. Ed. 2, p. 366, Springer-Verlag, Berlin, 1954.
9. Lamy, J., Louis, R., Michotey, G., Bricot, R., Sarles, J.C. Nouveau traité de technique chirurgicale. Vol. XI, p. 28. Masson et Cie., Paris, 1969.
10. Rumbo, H.G. Nutrición y cirugía. In Ortiz, F.E., Miranda, N.E., Moirano, J.J., Fassi, J.C. (Eds.) Cirugía. Ed. 3, p. 111. El Ateneo, Buenos Aires, 1993.
11. Sangster, W., Hunter, J.G. Surgical access for enteral nutrition. In Hunter, J.G., Sackier, J.M. Minimally invasive surgery. p. 113. McGraw-Hill, New York, 1993.
12. Schirmer, B., Scott, Jones, R. Small intestine. In Nora, P.F. (Ed.) Operative surgery. Ed. 3, p. 562. Philadelphia, 1990.
13. Torras, P.A., Nogueras, F.M. Enterostomías. In Pi Figueras, J. (Ed.) Práctica quirúrgica. Ed. 2, p. 356. Salvat, Barcelona, 1986.
14. Zollinger, R.M., Zollinger, R.M. Jr. Atlas of surgical operations. Ed. 4, p. 84. Macmillan, New York, 1975.

Section G
Small Intestine

CHAPTER 46
Meckel's Diverticulum

Meckel (12) was not the first surgeon to describe the diverticulum that carries his name, but he did carry out a very complete study of this anomaly and investigated its embryologic origin. Meckel's diverticulum is the most frequent malformation of the digestive tract and is made up of all the layers of the small bowel: mucosa, submucosa, muscularis, and serosa. This means that it is a true diverticulum. Meckel's diverticulum is always found on the antimesenteric border of the ileum, most frequently 40 to 50 cm from the ileocecal valve. According to Jay and colleagues (9), 28% of the Meckel's diverticula are located over 91 cm from the ileocecal valve. These authors were able to prove in their studies that the most distant diverticulum from the ileocecal valve was 167 cm away. Williams (23) observed the presence of diverticula up to 180 cm from the ileocecal valve.

The most frequent length of Meckel's diverticulum varies between 3 and 6 cm, with a medium transverse diameter of 2 cm (5, 9). Wansbrough and colleagues (22) have affirmed that the length of Meckel's diverticulum may vary between 1 and 26 cm but that 75% of cases have a length of 1 to 5 cm. The author has seen a case of a patient with a Meckel's diverticulum 34 cm long, which presented abdominal symptoms due to its size. The shape of a Meckel's diverticulum has been compared to that of a finger of a glove (5, 6). This embryonic abnormality is seen in from 1 to 2% of persons, according to several statistics.

The mucosa of a Meckel's diverticulum has the same structure as the mucosa of the ileum. However, the exclusive presence of ileal mucosa in the diverticulum is only found in 50% of cases (1, 5, 7, 9, 18). Frequently, heterotopic gastric mucosa coexists with ileal mucosa in the diverticulum (1, 5, 6, 8, 9). This gastric mucosa is of the fundic type and secretes acid. Less frequently, the ileal mucosa in the diverticulum coexists with duodenal, jejunal, or colonic mucosa. On the other hand, in 4 to 5% of cases (1, 9), nodules of pancreatic heterotopic tissue are found. The presence of peptic ulcer in a Meckel's diverticulum due to the presence of heterotopic gastric mucosa was discovered by Hübschmann in 1913 (8). The blood supply of a Meckel's diverticulum comes from the superior mesenteric artery. This artery, which irrigates the diverticulum, arises in the same vascular arcade from which other straight vessels arise, but runs in a different trajectory than the other straight vessels.

Meckel's diverticulum is a remnant of the vitelline duct from the embryonic stage. In the embryo the middle portion of the small bowel is connected to the vitelline sac by means of the vitelline duct, also known as the omphalomesenteric duct. As the embryo develops, the vitelline duct becomes obliterated, becoming a chord or fibrous band, which is later reabsorbed (5–7, 11, 21, 22). Obliteration of the vitelline duct takes place in the seventh week of embryonic development, at the time that the communication which existed between the midintestine and the vitelline sac was interrupted. If the vitelline duct does not become occluded or only becomes partially occluded, it can lead to a series of pathologic alterations (24 in all). We will only cover the most frequent alterations that are observed:

1. *Omphaloileal Fistula.* This is caused by persistence of the vitelline duct, which is not obliterated in any of its segments, for which reason a communication between the ileum and the skin of the abdomen, at the level of the umbilicus, persists (4–6). This anomaly is found in 2 to 6% of cases (Fig. 46.1).
2. *Umbilical Sinus.* This pathologic alteration is found in cases in which a limited segment of the vitelline duct is not occluded in the vicinity of the umbilicus, for which reason there is a cutaneous umbilical opening that communicates the sinus to the outside. Mucus secretions are observed, but no ileal content is observed because there is no communication between the umbilical sinus and the ileum. This alteration is seen in 1% of cases (Fig. 46.2).
3. *Vitelline Cyst.* This malformation originates when a segment of the vitelline duct, near the umbilicus, has been obliterated and a segment of this duct near the ileum has also been obliterated, but there remains a persistent portion in the midportion of the duct, giving origin to a cystic formation which accumulates mucus secretions. This alteration is found in 1% of cases (Fig. 46.3).
4. *Fibrous Band or Chord.* If the vitelline duct is obliterated but not reabsorbed, a fibrous band or chord is formed joining the ileum with the umbilicus. A similar fibrous chord may develop in cases in which the vitelline duct is obliterated and reabsorbed but the omphalomesenteric vessels are not reabsorbed. In both situations the fibrous band may give rise to obstructive complications of the small bowel. This malformation is seen in 10% of cases.
5. *Meckel's Diverticulum.* This malformation develops in cases in which a segment of the vitelline duct near the ileum remains permeable, while the rest of the vitelline duct is obliterated. This anomaly occurs in between 82 and 96% of the cases, according to several statistics (5, 6, 9, 11, 17, 18, 21–23). A Meckel's diverticulum may present in two ways: (a) The diverticulum is free, that is, not joined to the umbilicus by a fibrous chord. This condition is seen in 76% of the cases (5, 6, 22). (See Fig. 46-4) (b) The diverticulum is joined from its apex to the umbilicus by a fibrous chord, which represents the rest of the vitelline duct that has become obliterated but not reabsorbed. This anomalous condition represents about 24% of the cases (17, 18, 22). (See Fig. 46.5.)

In the great majority of patients, Meckel's diverticula are completely asymptomatic and are usually discovered during a surgical exploration of the abdomen for some other cause. Meckel's diverticulum produces symptoms only when complications have arisen. The most frequent complications of a Meckel's diverticulum, as well as other anomalies that are due to the embryologic development of the vitelline duct, are as follows:

1. *Peptic Ulcer.* Peptic ulcer originates due to the presence of a fundic type of heterotopic gastric mucosa. The peptic ulcer is usually located in the ileal mucosa, near the diverticulum. Less frequently, the peptic ulcer is located inside the diverticulum. Heterotopic gastric mucosa is found in a Meckel's diverticulum about 50% of the time. (See Figs. 46.15 and 46.16.) The most frequent complication of a peptic ulcer in this location is massive bleeding with passage of red blood from the rectum or melena. In some cases there is less loss of blood and it is intermittent. This complication occurs in about 40% of the cases. Hemorrhage due to peptic ulcer in this location is generally seen in children and young patients, although less frequently it can occur in adults. Endoscopy and a negative radiographic gastroduodenal examination in children or young people with hemorrhage through the rectum should lead to a suspicion of the diagnosis of peptic ulcer in a Meckel's diverticulum. Study of patients with technetium has given good results in the demonstration of fundic heterotopic gastric mucosa in the diverticulum. Less frequently, peptic ulcer in this location may be complicated by perforation.
2. *Intestinal Obstruction.* Intestinal obstruction is next in frequency to hemorrhage caused by peptic ulcer. This complication is seen in 32% of cases (5, 6). The obstruction of the bowel may develop in several ways, one of them being intestinal invagination with the diverticulum as the head of the invagination (Fig. 46.8). Intestinal obstruction can also be produced by incarceration of a Meckel's diverticulum in

an inguinal hernia. This alteration was described by Littré in 1701 (10). Meckel described it in 1809. Herniation of a Meckel's diverticulum is usually designated as a Littré's hernia (Fig. 46.9). Obstructive complications can develop in cases in which the Meckel's diverticulum is connected to the umbilicus by a fibrous chord (Fig. 46.6). Obstructive complications can develop without the presence of a Meckel's diverticulum in cases in which the vitelline duct has become occluded but has not been reabsorbed.

3. *Inflammation of Meckel's Diverticulum.* Acute inflammation of Meckel's diverticulum (acute diverticulitis) occupies the third place in the complications caused by the presence of a Meckel's diverticulum. It has a frequency of 17.6% (Fig. 46.10). It is very difficult to clinically differentiate acute Meckel's diverticulitis from acute appendicitis, with which it is usually confused. This diagnosis is generally made during surgical exploration of the abdomen. If a laparotomy has been performed with a diagnosis of acute appendicitis, but exploration shows that the appendix appears to be normal, one should not forget to explore the distal 160 cm of the ileum in search of an acute Meckel's diverticulitis.
4. *Neoplasms of Meckel's Diverticulum.* A Meckel's diverticulum can be the seat of benign or malignant neoplasms. This occurs in 2 to 6% of cases (5, 6). The following are some of the tumors that can develop in a Meckel's diverticulum: leiomyoma, leiomyosarcoma, carcinoid, and adenocarcinoma. Logically, surgical treatment of malignant lesions of a Meckel's diverticulum should be radical. The ileum should be resected, dividing it some 20 to 30 cm proximal to the tumor and including the right colon in the resected specimen.

SURGICAL TREATMENT OF MECKEL'S DIVERTICULUM

Even though, as stated previously, the great majority of Meckel's diverticula occur in completely asymptomatic fashion and are generally a surgical finding while the abdomen is being explored for some other cause, they can lead to serious and even mortal complication such as hemorrhage, intestinal obstruction, perforated acute diverticulitis, and so on. Mortality of resection of complicated Meckel's diverticulum is from 5 to 10%. This elevated mortality is usually due to delay in making the diagnosis and deciding on surgery.

Some surgeons (5, 6) believe that resection of a Meckel's diverticulum should be performed even if it is healthy, simply because it may lead to complications in the future and the mortality of resection of a healthy Meckel's diverticulum is infinitesimal. Other surgeons believe that although the possibility of a Meckel's diverticulum developing complications is remote, they do not accept its routine resection. The author believes that all asymptomatic Meckel's diverticula should be resected in the following cases:

1. Diverticula with a narrow neck in children or young patients.
2. When palpation of the diverticulum reveals increased thickening of its walls due to the presence of heterotopic gastric mucosa or nodules (heterotopic pancreas). The presence of heterotopic gastric mucosa usually produces an increase in the consistency of the wall of the diverticulum.
3. Meckel's diverticulum joined from its vertex to the umbilicus by a fibrous band. On the other hand, if a Meckel's diverticulum has a wide neck and does not present changes in the consistency of its walls, especially in adults, it is not necessary to carry out its resection.

Simple resection of a Meckel's diverticulum can be performed in cases in which it is not complicated by an ulcerative process, inflammation, or obstruction. The technique for the resection of an uncomplicated Meckel's diverticulum will be described later. In cases in which the diverticulum is complicated by an ulcerative process, the ulcer is frequently in the ileum and not in the diverticulum itself. For this reason, resection of the diverticulum will not include resection of the ulcer. In these cases, it is necessary to carry out a segmental resection of the ileum, which will permit resection of the diverticulum and the ulcer. This technique will be described later.

In patients with acute diverticulitis, it is frequent that the acute inflammation of the diverticulum extends to the walls of the ileum, which also makes it necessary to carry out a resection of a segment of ileum together with the diverticulum. In patients with an acute intestinal obstruction caused by the presence of a fibrous band, in patients with intestinal invagination due to the diverticulum, or in cases with a Littré hernia, the surgeon will determine after reduction of the obstruction the extent of intestinal resection to be carried out. This means that the surgical procedure should be adapted not only to the presence of a Meckel's diverticulum, but to the nature of the complication, its extent, the presence of intestinal obstruction, and the possibility of other simultaneous embryologic complications.

FIGURE 46.1 OMPHALOILEAL FISTULA
The vitelline duct or omphalomesenteric duct has not been obliterated, leaving a communication open between the ileum and the skin at the level of the umbilicus.

Surgical Treatment of Meckel's Diverticulum

FIGURE 46.2 UMBILICAL SINUS
The vitelline duct has been obliterated in almost its entire extension except at the level of the umbilicus where it remains open.

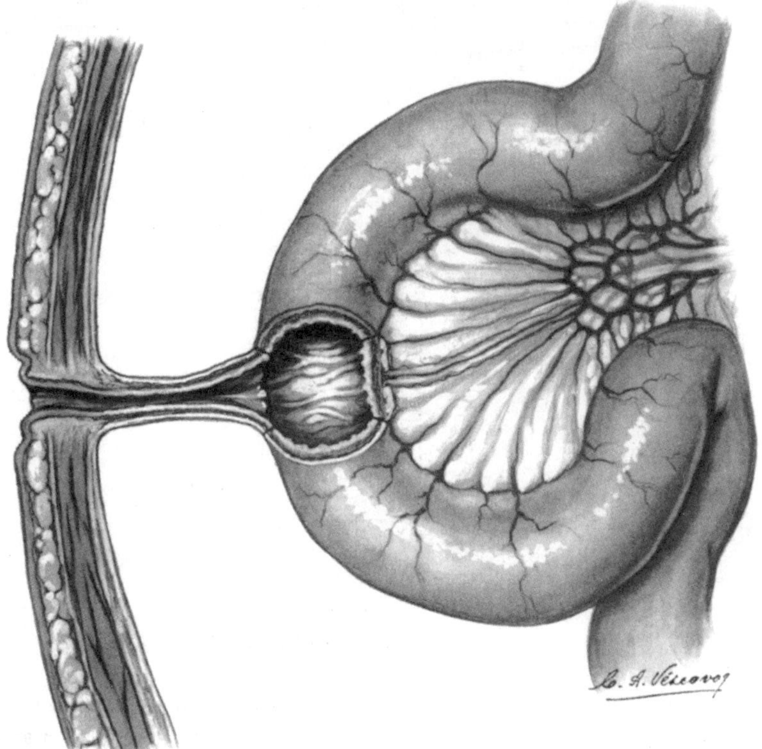

FIGURE 46.1 OMPHALOILEAL FISTULA

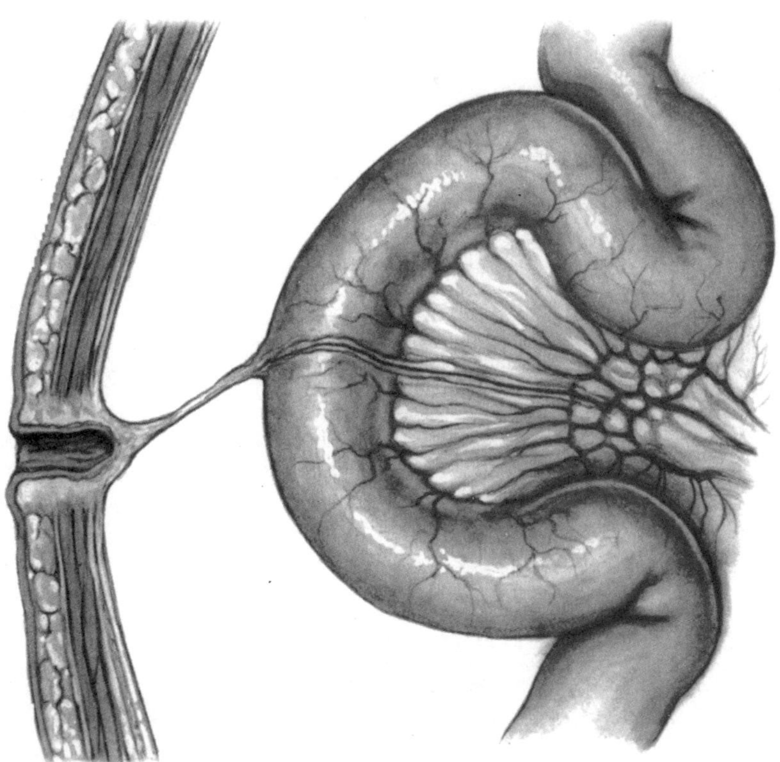

FIGURE 46.2 UMBILICAL SINUS

FIGURE 46.3 VITELLINE CYST
The vitelline duct has become obliterated in the segment near the umbilicus as well as in the segment near the ileum. Only the middle portion of the duct remains patent. This leads to the formation of a cyst with accumulation of mucus secretion.

Surgical Treatment of Meckel's Diverticulum

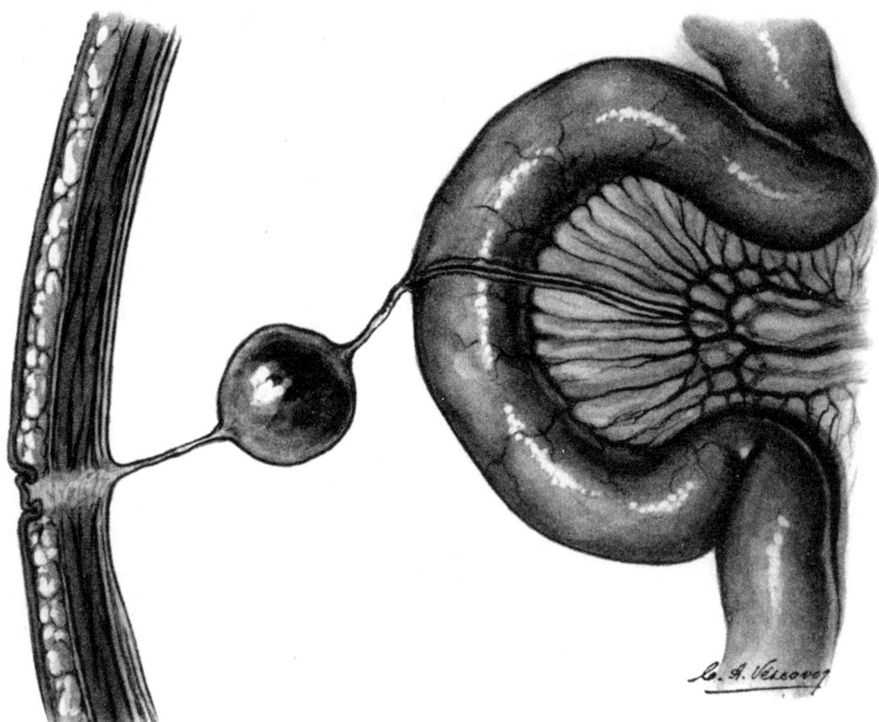

FIGURE 46.3 VITELLINE CYST

FIGURE 46.4 MECKEL'S DIVERTICULUM
This diverticulum is due to a malformation of a vitelline duct, which, as a result, has remained patent only in the segment of the duct near the ileum. The rest of the vitelline duct has been obliterated and reabsorbed. The diverticulum is free and can be seen to have its blood supply coming from a branch of the superior mesenteric artery, running subserosally up to the vertex of the diverticulum.

Surgical Treatment of Meckel's Diverticulum

FIGURE 46.5 MECKEL'S DIVERTICULUM JOINED TO THE UMBILICUS BY A FIBROUS BAND
This malformation may lead to small bowel obstruction.

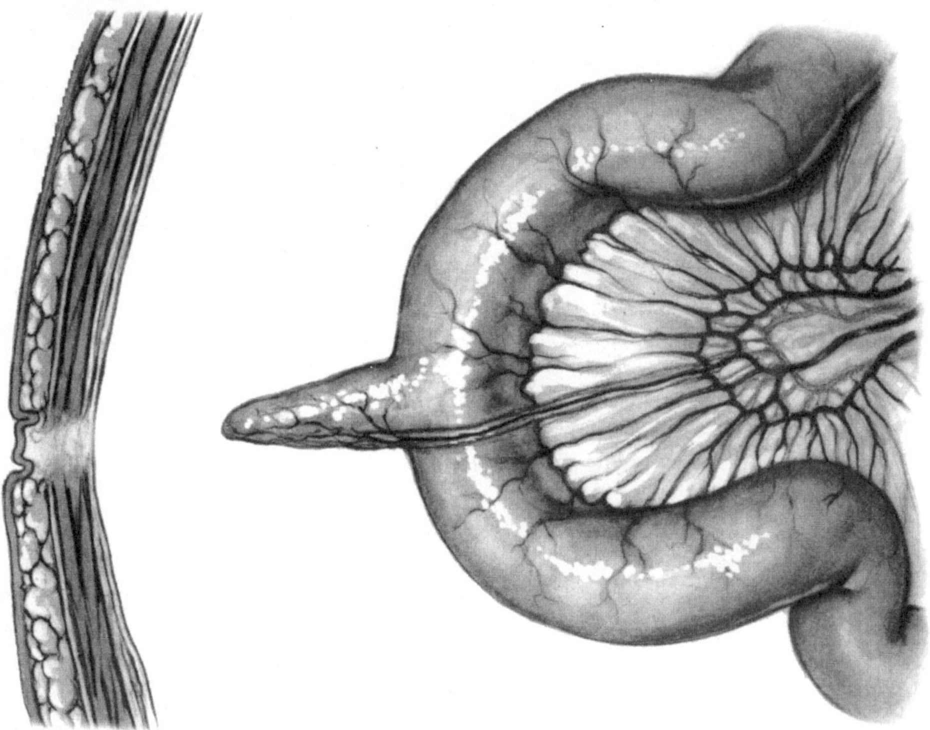

FIGURE 46.4 MECKEL'S DIVERTICULUM

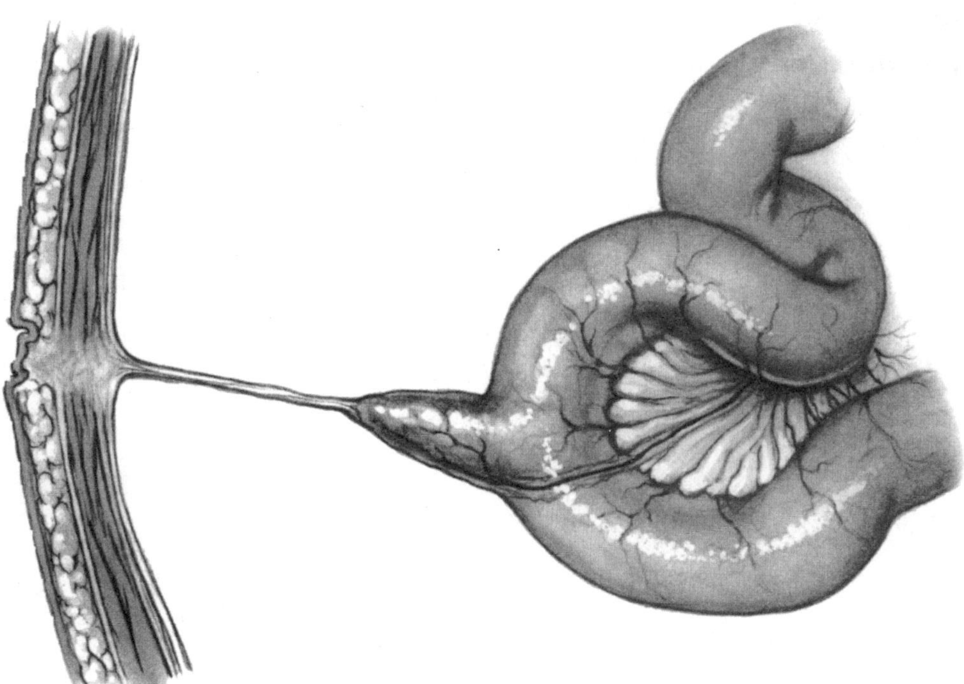

FIGURE 46.5 MECKEL'S DIVERTICULUM JOINED TO THE UMBILICUS BY A FIBROUS BAND

FIGURE 46.6 MECKEL'S DIVERTICULUM JOINED TO THE UMBILICUS BY A FIBROUS BAND

This arrangement has given rise to a bowel obstruction with strangulation due to twisting of the small bowel around the fibrous band.

Surgical Treatment of Meckel's Diverticulum

FIGURE 46.7 MECKEL'S DIVERTICULUM JOINED TO THE POSTERIOR ABDOMINAL WALL BY A FIBROUS BAND

This arrangement has given origin to obstruction of the bowel.

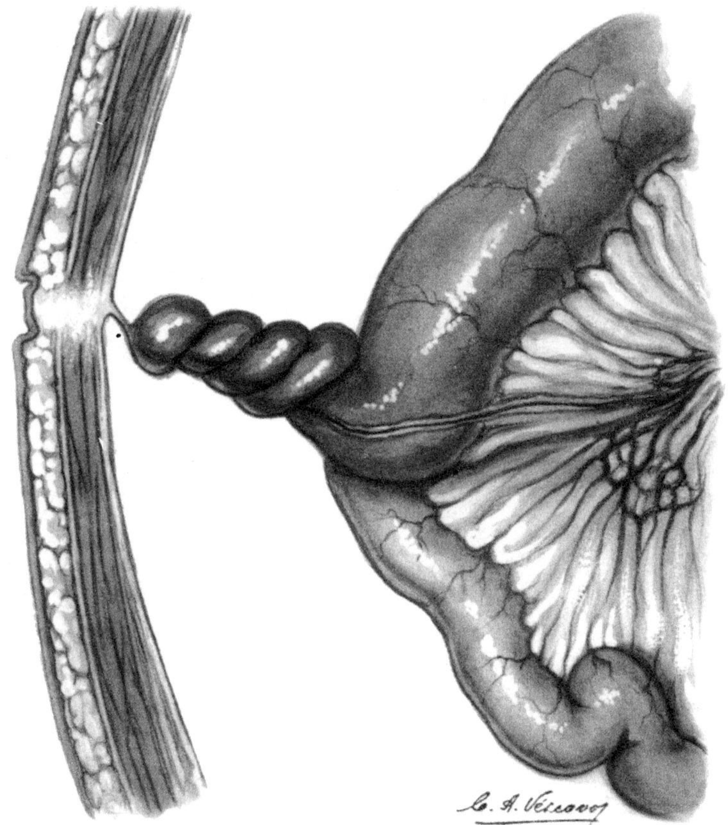

FIGURE 46.6 MECKEL'S DIVERTICULUM JOINED TO THE UMBILICUS BY A FIBROUS BAND

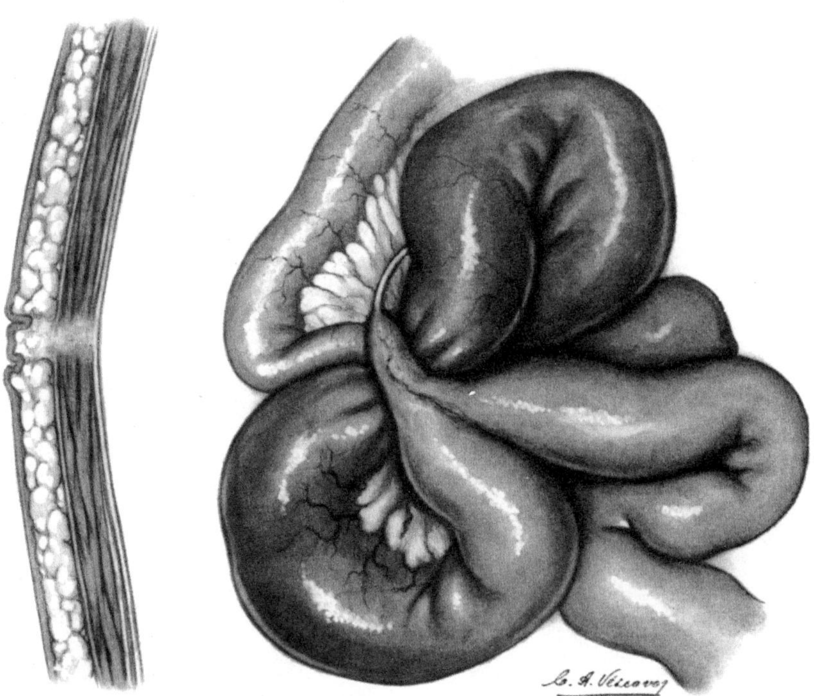

FIGURE 46.7 MECKEL'S DIVERTICULUM JOINED TO THE POSTERIOR ABDOMINAL WALL BY A FIBROUS BAND

Surgical Treatment of Meckel's Diverticulum

FIGURE 46.8 INTESTINAL OBSTRUCTION DUE TO INVAGINATION

The Meckel's diverticulum acts as the lead for the invagination.

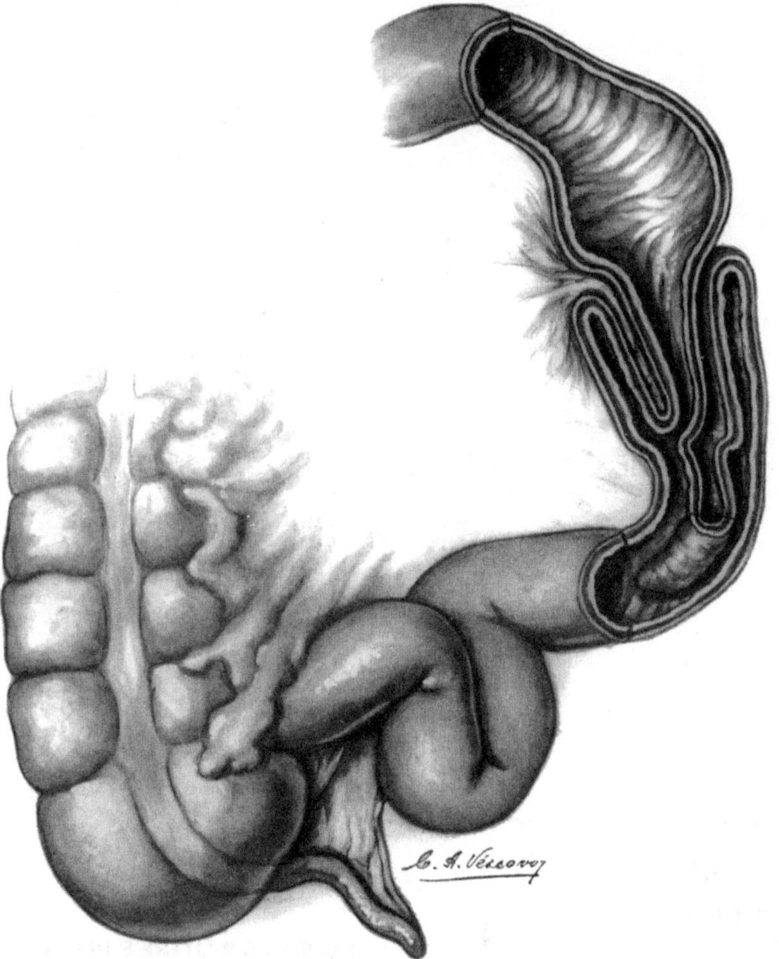

FIGURE 46.8 INTESTINAL OBSTRUCTION DUE TO INVAGINATION

Surgical Treatment of Meckel's Diverticulum

FIGURE 46.9 LITTRE'S HERNIA
A Meckel's diverticulum has become incarcerated in the hernial sac of a right inguinal hernia, giving rise to intestinal obstruction.

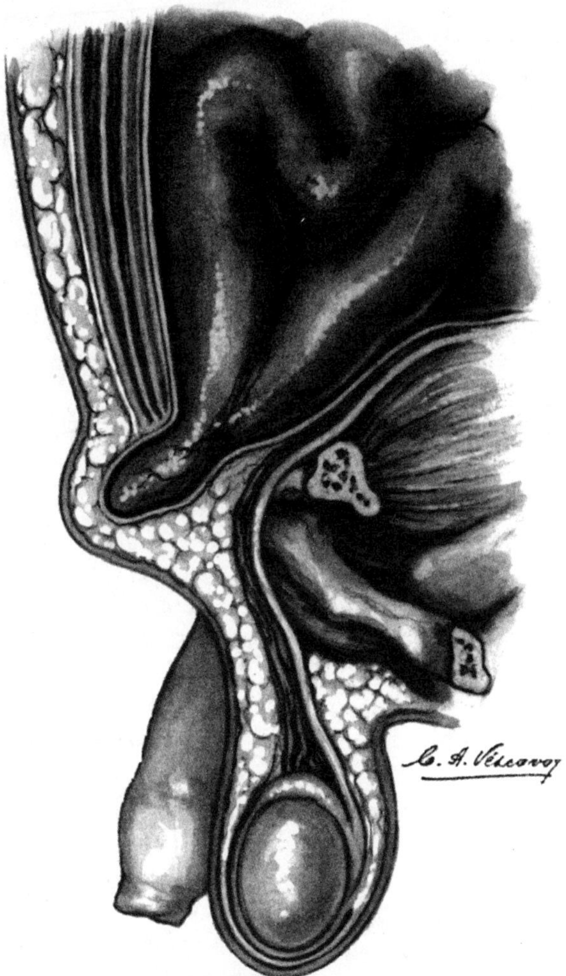

FIGURE 46.9 LITTRE'S HERNIA

FIGURE 46.10 ACUTE MECKEL'S DIVERTICULITIS
The Meckel's diverticulum has undergone an acute inflammatory process. Meckel's diverticulitis can be very difficult to differentiate clinically from acute appendicitis.

Surgical Treatment of Meckel's Diverticulum

FIGURE 46.11 RESECTION OF A MECKEL'S DIVERTICULUM
The apex of the diverticulum is grasped by a Babcock clamp. Two traction sutures are placed on the antimesenteric border of the ileum on each side of the base of the diverticulum. The artery supplying the diverticulum, coming from the superior mesenteric artery, is ligated. This artery is clearly distinguished from the other arterial branches irrigating the ileum.

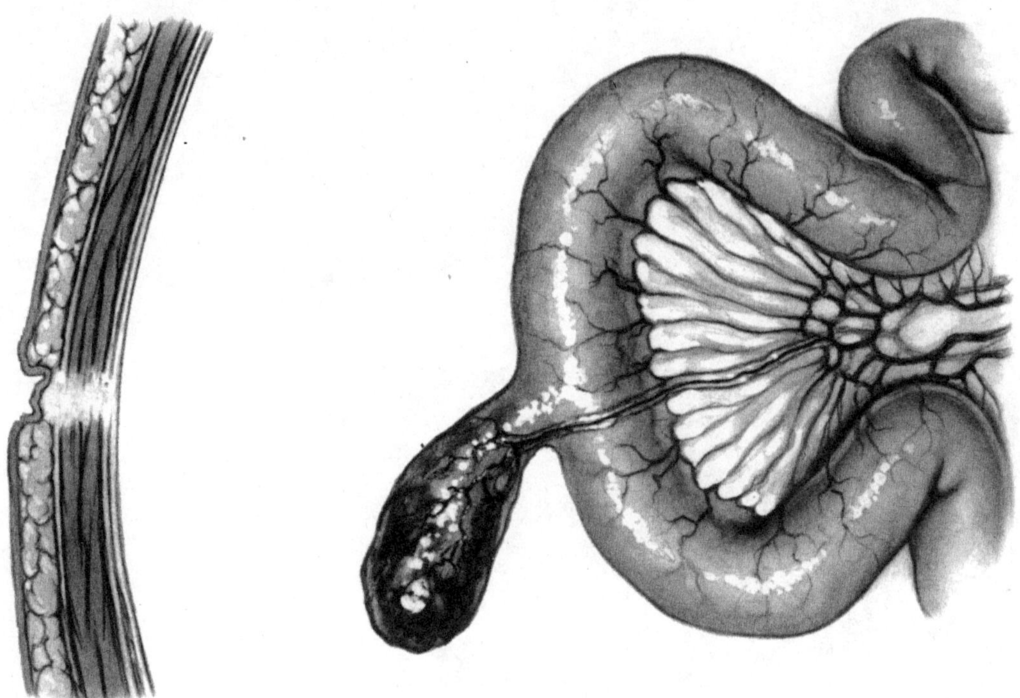

FIGURE 46.10 ACUTE MECKEL'S DIVERTICULITIS

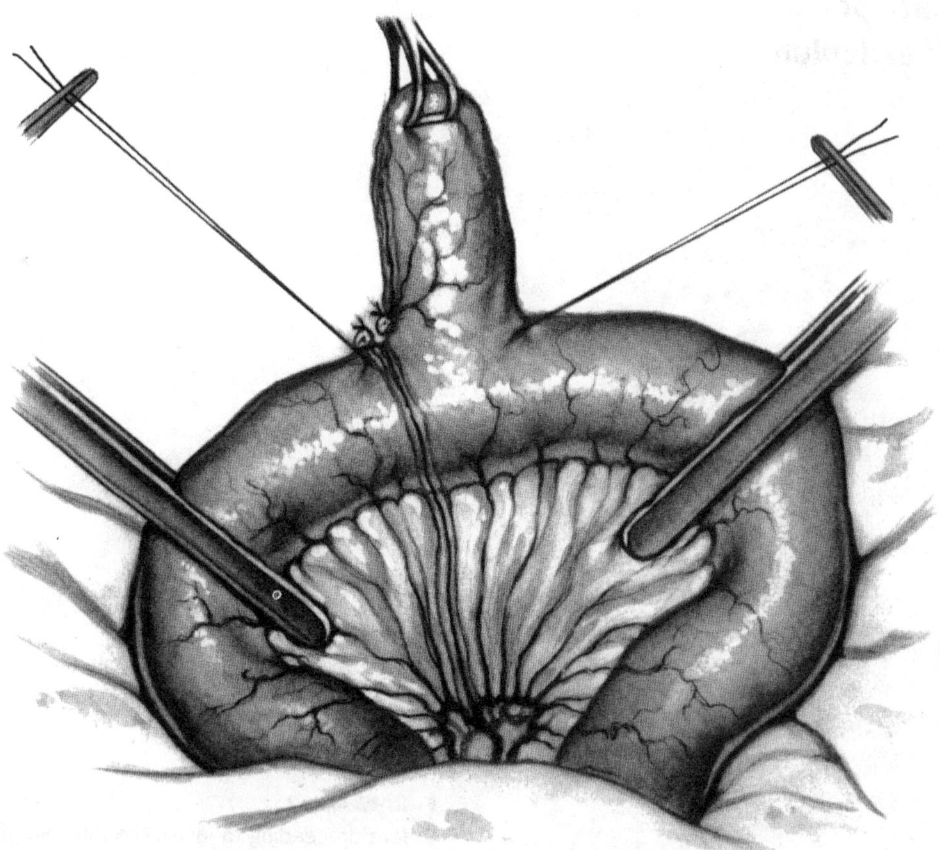

FIGURE 46.11 RESECTION OF A MECKEL'S DIVERTICULUM

FIGURE 46.12
The seromuscular layer at the base of the diverticulum has been divided with a scalpel.

Surgical Treatment of Meckel's Diverticulum

FIGURE 46.13
Before proceeding to incise the mucosa of the Meckel's diverticulum, two atraumatic clamps are placed on each side of the diverticulum.

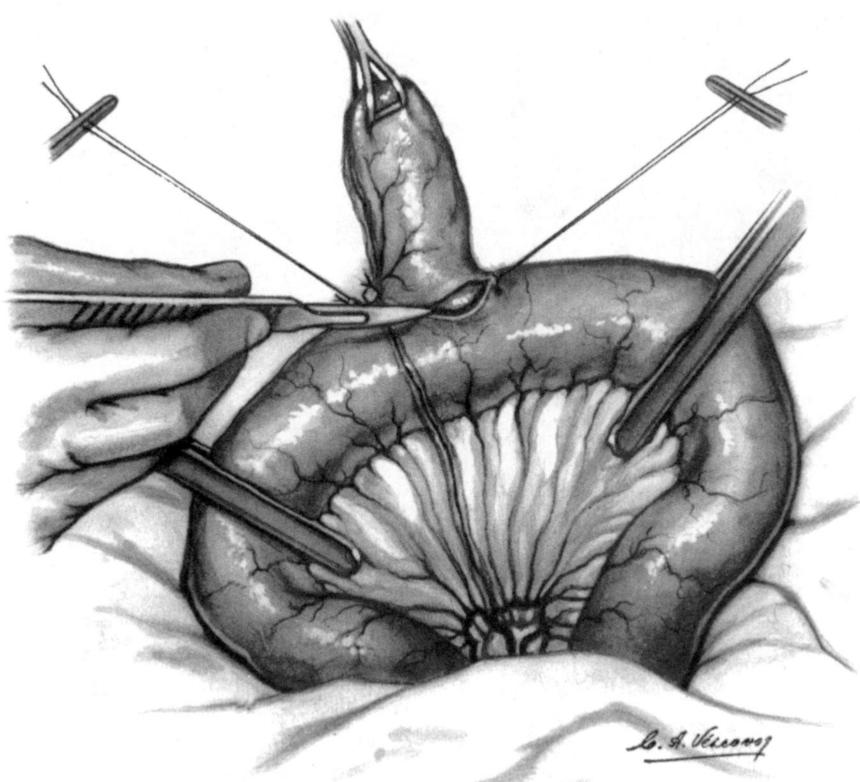

FIGURE 46.12

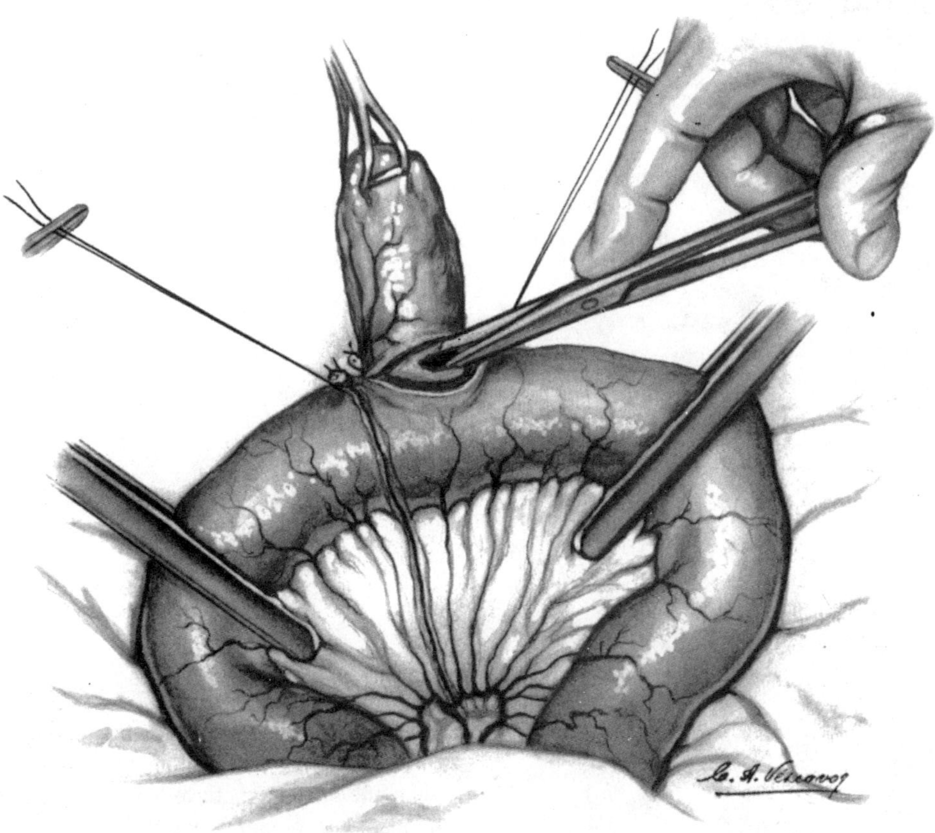

FIGURE 46.13

FIGURE 46.14

Once the diverticulum has been excised, the opening left by its resection is closed. This is carried out in two layers using interrupted sutures. The mucosal layer is closed with 3-0 chromic catgut and the seromuscular layer with nonabsorbable material. This technique is only used when the pathologic process is strictly limited to the diverticulum.

Surgical Treatment of Meckel's Diverticulum

FIGURE 46.15

A peptic ulcer can be seen at the junction of the diverticulum with the ileum, in the ileal mucosa near the diverticulum. If the technique described above is used to resect this diverticulum, the ulcer will remain in the ileum.

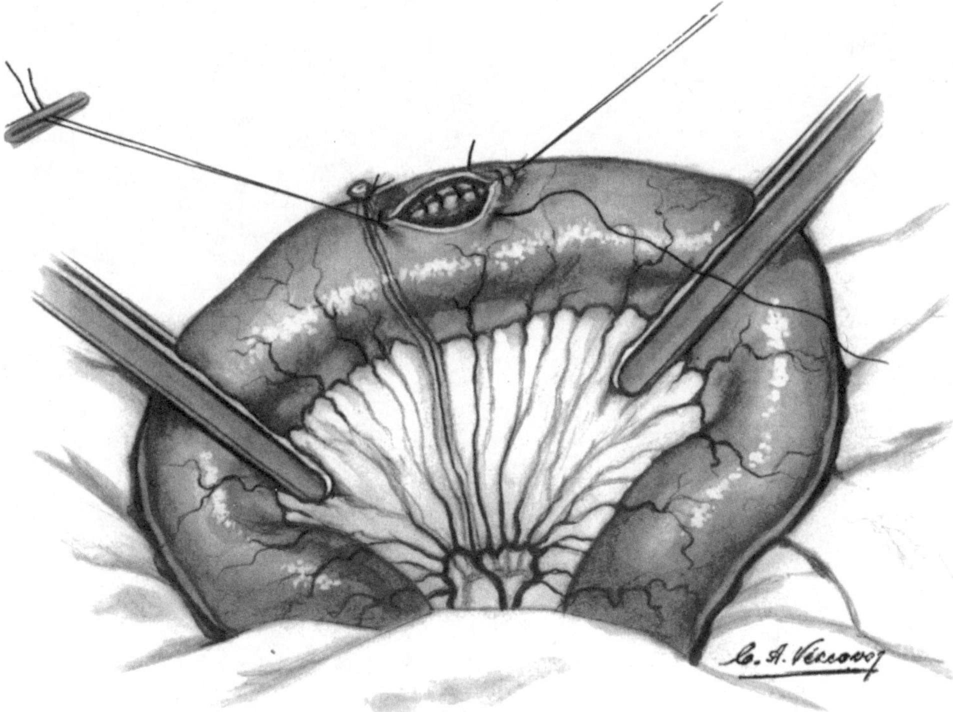

FIGURE 46.14

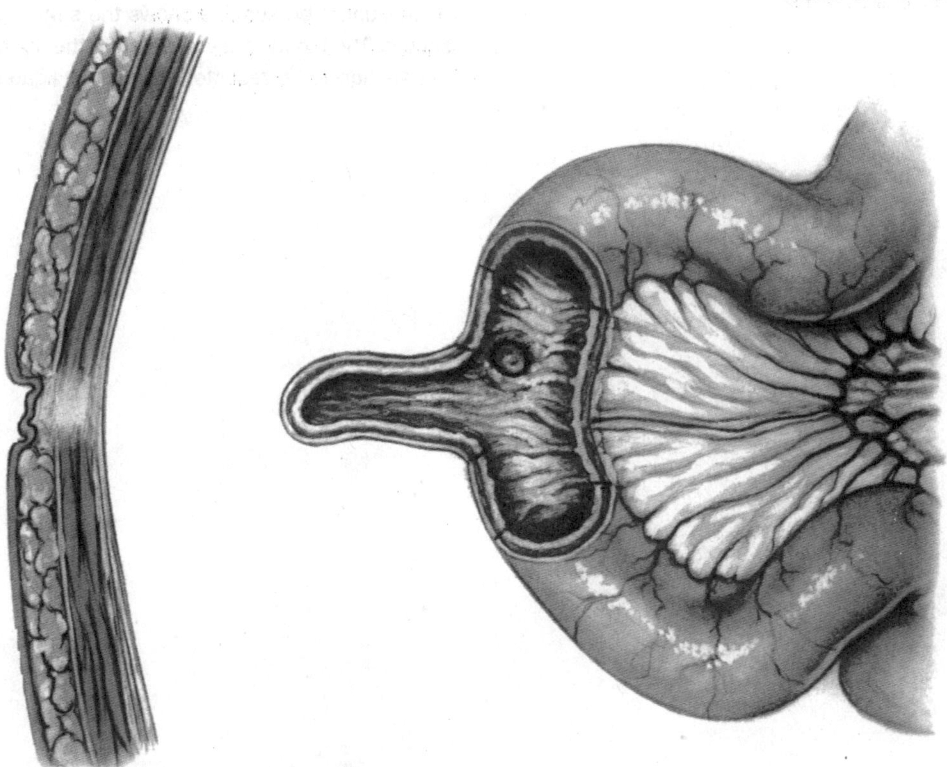

FIGURE 46.15

Surgical Treatment of Meckel's Diverticulum

FIGURE 46.16
In these cases a resection of a segment of ileum including the diverticulum and the peptic ulcer should be carried out. Two atraumatic clamps should be placed on both sides of the diverticulum. A broken line shows the segment of ileum to be resected. The blood vessels irrigating the ileum corresponding to the section to be resected have been ligated.

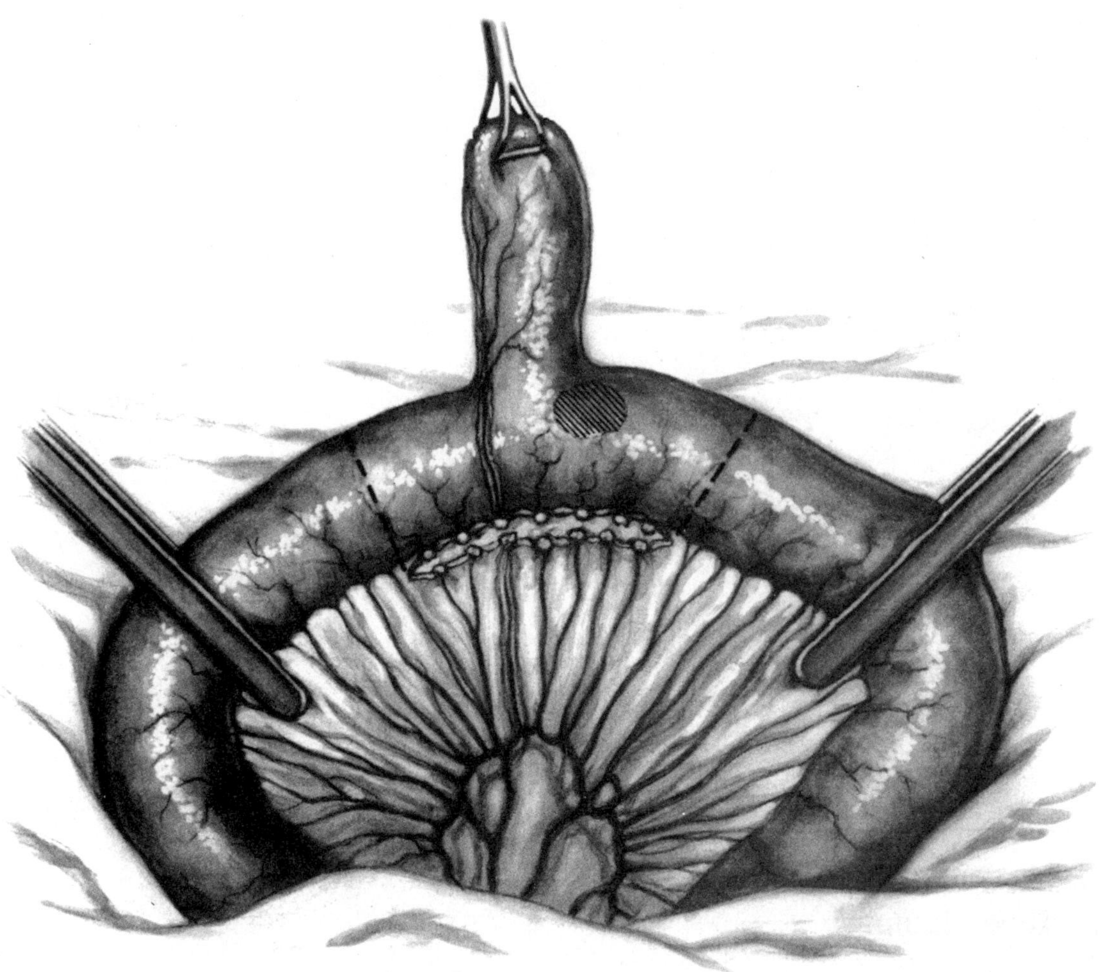

Surgical Treatment of Meckel's Diverticulum

FIGURE 46.17
The ileal segment including the Meckel's diverticulum and the peptic ulcer have been removed. The ileal ends are being sutured in end-to-end fashion, using interrupted sutures. The mucosal plane is closed with 3-0 chromic catgut, and the seromuscular layer is closed with nonabsorbable suture material.

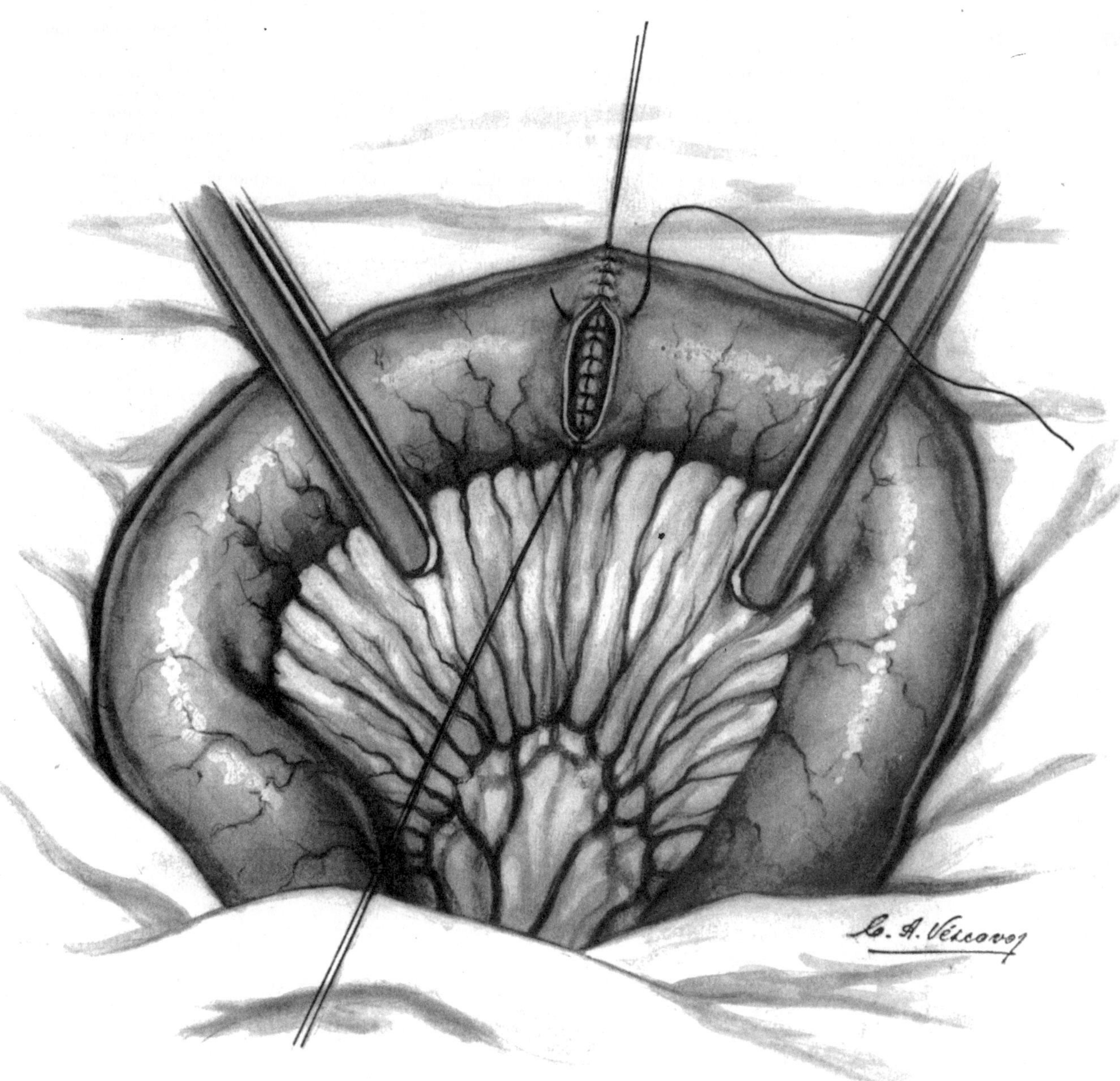

FIGURE 46.17

References

1. Berman, E.J., Schneider, A., Potts, W.J. Importance of gastric mucosa in Meckel's diverticulum. J.A.M.A. 156:6, 1957.
2. Cooney, D.R., Duszynski, D.O., Camboa, E., Karp, M.P., Jewet, T.C. Jr. The abdominal technetium scan (a decade of experience) J. Pediatr. Surg. 17:611, 1982.
3. De Bartolo, H.M. Jr., van Heerden, J.A. Meckel's diverticulum. Ann. Surg. 183:30, 1976.
4. Etala, E. Divertículo de Meckel. In Boretti, J.J., Lovesio, C. (Eds.) Cirugía. Vol. III, p. 1167. El Ateneo, Buenos Aires, 1989.
5. Gray, S.W., Skandalakis, J.E. Embriology for surgeons. p. 156. W.B. Saunders, Philadelphia, 1972.
6. Gray, S.W., Skandalakis, J.E. Atlas of surgical anatomy for general surgeons. p. 209. Williams & Wilkins, Baltimore, 1985.
7. Griffen, W.O. Jr. Meckel's diverticulum. In Sabiston, D.C. Jr. (Ed.). Textbook of surgery. Ed. 14, p. 866. W.B. Saunders, Philadelphia, 1991.
8. Hübschmann, N. Späperforation eines Mecklschen divertikels nach trauma. München Med. Wochenschr. 11:2051, 1913.
9. Jay, G.D. III, Margulis, R.R., McGraw, A.B., Northrip, R.R. Meckel's diverticulum: A survey of one hundred and three cases. Arch. Surg. 61:158, 1950.
10. Littré, A. Observation sur une nouvelle espèce de hernie. Mém. Acad. R. Sci. P. 300, 1700.
11. Mackey, W.C., Dinee, P. A fifty year experience with Meckel's diverticulum. Surg. Gynecol. Obstet. 156:56, 1983.
12. Meckel, J.F. Ueber die divertikel am darmkanal. Arch. Physiol. 9:421, 1809.
13. Moll, H.H. Giant Meckel's diverticulum (33½ inches long). Br. J. Surg. 14:176, 1926.
14. Netter, F.H. The Ciba collection of medical illustrations. Vol. III, p. 127. Ciba Pharmaceutical Company, New York, 1962.
15. Passaro, E. Jr., Richmond, D., Gordon, H.E. Surgery for Meckel's diverticulum in the adult: Factors in morbidity and mortality. Arch. Surg. 93:315, 1966.
16. Rumbo, H.G. Enfermedades quirúrgicas del intestino delgado. In Ortiz, F.E., Miranda, N.E., Moirano, J.J., Fassi, J.C. (Eds.) Cirugía. Ed. 3, p. 531. El Ateneo, Buenos Aires, 1993.
17. Rutherford, R.B., Akers, D.R. Meckel's diverticulum: A review of 148 pediatric patients with special reference to the pattern of bleeding and to mesodiverticular bands. Surgery 59:618, 1966.
18. Söderlund, S. Meckel's diverticulum: A clinical and histological study. Acta Chir. Scand. Suppl. 118:1, 1959.
19. Soltero, M.J., Bill, A.H. The natural history of Meckel's diverticulum and its relation to incidental removal. Am. J. Surg. 132:168, 1976.
20. Stewart, J.H., Storey, C.F. Meckel's diverticulum: A study of 141 cases. South. Med. J. 55:16, 1962.
21. Vane, D.W., West, K.W., Grosfeld, J.L. Vitelline duct anomalies. Experience with 217 childhood cases. Arch. Surg. 122:542, 1987.
22. Wansbrough, R.M., Thomson, S., Leckey, R.G. Meckel's diverticulum. A 42 year review of 273 cases at the Hospital for Sick Children. Can. J. Surg. 1:15, 1957.
23. Williams, R.S. Managment of Meckel's diverticulum. Br. J. Surg. 68:477, 1981.
24. Wine, C.R., Nahrwold, D.L., Waldhausen, J.A. Role of the technetium scan in diagnosis of Meckel's diverticulum. J. Pediatr. Surg. 9:885, 1974.

Section H

Colon, Rectum, and Anus

CHAPTER **47**

Surgical Anatomy of the Colon

The large intestine extends from the ileocecal junction to the anus, measuring an average of 150 cm. The caliber of the large intestine is quite variable and additionally varies according to its functional state. The segment that is greatest in diameter is the cecum, and the segment of smallest diameter is the sigmoid colon (16, 26). The large intestine becomes wider at the rectal ampulla and later diminishes in size in the anal canal.

Taken as a whole, the large intestine has the shape of a horseshoe with its concavity directed downward (23). The cecum, ascending colon, and part of the transverse colon originate embryologically from the midgut and are supplied by the superior mesenteric artery. The left colon and the rectum originate from the hind gut and are irrigated by the inferior mesenteric artery.

The ileum communicates with the colon through the ileocecal valve, which is located in its posterior medial border about 6 cm from the bottom of the cecum (16, 23, 26).

The large intestine is distinguished from the small intestine by several peculiarities:

1. Its caliber, which is greater.
2. By the presence of muscular ribbons, bands, or tenias in which longitudinal muscular fibers are concentrated, even though there is always a fine longitudinal muscular layer that is found along the entire colon (32).
3. The muscular ribbonlike structures lead to the formation of colonic dilations, which are separated from each other by transverse depressions (16, 26).
4. By the presence of epiploic appendices, which are made up of accumulations of fat, wrapped in peritoneum. When the epiploic appendices are ligated, they can lead to a local necrosis of the wall of the colon if the vascularity at their base is not preserved (31).

The ascending colon arises above the ileocecal junction. It runs upward from its origin, followed by the hepatic flexure of the colon. The ascending colon has an approximate length of 15 to 20 cm (23, 25, 26). The transverse colon arises from the hepatic flexure, has a length that varies between 30 and 60 cm, and follows a transverse direction from right to left, toward the splenic flexure. In reality, the direction of the transverse colon depends on the length of its mesocolon. If the mesocolon is long, the transverse colon may descend down to the pelvis. Once beyond the splenic flexure the descending colon begins. It generally has a vertical direction some 20 to 25 cm in length, ending at the left iliac crest and, in some patients, in the left iliac fossa (23, 24, 26). The descending colon is continuous with the sigmoid colon, which begins when a mesocolon is again noted. The sigmoid colon has a medium length of 40 cm, although great variations may occur and it may be either very short or excessively long. It occupies the left iliac fossa, the pelvis, and sometimes the right iliac fossa. The sigmoid colon ends anatomically at the third sacral vertebra, where the sigmoid colon loses its mesocolon as well as its ribbonlike longitudinal muscle fibers. These ribbons of longitudinal muscle spread at this point over the entire surface of the rectum as a continuous layer.

CECUM; ILEOCECAL VALVE; CECAL APPENDIX

The usual location of the cecum is in the right iliac fossa, resting on the iliopsoas muscle. This position may vary greatly, with location in the pelvis or in the upper abdomen. The junction of the ileum and the cecum forms an angle that opens downward (26). In 30% of individuals the cecum is intraperitoneal in location. In other cases, it may have a mesentery or be held to the posterior abdominal wall by the posterior parietal peritoneum (24). The cecum presents very visible longitudinal muscle bands, which arise in the base of the cecal appendix. From the base of the appendix the bands are distributed as follows: One band is directed toward the anterior wall of the cecum, while the other two are directed toward the posterior wall, one posterolaterally, and the other posteromedially (23, 26).

The ileocecal valve, when observed in the cadaver, appears to be made up of two folds, a superior and an inferior fold. Investigations carried out by several authors (2, 4, 5, 11, 16, 17, 23, 28, 33) have proven that in the structure and function of the ileocecal valve, muscular fibers intervene. According to Hollinshead (16), the ileocecal valve should be considered as a protrusion of the circular muscular layer and the submucosa of the ileum into the lumen of the cecum. Beattie (4) has shown the presence of a muscular sphincter that is very well developed and is an essential element of the valve. Bargen, Wesson, and Jackmann (2) have proven that both the circular muscle fibers and the longitudinal fibers of the ileum and colon are involved in the folds, provoking an action similar to that of a sphincter. Di Didio, quoted by Netter (23), has proven that the structure and function of the ileocecal valve involves muscular fibers that arise in the posterior medial muscular band, as well as from the terminal ileum. According to the quoted investigators, in a live patient, the communication between the ileum and the cecum is not by means of a valve, but by means of a sphincter, which is controlled by neural and hormonal factors (11, 16, 23). Examination of the ileocecal valve with a fiberoptic colonoscope would confirm the quoted investigations.

The cecal appendix, whose base is 2 to 3 cm below the ileocecal junction, is quite variable in its length as well as its position. The cecal appendix may be directed downward, entering into contact with the uterus and the adnexa, or upward, passing behind or in front of the cecum. Some posterior cecal appendices, because of their extension, should be considered more retrocolonic than retrocecal. The cecal appendix is wrapped by the peritoneum and invariably has a mesoappendix where the appendiceal artery runs, which in some cases is double. Even though the longitudinal tenias originate in the base of the cecal appendix, this organ presents both muscular layers, a longitudinal and a circular one, which are disposed in a continuous fashion. The submucosal layer of the appendix is very rich in lymphoepithelial tissue (22). The mucosa is similar to that which lines the colon, but it harbors a greater amount of cells with argentaffin granulations, which may give origin to carcinoid tumors (22).

ASCENDING COLON

This part of the colon is the continuation of the cecum above the ileocecal valve. This segment of colon is attached to the posterior wall of the abdomen by the posterior parietal peritoneum. In some 10% of patients, it is covered by peritoneum and has a mesocolon, which is fixed to the posterior abdominal wall. The longitudinal muscular ribbons have the same anatomic location as in the cecum. The ascending colon is related from below upward with the iliopsoas muscle, the quadratus lumborum muscle, the duodenum, and the lower pole of the right kidney. Its posterior wall is also in relation with the right ureter and the gonadal vessels. When the right colon is resected, care should be taken to prevent injuring the duodenum, the right ureter, and the gonadal vessels. When the hepatic flexure of the colon is mobilized, injury to some of the veins that constitute Henle's trunk should be avoided because hemostasis is difficult to carry out when this occurs.

TRANSVERSE COLON

The transverse colon is wrapped in peritoneum and joined by its mesocolon to the posterior wall of the abdomen, following a line from right to left that crosses over the second portion of the duodenum, the anterior surface of the head of the pancreas, and the inferior border of the body of the pancreas. The first 5 to 10 cm of the transverse colon, however, are not covered by peritoneum and are adjacent to the posterior wall, making this section of the transverse colon extraperitoneal. The greatest length of the transverse colon is seen in its middle third. It is joined to the greater curvature of the stomach by the gastrocolic ligament. The greater omentum hangs from the greater curvature of the stomach and then descends in front of the transverse colon to again return upward and become adherent to the transverse colon. The greater omentum can be separated from the transverse colon easily and without loss of blood. The transverse colon ends its tract at the splenic flexure of the colon. The splenic flexure is in a higher plane and more lateral than the hepatic flexure, making surgical approach more difficult. The splenic flexure is in relation to the inferior pole of the left kidney and at times, to the hilus of the kidney. The splenic flexure is also in relation with the spleen, and during mobilization of this flexure, this organ can be injured. The splenic flexure is joined to the diaphragm by the left phrenocolic ligament.

The transverse colon and its mesocolon divide the abdominal cavity into two compartments: a superior or supramesocolic compartment, also known as the gastrosplenohepatic compartment, and an inferior or inframesocolic compartment also known as the intestinal compartment (26).

DESCENDING COLON

This segment of colon runs vertically downward, extending from the splenic flexure to the left iliac crest or the left iliac fossa, varying according to where the sigmoid mesocolon starts. The descending colon is applied to the posterior wall of the abdomen and held there by the posterior parietal peritoneum. The relations of the posterior wall of the descending colon are similar on the left as those of the ascending colon on the right. The muscular tenias have the same disposition as in the ascending colon.

SIGMOID COLON

The sigmoid colon is the narrowest portion of the colon. It adopts an S shape as its name indicates. In the same fashion as the transverse colon, it is wrapped by the peritoneum and has a mesocolon, which is usually disposed in V fashion over the psoas muscle, the gonadal vessels, and the left ureter. Upon reaching the third sacral vertebra, it is continuous with the rectum as its mesocolon disappears and the muscular tenias are replaced by the continuous longitudinal muscular layer, which is wrapped around the entire rectum. The sigmoid colon has many variations in its length and its trajectory.

BLOOD SUPPLY OF THE COLON

As was said before, the cecum, ascending colon, and part of the transverse colon, which originate embryologically from the midgut, are supplied by the superior mesenteric artery. The descending colon, sigmoid colon, and rectum are supplied by the inferior mesenteric artery.

The superior mesenteric artery arises from the anterior wall of the aorta about 10 to 15 cm below the celiac trunk and passes behind the pancreas and in front of its uncinate process and the second portion of the duodenum. The middle colic artery arises from the superior mesenteric artery. In some patients, this artery arises from a common trunk with the right colic artery. According to Steward and Rankin (31), the middle colic artery is absent in 5% of patients. Griffiths (14) reported that it is absent in 22% of cases. Sonneland et al. (30), as well as Steward and Rankin, have also reported its absence in only 5% of cases. In 10% of individuals, there is a middle colic artery arising directly from the aorta (24). From its origin, the middle colic artery runs obliquely toward the hepatic flexure of the colon. Less frequently, it runs vertically toward the transverse colon, and more rarely, it runs obliquely toward the left side. After a trajectory of some 5 to 7 cm along the border of the colon, the middle colic artery divides into two branches: a right branch, which anastomoses with the ascending branch of the right colic artery, and a left branch, which anastomoses with the ascending branch of the left colic artery, which arises in the inferior mesenteric artery (7, 16, 24, 25, 26).

The right colic artery has a very variable origin, since it may arise from the superior mesenteric artery below the middle colic artery, in a common trunk with this artery, or from the ileocolic artery. According to Steward and Rankin (31), the right colic artery is absent in 18% of cases. Michels et al. (21) have found it absent in only 2% of patients. This artery, after running a variable course in the right mesocolon, divides into two branches, a superior one, which anastomoses with the right branch of the middle colic artery, and an inferior one, which anastomoses with the colic branch of the ileocolic artery. The superior mesenteric artery also gives rise to the ileocolic artery, which, after a variable course toward the ileocecal region, divides into two branches. These are an ascending or colonic branch, which anastomoses with a descending branch of the right colic artery, and a descending or ileal branch, which anastomoses with the terminal section of the superior mesenteric artery. The ileocolic artery enters into the ileocecal junction as an arcade from which the anterior cecal, the posterior cecal, and the appendicular arteries arise. The latter runs a very constant trajectory but is very irregular in its origin, and in 30% of cases, it is double (24).

The inferior mesenteric artery arises from the aorta about 3 or 4 cm above its bifurcation, some 10 cm from the sacral promontory, and 3 to 4 cm below the third portion of the duodenum (16, 23, 24, 26). About 3 or 4 cm from its origin in the aorta, it gives rise to a left colic artery, which later bifurcates into an ascending branch, which runs obliquely to the splenic flexure, where it anastomoses to the left branch of the middle colic artery, and a descending branch, which anastomoses with the ascending branch of the first sigmoidal artery. The number of sigmoidal arteries is quite variable, there being usually three or four, but at times as many as six. The first sigmoidal arteries arise from the ascending branch of the left colic artery; the rest arise directly from the inferior mesenteric artery. After giving off the sigmoidal branches the inferior mesenteric artery runs downward, passing in front of the common iliac artery and becoming the superior hemorrhoidal artery or superior rectal artery. When it reaches the third sacral vertebra, it divides into two branches, a right and a left branch (1, 7, 16, 21, 24).

The marginal artery of Drummond (8) is made up of the junction of the arterial arcades originating from the bifurcation of the middle colic, right colic, ileocolic, left colic, and sigmoidal arteries. The marginal artery or marginal artery of Drummond runs parallel to the mesenteric border of the colon. This artery supplies a connection of arterial blood from the superior mesenteric to the inferior mesenteric artery (19). The marginal artery of Drummond begins at the bifurcation of the ileocolic artery and ends in the sigmoidal arteries. The marginal artery of Drummond gives rise to the straight arteries that irrigate the colon, also known as the vasa recta. Each one of these vessels divides into two branches, an anterior and a posterior branch. These arteries run in the subserosa of the colon and later in the submucosa. The short vessels or vasa brevia are branches of the vasa recta. If the inferior mesenteric artery becomes occluded by arteriosclerosis or is ligated during a resection of an aneurysm of the abdominal aorta, the superior mesenteric artery maintains the viability of the left colon and sigmoid colon by means of the marginal artery of Drummond (9, 14, 21, 24, 31).

The arch known as Riolano is made up of an artery that joins the origin of the superior mesenteric artery or one of its principal branches to the inferior mesenteric artery or one of its principal branches. For this reason, the arch of Riolano does not constitute a marginal anastomosis. In the medical literature, it is frequently confused with the marginal artery of Drummond. The arch of Riolano is present in 7% of patients (24).

VEINS OF THE COLON

The veins of the colon have the same distribution as the arteries. The veins of the right colon and the transverse colon drain venous blood to the superior mesenteric vein, which is located to the right and in front of the superior mesenteric artery. The superior rectal vein (superior hemorrhoidal vein) is continuous with the inferior mesenteric vein, which receives venous blood from the rectum, the left colon, and the highest portion of the anal canal. The inferior mesenteric vein runs upward in a retroperitoneal plane, passing to the left of the ligament of Treitz, behind the body of the pancreas, where it joins the splenic vein (24, 26).

LYMPHATICS OF THE COLON

Knowledge of the distribution and lymphatic dissemination of the colon is of great importance in the treatment of malignant lesions of the colon. Jameson and Dobson (18) classified lymphatic nodes into four groups:

1. Epicolic lymph nodes located in the wall of the colon below the peritoneal layer and below the epiploic appendices. These epiploic lymph nodes are more numerous in the sigmoid colon.
2. Paracolic nodes, which are located between the mesenteric border of the colon and the marginal arcade of Drummond.
3. Intermediate nodes, situated along the principal arteries before they divide to form the arcade of Drummond.
4. Principal nodes, which are those that are located at the root of the superior mesenteric and inferior mesenteric arteries.

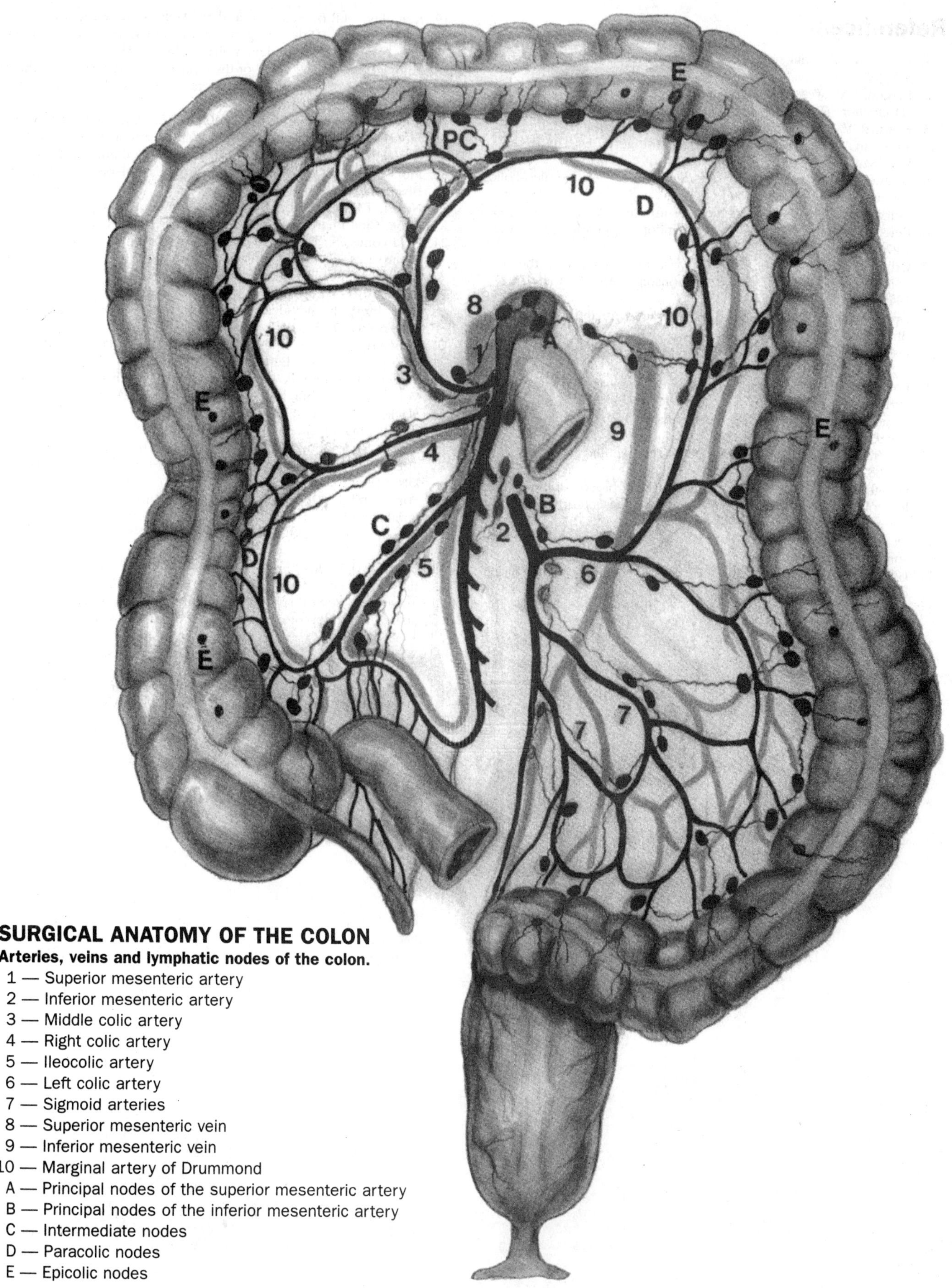

SURGICAL ANATOMY OF THE COLON

Arteries, veins and lymphatic nodes of the colon.

1 — Superior mesenteric artery
2 — Inferior mesenteric artery
3 — Middle colic artery
4 — Right colic artery
5 — Ileocolic artery
6 — Left colic artery
7 — Sigmoid arteries
8 — Superior mesenteric vein
9 — Inferior mesenteric vein
10 — Marginal artery of Drummond
A — Principal nodes of the superior mesenteric artery
B — Principal nodes of the inferior mesenteric artery
C — Intermediate nodes
D — Paracolic nodes
E — Epicolic nodes

References

1. Ayoud, S.F. Arterial supply to the human rectum. Acta Anat. 100: 317, 1978.
2. Bargen, J.A., Wesson, H.R., Jackmann, R.J. Studies on the ileocecal junction. (Ileocecus). Surg. Gynecol. Obstet. 71:33, 1940.
3. Beart, R.W. Jr., Nivatvongs, S., Wolff, B. The colon, rectum, and anus. In Nora, P.F. (Ed.) Operative surgery. Ed. 3, p. 610. W.B. Saunders, Philadelphia, 1990.
4. Beattie, J. The early stages of development of the ileo-colic sphincter. J. Anat. 59:56, 1924.
5. Berry, R.J.A. The anatomy of the caecum. Anat. Anz. 10:401, 1895.
6. Berry, R.J.A. The anatomy of the vermiform appendix. Anat. Anz. 10:761, 1895.
7. Caudwell, E.W., Anson, B.J. The visceral branches of the abdominal aorta. Topographical relationships. Am. J. Anat. 73:27, 1943.
8. Drummond, H. The arterial supply of the rectum and pelvic colon. Br. J. Surg. 1:677, 1913.
9. Fisher, D.F., Fry, W.I. Collateral mesenteric circulation. Surg. Gynecol. Obstet. 164:487, 1987.
10 Fozard, J.B.L., Pemberton, J.H. Applied surgical anatomy: Intra-abdominal contents. In Fielding, L.P., Goldberg, S.M. (Eds.) Surgery of the colon, rectum and anus. Ed. 5, p. 3. Butterworth-Heinemann, Oxford, 1993.
11. Gazet, J.C., Jarret, R.J. The ileocaeco-colic sphincter. Br. J. Surg. 51:368, 1964.
12. Goligher, J.C. The adequacy of the marginal blood supply to the left colon after high ligation of the inferior mesenteric artery during excision of the rectum. Br. J. Surg. 41:351, 1954.
13. Gray, S.W., Skandalakis, J.E. Atlas of surgical anatomy for general surgeons. p. 216. Williams & Wilkins, Baltimore, 1985.
14. Griffiths, J.D. Surgical anatomy of the blood supply of the distal colon. Ann. R. Coll. Surg. Engl. 19:241, 1956.
15. Harsha, W.T. Retrocecal appendix: Its diagnosis and surgical approach. Surg. Gynecol. Obstet. 74:180, 1942.
16. Hollinshead, W.H. Anatomy for surgeons. Vol. 2, p. 486. Hoeber-Harper, New York, 1956.
17. Hunter, R.H. The ileo-caecal junction. J. Anat. 68:264, 1934.
18. Jameson, J.K., Dobson, J.F. The lymphatics of the colon. Proc. R. Soc. Med. (Surg. Section) 2:149, 1909.
19. Keighley, M.R.B. Anatomy and physiology. In Keighley, M.R.B., Williams, N.S. (Eds). Surgery of the anus, rectum and colon. Vol. 1, p. 1. W.B. Saunders, Philadelphia, 1993.
20. Lindstrom, B.L. The value of the collateral circulation from the inferior mesenteric artery in obliteration of the lower abdominal aorta. Acta Chir. Scand. 1:677, 1950.
21. Michels, N.A., Siddarth, P., Kornblith, P.L., Park, W.W. The variant blood supply to the descending colon, rectosigmoid dissections: A review of medical literature. Dis. Colon Rectum 8:261, 1965.
22. Morson, B.C., Dawson, I.M.P. Gastrointestinal pathology. p. 391. Blackwell, Oxford, 1972.
23. Netter, F.H. The Ciba collection of medical illustrations. Vol. 3, p. 54. Ciba Pharmaceutical Company, New York, 1962.
24. Nivatvongs, S., Gordon, P.H. Surgical anatomy. In Gordon, P.H., Nivatvongs, S. (Eds,) Colon, rectum and anus. p. 3, Quality Medical Publishing, St. Louis, MO, 1992.
25. Robillard, G.L., Shapiro, A.L. Variational anatomy of the middle colic artery: Its significance in gastric and colonic surgery. J. Int. Coll. Surg. 10:157, 1947.
26. Rouvière, H. Compendio de anatomía y disección. Spanish edition, p. 552. Salvat, Barcelona, 1953.
27. Silling, L.F. Appendix. In Fromm, D. (Ed.) Gastrointestinal surgery. Vol. 2, p. 519. Churchill Livingstone, New York, 1985.
28. Slack, W.W. The anatomy, pathology and clinical features of diverticulitis of the colon. Br. J. Surg. 50:185, 1962.
29. Smith, L., Friend, W.G., Medwell, S.J. The superior mesenteric artery. The critical factor in the pouch pull through procedure. Dis. Colon Rectum 27:741, 1984.
30. Sonneland, J., Anson, B.J., Beaton, L.E. Surgical anatomy of the arterial supply to the colon from the superior mesenteric artery based upon a study of 600 specimens. Surg. Gynecol. Obstet. 106:385, 1958.
31. Steward, J.A., Rankin, F.W. Blood supply of the large intestine: Its surgical considerations. Arch. Surg. 26:843, 1933.
32. Torsoli, A., Remorino, M.L., Crucioli, V. The relationships between anatomy and motor activity of the colon. Am. J. Dig. Dis. 13:462, 1968.
33. Wakefield, E.G., Friedell, M.T. The structural significance of the ileocecal valve. J.A.M.A. 116:1889, 1941.
34. Wakeley, C.P.G. The position of the vermiform appendix as ascertained by an analysis of 10,000 cases. J. Anat. 67:277, 1933.

Section H

Colon, Rectum, and Anus

CHAPTER 48

Surgical Anatomy of the Rectum and Anus

The rectum is the continuation of the sigmoid colon. According to anatomists, it begins at the third sacral vertebra and ends at the anus. Surgeons, on the other hand, assert that the rectum begins at the sacral promontory and not at the third sacral vertebra (11, 20, 23, 25).

It must be admitted that the junction of the sigmoid with the rectum is not a sudden change but occurs gradually (23). The longitudinal tenias of the sigmoid colon begin to unite progressively until they form a longitudinal muscle layer in the anterior wall and another similar layer in the posterior wall, which later unite. These form a longitudinal muscular wrapping that encircles the rectum (23). The difficulty of establishing with precision the boundary between the sigmoid colon and the rectum has made it necessary to frequently use the term "rectosigmoid zone" instead of rectosigmoid junction. According to Goligher, the rectosigmoid zone corresponds to the last 5 to 8 cm of the sigmoid colon and the proximal 5 cm of the rectum (18–20). This implies that the limit between the sigmoid colon and the rectum is rather arbitrary, becoming only a problem of definition with no importance in surgical practice (23). The length of the rectum varies from 12 to 15 cm (21). The rectum does not have a mesentery, longitudinal bands, tenias, sacculations, transverse sulci, or epiploic appendices.

In general, surgical anatomists divide the rectum into two segments, a pelvic segment and a perineal segment. From the descriptive point of view, however, it is more useful to divide the rectum into three segments:

1. A superior segment covered by peritoneum on its anterior and lateral walls.
2. A middle segment covered by peritoneum only laterally.
3. An inferior segment that is completely extraperitoneal (subperitoneal).

The greatest portion of the rectum is subperitoneal. The portion of the rectum that is partially covered by peritoneum varies greatly in individuals and according to their sex. It is generally admitted that the anterior peritoneal reflection in the male is situated some 8 cm from the anal margin, while the posterior peritoneal reflection is situated about 12 to 15 cm from the anal margin (20, 21, 25).

In spite of its name, the rectum does not run in a straight line. A great part of its upper portion runs along the anterior wall of the sacrum and the coccyx, following its concavity as it passes the coccyx, where it changes abruptly in direction and runs downward and backward, converting itself into the anal canal (20, 21, 23, 25).

In addition, during its course, the rectum forms three lateral curves—the superior curve, which is convex to the right, the middle curve, which is convex to the left, and the inferior curve, which again is convex to the right. The inner aspects of these curves correspond to folds called the valves of Houston (20, 23). From the point of view of their structure, the valves of Houston consist of mucosa and submucosa of the rectum, but in some individuals, the circular muscular layer also participates in their structure (23). The middle valve of Houston corresponds in general with the anterior peritoneal reflection. The middle valve of Houston is known by the name of valve of Kohlrausch and is the most dominant of the three valves (20). Below the valve of Kohlrausch, the rectum presents a much larger lumen than its intraperitoneal segment and is known as the rectal ampulla. Due to the numerous variations presented by the valves of Houston, these should not be taken as fixed surgical landmarks (1, 20).

The three curves presented by the rectum in its descent toward the anus disappear when the rectum is mobilized surgically. This means that the surgeon can obtain a lengthening of the rectum, which in surgery to preserve the anal sphincter has a very important role.

Posteriorly, the rectum is related to the sacrum, the coccyx, the levator ani muscle, and the middle sacral artery. The relations of the anterior wall of the rectum vary in the male and the female. In the male, the intraperitoneal rectal segment is related to the small bowel loops and the sigmoid colon. The subperitoneal rectal segment in males is related to the prostate, seminal vesicles, deferent ducts, bladder, and ureters. In the female, the anterior wall of the intraperitoneal rectum is related to the uterus, the upper portion of the vagina, the adnexa, small intestinal loops, and the sigmoid colon. The rectal subperitoneal segment is related to the posterior wall of the vagina (12, 15, 23, 25).

ANAL CANAL

For anatomists, the anal canal begins at the pectinate line and ends at the anal margin (anatomic anal canal). For surgeons, the anal canal begins at the anal rectal ring and ends at the anal margin (surgical anal canal). The anatomic anal canal extends for a distance of 1.5 to 2 cm, while the surgical canal extends for 3 to 4 cm (12, 20, 21, 23).

Above the dentate line, the rectal mucosa forms 8 to 14 longitudinal folds called the columns of Morgagni. The base of each column of Morgagni is continuous with the anal crypts, into which empty some poorly developed glands. Foreign matter may become introduced into the crypts of Morgagni and lead to infection, also giving origin to anal fistulas (20, 23). The anorectal ring, which makes up the upper limit of the surgical canal, is constituted by the puborectalis muscle, which is the deepest fascicle of the levator ani muscle and is complemented by superior fibers of the deep fascicle of the external anal sphincter and by superior fibers from the internal anal sphincter. Transection of the anorectal ring inevitably leads to anal incontinence. The anorectal ring is easily palpable on rectal examination, in its posterior portion, but not in its anterior portion. This is explained by the arrangement of the puborectalis muscle, which forms a true sling surrounding the rectum posteriorly. The ends of this muscle, after surrounding the anorectal segment, insert on each side of the symphysis pubis, on its posterior aspect (9, 12, 15, 23, 25).

The pectinate or dentate line indicates the mucocutaneous junction. About 0.5 to 2 cm above this line, the mucosa is covered by cuboid epithelium, which is known as the transitional or cloacogenic zone (10). Above the transitional zone the epithelium is columnar (10, 30). Below the pectinate line, the epithelium is squamous, but is differentiated from the epithelium of the skin by being damp and not having any hairs, sebaceous glands, or sweat glands. The skin has all these elements and in addition has subcutaneous cellular tissue, which is lacking in the squamous epithelium of the anal canal (15, 21, 25).

The anal canal is related posteriorly with the coccyx, the puborectalis muscle, and the external and internal anal sphincters. In the male, the anterior wall of the anal canal is in relation to the urethral bulb, and in the woman to the perineal body and the vagina. The anal canal plays an important role in fecal continence and is normally kept closed by the tonic contraction of the anal sphincters.

Muscles of the Anal Canal

The anal canal is surrounded by muscles, which make up a tubular structure composed on the outside by the external anal sphincter and on the inside by the internal anal sphincter. The external anal sphincter is a voluntary muscle made up of three parts: (a) the subcutaneous part, (b) the superficial part, and (c) the deep part. The superior fibers of the deep part intermingle with the fibers of the puborectalis fascicle of the levator ani muscle (19, 28, 30, 32, 34).

The internal anal sphincter is an involuntary muscle about 25 to 35 mm long and is made up of a thickening of the anorectal circular muscle layer.

Levator Ani Muscle

The levator ani muscle separates the pelvis from the perineum, for which reason it is considered to be the diaphragm of the pelvis. The levator ani muscle as a whole has the form of a funnel, and through this funnel pass the urethra, the vagina, and the anal rectum. The levator ani muscle is made up of three portions:

1. The puborectalis muscle, which makes up the deepest portion of the levator ani and whose fibers surround the anal rectum above the anal sphincters and additionally surround the prostate in the male and the vagina in the female as they insert on the posterior aspect of both sides of the symphysis pubis.
2. The pubococcygeal muscle, which arises in the posterior portion of the pubis and the anterior portion of the obturator fascia. From its origin it runs horizontally backward, passing on both sides of the anal rectum as a thin band to insert into the coccyx.
3. The iliococcygeal muscle, which is a thin muscle that arises in the ischial spine and in the posterior surface of the obturator fascia, running down and backward to insert in the last two sacral vertebrae, the coccyx, and the anococcygeal raphe (12, 19, 23, 28).

PERIRECTAL SPACES AND FASCIAS (8, 12, 20, 23)

The subperitoneal portion of the rectum is surrounded by perirectal fat and by fascias arising from the pelvic fascia, which are of different density according to their localization. Knowledge of the different fascias as they are related to the rectum is of great surgical importance.

The wall of the subperitoneal rectum is surrounded by the fascia propria of the rectum. This fascia is not very dense, allowing the rectal ampulla to expand (23). The pelvic fascia becomes denser on the anterior wall of the sacrum, making up the thick presacral fascia. At the level of the fourth sacral vertebra, the retrosacral fascia arises from the presacral fascia. This fascia has good consistency and runs downward and forward to insert into the posterior portion of the rectum, just above the anorectal ring. To mobilize the posterior aspect of the rectum in order to arrive at the levator ani muscles, it is necessary to transect the retrosacral fascia. It is important to insist that division of the retrosacral fascia always be performed with a cutting instrument, scalpel or scissors, and not manually. Use of the hand to carry out transection of the retrosacral fascia may lead to severe complications such as rupture of the rectal wall or rupture of the presacral fascia, injuring the presacral venous plexus with consequent hemorrhage, which is very difficult to control.

The retrosacral fascia is also known as Waldeyer's fascia (8, 12, 20, 23). Because very different interpretations of the fascia of Waldeyer have been made, in order to avoid confusion, it is advisable to use the designation of retrosacral fascia (8, 20) instead of fascia of Waldeyer.

In its anterior portion the pelvic fascia becomes dense and becomes known as the fascia of Denonvilliers, which separates the anterior rectal wall from the prostate and from the seminal vesicles, extending from the bottom of the peritoneal sac to the floor of the pelvis. The fascia of Denonvilliers does not have the density of the presacral fascia and is rather easily invaded by tumors located in the anterior rectal wall at that level.

In carrying out a resection of the rectum the fascia of Denonvilliers should be transected in order to enter the correct plane between the anterior wall of the rectum and the seminal vesicles and prostate (12, 20, 23). Denonvilliers had designated this fascia as the prostatoperitoneal membrane.

The presence of the fascia of Denonvilliers between the rectum and the vagina in the woman is a controversial subject. Anyway, if the fascia of Denonvilliers is present in the woman, it lacks surgical importance (23, 36).

Laterally, there also exists a condensation of pelvic fascia made up of the lateral ligaments of the rectum, which fix this organ to both sides of the pelvis. Through these lateral ligaments the middle hemorrhoidal vessels and the lymphatic vessels run. In order to mobilize the rectum, laterally, down to the levator ani muscles, it is necessary to ligate and divide these ligaments.

Dissection of the rectum and its surrounding fascia must be carried out on an anatomic basis, performing smooth, careful maneuvers to prevent injury to the ureters and the prostate, the seminal vesicles, the prostatic urethra, and the nerves and nerve plexuses, injury to which may lead to impotence, and alterations of ejaculation as well as neurogenic bladder, and so on.

ARTERIES OF THE RECTUM AND ANUS

The rectum and the anus are supplied by the inferior mesenteric artery and the superior hemorrhoidal artery, which is its continuation, as well as the middle and inferior hemorrhoidal arteries.

The inferior mesenteric artery, after giving off the left colic and sigmoidal arteries, courses over the common iliac artery and vein, and changes its name to the superior hemorrhoidal artery. Upon reaching the vicinity of the third sacral vertebra, it bifurcates, giving off a right and a left branch. The right branch divides into an anterior and posterior branch. These branches anastomose with the middle rectal artery (hemorrhoidal).

The middle hemorrhoidal artery originates in the internal iliac artery and reaches the level of the rectum at the levator ani muscles, coursing through the lateral rectal ligaments. The middle rectal or hemorrhoidal artery anastomoses with the superior hemorrhoidal artery (2). A part of the rectum and the anal canal maintain adequate blood supply after ligation of the inferior mesenteric artery and the middle hemorrhoidal artery (5).

The inferior hemorrhoidal artery arises from the pudendal artery in Alcock's canal, passing to the anal rectum where it supplies the muscles of the anal sphincter.

VEINS OF THE RECTUM AND ANUS

The veins of the rectum and anus follow the same course as the arteries (20, 23). The superior rectal or hemorrhoidal vein carries venous blood from the rectum and the superior segment of the anal canal to the inferior mesenteric vein, which empties into the splenic vein. This means that the venous blood of the rectum and the superior segment of the anal canal (surgical anal canal) empties into the portal system (21, 25). The middle hemorrhoidal vein drains the inferior segment of the rectum and the superior segment of the anal canal, emptying into the internal iliac vein. This means that the venous drainage from this area runs to the systemic venous system. The drainage of the middle hemorrhoidal vein has little importance. The inferior hemorrhoidal vein drains the most inferior portion of the anal canal with its blood draining to the internal pudendal vein (20–23).

LYMPHATICS OF THE RECTUM AND ANUS

Lymphatic flow from the rectum and anus follows the course of the arteries. Knowledge of the lymphatic drainage of the rectum is very important because of the frequency of cancer in this location. Many investigators have studied the lymphatic drainage of the rectum (5, 6, 9, 13, 14, 29).

It is unanimously accepted at present that the lymphatic drainage of the rectum is by the following route: The lymphatics of the rectum from both the subperitoneal and intraperitoneal segments follow the trajectory of the superior and inferior hemorrhoidal arteries toward the precavoaortic lymph nodes. The lymphatic drainage of the surgical anal canal, above the pectinate line, runs toward the superior hemorrhoidal artery and the inferior hemorrhoidal artery upward, and laterally follows the course of the middle rectal vessels toward the internal iliac lymph nodes. The lymphatics located below the pectinate line run toward the inguinal lymph nodes.

NERVE SUPPLY OF THE RECTUM AND ANUS

The colon and rectum are innervated by the autonomous nervous system, with its sympathetic and parasympathetic components. The nerves follow the course of the blood vessels. Many investigators have studied the innervation of the colon and rectum, among them Learmonth (27), Woollard and Norrish (38), Telford and Stopford (35), Gask and Ross (12), and Hughes (24).

The levator ani muscles are supplied by fibers of the fourth sacral nerve, the superior rectal nerve, and the perianal nerves (24). Nerve supply of the external anal sphincter comes from the inferior rectal nerves.

Sympathetic innervation comes from the first, second, and third lumbar sympathetic ganglia. Their fibers descend to the inferior mesenteric plexus, and some of the fibers accompany the inferior mesenteric artery. The rest of the nerve fibers unite in the hypogastric plexus.

The parasympathetic innervation arises in the second, third, and fourth sacral nerves, which give origin to the nervi erigentes, which unite with the sympathetic nerves in the pelvic plexus. Several sympathetic and parasympathetic nerves of the pelvic plexus are distributed to the organs of the pelvis.

Dissection underneath the aortic bifurcation may injure the hypogastric plexus, leading to alterations in ejaculation.

Ligation and division of the lateral rectal ligaments may injure the sympathetic and parasympathetic nerves if the ligature and division is carried out too close to the wall of the pelvis. Dissection of the anterior rectal wall to separate it from the seminal vesicles and the prostate may lead to injury of the sympathetic and parasympathetic nerves. Injury to the above mentioned nerves may lead to sexual impotence and a neurogenic bladder.

Surgical Anatomy of the Rectum and Anus

FIGURE 48.1 CORONAL SECTION OF THE RECTUM, ANUS, AND PERINEAL REGION

1, Rectosigmoid junction; 2, superior valve of Houston; 3, middle valve of Houston; 4, inferior valve of Houston; 5, pectinate or dentate line; 6, pecten; 7, anal margin; 8, internal anal sphincter; 9, external anal sphincter; 10, levator ani muscle (puborectalis).

Surgical Anatomy of the Rectum and Anus

FIGURE 48.2 SAGITTAL SECTION SHOWING THE FASCIAL LAYERS RELATED TO THE RECTUM

1, Presacral fascia; 2, fascia propria of the rectum; 3, sacrorectal fascia (Waldeyer); 4, fascia of Denonvilliers.

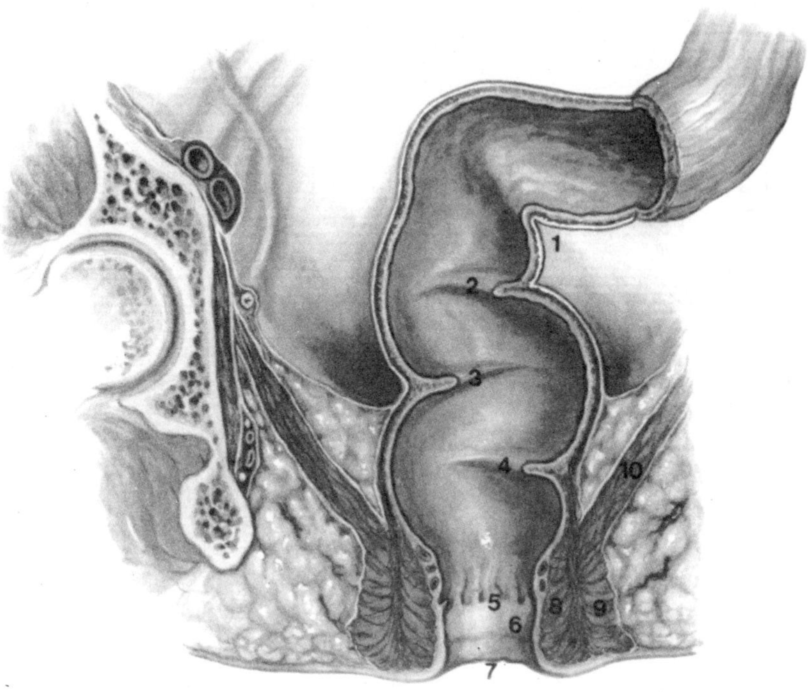

FIGURE 48.1 CORONAL SECTION OF THE RECTUM, ANUS, AND PERINEAL REGION

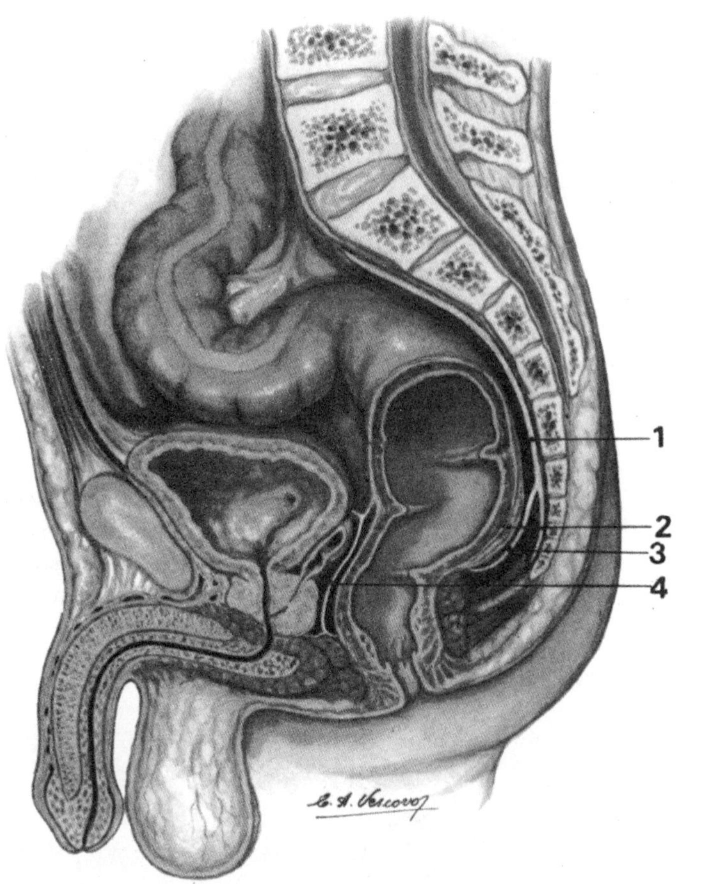

FIGURE 48.2 SAGITTAL SECTION SHOWING THE FASCIAL LAYERS RELATED TO THE RECTUM

Surgical Anatomy of the Rectum and Anus

FIGURE 48.3 ARTERIES OF THE RECTUM
1, Inferior mesenteric artery; 2, left colic artery; 3, sigmoidal arteries; 4, superior hemorrhoidal (rectal) artery; 5, right branch of the superior hemorrhoidal (rectal) artery; 6, left branch of the superior hemorrhoidal (rectal) artery; 7, middle sacral artery; 8, hypogastric (internal iliac) artery; 9, pudendal artery; 10, middle hemorrhoidal (rectal) artery; 11, inferior hemorrhoidal (rectal) artery.

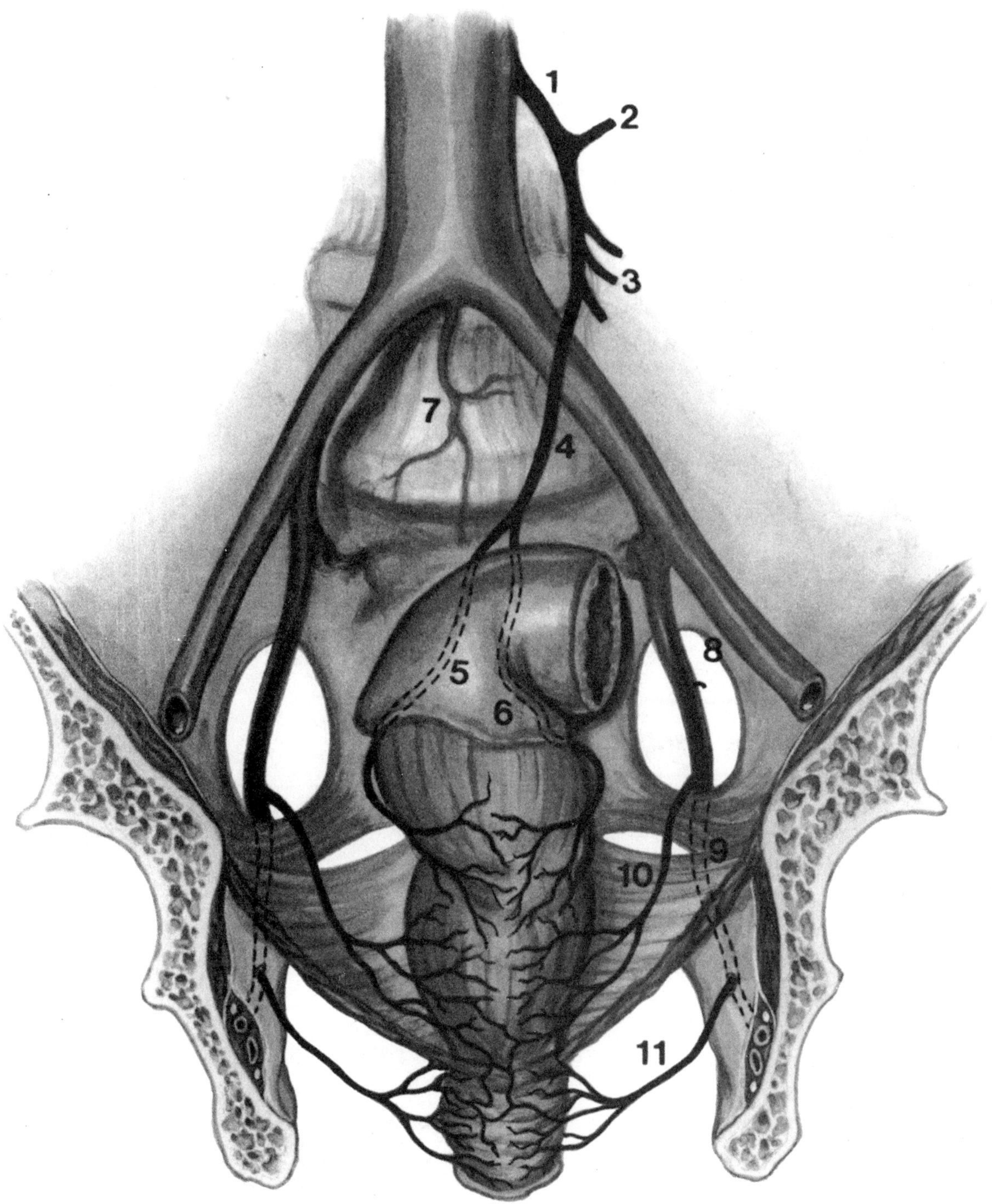

FIGURE 48.3 ARTERIES OF THE RECTUM

Surgical Anatomy of the Rectum and Anus

FIGURE 48.4
The lymphatics of both the intraperitoneal and the subperitoneal rectum follow the superior hemorrhoidal (rectal) artery toward the inferior mesenteric vessels, going on to the precaval preaortic lymph nodes. 1′, The lymphatic drainage of the segment of the anal canal between the pectinate line and the anorectal ring (superior limit of the surgical anal canal) runs toward the superior rectal (hemorrhoidal) artery and, from there, to the inferior mesenteric artery, laterally following the course of the middle rectal (hemorrhoidal) vessels toward the internal iliac lymph nodes. 2, The lymphatic vessels located below the pectinate line (anatomic anal canal) drain lymphatic fluid toward the inguinal nodes (see text).

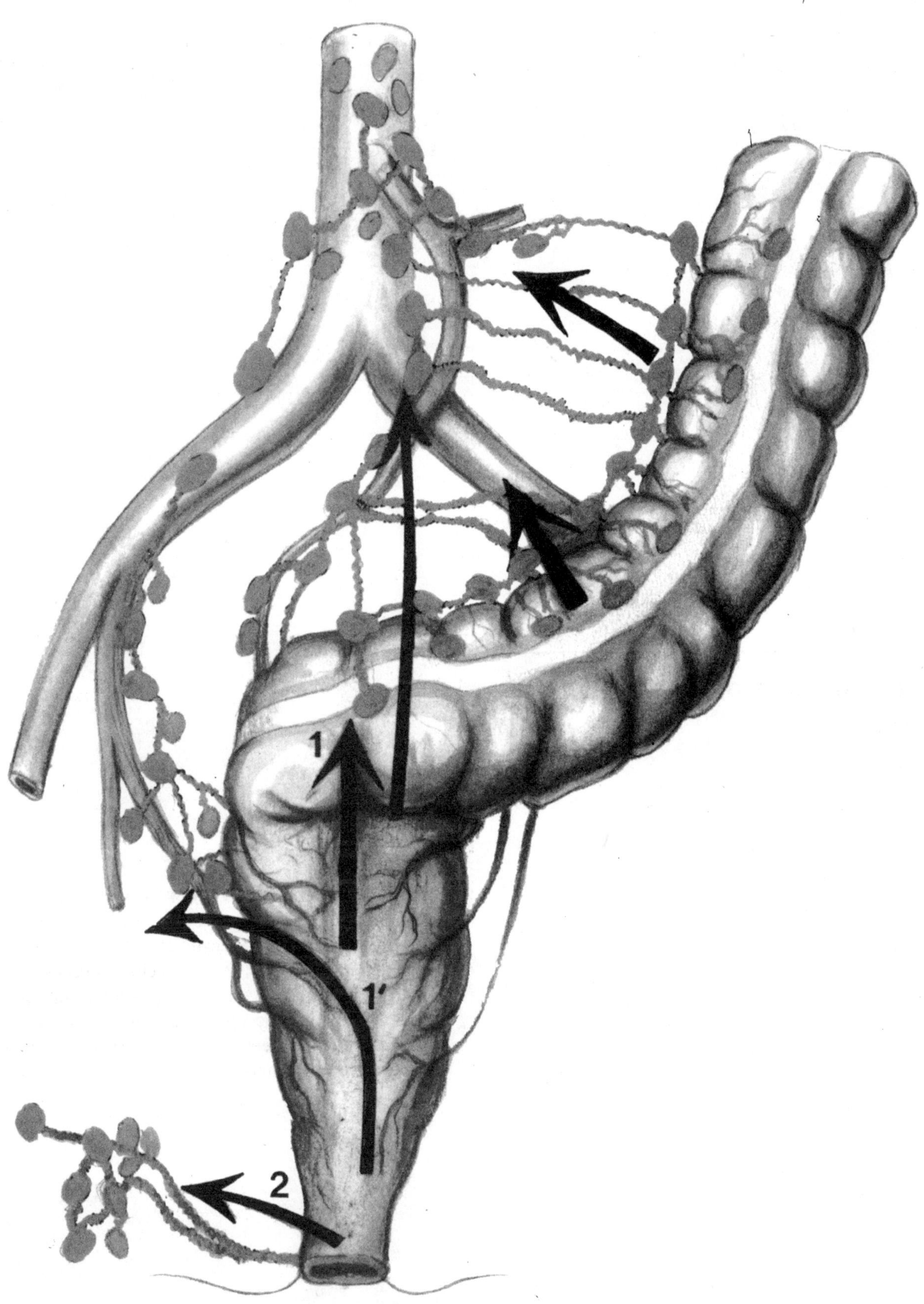

FIGURE 48.4

Surgical Anatomy of the Rectum and Anus

FIGURE 48.5 ANATOMY OF THE PERINEAL REGION

1, External anal sphincter (deep fascicle); 1′, External anal sphincter (superficial fascicle); 1″, External anal sphincter (subcutaneous fascicle); 2, puborectalis muscle (levator ani fascicle); 3, pubococcygeal muscle (levator ani muscle); 4, gluteus major; 5, anococcygeal ligament; 6, coccyx; 7, superficial transverse perineal muscle; 8, bulbocavernosus muscle; 9, ischiocavernosus muscle.

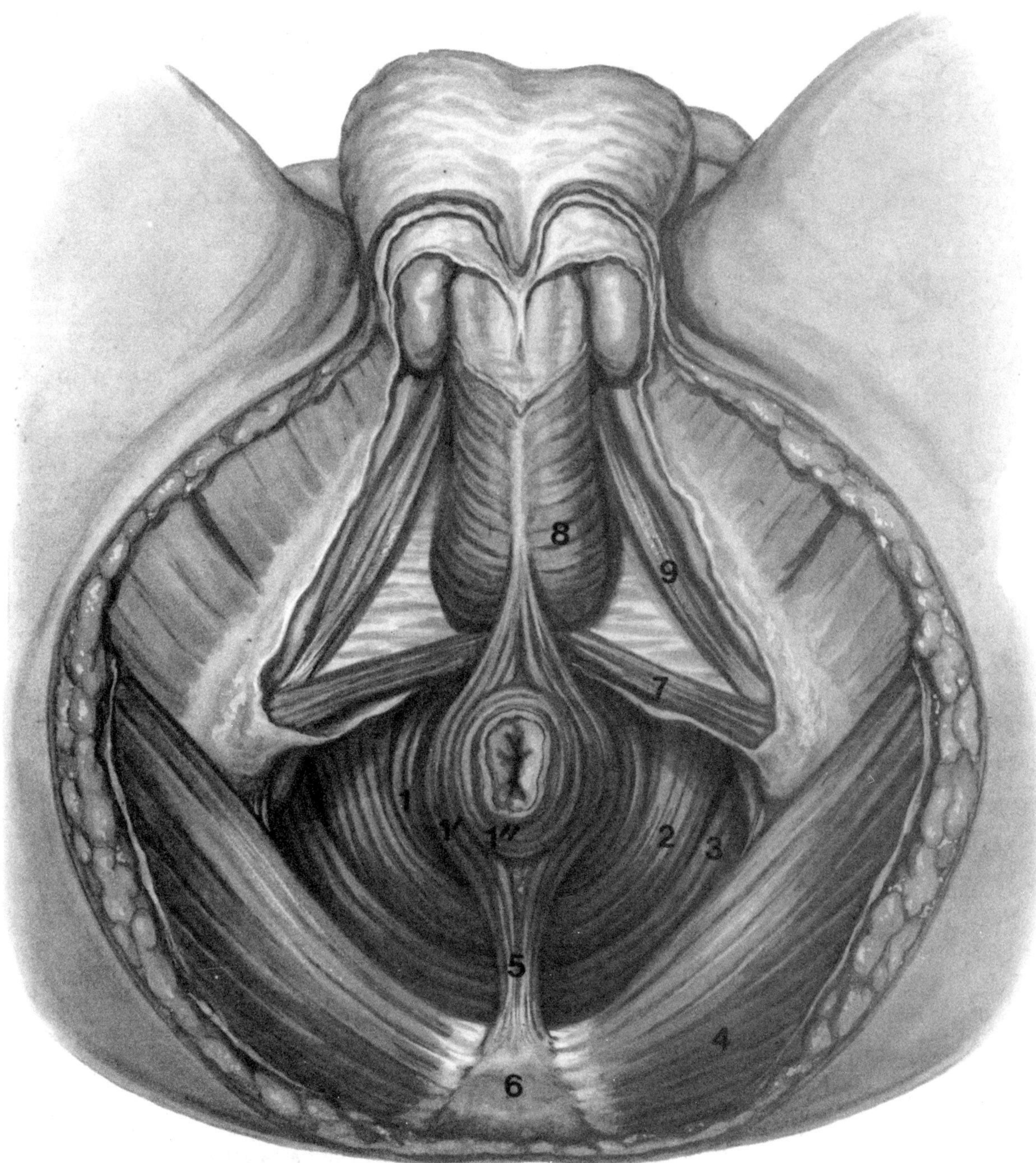

FIGURE 48.5 ANATOMY OF THE PERINEAL REGION

Surgical Anatomy of the Rectum and Anus

FIGURE 48.6 PERINEAL ARTERIES
1, Internal pudendal artery; 2, Alcock's canal; 3, inferior hemorrhoidal artery; 4, superficial perineal artery.

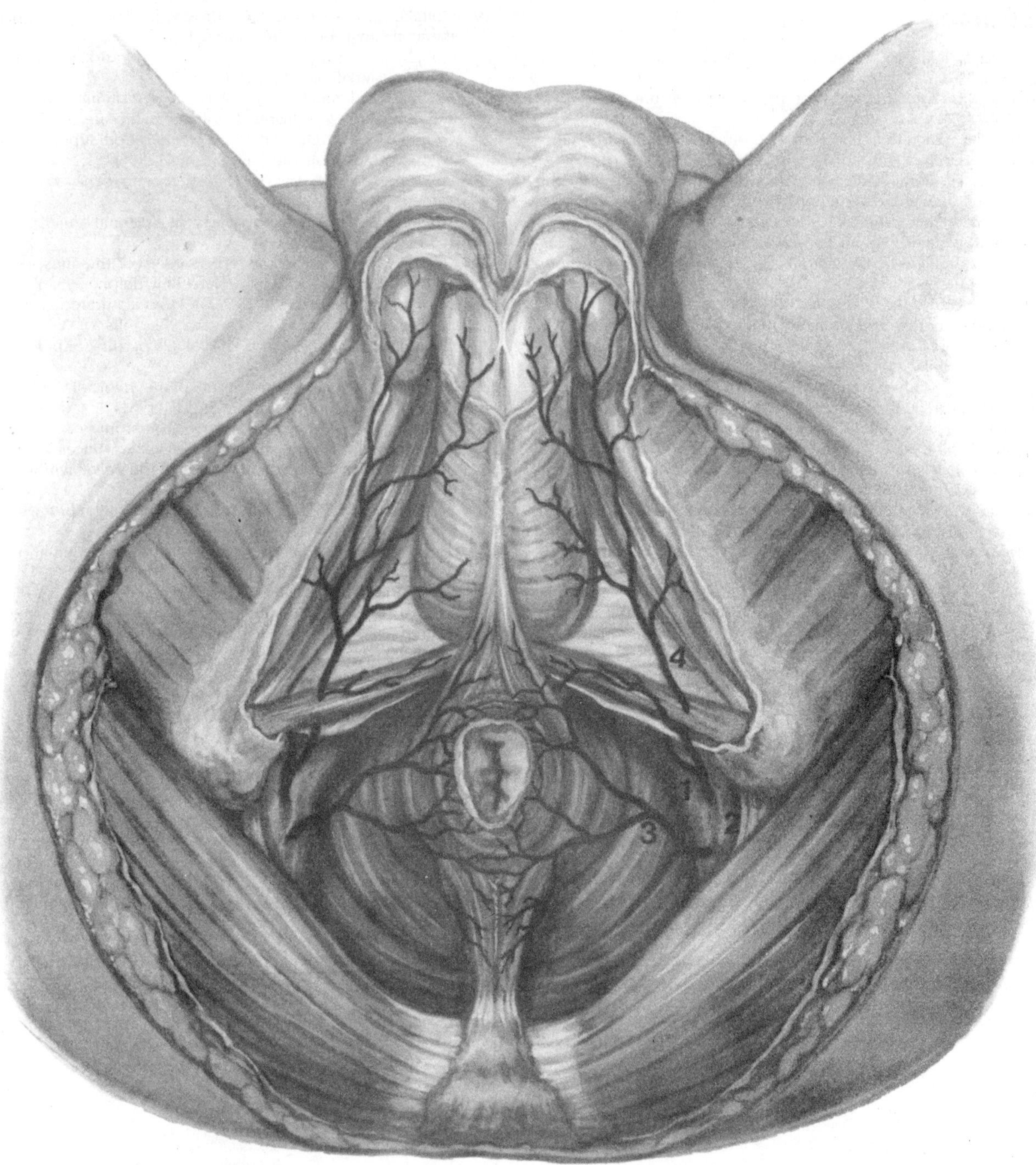

FIGURE 48.6 PERINEAL ARTERIES

References

1. Abramson, D.J. The valves of Houston in adults. Am. J. Surg. 136:334, 1978.
2. Ayoub, S.E. Arterial supply of the human rectum. Acta Anat. 100:317, 1978.
3. Babb, R.R., Kieraldo, J.H. Sexual dysfunction after abdomino-perineal resection. Am. J. Dig. Dis. 22:1127, 1971.
4. Bauer, J.J., Galernt, I.M., Salky, B., Kreel, I. Sexual dysfunction following protectomy for benign disease of the colon and rectum. Ann. Surg. 197:363, 1983.
5. Best, R.R., Blair, J.B. Sphincter preserving operations for rectal carcinoma as related to the anatomy of the lymphatics. Ann. Surg. 130:538, 1949.
6. Blair, J.B., Holyyoke, E.A., Best, R.R. A note on the lymphatics of the middle and lower rectum and anus. Anat. Rec. 108:635, 1950.
7. Corman, M.L. Colon and rectal surgery. Ed. 3, p. 596, 1993. Lippincott, Philadelphia, 1993.
8. Crapp, A.R., Cuthbertson, A.M. William Waldeyer and the rectosacral fascia. Surg. Gynecol. Obstet. 138:252, 1974.
9. D'Allaines, F. Traitement chirurgical du cancer du rectum. Flammarion, Paris, 1946.
10. Duthie, H.L., Gairns, F.W. Sensory nerve endings and sensation in the anal region of man. Br. J. Surg. 47:585, 1960.
11. Fozard, J.B.J., Pemberton, J.H. Applied surgical anatomy: Pelvic contents. In Fielding, L.P., Goldberg, S.M. (Eds.) Surgery of the colon, rectum and anus. Ed. 5, p. 11. Butterworth-Heinemann, Oxford, 1993.
12. Gask, G.E., Ross, J.P. The surgery of the sympathetic nervous system. Ed. 2. Bailliere Tindall, London, 1937.
13. Gilchrist, R.R., David, V.C. Lymphatic spread of carcinoma of the rectum. Ann. Surg. 108:621, 1938.
14. Glover, R.P., Waugh, J.M. The retrograde lymphatic spread of carcinoma of the "rectosigmoid region": Its influence on surgical procedures. Surg. Gynecol. Obstet. 82:434, 1946.
15. Goligher, J.C. The blood supply to the sigmoid and rectum. Br. J. Surg. 37:157, 1949.
16. Goligher, J.C., Hughes, E.S.R. Sensibility of the rectum and colon: Its role in the mechanism of anal continence. Lancet 1:543, 1951.
17. Goligher, J.C. Discussion on urological complications of excision of the rectum. Proc. R. Soc. Med. 44:824, 1951.
18. Goligher, J.C. The adequacy of marginal blood supply to the left colon after high ligation of the inferior mesenteric artery during excision of the rectum. Br. J. Surg. 41:351, 1954.
19. Goligher, J.C., Leacock, A.G., Brossy, J.J. The surgical anatomy of the anal canal. Br. J. Surg. 43:51, 1955.
20. Goligher, J.C. Surgery of the anus, rectum and colon. Ed. 4, p. 1. Bailliere Tindall, London, 1980.
21. Gray, S.W., Skandalakis, J.E. Atlas of surgical anatomy for general surgeons, P. 232. Williams & Wilkins. Baltimore, 1985.
22. Griffiths, J.D. Surgical anatomy of the blood supply of the distal colon. Ann. R. Coll. Surg. Engl. 19:241, 1956.
23. Hollinshead, W.H. Anatomy for surgeons. Vol. 2, p. 693. Hoeber-Harper, New York, 1956.
24. Hughes, E.S.R. Surgical anatomy of the anal canal. Aust. N. Z. J. Surg. 26:48, 1959.
25. Keighley, M.R.B., Williams, N.S. Surgery of the anus, rectum and colon. Vol. 1, p. 1. W.B. Saunders, Philadelphia, 1993.
26. Kodner, I.J., Fleshman, J.W., Fry, R.D. Anal and rectal cancer: Principles of management. In Schwartz, S.I., Ellis, H. (Eds.). Maingot's abdominal operations. Ed. 9, vol. 2, p. 1107. Appleton Lange, Norwalk, CT, 1985.
27. Learmonth, J.R. A contribution to the neurophysiology of the urinary bladder in man. Brain 54:147, 1931.
28. Milligan, E.T.C., Morgan, N. Surgical anatomy of the anal canal: With special reference to anorectal fistulae. Lancet 2:1150, 1934.
29. Nesselrod, J.P. An anatomic restudy of the pelvic lymphatics. Ann. Surg. 104:905, 1936.
30. Nivatvongs, S., Stern, H.S., Fryd, D.S. The length of the anal canal. Dis. Colon Rectum 24:600, 1982.
31. Parks, A.G. Pathogenesis and treatment of fistula-in-ano. Br. Med. J. 1:463, 1961.
32. Roslyn, J.J., Zinner, M.J. The colon and rectum. Surgical anatomy and operative procedure. In Sabiston, D.C. (ed). Textbook of surgery. Ed. 14, p. 899. W.B. Saunders, Philadelphia, 1991.
33. Shafik, A. A new concept of the anatomy of the anal sphincter mechanism of the physiology of defecation. The external anal sphincter: A triple-loop system. Invest. Urol. 12:412, 1975.
34. Siddhart, P., Ravo, B. Colorectal neovasculature and anal sphincter. Surg. Clin. North Am. 68:1195, 1988.
35. Telford, E.D., Stopford, J.S.B. Autonomic nerve supply of the distal colon; anatomical and clinical study. Br. Med. J. 1:572, 1934.
36. Tobin, C.E., Benjamin, J.A. Anatomical and surgical restudy of Denonvilliers' fascia. Surg. Gynecol. Obstet. 80:373, 1945.
37. Weinstein, M., Roberts, M. Sexual potency following surgery for rectal carcinoma. A follow-up of 44 patients. Ann. Surg. 185:295, 1977.
38. Woollard, H., Norrish, R.E. The anatomy of the peripheral sympathetic nervous system. Br. J. Surg. 21:83, 1933.

Section H

Colon, Rectum, and Anus

CHAPTER **49**

Colectomy for Cancer

GENERAL PRINCIPLES

In resections for carcinoma of the colon, it is necessary to fulfill several requirements to obtain the best late results with low mortality and morbidity. Other factors related to oncologic surgery should be taken into consideration with the object of obtaining a high survival index and offering the patient a maximum of well-being. Before proceeding with the analysis of these factors, we feel it is useful to make a short description of the most important pathologic characteristics of cancer of the colon and how it spreads, since these are related to surgical therapy.

In men, colorectal carcinoma is the most frequent cause of death due to cancer, after carcinoma of the lung and prostate. In addition, carcinomas of the colon and rectum constitute the most common form of cancer of the digestive tract (9, 22, 50, 66, 73, 96). In females, colorectal cancer is second in frequency, after breast cancer.

In 1987 there were 145,000 new carcinomas of the colon in the United States, and about 60,000 patients died due to these cancers. In the same year, there were 150,000 new cases of cancer of the lung, which led to 136,000 deaths (9, 22, 66, 96). At the same time as the increase in frequency of colorectal cancer there has been a modification of the location of carcinoma of the colon (88). According to Morgenstern and Lee (73), in 1009 patients, the carcinoma was located in the rectum in 15% of cases, and in the right colon in 24%. Previously there used to be 12 to 15% of patients who had carcinoma in the right colon. The increase in incidence of carcinoma of the right colon has been proven to occur in both Europe and in America, without any obvious cause being present for this change.

GROSS AND MICROSCOPIC CARCINOMA OF THE COLON AND ITS SPREAD

The most common gross appearance of cancer of the colon is an ulcerated tumor, with a polypoid tumor next in frequency. Less frequently, one observes an annular or stenosing form of tumor, which is most common in the left colon. Finally, there occurs the infiltrated form of tumor, which is more malignant than previous forms and appears grossly to be very much like the linitis plastica form of stomach carcinoma (74).

From the microscopic point of view, it is accepted that about 20% of carcinomas of the colon are histologically well differentiated, 60% are moderately differentiated, and in the remaining 20% the tumors are undifferentiated, according to Morson and Dawson (74).

The spread of carcinoma of the colon may occur in the following forms:

1. By continuity.
2. By the lymphatic route.
3. By the hematogenous route.
4. Directly through the abdomen.
5. By implantation.

Direct dissemination, or by continuity, is most frequent following the transverse axis of the colon. Dissemination following the longitudinal axis of the colon is less important. Microscopic infiltration rarely extends for more than 10 mm from the macroscopic limit of the tumor (74, 84). Direct infiltration in the transverse direction extends an average of one quarter of the circumference of the bowel every 6 months. The characteristics of dissemination of colon cancer are very important at the moment of determining the extent of the length of segment to be resected.

According to Morson and Dawson (74), direct spread of carcinoma is through the planes of less resistance. Neoplastic infiltration starts in the mucosa, then passes to the submucosa, where it spreads rapidly due to structural characteristics of the submucosa, which is made up of rather loose tissue. The muscularis propia layer is an impediment for spread of the tumor through the wall itself because it is a dense tissue that offers great resistance to spread of the tumor. Invasion of the muscularis propia layer is through the spaces where blood vessels pass through it (74).

In all of the cases, the pathologist should include in his or her report an estimation of the degree of malignancy of the tumor and its microscopic extent along the length of the bowel because these have important prognostic value (74).

Lymphatic Dissemination. In cancer of the colon, lymphatic invasion is progressive, step by step from lymph node to lymph node, and not in jumps. The first nodes to be involved are the paracolic nodes closest to the carcinoma. From there, malignant cells spread to the intermediate ganglia and then to the principal or precavoaortic nodes. Only rarely can invasion of distant ganglia occur without previous infiltration of the nodes near the tumor. All of the resected nodes should be examined microscopically. Patient survival diminishes in direct relation to the number of lymphatic nodes invaded by the tumor. According to Morson and Dawson (74), if only one node in the immediate vicinity of the tumor has been invaded, 5-year survival is 60%. If the lymphatic invasion has involved 2 to 5 ganglia, 5-year survival falls to 35%. If the neoplastic invasion has affected 6 or more nodes, 5-year survival diminishes to 20%. In order to have a better approximation of the length of time the patient should survive, the lymphatic invasion should be related to the degree of malignancy of the primary tumor, its degree of penetration and extension, and other factors.

Hematogenous Spread. In 75% of patients, hematogenous spread is toward the liver, in 15% toward the lung, in 5% toward the bones, and in 5% toward the brain (5, 10, 27, 51, 74). It has been proven that during the induction of anesthesia in surgery for cancer of the colon, 28% of patients have circulating malignant cells. This number rises to 50% if the study is performed during the laparotomy. In spite of these findings, follow-up of these patients did not show any changes in the prognosis due to the presence of circulating neoplastic malignant cells.

Every specimen resected for carcinoma should be examined very carefully to determine if there is carcinomous invasion of the veins. This invasion may be macroscopic or microscopic. Careful dissection of the course of the mesenteric vessels may show the presence of venous invasion or permeation (74). In a study performed by Morson on 1000 specimens of patients with carcinoma of the colon and rectum, 35% presented a dissemination of the cancer in the regional veins. The submucosal veins were invaded in 10% of patients, and in 25% of patients extramural permeation of the veins was found to exist. The frequency of venous dissemination was greater in the specimens in which the regional lymph nodes were found to be invaded and in the surgical specimens that revealed tumors of greater malignancy. According to Morson and other authors (14, 74, 94, 100), venous invasion or invasion limited to the submucosa does not change the prognosis in the patients, but permeation of the extramural veins leads to severe consequences in the prognosis, reducing 5-year survival from 55% to 30%. The presence of permeation of the veins by the tumor does not have the significance of an embolization of malignant cells or metastases some distance away (74).

Transabdominal Dissemination. Carcinoma of the colon grows deeply, and if it invades the serosa, malignant cells can become detached from the primary tumor and implant themselves in any portion of the peritoneal cavity. One organ that is frequently a receptacle for detached malignant colonic cells is the ovary. This is what is known as Krukenberg tumor. Some surgeons (69) have proposed carrying out prophylactic bilateral oophorectomy in women with carcinoma of the colon in the premenopausal period. Consent for this additional procedure should be obtained.

Implantation of Malignant Cells. The detached malignant cells from the primary tumor implant themselves and colonize raw surfaces in a colonic or colorectal suture line, in anal fistulas, in surgical wounds of hemorrhoidectomy, in fissures and fistulas, around colostomies, or even, in some cases, in the incision in the abdominal wall (1, 7, 11, 12, 15, 58, 61, 65, 71, 92). In colonic resections for carcinoma performed by laparoscopy, it has been shown that malignant cells have been implanted in the abdominal wall as the tumor is removed from the abdomen.

The chance of cancer of the colon or rectum in the suture line by implantation of malignant cells detached from the primary tumor is a proven fact (1, 7, 11, 12, 15, 58, 61, 65, 92). In addition to this form of recurrence in the suture line, by implantation of malignant cells, there is another form of "recurrence" in the suture line, which is not due to implantation of malignant cells detached from the primary tumor, but is due to having left tumor behind, which, as it continues to grow, invades the suture line (60, 74, 75).

STAGING OF CARCINOMA OF THE COLON

In 1932 Dukes (29) proposed a staging of carcinoma of the rectum, which was later applied to carcinoma of the colon (30–32). The staging proposed by Dukes is simple and easy to apply. Dukes' A Class corresponds to malignant lesions that have not gone through the muscularis propia layer of the colon and do not show any lymph node invasion (74, 75). This stage of evolution of cancer of the colon is seen in 15% of the cases, all of them being cured by surgical treatment. Dukes' B stage is when the carcinoma has passed through the muscularis propia layer and invaded pericolonic tissue without invasion of regional lymph nodes. This stage of evolution is seen in 35% of patients, and these have the possibility of being cured by means of surgery in 70% of patients (74, 75). Dukes' C is the stage in which carcinoma of the colon has invaded the lymph nodes. According to Morson and Dawson, one in every three patients in group C subjected to surgery can survive 5 years. The same authors assert that this group includes 50% of the patients.

After Dukes, many authors have made great efforts to attempt to establish a staging that will be of real help in determining the prognosis as exactly as possible in patients with carcinoma of the colon and rectum. None of the staging methods that have been proposed have been able to replace the classical staging of Dukes. These staging methods are very complex, difficult to record and apply (48, 50, 108), and therefore impractical. According to Gordon et al. (50), a staging method is valuable when it is simple and can be recorded easily. The T N M (Tumor, Nodes, Metastasis) staging method is not used as often due to its complexity.

The diagnosis of carcinoma of the colon is made by means of a clinical history, physical examination of the patient, rectal examination, rectoscopy, sigmoidoscopy, colonoscopy, double contrast by an enema X-ray study, chest X-ray, ultrasonography, computed axial tomography, magnetic resonance, and determination of the carcinoembryonic antigen. This latter study is very useful in determining postoperative recurrences.

FACTORS TO BE ASSESSED IN SURGERY FOR CARCINOMA OF THE COLON

As determined previously, in surgery for carcinoma of the colon, several factors must be contemplated, not only to obtain the best operative results, but also to attain the longest possible survival of the patients.

Proceeding in didactic fashion, these factors will be analyzed in orderly fashion just as if an operation for carcinoma of the colon were being carried out, beginning with intestinal preparation, the abdominal incision, and so on, and ending with the closure of the abdominal wall.

1. ***Preparation of the colon:*** An adequate preparation of the colon is essential before surgery with the object of diminishing septic complications as well as dehiscence of sutures. There is no doubt that it is impossible to sterilize the colon, but its septic state can be diminished considerably. Progress of surgery of the colon was delayed for many years because of the impossibility of adequately preparing the colon. Preparation of the colon is by mechanical means and by means of antibiotics that are adequately selected to attack the intestinal flora.

The following method of preparation of the colon for surgery is frequently used:

a. The patient should be kept on a liquid diet during the entire day before the operation.
b. The afternoon of that same day, the patient should ingest 4 liters of an electrolytic hypertonic solution of Glycopolyethylene over a period of 2 to 4 hours. This solution is given in order to carry out an oral irrigation of the colon. For some patients, ingestion of 4 liters of these solutions is very difficult due to the volume and the taste, and because in some patients, they produce nausea. In order to avoid the nausea, 10 mg of metoclopramide is given one hour previously. Patients who are prepared with the

oral solution should be given an intravenous infusion to avoid dehydration. Oral irrigation of the colon is contraindicated in patients with colonic obstruction and in patients of advanced age.

c. Another method that is effective in mechanically irrigating the colon is the ingestion of one liter of 10% Mannitol solution over a period of 2 hours on the day prior to the operation (35, 45, 54). Mechanical irrigation of the colon with Golytely or with the 10% Mannitol solution is carried out without using laxatives or enemas.

d. In cases in which patients do not tolerate oral mechanical irrigation, classic laxatives and enemas should be used. One of the most commonly used laxatives is magnesium sulfate. The patient should take 10 grams three times a day beginning 48 hours before surgery. Magnesium citrate can also be used, taking it in the same way and amount as the magnesium sulfate. When preparation of the colon is performed using laxatives, it is necessary to add cleansing enemas.

e. If the patient is found to be insufficiently prepared while in the operating room the surgeon may resort to irrigation of the colon by the procedure proposed by Dudley (28).

f. Mechanical irrigation should be complemented by antibiotic preparation of the colon. Surgeons use several antibiotics and combinations of antibiotics. It is important to select the antibiotics that are active against Gram positive, Gram negative, and anaerobic bacteria.

g. A frequently used combination of antibiotics is as follows: one gram of erythromycin base and one gram of neomycin, which will be taken at 1 P.M., at 2 P.M., and at 11 P.M. the day before surgery. To this combination, an injection of cephalosporin of the second generation antibiotics is added. Additionally, an intravenous injection of metronidazole, 500 mg, is added one hour before the surgery. In order to be able to prepare the colon adequately, the patient should be hospitalized 24 hours before the operation. It is generally not necessary to give any more antibiotics after the first day following the surgery.

2. ***Abdominal incision:*** The incisions that are used to carry out colonic resections are numerous, the most frequent one being the midline supra- and infraumbilical incision. The author prefers the right paramedian incision for surgery of the right colon and the left paramedian incision for surgery of the left colon. Once the abdomen is open, the edges of the abdominal incision should be protected with adequate gauze packs.

3. ***Exploration of the abdominal cavity:*** Before beginning to explore the abdominal cavity, it should be determined if the greater omentum is adherent to the capsule of the spleen. If these adhesions are present, they should be transected before exploring the abdomen to prevent rupture of the splenic capsule and consequent bleeding.

   Exploration of abdominal viscera should be carried out completely, both visually and by palpation. The presence of hepatic metastases and metastases to the peritoneal surface, visceral or parietal, should be investigated. Attention should be given to the pouch of Douglas, where metastatic nodules can be felt (Blumer shelf) or to the ovaries (Krukenberg tumor). A synchronous colonic tumor should be searched for, and unsuspected pathology should also be investigated. The liver can be studied by operative ultrasonography in case there are liver metastases that cannot be seen or felt (79). If a single metastatic tumor of the liver is present, in an easy location, it can be resected after resecting the colon for the carcinoma, if the patient's condition permits it. The position of the nasogastric tube that has been introduced by the anesthesiologist should be determined. This tube should be placed with its distal end in the gastric antrum.

   Once the described requirements have been accomplished, the carcinoma is identified and its location, size, the existence of serosal invasion, fixation, adherence to other organs or to the anterior or posterior abdominal wall, the presence of nodes, and their size and consistency, are studied. Special attention should be given to the principal or precavoaortic nodes. If there are doubts about the presence of metastasis in the principal or precavoaortic nodes, suspicious nodes should be removed for frozen section study. Examination of the tumor should be carried out with a minimum of handling, which is possible in the great majority of patients.

   Once the surgeon has carried out the exploration, he or she can determine with adequate certainty if the surgery will be carried out with hope for a cure or only for palliation.

4. ***Technique of colonic resection:*** The most important act of the surgeon is to carry out a resection of the primary tumor with a margin of safety including the lymphatic areas according to the location of the tumor. Resection of a cancer of the colon can be done with a conventional or classic technique, which consists of mobilizing the colon with the tumor, carrying out the vascular ligatures, and then resecting the colon with the tumor.

   Resection of the colon with the tumor can also be carried out by means of the "no touch isolation technique." This technique was originally proposed by Barnes in 1952 (7), but popularized by Turnbull of the Cleveland Clinic in the United States, whose work was published in 1967 (100), revealing the results obtained by him. The "no touch isolation technique" procedure consists of disconnecting the tumor from the body by ligating the blood vessels and later mobilizing the colon with the tumor so as to prevent handling of the tumor leading to dissemination of malignant cells by the venous route. Turnbull and colleagues, in 664 cases of carcinoma of the colon, obtained a 5-year survival of 58% in Dukes' Group C, while another team from the Cleveland Clinic, operating by the classical technique obtained only 28% 5-year survival in Dukes' Group C cases.

Following Turnbull's publication, Glass, Fazio, and others (45), also of the Cleveland Clinic, published late results of the "no touch" technique in 564 patients, obtaining a similar result to that obtained by Turnbull, even though the 5-year survival in the Dukes' Group C was somewhat lower, although always superior to that obtained with the classical technique. Wiggers and colleagues (104) in a prospective controlled and randomized multicentric study of 236 cases of cancer of the colon, operated on by means of a classical and "no touch" technique, presented a slightly superior survival with the "no touch" technique. This difference was too small to give it importance. Wiggers and colleagues additionally came to the conclusion that hepatic metastases appeared later with the "no touch" technique and that angioinvasive carcinomas develop metastases with less frequency than with the classical technique. Fielding (40) confirmed that angioinvasive carcinomas are those that metastasize to the liver more frequently and that this variety of colon cancer is the one that is most benefited by the "no touch" technique. Other authors have also emphasized this about angioinvasive carcinomas (45, 56, 101, 104, 105).

The author has practiced the "no touch" technique since 1965, after remaining for one month in the colorectal surgery department directed by Dr. Turnbull in the Cleveland Clinic, where he appreciated the advantages of this procedure.

The "no touch" technique emphasizes basic oncologic principles of surgery for cancer of the colon. Several statistical studies have revealed that 5-year survival in Dukes Group C patients has been greater with this technique than with the classical technique (45, 101, 104, 105). In some of these reports, survival was slightly elevated (104, 105), and in others it was obviously superior (45, 101). In none of these statistical studies was it shown that the mortality, morbidity, and operative time were greater with this technique than with the classical technique. On the other hand, the "no touch" technique was shown to be a simple, clean, and logical anatomic procedure.

The author has shown that surgeons who have once undertaken the "no touch" technique have not again performed a colectomy by the conventional technique.

There are surgeons who maintain a position contrary to the "no touch" technique because it does not increase the 5-year survival in Dukes' Group C, as had been reported by Turnbull. It is acceptable that the "no touch" technique may not be practiced by some surgeons because of lack of habit, lack of conviction, or some other reason, but it is difficult to accept that they have opposed the "no touch" technique, attacking its being carried out.

5. ***Ligature of the colonic lumen,*** proximal and distal to the carcinoma, is carried out to prevent the passage of malignant cells, which, if they are viable, may colonize raw surfaces. Ligatures should be placed around the colon. Viability of malignant cells that have become separated from the primary tumor lasts an average of 20 minutes (1, 8, 16, 33, 61, 65, 68, 75).
6. ***Ligature of colonic vessels:*** Ligature of the ileocolic and the right colic arteries should be carried out at their origin from the superior mesenteric artery. Ligature of the middle colic artery should be carried out at the inferior border of the pancreas. Ligature of the left colic artery should be carried out at its origin from the inferior mesenteric artery. The sigmoidal arteries should be ligated at their origin in the inferior mesenteric artery or in the left colic artery. Before transecting the colic arteries, it is advisable to place ligatures around the colon, proximally and distally, which are to be resected with the surgical specimen.

   In order to carry out the ligature of the colic arteries, the surgeon should know the anatomic distribution of the arteries of the colon and their anatomic variations. A great proportion of the surgical failures in surgery for carcinoma of the colon are due to the circulatory factor (25), because the blood supply of the colon is inferior to the blood supply of the stomach, small bowel, and rectum (85).
7. ***Ligature of the epiploic appendices:*** Incorrect ligature of the epiploic appendices may lead to local necrosis of the wall of the colon. This may be because the long, straight arteries that arise from the marginal artery of Drummond, before they enter underneath the muscular bands, run subserosally and sometimes have a loop in the base of the epiploic appendix. If the epiploic appendix is tied at or near its base, necrosis of the colonic wall may be pro-

duced. Therefore, ligature of the epiploic appendix should be carried out away from its base. It is therefore very important not to apply traction on the clamp that is grasping the epiploic appendix.

8. ***Mobilization of the colon:*** Mobilization of the colon is simple after having divided the parietocolic peritoneum, be it in the right or the left hemicolon.

In order to completely mobilize the transverse colon, the gastrocolic ligament should be divided. In mobilization of the cecum, as well as the sigmoid colon, care should be taken not to injure the ureter or the gonadal vessels. When the hepatic flexure is mobilized, care should be taken not to injure the duodenum. In the hepatic flexure, care should also be taken when applying traction to the mesocolon because the inferior pancreaticoduodenal vein, which together with the right gastroepiploic and the right superior colic veins makes up the trunk of Henle, which empties into the right lateral wall of the superior mesenteric vein, can be injured. Injury to the inferior pancreaticoduodenal vein may lead to hemorrhage, which is difficult to control due to retraction of the injured vein, which makes it difficult to grasp it with a hemostatic clamp. As will be seen later in the technique used to perform a right hemicolectomy, before mobilizing the hepatic flexure of the colon, the author ligates Henle's trunk at the inferior border of the neck of the pancreas. Ligation of the venous trunk of Henle allows exposure of the transverse mesocolon, the mesoduodenum, and the mesogastrium.

Mobilization of the splenic flexure of the colon may lead to injury of the spleen with its consequences.

9. ***Division of the colon:*** Before proceeding to transect the colon, it is very useful to cover the edges of the abdominal wound with a wound protector (25), which will be shown when the operative technique is described. The wound protector is removed at the end of the septic period in the surgery. If this appliance is not available, the wound edges should be protected with gauze pads. Atraumatic clamps are placed near the sites where the colon is to be transected to prevent, as much as possible, spillage of fecal contents. Additionally, the entire abdominal cavity is covered with gauze pads, leaving only the segment of the colon to be removed exposed.

10. ***Colocolic, ileocolic, or colorectal anastomosis:*** The great majority of surgeons agree that, if the anastomosis has been carried out correctly, results are similar with a manual suture, a mechanical suture, or a biofragmentable ring (Valtrac) (1, 20, 24, 25, 50, 53, 60, 77). Some surgeons carry out these anastomoses with only one layer of sutures, others in two layers, either continuously or with interrupted sutures.

The author prefers manual suturing in two layers using interrupted sutures, as will be shown later (71, 72). The mucosal layer is sutured with 3-0 chromic catgut; the seromuscular layer, which should include the submucosal layer, with cotton, silk, or nonabsorbable synthetic material. The results with this technique have been highly satisfactory. The edges of the colon to be anastomosed should be clean and well exposed, avoiding interposition of fatty tissue, mesentery, or an epiploic appendix.

In carrying out the anastomosis, inclusion of one or more diverticula should be avoided. If colonic diverticula are too numerous and their inclusion cannot be avoided, the technique should be changed to an end-to-side anastomosis (25). Care should be taken to avoid the formation of hematomas, whether in the colonic wall or in its mesocolon, to avoid a decrease in the blood supply to the colon. If the survival of one of the ends of the colon is suspect, another segment of the bowel should be selected to carry out the anastomosis. It is of great importance to start the anastomosis at the mesenteric border of the colon in order that this layer of sutures be carried out as correctly as possible, because the mesenteric border is the most difficult area to suture and is most exposed to dehiscence (92). It should be borne in mind when a colorectal or ileorectal anastomosis is performed that the longitudinal muscular layer of the rectum frequently retracts itself, and the suture of the colon may be performed without including this layer, which results in a suture line more prone to dehiscence.

11. ***Mechanical suture of the colon:*** This technique will be described later.
12. ***Colonic suturing with the biofragmentable ring*** (Valtrac): This technique will be described later.
13. ***Dehiscence of the colonic suture:*** In colonic surgery one should not be complacent because, if all the technical details are not carried out, a dehiscence of the suture line may occur, which is potentially fatal (60).

The possibility of dehiscence of the colonic suture line diminishes in the following situations:

1. The colon has been adequately prepared by mechanical means and with antibiotics.
2. There is no septic abdominal process present. Well-regarded surgeons (70), however, carry out resections and anastomoses of the colon with good results in the presence of peritoneal sepsis.
3. Healthy appearance of the colonic ends.
4. The colonic ends appear to be well supplied by blood.
5. The anastomosis has been correctly performed.
6. The anastomosis was not carried out under tension.

Schrock, Devenely, and Dunphy (92), in a very complete investigation of the causes of dehiscence of the colonic suture line, assert that if the above mentioned factors are respected, the incidence of dehiscence of the colonic suture line averages about 2%. There are other causes of dehiscence that may occur under special circumstances, such as surgical shock in the immediate postoperative period, emergency colonic surgery without preparation of the colon, the presence of carcinomatous tissue in the colonic ends to be anastomosed, preoperative X-ray therapy, and the presence of dead spaces (25, 92).

14. ***Proximal colostomy:*** It has been shown that a colostomy proximal to the suture line does not change the incidence of dehiscence but does improve the prognosis, due to a decrease in the mortality of dehiscence (25, 92). Proximal colostomy is only indicated in special cases—for example, when the evolution of the colorectal suture is doubtful, or in cases in which patients have been previously irradiated (25).
15. ***Cecostomy:*** A cecostomy does not carry out a complete deviation of the colonic contents and does not diminish the number of dehiscences or the mortality due to these dehiscences (25, 92).
16. ***End-to-end, end-to-side, and side-to-side anastomoses:*** The end-to-end anastomosis is the one most frequently used by surgeons. If the diameter of one of the ends to be anastomosed is less than the other, the Cheatle incision on the antimesenteric border can be resorted to in order to make both ends the same in diameter. The end-to-side anastomosis is carried out less frequently and is usually indicated in lower colorectal anastomoses, because the rectal ampulla has a greater diameter than the colon. The end-to-side is also indicated in cases in which it is not possible to carry out an end-to-end anastomosis due to the presence of many diverticula. A side-to-side colonic anastomosis is only rarely indicated.
17. ***Surgical control of the impermeability of the anastomosis:*** In all colonic anastomoses impermeability should be controlled. If mechanical suture is carried out, attention should be given to hemostasis of the edges of the colon in addition to control of the impermeability of the anastomosis.
18. ***Extent of colonic resection:*** The extent of colonic resection for carcinoma is related to the lymphatic areas that should be resected according to the location of the tumor. The drawings show the extent of resection of the colon to be carried out in different locations of the tumor. A segmental resection of the sigmoid colon in case of a localized tumor in a redundant sigmoid colon may be indicated. If the carcinoma is advanced and there is ample lymphatic dissemination, a resection of greater extent should be resorted to.
19. ***Extent of resection of the lymphatic areas:*** Extensive lymphatic resections have not improved the survival of patients with carcinoma of the colon (80). Some surgeons, however, are convinced that extensive resection of lymphatic areas improves the survival of the patient (38). It should be pointed out that extensive resection of nodes increases the morbidity and mortality of the procedures.
20. ***Closure of the mesentery:*** When the anastomosis of the colon is finished, the edges of the mesenteric border are sutured. The author prefers to suture the mesentery in two layers, suturing on one side the anterior, serosal layer and on the posterior side, the same serosal area, with nonabsorbable interrupted sutures. Using this technique, one avoids having to pass the sutures through the full thickness of the mesentery with the possibility of injuring a vessel and making further resection necessary. In addition, suturing of the peritoneum on both sides of the mesentery produces a better peritonealization.
21. ***Coverage of the colonic suture with the greater omentum:*** A correctly performed colonic anastomosis does not have to be covered with the greater omentum. A plastic procedure on the greater omentum may be indicated in subperitoneal colorectal anastomoses. This will both reinforce the suture lines between the colon, which is covered with peritoneum, and the rectum, which has no peritoneum, and fill the presacral dead space.
22. ***Drainage of the abdominal cavity:*** In anastomoses carried out within the peritoneal cavity, it is not necessary to leave an abdominal drain. A drain should be left in the pelvic cavity in patients with low subperitoneal colorectal anastomoses. Subperitoneal dissection of the rectum leads to a dead pelvic presacral space where serum and blood may accumulate, leading to suppuration and favoring dehiscence of the colorectal suture line. Drainage of the presacral space is carried out by means of a rubber tube connected to a closed suction apparatus (closed suction drain). The end of the drainage tube should be placed away from the suture line.
23. ***Closure of the abdominal wall:*** The abdominal wall is closed in layers. Before suturing the anterior rectal sheath and the subcutaneous cellular tissue, it is advisable to irrigate the wound with warm saline solution. If there happened to be considerable contamination during the procedure, the subcutaneous layer and the skin should not be sutured. Closure of the skin may then be carried out a week later using "steri-strips."

EXTENSION OF THE COLONIC RESECTION FOR CARCINOMA

The amplitude of resection of the lymph node bearing areas is done according to the location of the carcinoma in the colon, which will indicate the extent of colonic resection.

Extension of the Colonic Resection for Carcinoma

Extension of the Colonic Resection for Carcinoma

FIGURE 49.1
If the carcinoma is located in the cecum or the proximal portion of the ascending colon, the ileocolic, the right colic, and the right branch of the middle colic vessels should be ligated. Ligation of these vessels determines the need for the extent of resection: about 15 cm of the terminal ileum, the cecum, the ascending colon, the hepatic flexure, and the proximal half of the transverse colon (1). In carcinoma in this location, the lymphatic dissemination of the tumor follows the route of the ileocolic vessels. In some exceptional cases the lymphatic invasion extends toward the middle colic nodes. This may occur in cases of very advanced tumors that have obstructed the ileocolic and right colic lymph nodes (1). This right hemicolectomy is designated classical right hemicolectomy.

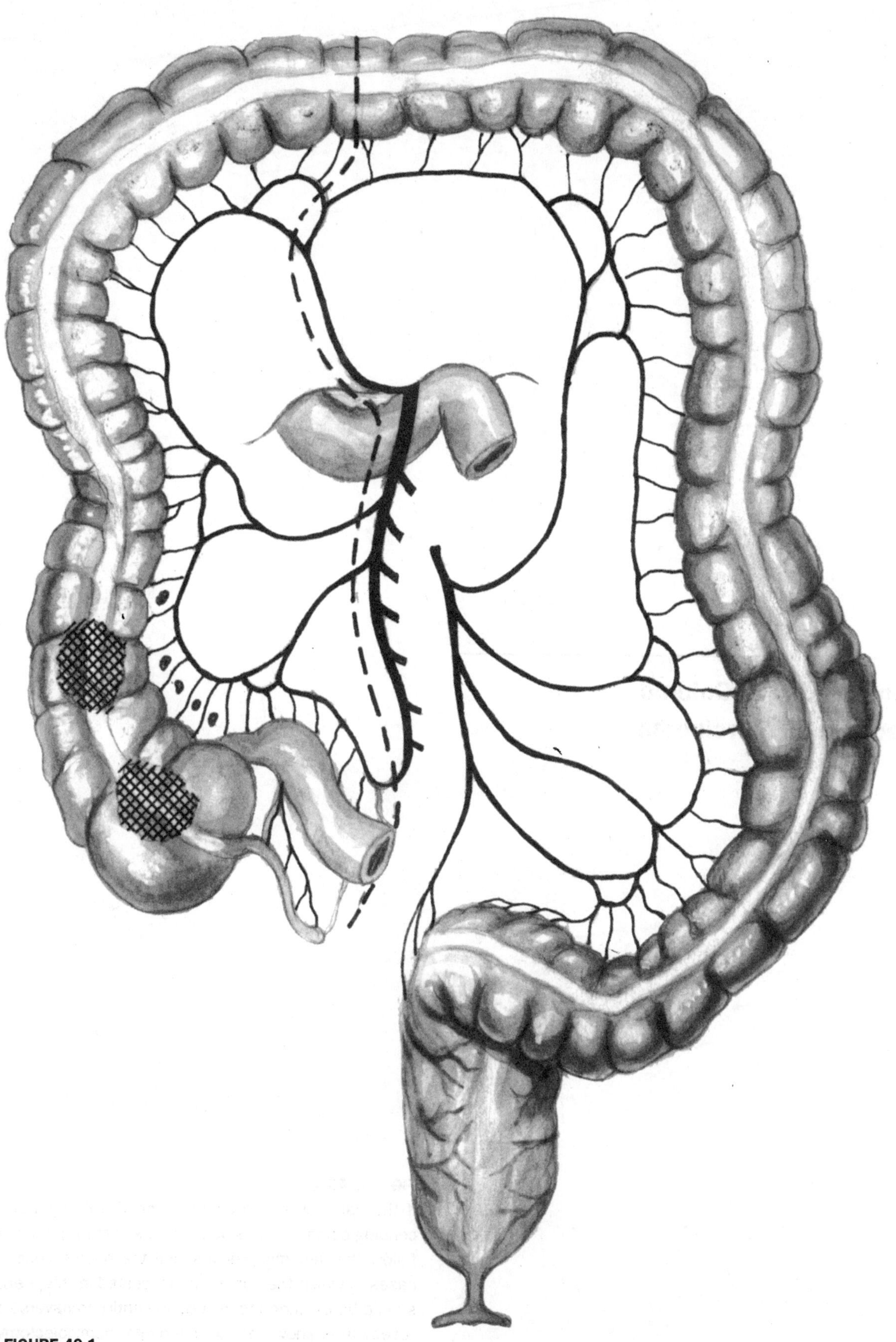

FIGURE 49.1

Extension of the Colonic Resection for Carcinoma

FIGURE 49.2

If the carcinoma is located in the distal segment of the ascending colon, the possibility exists that lymphatic spread may follow the ileocolic vessels and the middle colic vessels. In cases in which the carcinoma is located in this area, resection should be extended to include the entire transverse colon. This resection is known as extended right hemicolectomy.

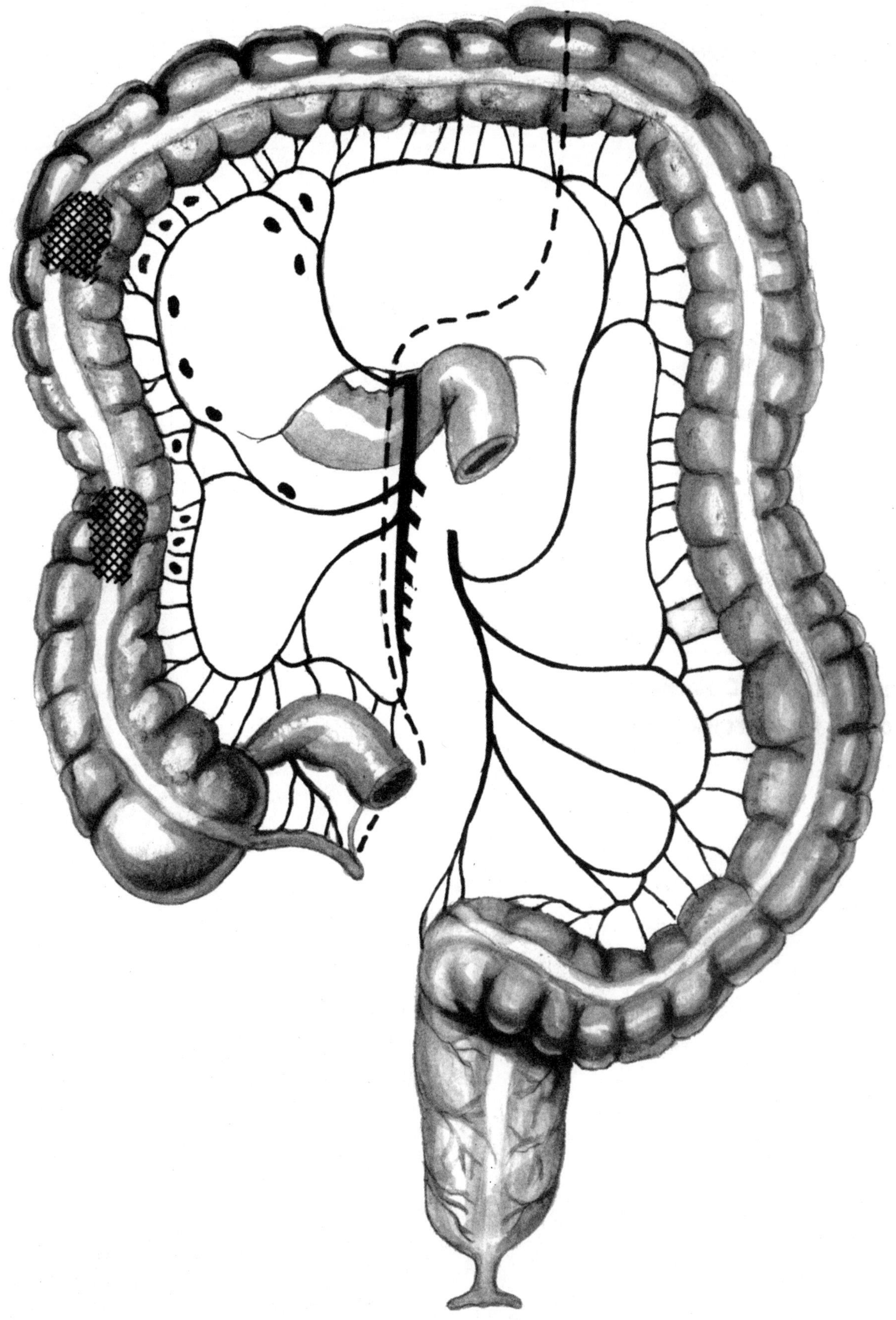

FIGURE 49.2

Extension of the Colonic Resection for Carcinoma

FIGURE 49.3
If the carcinoma is located in the proximal segment of the transverse colon a similar colonic resection is performed as the one described in Figure 49.2. In the carcinomas located in the middle third of the transverse colon, if this is redundant, it is usually possible to resect the entire transverse colon, ligating the middle colic vessels at the inferior border of the pancreas and reestablishing intestinal continuity by anastomosing the ascending colon to the descending colon. This is not always possible, however, because the colonic ends may not be approximated or the anastomosis will result in tension. In these cases it is convenient to perform an extended right hemicolectomy, anastomosing the ileum to the descending colon.

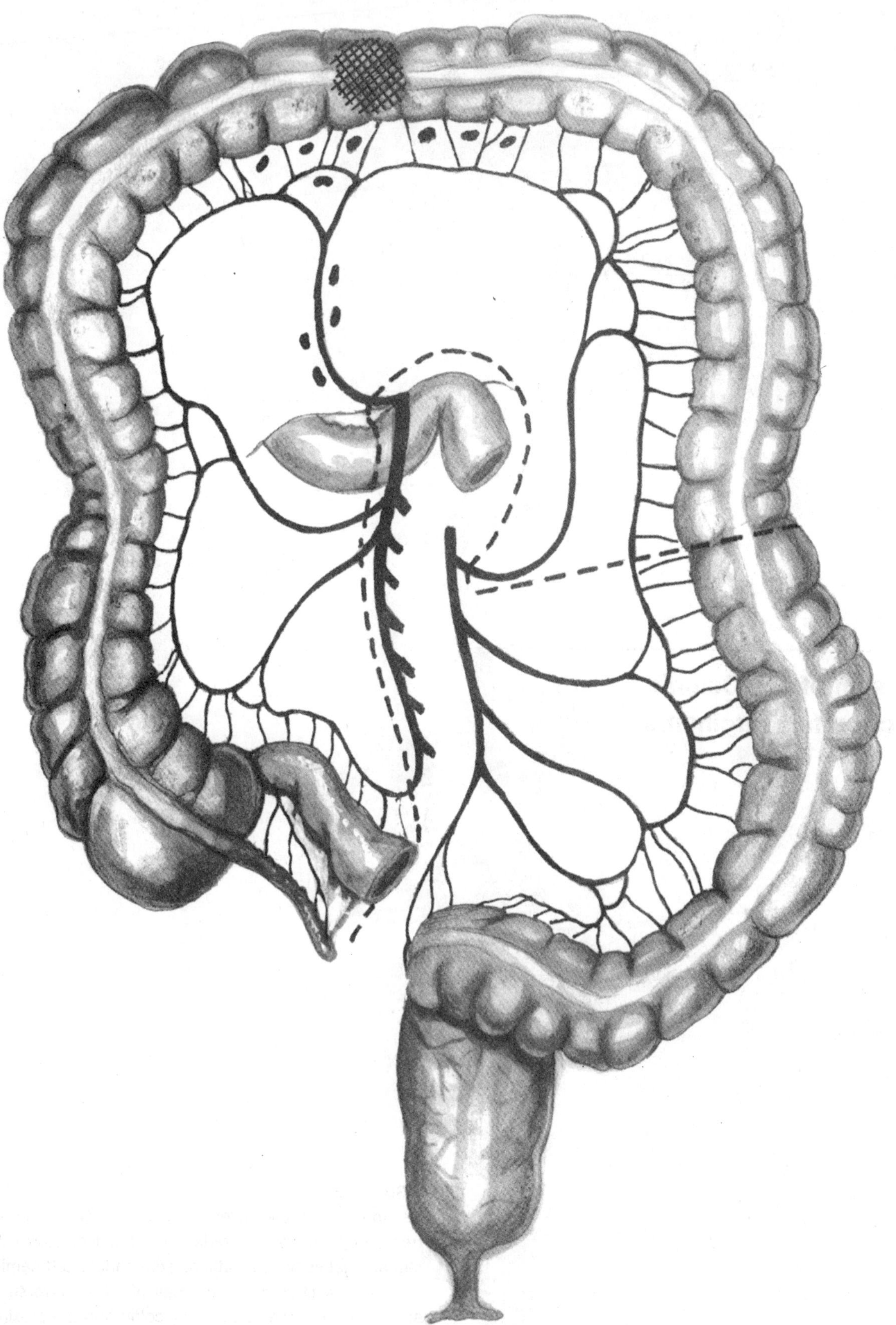

FIGURE 49.3

Extension of the Colonic Resection for Carcinoma

FIGURE 49.4
Carcinomas of the splenic flexure of the colon should be treated by means of a radical left hemicolectomy due to the characteristics of lymphatic dissemination. Left hemicolectomy involves resection of the left half of the transverse colon, the splenic flexure, the descending colon and the proximal half of the sigmoid colon, as shown in the drawing.

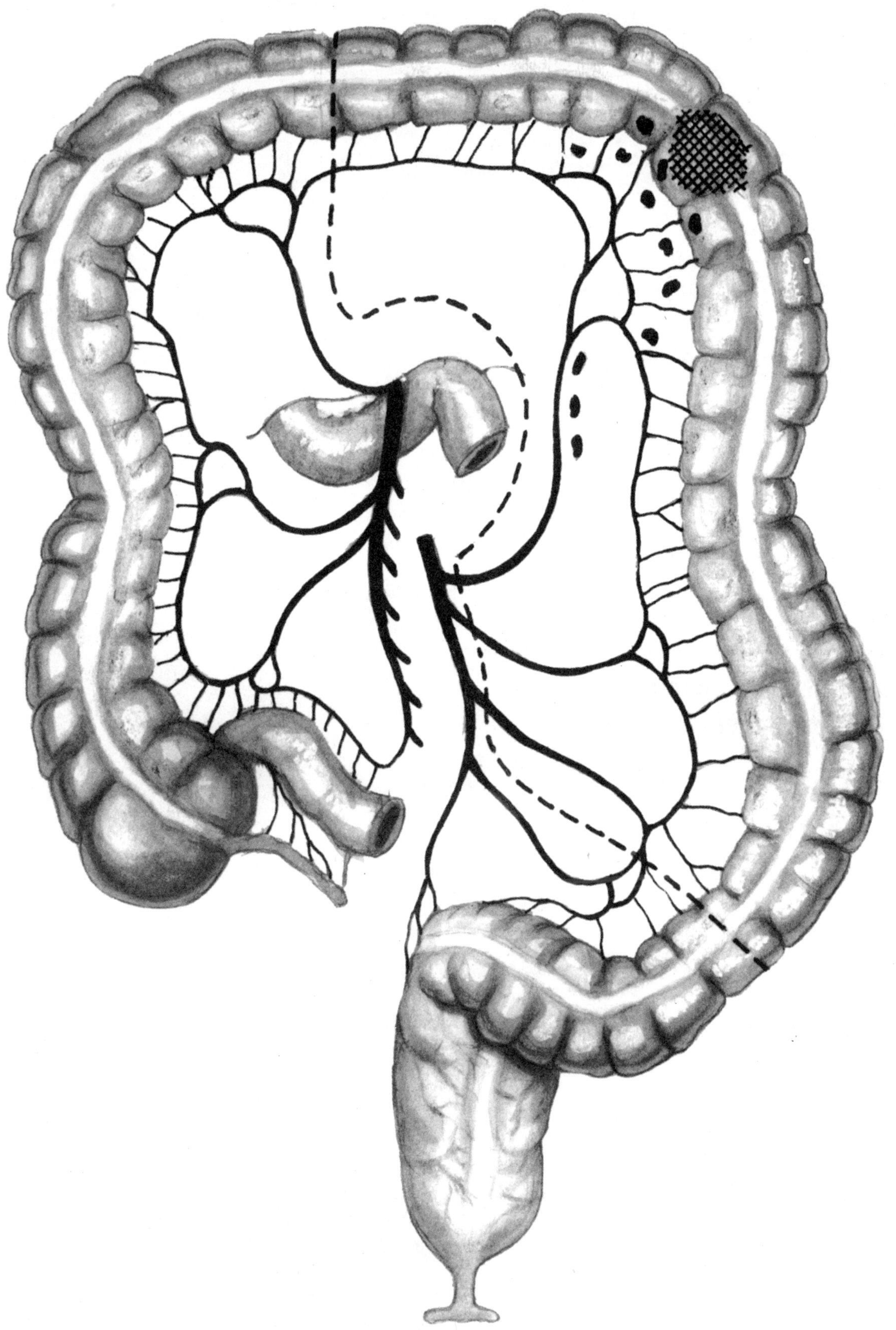

FIGURE 49.4

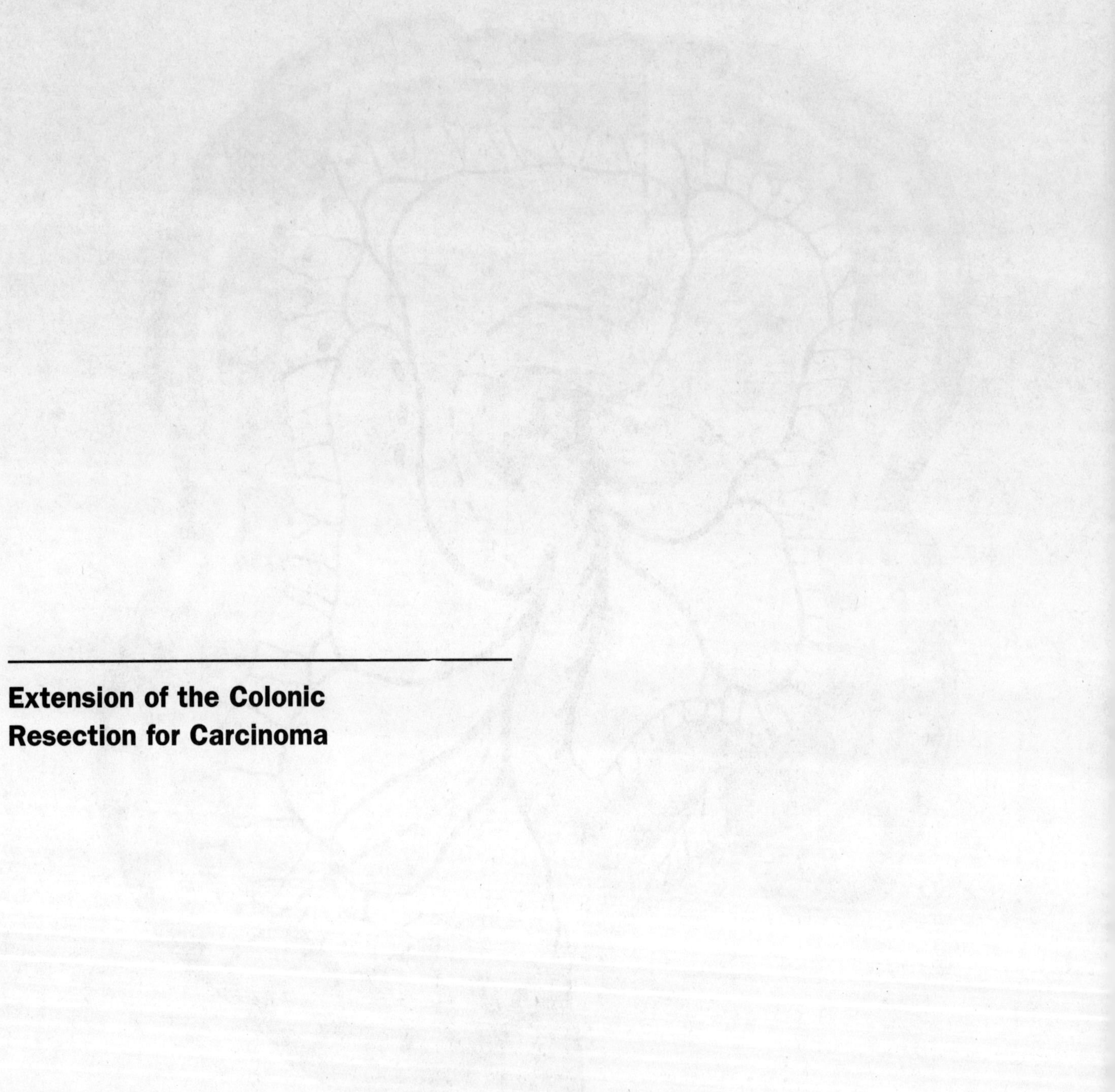

Extension of the Colonic Resection for Carcinoma

FIGURE 49.5
If the colonic carcinoma is located in the proximal part of the descending colon, resection should be similar to that described in Figure 49.4. If the carcinoma is located in the descending colon near the sigmoid colon, resection of the sigmoid colon should be added, anastomosing the transverse colon, which has been mobilized, to the rectum.

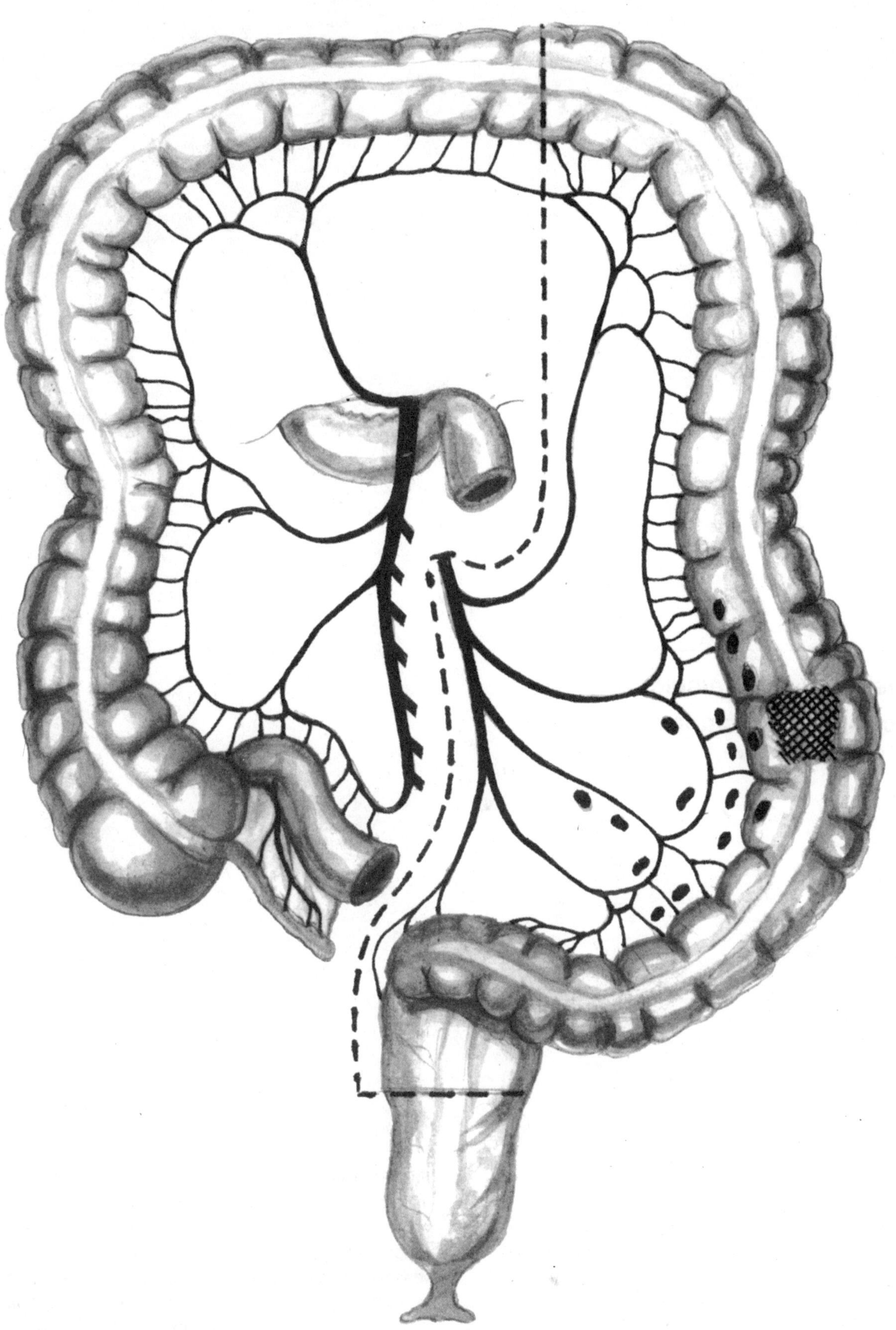

Extension of the Colonic Resection for Carcinoma

FIGURE 49.6

In carcinomas located in the sigmoid colon, two situations may occur. In the first, the tumor is rather advanced with invaded lymph nodes around the course of the left colic and sigmoidal vessels. In these cases it is necessary to ligate the inferior mesenteric artery at its origin in the aorta. Intestinal continuity is reestablished by anastomosing the transverse colon to the rectum.

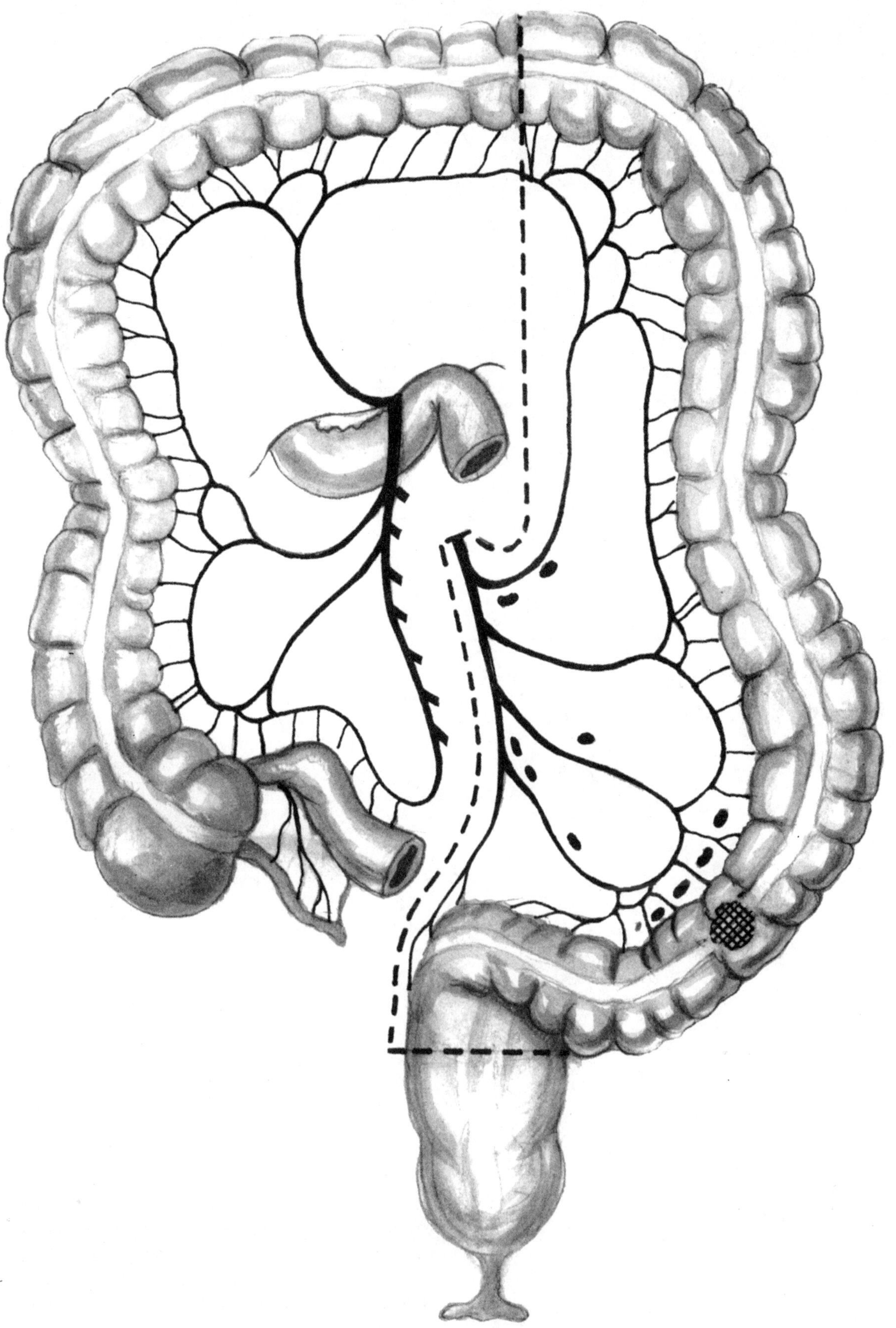

FIGURE 49.6

Extension of the Colonic Resection for Carcinoma

FIGURE 49.7
The other possibility is that the sigmoid carcinoma is not advanced, with only one or two invaded lymph nodes near the tumor and with a redundant sigmoid colon. This situation can be treated by limited segmental resection of the sigmoid colon. The results in this situation are similar to those that are obtained with an extended left hemicolectomy.

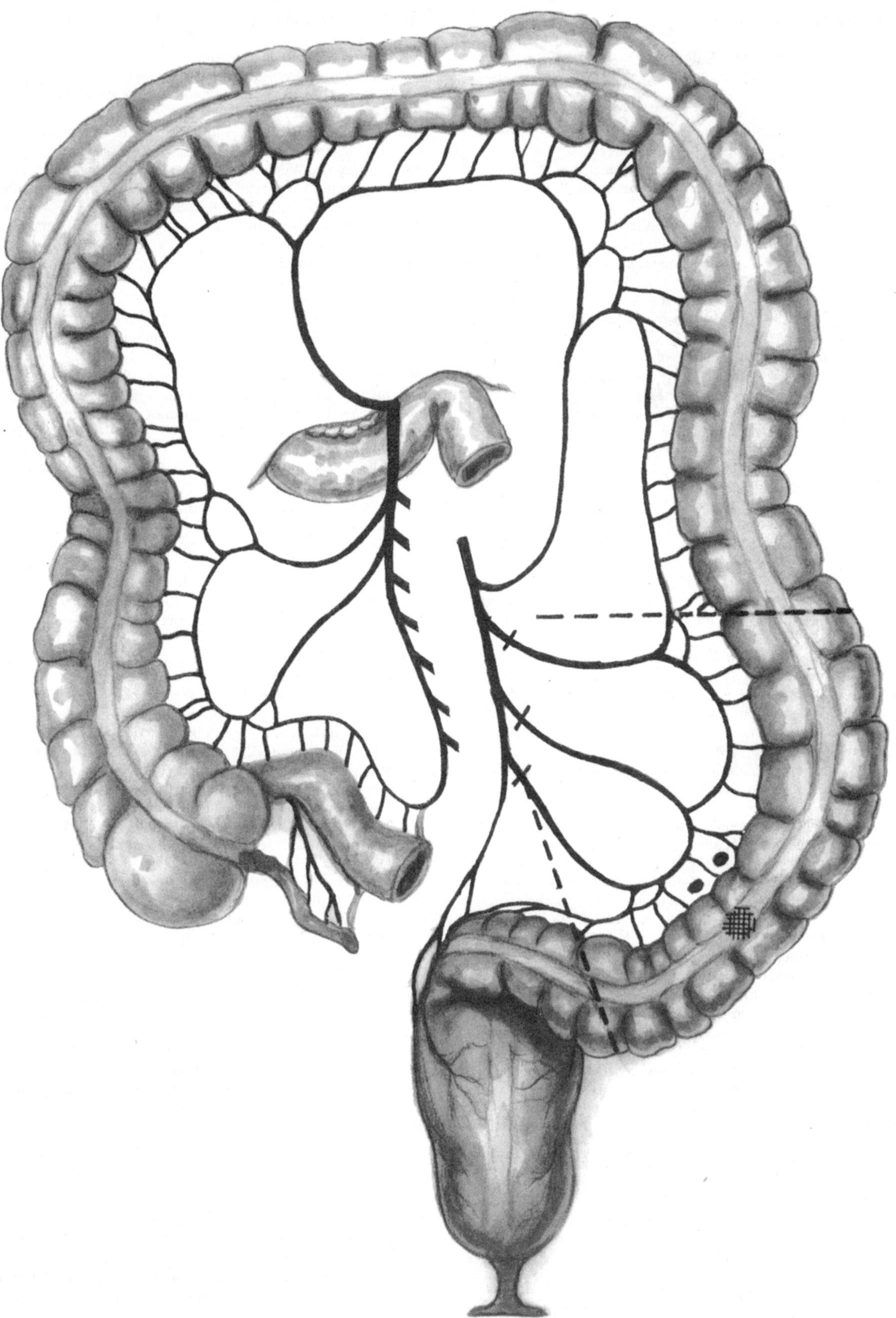

FIGURE 49.7

References

1. Akyol, A.M., McGregor, J.R., Galloway, D.J., et al. Recurrence of colorectal cancer after sutured and stapled bowel anastomosis. Br. J. Surg. 78:1297, 1991.
2. Beahrs, O.H., Myers, M.H. (Eds.) American Joint Committee for Cancer. Manual for staging of cancer. Ed. 2, p 73. Lippincott, Philadelphia, 1983.
3. Ackerman, N.B. Vascular influence on intestinal lymph flow and their relationship to operation for carcinoma of the intestine. Surg. Gynecol. Obstet. 137:801, 1973.
4. Ackerman, N.B. Primary arterial ligation in the resection of cancer of the colon. Am. J. Surg. 133:73, 1977.
5. Bacon, H.E., Jackson, C. Visceral metastases from carcinoma of distal colon and rectum. Surgery 33:495, 1953.
6. Baker, J.W., Margetts, L.H., Schutt, R.P. The distal and proximal margin of resection in carcinoma of the pelvic colon and rectum. Ann. Surg. 141:693, 1955.
7. Barnes, J.P. Physiological resection of the right colon. Surg. Gynecol. Obstet. 94:723, 1952.
8. Beal, J.M., Cornell, G.W. A study of the problem of recurrence of carcinoma at the anastomotic site following resection of the colon for carcinoma. Ann. Surg. 143:1, 1956.
9. Beart, R.W. Jr., Nivatvongs, S., Wolff, B. The colon, rectum and anus. In Nora, P.F. (Ed.) Operative surgery. Ed. 3, p. 610. W.B. Saunders, Philadelphia, 1990.
10. Beskin, C., Atwood, W. Peripheral bone metastases from carcinoma of the rectum. Surgery 31:273, 1952.
11. Black, W.A., Waugh, J.M. The intramural extension of carcinoma of the descending colon, sigmoid and rectosigmoid: A pathologic study. Surg. Gynecol. Obstet. 87:457, 1948.
12. Bonfanti, G., Rozetti, F., Doci, R., et al. Results of extended surgery for cancer of the rectum and sigmoid. Br. J. Surg. 69:305, 1982.
13. Boreham, P. Implantation metastases from cancer of the large bowel. Br. J. Surg. 46:103, 1958.
14. Carroll, S.E. The prognostic significance of gross venous invasion in carcinoma of the rectum. Can. J. Surg. 6:281, 1963.
15. Cohn, I. Jr. Control of tumor implantation during operations on the colon. Ann. Surg. 157:825, 1963.
16. Cole, W.H., Packard, D., Southwick, H.W. Carcinoma of the colon with special reference to the prevention of recurrence. J.A.M.A. 155:1549, 1954.
17. Coller, F.A., Kay, E.B., MacIntyre, R.S. Regional lymphatic metastases of carcinoma of the rectum. Surgery 8:294, 1940.
18. Cooke, R.V. Advanced carcinoma of the colon with emphasis on the inflammatory factor. Ann. R. Coll. Surg. Engl. 18:46, 1956.
19. Corman, M.L., Veidenheimer, M.C., Coller, J.A. Colorectal carcinoma. A decade of experience at the Lahey Clinic. Dis. Colon Rectum 22:477, 1979.
20. Corman, M.L., Prager, E.D., Hardy, T.G. Jr., Bubrick, M.F. Valtrac (B.A.R.) Study Group. Comparison of the Valtrac biofragmentable anastomosis in colon surgery: Results of a prospective, randomized clnical trial. Dis. Colon Rectum 32:183, 1989.
21. Corman, M.L. Principles of surgical technique in the treatment of carcinoma of the large bowel. World J. Surg. 15:592, 1991.
22. Correa, P., Haenszel, W. The epidemiology of large bowel cancer. Adv. Cancer Res. 26:1, 1978.
23. Capuis, P.H., Dent, M.F., Newland, R.C., et al. An evalulation of the American Joint Committee p. T.N.M. staging method for cancer of the colon and rectum. Dis. Colon Rectum 2:123, 1987.
24. Chassin, J.L., et al. The stapled gastrointestinal tract anastomosis: Incidence of postoperative complications compared with the sutured anastomosis. Ann. Surg. 188:689, 1978.
25. Chassin, J.L. Operative strategy in general surgery. Ed. 2, p. 291. Springer-Verlag, New York, 1994.
26. Deddish, M.R., Stearns, M.W. Anterior resection for carcinoma of the rectum and rectosigmoid area. Ann. Surg. 154:981, 1961.
27. Dionne, L. Pattern of blood-borne metastases from carcinoma of the rectum. Cancer 18:775, 1965.
28. Dudley, H.A.F., Radclife, A.G., McGeehan, D. Intraoperative irrigation of the colon to permit primary anastomoses. Br. J. Surg. 67:80, 1980.
29. Dukes, C.E. The classification of cancer of the rectum. J. Pathol. Bacteriol. 35:323, 1932.
30. Dukes, C.E. Cancer of the rectum: An analysis of 1000 cases. J. Pathol. Bacteriol. 50:527, 1940.
31. Dukes, C.E. The surgical pathology of tumours of the colon. Med. Press. 226:512, 1951.
32. Dukes, C.E., Bussey, H.J.R. The spread of rectal cancer and its effect on prognosis. Br. J. Surg. 12:309, 1958.
33. Durdey, P., Williams, N.S. The effect of malignant and inflammatory fixation on rectal carcinoma and on prognosis after rectal excision. Br. J. Surg. 71:787, 1984.
34. Ellis, H. Curative and palliative surgery in advanced carcinoma of the large bowel. Br. Med. J. 3:29, 1971.
35. Ellis, H. Resection of the colon. In Schwartz, S.I., Ellis, H. (Eds.) Maingot's abdominal operations. Ed. 9, vol. 2, p. 1049. Appleton Lange. Norwalk, CT, 1990.
36. El-Domeiri, A., Whiteley, H.W. Pronostic significance of abdominal wall involvement in carcinoma cecum. Cancer 26:552, 1970.
37. Engell, H.C. Cancer cells in the circulating blood: A clinical study on the occurrence of cancer cells in the peripheral blood and in venous blood drainage in tumor area at operation. Acta Chir. Scand. Suppl. 201, 1955.
38. Enker, W.E., Laffer, V.T., Black, G.E. Enhanced survival of patients with colon and rectal cancer is based upon wide anatomic resection. Ann. Surg. 190:350, 1979.
39. Fazio, V.W., Tjandra, J.J. Primary therapy of carcinoma of the large bowel. World J. Surg. 15:568, 1991.
40. Fielding, L.P. The portal vein and colorectal cancer. Br. J. Surg. 75:402, 1988.
41. Fisher, E.R., Turnbull, R.B. Jr. The cytologic demonstration and significance of tumor cells in the mesenteric venous blood in patients with colorectal carcinoma. Surg. Gynecol. Obstet. 100:102, 1955.
42. Gabriel, W.B., Dukes, C.E., Bussey, H.J.R. Lymphatic spread in cancer of the rectum. Br. J. Surg. 23:395, 1935.
43. Gilchrist, R.K., David, V.C. A consideration of pathological factors influencing five year survival in radical resection of the large bowel and rectum for carcinoma. Ann. Surg. 126:421, 1947.
44. Glass, R.L., Smith, L.E., Cochran, R.C. Subtotal colectomy for obstructing carcinoma of the left colon. Am. J. Surg. 145:335, 1983.
45. Glass, R.L., Fazio, V.W., Jagelman, D.G., Lavery, I.C., Weakley, F.L., Forsythe, S.R. The results of surgical treatment of cancer of the colon at the Cleveland Clinic from 1965–1975. Classification of the spread of colon cancer and long-term survival. Int. J. Colon Dis. 1:33, 1986.
46. Glover, R.P., Waugh, J.M. Retrograde lymphatic spread of carcinoma of the "rectosigmoid" region: Its influence on surgical procedures. Surg. Gynecol. Obstet. 80:434, 1945.
47. Goligher, J.C., Bussey, H.J.R. Local recurrence after sphincter-saving excisions for carcinoma of the rectum and rectosigmoid. Br. J. Surg. 39:155, 1951.
48. Goligher, J.C. The Dukes' A, B, and C categorization of the extent of spread of carcinomas of the rectum. Surg. Gynecol. Obstet. 146:793, 1976.
49. Goligher, J.C. Surgery of the anus, rectum and colon. Ed. 4, p. 424. Bailliere Tindall, London, 1980.
50. Gordon, P.H., Nivatvongs, S. Colon, rectum and anus. p. 501. Quality Medical Publishing, St. Louis, MO, 1992.
51. Griffiths, J.D., McKinna, J.A., Rowbothan, H.D., et al. Carcinoma of the colon and rectum: Circulating malignant cells and five-year survival. Cancer 31:226, 1973.
52. Grinnell, R.S. The grading and prognosis of carcinoma of the colon and rectum. Ann. Surg. 109:500, 1939.
53. Hardy, T.G. Jr., Pace, W.G., Maney, J.W., Katz, A.R., Kaganov, A.L. A biofragmentable ring for sutureless bowel anastomosis. Dis. Colon Rectum 28:484, 1985.
54. Hardy, T.G. Cancer of the colon. In Fazio, V.W. (Ed.) Current therapy in colon and rectal surgery. p. 301. B.C. Decker, Toronto, 1990.
55. Heald, R.H., Bussey, H.J.R. Clinical experiences at St. Mark's Hospital with multiple synchronous cancer of the colon and rectum. Dis. Colon Rectum 18:6, 1975.

56. Jagelman, D.G. Colectomy for malignant disease of the colon: The "no touch" isolation technique. In Fielding, L.P., Goldberg, S.M. (Eds.) Surgery of the colon, rectum and anus. Ed. 5, p. 359.
57. Jeekel, J. Curative resection of primary colorectal cancer. Br. J. Surg. 73:687, 1986.
58. Jeekel, J. Can radical surgery improve survival in colorectal cancer? World J. Surg. 11:412, 1987.
59. Jensen, H.E., Nielsen, J., Balslev, I. Extensive surgery in the treatment of carcinoma of the colon. Acta Chir. Scand. 136:431, 1970.
60. Keighley, M.R.B., Williams, N.S. Surgery of the anus, rectum and colon. Vol. 1, p. 830. W.B. Saunders, Philadelphia, 1993.
61. Keynes, W.M. Implantation from the bowel lumen in cancer of the large intestine. Ann. Surg. 153:357, 1961.
62. Killingback, M., Wilson, E., Hughes, E.S.R. Anal metastases from carcinoma of the rectum and colon. Aust. N. Z. J. Surg. 14:178, 1965.
63. Lamy, J., Louis, R., Michotey, G., Bricot, R., Sarles, J.C. Nouveau traité de technique chirurgicale. Vol. 11, p. 245. Masson et Cie, Paris, 1969.
64. Lasser, A. Synchronous primary adenocarcinoma of the colon and rectum. Dis. Colon Rectum 21:20, 1978.
65. LeQuesne, L.P., Thomson, A.D. Implantation recurrence of carcinoma of the rectum and colon. N. Engl. J. Med. 258:578, 1958.
66. Levin, K.E., Dozois, R.R. Epidemiology of large bowel cancer. World J. Surg. 15:562, 1991.
67. Long, L., Jonasson, O., Roberts, S., McGrath, R., McGrew, E., Cole, W.H. Cancer cells in blood: Results of simplified isolation technique. Arch. Surg. 80:910, 1960.
68. Long, R.T.L., Edward, R.H. Implantation metastases as a cause of local recurrence of colorectal carcinoma. Am. J. Surg. 157:194 1989.
69. Mackeigan, I.M., Ferguson, I.A. Prophylactic oophorectomy and colorectal cancer in pre-menopausal patients. Dis. Colon Rectum 222:401, 1979.
70. Madden, J.L., Tan, P.Y. Primary resection and anastomoses in the treatment of perforated lesions of the colon, with abscess or diffusing peritonitis. Surg. Gynecol. Obstet. 113:646, 1961.
71. Madden, J.L. Atlas of technics in surgery. Ed. 2, vol. 1, p. 384. Appleton Century Crofts, New York, 1964.
72. Madden, J.L. Large bowel resection. In Madden J.L. (Ed.) Abdominal wall hernia. p. 266. W.B. Saunders, Philadelphia, 1989.
73. Morgenstern, L., Lee, S.E. Spatial distribution of colonic carcinoma. Arch. Surg. 113:1142, 1978.
74. Morson, B.C., Dawson, I.M.P. Gastrointestinal pathology. p. 551. Blackwell Scientific Publications, Oxford, 1972.
75. Morson, B.C., Dawson, I.M.P. Gastrointestinal pathology Ed. 3, p. 423. Blackwell, Oxford, 1990.
76. Muir, E.G. Right hemicolectomy. Proc. R. Soc. Med. 40:831, 1947.
77. Muir, E.G. Safety in colonic resection. Proc. R. Soc. Med. 61:401, 1968.
78. Nicholls, R.J., Mason, A.Y., Morson, B.C., Dixon, A.K., Kelsey Fry, I. The clinical staging of rectal cancer. Br. J. Surg. 69:404, 1982.
79. Olsen, A.K. Intraoperative ultrasonography and the direction of liver metastases in patients with colorectal cancer. Br. J. Surg. 77:998, 1990.
80. Pezim, M.E., Nicholls, R.J. Survival after high or low ligation of the inferior mesenteric artery during curative surgery for rectal cancer. Ann. Surg. 200:729, 1984.
81. Phillips, R.K.S., Hittinger, R., Blesovsky, L., Fry, J.P., Fielding, L.P. Local recurrence following curative surgery for large bowel cancer: The overall picture. Br. J. Surg. 71:12, 1984.
82. Portnoy, J., Kagan, E., Gordon, P.H., et al. Prophylactic antibiotics in elective colorectal surgery. Dis. Colon Rectum 26:310, 1983.
83. Quénu, J., Loygue, J., Perrotin, J., Dubost, C., Moreaux, J. Operations sur les parois de l'abdomen et sur le tube digestive. p. 819. Masson et Cie, Paris, 1968.
84. Quer, E.A., Dahlin, D.C., Mayo, C.W. Retrograde intramural spread of carcinoma of the rectum and rectosigmoid. Surg. Gynecol. Obstet. 96:24, 1953.
85. Robillard, G.L., Shapiro, A.L. Variational anatomy of middle colic artery; its significance in gastric and colonic surgery. J. Int. Coll. Surg. 10:157, 1947.
86. Renkin, F.W. Curability of cancer of the colon, rectosigmoids and rectum. J.A.M.A. 101:491, 1933.
87. Rhodes, F.B., Holmes, F.F., Clark, G.M. Changing distribution of primary cancers in the large bowel. J.A.M.A. 238:1641, 1977.
88. Rosato, F.E., Marks, G. Changing site distribution patterns of colorectal cancer at Thomas Jefferson University Hospital. Dis. Colon Rectum 24:93, 1981.
89. Rothenberg, D.A. Conventional colectomy In Fielding, L.P., Goldberg, S.M. (Eds.). Surgery of the colon, rectum and anus. Ed. 5, p. 347. Butterworth-Heinemann, Oxford, 1993.
90. Scott, N.A., Taylor, B.A., Wolff, B.G., et al. Perianal metastases from sigmoid carcinoma. Objective evidence of a colonal origin. Report of a case. Dis. Colon Rectum 31:68, 1988.
91. Schoetz, D.J. Right hemicolectomy. In Bauer, J.J. (Ed.) Colorectal surgery illustrated. p. 63. Mosby–Year Book, St. Louis, 1993.
92. Schrock, T.R., DeVenely, C.W., Dunphy, J.E. Factors contributing to leakage of colonic anastomoses. Ann. Surg. 177:513, 1973.
93. Schrock, T.R. Cancer of the large intestine. In Way, L.W. Current surgical diagnosis and treatment. Ed. 9, p. 633. Appleton Lange, Norwalk, CT, 1991.
94. Shirouzu, K., Isomoto, H., Kakegawa, T. Prospective clinipathological study of venous invasion in colorectal cancer. Am. J. Surg 162:216, 1991.
95. Silverberg, E., Borin, C.C., Squires, T.S. Cancer statistics. CA Cancer J. Clin. 40:9, 1990.
96. Stearns, M.W., Schottenfeld, D. Techniques for the surgical management of colon cancer. Cancer 28:165, 1971.
97. Sugarbaker, P.H., Corlew, S. Influence of surgical technique on survival in patients with colorectal cancer. A review. Dis. Colon Rectum 25:545, 1982.
98. Sugarbaker, P.H. A perspective on clinical research strategies in carcinoma of the large bowel. World J. Surg. 15:609, 1991.
99. Talbot, I., Ritchie, S., Leighton, M.H., et al. Spread of rectal cancer within veins. Histological features and clinical significance. Am. J. Surg. 141:15, 1981.
100. Turnbull, R.B., Kyle, K., Watson, F.R., Spratt, J. Cancer of the colon: The influence of the "no touch isolation" technique on survival rates. Ann. Surg. 166:420, 1967.
101. Umpleby, H.C., Williamson, R.C. Anastomotic recurrence in large bowel cancer. Br. J. Surg. 74:873, 1987.
102. West of Scotland and Highland Anastomosis Study Group. Suturing or stapling in gastrointestinal surgery: A prospective randomized study. Br. J. Surg. 78:337, 1991.
103. Wiggers, T., Jeekel, J., Arends, J.W., Brinkhorst, A.P., Jörning, P.J.G., Kluck, H.M., et al. The no touch isolation technique in colon cancer (a prospective controlled multicentric trial). Surg. Oncol. Proc. A.S.C.O. 5:269, 1986.
104. Wiggers, T., Jeekel, J., Arends, J.W., et al. No-touch isolation technique in colon cancer: A controlled prospective trial. Br. J. Surg. 75:409, 1988.
105. Willet, C.G., Tepper, J.E., Cohen, M., Orlow, E., Welch, C.E. Failure patterns following curative resection for colonic adenocarcinoma. Ann. Surg. 200:685, 1984.
106. Wolmark, N., Fisher, B., Weland, H.S. The prognostic value of the modifications of the Dukes' C.E. of colorectal cancer. An analysis of the N.S.A.B.P. clinical trials. Ann. Surg. 203:115, 1986.
107. Zinkin, L.D. A critical review of the classifications and staging of colorectal cancer. Dis. Colon Rectum 26:37, 1981.

CHAPTER **50**

Right Radical Hemicolectomy

We will first describe the technique of the "no touch" right radical hemicolectomy and then the technique of the right radical hemicolectomy by the conventional or classic technique. A brief description will then be made of the right hemicolectomy in patients with acute obstruction and later in patients complicated by peritonitis.

Section H

Colon, Rectum, and Anus

Right Radical Hemicolectomy by the "No Touch" Technique

FIGURE 50.1
Right paramedian incision extending from a point 2 to 3 cm from the costal margin down to about 5 cm from the pubic spine. This incision allows ample access to the abdominal cavity for the performance of surgery for neoplasm.

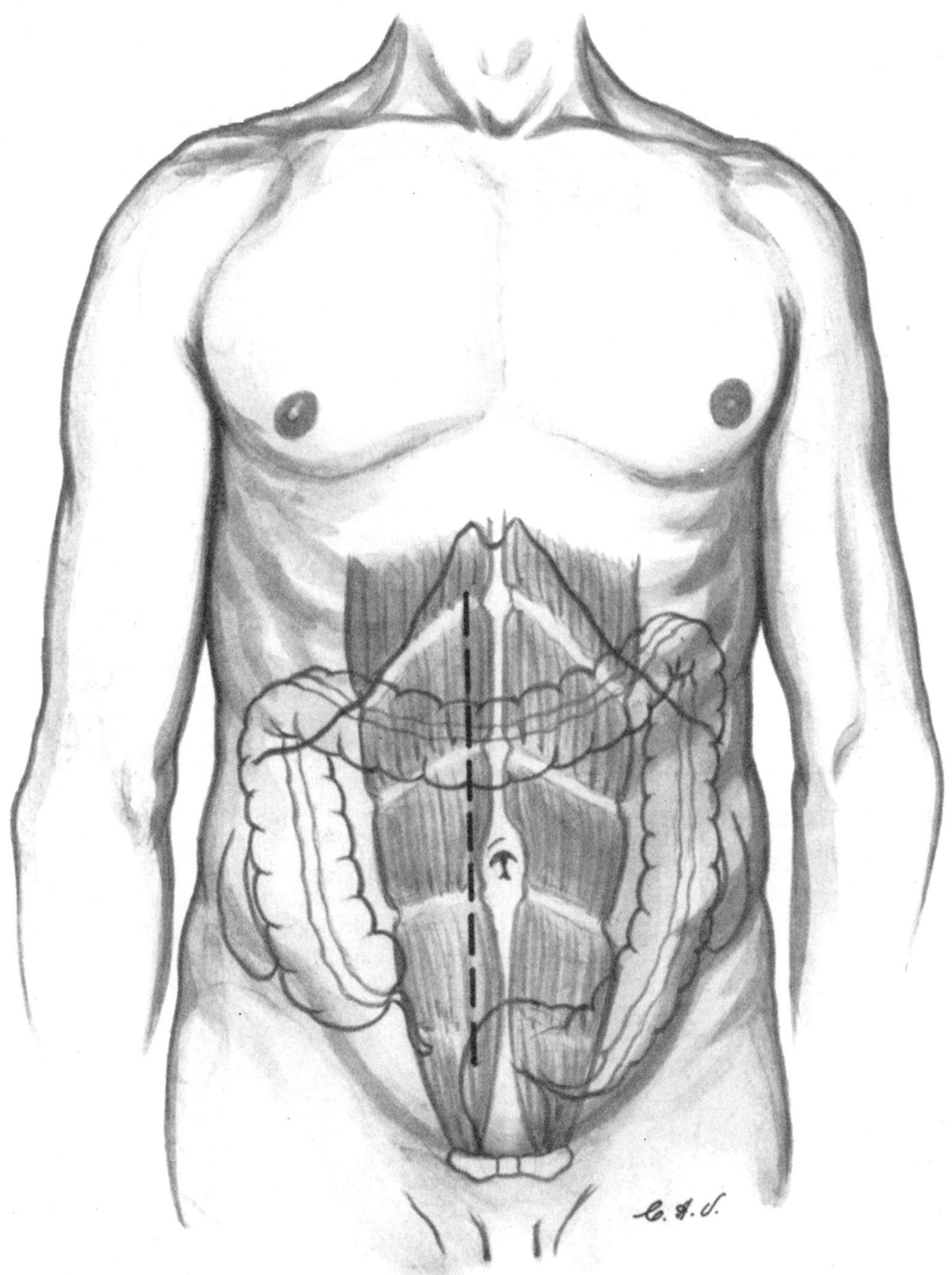

FIGURE 50.1

Right Radical Hemicolectomy by the "No Touch" Technique

FIGURE 50.2

The incision has been carried through the skin and the subcutaneous tissue. The anterior rectal sheath **(A)** has been incised at a point about 2 cm from the midline. The medial leaf of the rectal sheath is grasped with 3 hemostats and gentle traction applied to them by the second assistant, allowing the surgeon to free the medial border of the rectus muscle using curved scissors, as shown in the drawing. To carry out this maneuver correctly, the surgeon has to enter the cleavage plane between the muscle and the sheath, so as not to traumatize the muscle. In order to carry out an adequate liberation of the anterior rectus muscle, it is usually necessary to ligate and divide 3 or 4 blood vessels that are present in the aponeurotic insertions. Liberation of the medial border of the rectus muscle should be complete to facilitate its displacement toward the right.

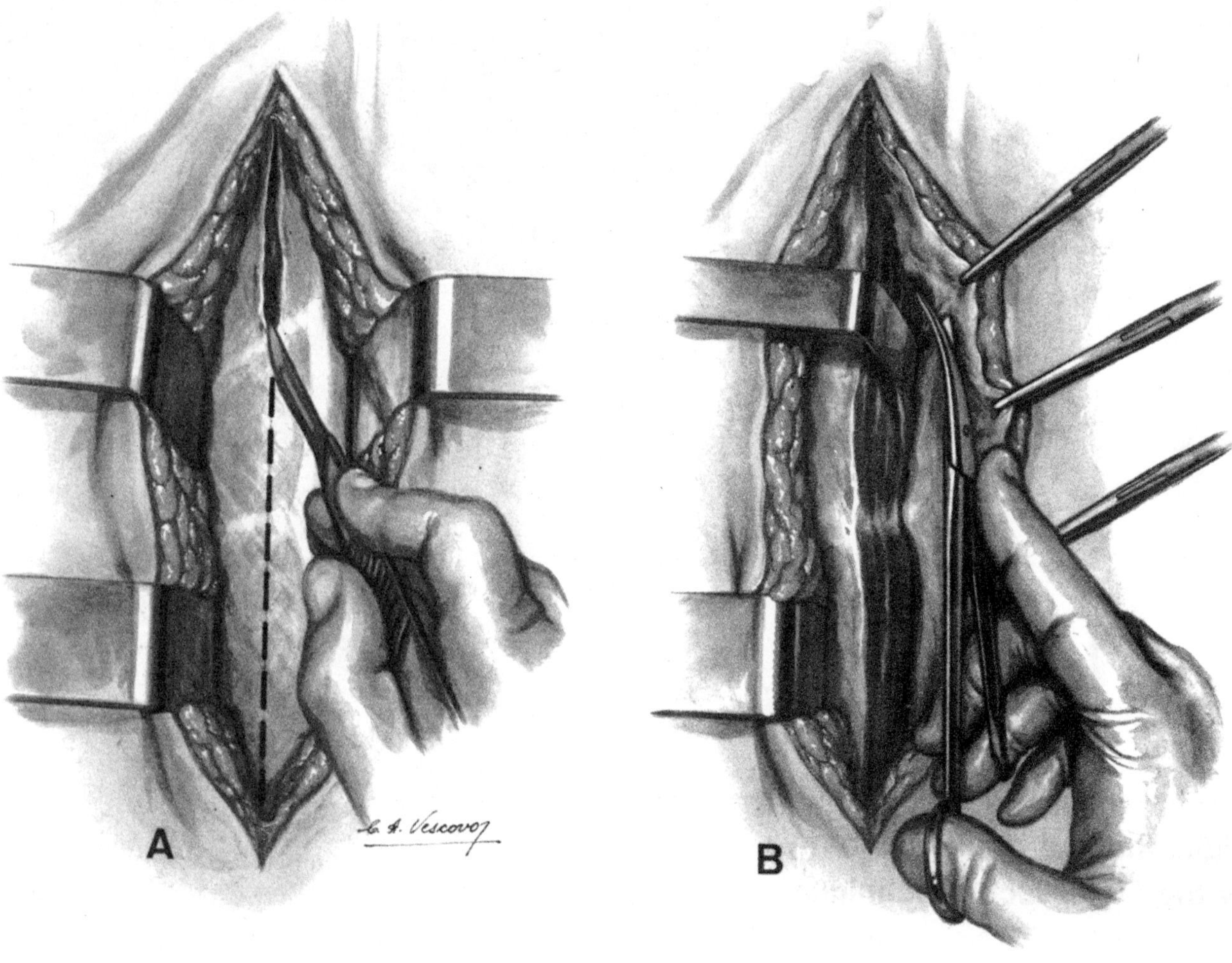

FIGURE 50.2

Right Radical Hemicolectomy by the "No Touch" Technique

FIGURE 50.3
The anterior rectus muscle has been retracted to the right, and the border of the transected anterior rectus sheath has been retracted toward the midline. Using two Allis clamps, the posterior rectus sheath and the anterior parietal peritoneum have been grasped. Care should be taken to avoid including the small bowel. The surgeon is about to incise the posterior rectus sheath with a scalpel, together with the parietal peritoneum, as shown in the drawing. Once the abdominal cavity has been opened, the incision is completed using several hemostatic clamps on both edges to apply traction in opposite directions while the peritoneal incision is carried upward using scissors and downward using a scalpel, and the first assistant continues to apply hemostatic clamps to the edges of the peritoneum.

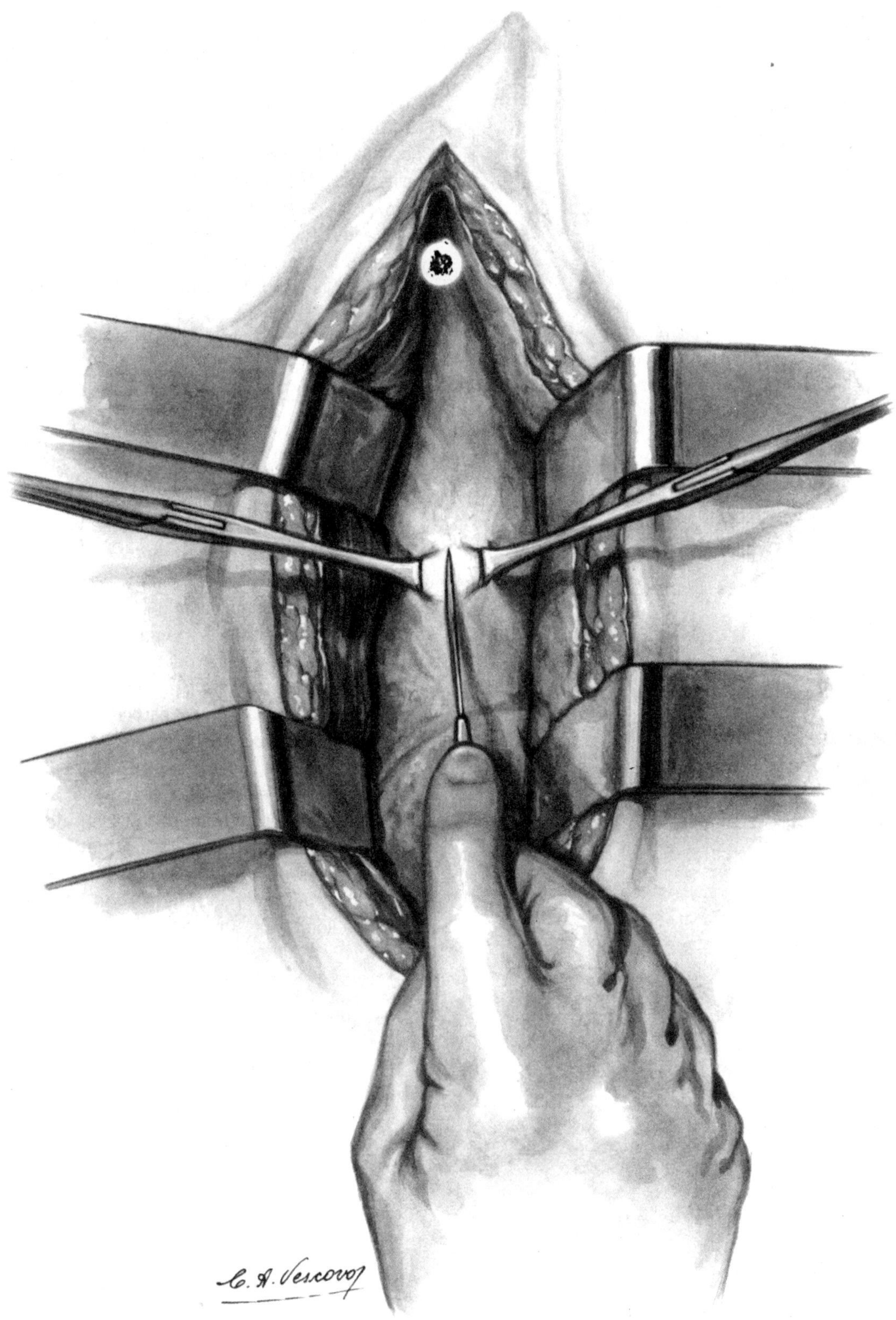

FIGURE 50.3

Right Radical Hemicolectomy by the "No Touch" Technique

FIGURE 50.4

Once the abdominal cavity has been opened, gauze pads are applied to protect the edges of the wound. A complete exploration of the abdominal cavity is then carried out to look for metastases. The carcinoma is then identified, its exact location and size are established, and the serosa of the colon inspected for invasion. The tumor is then observed to be fixed or mobile, with or without adhesions to other organs and to the anterior or posterior wall of the abdomen. Enlarged lymph nodes are searched for. All this information can be obtained without carrying out any major mobilization or handling of the tumor.

The illustration shows a carcinoma located in the proximal portion of the ascending colon. Simple traction on the cecum and the terminal ileum, using smooth Foerster clamps, is sufficient to obtain the required data to determine the resectability of the lesion. In the drawing to the left, the extent of resection of the colon for a carcinoma located in the proximal portion of the ascending colon is shown. The resection should include about 15 cm of the terminal ileum, the cecum, the ascending colon, and the proximal half of the transverse colon. To carry out this resection, it is necessary to ligate and divide the ileocolic vessels, the right colic vessels, and the right branches of the middle colic vessels. This extent of resection is known in medical literature as classic right hemicolectomy. If the carcinoma were located in the distal segment of the ascending colon or in the hepatic flexure, the extent of resection should be greater because it is necessary to ligate the middle colic vessels due to the location of the carcinoma and the possibility of lymphatic spread. The extent of this resection is what is known as extended right radical hemicolectomy.

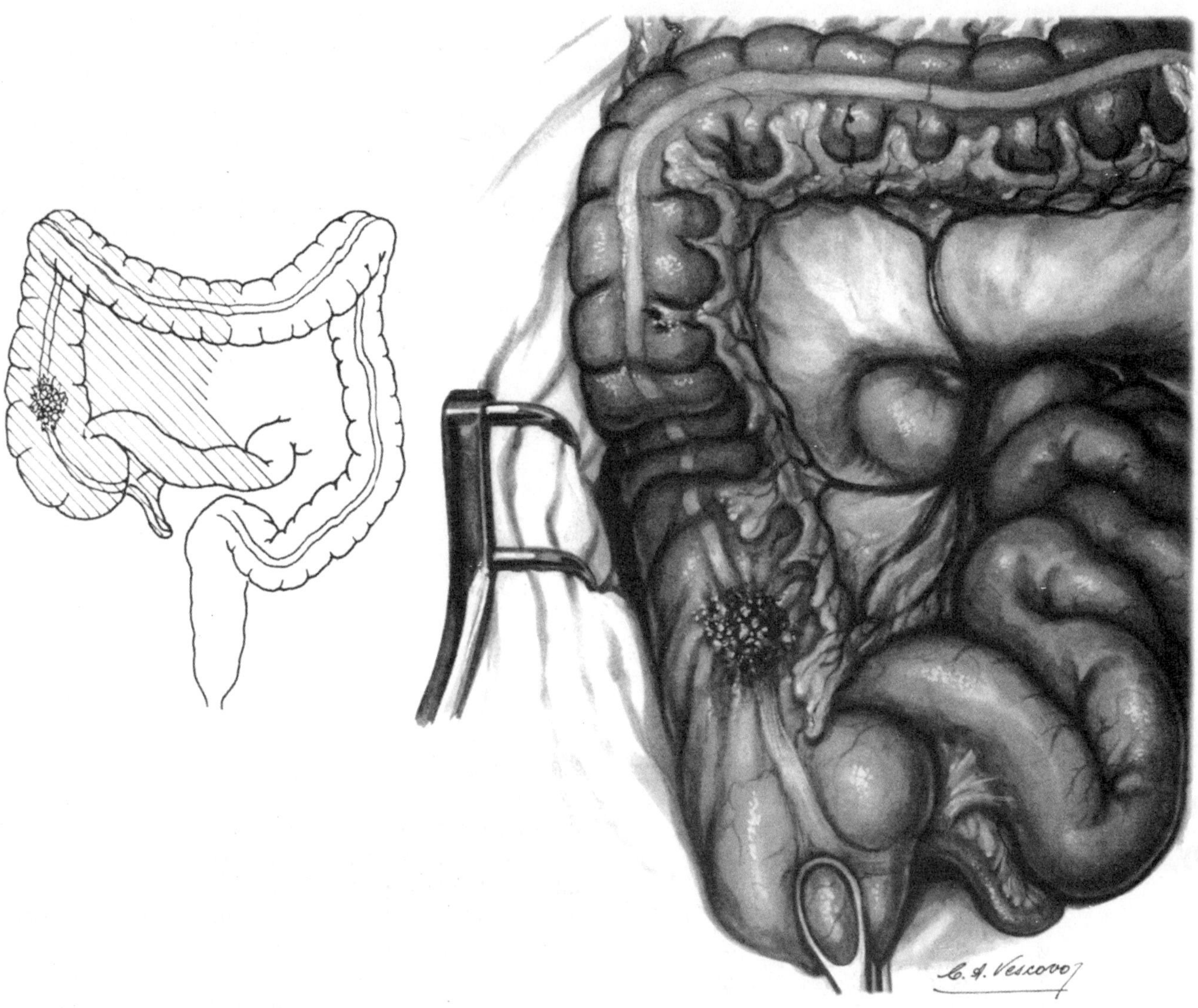

FIGURE 50.4

Right Radical Hemicolectomy by the "No Touch" Technique

FIGURE 50.5

To carry out a right radical hemicolectomy, it is not necessary to exteriorize the entire length of small bowel. Only the last 20 cm of the ileum should be exposed and retracted upward with the transverse colon and its mesocolon. The second assistant elevates the greater omentum with both hands to allow the surgeon, with the help of the first assistant, to proceed to carry out the necessary ligations and the division of the greater omentum at a point proximal to the midline. The drawing on the left shows, by means of a broken line, where the transection of the greater omentum and the gastrocolic ligament will be carried out.

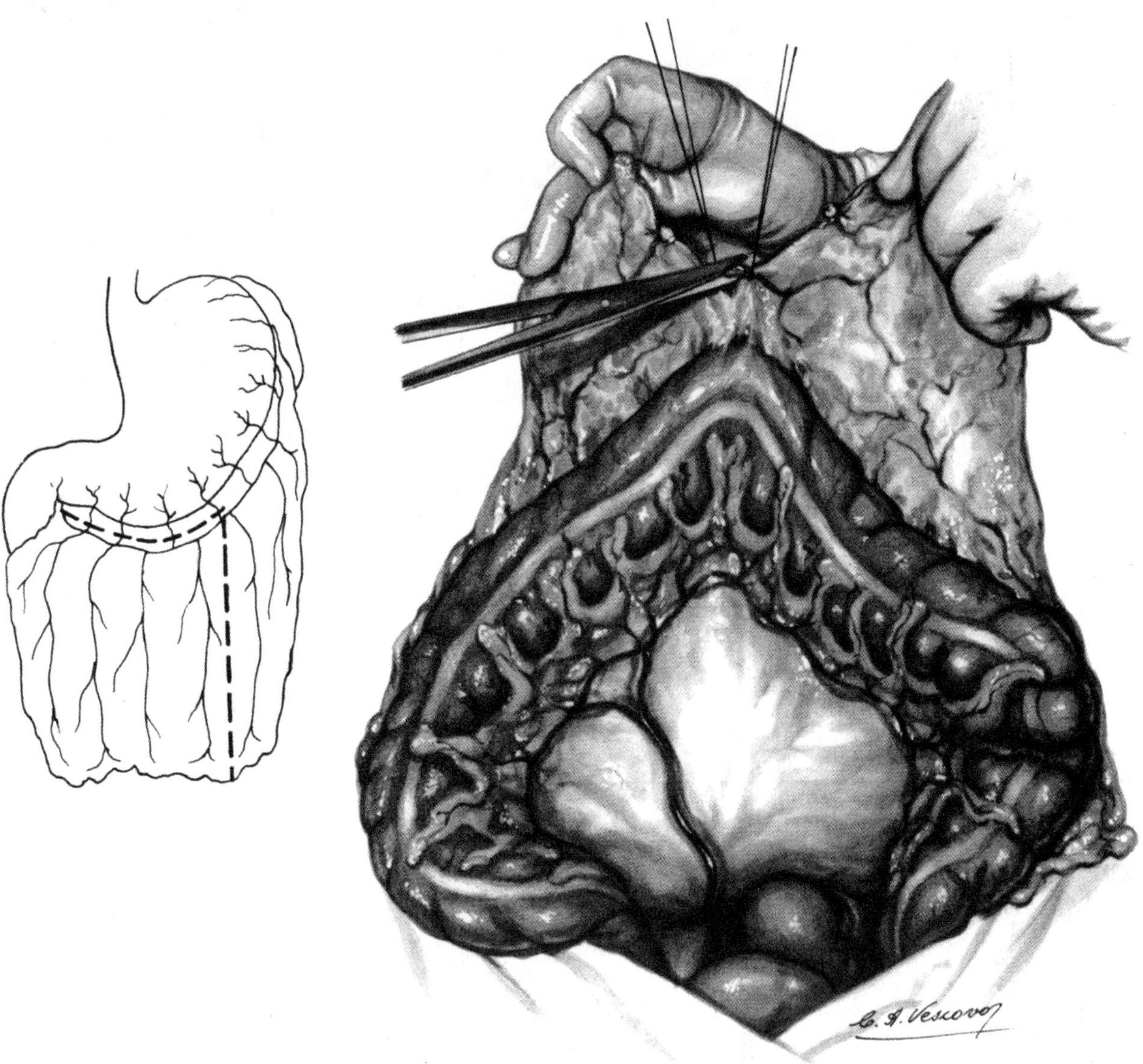

FIGURE 50.5

Right Radical Hemicolectomy by the "No Touch" Technique

FIGURE 50.6
The greater omentum has been transected, and the surgeon is preparing to carry out ligation of the gastroepiploic vascular arcade, as shown in the drawing.

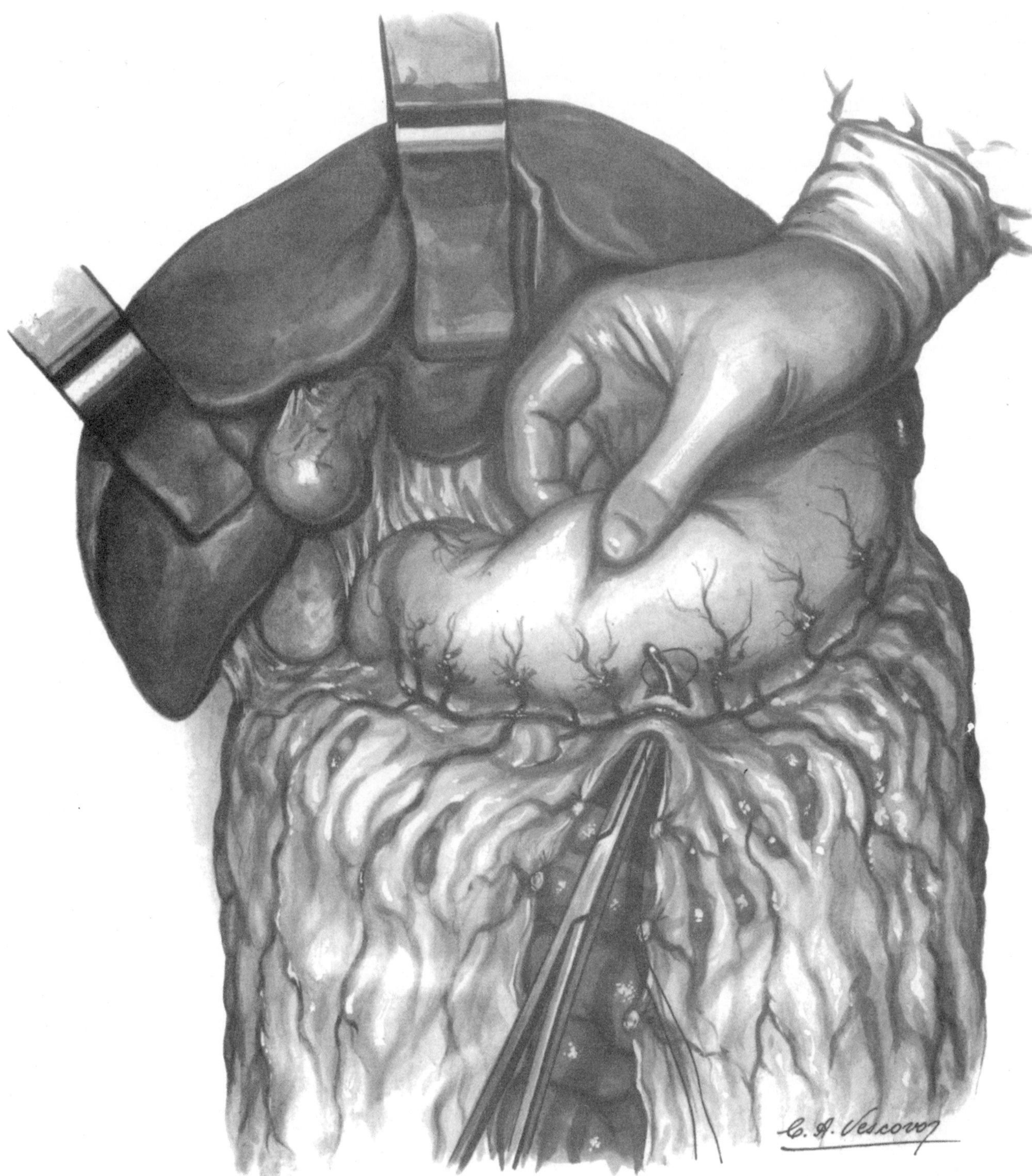

FIGURE 50.6

Right Radical Hemicolectomy by the "No Touch" Technique

FIGURE 50.7
Once the gastroepiploic arcade has been divided, the right portion of the gastrocolic ligament is divided above the arcade, allowing resection of the right gastroepiploic lymph nodes, especially when the carcinoma is located in the distal segment of the ascending colon or in the hepatic flexure.

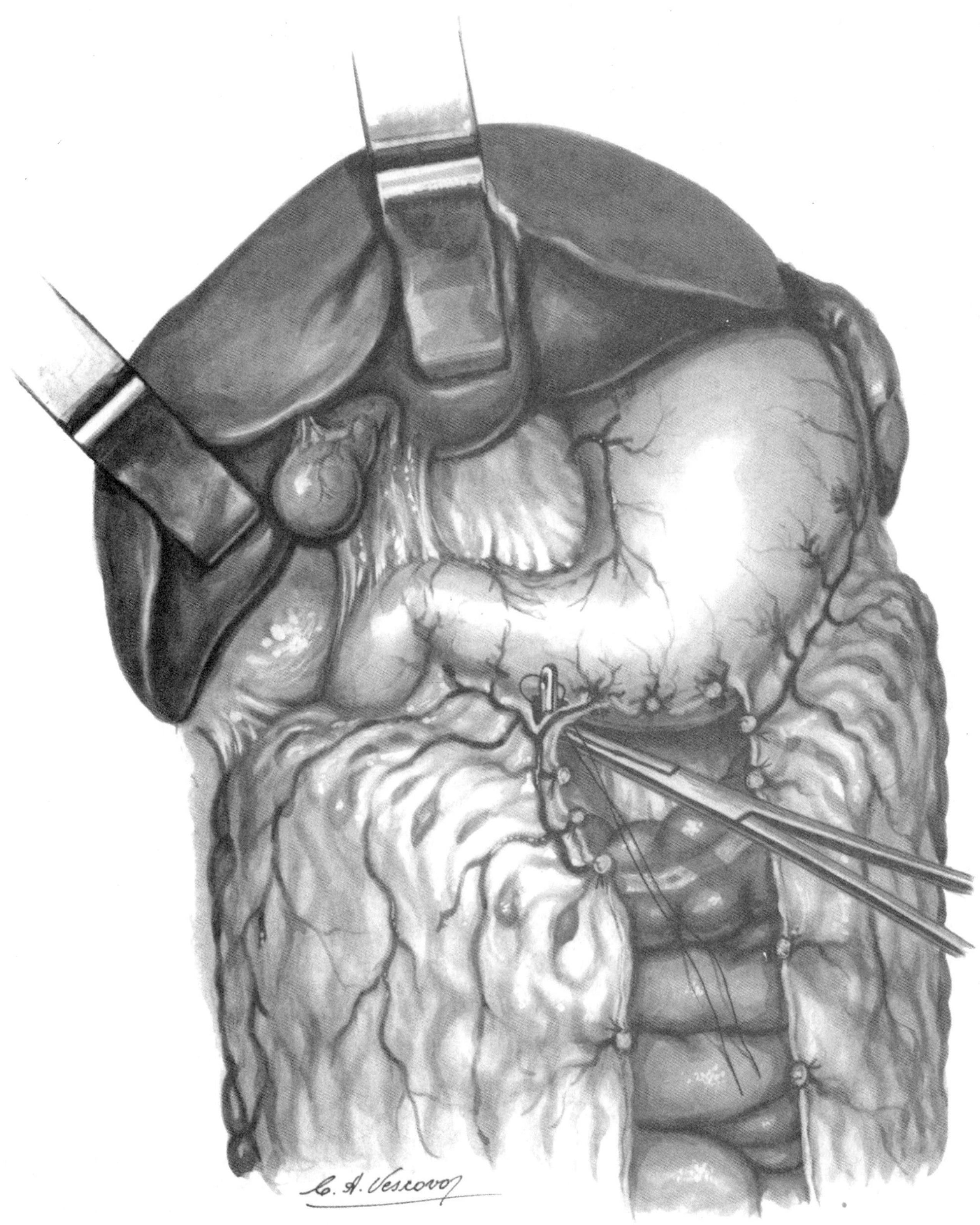

FIGURE 50.7

Right Radical Hemicolectomy by the "No Touch" Technique

FIGURE 50.8
This drawing shows the ligated gastroepiploic artery (A G E). The drawing also shows the right gastroepiploic vein (V G E), which, together with the right superior colic vein and the inferior and anterior pancreatoduodenal veins, will make up Henle's trunk (H). In some patients, simple traction on the colon and its mesocolon downward or to the right may produce avulsion of the inferior and anterior pancreatoduodenal veins with hemorrhage, which may be difficult to control and, in some cases, has been the cause of serious complications due to the unsuccessful attempt of the surgeon to apply hemostatic clamps and carry out hemostasis. The surgeon's technique in carrying out hemostasis due to avulsion of the inferior and anterior pancreatoduodenal veins is to carry out ligation of Henle's venous trunk, as shown in the next figure.

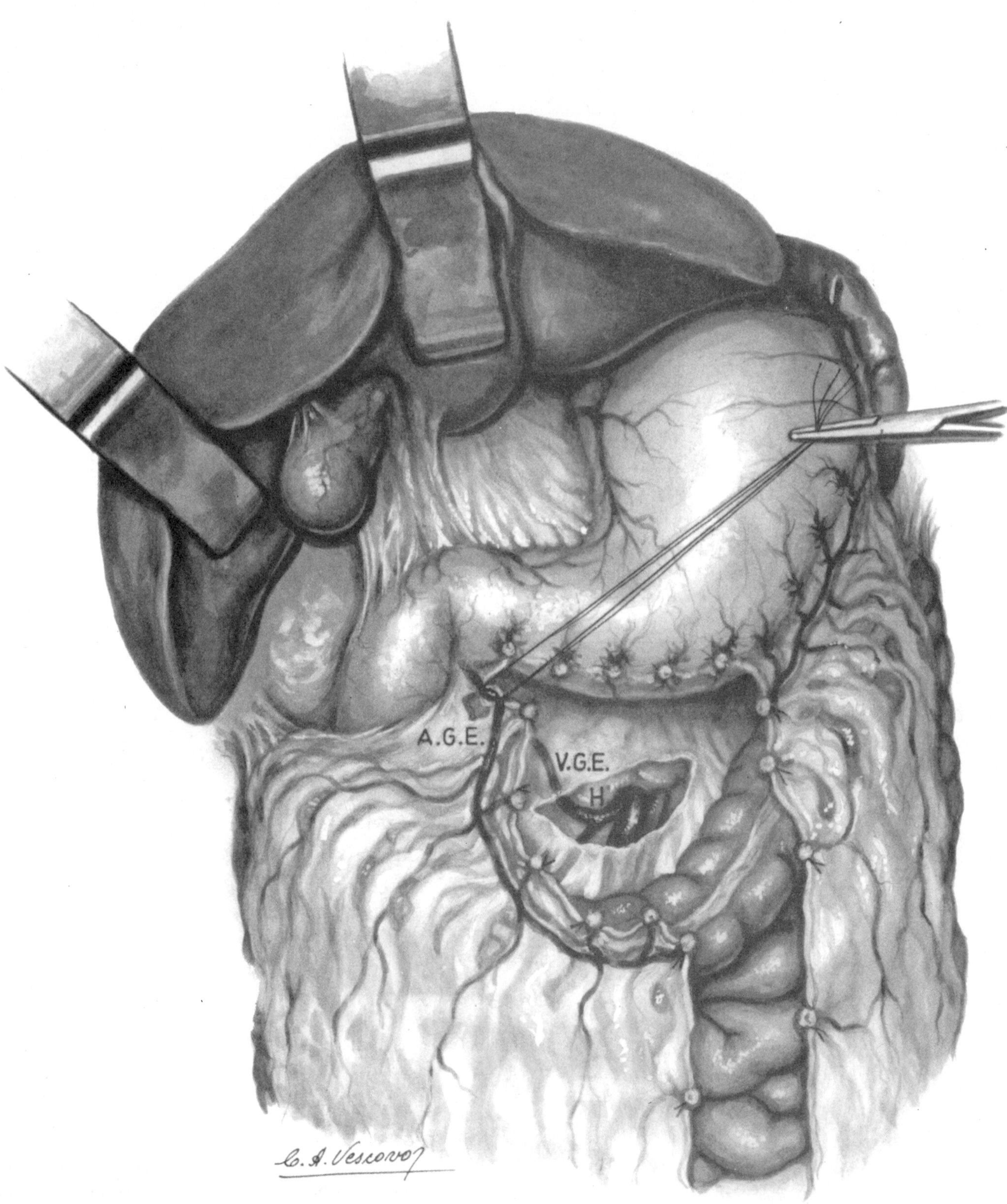

FIGURE 50.8

Right Radical Hemicolectomy by the "No Touch" Technique

FIGURE 50.9
This figure shows the ligation of Henle's venous trunk, which empties into the right side of the superior mesenteric vein and which should be looked for at the inferior border of the neck of the pancreas, once the posterior parietal peritoneum has been divided. To arrive with ease at Henle's trunk, the course of the right gastroepiploic vein should be followed to its convergence with Henle's trunk.

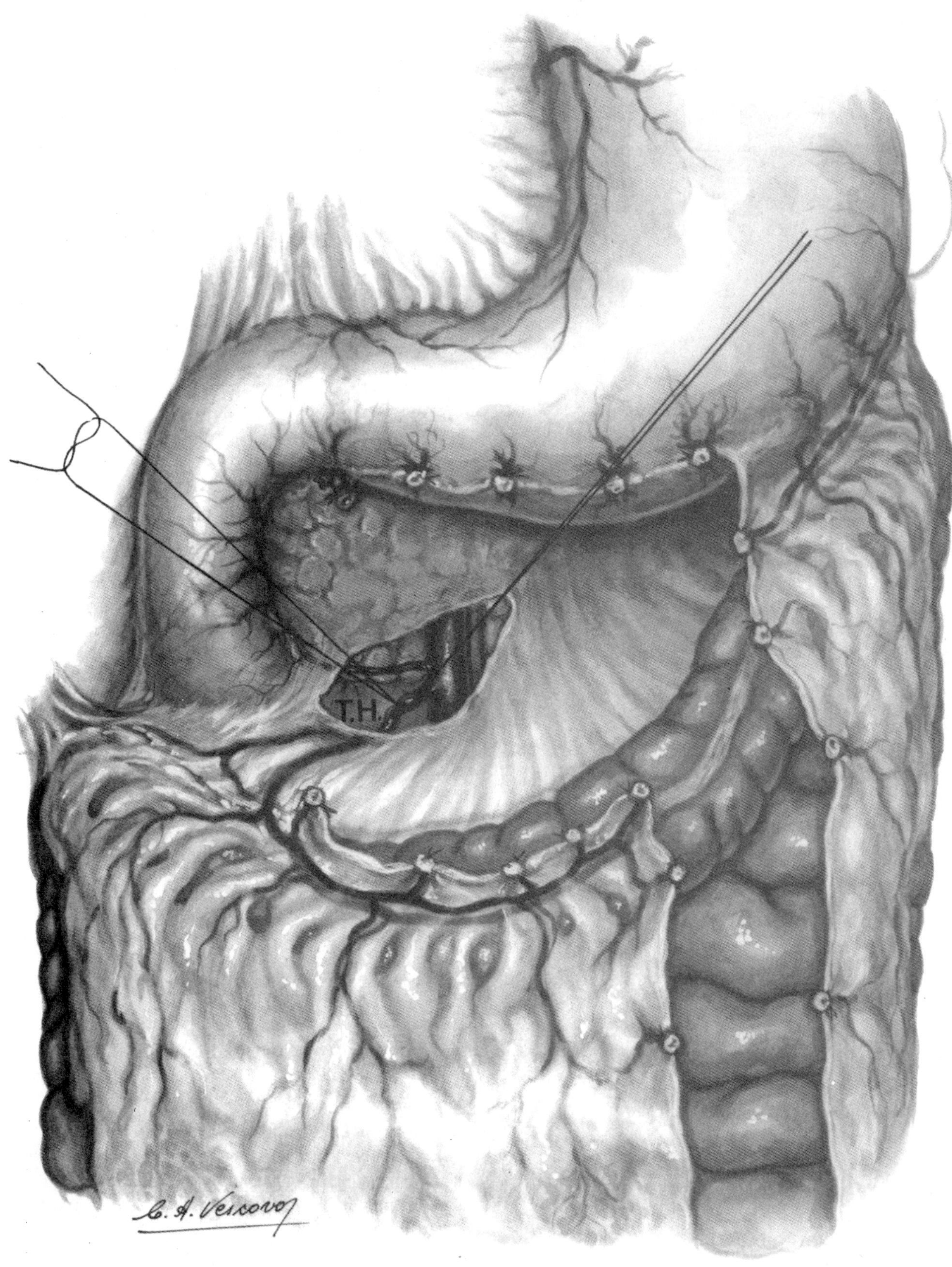

FIGURE 50.9

Right Radical Hemicolectomy by the "No Touch" Technique

FIGURE 50.10
The right half of the transverse colon has been freed together with the hepatic flexure after ligating and dividing the parieto-phrenohepatocolic ligament. The hepatic flexure of the colon has been carefully separated from the second and third portions of the duodenum.

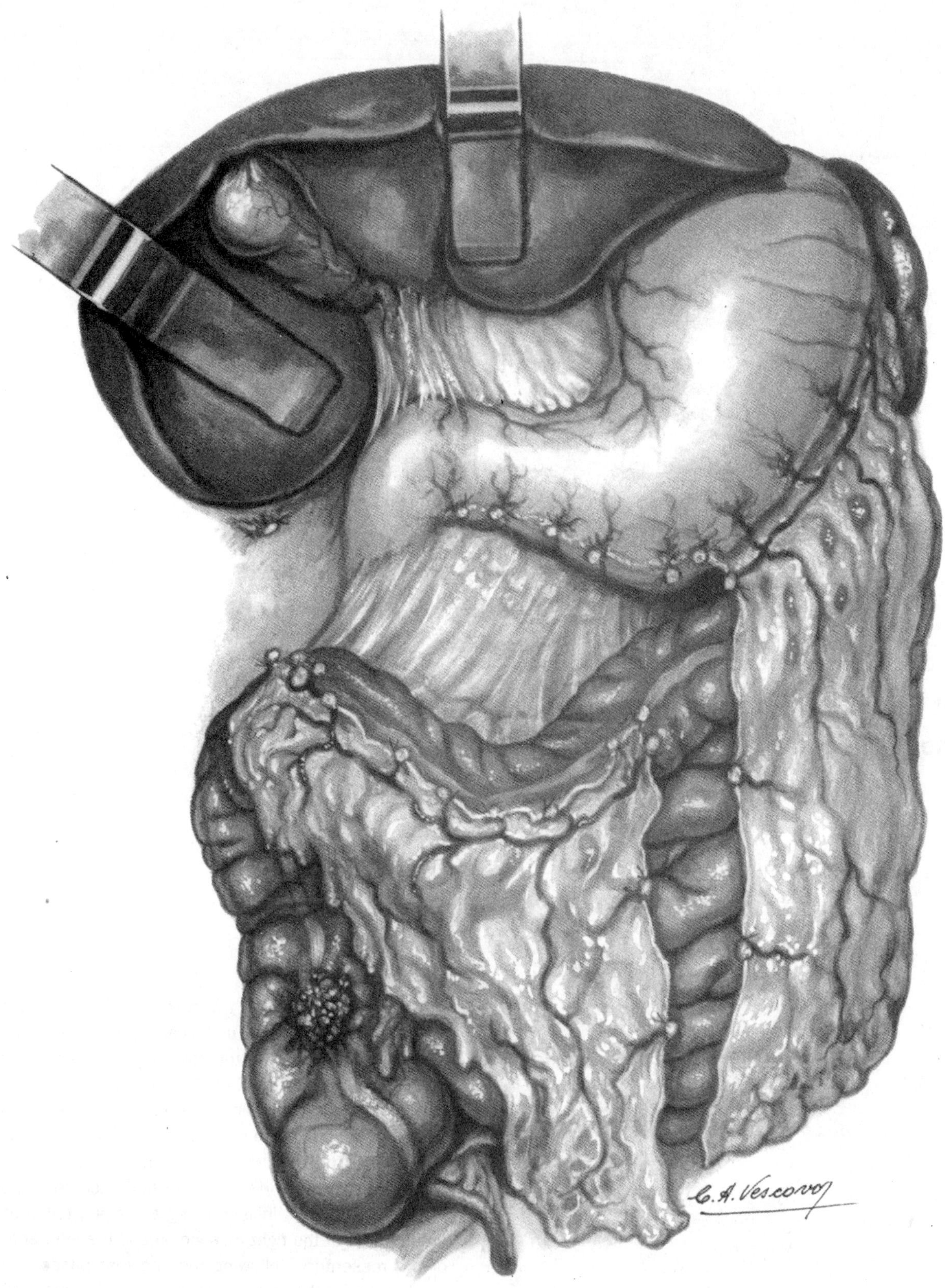

FIGURE 50.10

Right Radical Hemicolectomy by the "No Touch" Technique

FIGURE 50.11
Once the right half of the transverse colon has been freed, its lumen is occluded with umbilical tape, 3 mm wide, at the approximate level where the colon is to be transected. A similar maneuver is carried out in the terminal ileum. The object of occluding the colonic and ileal lumen is to prevent loose malignant cells that are still viable from colonizing the ileocolic suture line. The transverse colon and its mesocolon are then displaced upward, and the inferior peritoneal leaf of the transverse mesocolon is incised using a scalpel, together with the anterior leaf of the right mesocolon and the left peritoneal leaf of the mesentery, following the line that passes around the right border of the superior mesenteric vein and ending about 15 cm from the ileocecal valve. Transection of this serosa is carried out to facilitate visualization of the vascular pedicles, allowing their dissection and ligation in precise fashion at the level of the superior mesenteric vessels.

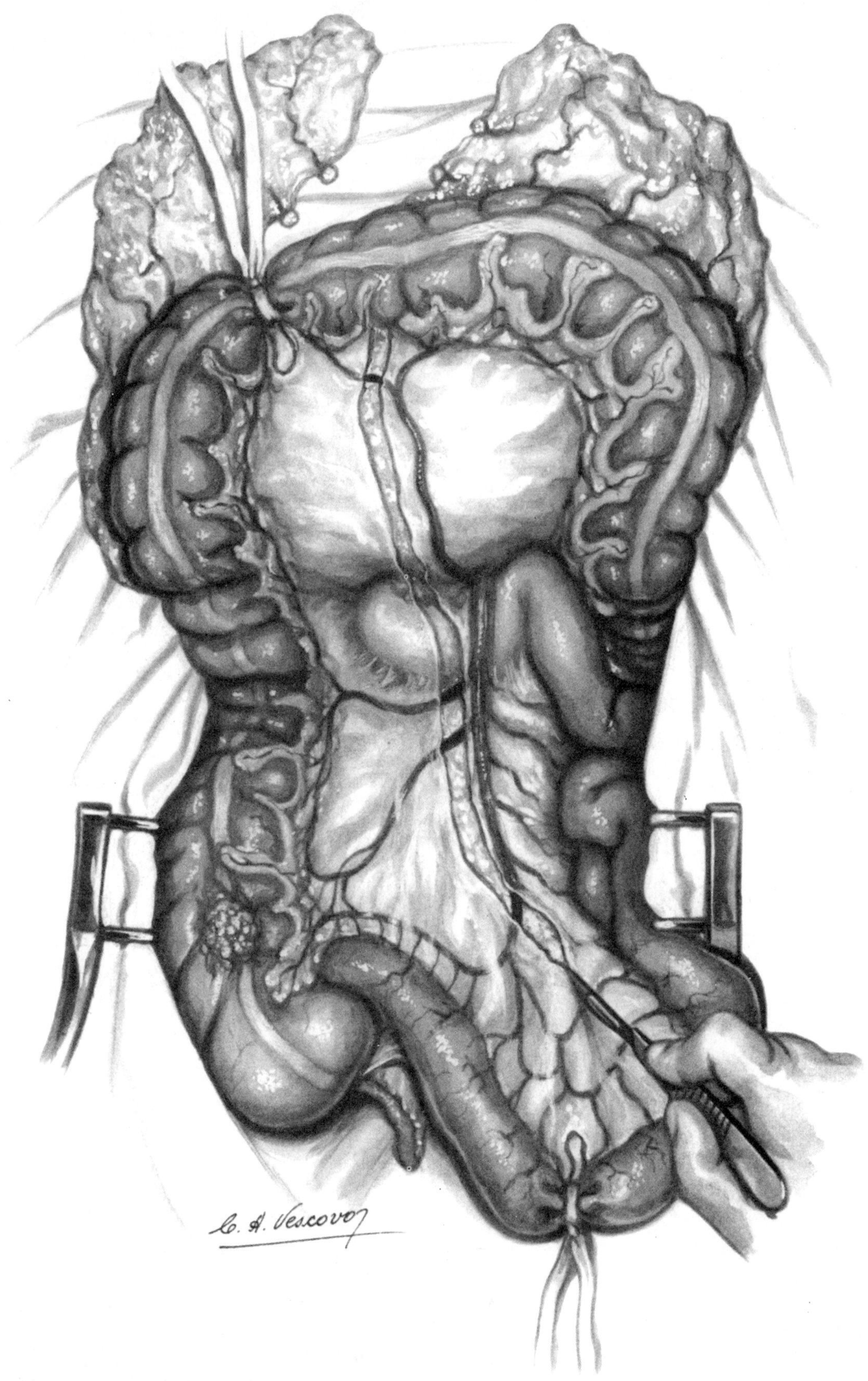

FIGURE 50.11

FIGURE 50.12
The dissection, ligation, and transection of the vascular pedicles of the right hemicolon has begun. Dissection of the ileocolic vascular pedicle has begun after ligating the right branch of the middle colic vascular pedicle and the right colic vascular pedicle. The peritoneal leaves have been divided, and traction is being applied in the opposite direction using Babcock clamps. The areolar tissue is being reflected using curved Mayo scissors, together with the lymphatic nodes to be resected en bloc with the surgical specimen.

Right Radical Hemicolectomy by the "No Touch" Technique

FIGURE 50.13
The ileocolic vascular pedicle has been dissected and is being ligated using nonabsorbable surgical material.

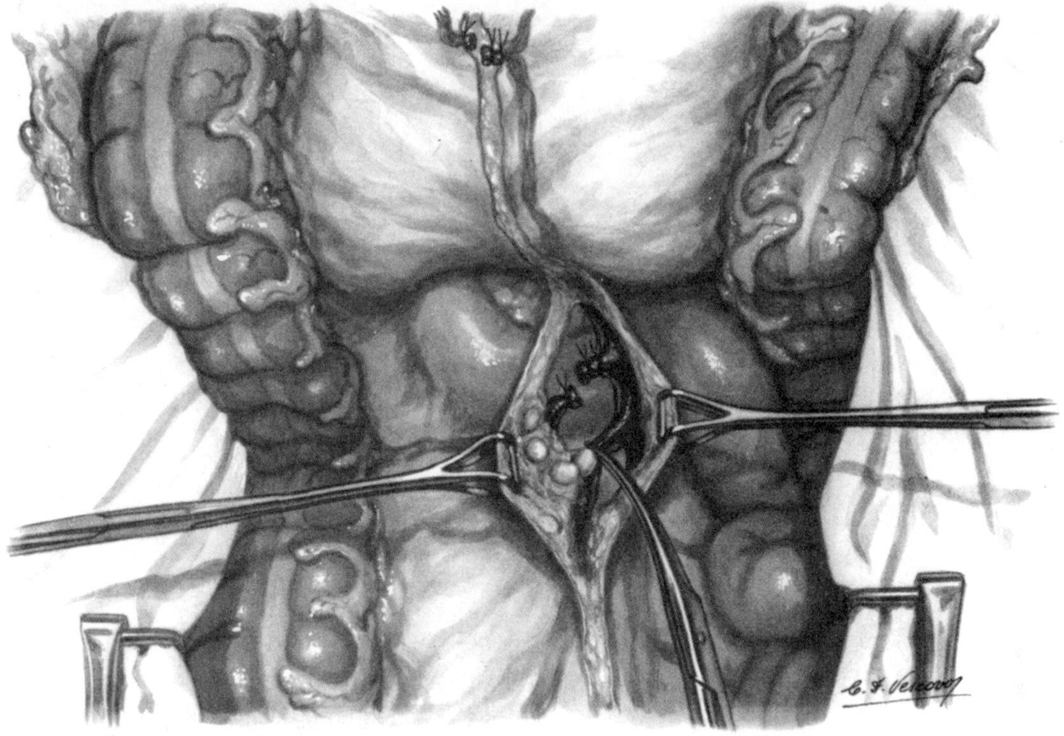

FIGURE 50.12

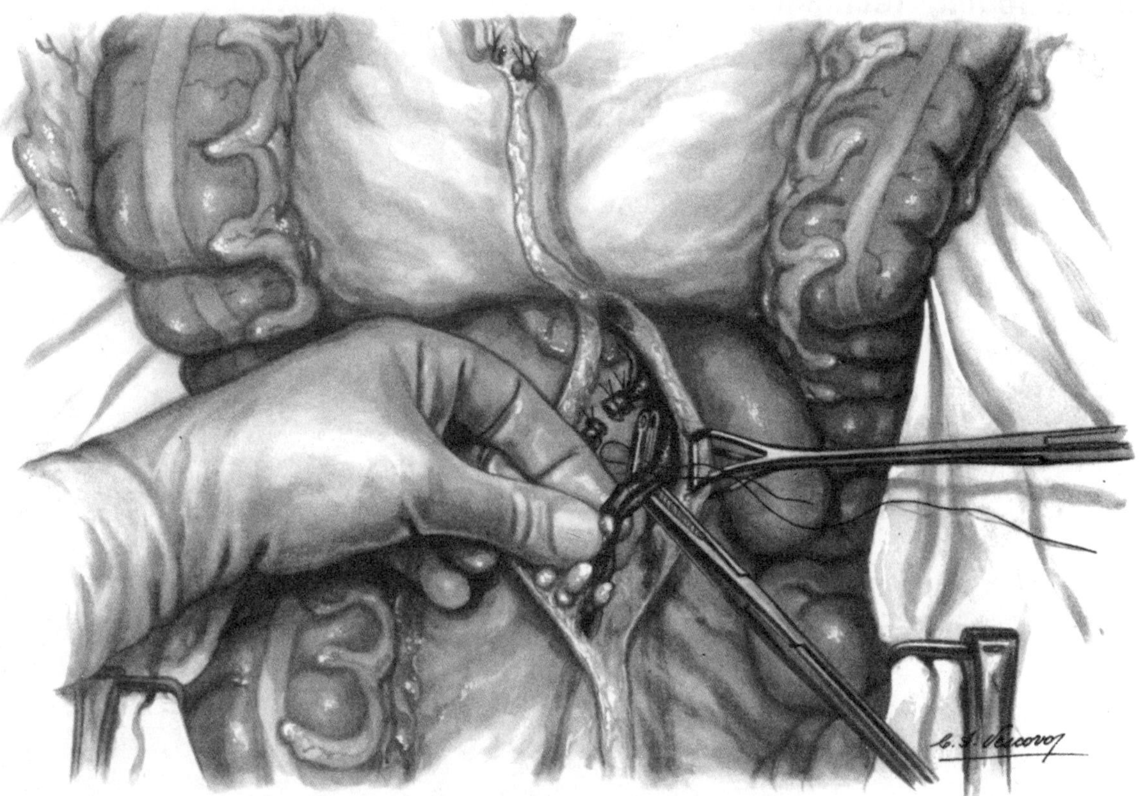

FIGURE 50.13

FIGURE 50.14
Two ligatures have been placed on the proximal side toward the superior mesenteric vessels and one ligature on the distal side, which will be resected with the specimen. The drawing shows the moment in which the ileocolic vascular pedicle is being transected, completely devoid of areolar tissue and lymph nodes.

Right Radical Hemicolectomy by the "No Touch" Technique

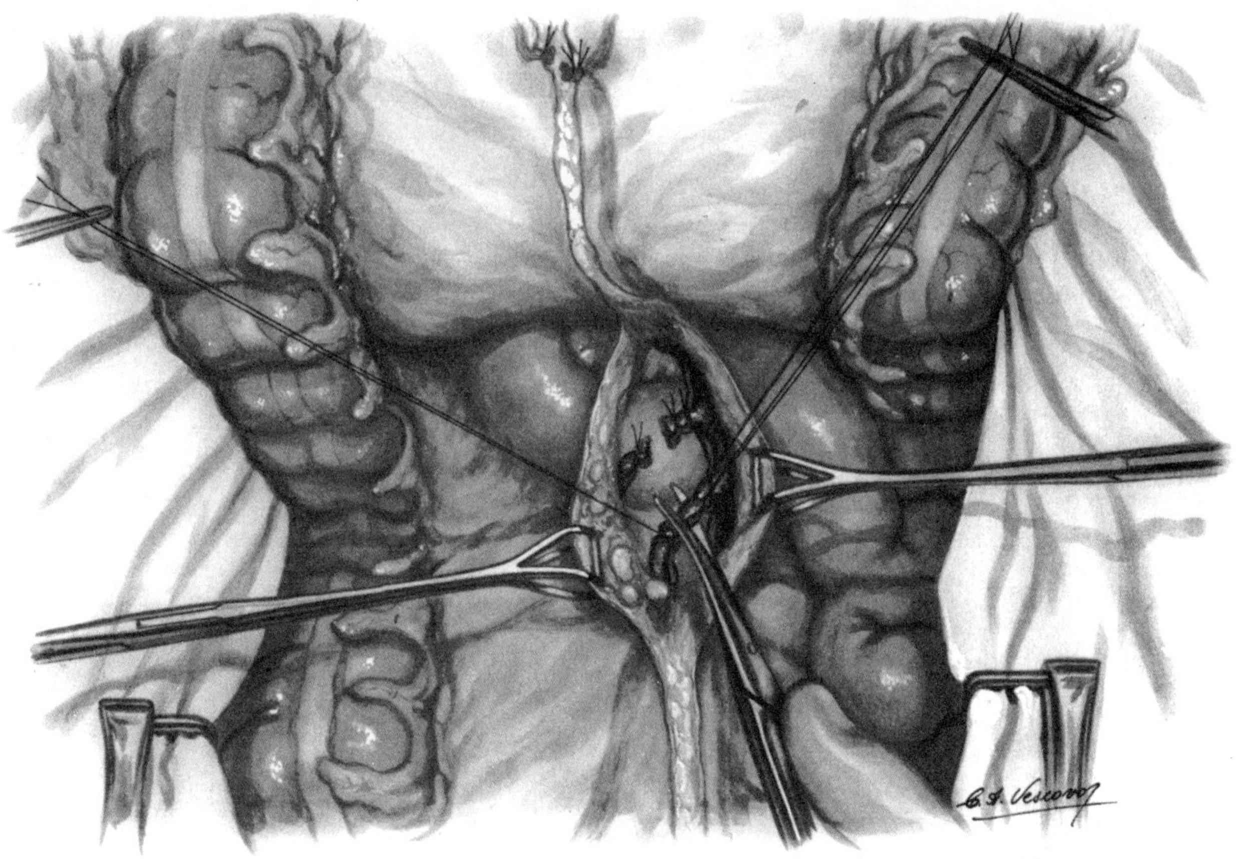

FIGURE 50.14

Right Radical Hemicolectomy by the "No Touch" Technique

FIGURE 50.15
Once the vascular pedicles of the right colon have been ligated, ligature of the mesentery of the ileum is carried out, as shown in the drawing. The broken line shows the site where the transverse mesocolon and the ileum will be divided.

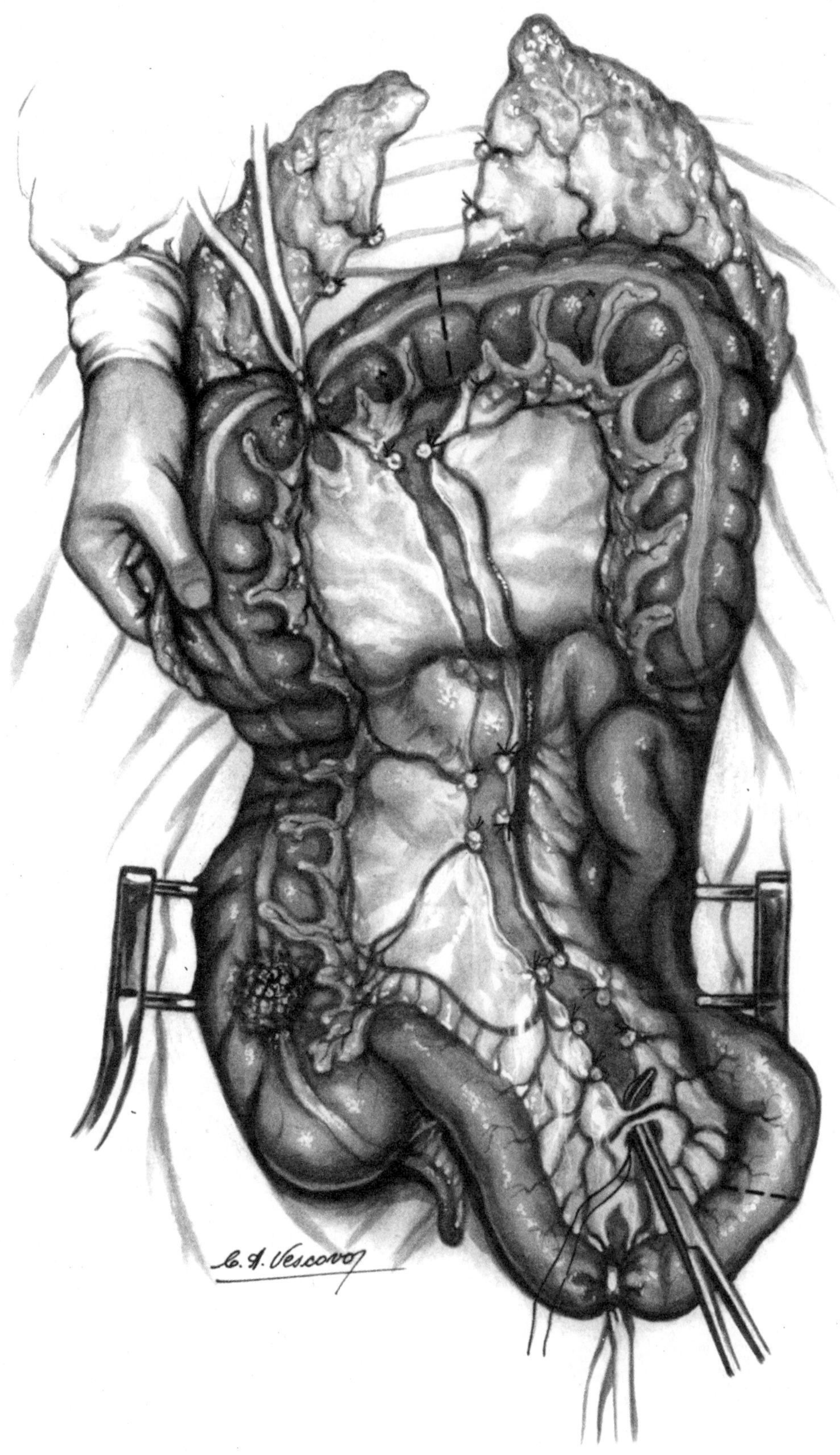

FIGURE 50.15

FIGURE 50.16
Before dividing the colon, which constitutes a septic stage in the operation, a wound protector is applied, which is made up of a layer of plastic joined to an arch, which adapts itself to the edges of the abdominal wound. Once the septic stage of the operation is completed, the wound protector is removed. If a wound protector is not available, the edges of the abdominal incision should be adequately protected with pads. 1, Wound protector; 2, large Balfour self-retaining retractor; 3, gauze pads placed at the beginning of the surgery to protect the surgical wound.

Right Radical Hemicolectomy by the "No Touch" Technique

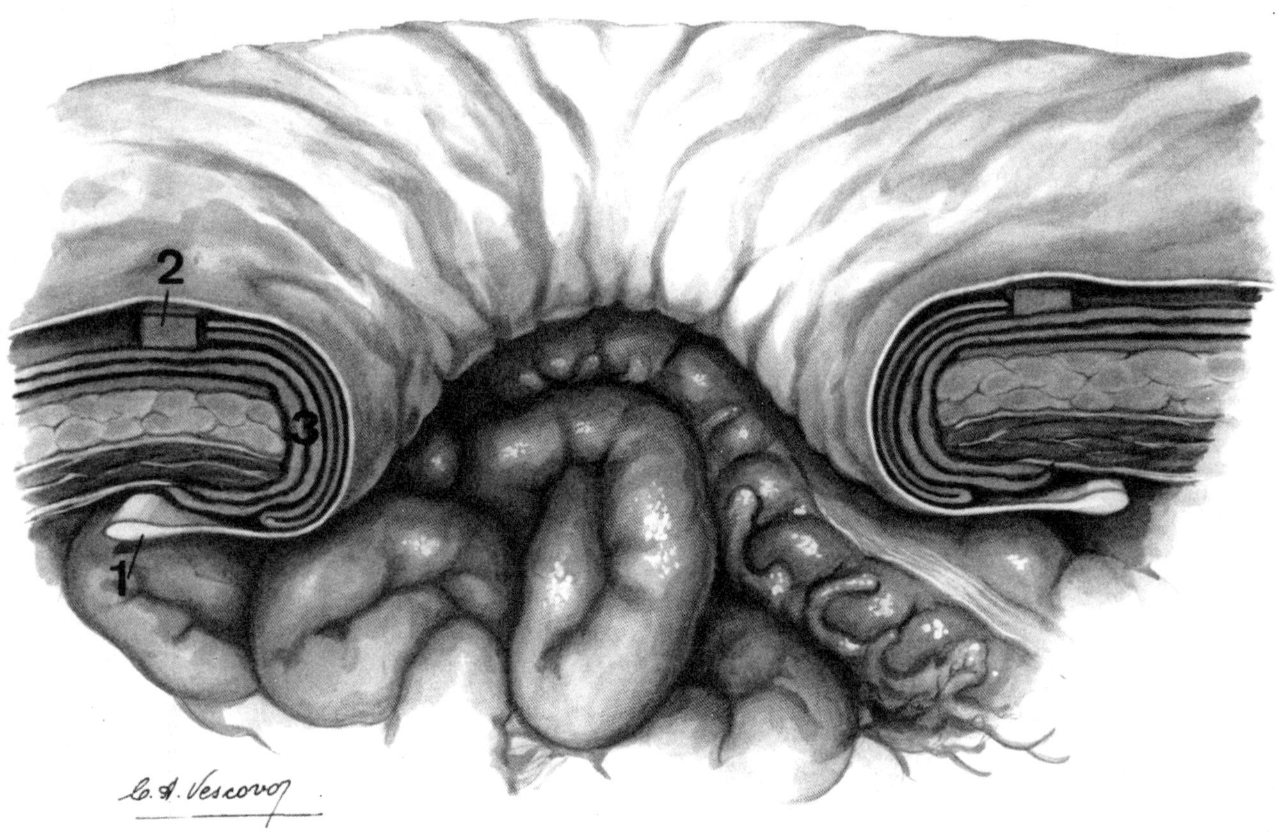

FIGURE 50.16

Right Radical Hemicolectomy by the "No Touch" Technique

FIGURE 50.17
Once the wound protector has been placed, it is necessary to occlude the colon with an atraumatic clamp about 10 cm from the line of transection to prevent fecal spillage into the abdominal cavity. The colonic end that is to be resected with the surgical specimen is wrapped into a gauze pad held in place by a large triangular Duval clamp, as shown in the drawing. Before the ileum is transected, a similar atraumatic clamp is applied. The ileal end to be resected is also covered with a gauze pad and held in place by a Duval clamp.

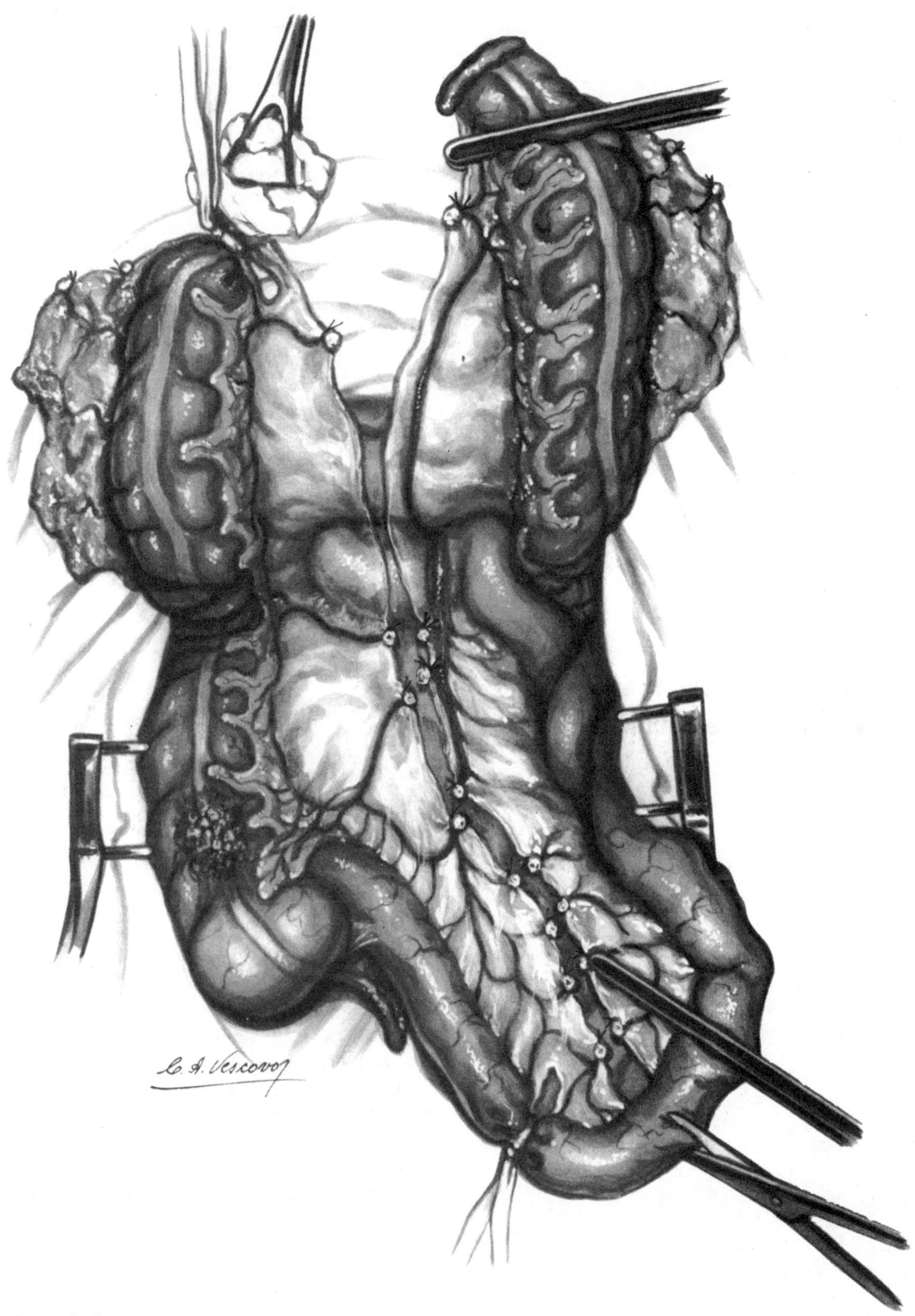

FIGURE 50.17

Right Radical Hemicolectomy by the "No Touch" Technique

FIGURE 50.18
Once the colonic segment to be resected has been separated from the organism, its mobilization and removal is carried out. The right colon is held to the organism by only the right parietocolic peritoneum, which has also been divided. The surgical specimen is ready to be removed. Once the parietocolic space has been dissected, the ureter and right gonadal vessels must again be identified. These usually rest on the psoas muscle, covered by a thin layer of urogenital fascia. While the parietocolic space is being dissected in order to remove the surgical specimen, the first assistant applies the palm of his or her right hand on the psoas muscle to protect the ureter and gonadal vessels.

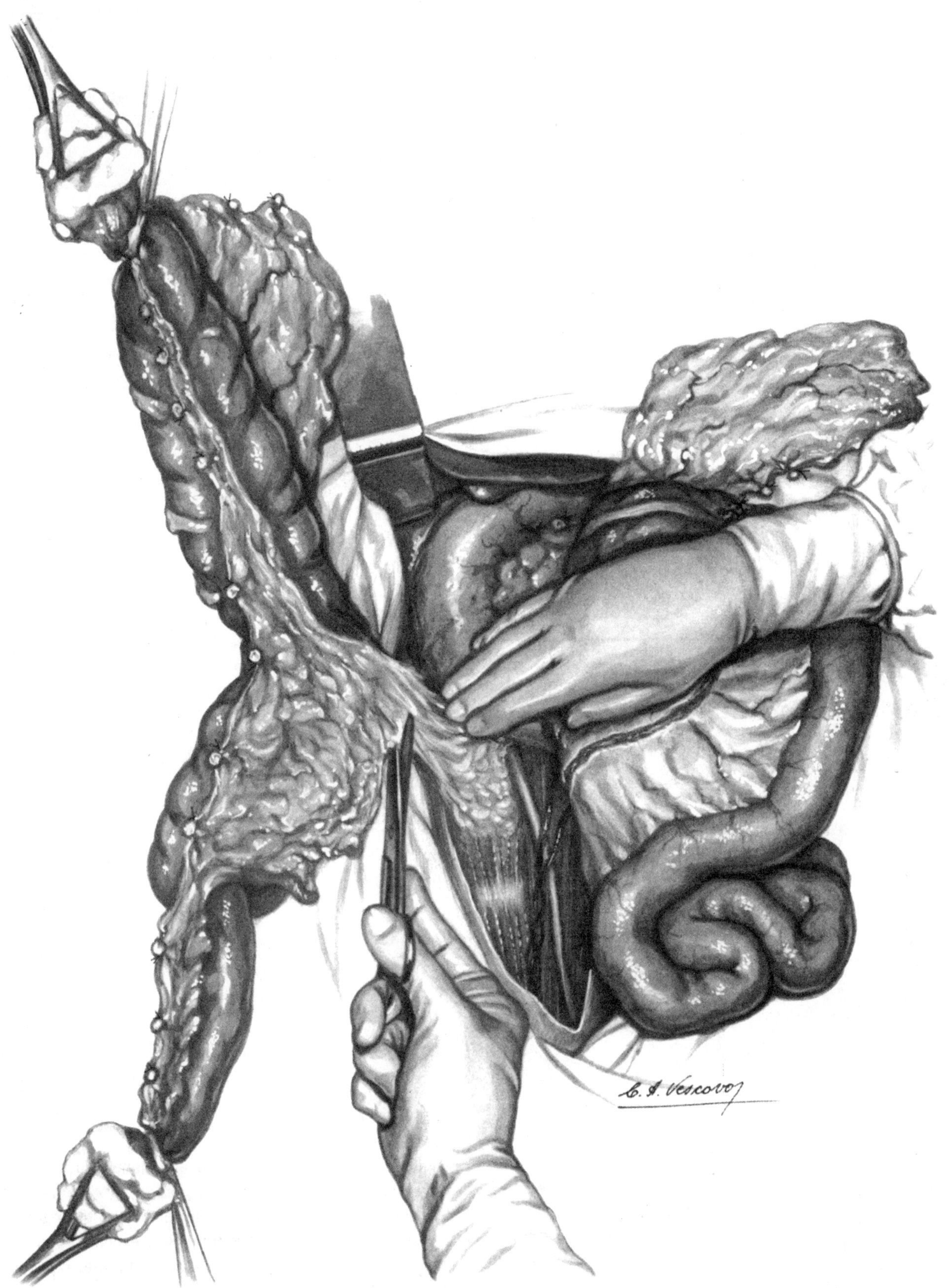

FIGURE 50.18

Right Radical Hemicolectomy by the "No Touch" Technique

FIGURE 50.19
This drawing is to show the cleavage plane through which the surgeon should pass in carrying out a right hemicolectomy. It is possible to appreciate 1, the relation to the right kidney; 2, the relation to the duodenum; 3, the right ureter and the gonadal vessels resting on the psoas muscle, covered by a thin layer of urogenital fascia.

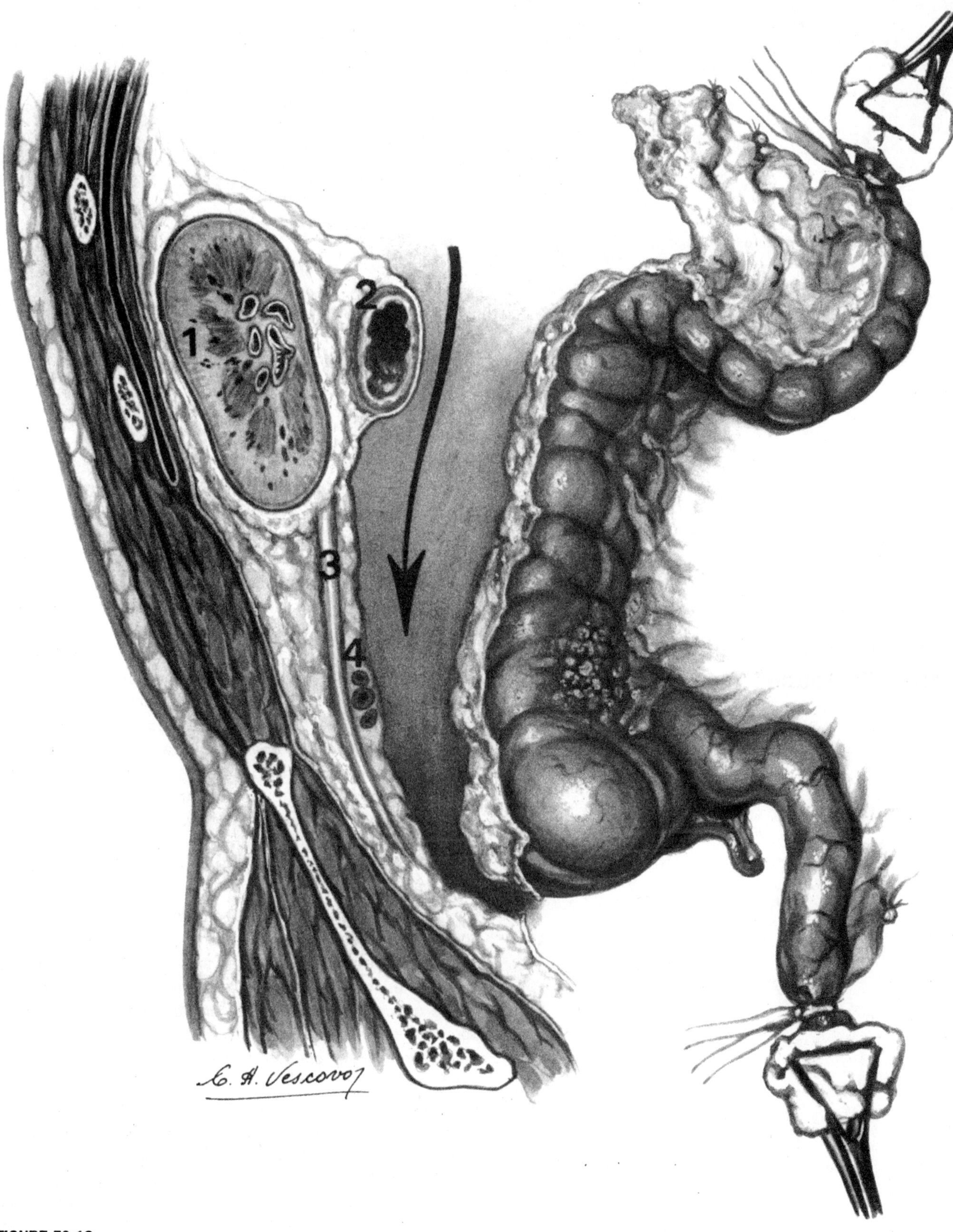

FIGURE 50.19

Right Radical Hemicolectomy by the "No Touch" Technique

FIGURE 50.20

Before starting to carry out the anastomosis of the ileum to the transverse colon in order to reestablish intestinal continuity, the ends to be anastomosed are again inspected to be sure they are adequately supplied by blood. Since the diameter of the ileum is smaller than that of the colon, it is necessary to increase it to make them more identical in diameter. For this purpose, the Cheatle procedure is carried out, which consists of performing a 25-mm-long straight line incision on the antimesenteric border of the ileum, as shown under **A.** The triangular corners of the end of the ileum are then trimmed off so that the ileum will acquire a rounded end, as shown under **B.** The ends to be anastomosed are then approximated. The atraumatic clamp that has been previously placed on the colon should be left in place until the anastomosis is completed to avoid septic contamination. If the atraumatic clamp that had been placed on the end of the ileum impedes the performance of the anastomosis, it can be removed as was done in this case.

The entire abdomen should be covered by gauze pads. The only visible organs should be the ends of the bowel to be anastomosed. It is advisable to begin the anastomosis by suturing the posterior or mesenteric hemicircumference, since it is more difficult to carry this out and this suture line is more prone to dehiscence. For this purpose, two seromuscular sutures are placed on both ends of the hemicircumference and another one in the middle, as shown under **C.** These sutures penetrate the seromuscular layer and come out to the free border of the same layer, as shown in the drawing. The material to be used for this layer may be cotton, silk, or nonabsorbable synthetic material. The three seromuscular sutures are tied as shown under **D. E,** The seromuscular layer of the mesenteric border has been sutured. **F,** The sutures for the posterior mucosal layer are being inserted. The material for the mucosal layer should be 3-0 chromic catgut.

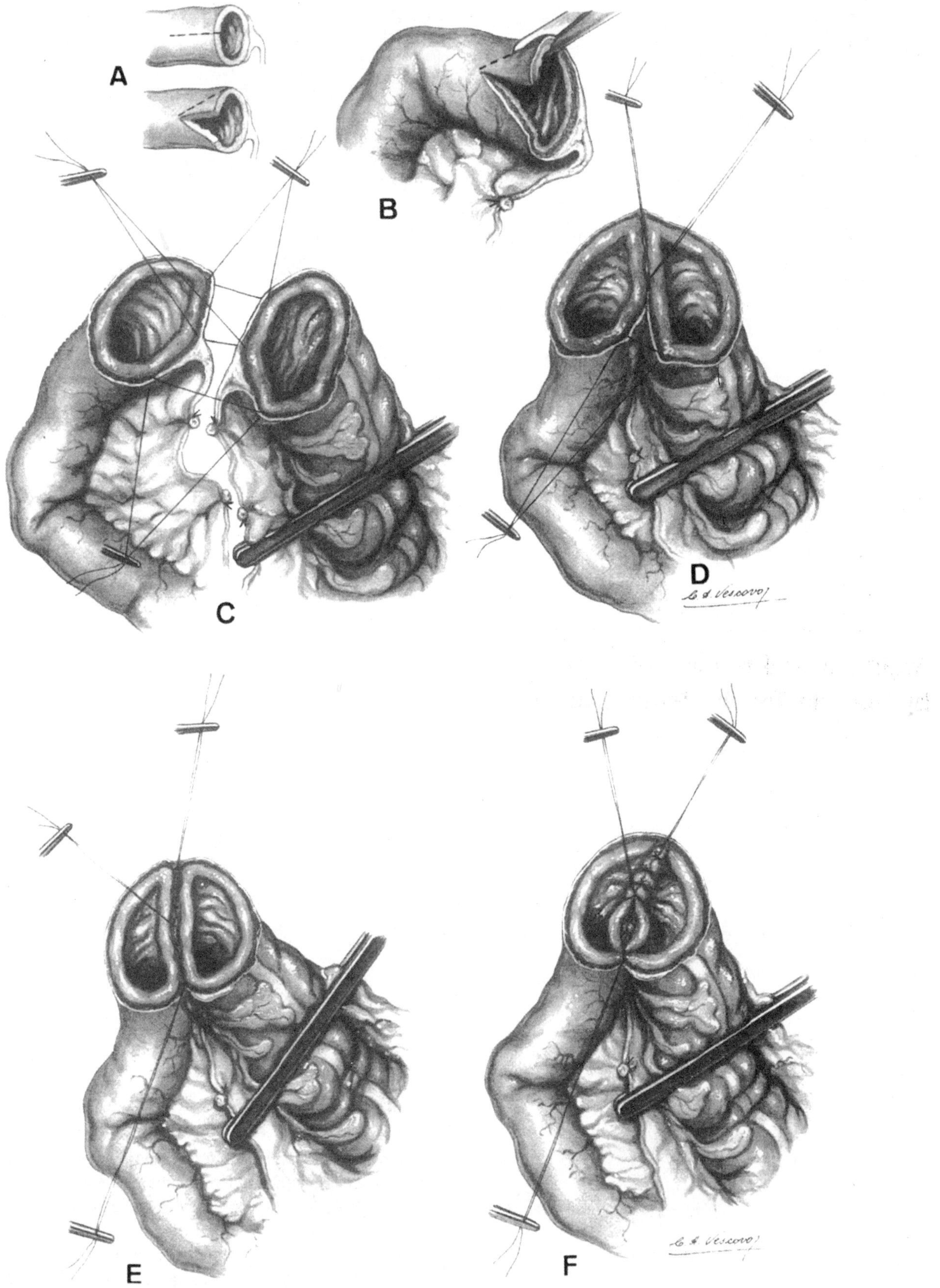
A
B
C
D
E
F

Right Radical Hemicolectomy by the "No Touch" Technique

FIGURE 50.20 (continued)
Once the two layers of the posterior hemicircumference or mesenteric layer have been completed, the mucosal layer of the anterior hemicircumference is sutured by placing sutures at each end and in the middle, as shown under **G** and **H.** **I,**The anterior mucosal layer is being completed. **J,** The seromuscular layer is being sutured. Please note that the sutures do not include a fold of the intestinal wall but are inserted through the edge of the transected border of the bowel, leading to very little inversion of the bowel wall into the intestinal lumen.

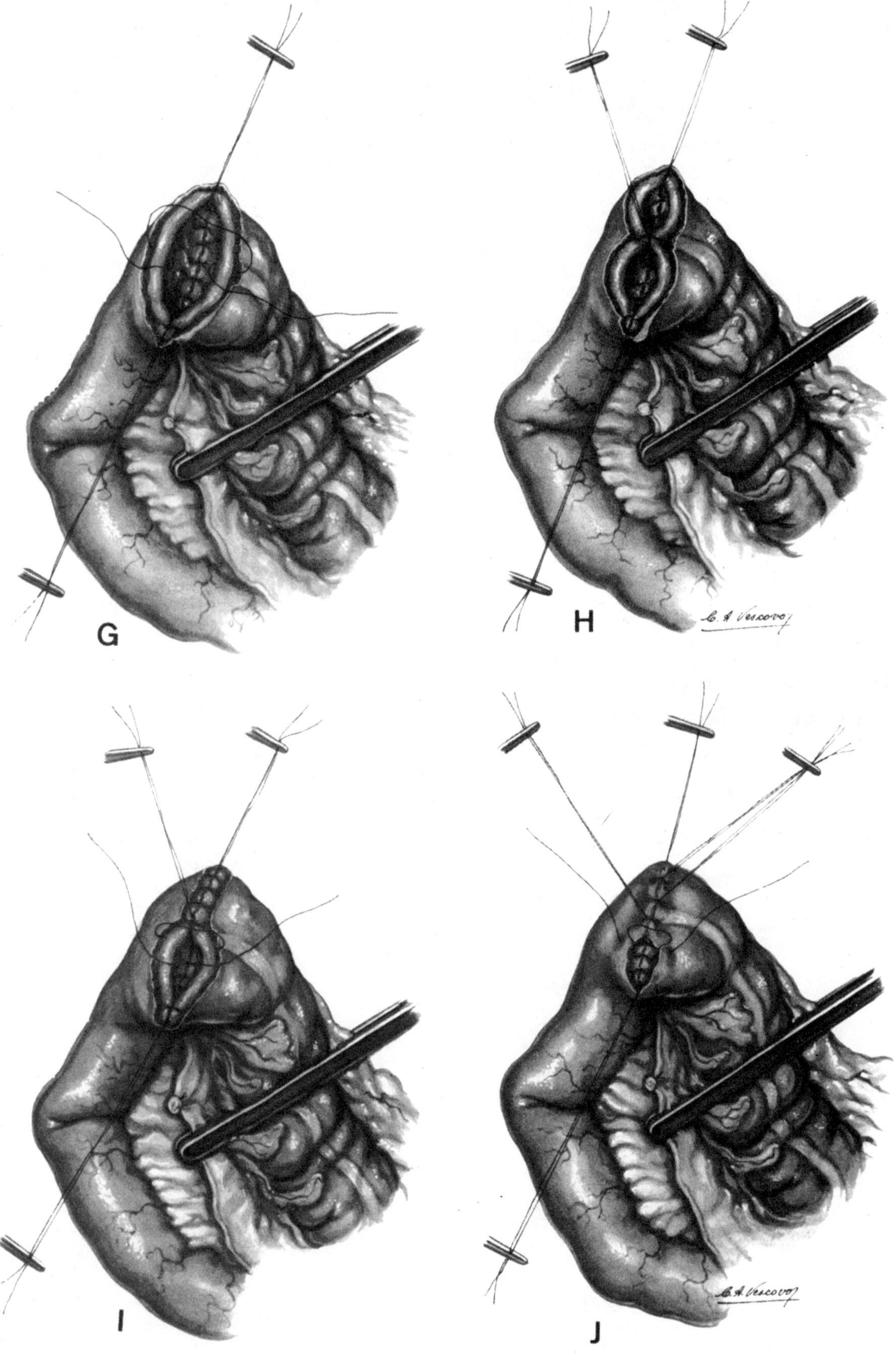
G
H
I
J

Right Radical Hemicolectomy by the "No Touch" Technique

FIGURE 50.21
The ileocolic anastomosis has been completed. The adequate diameter of this anastomosis can be seen. An opening remains between the mesentery and the mesocolon, which should be closed.

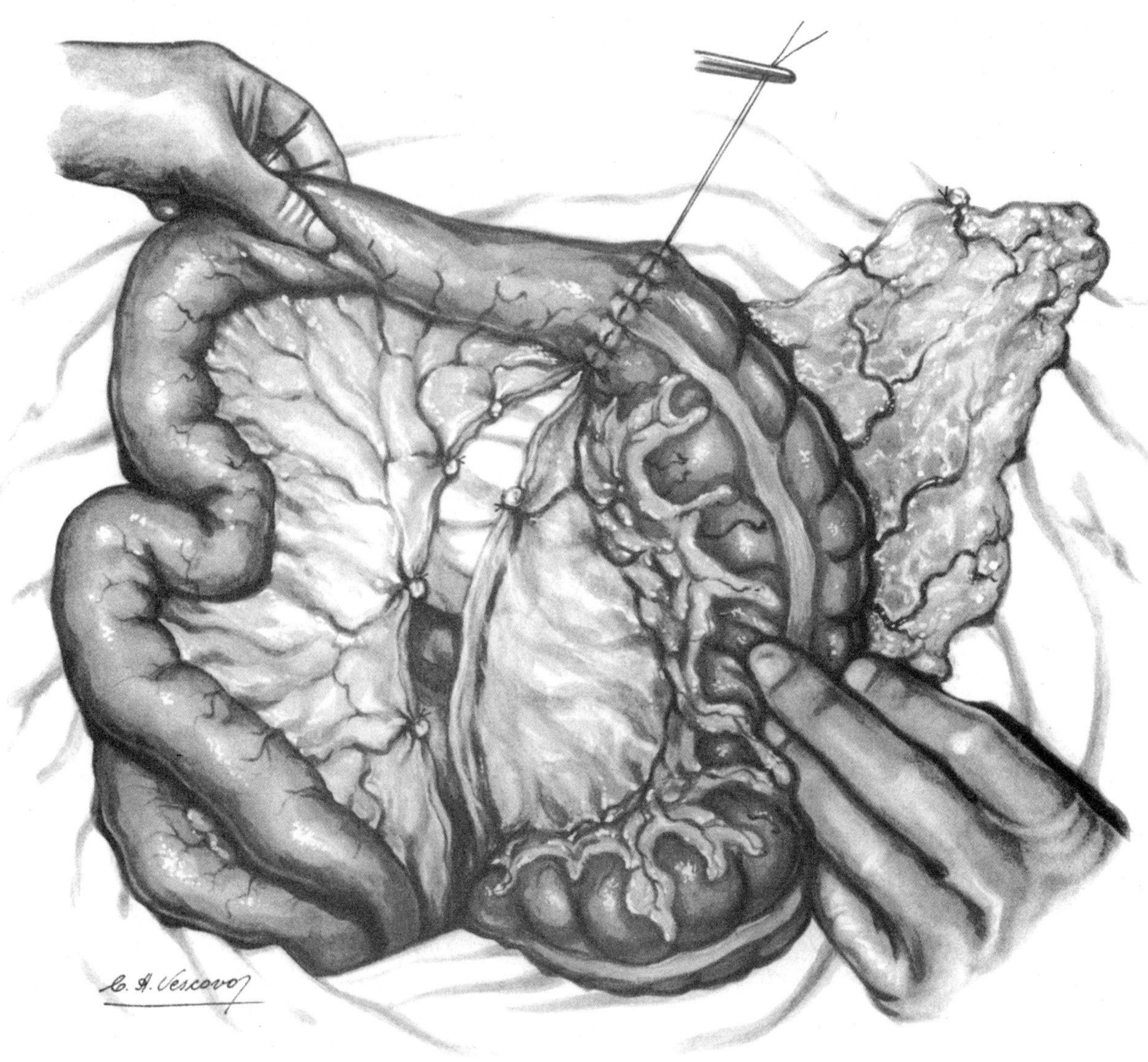

FIGURE 50.21

Right Radical Hemicolectomy by the "No Touch" Technique

FIGURE 50.22
The opening between the mesentery and the mesocolon is being sutured with interrupted nonabsorbable suture material. These sutures will grasp, on one side, the anterior serosal layer of the mesentery, and on the other side, the anterior serosal layer of the mesocolon. Sutures are not placed through the entire thickness of the mesentery to avoid injuring blood vessels.

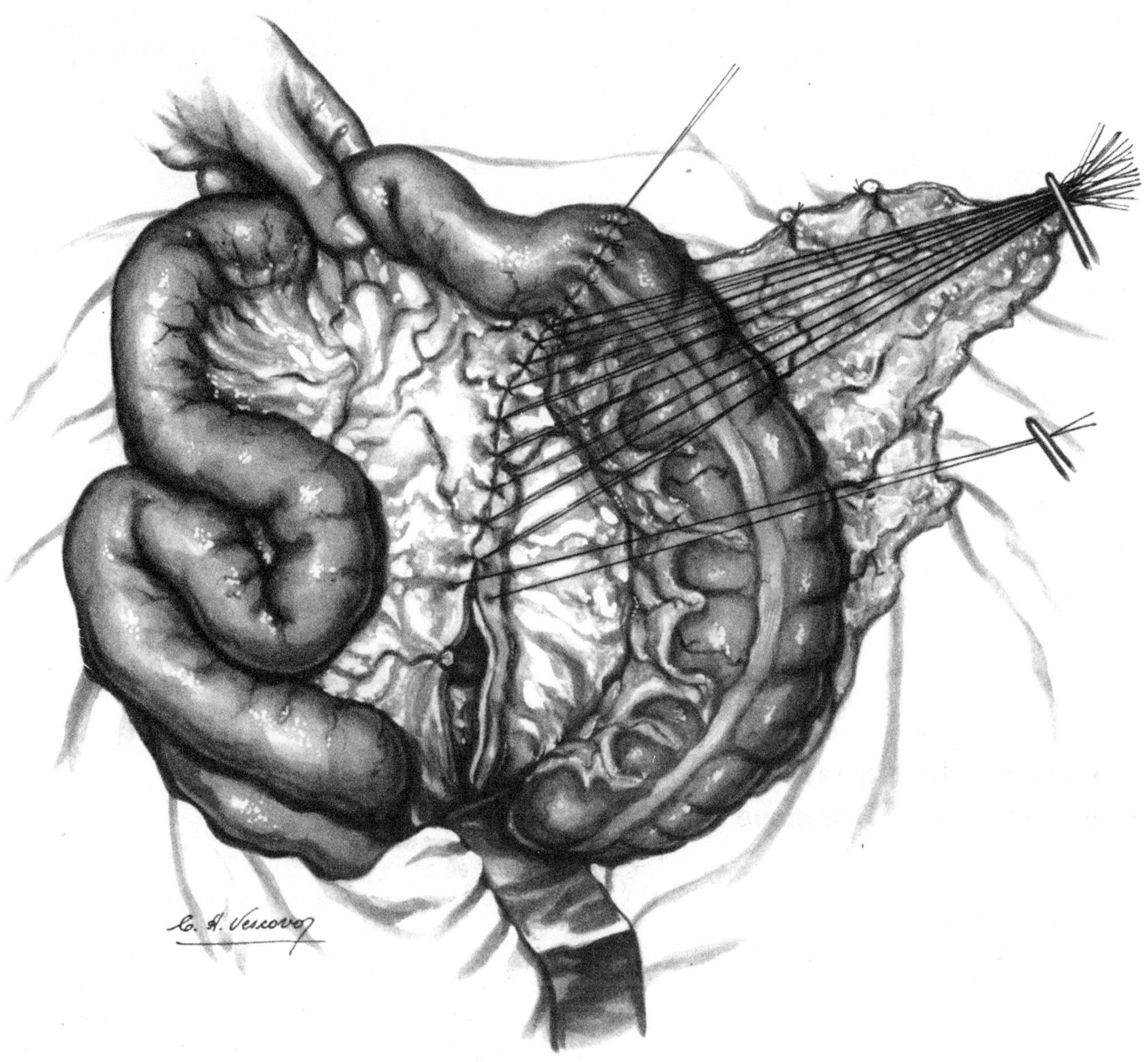

FIGURE 50.22

Right Radical Hemicolectomy by the "No Touch" Technique

FIGURE 50.23

Once the suture of the anterior serosal layer with the mesentery and the mesocolon is completed, the first assistant reflects the ileum and transverse colon downward and to the left to expose the posterior serosal layer, which is sutured in a way similar to the anterior serosal layer. The figure also shows that peritonealization of the space remaining after the resection of the right hemicolon is being carried out. Many surgeons will not peritonealize the posterior raw surface in order to prevent accumulation of blood or serum. The author always peritonealizes the posterior bed, and has never seen any complication. It must be pointed out that hemostasis of this bed should be carried out carefully. The drawing also shows the second and third portion of the duodenum, perirenal fat, the right ureter. and the gonadal vessels. The abdominal cavity is then profusely irrigated with warm saline and closure of the anterior abdominal wall is then carried out.

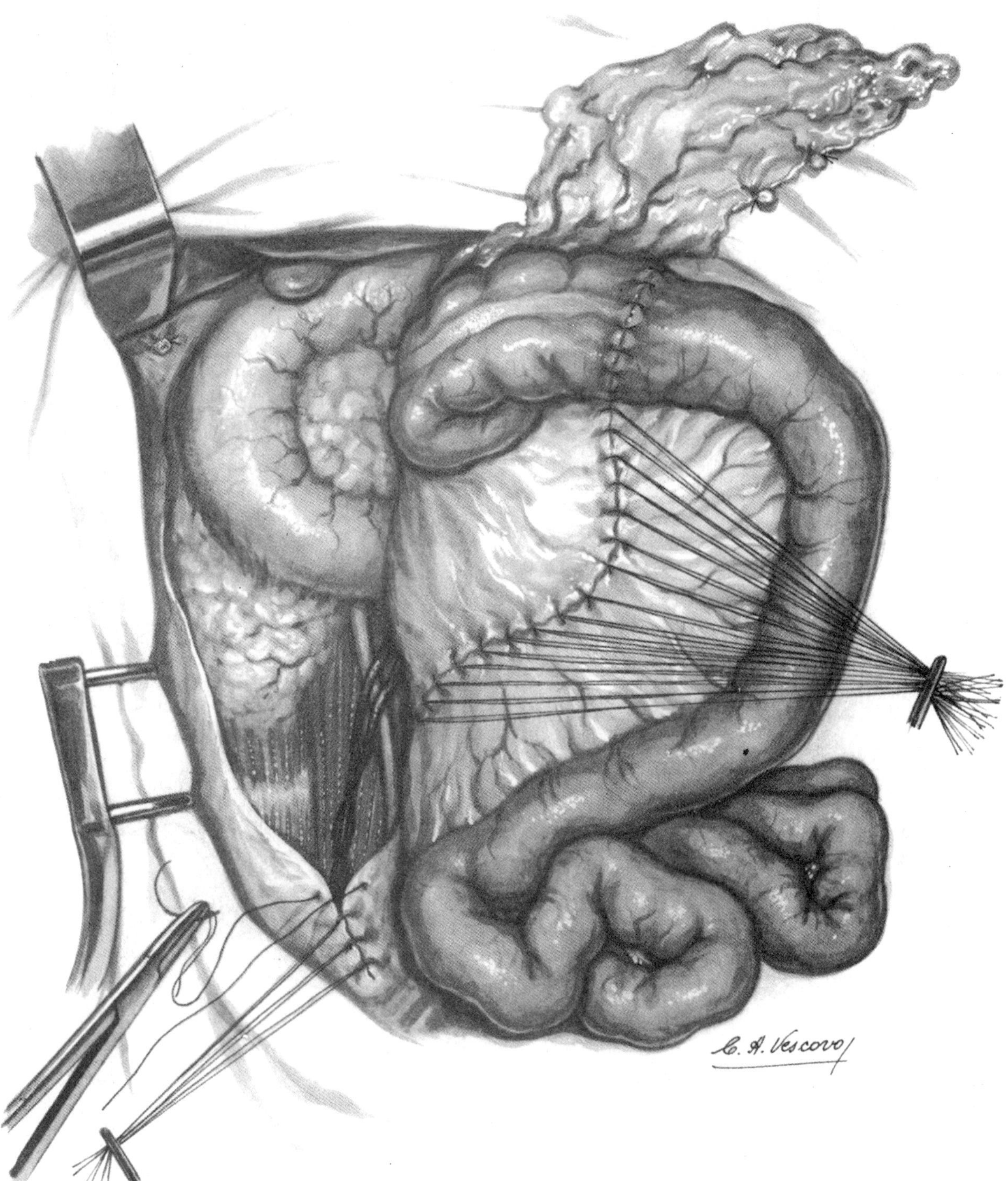

FIGURE 50.23

FIGURE 50.24
The abdominal wall is closed without drainage. **A,** Closure is being carried out of the posterior layer of the anterior abdominal wall, which is made up of parietal peritoneum and the posterior sheath of the anterior rectus abdominis muscle using interrupted sutures of synthetic material, of slow reabsorption. Before carrying out suturing of the anterior sheath of the rectus abdominis muscle, the wound is again irrigated with warm saline solution. **B,** The anterior sheath of the rectus abdominis muscle is being closed using interrupted sutures of linen, silk, or nonabsorbable synthetic material.

Right Radical Hemicolectomy by the "No Touch" Technique

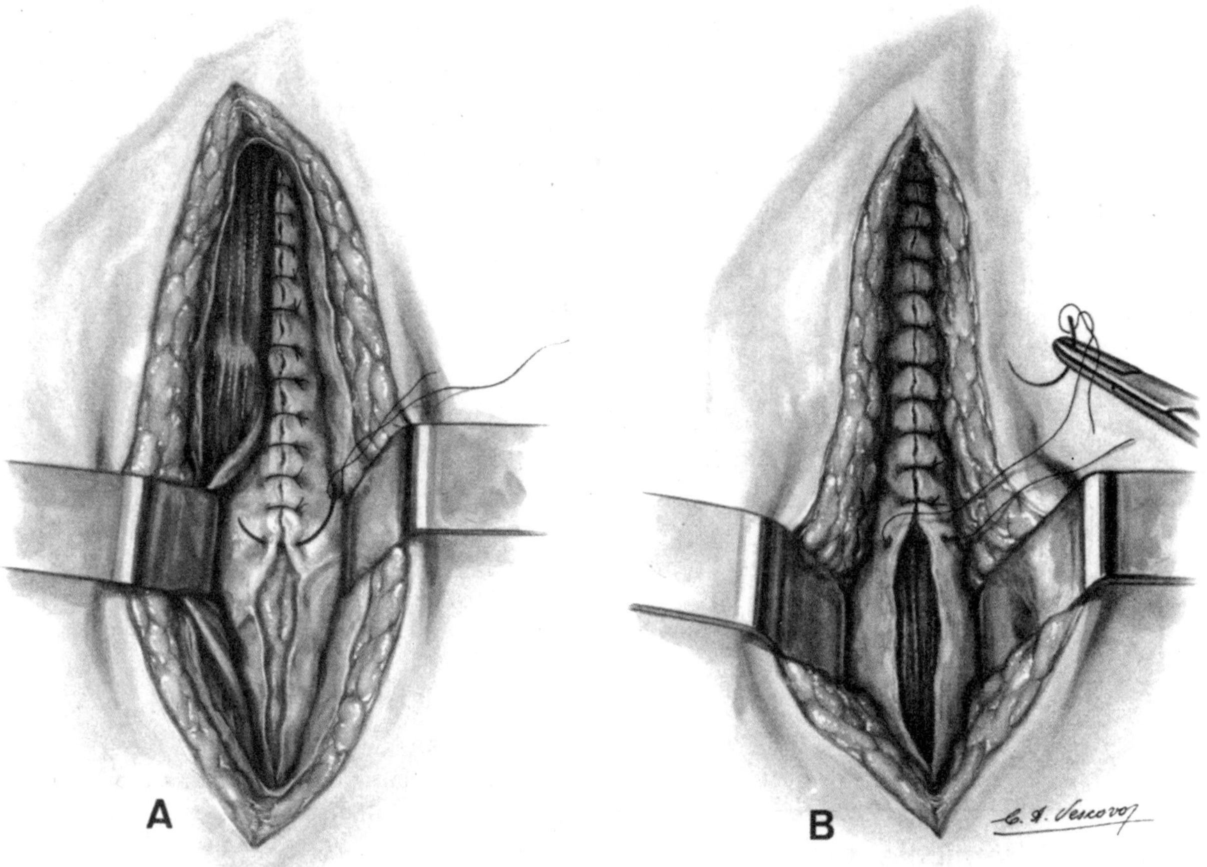

FIGURE 50.24

FIGURE 50.25

Before the subcutaneous layer is sutured, the wound should again be irrigated. The subcutaneous layer is closed with interrupted 3-0 catgut sutures and the skin is closed, using sutures on a straight needle. The ends of the thread are left long, tied in groups, as seen in the drawing, to facilitate their removal by applying traction so that they can be cut with a scissors or scalpel level with the skin.

Right Radical Hemicolectomy by the "No Touch" Technique

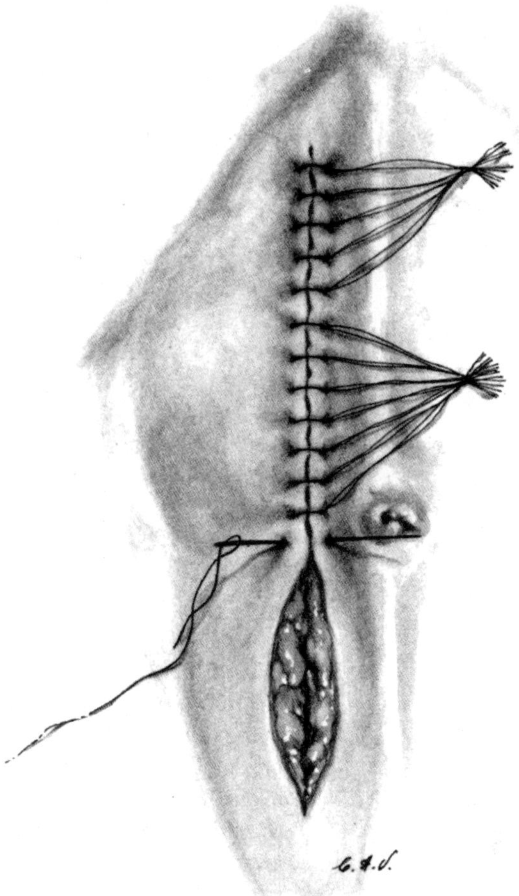

FIGURE 50.25

FIGURE 50.26

This drawing shows the surgical specimen made up of 15 cm of the terminal ileum, the cecum, the ascending colon, and the proximal half of the transverse colon. 1, Right branch of the middle colic vascular pedicle; 2, right colonic vascular pedicle with the intermediate and principal nodes that have not been invaded by the carcinoma (–); 3, ileocolic vessels with the intermediate and principal nodes that have not been invaded by the carcinoma

The carcinoma of the ascending colon had invaded the serosa. Histologic examination of all the resected nodes reveal that only three epicolic nodes (+) and two paracolic nodes near the tumor had been invaded by the tumor.

Right Radical Hemicolectomy by the "No Touch" Technique

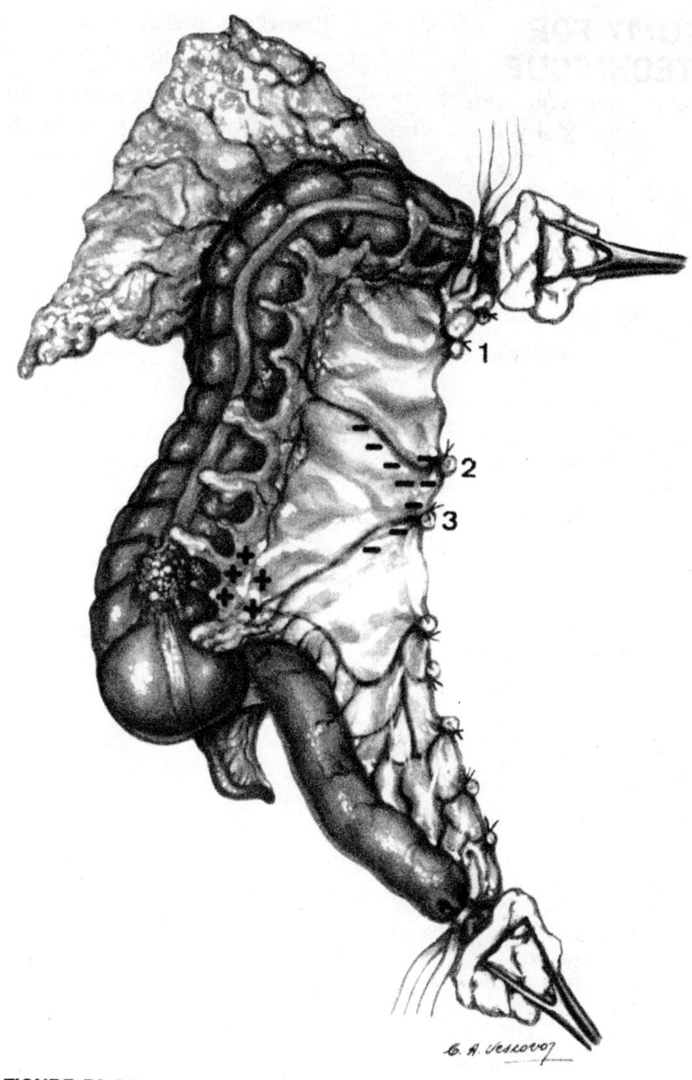

FIGURE 50.26

RIGHT HEMICOLECTOMY FOR CANCER: CLASSIC TECHNIQUE

The description of the classic right hemicolectomy by the no-touch technique, which is preferred by the author, has been made. The conventional technique is used more frequently, however. We will now describe this technique, with special emphasis on the stages that differ from the no touch technique, to avoid repetition.

Right Hemicolectomy for Cancer: Classic Technique

Right Hemicolectomy for Cancer: Classic Technique

FIGURE 50.27
The carcinoma is in a similar location. Using a broken line, the extent of resection of the right colon and greater omentum, which is no different from the no touch technique, is shown. The procedure begins by mobilizing the right colon with the tumor by dividing the right parietocolic peritoneum (see drawing). The right hemicolon and the tumor are reflected medially. The hepatic flexure of the colon is mobilized, and the gastrocolic ligament is transected, following the broken line.

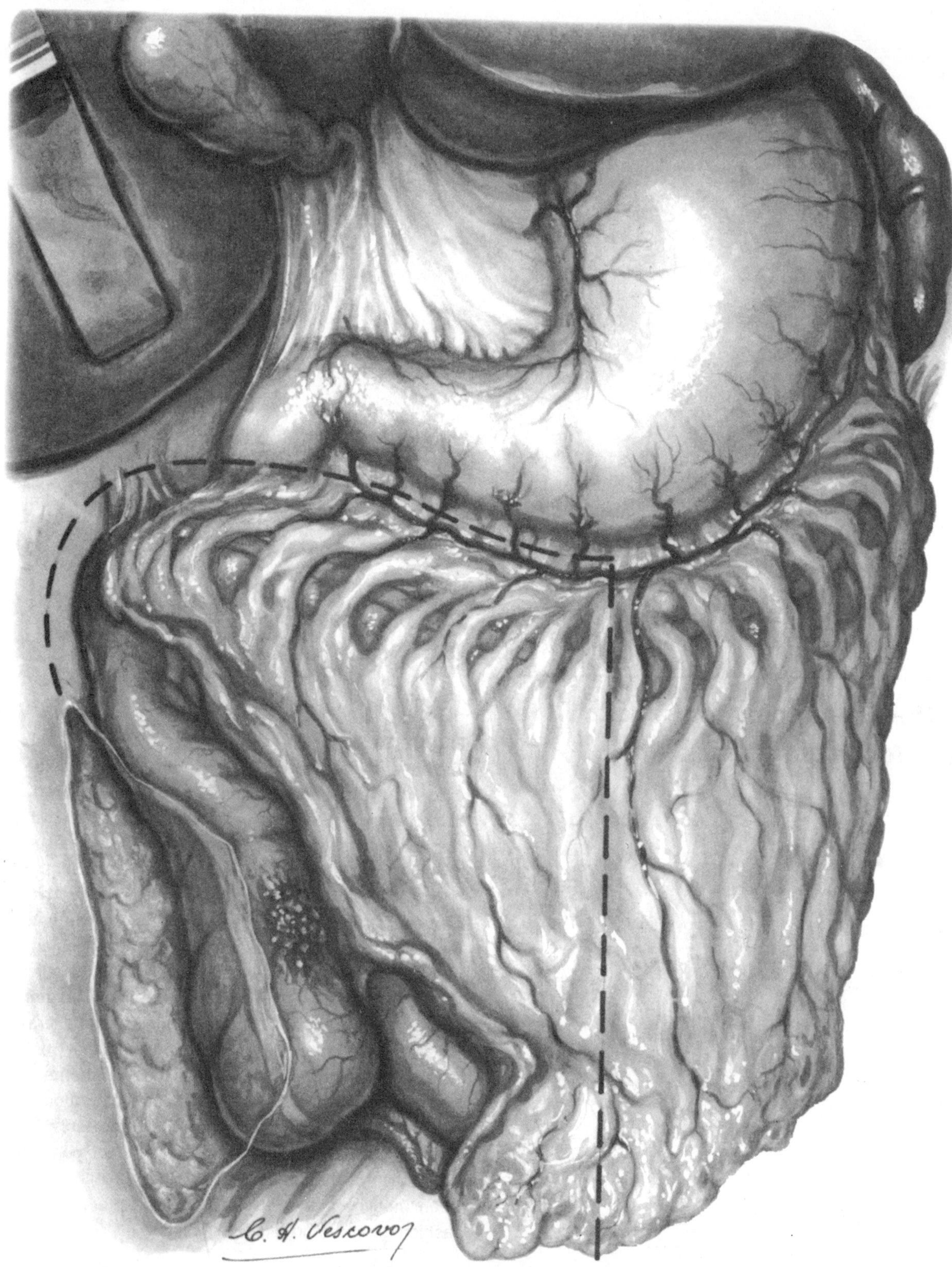

FIGURE 50.27

Right Hemicolectomy for Cancer: Classic Technique

FIGURE 50.28
The right hemicolon has been mobilized up to the midline, exposing the superior mesenteric vessels. The first assistant holds the mobilized colon with both hands or with two Babcock clamps. Care should be taken not to injure the second or third portions of the duodenum during dissection of the hepatic flexure, since the transverse mesocolon is very close to the duodenum. The same care should be taken in dissecting the ascending colon and cecum to avoid injuring the right ureter or gonadal vessels. In carrying out the dissection of the right hemicolon, the ureter may remain adherent to the posterior surface of the mesocolon, as in the drawing. The ureter should be carefully separated, manually or with scissors, in the same way as was described in the no touch technique. When traction is applied on the colon, downward or to the right, some of the veins that make up Henle's trunk may be ruptured, especially the anterior inferior pancreatoduodenal, since it is the most exposed. Once the right hemicolon has been mobilized, the vascular pedicles are ligated in similar fashion as in the no touch technique.

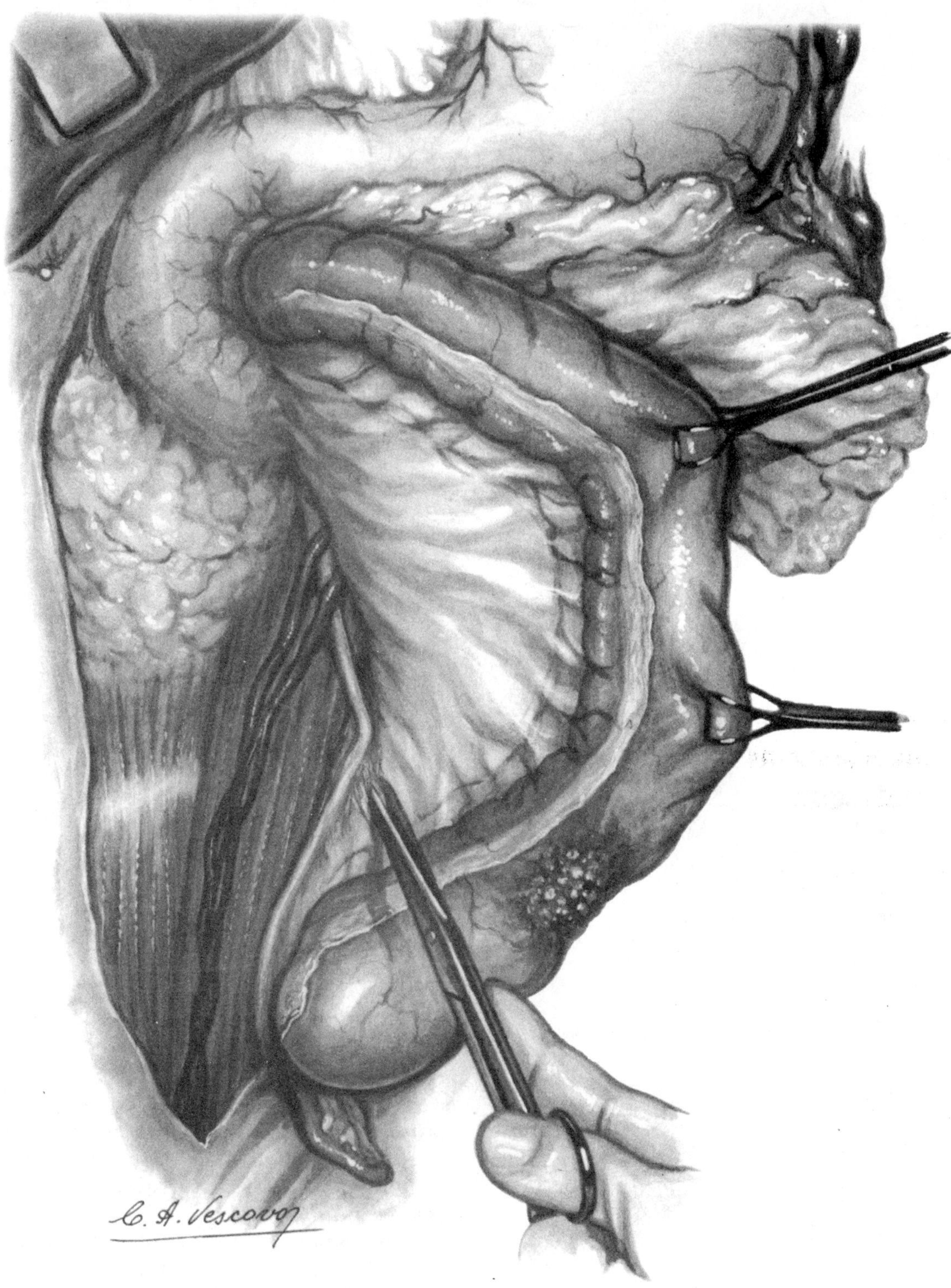

FIGURE 50.28

Right Hemicolectomy for Cancer: Classic Technique

FIGURE 50.29

An end-to-end ileocolic anastomosis is most frequently used to reestablish intestinal transit. Many surgeons, however, prefer the end-to-side anastomosis, while fewer surgeons use the side-to-side technique. The end-to-side anastomosis can be seen under **A.** The anastomosis of the ileum should be very near the closed end of the colon to avoid producing a blind loop syndrome. In the end-to-side anastomosis a second suture line is needed, to close the end of the colon, which means there is more probability of dehiscence. **B,** *Side-to-Side Ileocolic Anastomosis.* In this anastomosis the least extension of bowel should remain beyond the anastomosis to prevent development of a blind loop syndrome. In this technique, two additional suture lines are needed, to close the ends of the colon and the ileum, increasing the possibility of dehiscence.

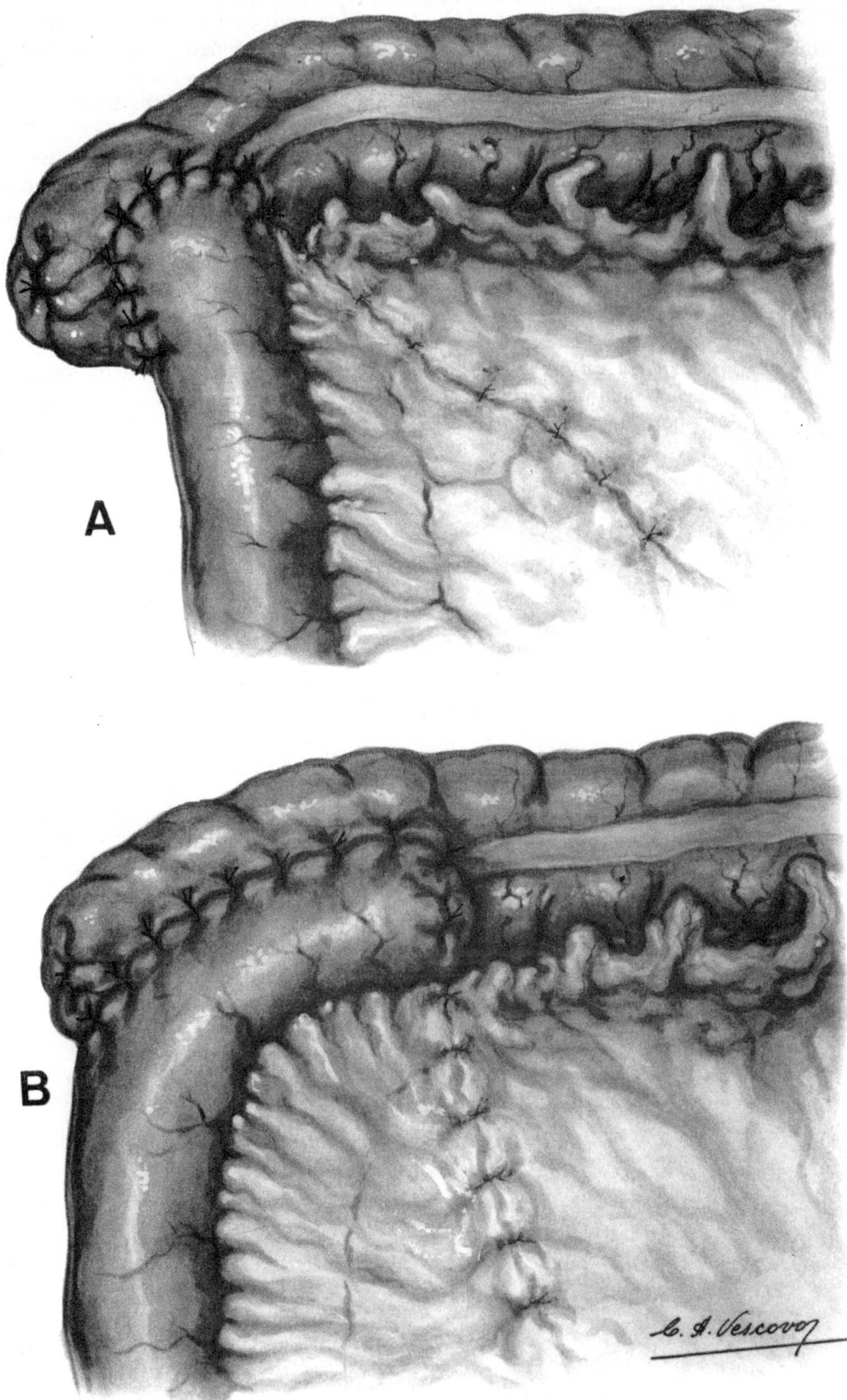

FIGURE 50.29

RIGHT HEMICOLECTOMY FOR CANCER COMPLICATED BY OBSTRUCTION

About 10% of carcinomas of the right hemicolon become complicated by obstruction. This is due to tumors of the ileocecal valve, ileocecocolic invagination caused by the carcinoma itself, or a stenosing tumor of the hepatic flexure or just proximal or distal to it.

Obstructive carcinomas of the right hemicolon are treated by one-stage resection and anastomosis, since statistics have shown that there are no differences in morbidity or mortality in nonobstructive carcinomas. On the contrary, in obstructive carcinomas of the left hemicolon, a one-stage resection and anastomosis significantly increases morbidity and mortality when compared with nonobstructed tumors of the same area. This difference can be explained by the following reasons:

1. The blood supply of the small bowel is much richer than that of the colon.
2. The wall of the small bowel has two well-constituted muscular layers, a longitudinal and a circular layer, while the colonic wall has only a circular layer, since the longitudinal layer consists of three ribbon bands.
3. The contents of the right colon are liquid whereas those of the left colon are usually solid.

Some surgeons leave a decompressive tube in place when they carry out a one-stage resection and anastomosis for obstructing carcinoma, as shown in the following figure.

Right Hemicolectomy for Cancer Complicated by Obstruction

FIGURE 50.30 RIGHT HEMICOLECTOMY FOR OBSTRUCTING CARCINOMA

A, A right hemicolectomy with end-to-side anastomosis of the ileum to the colon has been performed for obstructing carcinoma. A Pezzer tube has been inserted to decompress the transverse colon. The colonic stump has been closed with three layers of sutures, allowing the Pezzer tube to exit the colon and pass to the outside through a small incision in the abdominal wall. The tube is solidly fixed to the skin and connected to closed continuous suction. **B,** In this case decompression is carried out by means of a 16 F rubber tube with several openings along it, to decompress not only the colon but the ileum as well. Closure of the colonic stump, fixation of the decompression tube to the skin, and its attachment to a continuous suction apparatus is performed in a fashion similar to that explained under **A.** This type of decompression can only be carried out in end-to-side and side-to-side ileocolic anastomoses.

The decompression tube is removed about three weeks later. Once the tube has been removed, a fistula remains which closes spontaneously in a few days. Actually, decompression of right hemicolectomies is carried out very infrequently.

Right Hemicolectomy for Cancer Complicated by Obstruction

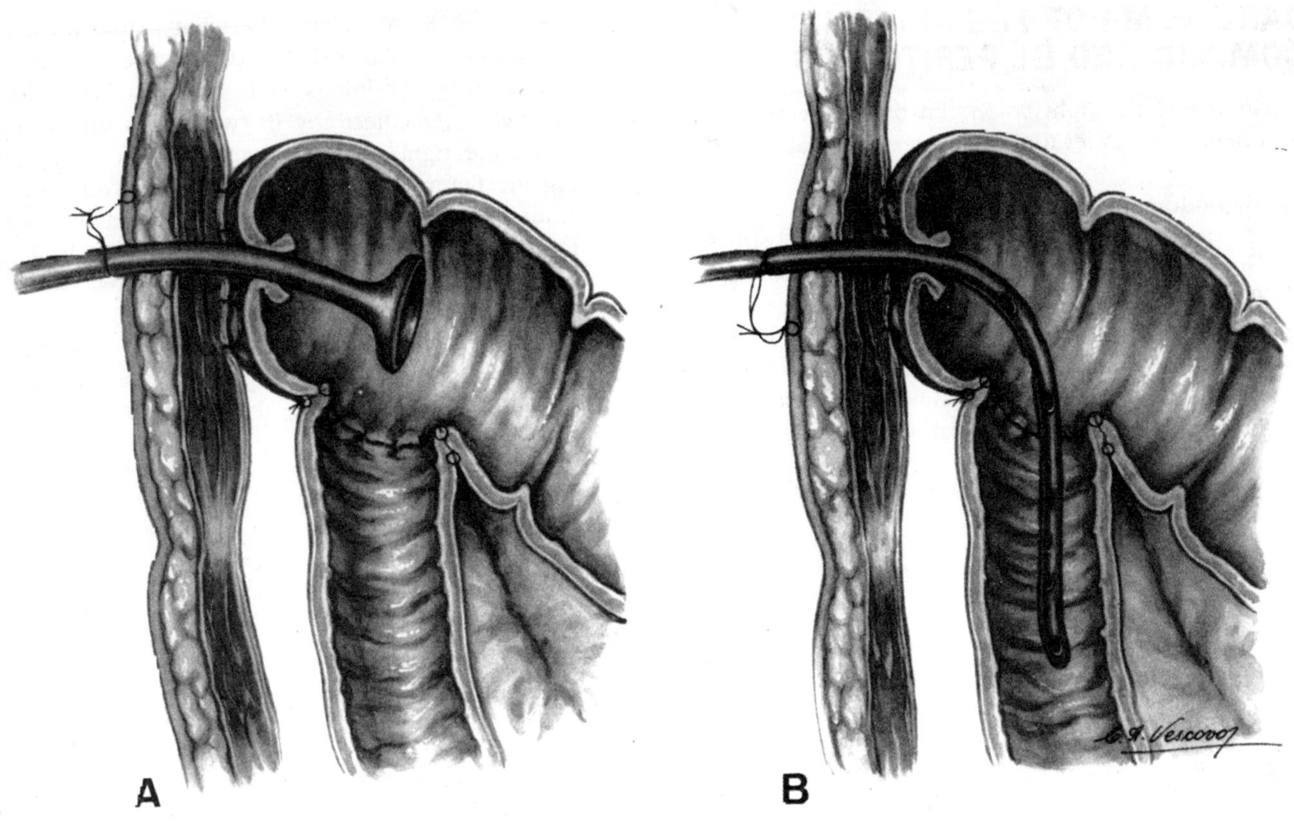

FIGURE 50.30 RIGHT HEMICOLECTOMY FOR OBSTRUCTING CARCINOMA

CARCINOMA OF THE RIGHT COLON COMPLICATED BY PERITONITIS

Carcinoma of the right colon can become complicated with peritonitis under the following circumstances:

1. By perforation of the carcinoma.
2. By perforation of the cecum due to an obstructing carcinoma of the ascending colon or the hepatic flexure of the colon with a competent ileocecal valve. This leads to the production of a closed intestinal obstruction with distension and ischemia of the cecal wall with the possibility of a perforation known as a diastatic perforation of the cecum. If a right hemicolectomy is carried out in the presence of peritonitis, the risk of dehiscence is serious. Under these conditions, it is advisable to perform the right hemicolectomy in two stages. In the first stage, the right hemicolectomy is performed leaving the ileum and the end of the transverse colon exiting the abdominal wall, as shown in the drawings. The abdominal cavity is profusely irrigated with warm saline, and the abdominal wall is closed. The septic process is adequately treated in the postoperative period. Intestinal continuity is reestablished when the septic process has been controlled, anastomosing the ileum to the transverse colon.

Carcinoma of the Right Colon Complicated by Peritonitis

FIGURE 50.31
Patient with an obstructing carcinoma located in the proximal portion of the ascending colon with a competent ileocecal valve. This closed obstruction led to a diastatic perforation of the anterior wall of the cecum and diffuse peritonitis. A right hemicolectomy has been carried out without reestablishing intestinal transit. The broken lines in the transverse colon and the terminal ileum show the site where the transection was carried out.

Carcinoma of the Right Colon Complicated by Peritonitis

FIGURE 50.32
Once the surgical specimen was removed, the abdominal cavity was profusely irrigated with warm saline and the ileal end was brought out the right iliac fossa by means of a Brooke ileostomy, which will make good management of the ileostomy easier postoperatively. The end of the transverse colon has been brought out in the left upper quadrant of the abdominal wall as a mucous fistula. Once the septic process has been controlled, intestinal transit is reestablished, anastomosing the ileal end to the colonic end.

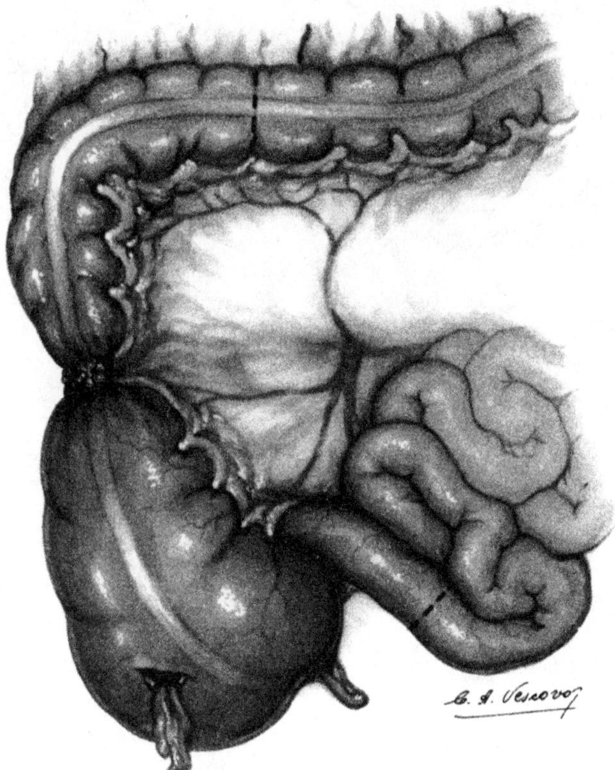

FIGURE 50.31

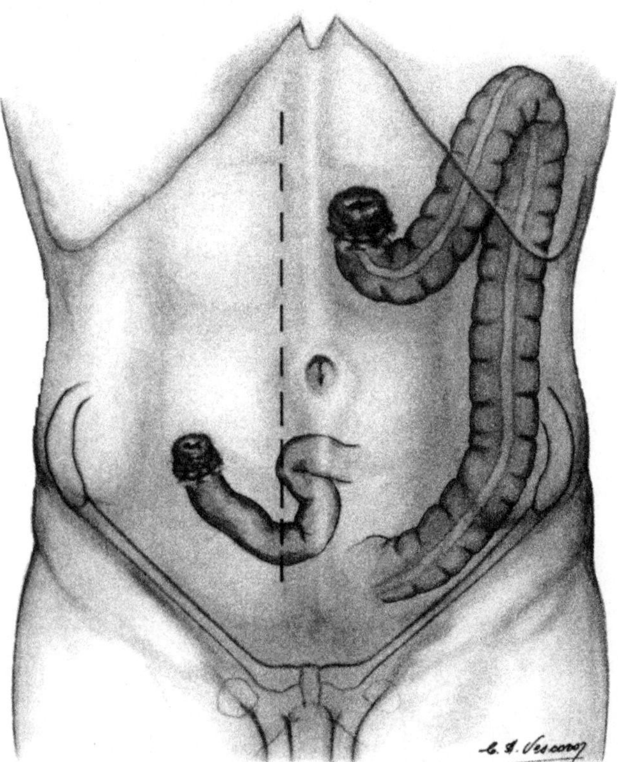

FIGURE 50.32

Section H

Colon, Rectum, and Anus

CHAPTER **51**

Left Radical Hemicolectomy

Left radical hemicolectomy is indicated in patients with carcinoma located in the splenic flexure of the colon, or distal to or proximal to it, either in the descending colon or in certain cases in the sigmoid colon. In left hemicolectomy for cancer, the distal half of the transverse colon, the splenic flexure, the descending colon, and part of the sigmoid colon or the complete sigmoid colon are resected.

The surgical technique is very similar in all the locations of the tumor in the left side of the colon except in cases of cancer located in the splenic flexure, which usually is more difficult to resect due to its deep location in the left hypochondrium and because of its close proximity to the spleen. Also, it is frequently in an advanced stage of development when it is diagnosed.

In the following, we will describe the surgical technique for left hemicolectomy in a carcinoma of the splenic flexure of the colon. We will then make a short description of the radical left hemicolectomy for carcinoma of the descending colon and of the sigmoid colon.

Left Radical Hemicolectomy for Carcinoma of the Splenic Flexure of the Colon

FIGURE 51.1

This is a schematic representation of a carcinoma of the splenic flexure of the colon and its possible lymphatic spread. As shown in the drawing, lymphatic spread of carcinoma of the splenic flexure of the colon follows the same course as other carcinomas of the colon—toward the paracolic lymph nodes and the intermediate and principal nodes, but also, simultaneously or successively, the lymphatic distribution may be toward the lymph nodes of the splenic hilus, 2, the left gastroepiploic nodes, 3, and the retropancreatic nodes, 4.

This multidirectional spread of carcinoma of the splenic flexure represented a serious challenge to surgeons in devising a surgical procedure that would make possible a more ample resection of lymphatics to improve patient survival. It was proposed that left radical hemicolectomy be carried out with resection of the tail and part of the body of the pancreas to remove the retropancreatic nodes, resection of the spleen to remove the splenic hilar nodes, and resection of the high segment of the greater curvature of the stomach to remove the left gastroepiploic nodes. This ample and aggressive procedure did not give the expected results, since it did not improve survival of the patients and it did increase morbidity and mortality, for which reason it was discontinued.

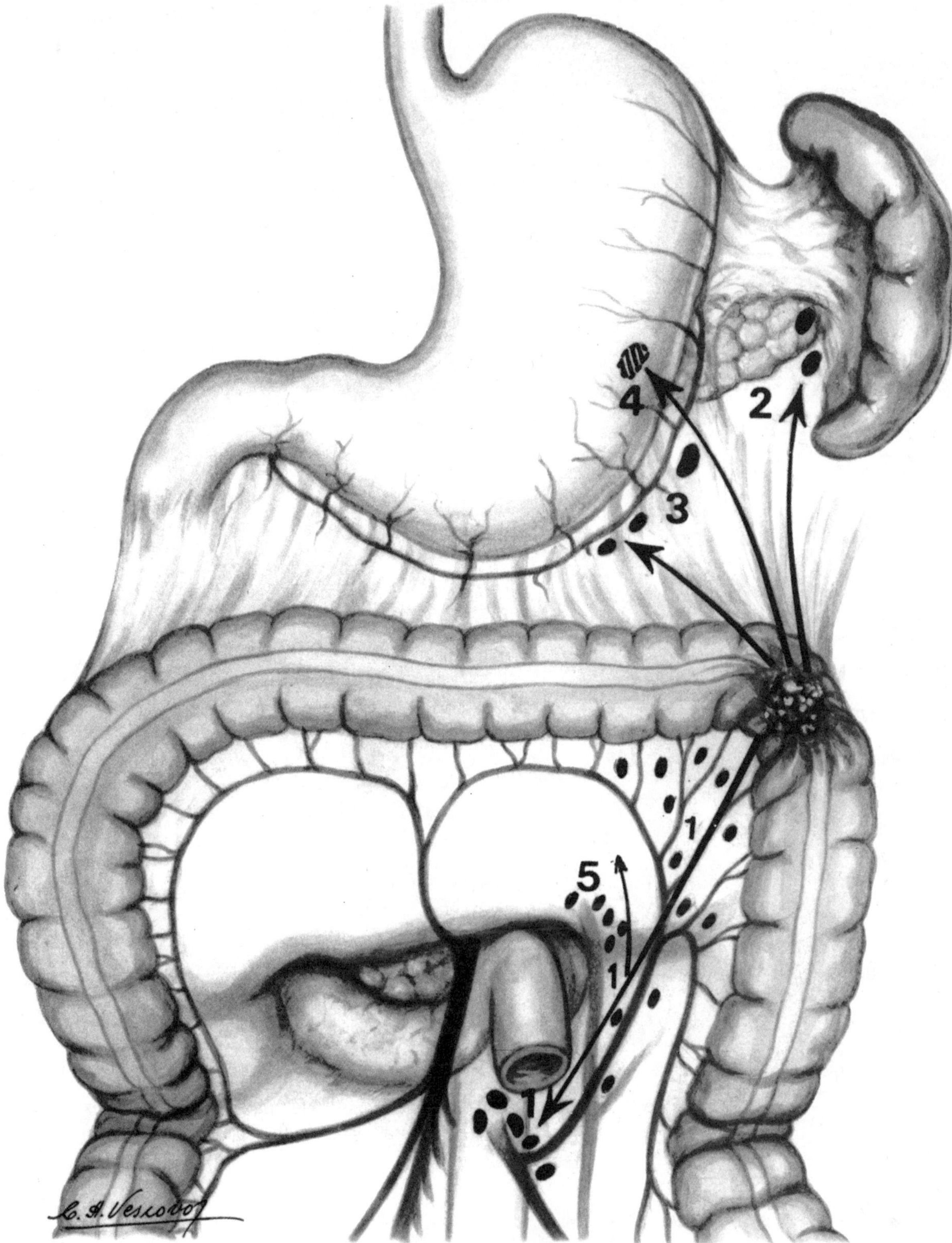

FIGURE 51.1

Left Radical Hemicolectomy for Carcinoma of the Splenic Flexure of the Colon

FIGURE 51.2
The author uses a left paramedian incision extending from the left costal margin to the spine of the pubis.

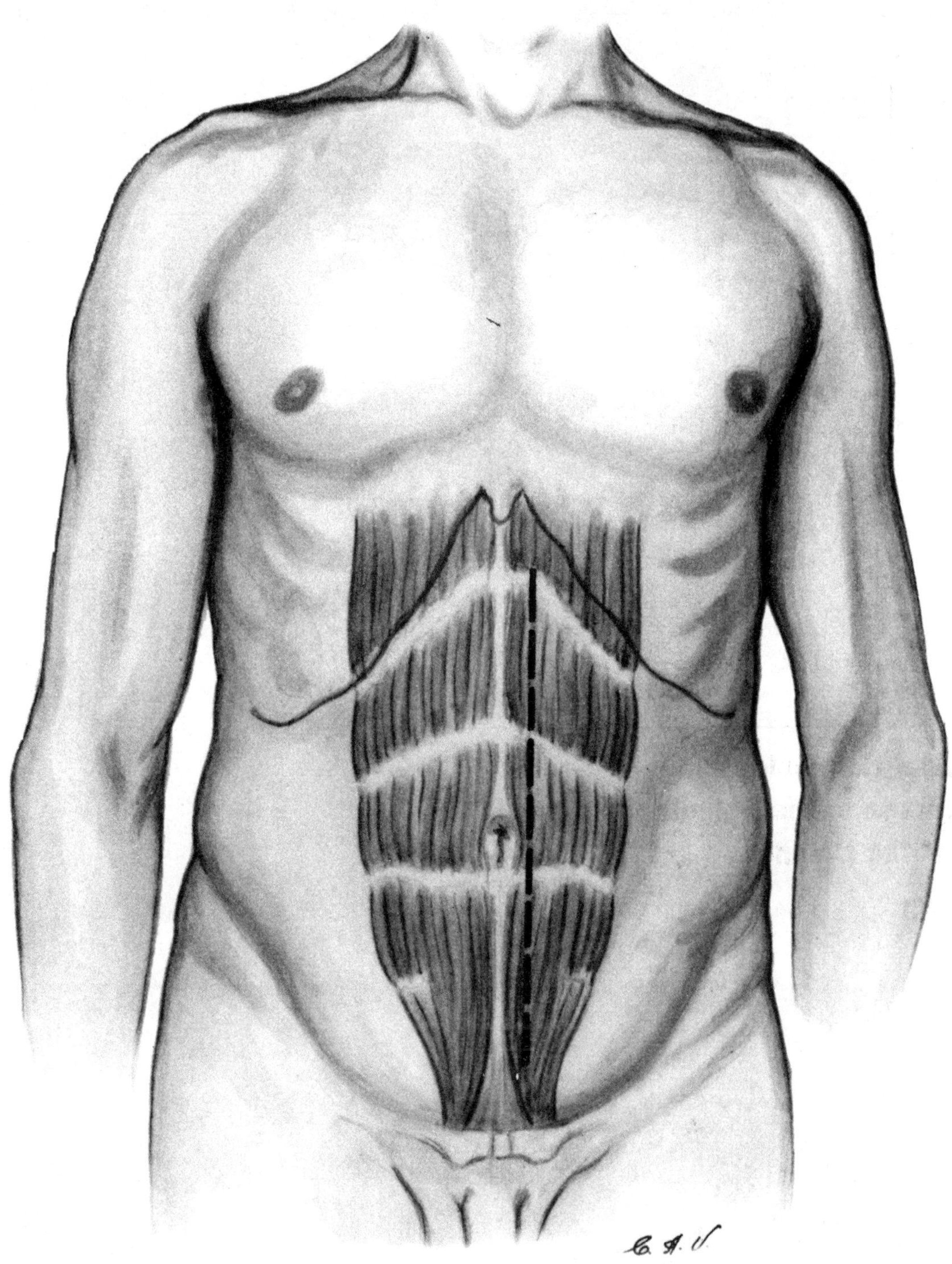

FIGURE 51.2

Left Radical Hemicolectomy for Carcinoma of the Splenic Flexure of the Colon

FIGURE 51.3
This drawing shows a carcinoma of the splenic flexure of the colon. Using a broken line, the extension of colonic resection with its mesocolon is shown, including the left half of the transverse colon, the splenic flexure, the descending colon, the proximal half of the sigmoid colon, and the left half of the greater omentum.

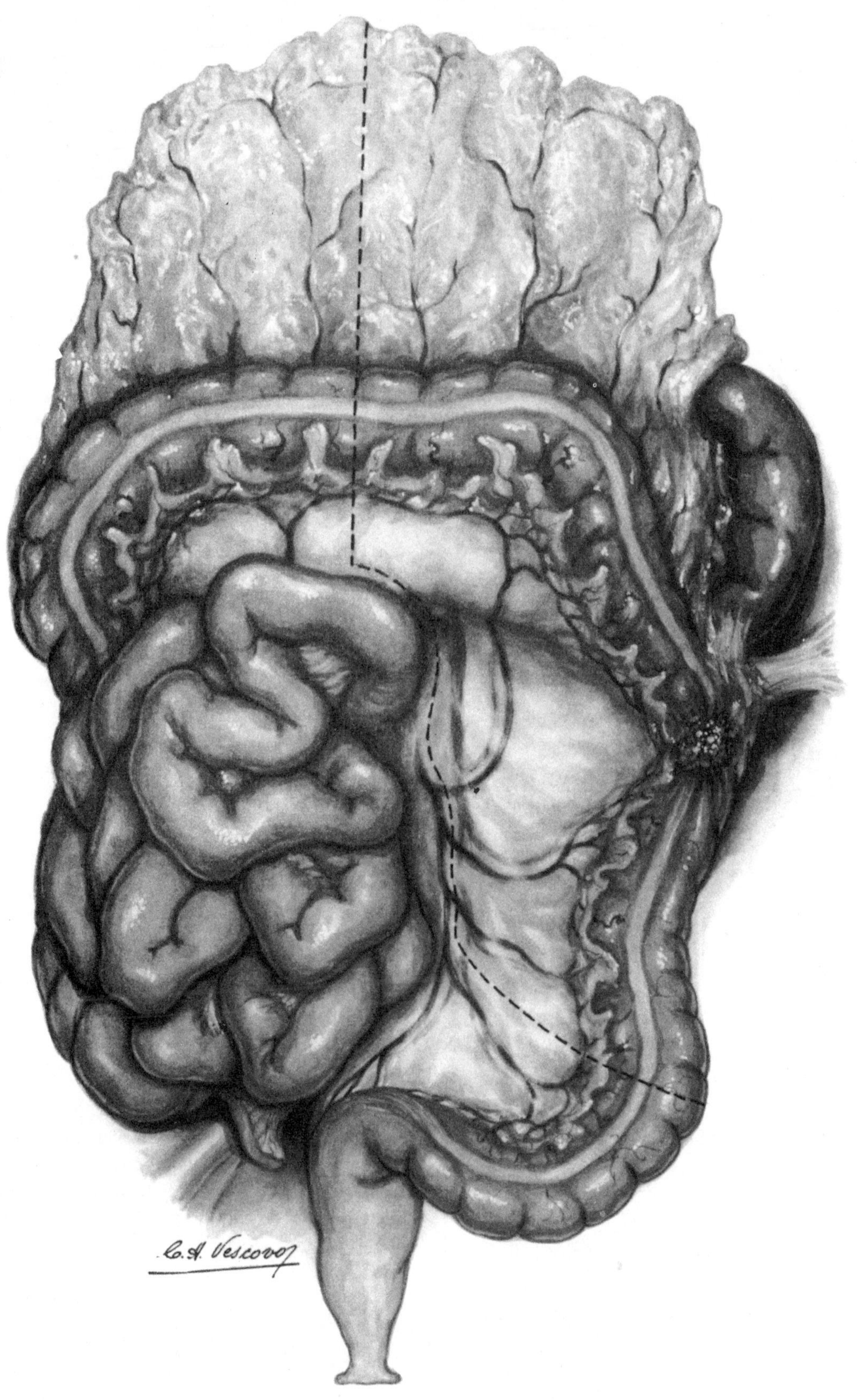

FIGURE 51.3

Left Radical Hemicolectomy for Carcinoma of the Splenic Flexure of the Colon

FIGURE 51.4
The greater omentum has been divided and ligated at the midline up to and including the left gastroepiploic arcade. The gastrocolic ligament has begun to be divided and ligated above the gastroepiploic arcade toward the proximal segment of the stomach.

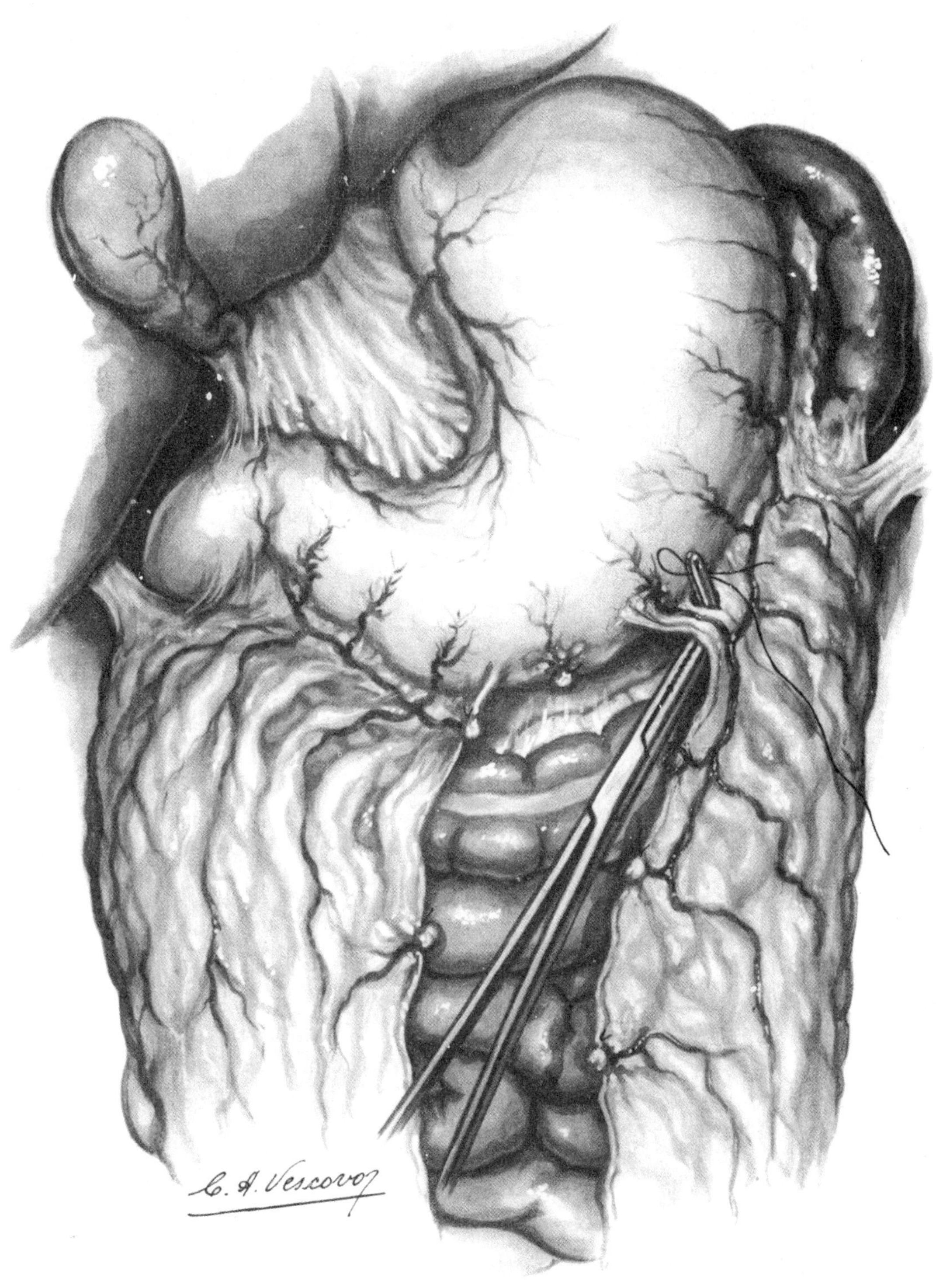

FIGURE 51.4

Left Radical Hemicolectomy for Carcinoma of the Splenic Flexure of the Colon

FIGURE 51.5
The colonic lumen has been obliterated above and below the tumor using 3-mm umbilical tape. The inferior peritoneal layer of the transverse mesocolon and the anterior peritoneal layer of the descending mesocolon as well as the proximal anterior layer of the sigmoid mesocolon have been divided following the broken line as shown in Figure 51.3. Division of the peritoneal layer facilitates identification and ligation of vascular pedicles. By means of the broken line we have also shown where the transverse colon and the sigmoid colon are to be transected.

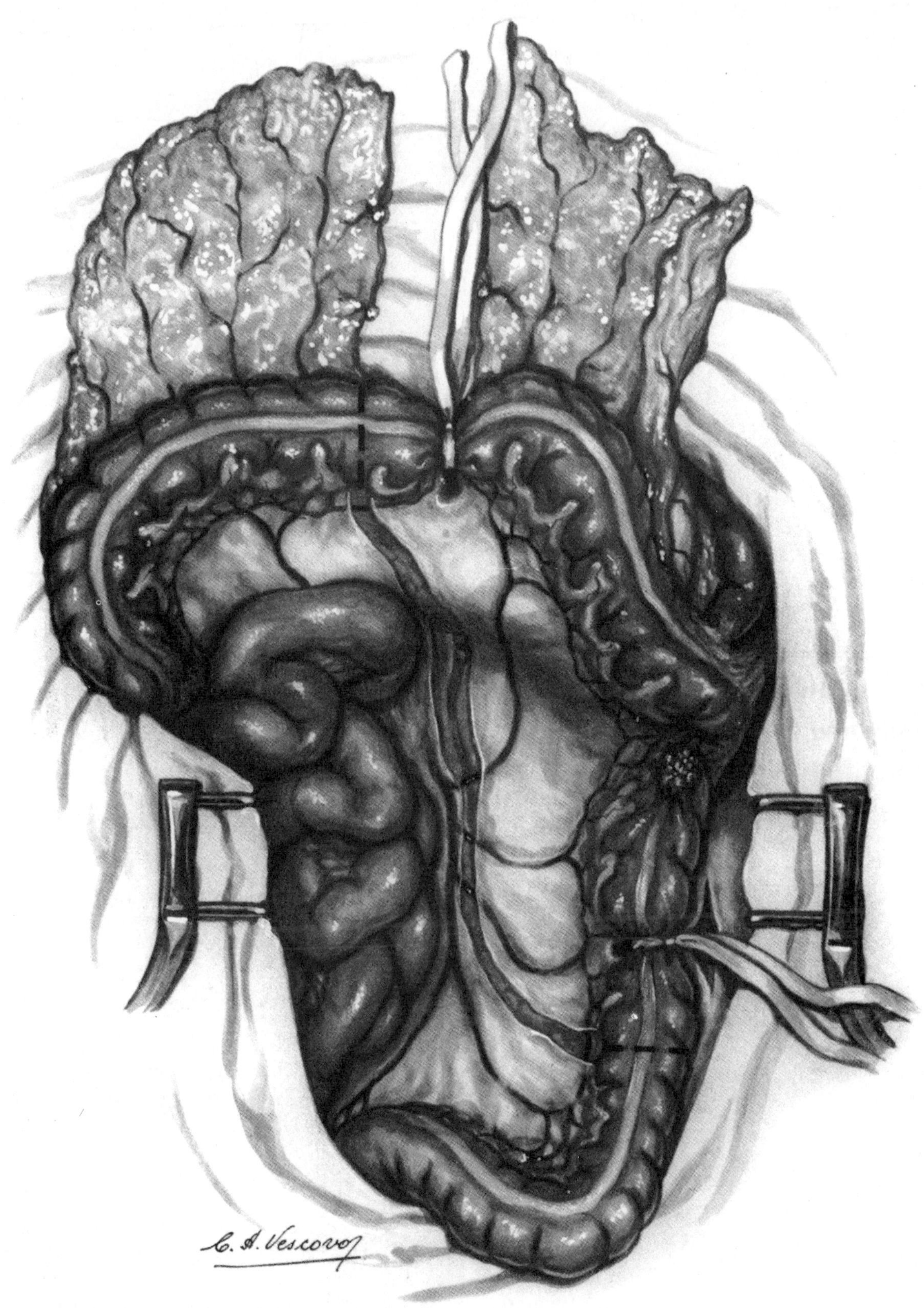

FIGURE 51.5

Left Radical Hemicolectomy for Carcinoma of the Splenic Flexure of the Colon

FIGURE 51.6
The vascular pedicles of the left hemicolon have been dissected, ligated, and transected. These are the left vascular pedicle and two proximal sigmoid pedicles. Before proceeding to divide the colon, two atraumatic straight clamps are placed about 5 cm from the site where the colon will be transected. A wound protector will also be applied to the borders of the incision to diminish, as much as possible, septic contamination. By means of the same wound protector, with the same object in mind, the entire abdominal cavity is protected by abdominal pads. The ends of the colonic segment that is to be resected are also wrapped in gauze pads held in place with large triangular Duval clamps.

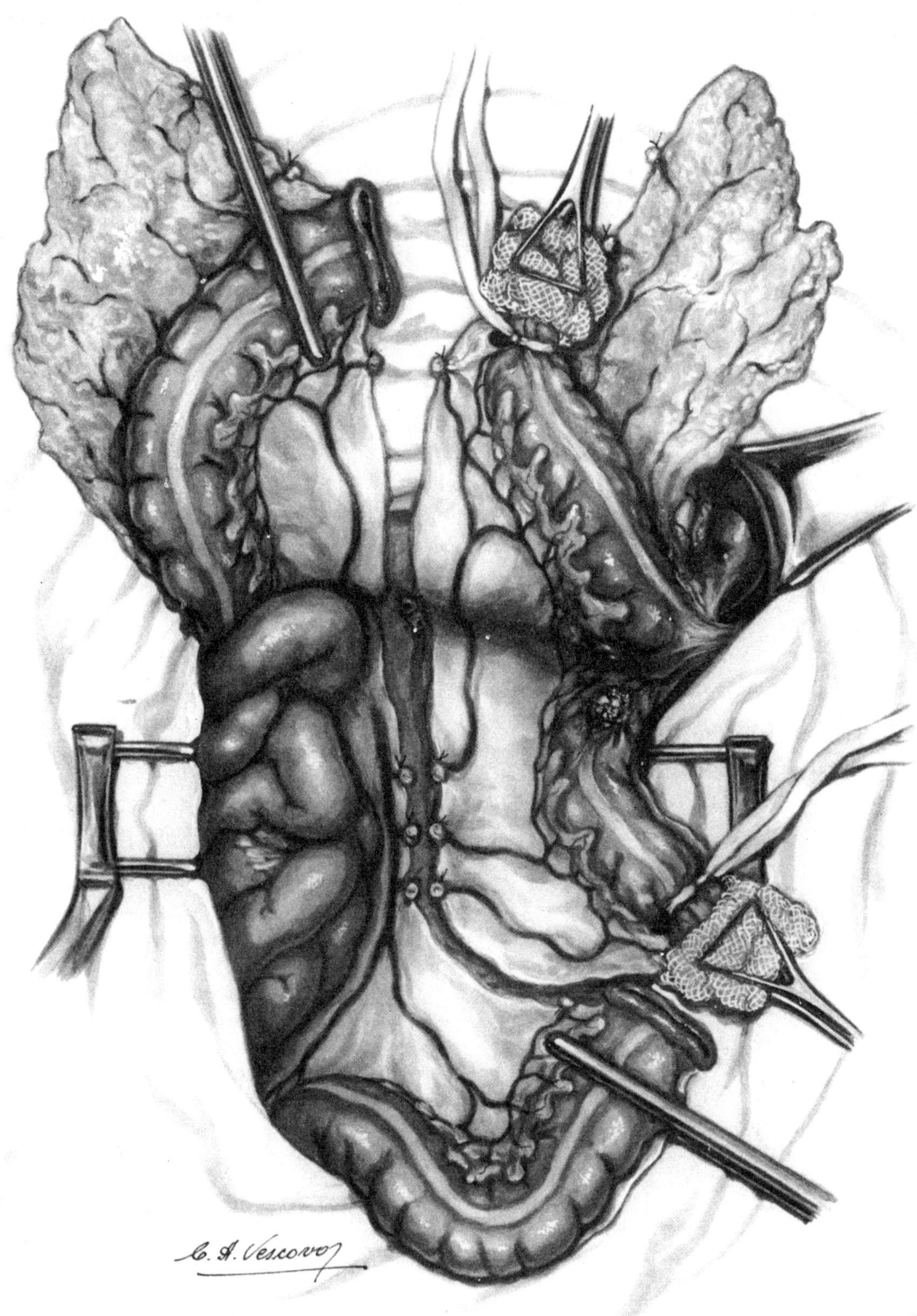

FIGURE 51.6

Left Radical Hemicolectomy for Carcinoma of the Splenic Flexure of the Colon

FIGURE 51.7

Once the vascular pedicles of the left hemicolon have been disconnected and the colon has been transected together with its mesocolon and the left parietal colic peritoneum from the sigmoid colon to the splenic flexure, ligation of the left phrenocolic ligament is carried out. Following this, ligation and transection of the splenocolic ligament will be carried out at a somewhat higher point, as shown by the broken line. Ligature and division of these ligaments should be carried out very carefully to avoid injuring the splenic capsule. If a lesion of the splenic capsule occurs, hemostasis with Surgicel, Avitene, gelatin sponge, oxicelulose, or other topical hemostatic agents can be tried.

In some patients, splenorrhaphy may be indicated using very fine atraumatic needles. It has been shown that the spleen has an important immunologic protective function, for which reason splenectomy should not be carried out in all patients with splenic hemorrhage, as it used to be done several years ago. In case of small hemorrhages, local treatment should always be tried. If the local treatment fails, one should not then hesitate to carry out the splenectomy. In cases of important lesions of the spleen, the best solution, because it is safer, is that of splenectomy. The abdominal wall should never be closed if there exists any doubt as to hemostasis when local hemostatic procedures are carried out. If a splenectomy has been carried out, the special precaution of vaccinating the patient against pneumococcus, to avoid possible septicemia by this bacteria, should be taken.

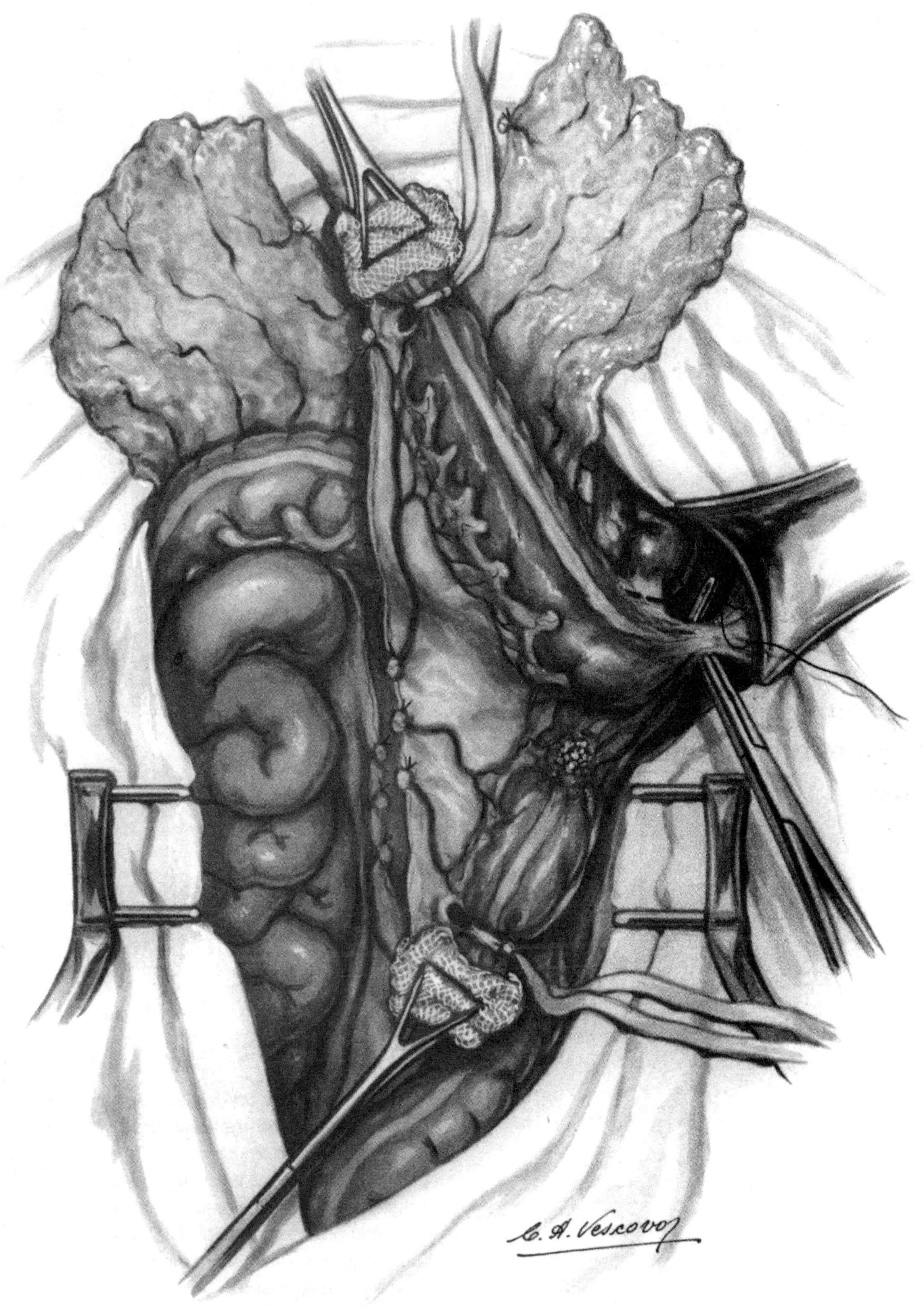

FIGURE 51.7

Left Radical Hemicolectomy for Carcinoma of the Splenic Flexure of the Colon

FIGURE 51.8

The drawing shows that an end-to-end anastomosis has been performed between the transverse colon and the distal segment of the sigmoid colon. This has been done in two layers using interrupted sutures, the mucous layer with 3-0 chromic catgut, and the seromuscular layer with nonabsorbable synthetic or other material. The space left by the resection of the mesocolon has been sutured, and the left parietocolic space is being closed.

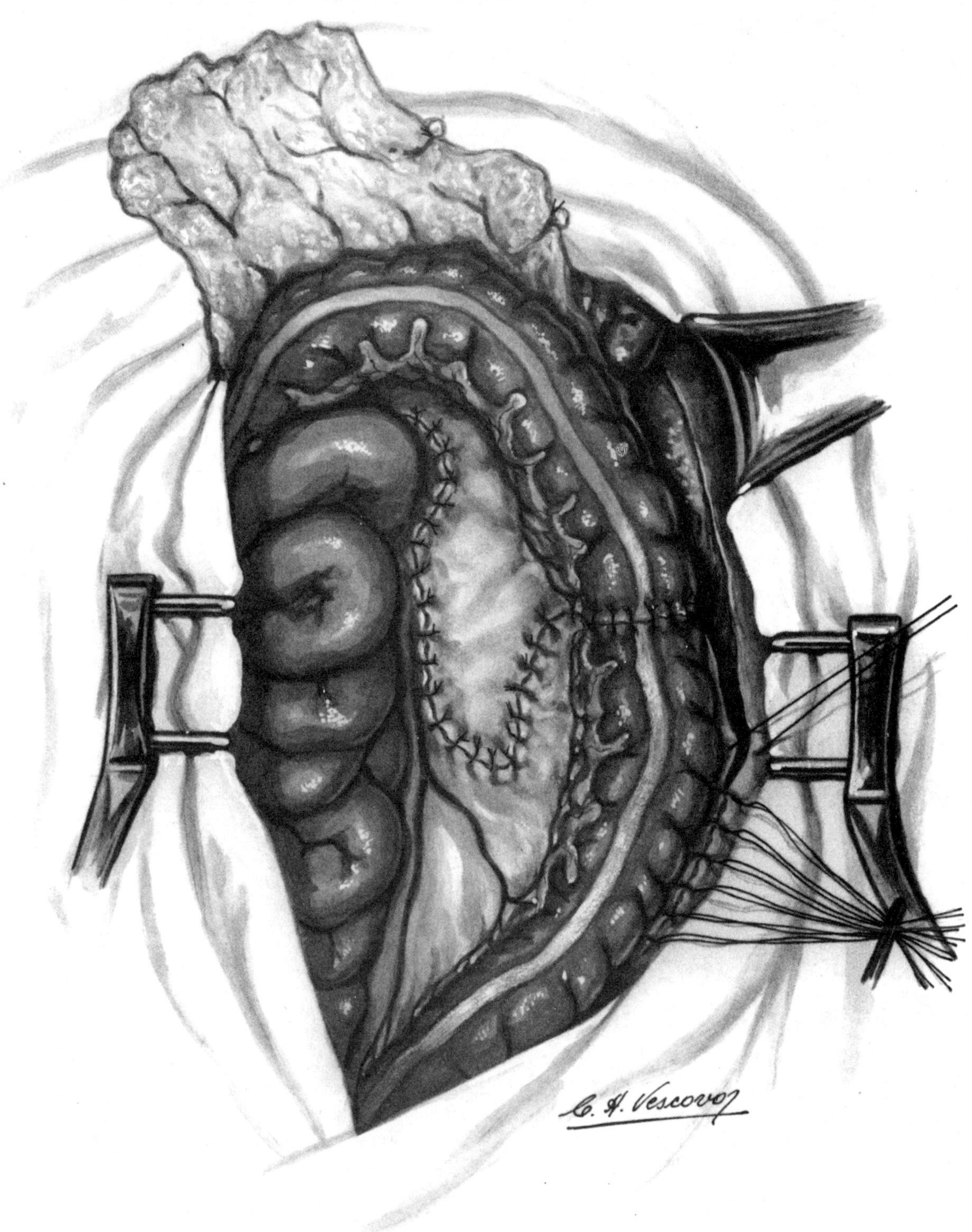

FIGURE 51.8

Left Radical Hemicolectomy for Carcinoma of the Splenic Flexure of the Colon

FIGURE 51.9
If the carcinoma of the splenic flexure has infiltrated the distal pancreas, the invaded distal segment of the pancreas should be resected together with the spleen, to facilitate resection of the left hemicolon. This amplification of the colonic resection is done by necessity and not to amplify the lymphadenectomy. In the great majority of patients, this amplified resection is palliative in nature. To facilitate resection of the infiltrated pancreatic segment, the proximal segment of the greater curvature of the stomach should be liberated by ligating the short vessels, as shown in the drawing.

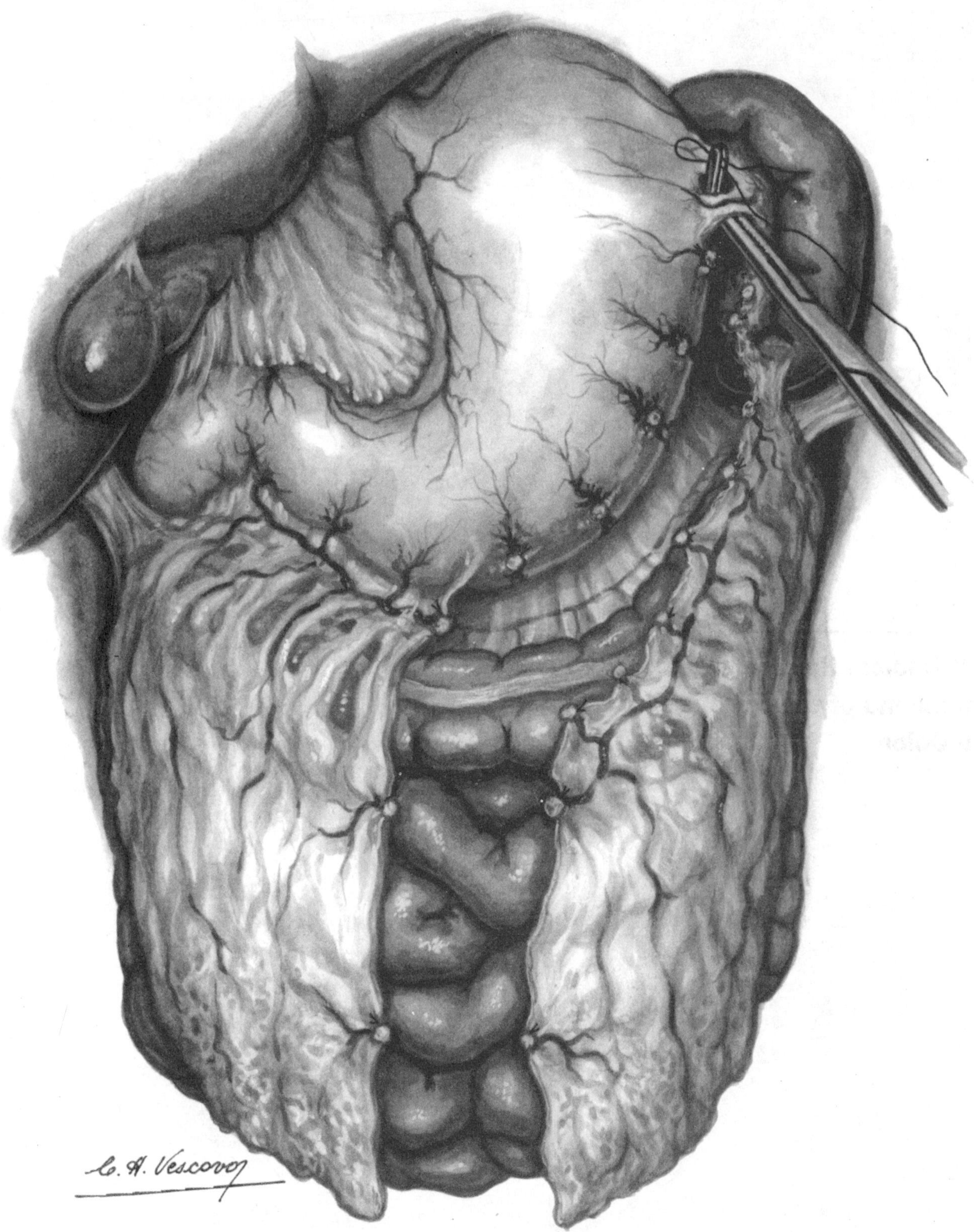

FIGURE 51.9

FIGURE 51.10
A, The proximal portion of the greater curvature of the stomach has been liberated and reflected upward, using two atraumatic triangular Duval clamps, exposing the body and tail of the pancreas as well as the hilus of the spleen. Using a broken line, the limits of the pancreatic resection have been shown. **B,** The splenic artery and vein have been ligated and divided. The pancreatic duct has been closed with two sutures using nonabsorbable material. The edge of the distal segment of the divided pancreas that is to be resected has been grasped with a large Duval clamp.

Left Radical Hemicolectomy for Carcinoma of the Splenic Flexure of the Colon

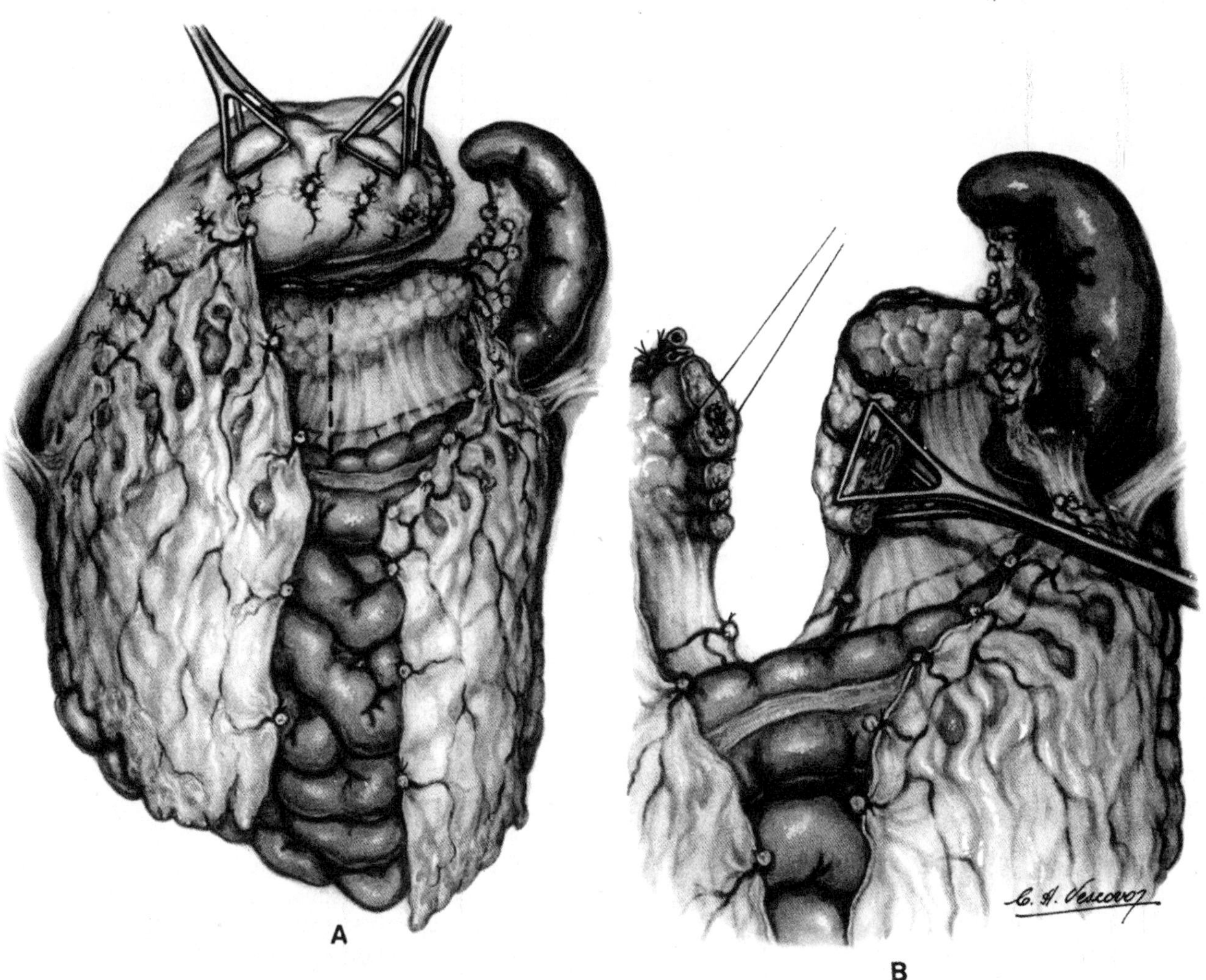

FIGURE 51.10

FIGURE 51.11
A, The left hemicolectomy has been carried out, including the tail and part of the body of the pancreas, together with the spleen. The colonic anastomosis has been performed in two layers using interrupted sutures, and the left parietocolic space is being closed with interrupted sutures. **B,** Using a Babcock clamp, a segment of the gastrocolic ligament that had been previously separated from the greater curvature of the stomach is grasped to cover the suture line of the transected end of the pancreas. **C,** The segment of gastrocolic ligament has been sutured over the transected end of the pancreas, using several nonabsorbable sutures.

Left Radical Hemicolectomy for Carcinoma of the Splenic Flexure of the Colon

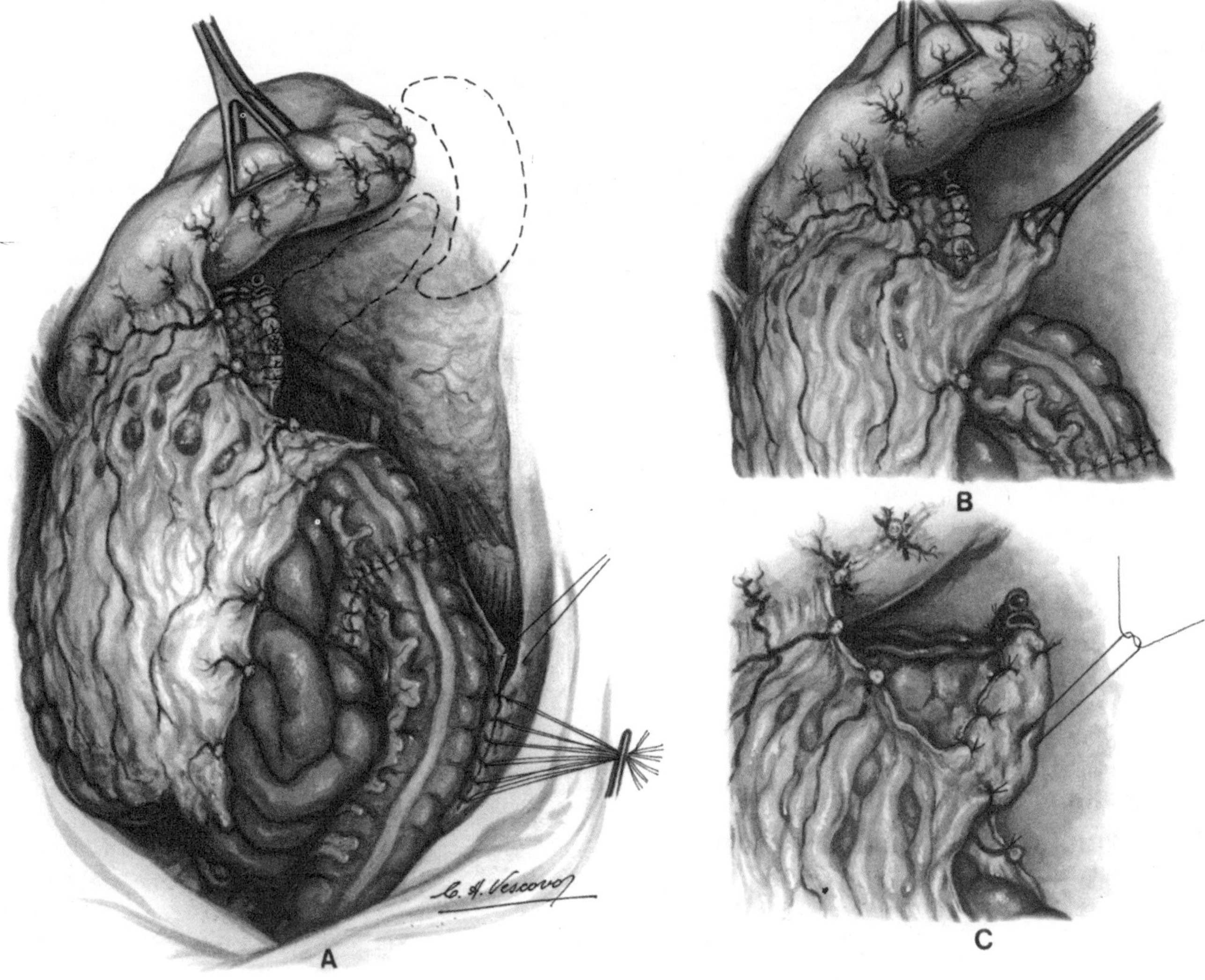

FIGURE 51.11

Left Radical Hemicolectomy for Carcinoma of the Descending Colon

FIGURE 51.12
The drawing shows a carcinoma of the middle third of the descending colon. The extent of resection of the left hemicolon with its mesocolon and lymphatic areas is shown by a broken line. The extent of resection is very similar to that carried out for carcinoma of the splenic flexure of the colon. If the carcinoma is located in the distal third of the descending colon, the resection should be extended to include the proximal segment of the rectum.

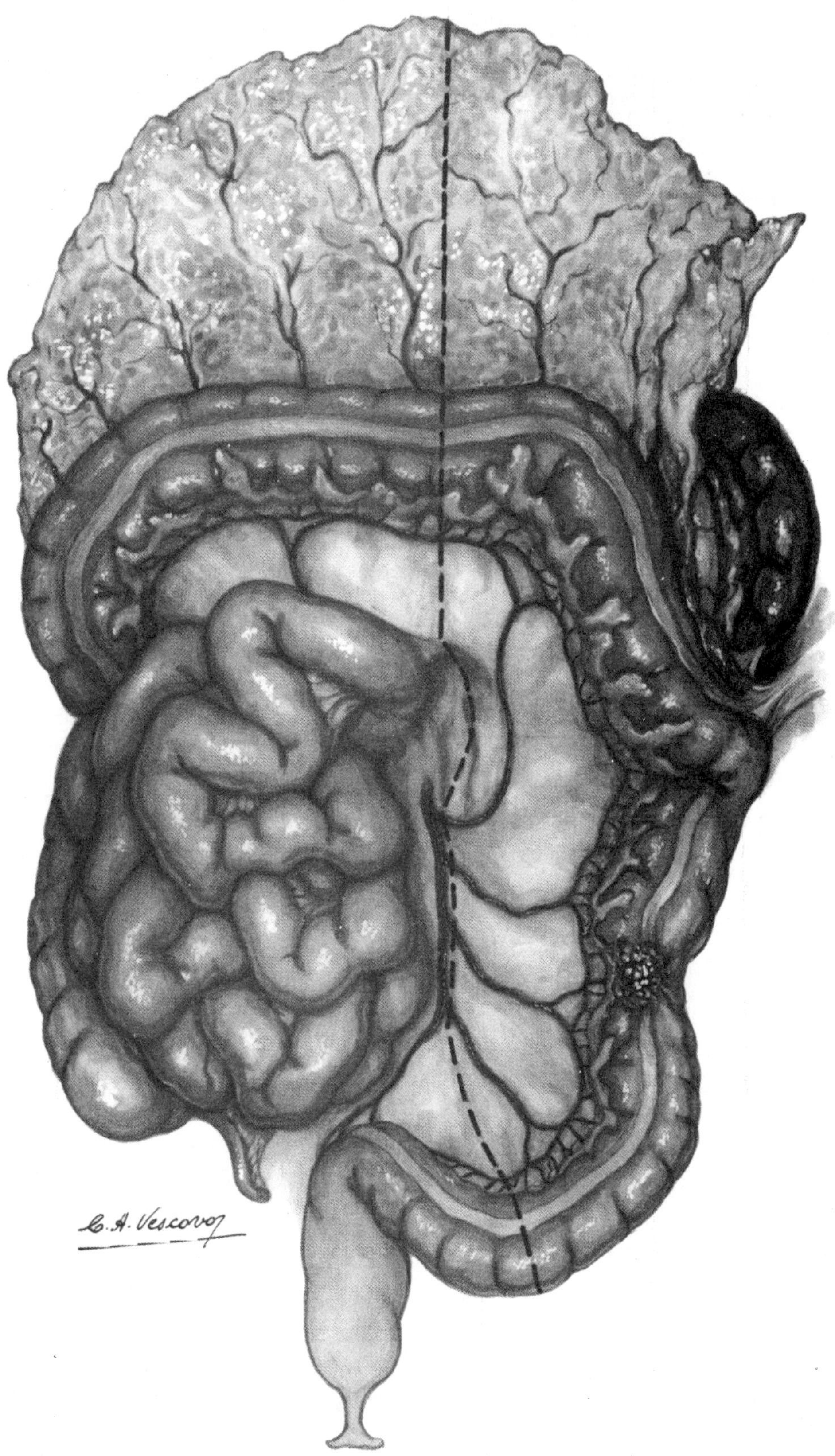

FIGURE 51.12

Left Radical Hemicolectomy for Carcinoma of the Descending Colon

FIGURE 51.13
The lumen of the left colon has been occluded above and below the tumor, using 3-mm-wide umbilical tape. The left colic vascular pedicle and the proximal three sigmoidal vessels have been ligated and divided. A broken line shows the site where the transverse colon and the sigmoid colon will be transected.

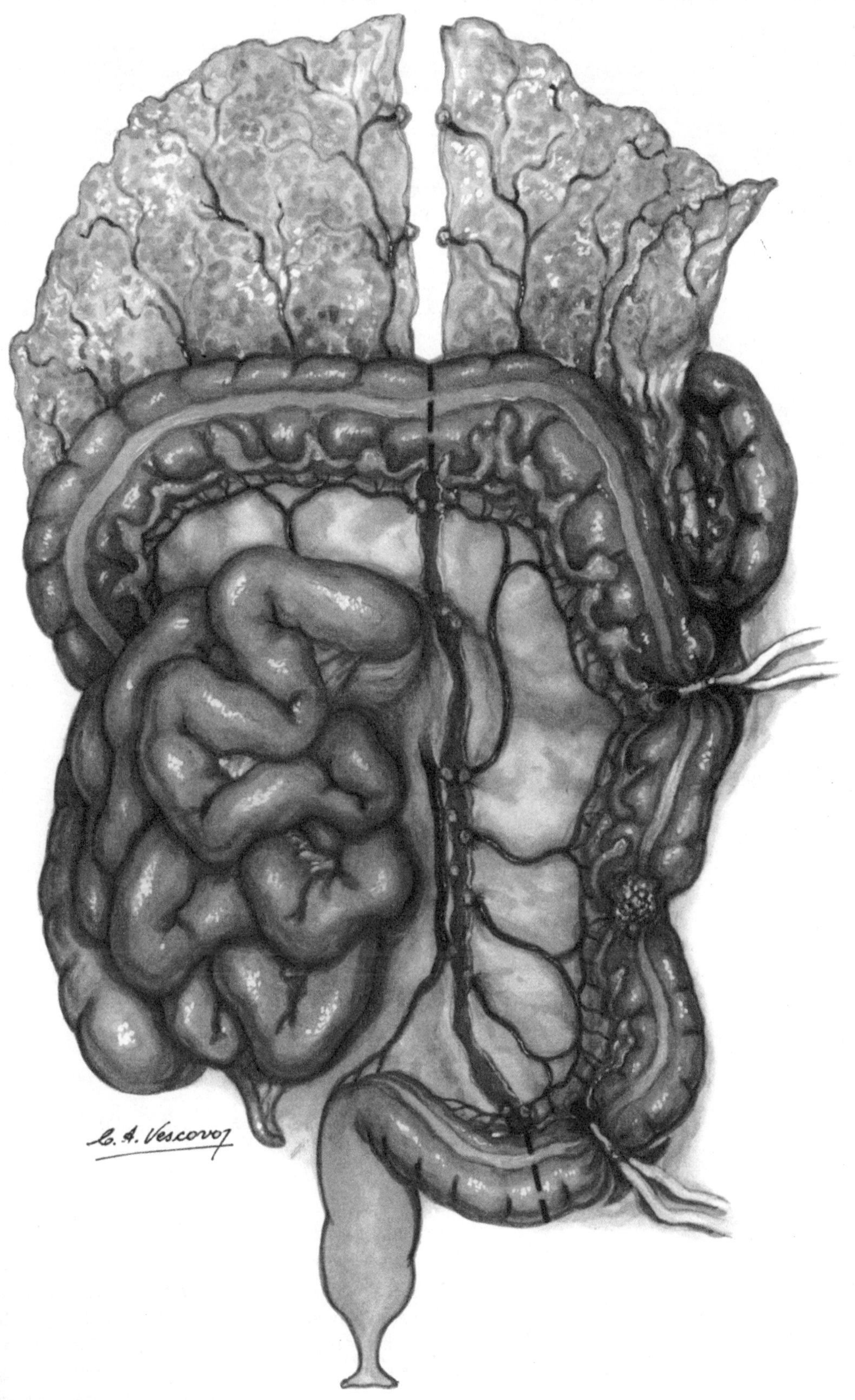

FIGURE 51.13

Left Radical Hemicolectomy for Carcinoma of the Descending Colon

FIGURE 51.14
The right half of the transverse colon including the hepatic flexure has been mobilized. The transverse colon has been anastomosed to the distal end of the sigmoid colon. The defect in the mesocolon has been closed with nonabsorbable interrupted sutures. The left parietocolic space is being closed. Above the colocolonic anastomosis, peritonealization is carried out using the greater omentum.

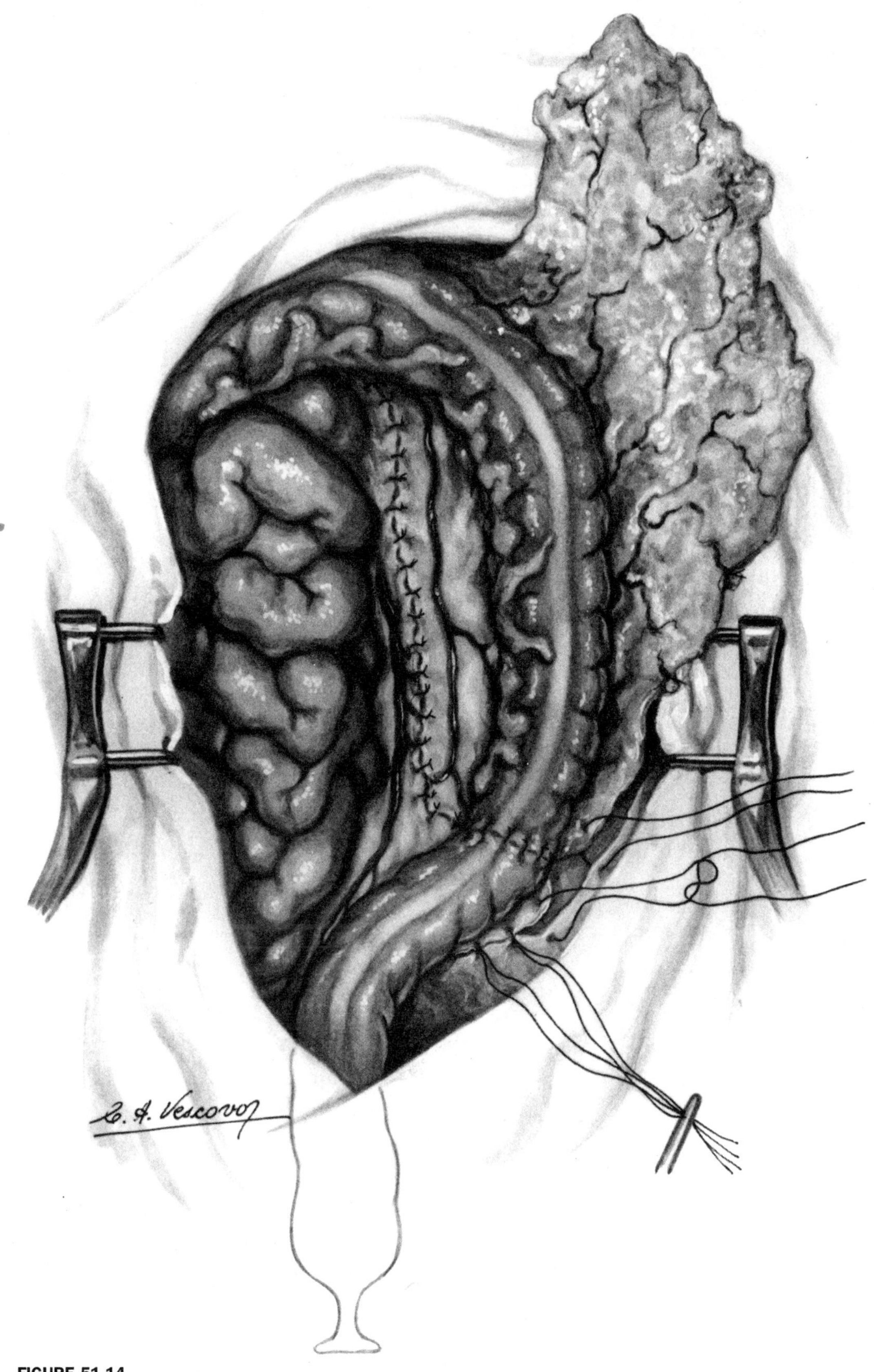

FIGURE 51.14

LEFT RADICAL HEMICOLECTOMY FOR CARCINOMA OF THE SIGMOID COLON

Many surgeons carry out a left radical hemicolectomy for carcinoma of the sigmoid colon, especially if the lesion is rather advanced, with nodes having been invaded by the tumor, and the sigmoid colon is not redundant. In older patients who present a limited invasion with a redundant sigmoid, a segmental resection of the sigmoid will give results similar to those of a left radical hemicolectomy.

Section H

Colon, Rectum, and Anus

CHAPTER 52

Colon Resection with Mechanical Anastomosis

FIGURE 52.1
The anastomosis is begun by using a monofilament suture and carrying out a purse string suture at the end of the proximal colon. This purse string suture can be performed manually or with the special clamp to construct purse strings. About 4 cm from the proximal colonic end, an incision is made that is large enough to introduce the EEA instrument. Once it is introduced to the lumen of the colon, the instrument is opened to advance the anvil and adjust the purse string at the end of the proximal colon over the central rod of the instrument. The purse string suture is being prepared using a special clamp, to construct the purse string in the distal end of the colon.

End-to-End Colocolonic Anastomosis (2, 10, 19)

FIGURE 52.2
The anvil of the EEA instrument is being introduced into the distal colon. The entrance of the anvil is facilitated if the posterior portion of the anvil is introduced first.

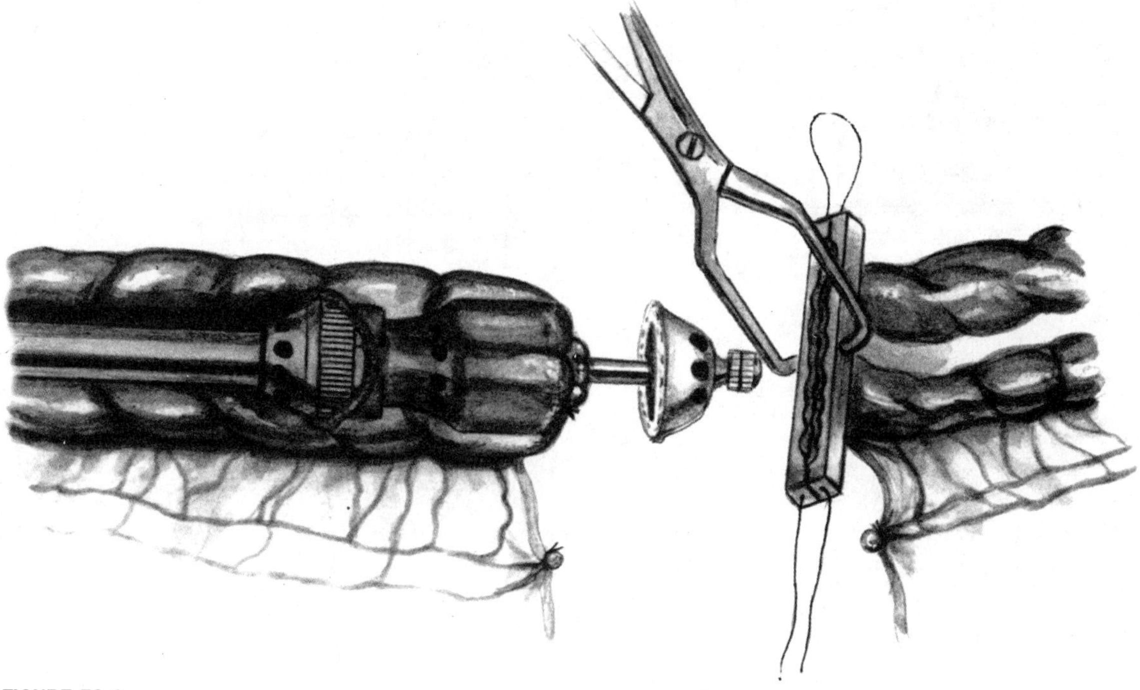

FIGURE 52.1

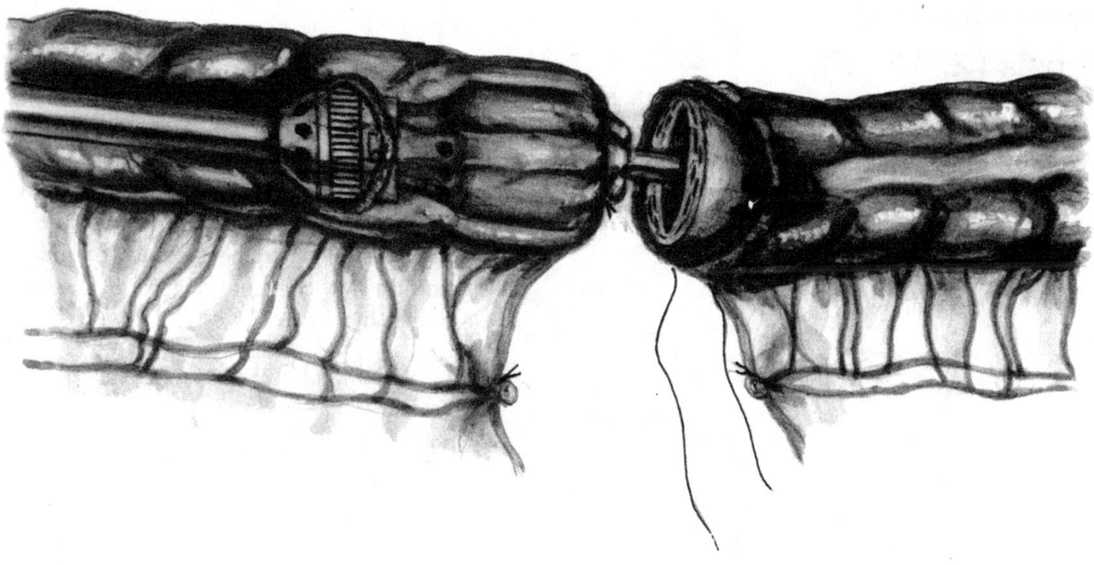

FIGURE 52.2

FIGURE 52.3
The anvil has been completely introduced into the lumen of the distal colonic segment and the purse string tied over the central rod. Closure of the EEA instrument is begun to approximate both ends of the colon.

End-to-End Colocolonic Anastomosis (2, 10, 19)

FIGURE 52.4
The instrument has been fired and is now being removed, as seen in the drawing. Once the EEA instrument has been removed, the anastomosis should be examined for bleeding, in order to carry out hemostasis before closure of the colotomy. Additionally, the EEA instrument has to be examined to confirm the removal of two complete rings of tissue including all the layers of the colonic walls.

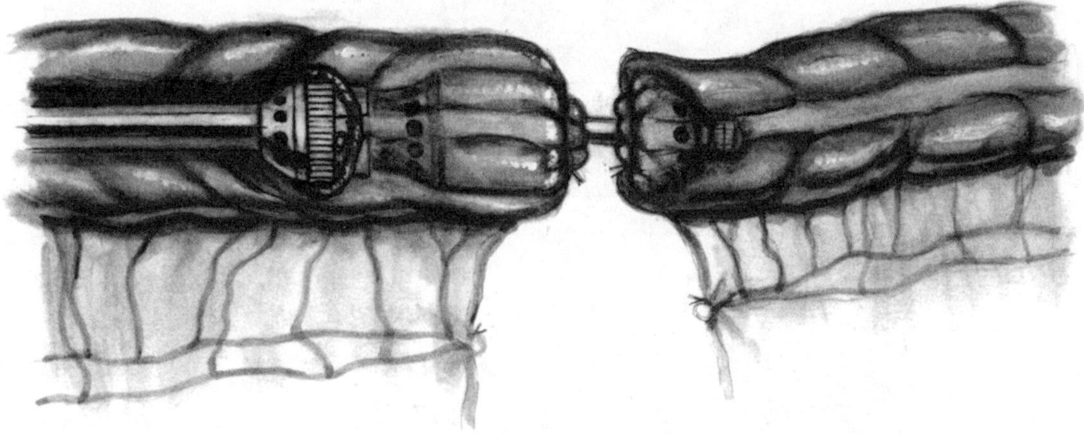

FIGURE 52.3

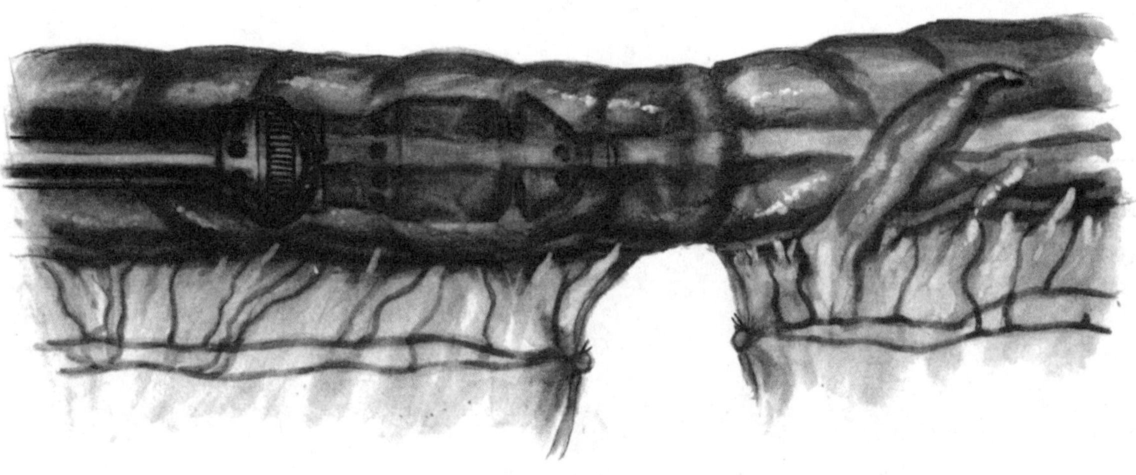

FIGURE 52.4

FIGURE 52.5

The colotomy is being closed after applying tracticn upward with two or three Allis clamps to allow closure, using the TA 55 instrument. This end-to-end colocolonic anastomosis is carried out frequently. Most surgeons, however, prefer to use natural orifices or the orifices made by resection of the segment of colon and do not perform a colotomy to introduce the EEA instrument, as in the described case (15, 18, 19).

End-to-End Colocolonic Anastomosis (2, 10, 19)

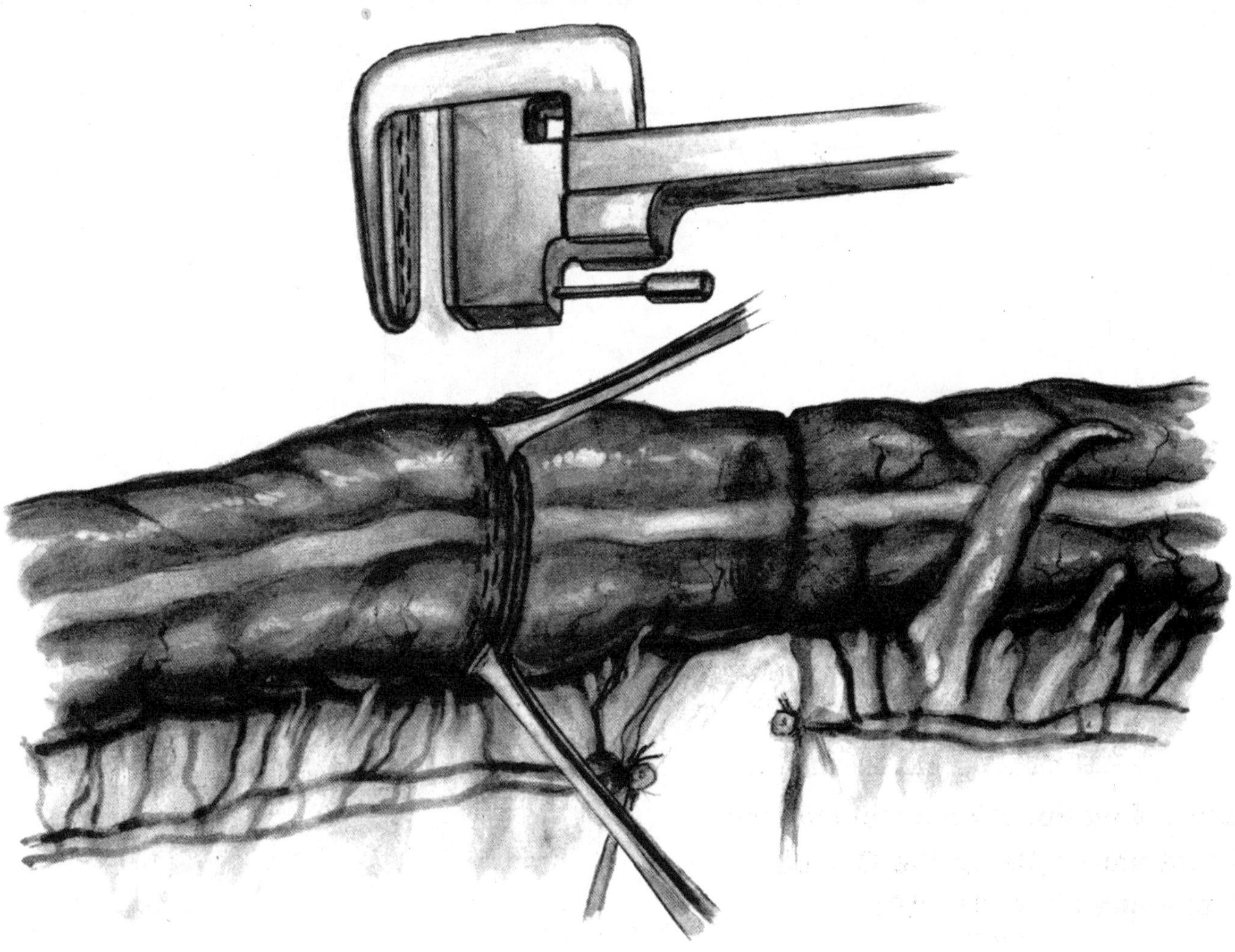

FIGURE 52.5

End-to-End Functional Colocolonic Anastomosis Using the Closed Technique (2–4, 15, 19)

FIGURE 52.6
The colon has been sutured and transected using the GIA instrument, and a functional end-to-end anastomosis is about to be performed to reestablish intestinal continuity. In the antimesenteric angles of the proximal and distal colon, a small segment is resected to permit the introduction of the arms of the GIA instrument, with the object of carrying out a side-to-side anastomosis between the proximal and the distal colon.

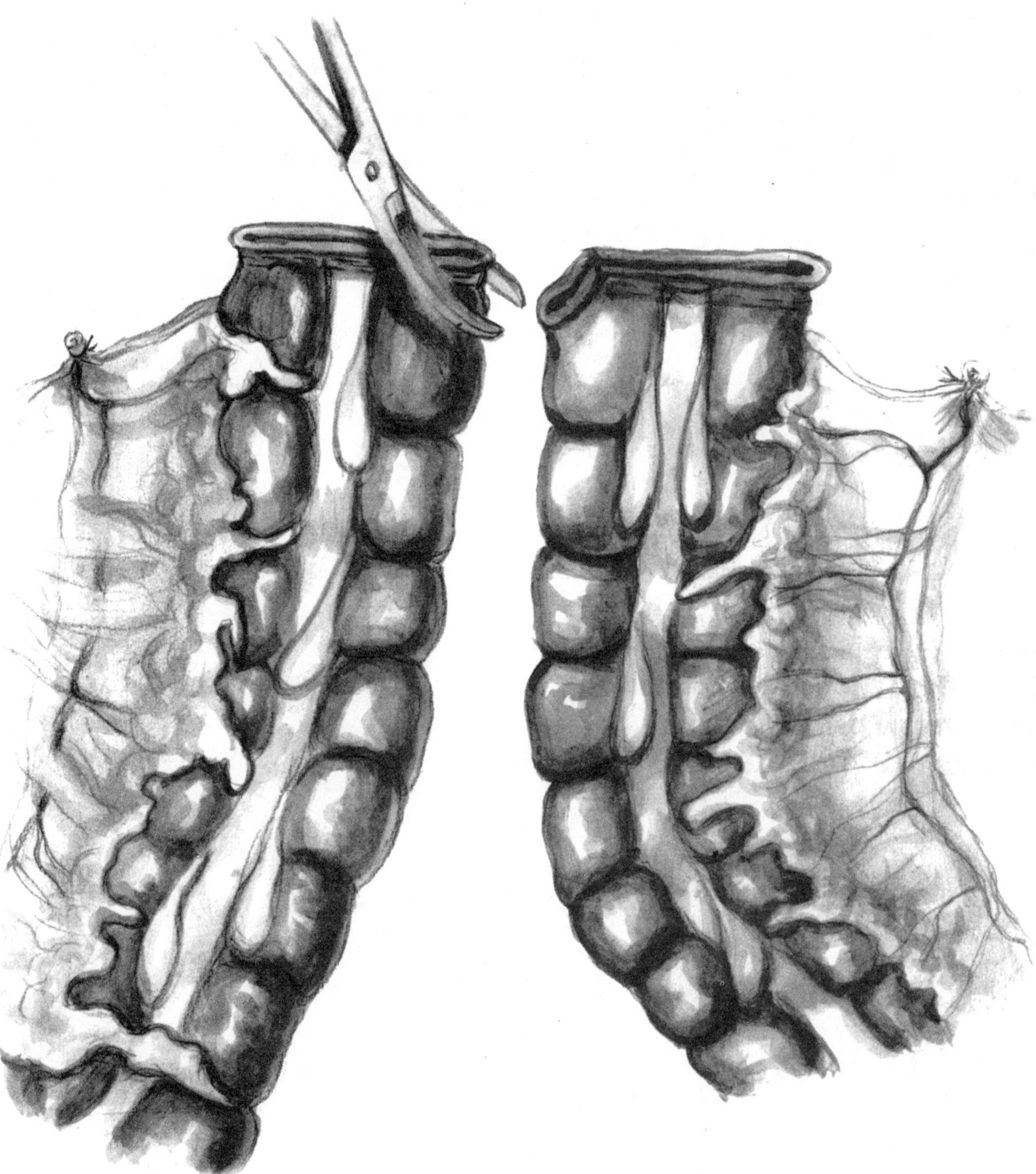

FIGURE 52.6

End-to-End Functional Colocolonic Anastomosis Using the Closed Technique (2–4, 15, 19)

FIGURE 52.7
The arms of the GIA instrument have been brought together after they are introduced into the ends of both colonic segments and rested against its antimesenteric walls. They are now prepared to be fired in order to carry out the suture and anastomosis in a side-to-side fashion between both colonic segments.

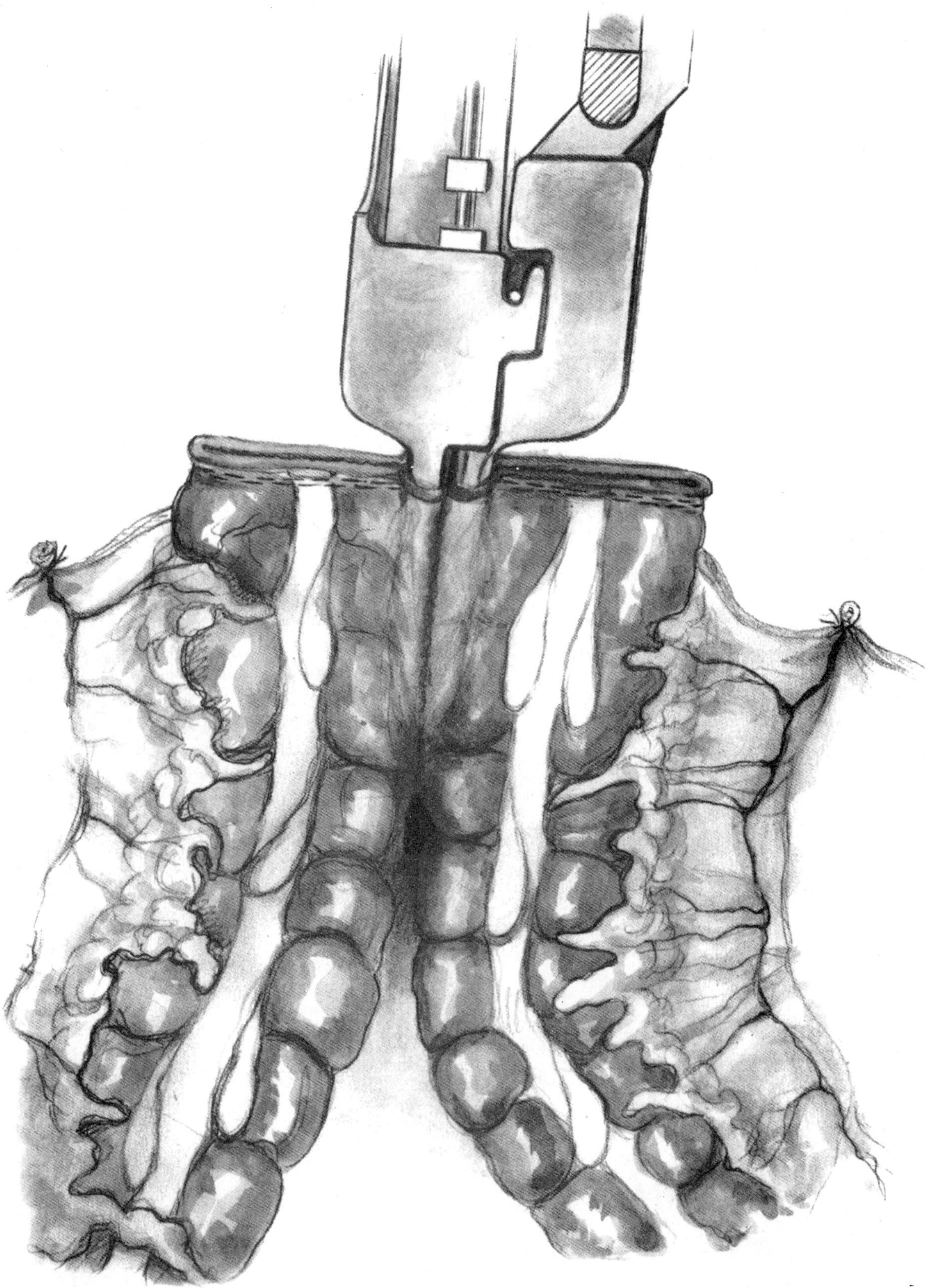

FIGURE 52.7

FIGURE 52.8
View of a section of the suture and the antimesenteric colonic walls in which one can see the side-to-side anastomosis between the proximal and distal colon. The anastomosis has the same diameter of the colon. According to Steichen and Ravitch, this side-to-side colocolonic anastomosis acquires a circular shape similar to the lumen of the colon with the passage of time. The external scar of the colocolonic suture, according to the same authors, as it heals, transforms the side-to-side anastomosis into an end-to-end anastomosis. This is the origin of the designation of end-to-end functional colocolonic anastomosis.

End-to-End Functional Colocolonic Anastomosis Using the Closed Technique (2–4, 15, 19)

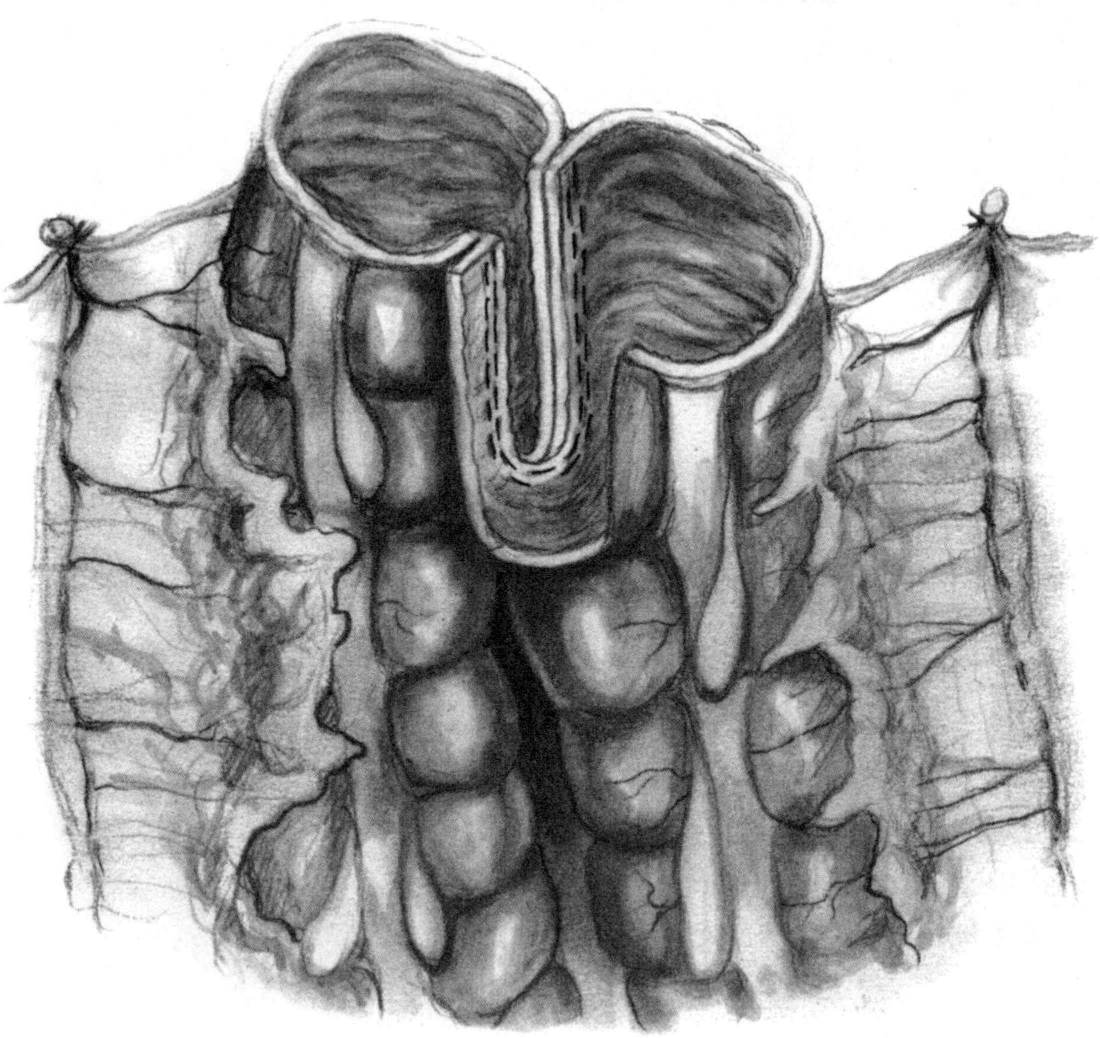

FIGURE 52.8

Functional Ileocolic End-to-End Anastomosis by the Closed Technique

FIGURE 52.9

The angles of both colonic segments through which the branches of the GIA instrument were introduced are being sutured. These segments are grasped by Allis clamps, and the TA 55 instrument is being used to suture them.

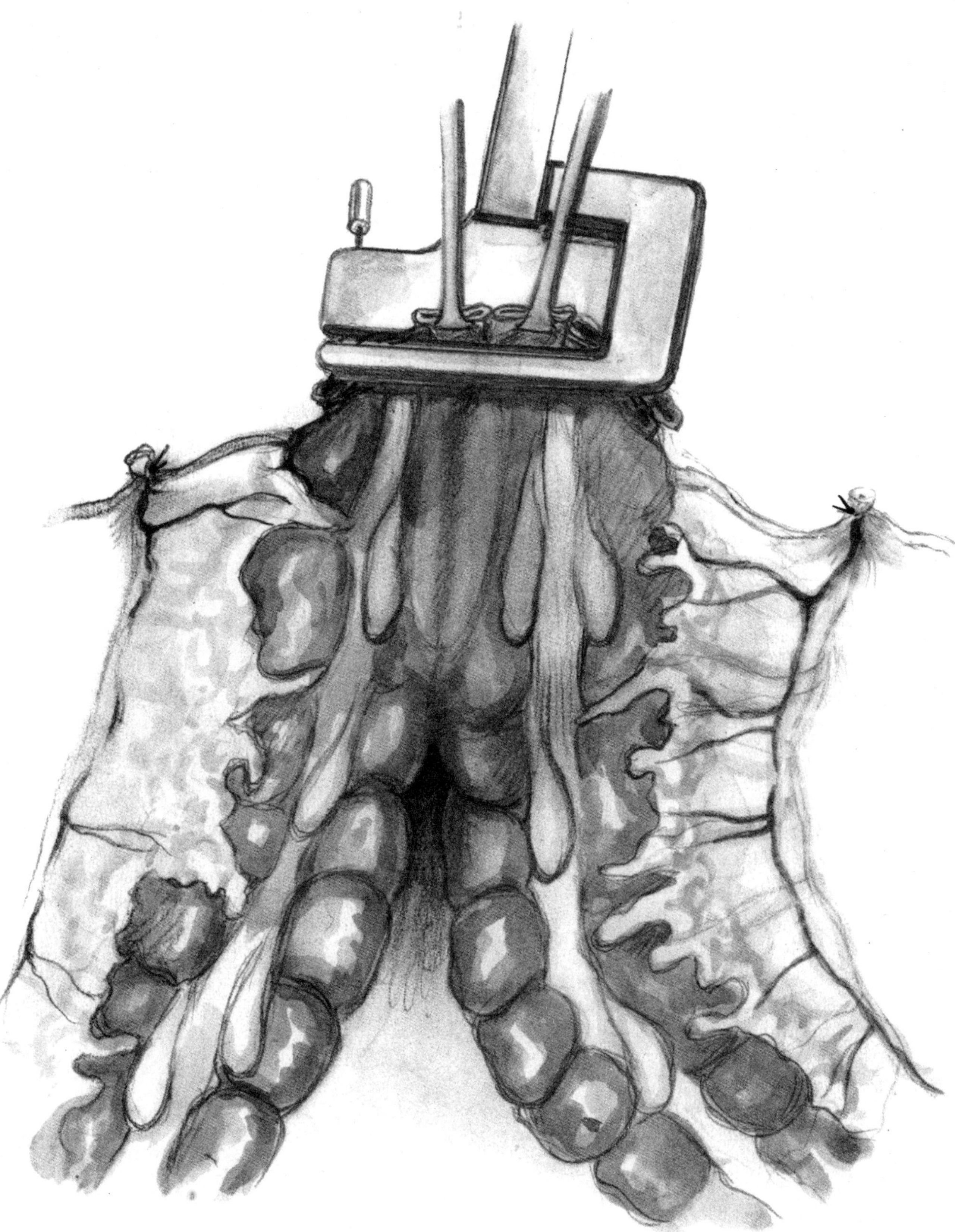

FIGURE 52.9

Functional Colocolonic End-to-End Anastomosis by the Closed Technique

FIGURE 52.10
The functional terminal colocolonic anastomosis has been completed, reestablishing intestinal continuity. We have shown the establishment of digestive transit with both colonic ends previously closed, using the GIA instrument. The same technique can be applied without closing both colonic ends. When intestinal continuity is reestablished with the colonic ends open, this technique is known as end-to-end functional colocolonic anastomosis by the open technique (4, 10, 14, 19).

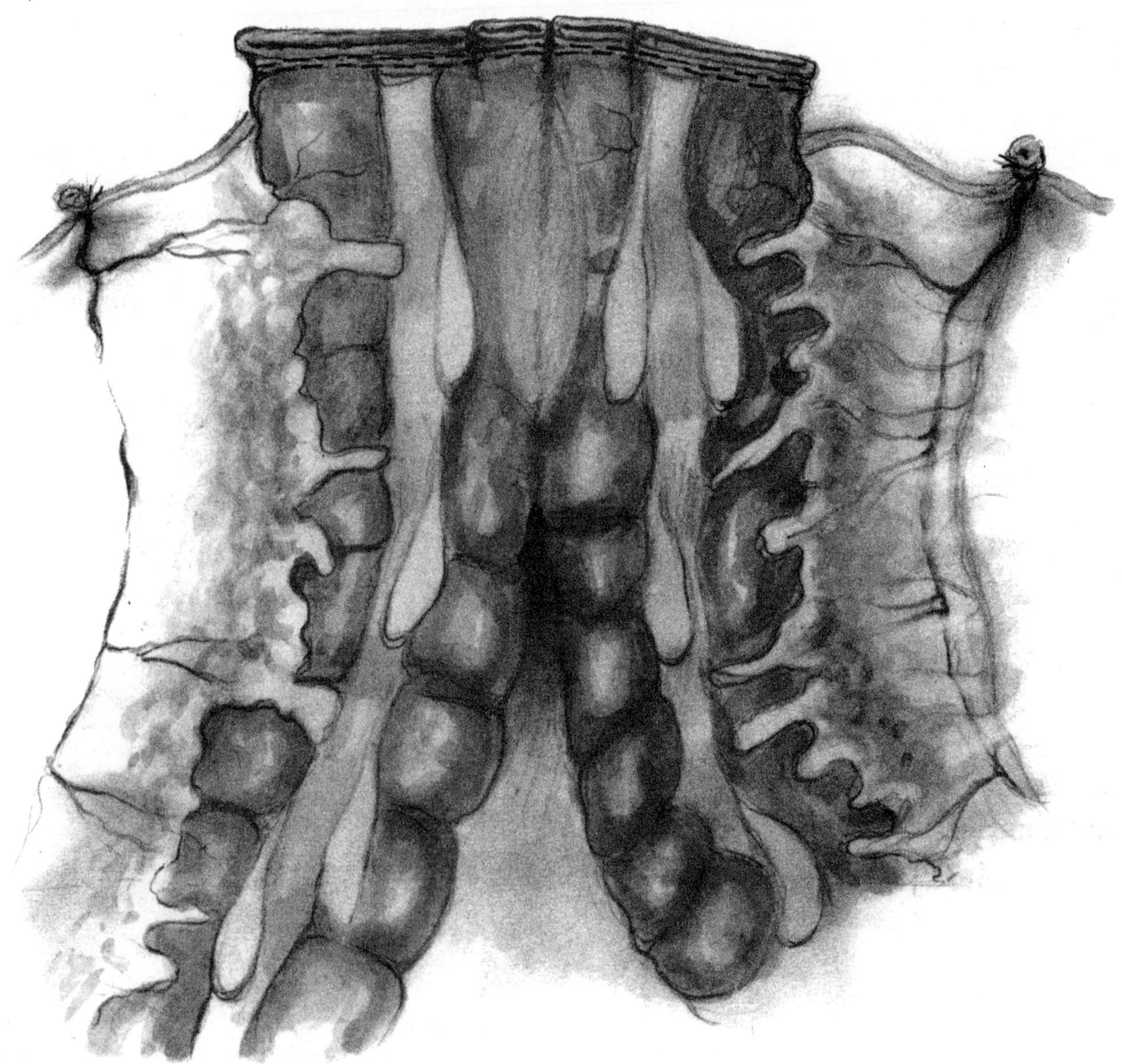

FIGURE 52.10

Functional Ileocolic End-to-End Anastomosis by the Closed Technique

FIGURE 52.11
The ends of the ileum and the transverse colon that have been previously sutured and transected using the GIA instrument are exposed.

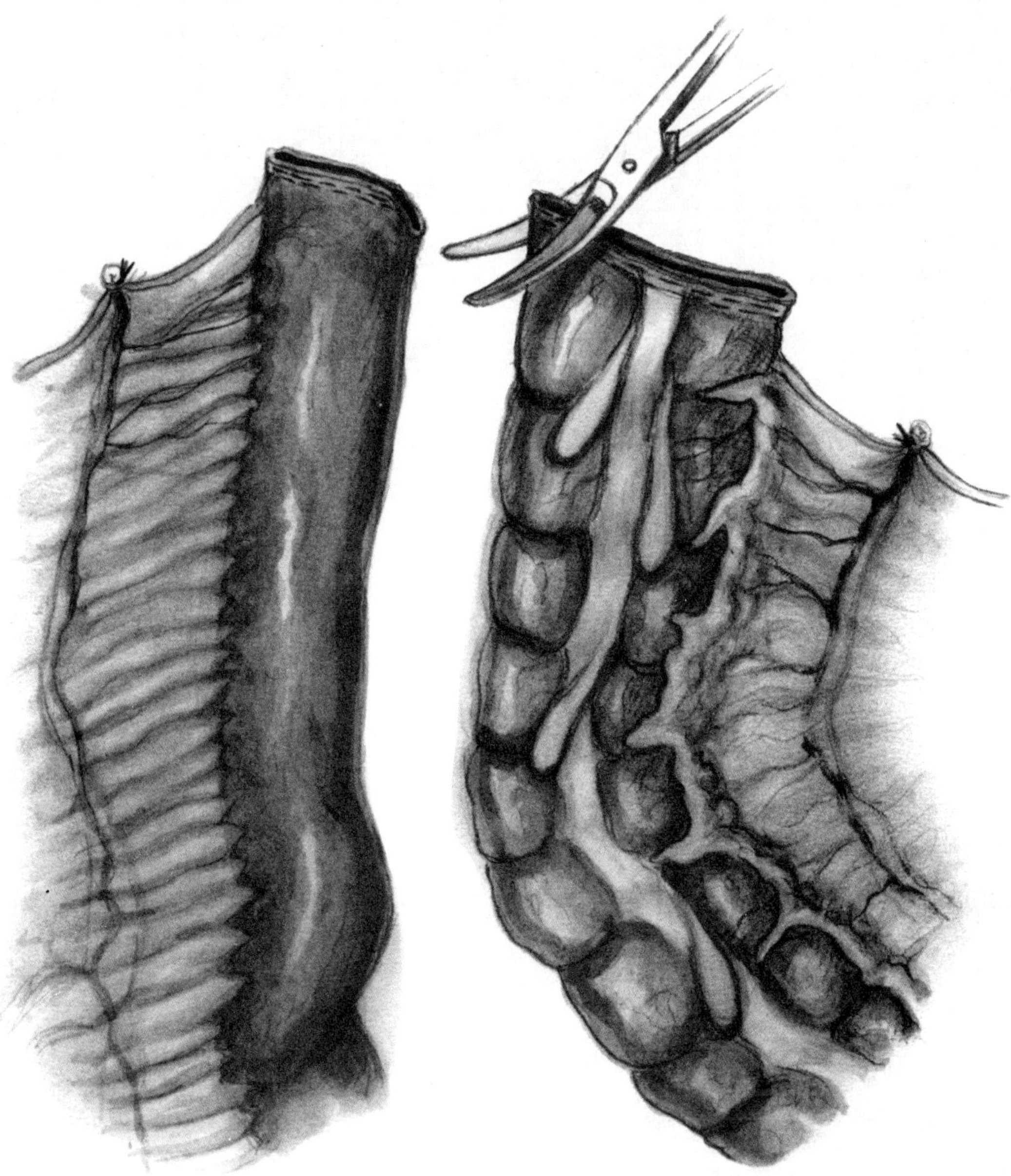

FIGURE 52.11

Functional Ileocolic End-to-End Anastomosis by the Closed Technique

FIGURE 52.12
The arms of the GIA instrument have been introduced separately and are then joined and fired to establish the anastomosis between the ileum and the colon through their antimesenteric walls.

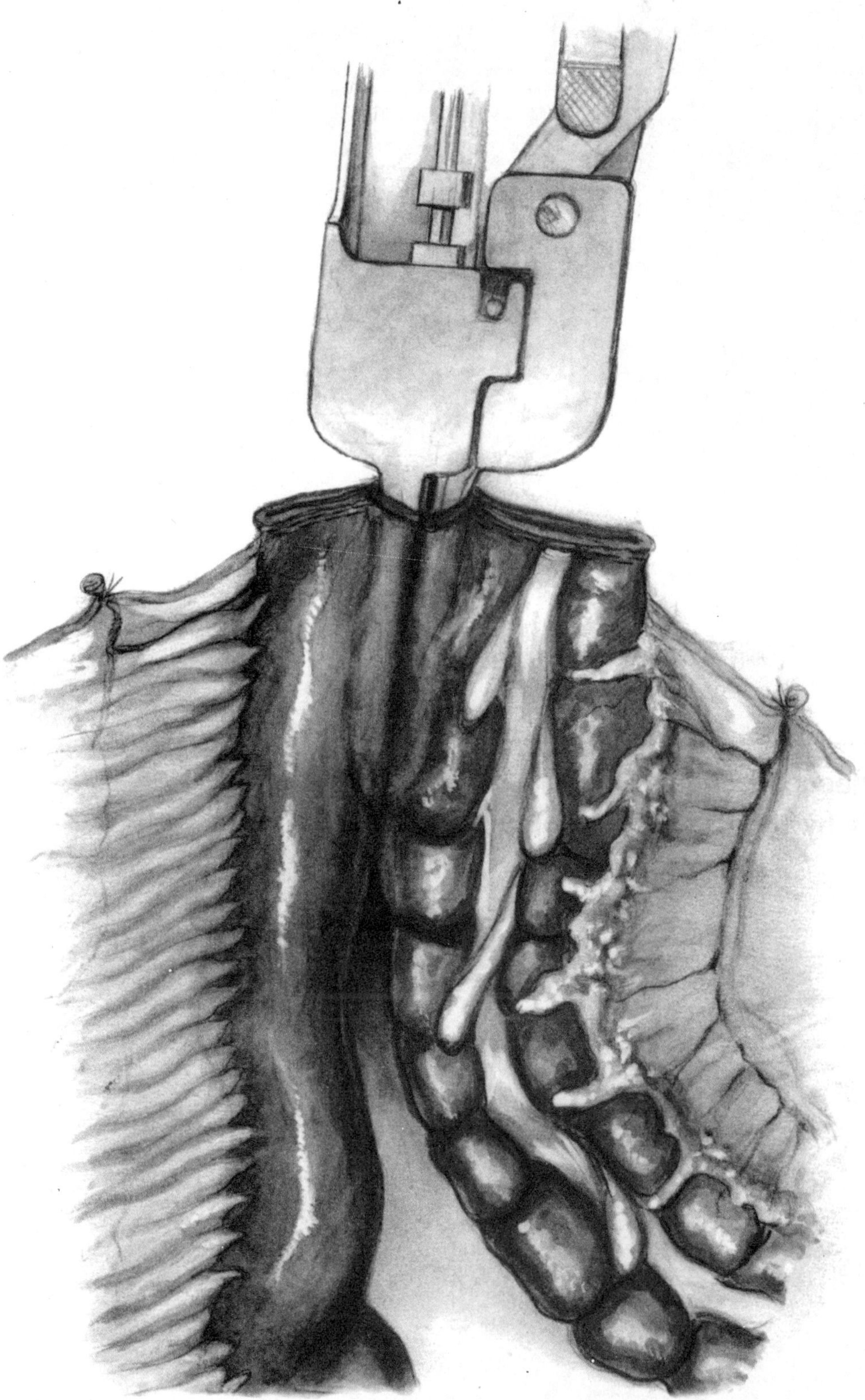

FIGURE 52.12

Functional Ileocolic End-to-End Anastomosis by the Closed Technique

FIGURE 52.13
View of a section of an end-to-end anastomosis between the ileum and the colon performed with the GIA instrument.

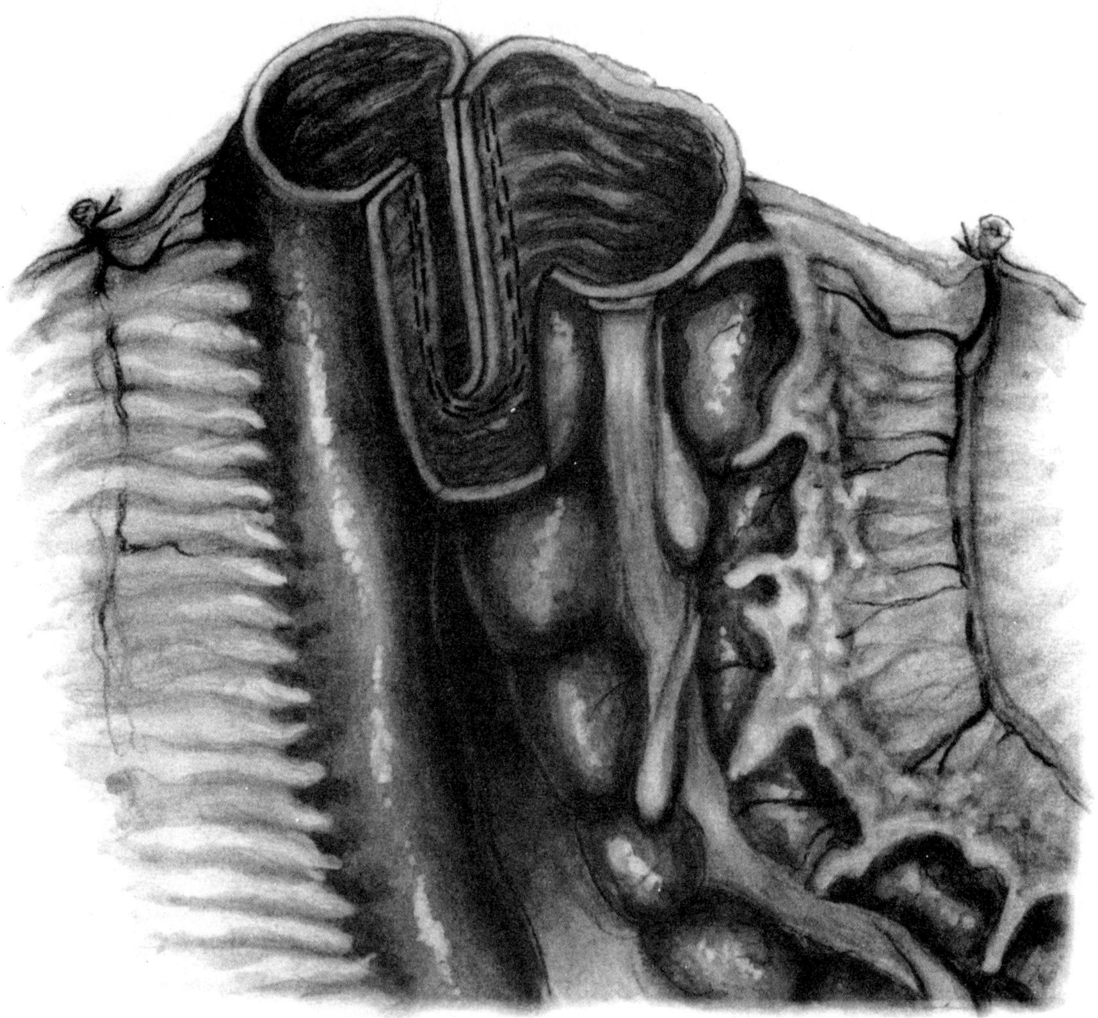

FIGURE 52.13

Functional Ileocolic End-to-End Anastomosis by the Closed Technique

FIGURE 52.14

Using a TA 55 instrument, suturing of the angles through which the arms of the GIA instrument were introduced to perform the side-to-side ileocolic anastomosis is being carried out. Using Allis clamps, the segments to be closed are grasped and by means of a TA 55 instrument, closure is carried out. The mucosa, which protrudes through the staples placed by the GIA instrument, is resected with scissors.

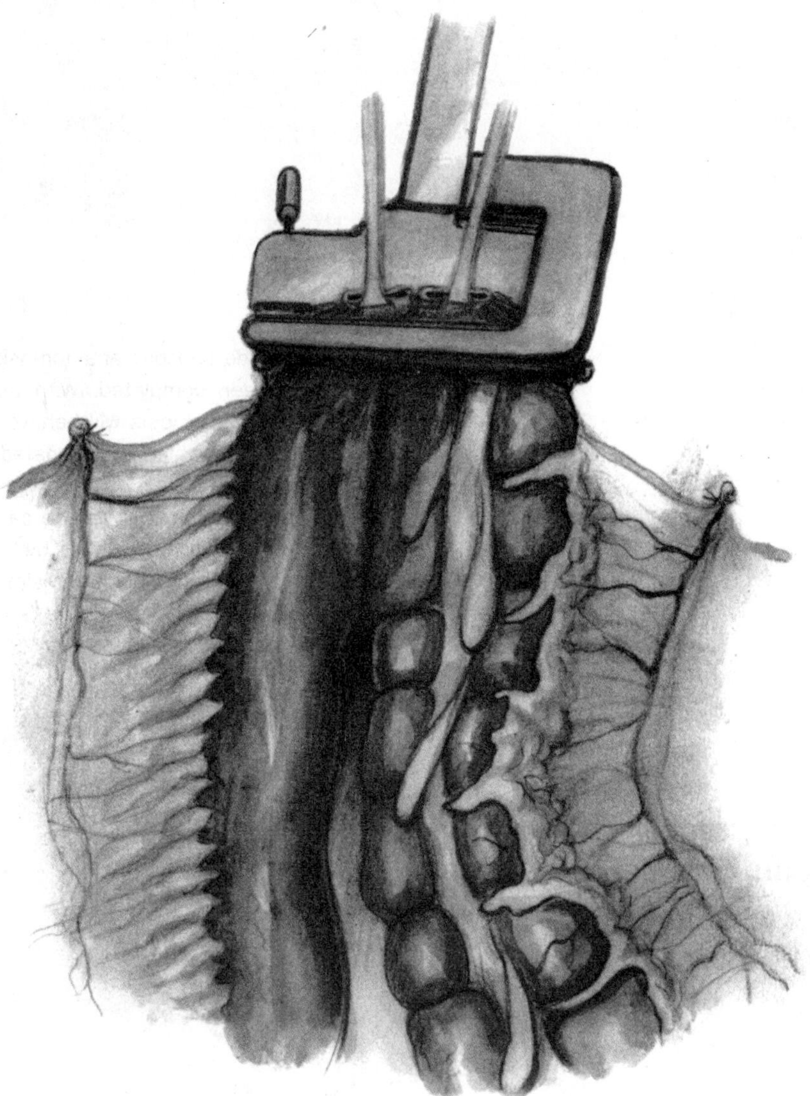

FIGURE 52.14

FIGURE 52.15
The side-to-side ileocolic anastomosis using the closed technique has been completed. With the passage of time, the side-to-side anastomosis will behave like an end-to-end anastomosis, which is why it is designated as functional end-to-end ileocolic anastomosis. Just as in the colonic anastomosis, the ileocolic anastomosis can be carried out with the colonic and ileal ends previously closed by the GIA instrument or with the ends open. The technique is similar in both cases. In this case it is designated a functional end-to-end ileocolic anastomosis by the open technique (19).

Functional Ileocolic End-to-End Anastomosis by the Closed Technique

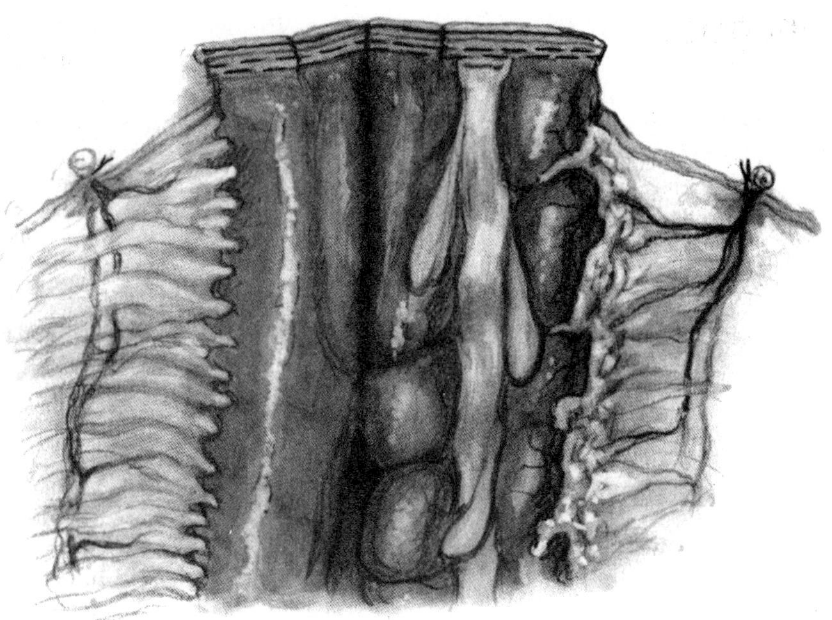

FIGURE 52.15

END-TO-SIDE ILEOCOLIC ANASTOMOSIS

Anastomosis of the ileum to the colon can be performed in end-to-end and end-to-side fashion using mechanical sutures. This technique can be carried out anastomosing the colon to the end of the ileum or the side of the ileum using the end of the colon.

Following is a description of the lateral anastomosis of the end of the colon to the end of the ileum (2, 4, 19).

End-to-Side Ileocolic Anastomosis

FIGURE 52.16

The end of the transverse colon is kept open with three Allis clamps based equidistant from each other to facilitate the introduction of the EEA instrument from which the anvil has been removed. The EEA instrument is introduced obliquely through a small incision in the colon toward its antimesenteric border. The central rod has been inserted through the small incision with a purse string suture around it, using a monofilament suture that is adjusted and tied down once the central rod of the EEA instrument has been introduced.

End-to-Side Ileocolic Anastomosis

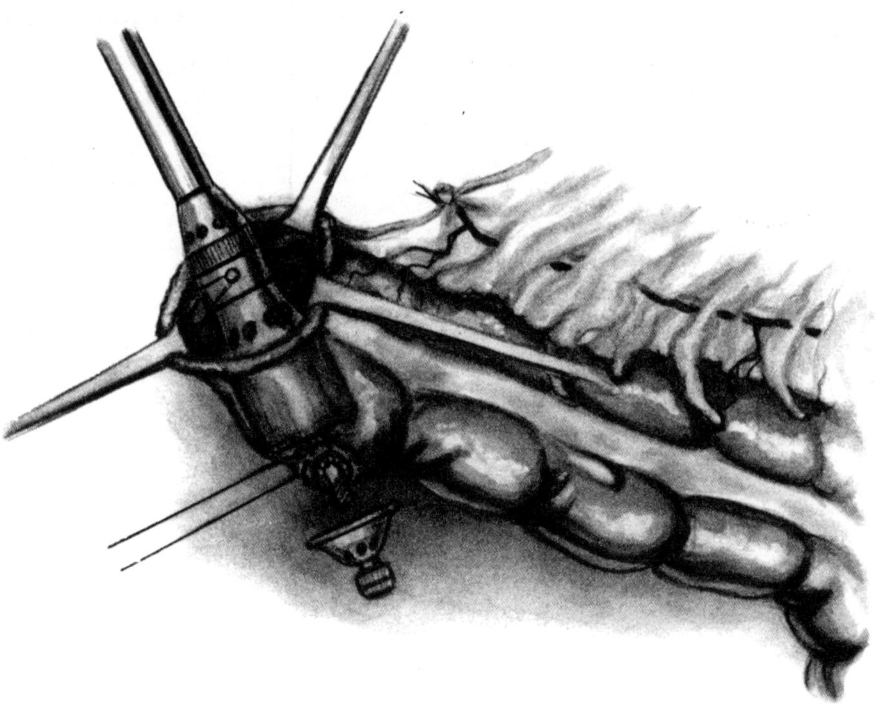

FIGURE 52.16

End-to-Side Ileocolic Anastomosis

FIGURE 52.17
The terminal ileum is held in place with three Allis clamps placed equidistantly. The caliber of the ileum has been previously measured by a sizer. Around the end of the ileum, a purse string has been constructed using a monofilament suture. The anvil has again been attached to the central rod of the EEA instrument.

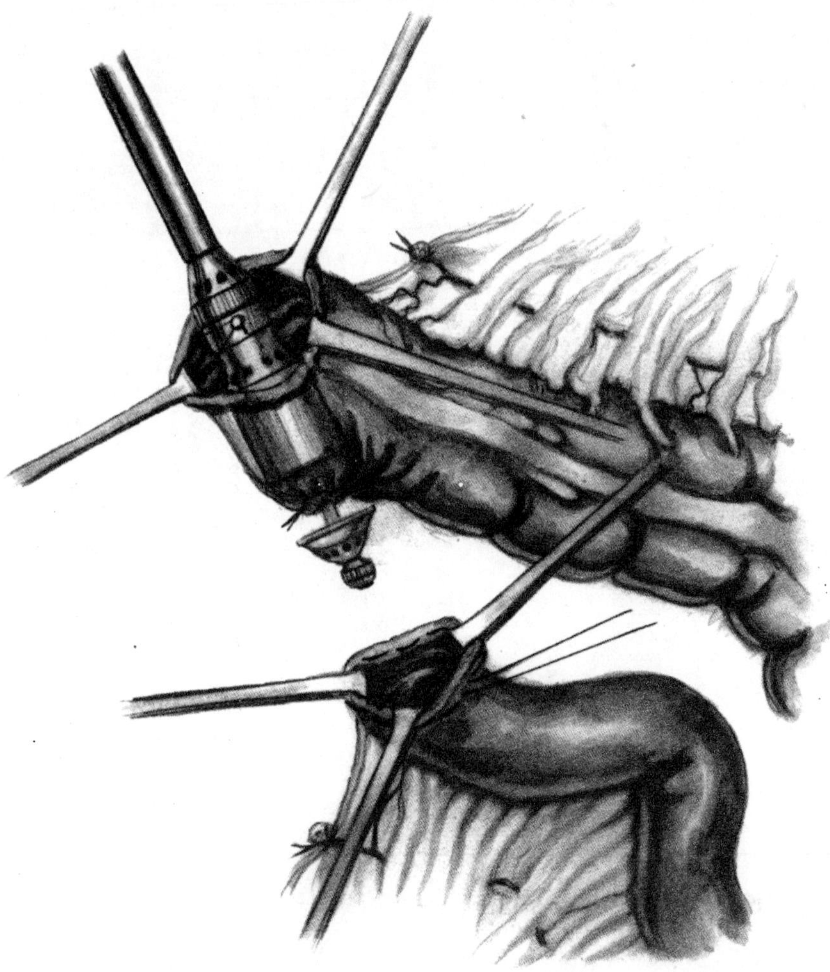

FIGURE 52.17

End-to-Side Ileocolic Anastomosis

FIGURE 52.18
The anvil of the instrument is being introduced into the lumen of the ileum. The entrance of the anvil into the ileum is facilitated if its posterior segment is introduced first.

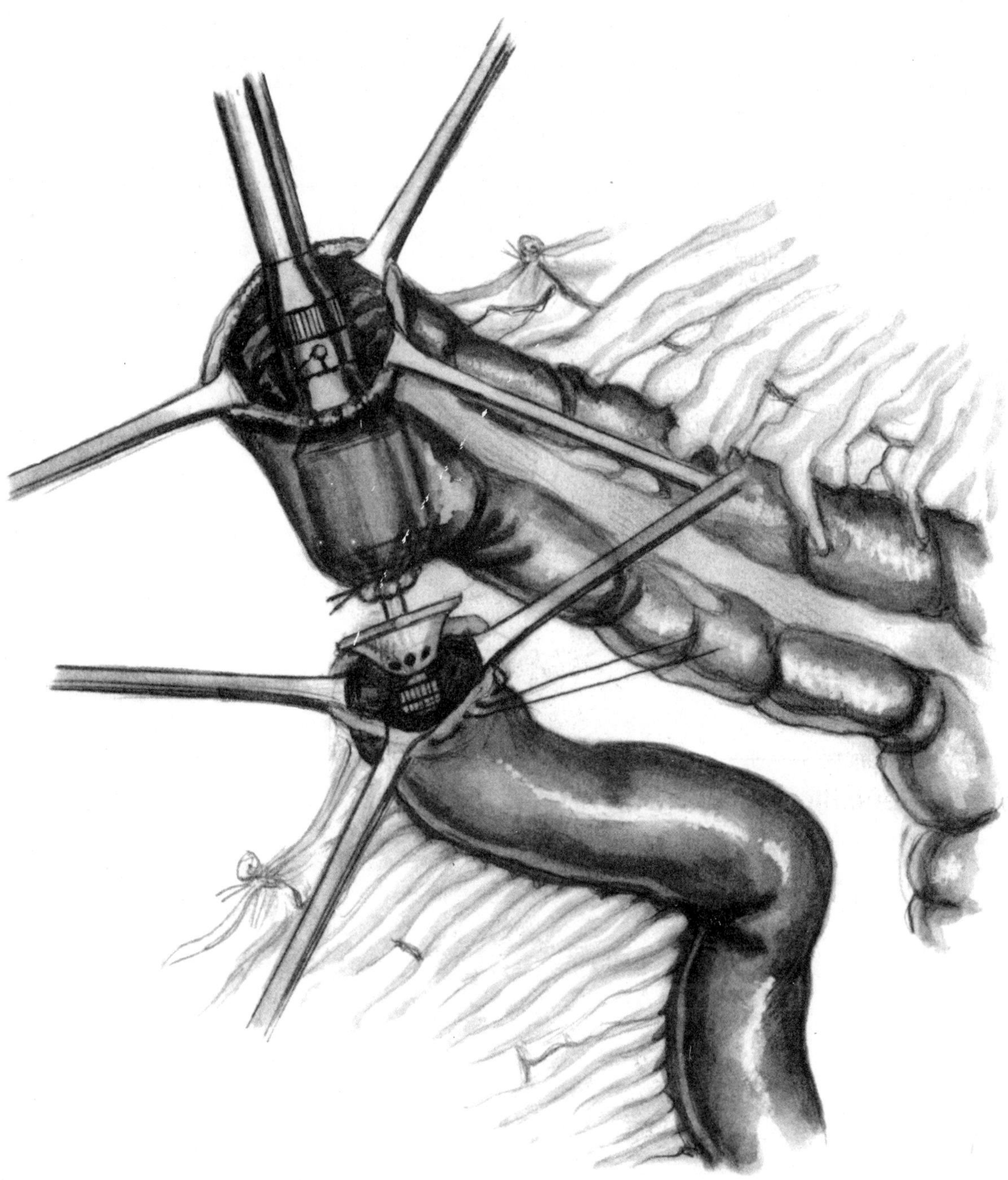

FIGURE 52.18

FIGURE 52.19
The anvil has been introduced into the lumen of the ileum after the purse string in the end of the ileum has been adjusted and the ileum has been approximated to the transverse colon.

End-to-Side Ileocolic Anastomosis

FIGURE 52.20
The EEA instrument has been fired, allowing the construction of the lateral anastomosis of the transverse colon to the end of the ileum. The integrity of the resected rings of tissue is confirmed, and the lack of bleeding at the site of the anastomosis is also confirmed. The end of the colon is then closed with a TA 55 instrument, as shown in the drawing.

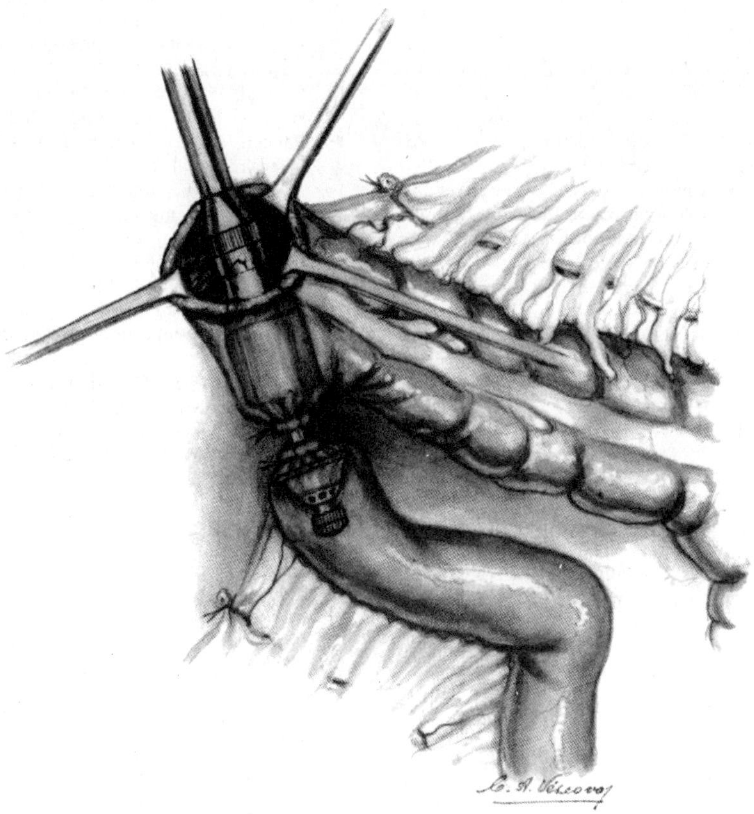

FIGURE 52.19

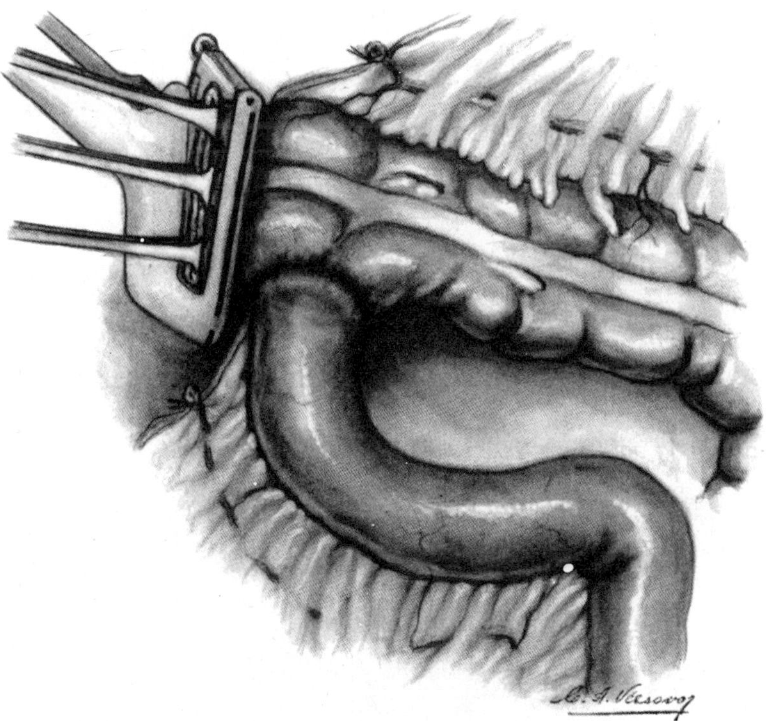

FIGURE 52.20

References

1. Beart, R.W., Kelly, K.A. Randomized prospective evaluation of the EEA stapler for colorectal anastomoses. Am. J. Surg. 141:143, 1981.
2. Beart, R.W. Jr. Stapling in colorectal surgery. In Fielding, L.P., Goldberg, S.M. (Eds.) Surgery of the colon, rectum and anus. Ed. 5, p. 74. Butterworth-Heinemann, Oxford, 1993.
3. Chassin, J.L., Rifkind, K.M., Sussman, B., Kassel, B., Fingaret, A., Orager, S., Chassin, P.S. The stapled gastrointestinal tract anastomosis. Incidence of postoperative complications compared with the sutured anastomosis. Ann. Surg. 188:689, 1978.
4. Chassin, J.L. Operative strategy in general surgery. Ed. 2, p. 11. Springer-Verlag, New York, 199.
5. Everett, W.G., Friend, P.J., Forty, J. Comparison of stapling and hand suture for left-sided large bowel anastomosis. Br. J. Surg. 73:345, 1986.
6. Fraser, I. An historic perspective on mechanical aids in intestinal anastomosis. Surg. Gynecol. Obstet. 155:566, 1982.
7. Gertsch, P., Baer, H., Kraft, R., Madden, G.L., Altermatt, H.J. Malignant cells are collected on circular staplers. Dis. Colon Rectum 35:238, 1992.
8. Gordon, P.H. Malignant neoplasms of the colon. In Gordon, P.H., Nivatvongs, S. (Eds.) Principles and practice of surgery for the colon, rectum and anus. Quality Medical Publishing, St. Louis, 1992.
9. Hurst, P.A., Prout, W.G., Kelly, J.M., Bannister, J.J., Walker, R.T. Local recurrence after low anterior resection using the staple gun. Br. J. Surg. 69:275, 1982.
10. Khoury, G.A., Waxman, B.P. Large bowel anastomoses. A review. Br. J. Surg. 70:61, 1983.
11. Phillips, R.K.S., Cook, H.T. Effect of steel wire sutures on the incidence of chemically induced rodent colonic tumours. Br. J. Surg. 73:671, 1986.
12. Ravitch, M.M., Rivarola, A. Enteroanastomosis with an automatic stapling instrument. Surgery 59:270, 1966.
13. Ravitch, M.M., Steichen, F.M. Techniques of staple suturing in gastrointestinal tract. Ann. Surg. 175:815, 1972.
14. Ravitch, M.M., Ong., T.H., Gazzola, I. A new precise and rapid technique of intestinal resection and anastomosis with staples. Surg. Gynecol. Obstet. 139:6, 1974.
15. Ravitch, M.M., Steichen, F.M. Principles and practice of surgical stapling. Year Book, Chicago, 1987.
16. Reiling, R.B., Reiling, W.A. Jr., Bernie, W.A. Prospective controlled study of gastrointestinal stapled anastomoses. Am. J. Surg. 139:147, 1980.
17. Scher, K.S., Scott-Conner, C., Jones, C.W., Leach, M. A comparison of stapled and sutured anastomoses in colon operations. Surg. Gynecol. Obstet. 155:489, 1982
18. Steichen, F.M., Ravitch, M.M. Mechanical sutures in surgery. Br. J. Surg. 70:191, 1973.
19. Steinchen, F.M., Ravitch, M.M. Staplers in gastrointestinal surgery. In Schwartz S.I., Ellis, H. (Eds.) Maingot's abdominal operations. Ed 9, vol. II, p. 1173. Appleton Lange, Norwalk, CT, 1990.
20. Waxman, B.P. Large bowel anastomoses. II The circular staplers. Br. J. Surg. 70:64, 1983.
21. Welter, R., Patel, J. Chirurgie mécanique digestive. Masson et Cie, Paris, 1985.
22. Wessner, J.D., Yohai, E., Heimlich, H.J. Complications of stapling devices. Surgery 82:395, 1977.

Section H

Colon, Rectum, and Anus

CHAPTER 53

Colonic Resection and Anastomosis with Biofragmentable Ring (VALTRAC)

In 1985, Hardy and colleagues (9, 10) proposed a procedure to carry out an intestinal anastomosis by means of a biofragmentable ring made up of polyglycolic acid (Dexon) and barium sulfate. The Dexon constituted 87.5% and the barium sulfate 12.5% by weight. Polyglycolic acid is a synthetic substance, light in weight and absorbable, to which the organism reacts very little. Barium sulfate is a radiopaque substance that permits radiographic control of the biofragmentable ring. This ring is known by the commercial name of Valtrac (Davis and Geck Medical Devices Division—American Cyanamid Co., Wayne, NJ). In practice, this ring is designated by the name of BAR (Biofragmentable Anastomotic Ring).

The BAR is made up of two identical interdigitated rings which, when in an open position (separated), leave a 6 mm space between them while, when in a closed position, the space between both rings is between 1.5 and 2.5 mm. The 1.5- to 2.5-mm space between the rings in the closed position avoids production of necrosis of the intestinal wall of the anastomotic site. To facilitate the adaptation of the BAR to anatomic variations in the bowel, there are several combinations of diameter and space between the rings in these rings. The festooned edges of the rings were designed to avoid changes in the blood supply of the intestinal wall. There are three sizes of rings: 28, 31, and 34 mm in external diameter. The lumen of all the rings is 14 mm less than the external diameter of the ring (1, 3, 6, 8, 9). In the third postoperative week, the rings become fragmented by hydrolysis and are eliminated with the feces, without the patient noticing it because they are soft in consistency.

To adequately select the BAR that is most serviceable in each case, it is necessary to measure the caliber of both intestinal ends that are to be anastomosed. For this purpose, a sizer is introduced into the intestinal lumen with the same object in mind as in the end-to-end anastomosis using the EEA instrument.

The intestinal anastomosis using the BAR is simple in its performance, since it is only necessary to perform a purse string suture on each end of the intestinal ends to fix the rings in place. The purse string suture can be performed manually or using the special clamp known as the purse string instrument. The material to be used to carry out the suturing should be synthetic, monofilament, and absorbable. To place the first ring of the BAR in the intestinal lumen, an instrument should be used that holds the ring to facilitate its introduction, known as an inserter. In addition, placement of the rings is facilitated if the intestinal borders are grasped with three Allis clamps (2, 4, 5). Once the rings are in place in both intestinal ends that are to be anastomosed and the purse string is adjusted, the surgeon approximates the rings with his or her fingers. The correct adjustment of the rings is recognized by a clicking noise.

The BAR ring should not be used to anastomose intestinal ends of different diameters. The BAR should not be used in low extraperitoneal colorectal anastomoses (4).

Anastomosis with the BAR should respect the fundamental principles of a colonic anastomosis:

1. Well vascularized intestinal ends that look healthy.
2. No tension in the suture line.
3. Correct serosal apposition.
4. Adequate caliber to the anastomosis.
5. The anastomosis should be waterproof.

Various authors have proven the efficacy and safety of the BAR anastomosis (1, 10).

COMPLICATIONS OF ANASTOMOSIS CARRIED OUT WITH THE BAR

According to the experience of several authors, the complications of this anastomosis can occur either during the surgical procedure or postoperatively.

Complications during surgery are narrowing of the intestinal lumen, rupture of the mucosa or the serosa of the bowel, errors in carrying out the adjustment of the purse strings, and rupture of the bowel, making it necessary to repair it by manual suture. The postoperative complications are especially intestinal stricture, dehiscence of the anastomosis, fistula, and so on (1, 2, 6, 8). Most authors agree that these complications are seen with the same incidence in manual, stapled, or BAR anastomoses (3–8).

The concept of carrying out intestinal anastomoses without sutures was originated in France in the past century. The best known procedure was the Murphy button (11). In the United States, the Murphy button was not very well accepted because it introduced into the organism a heavy foreign body, which, because it approximated the edges of the intestine too tightly, led to necrosis of the intestinal wall. With some frequency, a stricture of the bowel occurred postoperatively due to its reduced diameter and due to the complications that the Murphy button provoked in the intestinal wall.

The biofragmentable ring was introduced by Hardy and colleagues (9, 10), with the object of preventing the complications produced by the Murphy button because the BAR was lighter, produced very little reaction in the organism, and had an ample lumen to prevent strictures, and the festooned borders of the rings prevented necrosis of the borders of the bowel. Additionally, it is biofragmentable.

Surgical Technique

FIGURE 53.1
It can be observed that the BAR is made up of two identical rings with festoon borders, separated one from the other by a space 6 mm wide and held by the inserting handle. One of the rings is being introduced into the colonic lumen proximally, where a circular purse string has been inserted using reabsorbable monofilament synthetic material.

Surgical Technique

FIGURE 53.2
One of the rings of the BAR has been introduced into the proximal lumen and the purse string adjusted.

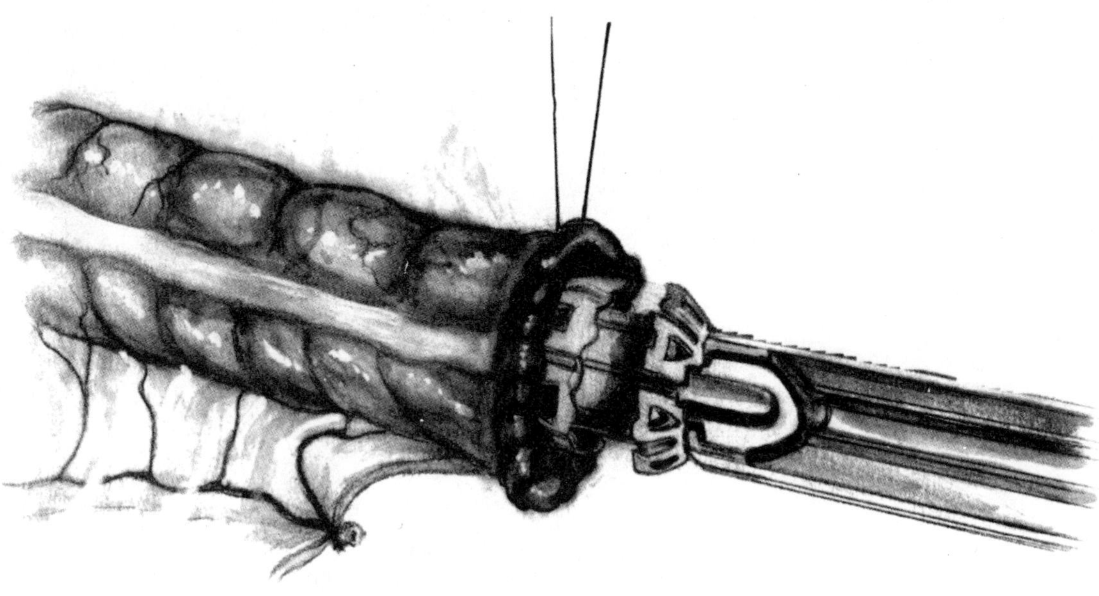

FIGURE 53.1

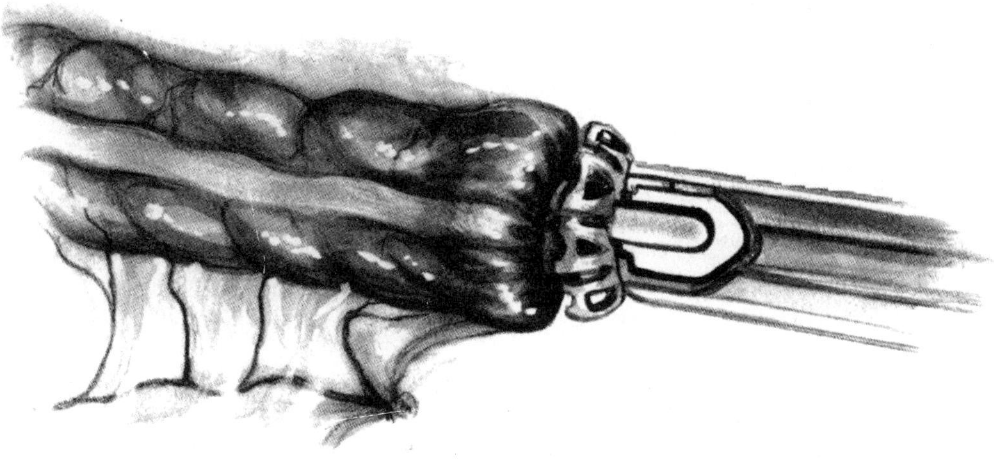

FIGURE 53.2

FIGURE 53.3
Once the purse string is adjusted on the proximal colon, the inserting handle is removed and the second ring is introduced directly into the lumen of the distal colon, where another purse string has been inserted.

Surgical Technique

FIGURE 53.4
The second purse string has been tied around the second ring in the lumen of the distal end of the bowel.

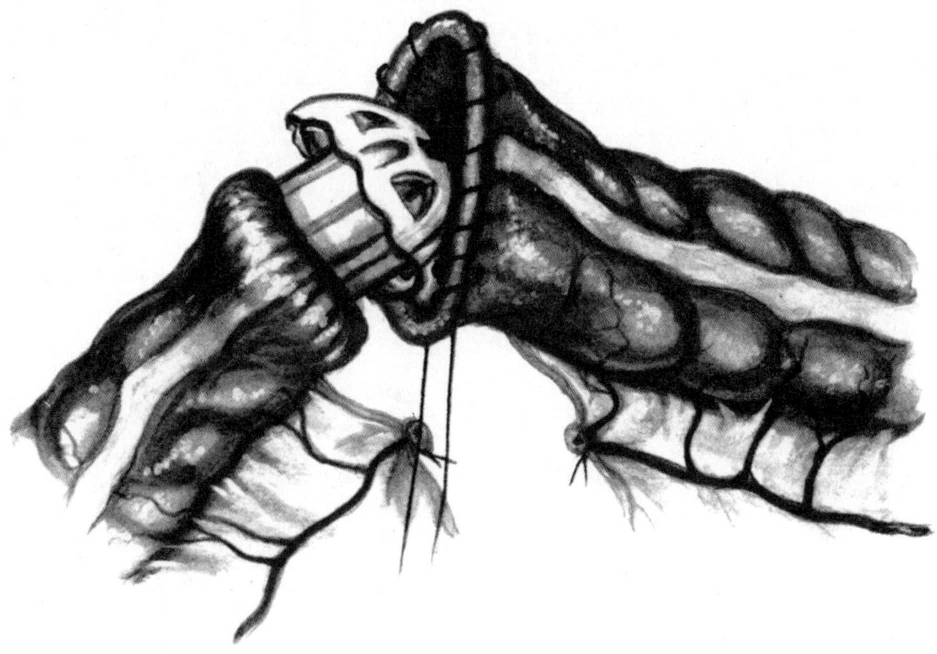

FIGURE 53.3

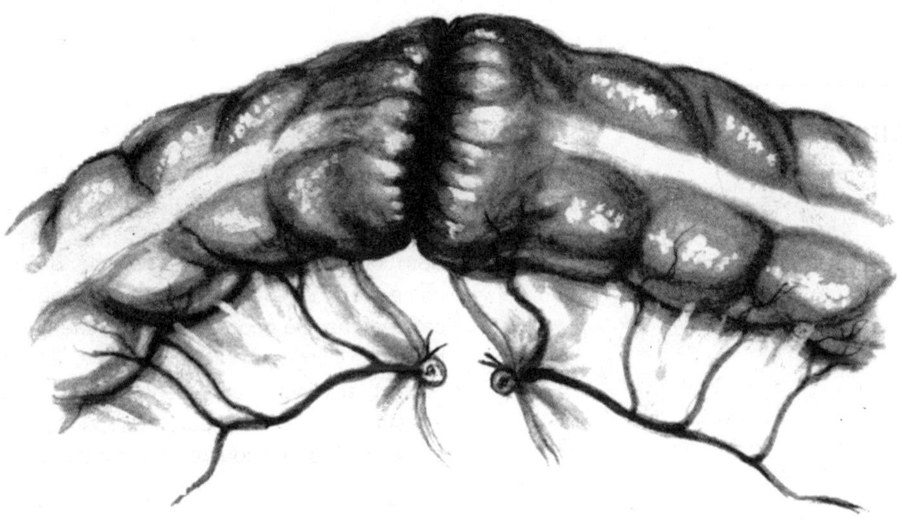

FIGURE 53.4

Surgical Technique

FIGURE 53.5

Both biofragmentable rings of the BAR are being adjusted using the index and middle fingers against the thumb. In some cases it may be necessary to use the index and thumb of both hands to carry out the adjustment. When the adjustment is correct, a clicking noise should be heard. Once the colonic anastomosis is finished, the opening in the mesocolon is closed with continuous or interrupted sutures.

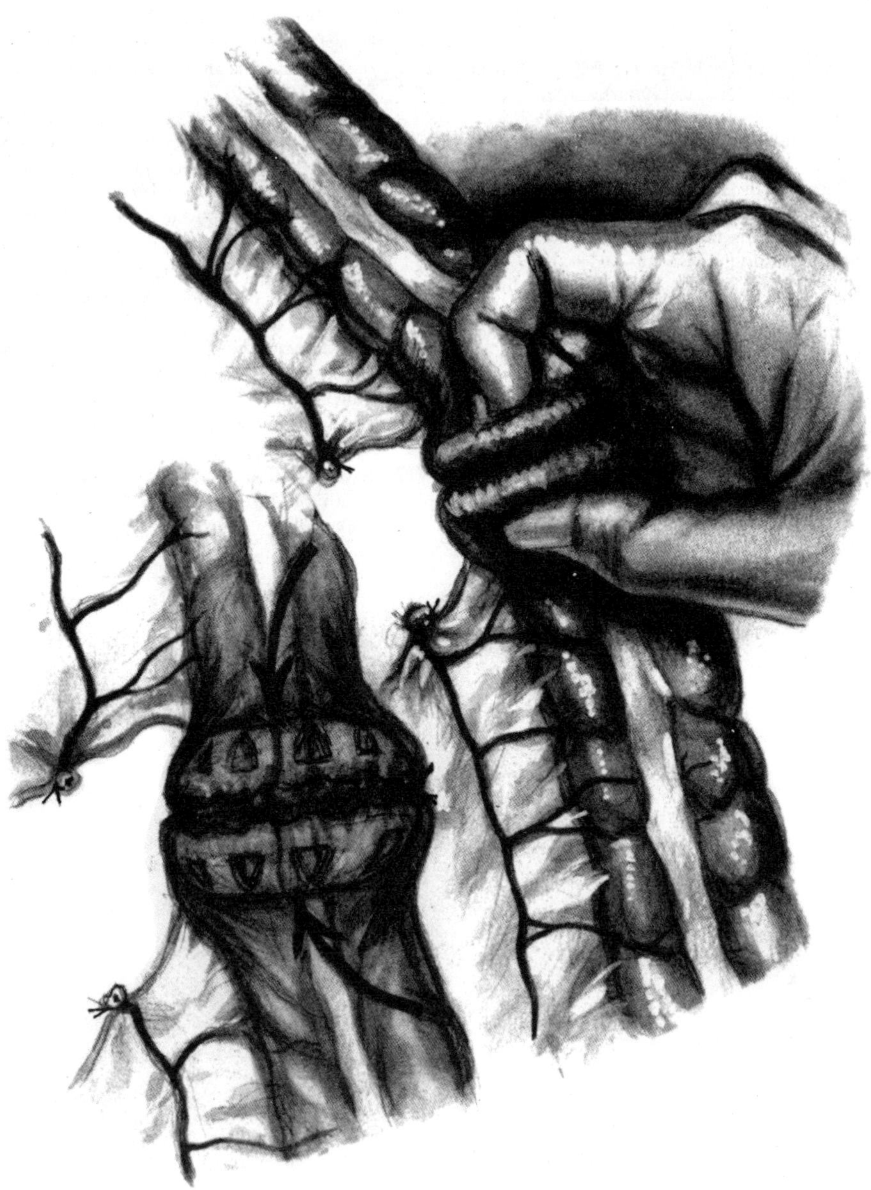

FIGURE 53.5

References

1. Bubrick, M.P., Corman, M.L., Cahil, C.J., Hardy, T.G. Jr., Carter Nance, F., Shatney, C.H. Prospective, randomized trial of the biofragmentable ring anastomosis. Am. J. Surg. 161:136, 1991.
2. Bubrick, M.P. Biodegradable anastomotic ring (BAR) technique. In Fielding, L., Goldberg, S.M. (Eds.) Surgery of the colon, rectum and anus. Ed. 5, p. 84. Butterworth-Heinemann, Oxford, 1993.
3. Cahil, C.J., Betzler, M., Gruwez, J.A., Jeekel, J., Patel, J.C., Zederfeldt, B. Sutureless large bowel anastomosis: European experience with the biofragmentable anastomosis ring. Br. J. Surg. 76:344, 1989.
4. Corman, M.L., Prager, E.D., Hardy, T.G. Jr., Bubrick, M.F., Valtrac (BAR) Study Group. Comparison of the Valtrac biofragmentable anastomosis ring with conventional suture and stapled anastomosis in colon surgery. Results of a prospective, randomized clinical trial. Dis. Colon Rectum 32:183, 1989.
5. Corman, M.L. Colon and rectal surgery. Ed. 3, p. 539. Lippincott, Philadelphia, 1993.
6. Dyess, D.L., Curreri, P.W., Ferrara, J.J. A new technique for sutureless intestinal anastomosis: A prospective randomized, clinical trial. Am. Surgeon 56:71, 1990.
7. Gullichsen, R., Ovaska, J., Brasken, P., Havia, T., Ekfors, T. Large bowel anastomosis in dogs: A comparative study with the biofragmentable ring, manual suture and mechanical stapler. Res. Surg. 3:162, 1991.
8. Gullichsen, R., Ovaska, J., Havia, T., Rantala, T. Colonic anastomosis with the biofragmentable anastomosis ring and manual suture: A prospective, randomized study. Br. J. Surg. 79:578, 1992.
9. Hardy, T.G. Jr., Pace, W.G., Maney, J.W., Katz, A.R., Kaganov, A.L. A biofragmentable ring for sutureless bowel anastomoses: An experimental study. Dis. Colon Rectum 28:484, 1985.
10. Hardy, T.G. Jr., Aguilar, P.S., Steward, W.R.C., Katz, A.R., Maney, J.W., Costanzo, J.T., Pace, W.G. Initial clinical experience with a biofragmentable ring for sutureless bowel anastomoses. Dis. Colon Rectum 30:55, 1987.
11. Murphy, J.B. Cholecysto-intestinal, gastro-intestinal, entero-intestinal anastomosis and approximation without sutures. Med. Rec. 42:665, 1892.
12. Ravitch, M.M. Development of intestinal anastomotic devices. South. Med. J. 75:1520, 1982

Section H

Colon, Rectum, and Anus

CHAPTER 54

Laparoscopic Resection of the Colon

It has been established that resection of the colon by laparoscopy is technically feasible (1-5, 7-9, 11-18). However, this does not mean that this procedure should be used without demonstrating its benefits over the classical technique. A new technique to treat an illness as serious as cancer of the colon cannot be based exclusively on simple arguments such as that with this technique patients ingest liquids and pass gases several hours earlier than with the conventional type of surgery, that the hospital stay is somewhat shorter, and that the operation is more cosmetic. When facing a diagnosis of cancer, these apparent advantages cannot be decisive.

There is no doubt that video laparoscopy has provoked a marked technologic progress and has stimulated the development of numerous instruments to overcome the great difficulty that this technique presents. If laparoscopic surgery of the colon improves or at least provides the same postoperative survival of patients with cancer of the colon and diminishes mortality and morbidity, then it will be time to consider this technique as real progress in the treatment of cancer of the colon. In the meantime, it should only be considered as a progress of technology.

It is well known that in the great majority of cases, resection of cancer of the colon is carried out with the assistance of laparoscopy (laparoscopic-assisted colectomy). This means that, with the help of laparoscopy, the colonic segment to be resected is mobilized and its vascular pedicles along the mesocolon are ligated, but the actual resection of the tumor and the anastomosis of the colonic ends is performed outside the abdominal cavity, after these have been exteriorized through an incision in the anterior abdominal wall. Once the resection and anastomosis of the colon has been performed, the remaining segments of the colon are replaced in the abdomen and the abdominal wound through which the colon was exteriorized is closed. The abdominal cavity is then reinsufflated to reestablish the pneumoperitoneum, and the entire abdomen is explored by means of a laparoscope to identify any bleeding points and complete the closure of the mesocolon that had been begun with the colon exteriorized. Finally, a thorough irrigation of the abdominal cavity with warm saline solution is carried out.

Another fact that acquires great importance in cancer surgery by means of the laparoscope is the impossibility for the surgeon to use his or her tactile sense. Tumors that have not invaded the serosal layer are difficult to detect by laparoscopic means, there having been cases in which the surgeon resected a healthy segment of the colon and left the involved segment in the abdomen. To prevent this serious mistake, patients should be placed on the operating table in the modified lithotomy position (Lloyd-Davies) so that the site of the tumor can be located exactly by means of a colonoscope during the operation.

In conclusion, it is possible to assert that resection of cancer of the colon with laparoscopic assistance is a new technique that is in the process of evolution and the results of which have not yet been evaluated. It is necessary to carry out prospective studies by experienced surgeons with the object of determining the future of laparoscopic surgery in the treatment of cancer of the colon. It is necessary to assert, in addition, that surgery for cancer of the colon by the laparoscopic approach should be in the hands of surgeons of great experience in colonic surgery and with special training in laparoscopic surgery who are willing to convert laparoscopic procedures to an open procedure whenever any difficulty arises.

PREPARATION OF THE PATIENT

The preparation of patients to be submitted to a colonic laparoscopic resection is similar to the preparation of the colon for open surgery (1, 2, 8, 11, 18).

In the first place, it is necessary to establish an exact diagnosis of the location of the cancer by means of endoscopic and radiographic studies, always considering that cancer of the colon that has not invaded the serosal layer is difficult to recognize by laparoscopy.

The day prior to surgery, the patient should ingest only liquids and carry out a mechanical cleansing of the colon by the oral route. The most efficient method of mechanical cleansing of the colon is that which is used at present, having the patient drink in a period of 2-4 hours, 4 liters of an electrolytic iso-osmotic solution of Glycolpoly ethylene, known commercially by the name of Golytely or Colyte. Not all patients are able to ingest these solutions because of their large volume, their salty flavor, and the frequent incidence of nausea. To diminish the nausea, 10 mg of Metoclopramide are given orally, 1 hour before the ingestion of the electrolytic solution. At present there is an electrolytic solution that is just as efficient as previous ones and better in taste, known as Nulytely. Patients who ingest these electrolytic solutions should receive an intravenous infusion to prevent dehydration.

Mechanical cleansing of the colon by the oral route should be completed with the administration of antibiotics against Gram positive and Gram negative bacilli as well as aerobic and anaerobic organisms. A combination of antibiotics, which should be ingested the day before the surgery, used frequently to prepare the colon is as follows: 3 doses of 1 gm of erythromycin base together with 1 gm of neomycin taken at 1 P.M., 2 P.M., and 11 P.M. the day before surgery. One hour before the start of the surgery, an intravenous injection of a second generation cephalosporin and 500 mg of Metronidazol are given.

The operating room and the instruments to be used should be prepared for conventional surgery as well as for laparoscopic surgery, in case a need should arise to convert the operation from a laparoscopic to an open procedure.

The patient is placed on the operating table in a modified lithotomy position (Lloyd-Davies) for either the laparoscopic right hemicolectomy or the laparoscopic left hemicolectomy. By placing the patient in this position, it is possible to introduce a colonoscope in cases in which there is doubt as to the topographic location of the tumor. This position, also allows an assistant to be placed between the legs of the patient, in case of need. Finally, the Premium CEEA (U.S. Surgical) or the Proximate ILS (Ethicon) can be introduced to carry out the colorectal anastomosis in low left hemicolectomies.

The operating table should be placed with a slight tilt of 20° (Trendelenburg position) to favor displacement of the small bowel upward. In right hemicolectomies, the table is also tilted 20° to the left to favor displacement of the small bowel to the left, while the opposite is done in left hemicolectomies.

SURGICAL TECHNIQUE

We will now describe the surgical technique for a laparoscopic right hemicolectomy and later we will describe the technique for a laparoscopic left hemicolectomy. Description of both techniques will be done in a limited fashion, only disclosing a very simple procedure and the steps that have to be carried out in this new surgery.

Laparoscopic Right Hemicolectomy

Laparoscopic Right Hemicolectomy

FIGURE 54.1

The circles drawn on the abdomen are the ports through which trocars will be inserted. Through these ports, the video laparoscopic instrument and other instruments necessary to carry out the right hemicolectomy with laparoscopic assistance will be introduced. The technique for the introduction of the Veress needle and the details of carrying out the pneumoperitoneum were described previously in Chapter 9. The placement and number of ports varies according to the criteria of the surgeon. The several ports shown in the drawing are those frequently used by several surgeons (2, 8, 9, 11). Once the pneumoperitoneum has been carried out, the first trocar, measuring 10-11 mm in diameter, is introduced to the same subumbilical incision through which the Veress needle was introduced. Through this port, the video laparoscopic instrument will be introduced. Once the instrument is introduced, the abdominal cavity is explored to investigate if the Veress needle or the subumbilical trocar (which are introduced blindly) caused any visceral or vascular injury. The liver is then explored to determine if there are metastases present. Other illnesses or pathologic conditions are investigated also.

It is important that the trocars to be used be at least 10-11 mm in diameter so that the surgeon will not be limited in the instruments that he or she can use. In patients in whom mechanical laparoscopic suturing is to be carried out, the trocars should be 12, 15, or even 18 mm in diameter.

The second trocar to be introduced is the suprapubic trocar. Then the subxiphoid trocar is introduced to the right of the midline to avoid the falciform ligament. In some patients it may be necessary to introduce a fourth trocar (8) to facilitate mobilization of the hepatic flexure of the colon. This trocar is placed below the right costal margin, in the midclavicular line. Another trocar is usually introduced in the right iliac fossa. Precise location of these ports in laparoscopic surgery has the same importance as the location of incisions in the abdominal wall in open surgery (18).

In laparoscopic surgery of the colon, the laparoscope is introduced in several ports of entry during the same surgical procedure, to facilitate some surgical maneuvers.

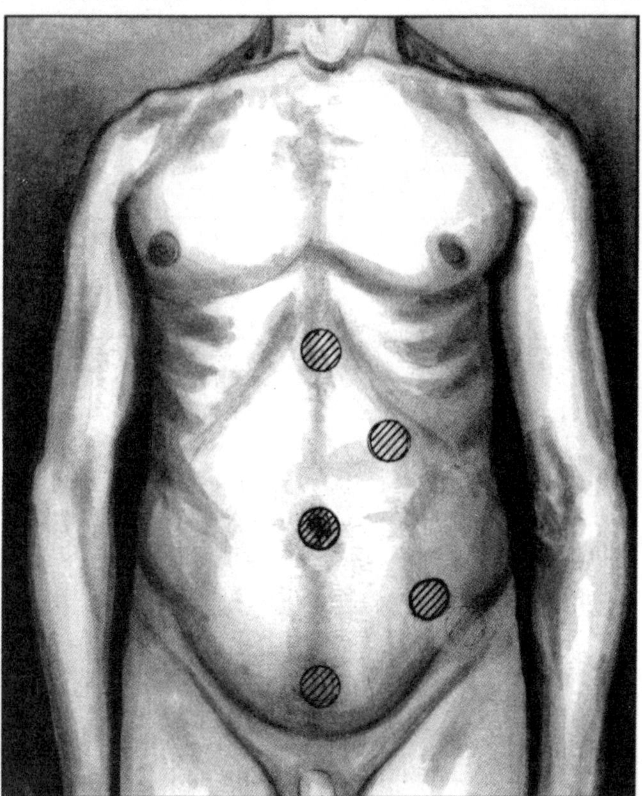

FIGURE 54.1

Laparoscopic Right Hemicolectomy

FIGURE 54.2

Through the same suprapubic port, a laparoscopic Babcock clamp is introduced to apply traction on the cecum toward the midline, exposing the right parietocolic gutter and proceeding with the sectioning of the peritoneum along the white line of Toldt, using curved laparoscopic scissors, connected or not to a monopolar electrocautery unit. The scissors are introduced through the right iliac fossa port. To facilitate visualization of the hepatic flexure of the colon, it is useful to use a lens with an angle of 30-50°. Through the right subcostal port, instruments can be introduced to facilitate mobilization of the hepatic flexure of the colon.

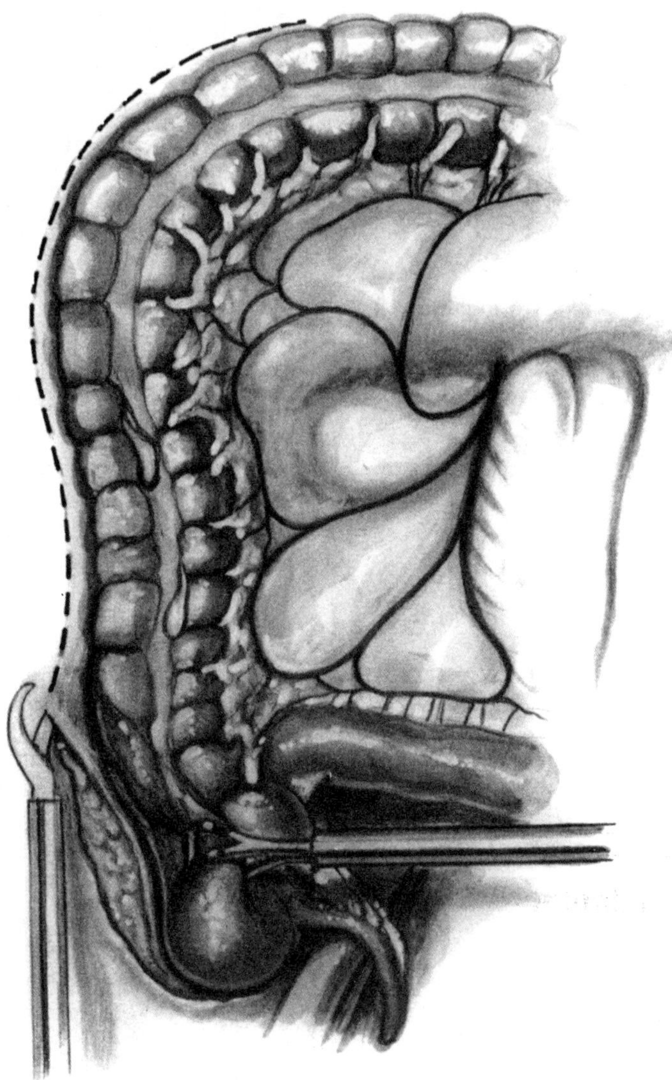

FIGURE 54.2

FIGURE 54.3
Once mobilization of the right hemicolon has been performed, the blood vessels of the mesocolon are identified in order to proceed with their dissection and ligation. Dissection is carried out with curved laparoscopic clamps, as advised by Jacobs and colleagues (8). Vascular ligatures are performed with clips, two on the proximal side of the vascular pedicle and two on the distal side. Ligation of the vessels in the mesocolon should be carried out as proximally as possible. Division of the pedicle is carried out with laparoscopic scissors. To carry out a safer procedure, the proximal vascular stump is ligated with a pretied surgical ligature (Endoloop). Laparoscopic stapling instruments can also be used to ligate the mesocolic vascular pedicles. This instrument introduces rows of staples and divides the tissues. It is introduced through the suprapubic port (8). In a right hemicolectomy, the right branch of the midcolic vessels, the right colic vessels, and the ileocolic vessels should be ligated and divided.

Laparoscopic Right Hemicolectomy

In a colon resection by laparoscopy, the pneumoperitoneum is maintained at a pressure of 10-12 mm of mercury. In laparoscopic cholecystectomy, the pressure of the pneumoperitoneum is kept at a slightly higher level. With the low pressure of the pneumoperitoneum in laparoscopic colectomy, it is possible to avoid dissection of the retroperitoneum by carbon dioxide, which may lead to subcutaneous emphysema.

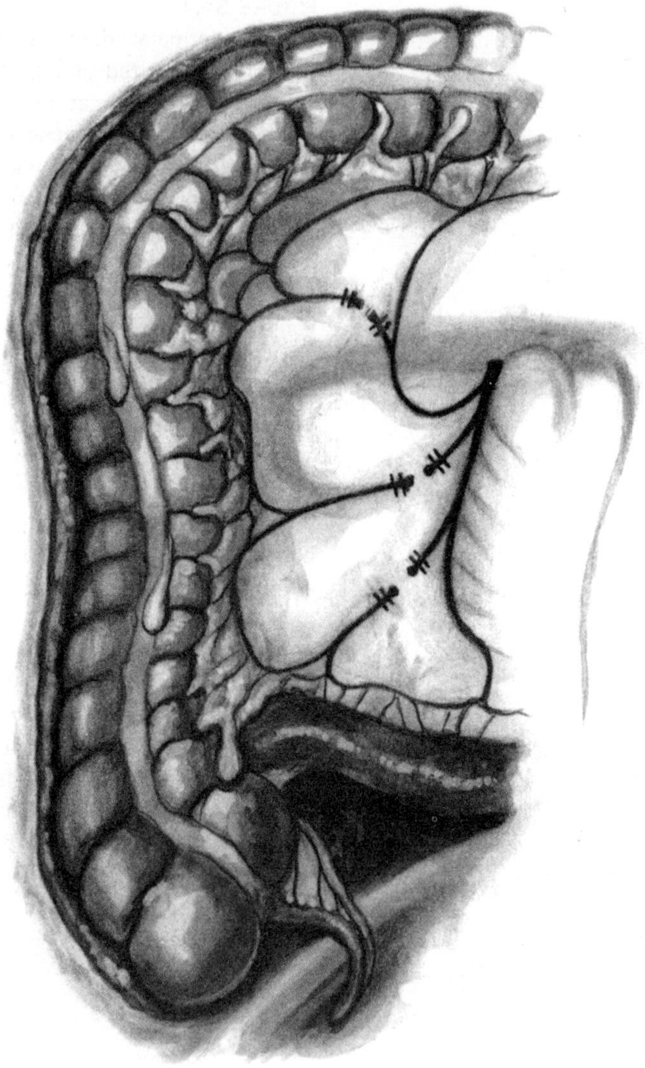

FIGURE 54.3

FIGURE 54.4

Once the terminal ileum and right hemicolon have been freed, they are exteriorized through a horizontal incision in the right side of the abdomen, at the level of the umbilicus, to the right of the anterior rectus muscle. Some surgeons carry out this ileocolic exteriorization through an amplification of the subumbilical incision. If the carcinoma has invaded the serosa of the colon, a waterproof bag is introduced and the colon inserted into it, to prevent possible seeding of the tumor along the edges of the abdominal incision, as has been observed in some cases. Once the terminal ileum and colon have been exteriorized, transection of the ileum and the colon using a GIA instrument is performed. This instrument sutures and divides both intestinal segments, making it possible to remove the surgical specimen. Intestinal continuity is reestablished by suturing the ileum to the colon in end-to-end or side-to-side fashion, using manual or mechanical technique. The drawing shows the establishment of ileocolic intestinal continuity using manual suturing in a side-to-side fashion, which will function as an end-to-end anastomosis.

Once the digestive transit has been reestablished, the intestine is reintroduced into the abdominal cavity. The incision in the abdominal wall that had been carried out to exteriorize the bowel is closed. The pneumoperitoneum is then reestablished. A new exploration of the abdomen is carried out to be sure there are no bleeding points, and the surgery is then completed by carrying out an extensive irrigation using warm saline solution.

Laparoscopic Right Hemicolectomy

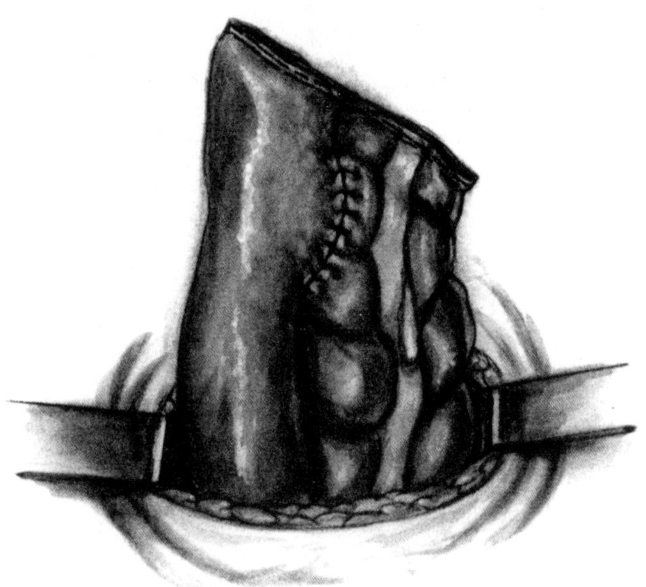

Laparoscopic Left Hemicolectomy

FIGURE 54.5

In order to carry out a left hemicolectomy for cancer using laparoscopy, four ports are usually made. In order to mobilize the splenic flexure of the colon, a fifth port is added (8). As usual, the first trocar is introduced in the lower border of the umbilicus, through which the video laparoscope will be introduced. Once the laparoscope has been introduced, a thorough exploration of the abdominal cavity is carried out to determine if the introduction of the Veress needle or the trocar led to any vascular or visceral lesion. The abdomen is explored for metastases to the liver or other viscera and for the presence of some other pathologic condition that had not been recognized. The suprapubic trocar is introduced to the right of the midline. Another trocar is introduced into the left lower quadrant of the abdomen. A fourth trocar is introduced under the right costal margin, in the midclavicular line. If necessary, a fifth trocar is introduced under the left costal margin, in the midclavicular line. This latter port is very useful in mobilization of the splenic flexure of the colon.

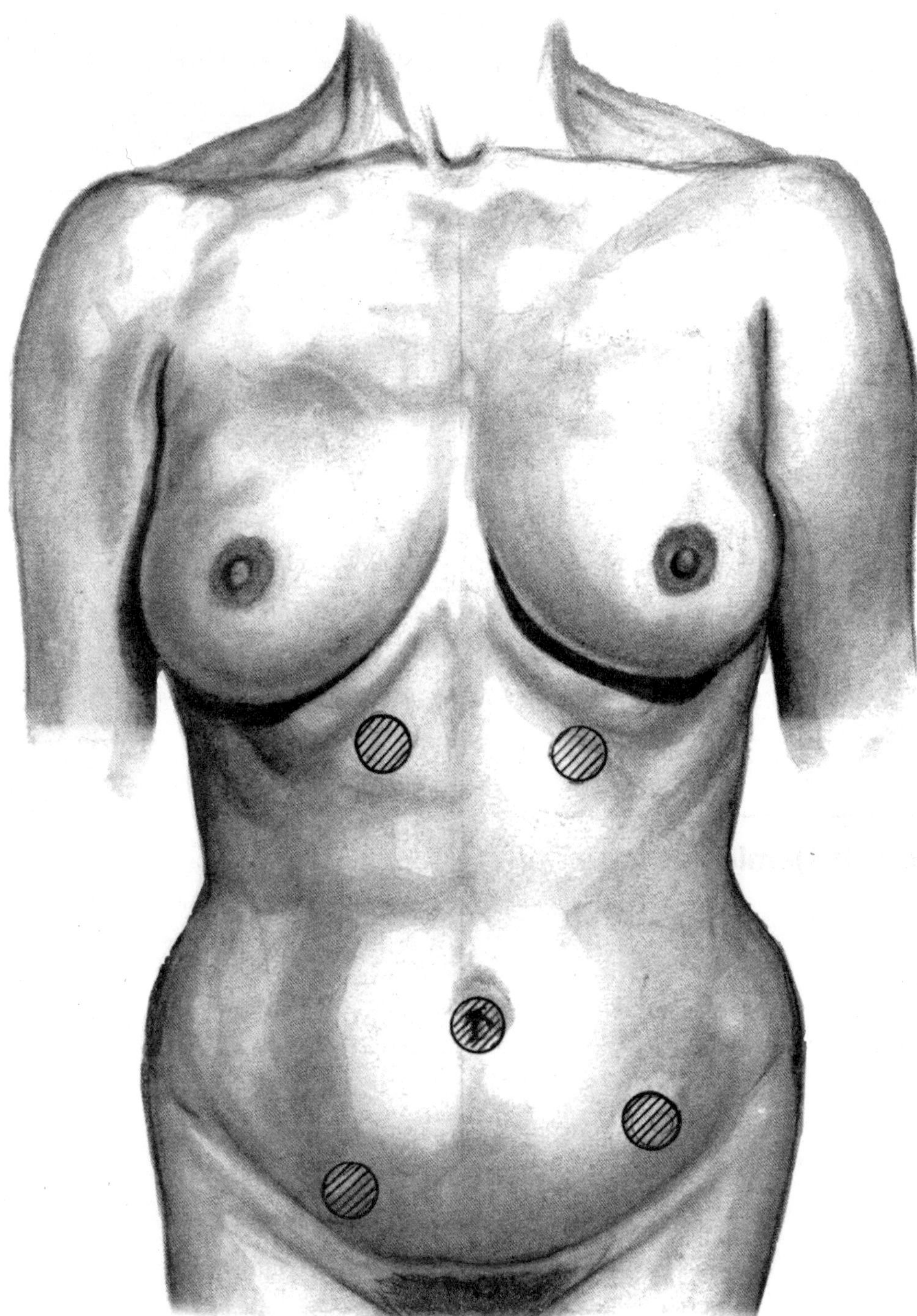

FIGURE 54.5

Laparoscopic Left Hemicolectomy

FIGURE 54.6
The first stage of a laparoscopic left hemicolectomy consists in division of the left parietocolic peritoneum. Using a laparoscopic Babcock clamp introduced through the suprapubic port, traction is applied to the sigmoid colon toward the midline in order to expose the left parietocolic peritoneum, which is then divided along the white line of Toldt, using curved laparoscopic scissors introduced through the port in the left iliac fossa. Division of this parietocolic peritoneum allows mobilization of the left hemicolon.

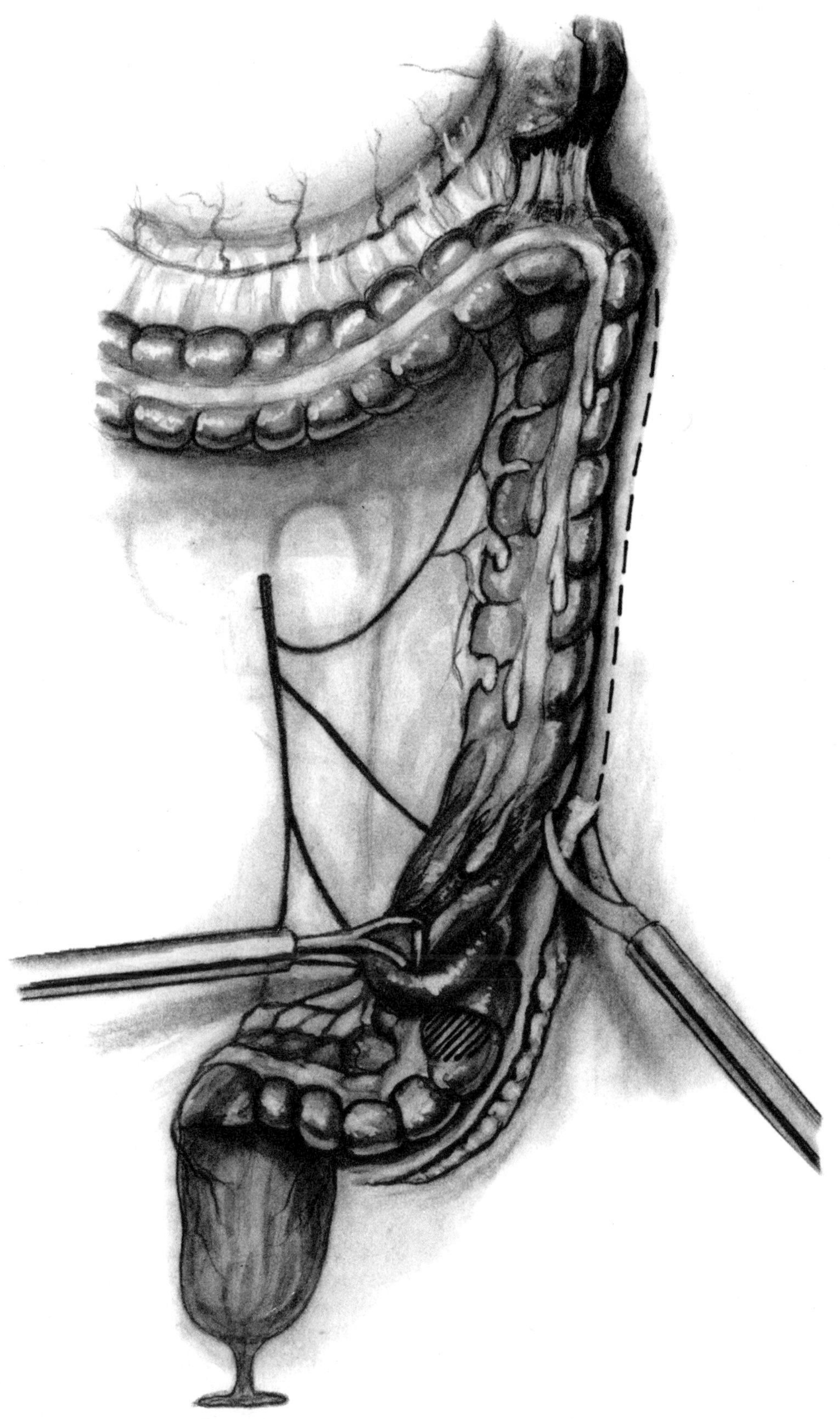

FIGURE 54.6

Laparoscopic Left Hemicolectomy

FIGURE 54.7
Once the left hemicolon has been mobilized, dissection of the vessels in the mesocolon using a curved laparoscopic clamp is carried out. These vessels are then ligated with clips. Two clips are placed proximally and two are placed distally with a 10-mm space between them. With curved laparoscopic scissors, the vascular pedicles between the clips are transected. In order to carry out a safer procedure, the proximal stump is ligated with an Endoloop (8). The vessels to be ligated and divided in a left hemicolectomy are pointed out in the drawing.

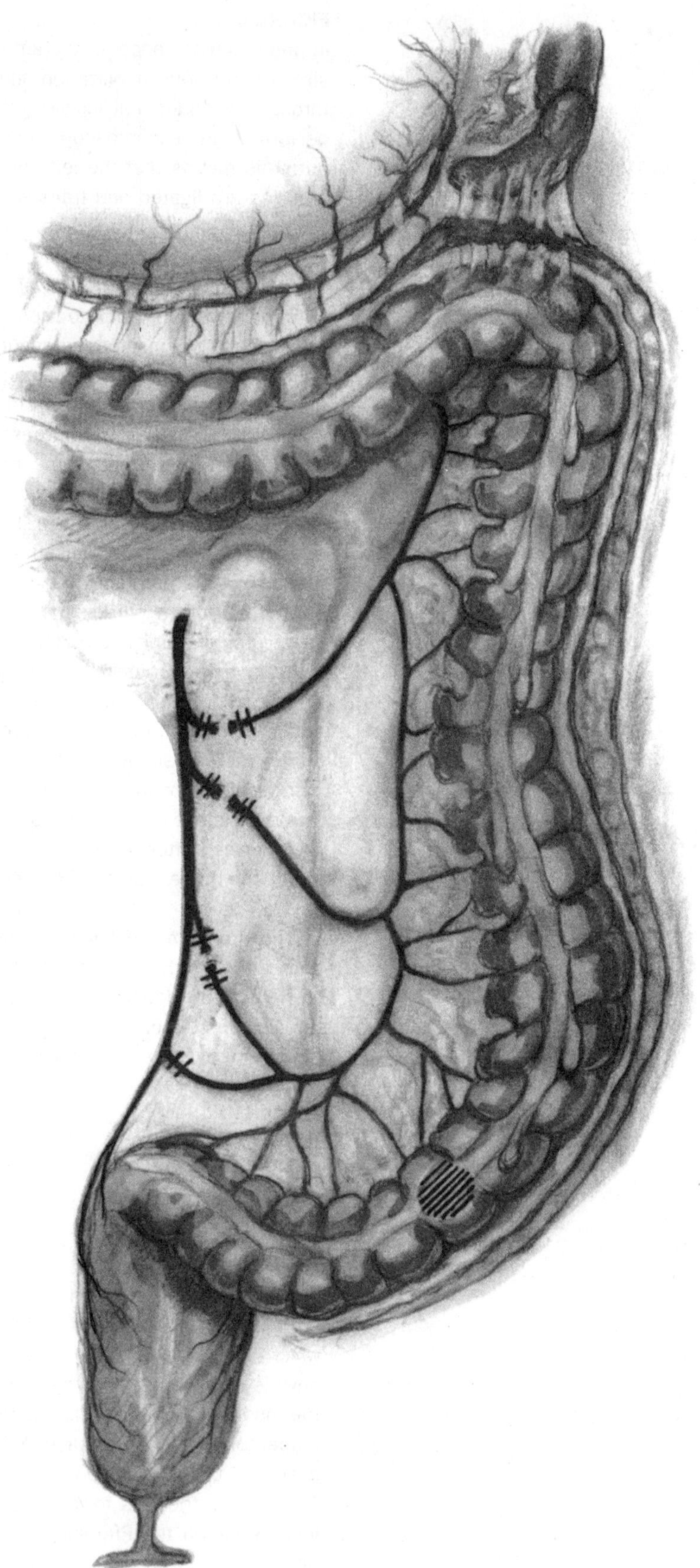

FIGURE 54.7

FIGURE 54.8

In patients with cancer of the left hemicolon in which it is possible to carry out mobilization and exteriorization of the colon through an abdominal incision, the same procedure as that performed in a laparoscopic right hemicolectomy is carried out. This means that the left colon is mobilized, the vascular pedicles are ligated and transected, the colon is exteriorized, and the segmental hemicolon with the tumor is removed. The colonic ends are then sutured manually or by means of mechanical suture, and the bowel is reintroduced into the abdominal cavity in order to close the abdominal wound and reestablish the pneumoperitoneum. In patients in whom it is impossible to exteriorize the colon with the tumor because it is located in the inferior segment of the sigmoid colon (rectosigmoid area), or in the rectum, reestablishment of intestinal transit should be performed by means of a circular Premium CEEA (U.S. Surgical) instrument or using the Proximate ILS (Ethicon) instrument introduced through the anus without the anvil. The anastomosis is carried out after resecting the colon with the tumor. For this purpose, the suprapubic trocar is replaced by an 18-mm trocar in order to allow the introduction of an endolineal stapler (Endoscopic linear cutter). This instrument simultaneously carries out suturing of the rectal sigmoid and transection of the bowel below the tumor. The transected and sutured proximal colon is exteriorized through an incision in the abdominal wall about 5-6 cm long. Once the colon with the tumor has been exteriorized, it is resected and a purse string suture carried out in the proximal colon end into which the anvil is introduced after it is removed from the Premium EEA instrument. The purse string is then tied down around the axis of the anvil.

Laparoscopic Left Hemicolectomy

The Premium CEEA instrument, without the anvil, is introduced through the rectum until its end is above the suture line carried out previously with the endolineal stapler. The stem of the EEA instrument should perforate the sutured rectal sigmoid end, either above, below, or through the previously performed suture line.

FIGURE 54.9

The proximal colon contains the anvil held in place by the purse string, which has been adjusted around the axis of the anvil, which has been removed from the stem. The colon with the anvil is reintroduced into the abdominal cavity. The incision in the abdominal wall is closed in two layers, and the pneumoperitoneum is reestablished. Through the suprapubic port, a special clamp is introduced to grasp the axis of the anvil. This directs the axis toward the rectum in order to introduce into its lumen the Premium EEA instrument. The axis of the anvil functions as a female instrument while the axis of the EEA instrument functions as a male instrument. Once the axis of the EEA instrument is introduced into the axis of the anvil, the cartridge is approximated to the anvil.

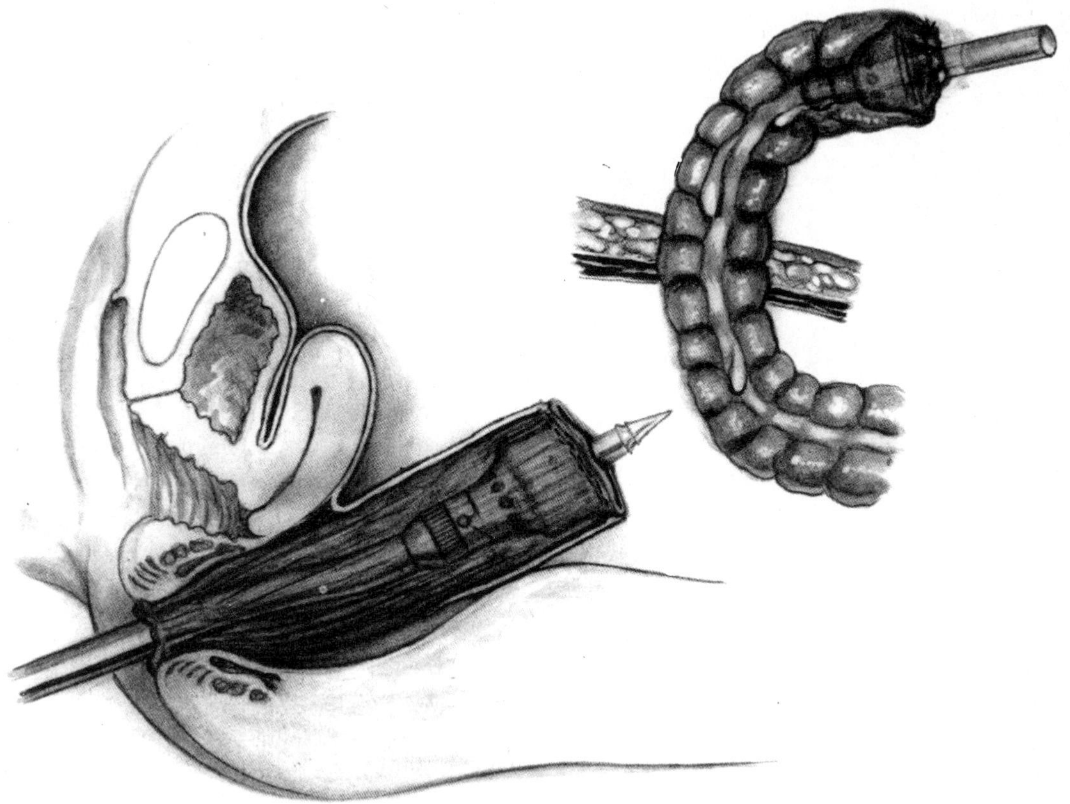

FIGURE 54.8

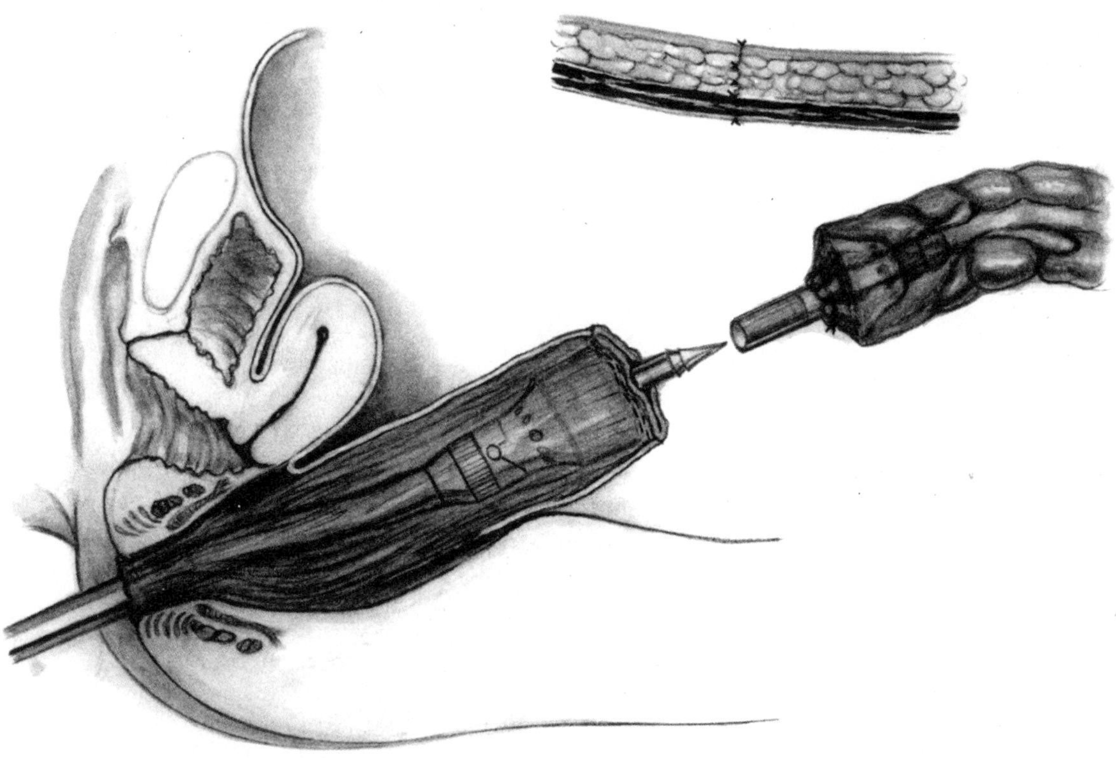

FIGURE 54.9

FIGURE 54.10
Once the cartridge of the EEA instrument has been approximated to the anvil, the instrument is fired, producing an anastomosis of the rectosigmoid to the colon. The instrument is removed from the rectum and the resected rings of intestine are investigated to be sure they are complete. The adequacy of the stapled anastomosis is then investigated. The abdominal cavity is then profusely irrigated with warm saline solution. The colorectal anastomosis can be performed using a rigid Premium EEA instrument or with a Proximate ILS instrument or the flexible and rechargeable 3M stapler.

Laparoscopic Left Hemicolectomy

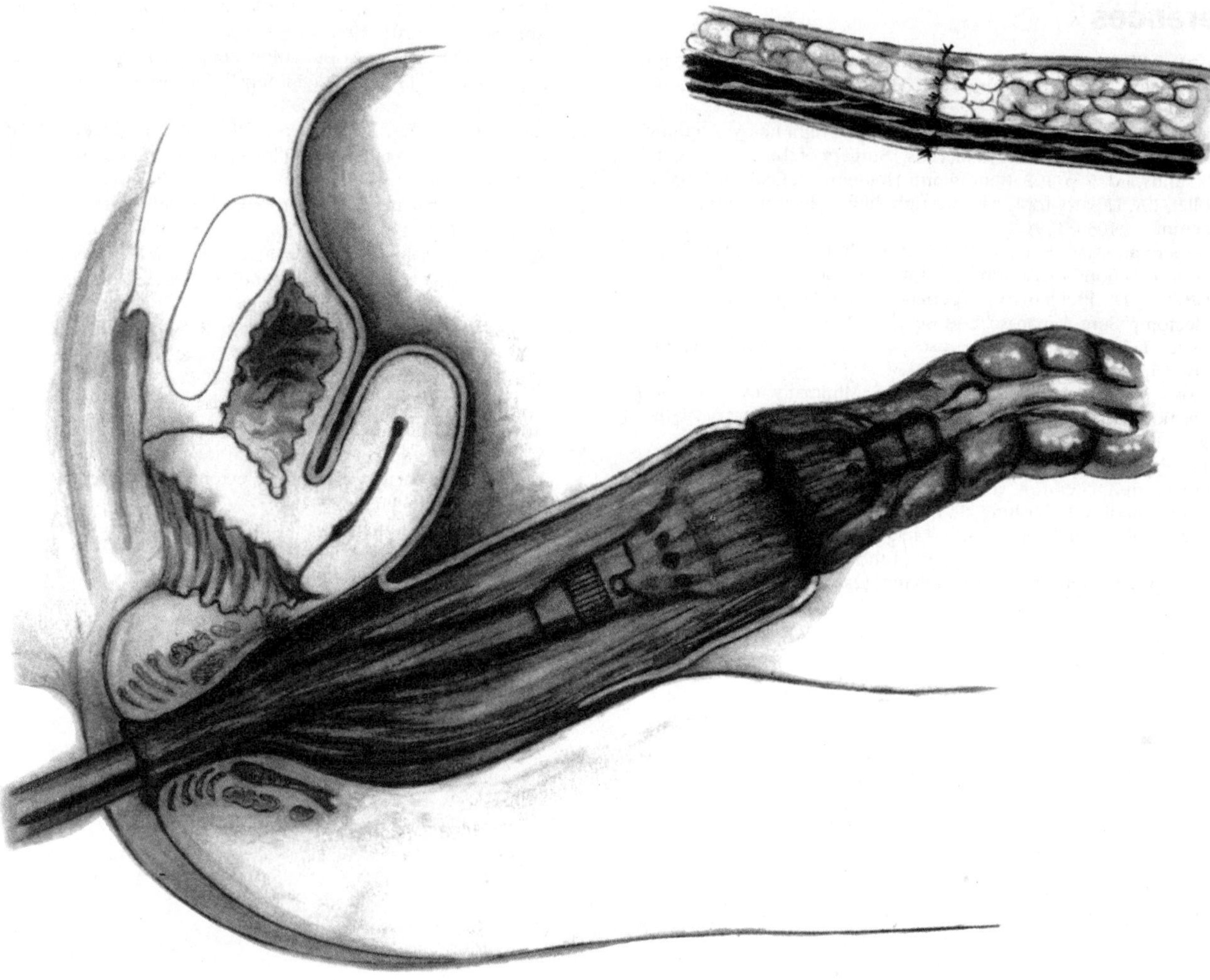

FIGURE 54.10

References

1. Beart, R.W. Jr. Laparoscopic-assisted colon resection. In Corman, M.L. Colon and rectal surgery. Ed. 3, p. 556. J.B. Lippincott, Philadelphia, 1993.
2. Beart, R.W. Jr., Lee, H. Laparoscopic-assisted right hemicolectomy. In Fielding, L.P., Goldberg, S.M. (Eds.) Surgery of the colon, rectum and anus. Ed. 5, p. 192. Butterworth-Heinemann, Oxford, 1993.
3. Coller, J.A. Laparoscopic-assisted right hemicolectomy. Dis. Colon Rectum. 34:1030, 1991.
4. Cooperman, A.M., Katz, V., Zimmon, D., Botero, G. Laparoscopic colon resection: A case report. J. Laparosc. Surg. 1:221, 1991.
5. Corbitt, J.D. Preliminary experience with laparoscopic-guided colectomy. Surg. Laparosc. Endosc. 2:79, 1992.
6. Fowler, D.L., White, S.A. Laparoscopic-assisted sigmoid resection. Surg. Laparosc. Endosc. 1:183, 1991.
7. Jacobs, M., Verdeja, J.C., Goldstein, H.S. Minimally invasive colon resection (laparoscopic colectomy). Surg. Laparosc. Endosc. 1:144, 1991.
8. Jacobs, M., Verdeja, J.C., Placencia, G. Laparoscopic colonic surgery. In Zucker, K.A. (Ed.) Surgical laparoscopy update. p. 327. Quality Medical Publishing, St. Louis, 1993.
9. Leahy, P.F. Laparoscopic-assisted left hemicolectomy. In Fielding L.P., Goldberg, S.M. (Eds.) Surgery of the colon, rectum and anus. Ed. 5, p. 196. Butterworth-Heinemann, Oxford, 1993.
10. Papas, T.N. Laparoscopic colectomy, the innovation continues. Ann. Surg. 216:701, 1992.
11. Sackier, J.M. Laparoscopic colon and rectal surgery. In Hunter, J.G., Sackier, J.M. (Eds.) Minimally invasive surgery. p. 179. McGraw-Hill, New York, 1993.
12. Salky, B.A., Bauer, J.J. Laparoscopic sigmoid resection. In Bauer, J.J. (Ed.). Colorectal surgery illustrated. p. 79. Mosby–Year Book, St. Louis, 1993.
13. Scoggin, S., Frazer, R.C. Laparoscopic bowel resection. Dis. Colon Rectum. 35:20, 1992.
14. Stolfi, V.M., Wilson, J.W., Fazie, V.W., Church, J.M. Laparoscopic intestinal sugery: A preliminary report. Dis. Colon Rectum 38:21, 1992.
15. Thorson, A.G., Wexner, S.D., Beart, R.W., Jagelman, D.G., Falk, P.M., Fitsggibon, R.J. Jr. Laparoscopic colectomy—A critical appraisal. Dis. Colon Rectum 35:21, 1992.
16. Wexner, S.D., Johansen, O.B. Laparoscopic bowel resection: Advantages and limitations. Ann. Med. 24:105, 1992.
17. Wexner, S.D., Johansen, O.B., Nogueras, J.J., Jagelman, D.G. Laparoscopic total abdominal colectomy: A prospective trial. Dis. Colon Rectum 35:651, 1992.
18. Wexner, S.D. Laparoscopic colectomy. In Keighley, M.R.B., Williams, N.S. (Eds.) Surgery of the anus, rectum and colon. Vol. 2, p. 2434. W.B. Saunders, London, 1993.

Section H

Colon, Rectum, and Anus

CHAPTER 55

Appendectomy

Even though the frequency of acute appendicitis has diminished in recent years, it continues to be the most common cause of acute abdomen (23, 26). Acute appendicitis may occur at any age but does so more frequently between 10 and 30 years of age. Patients with appendicitis at that stage of life are usually easier to diagnose than children under 5 years of age and old people, who frequently present a confusing, atypical clinical picture, which may make the diagnosis of appendicitis difficult. It is also difficult to make the diagnosis of appendicitis in immunosuppressed patients and in pregnant women. In these atypical cases the morbidity and mortality of acute appendicitis is increased due to delays in diagnosis and treatment (24, 27).

The appendix presents numerous variations in position, in relation to the cecum. In addition, the cecum also presents numerous variations in position due to its embryologic development and incomplete rotation of the colon. The most frequent position of the cecum is in the right iliac fossa, but it can be located in different parts of the abdomen, in the subhepatic region, in a submesenteric position, in the lesser pelvis, in the left iliac fossa, and so on (30). These variations in the position of the cecum and the appendix explain the surgical difficulties that occur in some patients during appendectomy. In spite of these variations in the position of the appendix in relation to the cecum, two facts do not vary:

1. The base of the appendix is always located at the point of convergence of the three cecal tenias.
2. The appendix is situated 2 to 2.5 cm below the ileocecal valve.

Both characteristics acquire great importance in identification of the appendix during surgery in difficult cases (10).

Originally the appendix is located at the vertex of the cecum. However, because the embryonic evolution of the cecum is asymmetrical, the appendix appears to be situated posteromedially, and not in the fundus of the cecum. The functions of the cecal appendix remain unknown (9). Histologic examination of the appendix usually shows a large quantity of lymphatic tissue. This remains constant up to 30 years of age but then gradually disappears until it is all gone in old age (9).

In more than 70% of cases, the determining factor in appendicitis is obstruction of the appendiceal lumen. In the remaining 30% of cases, acute appendicitis is not obstructive but catarrhal in origin (9).

The diagnosis of acute appendicitis is made by investigating the location and characteristics of the pain, the presence of signs of peritoneal irritation in the right iliac fossa, the presence of spasm of the muscles of the abdominal wall in the site of the pain, moderate fever, leukocytosis, and so on. The variable locations of the cecal appendix make diagnosis difficult and test the most experienced clinician. At present, many additions have been made in the clinical diagnosis such as high-resolution ultrasonography, computed tomography, and laparoscopy. Ultrasonography is important in diagnosing appendiceal and tuboovarian abscesses (17). It should be pointed out that ultrasonography is not useful in acute appendicitis if an abscess or diffuse peritonitis has not developed. Rectal examination is of great diagnostic importance to exclude a pelvic abscess. A plain abdominal x-ray of the abdomen should be taken to determine the position of the cecum in the abdomen.

In 25% of cases acute appendicitis leads to perforation. The number of perforations is larger in patients under 10 years of age and even larger in patients over 60 years old (9, 10, 26).

APPENDICEAL PHLEGMON

An appendiceal phlegmon is a palpable mass produced by an acute inflammatory process in the appendix, which has usually begun 4 to 5 days previously, and which produces an inflammatory mass made up of a conglomerate of small bowel loops joined to each other and adherent to the greater omentum, without the development of a purulent collection or abscess. This inflammatory process develops in 2 to 8% of cases of acute appendicitis and may be reabsorbed and disappear or become complicated by the development of an abscess or generalized peritonitis. In patients with an appendiceal phlegmon, appendectomy is not indicated if the patient is stable, afebrile, and has a soft abdomen and no leucocytosis (4, 7, 9, 12, 13). The appendix should be removed after more than 30 days have passed. If the clinical picture of a phlegmon of the appendix becomes complicated with an abscess or generalized peritonitis, surgery should not be delayed (4, 7, 9, 10, 12, 13, 18, 26, 28).

APPENDICEAL ABSCESS

This is a purulent collection blocked off by small bowel loops together with the greater omentum around an acutely inflamed appendix, which is usually perforated. Location of an appendiceal abscess is directly related to the topography of the cecum and the appendix. Therefore, any appendiceal abscess may be located in the right iliac fossa, in the right subhepatic space, in the pouch of Douglas, and so on. The initial treatment of an appendiceal abscess is medical, with antibiotics. If significant improvement with medical treatment occurs in 24 hours, the treatment should be continued. If the pain persists or becomes worse, however, or if the abscess increases in size, the temperature remains elevated, and the leukocytes in the blood rise or the palpable mass becomes fluctuant, surgical intervention should be carried out without delay, before spontaneous rupture of the abscess into the peritoneal cavity occurs. Surgical treatment of an appendiceal abscess consists of aspiration of the purulent contents and the sloughed tissue in the abscess, using an electric aspirator. The pathologic appendix can be removed during the intervention, if its removal is easy. Appendectomy should be avoided if it is necessary to separate inflamed loops of small bowel that are adherent to each other, with danger of injuring the bowel or rupturing the abscess. The abscess is drained to the outside by means of a Penrose drain brought out through a small stab wound. Some appendiceal abscesses, because of their location, should be drained through the rectum or the vagina.

Before intervening surgically, the patient should be reexamined, once anesthetized and relaxed. This palpation allows the surgeon to locate the abscess more exactly and place the incision in the most adequate site. If the appendix is not resected at the time the abscess is drained, because it is not advisable, the appendectomy should be done once the inflammatory process is over. If the appendix is not removed, recurrence of acute appendicitis, with or without abscess, will occur in 10% of patients (3, 26, 31). The appendiceal abscess can also be drained percutaneously under sonographic control or using computed tomography. If percutaneous drainage fails, surgical drainage can be used.

INCISIONS FOR APPENDECTOMY

Numerous incisions have been proposed to perform an appendectomy. Among them, the most used is the McArthur-McBurney incision (13), proposed by these New York surgeons in 1893. This incision is known as the McBurney incision. Another incision that is used is the Murphy incision, from the United States, known in France as the Jalaquier incision and in other countries as the Battle-Jalaguier-Kammerer incision. Many other incisions have been used in appendectomies. Some of them are the Rocky-Davis incision, the Sonnenburg incision, the Roux incision, the Lecène incision, the Chaput incision, and so on.

McBurney Incision

This incision is also known as a gridiron incision. It has the characteristic of entering the abdomen without transecting any muscle, simply splitting their fibers. The McBurney incision has several advantages (7):

1. It does not transect any muscles, as has been pointed out.
2. It does not injure any important vessels or nerves.
3. The incision is carried out at the site where the appendix is usually located.
4. Since no muscles are transected, the incision has a great tendency to close spontaneously, leaving a strong scar.
5. To close this incision, minimal suture material is used.

Besides these advantages, McBurney's incision presents some inconveniences:

1. The operative field is limited and insufficient in complex cases.
2. The abdomen cannot be satisfactorily explored through this incision.
3. In cases in which the incision's extension is insufficient, it can result in a weakened abdominal wall and an incisional hernia.
4. In cases with a doubtful diagnosis of appendicitis or in the presence of peritonitis of appendiceal origin, it is not advisable to use a McBurney incision, and an infraumbilical midline or paramedian incision should be used.

Extension of the McBurney Incision

The McBurney incision can be extended medially by transecting the anterior fascia of the rectus abdominis muscle for a distance of 2 cm. A Farabeuf or Richardson retractor is then inserted to retract the rectus muscle medially, allowing transection of the fascia of the posterior rectus muscle transversely for a distance of 2 cm, the same extent as the anterior fascia. During this maneuver, care should be taken to avoid injuring the epigastric vessels that run behind the anterior rectus muscle, wrapped in a thin fascia (7). In some cases the anterior rectus muscle itself can be transected transversely (6).

The McBurney incision can be extended laterally and upward, transecting the wide muscles of the abdomen, after splitting them, in some cases of ascending retrocecal or subhepatic appendicitis. This extension, however, produces a lot of weakness of the abdominal wall. In these cases it is better to close the McBurney incision and perform another, better adapted incision.

Murphy Incision

Murphy performed the first appendectomy on March 2, 1889, using the incision favored by him during his whole active life as a surgeon. The technique of this incision will be described later.

OTHER INDICATIONS FOR APPENDECTOMY

The great majority of appendectomies are done for acute appendicitis. On very few occasions appendectomy is done for other diagnoses. These could be recurring appendicitis and, exceptionally, chronic appendicitis, the existence of which is controversial. Other indications for appendectomy are mucocele or carcinoid tumor.

Appendiceal mucocele is characterized by marked increase in the diameter of the appendiceal lumen and changes in the appendiceal mucosa with hypersecretion of mucus. In some cases this process may extend outside the cecal appendix, causing appendiceal pseudomyxoma. When the mucocele is strictly localized to the appendix, appendectomy is the only treatment. If the mucocele has extended beyond the appendix, a more extensive operation should be performed.

The cecal appendix is the seat of the majority of carcinoid tumors. Carcinoid tumors of the appendix are usually small and asymptomatic, and are incidental histologic findings. In the majority of cases, appendectomy is enough treatment. There are a few exceptions:

1. Patients with a carcinoid 2 cm or larger in diameter.
2. Presence of metastases in regional lymph nodes.
3. Presence of tumor infiltration at the site of transection of the appendix, which means that there is residual neoplastic tissue.

In these cases a right hemicolectomy is indicated. Some surgeons also perform a right hemicolectomy in cases in which the appendiceal serosa or the mesoappendix are invaded, or when the carcinoid is located in the base of the appendix. Some surgeons will perform a hemicolectomy for tumors over 10 mm and under 20 mm in diameter. Invasion of the muscular layer or the serosa is frequent, but an increase in the incidence of distant metastases has not been proven when a simple appendectomy is performed.

Surgical Technique: Incisions for Appendectomy

FIGURE 55.1

1, McArthur-McBurney incision. Incision in the skin, 5 to 6 cm long, perpendicular to an imaginary line from the umbilicus to the anterior superior ileal spine, about 4 cm medial to the iliac spine. Half of the incision extends above the umbilicospinal line, and the other half extends below it. 2, Drawing of the John B. Murphy incision, called the Jalaguier incision in France and by others the Battle-Jalaguier-Kammerer incision. The Murphy incision is a longitudinal incision parallel to the lateral border of the anterior rectus muscle of the abdomen, 2 cm medial to it, and measuring 6 cm. This incision can be easily extended up or down. The midpoint of the Murphy incision is at the umbilicospinal line.

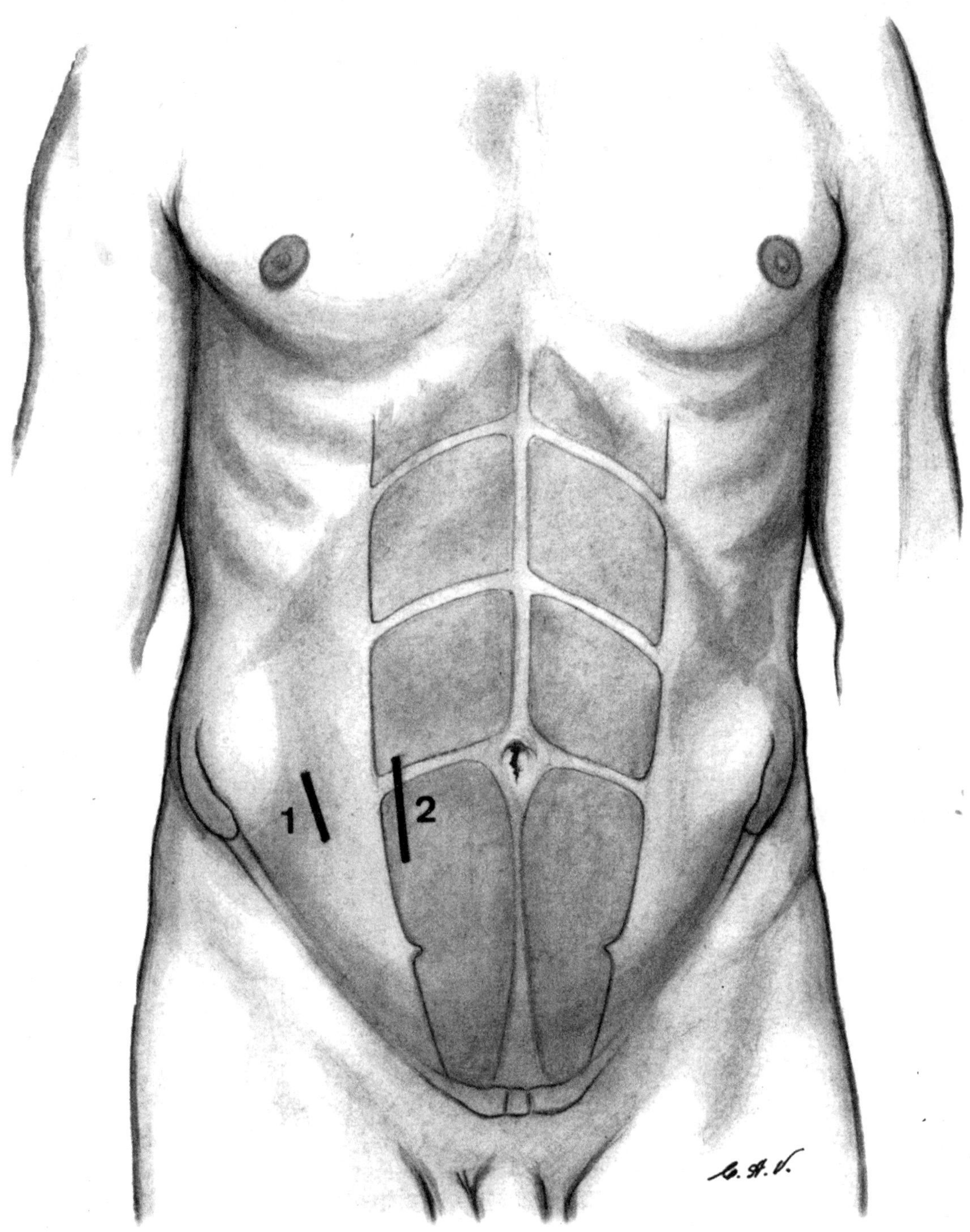

FIGURE 55.1

FIGURE 55.2 TECHNIQUE OF THE MCBURNEY INCISION
The skin and subcutaneous tissue have been incised with a scalpel down to the musculoaponeurotic layer of the major oblique muscle, whose fibers run in the same direction. The inferior tendinous portion is transected with a scalpel, while the muscular portion is split with a closed hemostat, which is opened to make room for the introduction of two Farabeuf, Richardson, or Finochietto retractors. Traction in opposite directions is applied to the retractors to separate the muscle fibers of the major abdominal oblique muscle, as shown in the drawing. Once the fibers of the major oblique have been separated, the muscular fibers of the minor abdominal oblique muscle can be seen running practically transversely.

Surgical Technique: Incisions for Appendectomy

FIGURE 55.3
The fibers of the minor abdominal oblique muscle have been split and separated in the opposite direction by two Farabeuf retractors. In the depth the fibers of the transversus abdominis muscle are seen, running transversely in a direction similar to the fibers of the minor oblique. Under the transversus abdominis is the layer of the fascia transversalis and then the peritoneum.

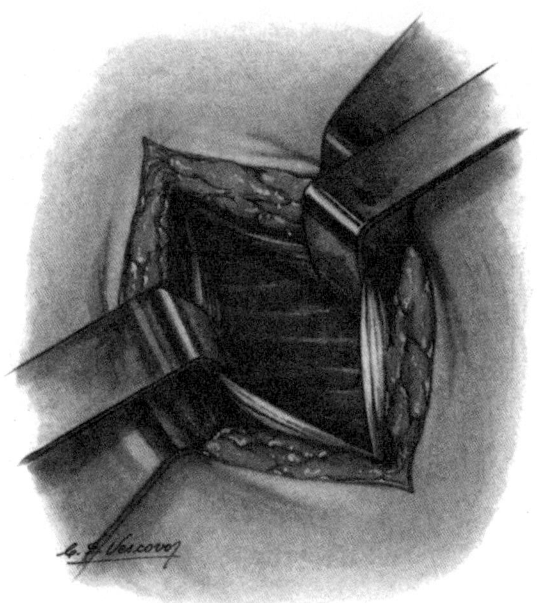

FIGURE 55.2 TECHNIQUE OF THE MCBURNEY INCISION

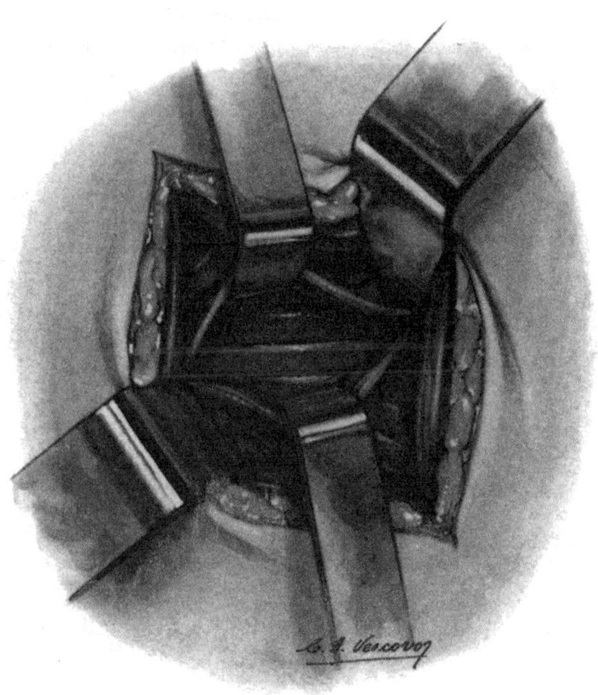

FIGURE 55.3

FIGURE 55.4
The layer formed by the transversalis fascia and the peritoneum has been grasped with two Allis clamps, making sure that an intestinal loop has not been grasped by an Allis clamp. This layer is then incised between the Allis clamps with a scalpel. With the peritoneum opened, the incision is extended upward with scissors and downward with a scalpel.

Surgical Technique: Incisions for Appendectomy

FIGURE 55.5
The transversalis fascia and peritoneum have been incised and Finochietto retractors inserted to amplify the operative field. In cases of normal location of the cecum and appendix, the McBurney incision falls on the most adequate site. The typical characteristics of the cecum can be seen, with its anterior tenia converging to the base of the appendix. The appendix extends in a descending internal direction.

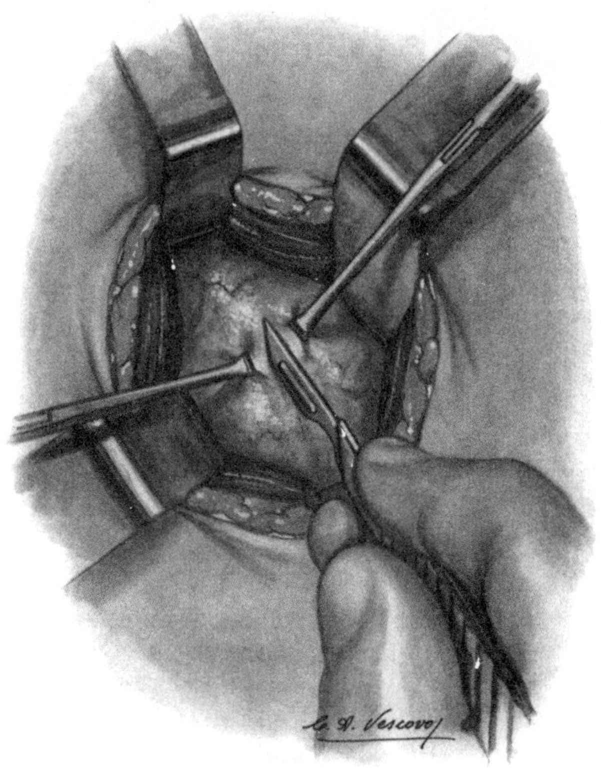

FIGURE 55.4

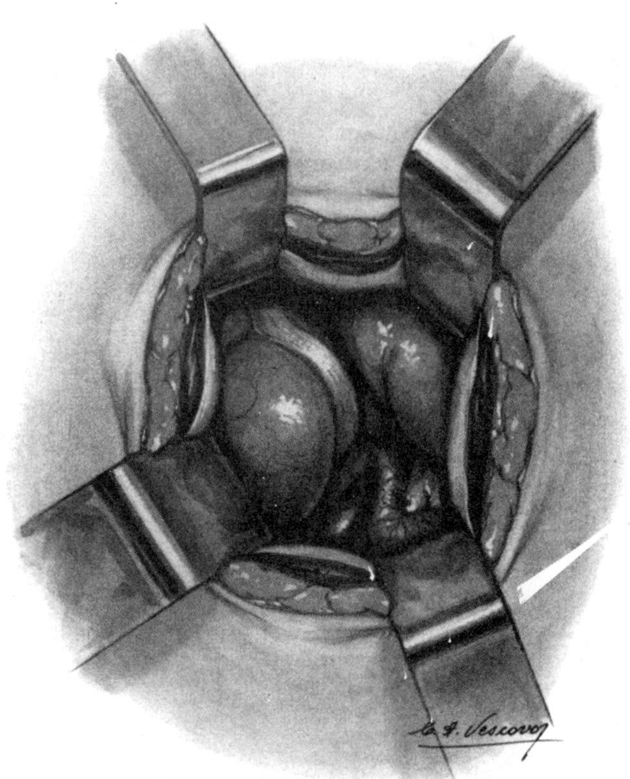

FIGURE 55.5

FIGURE 55.6 CLOSURE OF THE MCARTHUR-MCBURNEY INCISION

The drawing shows the closure of the peritoneum together with the transversalis fascia, using interrupted sutures of synthetic slow absorption material. This layer can also be closed with a continuous suture.

Surgical Technique: Incisions for Appendectomy

FIGURE 55.7

The transverse abdominal muscle has been sutured, and the minor oblique muscle is being closed with two or three sutures, using slow reabsorption synthetic material or chromic catgut. To avoid necrosis of the muscle fibers, the sutures should not be tied too tightly.

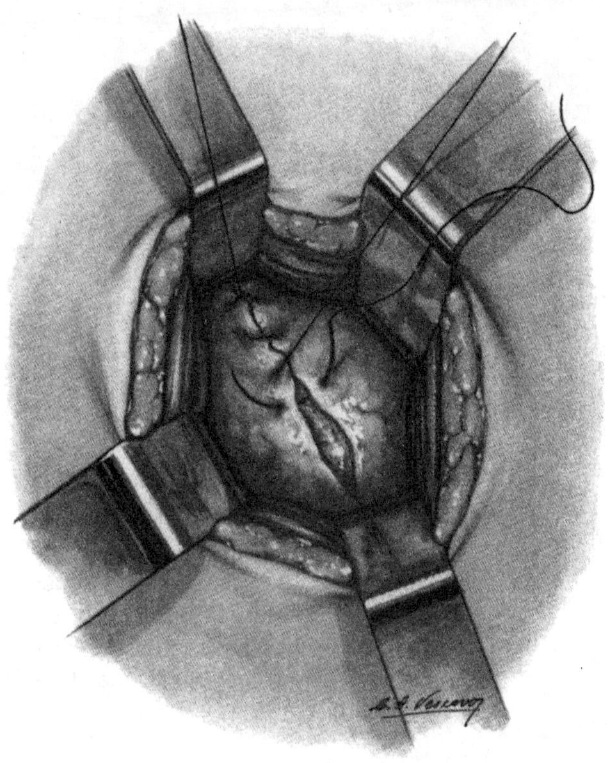

FIGURE 55.6 CLOSURE OF THE MCARTHUR-MCBURNEY INCISION

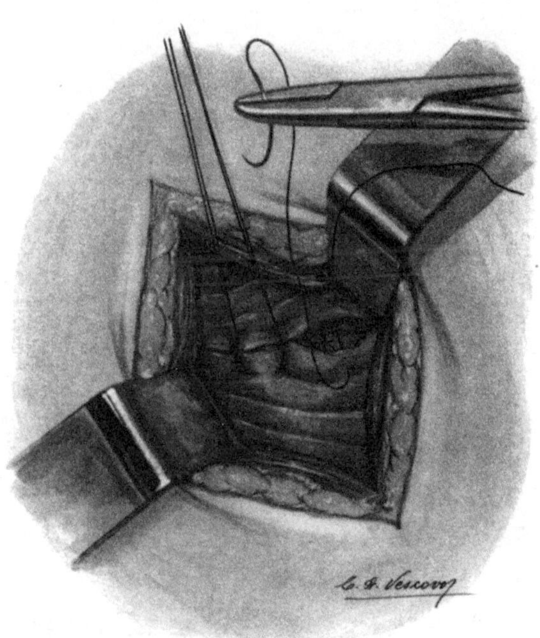

FIGURE 55.7

FIGURE 55.8
The major oblique muscle layer is being sutured, together with its aponeurosis, using the same technique and suture materials as in the minor oblique muscle. The layer of subcutaneous tissue and the skin are then closed.

Surgical Technique: Incisions for Appendectomy

FIGURE 55.9 MURPHY INCISION (JALAGUIER)
Once the skin and subcutaneous tissue are incised, the anterior fascia of the rectus muscle is exposed and, at 2 cm medial to its external border, a longitudinal incision is made to transect the anterior rectus fascia, as shown in the drawing.

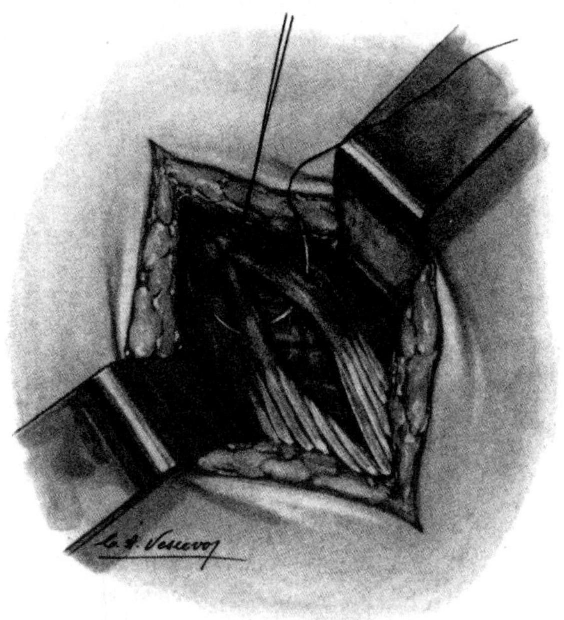

FIGURE 55.8

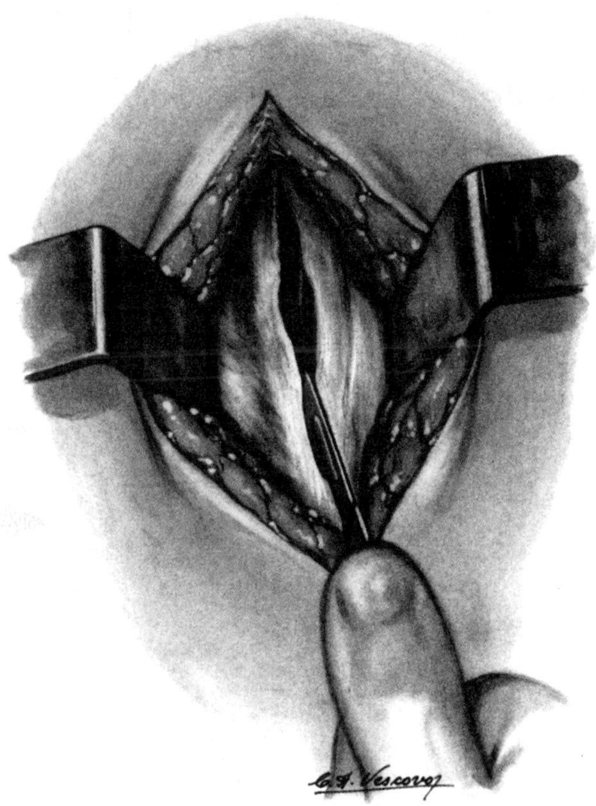

FIGURE 55.9 MURPHY INCISION (JALAGUIER)

FIGURE 55.10
After the anterior rectus fascia has been incised, its lateral border is grasped with two Allis clamps and a Finochietto retractor inserted to apply traction medially on the anterior rectus muscle. The thin layers of tissue around the epigastric vessels behind the muscle are also retracted medially, taking care not to injure them. Retraction of the anterior rectus muscle exposes the posterior fascia of the rectus muscle as well as the semilunar line, as seen in the drawing.

Surgical Technique: Incisions for Appendectomy

FIGURE 55.11
The transversalis fascia and the peritoneum have been grasped with two Allis clamps above the semilunar line, and this layer is about to be incised.

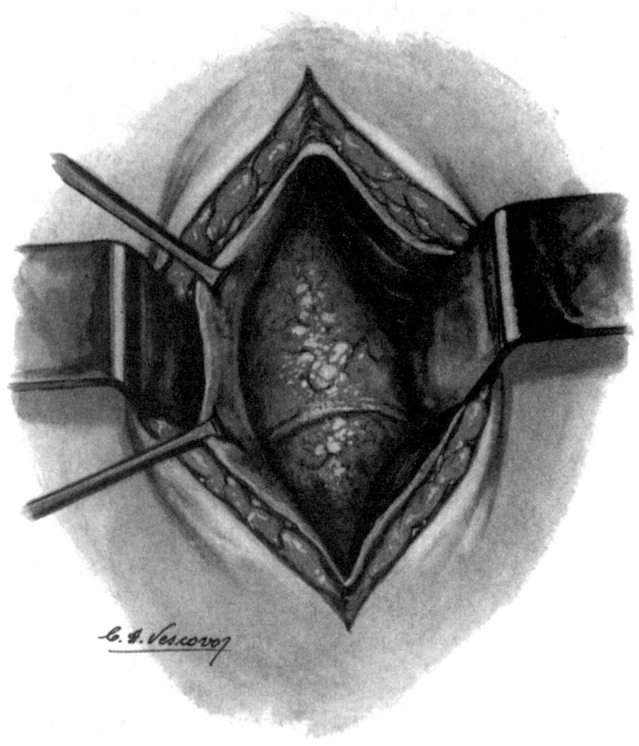

FIGURE 55.10

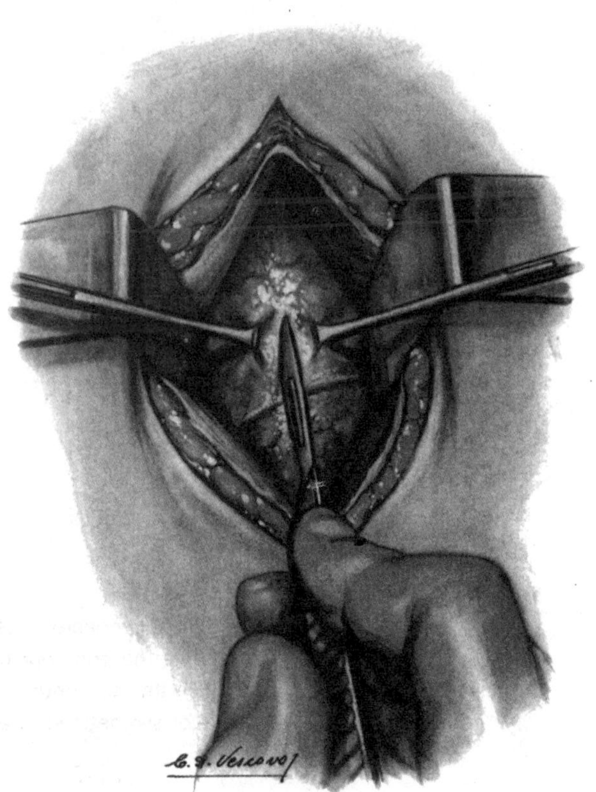

FIGURE 55.11

FIGURE 55.12
The peritoneal cavity has been opened and traction is being applied to the edges of the peritoneum with Allis clamps, exposing the cecum and appendix in normal position. The anterior tenia of the cecum is clearly visible, converging to the base of the appendix, which extends downward.

The Murphy incision is easy to carry out, offers a good surgical field, and can be extended upward or downward, as needed, without having to transect any muscles.

Surgical Technique: Incisions for Appendectomy

FIGURE 55.13
Once the appendectomy is concluded, the incision is closed by suturing the posterior fascia of the anterior rectus muscle together with the peritoneum using interrupted or continuous sutures of synthetic slow absorption material.

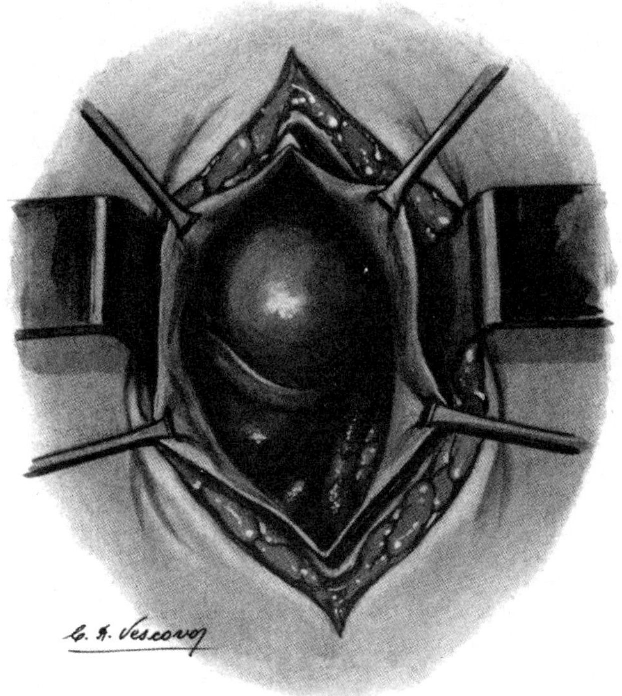

FIGURE 55.12

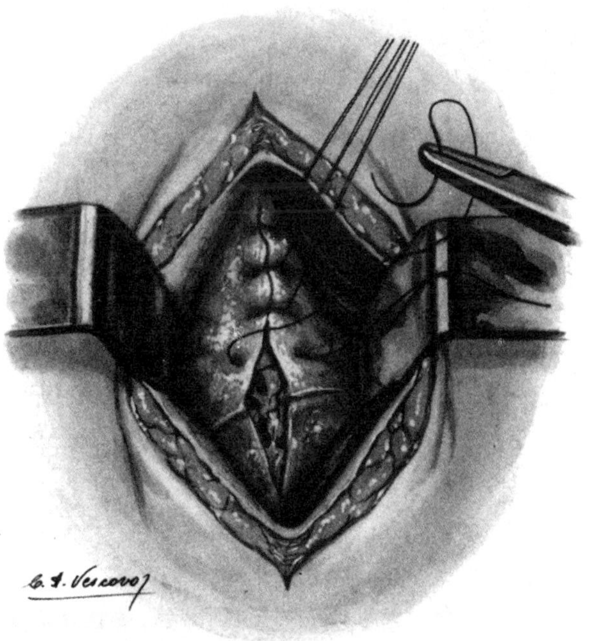

FIGURE 55.13

FIGURE 55.14

The anterior fascia of the anterior rectus muscle is being sutured with interrupted sutures, using synthetic slow absorption material. The subcutaneous layer and the skin are then closed. As shown, closure of the Murphy incision is very simple. If drainage is necessary, it is brought out through a counter incision.

Technique of Appendectomy

FIGURE 55.15 BLOOD SUPPLY OF THE ILEOCECAL REGION

The blood supply of the ileocecal region has numerous variations. This drawing shows one of the most frequent arrangements: 1, ileocolic artery; 2, colic artery; 3, cecal artery, dividing in two branches; 4, anterior cecal artery; 5, posterior cecal artery; 6, appendiceal artery; 7, ileal artery. In more than 30% of cases there is more than one appendiceal artery.

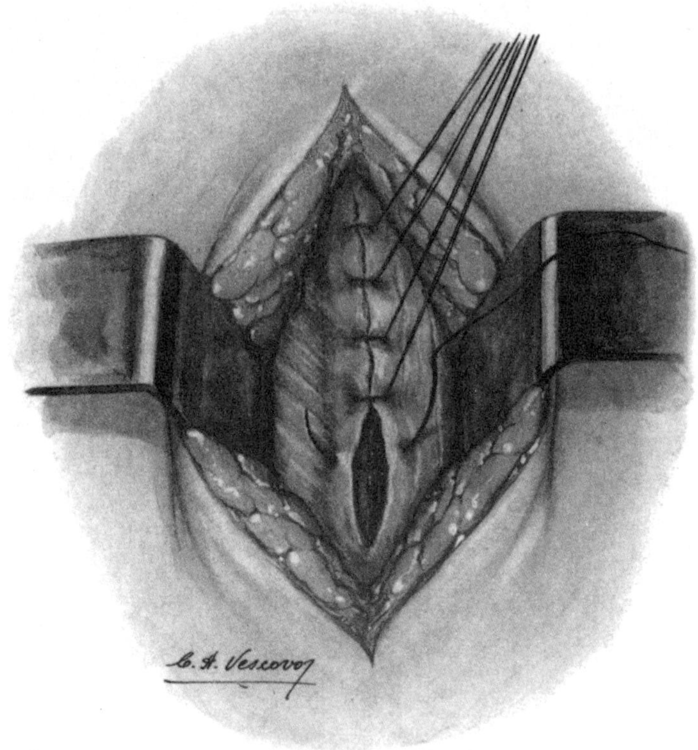

FIGURE 55.14

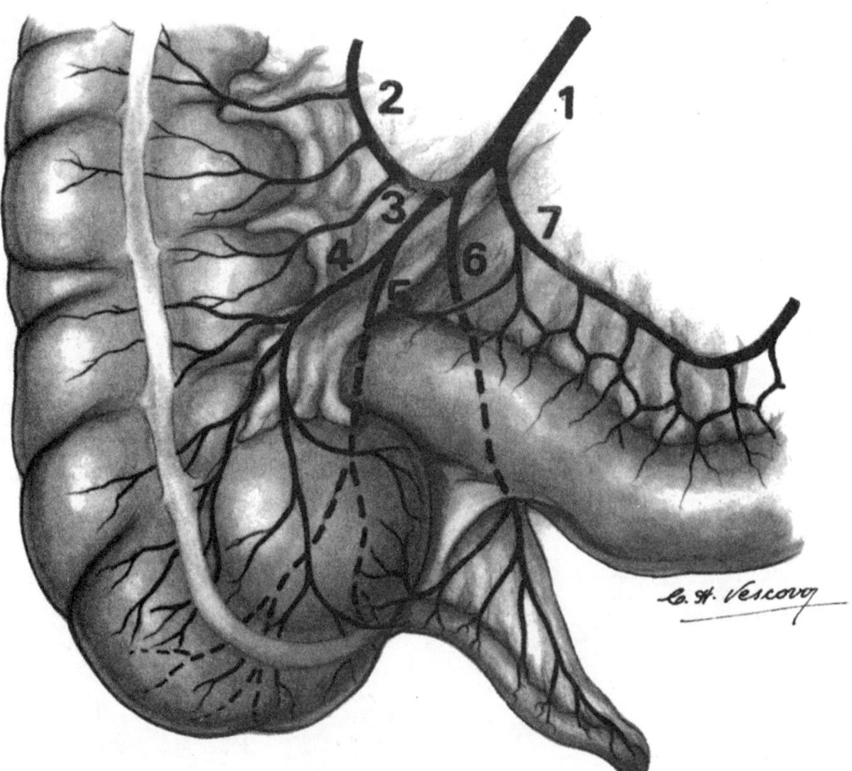

FIGURE 55.15 BLOOD SUPPLY OF THE ILEOCECAL REGION

Technique of Appendectomy

FIGURE 55.16
Schematic drawing showing the cecum in the right liliac fossa, with some of the many variations in position of the cecal appendix: 1, descending appendix; 2, internal lateral appendix; 3, external lateral appendix; 4, ascending retrocecal appendix.

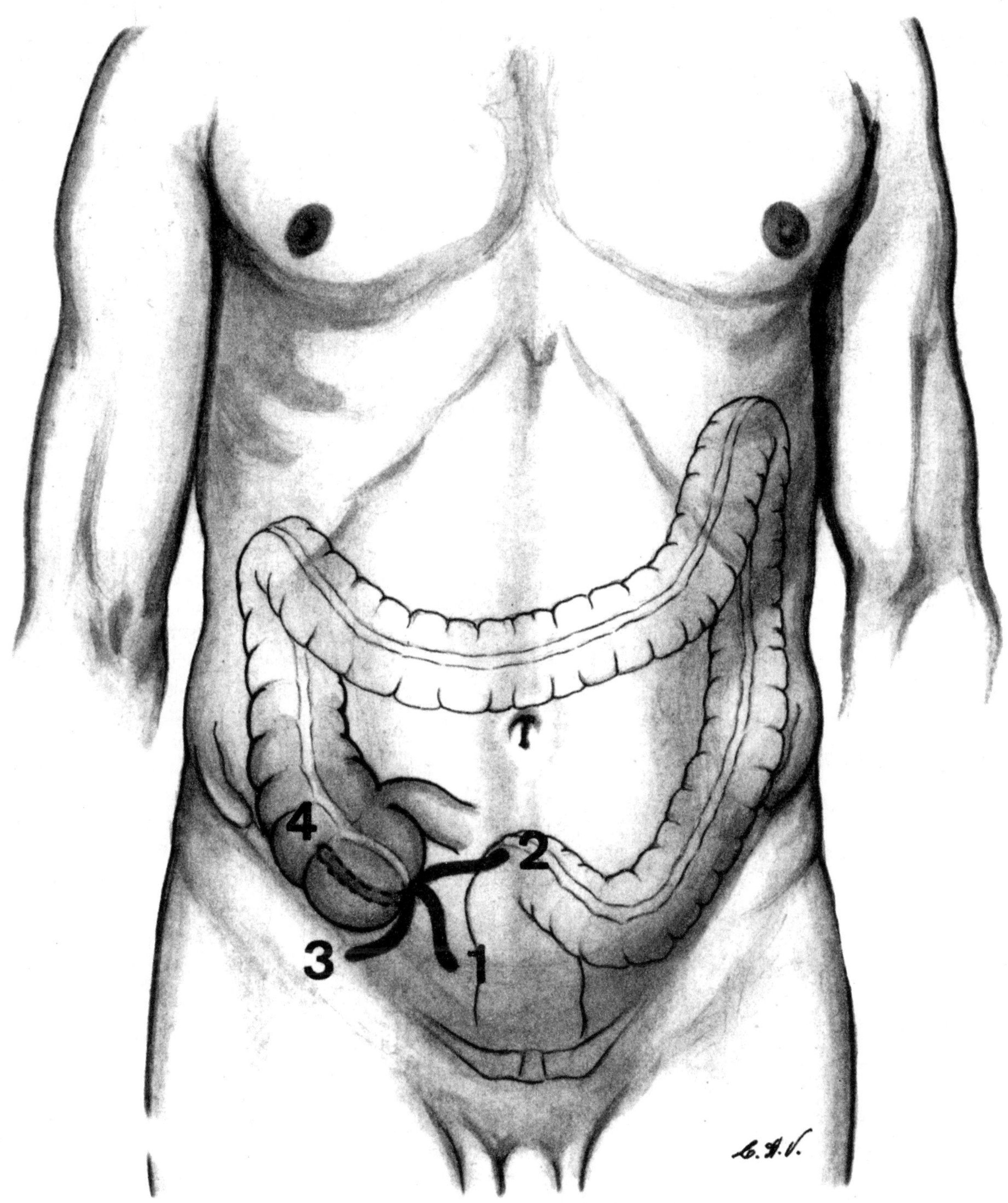

FIGURE 55.16

Technique of Appendectomy

FIGURE 55.17

Once the peritoneum is open, the cecum should be identified. In many cases this is easily done, but in others it may be confusing. The right iliac fossa may be occupied by the transverse or sigmoid colon. The cecum stands out by its prominent anterior tenia. The transverse colon is characterized by its adherent greater omentum, the sigmoid colon by its epiploic appendices, and the small intestine by its smaller caliber and by the absence of tenias or haustrations. If the cecal appendix is not readily found, traction is applied on the cecum with the index and middle fingers, following the cecum to its fundus. This will frequently show the appendix easily if it is free. In some cases the appendix is palpated but cannot be exteriorized due to adhesions holding it to the cecal wall or the mesentery. In these cases the appendix will only be exteriorized after dividing these adhesions. In other cases it is necessary to identify the site of convergence of the three tenias on the cecum and, from there, identify the cecal appendix. In addition, it should always be kept in mind that the base of the appendix is located 2.5 cm below the ileocecal junction. If the appendix does not appear diseased, the possibility of the presence of a Meckel's diverticulum should be investigated. For this purpose at least 90 cm of the terminal ileum should be examined. In the female, the presence of an inflammatory process of the adnexa has to be excluded by digital palpation of the right fallopian tube.

If the appendix presents characteristics of acute appendicitis, its resection will be undertaken. The cecum is delivered out of the surgical wound and held by the assistant's hands or with Babcock clamps. The distal end of the mesoappendix is pulled upward with a hemostatic clamp. The hemostatic clamp should never grasp the inflamed, fragile appendix. The appendiceal artery is ligated by passing a nonabsorbable suture around the base of the mesoappendix, as shown.

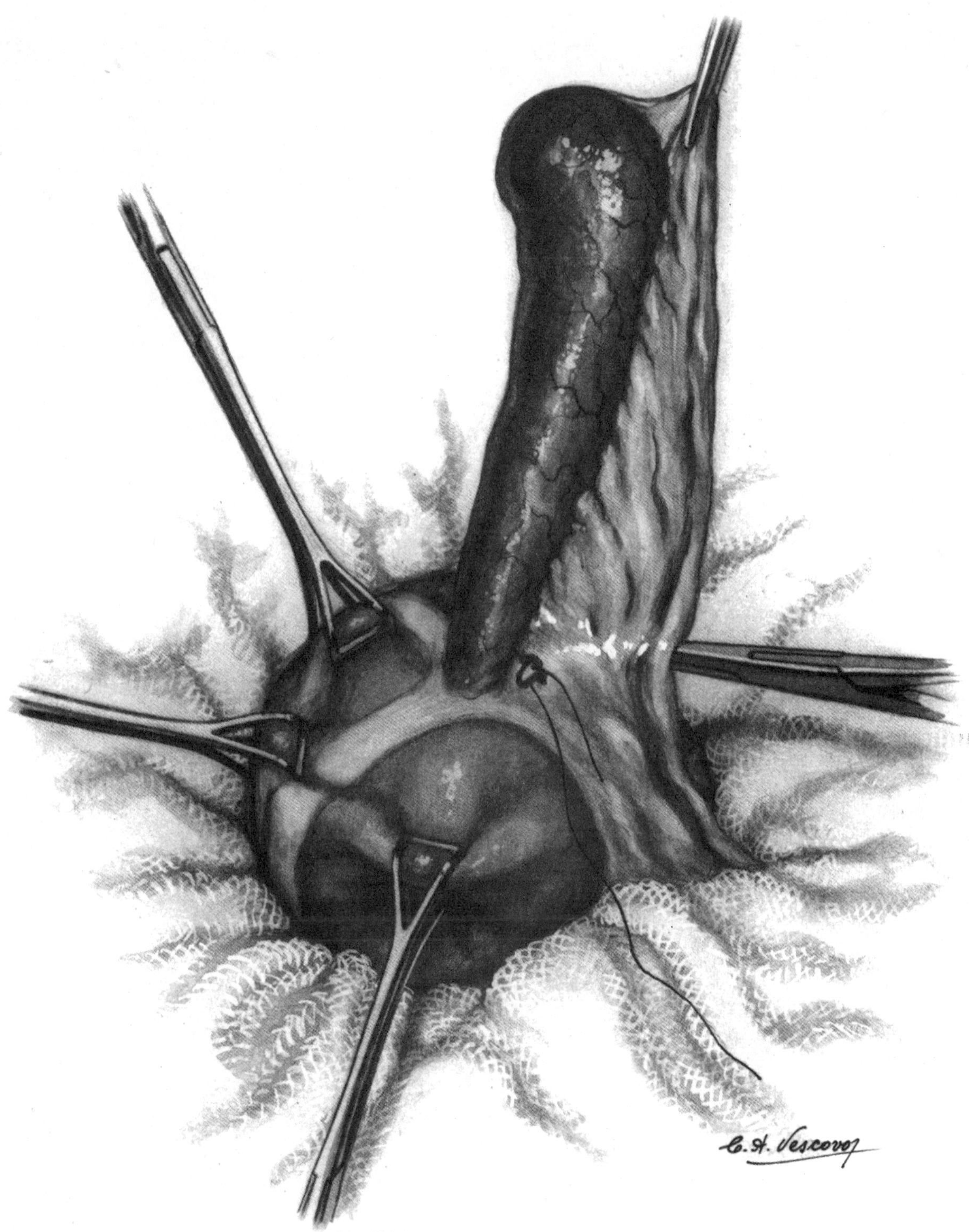

FIGURE 55.17

Technique of Appendectomy

FIGURE 55.18
The appendiceal artery has been ligated and the mesoappendix is being transected above the ligature, with scissors.

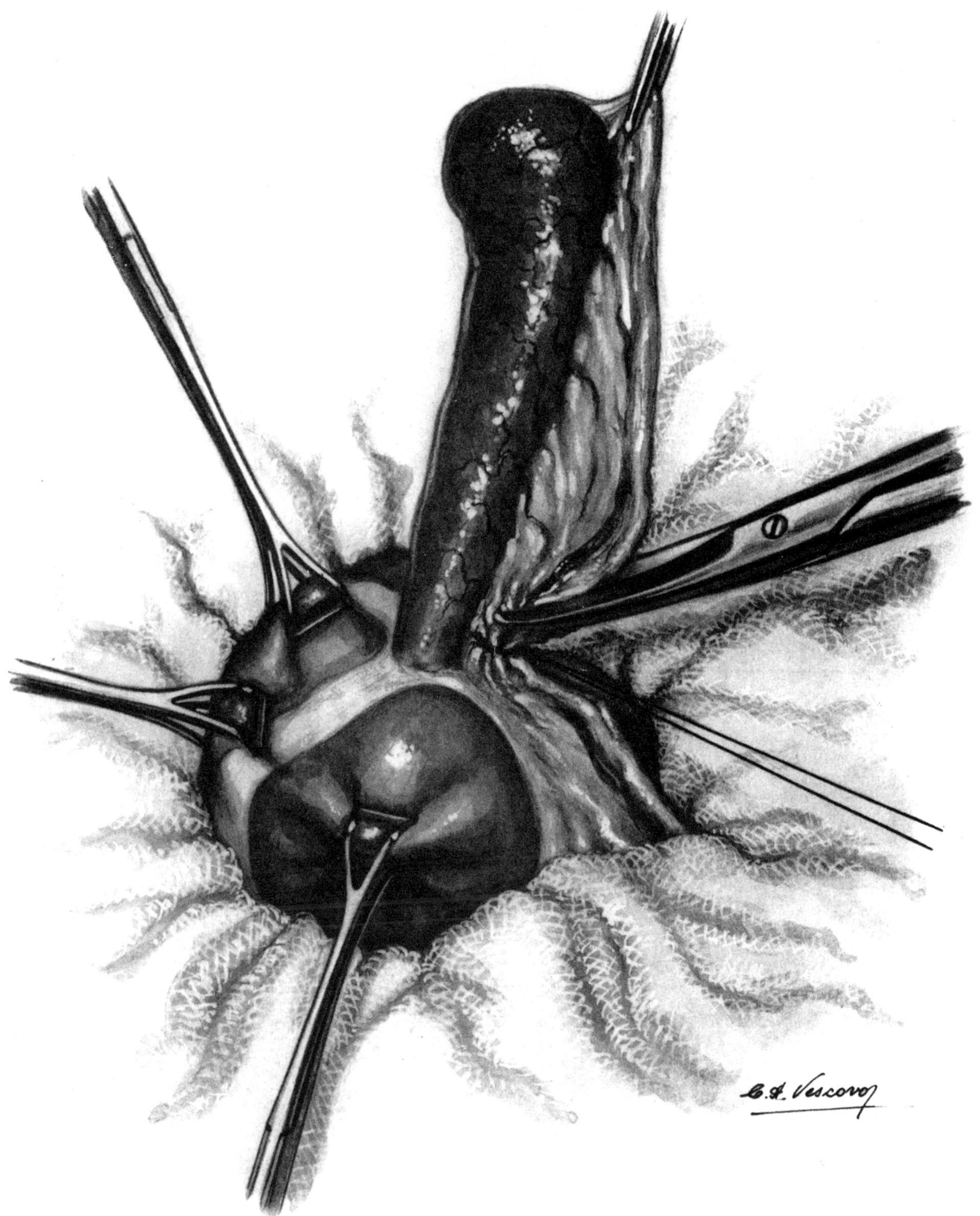

FIGURE 55.18

Technique of Appendectomy

FIGURE 55.19
The stump of the appendiceal artery has been grasped with a curved hemostat and the mesoappendix transected at the base. Using a straight clamp, the base of the appendix has been doubly crushed, as seen.

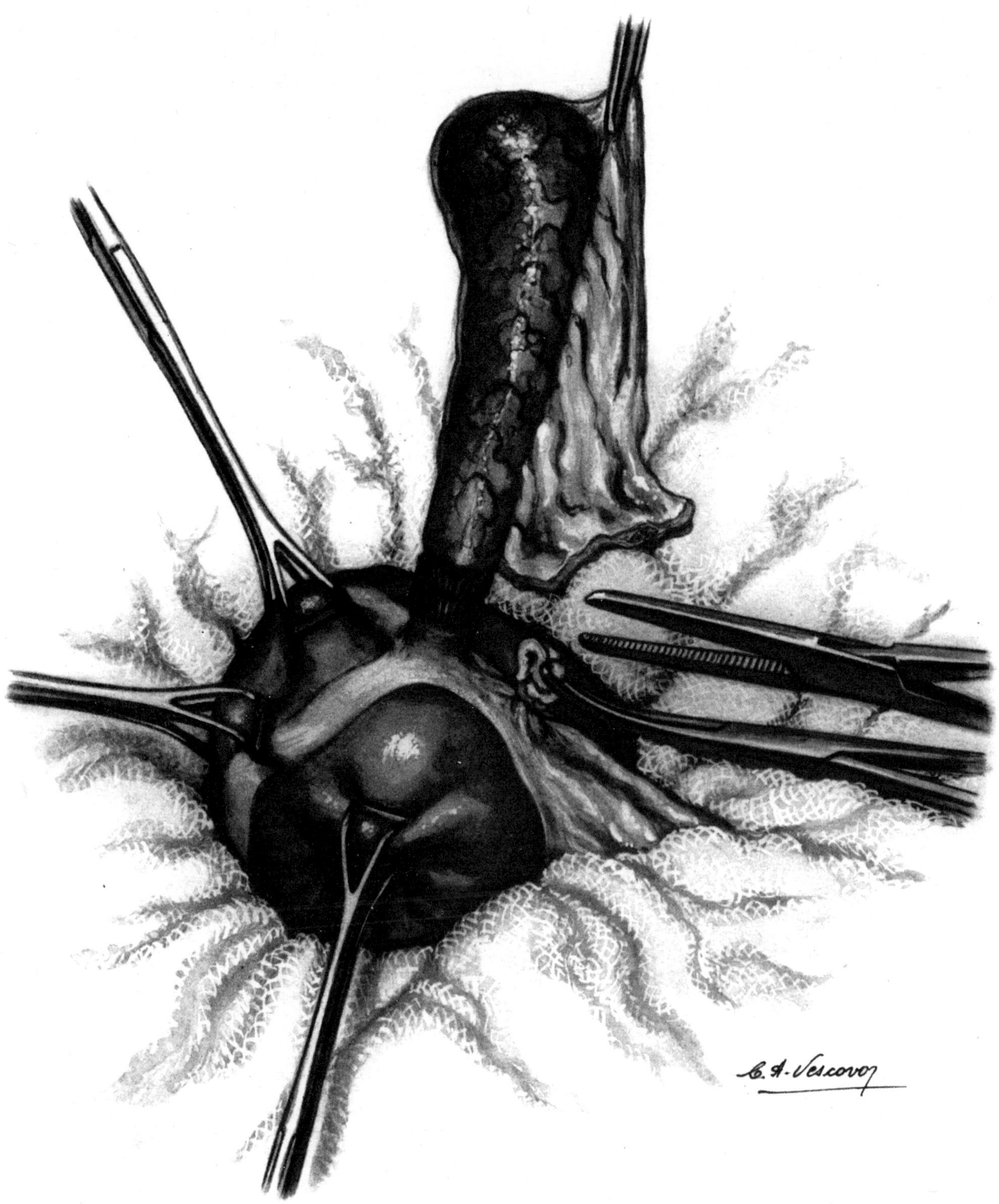

FIGURE 55.19

Technique of Appendectomy

FIGURE 55.20
A purse string suture has been placed around the base of the appendix using a nonabsorbable suture, including only the seromuscular layer of the cecum, about 8 to 10 mm from the base of the appendix.

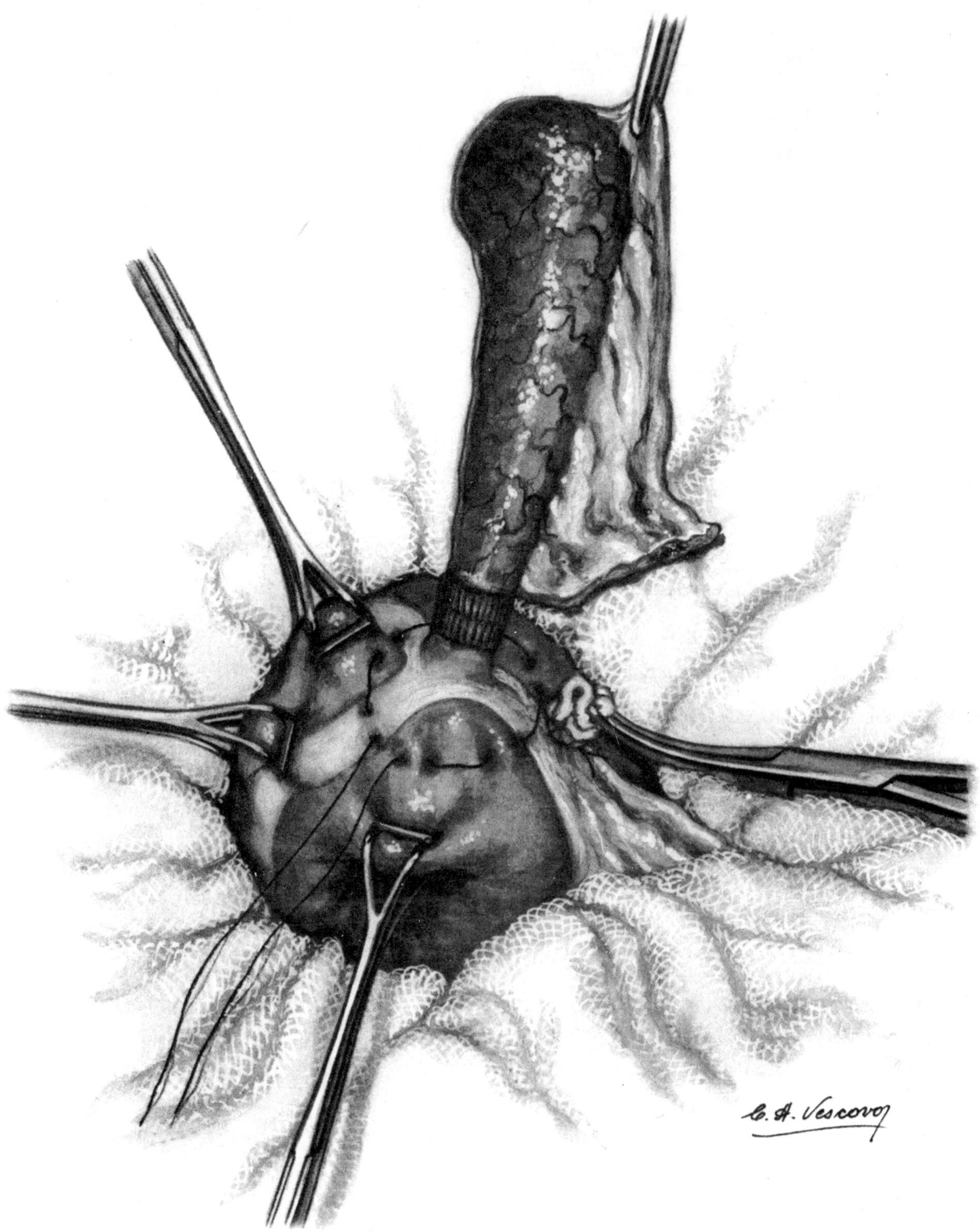

FIGURE 55.20

Technique of Appendectomy

FIGURE 55.21
The base of the appendix is ligated with a nonabsorbable suture.

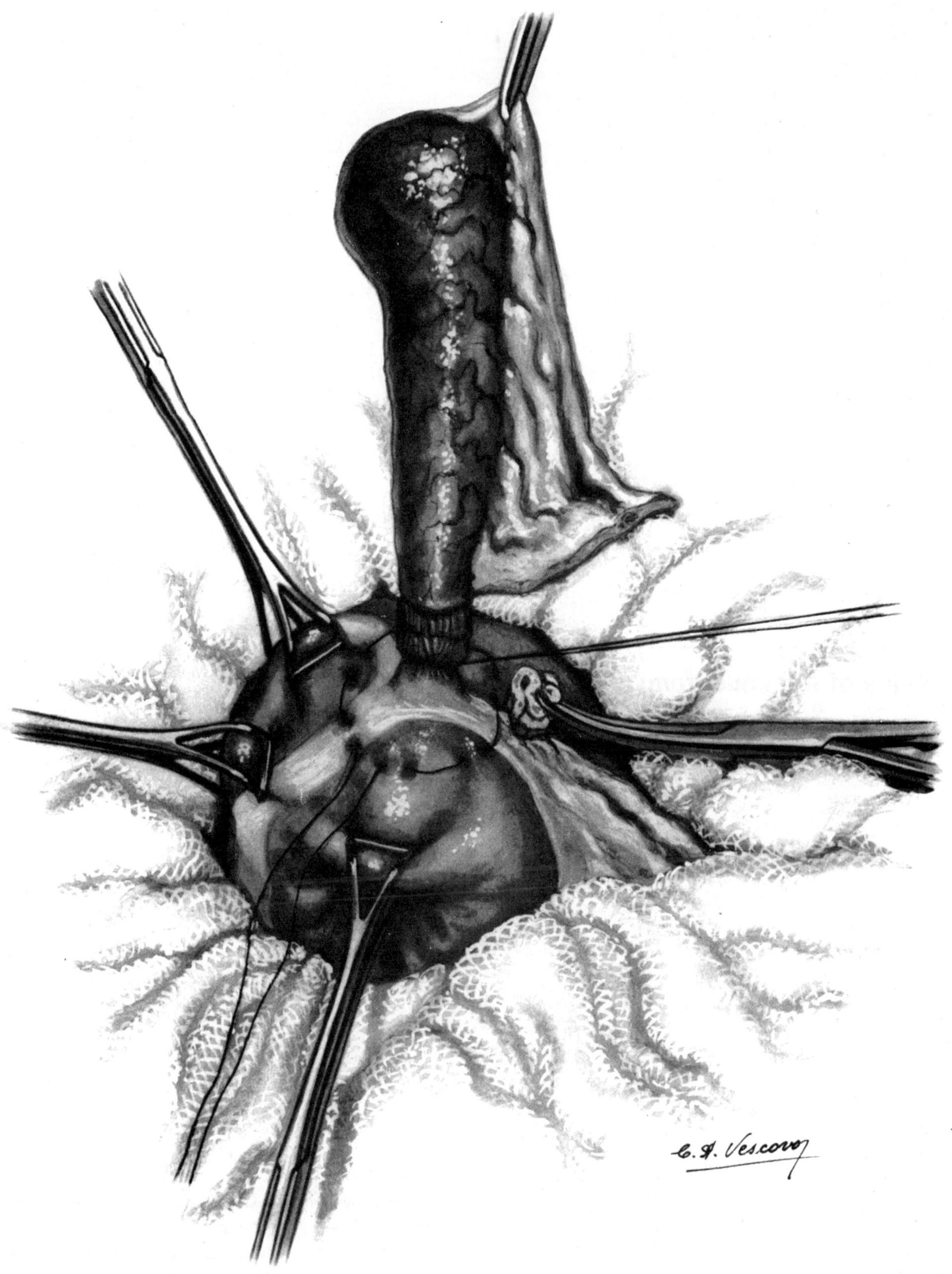

FIGURE 55.21

Technique of Appendectomy

FIGURE 55.22
The previously ligated base of the appendix is grasped with a dissection forceps. In addition, a hemostatic clamp has been placed distal to the crushed area and the appendix is then transected above the ligature, using a scalpel.

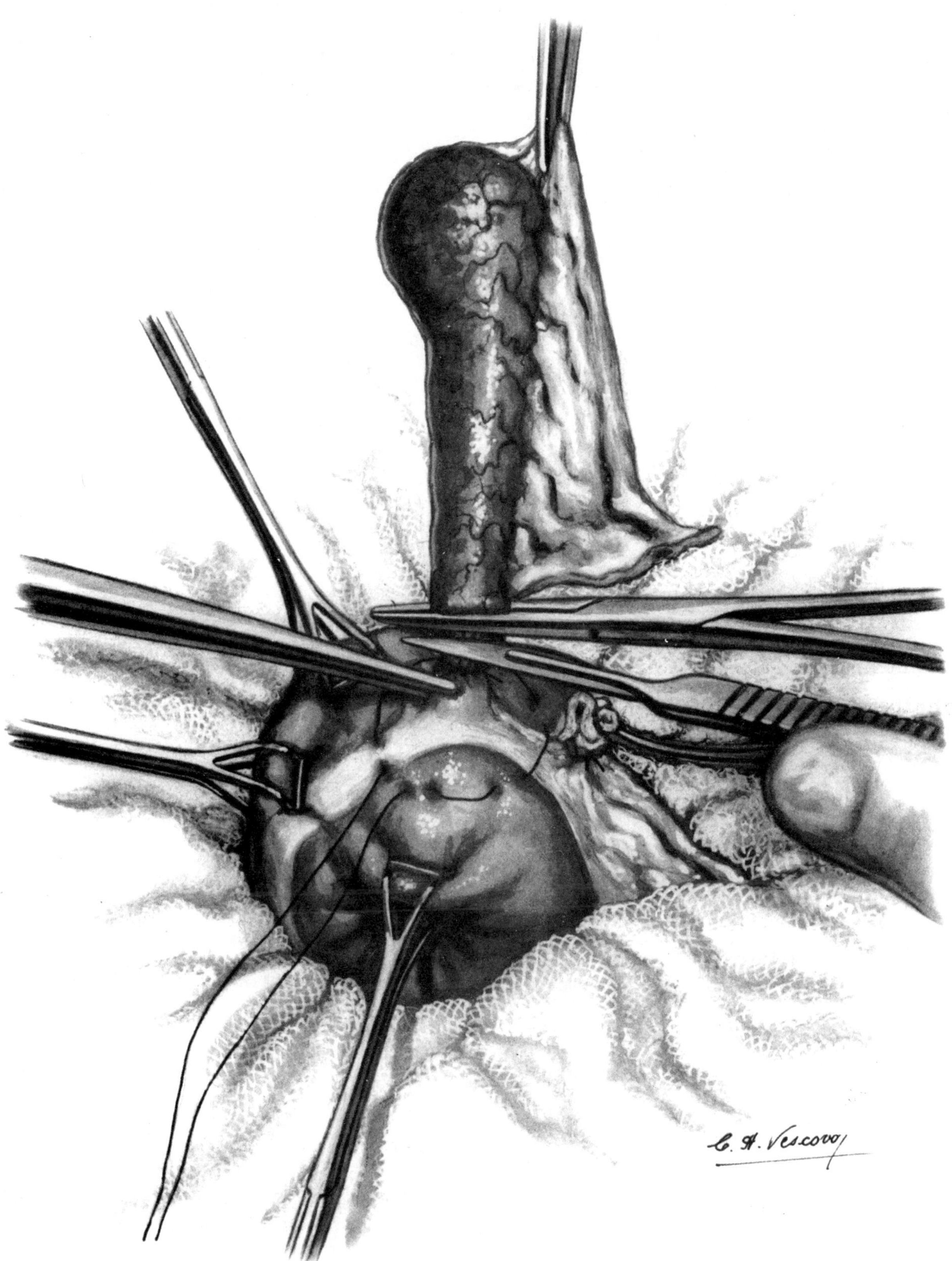

FIGURE 55.22

Technique of Appendectomy

FIGURE 55.23
The cecal appendix has been resected and removed from the operative field. A gauze pledget, soaked in povidone-iodine, has been passed over the appendiceal stump.

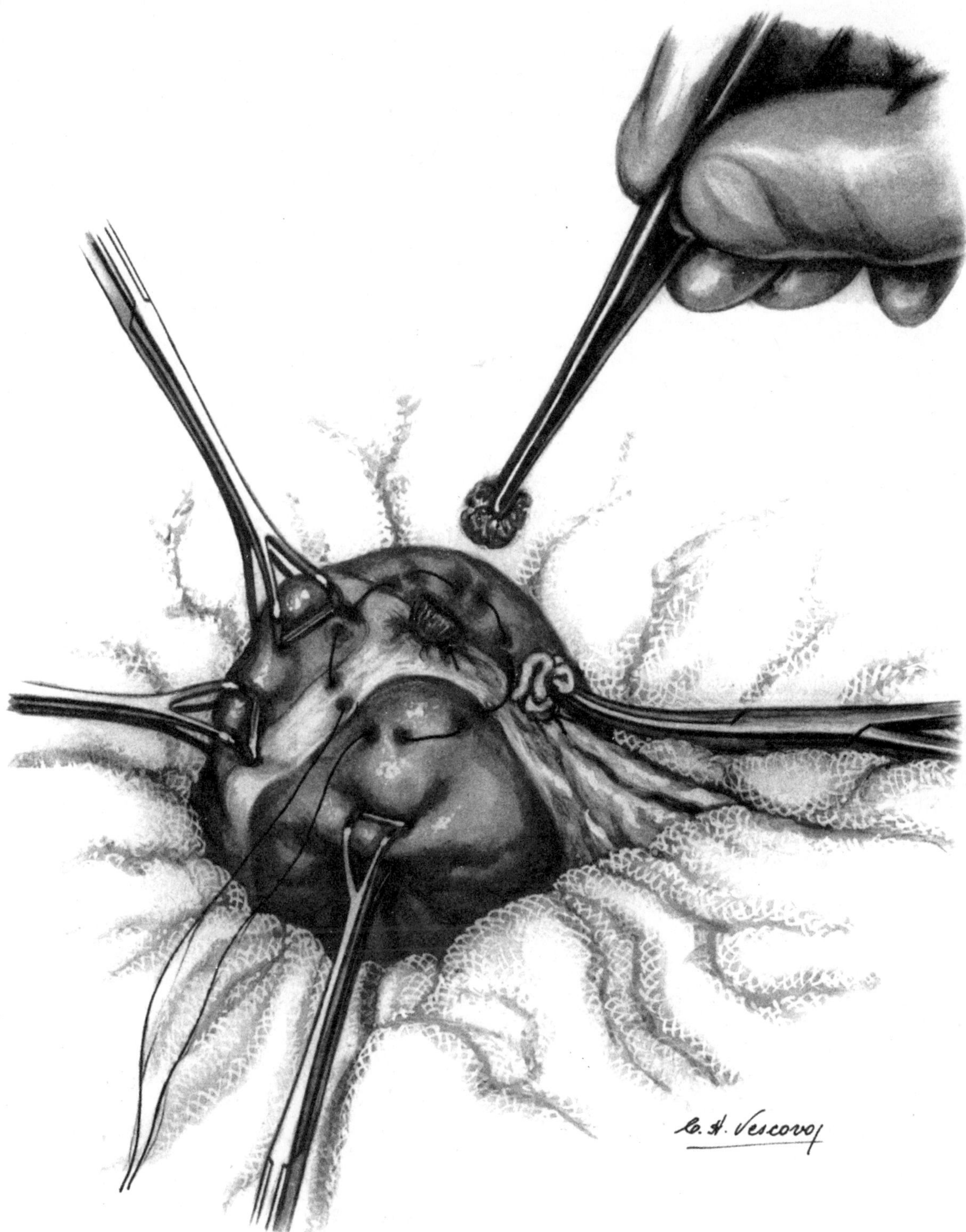

FIGURE 55.23

Technique of Appendectomy

FIGURE 55.24
The surgeon has grasped the ends of the purse string with the left hand and, with the right hand has grasped the appendiceal stump and introduced it into the cecal lumen, while pulling up on the purse string with the left hand. The insert shows the tied off purse string. Inversion of the duodenal stump is not indispensable, as has been established by various authors.

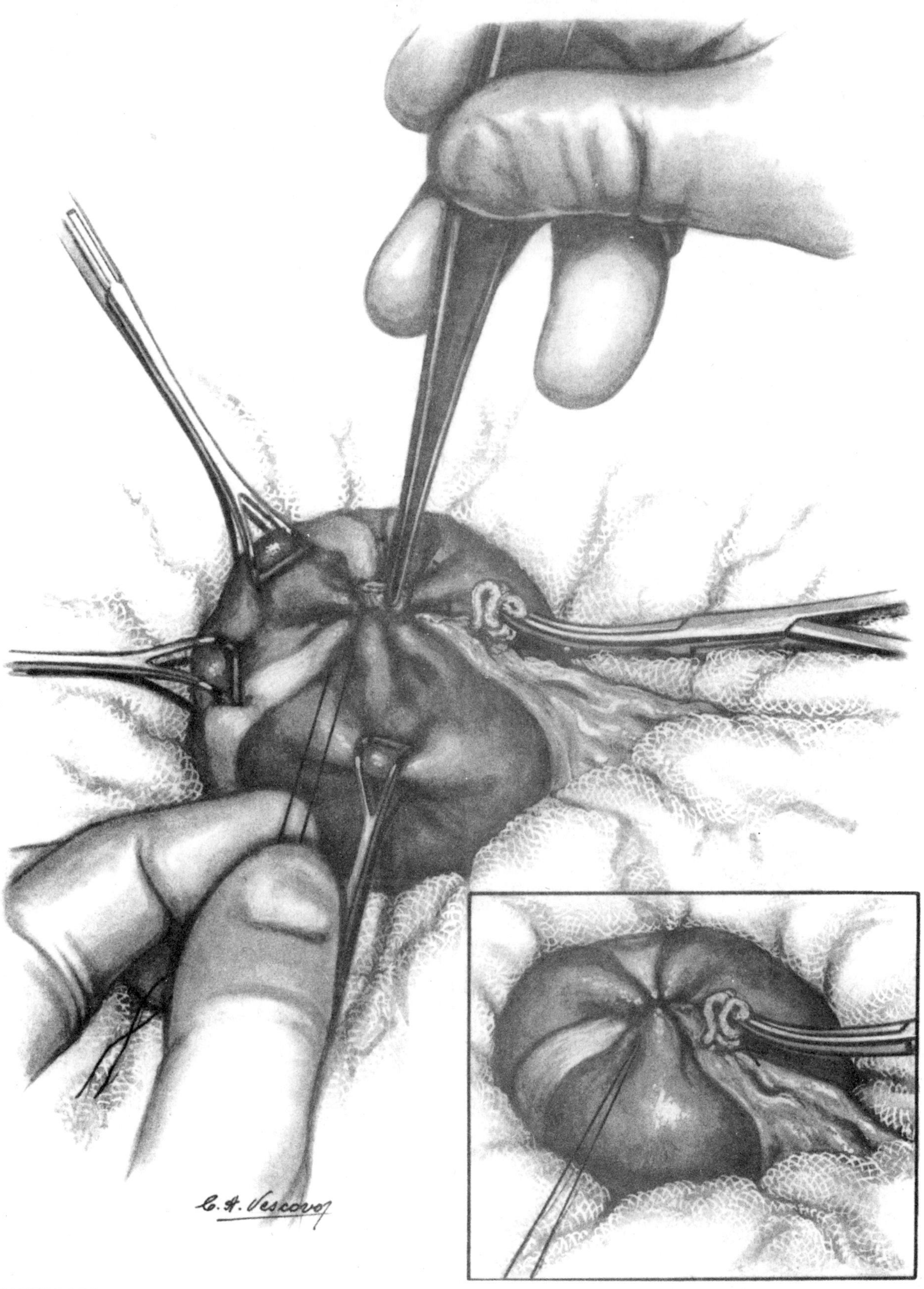

FIGURE 55.24

FIGURE 55.25
The stump of the appendiceal artery that had been grasped with a curved hemostat is applied over the inverted appendiceal stump to give more protection to the site of the inverted appendix.

Technique of Appendectomy

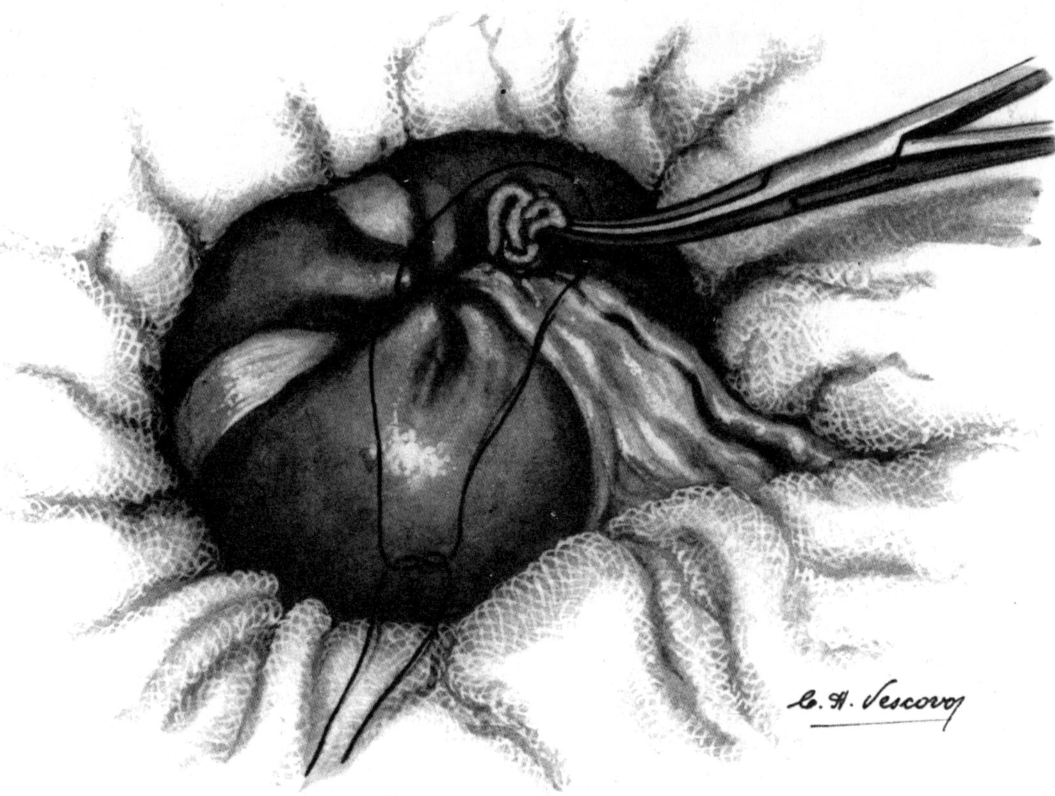

FIGURE 55.25

FIGURE 55.26
This ends of the appendiceal purse string have been tied around the stump of the appendiceal artery.

Technique of Appendectomy

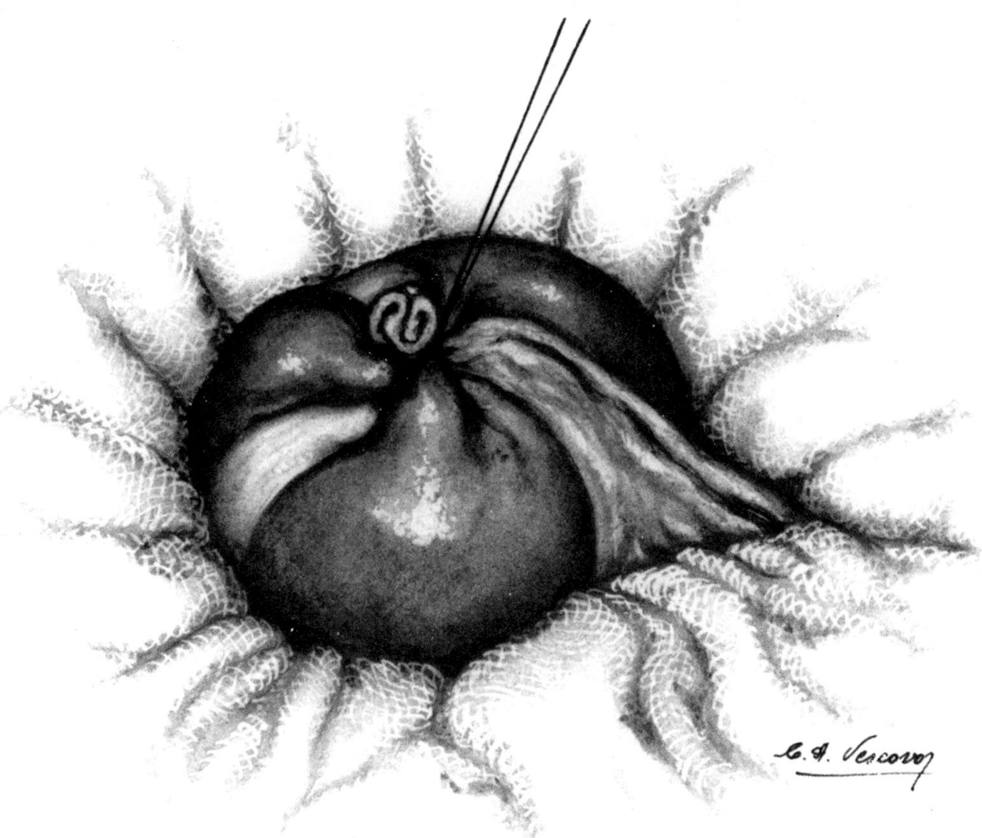

FIGURE 55.26

Technique of Appendectomy

FIGURE 55.27
In patients with an ascending retrocecal appendix joined to the posterior wall of the cecum by adhesions a different technique should be used. In this situation it is necessary to identify the base of the appendix and the appendiceal artery. The appendiceal artery is ligated and transected, the appendiceal base is crushed, and the transected appendix is inverted into the cecal lumen. Then liberation of the appendix is continued, dividing and tying off segments of the mesoappendix and the adhesions until the entire appendix is completely freed and resected. In cases in which the appendix is located behind the peritoneum of the cecum, the posterior parietal peritoneum should be incised in order to carry out the appendectomy.

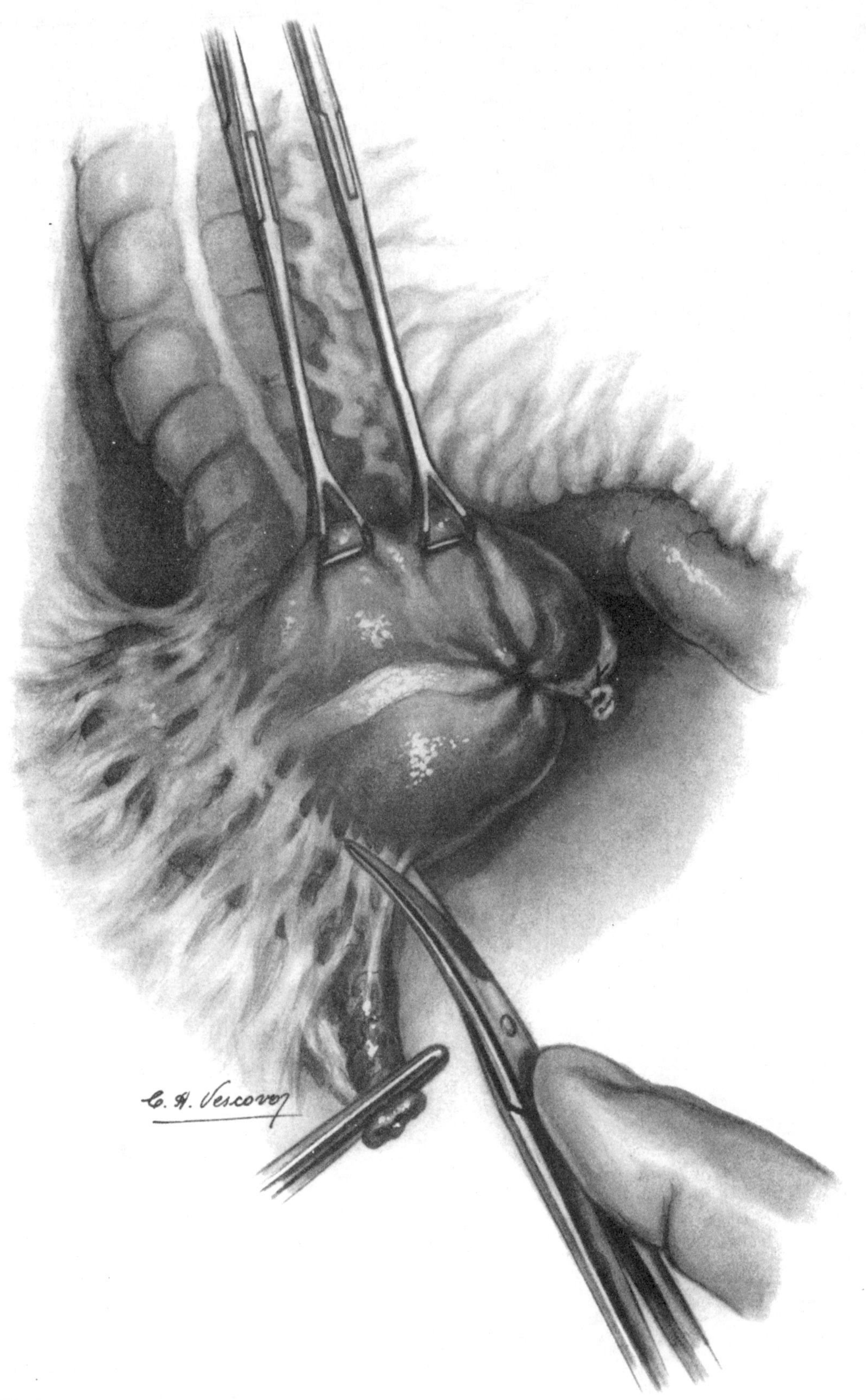

FIGURE 55.27

References

1. Berry, J. Jr., Malt, R.A. Appendicitis near its centenary. Ann. Surg. 200:567, 1984.
2. Black, W.P. Acute appendicitis in pregnancy. Br. Med. J. 1:1938, 1960.
3. Bradley, E.L., Isaacs, J. Appendiceal abscesses revisited. Arch. Surg. 113:130, 1978.
4. Bricot, R., L'appendice iléo-caecal. In Lamy, J., Louis, R., Michotey, G., Bricot, R., Sarles, J.C. (Eds.) Nouveau traité de technique chirurgicale. Vol. XI, p. 80. Masson et Cie, Paris, 1969.
5. Condon, R.E., Telford, G.L. Appendicitis. In Sabiston, D.C. Jr. (Ed.) Textbook of surgery. Ed. 14, p. 884. W.B. Saunders, Philadelphia, 1991.
6. Chassin, J.L. Operative strategy in general surgery. Ed. 2, p. 280. Springer-Verlag, New York, 1994.
7. Christmann, F.E., Ottolenghi, C.E., Raffo, J.M., von Grolman, G. Técnica quirúrgica. Ed. 10, p. 836. El Ateneo, Buenos Aires, 1970.
8. Doberneck, R.C. Appendectomy during pregnancy. Am. Surg. 51:265, 1985.
9. Doolas, A., Caldwell, R.G., Roseman, D.L., de Peyster, F.A. Appendix. In McCredie, J.A. (Ed.) Basic surgery. Ed. 2, p. 357. Macmillan, New York, 1986.
10. Ellis, H. Appendix. In Schwartz, S.I., Ellis, H. (Eds.) Maingot's abdominal operations. Ed. 9, vol. 2, p. 953. Appleton Lange, Norwalk, CT, 1990.
11. Engstrom, L., Fenyo, G. Appendicectomy: Assessment of stump invagination versus simple ligation: A prospective randomized trial. Br. J. Surg. 154:123, 1988.
12. Fassi, J.C. Apendicitis aguda y crónica. In Ortiz, F.E., Miranda, N.E., Moirano, J.J., Fassi, J.C. (Eds.) Cirugía. Ed. 3, p. 55. El Ateneo, Buenos Aires, 1993.
13. Giuliano, A. Clínica y terapéutica quirúgica. Urgencias en cirugía. Ed. 3, p. 23. El Ateneo, Buenos Aires, 1978.
14. Gómez, A., Wood, M. Acute appendicitis during pregnancy. Am. J. Surg. 137:180, 1979.
15. Gray, S.W., Skandalakis, J.E., McClusky, D.A. Atlas of surgical anatomy for general surgeons. p. 204. Williams & Wilkins, Baltimore, 1986.
16. Horowitz, M.D., Gómez, G.A., Santiesteban, R., Burkett, G. Acute appendicitis during pregnancy: Diagnosis and management. Arch. Surg. 120:1362, 1985.
17. Hubbell, D.S., Barton, W.K., Salomón, Q.D. Leukocytosis in appendicitis in older persons. J.A.M.A. 175:139, 1961.
18. Lewis, F.R., Holcroft, J.W., Boey, J., Dunphy, J.E. Appendicitis: A critical review of diagnosis and treatment in 1,000 cases. Arch. Surg. 110:677, 1975.
19. Madden, J.L. Atlas of technics in surgery. Ed. 2, vol. I, p. 356. Appleton Century Crofts, New York, 1964.
20. Moertel, C.G., Weiland, L.H., Nagorney, D.M., Dockerty, M.B. Carcinoma tumor of the appendix. Treatment and prognosis. N. Engl. J. Med. 317:1699, 1987.
21. Newstead, G.L. Open appendectomy. In Fielding, L.P., Goldberg, S.M. (Eds.) Surgery of the colon, rectum and anus. Ed. 5, p. 337. Butterworth-Heinemann, Oxford, 1993.
22. Owens, B.J. III, Hamit, H.F. Appendicitis in the elderly. Ann. Surg. 187:392, 1978.
23. Palumbo, L.T. Appendicitis—Is it on the wane? Am. J. Surg. 98:702, 1959.
24. Peltokallio, P., Jauhianen, K. Acute appendicitis in the aged patient: Study of 300 cases after the age of 60. Arch. Surg. 100:140, 1970.
25. Pieper, R., Forsell, P., Kager, L. Perforating appendicitis. A nine-year study of treatment and results. Acta Chir. Scand. (Suppl.) 530:51, 1986.
26. Shackelford, R.T., Zuidema, G.T. Surgery of the alimentary tract. Ed. 2, vol. 3, p. 57. W.B. Saunders, Philadelphia, 1982.
27. Stone, H.H., Sanders, S.R., Martin, J.D. Jr. Perforated appendicitis in children. Surgery 69:673, 1971.
28. Tammaro, J.C. Appendicitis aguda. In Boretti, J.J., Lovesio, C. (Eds.) Cirugía. Vol. III, p. 1401. El Ateneo, Buenos Aires, 1989.
29. Thorbjarnarson, B., Loehr, W.J. Acute appendicitis in patients over the age of sixty. Surg. Gynecol. Obstet. 125:1277, 1967.
30. Wakely, C.P.G. Position of vermiform appendix as ascertained by analysis of 10,000 cases. J. Anat. 67:277, 1933.
31. Walt, A.J. The appendix. In Nora, P.F. (Ed.) Operative surgery. Ed. 3, p. 606. W.B. Saunders, Philadelphia, 1990.
32. Zollinger, R.M., Zollinger, R.M. Jr. Atlas of surgical operations. Ed. 4, p. 92. Macmillan, New York, 1975.

Section H

Colon, Rectum, and Anus

CHAPTER **56**

Laparoscopic Appendectomy

In 1983, Semm (23), a German gynecologist, did the first endoscopic incidental removal of a cecal appendix in a patient with extensive endometriosis that affected the cecum and the appendix, among other organs (15). In his publication, Semm affirmed that the laparoscopic surgical procedure should not be done for acute appendicitis. Schreiber (22), also German, presented the first series of laparoscopic appendectomies in 1987, referring to 70 female patients, 24% of which had acute appendicitis. Schreiber concluded that laparoscopic appendectomy was not only efficacious but safe. Pier and colleagues (16) presented, in Germany, in 1925, 625 cases of appendectomies performed laparoscopically of which only 2% had to be converted to open surgery. From the above, it can be concluded that the practice of laparoscopic appendectomy had been carried out mainly in Germany.

With the passage of time this procedure began to be used in other surgical centers of Europe and America. Videolaparoscopy, by better visualization, permitted exploration of both the upper and the lower abdomen, which resulted in great efficiency in making the correct diagnosis of appendicitis (3, 5, 13). If during exploration the surgeon finds that the appendix is not giving rise to the patient's symptoms, laparoscopy will permit exploration of the rest of the abdomen to determine if there is any other affliction—be it in the gallbladder, in the stomach or duodenum, in a Meckel's diverticulum, in the adnexa, and so on—that would explain the symptomatology. This possibility that laparoscopy offers avoids the need of intense traction on the wound edges of an incision during open surgery or the need to extend the incision or make another incision to make a diagnosis (3, 5, 13).

In spite of these advantages, laparoscopic appendectomy has not been accepted by surgeons as well as laparoscopic cholecystectomy has, even though the latter was performed 5 years earlier. This attitude on the part of surgeons has been influenced by the fact that open appendectomy is an easy procedure, well controlled, and with very good results. At the same time, the incision for an open appendectomy does not cause more postoperative disability than the disability due to the sum of the various incisions needed to introduce the trochars (5, 15). Additionally, if the appendix should rupture during laparoscopic appendectomy, this could lead to a more serious problem than in an open procedure, and it would be much more difficult to control. The postoperative recovery time of both procedures is also quite similar (2, 15). Up to now there has been no incontrovertible proof that laparoscopic appendectomy is safer, is less costly, and has a shorter recovery period (2, 15). It is very possible that these reasons have led to the lack of enthusiasm of surgeons for this procedure, which explains its limited spread (2, 15). There is no doubt, however, as to its value in making certain the diagnosis of appendicitis.

CONTRAINDICATIONS OF LAPAROSCOPIC APPENDECTOMY

Most of the contraindications of laparoscopic appendectomy are relative, such as previous lower abdominal surgery, appendiceal abscess/or phlegmon, pregnancy, and so on. In these cases the indication for laparoscopic appendectomy will be directly related to the capacity and experience of the surgeon.

SURGICAL TECHNIQUE

The operating room, the patient, and the instruments should be prepared to carry out not only a laparoscopic appendectomy, but an open procedure, if the need arises.

The patient is placed in the dorsal decubitus position, slightly inclined to the left.

The video monitor is placed at the foot of the patient. The surgeon stands to the left of the patient and the first assistant stands on the right, in front of the surgeon.

A nasogastric tube is passed and a Foley catheter is inserted into the bladder, to be removed before the patient wakes up.

The pneumoperitoneum is carried out using the same technique described in Chapter 9.

Wide spectrum antibiotics should be given intravenously before starting the procedure. These should be continued for at least a few hours, postoperatively.

There are several ways to perform a laparoscopic appendectomy. There are also variations as to the number of ports of entry used, as well as the caliber of the trocars and cannulas, which should be according to the instruments the surgeon usually uses. In case of doubt, it is preferable to use 10 to 11 mm trocars and cannulas, which will allow the use of larger instruments, if this becomes necessary during the procedure. If Endo instruments (GIA—United States Surgical Corporation) are used, the trocars should be of the 12 mm size.

CONVERSION

Conversion to open surgery may be necessary in patients with marked anatomic variations, in patients with a very severely inflamed appendix, in the presence of multiple adhesions, in cases of appendiceal abscess, and so on.

Technique of Laparoscopic Appendectomy

FIGURE 56.1

The drawing on the left shows the ports of entry of the trocars and cannulas (8, 10, 19). It is convenient to use four ports of entry for appendectomy (8, 10, 19), which are as follows:

1. A subumbilical port, 10 mm in diameter, to insert the laparoscope.
2. A 5 mm suprapubic port to insert the grasper, which will be used to hold the distal end of the mesoappendix.
3. A port in the right upper quadrant of the abdomen, outside the lateral border of the anterior rectus muscle, 10 mm in diameter. Through this port a clamp will be passed to grasp the distal end of the appendix. In addition, this port will be used to extract the resected appendix.
4. A 5 mm port in the left iliac fossa, which will be used only to insert a hook or laparoscopic scissors. If an Endo-GIA instrument is to be used, this port should be 12 mm in diameter. The drawing on the left shows the cecum, the terminal ileum, and the appendix. A grasping forceps, passed through the suprapubic port, is holding the distal end of the mesoappendix. Another forceps has been passed through the right upper quadrant port and is holding the distal end of the appendix (19).

Technique of Laparoscopic Appendectomy

FIGURE 56.2

Traction is maintained on the appendix and its mesoappendix (19). The mesoappendix has been dissected using the hook, until the ileocecal junction and the base of the appendix are clearly seen. Two clips are applied to the appendiceal artery near the cecum and, using a laparoscopic scissors, passed through the left iliac port. The appendiceal artery and the mesoappendix are transected near the cecum, along the dotted line.

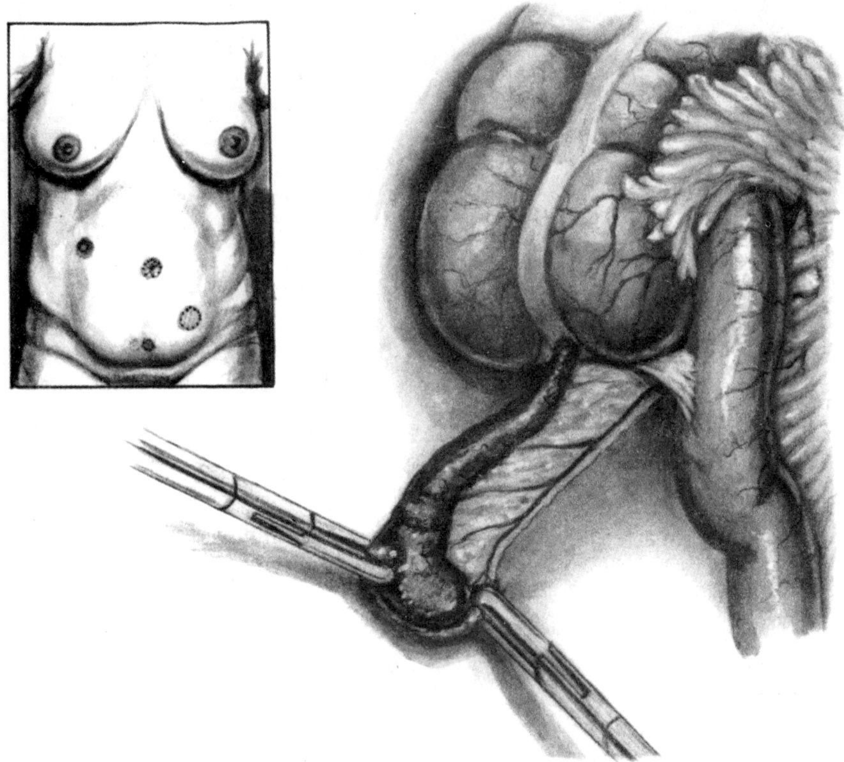

FIGURE 56.1

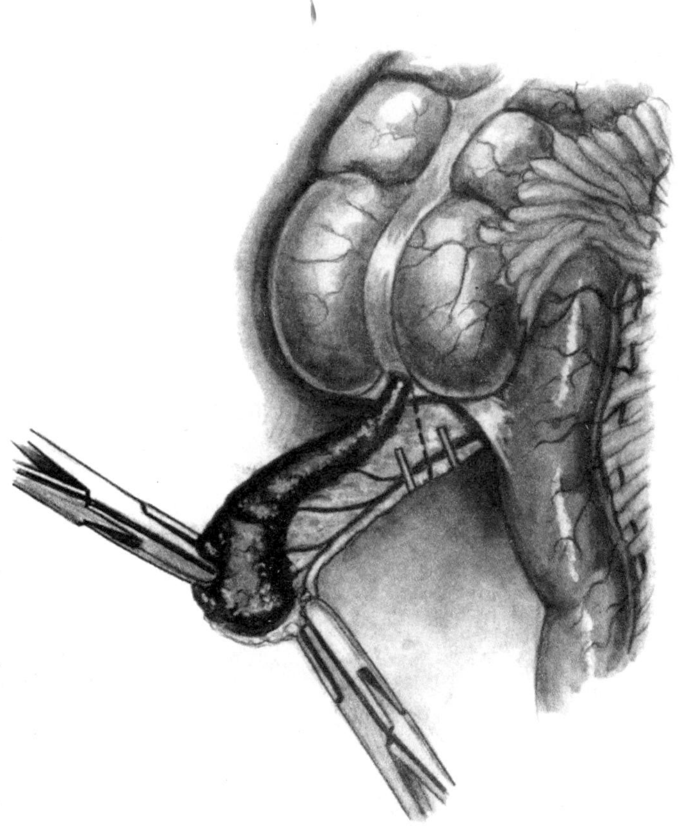

FIGURE 56.2

FIGURE 56.3
If, instead of ligating the appendiceal artery with clips, ligation is performed with an Endo-GIA instrument, the instrument should be introduced through a 12 mm port in the left iliac fossa.

Technique of Laparoscopic Appendectomy

FIGURE 56.4
Once the artery has been ligated and divided with the mesoappendix, the appendix should be ligated using three pretied surgical loops (Endo-Loop). Two Endo-Loops are placed on the base of the appendix, very close to the cecum, and the third Endo-Loop, which will be removed with the appendix, is placed 1 cm distally. Using laparoscopic scissors the appendix is being transected between the two Endo-Loops at the appendiceal base and the loop that is to be extracted with the appendix (2, 5, 15). The appendix is placed in a small plastic bag to avoid contamination and is then removed through the right upper quadrant port. Some surgeons invert the appendiceal stump into the cecum using a purse string or a Z suture. Some surgeons have proven that results are the same with or without inversion of the stump (6).

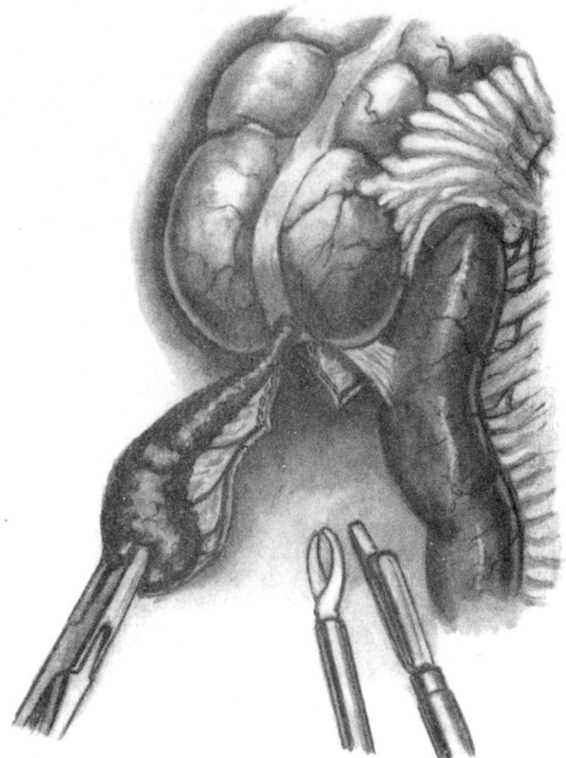

FIGURE 56.3

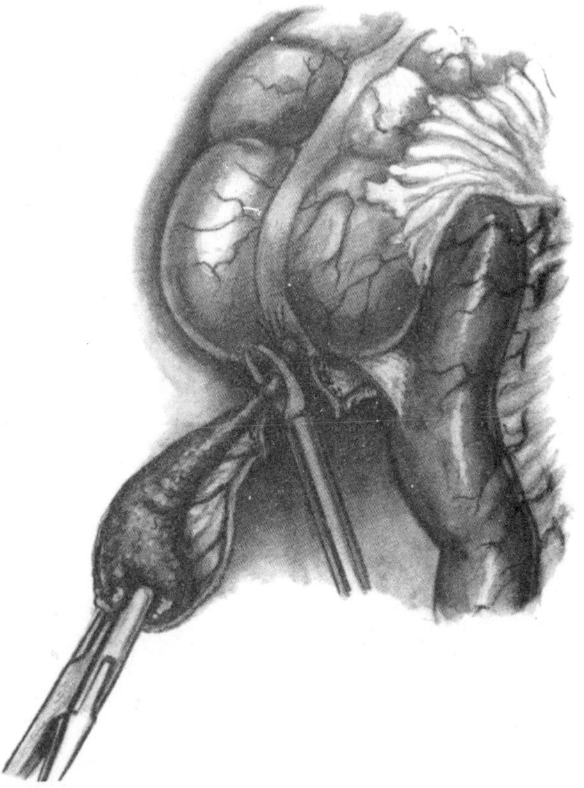

FIGURE 56.4

References

1. Atwood, S.E.A., Hill, A.D.K., Murphy, P.G., Thorton, J., Stephens, R.B. A prospective randomized trial of laparoscopic versus open appendectomy. Surgery 112:497, 1992.
2. Bailey, R.W., Zucker, K.A. Laparoscopic-assisted appendectomy. In Fielding, L.P., Goldberg, S.M. (Eds.) Surgery of the colon, rectum and anus. Ed. 5, p. 177. Butterworth-Heinemann, Oxford, 1993.
3. Clark, P.J., Hands, L.J., Couch, M.H. The use of laparoscopy in the management of right iliac fossa pain. Ann. R. Coll. Surg. 68:68, 1986.
4. Dubois, F. Appendicectomie. In Bruhat, M.A., Dubois, F. (Eds.) La chirurgie abdominopelvienne par celioscopie. p. 139. Springer-Verlag, Paris, 1992.
5. Easter, D.W. Diagnosis and treatment of acute appendicitis with laparoscopic methods. In Hunter, J.G., Sackier, J.M. (Eds.) Minimally invasive surgery. p. 171. McGraw-Hill, New York, 1993.
6. Engstrom, L., Fenyö, G. Appendectomy assessment of stump invagination versus simple ligation, a prospective randomized trial. Br. J. Surg. 72:971, 1985.
7. Gangal, M.I., Gangal, M.H. Laparoscopic appendectomy. Endoscopy 19:127, 1987.
8. Götz, F., Pier, A., Bacher, C. Modified laparoscopic appendectomy in surgery: A report on 388 operations. Surg. Endosc. 4:6, 1990.
9. Kelling, G. Zur coelioscopie. Arch. Klin. Chir. 126:226, 1923.
10. Leahy, P.F. Technique of laparoscopic appendectomy. Br. J. Surg. 76:616, 1989.
11. Loh, A., Taylor, R.S. Laparoscopic appendectomy. Br. J. Surg. 79:289, 1992.
12. McAnena, O.J., Austin, O., O'Connell, P.R., Hederman, W.P., Gorey, T.F., Fitzpatrick, J. Laparoscopic versus open appendectomy: A prospective evaluation. Br. J. Surg. 79:818, 1992.
13. Navez, B., d'Udekem, Y., Cambier, E., Richir, C., de Pierpont, B., Guiot, P. Laparoscopy for management of nontraumatic acute abdomen. World J. Surg. 19:382, 1995.
14. Olsen, D.O. Laparoscopic appendectomy using a linear stapling device. Surg. Rounds 14:873, 1991.
15. O'Reilly, M.J., Reddick, E.J., Miller, W.D., Saye, W.B. Laparoscopic appendectomy. In Zucker, K.A. (Ed.) Surgical laparoscopic update. p. 301. Quality Medical Publishing, St. Louis, 1993.
16. Pier, A., Götz, F., Bacher, C. Laparoscopic appendectomy in 625 cases from innovation to routine. Surg. Laparosc. Endosc. 1:8, 1991.
17. Pier, A., Götz, F. Laparoscopic appendicectomy. In Cuschieri, A., Buess, G., Perissat, J. (Eds.) Operative manual of endoscopic surgery. p. 194. Springer-Verlag, Berlin, 1992.
18. Saye, W.B., Rives, D.A., Cochran, E.B. Laparoscopic appendectomy: Three years' experience. Laparosc. Endosc. 2:109, 1991.
19. Salky, B.A. Laparoscopic appendectomy. In Bauer, J.J. (Ed.) Colorectal surgery illustrated. p. 223. Mosby–Year Book, St. Louis, 1993.
20. Scott-Conner, C.E.H., Hall, T.J., Anglin, B.L., Muakkassa, F.F. Laparoscopic appendectomy: Initial experience in a teaching program. Ann. Surg. 215:660, 1992.
21. Schiaffino, L., Mouro, J., Karagel, M., Levard, H., Berthelot, G., Dubois, F. Laparoscopic appendectomy. A study of 154 consecutive cases. Intern. Surg. 78:280, 1993.
22. Schreiber, J.H. Early experience with laparoscopic appendectomy in women. Surg. Endosc. 1:211, 987.
23. Semm, K. Endoscopic appendectomy. Endoscopy 15:59, 1983.

Section H

Colon, Rectum, and Anus

CHAPTER 57

Transverse Colostomy and Closure

A loop transverse colostomy is a surgical procedure designed to temporarily shunt the fecal stream. In spite of all the controversies it is the most commonly used procedure at present. The most common indications for this procedure are the following:

1. Obstruction or threatening obstruction of the distal colon.
2. Inflammatory process of the distal colon, usually due to sigmoid diverticulitis.
3. Colorectal trauma.
4. Perineal wounds.
5. To protect colorectal anastomoses.
6. In colorectal lesions due to irradiation etc. (1, 6–9, 11, 12, 18, 21, 23).

At present, transverse loop colostomy is recommended infrequently to protect low colorectal anastomoses and, in cases of sigmoid inflammation, because surgeons more frequently perform one stage resections and anastomosis, either manually or mechanically (9, 12, 17, 18, 22, 23, 32). On the other hand, there are surgeons who have stopped doing transverse colostomies as temporary shunts, preferring a loop ileostomy with the conviction that this procedure adapts itself better to collecting bags (7, 18, 22). They also affirm that with this procedure, it is frequently not necessary to use a rod to hold the ileal loop and that, if a rod has to be used, closure of these diverting ileostomies leads to less morbidity than transverse loop colostomies (13, 31, 32). According to some authors (14, 18, 22, 26, 27), a loop ileostomy completely diverts the fecal stream, which is not always the case in a transverse colostomy. For some authors (18, 22, 23, 26), a transverse colostomy is difficult to manage because of its large size and because collecting bags are not always reliable. It has also been asserted (18, 32) that transverse colostomies are frequently complicated by prolapse, retraction, obstruction, and protrusion. Additionally, their closure is difficult and complications are frequent. Some authors (8, 14) believe that the transverse colostomy will frequently retract and, after 6 months, cease to completely divert the fecal stream. Because of this, some surgeons prefer a double barrel colostomy instead of a loop colostomy. There are authors (32) who do not recommend a loop colostomy because many of these have to be left as permanent colostomies, especially when hepatic metastases and ascites develop. Another disadvantage attributed to loop colostomy is that the marginal artery of Drummond may be obliterated by the surgeon during the procedure or its closure, which may alter the blood supply to the distal colon if the need arises to ligate the inferior mesenteric artery at its origin in the aorta.

The author believes that the loop colostomy is a good operation, easy to carry out and easy to close. Complications are few if the colostomy is done correctly and in the correct site. Postoperative complications of this operation are usually due to errors in technique. Complications occur more frequently when the operation is done as an emergency procedure. Rombeau and colleagues (24) have shown that a transverse loop colostomy produces complete shunting of the fecal stream. On the other hand, a transverse colostomy is designed to shunt the fecal stream only temporarily. Permanent colostomies should be performed using different techniques. Closure of a transverse colostomy does not present any difficulty if it has been performed correctly. Closure of a transverse colostomy is much easier if at least 6 weeks have gone by since it was performed. The author has never encountered any difficulty in the patient becoming adapted to a loop colostomy while awaiting definitive colonic resection. If leakage should occur in a loop colostomy, it is never as serious as leakage from an ileostomy. On the other hand, closure of a loop ileostomy is not simpler than closure of a loop colostomy.

Some authors (8, 9) prefer to perform a transverse loop colostomy on the left side rather than the right side, because the colonic contents are thicker on the left. The author agrees with this as long as the left transverse colostomy does not present any difficulty in case it becomes necessary to mobilize and bring down the left transverse colon and the splenic flexure to carry out a low colorectal or coloanal anastomosis.

The author has proven that, when the transverse colostomy is carried out near the fixed segment of the transverse colon, the possibility of postoperative prolapse is much less frequent. In regard to the technique used to close a transverse colostomy, as will be seen later, it is important to point out that the closure should be intraperitoneal, since extraperitoneal closure may lead to traction and eventration.

SURGICAL TECHNIQUE

We will now describe the technique for a right transverse loop colostomy, which is performed more frequently. The technique for closure of this colostomy will be described later.

Surgical Technique

FIGURE 57.1
Transverse incision over the right rectus abdominis muscle halfway between the costal arch and the umbilicus. **A,** Incision for the performance of a right transverse loop colostomy. **B,** Incision for a left transverse loop colostomy. The incision should cover the entire width of the anterior rectus muscle.

Transverse Loop Colostomy

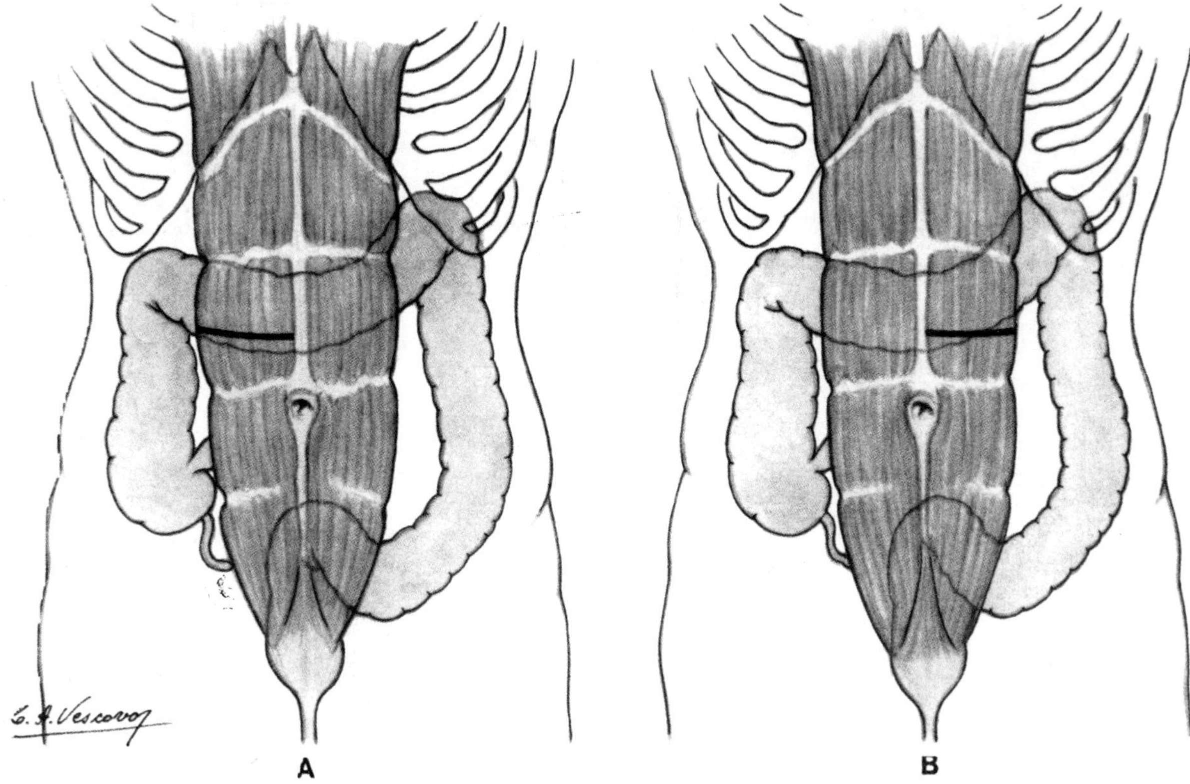

FIGURE 57.1

FIGURE 57.2

The skin and subcutaneous tissue have been incised. **A,** The anterior fascia of the rectus muscle is transected. **B,** The anterior rectus muscle is divided in the same direction. Some surgeons split the muscle fibers instead of transecting them; others transect only part of the rectus muscle. The author prefers to transect the entire rectus muscle so that the surgeon's hand can be introduced in order to locate the lesion, determine its extent and its resectability, and so on, avoiding a "blind" transverse colostomy. **C,** Transection of the posterior rectus sheath together with the peritoneum. **D,** Once hemostasis of the rectus muscle has been completed, both sides of the transected rectus muscle are covered by suturing the anterior and posterior rectus sheaths, including the peritoneum, using interrupted sutures. This is done to cover the muscle and diminish the fibrosis and adhesions that the muscle fibers frequently produce, making closure of the colostomy more difficult.

Transverse Loop Colostomy

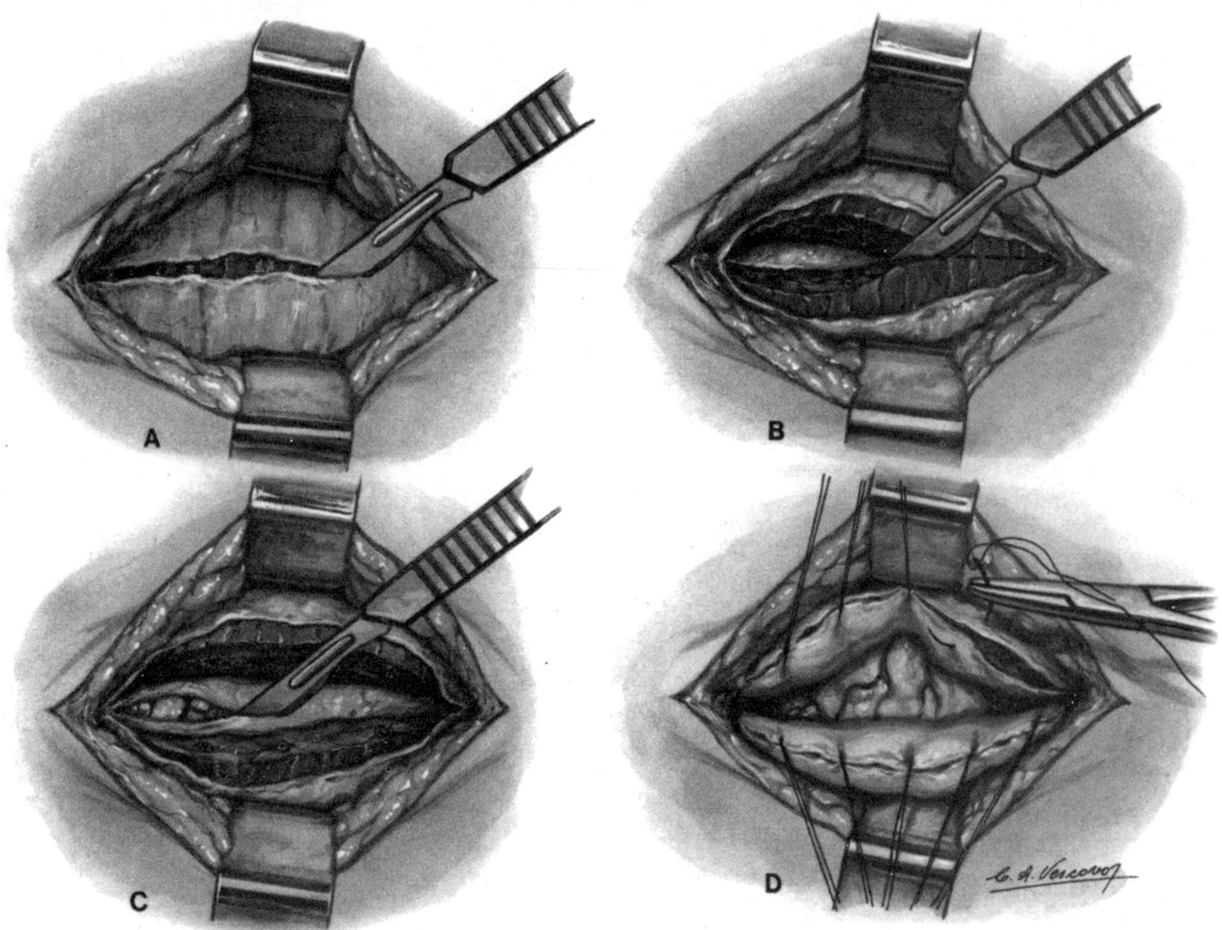

FIGURE 57.2

Transverse Loop Colostomy

FIGURE 57.3

It is important that the surgeon insert a hand, usually the left, to locate the lesion. In order to make this maneuver easier, the first assistant should pull apart the long suture ends used to cover the sheath of the transected rectus muscle. The introduction of the hand is facilitated if it is placed as in the delivery of a baby.

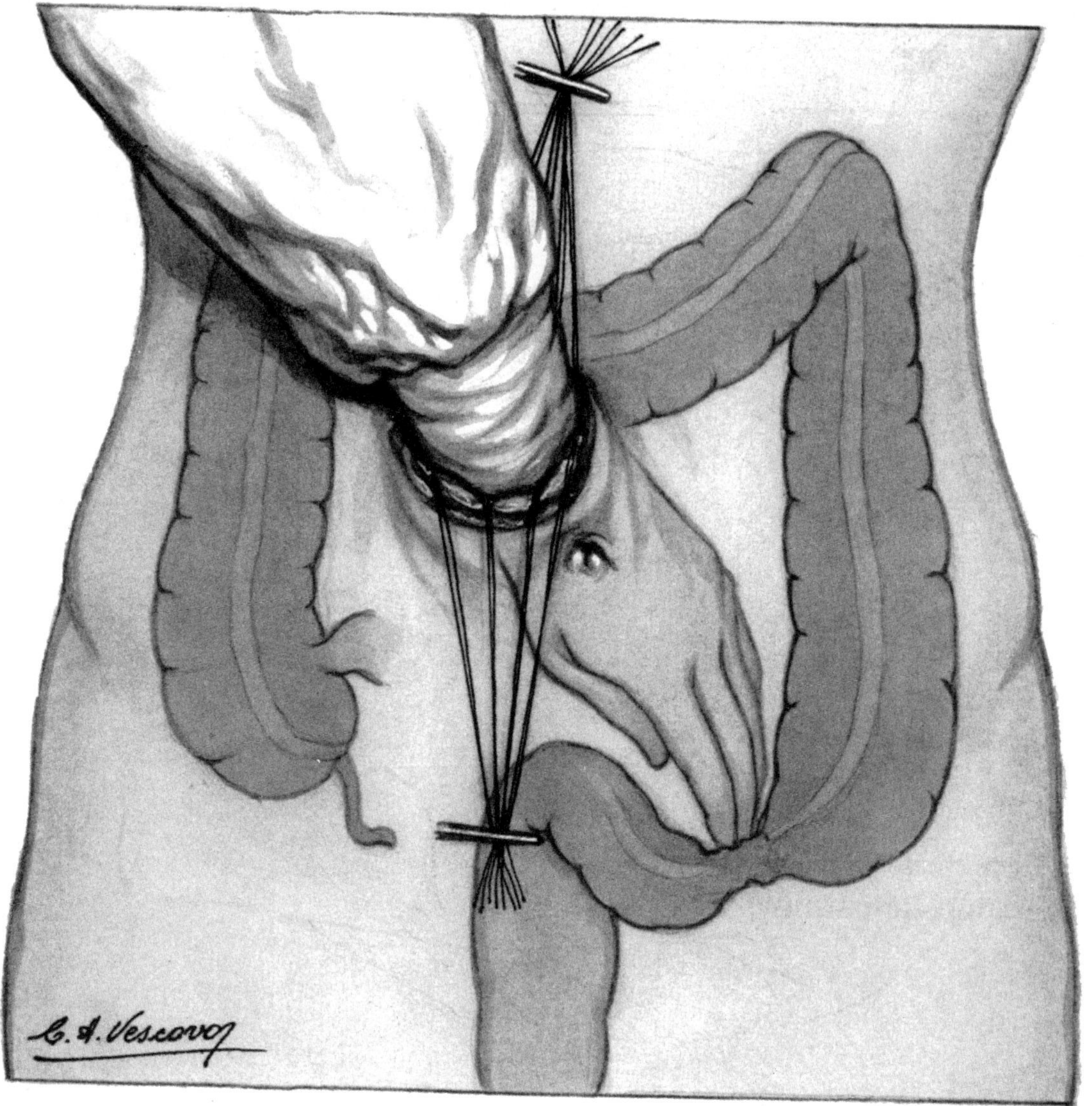

FIGURE 57.3

Transverse Loop Colostomy

FIGURE 57.4

A, The greater omentum is being separated from the transverse colon to completely mobilize the portion of the colon that is going to be used to construct the colostomy. This segment of colon should be contiguous to the fixed portion of the colon (hepatic flexure). **B,** A curved clamp is passed through an avascular portion of mesentery, close to the mesenteric border of the colon, to grasp a soft rubber catheter or Penrose drain. Care should be taken to avoid injury to the marginal artery of Drummond in passing the clamp. The insert shows the clamp passing through the mesocolon. The marginal artery of Drummond can be observed, passing far from the clamp.

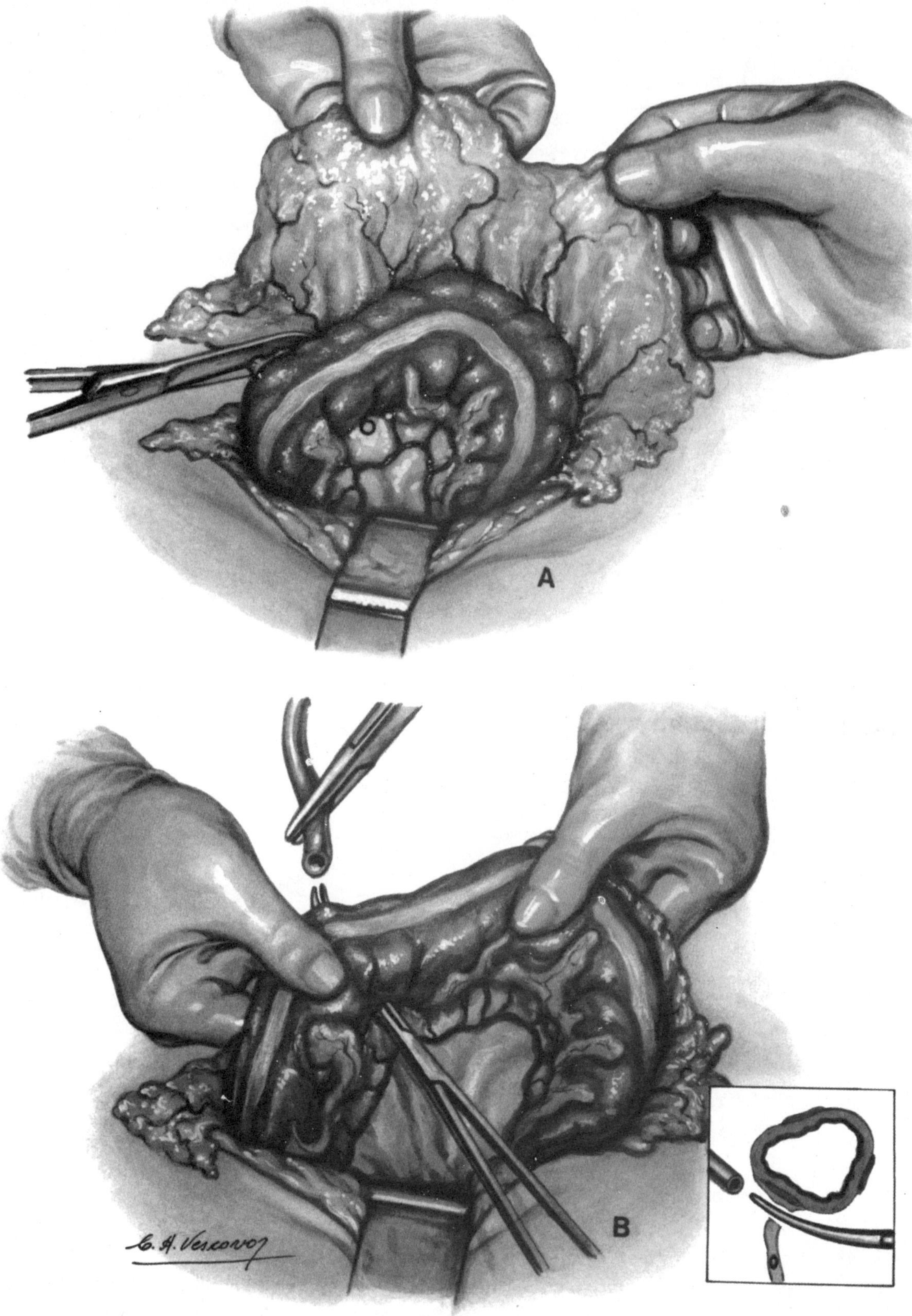

FIGURE 57.4

Transverse Loop Colostomy

FIGURE 57.5
A, This shows where the rubber catheter will pass, near the fixed segment of the transverse colon. Performing the colostomy near the fixed segment of the colon produces a lower incidence of prolapse. **B,** Traction is applied to the catheter surrounding the transverse colon.

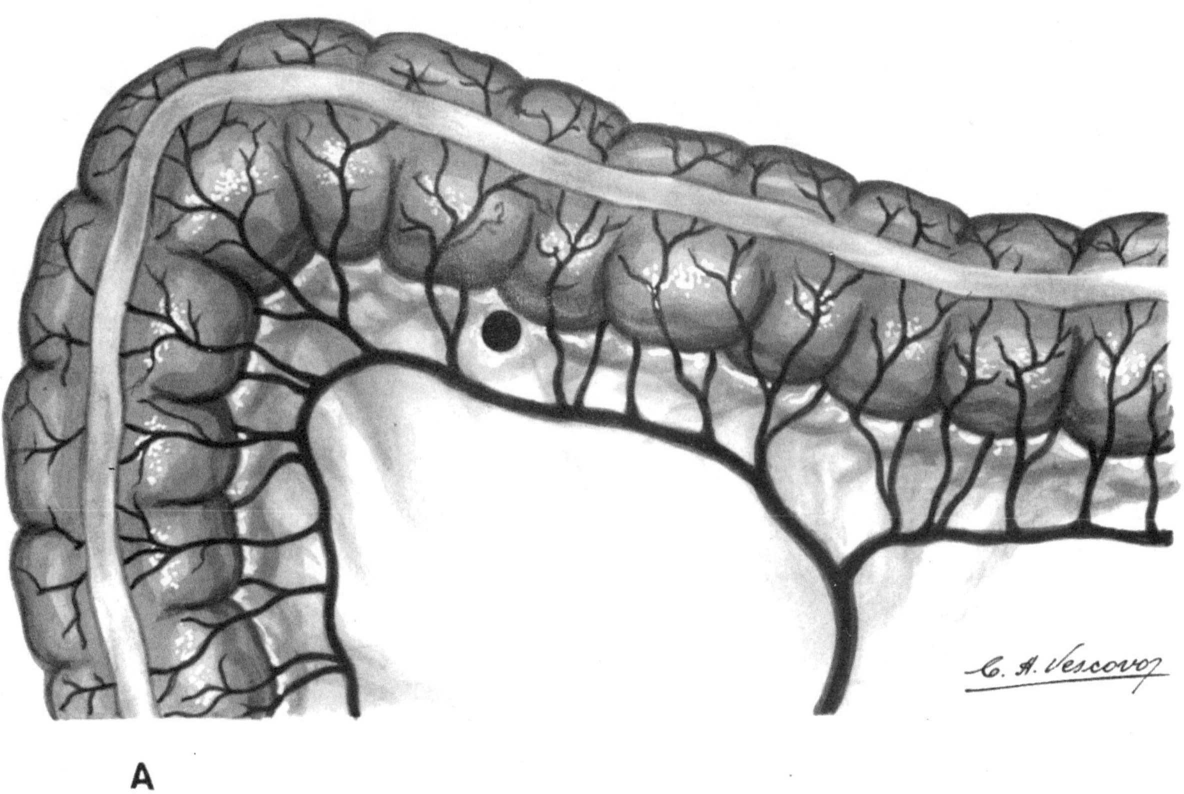

A

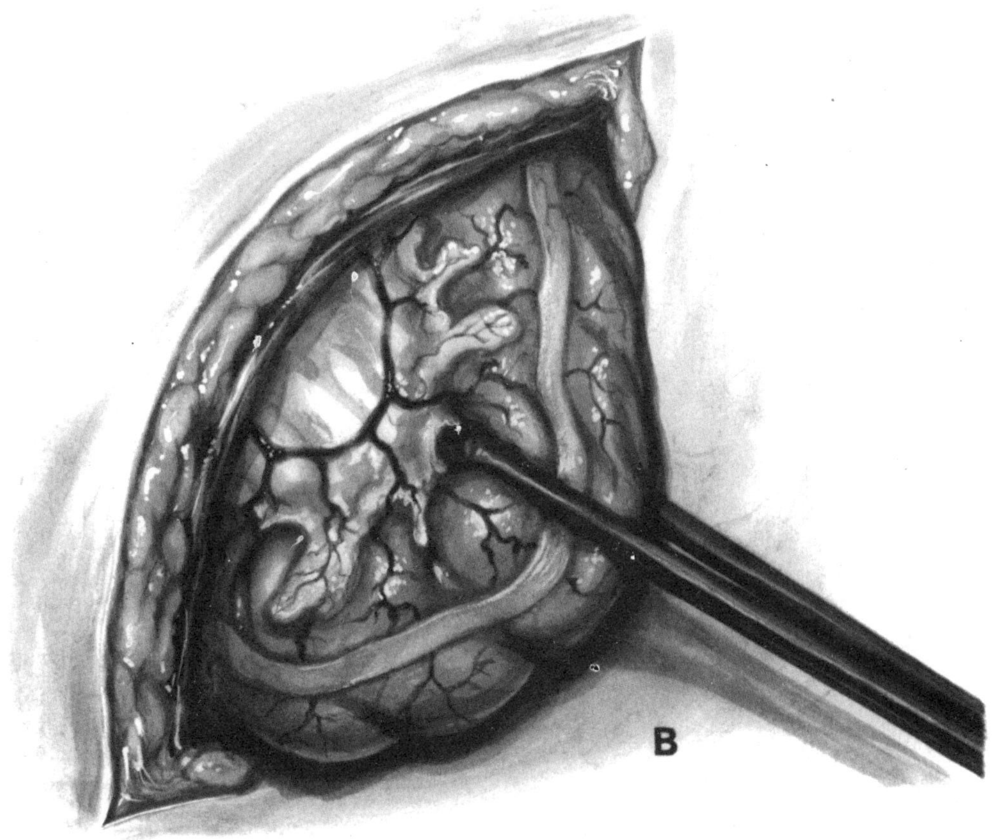

B

FIGURE 57.5

Transverse Loop Colostomy

FIGURE 57.6
A, Several epiploic appendices are sutured to the parietal peritoneum in order to keep intestinal loops from prolapsing between the colon and the edges of the wound. This will also fix the colon in the wound. Care should be taken that the sutures in the epiploic appendices pass far from the colon itself so as not to compromise the blood supply. **B,** The same procedure is being carried out in the superior border of the incision.

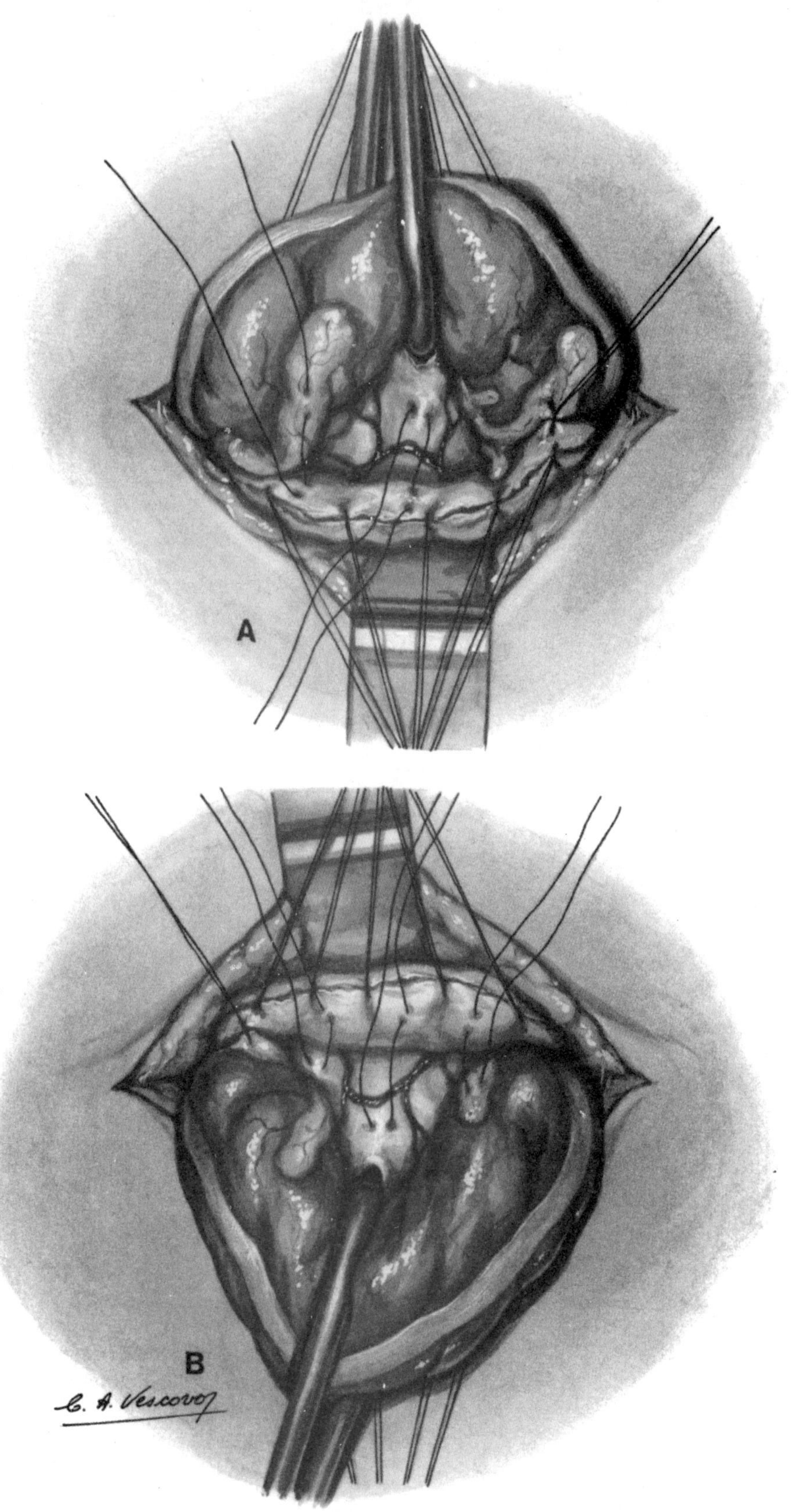

FIGURE 57.6

Transverse Loop Colostomy

FIGURE 57.7
A, The loop of transverse colon has been fixed to the parietal peritoneum wall, using the epiploic appendices, and the skin and subcutaneous tissue is being sutured to both sides of the colonic loop. **B,** The rod that will help hold the loop of colon in place is being inserted.

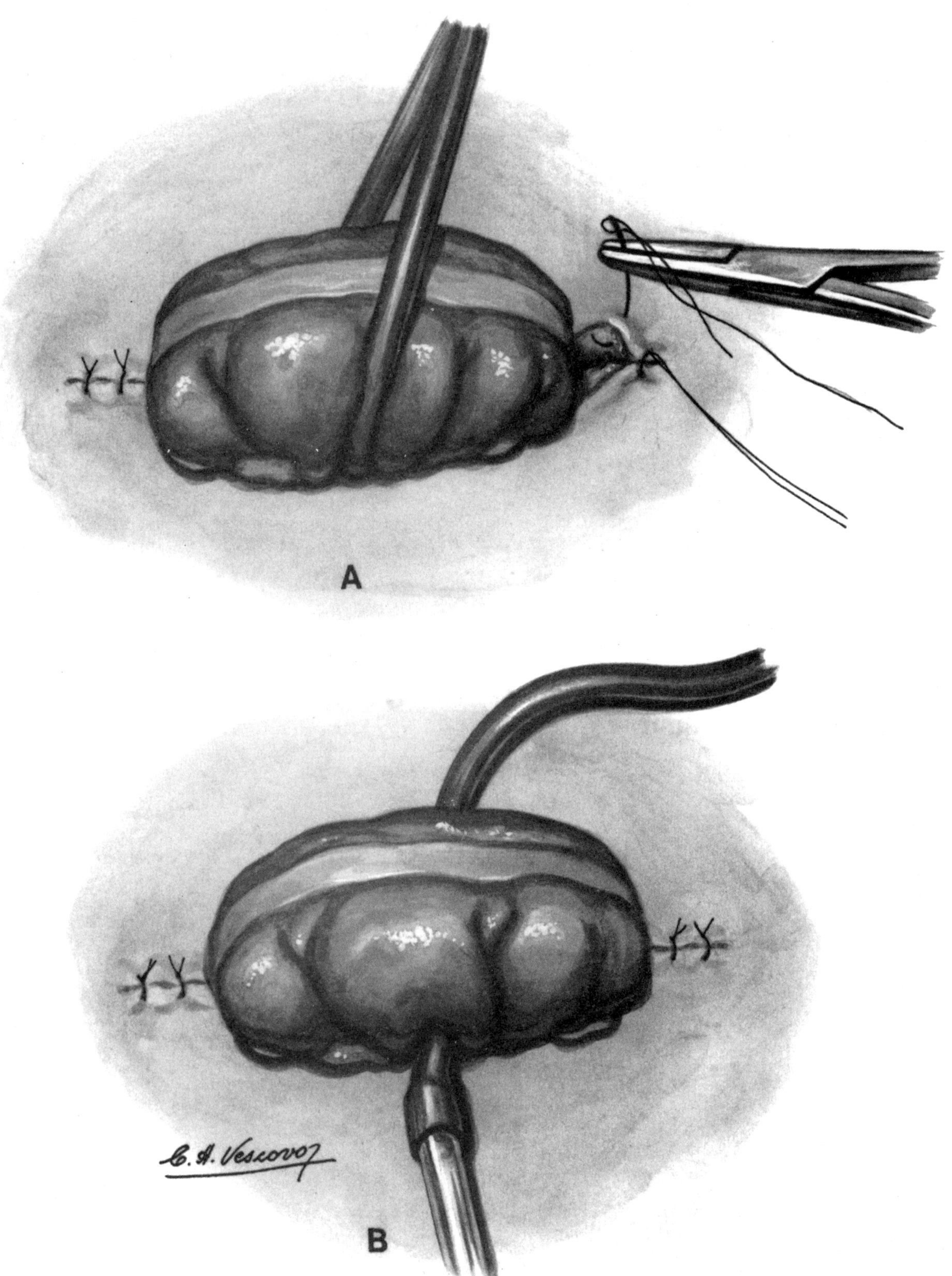

FIGURE 57.7

Transverse Loop Colostomy

FIGURE 57.8

A, Using an electric scalpel, the transverse colon is being incised along a longitudinal tenia. The colon can also be incised transversely to "mature" the colostomy. **B,** The edge of the colon is being sutured to the skin with interrupted 2-0 catgut. **C,** The colostomy has been matured. A colostomy bag should be applied before the patient leaves the operating room.

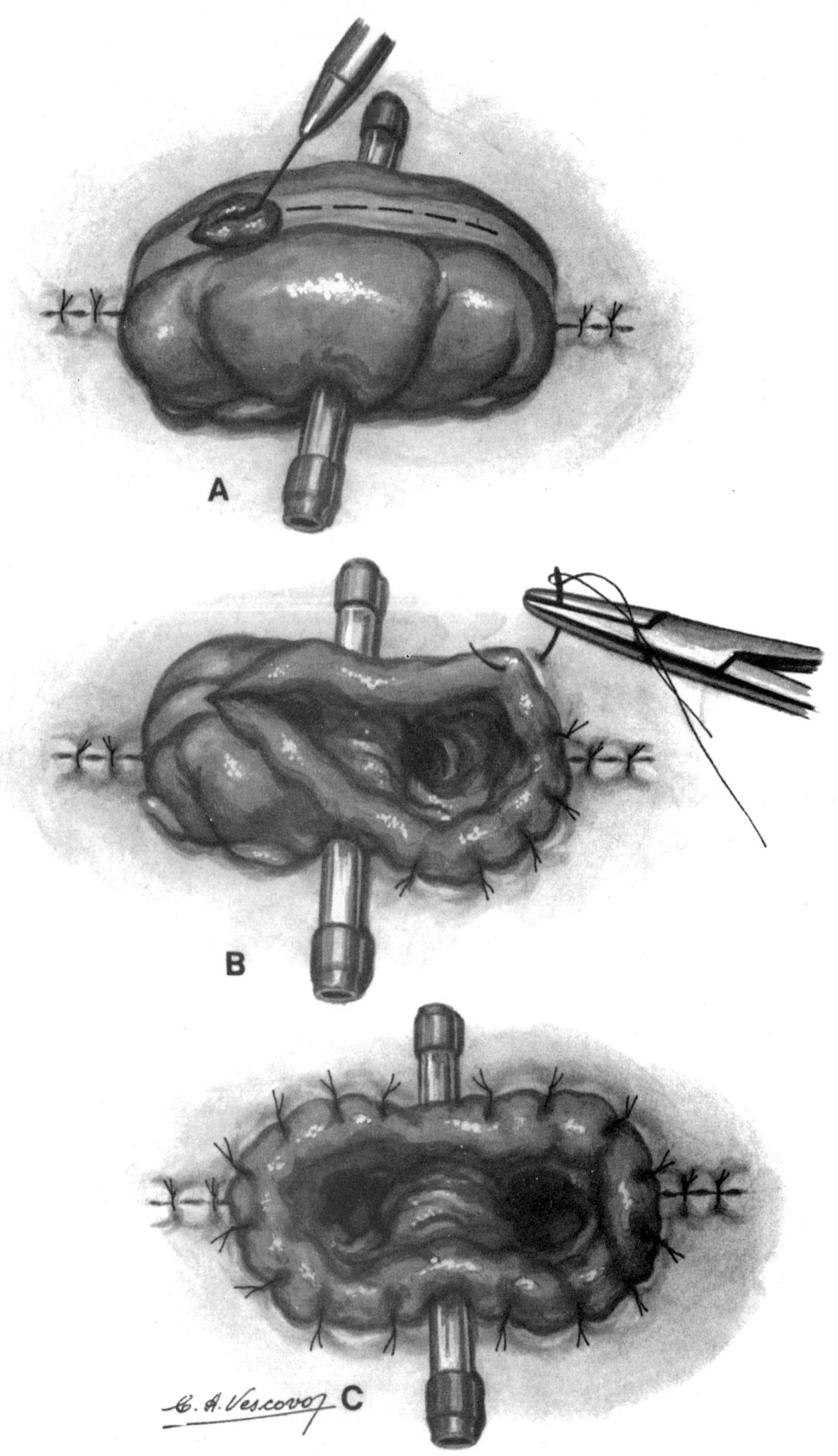

FIGURE 57.8

Transverse Loop Colostomy

FIGURE 57.9

If the patient is very distended due to distal colonic obstruction, the gaseous contents of the colon can be aspirated, as shown in the insert, to diminish the tension in the colon. The surgeon can then proceed with maturation of the colostomy. If the colonic contents are liquid, instead of mostly gaseous, maturation may be done during the same procedure. It is preferable, however, to insert a Pezzer or a Foley catheter held in place with a purse string to aspirate colonic contents. The colostomy is then opened the following day with an electric scalpel, without maturing it. It is preferable that the spillage of fecal material occur outside the operating room. **A,** A purse string suture has been applied and a Pezzer catheter is about to be introduced. **B,** The Pezzer catheter has been introduced and the purse string suture tied around it.

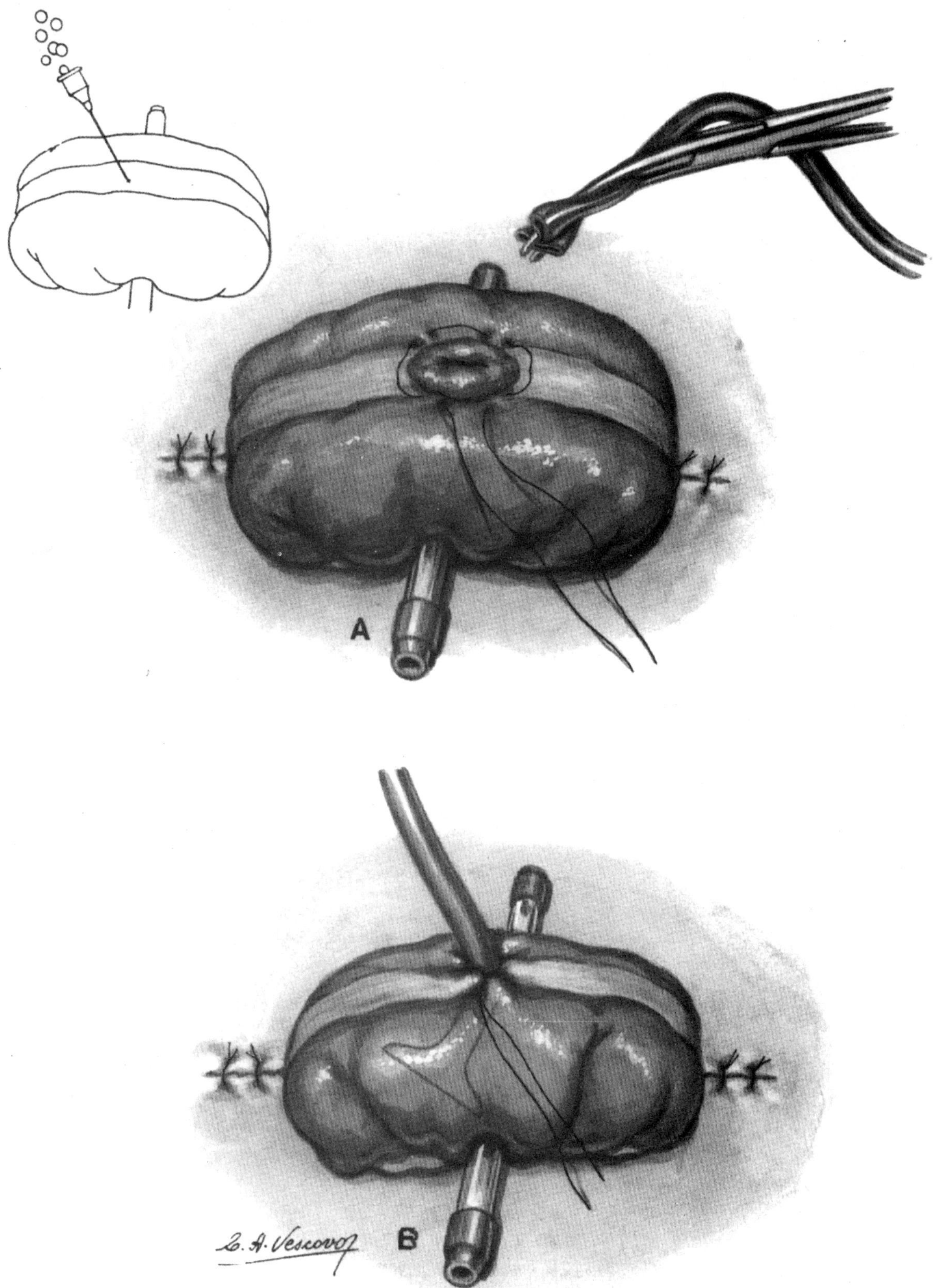

FIGURE 57.9

Transverse Colostomy Closure

FIGURE 57.10
A, An incision is made in the skin around the colostomy. **B,** The skin and subcutaneous tissues are incised and the edges grasped with Allis clamps. **C,** The skin and subcutaneous tissue incision has been completed.

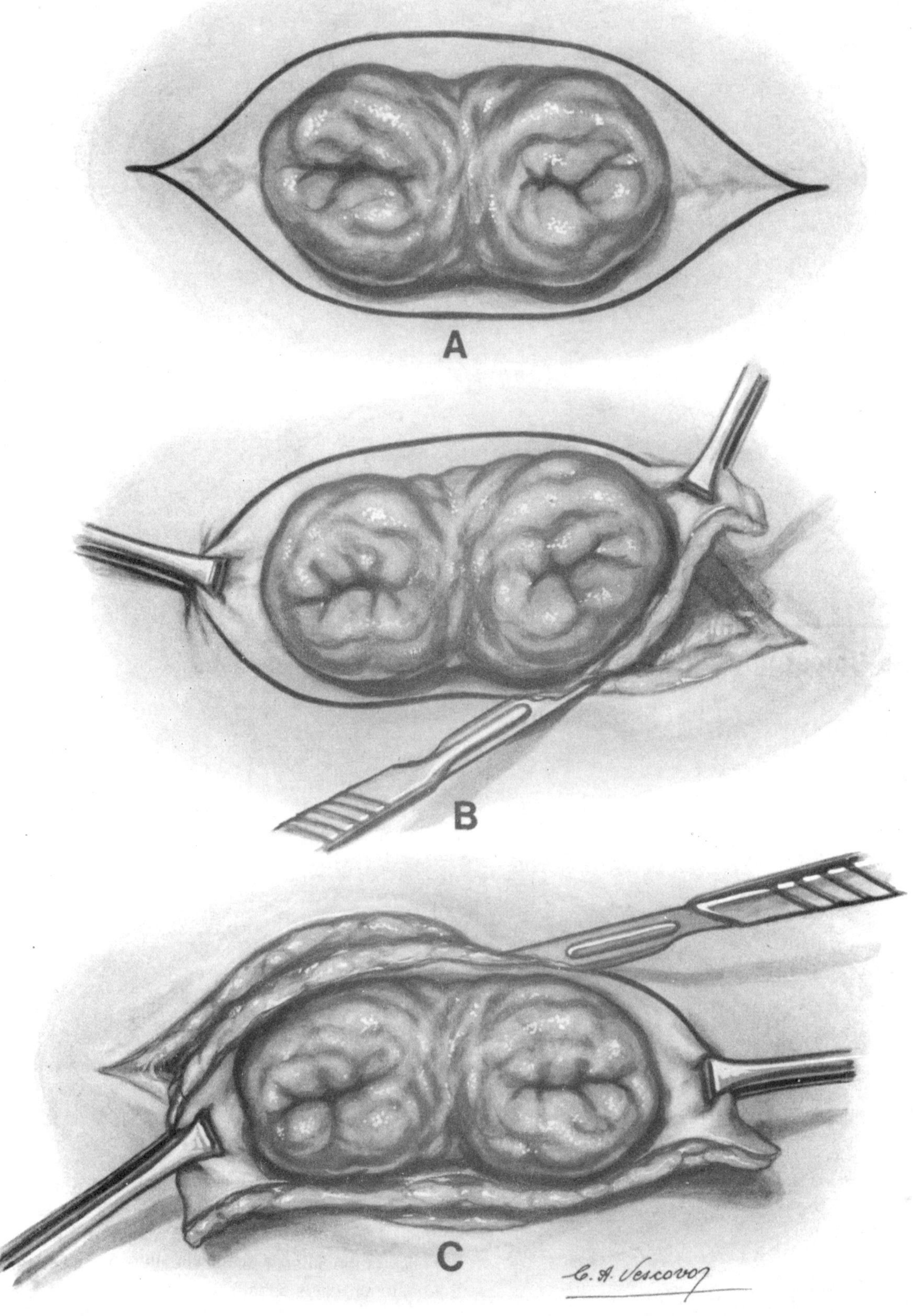

FIGURE 57.10

Transverse Colostomy Closure

FIGURE 57.11

A, The edges of the incision are being held with Allis clamps and traction is being applied upward. The tissue incision is continued down to the edge of the wound. **B,** Using a scalpel, the edge of the anterior rectus sheath is being separated from the posterior rectus sheath.

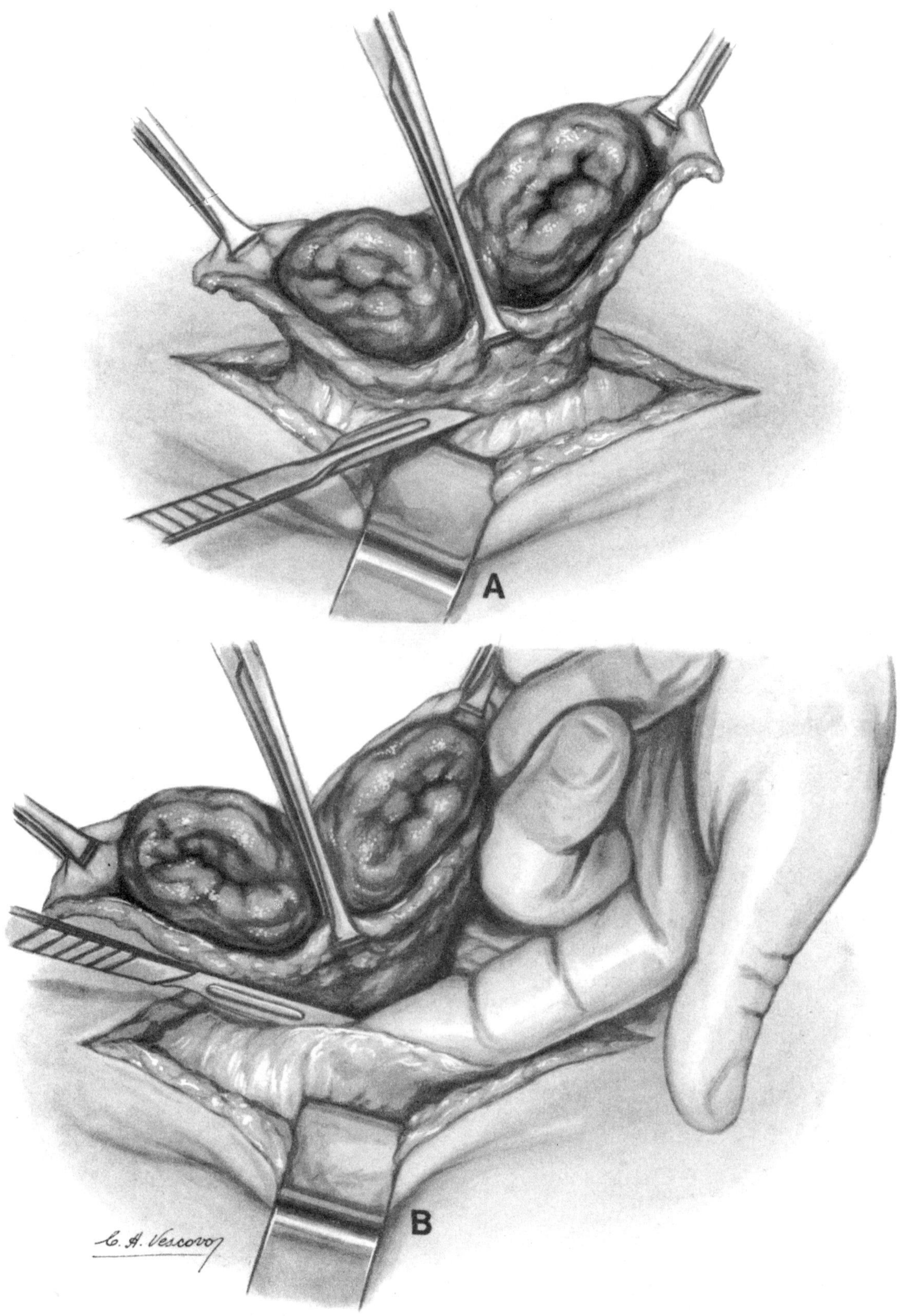

FIGURE 57.11

Transverse Colostomy Closure

FIGURE 57.12

A, The transverse colon is being pulled up with Allis clamps after freeing it from the wound edges. **B,** The skin and subcutaneous tissues are removed from around the colostomy, using scissors.

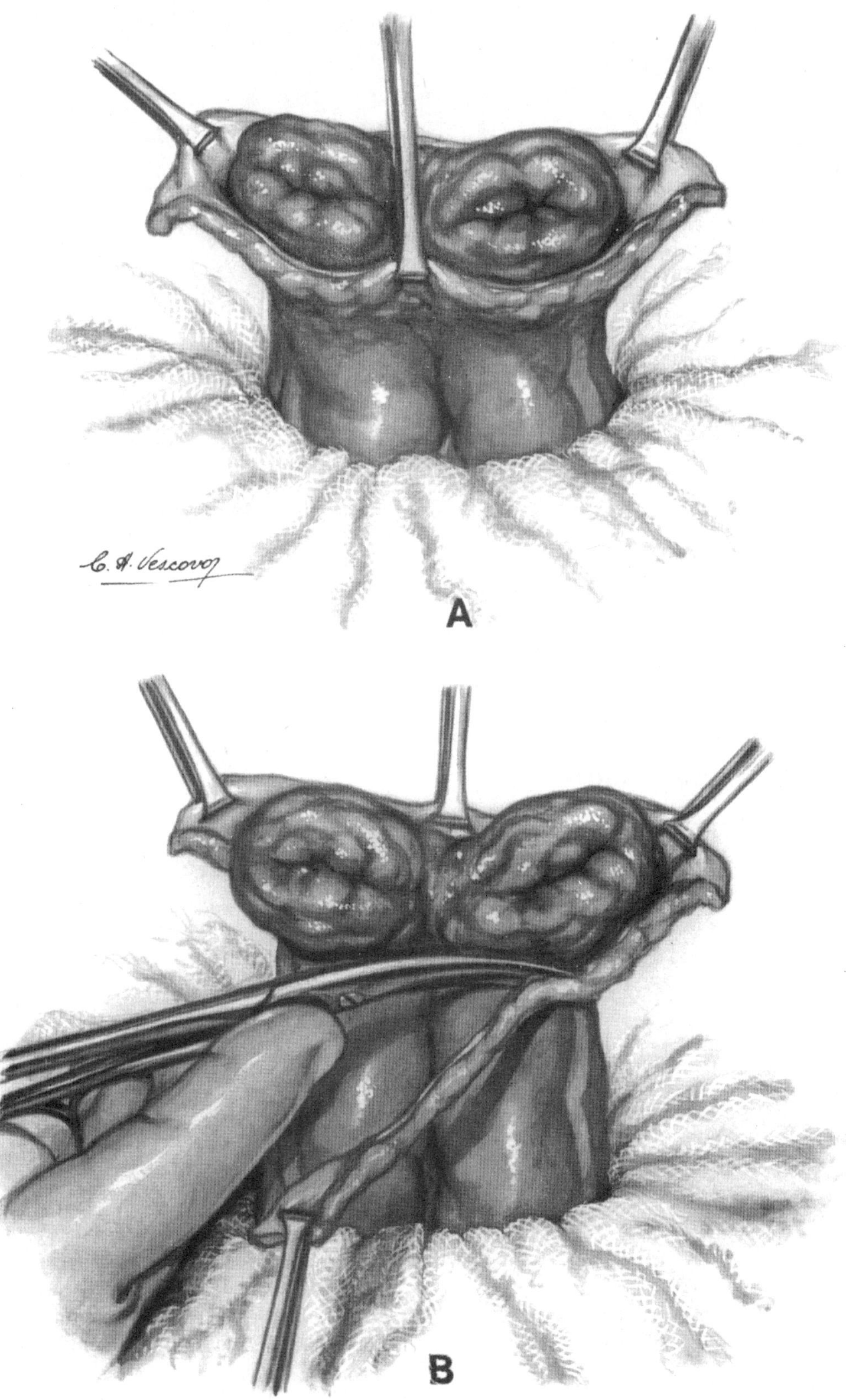

FIGURE 57.12

Transverse Colostomy Closure

FIGURE 57.13
Once the entire colonic circumference has been freed, its edges are examined to be sure their blood supply is adequate before the colon is sutured. **A,** The mucosa on both sides of the colon is being sutured with interrupted 3-0 chromic catgut. **B,** The Allis clamps have been replaced by traction sutures, continuing the mucosal closure, with the knots turned in. **C,** Once the mucosal layer is completed, the seromuscular layer is closed with nonabsorbable sutures.

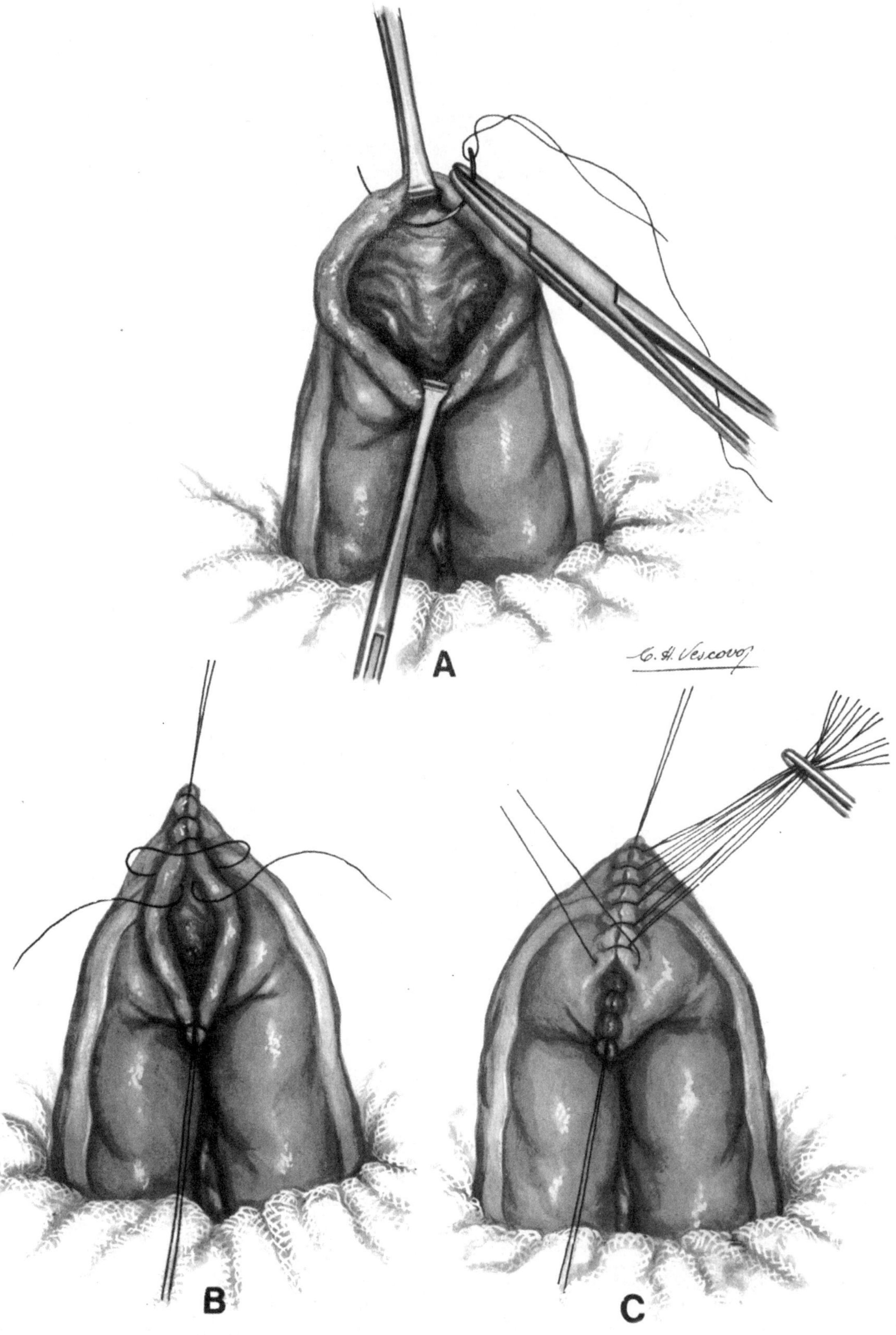

FIGURE 57.13

Transverse Colostomy Closure

FIGURE 57.14
A, Once the colon is closed, the fibrous tissue that frequently develops in the mesocolon and holds the proximal and distal limbs of the colostomy together is removed. This avoids angulations and possible colonic obstruction. **B,** Using a smooth Foerster clamp, the colonic loop is being introduced into the abdominal cavity to begin closing the abdominal incision.

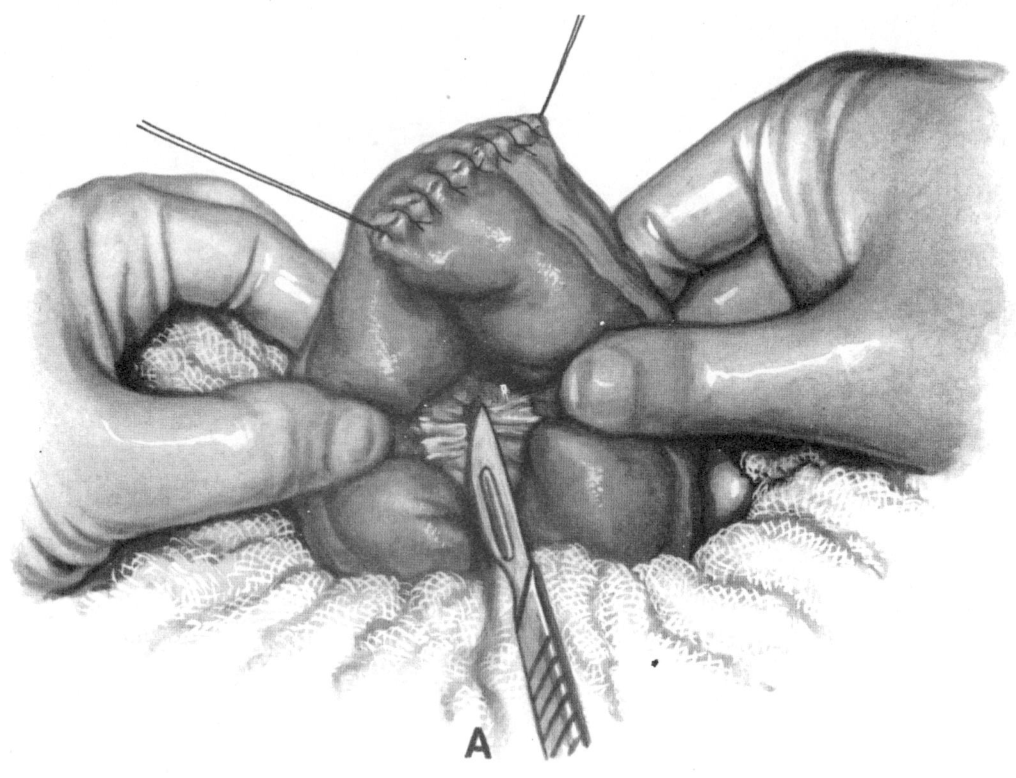

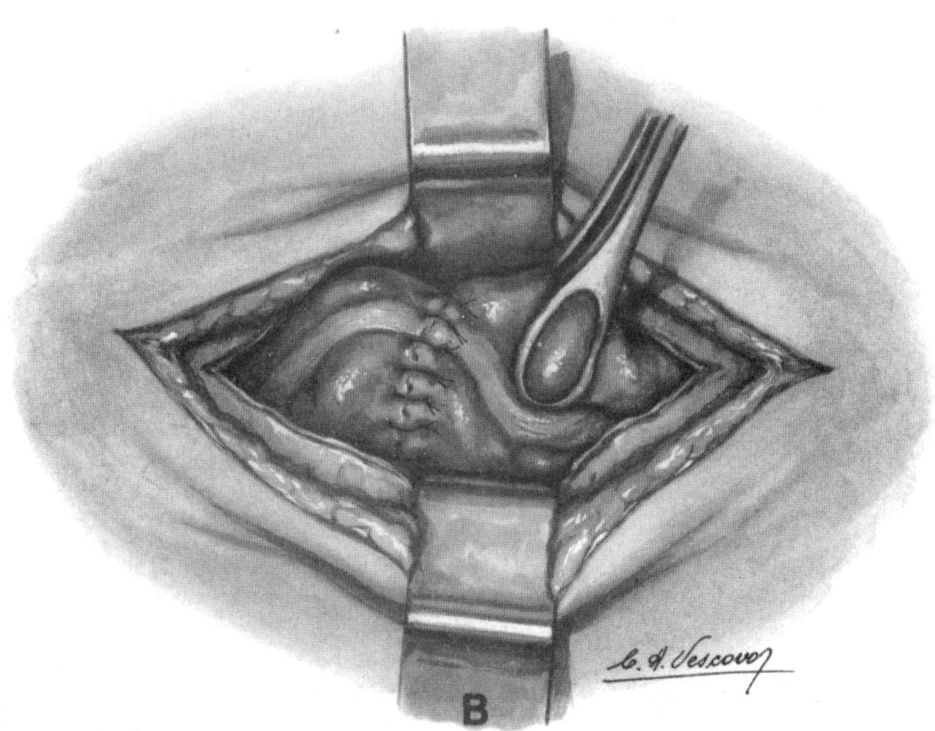

FIGURE 57.14

Transverse Colostomy Closure

FIGURE 57.15
When the loop colostomy was carried out, the anterior and posterior rectus sheaths were sutured together so as to construct a sort of envelope surrounding the transected muscle fibers. **A,** The anterior rectus fascia that had been sutured to the posterior rectus fascia has been incised in order to begin closing the abdominal wall in layers. **B,** In some patients retraction of the transected rectus abdominis muscle prevents suturing the abdominal incision without tension. In these cases it is advisable to carry out a relaxing incision in the anterior rectus sheath about 4 or 5 cm above the upper border of the incision. This will facilitate the approximation of the wound edges for the closure.

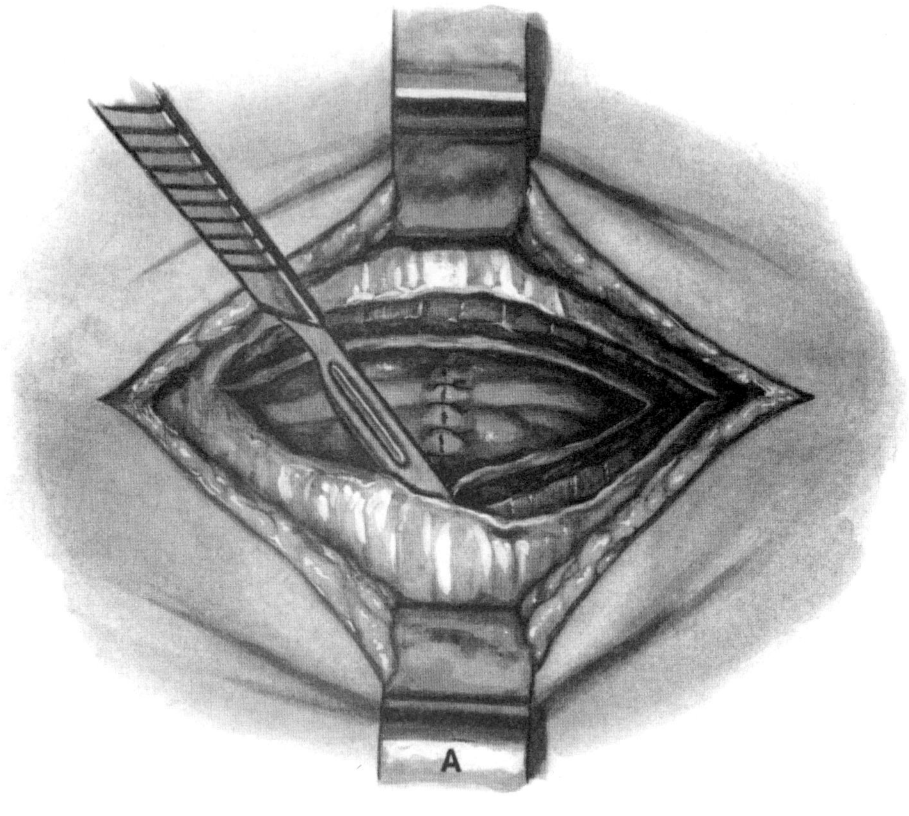

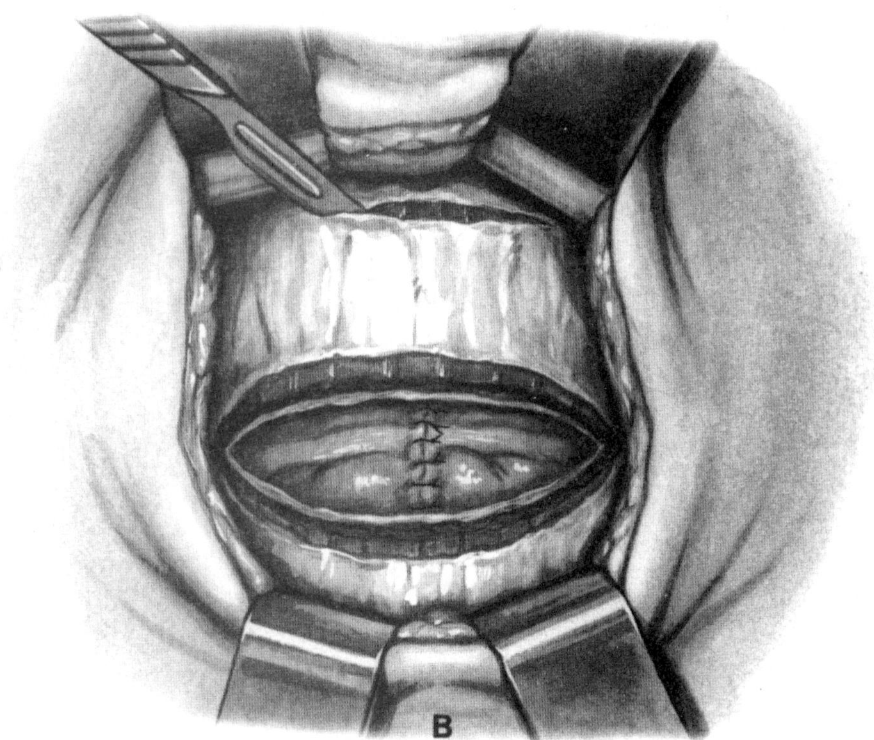

FIGURE 57.15

Transverse Colostomy Closure

FIGURE 57.16

A, If this relaxing incision is not sufficient to permit closure of the wound without tension, another relaxing incision can be made below the wound in similar fashion. **B,** The peritoneum is being closed together with the posterior fascia of the rectus abdominis muscle, using slow absorption interrupted sutures.

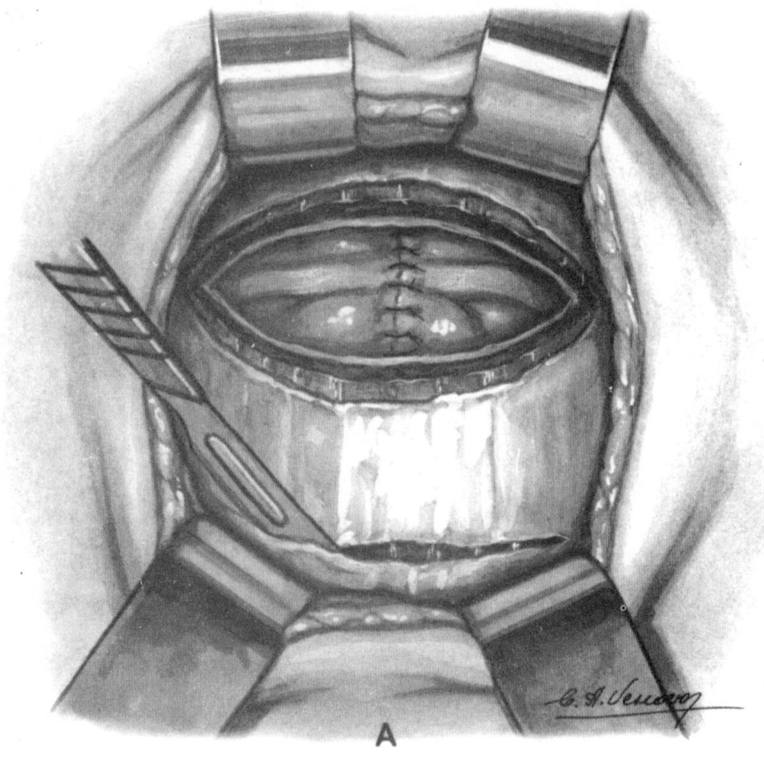

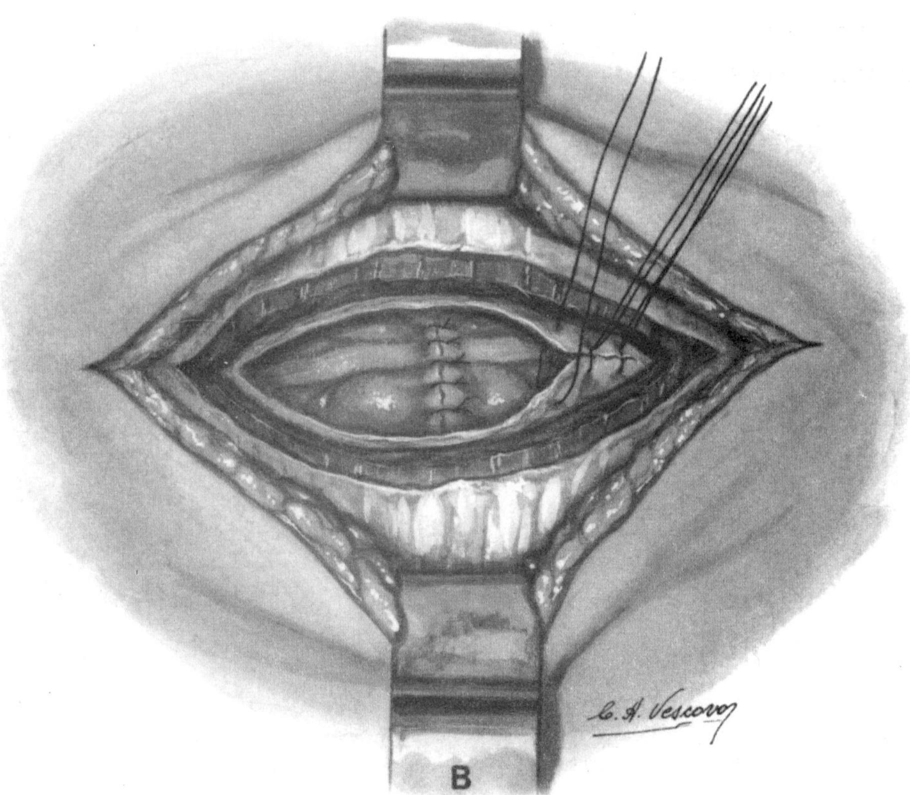

FIGURE 57.16

Transverse Colostomy Closure

FIGURE 57.17

A, Once the deep layer is closed, the anterior layer of the rectus fascia is closed with synthetic slow absorption sutures. **B,** The wound is irrigated with warm saline solution.

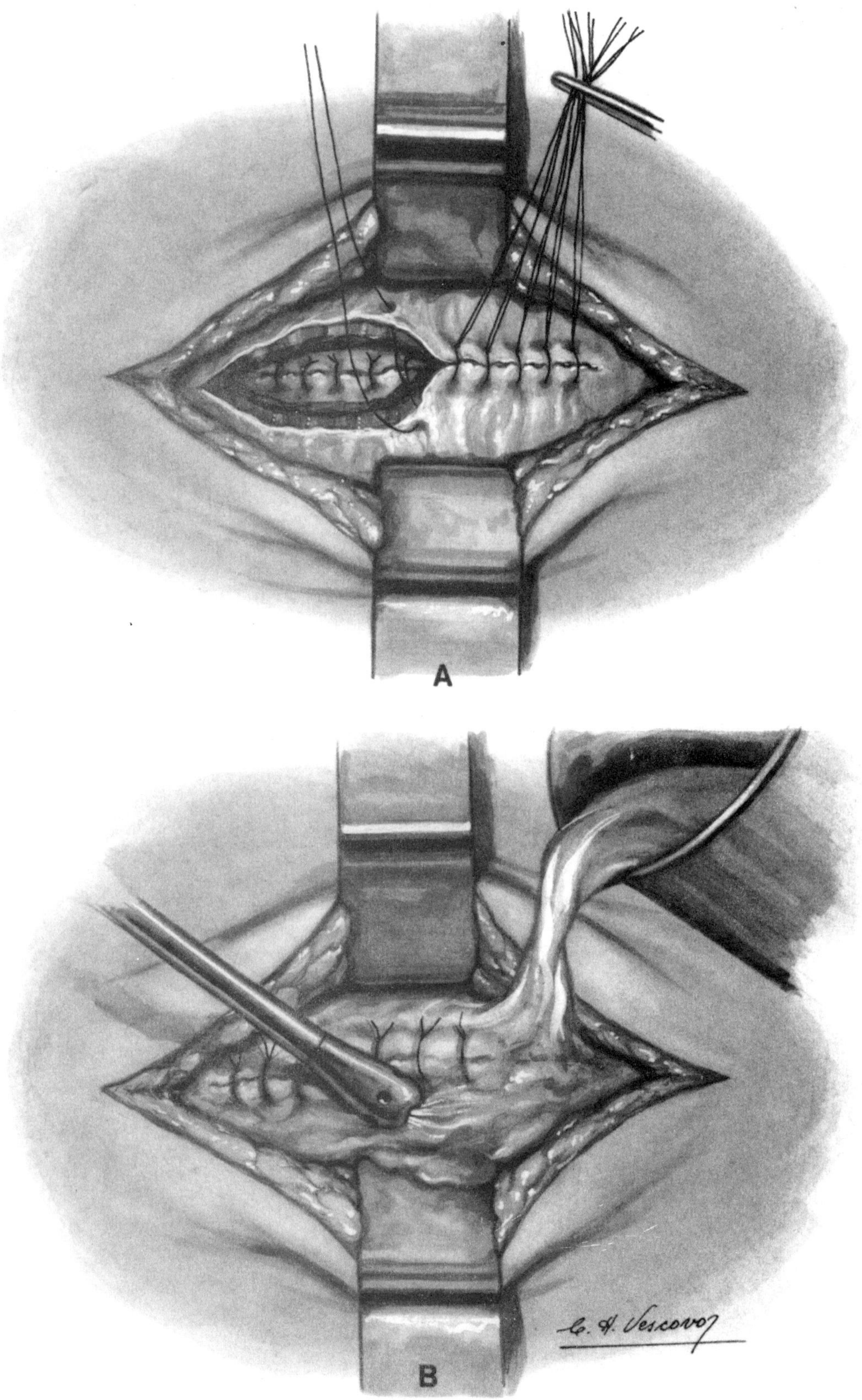

FIGURE 57.17

FIGURE 57.18
The skin and subcutaneous tissue are being sutured using interrupted somewhat separated sutures and leaving a Penrose drain in place. In some patients it may be convenient to pack the wound open for 6 or 7 days using iodoform gauze, then closing the wound with Steri-Strips.

Transverse Colostomy Closure

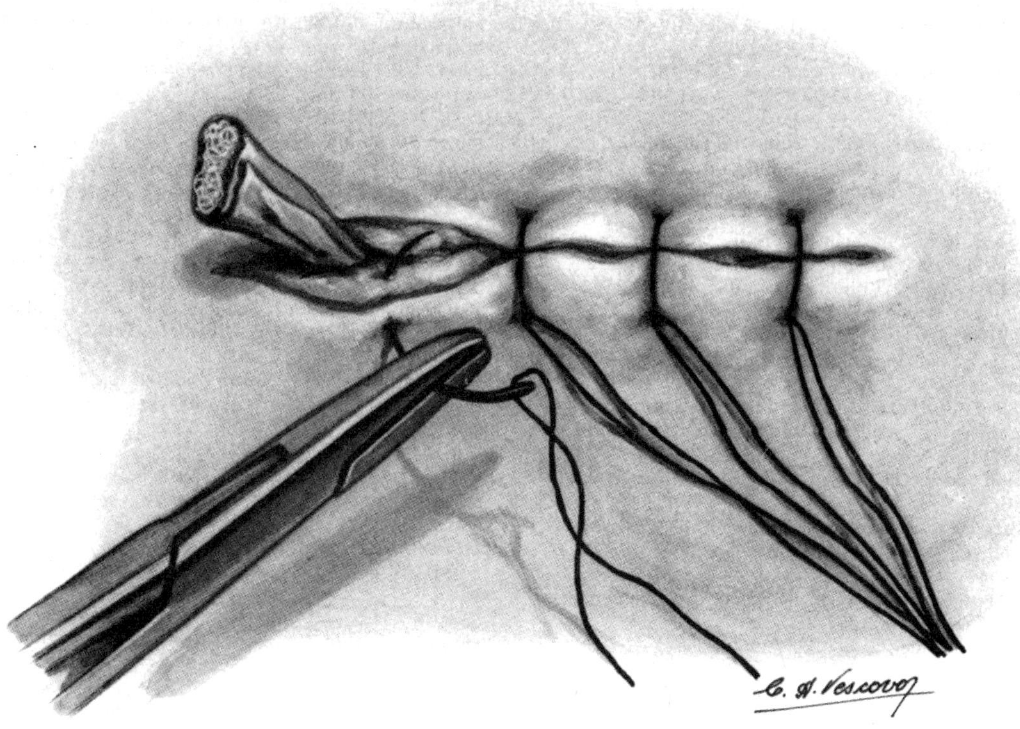

FIGURE 57.18

References

1. Abcarian, H., Pearl, R.K. Stomas. Surg. Clin. North. Am. 68:1295, 1988.
2. Aitken, R.J., Stevens, P.J., Preez, N., Elliot, M.S. Raising a colostomy, results of a prospective surgical audit. Int. J. Colorectal Dis. 1:244, 1986.
3. Aston, C., Everett, W.G. Comparison of early and late closure of transverse loop colostomies. Ann. R. Coll. Surg. Engl. 66:331, 1984.
4. Baker, F.S. The rodless loop colostomy. Dis. Colon Rectum 18:528, 1975.
5. Barron, J., Fallis, L.S. Colostomy, closure by the intraperitoneal method. Dis. Colon Rectum 1:466, 1958.
6. Boman-Sandelin, K., Fengo, G. Construction and closure of transverse loop colostomy. Dis. Colon Rectum 28:774, 1985.
7. Bubrick, M.P., Rolstad, B.S. Intestinal stomas. In Gordon, P.H., Nivatvongs, S. (Eds.) Colon, rectum and anus. p. 855. Quality Medical Publishing, St. Louis, 1992.
8. Corman, J.M., Odenheimer, D.B. Securing the loop. Historic review of the method used for creating a loop colostomy. Dis. Colon Rectum 34:1014, 1991.
9. Corman, M.L. Colon and rectal surgery. Ed. 3, p. 1097. Lippincott, Philadelphia, 1993.
10. Chandler, J.G., Evans, B.P. Colostomy prolapse. Surgery 84:577, 1978.
11. Chassin, J.L. Operative strategy. In General surgery. Ed. 2, p. 432. Springer-Verlag, New York, 1994.
12. Devlin, H.B. Colostomy. Indications, management and complications. Ann. R. Coll. Surg. Engl. 52:392, 1973.
13. Feinberg, S.M., Mc.Leod, R.S., Cohen, Z. Complications of loop ileostomy. Am. J. Surg. 153:102, 1987.
14. Fontes, B., Fontes, W., Utiyama, E.M., et al. The efficacy of loop colostomy for complete fecal diversion. Dis. Colon Rectum 31:298, 1988.
15. Hurwitz, A. Transverse colostomy. Ann. Surg. 122:834, 1971.
16. Irvin, T.T. Recent results of colostomy closure: A prospective study of 98 operations. J. R. Coll. Surg. Edinb. 32:357, 1987.
17. Jarpa, S. Transverse or sigmoid loop colostomy. Surg. Gynecol. Obstet. 163:372, 1986.
18. Keighley, M.R.B., Williams, N.S. Surgery of the anus, rectum and colon. Vol. I, p. 200. W.B. Saunders, Philadelphia, 1993.
19. Miles, R.M., Greene, R.S. Review of colostomy in a community hospital. Am. J. Surg. 49:182, 1983.
20. Parks, S.E., Hastings, P.R. Complications of colostomy closure. Am. J. Surg. 149:672, 1985.
21. Pearl, R.K., Prasad, M.L., Orsay, C.P., et al. Early local complications from intestinal stomas. Arch. Surg. 120:1145, 1985.
22. Pearl, R.K., Abcarian, H. Diverting stomas. In Mackeigan, J.M., Cataldo, P.A. (Eds.) Intestinal stomas. Quality Medical Publishing, St. Louis, 1993.
23. Phillips, R.K.S., Thomson, J.P.S. Colostomy. In Fielding, L.P., Goldberg, S.M. (Eds.) Surgery of the colon, rectum and anus. Ed. 5, p. 274 Butterworth-Heinemann, Oxford, 1993.
24. Rombeau, J.L., Wilk, P.J., Turnbull, R.B., et al. Total fecal diversion by the temporary skin-level loop transverse colostomy. Dis. Colon Rectum 21:223, 1978.
25. Rosen, L., Friedman, I.H. Morbidity and mortality following intraperitoneal closure of transverse loop colostomy. In Turnbull, R.B., Weackley, F.L. (Eds.) An atlas of intestinal stomas. p. 97. C.V. Mosby, St. Louis, 1967.
26. Rutegard, J., Dahlgren, S. Transverse colostomy or loop ileostomy as diverting stoma in colorectal surgery. Acta Chir. Scand. 153:229, 1987.
27. Schifield, P.F., Cade, D., Lambert, M. Dependent proximal loop colostomy. Does it defunction the distal colon? Br. J. Surg. 67:201, 1980.
28. Smit, R., Walt, A.J. The morbidity and cost of the temporary colostomy. Dis. Colon Rectum 21:558, 1978.
29. Unti, J.A., Abcarian, H., Pearl, R.K., et al. Rodless end-loop stomas. A seven year experience. Dis. Colon Rectum 34:999, 1991.
30. Wangensteen, O.H. Complete fecal diversion achieved by a simple loop colostomy. Surg. Gynecol. Obstet. 84:409, 1947.
31. Williams, N.S., Nasmyth, D.G., Jones, D., et al. Defunctioning stomas: A postoperative controlled trial comparing loop ileostomy with loop transverse colostomy. Br. J. Surg. 74:566, 1986.
32. Winkler, M.J., Volpe, P.A. Loop transverse colostomy. The case against. Dis. Colon Rectum 25:321, 1982.

Section H

Colon, Rectum, and Anus

CHAPTER **58**

Cecostomy

A cecostomy is an operation that, at present, is very controversial. A cecostomy does not completely divert the fecal stream, for which reason it is not indicated as an operation to protect colorectal anastomoses. On the other hand, care of the cecostomy catheter must be very rigorous to keep it from becoming obstructed (5, 18). Manometric studies have shown that a cecostomy will not protect rectal anastomoses from proximal high-pressure peristaltic waves. There is a group of surgeons who believe that a cecostomy is important in protecting distal colonic anastomoses (7, 8, 10, 12, 25, 26).

At present, cecostomy is practically reserved for patients with Ogilvie syndrome, in whom decompressive fiberoptic colonoscopy has failed. Decompressive endoscopic colonoscopy is successful in 61 to 91% of patients, with an incidence of recurrence of 22% and risk of perforation in some patients (21, 23). Another indication for cecostomy is to fix the bowel in place in patients with cecal volvulus (1, 5, 16, 17, 21–23).

The cecostomy tube has to be carefully controlled to keep it from becoming obstructed. Thirty-six to forty-eight hours after the cecostomy, the tube should be irrigated with warm isotonic saline and the irrigant then aspirated. This should be done every 6 hours. On the 7th day the suture holding the tube in place is cut. Usually the tube will fall out on about the 9th or 10th day. If the cecostomy was done with a Foley catheter, the balloon should be deflated to facilitate its expulsion.

The most common complications of cecostomy are suppuration of the wound due to contamination and filtration of fecal fluid around the tube. After the cecostomy tube has been removed, the wound usually closes spontaneously, but in some cases it shows no tendency to close.

Recently, cecostomy tubes have been introduced percutaneously using computed tomography (4, 9, 15, 19, 21). Tubes inserted using this technique are usually 12 F in caliber. These procedures are done under local anesthesia. Morrison et al. (15) have described a transperitoneal approach using radioscopic means, without having to use computed tomography.

Operative Technique

FIGURE 58.1
McBurney incision, 5 to 6 cm long, in the right iliac fossa. The cecum is identified by its anatomic characteristics. The edges of the incision are protected with gauze. A purse string suture is inserted using nonabsorbable material.

FIGURE 58.2
If the cecal distension does not permit correct insertion of the purse string suture, the cecum can be aspirated using a trocar inserted through the anterior tenia. After gas and fluid are aspirated, three Babcock clamps are applied to exert traction in order to avoid retraction of the cecum into the abdomen.

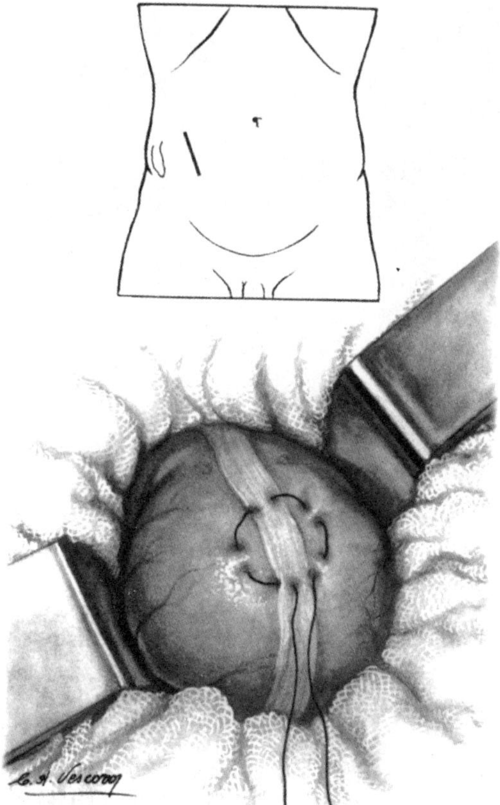

FIGURE 58.1

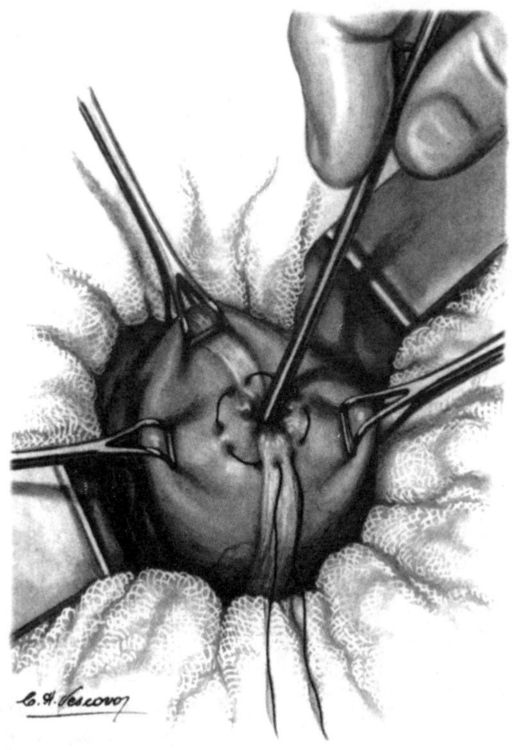

FIGURE 58.2

FIGURE 58.3
An incision has been made in the anterior cecal wall, through the anterior tenia, and a 24 to 30 F Pezzer tube, held by a curved clamp, is about to be inserted. Several perforations can be made in the Pezzer tube to facilitate drainage. A Foley tube of the same caliber can also be used. The Foley balloon should be inflated after the purse string has been tied.

Operative Technique

FIGURE 58.4
The Pezzer tube has been inserted and the purse string adjusted. A second purse string is then inserted around the tube for greater security.

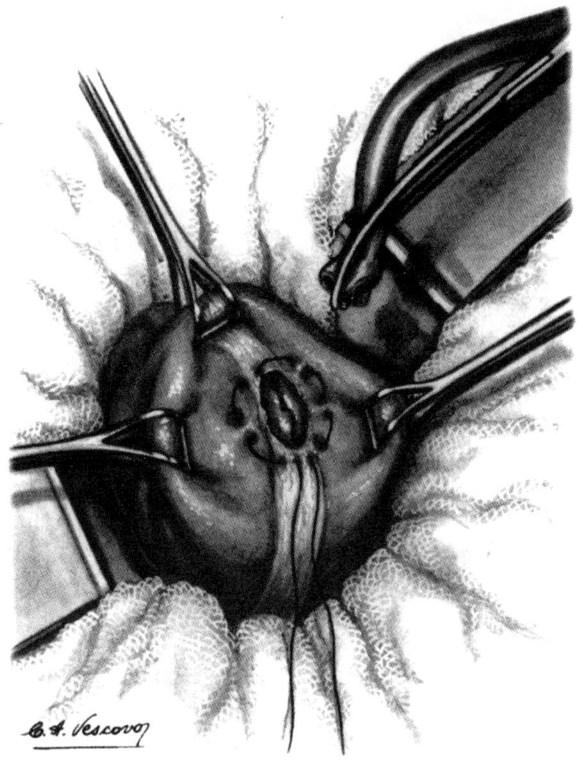

FIGURE 58.3

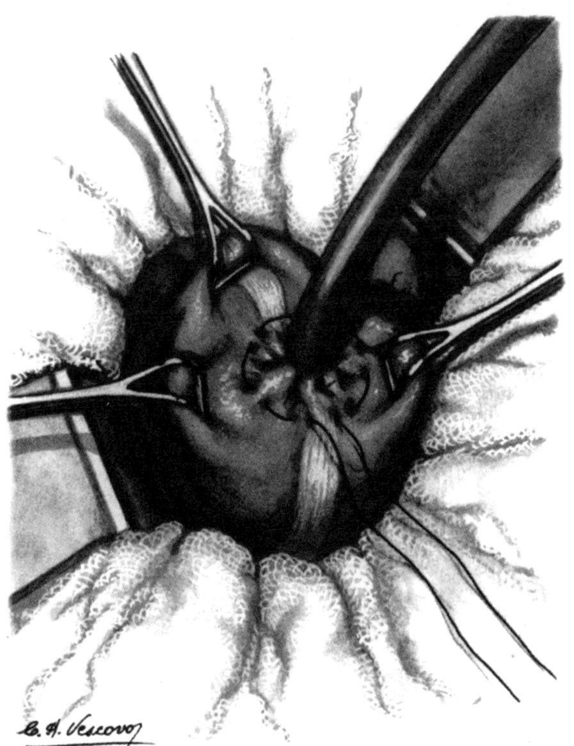

FIGURE 58.4

FIGURE 58.5
The second purse string has been tied and its loose ends transected in order to proceed with fixation of the cecum to the parietal peritoneum around the tube, using nonabsorbable sutures.

Operative Technique

FIGURE 58.6
Once the cecum has been fixed to the parietal peritoneum, the peritoneal closure is done using interrupted, nonabsorbable sutures.

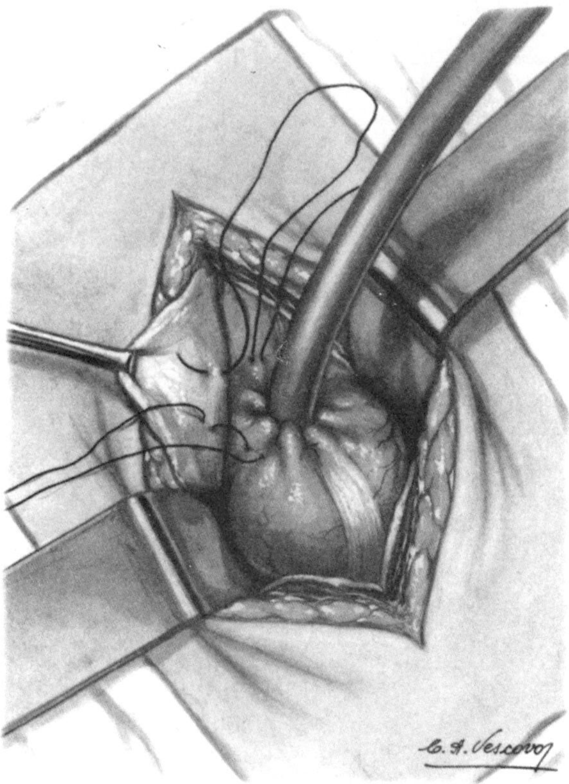

FIGURE 58.5

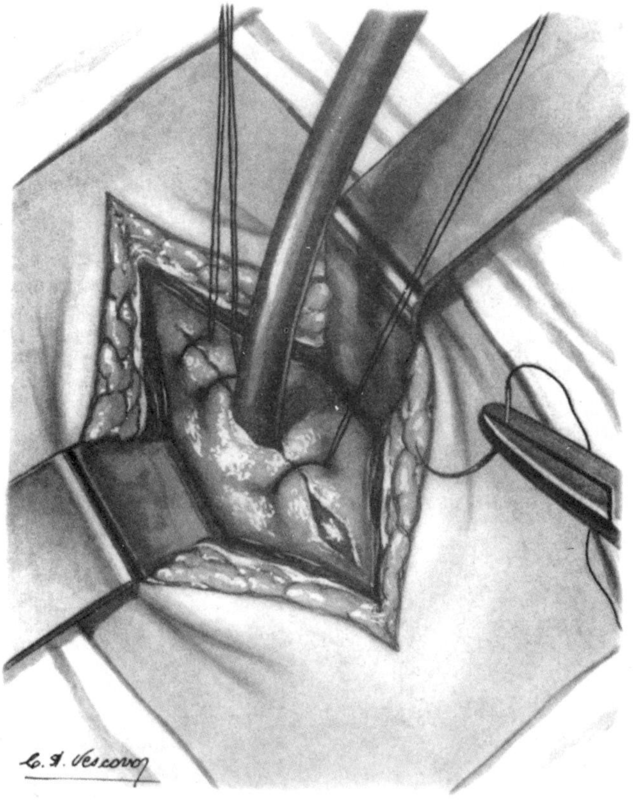

FIGURE 58.6

FIGURE 58.7
The major oblique muscle is being closed with interrupted, nonabsorbable sutures.

Operative Technique

FIGURE 58.8
The subcutaneous tissue has been closed with 2-0 catgut, and the skin is being closed with nonabsorbable material. The cecostomy tube has been solidly fixed to the skin to prevent its expulsion due to some movement by the patient.

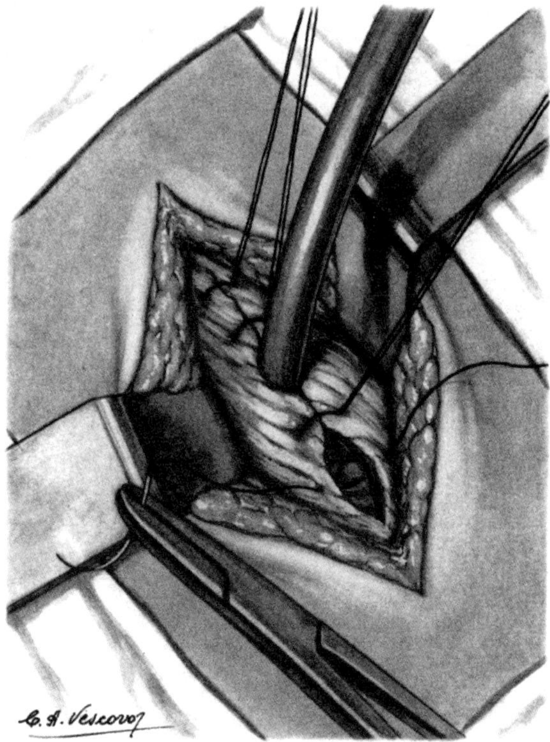

FIGURE 58.7

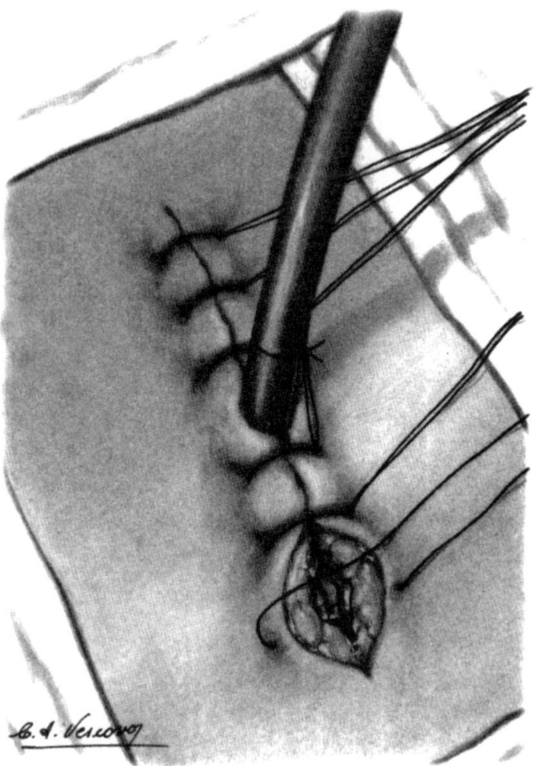

FIGURE 58.8

Operative Technique

FIGURE 58.9
Sectional view of the completed cecostomy. The two purse string sutures are seen holding the Pezzer tube. Also seen are the fixation of the cecum to the anterior parietal peritoneum and fixation of the tube to the skin.

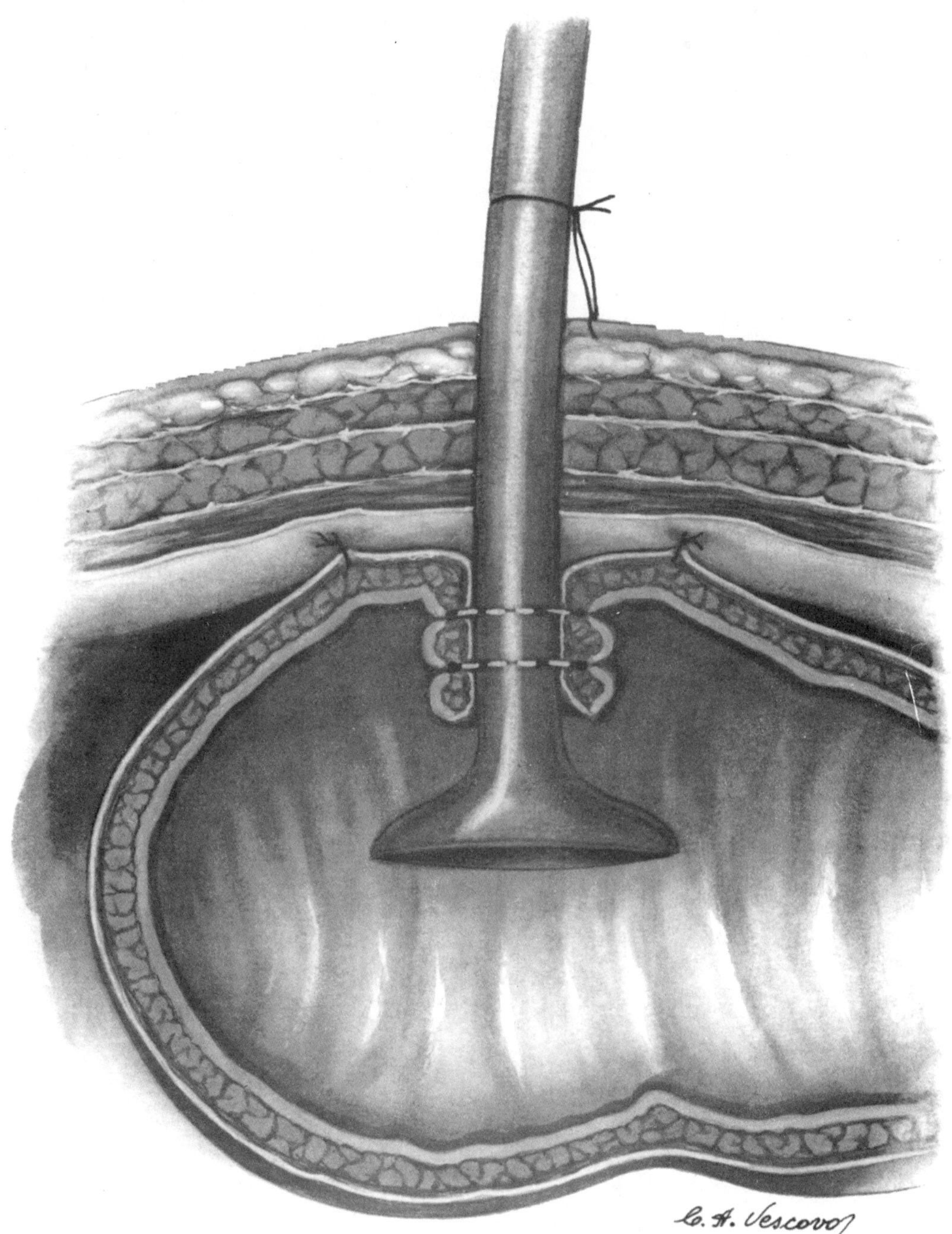

FIGURE 58.9

Operative Technique

FIGURE 58.10

If the patient has undergone an abdominal procedure and the surgeon believes a complementary cecostomy is necessary, the tube is placed in exactly the same manner and brought out through a small incision in the anterior abdominal wall. The cecum is then fixed to the anterior peritoneum, around the tube. The tube is then fixed to the skin, as shown in the drawing and in the upper and lower inserts.

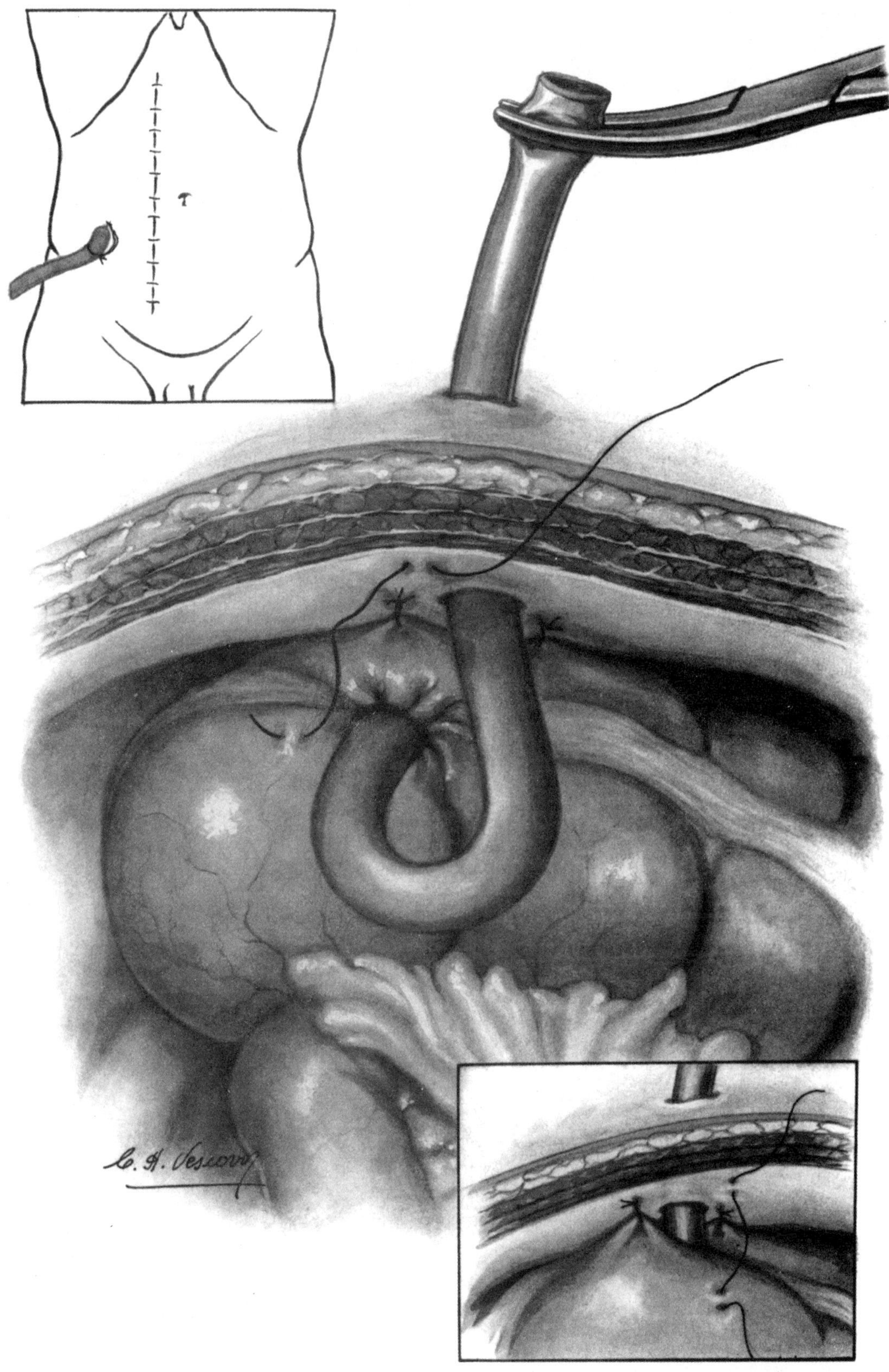

FIGURE 58.10

References

1. Anderson, J.R., Welch, G.H. Acute volvulus of the right colon: an analysis of 59 patients. World J. Surg. 10:336, 1986.
2. Bubrick, M.P., Rolstad, B.S. Intestinal stomas. In Gordon, P.H., Nivatvongs, S. (Eds.) Colon, rectum and anus. p. 855. Quality Medical Publishing, St. Louis, 1992.
3. Casola, G., Withers, C., van Sonnenberg, E., et al. Percutaneous cecostomy for decompression of the massive distended cecum. Radiology 158:793, 1986.
4. Crass, J.R., Simmons, R.L., Frick, M.P., et al. Percutaneous decompression of the colon using C. T. guidance in Ogilvie Syndrome. Am. J. Roentgenol. 144:475, 1985.
5. Chassin, J.L. Operative strategy in general surgery. Ed. 2, p. 429. Springer-Verlag, New York, 1994.
6. Florer, R.E. Cecostomy: Indication and technique. Am. J. Surg. 93:865, 1957.
7. Gerber, A., Thompson, R.J. Jr. Use of a tube cecostomy to lower the mortality in acute large intestinal obstruction due to carcinoma. Am. J. Surg. 110:893, 1965.
8. Goldstein, S.D., Salvati, E.P., Rubin, R.J., et al. Tube cecostomy with cecal extraperitonealization in the management of obstructing left sided carcinoma of the large intestine. Surg. Gynecol. Obstet. 162:379, 1986.
9. Haaga, J.R., Bick, R.J., Zollinger, R.M. Jr. C. T. Guided percutaneous catheter cecostomy. Gastrointest. Radiol. 12:166, 1987.
10. Hughes, E.S.R. Cecostomy: A part of an efficient method of decompressing the colon obstructed by cancer. Dis. Colon Rectum 6:454, 1963.
11. Ingoldby, C.J.H., Dawson, A., Addison, N.V. A new technique of cecostomy using endotracheal tubes. Ann. R. Coll. Surg. Engl. 71:211, 1989.
12. Jackson, P.J., Baird, R.M. Cecostomy: An analysis of 102 cases. Am. J. Surg. 114:297, 1967.
13. Kodner, I.J. Colostomy and ileostomy. Clin. Symp. 30:2, 1978.
14. Maynard, A. de L., Turrell, R. Acute left colon obstruction with special reference to cecostomy versus transversostomy. Surg. Gynecol. Obstet. 100:667, 1955.
15. Morrison, M.C., Lee, M.J., Stafford, S.A., et al. Percutaneous cecostomy: Controlled transperitoneal approach. Radiology 176:574, 1990.
16. Nanni, G., Garbini, A., Luchetti, P., et al. Ogilvie's syndrome (acute colonic pseudo-obstruction); review of the literature and a report of four additional cases. Dis. Colon Rectum 25:157, 1982.
17. Nivatvongs, S., Vermeulen, J.D., Fang, D.T. Colonoscopic decompression of acute pseudo-obstruction of the colon. Ann. Surg. 196:598, 1982.
18. Phillips, R.K.S., Thomson, J.P.S. Tube caecostomy. In Fielding, L.P., Goldberg, S.M. (Eds.) Surgery of the colon, rectum and anus. Ed. 5, p. 270. Butterworth-Heinemann, Oxford, 1993.
19. Ponsky, J.L., Aszoki, A., Perse, D. Percutaneous endoscopic cecostomy: A new approach to nonobstructive colonic dilatation. Gastrointest. Endosc. 32:108, 1982.
20. Quinn, S.F., Jones, E.N., Maroney, T. Percutaneous cecostomy in the management of cecal volvulus: Report of a case. J. Intervent. Radiol. 2:137, 1987.
21. Senagore, A. Cecostomy. In Mackeigan, J.M., Cataldo, P.A. (Eds.) Intestinal stomas. p. 127. Quality Medical Publishing, St. Louis, 1993.
22. Strodel, W.E., Nostrant, T.T., Eckhauser, F.E., et al. Therapeutic and diagnostic colonoscopy in nonobstructive colonic dilatation. Ann. Surg. 194:416, 1983.
23. Vanek, V.W., Al-Salti, M. Acute pseudo-obstruction of the colon (Ogilvie's syndrome). An analysis of 400 cases. Dis. Colon Rectum 29:203, 1986.
24. Wheeler, M.H., Barker, J. Closure of colostomy, a safe procedure. Dis. Colon Rectum 20:29, 1977.
25. Westdahel, P.R. A comparison of cecostomy and colostomy in the management of acute obstruction of the left colon. Am. J. Surg. 96:324, 1958.
26. Westdahel, R.P., Russell, T. In support of blind tube cecostomy in acute obstruction of the descending colon: Analysis of ninety-three emergency colostomies. Am. J. Surg. 118:577, 1969.

Section H

Colon, Rectum, and Anus

CHAPTER **59**

Surgery of Cancer of the Rectum

The incidence of carcinoma of the rectum remains stable while the incidence of carcinoma of the colon continues to increase. Studies of the pathology of cancer of the rectum and its spread have proven that its distal spread rarely extends beyond 10 mm from the macroscopic limit of the tumor. Based on this fact, at present, a greater number of operations with preservation of the anal sphincter are being performed without altering the figures for morbidity, mortality, and 5 year survival (6–8, 15, 17, 21, 23, 40, 56, 74, 83, 84, 87–89). According to Heald (44), up to several years ago, anterior resection of the rectum was performed in only 30 to 50% of patients with rectal cancer, because this procedure was recommended only for tumors of the upper third of the rectum and the rectosigmoid. According to the same author, anterior resection of the rectum is now performed in 80 to 90% of cases of rectal carcinoma.

Anatomic studies of the rectum have led to better knowledge of its innervation. This has made possible resections of the rectum for cancer with a lower percentage of male patients having loss of erection and ejaculation, and with functional alterations of the bladder.

Technological progress has led to the creation of new and ingenious instruments that make it easier to carry out rectal resections, preserving sphincteric continence. Better preparation and postoperative care of patients has contributed to their recuperation and offered them a better quality of life.

It is very probable that in the near future, advances will be made that will result in improvement in both immediate as well as late surgical results.

SURGICAL ANATOMY OF THE RECTUM

Knowledge of the surgical anatomy of the rectum is very important in performing correct surgery and in the adoption of the procedure that is most adequate, according to the location of the tumor and other factors that will be analyzed later. We will only point out basic notions of the surgical anatomy of the rectum, since this subject has been covered in a previous chapter.

The length of the rectum varies greatly, according to variations in the patient's constitutional habitus, sex, and age. It is generally accepted that the rectum is about 15 cm long, from the third sacral vertebra to the anal margin. The rectum has one intraperitoneal and another extraperitoneal segment, for which reason some authors divide it into the intraperitoneal rectum and the extra- or subperitoneal rectum (85). However, division of the rectum into three segments is more useful and more practical. The inferior segment or lower third of the rectum is 7 cm long and completely extraperitoneal. The middle segment extends from 7 to 11 cm from the anal margin and is partially covered with peritoneum. The superior segment is above the 11-cm level and extends to its junction with the sigmoid colon. The distal 4 cm of the rectum correspond to the surgical anal canal, the superior limit of which is the anorectal ring and the inferior limit, the anal margin. The anatomic anal canal extends from the pectinate line to the anal margin and is 2 cm long. Anal continence is preserved if the rectum is transected 1 or 2 cm above the pectinate line. The anorectal ring is located 4 cm from the anal margin and is made up of the puborectalis muscle, complemented by superior fibers of the deep fascicle of the external anal sphincter and superior fibers of the internal anal sphincter. Transection of the anorectal ring inevitably leads to anal incontinence.

The rectum, which is the continuation of the sigmoid colon, extends from the third sacral vertebra to the margin of the anus. For practical reasons, surgeons generally consider the upper limit of the rectum to be at the level of the sacral promontory, a more significant landmark. It should be pointed out that the junction of the sigmoid with the rectum is not sudden, but gradual, making it difficult to precisely establish the limit between the sigmoid and the rectum. For this reason, it is more appropriate to use the term "rectosigmoid zone" instead of "junction," since the limit between rectum and sigmoid is rather arbitrary.

The upper segment of rectum has peritoneum covering its anterior and lateral walls. The middle segment is only covered by peritoneum on its lateral walls, and the inferior segment of the rectum is completely extraperitoneal.

Valves of Houston

In its course, the rectum has three curves, which internally correspond to the valves of Houston. The middle valve of Houston is usually at the level of the anterior peritoneal reflection. Below the middle valve of Houston, the lumen of the rectum widens considerably, constituting the rectal ampulla.

When dissection and surgical mobilization of the rectum is performed, its curves are straightened out, making it 4 to 5 cm longer, a fact of great importance in surgery for cancer of the rectum with preservation of sphincteric function.

The anal canal is surrounded by muscles, the external anal sphincter on the outside, and the internal sphincter on the inside. The external sphincter is voluntary and made up of three parts: (a) the subcutaneous portion, (b) the superficial portion, and (c) the deep portion. The internal anal sphincter is involuntary and consists of thickening of the circular muscular anorectal layer.

Pelvic Fascia

The subperitoneal rectum is lodged inside the pelvis, surrounded by perirectal fat and by fascias arising from the pelvic fascia, which has different densities according to its topography. Knowledge of the location and density of perirectal fascias is very important in rectal surgery, so that this organ can be mobilized along more adequate planes.

PREOPERATIVE DETERMINATION OF THE LOCATION OF RECTAL CANCER

The first maneuver performed by the surgeon to determine the localization of a rectal cancer is digital palpation. This procedure is useful but in no way conclusive in determining the level of the cancer, because the tumor may be prolapsed and appear to be located at a lower level. On the other hand, if the tumor is infiltrating, it may retract into the rectal wall and appear to be at a higher level. Digital rectal examination may furnish some other important data about the rectal cancer, proving it to be flat, polypoid, ulcerated, or infiltrating. In addition, rectal examination may determine its mobility, degree of fixation, and circumferential extension; prostatic or bladder invasion in the male, or invasion of the vagina in the female; invasion of the pouch of Douglas; the presence of lymphadenopathy; and so on.

The best procedure to determine the level at which a rectal tumor is located is by means of a rigid scope, with the patient in the left lateral decubitus position. Measurement should be taken from the inferior border of the tumor to the anal margin. The length of the tumor is determined by measuring the distance between the superior border of the base of the cancer and the anal margin. The difference between the two measurements is the length of the carcinoma.

Several biopsies should be taken during endoscopic examination of a rectal cancer to confirm the diagnosis and to determine the degree of cellular differentiation.

An endorectal sonographic study is valuable in patients with rectal cancer to show the extent of the tumor, its penetration, and the possibility of showing the presence of adenopathy without affirming it to be inflammatory or neoplastic (46, 51).

Functional Study of the Anal Sphincter

In patients who may be subjected to surgery for rectal cancer with preservation of the sphincter, it is important to know beforehand the functional status of the anal sphincter. In patients with a weak sphincter, the therapeutic plan of conservation of the sphincter may have to be changed. In order to have normal sphincteric continence, it is necessary to have (17) (a) the presence of 1 or 2 cm of rectal wall above the pectinate line, (b) good functioning of the puborectalis muscles, and (c) normal function of the internal and external anal sphincters. Some surgeons (93) recommend manometric studies of the function of the anal sphincter in all patients who may be subjected to anterior resection of the rectum. Some surgeons believe rectal examination is enough to determine the functional status of the anal sphincter. Others (93) believe rectal examination is insufficient because it is subjective, demonstrating many variations in the same patient when examined by different examiners.

In addition to evaluation of the functional status of the anal sphincter, the defecatory habits of the patient should be studied to determine the number of daily bowel movements, as well as the presence of frequent diarrhea due to accelerated intestinal transit. Patients with frequent diarrhea or several bowel movements daily are not good candidates for low anterior resection. Study of the patient will be completed by a general examination with X-rays of the colon and chest, colonoscopy, ultrasonography, computed tomography of the abdomen and pelvis, and so on.

If there are no contraindications to the operation, resectability of the rectal cancer will ultimately depend on surgical exploration. The possibility of performing a low anterior resection can only be determined after ample mobilization of the rectum posteriorly, freeing it from the sacral concavity, and liberation of the anterior and lateral walls with transection of its ligaments. The finding of a fixed rectum on digital rectal examination is not an absolute indication of nonresectability, because, in 25% of fixed rectal tumors, fixation is due to an inflammatory process, not neoplastic (29).

PREPARATION OF THE COLON FOR SURGERY

Colorectal preparation of patients to be subjected to surgery for rectal cancer is similar to that used in surgery of the colon. The patient should take only liquids on the day before surgery and carry out cleansing of the colon and rectum by the oral route. One of the methods for mechanical colorectal cleansing is as follows: The day before the operation, the patient should drink 4 liters of an iso-osmotic electrolytic solution of glycol polyethylene, known as Golytely or Colyte, over a period of 4 hours. There is another electrolytic solution known as Nulytely, better tasting and just as efficient as the others. Oral mechanical colorectal cleansing should be complemented orally by administration of antibiotics that are active against Gram positive and Gram negative as well as aerobic and anaerobic flora. Frequently used combination of antibiotics the day before surgery is three 1-gm doses of erythromycin base together with 1 gm of neomycin at 1:00 P.M., 2:00 P.M., and 11:00 P.M. One hour before surgery, the patient is given a second generation cephalosporin by intravenous injection and 500 mg of Metronidazol.

SELECTION OF THE SURGICAL TECHNIQUE

Selection of the technique to be used in treating cancer of the rectum is based on several factors, some of which will be analyzed as follows:

1. Level at which the rectal cancer is located. Carcinomas located about 11 cm from the anal margin can usually be treated with a high anterior resection. In this location it is not necessary to mobilize the rectum widely. The partial presence of serosa permits a safer suture, the ends of the colon are similar in diameter, there is no need for presacral drainage, primary healing of the anastomosis is frequent, and continence remains intact. In general, surgical results in this tumor location are superior to those for tumors of the middle third. Some surgeons use only one-layer anastomosis. The anastomosis can also be performed by mechanical means, using the circular stapler (1, 3, 12, 17, 37, 49). Most of the tumors of the rectum located in its middle third can be treated with a low anterior resection. In order to do this, it is necessary to carry out an ample mobilization of the rectum posteriorly, anteriorly, and laterally. Transection of the rectum distal to the macroscopic limit of the tumor should be performed no less than 2 cm away. In patients with voluminous undifferentiated infiltrative tumors, transection of the rectum should be further away. The surgical procedure used for tumors in this location has been discussed for many years, because it was thought that transection of the rectum had to be performed no less than 5 cm from the tumor. At present, this concept has changed, for which reason only few of the rectal cancers of this

location are subjected to an abdominoperineal resection (2, 17, 32, 38, 44, 47, 88, 89, 93).

Some surgeons use a protective transverse colostomy in patients with a doubtful suture line after a low anterior resection. Others prefer a loop ileostomy for protection. Neither the transverse colostomy nor a loop ileostomy will prevent dehiscence of the anastomosis, but they will facilitate its healing. A loop ileostomy may cause stenosis and intestinal obstruction when it is closed, complications that are much less frequent after closure of a transverse colostomy, since it is in the supramesocolic portion of the abdomen. Tumors of the distal third of the rectum are usually treated by an abdominoperineal resection. Nevertheless, if tumors are small, of a polypoid type, and histologically differentiated, they can be treated by a low anterior resection with results similar to the abdominoperineal without the inconvenience of a permanent colostomy (88, 90, 93).

2. Macroscopic type of the carcinoma. In infiltrative tumors, transection of the rectum distal to the tumor should be performed at a distance greater than 2 cm.
3. Size of the lesion. In well-developed lesions, transection of the rectum distal to the tumor should be performed more than 2 cm away.
4. Infiltration of neighboring organ. Infiltration by the neoplasm of organs next to the rectal tumor, such as the prostate, pouch of Douglas, bladder, or vagina, will make the surgeon vary his or her technique. Surgical excesses, resecting organs at any cost, should be avoided.
5. Histology of the tumor. The margin used in histologically undifferentiated tumors should be larger than that in differentiated tumors.
6. Endorectal ultrasonography. The image seen in endorectal ultrasonography may change the surgical procedure.
7. Constitutional habitus. Patients, especially men, with a hypersthenic habitus are less suitable than those with an asthenic habitus for a low anterior resection.
8. Sex. Low anterior resection is easier in women than in men because of their wider pelvis. Also, the pelvic operative field can be increased by resection of the uterus.
9. Obesity. Obese patients present greater difficulty than thin patients in low anterior resections.
10. Age. Patients of advanced age, in addition to being a greater surgical risk, may have a weak anal sphincter, which may make it necessary to vary the surgical procedure to be employed.
11. Patients who are blind and have mental changes and difficulty moving their arms may present problems in the selection of the surgical technique.

Anterior Resection of the Rectum: Surgical Techniques

FIGURE 59.1

The best position for performing resection of a rectal cancer is the Lloyd-Davies (54) modified lithotomy position using the Lloyd-Davies stirrups or other stirrups with the same purpose. A small pillow or sand bag is placed under the sacrum to elevate the sacrum above the level of the operating table. The Lloyd-Davies position allows simultaneous action by an abdominal surgical team and a perineal team, to carry out a colorectal anastomosis with the circular stapler or an abdominoperineal operation without having to change the patient's position. A Foley catheter is inserted into the bladder. Urine should be collected in a bag within view of the anesthesiologist.

Anterior Resection with Manual Suture: High Anterior Resection

FIGURE 59.2 ABDOMINAL INCISION

In patients in whom the rectal carcinoma is more than 11 cm from the anal margin, a location in which an anterior resection is frequently performed, the author prefers a left paramedian incision extending from the pubis to about 8 cm above the level of the umbilicus. If it is necessary to mobilize the splenic flexure of the colon, the incision can be extended to the costal margin. In patients with cancer of the lower third of the rectum in whom there is a great probability of having to do an abdominoperineal Miles operation, the author prefers a right paramedian incision. The right paramedian incision is further away from the colostomy, which should be brought out through the left anterior rectus muscle. In patients in whom there is doubt about doing an anterior resection or a Miles abdominoperineal operation, a midline incision is preferable, starting at the pubis and extending about 8 cm above the umbilicus.

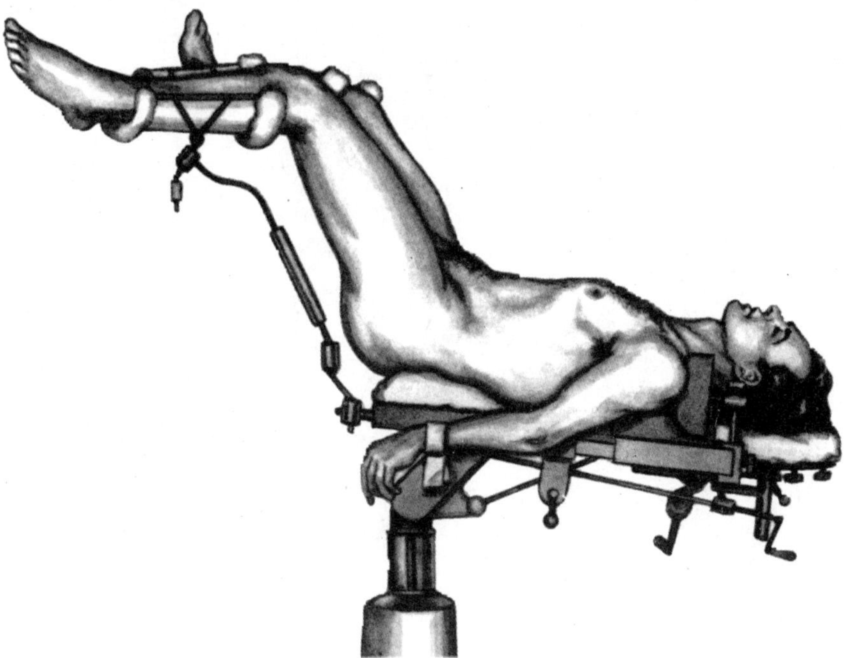

FIGURE 59.1

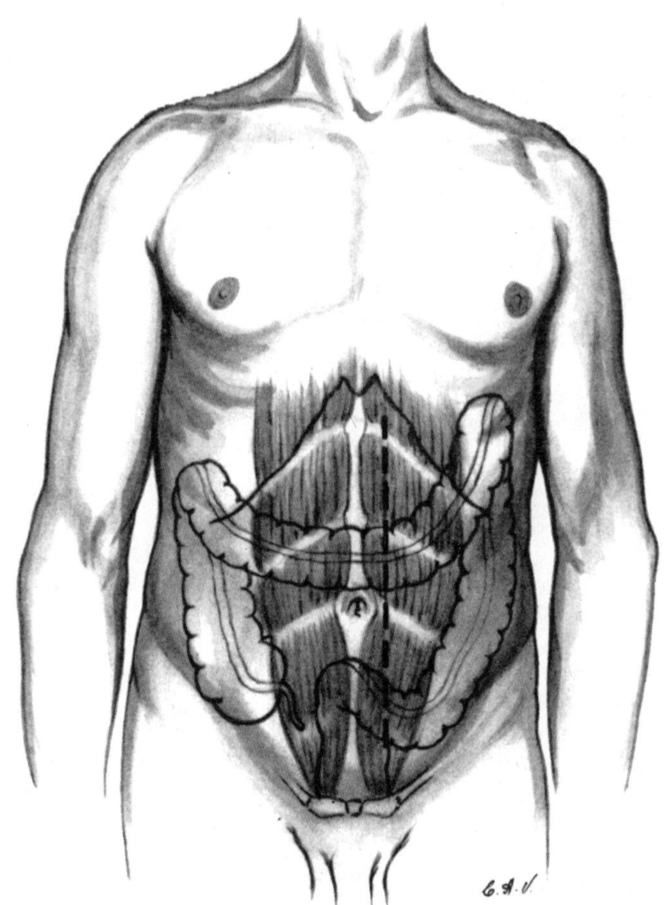

FIGURE 59.2 ABDOMINAL INCISION

Anterior Resection with Manual Suture: High Anterior Resection

FIGURE 59.3
The skin and subcutaneous tissue have been incised, and the anterior fascia of the left anterior rectus muscle is being incised, with a scalpel, about 2 cm from the midline.

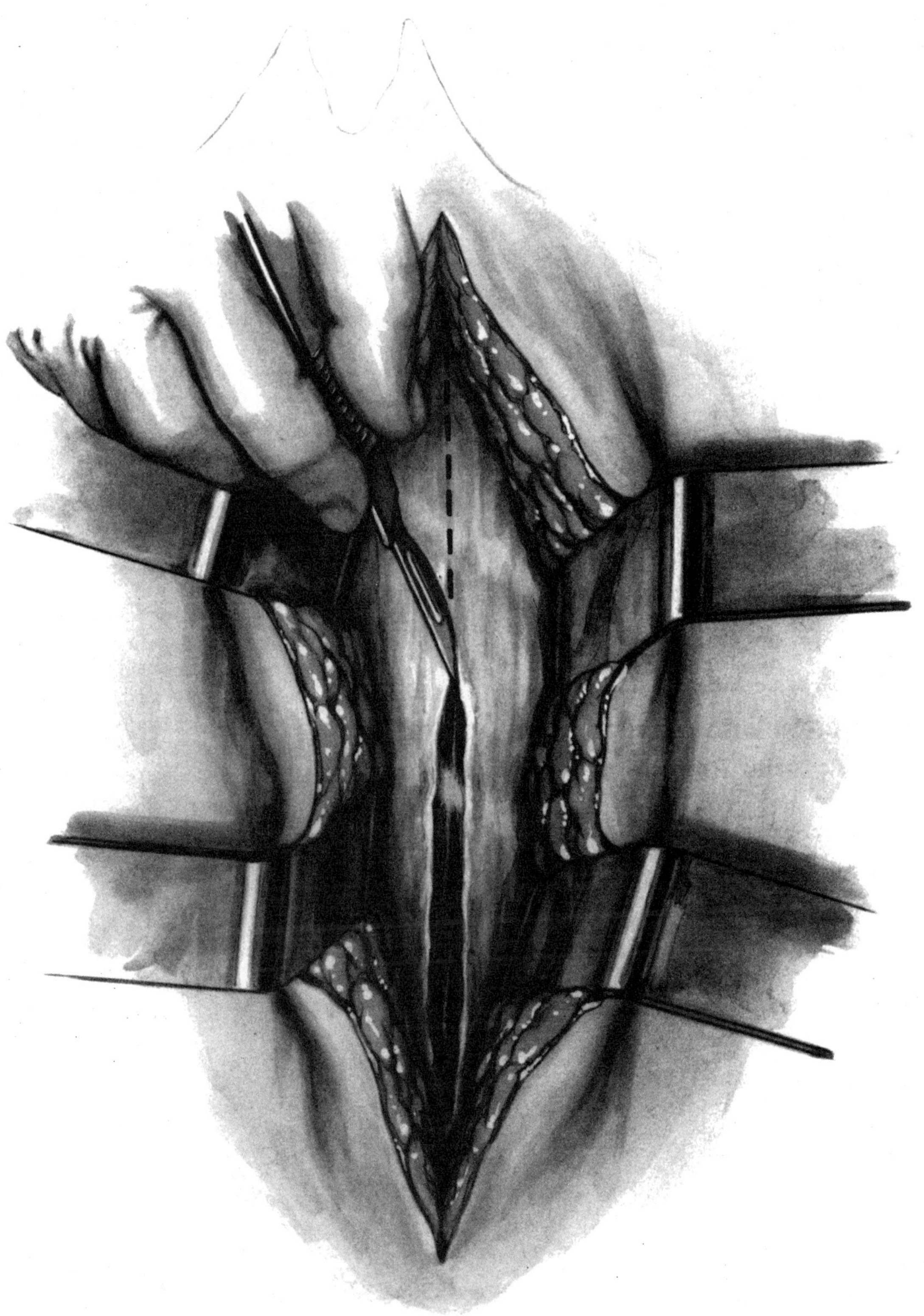

FIGURE 59.3

FIGURE 59.4

Once the anterior fascia of the left anterior rectus muscle has been incised, as shown, the medial border of the rectus muscle is separated from the angle formed by the two rectal fascias, using scissors. The aponeurotic insertions are clamped and ligated. Once the rectus muscle has been separated, the posterior fascia is incised, together with the peritoneum. A large Balfour or other self-retaining retractor is inserted into the abdominal cavity. The entire abdomen is explored to search for metastases in the liver or other organs. In addition, the presence of some other pathologic process or a synchronous carcinoma of the colon is searched for. If no hepatic metastases are palpable, the search can be extended by means of intraoperative ultrasonography. The level of the rectal cancer is investigated, to determine if it is located above or level with the peritoneal reflection, or in a subperitoneal location. Not all of the subperitoneal tumors are palpable through the abdomen.

Anterior Resection with Manual Suture: High Anterior Resection

If the tumor is in the peritoneal cavity, if it is not too big, if it is polypoid and movable, it is very probable that a high anterior resection can be performed with good immediate as well as late results. If the tumor is fixed or there is adenopathy, this possibility is much less. If the tumor is located below the peritoneal reflection and is not palpable, the possibility of performing an anterior resection cannot be predicted until the peritoneum is opened and the rectum mobilized. The loops of small bowel are elevated to the upper part of the abdomen, wrapped in moist, warm saline compresses and held in place by the second assistant.

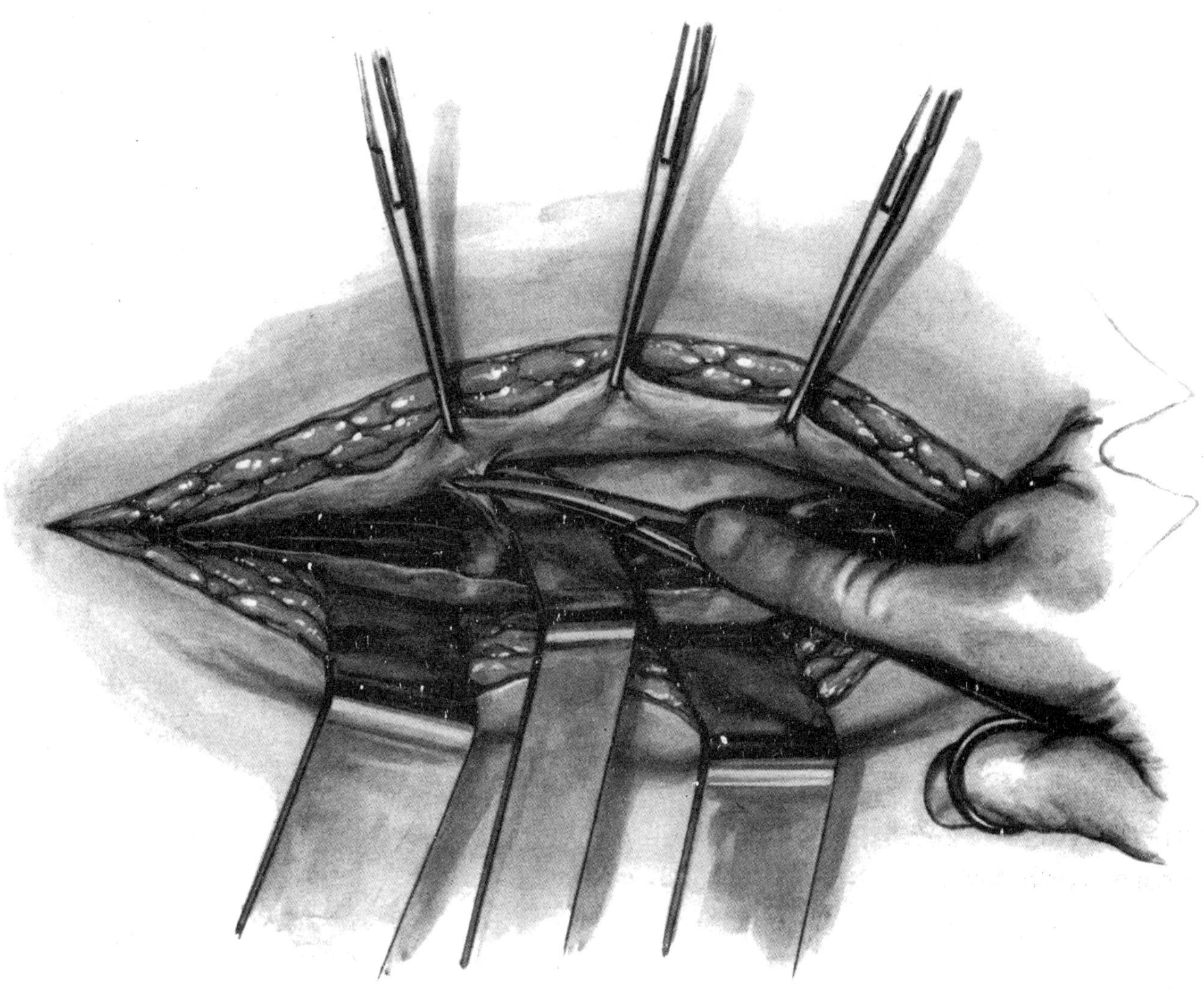

FIGURE 59.4

Anterior Resection with Manual Suture: High Anterior Resection

FIGURE 59.5
The surgeon applies upward traction to the rectum with his left hand, confirming that the carcinoma is limited to the intraperitoneal wall of the rectum without infiltrating the peritoneum.

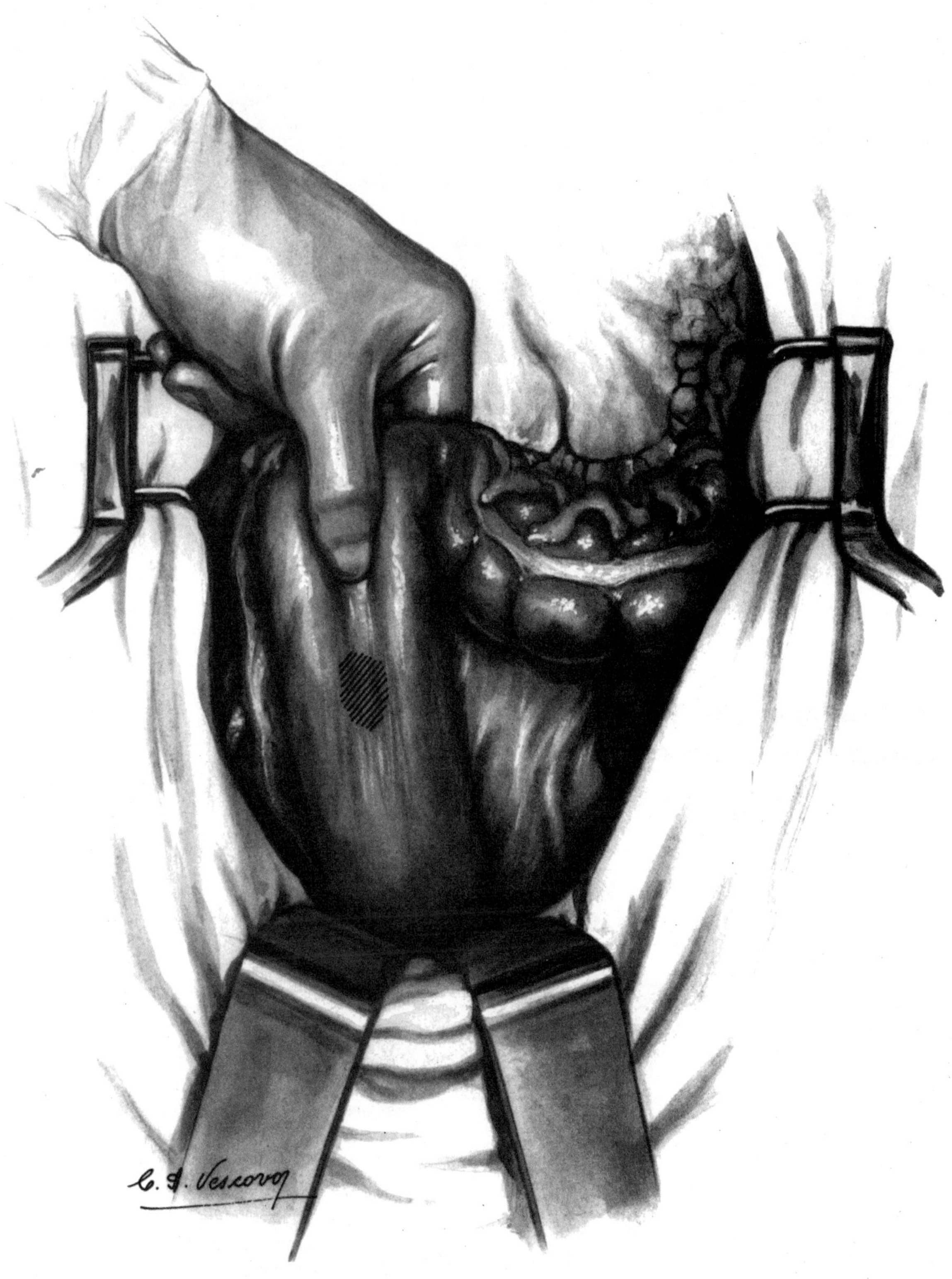

FIGURE 59.5

Anterior Resection with Manual Suture: High Anterior Resection

FIGURE 59.6
The first assistant retracts the sigmoid colon to the right, exposing the left lateral peritoneal gutter. Some congenital adhesions that are usually present between the mesosigmoid and the parietal peritoneum are divided. The left parietal peritoneum is transected, using scissors, and the entire left ureter is identified, to avoid injuring it. The gonadal vessels are also identified. The incision of the peritoneum is then continued down to the bladder, as shown by the broken line.

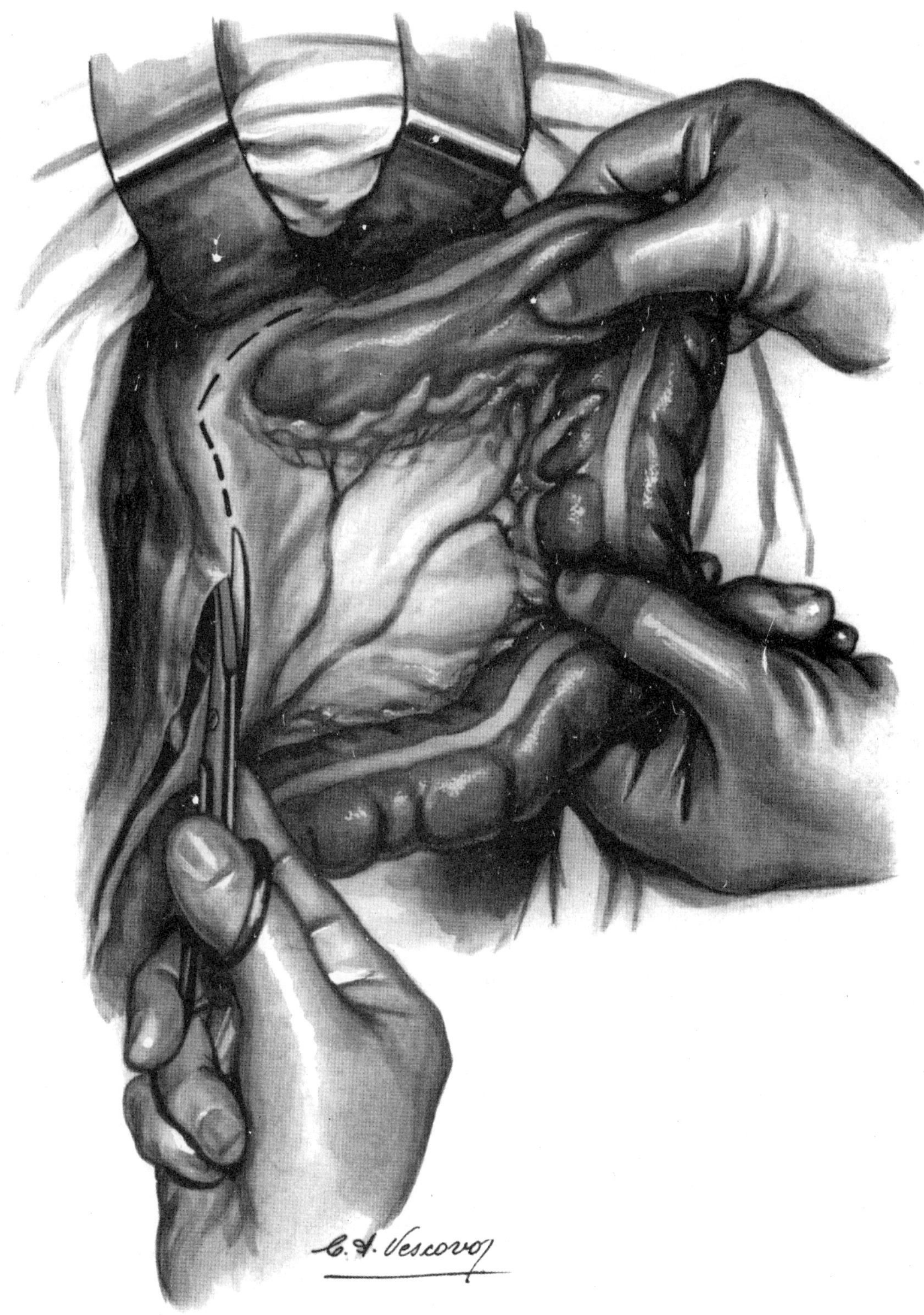

FIGURE 59.6

FIGURE 59.7
The drawing shows the course of the ureter and the left gonadal vessels. The lumen of the colon has been occluded with umbilical tape at the junction of the sigmoid colon and the descending colon. Using scissors, the parietocolic peritoneum is incised proximally. The extent of mobilization of the proximal colon depends on the redundancy of the sigmoid colon. If the sigmoid colon is long and has a good blood supply, it is not necessary to mobilize the proximal colon, but if the sigmoid colon is short, it is necessary to mobilize the colon and even the splenic flexure.

Anterior Resection with Manual Suture: High Anterior Resection

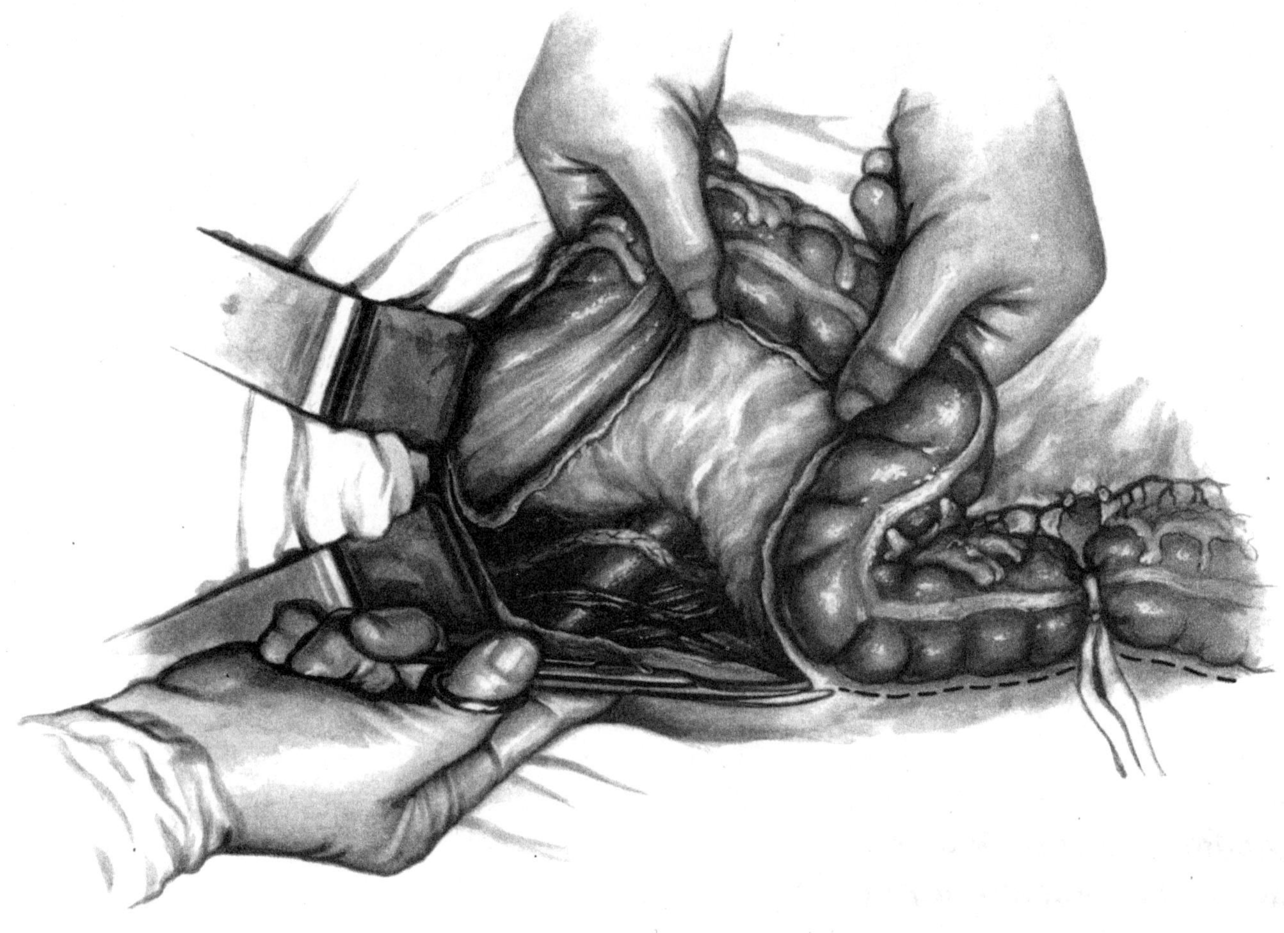

FIGURE 59.7

Anterior Resection with Manual Suture: High Anterior Resection

FIGURE 59.8
The surgeon applies upward traction to the rectosigmoid region and proceeds with division of the peritoneum on the right side, toward the bladder, to meet the peritoneal incision on the left side.

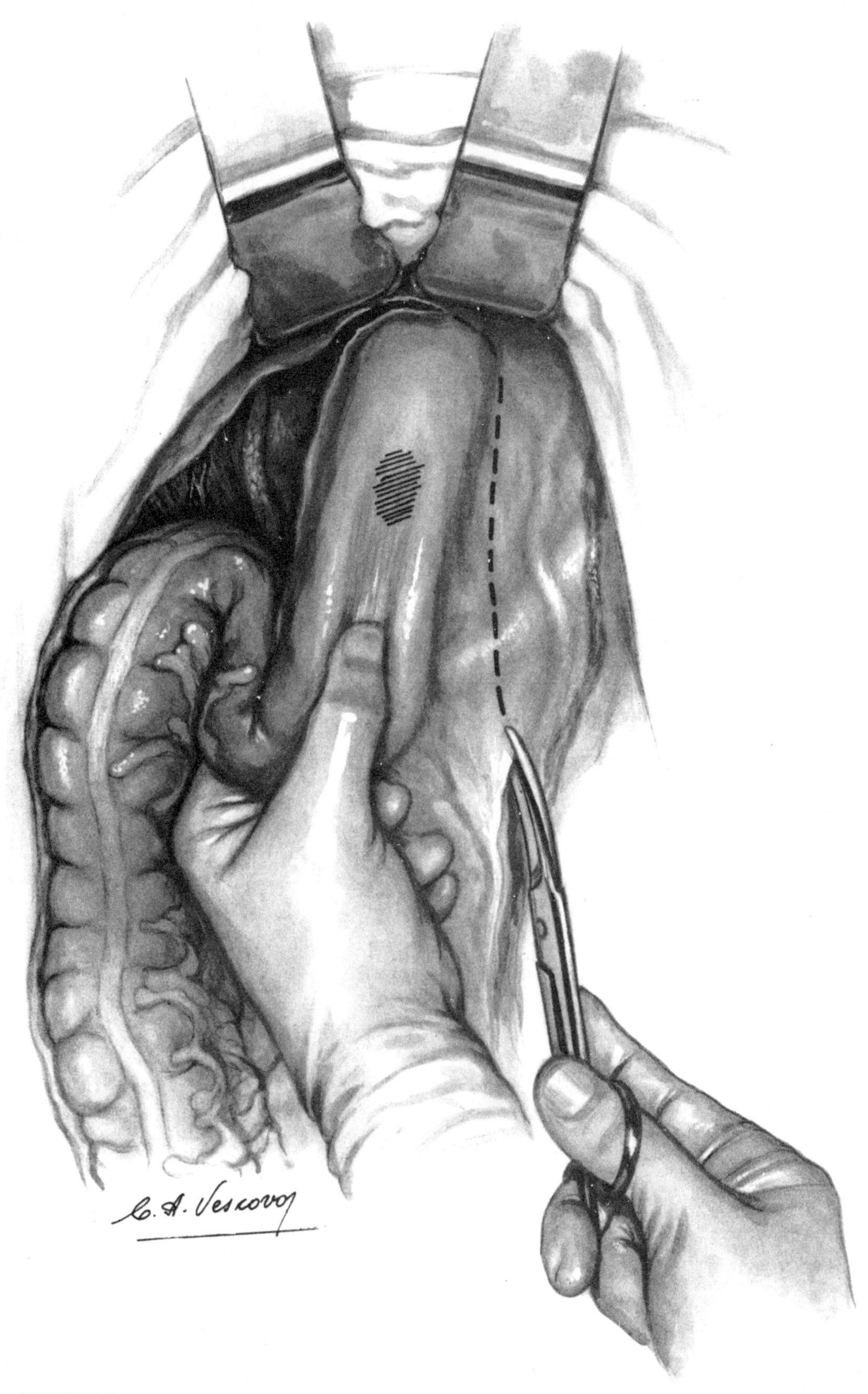

FIGURE 59.8

Anterior Resection with Manual Suture: High Anterior Resection

FIGURE 59.9

1, The inferior mesenteric artery has been doubly ligated and divided at its origin from the aorta. 2, Ligature and division of the inferior mesenteric artery can also be done after the origin of the left colic artery. The inferior mesenteric vein has been ligated and divided below the lower edge of the body of the pancreas, to the left of the duodenojejunal junction. As stated before, the peritoneal incision is continued down to meet the peritoneal incision on the left side.

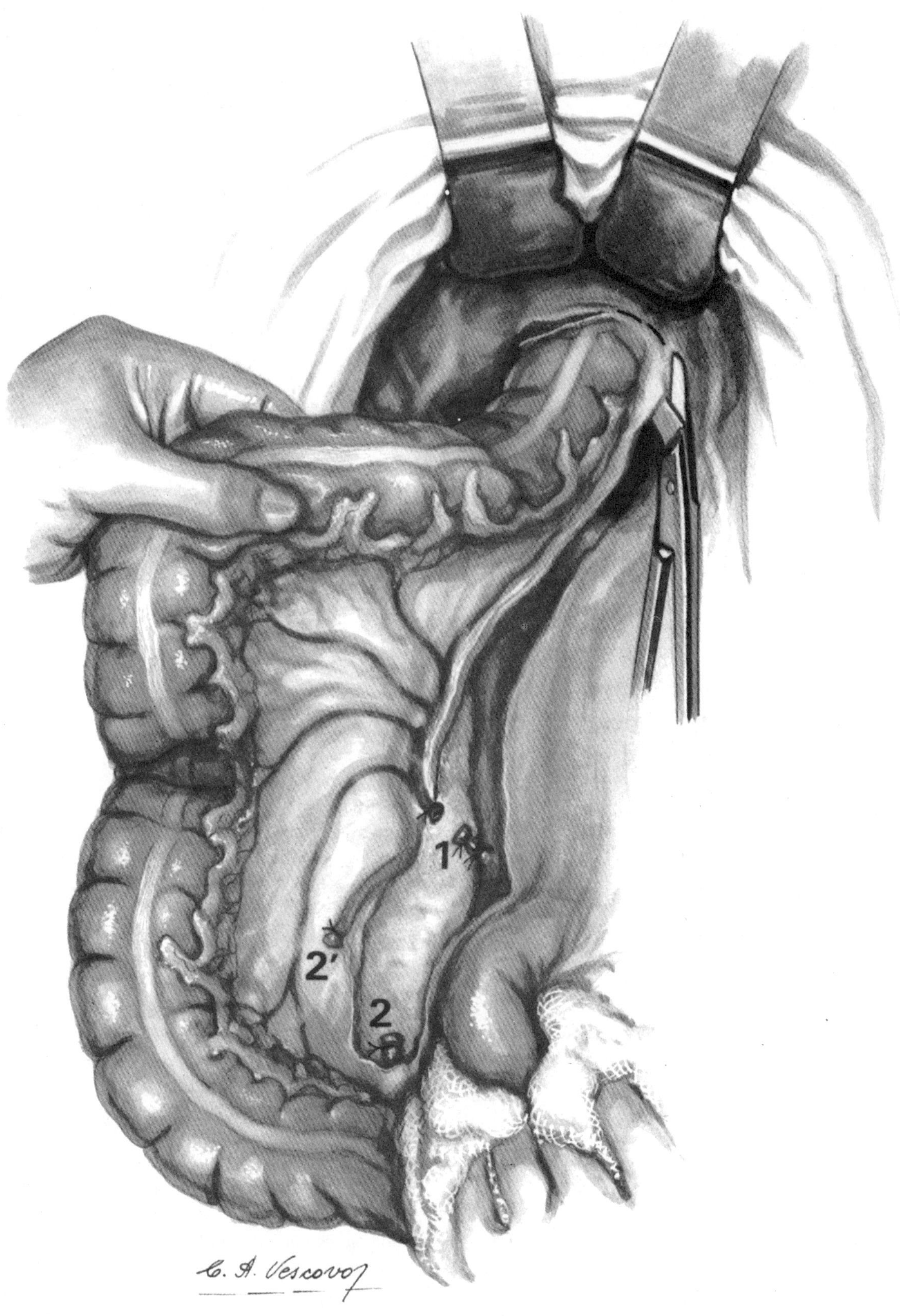

FIGURE 59.9

Anterior Resection with Manual Suture: High Anterior Resection

FIGURE 59.10

The figure shows that the small bowel loops have been wrapped in pads moistened with warm saline and are held by the second assistant. The ligature and division of the inferior mesenteric vessels can be observed. An atraumatic anterior resection clamp, designed by the author, has been placed in the pelvis, about 5 cm distal to the tumor. A rectal tube is introduced through the anus and the rectum irrigated with one liter of a 1% solution of cetrimide to kill any viable neoplastic cells that have been shed by the tumor. After the irrigation, the rubber tube is removed and, as shown in the drawing, another anterior resection clamp is placed 2 or 3 cm below the first clamp. The broken line shows the level of transection of the rectum, free of viable neoplastic cells. An umbilical tape has been placed to occlude the lumen of the proximal sigmoid colon. Above this ligature, a straight atraumatic clamp is placed to occlude the colonic lumen when it is transected to remove the surgical specimen. Another anterior resection clamp has been placed above the straight clamp. The colon will be transected along the broken line, between the anterior resection clamp and the straight clamp. A wound protector is inserted, as described in the chapter on colon surgery.

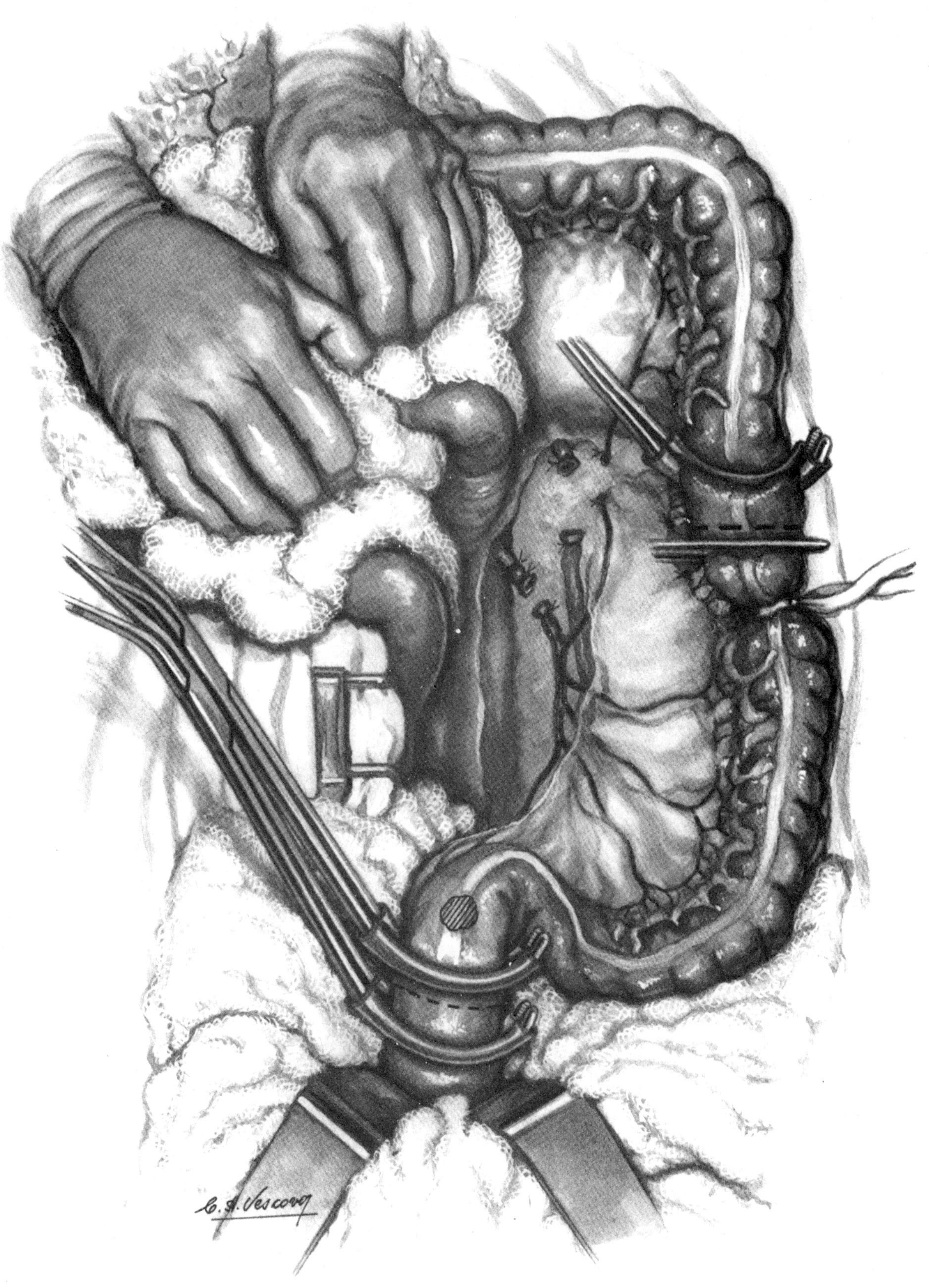

FIGURE 59.10

Anterior Resection with Manual Suture: High Anterior Resection

FIGURE 59.11
The proximal colon has been transected. An assistant pulls the colon upward by means of the straight clamp. The surgeon, using a right angle scissors, transects the rectum between the two anterior resection clamps.

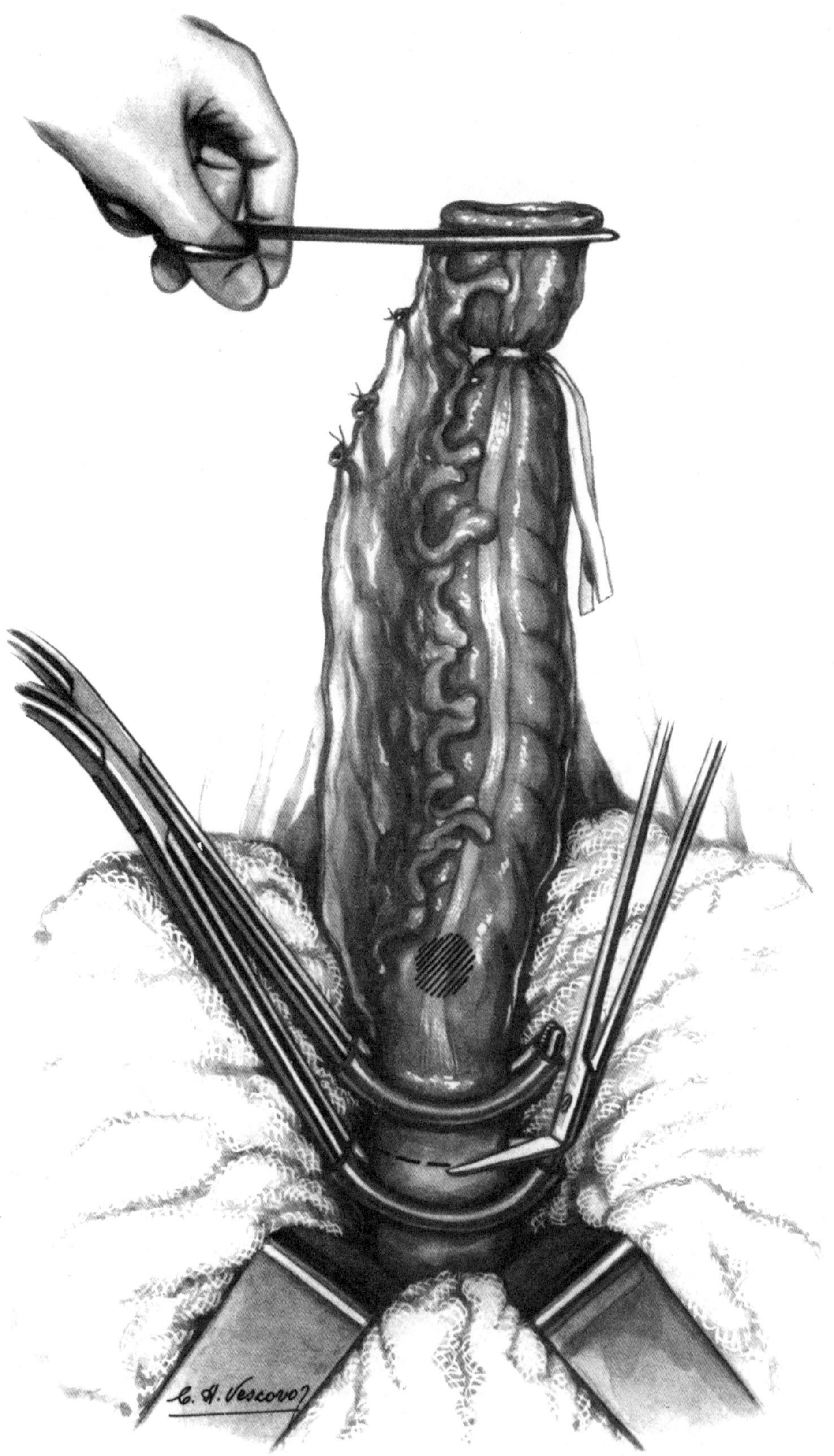

FIGURE 59.11

FIGURE 59.12
The surgical specimen has been removed and given to the pathologist for study. There were three lymph nodes near the tumor, invaded by the carcinoma.

Anterior Resection with Manual Suture: High Anterior Resection

FIGURE 59.13
The anterior resection clamps have been approximated to anastomose the colon to the rectum. The author prefers a two-layer anastomosis. Suturing can also be done in one layer. The anastomosis has begun with the posterior seromuscular layer. In some patients, even though it is a high anterior resection, suturing should be done between the seromuscular layer of the colon and the muscular layer of the rectum, which is devoid of peritoneum, the same as in a low anterior resection. The posterior layer is sutured with nonabsorbable material. The anterior resection clamps have been placed on the right side of the patient. These clamps can be placed from either side of the patient, whichever is more convenient for the surgeon.

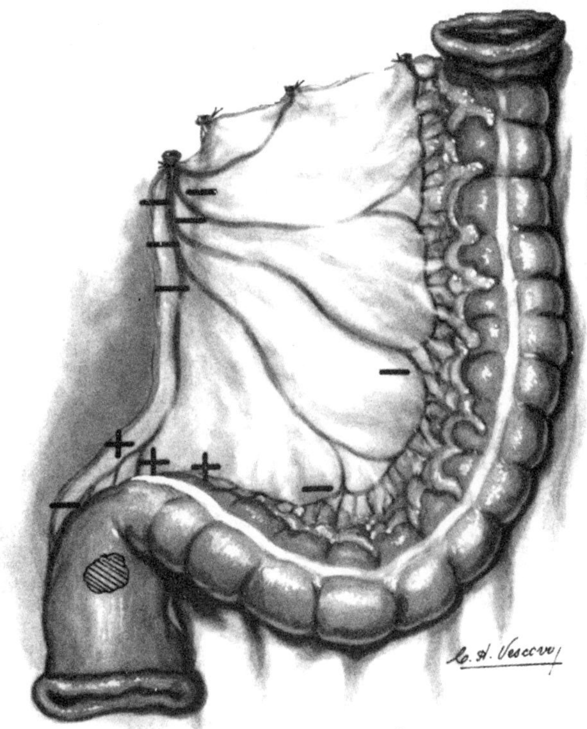

FIGURE 59.12

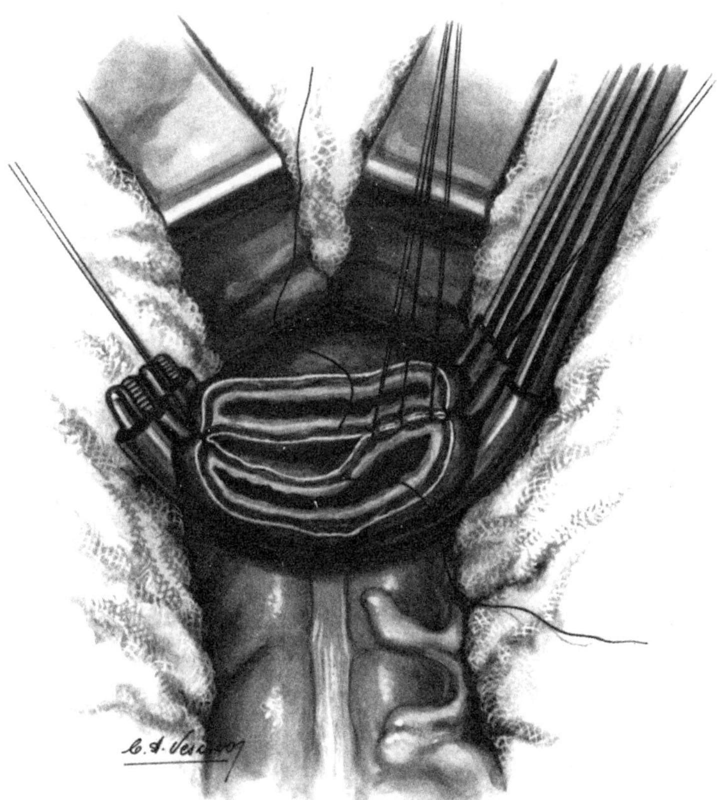

FIGURE 59.13

Anterior Resection with Manual Suture: High Anterior Resection

FIGURE 59.14
The posterior mucosal layer is being sutured using absorbable synthetic sutures or 2-0 chromic catgut.

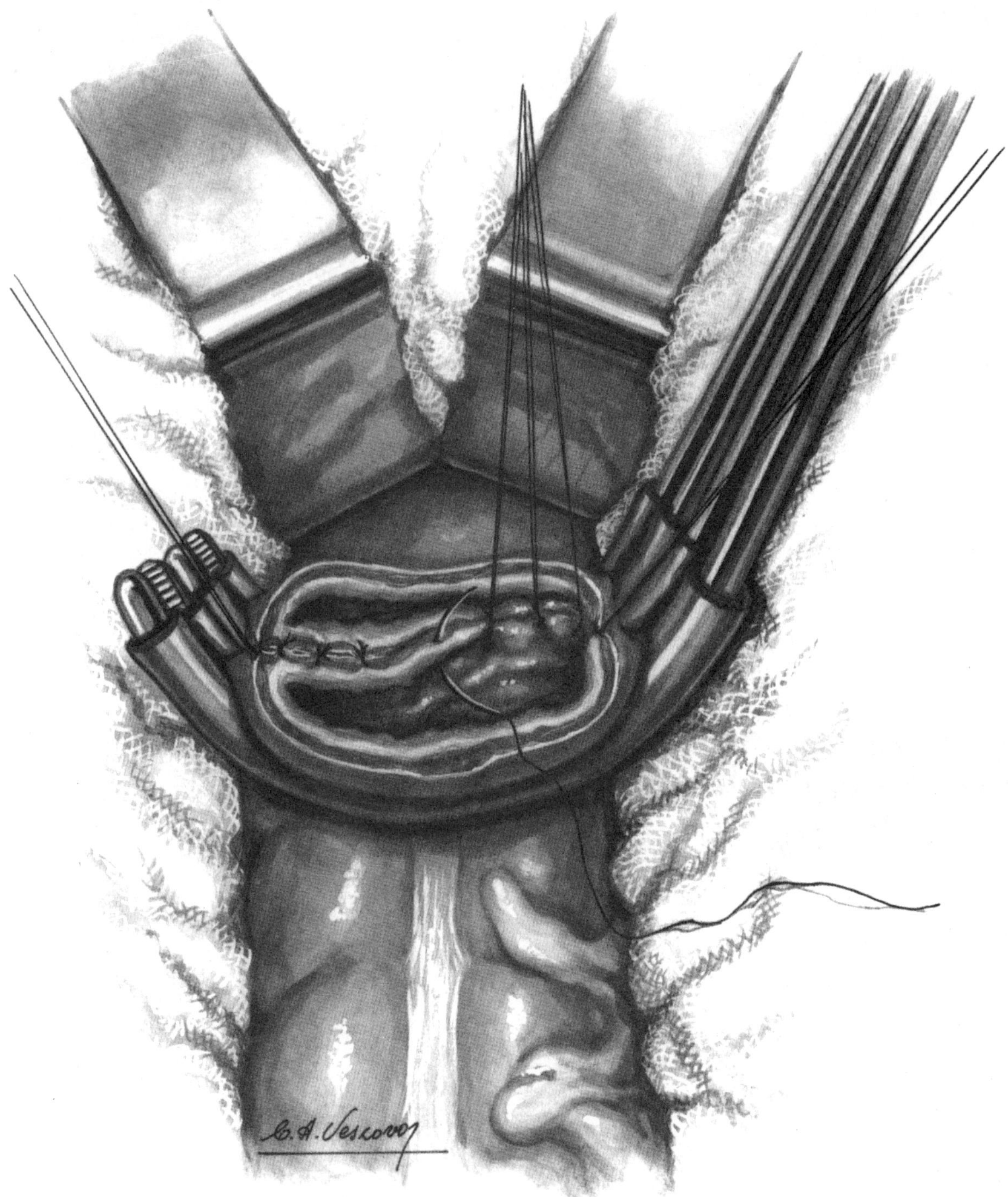

FIGURE 59.14

Anterior Resection with Manual Suture: High Anterior Resection

FIGURE 59.15
The anterior mucosal layer is being sutured with the knots on the inside.

FIGURE 59.16
The anterior seromuscular suture line has been completed with nonabsorbable material. The pelvic floor is peritonealized and the abdominal wall is closed without drainage.

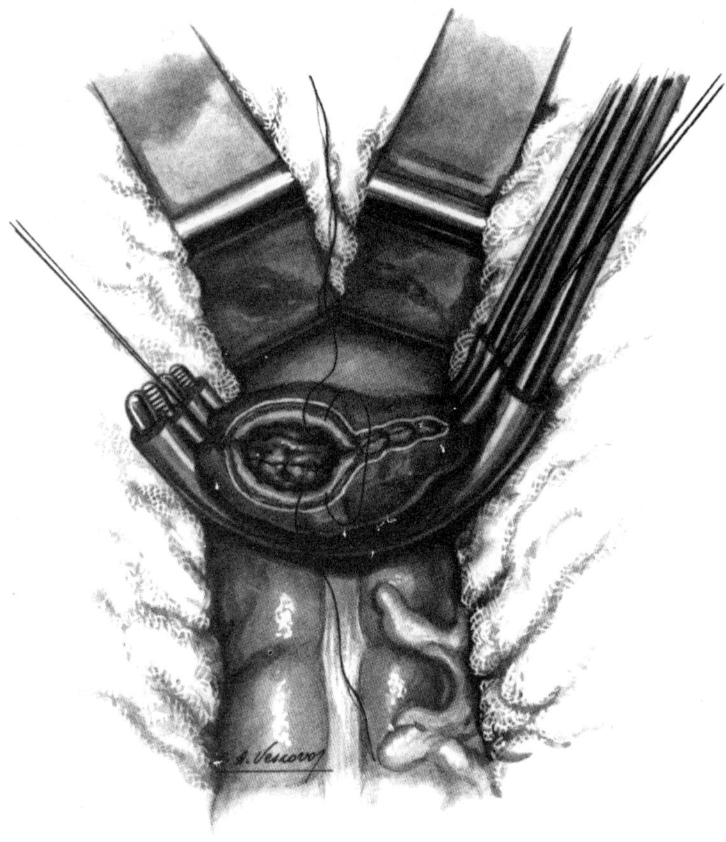

FIGURE 59.15

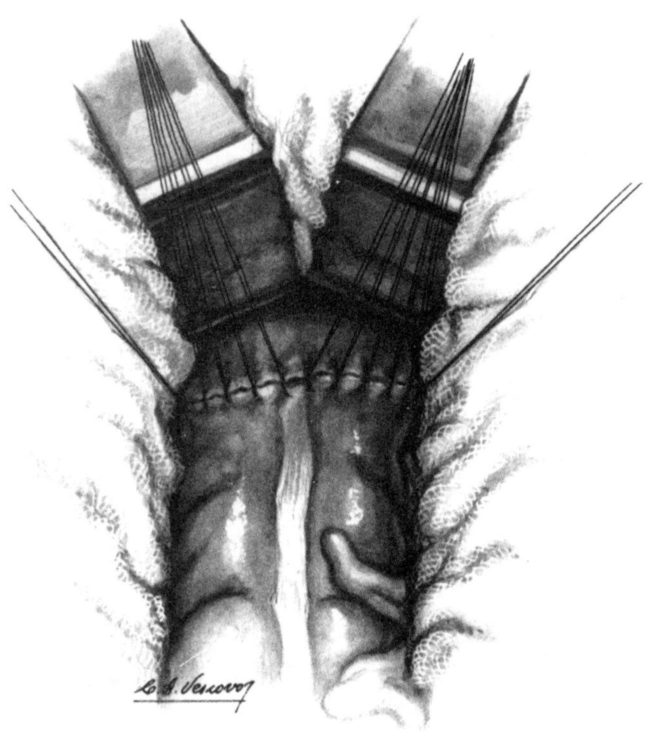

FIGURE 59.16

FIGURE 59.17
The peritoneum of the abdominal wall is being closed with interrupted absorbable synthetic sutures. This layer can be closed with a continuous suture, as preferred by many surgeons.

Anterior Resection with Manual Suture: High Anterior Resection

FIGURE 59.18
Closure of the anterior rectus sheath with interrupted nonabsorbable sutures. This layer can also be closed with a continuous suture.

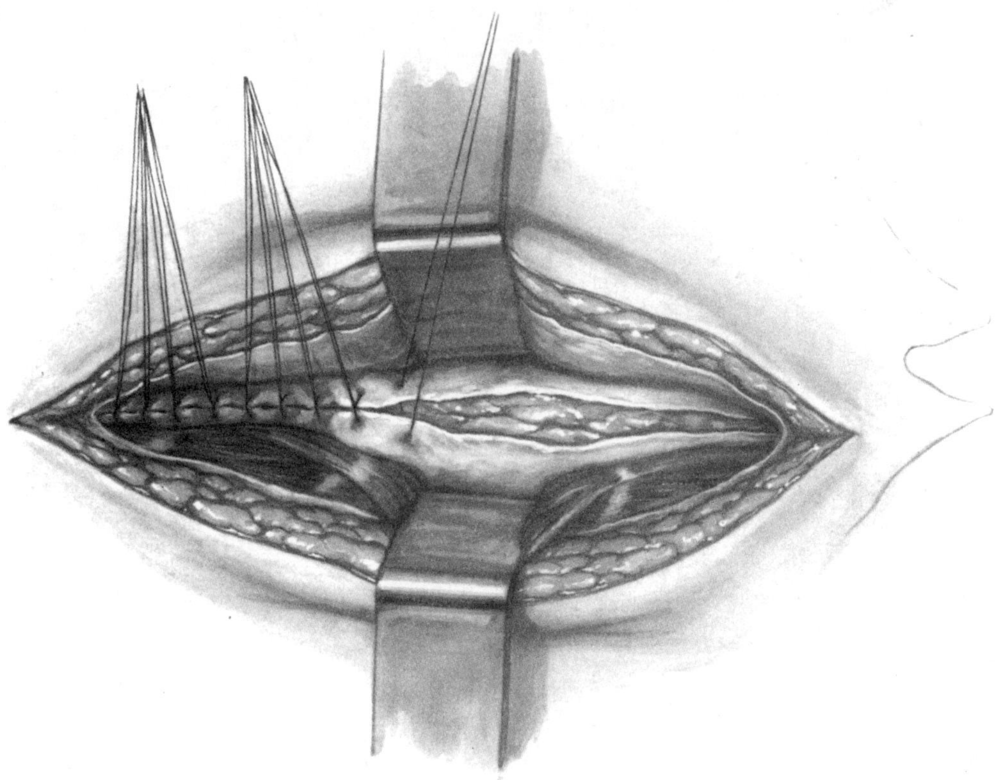

FIGURE 59.17

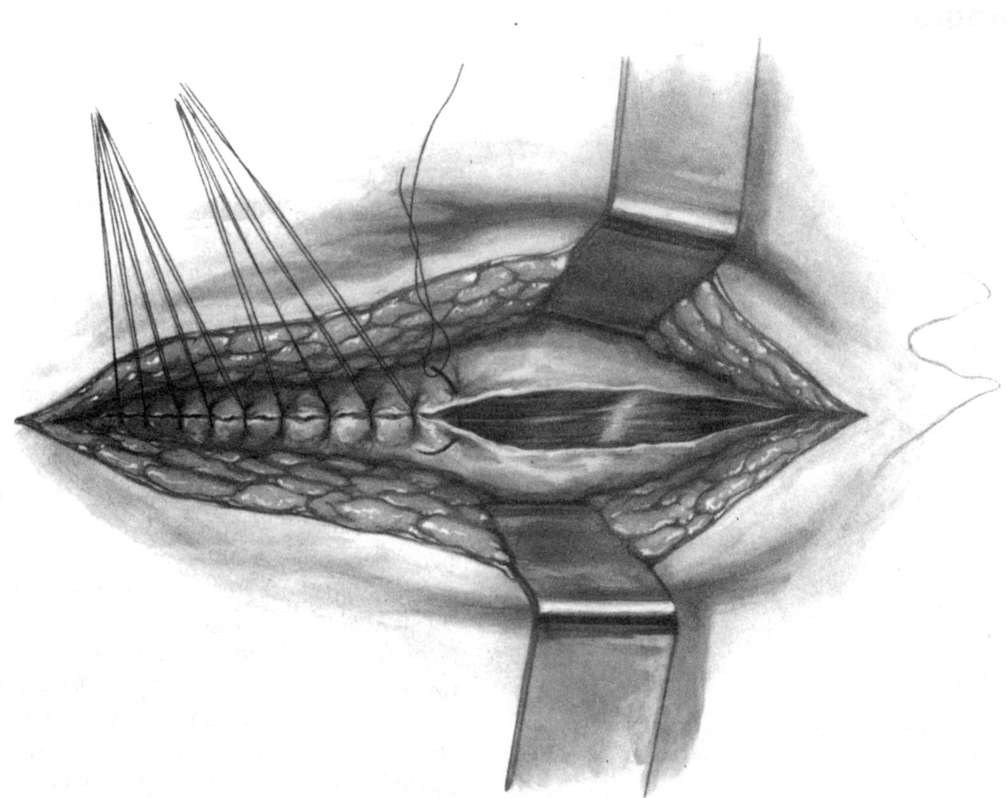

FIGURE 59.18

Low Anterior Resection with Manual Suture

FIGURE 59.19

In general, the technique of a low anterior resection for rectal cancer is similar to that for a high anterior resection. The most important difference is that in a low anterior resection, an extensive mobilization of the rectum is performed in front, behind, and laterally, with transection of the lateral ligaments. This mobilization makes this operation more complex and prone to greater morbidity than a high anterior resection. In a low anterior resection it is frequently necessary to mobilize the splenic flexure of the colon to avoid a colorectal anastomosis under tension in the pelvic cavity. The drawing shows the small bowel wrapped in compresses, moistened in warm saline solution, held in place by the second assistant in the upper abdomen. The inferior mesenteric artery has been doubly ligated about 2 cm from its origin in the aorta. Using scissors, the inferior mesenteric artery is being divided between the proximal two ligatures and the distal one. Many surgeons prefer to ligate the inferior mesenteric artery below the origin of the left colic artery, as shown in the inset. The drawing also shows the subperitoneal location of the rectal carcinoma.

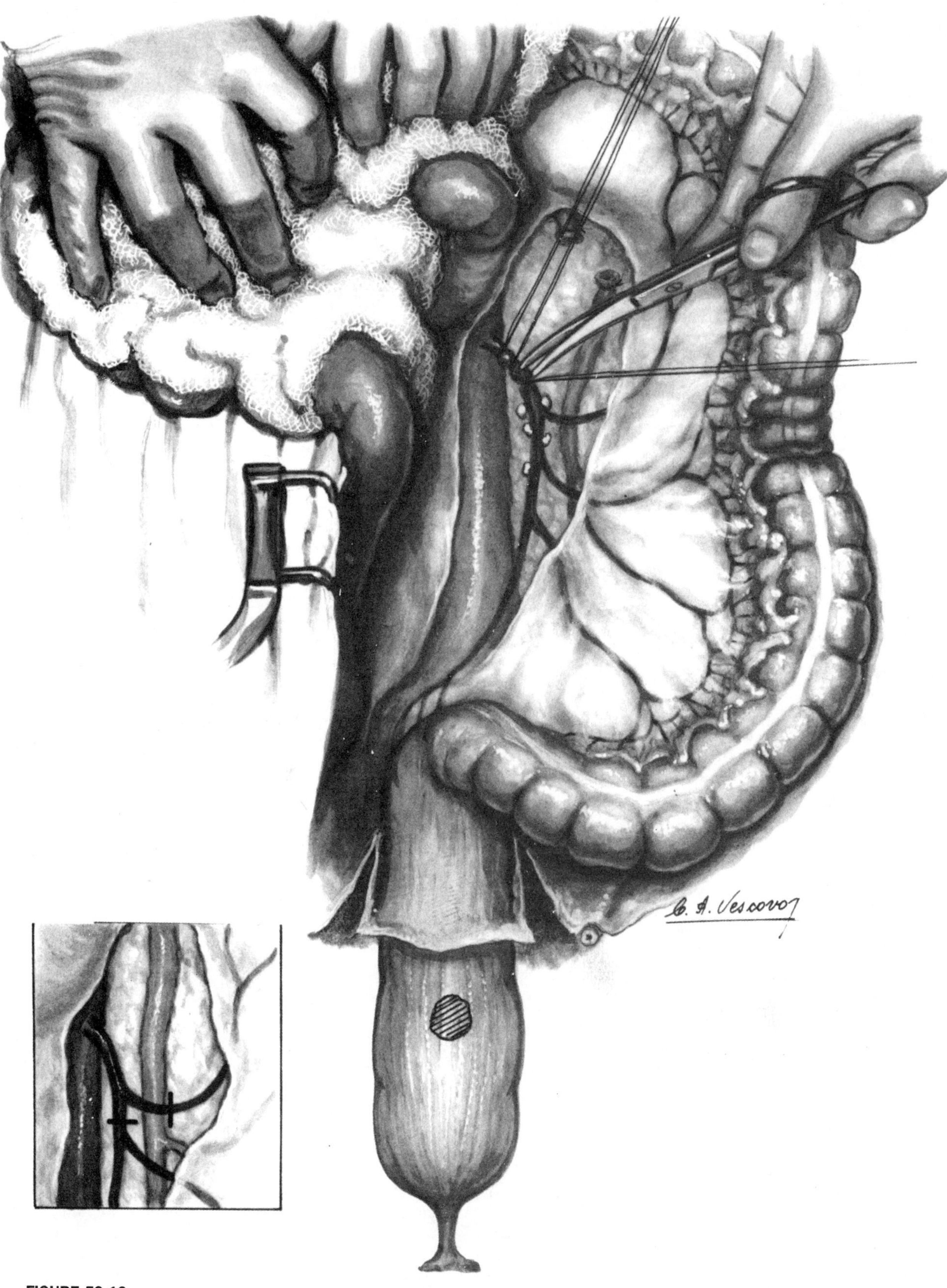

FIGURE 59.19

Low Anterior Resection with Manual Suture

FIGURE 59.20

1. The sigmoidorectal peritoneum has been incised in similar fashion as in a high anterior resection, and the ureter and gonadal vessels have been identified. Dissection of the posterior rectal wall has begun at the sacral promontory, using long curved scissors. At the sacral promontory there is a layer of areolar tissue, which is more prominent laterally than in the midline. In the midline the tissue is denser, and within it run some small arteries, branches of the middle sacral. Dissection with scissors should be anterior to the presacral fascia, avoiding injuring it. A Jones scissors is well suited for this dissection. In the distal pelvic cavity the surgeon will encounter the rectosacral or Waldeyer fascia, which is dense and should be incised with the same scissors. The rectosacral fascia should not be ruptured with the fingers because this may injure the rectal wall or rupture the presacral fascia, rupturing some veins of the presacral venous plexus, which can retract into the sacral foramina, making hemostasis difficult. In this situation, hemostasis can be attained with bone wax, Surgicel, Avitene, or with a titanium thumbtack of Nivatvongs and Fang (66).

Presacral dissection can be performed well without injuring the hypogastric nerves. Preservation of these nerves prevents alterations in ejaculation in male patients. The hypogastric nerves run along the posterolateral pelvic wall and are constituted by two or three branches running near the hypogastric artery. These nerves can be preserved without compromising curability of the patients (17, 31, 93). The S-2 to S-4 parasympathetic fibers that have to do with erection are not as visible as the hypogastric nerves and emerge distal to the pyriform muscles (31). The possibility of carrying out a low anterior resection depends considerably on the correctness of the rectal mobilization. Dissection of the rectum should be done with scissors, freeing it posteriorly down to the tip of the coccyx, in front to the level of the pubis, and laterally to the levator ani muscles. The hand should be introduced only to determine the degree of liberation of the rectum posteriorly and to define the lateral ligaments of the rectum. The mesorectum, located posteriorly, should be divided between clamps if at all possible. If not, it should be divided with electrocautery. The posterior rectal wall should be clean down to 3 or 4 cm below the tumor (41–44, 93).

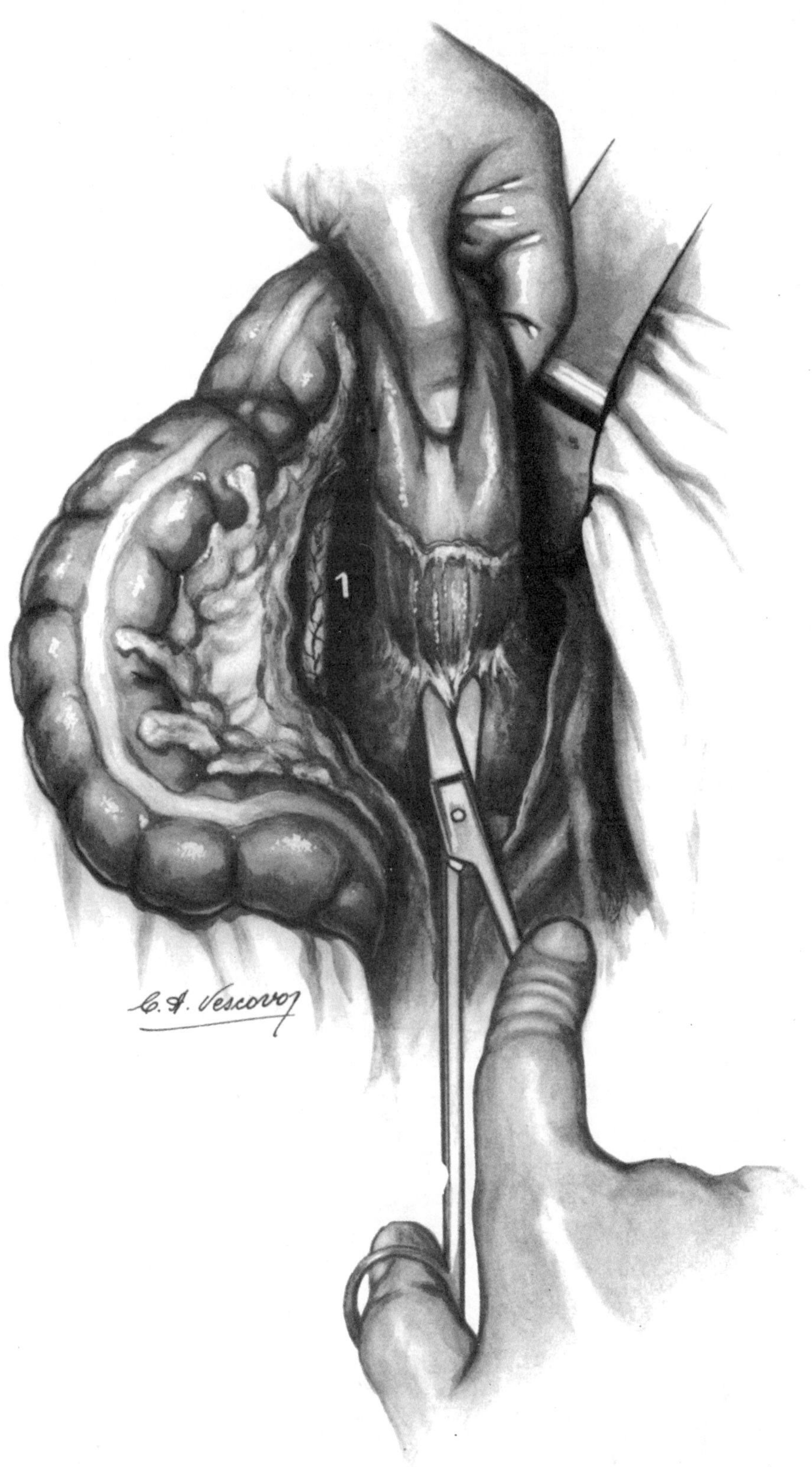

FIGURE 59.20

FIGURE 59.21
Sectional view of the dissection of the posterior wall of the rectum, which is being separated from the sacral concavity. The curved scissors transects the tissue in front of the presacral fascia. Upon arrival at the level of the fourth sacral vertebra, the rectosacral or Waldeyer's fascia will be encountered. This should be transected with scissors to prevent serious complications.

Low Anterior Resection with Manual Suture

FIGURE 59.22
Once the posterior rectal wall has been liberated from the sacral concavity, the surgeon introduces a hand behind the rectum and defines, toward both sides, the lateral ligaments of the rectum.

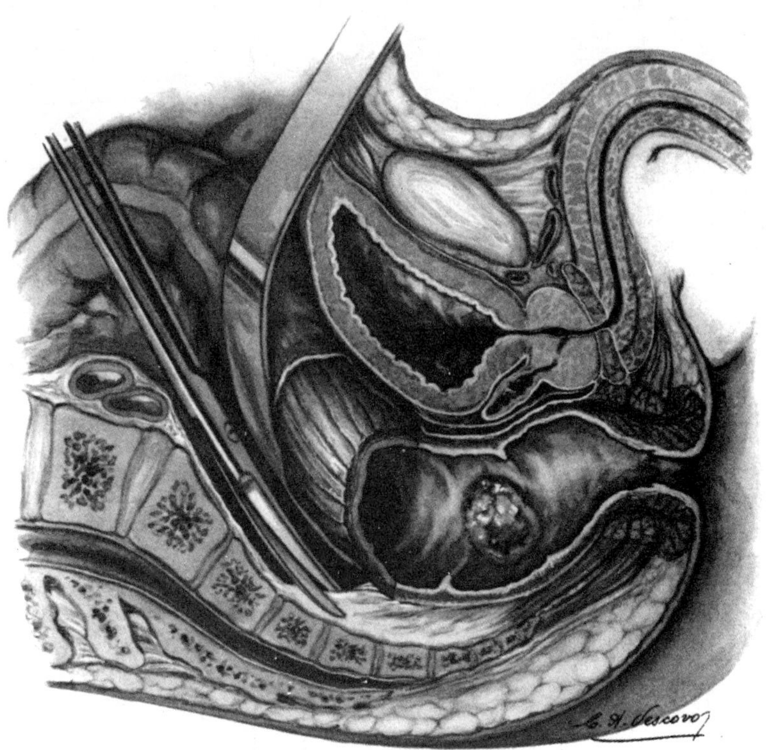

FIGURE 59.21

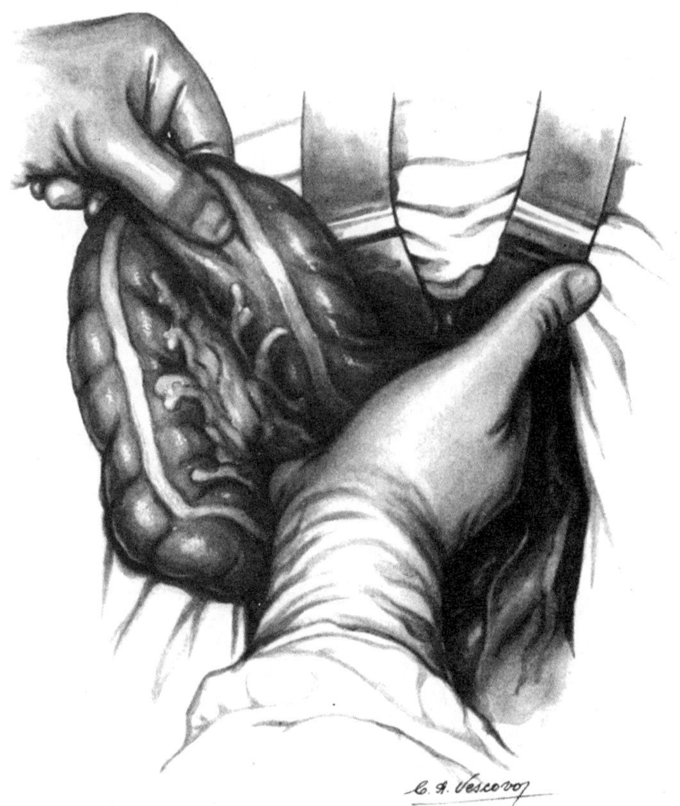

FIGURE 59.22

Low Anterior Resection with Manual Suture

FIGURE 59.23
Traction is applied upward, with two Allis clamps, to the previously sectioned peritoneum covering the bladder. Using blunt curved scissors, the plane between the bladder and anterior rectal wall is developed to separate both organs.

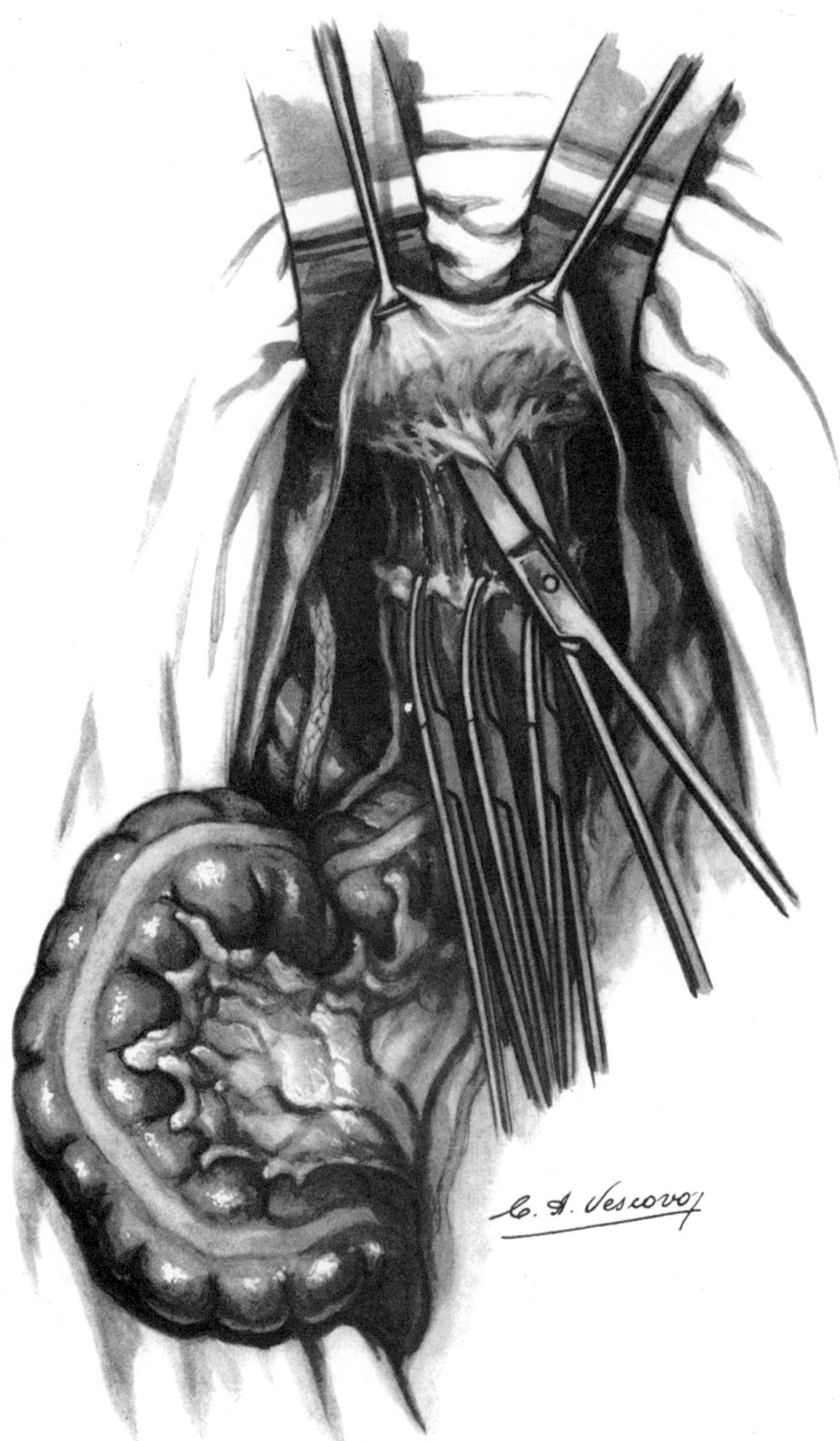

FIGURE 59.23

Low Anterior Resection with Manual Suture

FIGURE 59.24

Using two retractors, both seminal vesicles are reflected upward. The Lloyd-Davies retractor, created for this purpose, is very useful. In order to continue with the separation of the seminal vesicles and the prostate from the rectal wall, it is necessary to incise the fascia of Denonvilliers, using straight scissors, as seen in the drawing. Transection of the fascia of Denonvilliers should not be extended too far laterally, to avoid injuring the nerves that control sexual potency in the male. Dissection of the anterior rectal wall is much easier in the female.

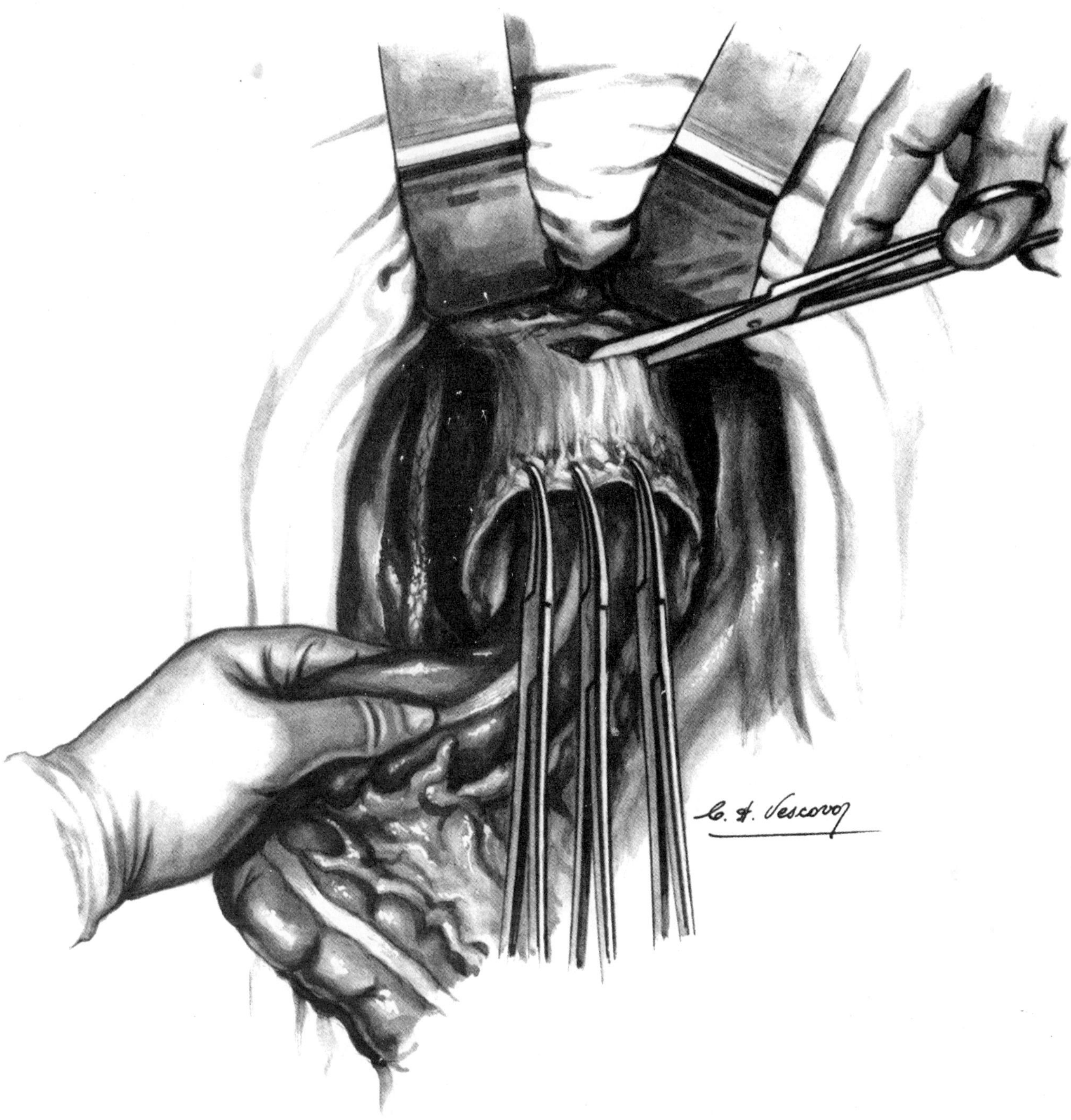

FIGURE 59.24

Low Anterior Resection with Manual Suture

FIGURE 59.25
Separation of the seminal vesicles and the prostate from the rectal wall is completed digitally. If any bleeding develops during dissection of the anterior wall of the rectum, it is controlled with electrocautery.

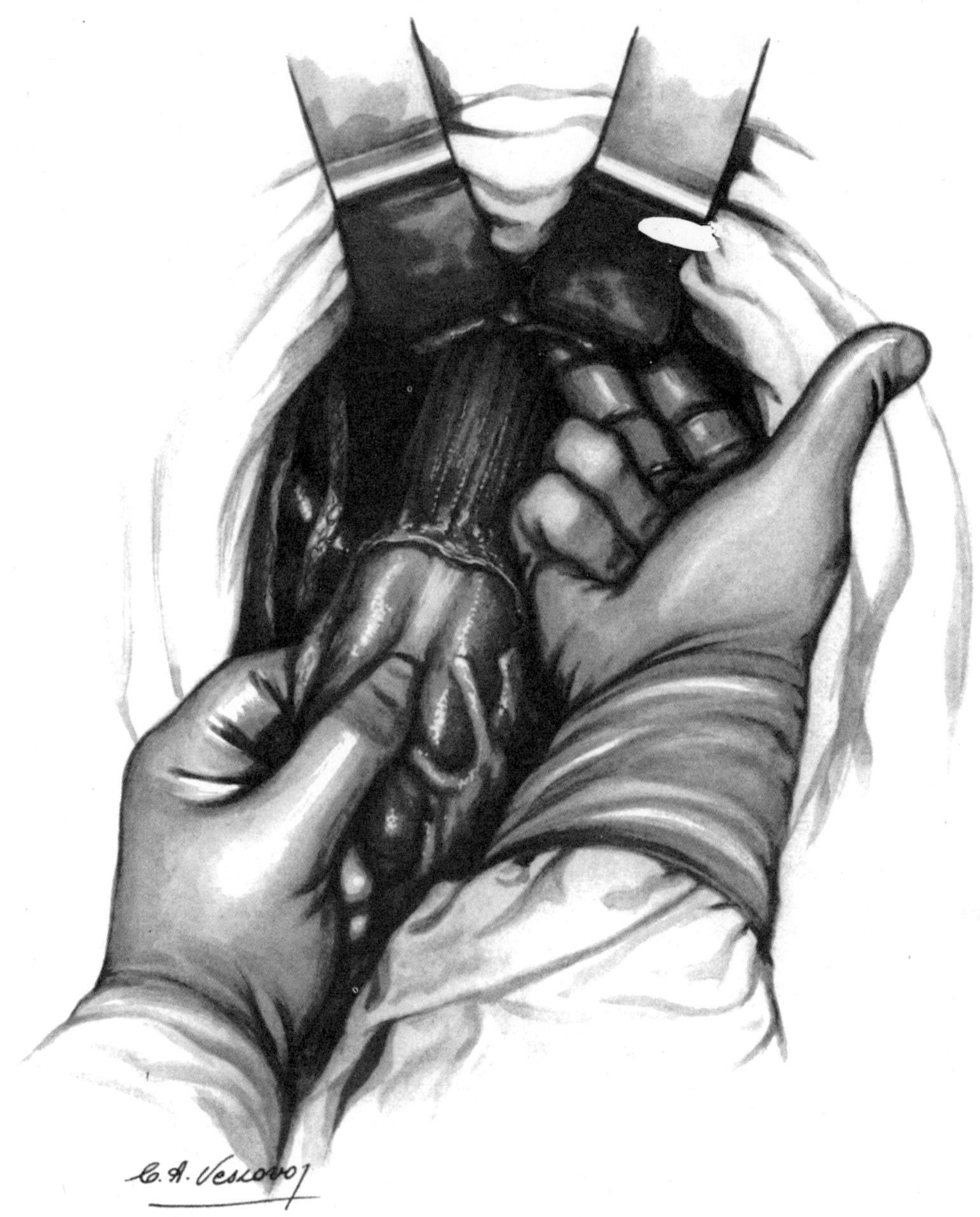

FIGURE 59.25

Low Anterior Resection with Manual Suture

FIGURE 59.26

After posterior and anterior liberation of the rectum is complete, only lateral liberation is left. For this purpose, the lateral ligaments have to be ligated and transected. The middle hemorrhoidal vessels or some of its branches run in the lateral ligaments. They should be carefully identified before ligating them. The left ureter should be identified, and the ligature should not include the hypogastric nerve. To ligate the right lateral ligament, traction is applied to the left, and to ligate the left lateral ligament, traction is applied to the right. The upper drawing shows the identified right lateral ligament. A Finochietto clamp, with a nonabsorbable suture, has been passed around it to ligate it. On the left side, the site of the ligature of the lateral ligament is shown by a dotted line. Some surgeons ligate the lateral ligaments of the rectum with mechanical sutures, as is seen in the lower drawing. After the rectum has been liberated on all sides, its three curves straighten out, making it 4 to 5 cm longer. This is why tumors at the 7-cm level can be brought up to 11 to 12 cm from the anal margin, favoring low anterior resection.

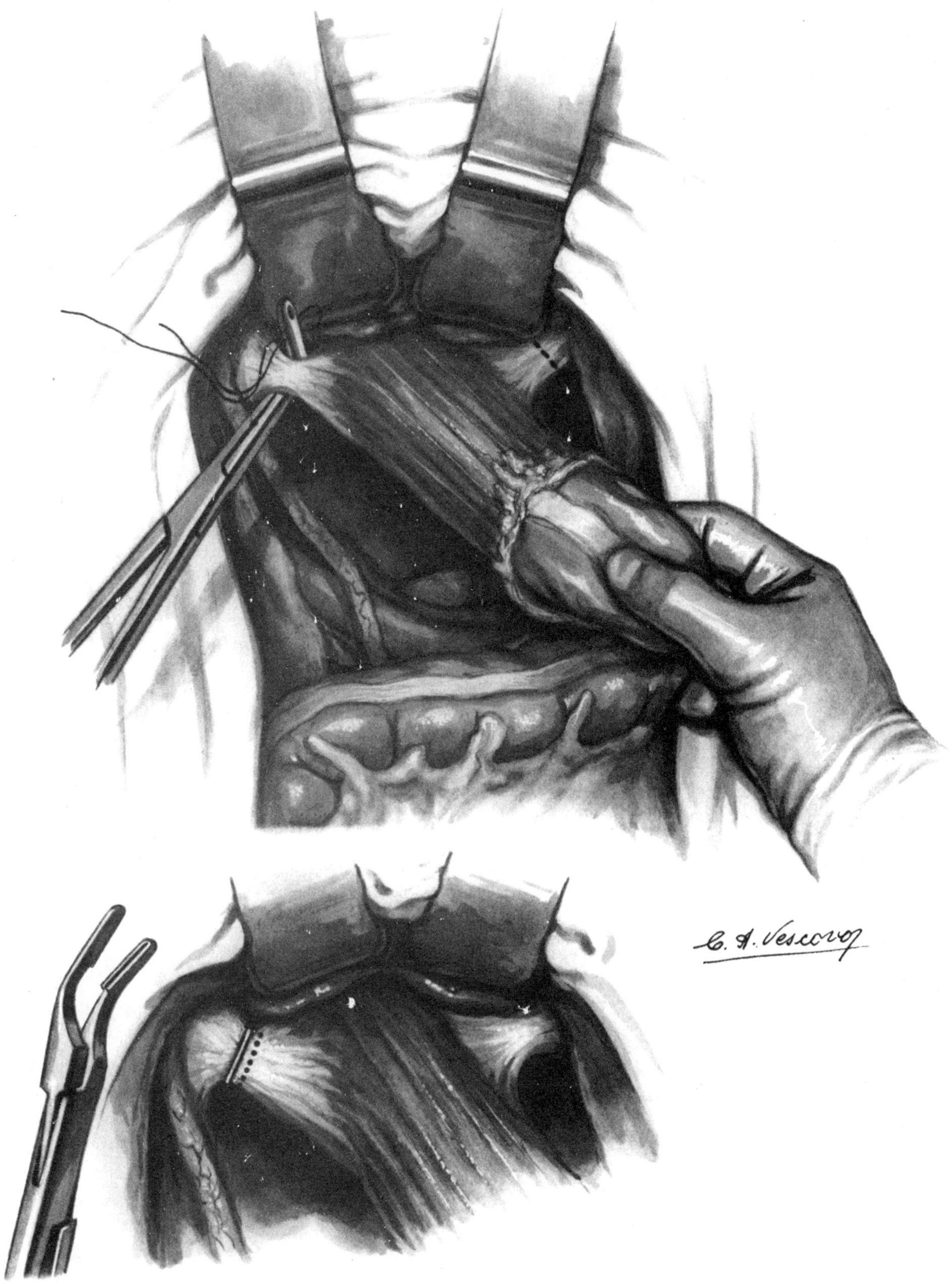

FIGURE 59.26

Low Anterior Resection with Manual Suture

FIGURE 59.27

In a low anterior resection, the need of mobilizing the left colon frequently arises, to facilitate bringing it down in order to carry out a colorectal anastomosis in the pelvis without tension. Mobilization of the left hemicolon starts by ligating and dividing the left half of the gastrocolic ligament below the gastroepiploic arcade, as shown.

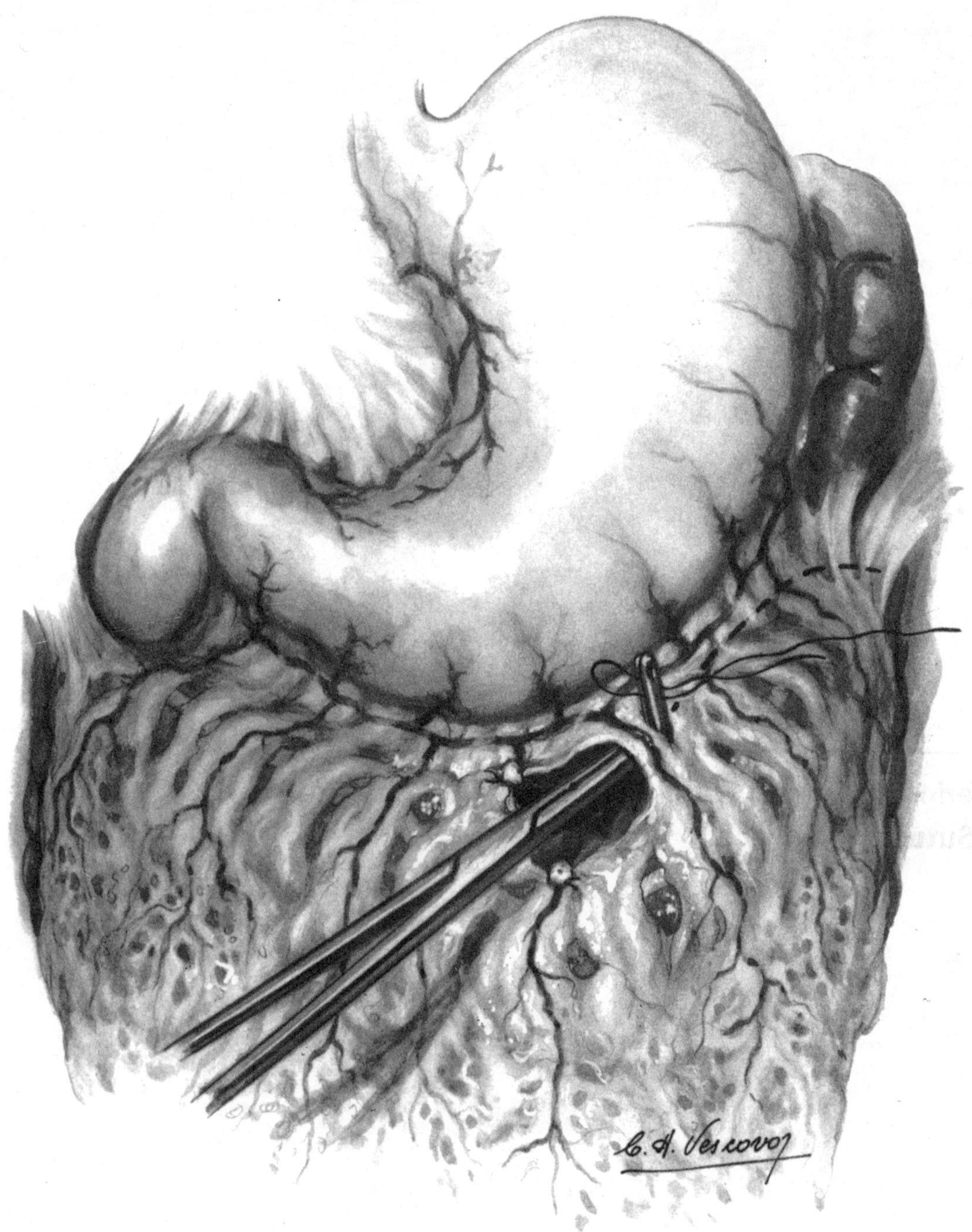

FIGURE 59.27

Low Anterior Resection with Manual Suture

FIGURE 59.28
Once the transection of the gastrocolic ligament is complete, the left parietocolic peritoneal incision is completed, up to the vertex of the splenic flexure.

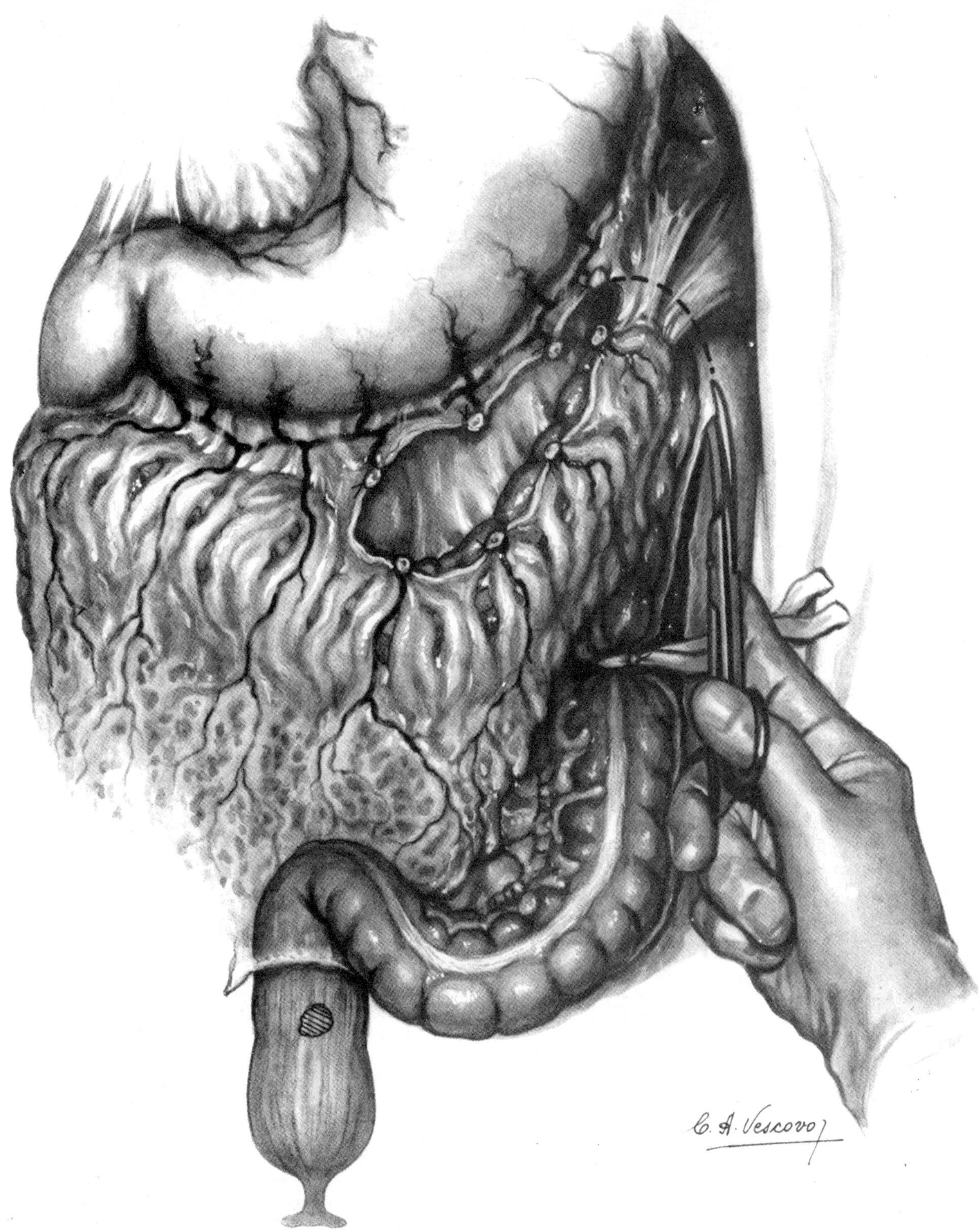

FIGURE 59.28

Low Anterior Resection with Manual Suture

FIGURE 59.29
The surgeon applies gentle traction, downward and to the right, to the transverse and descending colon, exposing the phrenocolic and splenocolic ligaments that are to be divided.

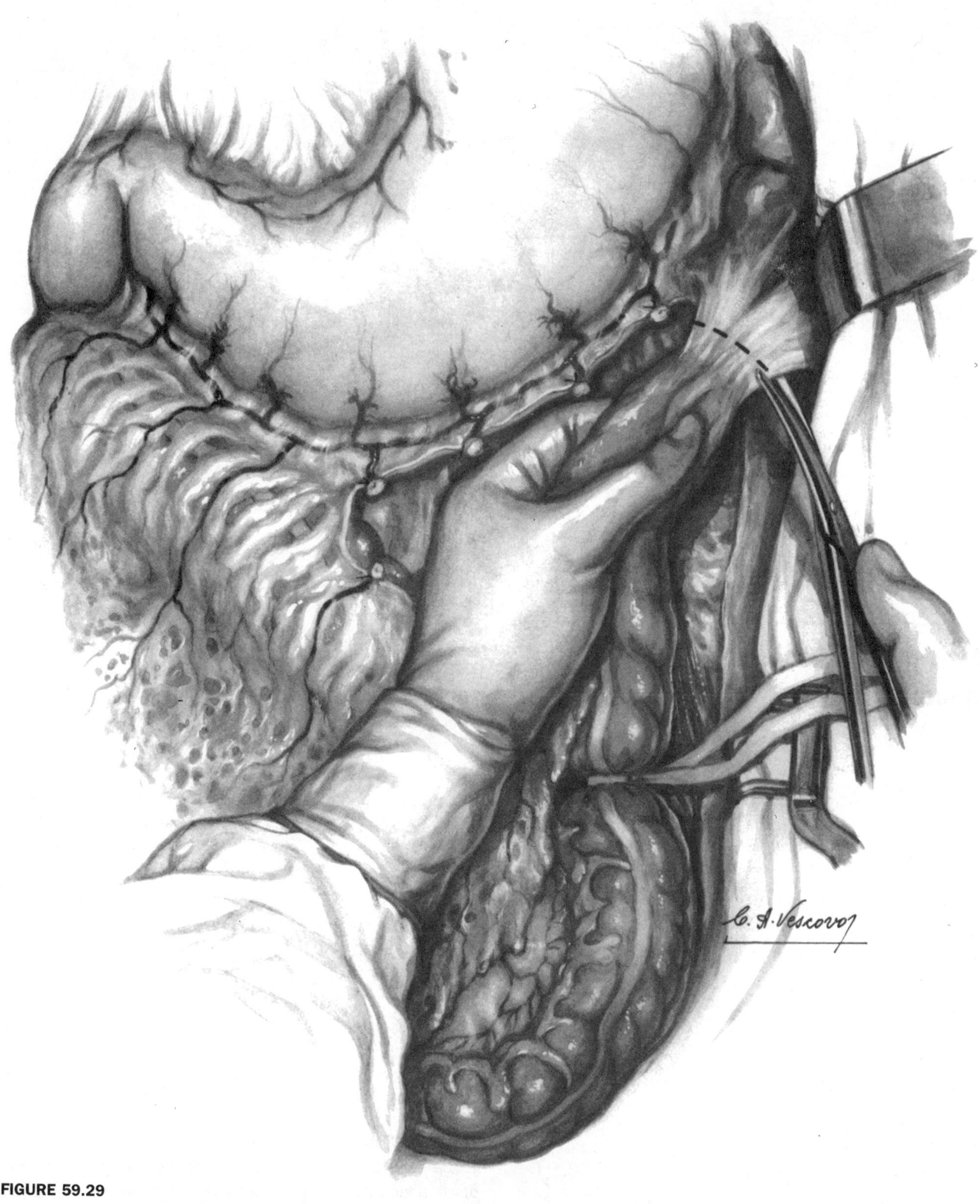

FIGURE 59.29

Low Anterior Resection with Manual Suture

FIGURE 59.30
To be able to bring the distal transverse segment of colon down adequately, it is necessary to divide the peritoneum along the lower border of the body and tail of the pancreas, as shown.

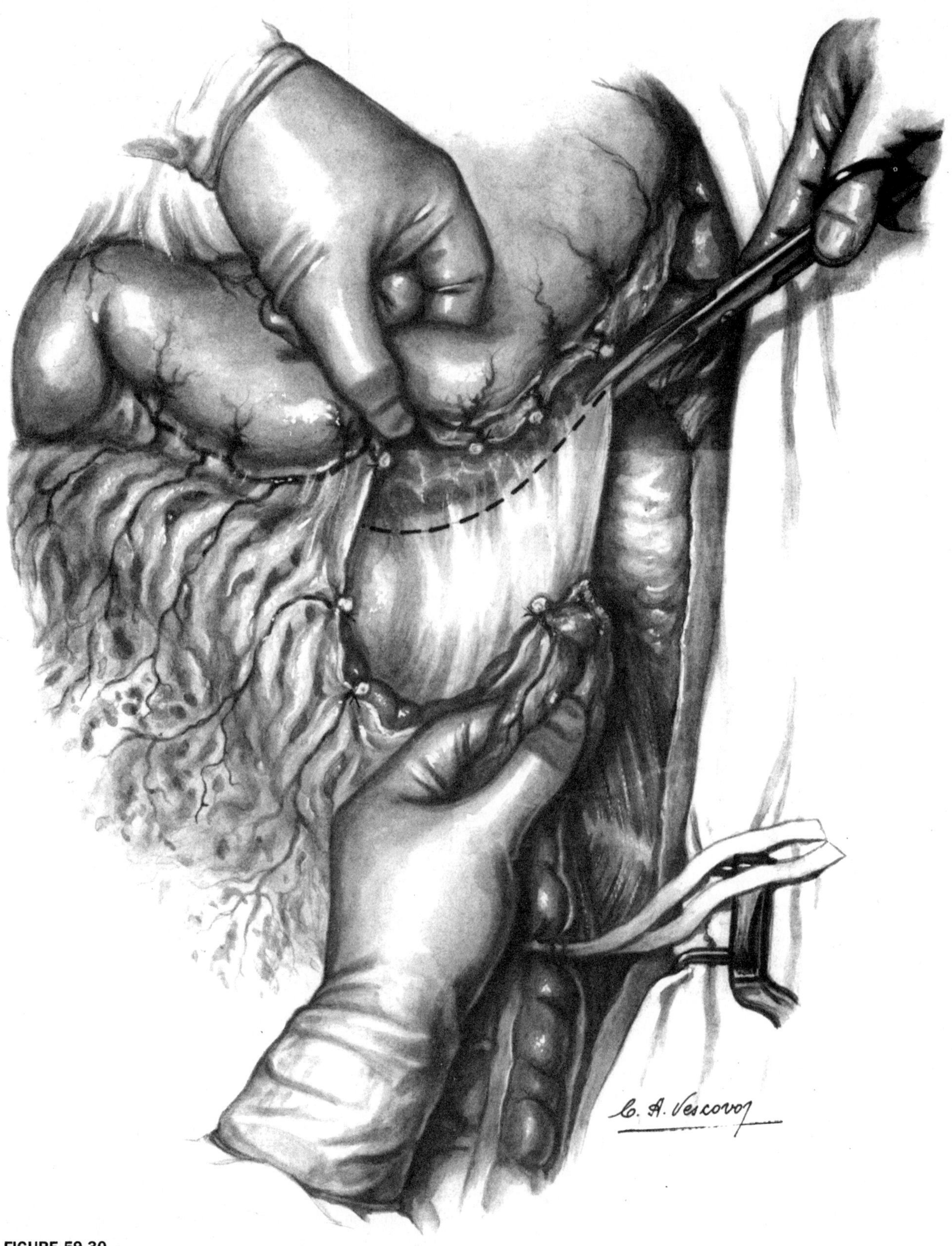

FIGURE 59.30

Low Anterior Resection with Manual Suture

FIGURE 59.31

Once mobilization of the left colon is complete, an anterior resection clamp, designed by the author, is placed just distal to the rectal tumor.

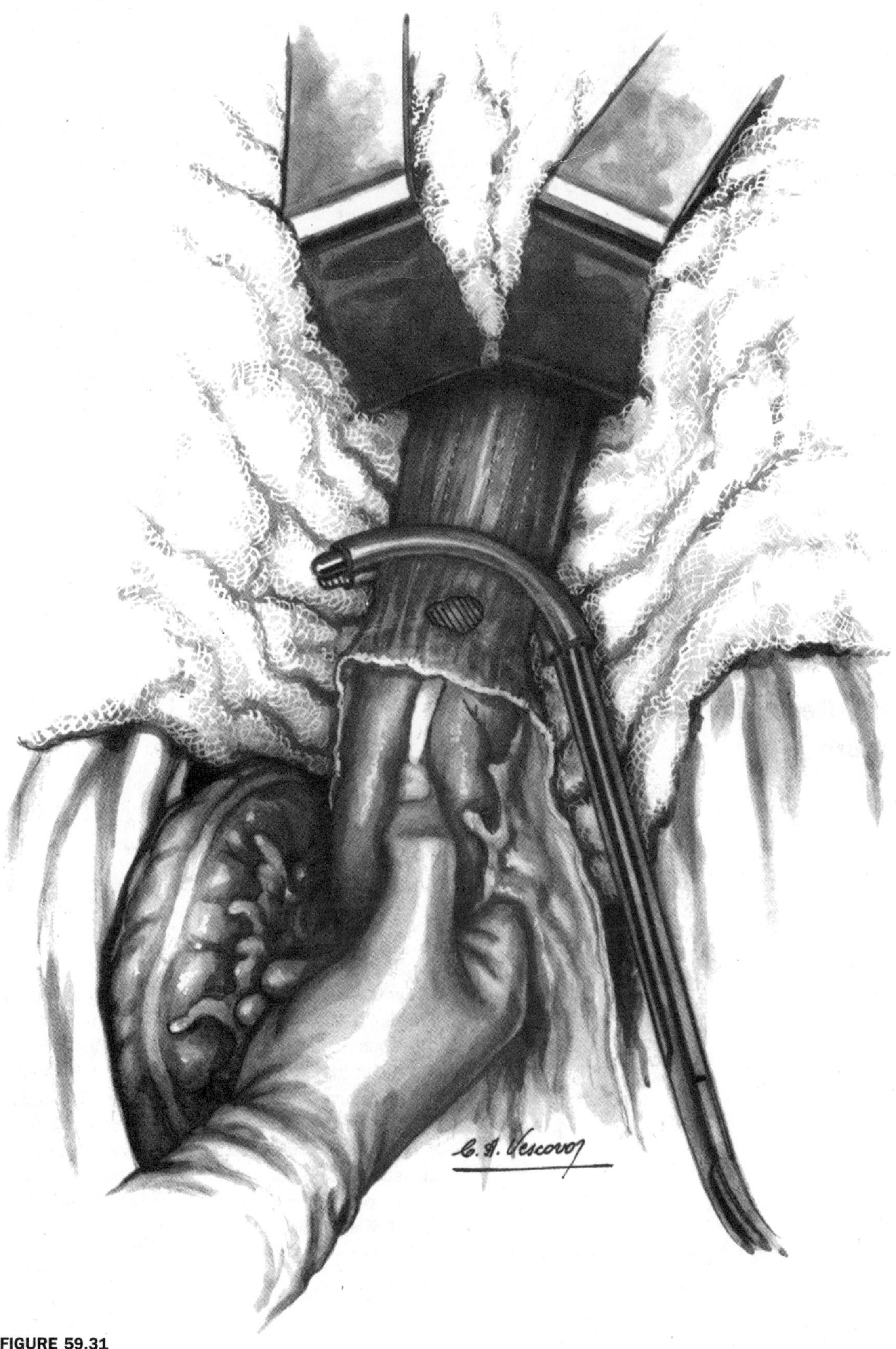

FIGURE 59.31

Low Anterior Resection with Manual Suture

FIGURE 59.32
A rubber tube has been introduced through the anus to irrigate the rectum below the anterior resection clamp with one liter of a 1% aqueous solution of cetrimide. After the rectum is washed with the cancericidal solution, one liter of saline solution is introduced through the same tube. The interior of the rectum is then aspirated to remove any residual fluid. Irrigation with the 1% cetrimide solution is done to destroy any viable neoplastic cells. Other cancericidal solution are also used for the same purpose, such as 1% mercury bichloride, Dakin's solution, 40% ethyl alcohol, and so on.

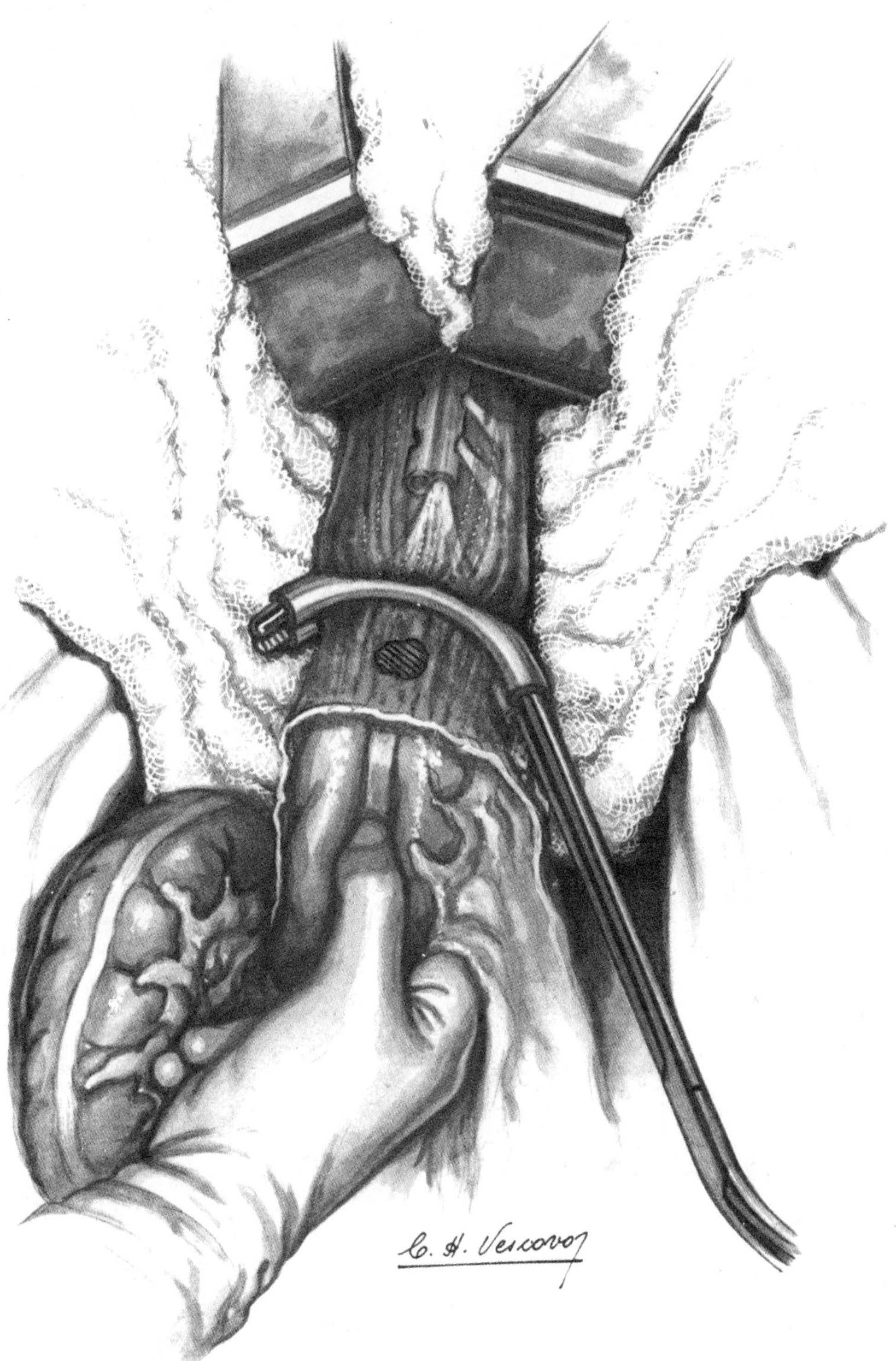

FIGURE 59.32

Low Anterior Resection with Manual Suture

FIGURE 59.33
Once the rectum has been washed, another anterior resection clamp is placed distal to the first clamp in the zone free of viable neoplastic cells. Using an angled scissors, the rectum is transected between both clamps. To make it clearer, the drawing shows the anterior resection clamps further apart than the distance they can actually be placed in a low anterior resection. The rectum should be transected no less than 2 cm beyond the distal limit of the tumor.

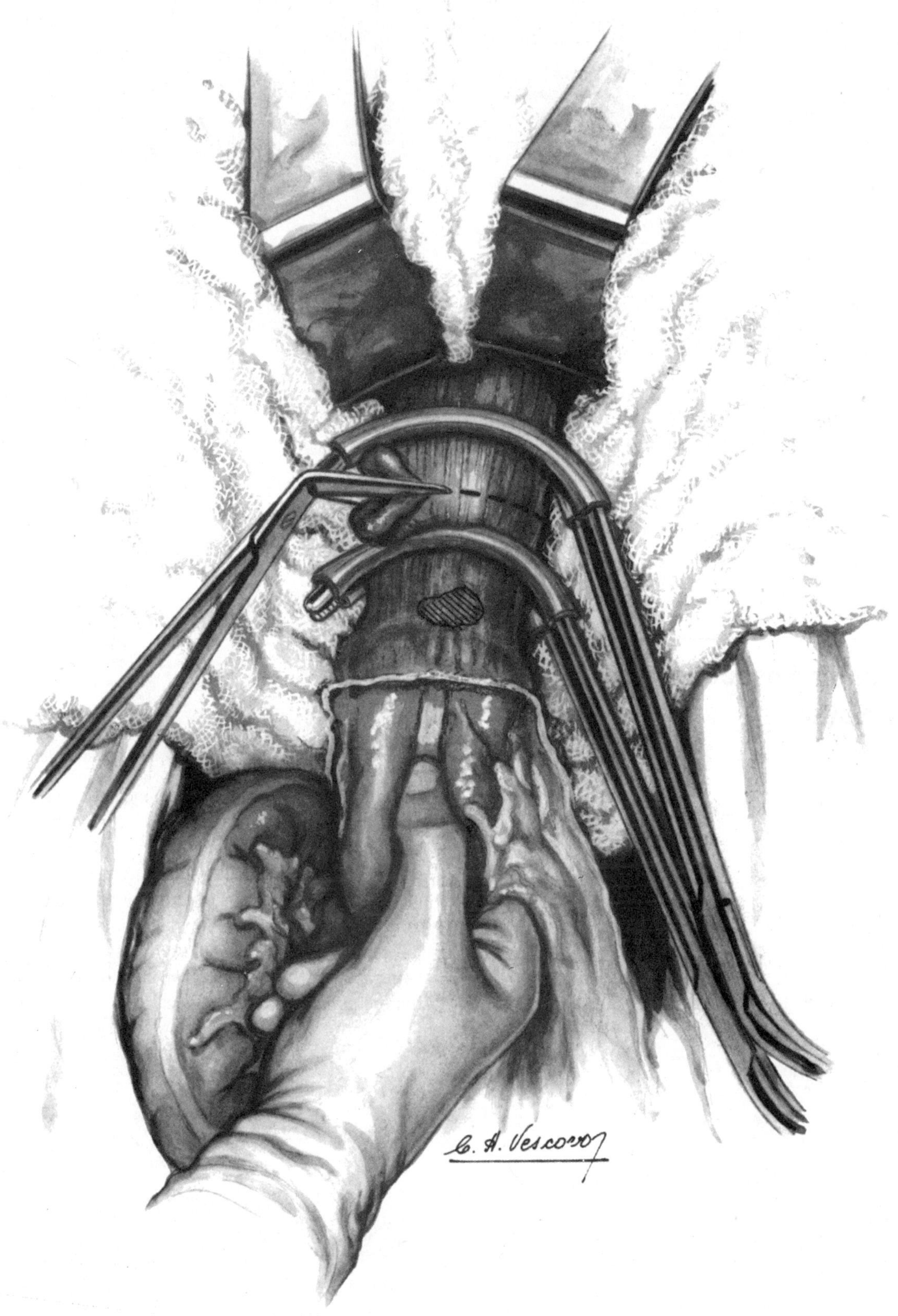

FIGURE 59.33

Low Anterior Resection with Manual Suture

FIGURE 59.34

The rectum and the distal descending colon have been transected, and the surgical specimen, consisting of the distal descending colon, the sigmoid colon, and the proximal segment of the rectum, has been removed. The end of the descending colon, to be anastomosed to the rectum, has another anterior resection clamp. This clamp has been approximated to the rectal clamp, and the posterior seromuscular layer of the colon is being sutured to the muscular layer of the rectum with interrupted nonabsorbable sutures.

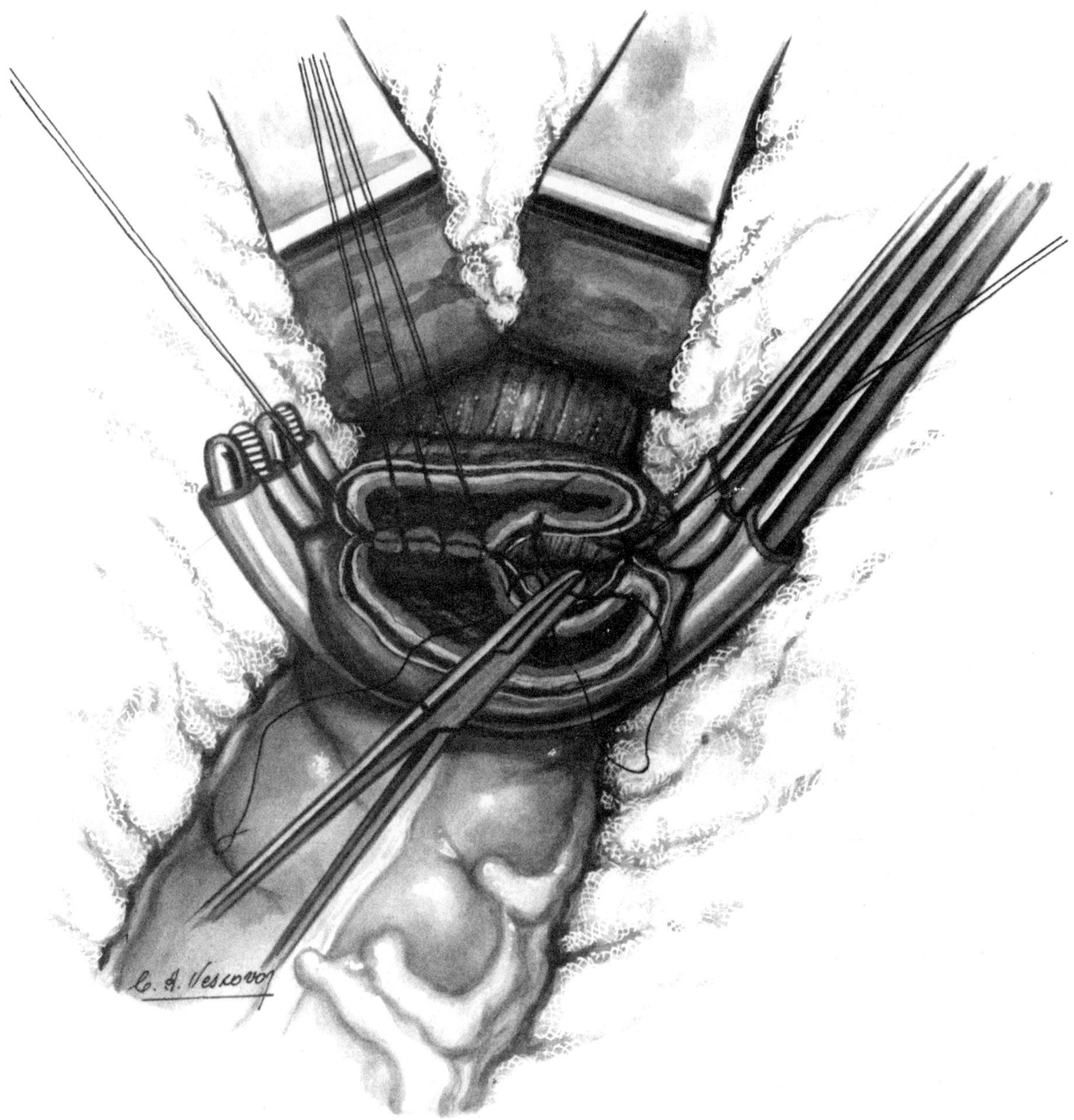

FIGURE 59.34

Low Anterior Resection with Manual Suture

FIGURE 59.35

When this seromuscular-muscular layer is complete, the posterior mucosal layer is sutured with interrupted synthetic absorbable sutures.

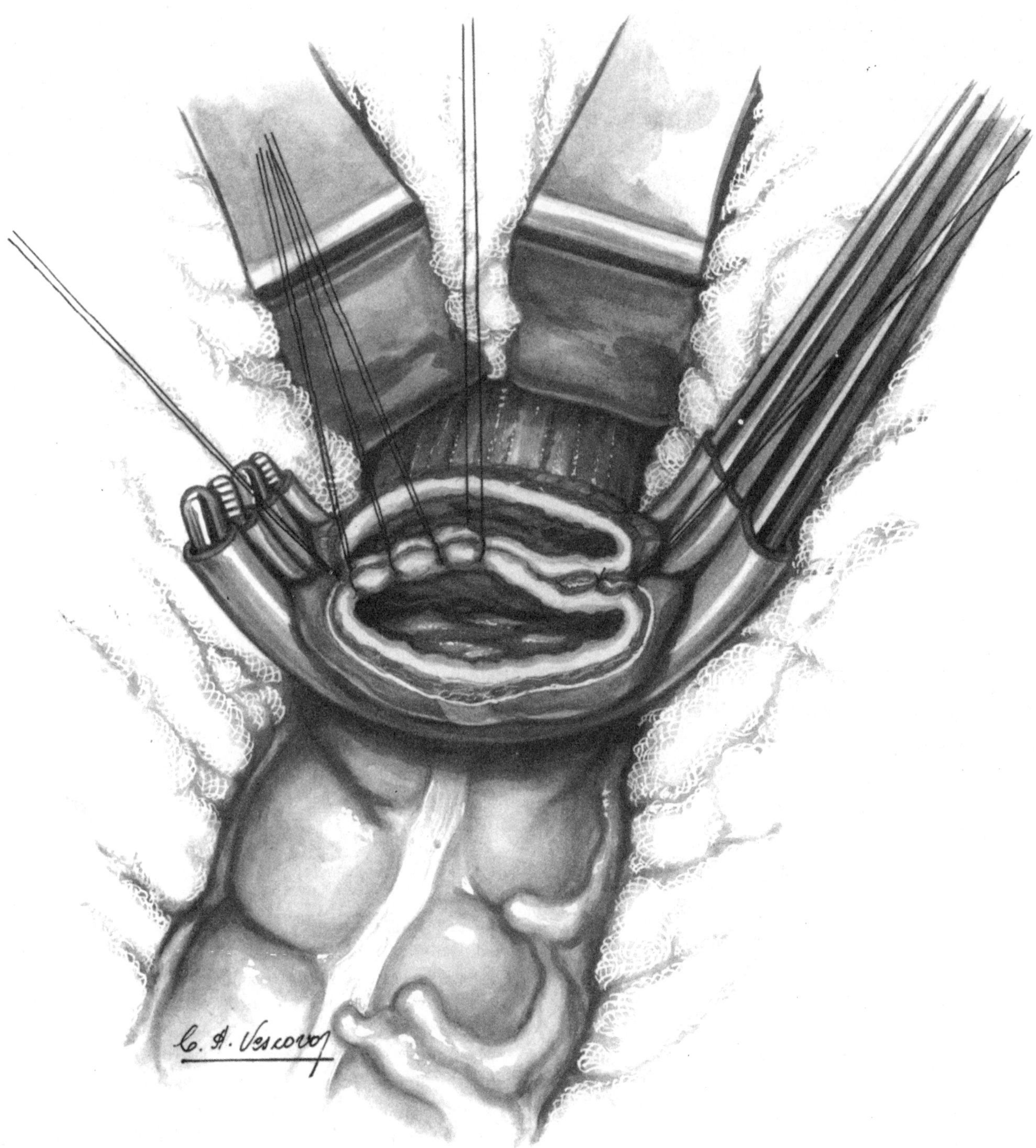

FIGURE 59.35

FIGURE 59.36
The anterior mucosal layer is being sutured with reabsorbable synthetic material, leaving the knots on the inside.

Low Anterior Resection with Manual Suture

FIGURE 59.37
The anterior seromuscular-muscular layer has been sutured, reestablishing intestinal continuity. The pelvic floor is peritonealized in patients with a low anterior resection. Usually, serosanguinous fluid accumulates in the presacral space, which later suppurates and may give rise to a dehiscence of the anastomosis. To prevent this complication, a continuous closed drainage tube is left in the presacral space, brought out through a small incision in the anterior abdominal wall. This tube is removed 4 or 5 days later. Some surgeons either do not peritonealize the pelvis or drain the presacral space. This conduct is based on allowing the serosanguinous fluid to enter freely into the abdominal cavity, preventing suppuration. In patients with a low anterior resection, it is usually unnecessary to perform a protective transverse colostomy if the anastomosis has been satisfactory. If the suture line is not satisfactory, a colostomy should be made without hesitation. A transverse colostomy does not prevent dehiscence or formation of a fistula, but does help it to heal. Some surgeons (93) use a loop ileostomy instead of a protective transverse colostomy.

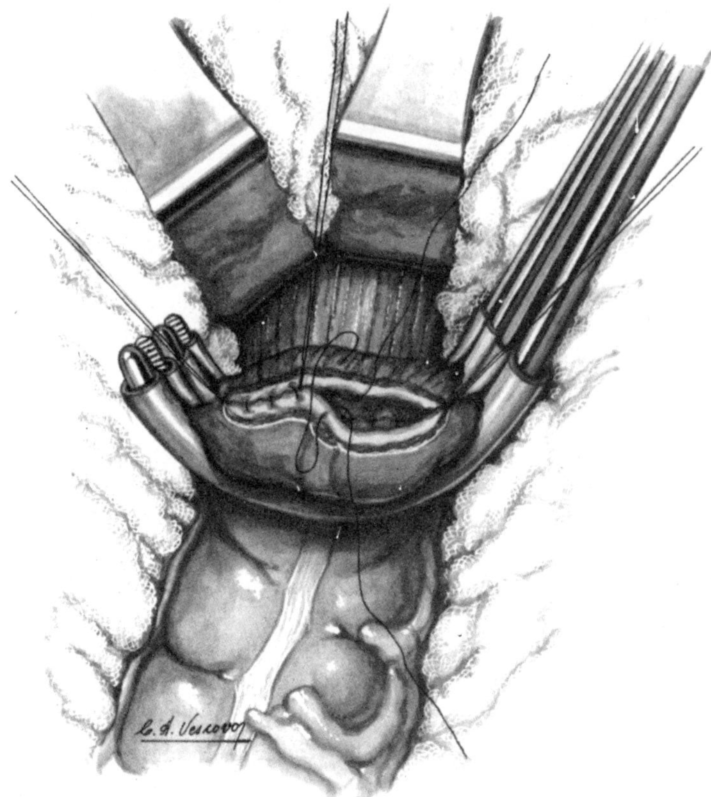

FIGURE 59.36

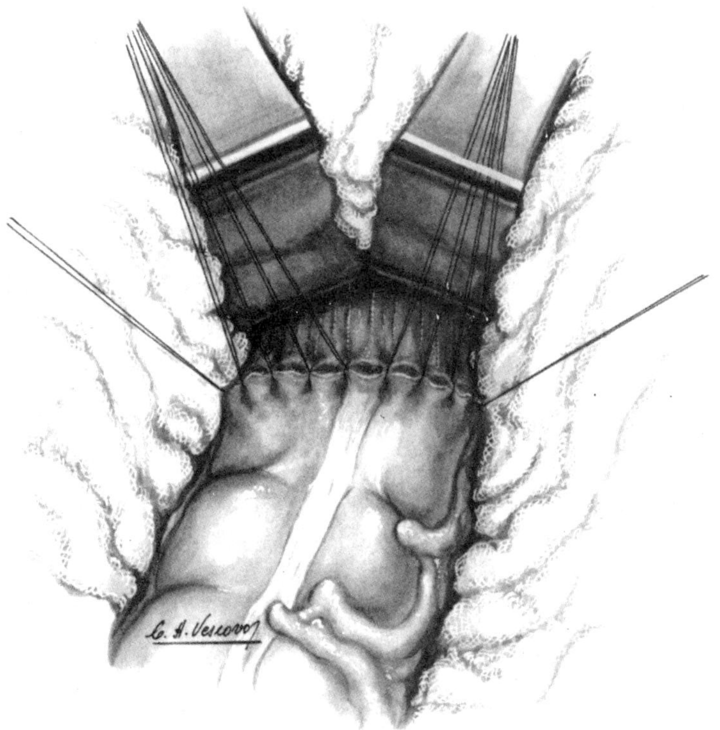

FIGURE 59.37

Low Anterior Resection with Manual Suture

FIGURE 59.38

In cases in which the colon has to be anastomosed to the rectal ampulla, which has a diameter two or three times that of the colon, instead of an end-to-end anastomosis, it is necessary to anastomose the side of the colon to the end of the rectum (10, 11), as shown in the drawing. This anastomosis has afforded very good results. Care should be taken that the colonic stump be short to avoid a blind loop syndrome.

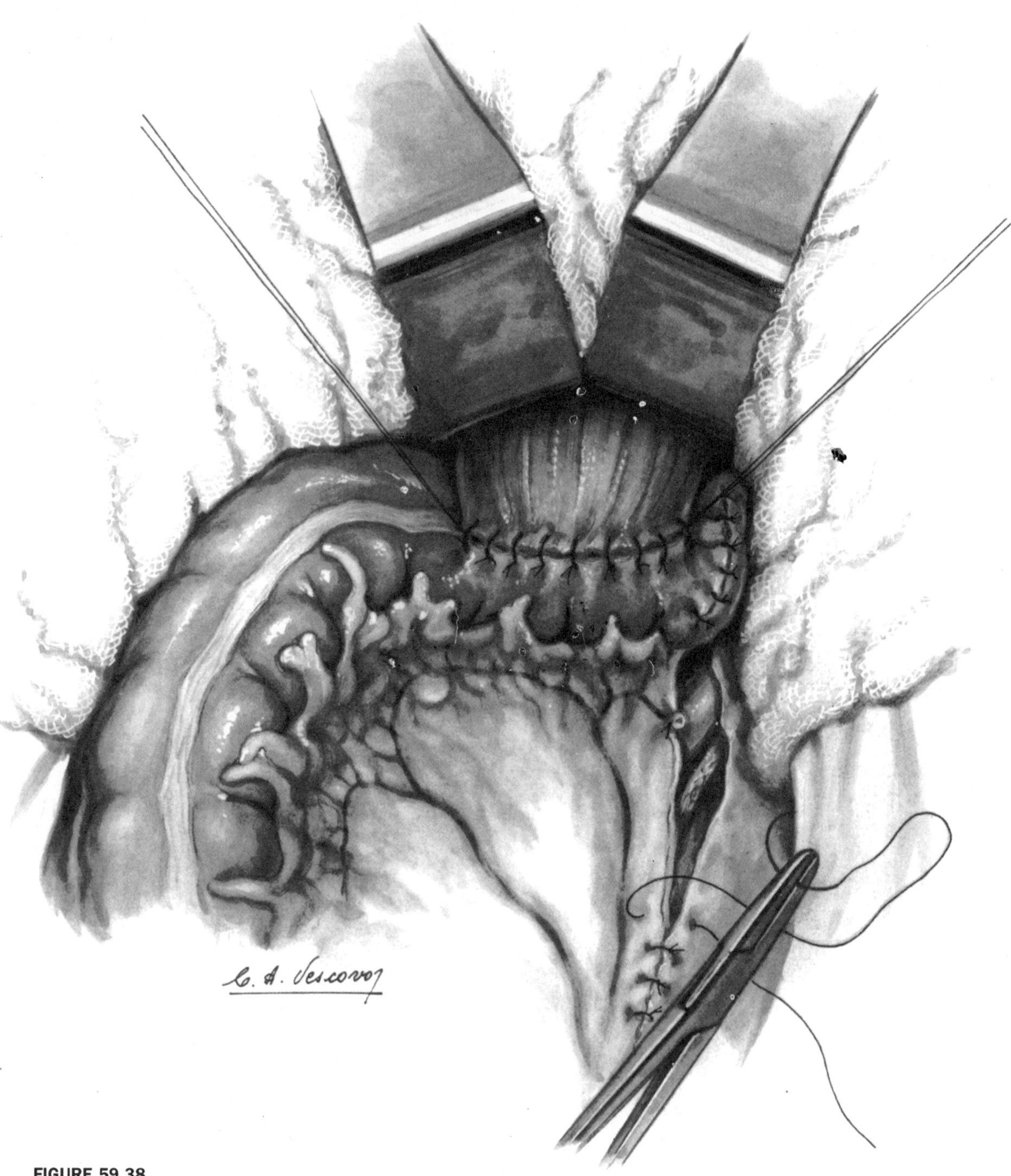

FIGURE 59.38

Low Anterior Resection with Manual Suture

FIGURE 59.39

Once the anastomosis is finished, the operation is completed by suturing the peritoneum of the left parietocolic space using interrupted sutures or a running suture. The mesentery is then closed. Some surgeons do not peritonealize the parietocolic space.

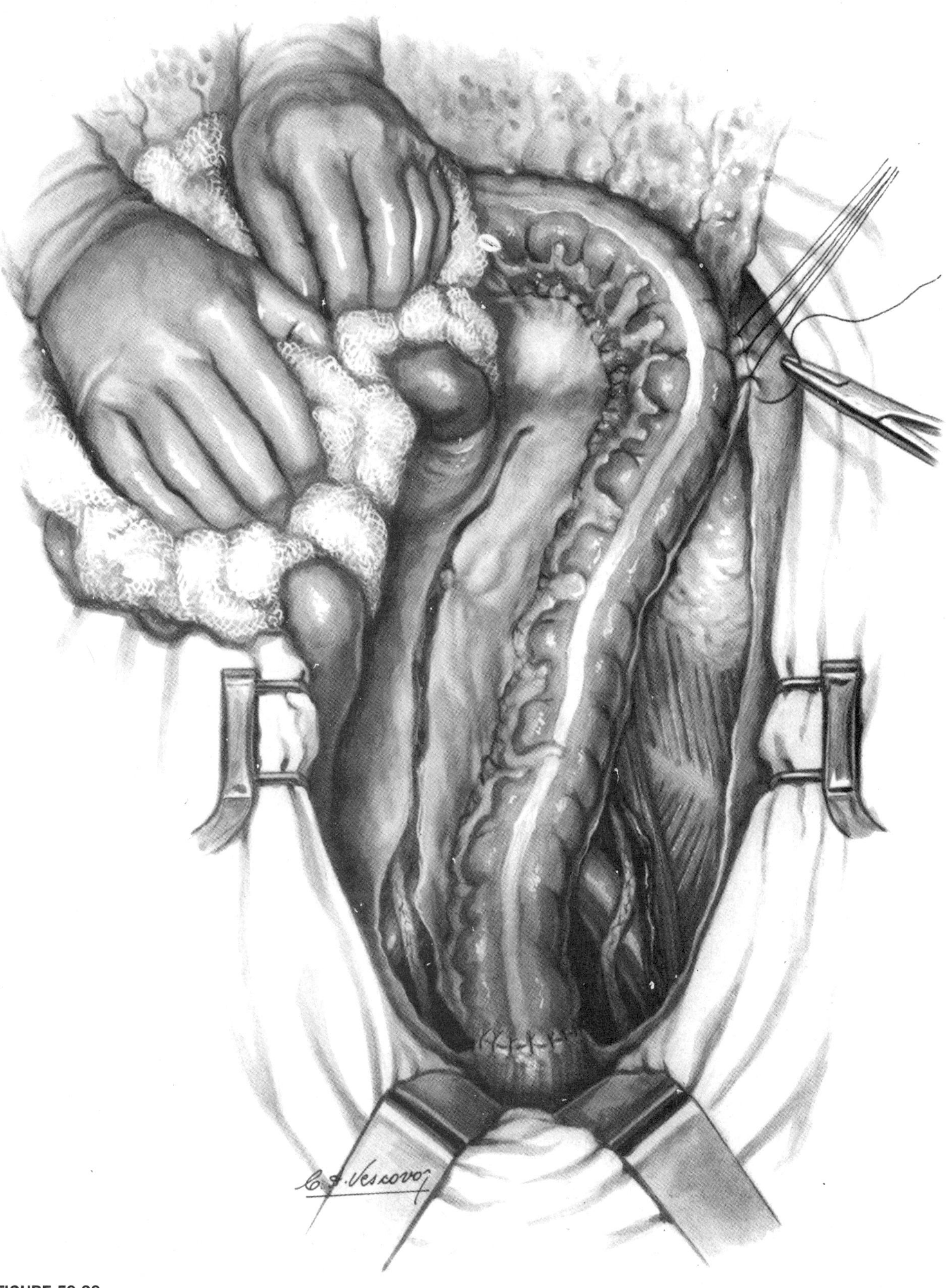

FIGURE 59.39

Low Anterior Resection with Manual Suture

FIGURE 59.40

In cases in which it is difficult or impossible to close the peritoneum of the parietocolic space, the greater omentum may be used, as shown. The drawing also shows that the mesentery is being sutured.

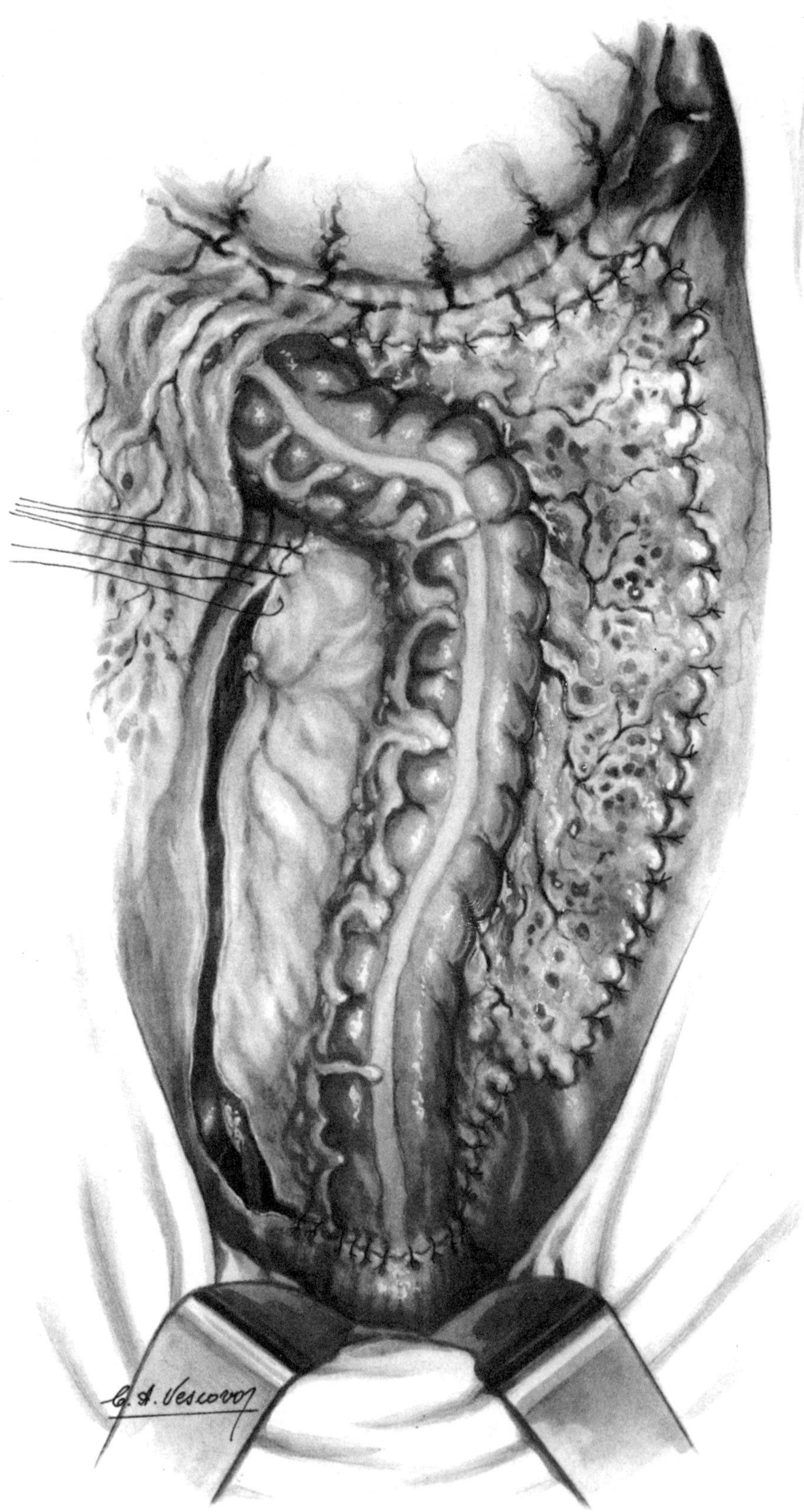

FIGURE 59.40

Low Anterior Resection with Manual Suture

FIGURE 59.41
Semischematic drawing showing the final aspect of the completed operation.

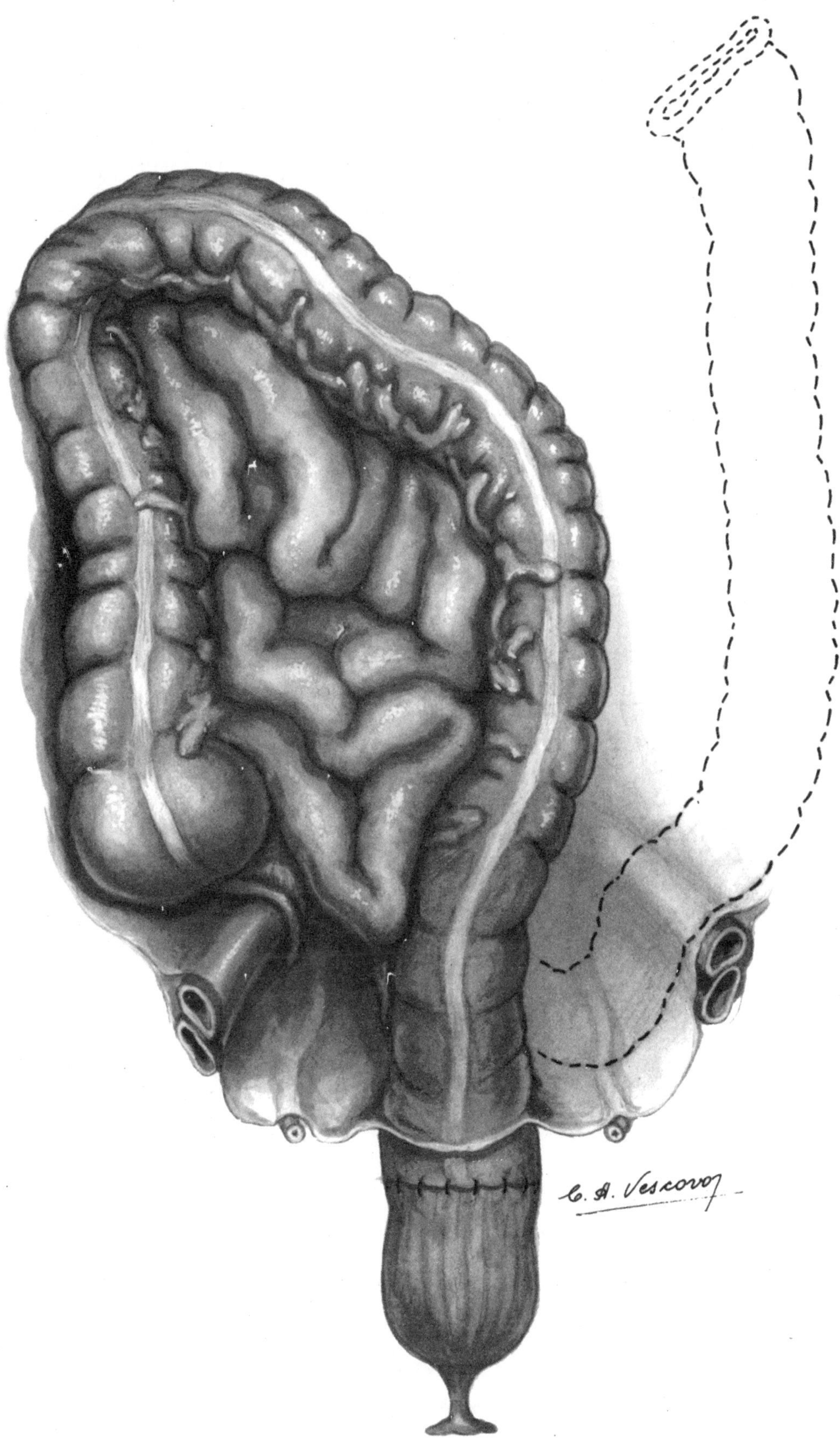

FIGURE 59.41

Low Anterior Resection with Manual Suture

FIGURE 59.42

In a few cases the left colon cannot be brought down to the pelvic cavity and sutured to the rectum without traction. In this situation the colon can be made to traverse a shorter course to the pelvic cavity by passing it through the mesentery, as seen in the drawing, between the superior mesenteric artery and the ileocolic artery (81).

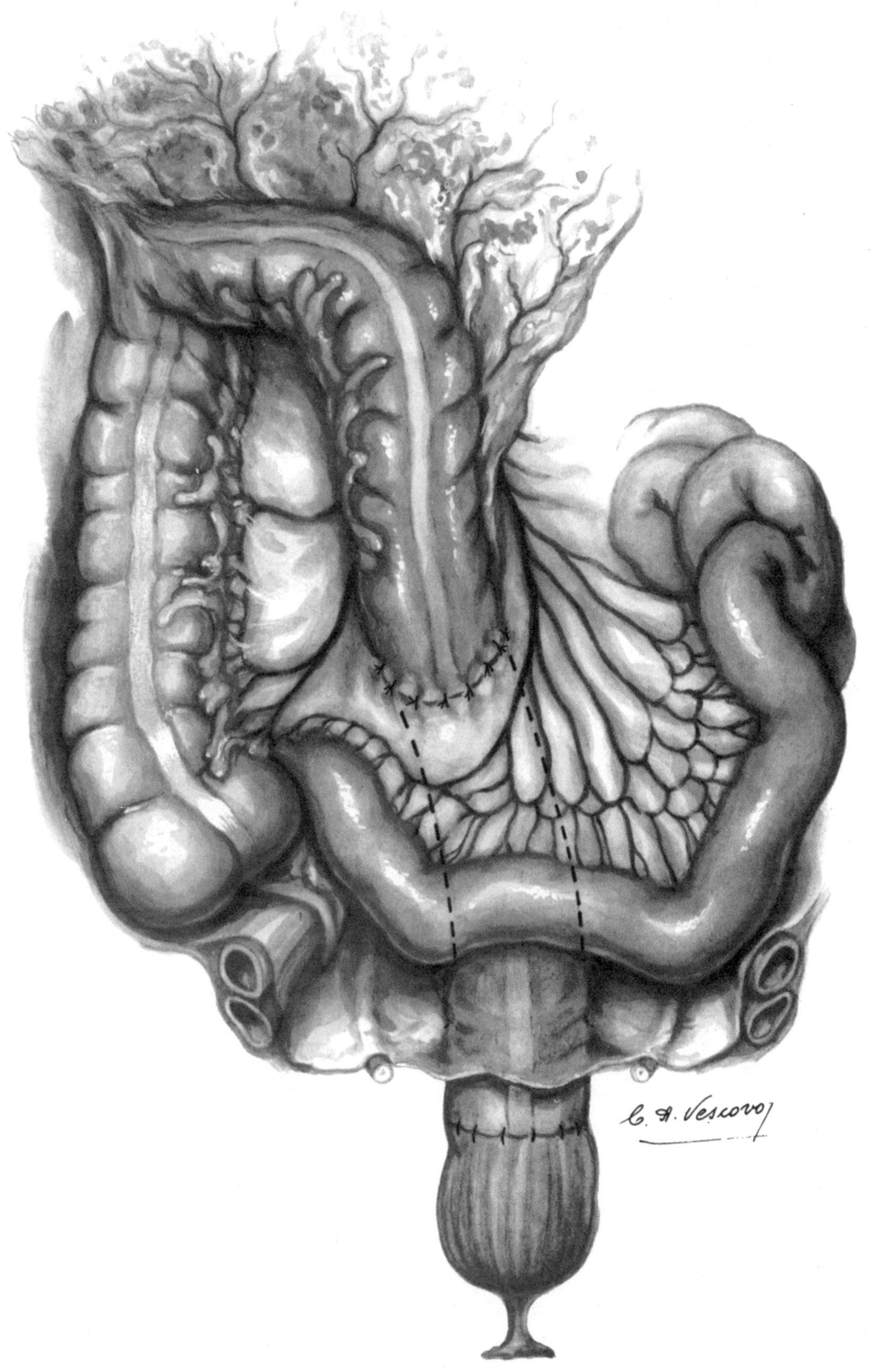

FIGURE 59.42

Low Anterior Resection with Anastomosis Using the Circular EEA Stapler

Anastomosis with the EEA stapler has increased the indications for low anterior resection in rectal cancer and has simplified its execution. With this procedure it is possible to perform a colorectal anastomosis with the double stapler, using the premium disposable CEEA instrument with a removable anvil and the Roticulator (U.S. Surgical) or the Proximate ILS instrument with a removable anvil (Ethicon).

Low Anterior Resection with Anastomosis Using the Circular EEA Stapler

Low Anterior Resection with Anastomosis Using the Circular EEA Stapler

FIGURE 59.43 REGULAR EEA INSTRUMENT
1, Shaft; 2, wing nut; 3, cartridge tie; 4, safety device; 5, trigger handles; 6, 6', cartridge; 7, 7', anvil; 8, two concentric circular rows of staggered staples; 9, staples.

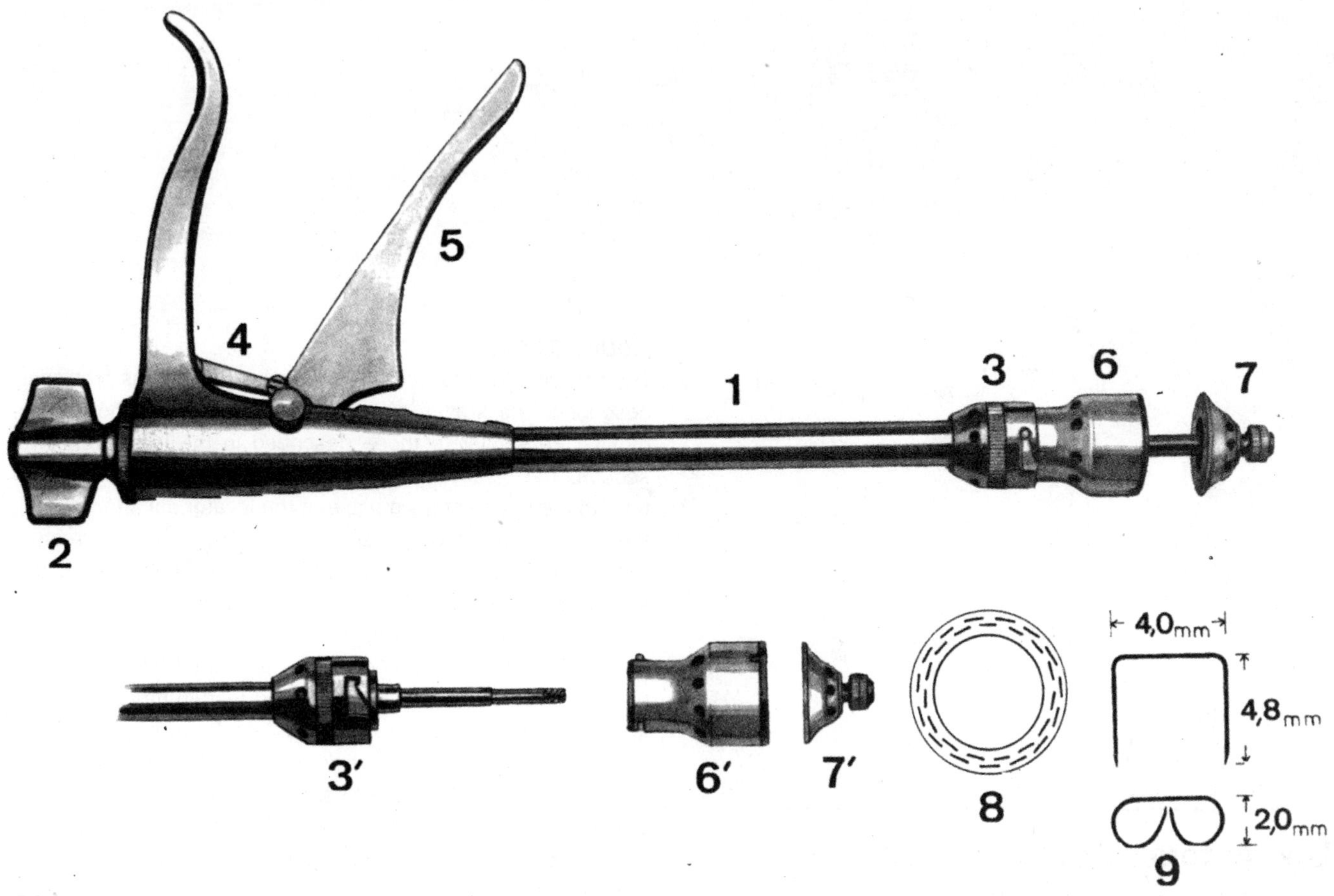

FIGURE 59.43 REGULAR EEA INSTRUMENT

Low Anterior Resection with Anastomosis Using the Circular EEA Stapler

FIGURE 59.44

The patient is placed in the Lloyd-Davies position as previously described. The stages of the procedure, prior to the anastomosis, are similar to those described in the low anterior resection. The dissection of the posterior rectal wall should extend to the puborectalis muscle of the levator ani after incising the rectosacral or Waldeyer's fascia. Anteriorly, the rectum should be dissected beyond the prostate. Laterally, the dissection should extend to the levator ani muscles, after transecting the lateral rectal ligaments. Selection of the surgical procedure to be used can only be determined after mobilizing the rectum (17, 50, 65, 93). Once the rectum has been mobilized, a right-angle clamp is placed 1 to 2 cm beyond the tumor. The author uses the previously described anterior resection clamp instead of the right-angle clamp. This clamp is very practical because its arms extend obliquely out of the surgical field without obstructing the surgeon's view during insertion of the purse string suture.

The rectum is washed with one liter of a 1% cetrimide solution to destroy any residual viable neoplastic cells (93). The rectum is immediately washed with one liter of saline solution. Traction is applied to the clamp to stretch the rectum and make it easier to insert the purse string, which should be done gradually (17, 93). This means that, as the rectum is transected, the purse string suture is begun in the distal edge with a continuous 2-0 prolene suture. The entire anterior wall of the rectum is transected and the purse string suture completed in the distal border. The same technique is used in the posterior rectal wall (see inset). This technique facilitates insertion of the purse string manually. If the rectum is completely transected, it would retract into the bottom of the pelvic cavity, making it difficult or impossible to insert the purse string in the rectal stump. These same difficulties present themselves if the purse string insertion is attempted with a purse string instrument (autosuture). Some surgeons (93) have an assistant push up on the perineum with a fist, toward the abdominal cavity. This maneuver may elevate the rectal border 2 or 3 cm.

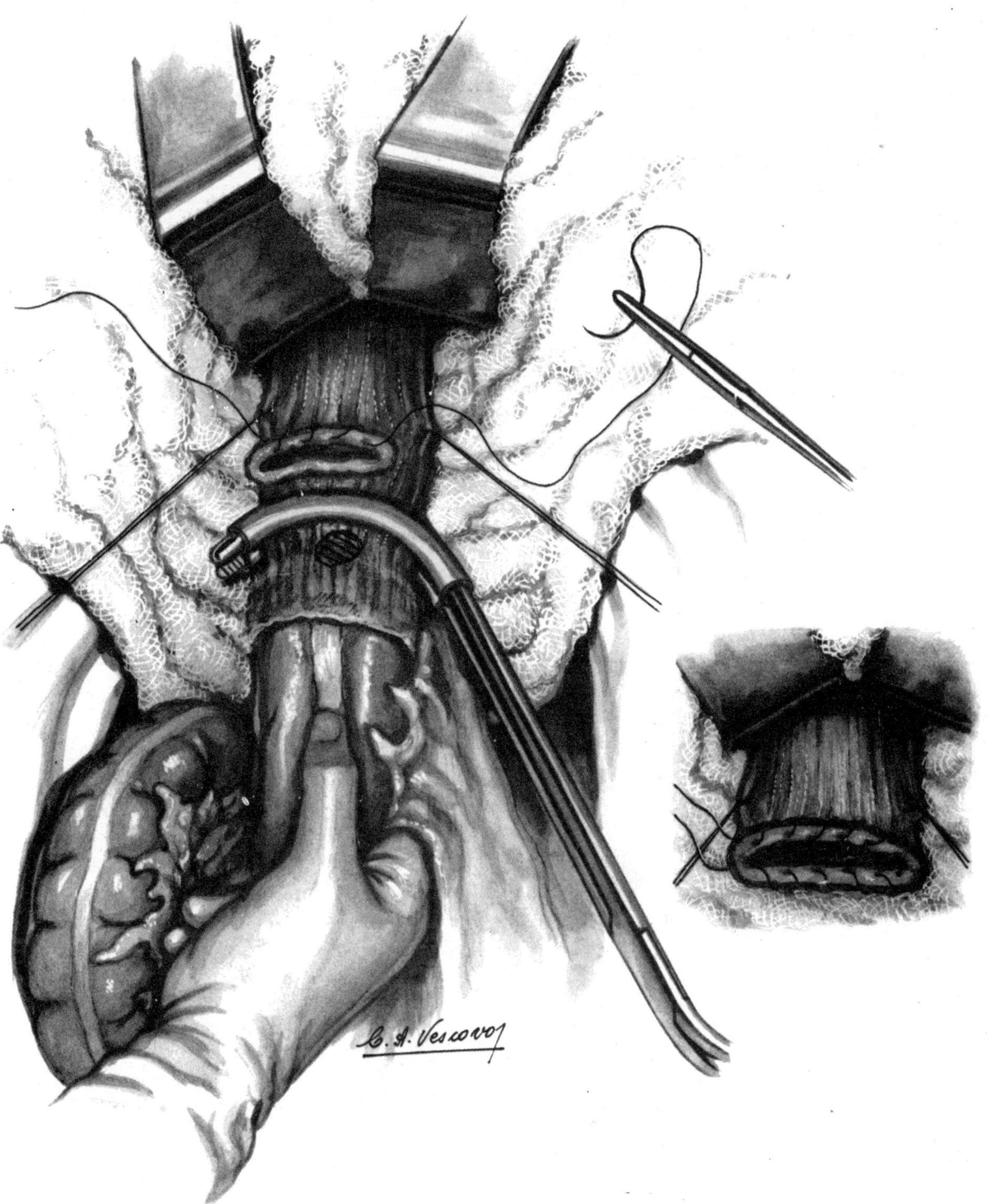

FIGURE 59.44

Low Anterior Resection with Anastomosis Using the Circular EEA Stapler

FIGURE 59.45

To carry out the purse string in the distal rectum, some surgeons use a purse string applicator (U.S. Surgical). This instrument inserts a purse string into the muscular layer of the rectum, since this instrument has the purse string suture in it, and the suture remains in the rectal wall.

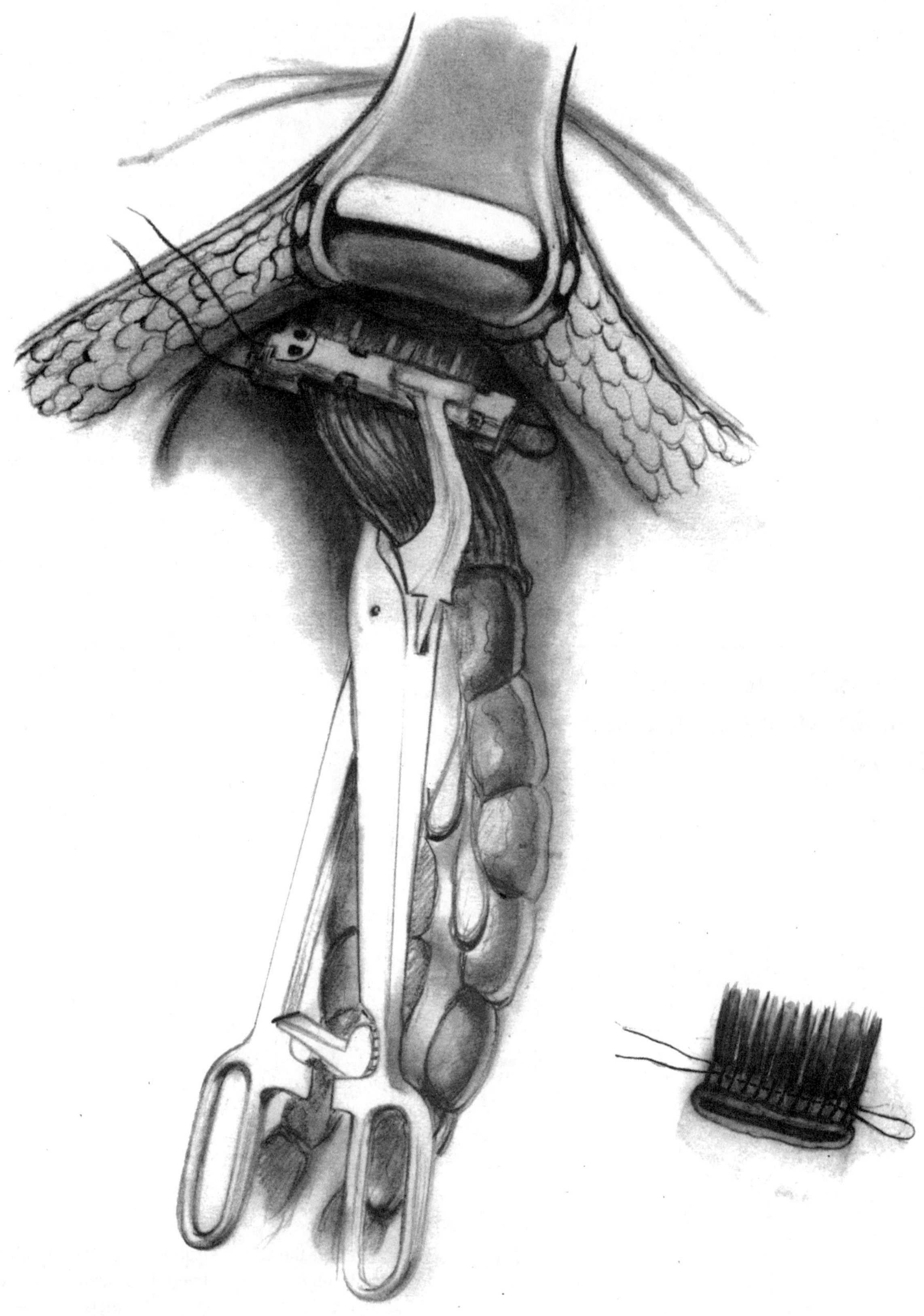

FIGURE 59.45

FIGURE 59.46
The surgical specimen has been removed. An anterior resection clamp has been placed in the colon to prevent any spillage of the intestinal contents, and a purse string suture has been placed in its end, using 2-0 Prolene, after confirming that its caliber was adequate to permit introduction of an EEA 31 instrument. The ends of the colon and rectum must be clean of fat, areolar tissue, and mesentery for a distance of at least 15 mm. In the drawings on the left, it can be seen that a purse string suture is being carried out on the distal colonic end, using the special purse string instrument similar to the Furniss clamp. There is no difficulty with the purse string of the colonic end. It can be done manually as well as with the purse string instrument.

Low Anterior Resection with Anastomosis Using the Circular EEA Stapler

FIGURE 59.47
The wing nut of the EEA instrument has been rotated counter clockwise to open the instrument and separate the anvil from the cartridge. The purse string on the rectal end has been adjusted around the shaft. The anvil is about to be inserted into the colonic end. To carry out this maneuver it is useful to place three Babcock or Allis clamps on the edge of the colonic circumference to facilitate introduction of the anvil.

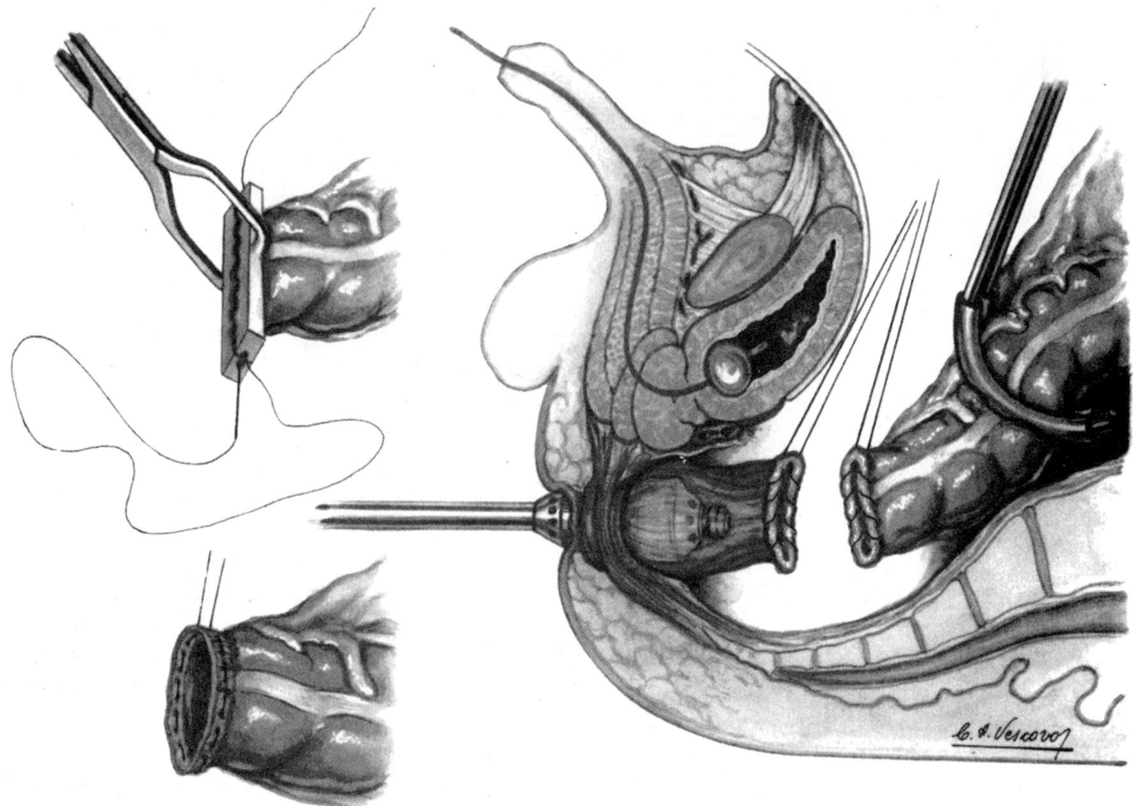

FIGURE 59.46

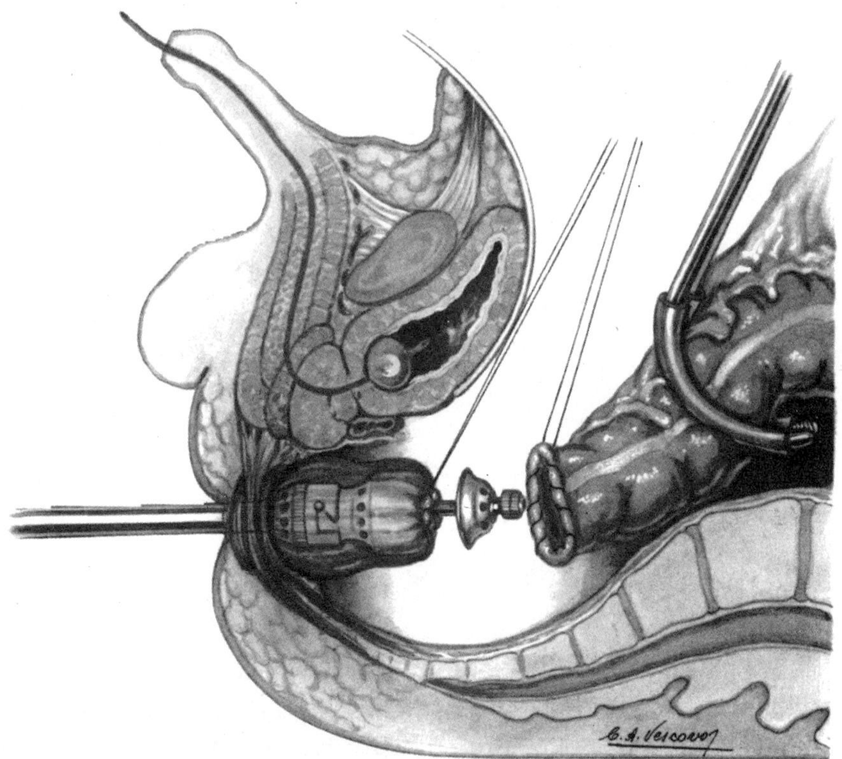

FIGURE 59.47

FIGURE 59.48

The anvil of the EEA instrument has been introduced inside the colonic end and the purse string adjusted around the shaft. The ends of the purse string sutures of the rectum and the colon have been tied and cut less than 5 mm from the knot. The caliber of the colon should admit the anvil of the EEA 31 instrument. If the anvil cannot be introduced, the colon can be dilated with Hegar bougies (93). If it cannot be dilated enough, an EEA 28 instrument can be used. It should be pointed out that the best functional results are obtained with the EEA 31 instrument. Smaller EEA instruments are prone to stricture of the anastomosis. This inconvenience can be avoided by bringing down the splenic flexure and performing the colorectal anastomosis with a segment of the distal descending or sigmoid colon.

Low Anterior Resection with Anastomosis Using the Circular EEA Stapler

FIGURE 59.49

The wing nuts of the instrument are rotated clockwise until the arrows indicate that the anvil and the cartridge are solidly against each other. This is confirmed by observing the instrument.

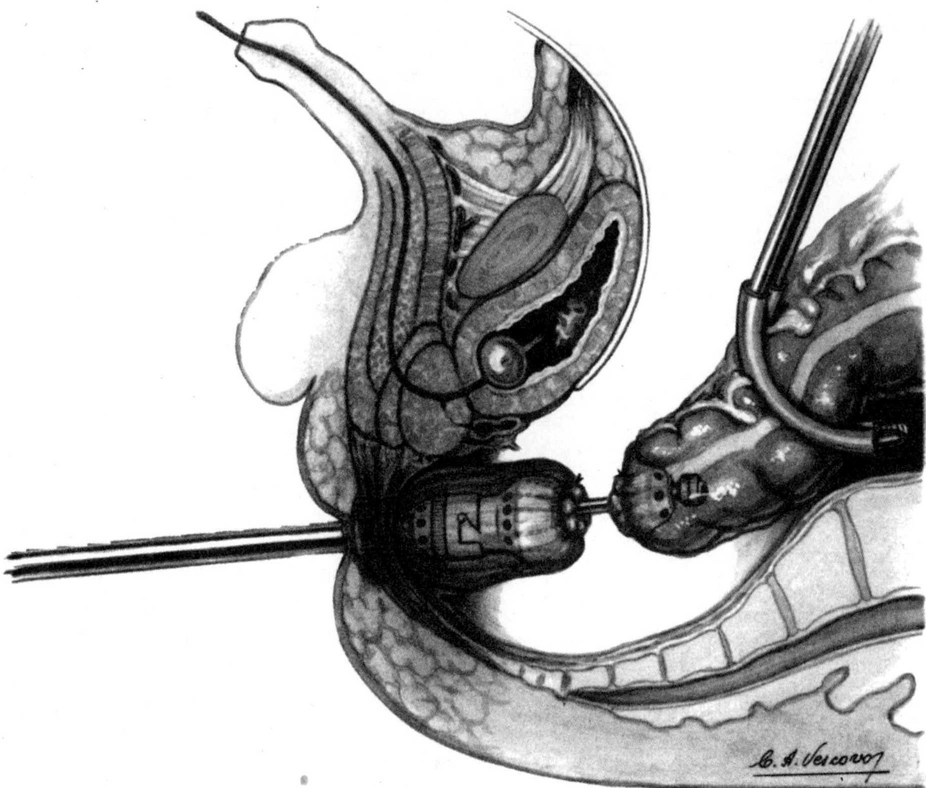

FIGURE 59.48

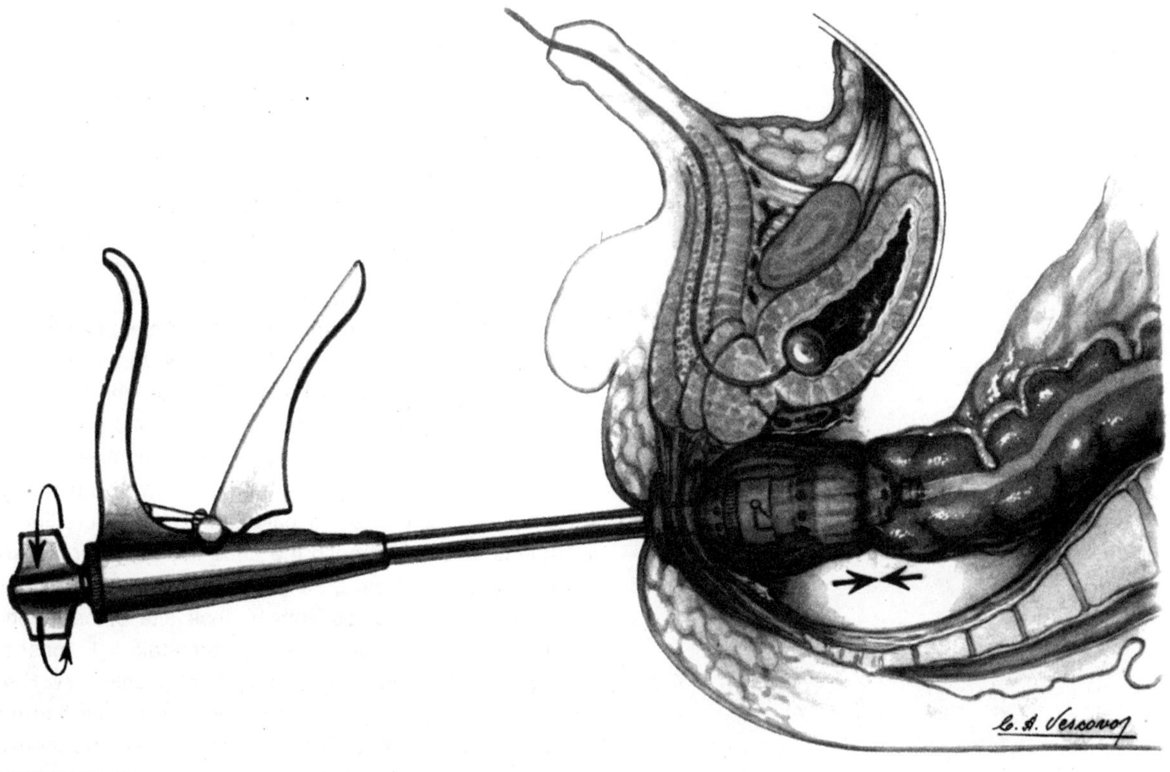

FIGURE 59.49

FIGURE 59.50
The instrument has been completely closed and the signal indicates it is perfectly adjusted, so it can be fired by squeezing the trigger handle of the instrument (arrow). Firing the instrument places two concentric circular rows of staples in staggered fashion. Simultaneously, a circular scalpel transects two rings of tissue inside the lines of staples, creating an end-to-end colorectal anastomosis. The diameter of the lumen of the anastomosis is 21 mm.

Low Anterior Resection with Anastomosis Using the Circular EEA Stapler

FIGURE 59.51
Once the colorectal anastomosis is complete, the EEA instrument is extracted. This should be done delicately and with precision. Once the instrument has been removed, it should be confirmed that the doughnuts of tissue from the rectal and colonic ends are complete and made up of all their layers (see inset). If the rings are not complete, attempts should be made to locate the defect to correct it with sutures. To determine if the anastomosis is waterproof, the following test should carried out: The pelvis is filled with saline and a few minutes allowed to pass so that the remaining air bubbles, which are always present, disappear. Simultaneously, an atraumatic clamp is placed on the proximal colon above the suture line. A rectal tube is inserted through the anus and a moderate amount of air introduced. If no bubbles are seen, the suture line is impermeable. If bubbles appear, their site of origin should be searched for and corrective measures taken. In most cases, a protective transverse colostomy is not necessary. However, if the anastomosis is doubtful or there was a need to repair the anastomosis, a protective transverse colostomy should be performed.

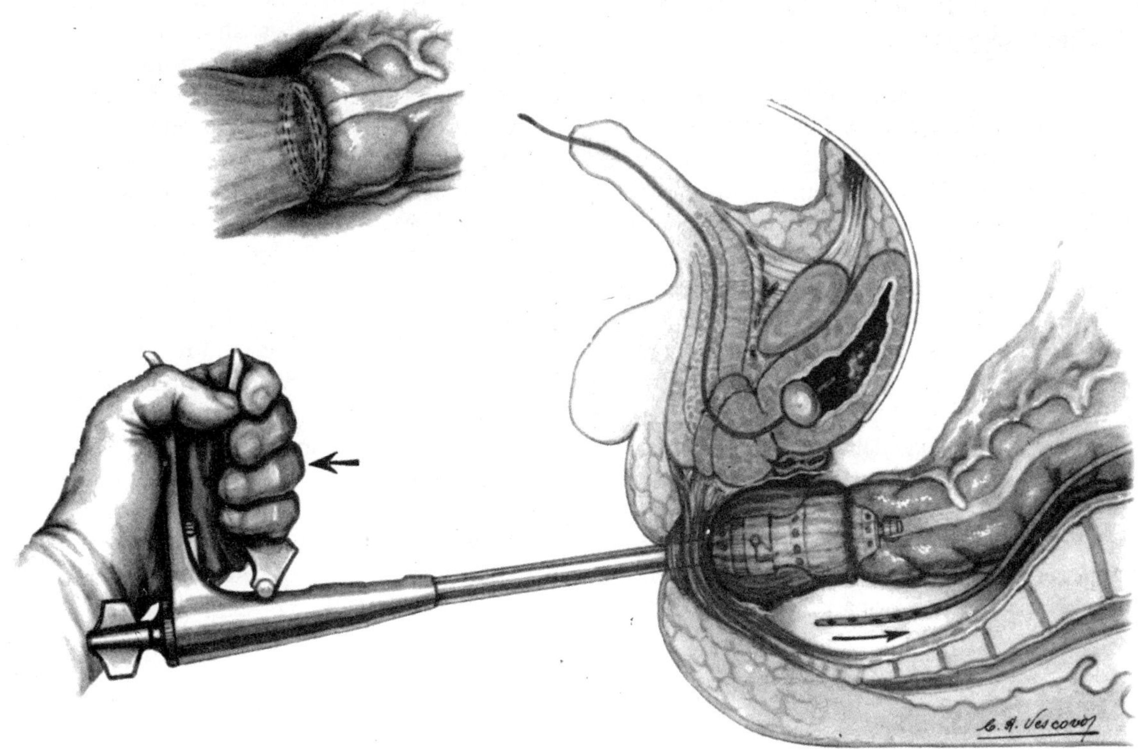

FIGURE 59.50

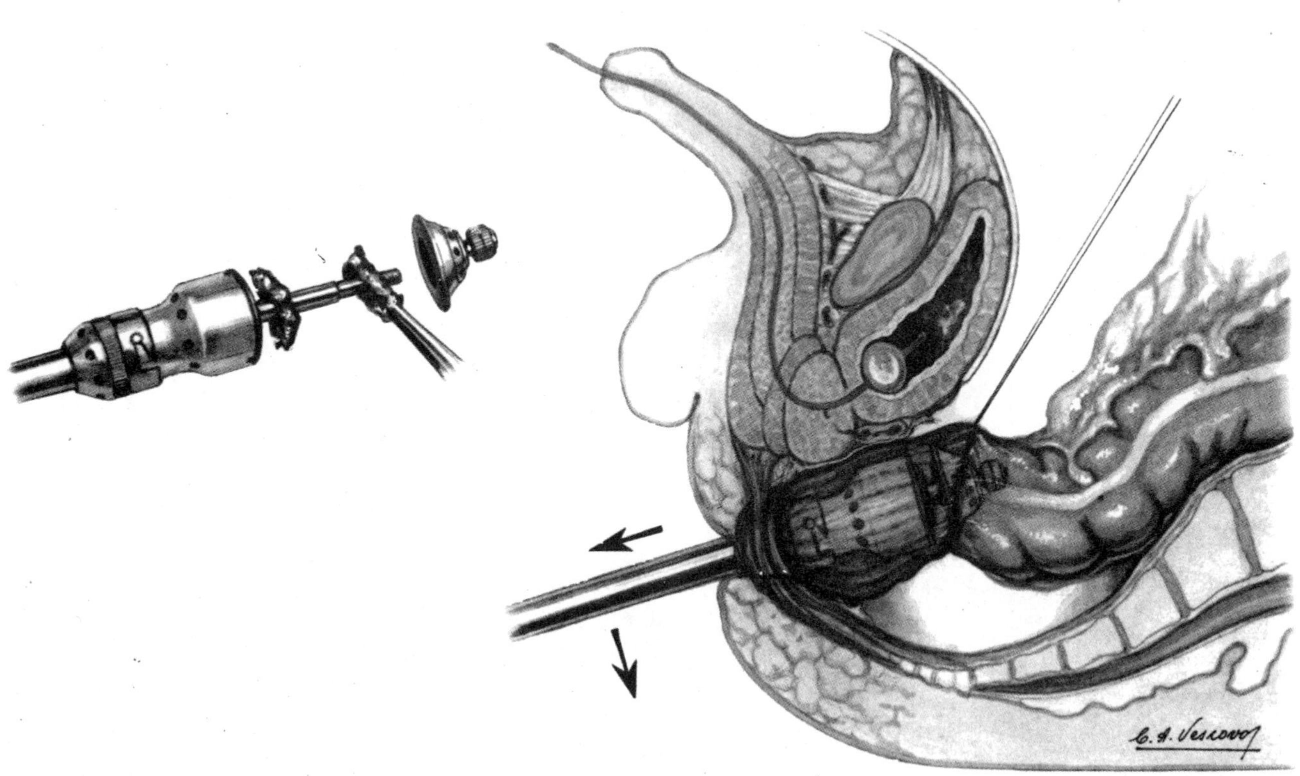

FIGURE 59.51

Low Anterior Resection with Double Suture Using Staplers

To perform a low colorectal anastomosis, Knight and Griffen (50), proposed the Premium CEEA (U.S. Surgical) instrument, characterized by having a removable anvil and shaft. Together with this instrument a Roticulator TA 55 (U.S. Surgical) is used. This can carry out a linear suture very low in the rectum because of its ability to rotate and introduce it to the bottom of the pelvis. This instrument closes the rectum, down low, very near the anal canal, placing two rows of staples distal to the tumor. By using the Roticulator, placement of a purse string low in the rectum, which is always difficult, can be avoided. In addition, closure with the Roticulator is safer than a purse string. Additionally, the Roticulator can be used in a very wide rectum with thick walls, conditions that contraindicate the use of purse string sutures.

The Roticulator closes the rectum with two layers of staplers, and the anastomosis is made with the CEEA instrument. The first step of the anastomosis consists in removing the anvil with its shaft, replacing it with a trochar introduced into the shaft of the cartridge, which remained empty when the anvil and its shaft were removed. The trochar is retracted into the cartridge to let the CEEA instrument advance through the rectum. The anvil, with its shaft, is inserted into the colonic end, where a purse string suture had been previously placed, using the purse string instrument, with 2-0 Prolene suture. This method is usually known as a double stapling technique because it realizes a linear row of staples in the rectum with the Roticulator and a second circular suture line with staples, using the CEEA instrument. This procedure is also known as the CEEA-Roticulator technique (17). Some authors (93) believe the two suture lines with staples close to each other may cause ischemia of the tissues in some cases. However, this complication has rarely been reported.

We will now describe the technique of a low colorectal anastomosis using the Roticulator and the CEEA instrument.

Low Anterior Resection with Double Suture Using Staplers

Low Anterior Resection with Double Suture Using Staplers

FIGURE 59.52

The Roticulator has been introduced deep into the pelvic cavity to apply two linear rows of staples after it is fired. A right-angle clamp is then placed on the rectum, distal to the tumor, and the rectum transected transversely with a scalpel, following the inferior border of the Roticulator (17).

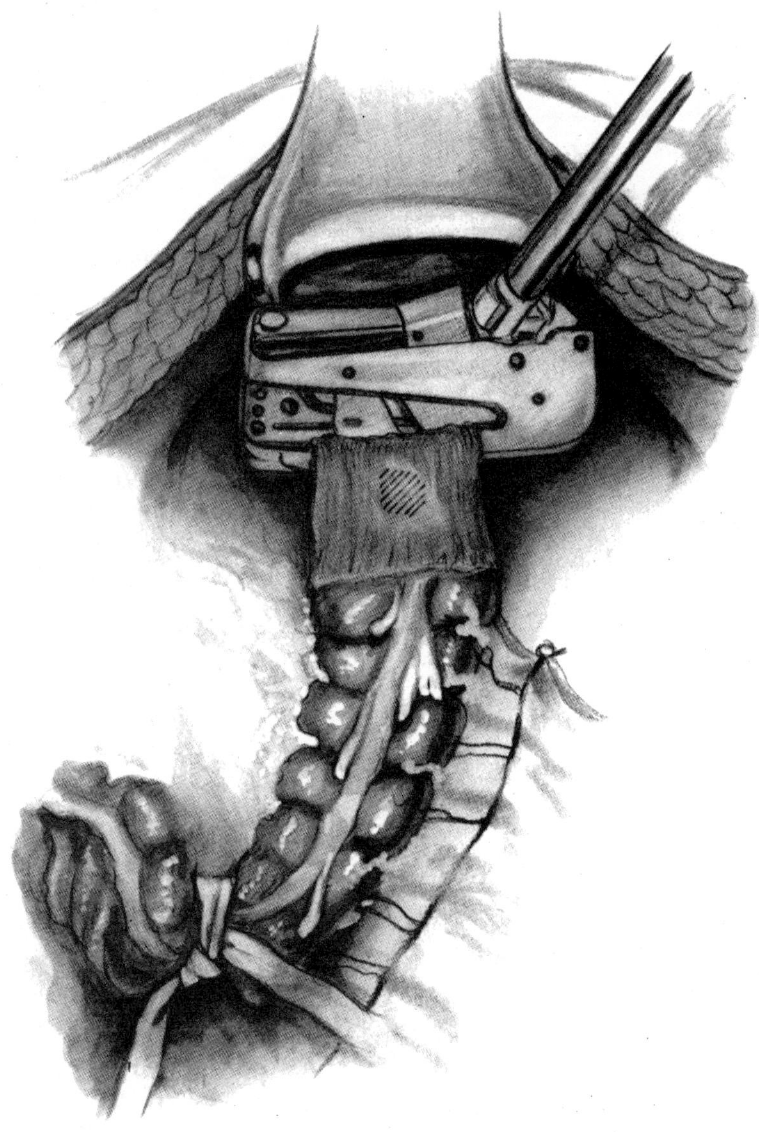

FIGURE 59.52

FIGURE 59.53
The anvil and its shaft are removed from the CEEA instrument. To replace the anvil and its shaft, a trochar is introduced into the hollow shaft of the cartridge, which is then retracted into the interior of the cartridge to allow passage of the CEEA instrument through the rectum. The CEEA instrument has been inserted and, as it approaches the line of staples introduced by the Roticulator, the wing nut on the back of the instrument is rotated to advance the trochar, which was retracted inside the cartridge. The trochar should extend beyond the line of staples, either through the line itself, which is facilitated by making a small incision in it, or through the anterior rectal wall, about 2 cm below the line of staples.

Low Anterior Resection with Double Suture Using Staplers

FIGURE 59.54
Once the trochar has passed beyond the staple line, it is removed, leaving the shaft of the cartridge empty again.

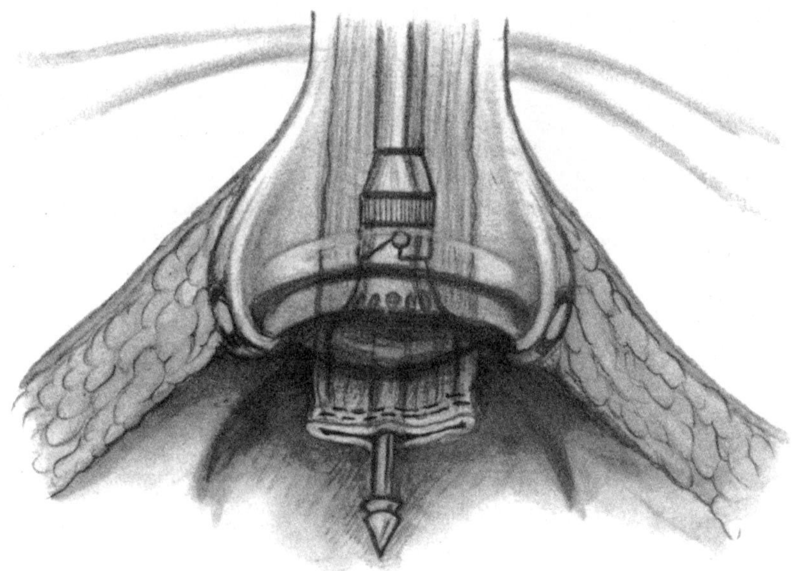

FIGURE 59.53

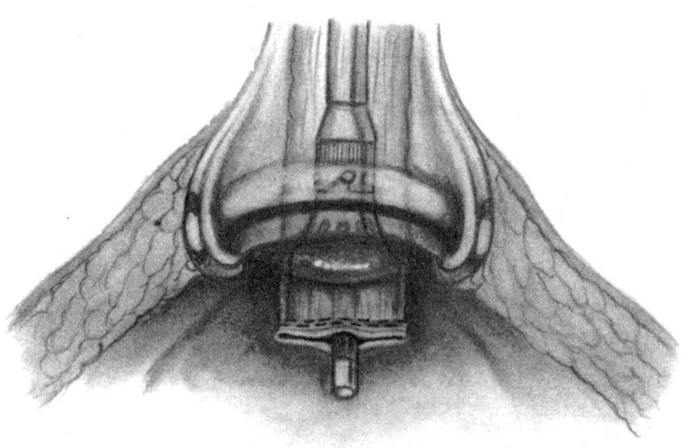

FIGURE 59.54

FIGURE 59.55
The proximal colon has been transected and the surgical specimen removed. A purse string suture has been placed in the colonic end, using the purse string instrument, with 2-0 Prolene. The drawing shows that the anvil is being inserted into the colonic end.

Low Anterior Resection with Double Suture Using Staplers

FIGURE 59.56
The anvil has been completely inserted into the colonic lumen and the purse string suture adjusted around the shaft of the anvil.

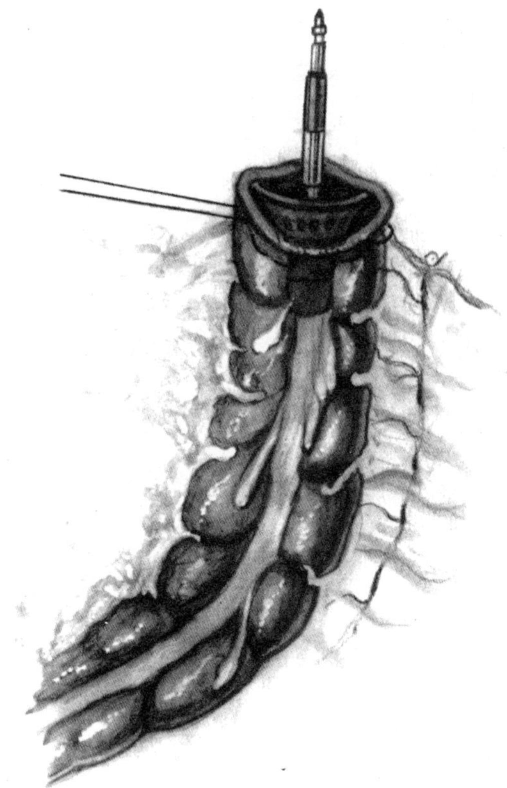

FIGURE 59.55

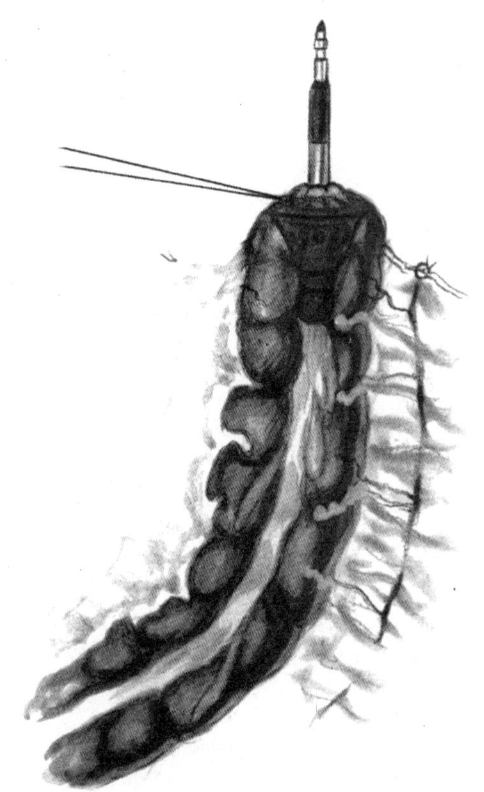

FIGURE 59.56

Low Anterior Resection with Double Suture Using Staplers

FIGURE 59.57
The shaft of the anvil is about to be inserted into the hollow shaft of the cartridge.

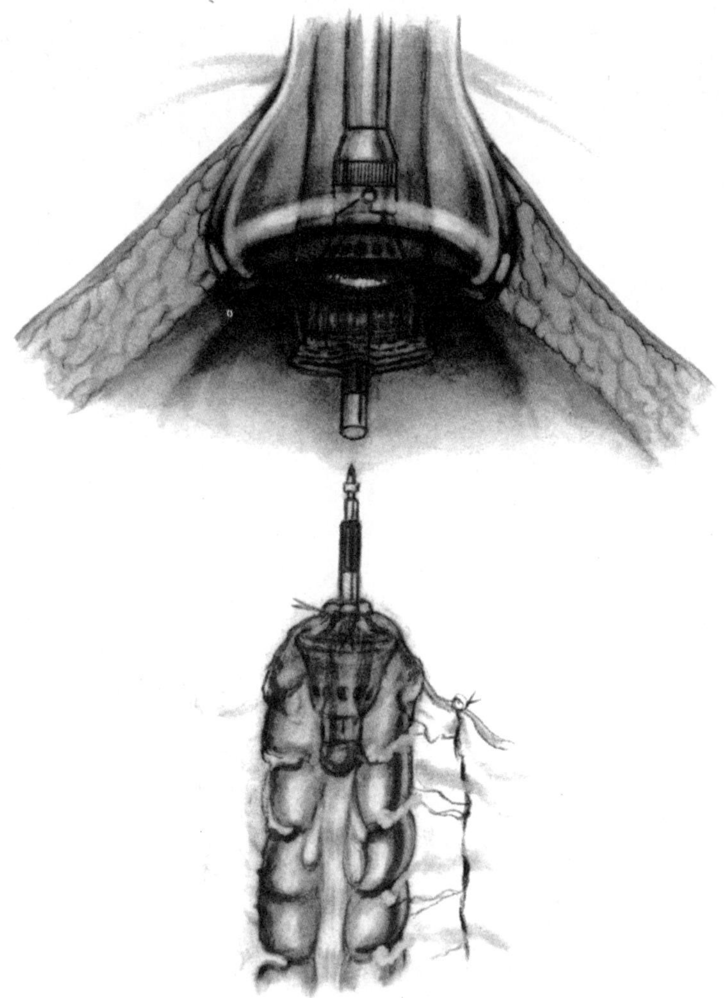

FIGURE 59.57

FIGURE 59.58
The shaft of the anvil has been inserted into the hollow shaft of the cartridge.

Low Anterior Resection with Double Suture Using Staplers

FIGURE 59.59
The wing nut has been turned, bringing the anvil firmly against the cartridge in order to fire it, executing the low colorectal anastomosis. The CEEA instrument is removed from the rectum, and the tissue rings in the instrument are examined to confirm if they are complete and made up of all the layers of the colon and rectum. The impermeability of the anastomosis is then confirmed. This is done by applying an atraumatic clamp to the colon near the anastomosis. The pelvic cavity is filled with saline solution, and air is injected through a catheter inserted into the rectum. If no air bubbles are seen, the suture line is impermeable. If bubbles appear, the suture line is incomplete and the site of leakage should be searched for, in order to correct it. A closed suction drainage catheter is left in the sacral cavity and brought out through a small counterincision in the anterior abdominal wall. This catheter is usually removed in 5 to 6 days.

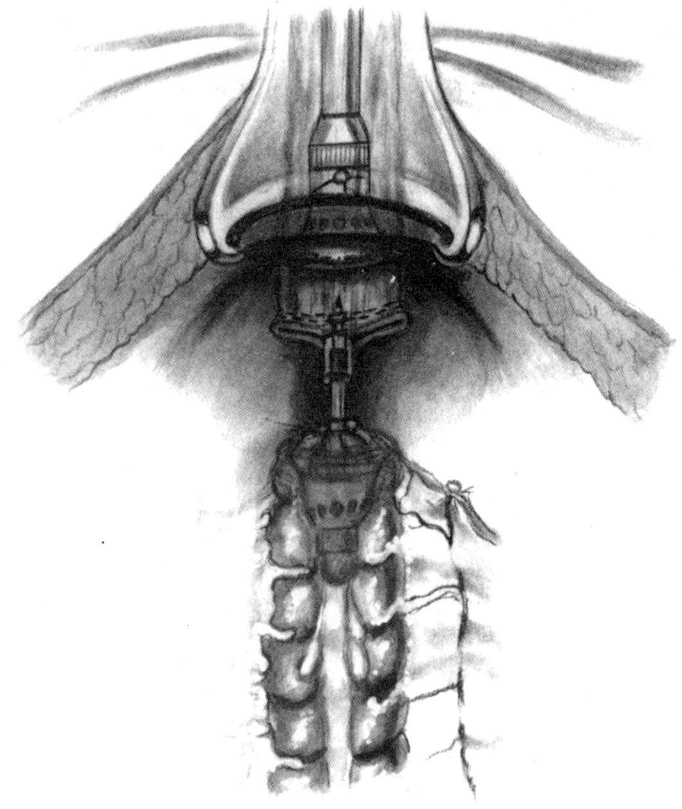

FIGURE 59.58

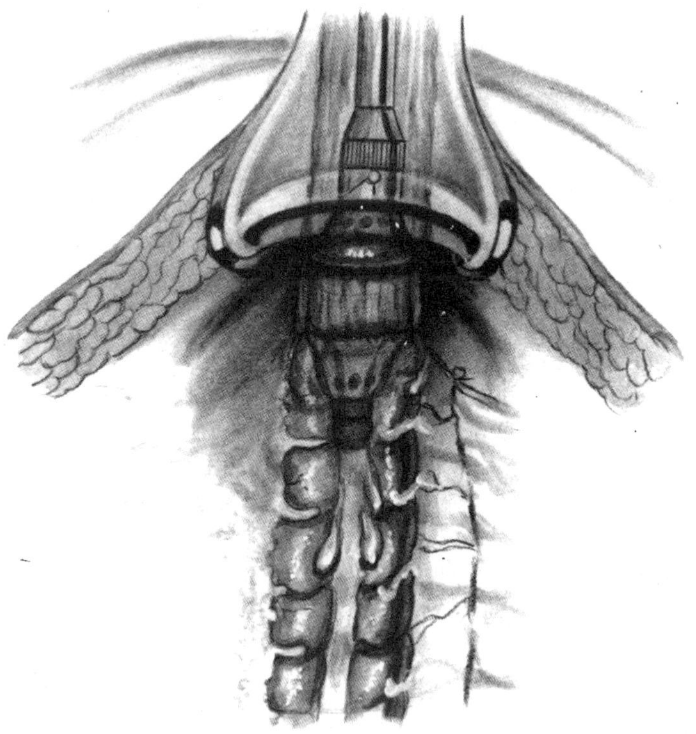

FIGURE 59.59

ABDOMINOPERINEAL RESECTION OF RECTAL CANCER

Abdominoperineal resection of rectal cancer was proposed by Ernest Miles of London in 1908. At first, the Miles operation was used for all locations of rectal cancer. At present, this operation is performed much less frequently, since it has been progressively replaced by anterior resection of the rectum and by local excision of the cancer, by electrofulguration, or by intracavitary irradiation. At present, only 15% of rectal cancers are treated by abdominoperineal resection.

The Miles operation consists of removal of the entire rectum with both anal sphincters, removal of the distal half or the entire sigmoid colon with its mesentery, and the establishment of a permanent colostomy in the left iliac fossa.

Some of the indications of the Miles procedure, now significantly reduced, are the following: (a) with some exceptions, cancers of the distal third of the rectum; (b) in voluminous, infiltrative, or poorly differentiated cancers of the middle third of the rectum; and (c) in carcinomas of the anal canal in which local resection combined with medical therapy have failed.

The technique of abdominoperineal resection used at present in most surgical centers is a modification of the classical Miles technique. This technique was proposed in 1939 by Lloyd-Davies (54) and consists of placing the patient in a lithotomy-Trendelenburg position, allowing two surgical teams to operate synchronously, one in the abdomen and the other in the perineum (synchronous combined abdominoperineal excision of the rectum) (79, 80, 86, 88, 94).

The Lloyd-Davis technique has definite advantages over the classical Miles technique, among them: (a) With this technique it is not necessary to change the patient's position, with all the inconveniences this presents in the operating room; (b) this technique significantly shortens operative time; (c) hemostasis in the pelvic cavity is easier; and (d) resection of voluminous rectal tumors is easier.

Some surgeons place the patient in the Lloyd-Davies position but carry out the operation with only one team, operating first in the abdomen and then going down to the perineum. Other surgeons are faithful to the classical technique, carrying out the abdominal stage with the patient in decubitus position, changing the patient for the perineal stage. The technique used to mobilize the rectum in an abdominoperineal resection is the same as the technique used in an anterior resection.

In the operation with two synchronous teams, the abdominal surgeon starts the procedure. The perineal surgeon, with similar experience as the abdominal surgeon, starts to operate when the abdominal surgeon starts to mobilize the rectum. The abdominal surgeon mobilizes the rectum posteriorly, down to the puborectalis muscle of the levator ani after having sectioned the rectosacral or Waldeyer fascia. If the abdominal surgeon has not sectioned Waldeyer's fascia, it can be comfortably transected by the perineal surgeon, after dividing the levator ani muscle posteriorly and laterally, as will be shown in later drawings.

It is important to transect Waldeyer's fascia with a cutting instrument, scissors, or scalpel, and not bluntly with the hands, to avoid injuring the presacral venous plexus and causing hemorrhages that are difficult to control. Once posterior mobilization of the rectum is complete, the rectum is mobilized anteriorly to separate the anterior rectal wall from the bladder, the seminal vesicles and prostate in males, and the vagina in women. To mobilize the rectum anteriorly, the fascia of Denonvilliers has to be transected. Frequently, anterior mobilization of the rectum has to be completed by the perineal surgeon. Laterally, the abdominal surgeon identifies, ligates, and transects the lateral ligaments. Frequently, this has to be completed distally by the perineal surgeon.

Once the rectum has been completely mobilized, the abdominal surgeon transects the sigmoid colon and covers the distal end to diminish contamination. The distal colonic end is delivered to the perineal surgeon. The abdominal surgeon sutures the pelvic floor with interrupted or continuous sutures and proceeds with the realization of the colostomy at the previously chosen site.

The abdominal wall is then closed, the colostomy is matured and covered with a colostomy bag. The perineal surgeon, who has already removed the rectum, controls bleeding and places two Jackson-Pratt closed continuous drainage tubes. Then he closes the perineum with one layer of interrupted sutures, including the skin and the subcutaneous tissue.

Surgical Technique

FIGURE 59.60

The drawing shows the ideal location of the colostomy site in an abdominoperineal resection for rectal cancer. As can be seen, the site chosen for the colostomy is located in the left lower quadrant of the abdomen, through the anterior rectus muscle. The colostomy should be away from osseous prominences, scars, the umbilicus, and the site of drainage tubes, and below the waistline. The site for the colostomy should be selected before the operation. A stoma therapist is very valuable. A practical test should be carried out, placing a colostomy bag with its strap and then having the patient adopt various positions in order to carefully observe modifications the colostomy disk may need in a sitting, standing, or supine position. In addition to being comfortable, the site selected for the colostomy should also be accessible and visible for the patient. The site for the colostomy should be clearly marked so that it is visible during the operation.

Obese patients present difficult problems caused by abdominal folds, which hide the colostomy stoma or make it difficult to adapt colostomy bags. In obese patients, it is not advisable to select a low position for the colostomy because it will frequently be hidden by an abdominal fold. In these patients, a high place on the abdomen should be selected, such as the left abdomen, 5 to 6 cm below the costal arch where abdominal folds rarely develop.

Surgical Technique

FIGURE 59.61

The rectum has been mobilized using the same technique as in a low anterior resection. A broken line shows the site where the inferior mesenteric artery will be ligated, distal to the origin of the left colic artery. The same line shows where the surgeon will transect the sigmoid colon and its mesentery. The end of the colon at the site of the colostomy has to be checked to be sure it has a good blood supply. If the marginal artery is not pulsating, it is advisable to transect it to determine if it has an adequate flow of blood.

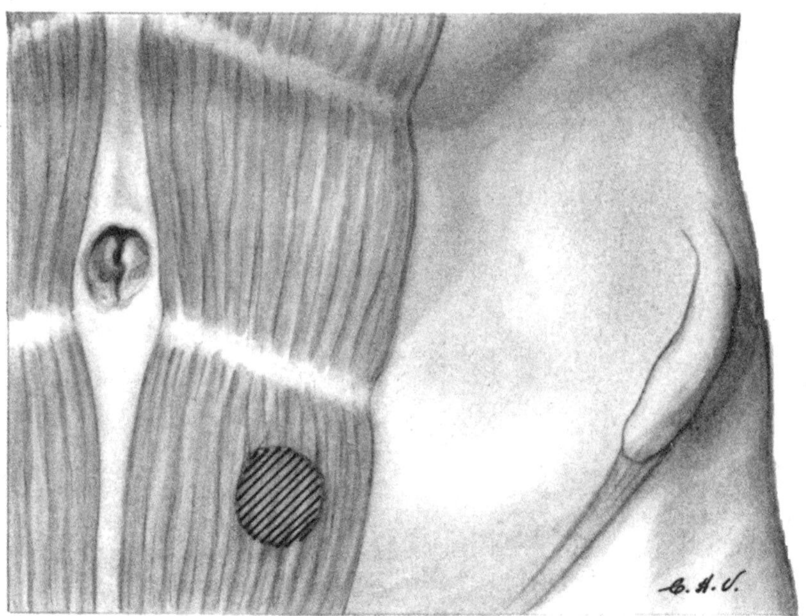

FIGURE 59.60

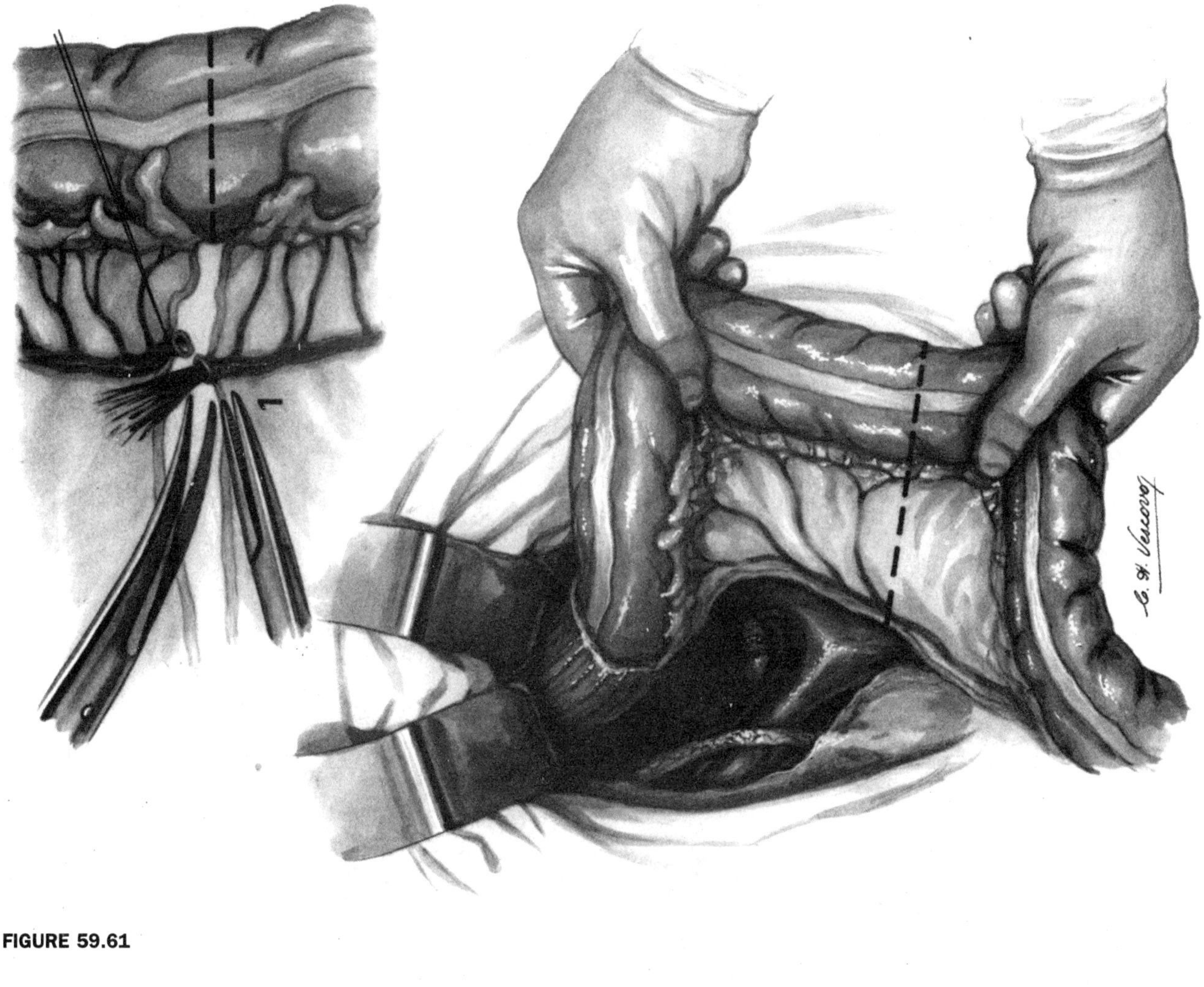

FIGURE 59.61

FIGURE 59.62
An extraperitoneal tunnel is being developed manually through which the colon will pass to construct the colostomy at the previously marked site on the skin, as shown in the drawing. The extraperitoneal colostomy is an excellent site for a permanent iliac colostomy. This technique diminishes the number of small bowel obstructions, pericolostomy hernias, and prolapse of bowel, compared to patients with intraperitoneal colostomies. It should be pointed out that an extraperitoneal colostomy should not be done for temporary iliac colostomies, since taking down an extraperitoneal colostomy to perform a colorectal anastomosis is much more complicated than in an intraperitoneal colostomy (38).

Surgical Technique

FIGURE 59.63
A 2 cm disk of skin and subcutaneous tissue is removed at the previously marked colostomy site. The anterior fascia of the anterior rectum muscle is incised in cruciate form and each of the quadrants removed separately, as shown. The muscle fibers are then split and some of them are cut. The posterior rectus fascia and peritoneum are incised in the same way.

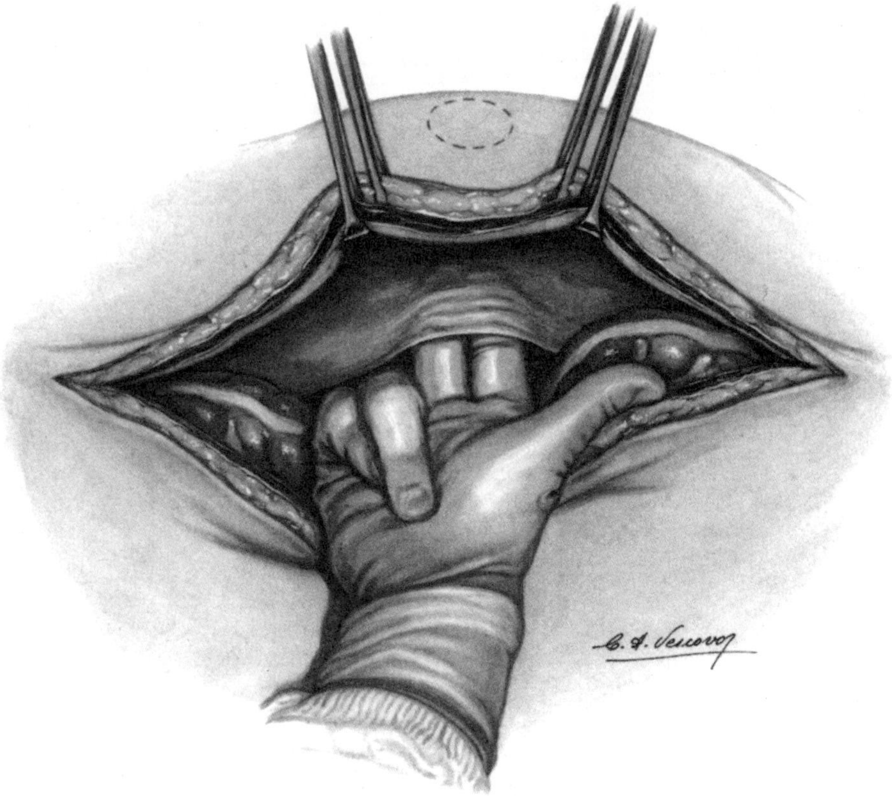

FIGURE 59.62

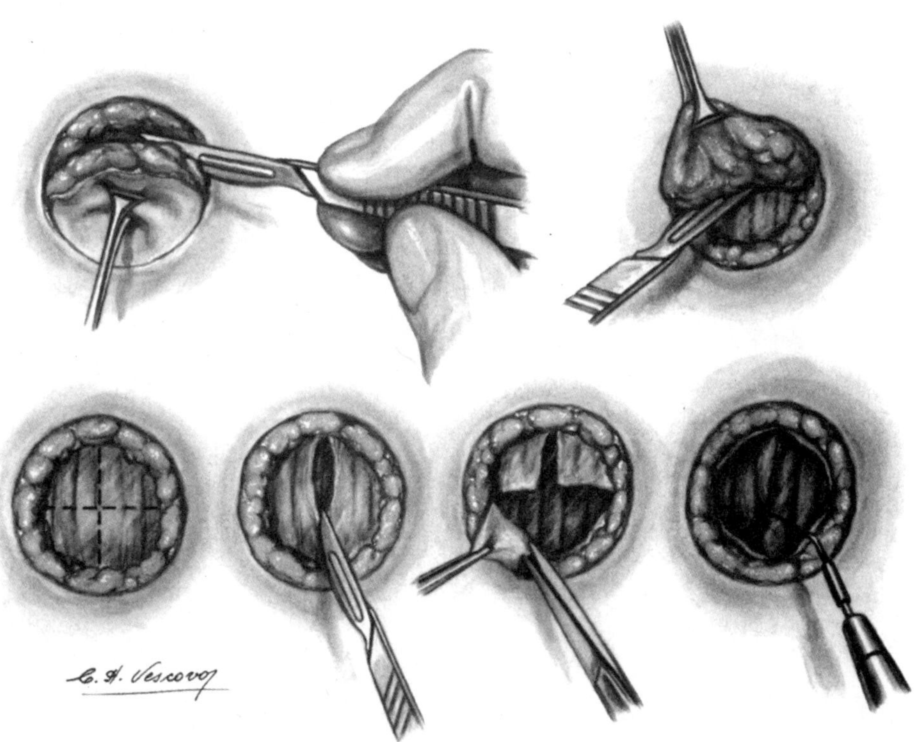

FIGURE 59.63

Surgical Technique

FIGURE 59.64
Once the opening in the abdominal wall and the tunnel are complete, the surgeon confirms that two fingers can pass readily through them, as shown in the drawing.

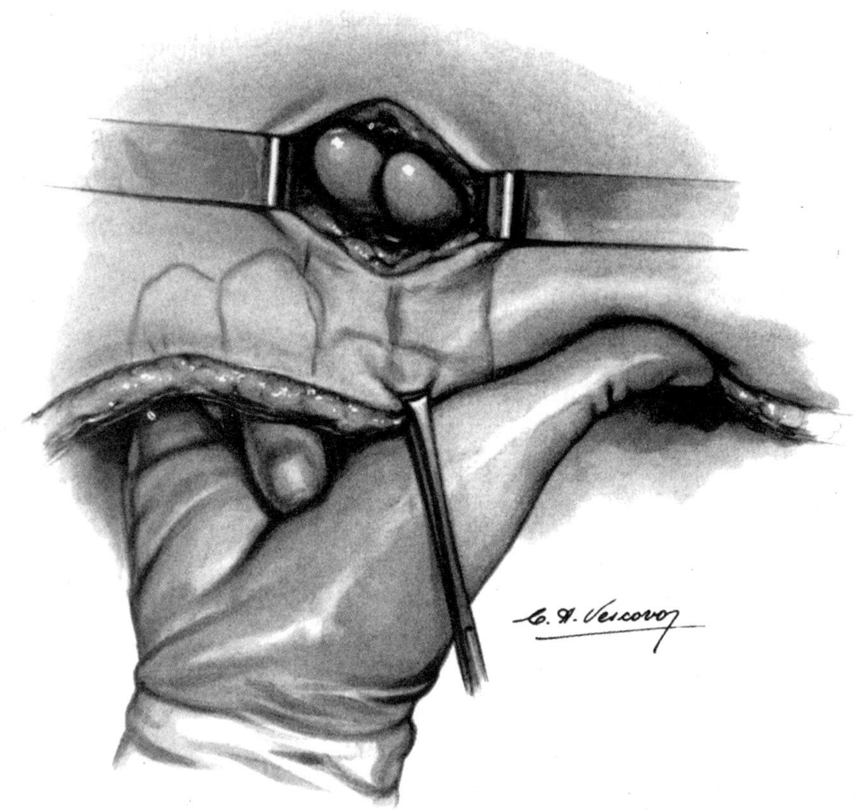

FIGURE 59.64

Surgical Technique

FIGURE 59.65

A long, curved atraumatic clamp designed by the author is passed through the skin opening and tunnel constructed for the colostomy. This clamp grasps the proximal colon at the site chosen for its transection. On the distal side of the colon that is about to be removed with the specimen, a clamp is placed to prevent any spillage of colonic contents. A broken line shows the site where the colon is to be transected.

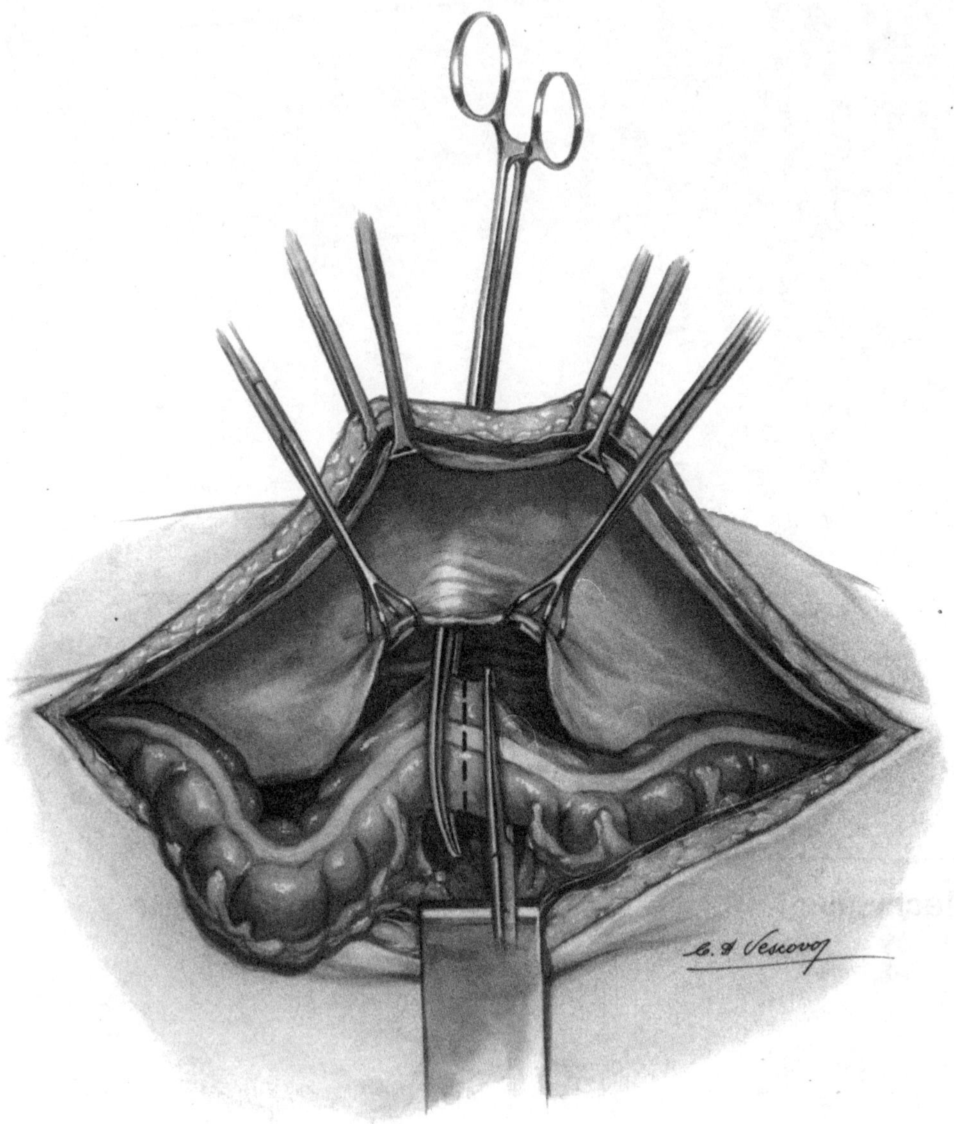

FIGURE 59.65

Surgical Technique

FIGURE 59.66
The sigmoid colon has been divided. The distal side is wrapped in plastic, which is tied around the clamp to prevent contamination. The proximal end, which had been grasped with the author's atraumatic clamp, is covered with the metallic sheath that is part of the instrument and is used during this part of the procedure to bring the end of the colon through the tunnel without contaminating the tissues along the tract. In the upper part of the drawing, the instrument is shown with its two parts: the curved clamp and its protective metallic sheath.

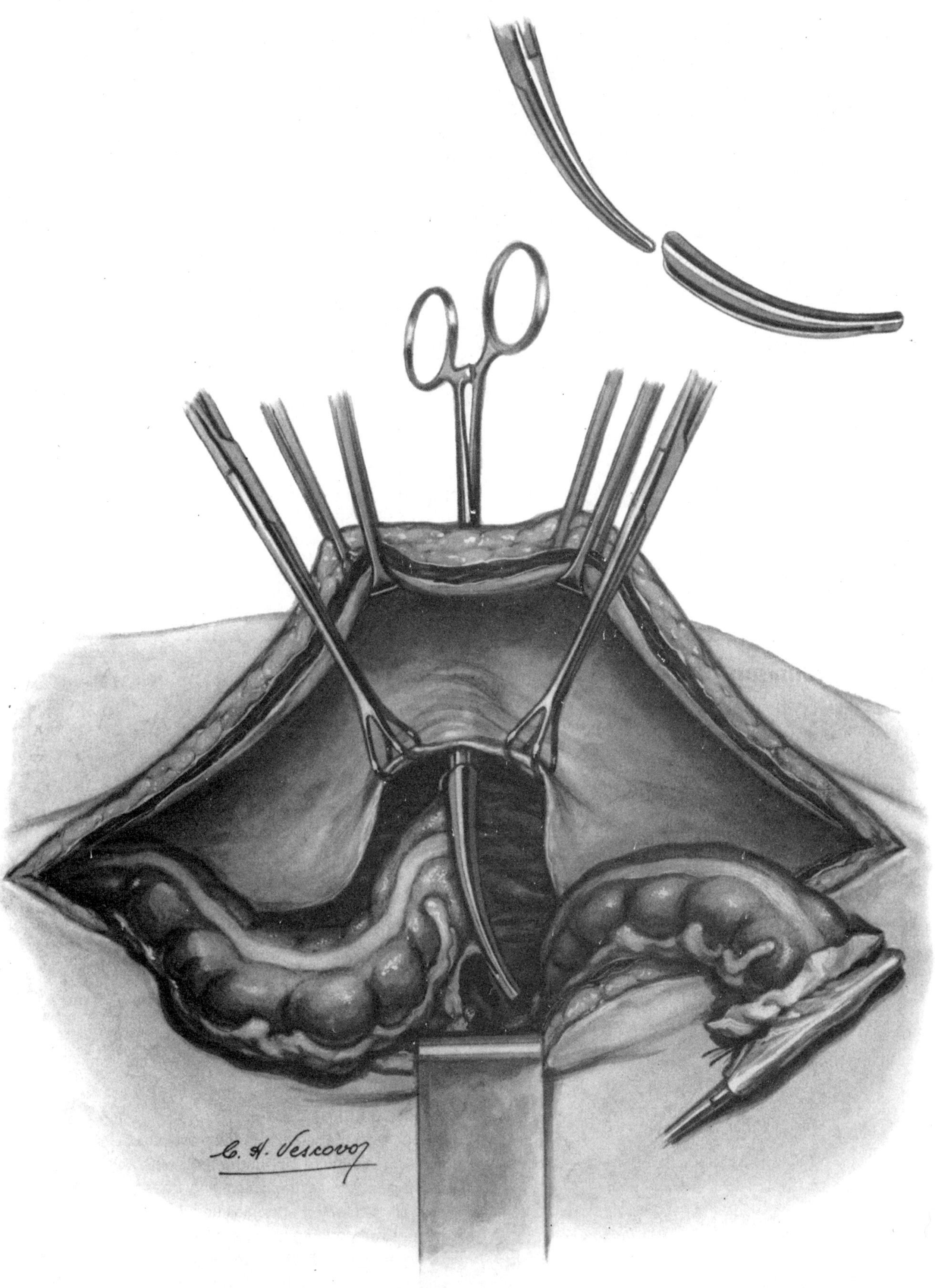

FIGURE 59.66

FIGURE 59.67
The proximal colonic end has been passed through the extraperitoneal tunnel and exteriorized through the parietal orifice made for the colostomy. The metallic sheath is removed, and then the clamp is removed. Since the clamp is atraumatic, none of the clamped tissue will have to be excised.

Surgical Technique

FIGURE 59.68
If the author's clamp is not available, the colon can be transected with TA 55 instrument, which places a double row of staples across the colon and transects it. The colon can also be transected after placing a De Martel, Zachary-Cope, or other similar clamp across it. The drawing shows the colon being transected after applying a De Martel clamp. Both colonic ends have been wrapped in plastic to prevent contamination.

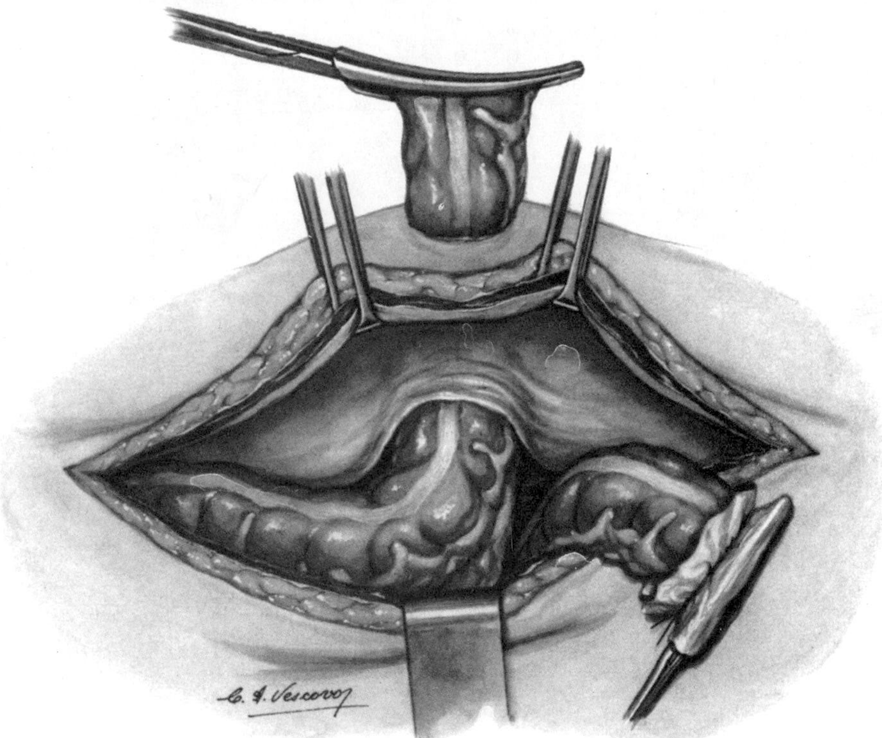

FIGURE 59.67

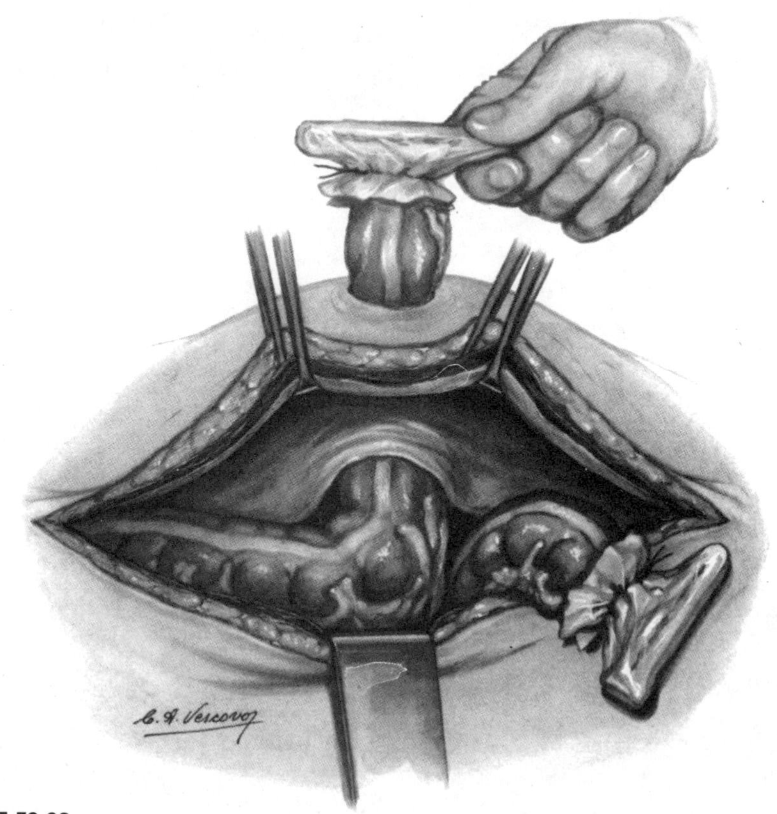

FIGURE 59.68

Surgical Technique

FIGURE 59.69
An easy and practical method that does not require any special instrument is the Valdoni technique. The divided colonic ends are covered with rubber or plastic sheeting, as shown, which does not require any explanation.

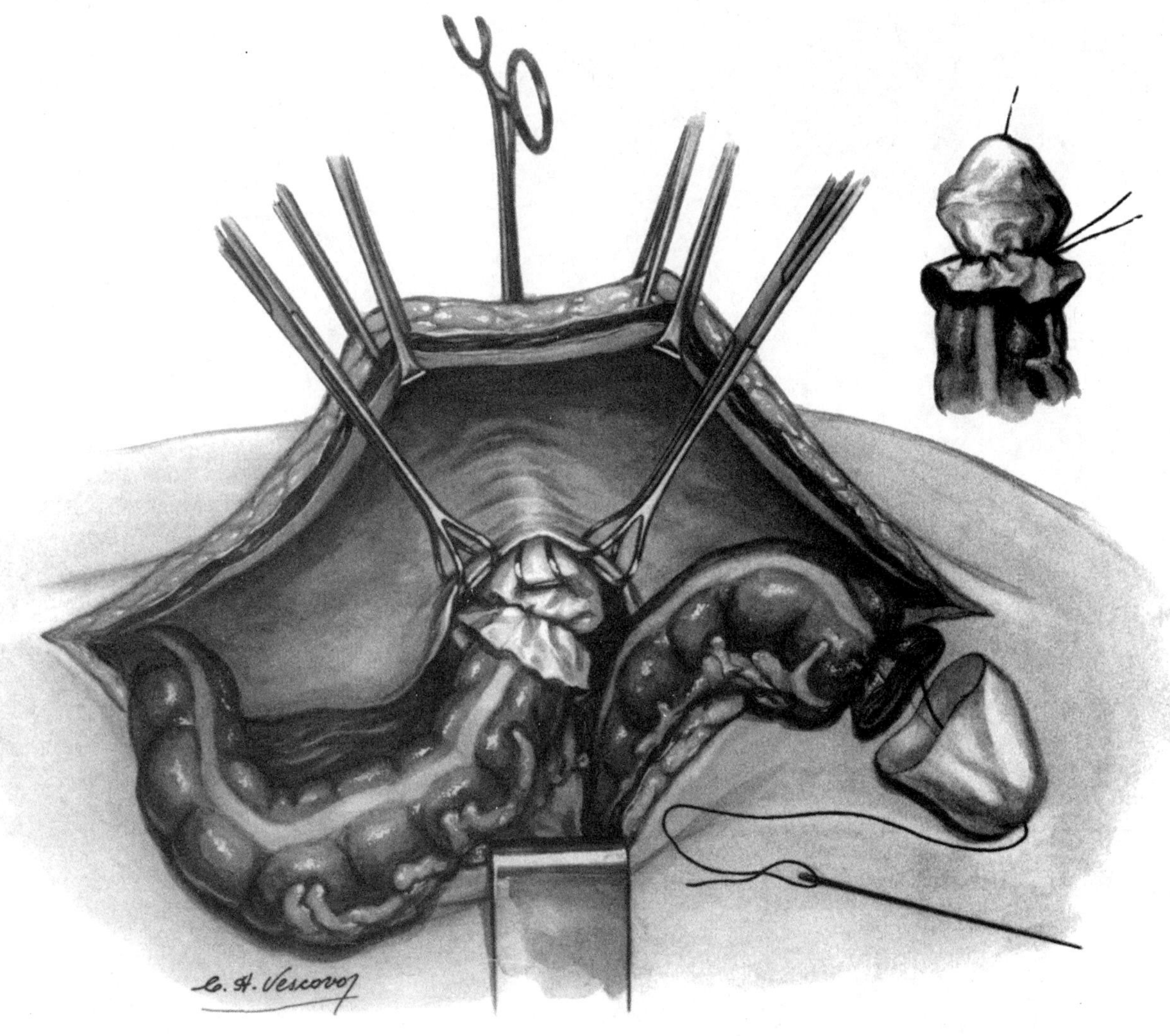

FIGURE 59.69

FIGURE 59.70

The abdominal surgeon, after exteriorizing the proximal colon through the tunnel and after delivering the distal end to the perineal surgeon, proceeds with peritonealization of the pelvis and the abdomen, as can be seen in the drawing. The author uses interrupted nonabsorbable sutures, but many surgeons use a continuous suture.

Surgical Technique

FIGURE 59.71

Some surgeons prefer to exteriorize the colostomy by the intraperitoneal route. If this technique is used, either because of preference or because the extraperitoneal route cannot used, it is necessary to close the left parietocolic space to prevent small bowel loops from passing through this space and causing small bowel obstruction. To carry this out, the author's clamp is very useful, though not indispensable. The left parietocolic space is closed with a purse string suture, or sometimes with two purse strings or with interrupted sutures. The inset shows how the left parietocolic space is blocked off once the purse string is tied.

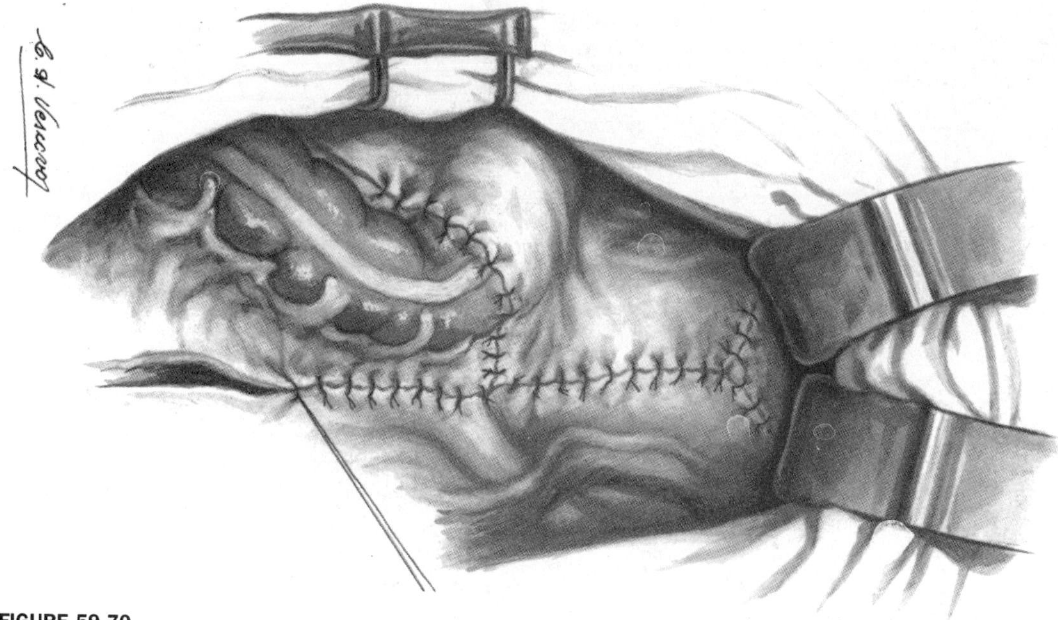

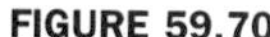

FIGURE 59.70

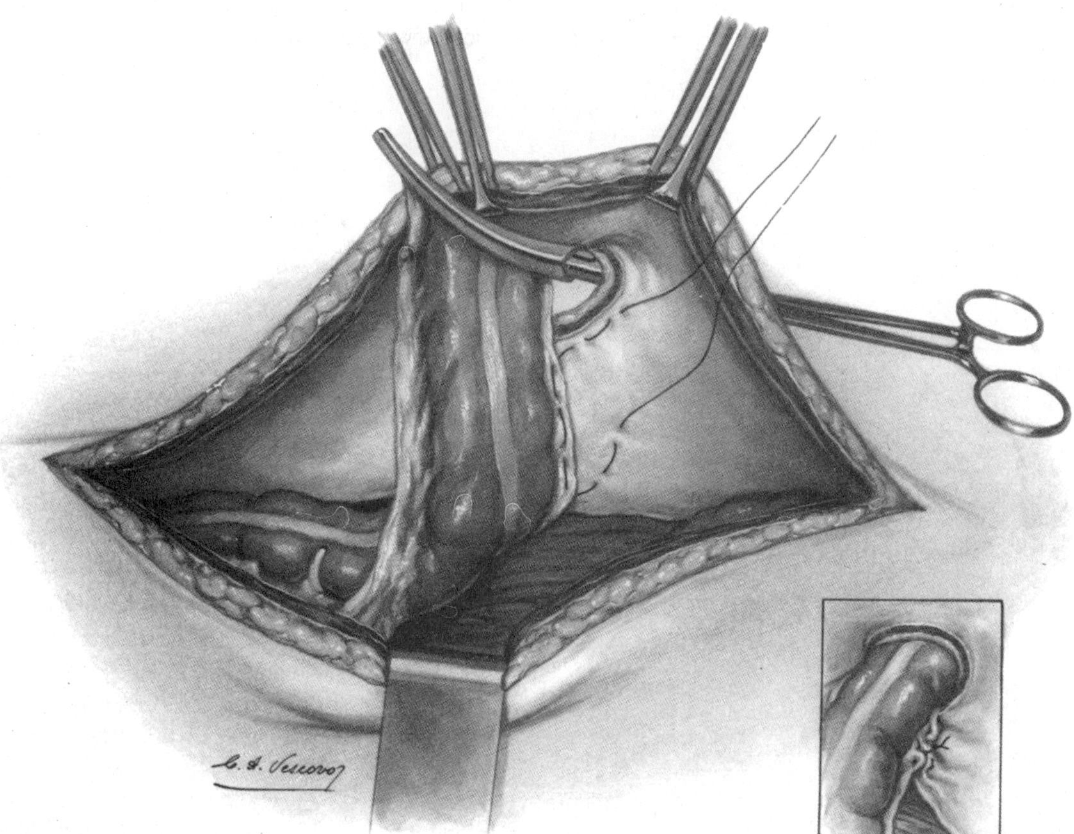

FIGURE 59.71

FIGURE 59.72
The exteriorized colonic end used for the colostomy should measure 3 or 4 cm above the skin level. It should be brought out without any traction. If there is any traction, the colon should be liberated more. Once exteriorized, the colostomy should be matured by suturing the edge of the colon to the skin at the four cardinal points. Later, intermediate sutures are placed, as seen. These sutures should be 2-0 chromic catgut. A colostomy bag is finally applied.

Surgical Technique

FIGURE 59.73
The perineal surgeon closes the anus with one or two purse string sutures, leaving the ends long to apply traction to them. The skin and subcutaneous tissue is then incised in elliptical fashion with the greater diameter oriented in an anteroposterior direction, extending from a point halfway from the urethral bulb to the anal margin, back to the tip of the coccyx. Laterally, the incision should pass about 3 cm from the anal margin. In cases with low rectal cancer, the resection of skin and subcutaneous tissue can be more extensive. The incision is deepened laterally in the ischiorectal fossa where the hemorrhoidal or inferior rectal vessels are found. These are usually divided into two branches, which should be ligated. The borders of the skin on both sides are grasped with several Littlewood, Allis, or Babcock clamps for traction purposes, as seen in the drawing on the right. The anococcygeal raphe is transected with a scalpel.

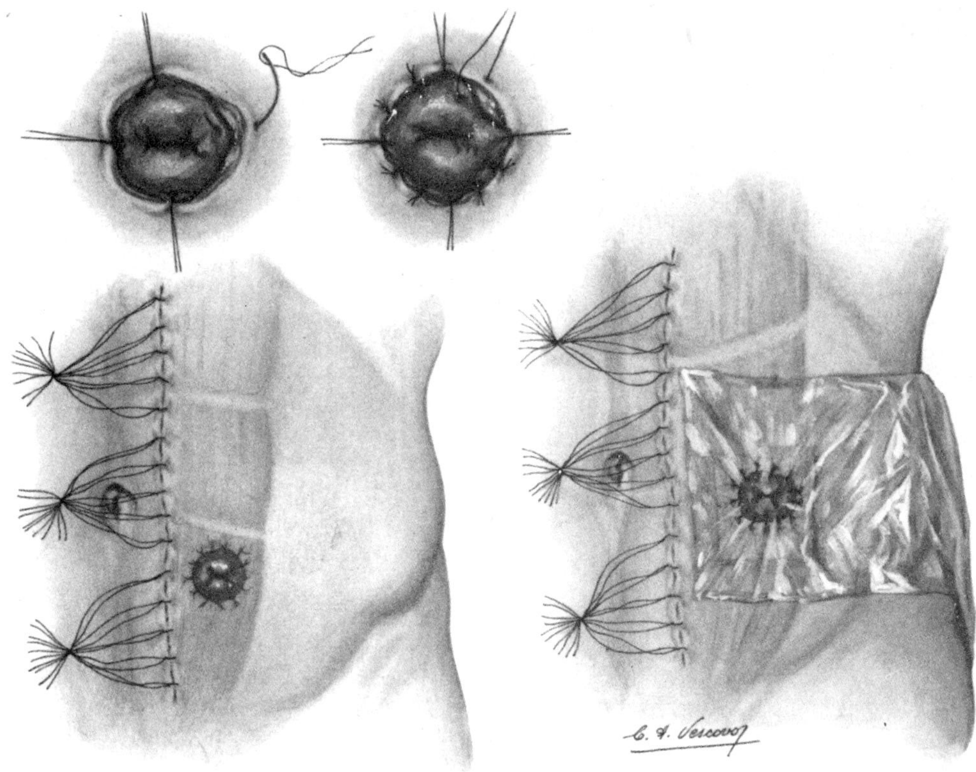

FIGURE 59.72

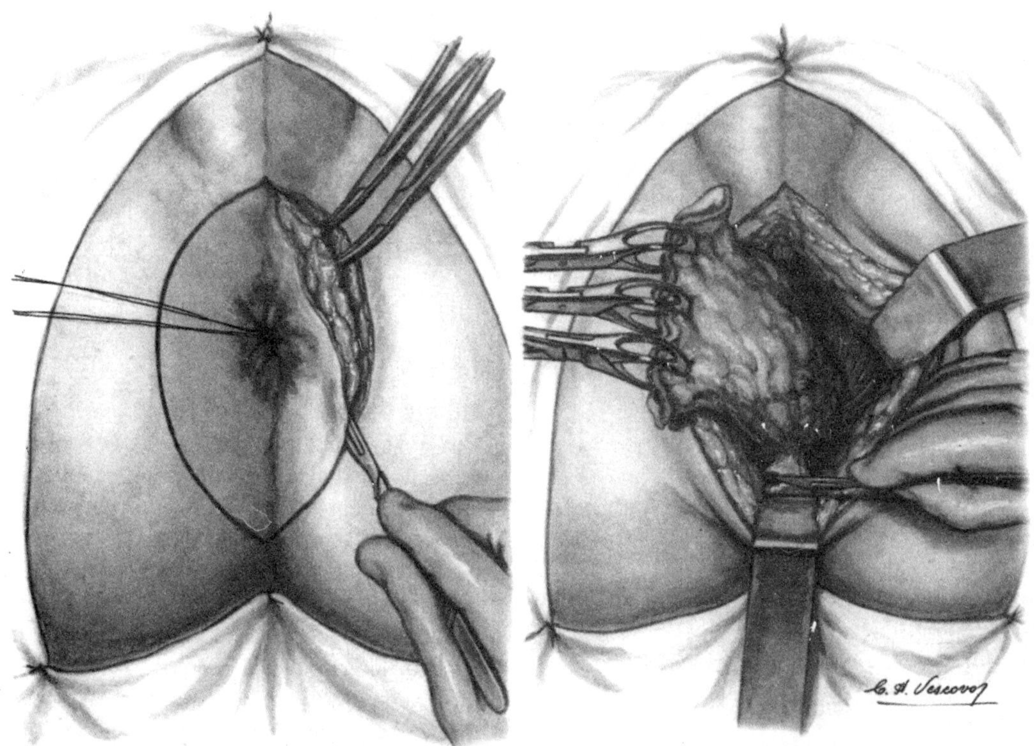

FIGURE 59.73

FIGURE 59.74
Once the raphe is transected, the surgeon makes a small opening between it and the levator ani muscle, through which he or she introduces the left index finger, elevating the levator and transecting it posteriorly and laterally with curved scissors This maneuver is repeated on the other side. If the abdominal surgeon has not incised Waldeyer's fascia, the perineal surgeon can do it easily, as seen in the drawing on the right.

Surgical Technique

FIGURE 59.75
The most difficult and dangerous segment of the rectum to be freed is the anterior rectal segment in the male. The Foley catheter inserted into the bladder facilitates identification of the urethra to avoid injuring it. The puborectalis and pubococcygeus muscles are transected on both sides of the midline by passing a finger under them. The anterior midline raphe should be transected and the rectouretralis muscle cut in the midline, along a place parallel to the base of the prostate. Dissection of the anterior portion of the rectum should always follow a plane posterior to the transverse perineal muscles. Frequently, the perineal surgeon completes the transection of the distal part of the lateral rectal ligaments.

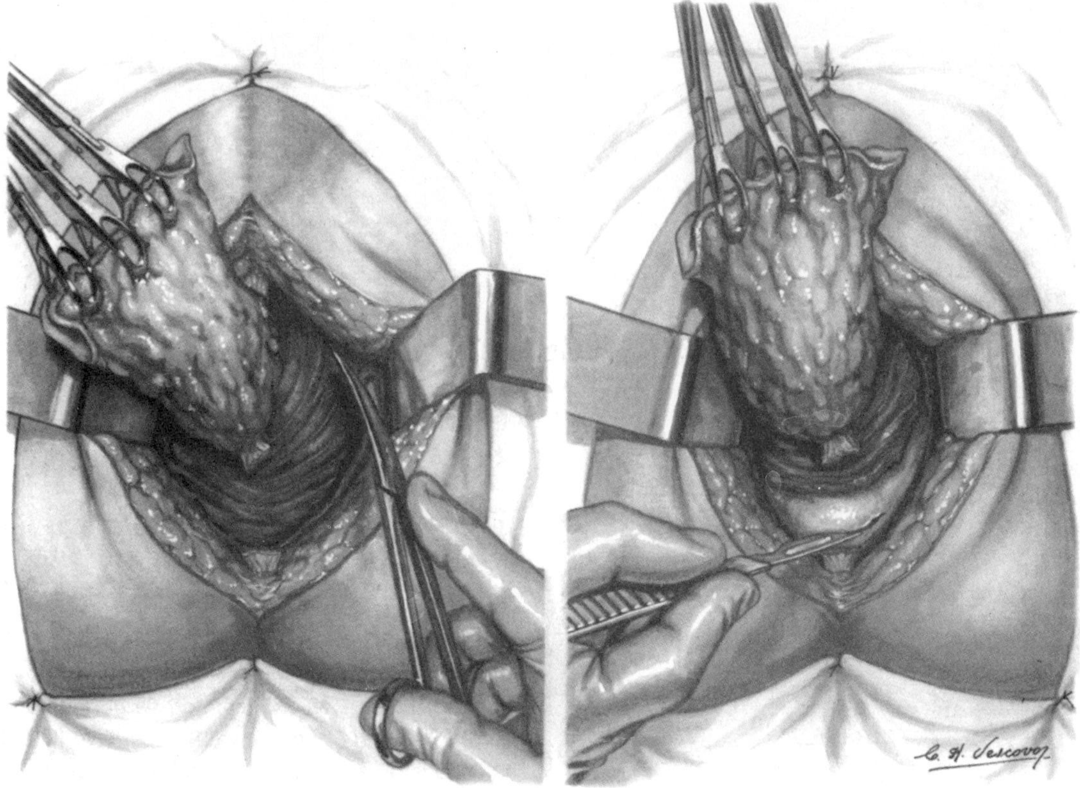

FIGURE 59.74

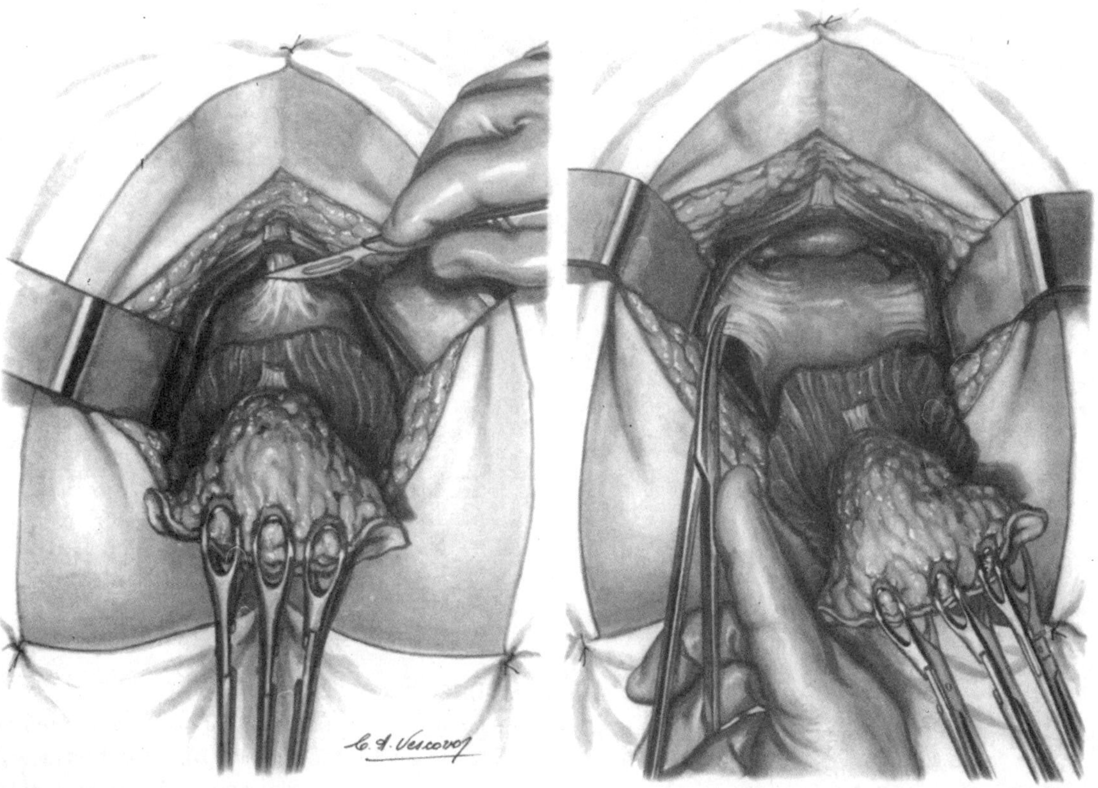

FIGURE 59.75

FIGURE 59.76
The abdominal surgeon delivers the transected end of the colon to the perineal surgeon, so he or she can complete its liberation and remove it from the operative field. In more difficult cases, it is convenient to deliver the colon earlier to facilitate dissection of the anterior portion of the rectum.

Surgical Technique

FIGURE 59.77
Sectional view of the planes of dissection of the rectum in the male (**A**) and in the female (**B**). In 1, transection of Denonvilliers' fascia is shown, and in 2, transection of the rectosacral or Waldeyer's fascia is seen.

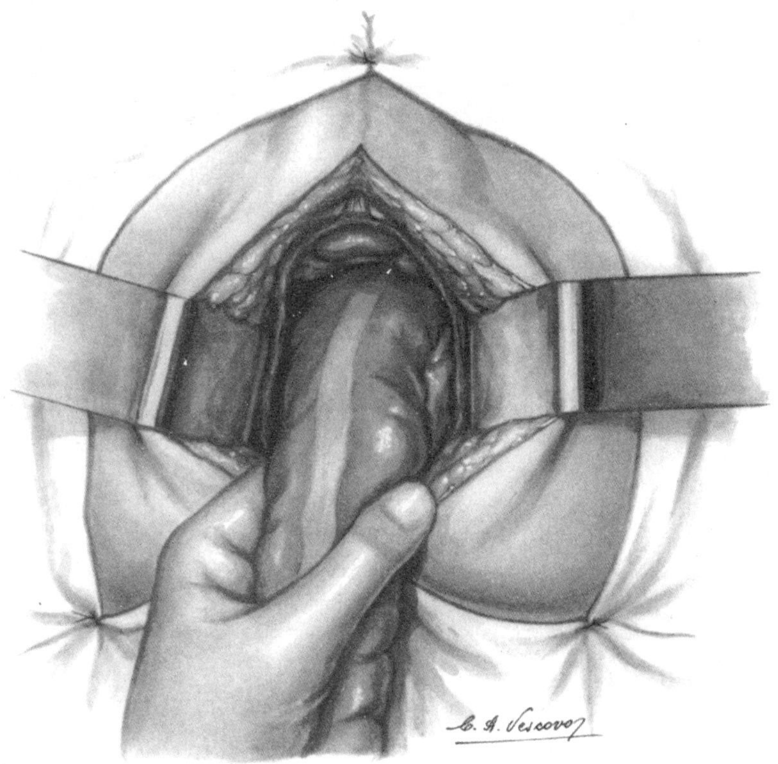

FIGURE 59.76

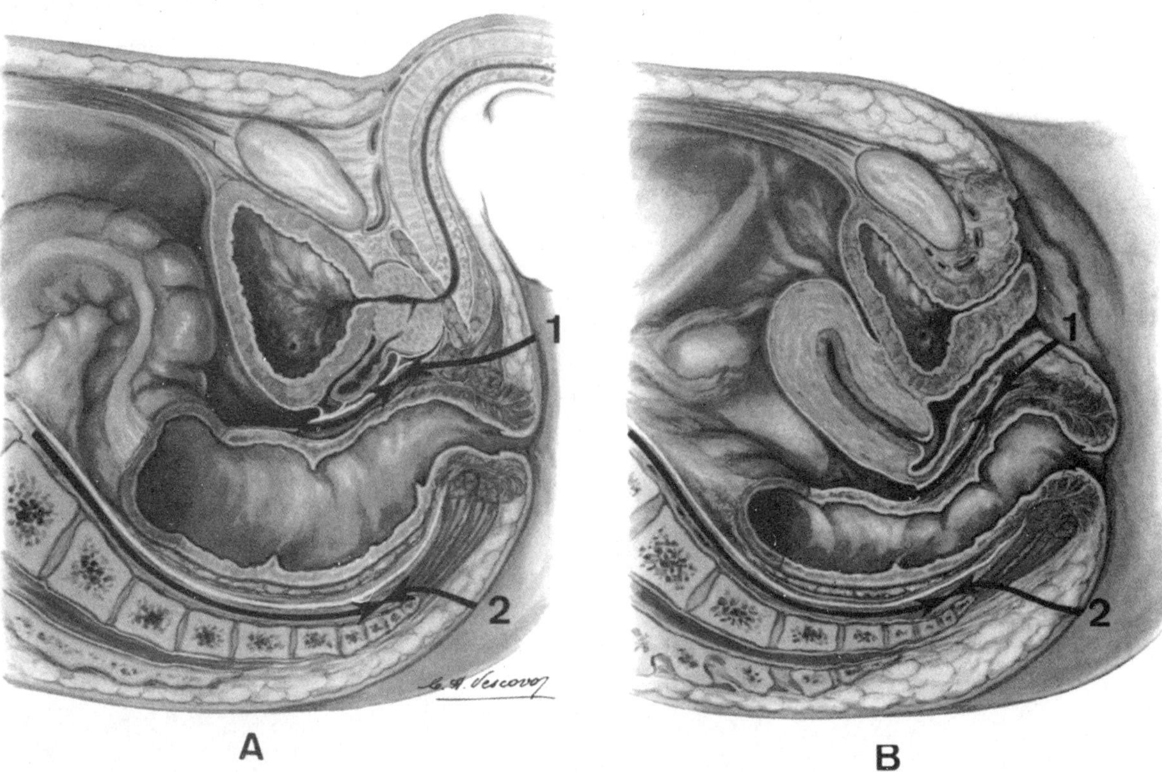

FIGURE 59.77

Surgical Technique

FIGURE 59.78
After the rectum is removed, the perineal skin and subcutaneous tissue is sutured, with interrupted sutures, leaving two Jackson-Pratt drainage tubes connected to a closed continuous suction system.

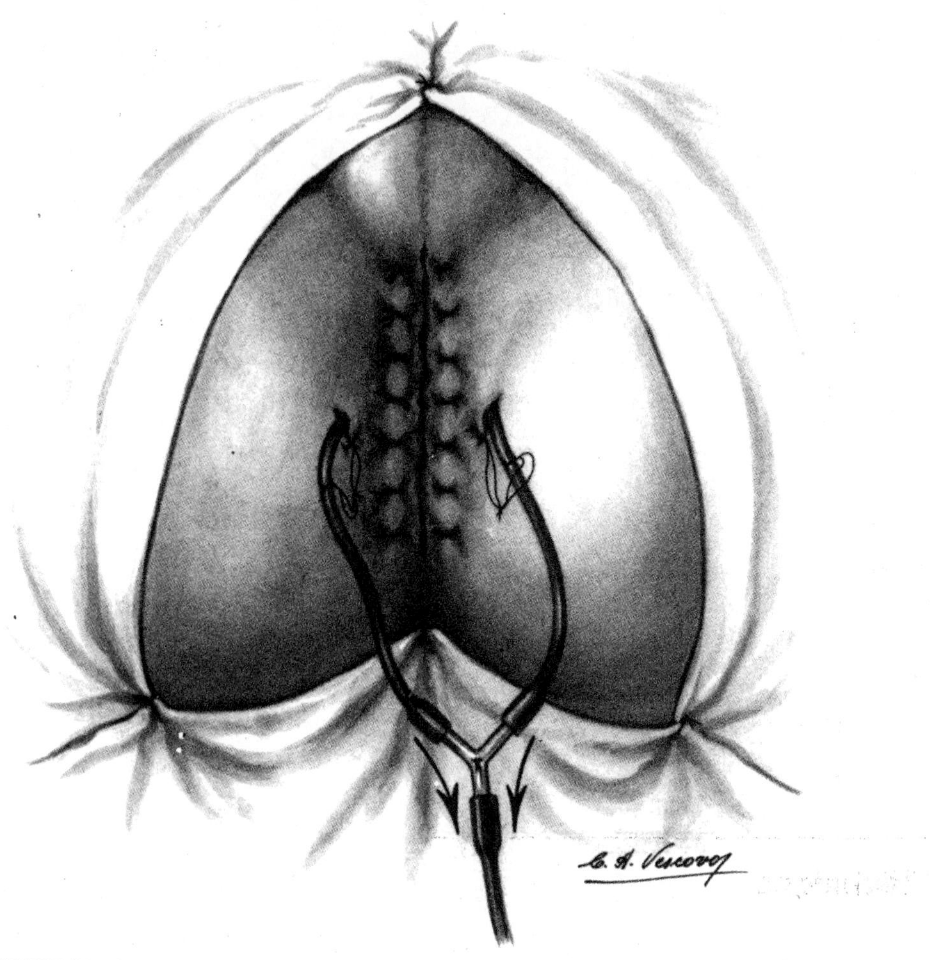

FIGURE 59.78

Surgical Technique

FIGURE 59.79
In cases of severe uncontrollable bleeding due to injury to the presacral venous plexus, gauze packing can be resorted to, after inserting plastic sheeting to prevent adhesion of the gauze to the patient's tissues. The abdominal surgeon can determine when the pelvic cavity has been completely packed.

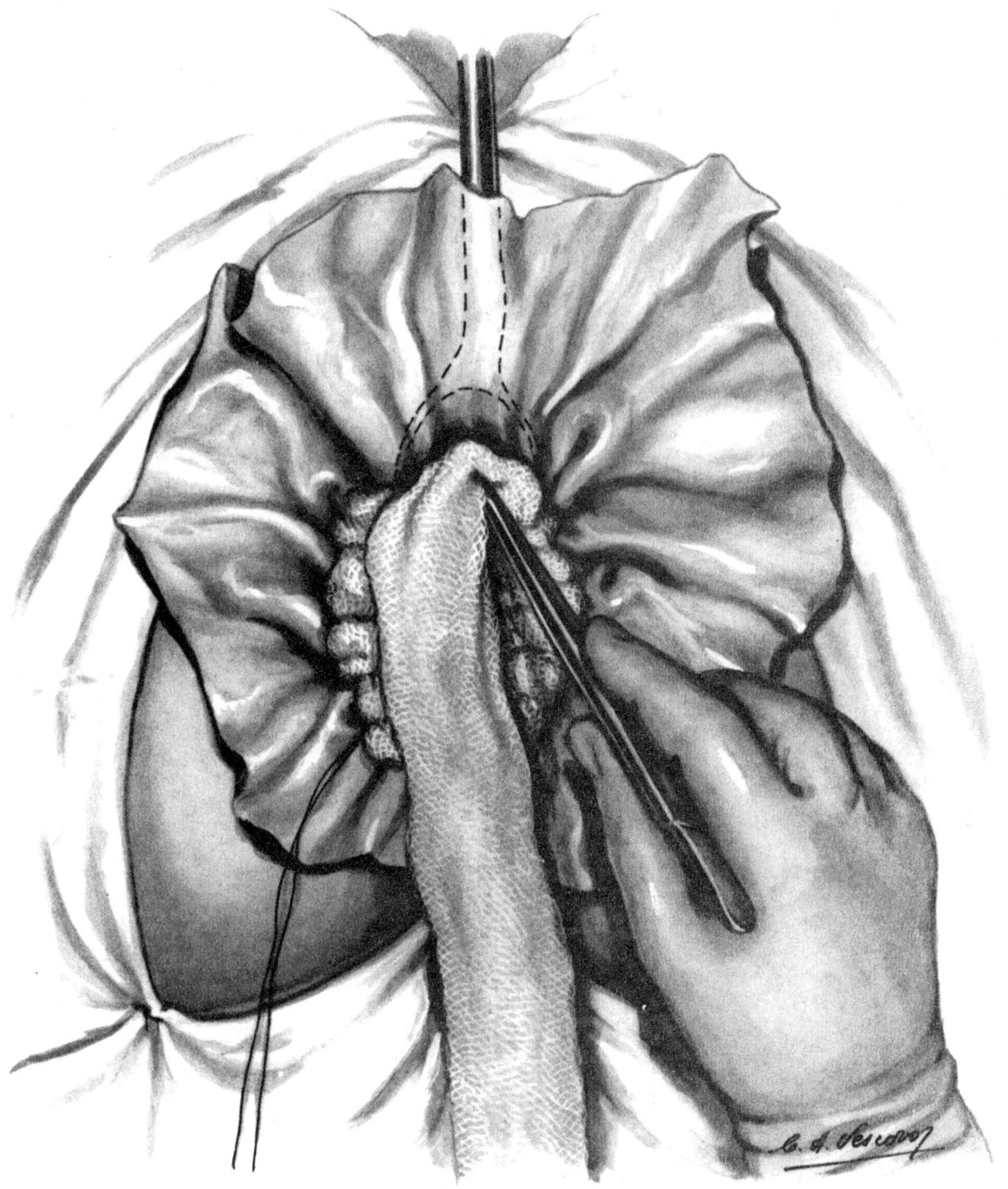

FIGURE 59.79

FIGURE 59.80
After the packing with gauze, the excess plastic sheeting is removed and the skin and subcutaneous tissue is partially closed so that the gauze packing is more effective.

Surgical Technique

FIGURE 59.81
This is a sectional view showing the gauze packing in the pelvic cavity, staying out of the abdominal cavity.

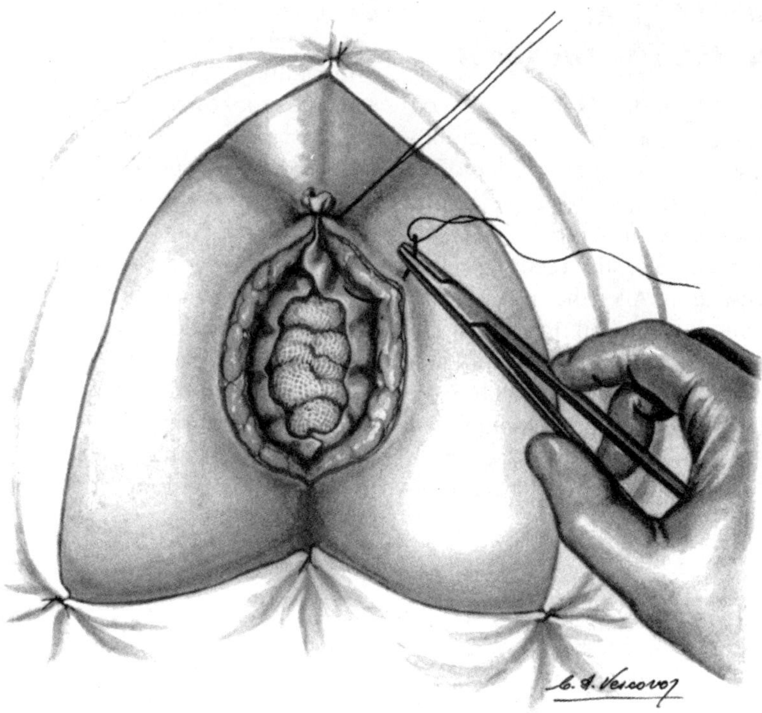

FIGURE 59.80

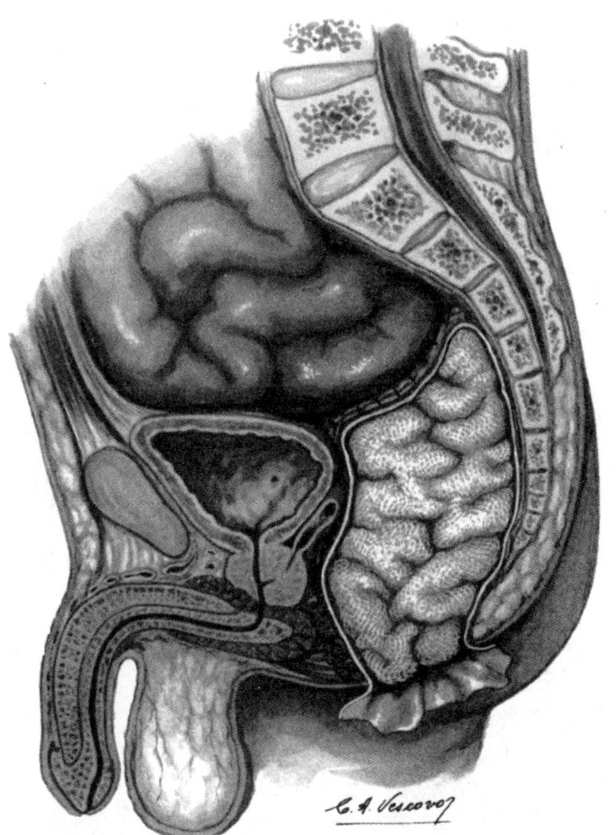

FIGURE 59.81

RESECTION AND COLOANAL ANASTOMOSIS IN RECTAL CANCER

In 1972 (70), Parks described the abdominotransanal technique in resection of the rectum for cancer with reestablishment of intestinal transit by performing a coloanal anastomosis, through the anal canal, without eversion of the rectal mucosa, which was done in previous procedures (8, 9, 22, 23). In this technique, the rectum is liberated as in a low anterior resection. After the rectum is liberated, it is transected above the anorectal ring. A cylinder of rectal mucosa above the pectinate line is resected transanally. Adequate exposure is obtained with Parks or Gelpi self-retaining retractors. Intestinal continuity is reestablished anastomosing the end of the colon to the mucosa of the anal canal, above the pectinate line with interrupted synthetic slow absorption sutures. End-to-end coloanal anastomosis frequently results in diarrhea or anal incontinence. Lazorthes and colleagues (53), in 1986, proposed construction of a J-pouch reservoir, with colon, using manual or mechanical suturing, with the object of reducing the frequency of diarrhea or incontinence.

Parc et al. (69) proposed a similar technique. The colonic reservoir is also sutured to the anal canal mucosa through the transanal route. There are controversial opinions over the benefits of the colonic pouch over an end-to-end coloanal anastomosis. The coloanal anastomosis is not easy, and it is only necessary on a few occasions when the use of another technique to reestablish intestinal transit is not possible (31). The end-to-end coloanal anastomosis should be protected by a transverse colostomy or a loop ileostomy.

Surgical Technique

Surgical Technique

FIGURE 59.82 COLOANAL ANASTOMOSIS FOR LOW RECTAL CANCER

The rectal cancer has been resected, and a J-pouch reservoir has been constructed with colon. A cylinder of mucosa has been excised from the anal canal, above the pectinate line, and the wall of the colonic reservoir is being sutured to the anal canal mucosa, above the pectinate line, using interrupted, synthetic, slow absorbing sutures, through the transanal route.

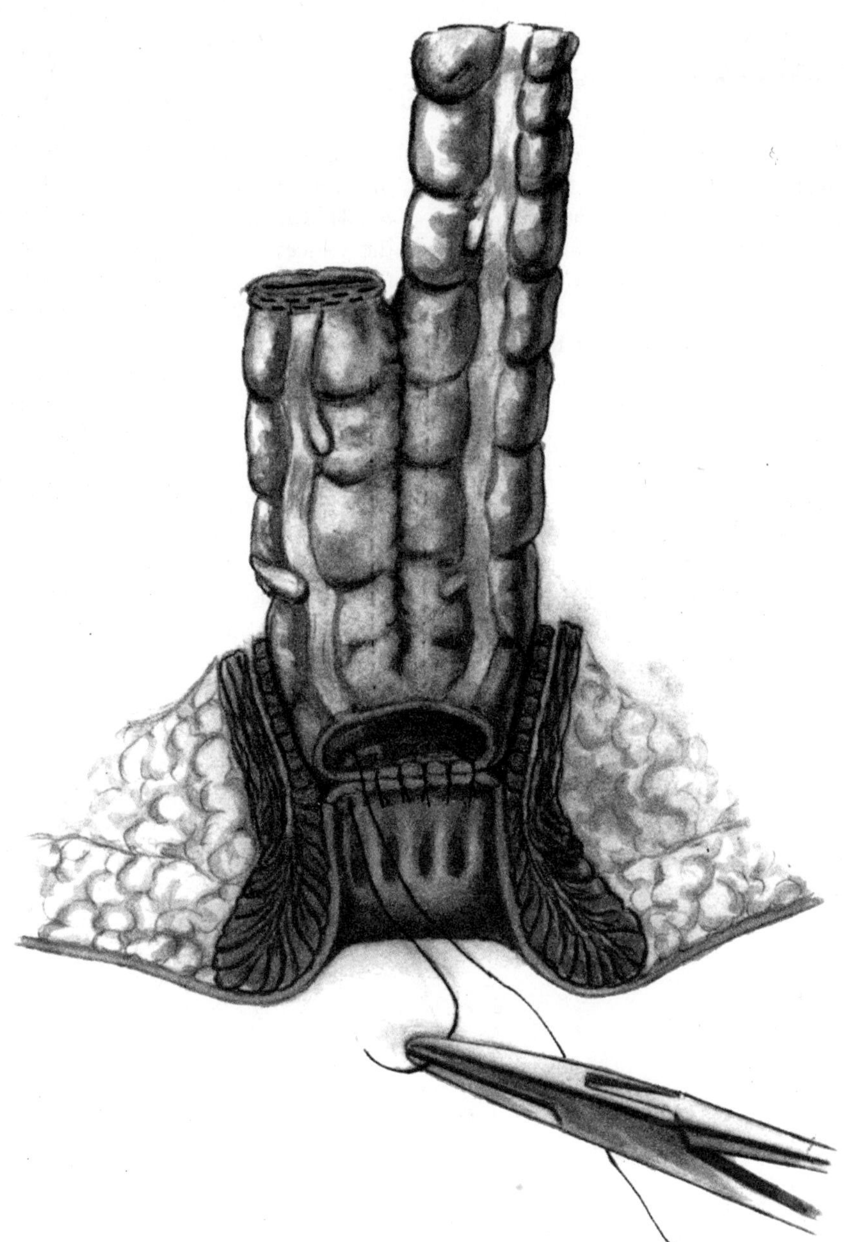

FIGURE 59.82 COLOANAL ANASTOMOSIS FOR LOW RECTAL CANCER

RECTAL CANCER—HARTMANN PROCEDURE

Henri Hartmann, a surgeon from the Hotel Dieu, Paris, presented a new operation for resection of rectal cancer, later known as the Hartmann procedure, to the 30th French Congress of Surgery in Strasbourg, in 1921. The Hartmann procedure consists of (a) segmental colorectal resection, including the carcinoma, (b) terminal colostomy, and (c) closure of the distal rectal stump (17). It should be noted that anterior resection of the rectum was not done when Hartmann presented his technique (24, 25).

The Hartmann procedure in the treatment of rectal cancer is actually used very infrequently and its indications are limited to special cases. Some of the indications are the following: (a) patients with rectal cancer in whom the anastomosis is very risky; (b) perforated rectosigmoidal cancer; (c) patients with systemic diseases that contraindicate a low anterior resection; (d) patients with rectal cancer with metastases; (e) patients in whom local recurrence is inevitable; (f) the surgeon avoids a low anterior resection due to the presence of a functionally weak anal sphincter; and (g) cases in which it was impossible to perform a mucous fistula because of the shortness of the segment distal to the colorectal resection (44, 93).

Though the Hartmann procedure was originally proposed for rectal cancer, at present, its most frequent indication is in peritonitis due to perforated acute diverticulitis.

The most important advantage of the Hartmann procedure is that it resects the cancer or the septic process in cases of acute perforated diverticulitis. Even though the Hartmann procedure has the advantage of resecting the cancer or the septic focus, it has an inconvenience that becomes apparent during reestablishment of intestinal transit, which is usually difficult. The level of transection of the rectum depends on the localization of the cancer. In some patients the rectum has to be transected very low, and the surgeon must resort to a Roticulator for the suturing. The rectum should be transected at least 2 cm distal to the tumor (17, 39, 93).

In patients with acute perforated diverticulitis, transection of the rectum can be done at a higher level, at the sacral promontory, because it is extremely rare for a phlegmonous process to extend below the promontory. Higher rectal transection makes reconstruction of intestinal transit easier.

Identification of the rectum can be facilitated by placing two or three 2-0 Prolene sutures. These sutures are fixed to the sacral promontory and its ends are left long. In this way, folding of the rectal stump with its consequent fall into the pelvic cavity, where it usually adheres to the bladder in males or to the uterus or vagina in females, can be avoided.

Surgical Technique

Surgical Technique

FIGURE 59.83

The upper drawing shows in schematic fashion the extent of the colorectal resection in patients with rectal cancer who are to be subjected to a Hartmann operation. The lower left drawing shows, by means of a broken line, the level of transection of the rectum, situated between two anterior resection clamps. The lower right drawing is a schematic presentation of the finished Hartmann procedure. The colorectal segment shown in the upper figure has been resected. In addition, a terminal colostomy has been realized. The rectum has been transected, and its distal end has been sutured manually. This can also be carried out with staplers. In the latter cases it is advisable to invert the rectal border with manual sutures, because fistulas have been known to develop when only staplers are used, due to rectal mucosal secretion. If transection of the rectum has to be done lower, the Roticulator can be used.

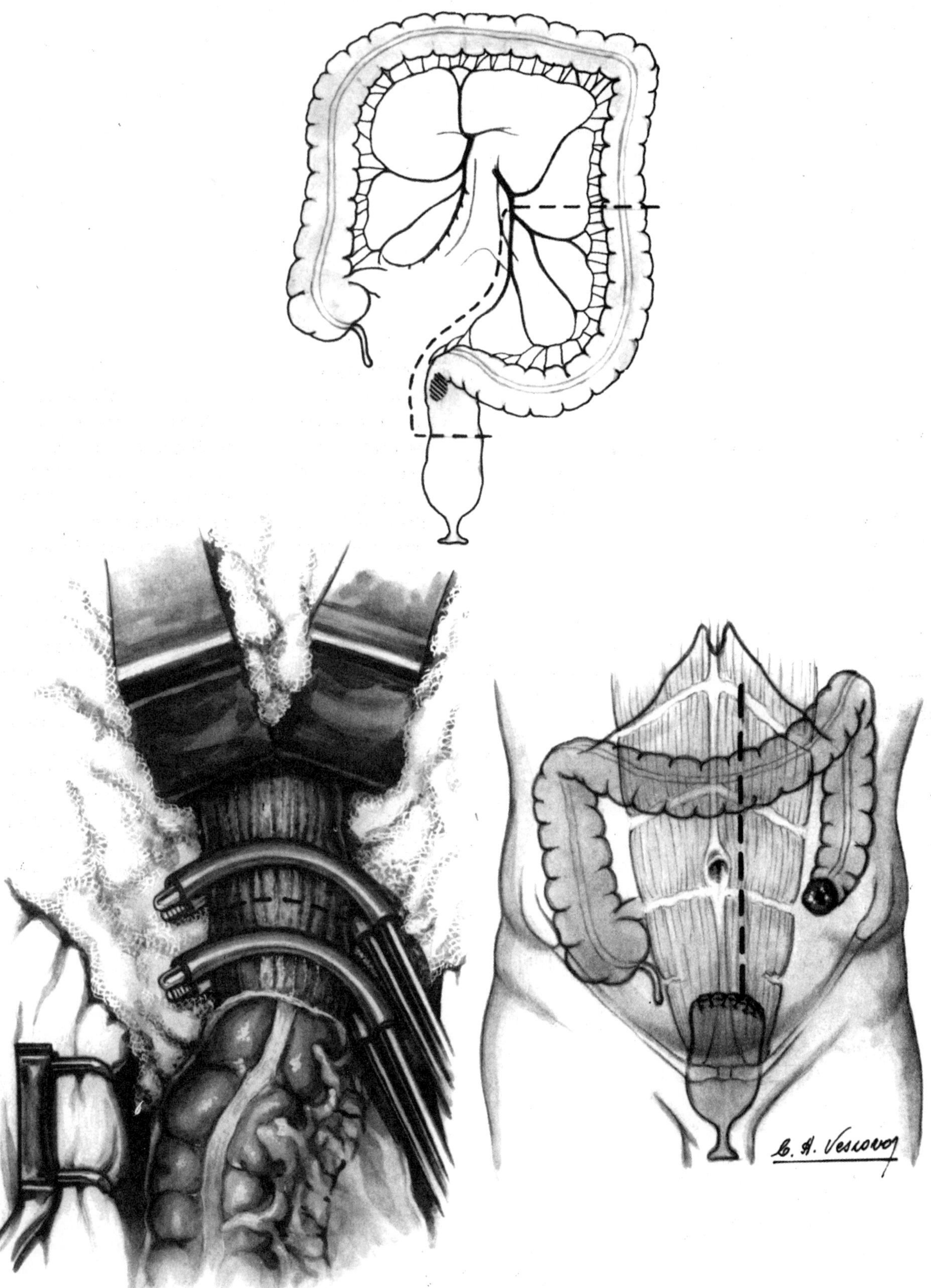

FIGURE 59.83

FIGURE 59.84

Reestablishment of colorectal transit after a Hartmann procedure can be very difficult. Manual or mechanical suturing can be used. In the latter, an EEA or a CEEA instrument can be used. The CEEA instrument is being used more frequently because of its definite advantages (39). In the following we will describe the technique for reestablishment of intestinal transit after a Hartmann procedure, using the EEA instrument (17, 33, 37, 93).

Surgical Technique

The patient is placed in a lithotomy Trendelenburg position (54). The most frequently used incision is over the previous incision. After entering the abdomen, the surgeon identifies the rectal stump and partially frees it from its adhesions. To facilitate its identification, a lighted rectoscope is introduced through the anus. Then, an EEA instrument is inserted through the anus, without its anvil. The central shaft of the instrument is inserted so that it pushes the anterior rectal wall. At this site, the surgeon makes a small incision with a scalpel in the anterior rectal wall (see drawing) and the central shaft is exteriorized. The abdominal surgeon frees the colon enough that a colorectal anastomosis without traction can be performed. The colonic end has been clamped with an atraumatic anterior resection clamp after inserting a purse string suture in its end.

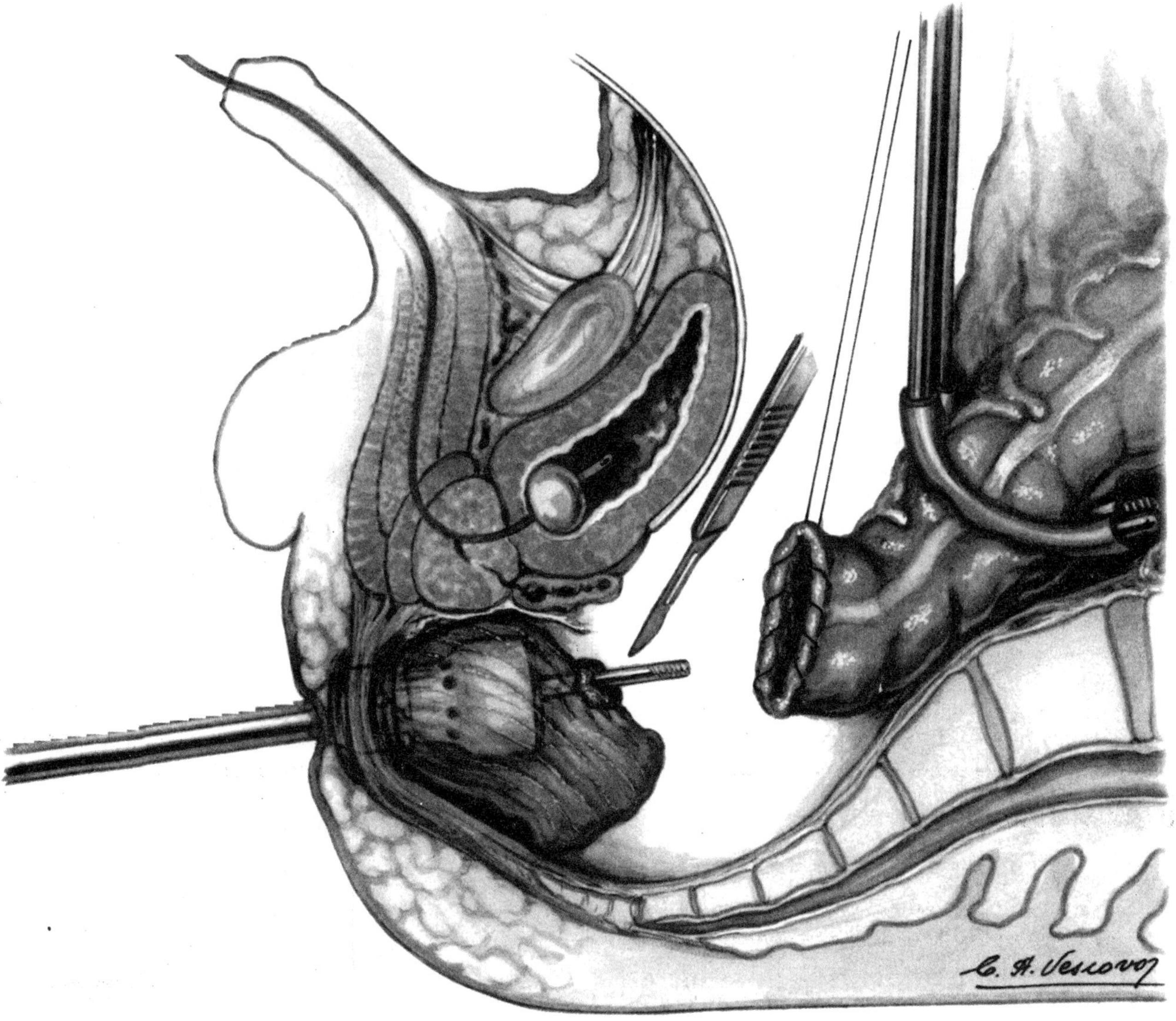

FIGURE 59.84

FIGURE 59.85
The anvil is reinserted into the central shaft of the EEA instrument being introduced into the colonic lumen.

Surgical Technique

FIGURE 59.86
The anvil has been approximated to the cartridge of the EEA instrument, and by firing it, colorectal transit has been reestablished. As stated previously, at present reestablishment of intestinal transit in a Hartmann operation is frequently done using the double stapling technique described in the low anterior resection with staplers (39). Once the anastomosis is complete, the pelvic cavity is drained with a Jackson Pratt catheter connected to closed, continuous drainage.

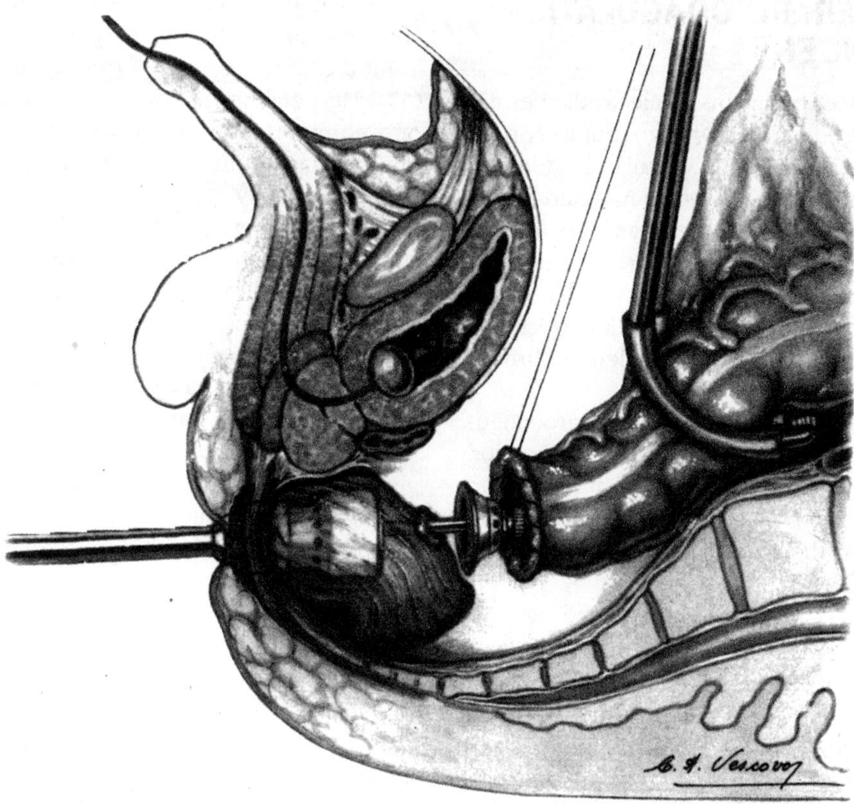

FIGURE 59.85

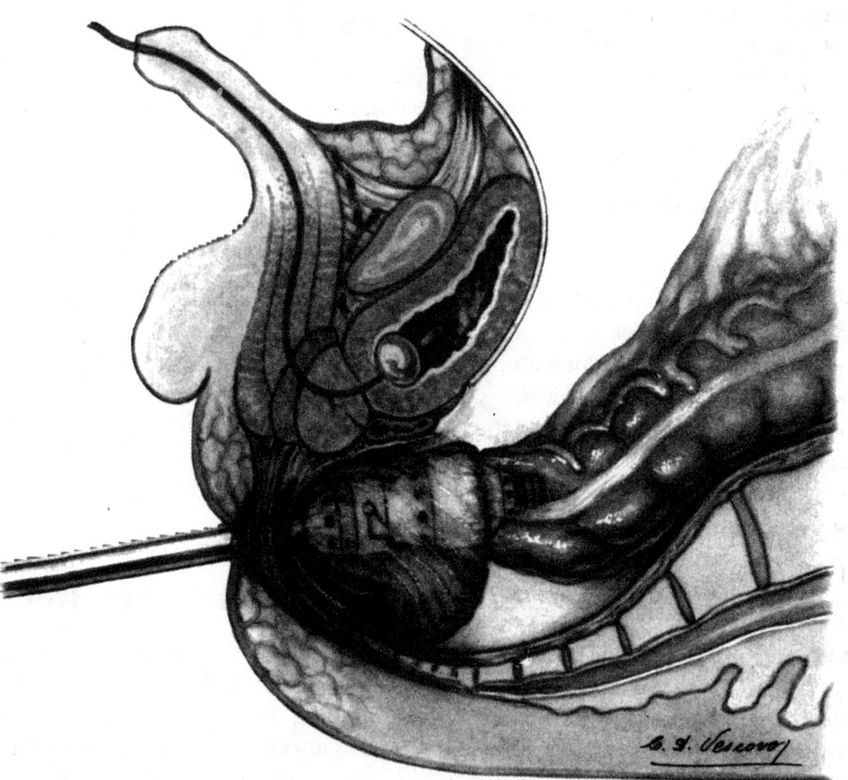

FIGURE 59.86

ELECTRODIATHERMIC COAGULATION OF RECTAL CANCER

Treatment of rectal cancer by means of electrodiathermic coagulation was proposed many years ago, but its spread among surgeons did not begin until John L. Madden of New York wrote about it in 1967. Madden again wrote about it in 1983 and 1990 (57, 58). After Madden's first article, articles by other surgeons appeared (20, 30, 76) confirming the good results reported by Madden using this technique. In a personal communication (October 19, 1995), and with vast experience, Madden confirmed his previous good results.

It is obvious that there are advantage of electrocoagulation over abdominoperineal resection for rectal cancer. These advantages are avoidance of a major operation such as abdominoperineal resection and its definitive colostomy. In addition, the mortality of electrocoagulation is practically nil (38).

Electrocoagulation has some disadvantages, however, because this procedure may not destroy the entire malignancy, and if the carcinoma has produced lymphatic metastases, this treatment is not curative. At present, endorectal ultrasonography is undoubtedly beneficial to determine the degree of penetration of a carcinoma into the rectal wall and, in some cases, it can also show enlarged lymph nodes, suspicious of being invaded by the neoplasm.

The majority of those that practice electrocoagulation to treat rectal cancer carry out a very strict selection of the patients to be subjected to this therapy (93). Some of the indications for this treatment are the following: (a) the rectal cancer should be polypoid and well differentiated histologically; (b) the rectal carcinoma should extend less than half of the rectal circumference; other authors (76) believe that the carcinoma should be less than 4 cm in diameter; (c) electrocoagulation can be used in patients whose general condition does not tolerate an abdominoperineal or low anterior resection; (d) electrocoagulation is indicated in patients that do not accept a permanent colostomy; (e) this treatment can be indicated in patients who are blind or incapacitated physically or mentally to care for their colostomy; (f) some surgeons only use electrocoagulation in tumors of the posterior and lateral rectal walls, avoiding tumors of the anterior wall due to the danger of injuring adjoining organs (vagina, bladder); and (g) electrocoagulation can be used as palliation of rectal cancer, to delay or avoid carrying out a permanent colostomy.

For this therapy, the rectal carcinoma should be located in the terminal 7.5 cm of the rectum, below the peritoneal reflection. Most surgeons do not advise electrofulguration of rectal tumors that are fixed or invade the entire rectal wall. In these cases the majority of surgeons recommend abdominoperineal resection.

As stated before, Dr. Madden has great experience with this technique, applying it more widely and adopting it as the primary, preferred treatment of rectal cancer (57). He does not believe it is contraindicated in tumors of the anterior wall of the rectum, male or female, or in undifferentiated tumors which are infiltrated or ulcerated circumferentially.

In electrofulguration of rectal cancer, a good relationship between the surgeon and the patient is necessary. The patient must realize the need to be hospitalized on several occasions for control examinations. In these examinations the patient should be anesthetized, either by general or spinal anesthesia. The patient must also know that, if electrocoagulation fails, he or she should be subjected to an abdominoperineal resection. An electrofulguration takes 1 to 4 hours to carry out, rarely less. Electrofulguration should not be performed in ambulatory patients. These should be hospitalized and anesthetized.

Preparation of the Patient

Before subjecting a patient to electrofulguration for rectal cancer, he or she should be hospitalized for 24 hours and kept on a liquid diet. Although some surgeons do not believe it is necessary, it is always convenient that the patient have a clean bowel and with the same preparation as that used in colorectal operations, which was described earlier.

Anesthesia

As previously stated, patients should be subjected to spinal or general anesthesia for electrofulguration of rectal cancer. Spinal anesthesia is preferable because it produces good muscular relaxation.

Position of the Patient

The patient should be placed in lithotomy position to treat lesions of the posterior rectal wall, and in the prone position to treat lesions of the anterior rectal wall. Both positions can be used in the same patient (Madden) to be able to visualize the carcinoma more completely and be able to carry out the treatment more effectively. Good exposure of the neoplasm is sine qua non for this treatment.

Instruments for Electrocoagulation

The instruments used in electrofulguration are relatively simple. There is no need for expensive, sophisticated equipment as some of those used in local treatment of rectal cancer. It is important to have an endorectal retractor (Madden) made up of three Deaver type narrow blades that can be fixed in the most convenient position, so that two assistant surgeons are not needed to hold them. One of the blades has fiberoptic illumination which provides clear vision of the lesion (see figures). The fulguration should be done with a needle electrode because this concentrates the temperature more and penetrates more deeply. A uterine curette is needed to remove electrocoagulated tissue. The fulguration should be repeated until all the neoplastic tumor is destroyed together with an additional 2 cm of apparently healthy tissue around the carcinoma, because of the possibility of microscopic submucosal focus of neoplasm around the tumor. A suction apparatus is necessary to remove the smoke generated during coagulation so as to maintain a clear view of the field.

TECHNIQUE OF ELECTRODIATHERMIC COAGULATION

Electrocoagulation is begun peripherally in the tumor, extending to the central portion, and introducing the needle well into the neoplasm. Once a segment of the neoplastic mass has been fulgurated, the uterine curette is used to remove the electrocoagulated tumoral rests. Electrocoagulation is continued until the neoplastic mass is completely destroyed. During the same session, electrocoagulation and curettage is repeated three to four times, until arriving at pliable, soft, elastic tissue, characteristic of healthy tissue. Tissue infiltrated by tumor is usually rigid, hard, and not pliable. To identify normal tissue, good visibility is indispensable as well as digital palpation of the area to distinguish normal tissue from tissue infiltrated by tumor. Aspiration of smoke should be continuous for good visualization of the procedure being carried out.

Neoplastic lesions below 7.5 cm of the posterior rectal wall can be electrofulgurated without fear because that segment is extraperitoneal and there are no inconveniences in going beyond the limits of the rectal wall and fulgurating perirectal areolar tissue.

Neoplastic lesions of the anterior rectal wall should be electrocoagulated much more carefully because of their relation to the vagina in the female and the bladder in the male. It should be noted that the anterior rectal wall is partially inside the peritoneal cavity.

After the fulguration, the patient should remain hospitalized because of the possibility of complications. About 8 to 10 days later, the patient should be examined under anesthesia for control of the lesion, to biopsy suspicious areas, and to complete the electrofulguration if this proves necessary. The patient is again examined 30 days later and every 3 months during the first year. One month after electrofulguration, it is useful to carry out an endorectal ultrasonography to evaluate the possibility of there being invaded lymph nodes, which can be seen by this method (38). If ultrasonography shows the possible existence of invaded lymph nodes, abdominoperineal resection should be advised. This operation should also be done in patients in whom electrofulguration has not been effective.

Complications

The most frequent complication of electrofulguration for carcinoma of the rectum is hemorrhage, which usually occurs 6 to 8 days later, with the patient still hospitalized. In about half of the cases, the hemorrhage stops spontaneously. If bleeding does not stop spontaneously, hemostasis should be carried out by performing a new electrofulguration, using a ball or disk electrode, and not a needle electrode (57, 58). Before this hemostatic electrofulguration, the rectum should be washed with hydrogen peroxide and warm saline solution (57) to remove clots and attain better visualization. Irrigation is repeated in five minutes. An abdominoperineal resection should be advised if the bleeding does not stop with a new electrocoagulation. Another complication that may occur is rectal stricture due to circular lesions or when it was necessary to carry out several electrocoagulations. Other complications include (a) rectovaginal fistula due to electrofulguration of lesions of the anterior rectal wall in females, (b) rectovesical fistulas in males, (c) perforation of the rectum into the peritoneal cavity, and (d) fever, following electrofulguration, which is treated with wide spectrum antibiotics.

The results obtained by Madden with this procedure are 5-year survival, 64%; in lesions less than 3 cm in diameter, survival was 62% (57). Other surgeons have reported similar results (20, 30, 76).

FIGURE 59.87

The patient. under spinal anesthesia, has been placed in lithotomy position. The Madden self-retaining retractor, made up of three narrow Deaver blades that can be fixed in the most adequate position, without having to be held by two assistants, has been placed. The upper blade has a fiberoptic illuminating system, which allows excellent visibility. This illuminated blade can be changed in position, if necessary. The surgeon holds the suction cannula in the left hand to remove the smoke produced by the electrocoagulation to maintain good visibility. With the right hand, the surgeon holds the coagulating electrode.

Complications

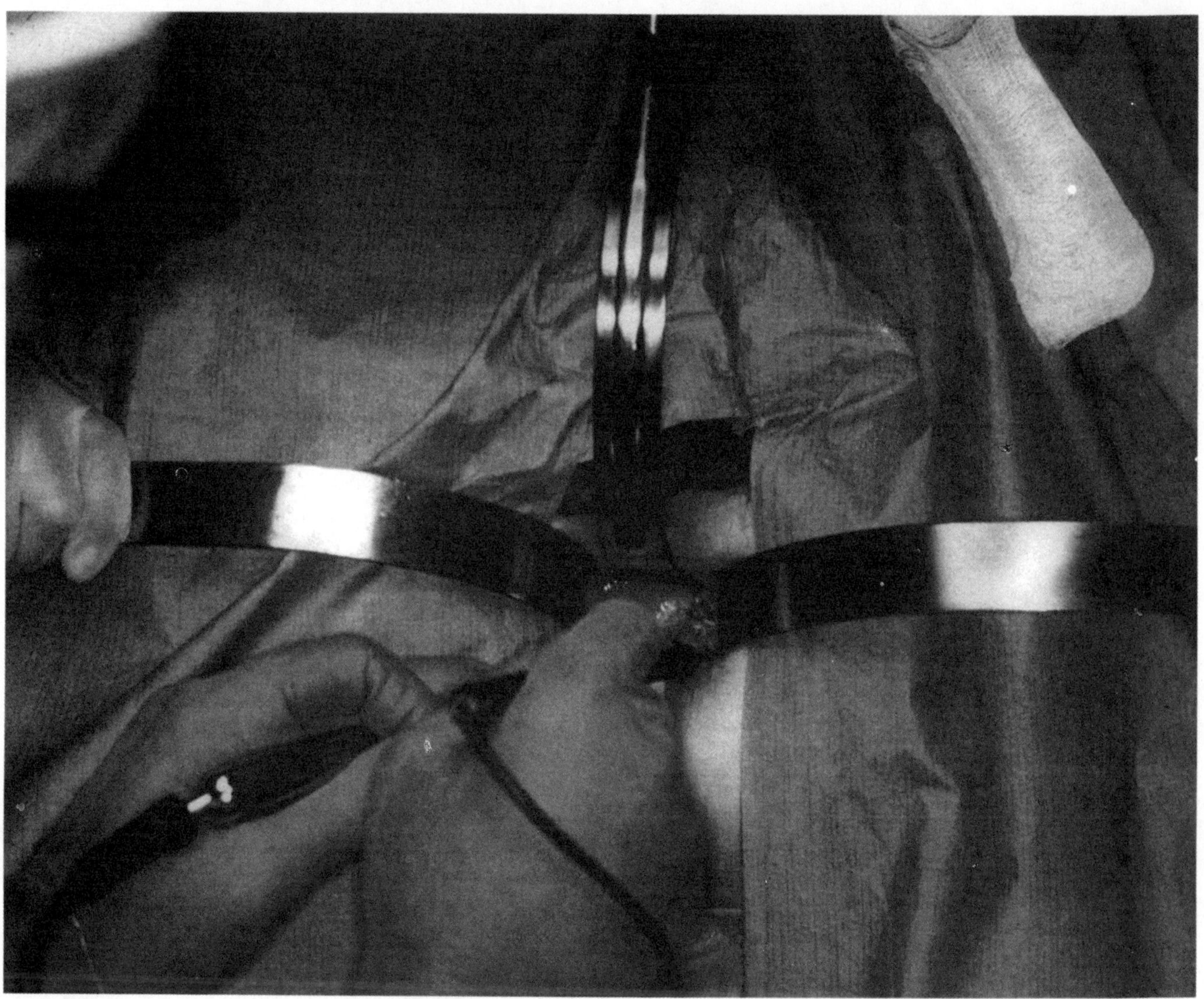

FIGURE 59.87

Complications

FIGURE 59.88
This drawing shows a patient with cancer of the posterior rectal wall, placed in lithotomy position. This is the best position for electrocoagulating neoplastic lesions in this location.

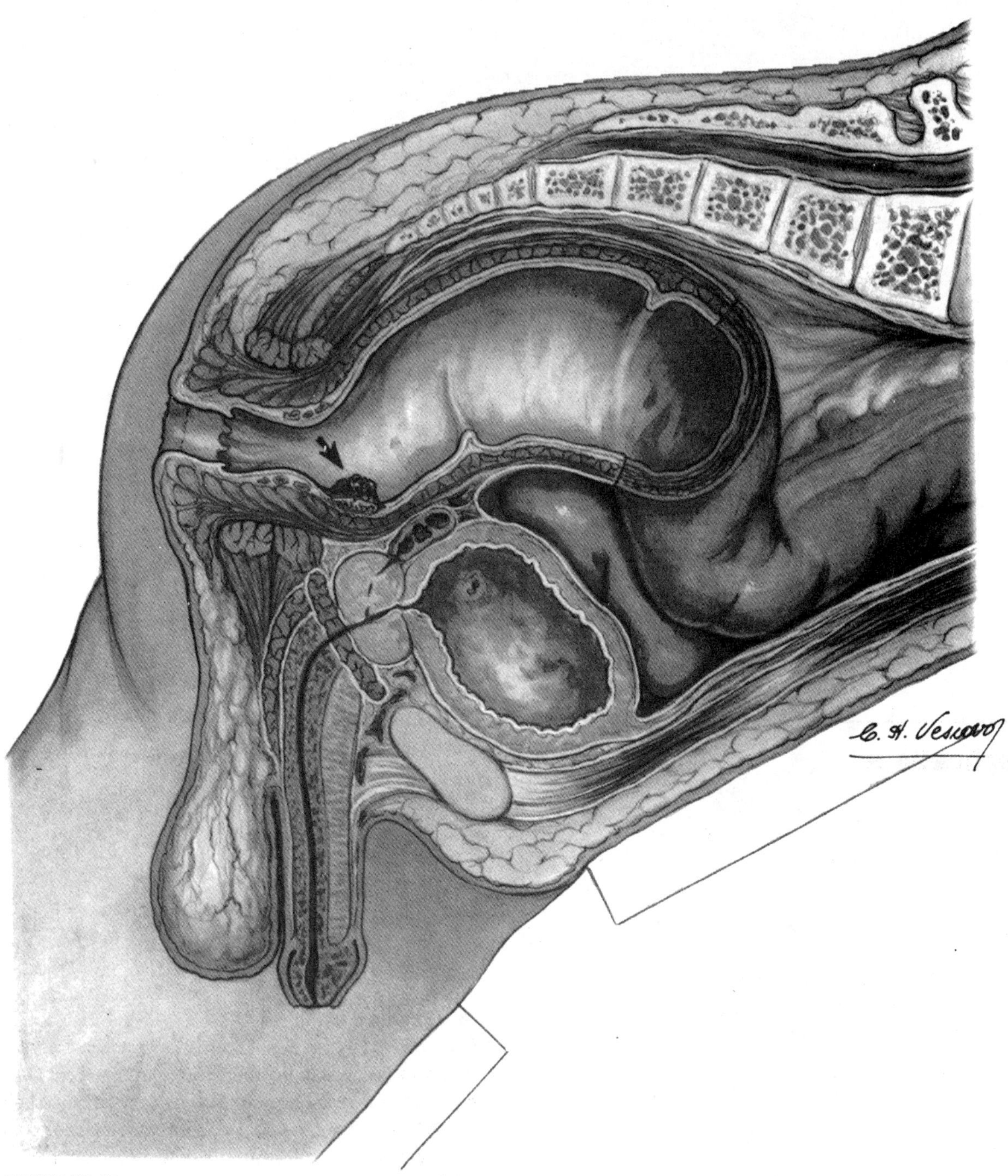

FIGURE 59.88

Complications

FIGURE 59.89

This drawing shows a patient with a carcinoma of the anterior rectal wall, placed in prone position, the best position for electrofulgurating carcinomas in this location. It should be pointed out that, in many cases, it is necessary to place the patient in both positions successively, in order to better visualize the lesion and facilitate its total destruction.

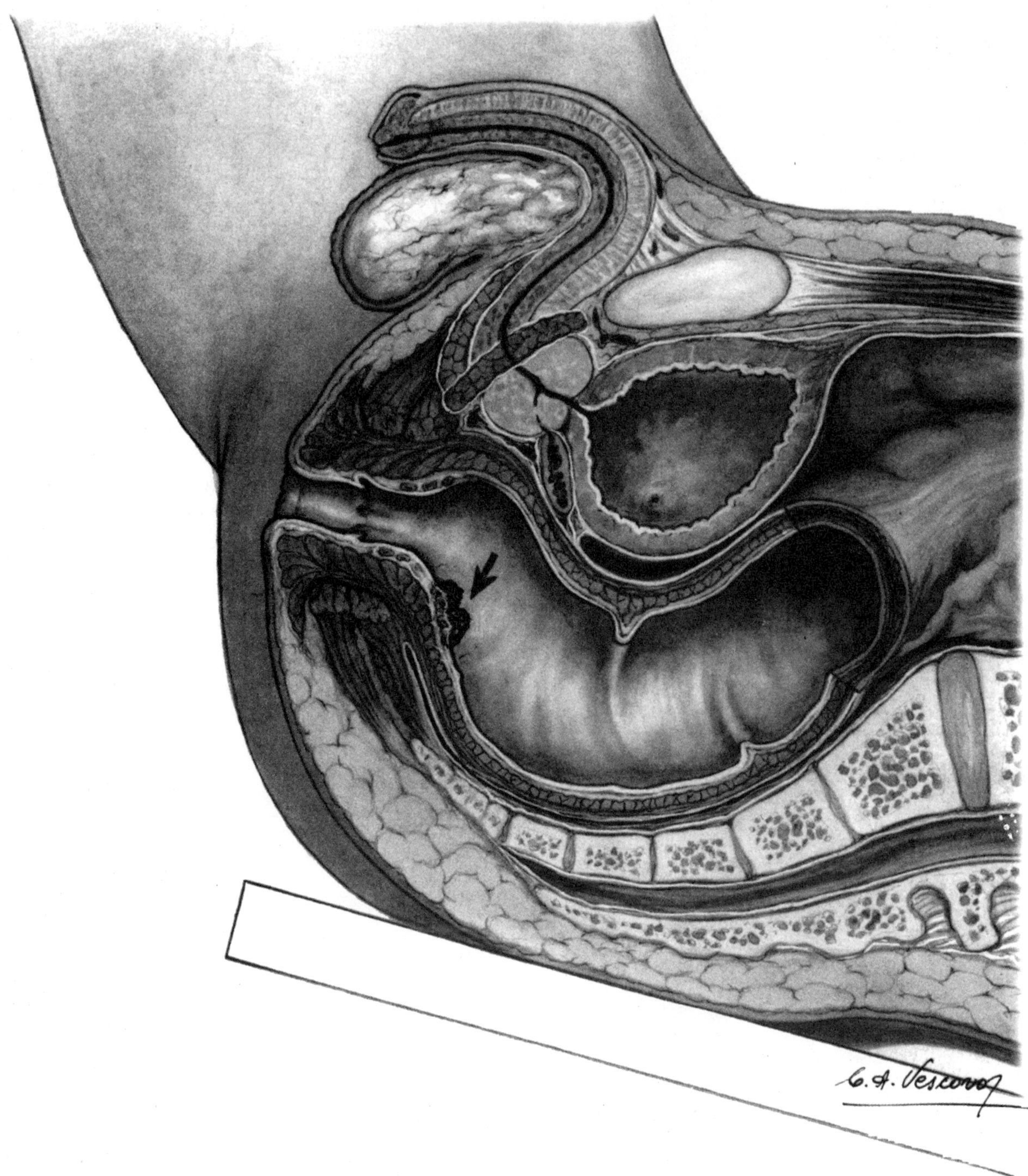

FIGURE 59.89

FIGURE 59.90
The drawing shows a carcinoma of the posterior rectal wall with moderate infiltration of the mucosa toward the patient's right side. The broken line shows the extent of electrofulguration to be carried out. The electrofulguration should extend about 2 cm into the healthy area around the carcinoma. The surgeon can be seen holding the aspiration cannula with the left hand and, in the right hand, the handle of the electrocoagulation equipment with a needle electrode.

Complications

FIGURE 59.91
The surgeon is electrocoagulating the rectal carcinoma.

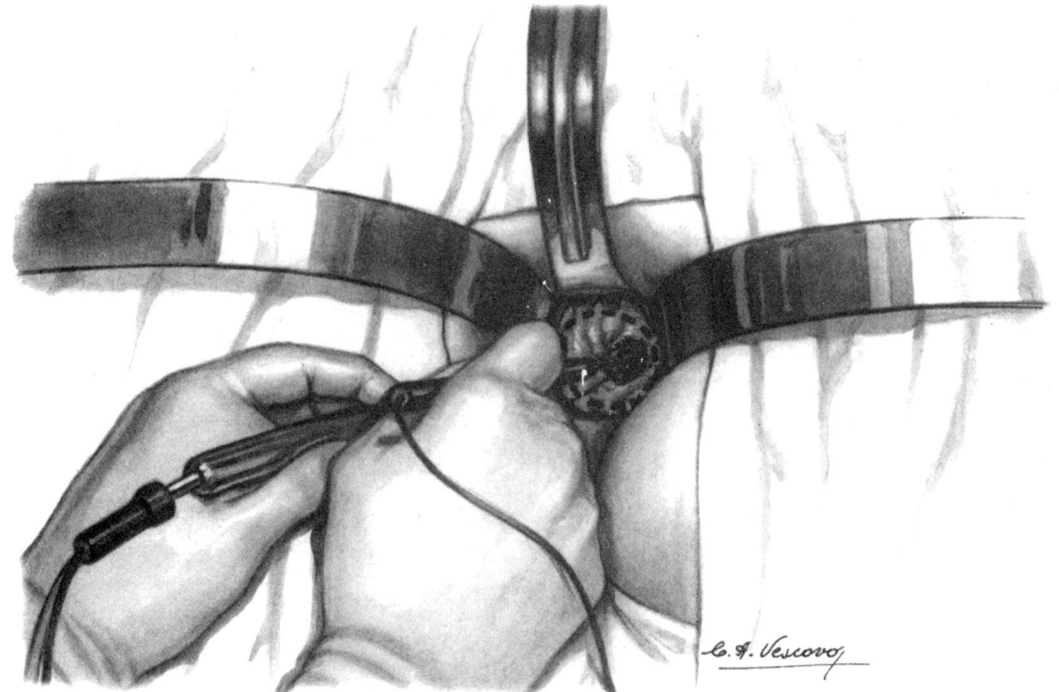

FIGURE 59.90

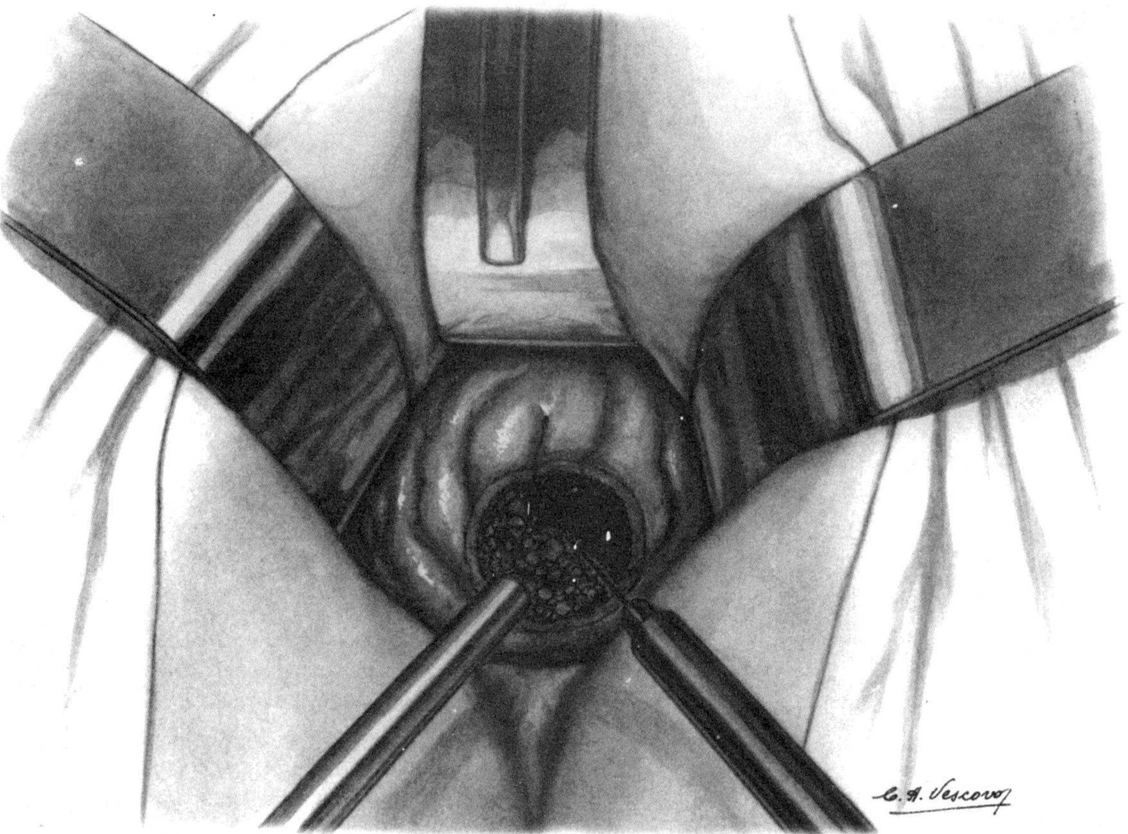

FIGURE 59.91

FIGURE 59.92
Using a uterine curette, the surgeon removes the electrocoagulated tumor remnants. The figure shows that the circular muscle layer has been electrocoagulated, exposing the muscle fibers of the longitudinal layer.

Complications

FIGURE 59.93
The entire circular muscle layer has been electrocoagulated, exposing the muscular fibers of the longitudinal layer. When the electrofulguration is done carefully, layer by layer, it is possible to determine approximately the degree of parietal penetration of the neoplastic process. Digital palpation is very useful in determining the presence of hard, infiltrated tissue or soft, pliable tissue corresponding to tissue not invaded by the carcinoma.

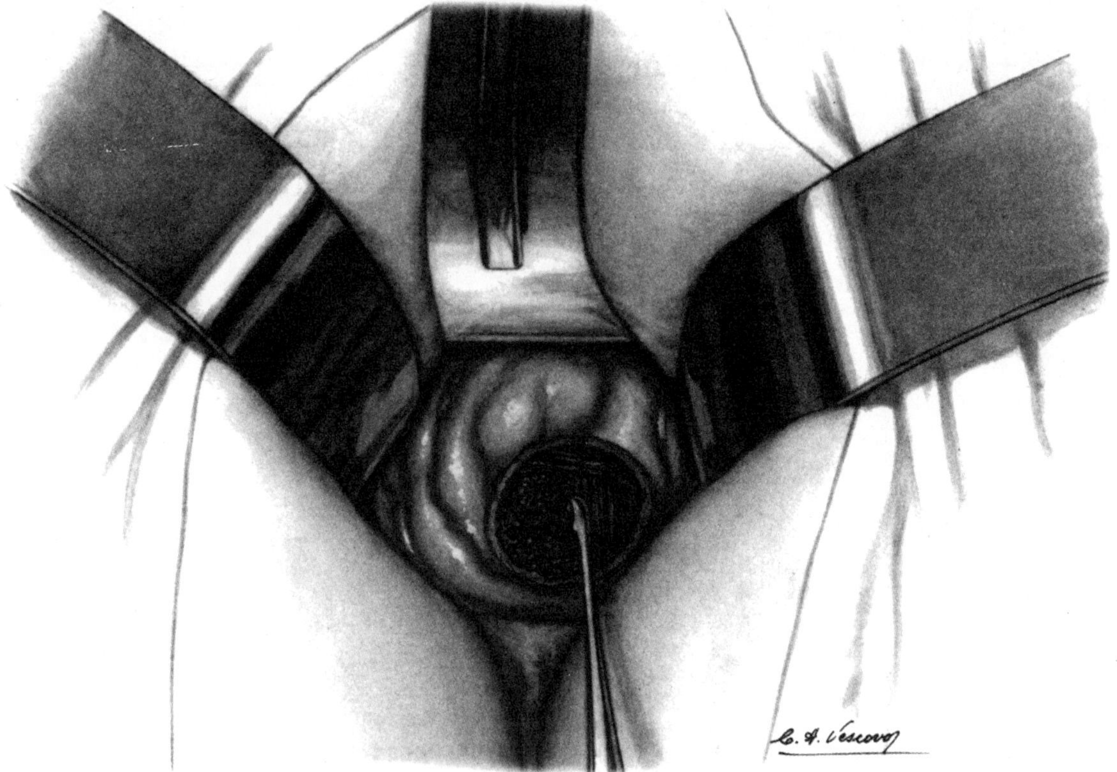

GURE 59.92

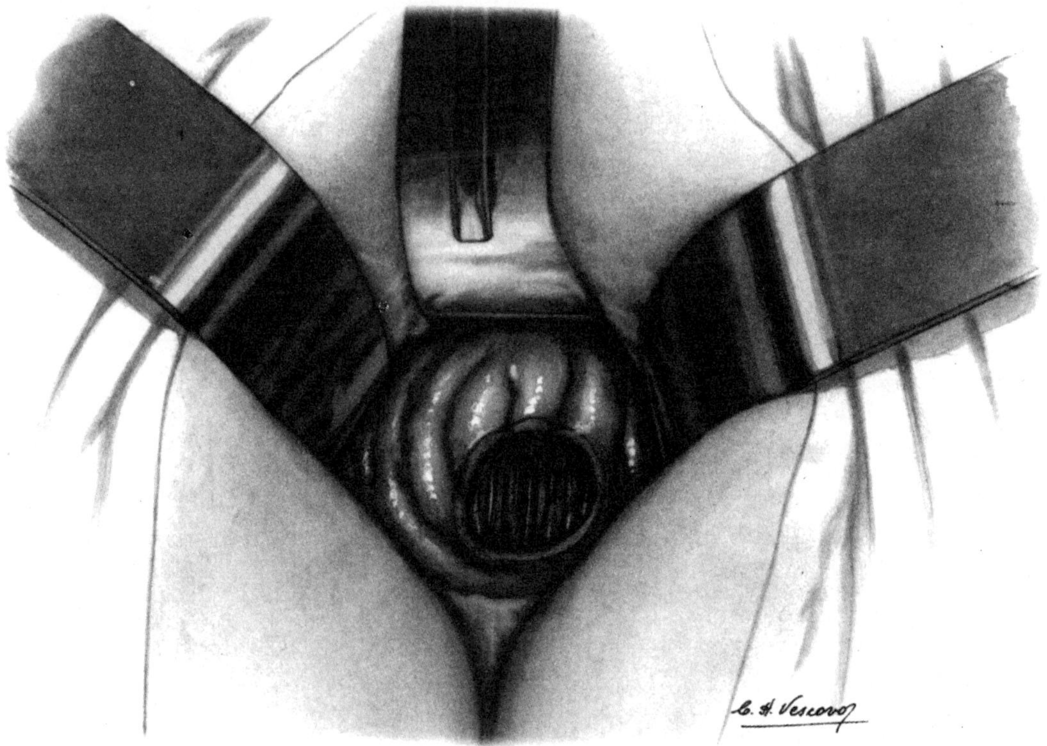

FIGURE 59.93

FIGURE 59.94
In cases of tumors localized in the posterior wall of the rectum, electrofulguration can be vigorously pursued without worrying if the electrofulguration has gone beyond the limits of the rectal wall and penetrated the perirectal areolar fat. Electrofulguration of the posterior perirectum is not associated with any important complications.

Complications

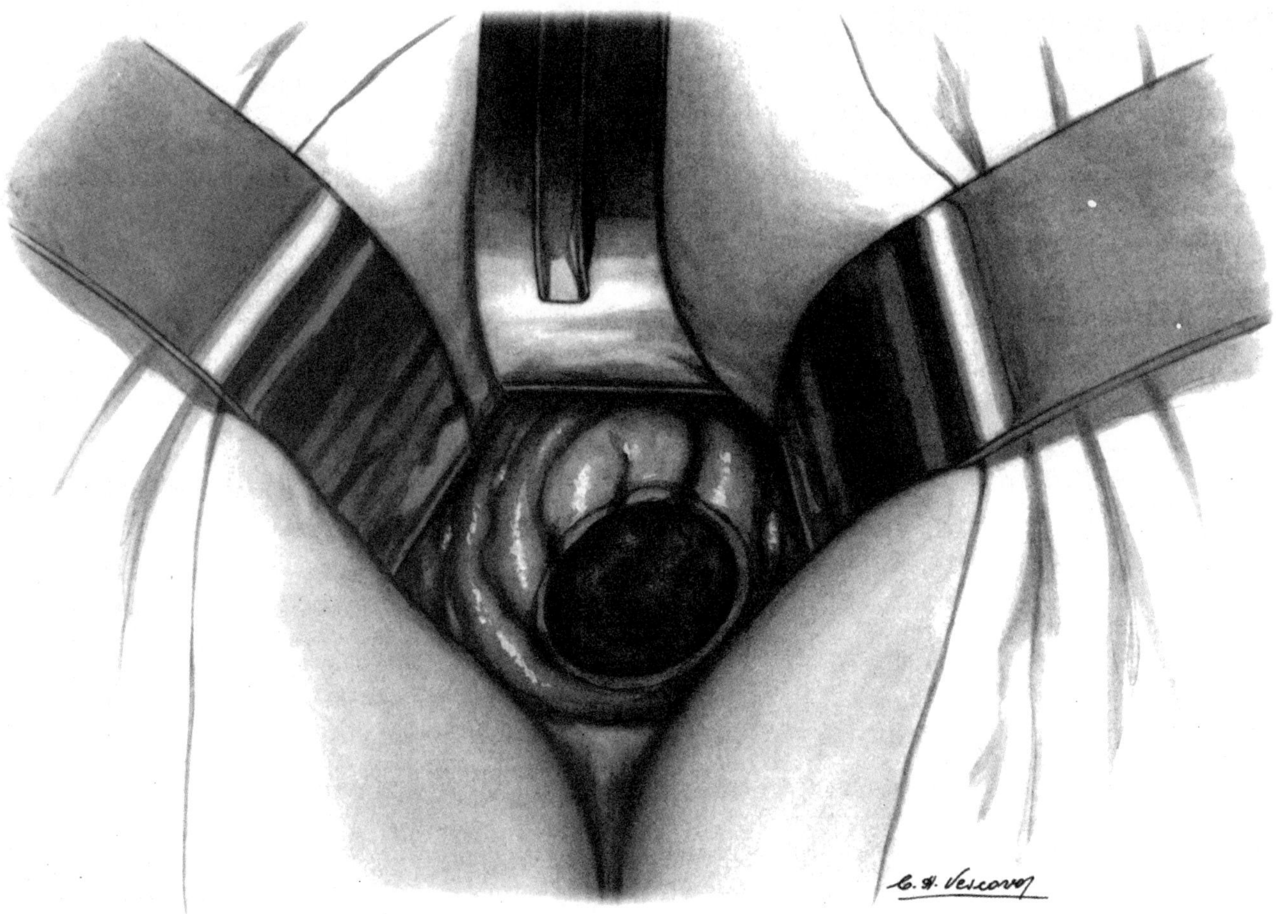

FIGURE 59.94

OTHER LOCAL TREATMENTS FOR RECTAL CANCER

There are other local treatments for rectal cancer, in addition to electrodiathermic coagulation (38, 58, 67, 93), which will be considered as follows: (a) local surgical excision of rectal cancer, (b) intracavity radiation (Papillon), (c) treatment with laser rays, and (d) cryotherapy.

Local Excision of Rectal Cancer

Local excision of rectal cancer can be done by the transanal route or the transsphincteric route.

Local Excision of Rectal Cancer by the Transanal Route

Surgeons who use this method usually recommend it for

1. tumors of the distal half of the rectum
2. small tumors, 2 to 3 cm in diameter
3. exophytic tumors
4. movable tumors
5. tumors that are not ulcerated
6. histologically well differentiated tumors, proven by several biopsies from different sites on the carcinoma. This confirmation is important because undifferentiated tumors, even though small in size, have frequently produced metastases to regional lymph nodes

The tumors should be limited to the rectal wall, preferably those that have not grown through the muscularis propia. Endorectal ultrasonography may clearly show the degree of penetration of the rectal wall by the carcinoma, and it may also show enlarged lymph nodes, raising suspicions that they have been invaded by tumor. Rectal examination and bimanual palpation under general or spinal anesthesia should raise the suspicion of the presence of palpable lymph nodes that may be invaded by the tumor. Computed tomography should also not raise suspicions of involved lymph nodes. Local excision of rectal cancer may be indicated in patients who should be treated by abdominoperineal resection, but whose general condition contraindicates this procedure.

Surgeons who favor transanal local excision of rectal cancer state that this procedure has the following advantages: (a) By means of this technique, the resected surgical specimen is preserved and not destroyed, as in other local treatments of rectal cancer, allowing a complete study by the pathologist; (b) local excision of rectal cancer avoids a major procedure such as an abdominoperineal resection; and (c) the rectal carcinomas, with the described characteristics, that can be selected for local excision, only have metastases to lymph nodes in 10% of cases (93).

Local surgical resection of rectal cancer, in spite of its apparent advantages, presents some weak points: (a) This procedure can only be performed in 3 to 5% of rectal cancers. In St. Mark's Hospital, London, only 3.3% of 2303 cases of rectal cancer (93) could be subjected to this procedure. (b) In spite of strict selection of cases for this operation, local recurrence is frequent, due to implantation of viable neoplastic cells desquamated from the primary tumor. (c) This evidence leads to the conclusion that electrocoagulation is preferable in these carcinomas, rather than local excision (58, 93).

Local Excision of Rectal Cancer by the Transphincteric Route

Local excision of rectal cancer by the transphincteric route was proposed by Bevan, of the United States, in 1917, to treat small tumors in this location (14). In 1970, York Mason of the United Kingdom again recommended this technique with great enthusiasm (59).

The Bevan-Mason operation, of local resection of rectal cancer by the transphincteric route, approaches the rectum posteriorly. This procedure is better adapted to treat tumors localized in the anterior or anterolateral rectal walls, from 7 to 10 cm from the anal margin, and whose diameter does not exceed 4 cm. This procedure has not been well accepted by surgeons in spite of the good results reported by York Mason. Unfavorable criticism of this technique is based on its transection of several layers of tissue, which predisposes the patient, more than the transanal route, to seeding of viable neoplastic cells desquamated from the primary tumor. In addition, this operation may give rise to other complications, some of which may compromise anal continence.

Preparation of Patients Who Are To Be Subjected to Local Excision of Rectal Cancer

Preparation of patients to be subjected to local excision of rectal cancer, either transanally or through the transsphincteric route, is similar to the preparation used in classic colorectal operations. The patient should be hospitalized the day before surgery and the large bowel prepared in similar fashion as previously described, both mechanically and with antibiotics. Anesthesia should be spinal, epidural, or general.

Position of the patient

If the operation is to be done transanally, the patient's position will vary according to the location of the carcinoma. If the tumor is located in the posterior wall, the patient should be placed in the lithotomy position. If the tumor is anterior in location, the patient should be placed in the prone position. Patients who are to be operated on by the transsphincteric approach should be placed in the prone position.

Surgical Technique

Transanal route

For this operation, self-retaining retractors such as the Parks, Gelpi, or Pratt retractors are convenient. The technique of excision of the carcinoma is similar to that used to remove villous adenomas of the rectum, but instead of entering the submucosal layer, the entire thickness of the rectal wall around the tumor should be transected, about 2 cm beyond the macroscopic border. The defect in the wall is closed transversely in one layer, with interrupted slow absorption sutures, including the entire thickness of the rectal wall.

Transphincteric route

The patient is placed in prone position and the operating table flexed at the hip joint. The buttocks are separated with adhesive tape. The incision is started in the midline of anus and extended upward, following the midline and continuing over the left sacral border to its midline, then continuing over the left sacral border to its middle third. Once the skin and soft tissues are incised, the mucocutaneous junction of the anal canal is identified and two sutures are placed, symmetrically, in the midline, leaving them long as guide sutures. Then, symmetrical sutures are placed into the posterior rectal wall, on each side of the midline, for traction and as guide sutures during closure of the rectal wall. The external anal sphincter is then transected in the midline, tagging each muscular bundle symmetrically with different colored sutures. The puborectalis muscle is then transected and its borders marked with different color sutures. The procedure is then repeated in the internal anal sphincter and its borders tagged with different colors, before or after transecting them. This is of great importance to avoid confusion during closure, which may lead to severe alterations of function.

Once the posterior rectal wall and the sphincter have been incised, the rectal carcinoma is resected. The tumor is usually localized in the anterior rectal wall, 7 to 10 cm from the anal margin. Once the carcinoma, which should be less than 4 cm in diameter, has been resected, the defect is closed using slow absorbing synthetic sutures in two layers, first the muscular and then the mucosal layer. The posterior rectal wall is closed in one layer of interrupted sutures, using the same material. Finally, the transected sphincters are sutured with the same material, being very careful to avoid confusion in suturing the ends held by the different color sutures.

Intracavitary Radiation of Rectal Cancer (Papillon)

In 1973, Papillon, from Lyon, France, proposed a procedure to administer radiotherapy to a small area over a short period of time, calling it contact radiotherapy or intracavitary radiotherapy (67). To carry this procedure out, it is not necessary to hospitalize the patient. The Papillon treatment should be limited to well-differentiated papillary tumors of less than 3 cm in diameter without evidence of lymph node invasion. Using these limitations, this treatment can only be applied to 10% of rectal carcinomas.

Intracavitary irradiation consists in administering 3000 to 4000 RAD in 3 minutes. Treatment is repeated in 7 to 10 days. A total of 9000 to 15,000 RAD are given in 4 to 6 weeks (58). Radiotherapy is administered through a proctoscope 3 cm or less in diameter.

In an article published in 1990 (68), the 5-year survival in 310 cases was 76%, with a local recurrence rate of 8.3% and a mortality rate of 7.7%. In 1987, however, Lavery (52) reported 18% recurrence rate in 62 patients followed for 31 months, with 29% recurrence rate in ulcerated cases, and 14% recurrence rate in polypoid tumors.

The Papillon technique has not been widely used. An interesting fact reported by Madden is that in cases with recurrence, the patient can still be treated with electrocoagulation.

Treatment of Rectal Cancer with Laser Rays

Laser rays are used in local treatment of rectal cancer for palliation or, in some selected cases, for cure. Laser rays are used for palliation to increase the rectal lumen in patients with obstruction and to control bleeding in some patients with bleeding tumors. Laser rays control bleeding at the same time that the tissues are incised. Because of this, they can be used to resect localized tumors of the distal half of the rectum that are small, movable, polypoid, well differentiated, and not ulcerated or infiltrating.

Cryotherapy

Destruction of rectal carcinoma by freezing is used infrequently. The temperature used in this treatment is 20 degrees below zero. The procedure consists of placing the contact catheter in close proximity to the tumor and then moving it to other areas of the tumor until the entire tumor is frozen. Freezing leads to necrosis of the carcinoma within several weeks (38, 93). During these weeks, the patient presents foul smelling rectal discharges and, occasionally, bleeding. One month later, the tumor is examined to determine the need for another freezing.

Some surgeons practice this procedure without general anesthesia. The majority of surgeons, however, believe that general or spinal anesthesia is indispensable because, even though application of cryotherapy to the tumor is not very painful, patients do not tolerate the necessary self-retaining anal retractors (93). It is felt that the palliation attained by cryotherapy is not as good as that attained in other local procedures used in the treatment of rectal cancer. In spite of this, Heberer, of Germany (45), asserts having attained satisfactory results with this procedure.

References

1. Adolff, M., Arnoud, J.P., Beehary, S. Stapled versus sutured colorectal anastomosis. Arch. Surg. 115:1436, 1980.
2. Akwari, O.E., Kelly, K. Anterior resection for adenocarcimona of the distal large bowel. Am. J. Surg. 139:88, 1980
3. Akyol, A.M., McGregor, J.R., Galloway, O.J., Murray, G., George, W.D. Recurrence of colorectal cancer after sutured and stapled large bowel anastomosis. Br. J. Surg. 78:1297, 1983.
4. Andersberg, B., Enblad, R., Stodahl, R. Recurrent rectal carcinoma after anterior resection and rectal stapling. Br. J. Surg. 70:104, 1983.
5. Astler, V.B., Coller, F.A. The prognostic significance of direct extension of carcinoma of the colon and rectum. Ann. Surg. 139:846, 1954.
6. Babcock, W.W. Operative treatment of carcinoma of rectosigmoid with methods for elimination of colostomy. Surg. Gynecol. Obstet. 55:627, 1932
7. Babcock, W.W. Experiences with resection of the colon and the elimination of colostomy. Am. J. Surg. 46:186, 1939.
8. Babcock, W.W. Radical simple-stage extirpation for cancer of the large bowel with retained functional anus. Surg. Gynecol. Obstet. 85:1, 1947.
9. Bacon, H.E. Evolution of sphincter muscle preservation and reestablishment of continuity in the operative treatment of rectal and sigmoidal cancer. Surg. Gynecol. Obstet. 81:113, 1945.
10. Baker, J.W. Low end to side rectosigmoidal anastomosis. Arch. Surg. 61:143, 1950.
11. Baker, J.W. Side-to-end colorectal anastomosis. In Malt, R.A. (Ed.) Surgical techniques illustrated. Vol. 2, no. 2, p. 31. Little, Brown, Boston, 1977.
12. Beart, R.W., Kelly, K.A. Randomized prospective evaluation of the E.E.A. stapler for colo-rectal anastomoses. Am. J. Surg. 141:143, 1981.
13. Becker, J. Abdominoperineal resection for cancer of the rectum. In Bauer, J.J. (Ed.) Colorectal surgery illustrated. p. 137. Mosby–Year Book, St. Louis, 1993.
14. Bevan, A.D., Carcinoma of the rectum: Treatment by local excision. Surg. Clin. North Am. 1:1233, 1917.
15. Block, W.A., Waugh, J.M. The intramural extension of carcimona of the descending colon, sigmoid and rectosigmoid: A pathological study. Surg. Gynecol. Obstet. 87:457, 1948.
16. Cady, J., Godfroy, J., Siband, O., et al. La désunion anastomotic en chirurgie colique et rectal. Etude comparative des procédés de suture manuelle et mécanique à propos d'une série de 149 résections. Ann. Chir. 34:350, 1980.
17. Chassin, J.L. Operative strategy in general surgery. Ed. 2, p. 337. Springer-Verlag, New York, 1993.
18. Cohen, A.M., Enker, W.E., Minsky, B.D. Proctectomy and coloanal reconstruction for rectal cancer. Dis. Colon Rectum 33:40, 1990.
19. Coller, F.A., Kay, E.B., MacIntyre, R.S. Regional lymphatic metastases of carcinoma of the rectum. Surgery 8:294, 1940.
20. Crile, G., Jr., Turnbull, R.B. Jr. The role of electrocoagulation in the treatment of carcinoma of the rectum. Surg. Gynecol. Obstet. 135:391, 1972.
21. Cullen, P.K., Mayo, C.W. A further evaluation of the one-stage low anterior resection. Dis. Colon Rectum 6:415, 1963.
22. Cutait, D.E., Figlioni, F.J. A new method of colo-rectal anastomosis in abdomino-perineal resection. Dis. Colon Rectum 6:415, 1963.
23. D'Allaines, F. Traitment chirurgical du cancer du rectum. Ed. 2, p. 27. Flammarion, Paris, 1946.
24. Dixon, C.F. Surgical removal of lesions occuring in sigmoid rectosigmoid. Am. J. Surg. 46:12, 1939.
25. Dixon, C.F. Anterior resection for malignant lesion of upper part of rectum and lower part of sigmoid. Ann. Surg. 128:425, 1948.
26. Dukes, C.E. The spread of cancer of the rectum. Br. J. Surg. 17:643, 1930.
27. Dukes, C.E. The classification of cancer of the rectum. J. Pathol. Bacteriol. 35:323, 1932.
28. Durdey, P., Williams, N.S. The effect of malignant and inflammatory fixation of rectal carcinoma as prognosis after rectal excision. Br. J. Surg. 70:150, 1983.
29. Durdey, P., Williams, N.S. The effect of malignant and inflammatory fixation of rectal carcinoma as prognosis after rectal excision. Br. J. Surg. 71:787, 1984.
30. Eisenstat, T.E., Deak, S.T., Rubin, R.J. et al. Five year survival in patients with caracinoma of the rectum, treated by electrocoagulation. Am. J. Surg. 143:127, 1982.
31. Enker, W.E. Cancer of the rectum: Operative management and adjuvant therapy. In Fazio, V.W. (Ed.) Current therapy in colon and rectal surgery. p. 120. B.C. Decker, Toronto, 1990.
32. Etala, E. Cirugia conservadora del esfinter anal en el cancer del recto. Dia. Med. 45:319, 1973.
33. Fain, S.N., Patin, S., Morgenstern, L. Use of mechanical suturing apparatus in low colorectal anastomosis. Arch. Surg. 110:1079, 1975.
34. Gabriel, W.B., Dukes, C.E., Bussey, H.J.R. Lymphatic spread in cancer of the rectum. Br. J. Surg. 23:395, 1935.
35. Gilchrist, R.K., David, V.C. Lymphatic spread of carcinoma of the rectum. Ann. Surg. 108:621, 1938.
36. Goligher, J.C., Graham, N.G., Dombal, F.T. Anastomotic dehiscence after anterior resection of rectum and sigmoid. Br. J. Surg. 57:9, 1970.
37. Goligher, J.C. Use of circular stapling gun with peranal insertion of anorectal purse-string suture for construction of very low colorectal or colo-anal anastomoses. Br. J. Surg. 66:501, 1979.
38. Gordon, P.H. Malignant neoplasms of the Rectum. In Gordon, P.H., Nivatvongs, S. (Eds.). Principles and practice of surgery for the colon, rectum, and anus. p. 591. Quality Medical Publishing, St. Louis, Missouri, 1992.
39. Griffen, F.D., Knight, C.D., Whitaker, J.M. The double stapling technique for low anterior resection. Ann. Surg. 211:745, 1990.
40. Grinnell, R.S. Distal intramural spread of carcinoma of the rectum and recto-sigmoid. Surg. Gynecol. Obstet. 99:421, 1954.
41. Heald, R.J., Husband, E.M., Gunselman, W., Ryall, R.D.H. The mesorectum in rectal cancer surgery, the clue to pelvic recurrence. Br. J. Surg. 69:613, 1982.
42. Heald, R.J., Ryall, R.D. Recurrence and survival after total mesorectal excision for rectal cancer. Lancet 1:1479, 1986.
43. Heald, R.J. Rectal cancer: Resection and local recurrence. A personal review. Perspect. Colon Rectal Surg. 1:1, 1986.
44. Heald, R.J. Anterior resection of the rectum. In Fielding, L.P., Goldberg, S.M. (Eds.) Surgery of the colon, rectum and anus. Ed. 5, p 456. Butterworth-Heinemann, Oxford, 1993.
45. Heberer, C., et al. Local procedure in the management of rectal cancer. World J. Surg. 11:499, 1987.
46. Hildebrandt, V., Feifel, G. Preoperative staging of rectal cancer by intrarectal ultrasound. Dis. Colon Rectum 28:42, 1985.
47. Jarvinen, H.J., Ovaska, J., Mecklin. J.P. Improvements in the treatment and prognosis of colorectal carcinoma. Br. J. Surg. 75:25, 1988.

48. Karanjia, N.D., Corder, A.P., Hodsworth, P.J., Heald, R.J. Risk of peritonitis and fatal septicemia and the need to defunction the low anastomosis. Br. J. Surg. 78:196, 1991.
49. Kirwan, W.D. Integrity of low colo-rectal E.E.A.-stapled anastomosis. Br. J. Surg. 68:539, 1981.
50. Knight, C.D., Griffen, F.D. Techniques for low rectal reconstruction. Curr. Probl. Surg. 20:391, 1983.
51. Konishi, F., Muto, T. Takahashic, et al. Transrectal ultrasonography for the assessment of invasion of rectal carcinoma. Dis. Colon Rectum 28:889, 1985.
52. Lavery, I.C., et al. Definitive management of rectal cancer by contact (endocavitary) irradiation. Dis. Colon Rectum 30:835, 1987.
53. Lazorthes, F., Fages, P., Chiotasso, P., Lemozy, J., Bloom, E. Resection of the rectum with construction of a colonic reservoir and colo-anal anastomosis for carcinoma of the rectum. Br. J. Surg. 73:136, 1986.
54. Lloyd-Davies, O.V. Lithotomy-Trendelenburg position for resection of rectum and lower pelvic colon. Lancet 2:74, 1939.
55. Localio, S.A., Eng, K., Coppa, G.F. Abdomino-sacral resection for mid rectal cancer. Ann. Surg. 198:320, 1983.
56. Lockhart-Mummery, H.D., Ritchie, J.K., Hawley, P.R. The results of surgical treatment for carcinoma of the rectum at St. Mark's Hospital from 1948 to 1972. Br. J. Surg. 63:673, 1976.
57. Madden, J.L., Kandalaft, S.I. Electrocoagulation as primary curative method in the treatment of carcinoma of the rectum. Surg. Gynecol. Obstet. 157:164, 1983.
58 Madden, J.L. Cancer of the rectum: Local treatment. In Fazio, V.W. (Ed.) Current therapy in colon and rectal surgery. p. 130. B.C. Decker, Toronto, 1990.
59. Mason, A.Y., The place of local resection in the treatment of rectal carcinoma. Proc. R. Soc. Med. 62:1259, 1970.
60. Mayo, C.W., Fly, O.A. Analysis of five year survival in carcinoma of the rectum and rectosigmoid. Surg. Gynecol. Obstet. 103:94, 1956.
61. McGinn, F.P., Gartell, P.C., Clifford, P.C., Brinton, F.J. Staples or suture for low colorectal anastomoses: A prospective randomized trial. Br. J. Surg. 72:603, 1985.
62. Morgan, L.N. Trends in the treatment of tumors of the rectum, rectosigmoid, and left colon. J. R. Coll. Surg. Edinb. 1:112, 1955.
63. Morson, B.C. Factors influencing the prognosis of early cancer of the rectum. Proc. R. Soc. Med. 59:607, 1966.
64. Morson, B.C., Dawson, I.M.P. Gastrointestinal pathology. p. 432 Blackwell, Oxford, 1972.
65. Murray, J.J., Veidenheimer, M.C. Abdominoperineal excision of the rectum. In Fielding, L.P., Goldberg, S.M. (Eds.) Surgery of the colon, rectum, and anus. Ed. 5, p. 472. Butterworth-Heinemann, Oxford, 1993.
66. Nivatvongs, S., Fang, D.T. The use of thumbtacks to stop massive presacral hemorrhage. Dis. Colon Rectum 29:589, 1986.
67. Papillon, J. Endocavitary irradiation in the curative treatment of early rectal cancer. Dis. Colon Rectum 17:172, 1974.
68. Papillon, J. Present status of radiation therapy in conservative management of rectal cancer. Radiother. Oncol. 17:275, 1990.
69. Parc, R., et al. Resection and coloanal anastomosis with colonic reservoir for rectal carcinoma. Br. J. Surg. 73:139, 1986.
70. Parks, A.G. Transanal technique in low rectal anastomosis. Proc. R. Soc. Med. 65:975, 1972
71. Parks, A.G., Percy, J.P. Resection and sutured coloanal anastomosis for rectal carcinoma. Br. J Surg 69:301, 1982.
72. Pezim, M.E., Nicholls, R. Survival after high or low ligation of the inferior mesenteric artery during curative surgery for rectal cancer. Ann. Surg. 200:729, 1984.
73. Philips, R.K.S., Hittinger, R., Blesovsky, I., Fry, J.S., Fielding, I.P. Local recurrence after curative surgery for large bowel cancer: The overall picture. Br. J. Surg. 71:12, 1983.
74. Quer, E.A., Dahlin, D.C., Mayo, C.W. Retrograde intramural spread of carcinoma of the rectum and rectosigmoid: A microscopic study. Surg. Gynecol. Obstet. 96:24, 1953.
75. Quirke, P., Dixon, M.F., Durdey, P., Williams, N,S. Local recurrence of rectal adenocarcinoma due to inadequate surgical resection. Lancet 2:996, 1986.
76. Salvati, E.P., Rubin, R.J. Electrocoagulation as primary therapy of rectal carcinoma. Am. J. Surg. 132:583, 1976.
77. Schrock, T.R., Devenely, C.W., Dunphy, J.E. Factors contributing to leakage of colonic anastomosis. Ann. Surg. 177:513, 1973.
78. Stearns, M.W., Bincley, G.E. The influence of location on prognosis in operable rectal cancer. Surg. Gynecol. Obstet. 96:368, 1953.
79. Stearns, M.W., Jr. The choice among anterior resection: The pull-through and abdominoperineal resection of the rectum. Cancer. 34:969, 1974.
80. Strauss, R.J., Friedman, M., Platt, M., Wise, L. Surgical treatment of rectal carcinoma: Results of anterior resection versus abdominoperineal resection at a community hospital. Dis. Colon Rectum 21:269, 1978.
81. Turnbull, R.B., Jr., Cuthbertson, F.M. Abdominorectal pull-through resection for cancer and for Hirschprung disease. Cleve. Clin. Q. 28:109, 1961.
82. Umpleby, H.C., Fermor, B., Symes, M.O., Williamson, R.C.N. Viability of exfoliated colo-rectal carcinoma cells. Br. J. Surg. 71:659, 1984.
83. Wangensteen, O.H. Primary resection (closed anastomosis) of rectal ampulla for malignancy with preservation of sphincteric function. Surg. Gynecol. Obstet. 81:1, 1945.
84. Waugh, J.M., Block, M.A., Gage, R.P. Three and five year survival following combined abdomino-perineal resection, abdomino-resection with sphincter preservation, and anterior resection for carcinoma of the rectum and lower part of the sigmoid colon. Ann. Surg. 142:752, 1955.
85. Welch, C.E., Ottinger, L.W., Welch, J.P. Manual of lower gastrointestinal surgery. p. 81. Springer Verlag, New York, 1980.
86. Whittaker, M., Goligher, J.C. The prognosis after surgical treatment for carcinoma of the rectum. Br. J. Surg. 63:384, 1976.
87. Williams, R.D., Yurko, A.A., Kerr, G., Zollinger, R.M. Comparison of anterior and abdomino-perineal resection for low pelvic colon and rectal cancer. Am. J. Surg. 111:114, 1966.
88. Williams, N.S., Durdey, P., Johnston, D. The outcome following sphincter-saving resection and abdominoperineal resection for low rectal cancer. Br. J. Surg. 72:595, 1983.
89. Williams, N.S., Dixon, M.E., Johnson, D. Reappraisal of the 5 cm rule of distal excision for carcinoma of the rectum: A study of distal intramural spread and of patient survival. Br. J. Surg. 70:150, 1983.
90. Williams, N.S., Johnston, D. Survival and recurrence after sphincter saving resection and abdomino-perineal resection for carcinoma of the middle third of the rectum. Br. J. Surg. 71:278, 1984.
91. Williams, N.S. The rationale for preservation of the anal sphincter in low rectal cancer. Br. J. Surg. 575:581, 1984.
92. Williams, N.S., Nasmyth, D.G., Jones, D., Smith, A.H. Defunctioning stomas: A prospective controlled trial comparing loop ileostomy with loop transverse colostomy. Br. J. Surg. 73:566, 1986.
93. Williams, N.S. Surgical treatment of rectal cancer. In Keighley, M.R.B., Williams, N.S. (Eds.) Surgery of the anus, rectum, and colon. Vol. 1, p. 939. W.B. Saunders, Philadelphia, 1993.
94. Wilson, S.M., Beahars, O.H. The curative treatment of carcinoma of the sigmoid, rectosigmoid, and rectum. Ann. Surg. 183:556, 1976.
95. Wolmark, N., Fisher, B. An analysis of survival and treatment failure following abdomino-perineal resection and sphincter-saving resection in Dukes B and C rectal carcinoma. Ann. Surg. 204:480, 1986.
96. Wood, W.Q., Wilkie, D.P.S. Carcinoma of the rectum: An anatomic pathological study. Edinb. Med. J. 40:321, 1933.
97. Zollinger, R.M., Sheppard, M.H. Carcinoma of the rectum and the rectosigmoid, a review of 729 cases. Arch. Surg. 102:335, 1971.

[illegible]

Section H

Colon, Rectum, and Anus

CHAPTER **60**

Ulcerative Colitis

GENERAL CONSIDERATIONS

Ulcerative colitis is a disease that affects the rectum and colon. The rectum is the site where the disease usually starts and where it may remain localized or extend to the colon partially (sigmoid colon, entire left colon) or completely up to the ileocecal valve (universal ulcerative colitis). The universal form of the disease affects 30% of patients. Spread of the disease in the colon is diffuse and continuous, without healthy intermediate areas, as are seen in Crohn's disease of the colon.

In 10% of patients with universal ulcerative colitis the terminal ileum may also present changes that are known as "backwash ileitis." This ileitis may extend up to the 35 cm above the ileocecal valve. However, ileitis due to ulcerative colitis does not have the clinicopathologic or prognostic importance of Crohn's disease. It is important to differentiate between both conditions to determine the most adequate therapy. It is possible to differentiate between ulcerative colitis and Crohn's disease of the colon in 85% of cases, but it is not possible in 15%. Under these circumstances the colitis is designated as indeterminate. A diagnosis of indeterminate colitis forces the adoption of a surgical posture different from that in ulcerative colitis. It has been proven that resection of the rectum and colon in ulcerative colitis definitely cures the illness, in contrast to Crohn's disease, which is a recurring illness.

Ulcerative colitis is an unspecific inflammatory process of unknown cause that in the great majority of cases only affects the mucosa and submucosa of the colon and rectum. Crohn's disease is also an inflammatory process of unspecified origin, but this inflammatory process is not limited to the mucosa and submucosa, but invades all layers of the bowel, either as a lymphoplasmocytic infiltration or in a transmural granulomatous form.

In patients with ulcerative colitis complicated by an acute, fulminating process known as toxic megacolon, the inflammatory colonic process is not limited to the mucosa and submucosa, but invades the other layers of the colon and can result in localized necrosis of the bowel with a free perforation walled off by the greater omentum, loops of small bowel, or parietal peritoneum.

From the microscopic point of view, ulcerative colitis is characterized by congestion and edema of the mucosa and submucosa with the formation of cryptic microabscesses made up by the accumulation of neutrophils that fill the crypts of Leiberkuhn. Expansion of these abscesses makes them join each other, giving rise to superficial ulcers with undermined borders. In cases of chronic ulcerative colitis with acute recurring inflammatory crises, the edges of the ulcers are invaded by an inflammatory process and granulation tissue making up the so-called pseudopolyps or inflammatory polyps that protrude from the borders of the ulcerations.

The clinical picture of ulcerative colitis is quite variable, but its most frequent presentation is that of a chronic process with alternating remissions and recurrences of variable severity and frequency. In some cases, illness or one of its reactivations may start acutely, in fulminating fashion or with a toxic megacolon.

Ulcerative colitis invades the rectum in almost all cases. It is extremely rare for the rectum to remain completely free, although it may appear to be. In Crohn's disease the rectum is involved in 50% of patients. Ulcerative colitis affects all ages but is undoubtedly more frequent from 15 to 30 years of age.

The most common symptoms of ulcerative colitis are bloody diarrhea with mucus and pus, large watery discharges with blood staining, colicky abdominal pains, fever, vomiting, weight loss, urgency, tenesmus, and, in some cases, anal incontinence. The symptomatology varies according to the extension and degree of activity of the disease.

Fifteen to twenty percent of patients affected with ulcerative colitis have anorectal complications. In Crohn's disease these complications are more frequent and more serious. Twenty-five percent of patients with ulcerative colitis have extracolonic symptoms such as erythema nodosum, pyogenic gangrenous dermatitis, arthritis, ankylosing spondylitis, ophthalmic complications, and so on.

The diagnosis of ulcerative colitis is made by the symptoms presented by the patient and by endoscopy, which usually shows a congested, granular, and very friable mucosa that bleeds easily. Rectal digital examination shows a granular or sandy mucosal surface. The finger is usually bloodstained. During periods of reactivation, the rectocolonic mucosa becomes more friable and reddish-purple in color. Biopsy of the rectocolonic mucosa, without being specific, contributes to the diagnosis. Radiographic examination, by barium enema, is of great importance in diagnosing ulcerative colitis. This examination should not be performed in patients with an acute clinical picture (acute fulminating colitis, toxic megacolon) because the colon may be perforated or become perforated by the pressure of the enema. The clinical picture is enough to make the diagnosis of toxic megacolon together with the evolution of the patient, laboratory data, and direct abdominal x-ray of the abdomen.

SURGICAL INDICATIONS

The most frequent indications for surgery in cases of ulcerative colitis are due to the patient becoming refractory to well-conducted medical treatment. In other cases the patient does not tolerate medications, is extremely weak, is very thin, has bloody diarrhea and anal incontinence, or is incapacitated in performing ordinary tasks. Children stop growing, there are intolerable perianal complications, there is severe progressive dysplasia of the colorectal mucosa or the presence of one or more colorectal carcinomas, and so on. Less frequently, surgery has to be done for an acute complication, such as fulminating acute colitis, toxic megacolon, colonic perforation, or massive bleeding.

Surgical Procedures Available in the Treatment of Ulcerative Colitis

The following procedures are available at present for the treatment of ulcerative colitis:

1. Total proctocolectomy with Brooke ileostomy.
2. Total colectomy with ileorectal anastomosis.
3. Subtotal colectomy with mucus fistula and Brooke ileostomy.
4. Total proctocolectomy with continent Kock ileostomy.
5. Lateral ileostomy and decompressive colostomy (Turnbull "blowhole" technique).
6. Colonic resection with upper part of rectum, anorectal mucosectomy, and ileal reservoir with ileoanal anastomosis (restorative proctocolectomy).

Total proctocolectomy with Brooke ileostomy

This procedure consists of resection of the entire colon and rectum with the construction of a permanent Brooke ileostomy. The procedure is a cure for patients with ulcerative colitis and has low morbidity and mortality. This is considered to be a classic procedure in the treatment of ulcerative colitis and is a model in the evaluation of other surgical procedures. Total proctocolectomy with Brooke ileostomy has stood the test of time.

At present the tendency is to perform this procedure less frequently and use restorative proctocolectomy more frequently, which is well accepted by patients since it reestablishes normal intestinal transit by anastomosing an ileal reservoir with the anal canal. For this reason total proctocolectomy with Brooke ileostomy is indicated less frequently. Some of these indications are the following:

1. Patients in very poor general condition.
2. Patients over 60 years old.
3. Patients with a weak anal sphincter.
4. Patients who are not willing to accept the possibility of reoperations.
5. Patients with a doubtful diagnosis of Crohn's disease.
6. Patients who want the safest, simplest, and most definitive procedures with the least number of complications.
7. Patients with many years of suffering with ulcerative colitis. These usually accept total proctocolectomy with Brooke ileostomy readily.

Total proctocolectomy with Brooke ileostomy will be described later.

Total colectomy with ileorectal anastomosis

This procedure is used infrequently in very selected patients. Aylett, of London (2, 3), has published very good results with this technique in 300 patients. If selection of patients for this procedure has not been very rigorous, the patients will undergo great suffering. This procedure is indicated in young patients with good anal continence, but, as previously stated, patients with ulcerative colitis rarely have a normal rectum and the inflammation may become reactivated, causing uncontrollable daily and nightly diarrhea, incontinence, loss of fecal matter and mucus, and so on. Patients with this procedure should be very carefully followed with endoscopy and biopsy because they may develop severe dysplasia or rectal cancer.

Subtotal colectomy with mucus fistula and Brooke ileostomy

This procedure is usually indicated in patients in poor general condition, particularly with acute complications, who need to be operated on urgently for fulminating colitis or toxic megacolon. This procedure consists of resection of the entire colon except the distal sigmoid colon, which will be used to establish a mucus fistula. The procedure is completed with a Brooke ileostomy. The advantages of this technique are several:

1. It is less complicated than total proctocolectomy.
2. It is less serious and risky.
3. Since it preserves the rectum and anus, the possibility always exists of reestablishment of normal intestinal transit by means of an ileoanal pouch.
4. Since the rectum is not resected, dissection of this organ during full inflammatory activity, with the possibility of injury to pelvic nerves and consequent problems with erection and functional bladder problems, can be avoided.
5. If a mucus fistula using the sigmoid colon is to be avoided, the sigmoid end can be closed manually or mechanically, implanting it in the abdominal wall, in the subcutaneous layer, suturing the aponeurosis of the abdominal wall under it and the skin over it.

This is the most indicated procedure if a mucus fistula using sigmoid colon is not established. It is not advisable to do a Hartmann procedure, which consists of suturing the sigmoid end (or the rectal end) and dropping it in the peritoneal or pelvic cavity, in ulcerative colitis. The colitis produces great secretion of mucus, which increases the pressure in the sigmoid colon with dehiscence of the suture line of the sigmoid colon into the peritoneal or pelvic cavity. If the colonic end is implanted in the subcutaneous tissue, dehiscence of the suture line and spillage of intestinal contents will not be serious. On the other hand, the rectum and colon should be examined periodically by endoscopy and biopsy for the possibility of development of severe dysplasia or cancer.

Total proctocolectomy with continent Kock ileostomy

This procedure was proposed by Nils Kock, of Sweden, in 1969, to replace the Brooke colostomy (12) with a continent ileostomy. The continent Kock ileostomy consists of a reservoir constructed from the terminal ileum (Kock's reservoir or Kock's pouch) and provided with a nipple valve to prevent spontaneous emptying of accumulated intestinal content from the pouch. The fundamental purpose pursued by Kock was that the patient would not have to wear a permanent ileostomy appliance, which is indispensable in the Brooke ileostomy.

The Kock reservoir was proposed with great enthusiasm by its author and was accepted in surgical centers of Europe and the United States, where patients with ulcerative colitis concentrate (28, 31, 39, 42, 45, 50, 51, 98). However, the Kock reservoir did not stand the test of time. Many complications developed with the procedure, and many modifications of the original Kock technique were introduced to diminish complications.

The Kock reservoir has a capacity of 500 to 600 mL. If the reservoir functions correctly, it should be emptied 3 or 4 times a day. According to Kock, if the patient has become adapted to the reservoir, it won't be necessary to empty it during the night.

Some of the numerous immediate and late complications of the continent Kock ileostomy are the following: peritonitis, dehiscence of the reservoir's suture lines, necrosis of the exit ileostomy, intestinal obstruction, malfunction of the valve, incontinence, obstruction, eversion, fistulas, separation of the reservoir from the abdominal wall, and so on. About 30% of cases with a Kock ileostomy have to be reoperated (19). At present it is difficult to justify a Kock reservoir. Most patients prefer an ileal pelvic reservoir anastomosed to the anal canal because it preserves normal sphincteric function (18, 19, 42, 44, 45, 98).

Some of the very limited indications for a continent Kock ileostomy at present are:

1. Patients who should be subjected to total proctocolectomy but do not accept wearing a permanent ileostomy bag.
2. Patients who have not been able to adapt to a previously performed total proctocolectomy with Brooke ileostomy.
3. Cases of failure of an ileocecal pouch.

The technique of a continent Kock ileostomy will be described later.

Lateral ileostomy and decompressive colostomy (Turnbull "blowhole" technique)

This technique was described by Turnbull and colleagues of the Cleveland Clinic in the United States (93) for the treatment of toxic megacolon with walled off perforation. The object of this procedure is to detour the fecal stream by means of a loop ileostomy and decompress the dilated transverse colon by means of a colostomy through a small incision in the abdominal wall. This simple, atraumatic, fast procedure (68) prepares the patient for a later resection of the perforated colon.

At present the diagnosis of toxic megacolon is usually made earlier. Early surgery is accepted if the patient does not improve with medical therapy. There is no doubt that powerful antibiotics against colonic flora are available. For these reasons we have become convinced that total colectomy is the best procedure for toxic perforated walled off megacolon and not the Turnbull procedure (69). However, a small number of patients can benefit from the Turnbull operation:

1. Patients with multiple walled off colonic perforations.
2. Patients in precarious general condition, which leads the surgeon to perform a lesser procedure.
3. Patients with a very high and dilated splenic flexure in addition to a walled off perforation.
4. Lack of experience by the surgeon. If the surgeon, upon entering the abdomen, senses a fecal odor or observes pus in the peritoneal cavity, he or she should proceed with resection of the perforated colon.

In conclusion, the surgeon should select the best procedure according to the findings, with the abdomen open (68).

The Turnbull technique, even though infrequently used, should be available to surgeons for urgent cases. Therefore, this technique will be described later.

Resection of the colon and upper rectum, anorectal mucosectomy, and ileal reservoir with ileoanal anastomosis (restorative proctocolectomy)

An alternative to classical proctocolectomy with permanent ileostomy that is becoming more widely accepted is the restorative proctocolectomy, which consists of total resection of the colon with mobilization of the proximal two thirds of the rectum, resection of 4 to 6 cm of rectal mucosa above the pectinate line, and construction of an ileal reservoir, which is anastomosed to the anal canal. As a precautionary procedure, a loop ileostomy is performed 25 to 30 cm above the ileal reservoir. This procedure removes diseased tissue, maintaining intestinal continuity and anal continence.

This operation is indicated in patients with ulcerative colitis who are in good general condition and whose anal sphincter functions normally. Patients with a weak anal sphincter and patients with perineal complications such as fistulas or abscesses cannot be subjected to this procedure. Patients with suspicion of Crohn's disease should also be excluded.

The patient should be informed that, after the procedure, anorectal function will be different. Once the period of adaptation is over, patients who undergo this procedure have 4 to 8 bowel movements daily, and frequently have diarrhea and fecal or mucoid discharges at night or during daytime, with incontinence at times. The period of adaptation may be prolonged, lasting 6 to 12 months, or even longer.

Reestablishment of ileoanal transit is done by construction of ileoanal reservoirs that are anastomosed to the anal canal. Many reservoirs have been designed, with multiple variations of shape and size. The most frequently used ileal reservoirs are the following:

1. J-pouch. Utsunomiya and colleagues (95, 96).
2. S-pouch. Parks and Nicholls (70, 71).
3. H-pouch. Fonkalsrud (33–37).
4. W-pouch. Nicholls and Lubowski (65).

The J-pouch is performed more frequently because it is easier, uses up less ileum, and empties easily, and because it is seldom necessary to empty it by transanal catheterization. The J-pouch can, however, present some inconveniences:

1. Because it is small, it may lead to 2 or 3 daily bowel movements more than the S- or W-pouch.

2. In some patients it is difficult or impossible to bring the elbow of the J-pouch down to the anal canal to be able to perform the anastomosis without tension.
3. In some cases mobilization of the mesentery may elongate it sufficiently to make an anastomosis, without tension, to the anal canal.
4. A different type of pouch should be used if it is not possible to carry out an anastomosis without tension. This is why it is necessary that the surgeon have some experience in constructing other pouches.

It is convenient that the surgeon know, at least, how to construct a J-pouch and an S-pouch, which rarely present any difficulty in reaching the anal canal without tension.

To construct a J-pouch, 30 cm of terminal ileum are needed, 15 cm for each arm of the J. The arms of the J should not be longer than 15 cm, since that may favor development of pouchitis. The anastomosis of the J-pouch to the anal canal is made with the elbow or bottom of the J, that is to the pouch itself. This is very important to make spontaneous emptying easier. The J-pouch can be realized with manual suturing or by mechanical means, with a GIA instrument. The instrument is introduced through a small enterotomy in each arm of the J and applied in both directions.

The S-pouch has greater capacity than the J-pouch and can usually be carried down to the pelvis without difficulty. However, the S-pouch may be difficult to empty and a transanal catheter may be necessary. It has been shown that the shorter the outlet arm, the less likely the need for catheterization. For this reason, the outlet arm should not be more than 2 cm long. The S-pouch uses 40 cm of terminal ileum pleated in three segments with an S configuration. Each segment of the S-pouch has a length of 12 cm. Parks made each segment 15 cm long. Some surgeons make each segment 10 cm long. Parks made the outlet arm 5 cm long. As previously stated, the shorter the outlet arm of the pouch, the lower the possibility of retention and the need for catheterization. For this reason the outlet arm is kept 2 cm long. Anastomosis of the pleated ileal segments is done manually or with mechanical sutures.

The H-reservoir is constructed by anastomosing, in side-to-side isoperistaltic fashion, two 12-cm-long loops of ileum. Fonkalsrud emphasizes that the loops be oriented in isoperistaltic fashion to make it possible to empty the pouch spontaneously, without having to catheterize it. The efferent segment of the pouch that is to be anastomosed to the anal canal is 1 to 2 cm long. Surgeons who use this pouch prefer it for the following reasons:

1. It is easier to construct.
2. It has less mesentery.
3. It uses a mobile segment of bowel to be anastomosed to the anal canal.
4. It rarely presents emptying problems.

The W-pouch uses the terminal 50 cm of ileum, pleated in four 12-cm-long segments each, which, when sutured, take up a W shape, making a pouch of greater capacity. It is also known as a quadruple W-pouch. According to Nicholls and Plezim (64), this pouch leads to less numerous daily evacuations.

Complications

Restorative proctocolectomy has a mortality similar to total proctocolectomy with Brooke ileostomy but with more complications. Some of these are bowel obstruction, dehiscence of suture lines, sepsis in the space between the reservoir and the muscular wall of the rectum, abscesses, perianal infections, pelvis infections, ileoperineal or ileovaginal fistulas, pelvic sepsis, strictures, pouchitis, nocturnal incontinence (5–6% of cases), and failure of the procedure (5–10% of cases). The technique for restorative proctocolectomy will be described later.

SURGICAL TECHNIQUE

Total Proctocolectomy with Brooke Ileostomy

This procedure is curative for ulcerative colitis but has the inconvenience of a permanent ileostomy. The operation consists of resection of the entire colon, rectum, and anus, and construction of a Brooke ileostomy.

The site for the ileostomy has to be carefully selected before the operation, making the necessary tests with the patient sitting and lying down. The ileostomy should be placed below the waistline, far from osseous prominences, skin folds, scars, and the umbilicus. During this selection the patient's constitutional habitus and occupation must be kept in mind. The best site for an ileostomy is the right ileal fossa, through the anterior abdominal rectus muscle. The colon should be prepared in similar fashion as that described in Chapters 48 and 49.

The patient is placed in a modified lithotomy position (Lloyd-Davies), which allows two surgical teams to operate simultaneously. Before the operation is begun, the anus is closed with two purse string sutures placed inside the intersphincteric sulcus to keep contamination to a minimum, since it is an important factor in healing of the perineal wound.

Total Proctocolectomy with Brooke Ileostomy

FIGURE 60.1
This figure shows that a left paramedian incision has been made, above and below the umbilicus, which is the incision used by the author in total proctocolectomy with Brooke ileostomy because this incision is father away from the ileostomy than the midline incision.

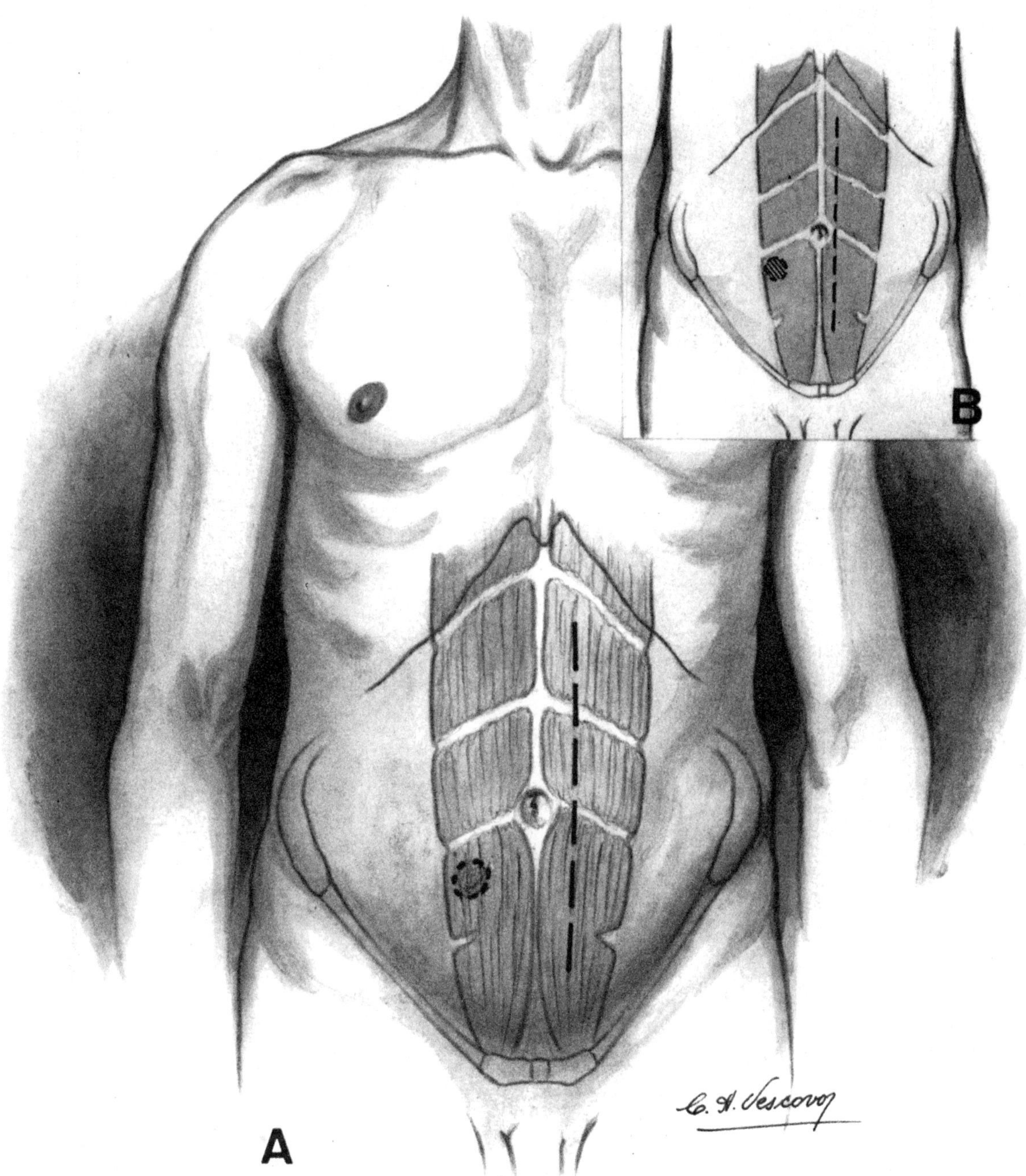

FIGURE 60.1

Total Proctocolectomy with Brooke Ileostomy

FIGURE 60.2
The extent of the total proctocolectomy with ileostomy is shown. The anal incision will pass through the intersphincteric sulcus.

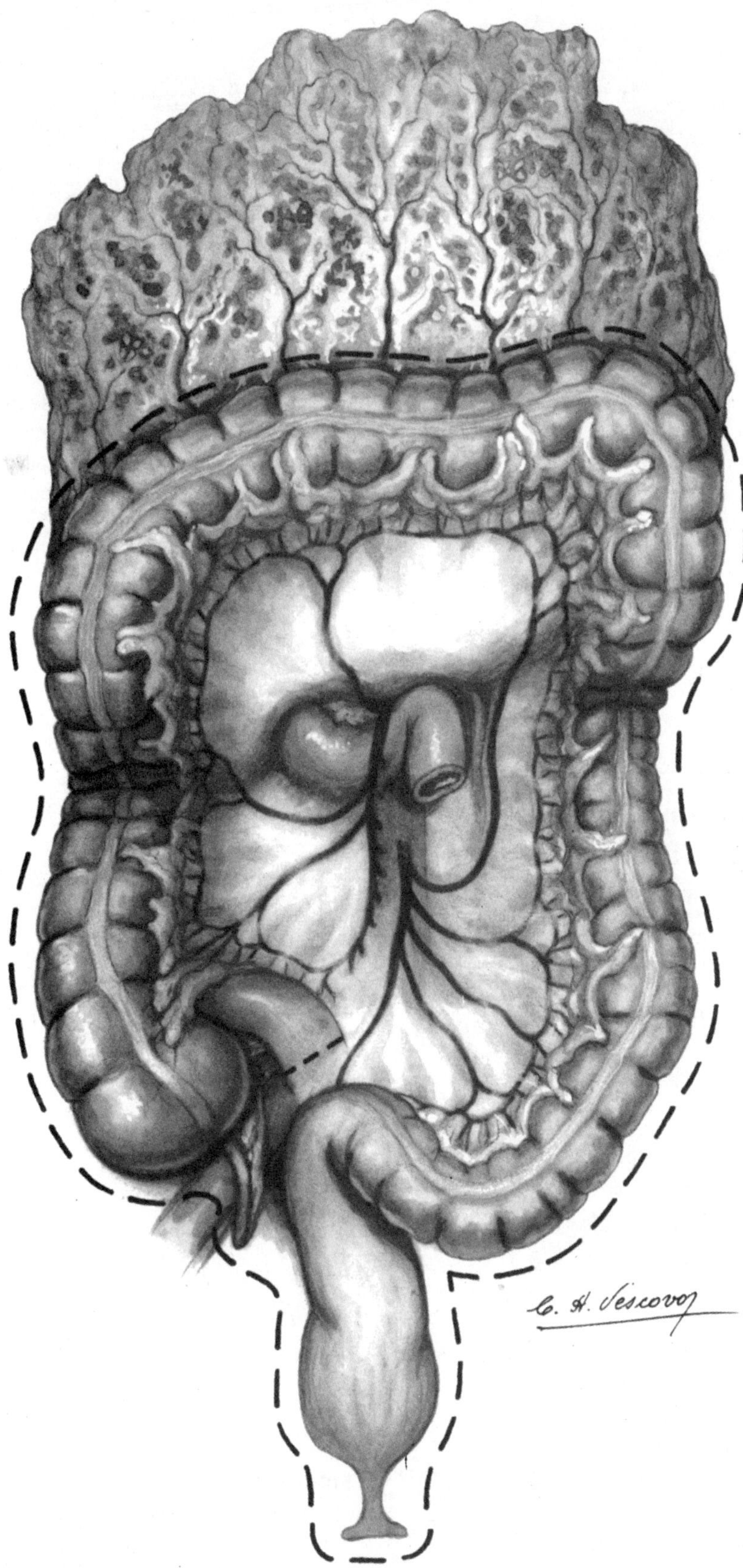

FIGURE 60.2

FIGURE 60.3
The greater omentum is being separated from the transverse colon, using scissors. If the surgeon uses the correct tissue plane, this separation is practically bloodless. Many surgeons prefer to remove the omentum because they believe it may increase the incidence of bowel obstruction, which has never proven to be true. On the other hand, the greater omentum's protective function is well known.

Total Proctocolectomy with Brooke Ileostomy

FIGURE 60.4
The total proctocolectomy is begun by freeing the right hemicolon. The first assistant applies traction to the right hemicolon toward the left side of the patient with both hands to expose the right parietocolic space. The surgeon transects the peritoneum along the white line of Toldt.

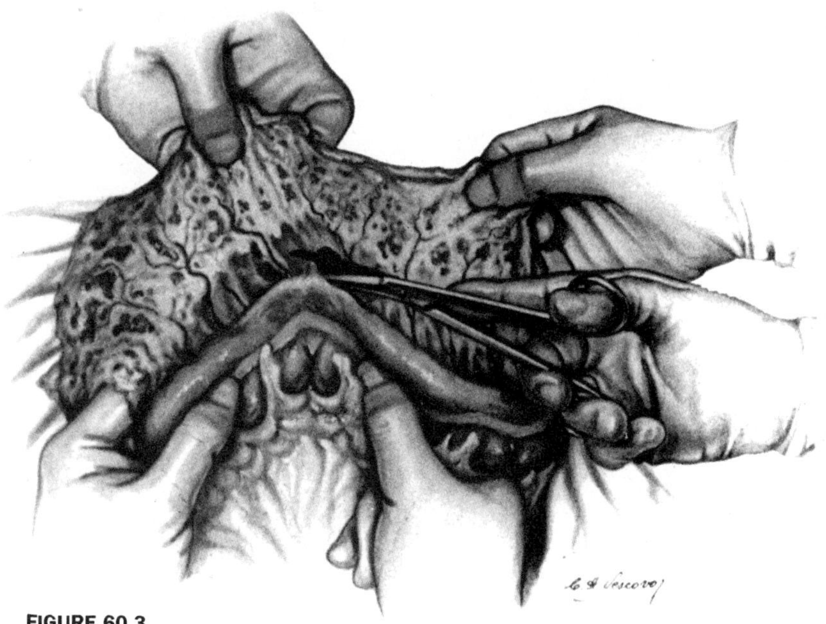

FIGURE 60.3

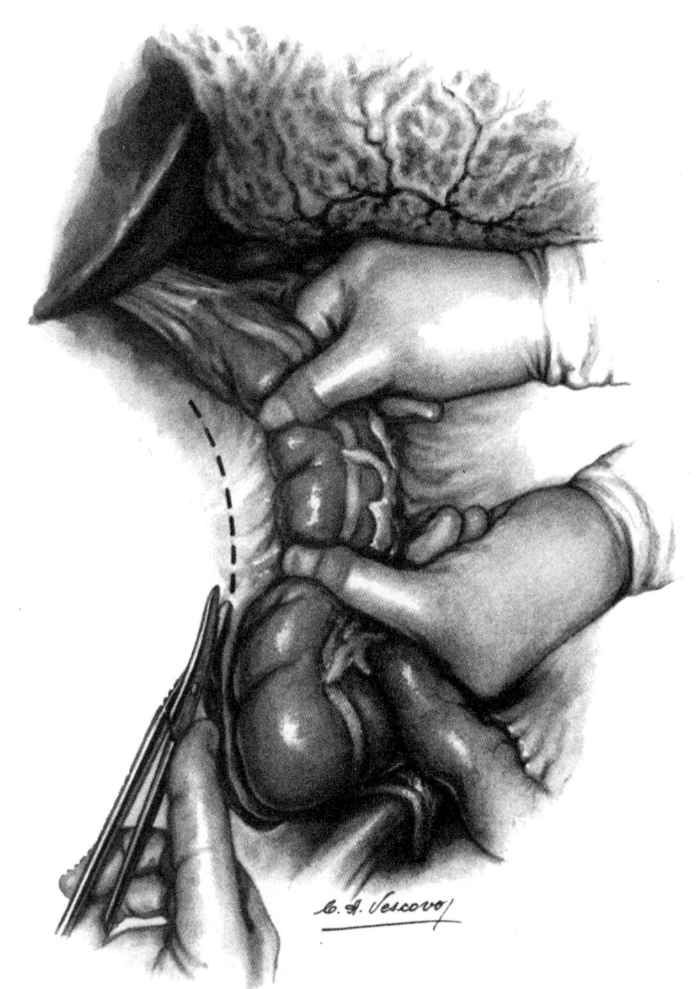

FIGURE 60.4

Total Proctocolectomy with Brooke Ileostomy

FIGURE 60.5
Once the cecum and ascending colon have been liberated, the surgeon proceeds with liberation of the hepatic flexure of the colon by transecting the hepatophrenocolic ligament with scissors.

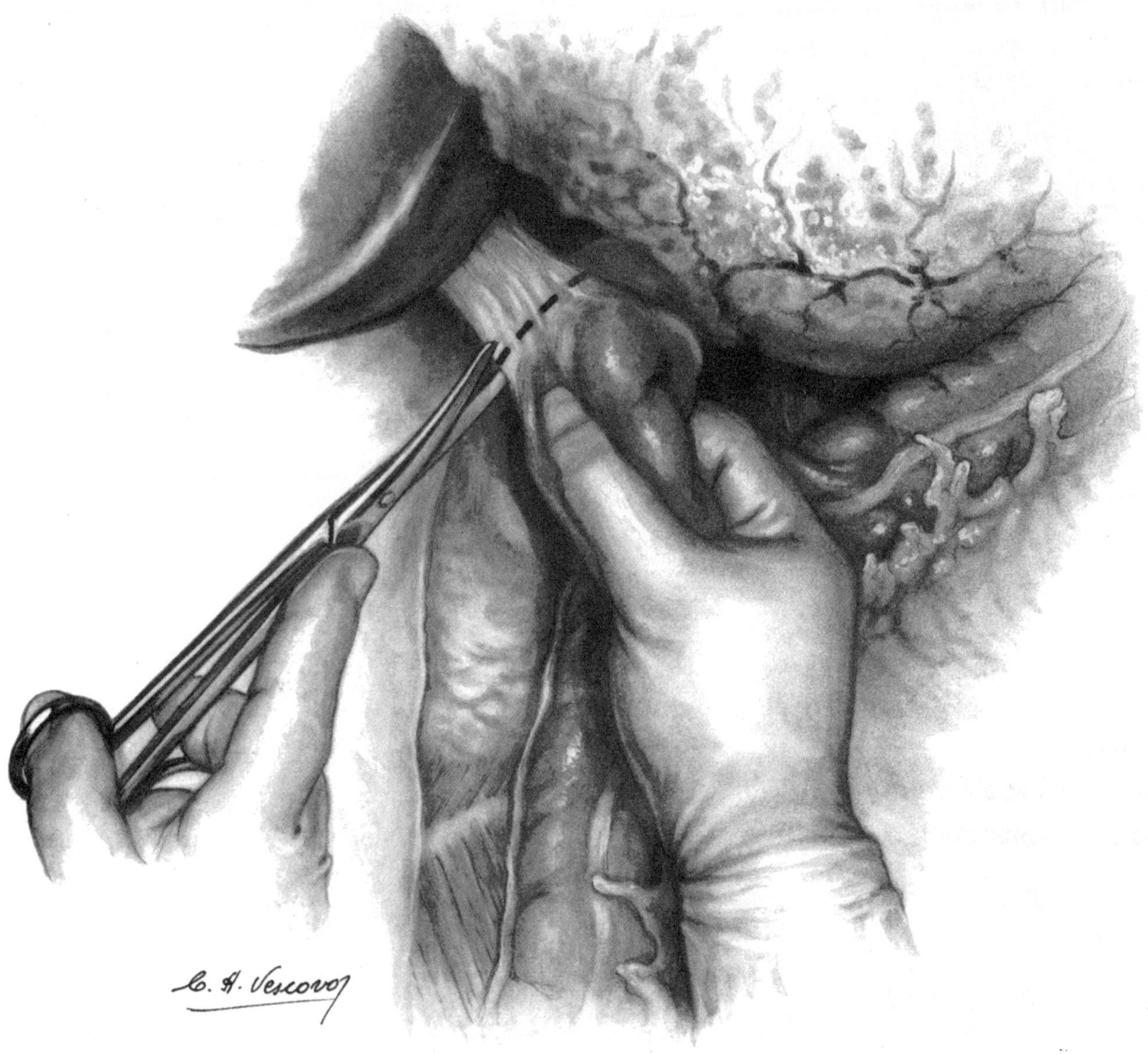

FIGURE 60.5

Total Proctocolectomy with Brooke Ileostomy

FIGURE 60.6
The left hemicolon has been liberated by transecting the left parietocolic peritoneum along the white line of Toldt. It is possible to observe the left ureter and gonadal vessels.

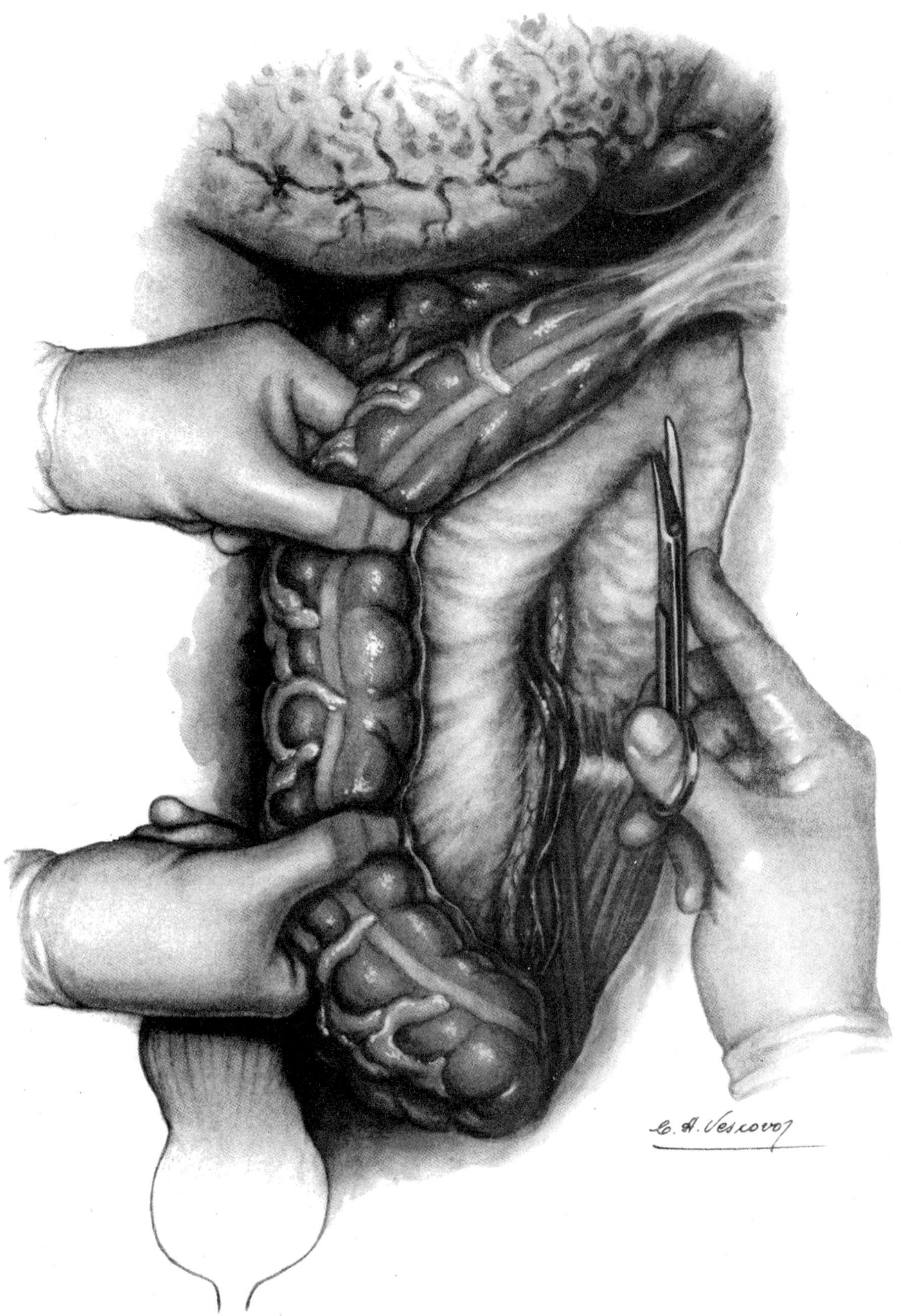

FIGURE 60.6

Total Proctocolectomy with Brooke Ileostomy

FIGURE 60.7

Before starting to liberate the splenic flexure, the transverse colon and the descending colon have been completely liberated. In addition, the splenocolic ligament has been previously ligated and transected to prevent rupture of the splenic capsule, by traction, with its consequent hemorrhage. The surgeon grasps the splenic flexure with the left hand and applies gentle traction downward and to the right, exposing the phrenocolic ligament, which is to be divided.

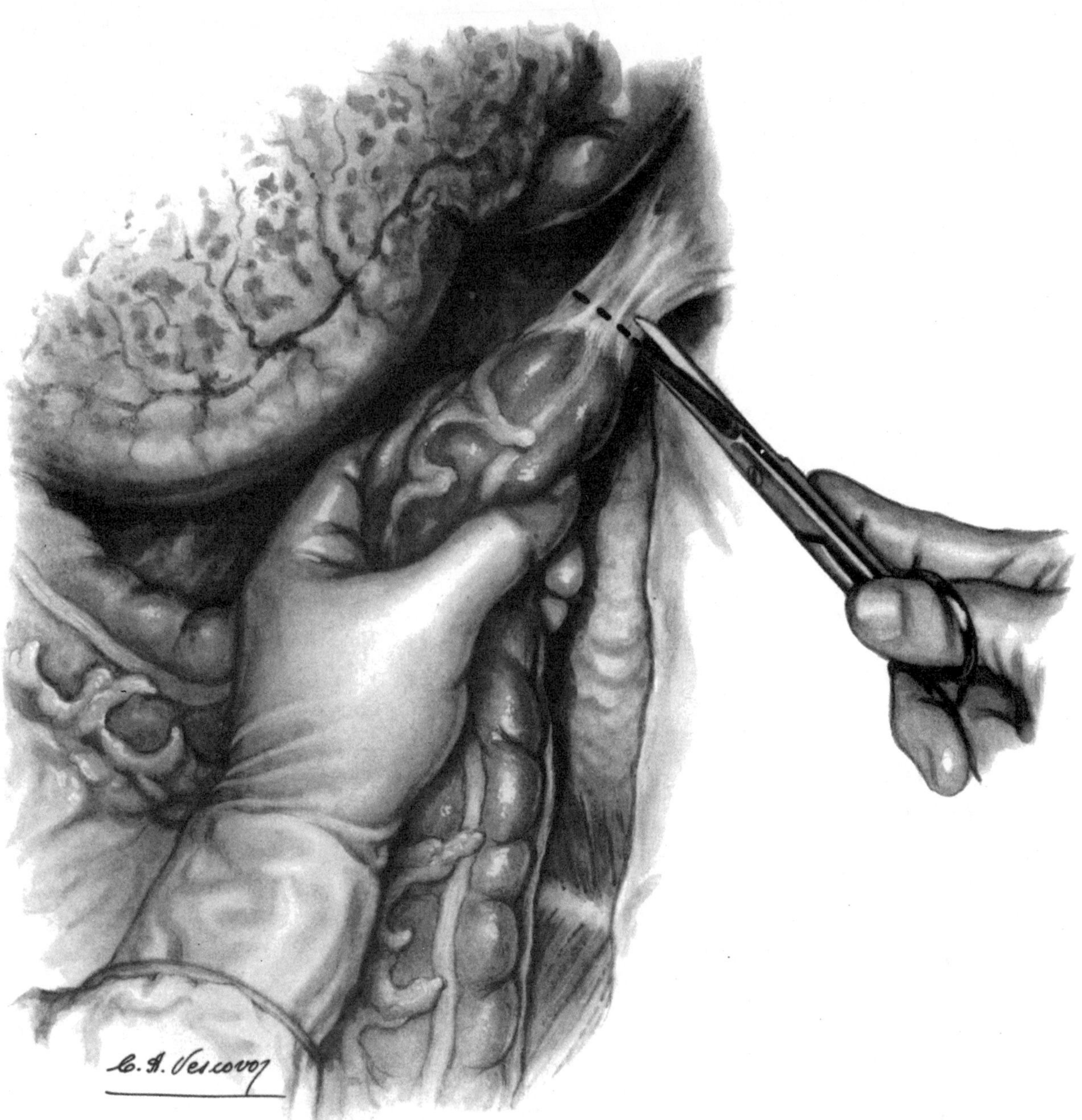

FIGURE 60.7

Total Proctocolectomy with Brooke Ileostomy

FIGURE 60.8
The drawing shows the blood vessels supplying the cecum and the ascending and transverse colon. Heavy lines show the site of ligation of the left hemicolon and the rest of the rectum. As can be seen, the vascular ligatures are not performed in the root of the mesentery as in rectocolonic cancer surgery.

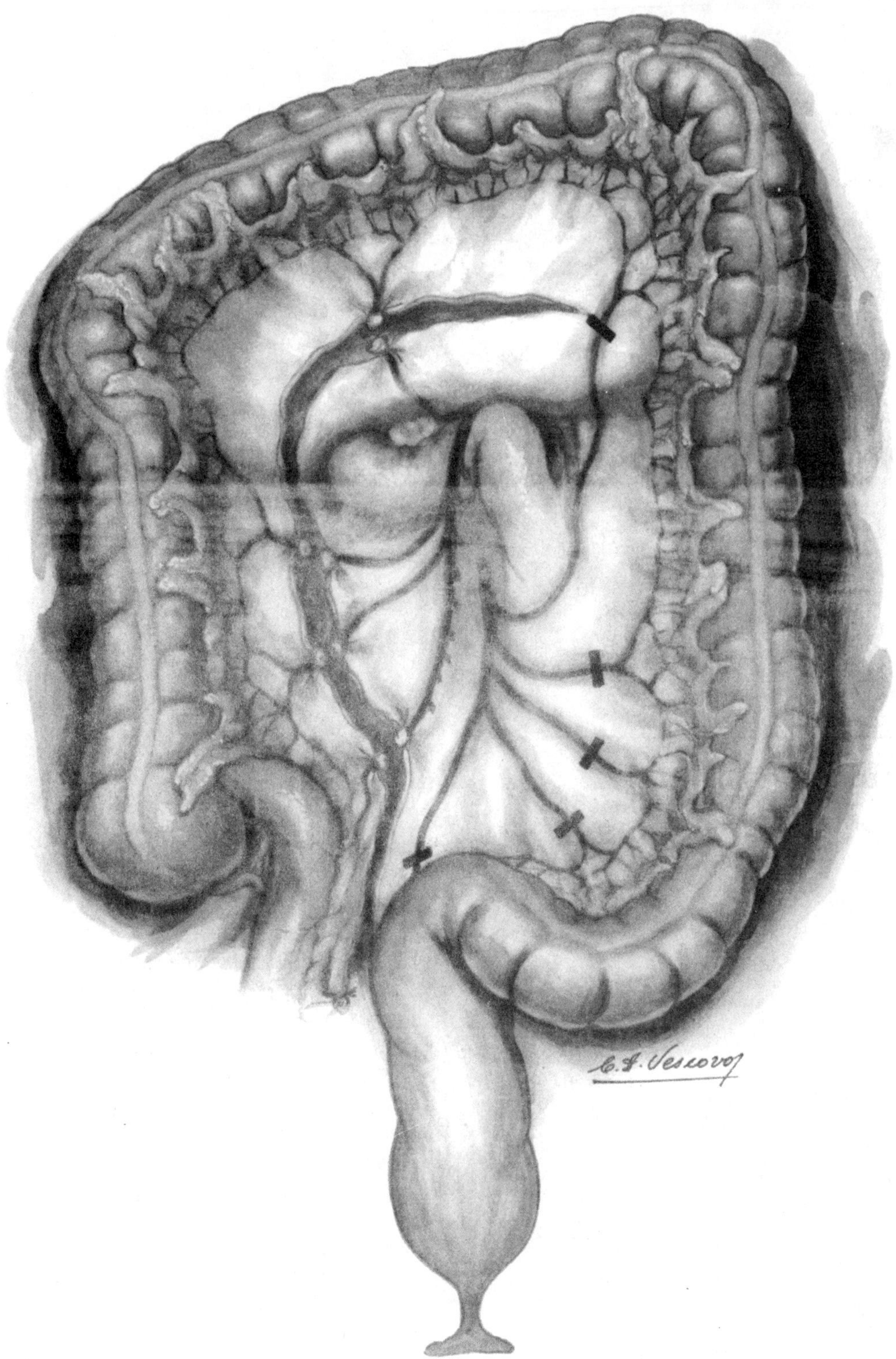

FIGURE 60.8

Total Proctocolectomy with Brooke Ileostomy

FIGURE 60.9

Liberation of the rectum is about to start. The inferior mesenteric artery should not be ligated at its origin in the aorta. The superior rectal (or hemorrhoidal) artery should be divided below the aortic bifurcation and near the rectal wall, to avoid injuring the superior pelvic sympathetic plexus and the nervi erigentes.

Dissection behind the rectum should be performed with scissors, down to the tip of the coccyx, after dividing Waldeyer's fascia, staying anterior to the nervi erigentes. Dissection anterior to the rectum is done transecting the fascia of Denonvilliers, staying close to the rectal wall. During this dissection, injury to the seminal vesicles should be avoided. Dissection should reach the prostate in the male and the vagina in the female. Laterally, rectal dissection is performed by dividing the lateral ligaments close to the rectal wall. Dissection of the rectum should extend down to the levator ani muscles.

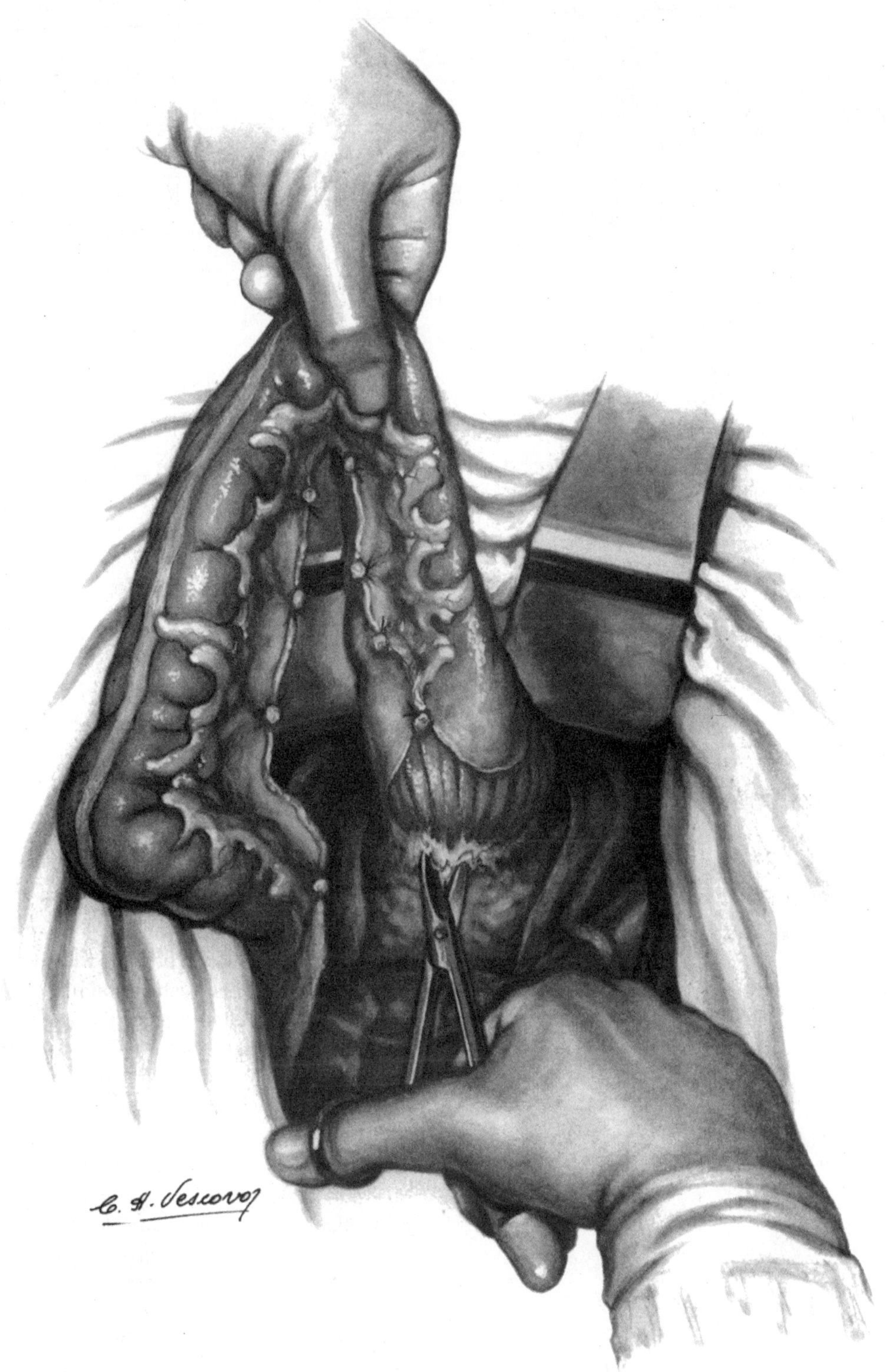

FIGURE 60.9

Total Proctocolectomy with Brooke Ileostomy

FIGURE 60.10

The perineal resection in patients with ulcerative colitis is done in much more limited fashion than in patients with cancer of the rectum. As stated before, the anus was closed with two purse string sutures placed inside the intersphincteric sulcus. An incision is made in the intersphincteric sulcus and the rectum dissected posteriorly and laterally up to the levator muscles. Anteriorly, rectal dissection should be kept inside the anterior border of the superficial transverse perineal muscle. In the lateral section shown in the drawing, the planes of dissection of the rectum for ulcerative colitis can be seen. Anorectal dissection is started at the intersphincteric line, marked with arrows running upward. The solid arrows pointing downward show the rectal dissection done by the abdominal surgeon. The levator ani muscles are transected close to the rectum. The broken lines show the plane of resection of the perineum in rectal cancer.

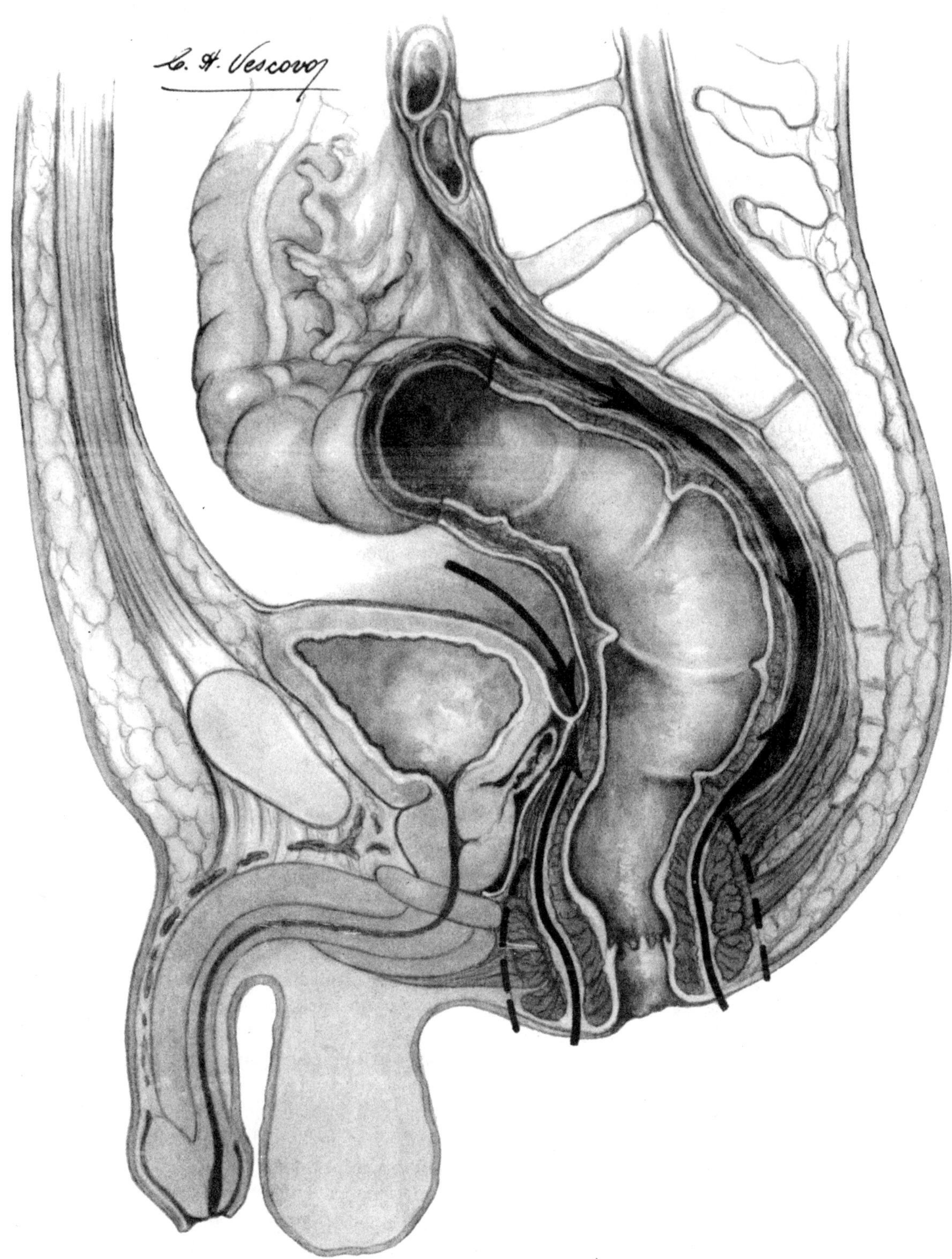

FIGURE 60.10

FIGURE 60.11
The drawing shows the dissection between the internal and external sphincter (intersphincteric division).

Total Proctocolectomy with Brooke Ileostomy

FIGURE 60.12
After liberating the colon and the upper rectum, the abdominal surgeon transects the terminal ileum (see Figure 60.13). After freeing the perineal rectum, the surgeon removes the surgical specimen. The abdominal surgeon sutures the pelvis peritoneum while the perineal surgeon thoroughly controls perineal bleeding. After the abdominal surgeon has completed suturing the pelvic peritoneum, the perineal surgeon thoroughly irrigates the perineal cavity, using warm saline solution to better visualize bleeding points so they can be more completely controlled. Two drainage tubes are then placed in the presacral space and are brought out the skin on both sides of the wound. The levator ani muscles are then sutured with absorbable material (A). Later, the skin is closed with interrupted sutures and the drainage tubes joined and connected to a closed continuous suction (B). When hemostasis has been satisfactory and contamination kept at a minimum, the levator ani muscles can be sutured, if continuous closed suction to the presacral space is added. If hemostasis was incomplete or if contamination could not be avoided, it is not advisable to suture the levator ani muscles or the perineal skin, and the wound should be left open, packed with gauze, so it will close by secondary intention. In cases in which there has been contamination, intersphincteric dissection of the perineum should not be performed and the dissection should be carried out on the outside of the external anal sphincter.

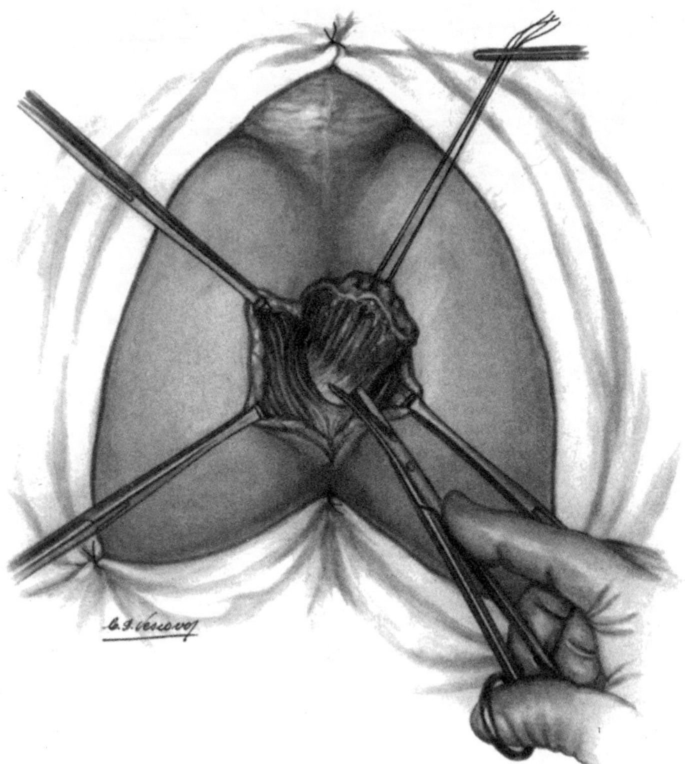

FIGURE 60.11

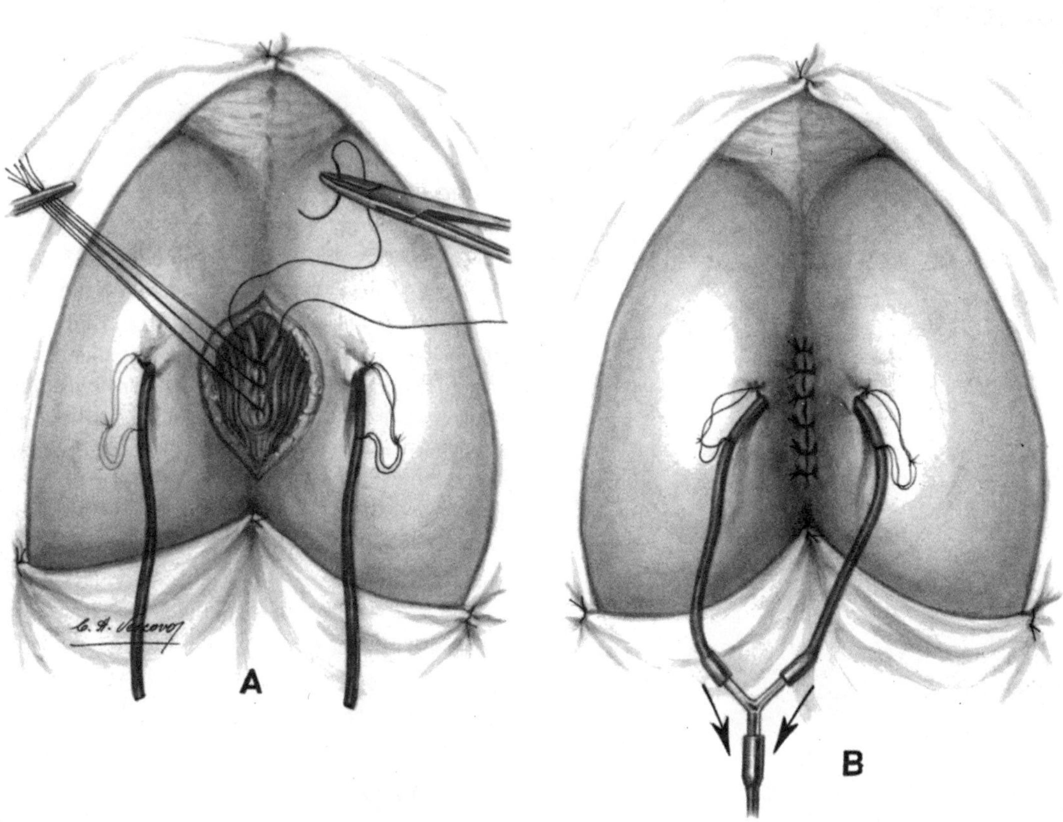

FIGURE 60.12

Total Proctocolectomy with Brooke Ileostomy

FIGURE 60.13

Once the colon and rectum have been liberated, the abdominal surgeon transects the terminal ileum 6 to 8 cm from the ileocecal valve. A clamp has been placed in the distal side of the ileum and an atraumatic clamp placed proximally. Some surgeons use the GIA instrument to transect and suture the ileum. Many surgeons transect the ileum more proximally. In cases of "backwash ileitis," some surgeons transect the ileum further away from the ileocecal valve. It has been shown that, if the patient has ulcerative colitis and the lesion in the ileum is "backwash ileitis," it is not necessary to get away from the ileocecal valve because the ileal lesion will heal readily after total proctocolectomy. If there is any doubt about the possible presence of Crohn's disease, the ileostomy should be performed in a healthy part of the terminal ileum.

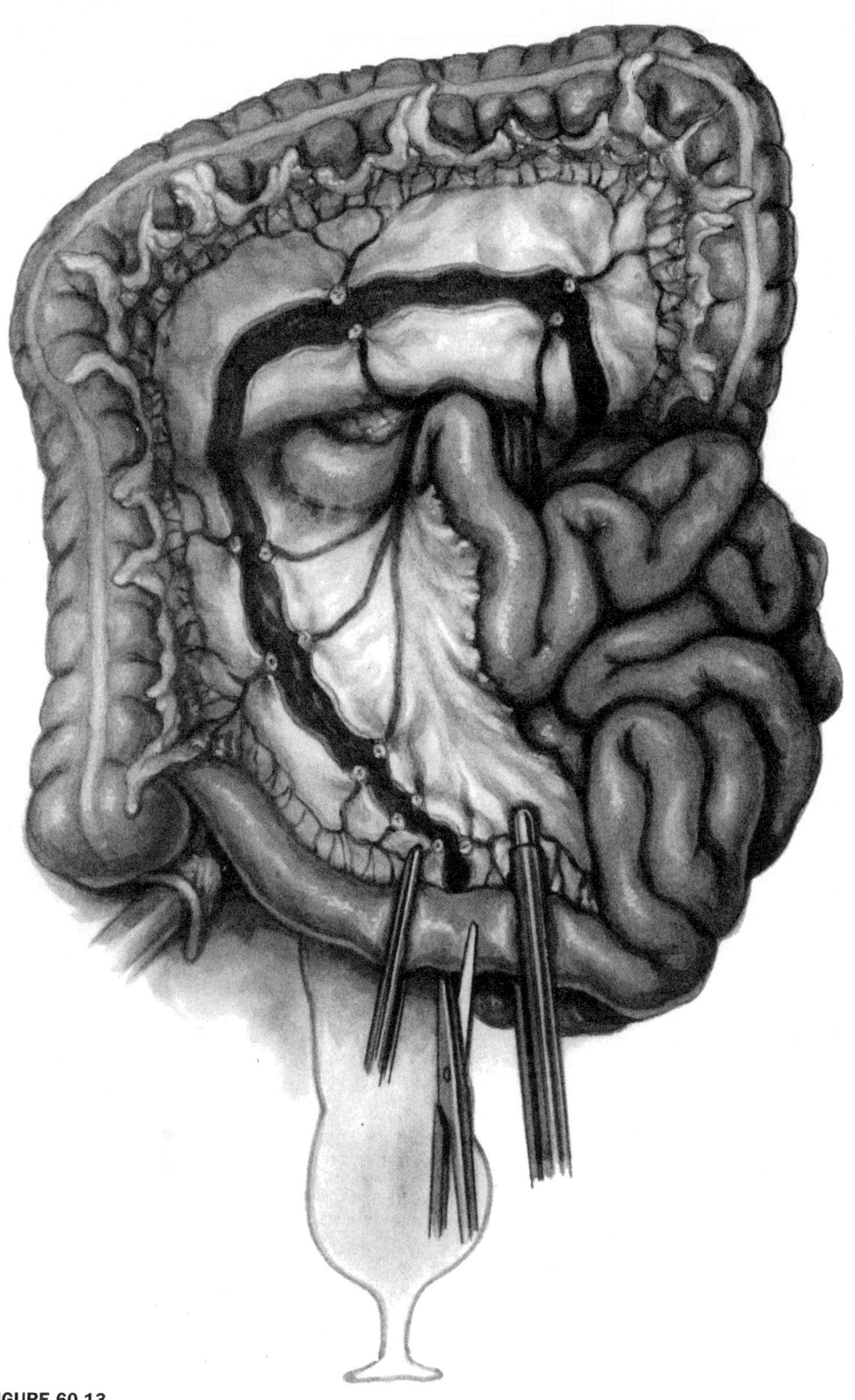

FIGURE 60.13

FIGURE 60.14

A, Once the ileum is transected, an opening is made at the selected site in the abdominal wall for the construction of a Brooke ileostomy. **B** and **C,** A disk of skin and subcutaneous tissue 2 cm in diameter is excised. **D,** The anterior fascia of the rectus muscle is incised longitudinally. **E,** The muscle fibers of the anterior rectus muscle are split and some are partially transected. **F,** Two fingers should pass comfortably through this opening.

Total Proctocolectomy with Brooke Ileostomy

FIGURE 60.15

The terminal ileum is passed through the opening, covered with a rubber sheet held in place with a Babcock clamp.

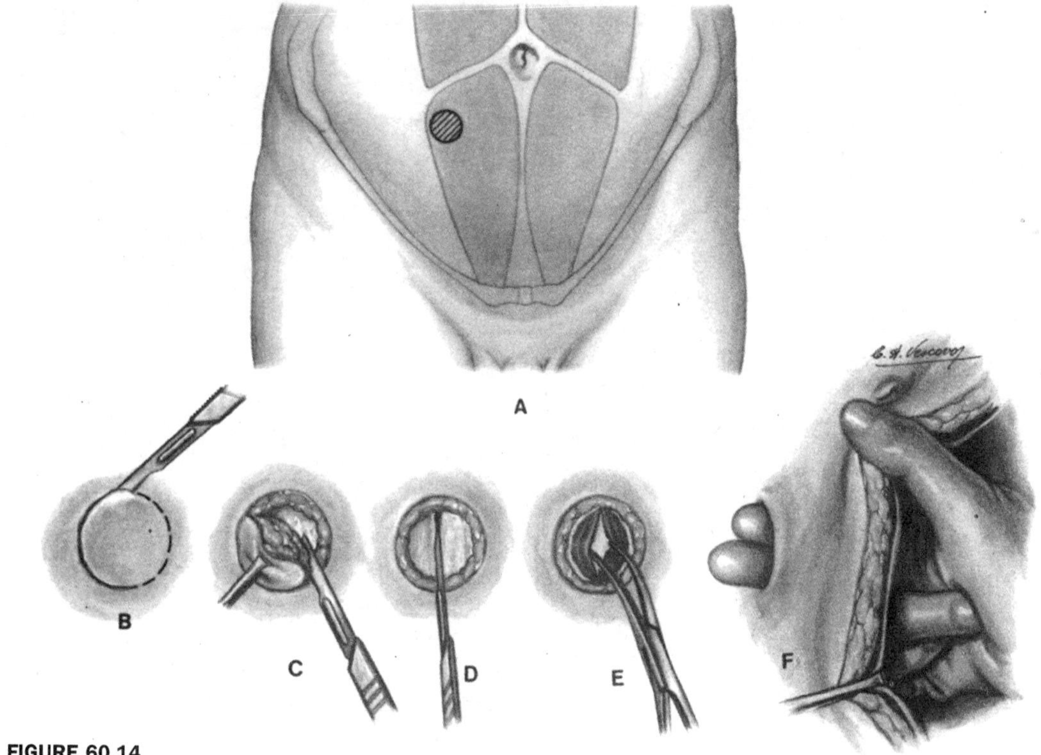

FIGURE 60.14

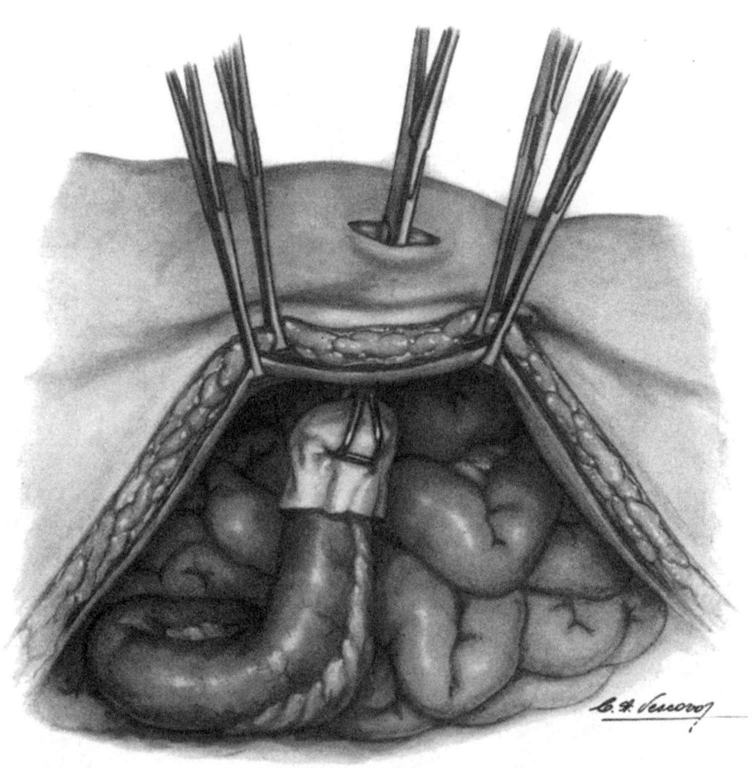

FIGURE 60.15

FIGURE 60.16
The ileum has been exteriorized 5 cm above the skin level, still covered with rubber sheet held with a Babcock clamp. The border of the peritoneum is being sutured to the edge of the mesentery with nonabsorbable interrupted sutures.

Total Proctocolectomy with Brooke Ileostomy

FIGURE 60.17
The ileum has been exteriorized about 5 cm above the skin level and is held by two Babcock clamps. **A,** The mesentery is sutured to the anterior rectus muscle fascia with two sutures. Two Babcock clamps have been introduced into the lumen of tne ileum to apply traction to the mucosa and evert the ileum. **B,** The edges of the ileum are being sutured to the edges of the skin using 2-0 chromic catgut. Some surgeons use the subcuticular layer of skin. **C,** The ileum has been sutured to the skin of the abdominal orifice. **D,** View of a section showing the eversion of the ileum.

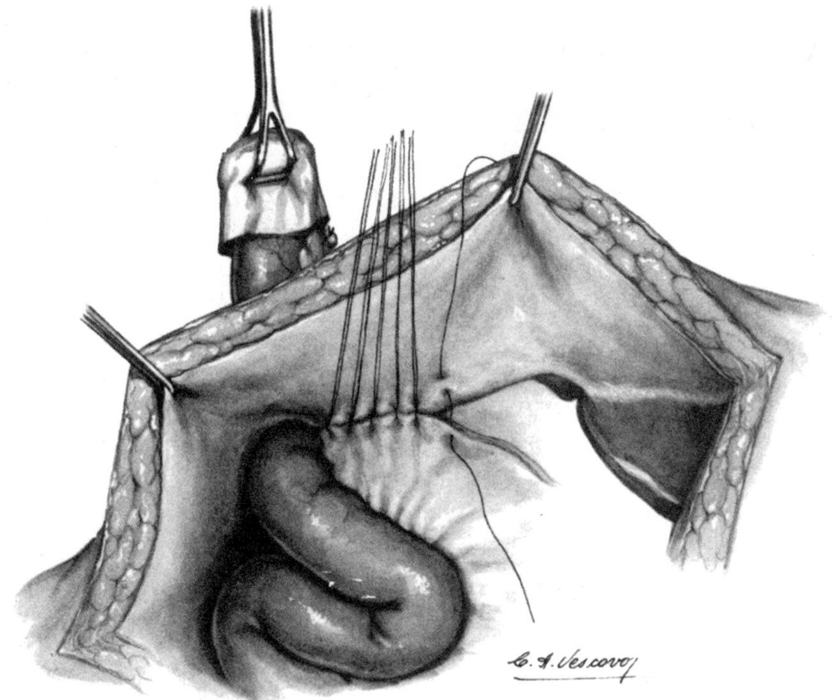

FIGURE 60.16

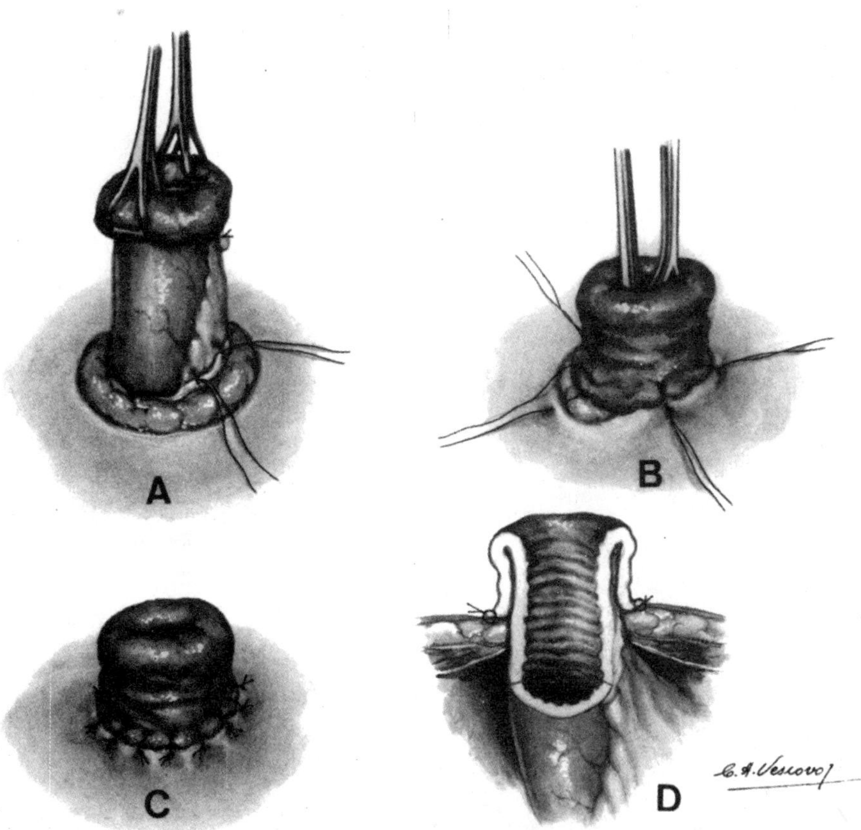

FIGURE 60.17

Total Proctocolectomy with Brooke Ileostomy

FIGURE 60.18
The left paramedian incision has been closed. The skin sutures have been left long to facilitate their removal. A transparent ileostomy bag covers the ileostomy to allow immediate postoperative follow-up.

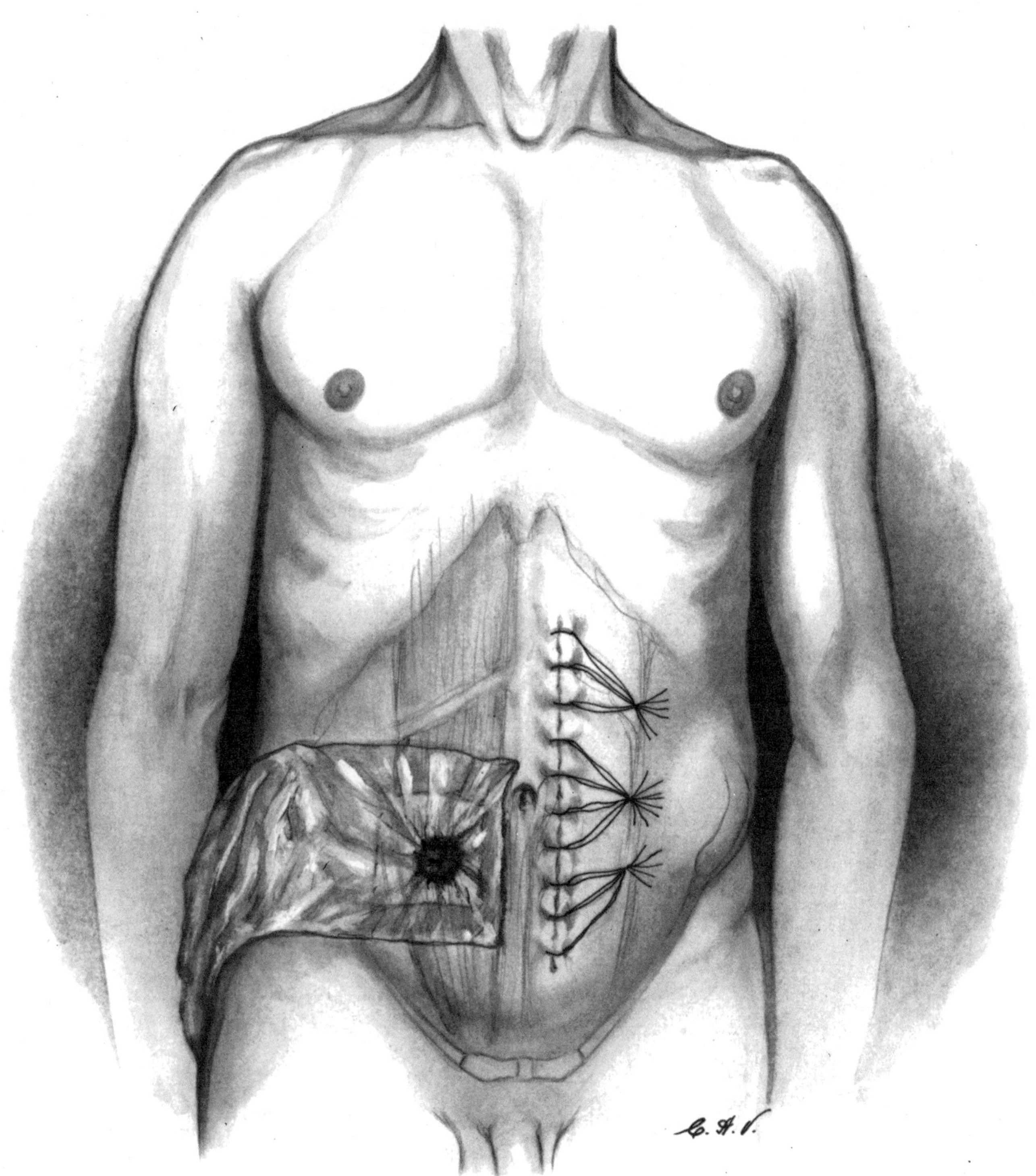

FIGURE 60.18

Total Proctocolectomy with Continent Kock Ileostomy

FIGURE 60.19

To construct a Kock reservoir, 45 to 50 cm of terminal ileum are needed: **A,** Five to ten centimeters are needed to construct the outlet of the reservoir, which is the segment to be brought out to the skin. A special catheter will be passed through this segment to empty the reservoir. If the abdominal wall is thin, 5 cm of ileum will be needed, but if the abdominal wall is thick, 10 cm of ileum will be needed. **B,** About 8 to 10 cm of ileum will be needed to construct the nipple valve, which will prevent spontaneous emptying of the reservoir. Some 30 cm of ileum, folded as a U with each limb 15 cm long, will be needed to construct the reservoir, as seen in the drawing. It is important to exteriorize the ileal segment to be used in constructing the Kock reservoir, orienting it so that the bottom of the U is oriented toward the left flank of the patient while the segment of ileum held by the Duval clamp is directed toward the head of the patient. The surgeon stands to the left of the patient. To construct the valve it is necessary to remove all the fat and serosa from a triangular segment of mesentery, avoiding ligating important vessels. This will permit invagination of the ileal wall, as will be shown in the next few drawings.

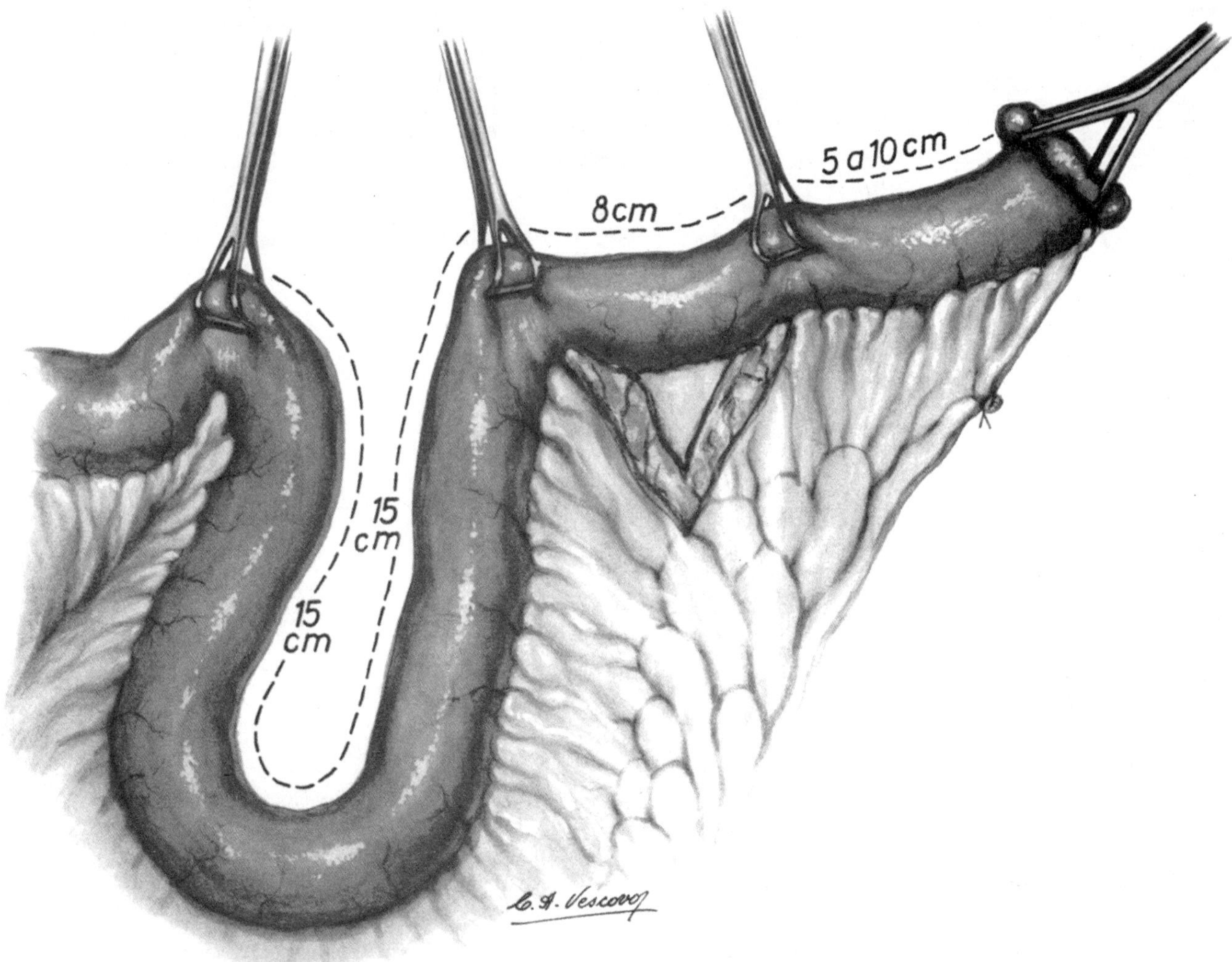

FIGURE 60.19

Total Proctocolectomy with Continent Kock Ileostomy

FIGURE 60.20
The reservoir is being constructed. For this purpose the limbs of the U are sutured to each other using a continuous seromuscular suture with nonabsorbable material, along the antimesenteric borders. The ileal wall is then incised along the broken line. As shown, the broken line of the proximal limb extends 2 to 3 cm higher than the distal limb.

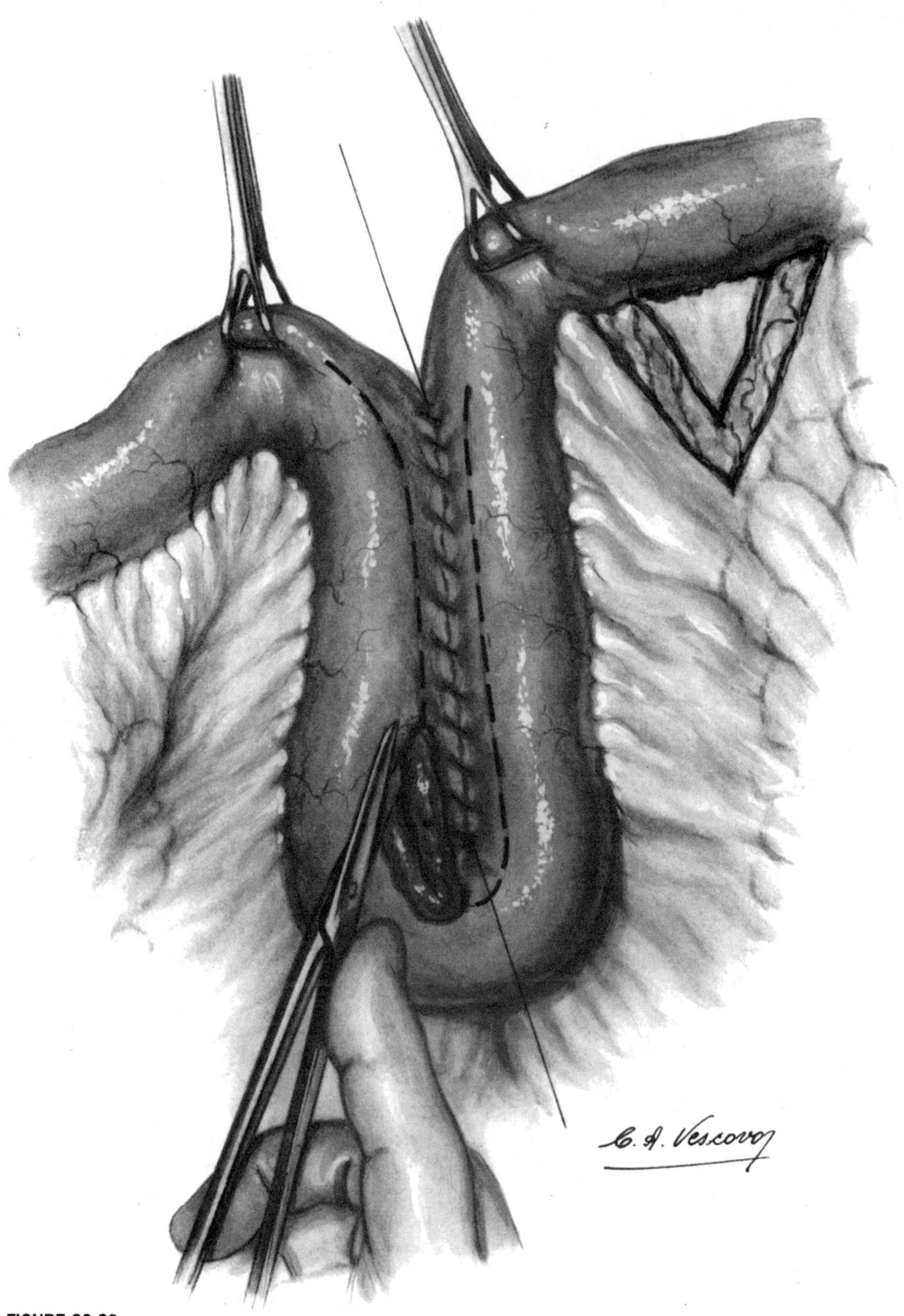

FIGURE 60.20

Total Proctocolectomy with Continent Kock Ileostomy

FIGURE 60.21
After the ileal segment arranged as a U has been opened, the reservoir is constructed by carrying out a through and through suture of the entire wall, from one side to the other, using slow absorbing material. It can again be seen that the opening of the reservoir extends more along the afferent than the efferent limb. This is done so as not to kink the afferent limb when the reservoir is fixed to the abdominal valve.

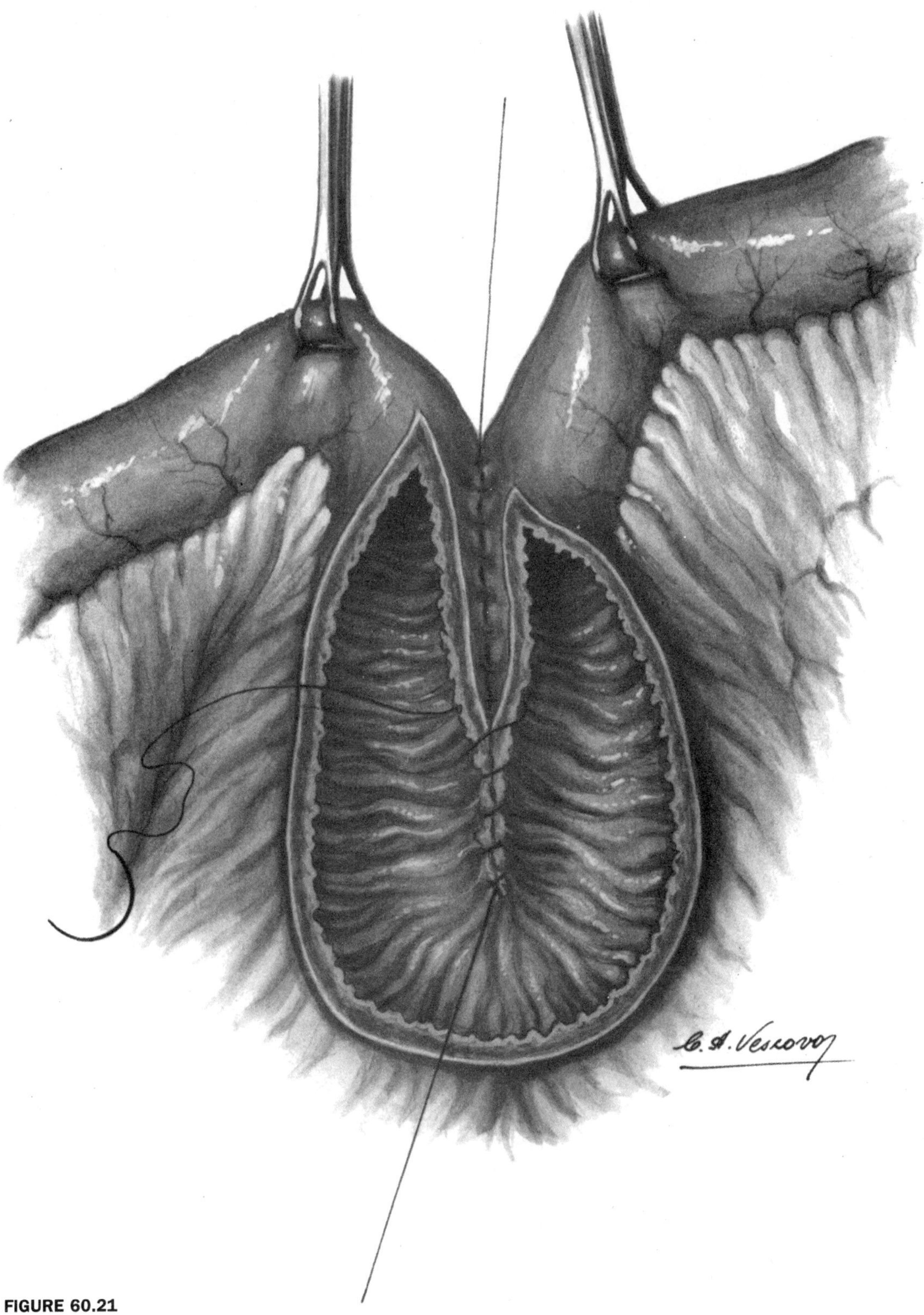

FIGURE 60.21

Total Proctocolectomy with Continent Kock Ileostomy

FIGURE 60.22

The nipple-shaped valve is being constructed. This must be done before completing the suturing of the reservoir. For this purpose, a Babcock clamp is introduced into the segment of ileum destined for the construction of the valve and the wall of that segment of ileum is grasped halfway down and invaginated into the interior of the reservoir.

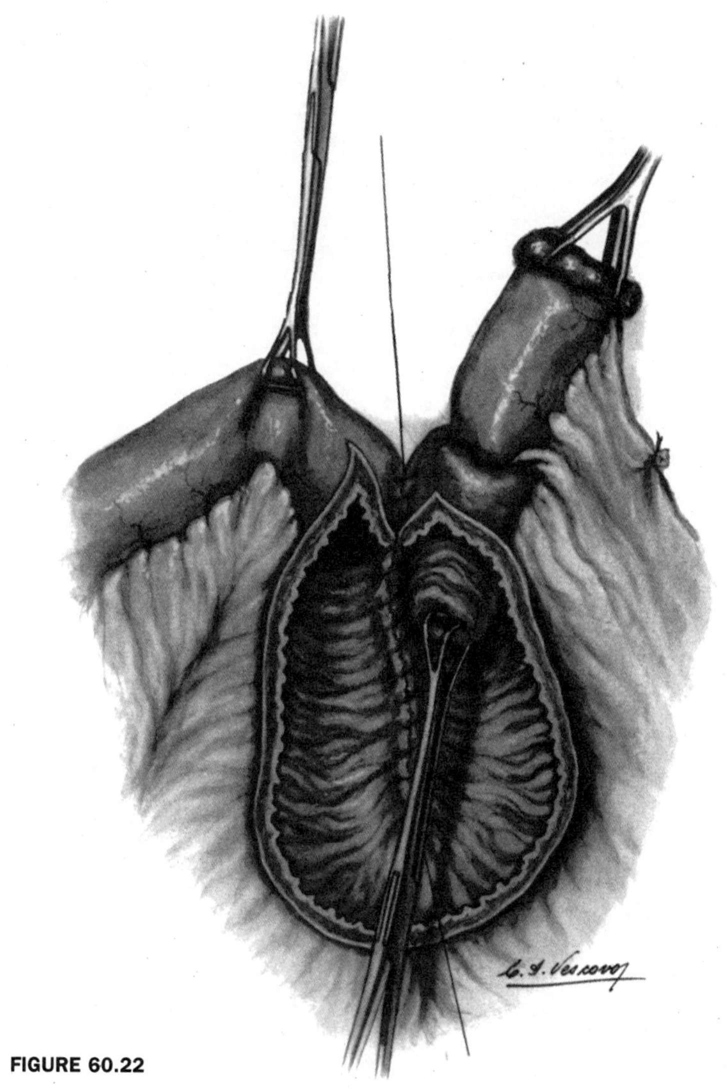

FIGURE 60.22

FIGURE 60.23
Once the wall of the ileum used to construct the nipple valve is invaginated, it is fixed with four rows of staples using the linear stapler, and avoiding the mesentery. The finished valve measures 5 cm in length.

Total Proctocolectomy with Continent Kock Ileostomy

FIGURE 60.24
A, Details of the invagination and fixation of the ileal segment to construct the valve; **B,** the four rows of staples placed to hold the valve in place respecting the mesentery.

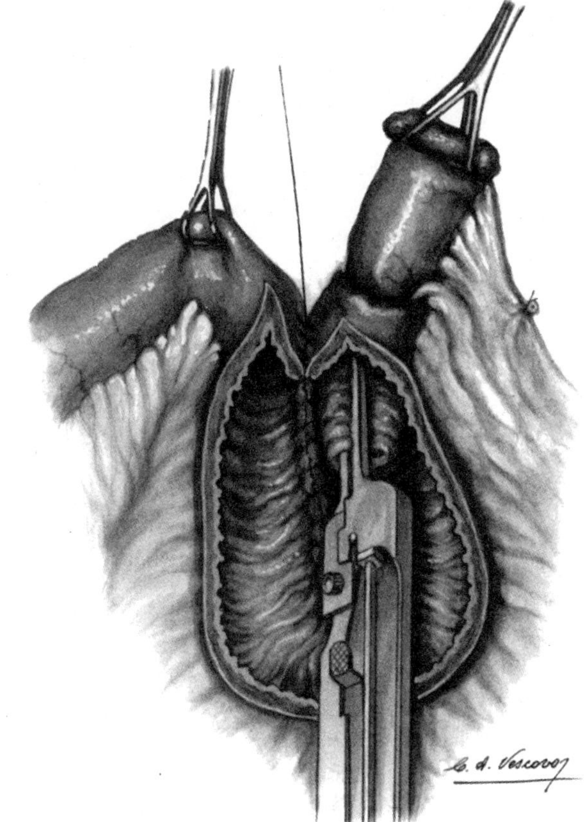

FIGURE 60.23

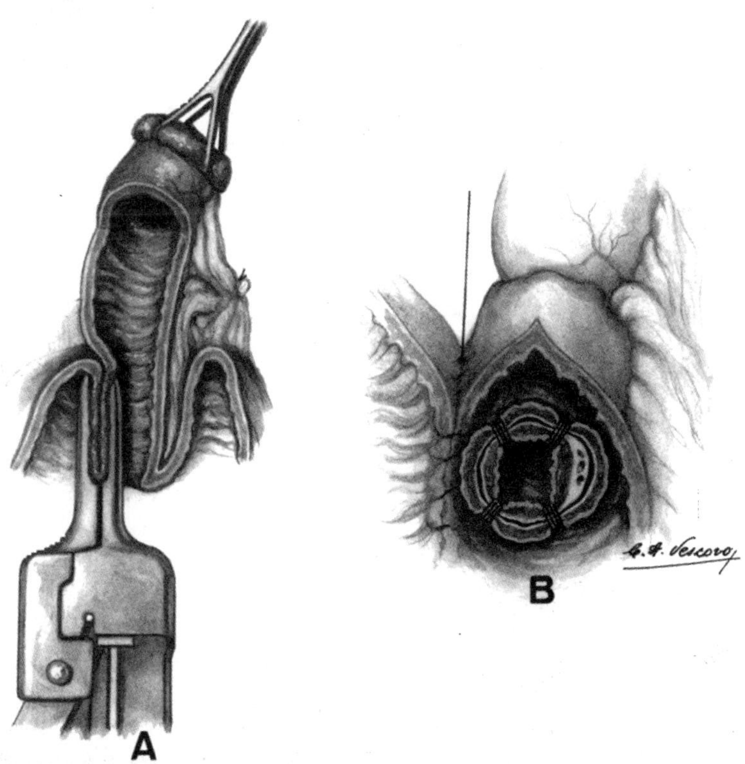

FIGURE 60.24

FIGURE 60.25
Once construction of the valve is complete, the anterior wall of the reservoir is closed in similar fashion as the posterior wall was closed.

Total Proctocolectomy with Continent Kock Ileostomy

FIGURE 60.26
With the valve completed together with the closure of the reservoir, the direction of the reservoir is changed so that its anterior wall becomes posterior. This change in direction allows the reservoir to be placed in the inferior portion of the abdominal cavity.

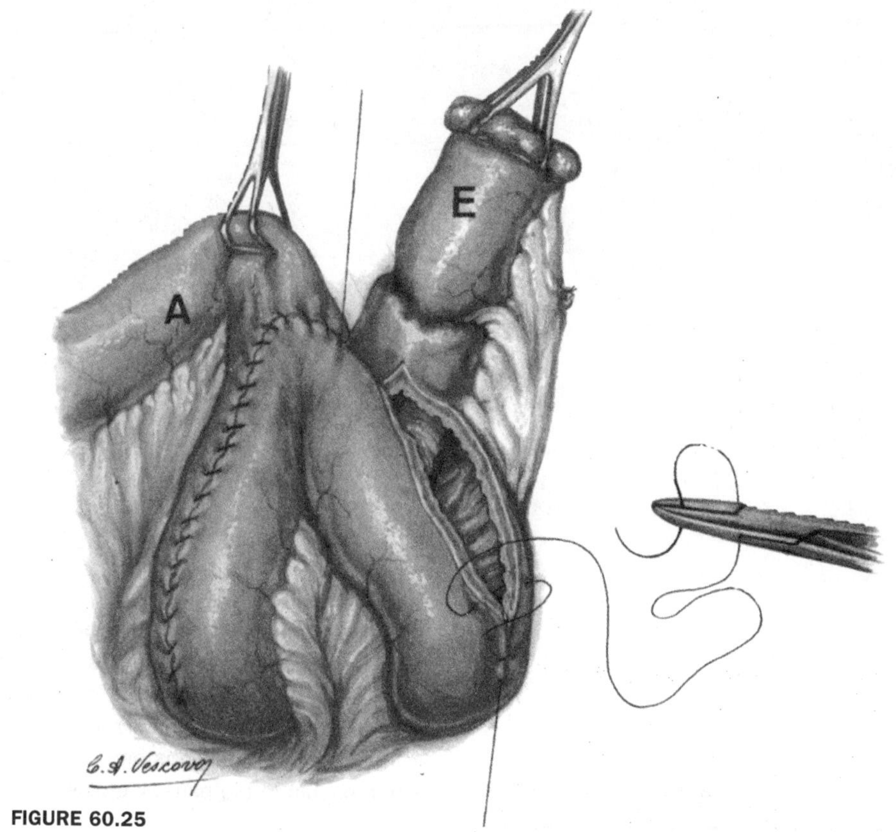

FIGURE 60.25

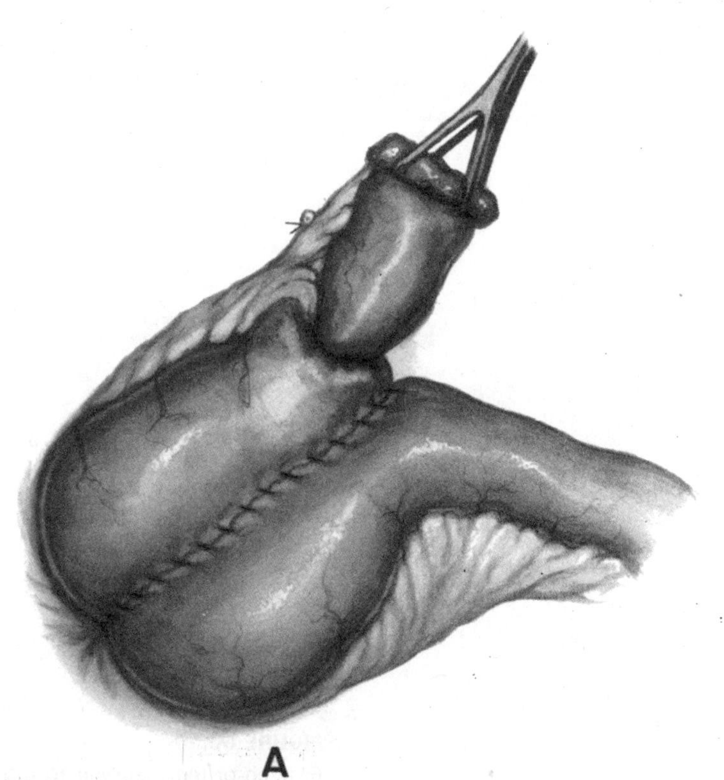

FIGURE 60.26

FIGURE 60.27
At the site in the abdominal wall selected before the operation for the ileostomy an opening is made that will allow two fingers to pass easily. The fascia is incised, and the muscular fibers of the anterior abdominal rectus muscle are split. The edges of the bag near the ileostomy are fixed to the edges of the peritoneum in the parietal orifice, as can be seen.

Total Proctocolectomy with Continent Kock Ileostomy

FIGURE 60.28
Fixation of the reservoir to the peritoneal edges of the orifice in the abdominal wall is being completed.

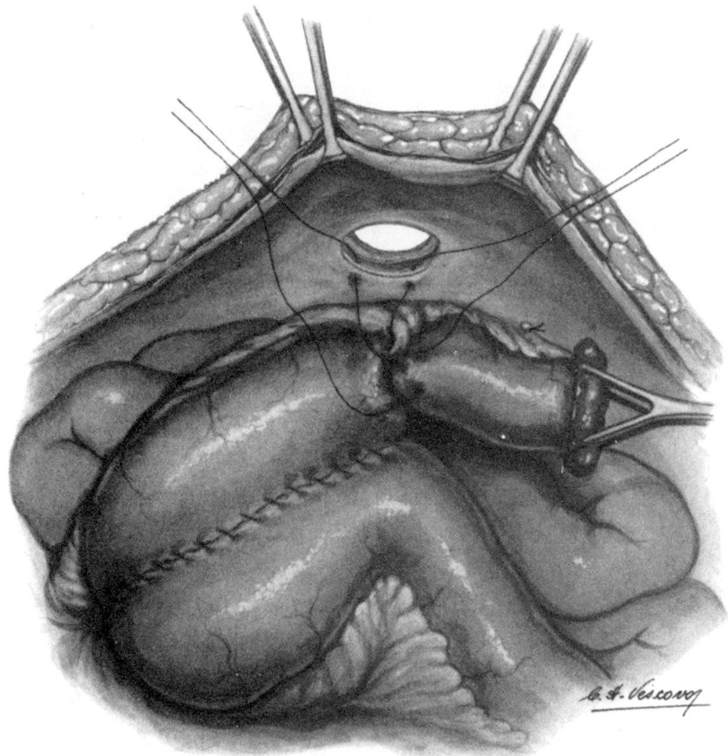

FIGURE 60.27

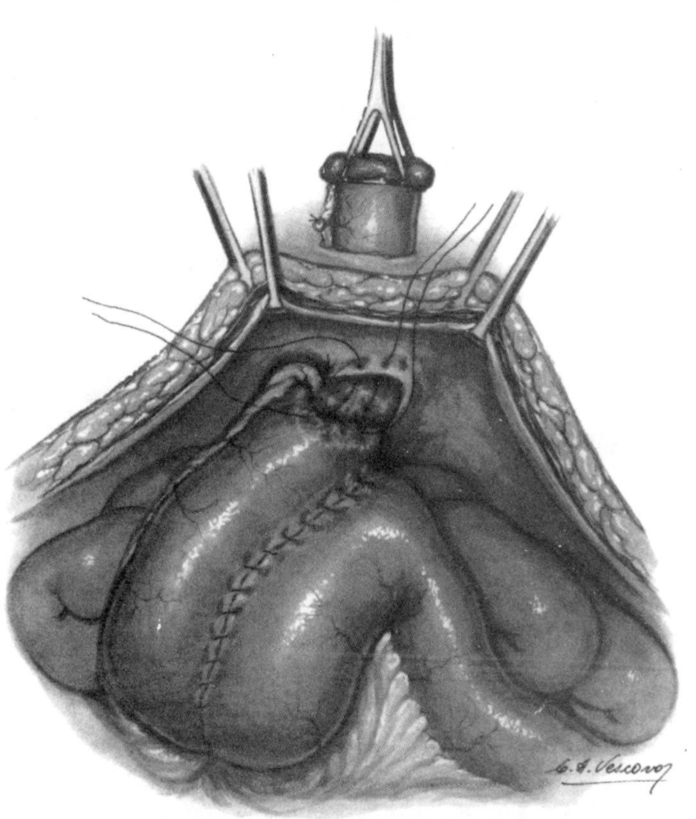

FIGURE 60.28

FIGURE 60.29
View of a section of the reservoir with the valve and the ileostomy. The end of the ileum has been sutured to the skin of the parietal orifice with interrupted 2-0 chromic catgut. A 28 F catheter is introduced down to the bottom of the reservoir and fixed in place, before closing the abdomen. Some surgeons perform a loop ileostomy, to protect the reservoir, which is closed 8 weeks later (45).

Total Proctocolectomy with Continent Kock Ileostomy

FIGURE 60.30
The 28 F catheter placed in the bottom of the reservoir is connected to a tube to drain the contents into a plastic bag, as seen in the drawing (45, 49).

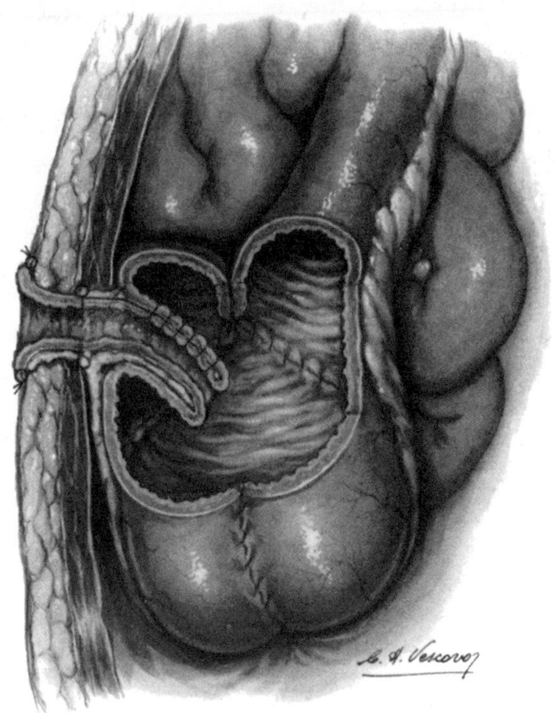

FIGURE 60.29

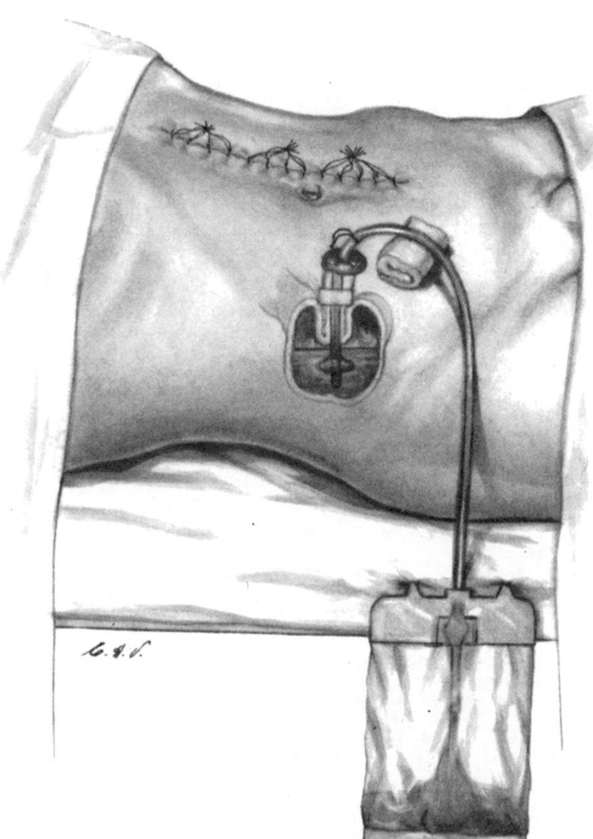

FIGURE 60.30

FIGURE 60.31
The 28 F catheter is removed 4 weeks later and the patient is taught how to empty the catheter. The reservoir is emptied 3 or 4 times a day (45). In general, if the Kock reservoir functions correctly, it is not necessary to empty it during the night.

Total Proctocolectomy with Continent Kock Ileostomy

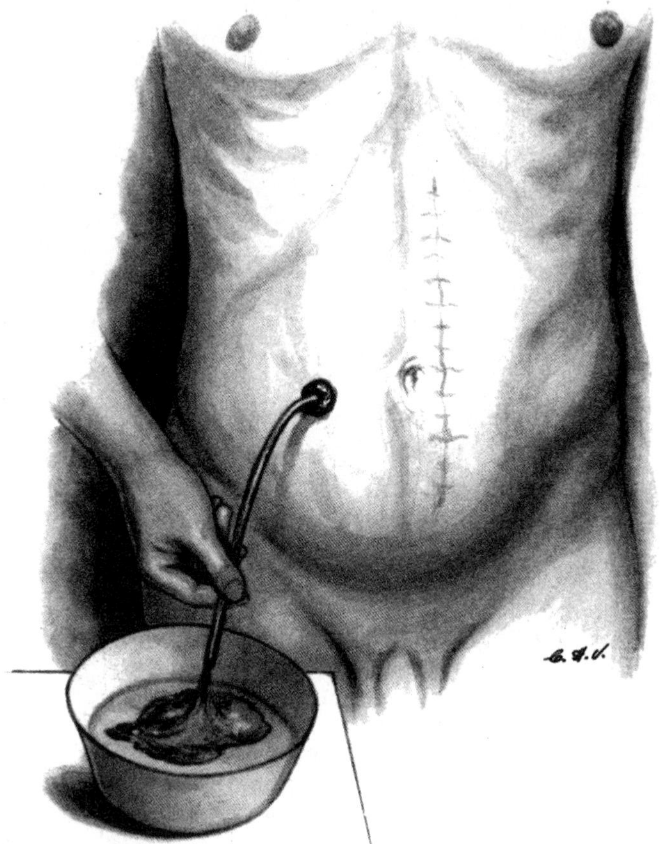

FIGURE 60.31

Loop Ileostomy with Decompressive Colostomy (Turnbull "Blowhole" Technique)

FIGURE 60.32

The drawing shows the two incisions usually made in the Turnbull "blowhole" technique. The lower, median or left paramedian, incision, about 6 to 8 cm long, is made to carry out a summary exploration of the abdomen, eliminate the presence of a free perforation into the peritoneal cavity, and perform a loop ileostomy. The loop ileostomy is performed 35 to 40 cm proximal to the ileocecal valve (68) with the object of leaving the terminal ileum free in case it becomes possible later to construct an ileal pouch and anastomose it to the anal canal. The loop ileostomy is constructed so that the proximal end of the ileum is in a caudal position while the caudal end is in a proximal position. This arrangement is used to prevent a change in the position of the distal ileum in a later possible resection of the colon. The lower incision is closed and the upper incision made along the indicated line. A decompressive colostomy of the transverse colon will be performed through this incision. Correct positioning of this incision should be based on the location of the dilated transverse colon, as determined by a previous plane x-ray of the abdomen.

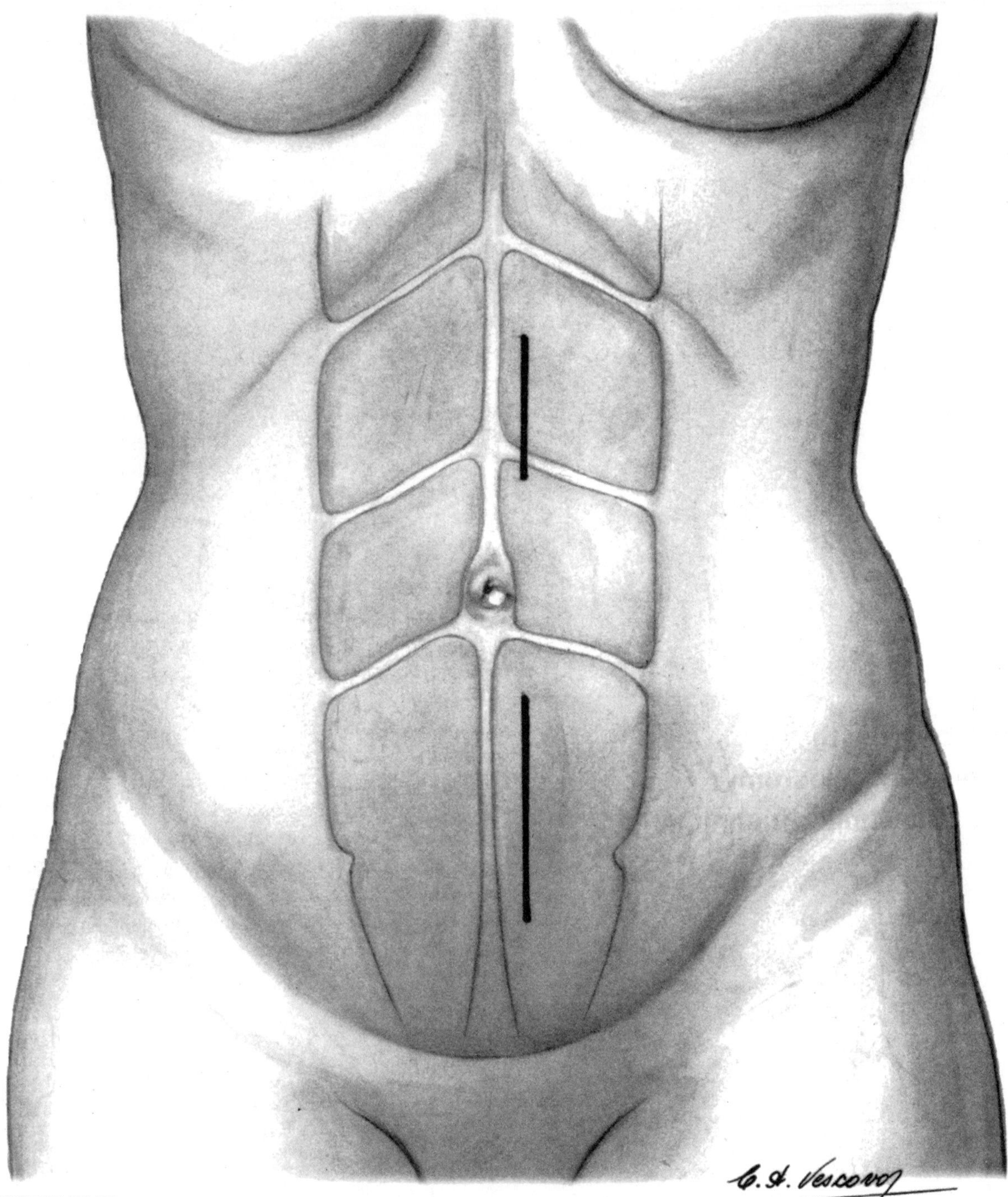

FIGURE 60.32

FIGURE 60.33
A, With the peritoneum open, the gastrocolic ligament and the greater omentum are visible. A vertical broken line shows where the gastrocolic ligament and the greater omentum will be incised to expose the transverse colon. **B,** Using several interrupted 2-0 catgut sutures, the wall of the transverse colon is attached to the previously incised greater omentum and parietal peritoneum. The transverse colon is then punctured through the small circle shown on the tenia. **C,** An incision is made with a scalpel in the anterior wall of the transverse colon. The decompressive colostomy is completed, suturing the wall of the colon to the skin with interrupted sutures of 2-0 chromic catgut. Handling and suturing of the colon must be very carefully done because of its great fragility.

Loop Ileostomy with Decompressive Colostomy (Turnbull "Blowhole" Technique)

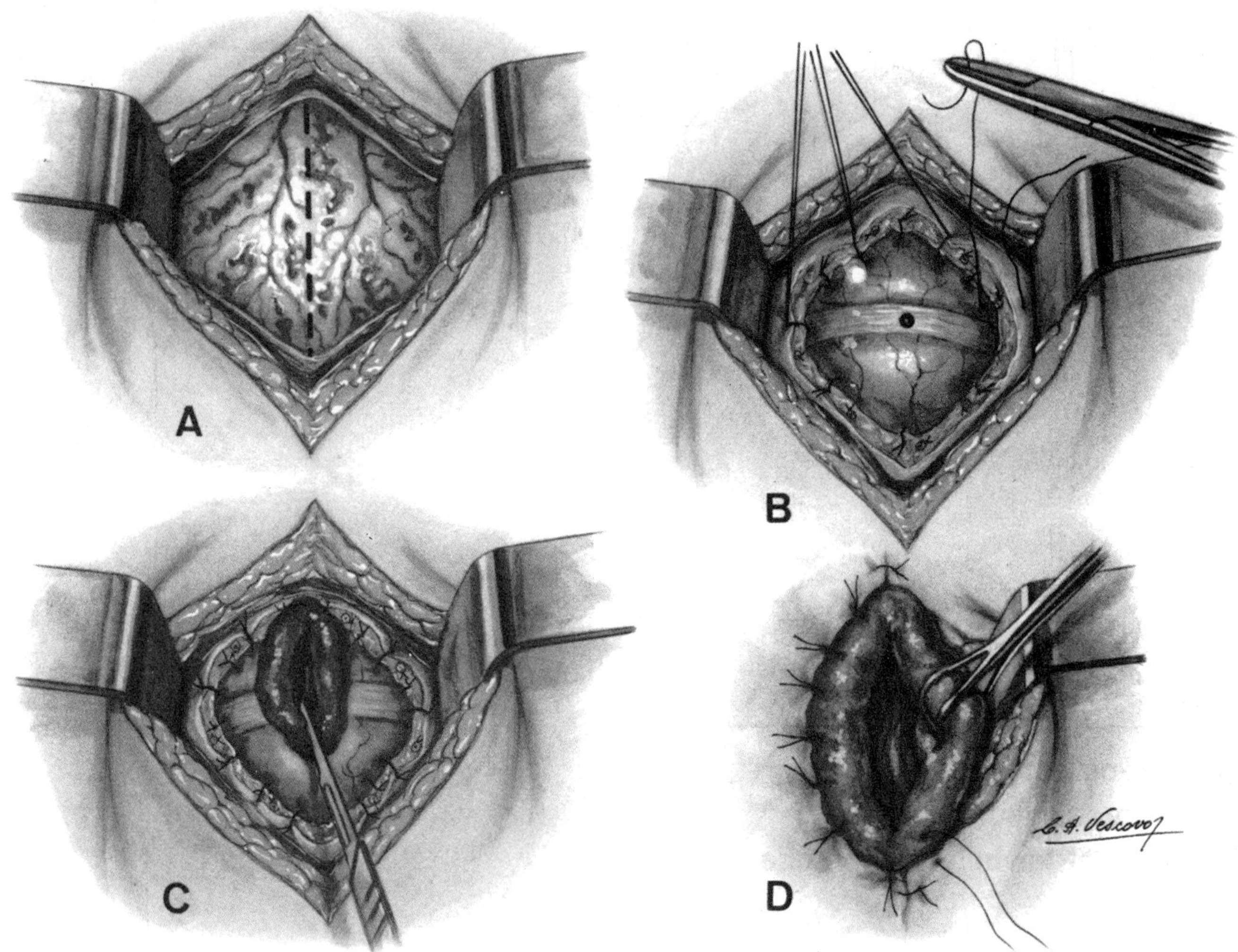

FIGURE 60.33

Loop Ileostomy with Decompressive Colostomy (Turnbull "Blowhole" Technique)

FIGURE 60.34
The drawing shows the completed Turnbull "blowhole" operation: 1, loop ileostomy; 2, decompressive transverse colostomy.

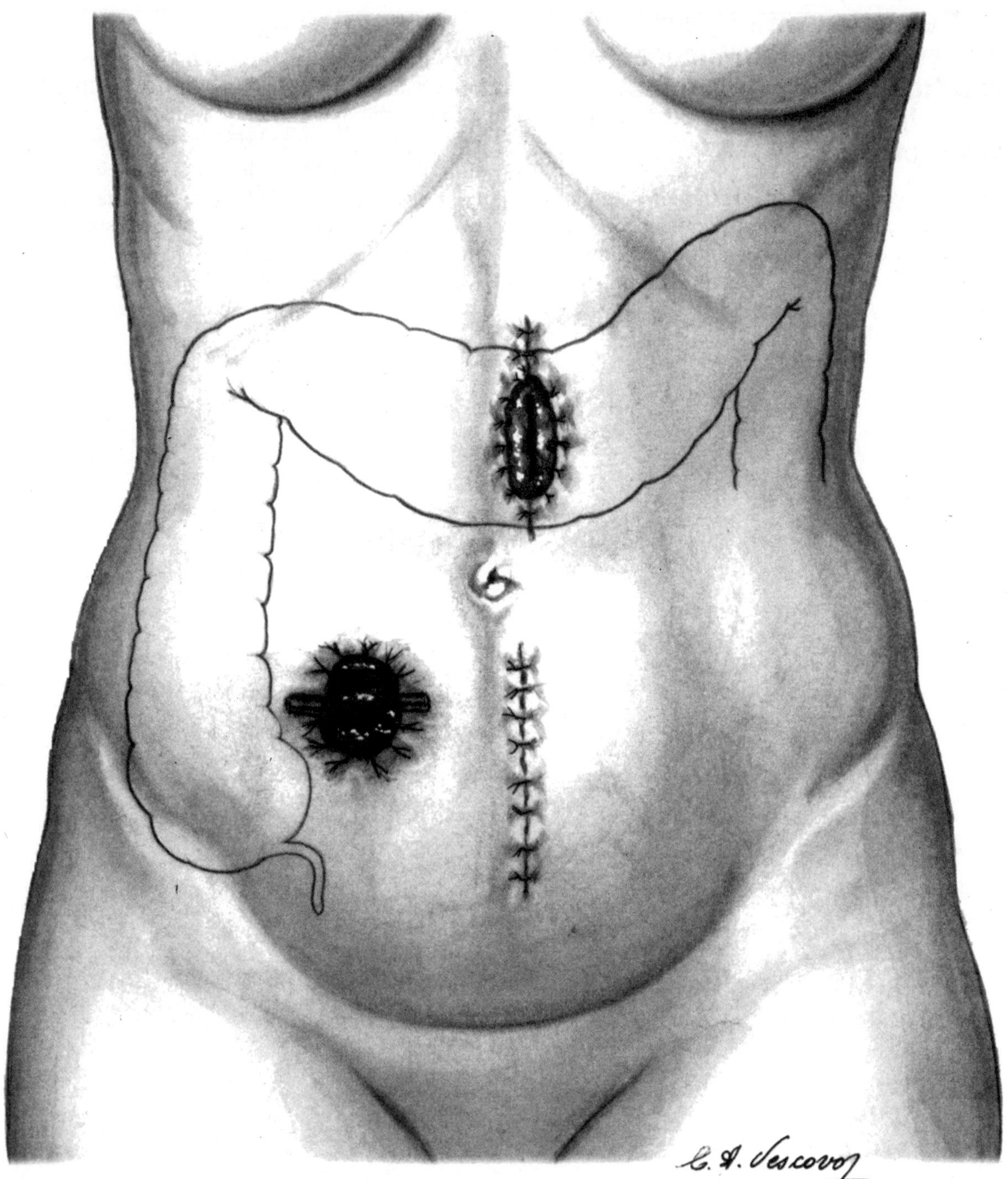

FIGURE 60.34

Colonic Resection with Upper Part of the Rectum, Anorectal Mucosectomy and Ileal Reservoir with Ileoanal Anastomosis (Restorative Proctocolectomy)

The patient is placed in a modified lithotomy position so that two surgical teams can operate simultaneously, one in the abdomen and another through the perineum. The abdominal surgeon will be in charge of resecting the entire colon and the proximal two thirds of the rectum, and constructing an ileal reservoir. The perineal surgeon will dissect the anorectal mucosa from the pectinate line to 4 to 6 cm above that line. In addition, the perineal surgeon will direct the abdominal surgeon during transection of the muscular cylinder of the rectum (after its mucosa has been removed) to be sure this incision is made in the correct position. The perineal surgeon will suture the ileal reservoir constructed by the abdominal surgeon to the pectineal mucosa to reestablish intestinal transit.

Restorative Proctocolectomy

FIGURE 60.35

The abdominal surgeon, after mobilization of the colon and upper rectum, resects it, preserving the distal rectum, the anus, and its sphincters. The drawing shows the abdominal surgeon at the moment of transection of the terminal ileum as close as possible to the ileocecal valve, using the GIA instrument or manual technique. After transection of the ileum, the ileal reservoir is constructed, in the form of a J, an S, an H, or a W. The most frequently used reservoir is the J-reservoir and the next in frequency is the S-reservoir. In the following, construction of the J-reservoir will be described and, later, construction of the S-reservoir will be described.

Restorative Proctocolectomy

To construct a J-pouch reservoir a segment of ileum 30 cm long is needed. The ileal segment is folded in the form of a J. Each limb of the J should be 15 cm long. If the limbs are over 15 cm long, this would favor development of the complication known as pouchitis. The elbow or bottom of the J should be directed downward. Before beginning construction of the reservoir it is indispensable to determine that the bottom of the J will reach the pectinate line without tension. It has been proven that, if the bottom of the J can be brought down to a point 6 cm below the pubic symphysis, it can be sutured without tension to the mucosa of the pectinate line (86). This test can be done directly if the segment of proximal rectum has been resected. If the elbow of the ileal reservoir does not reach the pectinate line easily, mobilization of the mesentery and ligation of some of its vessels can be done, taking care not to compromise the blood supply of the ileal reservoir. Before ligating any vessels it is essential to determine, using atraumatic vascular clamps, that ligating a vessel will not compromise the blood supply of the J-pouch.

Burnstein et al. (13) have proposed several maneuvers to make the J-pouch ileal limb longer. If it is not possible to anastomose the J-pouch to the pectinate line without tension, some other type of reservoir should be constructed. Frequently, an S-pouch, which can usually be anastomosed to the canal without tension, is resorted to. Once the colon and rectum are resected, they should be studied by the pathologist to confirm the diagnosis of ulcerative colitis. If there is still doubt as to the diagnosis of Crohn's disease, some other surgical procedure should be performed, because intestinal reservoirs are contraindicated in Crohn's disease.

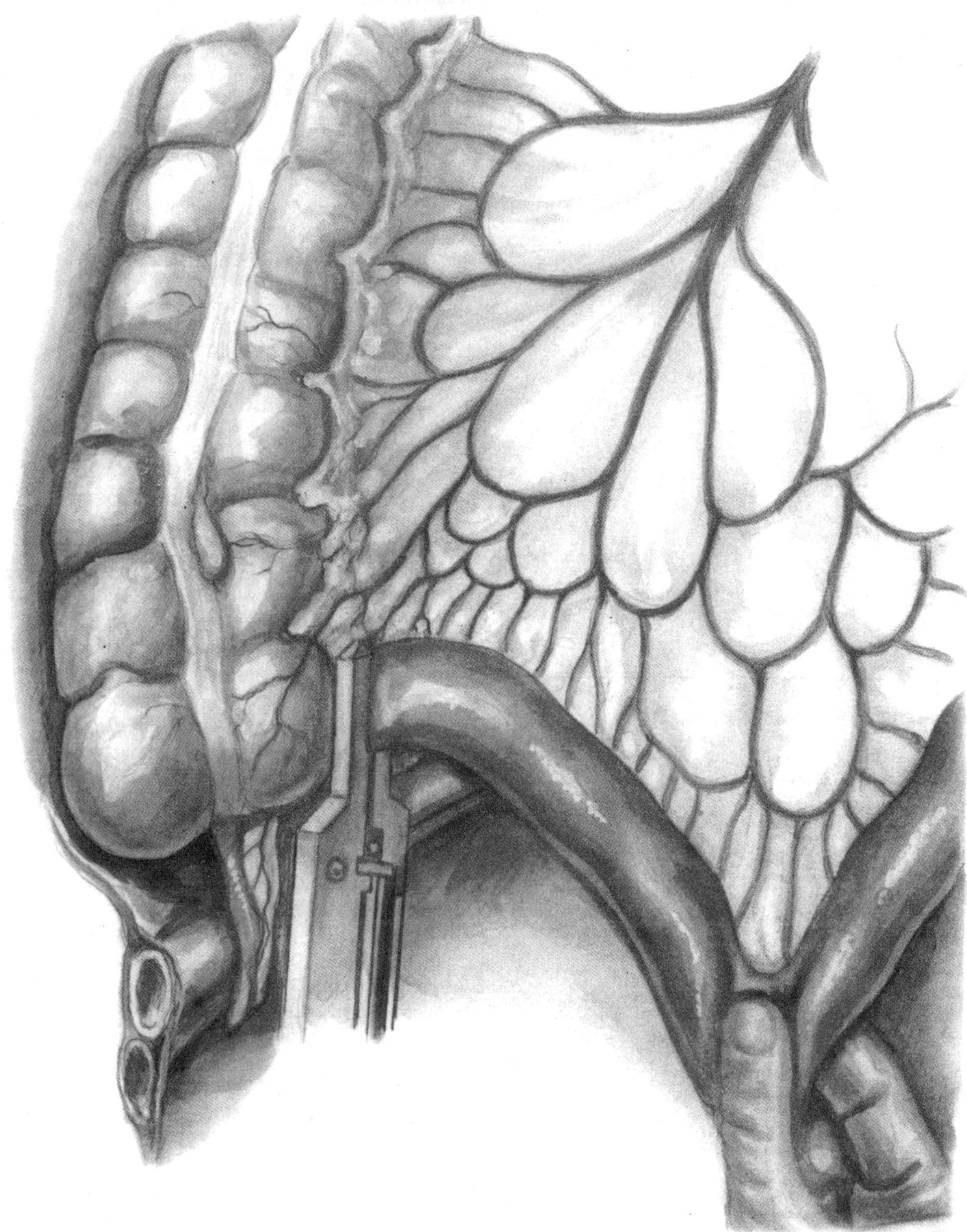

FIGURE 60.35

FIGURE 60.36
The ileum, whose terminal end has been closed with a GIA instrument, is folded in the shape of a J. Anastomosis of the two limbs that make up the J is also carried out with the GIA. The limbs of the instrument are introduced through two small transverse incisions in the medial side of the limbs of the J. The GIA instrument is directed downward and then upward to anastomose the antimesenteric borders of the J. The bottom or elbow of the J is preserved, to be anastomosed to the pectinate line by the perineal surgeon, without affecting its blood supply. Construction of the J-pouch can also be done manually.

Restorative Proctocolectomy

FIGURE 60.37
While the surgeon resects the colon and prepares the J-pouch, the perineal surgeon dissects the anorectal mucosa transanally starting at the pectinate line and extending upward about 4 to 6 cm. Self-retaining retractors should be used during dissection of the anorectal mucosa. The Parks retractors are more frequently used. The disposable Lon Star or Gelpi retractors are also used.

Dissection of the anorectal mucosa is a tedious, difficult process due to the inflammatory process of the ulcerative colitis. It is important to start the dissection in the correct submucosal plane. Mucosal dissection should be circumferential, resecting a cylindrical segment. Anorectal mucosal remnants should not be left behind, since they could give rise to rectal cancer later. The dissection should stay out of the muscular layer of the rectum in order to prevent functional alterations. Careful hemostasis should be done using the electrocautery with a needle point. To facilitate dissection it is advantageous to inject, into the submucosal plane at the level of the pectinate line, an 0.5% Novocain solution with epinephrine (1:200,000). This will diminish bleeding during the mucosal dissection and produce relaxation of the anal sphincters. Some surgeons perform the mucosal dissection with the patient in the prone position (80–82), which makes mucosal dissection easier. Once this dissection is completed, the patient is placed in the modified lithotomy position to continue the operation. On the other hand, it may be impossible to construct the ileal reservoir because of one of several reasons such as shortness of the mesentery, the presence of ischemia of the bottom of the reservoir, and so on, which would mean a waste of time. Other surgeons (43, 44) carry out the mucosal dissection by the abdominal route, convinced that through this approach there is less anal incontinence and less probability of infection.

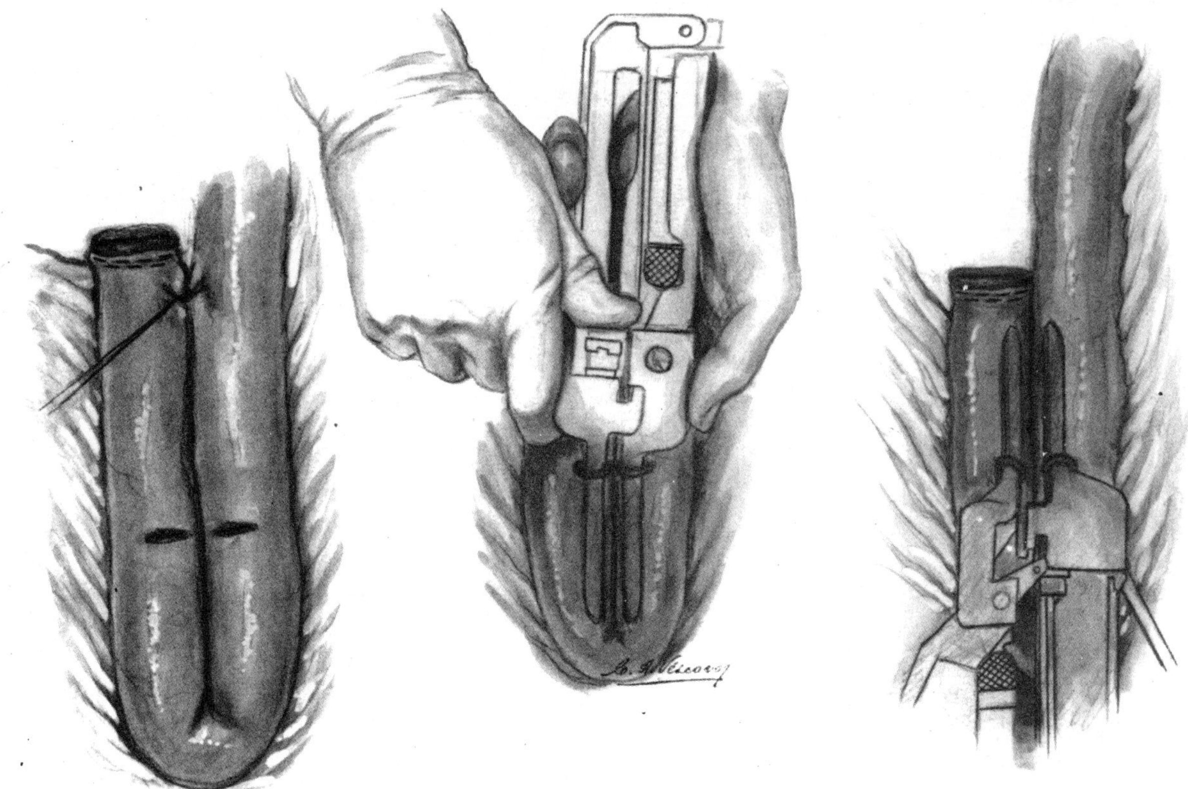

FIGURE 60.36

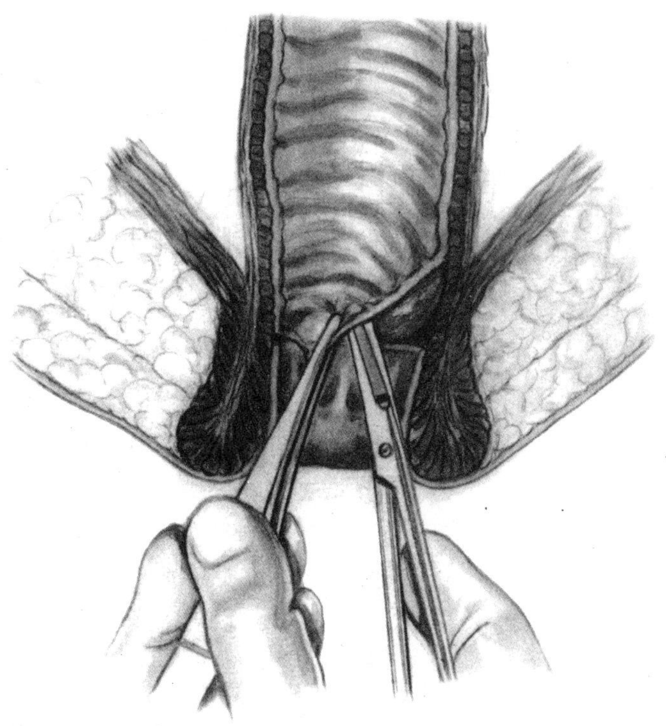

FIGURE 60.37

FIGURE 60.38
Once the anorectal mucosal dissection is completed, the lower end of the mucosal cylinder is closed by ligating it with a heavy suture or by using a purse string suture, as seen in the drawing. The mucosal stump can then be pushed upward with a blunt clamp or a gauze pledget on a clamp (5). The mucosal stump is pushed upward so the abdominal surgeon can feel it and be better oriented before incising the muscular wall of the rectum.

Restorative Proctocolectomy

FIGURE 60.39
Sectional view to show the anastomosis of the elbow of the J-pouch being sutured to the pectinate line including, in partial form, the muscular cylinder of the rectum.

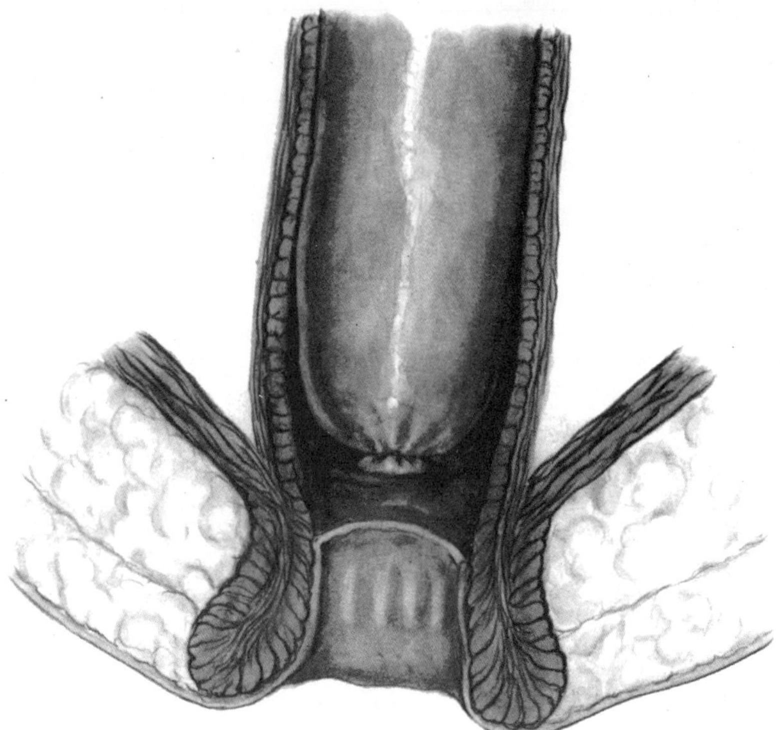

FIGURE 60.38

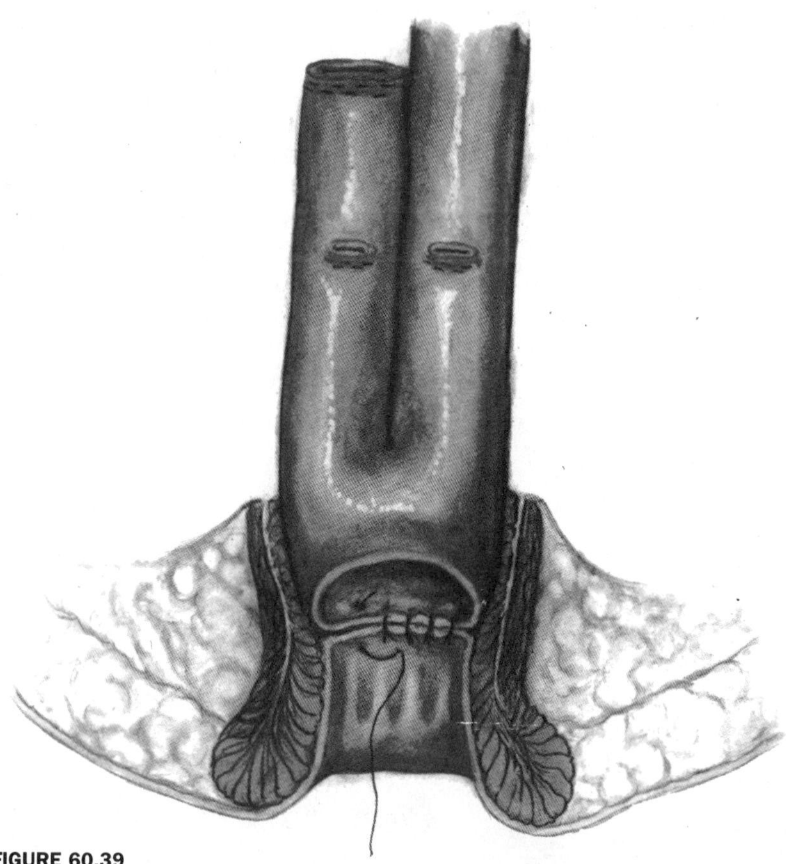

FIGURE 60.39

Restorative Proctocolectomy

FIGURE 60.40

This drawing shows the transanal suturing of the bottom of the ileal reservoir to the pectinate line. A pair of Gelpi retractors are being used. Some surgeons perform this anastomosis using double stapling (CEEA stapler). This latter method produces excessive invagination of tissue and leaves rectal mucosa behind, which could give rise to rectal carcinoma in the future.

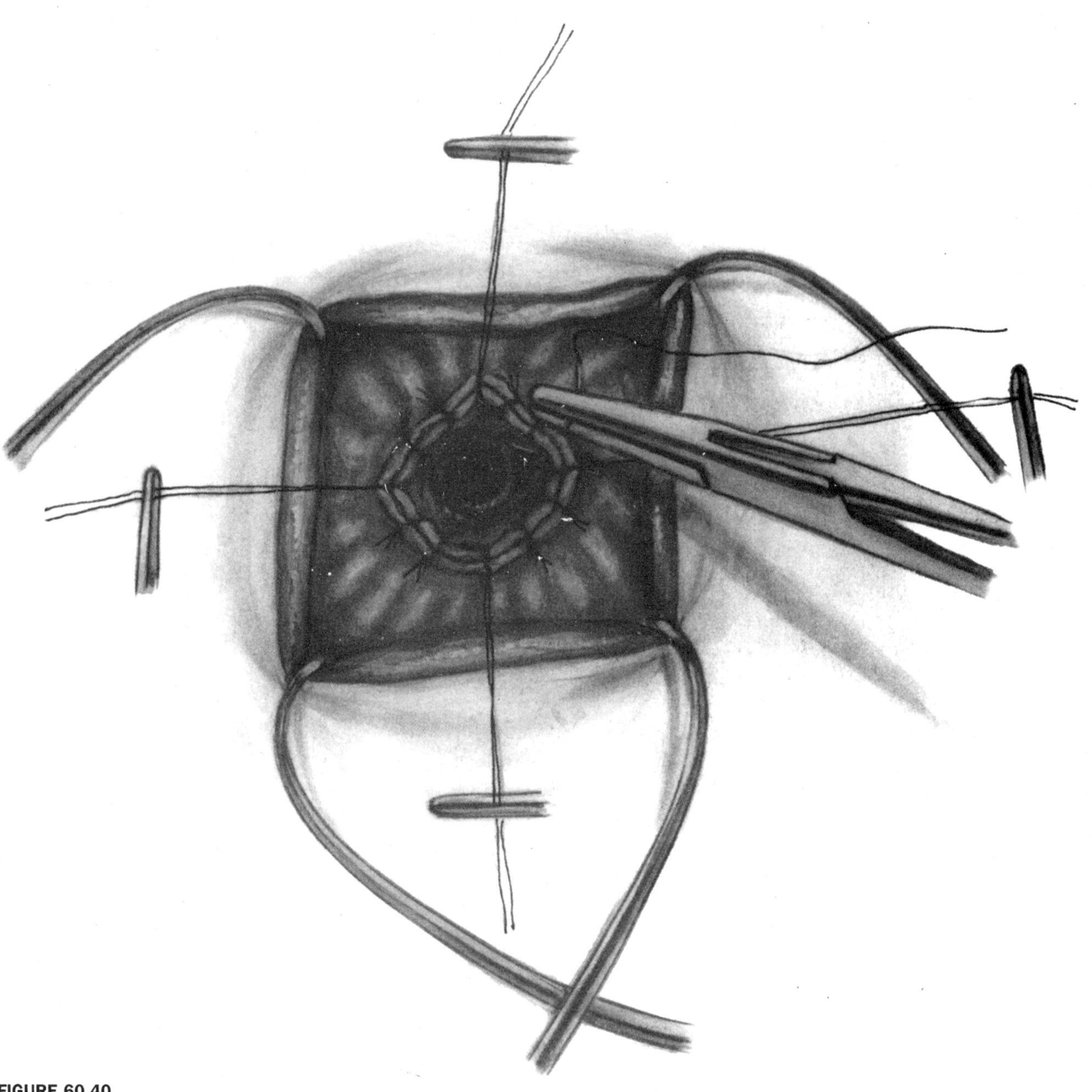

FIGURE 60.40

Restorative Proctocolectomy

FIGURE 60.41

Resection of the entire colon with the upper two thirds of the rectum and all the rectal mucosa above the pectinate line has been done. The J reservoir has been anastomosed to the pectinate line. A loop ileostomy has been made about 30 cm above the ileoanal anastomosis to protect it. This protective loop ileostomy is usually closed about 3 months after the procedure if follow-up shows that the reservoir is functioning correctly. Some surgeons (16, 38, 61, 88) do not perform a protective loop ileostomy.

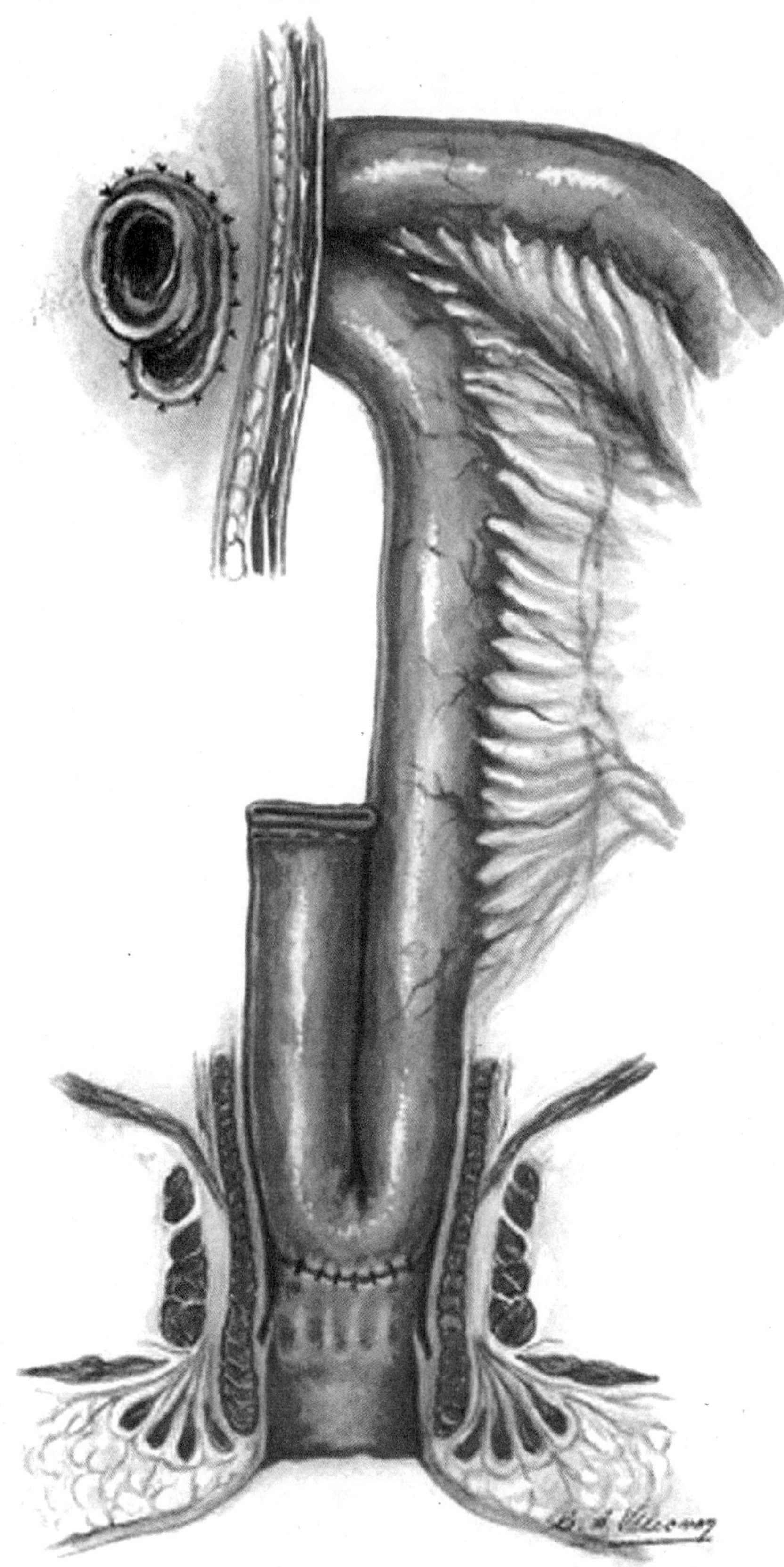

FIGURE 60.41

Restorative Proctocolectomy

FIGURE 60.42 CONSTRUCTION OF AN S RESERVOIR (PARKS; 70)

The ileal S is carried out with three folds of terminal ileum. Parks used 15 cm of ileum in each fold. At present these folds are made of 10 or 12 cm of ileum each. Originally Parks used 5 cm of ileum for the exit segment, as shown under **A.** At present the exit ileal segment is usually only 2 cm long to prevent retention of secretions in tne reservoir and make catheterization less frequent. **B,** Suturing of the seromuscular layer of the three folds has been done and (**C**) a broken line shows where the wall of the ileal limbs will be incised. **D** and **E,** The entire thickness of the wall of the ileal limbs are being sutured using interrupted sutures. The anastomosis can also be performed with a continuous suture or by mechanical means.

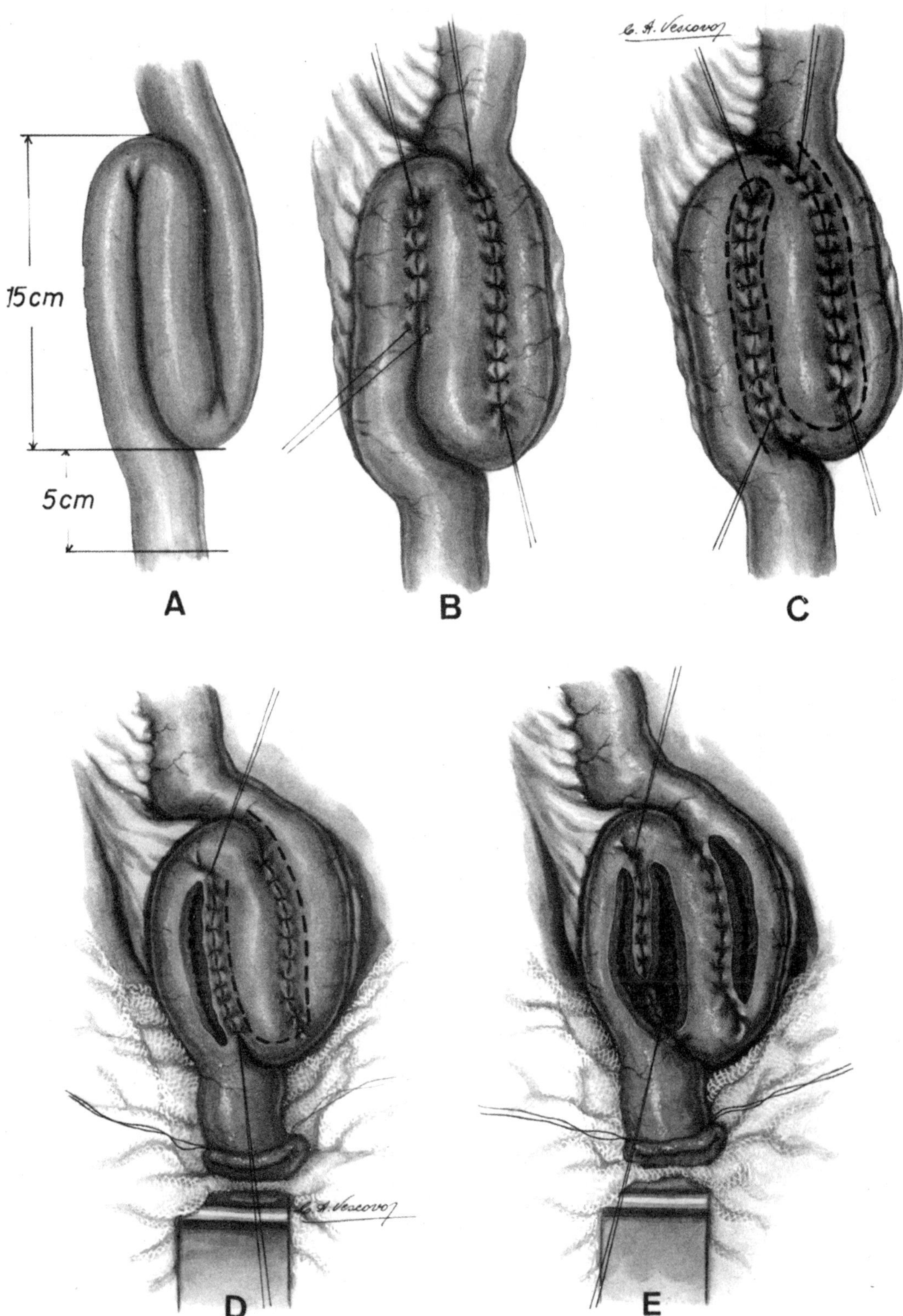

FIGURE 60.42 CONSTRUCTION OF AN S RESERVOIR (PARKS; 70)

Restorative Proctocolectomy

FIGURE 60.42 CONSTRUCTION OF AN S RESERVOIR (PARKS; 70)

G, The S pouch has been constructed. In **F,** one can observe the interior capacity of the reservoir. The exit end of ileum should not be longer than 2 cm. If it is too long, the excess should be resected before performing the anastomosis.

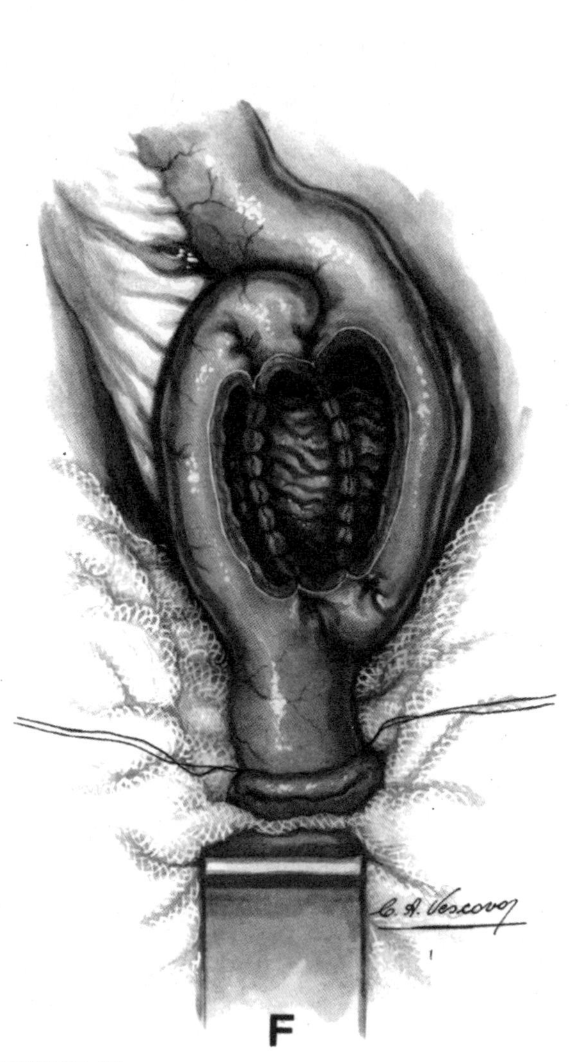

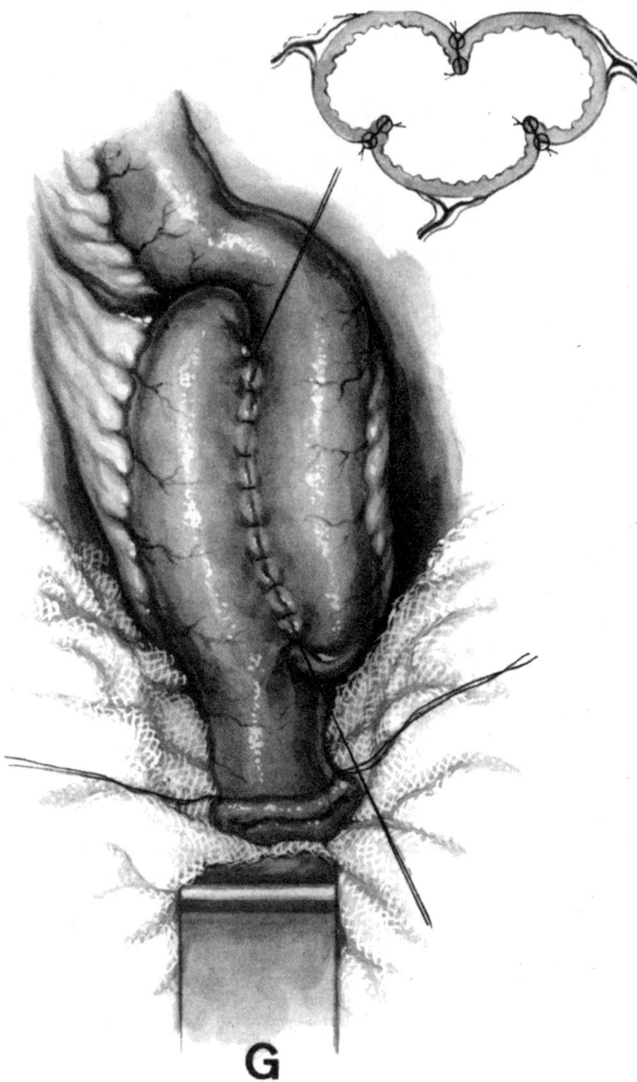

FIGURE 60.42

FIGURE 60.43
Once the S-pouch has been completed and sutured to the pectinate line, a protective loop ileostomy is made 30 to 35 cm from the reservoir. An opening is made in the right ileal fossa through the rectus abdominis muscle, through which the index and middle fingers of the surgeon should pass comfortably.

Restorative Proctocolectomy

FIGURE 60.44
The protective loop ileostomy has been completed. The drawing shows that the functioning end of the loop ileostomy (which is the one with the larger diameter) has been placed in the upper side.

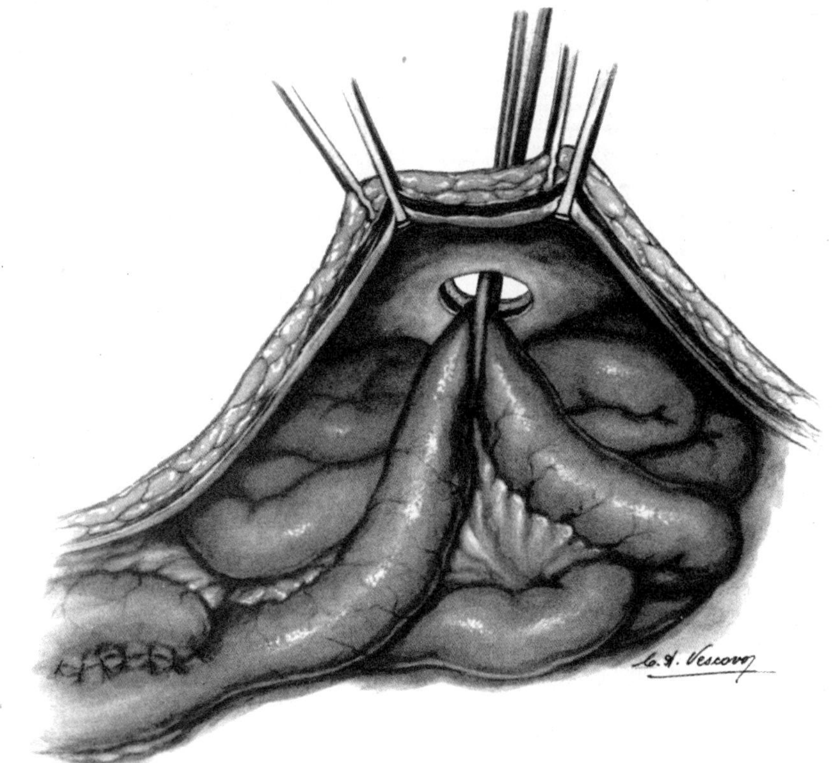

FIGURE 60.43

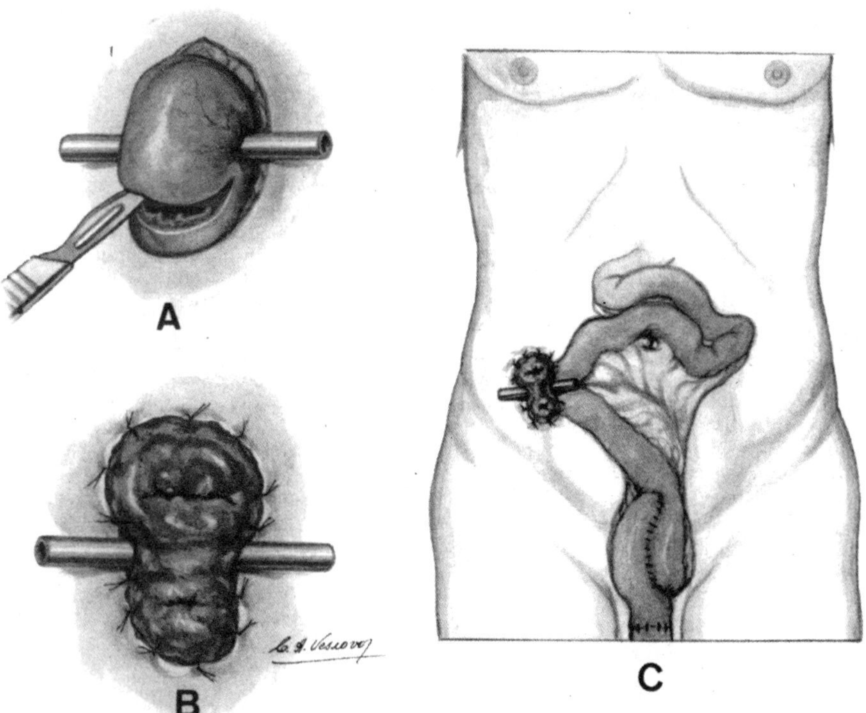

FIGURE 60.44

References

1. Albrechtsen, D., Bergan, A., Nigaard, K., Gjone, E., Flatmark, A. Urgent surgery for ulcerative colitis: Early colectomy in 132 patients. World J. Surg. 5:607, 1981.
2. Aylett, S.O. Diffuse ulcerative colitis and its treatment by ileorectal anastomosis. Ann. R. Coll. Surg. Engl. 27:260, 1960.
3. Aylett, S.O. Three hundred cases of diffuse ulcerative colitis treated by total colectomy and ileorectal anastomosis. Br. Med. J. 1:1001, 1966.
4. Bargen, J.A. Chronic ulcerative colitis associated with malignant disease. Arch. Surg. 17:561, 1928.
5. Bauer, J.J. Total abdominal colectomy with mucosal proctectomy and ileal J (or S) reservoir. In Bauer, J.J. (Ed.) Colorectal surgery illustrated. p. 209. Mosby–Year Book, St. Louis, 1993.
6. Beart, R.W. Jr., Dozois, R.R., Kelly K.A. Ileoanal anastomosis in the adult. Surg. Gynecol. Obstet. 154:826, 1982.
7. Beart, R.W. Jr. Proctocolectomy and ileoanal anastomosis. World J. Surg. 12:160, 1988.
8. Beart, R.W. Jr. Ulcerative colitis: Complications of pelvic pouch. In Fazio, V.W. (Ed.) Current therapy in colon and rectal surgery. p. 180. B.C. Decker, Toronto, 1990.
9. Becker, J.M. Anal sphincter function after colectomy, mucosal proctectomy, and endorectal ileoanal pull-through. Arch. Surg. 119:526, 1984.
10. Becker, J.M., Raymond, J.L. Ileal pouch-anal anastomosis: A single surgeon's experience with 100 consecutive cases. Ann. Surg. 204:375, 1986.
11. Block, G.E. Total proctocolectomy for inflammatory bowel disease. In Nyhus, L.M., Baker, R.J. (Eds.) Mastery of surgery. Ed. 2, vol. II, p. 1285. Little, Brown, Boston 1992.
12. Brooke, B.N. The management of an ileostomy including its complications. Lancet 2:102, 1952.
13. Burnstein, M.J., Shoetz, D.J. Jr., Coller, J.A., Veindenheimer, M.C. Technique of mesenteric lengthening in ileal reservoir–anal anastomosis. Dis. Colon Rectum 30:863, 1987.
14. Carter, F.M., McLeod, R.S., Cohen, Z. Subtotal colectomy for ulcerative colitis: Complications related to the rectal remnant. Dis. Colon Rectum 34:1005, 1991.
15. Cohen, Z., McLeod, R.S. Proctocolectomy and ileoanal anastomosis with J-shaped or S-shaped ileal pouch. World J. Surg. 12:164, 1988.
16. Cohen, Z., McLeod, R.S., Stephen, W., Stern, H.S., O'Connor, B., Reznick, R. Continuing evolution of the pelvic pouch procedure. Ann. Surg. 16:506, 1992.
17. Collins, R.H., Feidman, M., Fordtran, J.S. Colon cancer dysplasia and surveillance in patients with ulcerative colitis. A critical review. N. Engl. J. Med. 316:1654, 1987.
18. Corman, M.L. Colon and rectal surgery. Ed. 3, p. 901. Lippincott, Philadelphia, 1993.
19. Chassin, J.L. Operative strategy in general surgery. Ed. 2, p. 403. Springer-Verlag, New York, 1993.
20. Danovitch, S.H. Fulminant colitis and toxic megacolon. Gastroenterol. Clin. North Am. 18:73, 1989.
21. Danzi, J.T. Extraintestinal manifestations of idiopathic inflammatory bowel disease. Arch. Intern. Med. 148:297, 1988.
22. Dozois, R.R., Kelly, K.A. Newer operations for ulcerative colitis and Crohn's disease. In Kisner, J.B., Shorter, R.G. (Eds.) Inflammatory bowel disease. Ed. 3. London, Balliere Tindall, 1980.
23. Dozois, R.R. Pelvic and perianastomotic complications after ileoanal anastomosis. Perspect. Colon Rectal Surg. 1:113, 1988.
24. Dozois, R.R. Technique of ileal pouch–anal anastomosis. Perspect. Colon Rectal Surg. 2:85, 1989.
25. Dozois, R.R. Ulcerative colitis: Surgical alternatives. In Fazio V.W. (Ed.) Current therapy in colon and rectal surgery. p. 166, B.C. Decker, Philadelphia, 1990.
26. Ekbom, A., Helmick, C., Zack, M., Adami, H.O. Ulcerative colitis and colorectal cancer. A population-based study. N. Engl. J. Med. 323:1228, 1990.
27. Fazio, V.W. Toxic megacolon in ulcerative colitis and Crohn's colitis. Clin. Gastroenterol. 389:407, 1980.
28. Fazio, V.W., Church, J.M. Complications and function of the continent ileostomy at the Cleveland Clinic. World J. Surg. 12:148, 1988.
29. Fazio, V.W., Verschueren, R.C.J. Ileostomy. Colostomy for toxic megacolon. In Nyhus, L.M., Baker, R.J. (Eds.) Mastery of surgery. Ed. 2, vol. II, p. 1223. Little, Brown, Boston, 1992.
30. Bazio, V.W. Total colectomy with ileorectal anastomosis. In Nyhus, L.M., Baker, R.J. (Eds.) Mastery of surgery. Ed. 2, vol. II, p. 1273. Little, Brown, Boston, 1992.
31. Fazio, V.W., Tjandra, J.J. Technique for nipple valve fixation to prevent valve slippage in continent ileostomy. Dis. Colon Rectum 35:1177, 1992.
32. Ferrari, B.T., Fonkalsrud, E.W. Endorectal ileal pull-through operation with ileal reservoir after total colectomy. Am. J. Surg. 136:113, 1978.
33. Fonkalsrud, E.W. Total colectomy and endorectal ileal pullthrough with internal ileal reservoir for ulcerative colitis. Surg. Gynecol. Obstet. 150:1, 1980.
34. Fonkalsrud, E.W. Endorectal pullthrough with ileal reservoir for ulcerative colitis and polyposis. Am. J. Surg. 144:81, 1982.
35. Fonkalsrud, E.W. Endorectal ileoanal anastomosis with isoperistaltic ileal reservoir after colectomy and mucosal proctectomy. Ann. Surg. 199:151, 1984.
36. Fonkalsrud, E.W. Update on clinical experience with different surgical techniques on the endorectal pullthrough operation for colitis and polyposis. Surg. Gynecol. Obstet. 165:309, 1987.
37. Fonkalsrud, E.W., Stelzner, M., McDonald, N. Experience with the endorectal ileal pullthrough with lateral reservoir for ulcerative colitis and polyposis. Arch. Surg. 123:1053, 1988.
38. Galandiuk, S., Wolff, B.G., Dozois, R.R., Beart, R.W. Jr. Ileal pouch–anal anastomosis without ileostomy. Dis. Colon Rectum 34:870, 1991.
39. Goligher, J.C. Procedures conserving continence in the surgical management of ulcerative colitis. Surg. Clin. North Am. 63:49, 1983.
40. Hawley, P.R. Emergency surgery for ulcerative colitis. World J. Surg. 12:169, 1988.
41. Heppell, J., Farkough, E., Dube, S., Pelloquin Morgan, S., Bernard, D. Toxic megacolon. Analysis of 70 cases. Dis. Colon Rectum 29:789, 1986.
42. Hulten, L. The continent ileostomy (Kock pouch) versus the restorative proctocolectomy (pelvic pouch). World J. Surg. 9:952, 1985.
43. Keighley, M.R.B. Abdominal mucosectomy reduces the incidence of soiling and sphincter damage after restorative proctocolectomy and J-pouch. Dis. Colon Rectum 30:386, 1987.
44. Keighley, M.R.B. Ulcerative colitis. In Keighley, M.R.B., Williams, N.S. (Eds.) Surgery of the anus, rectum and colon. Vol. 2, p. 1239. W.B. Saunders, London, 1993.
45. Kewenter, J., Brevinge, H. Continent ileostomy (reservoir ileostomy). In Fielding, L.P., Goldberg, S.M. (Eds.) Surgery of the colon, rectum and anus. Ed. 5, p. 590. Butterworth-Heinemann, Oxford, 1993.
46. Kirsner, J.B., Shorter, R.G. Inflammatory bowel disease. Lea & Febiger, Philadelphia, 1988.
47. Kmiot, W.A., Keighley, M.R.B. Pouchitis: Defining and objective method of diagnosis. Int. J. Colorectal Dis. 4:222, 1989.
48. Kock, N.G. Intra-abdominal "reservoir" in patients with permanent ileostomy, Preliminary observations on a procedure resulting in fecal continence in five ileostomy patients. Arch. Surg. 99:223, 1969.
49. Kock, N.G., Brevinge, H., Operskoy, B. Continent ileostomy. Perspect. Colon Rectal Surg. 2(2):71, 1989.
50. Kock, N.G. Conversion from a standard ileostomy to a Kock pouch. In Bauer, J.J. (Ed.) Colorectal surgery illustrated. p. 193. Mosby–Year Book, St. Louis, 1993.
51. Köhler, L.W., Pemberton, J.H., Zinsmeister, A.R., Kelly, K.A. Quality of life after proctocolectomy. A comparison of Brooke ileostomy, Kock pouch and ileal pouch–anal anastomosis. Gastroenterology 101:679, 1991.
52. Lavery, I.C., Chiulli, R.A., Jagelman, D.G., Fazio, V.W., Weakley, F.L. Survival with carcinoma arising in mucosal ulcerative colitis. Ann. Surg. 195:508, 1982.
53. Lavery, I.C. Colectomy and ileorectal anastomosis. In Baurer, J.J. (Ed.) Colorectal surgery illustrated. p. 201. Mosby–Year Book, St. Louis, 1993.
54. Madoff, R. D. Ulcerative colitis. In Bell, R.H. Jr., Rikkers, L.F., Mulholland, M.W. (Eds.) Digestive tract surgery. p. 1339. Lippincott-Raven, 1996.

55. Mackeigan, J.M., Cataldo, P.A. Intestinal stomas. Quality Medical Publishing, St. Louis, 1993.
56. Martin, L.W., LeCoultre, C. Technical considerations in performing total colectomy and Soave endorectal anastomosis for ulcerative colitis. Ann. Surg. 186:477, 1977.
57. Martin, L.W., LeCoultre, C. Technical considerations in performing total colectomy and Soave endorectal anastomosis for ulcerative colitis. J. Pediatr. Surg. 13:762, 1978.
58. Martin, L.W., Fischer, J.V. Preservation of anorectal continence following total colectomy. Ann. Surg. 196:700, 1982.
59. Martin, L.W. Total colectomy with mucosal proctectomy for ulcerative colitis. In Nyhus, L.M., Baker, R.J. (Eds.) Mastery of surgery. Ed. 2, vol. II, p. 1246. Little, Brown, Boston, 1992.
60. Matikainen, M., Santavirta, J., Hiltunen, K.M. Ileoanal anastomosis without covering ileostomy. Dis. Colon Rectum 33:384, 1990.
61. Metcalf, A.M., Kelly, K.A., Beart, R.W. Jr., Dozois, R.R., Wolff, B.G., Istrup, D.M. Ileal pouch–anal anastomosis without temporary diverting ileostomy. Dis. Colon Rectum 21:33, 1986.
62. Monsen, V., Sorstad, J., Hellers, G., Johanson, C. Extracolonic diagnoses in ulcerative colitis: An epidemiological study. Am. J. Gastroenterol. 85:711, 1990.
63. Morson, B.C., Dawson, I.M.P. Gastrointestinal pathology. p. 458. Blackwell, Oxford, 1972.
64. Nicholls, R.J., Pezim, M.E. Restorative proctocolectomy with ileal reservoir for ulcerative colitis and familial polyposis: A comparison of three reservoir designs. Br. J. Surg. 72:470, 1985.
65. Nicholls, R.J., Lubowski, D.R. Restorative proctocolectomy: The four loop (W) reservoir. Br. J. Surg. 74:564, 1987.
66. Nissen, R. Demonstrationen aus der operativen chirurgie zunachst einige beobachtungen aus der platischen chirurgie Zentralbl. Chir. 60:888, 1933.
67. Nivatvongs, S. Ulcerative colitis. In Gordon, P.H., Nivatvongs, S. (Eds.) Colon, rectum and anus. p. 667. Quality Medical Publishing, St. Louis, 1992.
68. Oakley, J.R. Acute ulcerative colitis and toxic dilatation. In Fazio, V.W. (Ed.) Current therapy in colon and rectal surgery. p. 174. B.C. Decker, Toronto, 1990.
69. Parc, R., Tiret, E., Frileaux, P., Moszkowoski, E., Loygue, J. Resection and coloanal anastomosis with colonic reservoir for rectal carcinoma. Br. J. Surg. 73:139, 1986.
70. Parks, A.G., Nicholls, R.J. Proctocolectomy without ileostomy for ulcerative colitis. Br. Med. J. 2:85, 1978.
71. Parks, A.G., Nicholls, R.J., Belliveau, P. Proctocolectomy with ileal reservoir and anal anastomosis. Br. J. Surg. 67:533, 1980.
72. Pearl, R.K., Nelson, R.L., Prasad, M.L., Abcarian, H., Schuller, N. Ileoanal anastomosis 24 years after total proctocolectomy for ulcerative colitis. Dis. Colon Rectum 28:180, 1985.
73. Pemberton, J.H., Kelly, K.A., Beart, R.W. Jr., Dozois, R.R., Wolff, B.G., Ilstrup, D.M. Ileal pouch–anal anastomosis for chronic ulcerative colitis. Long-term results. Ann. Surg. 206:504, 1987.
74. Pemberton, J.H., Phillips, S.F., Ready, R.R., Zinsmeister, A.R., Beahrs, O.H. Quality of life after Brooke ileostomy and ileal pouch–anal anastomosis. Ann. Surg. 209:620, 1989.
75. Pena, J.L., Gemlo, B.T., Rothenberger, D.A. Ileal pouch–anal anastomosis: State of the art. Baillieres Clin. Gastroenterol. 6:113, 1992.
76. Ransohoff, D.F. Cancer in ulcerative colitis (Editorial). Gastroenterology 94:1089, 1988.
77. Ravitch, M.M., Sabiston, D.C. Anal ileostomy with preservation of the sphincter. A proposed operation in patients requiring total colectomy for benign lesions. Surg. Gynecol. Obstet. 84:1098, 1947.
78. Ravitch, M.M. Anal ileostomy with sphincter preservation in patients requiring total colectomy for benign conditions. Surgery 24:170, 1948.
79. Ravitch, M.M., Handelsman, J.C. One stage resection of entire colon and rectum for ulcerative colitis and polypoid adenomatosis. Bull. Johns Hopkins Hosp. 88:59, 1951.
80. Rothenberger, D.A., Verneulen, F.D., Christenson, C.E., Nivatvongs, S., et al. Restorative proctocolectomy with ileal reservoir and ileoanal anastomosis. Am. J. Surg. 145:82, 1983.
81. Rothenberger, D.A., Fazio, V.W., Keighley, M.R.B., Schoetz, D.J., Wolff, B.G. Ileal pouch-anal anastomosis: Current controversies. Perspect. Colon Rectal Surg. 4:233, 1991.
82. Rothenberger, D.A. Pouch procedures: Introductory comment. In Fielding, L.P., Golberg, S.M. (Eds.) Surgery of the colon, rectum and anus. Ed. 5. p. 589. Butterworth-Heinemann, Oxford, 1993.
83. Sagar, P.M., Lewis, W., Holdsworth, P.J., Johnston, D. One stage restorative proctocolectomy without temporary defunctioning ileostomy. Dis. Colon Rectum 35:582, 1992.
84. Schrock, T.R. Colitis. In Way, L.W. (Ed.) Current surgical diagnosis and treatment. Ed. 9, p. 666. Appleton Lange, Norwalk, CT, 1991.
85. Seow-Choen, S., Tsunoda, A., Nicholl, S. Prospective randomized trial comparing anal function after hand-sewn ileoanal anastomosis with mucosectomy versus stapled ileoanal anastomosis without mucosectomy. Br. J. Surg. 78:430, 1991.
86. Smith, L., Friend, W.G., Medwell, S.J. The superior mesenteric artery: The critical factor in the pouch pull-through procedure. Dis. Colon Rectum 27:741, 1984.
87. Soave, F.A. A new surgical technique for treatment of Hirschprung's disease. Surgery 56:1007, 1964.
88. Sugerman, H.J., Newsone, H.H., DeCosta, G., Zfass, A.M. Stapled ileoanal anastomosis for ulcerative colitis and familial polyposis without a temporary diverting ileostomy. Ann. Surg. 213:606, 1991.
89. Sullivan, E.S., Garnjobst, W.M. Advantage of initial transanal mucosal stripping in ileo-anal pull through procedures. Dis. Colon Rectum 25:170, 1982.
90. Taylor, B.M., Beart, R.W., Dozois, R.R., Kelly, K.A., Phillips, S.F. Straight ileoanal anastomosis V ileal pouch–anal anastomosis after colectomy and mucosal proctectomy. Arch. Surg. 118:696, 1983.
91. Telander, R.L., Perrault, J. Colectomy and ileoanal anastomosis in young patients. Arch. Surg. 116:623, 1981.
92. Turnbull, R.B. Jr., Weakley, F.L. Atlas of intestinal stomas. C.V. Mosby, St. Louis, 1967.
93. Turnbull, R.B. Jr., Hawk, W.A., Weakley, F.L. Surgical treatment of toxic megacolon: Ileostomy and colostomy to prepare patients for colectomy. Am. J. Surg. 122:325, 1971.
94. Tytgat, G.N., van Deventer, S.J. Pouchitis. Int. J. Colorectal Dis. 3:226, 1988.
95. Utsunomiya, J., Iwama, T., Inajo, M., et al. Total colectomy, mucosal proctectomy and ileoanal anastomosis. Dis. Colon Rectum 23:459, 1980.
96. Utsunomiya, J. Ileoanal anastomosis with ileal reservoir: J pouch. In Fielding, L.P., Goldberg, S.M. (Eds.). Surgery of the colon, rectum and anus. Ed. 5, p. 629. Butterworth-Heinemann, Oxford, 1993.
97. van Heerden, J.A., Beart, R.W. Jr. Carcinoma of the colon and rectum complicating chronic ulcerative colitis. Dis. Colon Rectum 23:155, 1980.
98. Vernava, A.M., Goldberg, S.M. Is the Kock pouch still a viable option? Int. Colorectal Dis. 3:135, 1988.
99. Wexner, S.D., Jagelman, A.G. The double-stapled ileal reservoir and ileo-anal anastomosis. Perspect. Colon Rectal Surg. 3:132, 1990.
100. Wexner, S.D., Wong, W.D., Rothenberger, D.A., Goldberg, S.M. The ileoanal reservoir. Am. J. Surg. 159:178, 1990.

Section H

Colon, Rectum, and Anus

CHAPTER 61

Crohn's Disease

Crohn's disease is a complex affliction of unknown cause that can affect any segment of the gastrointestinal tract, from the skin around the mouth to the perianal skin. Histologically, it is an unspecific, transmural inflammatory process of slow, insidious evolution (31, 41). The illness affects segments of the gastrointestinal tract except in some cases of Crohn's colitis in which the process extends diffusely through the entire extent of the colon and rectum, in continuous fashion. The evolution of Crohn's disease is variable and its prognosis unpredictable. This illness is characterized by production of internal or external fistulas, the latter usually due to previous surgical interventions (5, 6, 16, 18, 31). Crohn's disease is a recurring process with more recurrences the longer the follow-up of the patients (16, 30, 31, 34). Both medical and surgical treatment should be considered palliative, since the disease is incurable and recurrences mean more surgical procedures because the illness continues its course.

Surgical treatment of Crohn's disease is indicated when medical treatment has failed and symptoms persist or become worse. Indications for surgery should be based on symptoms and not on radiologic images. Surgical treatment does not cure patients but makes symptoms disappear, favoring the patient's recovery and allowing the patient to have a normal life for a variable period of time.

The most frequent site of recurrence of Crohn's disease is the distal ileum, with or without simultaneous lesions in the cecum or the ascending colon (6, 15, 28, 34, 41). This location of the illness is usually known as classic Crohn's disease (31).

CROHN'S DISEASE OF THE SMALL BOWEL

Crohn's disease of the small intestine begins with a small superficial soft ulcer that later invades the muscular and serosal layers, giving rise to an inflammatory process that affects the entire thickness of the intestinal wall. The inflammatory process of the serosa (serositis) favors the production of adhesions to other intestinal loops and, later, to internal fistulas and intraabdominal abscesses. The transmural inflammatory process of the bowel increases the consistency of the affected segment of bowel and narrowing of its lumen. The mesentery is also affected by Crohn's disease, which causes increased thickness and consistency with occasional severe infarction of its lymph nodes (6, 10, 14, 19, 21, 31, 34, 41). The mesenteric fat of the involved bowel segment advances on both sides of the intestinal wall, completely surrounding the bowel in many cases (Fig. 1).

The external appearance of the affected segment, its increased consistency, and the advancement of the mesenteric fat give the bowel an appearance that makes it easily distinguished from healthy bowel, making the site of transection in surgical cases obvious. The increase in thickness and consistency of the sick bowel frequently cause an obstructive clinical picture that is rarely acute and complete, more frequently partial.

In 55% of patients Crohn's disease involves the small and large bowel simultaneously, in 30% the disease is localized in the small bowel, and in 15% of cases it is localized in the large bowel. Patients who have Crohn's disease of the small and large bowel simultaneously have anorectal lesions in 41% of cases, while only 21% of patients with the disease limited to the small bowel present anorectal lesions (15, 16, 19, 22, 33, 34, 42).

The diagnosis of Crohn's disease of the small bowel is made by the clinical history and abdominal palpation. The affected small bowel has, as was previously stated, thickened walls, making it frequently palpable. To this are added the obstructive bowel sounds due to narrowing of the bowel. X-ray of the small bowel using radiopaque contrast material is of great importance, as dilated and narrowed segments of jejunum and, especially, ileum can be seen. The study is more revealing if it shows a Kantor string sign, which is of greater diagnostic value, although not pathognomonic of Crohn's disease of the distal ileum. The diagnosis of intraabdominal abscesses, thick bowel walls, phlegmons, and/or fistulas is frequently made by means of magnetic resonance, computed tomography, and ultrasonography.

The surgical procedure used in the treatment of Crohn's disease of the small bowel is resection of the affected segment. The line of resection should pass about 5 or 6 cm from the lesion. A sufficiently large segment of mesentery should be resected to permit adequate suturing of the bowel ends. This anastomosis is made in end-to-end fashion, using one or two layers of continuous or interrupted sutures. The author uses two layers of interrupted sutures, the mucosal layer with 3-0 chromic catgut, and the seromuscular layer with synthetic nonabsorbable sutures. If the distal end is narrower in caliber then the proximal end, its diameter can be increased using the Cheatle technique.

Transection of the bowel 5 cm from the macroscopic lesion may pass through tissue microscopically invaded by disease. Different statistics have shown that late results in these cases are similar to those where the bowel is sectioned through healthy tissue (8, 44, 53). Some authors affirm (51, 52) that recurrences are less frequent when the bowel is transected through healthy tissue. Most authors presently maintain that transection should be carried out 5 cm from the macroscopic lesion, be it invaded or not by the disease. If the disease involves the distal ileum and the cecum or ascending colon simultaneously, resection should include the cecum and ascending colon, transecting the colon 5 cm from the macroscopic lesion and reconstructing bowel transit by means of an ileocolic anastomosis.

If the patient has an enterocutaneous fistula, surgery may be indicated according to the amount of loss from the fistula. Surgery should be advised if there is a daily loss of more than 500 mL without any tendency to diminish with medical therapy for 6 to 8 weeks (5, 18, 29, 31). If there is a daily loss of less than 500 mL with a tendency to diminish under medical care, the operation can be postponed, sometimes definitively. In patients with external fistulas the nutritional and electrolytic balance of the patient should be strictly controlled. In addition, the abdominal skin should be protected with protective substances as well as special bags.

In patients with internal fistulas surgery is indicated if there are alterations in nutrition and loss of liquids and electrolytes due to uncontrollable diarrhea or other alterations. Patients with internal fistulas that are asymptomatic, or moderately symptomatic, do not have to be operated upon.

Patients that have been subjected to several small bowel resections run the risk of developing short bowel syndrome. This possibility also exists in patients with very extensive Crohn's disease (5, 15, 24, 30, 31, 37). Under these conditions indications for surgery and the extent of resection should be carefully considered.

Internal fistulas may be jejunoileal, ileocecal, ileosigmoidal, ileovesical, ileovaginal, and so on. Surgical treatment of fistulas consists of resection of the segment where the fistula arises together with the fistulous tract. The segment of bowel where the fistula empties does not have to be resected unless it is also affected by Crohn's disease. The operation should be limited to resection of only a few millimeters beyond the end of the fistula.

In patients with an intraabdominal abscess the most indicated treatment is percutaneous drainage of the abscess with computed tomography or ultrasonography. The intestinal lesion can be resected after sepsis has disappeared. Percutaneous drainage of the intraabdominal abscess may be insufficient or the abscess may recur. In these cases, surgical drainage may be necessary.

Bypass and bypass with exclusion of the area of Crohn's disease operations that were frequently used previously are, at present, rarely used, and only in cases in which it is impossible to resect the affected segment or in which resection presents a grave risk for the patient.

It must be kept in mind that bypass surgery frequently produces a blind loop syndrome. On the other hand, the intestinal segment that has been excluded by the bypass can develop into a carcinoma during the course of the disease without producing any symptoms. In these cases the problem is complicated because the segment with the carcinoma is excluded, which makes confirmation of the carcinoma difficult (26, 27).

In surgery for Crohn's disease the incision, if at all possible, should be made in the left side of the abdomen in order to leave the right iliac fossa free in case it should be necessary to perform a definitive Brooke ileostomy in the future.

Strictureplasty

This surgical procedure has begun to be practiced in recent years in selected cases of Crohn's disease of the small bowel. Strictureplasty was proposed by Katariya (32), a Hindu surgeon, to treat short fibrous obstructive lesions of the small bowel caused by tuberculosis. This procedure was first used in Crohn's disease by Lee (36). Later, Alexander-Williams, of Birmingham (England) (1–3), popularized the technique with his good results. The experiences of Fazio and colleagues (20), Dehn and colleagues (11), and Sharif and Alexander-Williams confirmed these good results. Indications for strictureplasty are as follows:

1. Previously operated patients with recurrence who present one or more short fibrous strictures.
2. Patients with short bowel syndrome with one or more short fibrous strictures of the small bowel. Intestinal resection is contraindicated in these patients, no matter how short the resection may be.
3. Strictureplasty should only be performed in short, fibrous strictures, not in strictures with active inflammation.

Strictureplasty may be complicated with intestinal fistula, recurrence of the stricture, and septic abdominal problems. Strictureplasty does not involve resection of the intestinal lesion and is, therefore, more prone to lead to cancer than when the lesion is resected.

CROHN'S DISEASE AND APPENDECTOMY

It is very infrequent that acute appendicitis occurs in a patient with ileal or ileocecal Crohn's disease (21). It has not been definitely proven that an acute ileitis or ileocolitis can evolve into a typical Crohn's disease with its prolonged evolution. Frequently, acute ileitis or ileocolitis is caused by enterocolitic *Yersinia*, producing a clinical picture frequently confused with acute appendicitis but that can be treated medically without any residuals in the ileum or the cecum.

In patients with ileal, ileocecal, or ileocolic Crohn's disease, removal of the appendix prophylactically exposes the patient to complications, especially fistulas. At times, without resecting the cecal appendix, a fistula may develop by simple handling of the ileocecal area. The fistulous complication may be cecal, due to the resection of the appendix, or ileal, with or without appendectomy, probably due to rupture of a deep fissure of the ileum or due to a microperforation of the terminal ileum (39). Many surgeons (9, 19, 21) will resect the appendix in cases of Crohn's disease with a normal appearing cecum. It is the author's opinion that, *when a laparotomy is performed with a diagnosis of acute appendicitis, and the appendix is normal but there is ileal or ileocecal Crohn's disease, it is not prudent to carry out a prophylactic appendectomy.*

In case the patient presents symptoms localized to the right iliac fossa of several days' duration, it is possible that an abscess is developing and surgery may lead to an enterocutaneous fistula (52).

CROHN'S DISEASE OF THE COLON AND RECTUM

Crohn's disease more frequently affects the right colon than the left, and it is usually segmental (6, 15, 31). Ulcerative colitis, on the contrary, predominantly affects the distal colon and rectum, and spreads proximally in the colon, in continuous fashion, and not segmentally. Crohn's disease, in 10 to 15% of cases, also affects the colon and rectum in continuity, making differential diagnosis difficult, even with microscopic examination, which may lead to a mistaken surgical procedure (50). About 80% of patients with Crohn's disease of the colon may eventually need surgical treatment for their illness during the course of their disease (6, 7, 15, 50).

The procedure of choice in Crohn's disease of the colon depends on several factors (50):

1. Location of the lesion.
2. Extension of the lesion.
3. Condition of the rectum, normal or diseased.
4. Condition of the anoperineal area.
5. Age of the patient.
6. Acceptance by the patient of a permanent Brooke ileostomy.

Crohn's disease, when located in the right colon, is usually associated with an ileal lesion that frequently produces obstructive symptoms. Patients with this localization of Crohn's disease have to be submitted to surgery in 90% of cases, at some time during the evolution of their illness (4, 13, 15, 50). When located in the left colon, Crohn's disease generally affects older patients than those with the disease in their right colon, and indications for surgery during the course of their illness are lower, about 50%.

Crohn's disease, located in the right colon, with a simultaneous ileal lesion, frequently develops intraabdominal abscesses or enterocutaneous fistulas. Patients with the disease restricted to the sigmoid may develop obstruction or uncontrollable diarrhea.

Total proctocolectomy with permanent Brooke ileostomy is the operation with less recurrences used in treating Crohn's disease of the colon. However, this operation is associated with a permanent Brooke ileostomy and involves resection of the anus and rectum, which is frequently associated with sexual dysfunction in men. Less major operations, however, are indicated in Crohn's disease that is limited to a segment of colon (4, 7, 37, 38, 50, 52). In patients with Crohn's disease limited to the right colon, with or without simultaneous disease in the ileum, the most frequently performed operation is a limited hemicolectomy.

If the disease is located in the transverse colon, the splenic flexure, or the descending or sigmoid colon, and the rectum and ileum are healthy, a segmental resection of colon can be done. If the ileum is affected or the patient has been previously operated on for the same affliction or presents rectal or anoperineal disease, a segmental resection should not be done.

In patients with segmental involvement of the right or left colon with healthy ileum, rectum, and anoperineal areas, a total colectomy with ileorectal anastomosis can be done. If the sigmoid is not affected, a subtotal colectomy with ileosigmoidal anastomosis may be indicated. Patients with segmental resection or with total colectomy and ileorectal anastomoses will develop recurrences in 50 to 60% of cases and will have to be subjected to a total colectomy with permanent Brooke ileostomy.

The position adopted by many surgeons is acceptable when they choose to carry out a segmental colectomy or a total or subtotal colectomy with ileorectal or ileosigmoidal anastomosis because it offers young patients the possibility of passing their young years with normal sexual activity and having children, even though they know it is very possible they may need a proctocolectomy with permanent ileostomy in the future.

OPERATIVE TECHNIQUE

The operative technique in resection and anastomosis of the small bowel for Crohn's disease is similar to the technique described in the chapter on resection and anastomosis of the small bowel. The surgical techniques for colectomy, proctocolectomy with permanent Brooke ileostomy, and Miles abdominoperineal resection are described in the chapters covering surgery in ulcerative colitis and carcinoma of the colon and rectum.

Operative Technique

FIGURE 61.1
Surgical photograph of a patient with Crohn's disease of the ileum in which it is possible to observe an area of bowel with a pronounced stenosis, a marked thickening of the mesentery, and very enlarged nodes. The mesenteric fat has practically surrounded the entire circumference of the affected bowel. The right hand of the surgeon is holding a segment of ileum proximal to the lesion with normal appearing walls, allowing the macroscopic differences between the affected segment and the apparently healthy segment to be seen.

Operative Technique

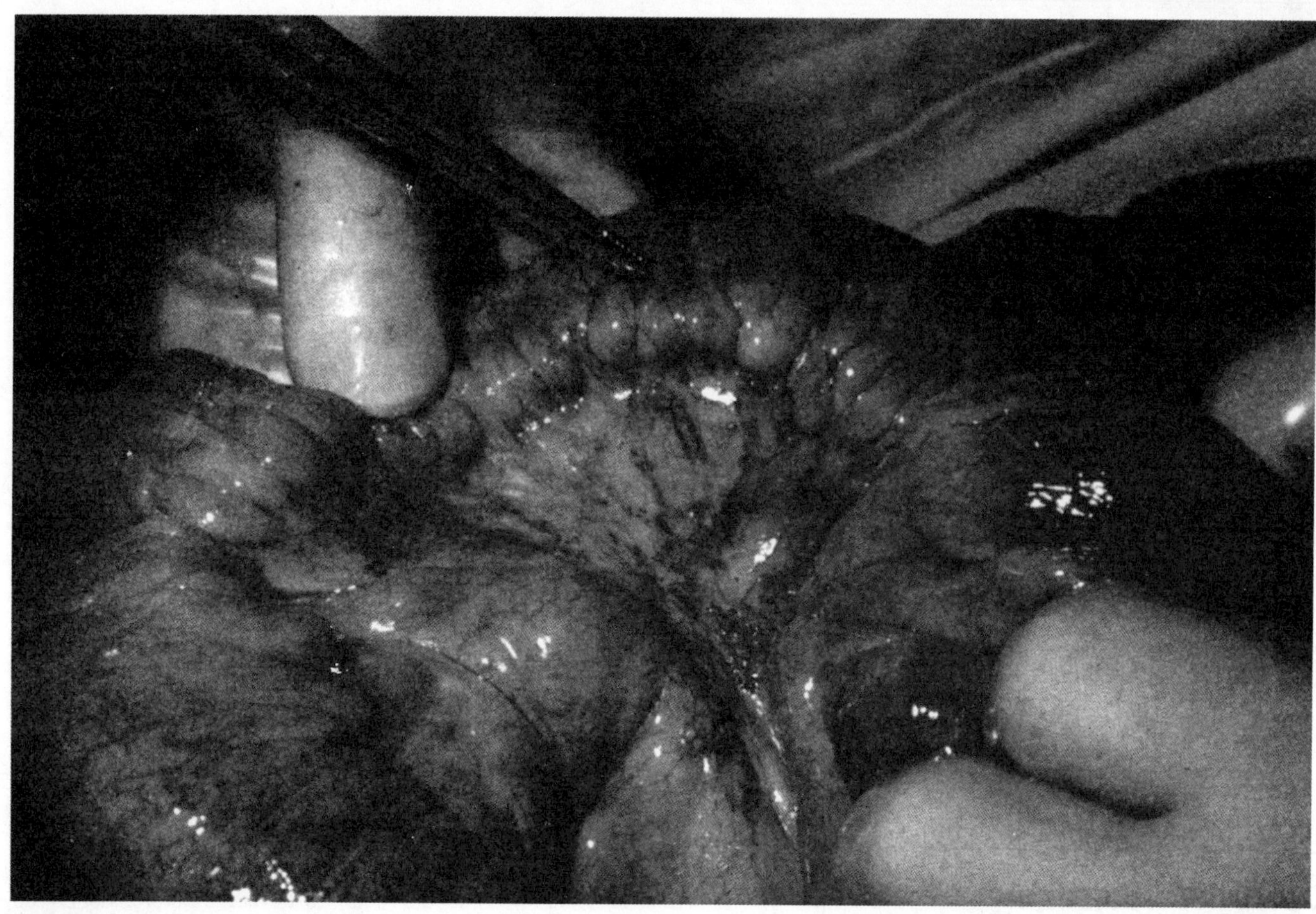

FIGURE 61.1

Operative Technique

FIGURE 61.2 HEINEKE-MIKULICZ (ALEXANDER-WILLIAMS) STRICTUREPLASTY (1–3)

Two traction sutures have been placed, one on each side, in the center of the stenotic lesion of the small intestine. With an electric scalpel, the antimesenteric border of the bowel is incised longitudinally, The incision is begun in the distal healthy bowel and then extended through the stenotic area and finally the healthy proximal segment. The open bowel is inspected and explored for possible additional strictures, not obvious on inspection and palpation, so that they can be treated in the same operation. For this purpose a 30 F catheter with a balloon at its end is used. Frequently several strictureplasties are done during one operation.

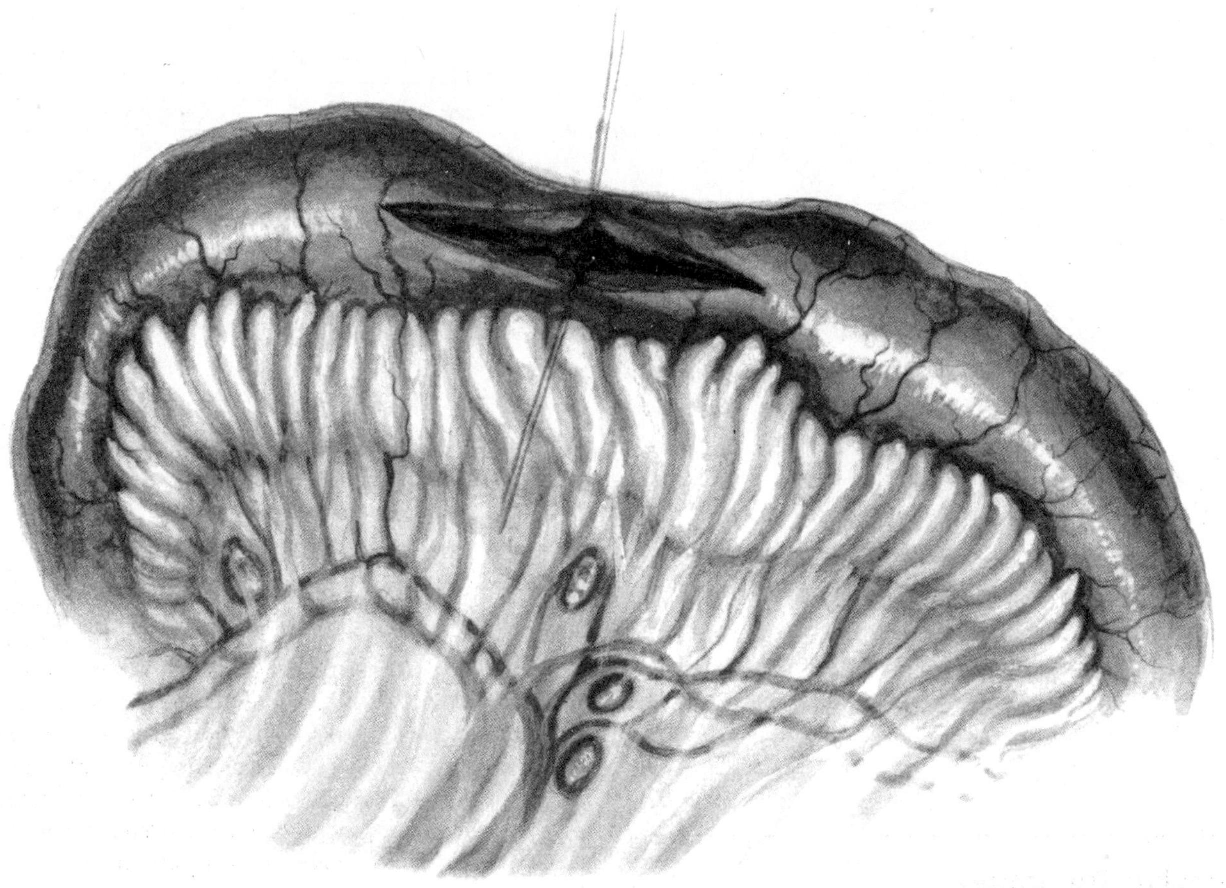

FIGURE 61.2 HEINEKE-MIKULICZ (ALEXANDER-WILLIAMS) STRICTUREPLASTY (1–3)

FIGURE 61.3
The longitudinal incision is closed transversely with interrupted Vicryl (Ethicon) sutures, in the same way as in a Heineke-Mikulicz pyloroplasty. Some surgeons use two layers of interrupted or continuous sutures, which is not easy to do because of the fibrosis of the intestinal wall. Alexander-Williams advises that the adequacy of this closure be tested by insufflation, with carbonic anhydrase, to test for leakage. If there is any doubt, some surgeons recommend covering the suture line with a jejunal serosal patch. Before closing, the abdominal cavity should be irrigated with several liters of warm saline solution. The Heineke-Mikulicz strictureplasty is used for short fibrous strictures. Longer strictures should be treated using the Finney technique.

Operative Technique

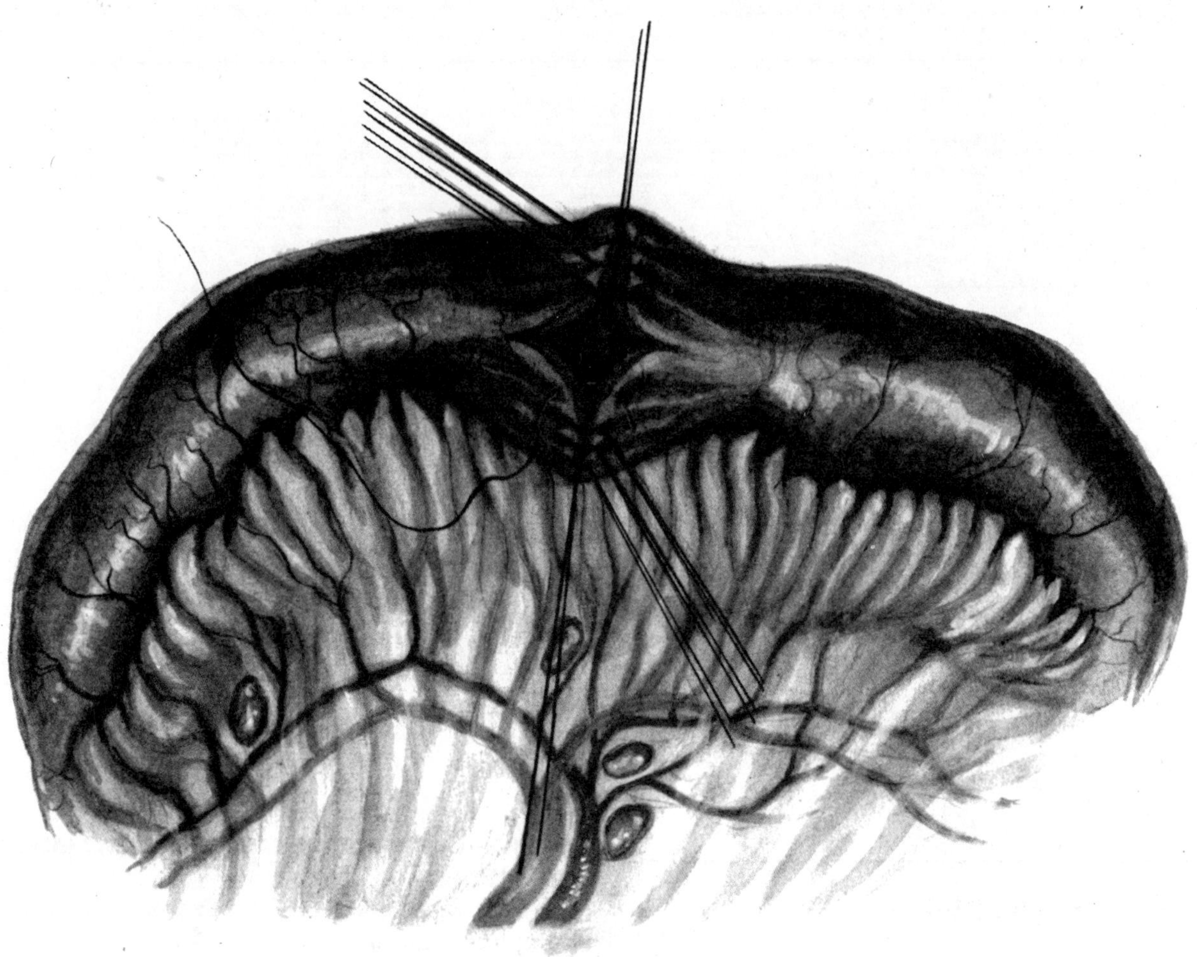

FIGURE 61.3

Operative Technique

FIGURE 61.4 FINNEY-TYPE STRICTUREPLASTY (ALEXANDER-WILLIAMS) (1–3)

The long fibrous stricture is due to Crohn's disease. **A,** The stenosed segment is being incised using a conventional scalpel, extending this incision 3 or 4 cm beyond the stricture both proximally and distally. The bowel can be incised with a conventional scalpel, since hemostasis will be done with the bowel suture. With the bowel open, its lumen will be explored, distally and proximally, with a 30 F catheter with a balloon at its end, so as to search for the possibility of other strictures that are not obvious on inspection or palpation, to be able to treat them during the same surgical procedure. **B,** Three traction sutures have been placed and the bowel has been folded in preparation for the Finney technique. **C,** The posterior borders of the intestine have been sutured with interrupted Vicryl sutures, and the anterior borders are being sutured with the same material, using interrupted or continuous sutures.

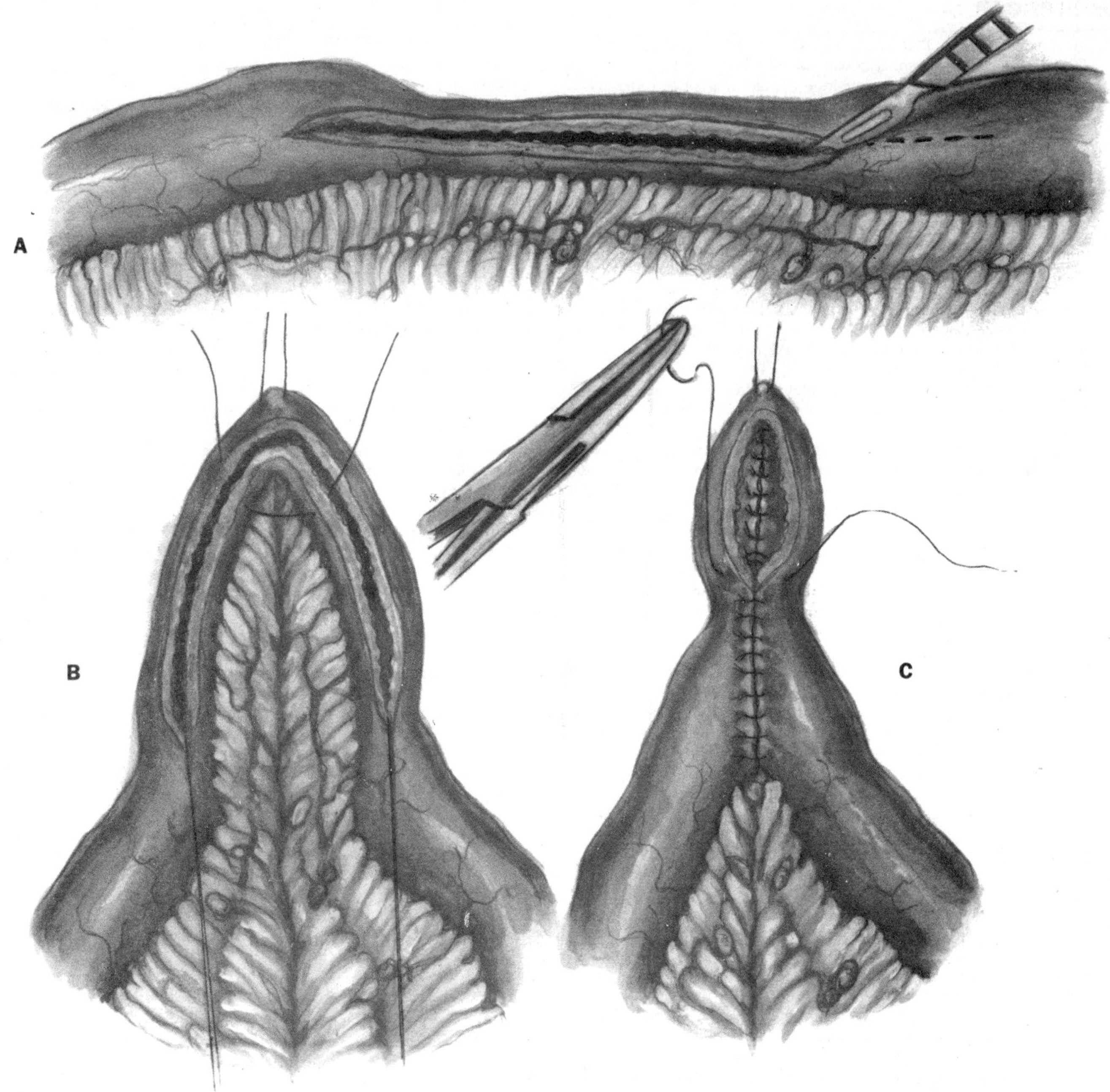

FIGURE 61.4 FINNEY-TYPE STRICTUREPLASTY (ALEXANDER-WILLIAMS) (1–3)

References

1. Alexander-Williams, J., Haynes, I.G. Conservative operations for Crohn's disease of the small bowel. World J. Surg. 9:945, 1985.
2. Alexander-Williams, J. The technique of intestinal strictureplasty. Int. J. Colorectal Dis. 1:54, 1986.
3. Alexander-Williams, J. Intestinal stricturoplasty. In Fielding, L.P., Goldberg, S.M. (Eds.) Surgery of the colon, rectum and anus. Ed. 5, p. 320. Butterworth-Heinemann, Oxford, 1993.
4. Allan, A., Andrew, H., Hilton, C., Keighley, M., Allan, R., Alexander-Williams, J. Segmental colonic resection is appropriate operation for short skip lesions due to Crohn's disease in the colon. World J. Surg. 13:611,1989.
5. Annibali, R., Pietri, P. Fistulous complications of Crohn's disease. Int. Surg. 77:19, 1992.
6. Bernell, O., Hellers, G. Resection of the small intestine for inflammatory bowel disease. In Fielding, L.P., Goldberg, S.M. (Eds.) Surgery of the colon, rectum and anus. Ed. 5, p. 308. Butterworth-Heinemann, Oxford, 1993.
7. Buchmann, P., Weterman, I.T., Keighley, M.R.B., et al. The prognosis of ileorectal anastomosis in Crohn's disease. Br. J. Surg. 68:7, 1981.
8. Cooper, J.C., Williams, M.S. The influence of microscopic disease at the margin of resection on recurrence rates in Crohn's disease. Ann. R. Coll. Surg. Engl. 68:23, 1986.
9. Corman, M.L. Colon and rectal surgery. Ed. 3, p. 1012. Lippincott, Philadelphia, 1993.
10. Crohn, B.B., Ginzburg, I., Oppenheimer, G.D. Regional enteritis: A pathological and clinical study. J.A.M.A. 99:1323, 1932.
11. Dehn, T.C.B., Kettlewel, M.G.W., Mortensen, N.J., et al. Ten year experience of strictureplasty for obstructive Crohn's disease. Br. J. Surg. 76:339, 1991.
12. Etala, E. Enteritis regional. Rev. Argent. Cirug. 9:200, 1965.
13. Etala, E., Romero, L.M. Colitis ulcerosas segmentarias. Bull. Soc. Internat. Chirurg. 5:118, 1968.
14. Etala, E., Zuckerberg, C., Bonini, E.H. La patología del íleon terminal en la colitis ulcerosa y en la Enfermedad de Crohn del colon. Pren. Méd. Argent. 68:339, 1981.
15. Farmer, R.G., Hawk, W.A., Turnbull, R.B. Jr. Indication for surgery in Crohn's disease, Analyses of 500 cases. Gastroenterology 71:245, 1976.
16. Farmer, R.G., Whelan, G., Fazio, V.W. Long-term follow-up of patients with Crohn's disease. Gastroenterology 88:1818, 1985.
17. Fazio, V.W. Toxic megacolon in ulcerative colitis and Crohn's colitis. Clin. Gastroenterol. 9:389, 1980.
18. Fazio, V.W., Coutsoftides, T., Steiger, E. Factors influencing the outcome of treatment of small bowel cutaneous fistula. World J. Surg. 7:481, 1983.
19. Fazio, V.W. Regional enteritis (Crohn's disease): Indication for surgery and operative strategy. Surg. Clin. North Am. 63:27, 1983.
20. Fazio, V.W., Galandiuk, S., Jagelman, D.G., Lavery, I.C. Strictureplasty in Crohn's disease. Ann. Surg. 210:621, 1989.
21. Fromm, D. Small intestine. In Fromm, D. (Ed.) Gastrointestinal surgery. Vol. 1, p. 371. Churchill Livingstone, New York, 1985.
22. Fry, R.D., Shemesh, E.L., Kodner, I.J. The management of anal and perineal Crohn's disease. Technique and results. Surg. Gynecol. Obstet. 168:42, 1989.
23. Goligher, J.C. Surgery of the anus, rectum and colon. Ed. 4, p. 827. Balliere Tindall, London, 1980.
24. Goligher, J.C. The long-term results of excisional surgery in primary and recurrent Crohn's disease after resection. Dis. Colon Rectum 28:51, 1985.
25. Gordon, P.H., Nivatvongs, S. Colon, rectum and anus. p. 719. Quality Medical Publishing, St. Louis, 1962.
26. Greenstein, A.J., Sachar, D., Pucilo, A., et al. Cancer in Crohn's disease after diversionary surgery. A report of seven carcinomas occurring in excluded bowel. Am. J. Surg. 135:86, 1978.
27. Hawker, P.C., Gyde, S.N., Thompson, H., Allan, R.N. Adenocarcinoma of the small intestine complicating Crohn's disease. Gut 23:188, 1982.
28. Higgens, C.S., Allan, R.N. Crohn's disease of the ileum. Gut 21:933, 1980.
29. Hill, G.L. Operative strategy in the treatment of enterocutaneous fistulas. World J. Surg. 7:495, 1983.
30. Homan, W.P., Dineen, P. Comparison of the results of resection, bypass and bypass with exclusion for ileocecal Crohn's disease.
31. Hulten, L. Surgical management and strategy in classical Crohn's disease. Int. Surg. 77:2, 1992.
32. Katariya, R.N., Sood, S., Rao, P.G., Rao, P.L.N.G. Stricture-plasty for tubercular structures of the gastro-intestinal tract. Br. J. Surg. 64:496, 1977.
33. Kelly, K.A., Wolf, B.G. Crohn's disease (regional enteritis). In Sabiston, D.C. (Ed.) Textbook of surgery. Ed. 14, p. 843. W.B. Saunders, Philadelphia, 1991.
34. Kyle, J., Crohn's disease. p. 1. William Heinemann Medical Books, London, 1972.
35. Kovalcik, P., Simstei, L., Weiss, M., Mullen, J. The dilemma of Crohn's disease: Crohn's disease and appendectomy. Dis. Colon Rectum 20:377, 1977.
36. Lee, E.C.G., Papainnou, N. Minimal surgery for chronic obstruction in patients with extensive or universal Crohn's disease. Ann. R. Coll. Surg. Engl. 64:229, 1982.
37. Lock, M.R., Farmer, R.C., Fazio, V.W., et al. Recurrence and reoperation for Crohn's disease. N. Engl. J. Med. 304:1586, 1981.
38. Longo, W.E., Ballantyne, G.H., Cahow, E. Treatment of Crohn's colitis: Segmental or total colectomy. Arch. Surg. 123:588, 1988.
39. Marx, F.W. Jr. Incidental appendectomy with regional enteritis. Arch. Surg. 88:546, 1964.
40. Mekhjian, H.S., Seitz, D.M., Watts, H.D., et al. National Cooperative. Crohn's disease study: Factors determining recurrence of Crohn's disease after surgery. Gastroenterology 77:907, 1979.
41. Morson, B.C., Lockhart-Mummery, H.E. Crohn's disease of the colon. Gastroenterología 92:168, 1959.
42. O'Brien, J.J., Bayless, T.M. Crohn's disease: Medical treatment. In Fazio, V.W. (Ed.) Current therapy in colon and rectal surgery. p. 188. B.C. Decker, Toronto, Philadelphia, 1990.
43. Petit, S.H., Irving, M.H. The operative management of fistulous Crohn's disease. Surg. Gynecol. Obstet. 167:223, 1988.
44. Pennington, L., Hamilton, S.R., Bayless, T.M., Cameron, J.L. Surgical management of Crohn's disease: Influence of disease at margin of resection. Ann. Surg. 192:311, 1980.
45. Rawlinson, J., Hughes, R.G. Acute supurative appendicitis: A rare associate of Crohn's disease. Dis. Colon Rectum 28:608, 1985.
46. Sharif, H., Alexander-Williams, J. The role of strictureplasty in Crohn's disease. Int. Surg. 77:15, 1992.
47. Simonowitz, D.A., Rusch, V.W., Stevenson, J.K. Natural history of incidental appendectomy in patients with Crohn's disease who required subsequent bowel resection. Am. J. Surg. 143:171, 1982.
48. Soylan, J., Wilson, D.A.L., Allan, A., et al. Recurrence after strictureplasty or resection for Crohn's disease. Br. J. Surg. 76:335, 1989.
49. Thompson, J.S. Strategies for preserving intestinal length in short-bowel syndrome. Dis. Colon Rectum 30:208, 1987.
50. Tjandra, J.J., Fazio, V.W. Surgery for Crohn's colitis. Intern. Surg. 77:2, 1992.
51. Wolff, B.G., Beart, R.W. Jr., Dozois, R.R., et al. The importance of disease free margins in resection for Crohn's disease. Dis. Colon Rectum 26:239, 1983.
52. Wolff, B.G. Crohn's colitis. In Fazio, V.W. (Ed.) Current therapy in colon and rectal surgery. p. 195. B.C. Decker, Toronto, Philadelphia, 1990.
53. Wolfson, D.M., Sachar, D.B., Cohen, A., et al. Granulomas do not affect postoperative recurrence rates in Crohn's disease. Gastroenterology 83:405, 1982.

Section H

Colon, Rectum, and Anus

CHAPTER **62**

Surgery of Non-neoplastic Anorectal Diseases

In this chapter we will describe the surgical treatment of the following nonneoplastic afflictions of the anoretal area:

1. Hemorrhoids.
2. Anal fissure.
3. Anorectal abscesses.
4. Anal fistula.
5. Rectal prolapse.
6. Pilonidal disease.

HEMORRHOIDS

Hemorrhoids are frequently seen in women as well as in men, but predominate in males (10). Though they occur at any age, hemorrhoids are more frequent after 50 years of age. Many people with hemorrhoids remain completely asymptomatic (19, 24).

Classification

Hemorrhoids are classified in two groups: internal hemorrhoids and external hemorrhoids. Internal hemorrhoids are made up of a vascular tissue arising from the internal submucosal hemorrhoidal plexus made up of branches of the superior rectal (superior hemorrhoidal) vein (18, 19, 24). They are located above the pectineal line (dentate line) and are therefore covered by mucosa or transitional epithelium. External hemorrhoids are made up of a dilated vascular plexus arising from the inferior hemorrhoidal plexus. They are located below the pectinate line and are covered with squamous epithelium (anoderm) or perianal skin. Hemorrhoids are said to be mixed when internal and external hemorrhoids are simultaneously found in the same patient.

Classification of internal hemorrhoids

According to their extent of projection into the lumen of the anal canal, internal hemorrhoids are divided into four degrees (9, 10, 18, 24):

First Degree. The hemorrhoids project into the lumen of the anal canal during defecation.
Second Degree. The hemorrhoids project outside the anal margin during the act of defecation but are reduced spontaneously once defecation is over.
Third Degree. Same as second degree but the hemorrhoids do not become reduced spontaneously and have to be reduced manually once defecation is over.
Fourth Degree. The hemorrhoids project outside the anal margin permanently and are not reducible.

Distribution of the internal hemorrhoidal groups

In the majority of patients with internal hemorrhoids the groups of hemorrhoids are distributed as follows, with the patient in the lithotomy position (9, 10, 15–17).

1. Left lateral hemorrhoidal group, located at 3 o'clock.
2. Right posterior hemorrhoidal group, located between 7 and 8 o'clock.
3. Right anterior group, located between 10 and 11 o'clock. This group is usually less prominent.

Between these groups, other accessory groups can be seen.

Symptoms

The most frequent symptoms of internal hemorrhoids are bleeding and prolapse of the groups. Infrequently the patients may present pain due to prolapse and inability to reduce the hemorrhoids. Frequent bleeding may lead to severe anemia.

Diagnosis

The diagnosis of hemorrhoids is made by the symptoms presented by the patient, which should be confirmed by rectal examination, which should be done first, to rule out a low rectal carcinoma or one in the anal canal. Endoscopy should be added to confirm the presence of hemorrhoids or some other pathologic process. Endoscopic examination of the rectum and colon is indispensable to exclude a carcinoma or an inflammatory disease of the colon. Additionally, a radiographic examination of the colon should be performed to eliminate other conditions.

Therapeutic Procedures

The therapeutic procedures used to treat symptomatic internal hemorrhoids are various, but the most used are the following:

1. Sclerotherapy.
2. Rubber band ligation.
3. Infrared photocoagulation.
4. Surgical excision.

Sclerotherapy

In 1869, John Morgan, of the United Kingdom, initiated sclerotherapy of veins. This procedure, which is still used, though less frequently, particularly in the United Kingdom, has the object of producing fibrosis to prevent hemorrhoidal prolapse (6, 9, 10). Injection of the sclerosing substance should be carried out in the submucosa of the proximal part of the hemorrhoid, at the level of the anorectal ring. The sclerosing substance should not be injected into the vein itself and should not be used to treat external hemorrhoids. Sclerotherapy is usually indicated in first or second degree symptomatic hemorrhoids. Sclerotherapy has been partially replaced by rubber band ligation and photocoagulation.

Rubber band ligation

This procedure was proposed in 1954, by Blaisdell, and later modified by Barron in 1963 (3). Simple, fast, and effective (18, 19), it is used in first or second degree and in very selected cases with third degree hemorrhoids. Rubber band ligation can be done in the office, without need for anesthesia. Ligation can be done with the primitive Barron instrument or other ligators such as the McGuney, Lurz-Goltner, or McGown instruments.

In order to perform rubber band ligation, an anoscope that will allow a ligator to be introduced has to be inserted. Once the scope and the ligator are in place, an Allis clamp is passed through the ligator's drum and the hemorrhoidal mass to be ligated is grasped. The tissue should be grasped above the dentate line so as not to produce any pain. Traction is applied to the Allis clamp so the hemorrhoid enters the drum. The handles of the ligator are adjusted and the mechanism is fired. The two previously inserted rubber rings adjust themselves in the neck of the hemorrhoidal mass. These rings should fall above the pectinate line, so as not to be painful (5, 18, 19, 24). The tissue included in the elastic bands is fixed and then becomes necrotic, later producing an eschar that sloughs off spontaneously. It should be pointed out that the elastic band does not cure the hemorrhoid as well as surgical excision, but it does alleviate symptoms.

Infrared photocoagulation

This procedure is simple and inexpensive. It should be used above the pectinate line so as not to produce pain. Infrared photocoagulation leads to coagulation of proteins and evaporation of the water in the cells (5, 6, 18, 19, 24).

Surgical resection of internal hemorrhoids

This is the most adequate treatment for permanent cure (9, 10, 13). It is indicated in well-developed third degree hemorrhoids, in prolapsing hemorrhoids that must be reduced manually, in some cases of second degree hemorrhoids (2), and in patients in whom the above treatments have failed. According to Williams (25), surgical resection of symptomatic internal hemorrhoids is indicated in 10% of patients. The surgical technique for this procedure will be described later.

Acute Thrombosis of External Hemorrhoids

Up to now, the exact cause of acute thrombosis of external hemorrhoids has not been proven. In some cases it has been shown that it is due to severe constipation or diarrhea. Numerous patients, neither with constipation or diarrhea, who were asymptomatic and did not know they had external hemorrhoids, have developed acute thrombosis (6, 18, 24). Acute hemorrhoidal thrombosis is manifested by sudden, persistent, intense, burning pain, made worse by attempts to defecate. The pain is directly related to the size of the thrombosis. A tense, very painful swelling appears in the anoderm. If the pain is severe and of less than 48 hours' duration, surgical treatment is indicated. If the patient consults the surgeon after 72 hours, the pain is usually receding, making surgery unnecessary. The later the patient with this problem is seen, the lower the probability of surgery, since the operation only alleviates pain and the condition is self-limited. External hemorrhoidal thrombosis has been proven to have intravascular clots. Surgical treatment of this condition consists of resection of the painful mass, including skin, subcutaneous tissue, and the clot. Simple incision and evacuation of the clot does not always relieve pain and may lead to abscess formation. The surgical technique for this condition will be described later.

FIGURE 62.1
Section showing localization of internal and external hemorrhoids. Internal hemorrhoids are located above the pectinate line and are covered by mucosa or transitional epithelium. External hemorrhoids are located below the pectinate line and are covered by squamous epithelium (anoderm) or perianal skin.

Surgical Technique

FIGURE 62.2 INTERNAL HEMORRHOIDS
Local, caudal, or general anesthesia is used to operate on internal hemorrhoids. The author uses the lithotomy position. Many surgeons use the prone position, which facilitates visualization of the anal canal, but is very uncomfortable for the patient and for the anesthesiologist if general anesthesia is used. In most patients, internal hemorrhoids are arranged in three groups. With the patient in the lithotomy position the groups are located as follows: left lateral group at the 3 o'clock position; right posterior group, between 7 and 8 o'clock; right anterior group between 10 and 11 o'clock. Resection of internal hemorrhoids by the classical Milligan and Morgan technique (13, 15–17) is begun by placing a hemostatic clamp on the skin next to each group of hemorrhoids to be resected (see drawing). Using gentle traction on the clamps exposes the hemorrhoids so that they can be clearly seen. Making use of this exposure, three additional hemostatic clamps are placed on each of the three groups of hemorrhoids, exposing the pedicles of each group by applying traction to them. The figure of a triangle appears. To keep the drawing clear, the last three clamps are not shown.

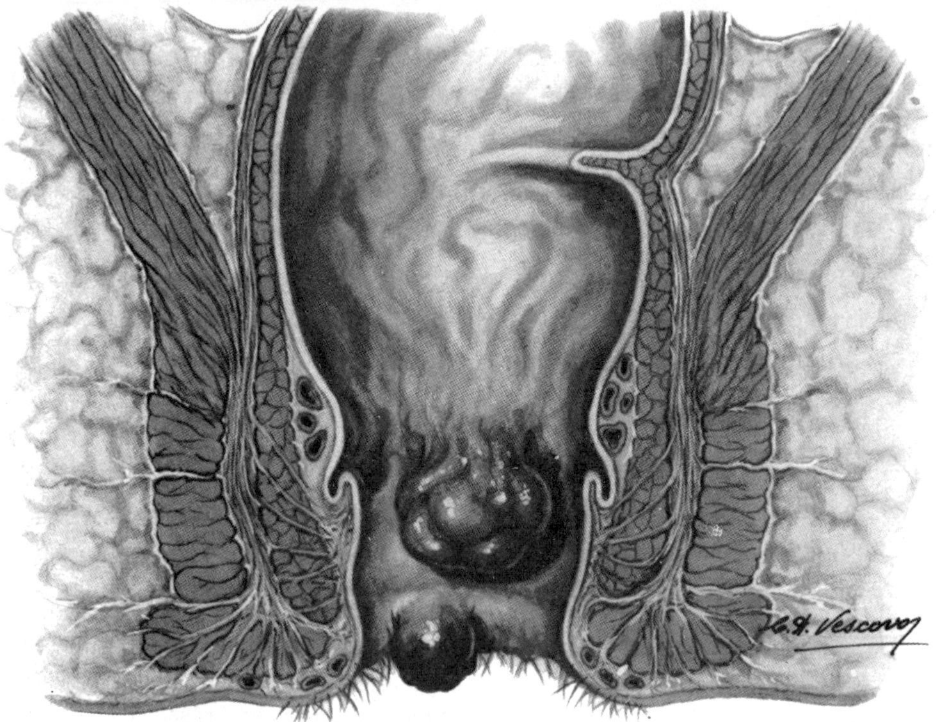

FIGURE 62.1

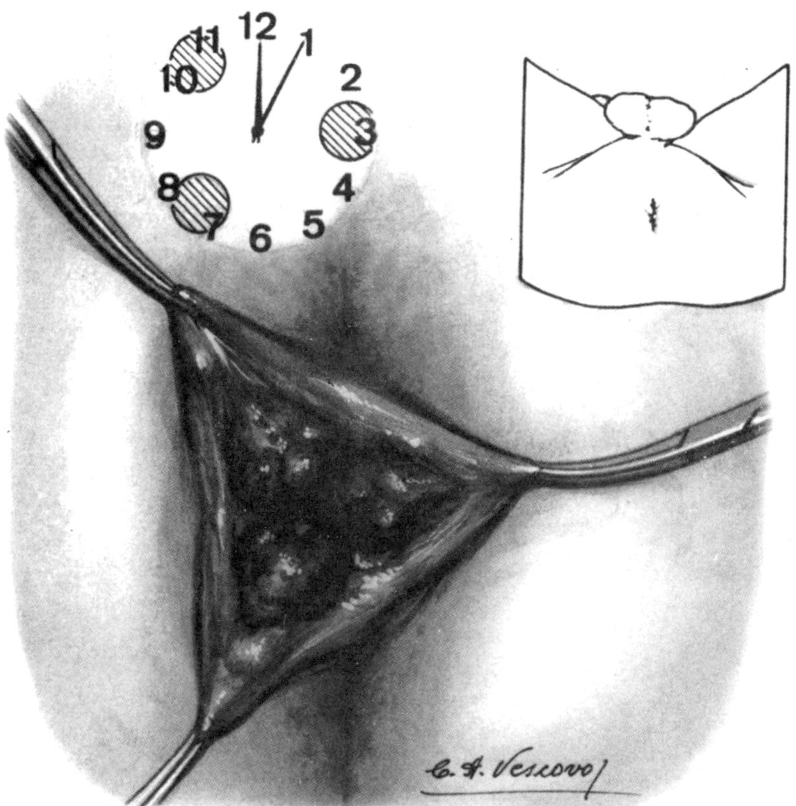

FIGURE 62.2 INTERNAL HEMORRHOIDS

FIGURE 62.3
The procedure is begun by resecting the left lateral group first. The skin near the hemostatic clamp is incised first, and then the incision is continued around the hemorrhoidal group. Once the skin has been incised, the subcutaneous fibers of the external anal sphincter can be seen and preserved. Dissection of the mucosa is then carried out, entering the submucosal plane, where the pale fibers of the internal anal sphincter can be observed.

Surgical Technique

FIGURE 62.4
The hemorrhoidal mass is being dissected, using blunt scissors, following the submucosal layer.

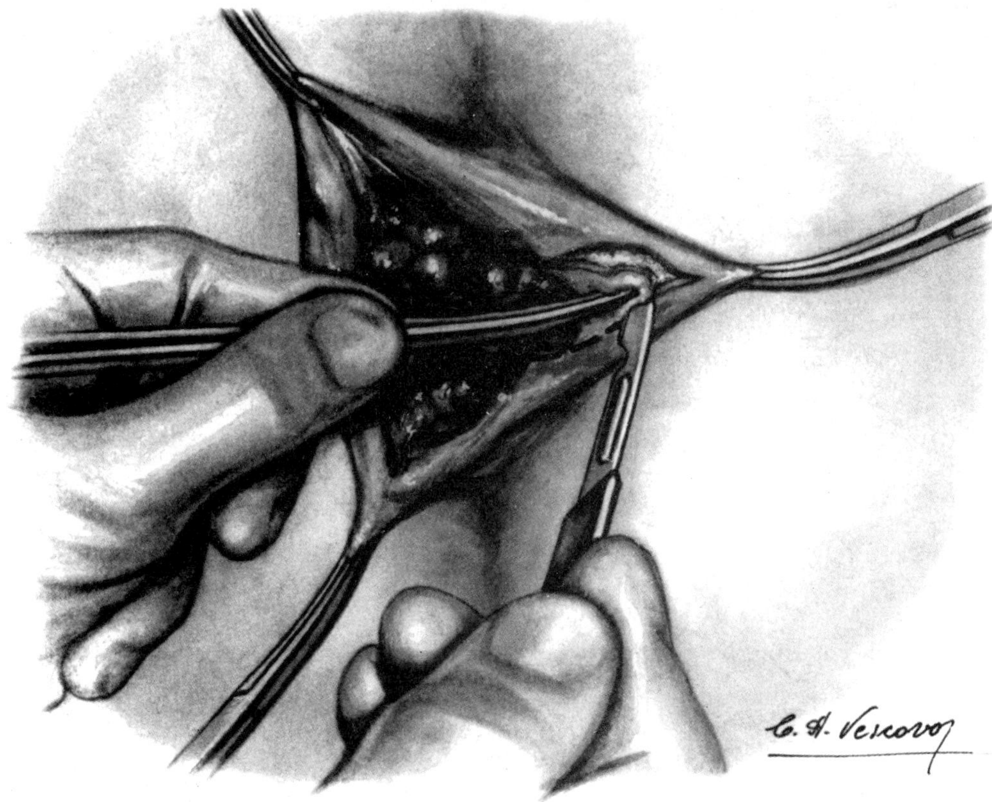

FIGURE 62.3

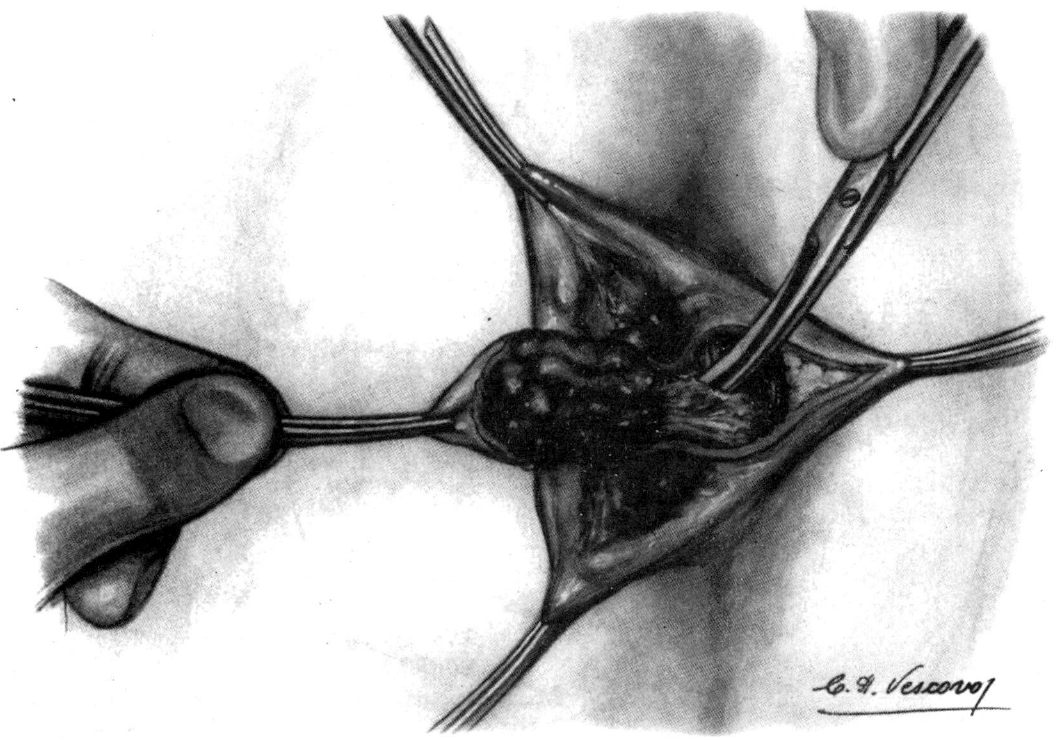

FIGURE 62.4

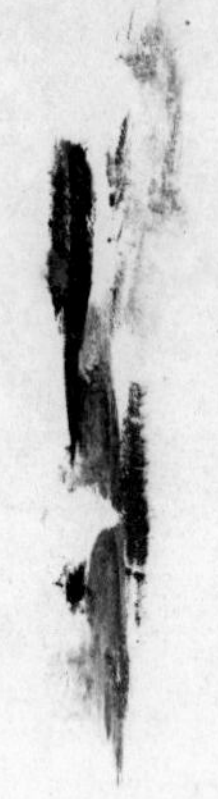

FIGURE 62.5
This section shows the completed dissection of the hemorrhoid, arriving at its pedicle, protecting the muscular fibers of the internal anal sphincter.

Surgical Technique

FIGURE 62.6
The hemorrhoidal pedicle is being sutured, using 2-0 Vicryl transfixion ligature. This suture is left long temporarily to facilitate prompt identification of the stump if it happens to bleed.

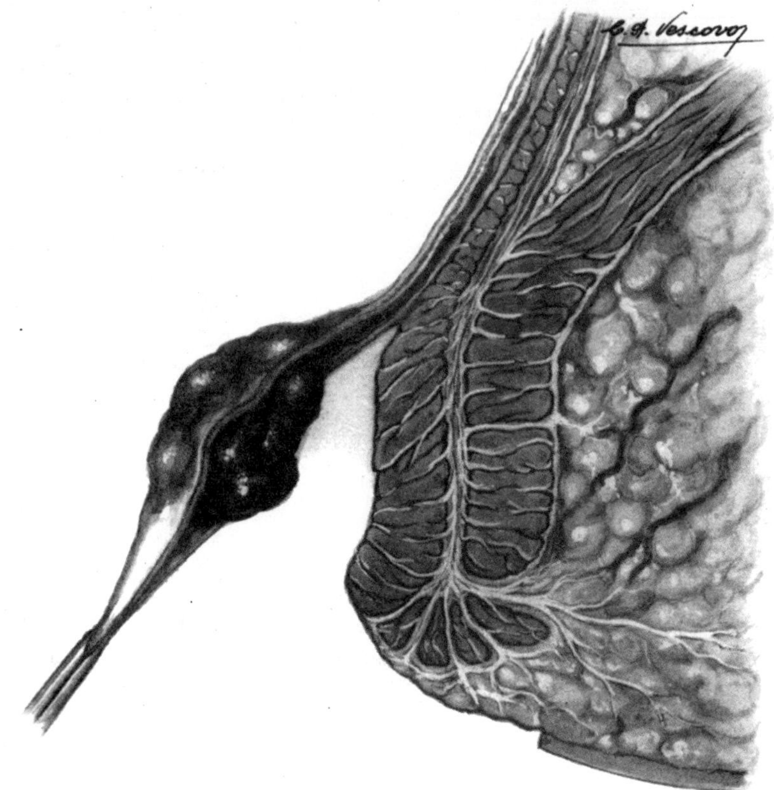

FIGURE 62.5

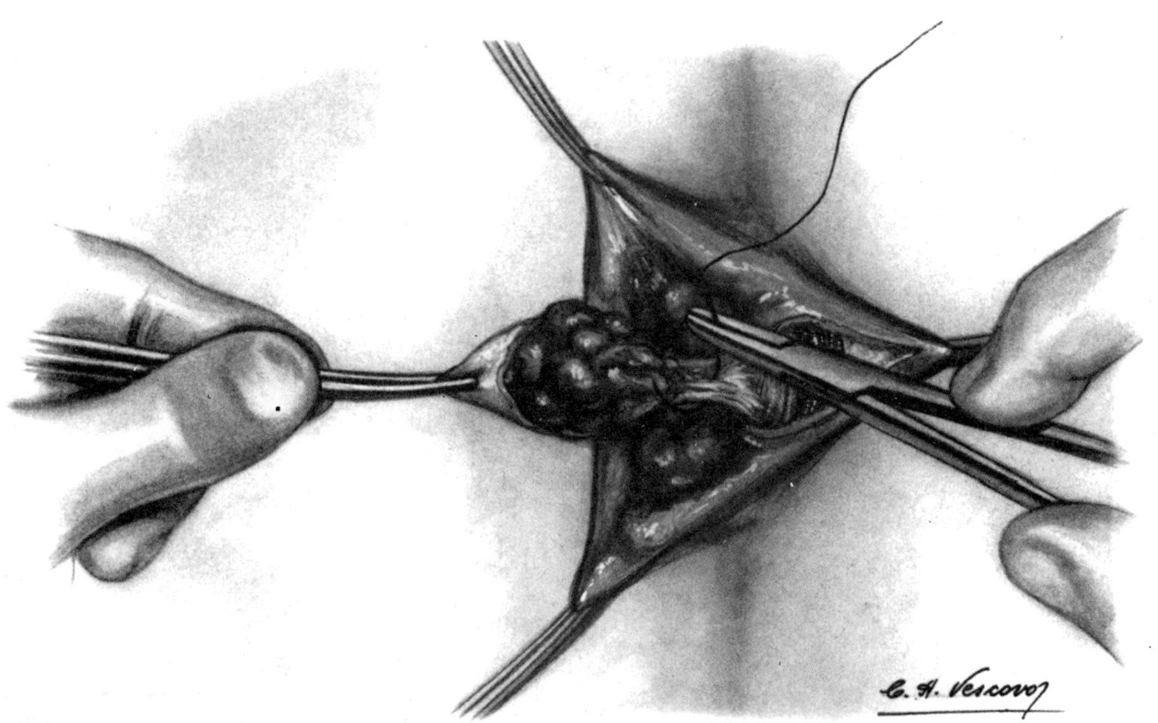

FIGURE 62.6

FIGURE 62.7
The pedicle of the left lateral hemorrhoidal group has been ligated and divided. The drawing shows the integrity of the muscle fibers of the subcutaneous portion of the external anal sphincter, the fibers of which are darker (striated muscle). The muscle fibers of the internal anal sphincter can also be seen. These are lighter in color (smooth muscle).

Surgical Technique

FIGURE 62.8
Once the lateral internal hemorrhoidal group has been removed, the right posterior group is resected, using the same technique. Finally the right anterior group, which is the least important, is resected.

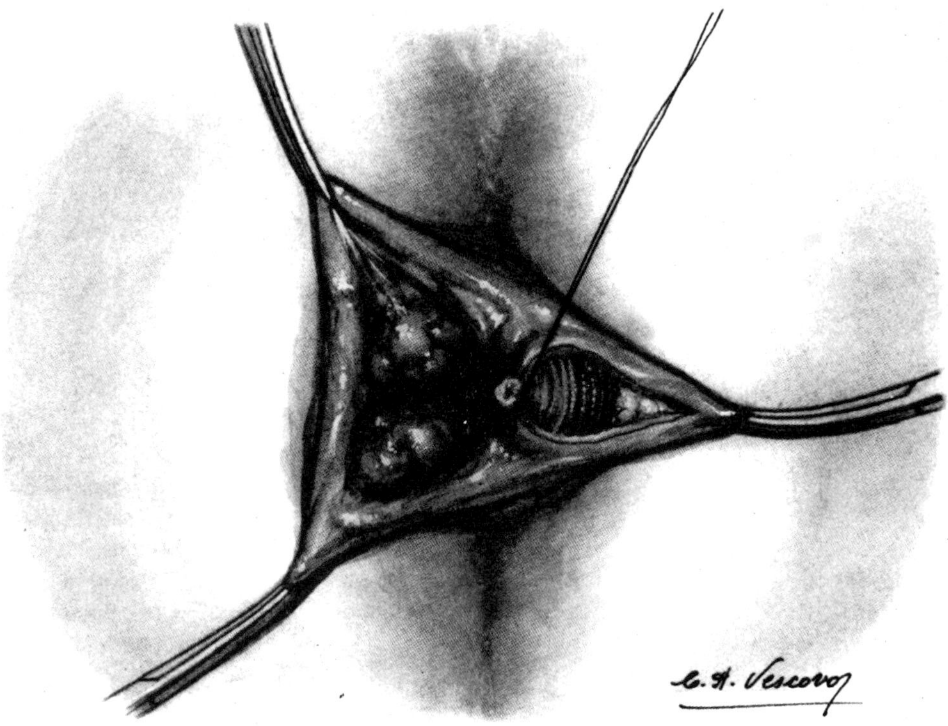

FIGURE 62.7

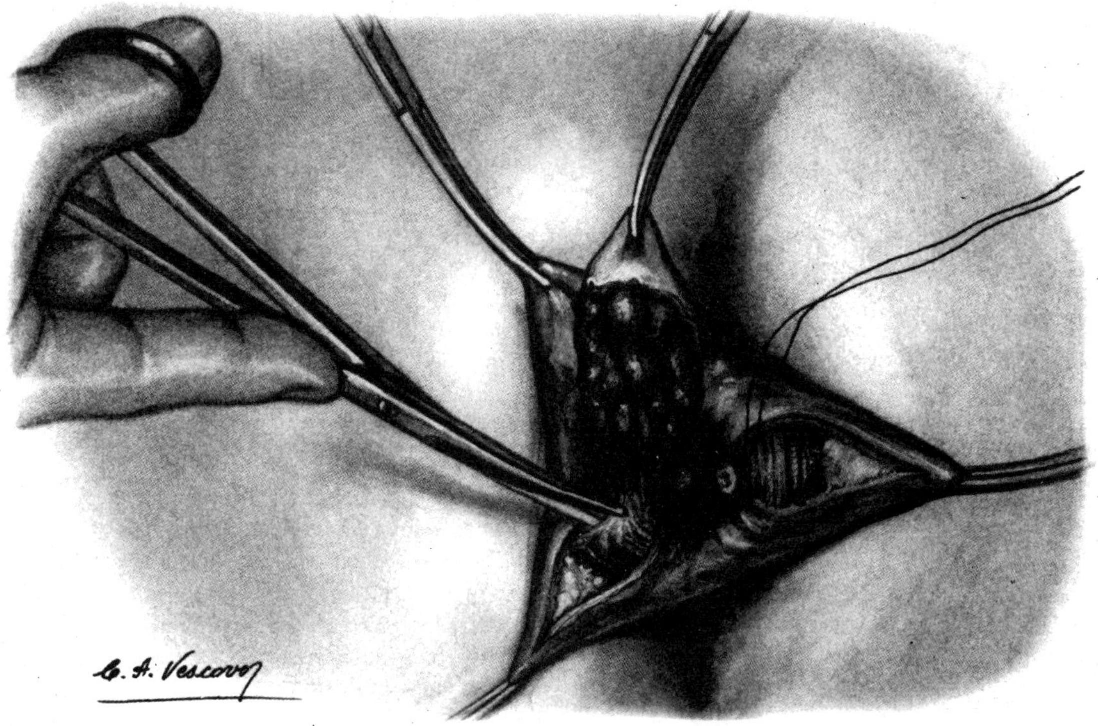

FIGURE 62.8

FIGURE 62.9
The drawing shows that the three most important hemorrhoidal groups have been removed. Lateral traction exerted by the surgeon exposes the hemorrhoidal pedicles, as well as the subcutaneous fibers of the external anal sphincter and the internal sphincter. One can observe that wide enough mucocutaneous bridges have been left between the resected hemorrhoidal groups to avoid postoperative anal stricturing. Each mucocutaneous bridge should measure at least 10 mm. The long ends of the ligatures are then cut.

Surgical Technique

FIGURE 62.10
If the Milligan-Morgan technique is used, the mucocutaneous wounds are not closed. In 1959, Ferguson (7, 8) proposed carrying out resection of hemorrhoidal groups suturing the skin and mucosa. If this is done, the edges of the mucocutaneous wounds should not be too wide, to avoid tension on the suture line. At present, most surgeons use this technique. Results are very good in both techniques. Suturing of the mucocutaneous wound is done with interrupted or continuous 2-0 catgut sutures.

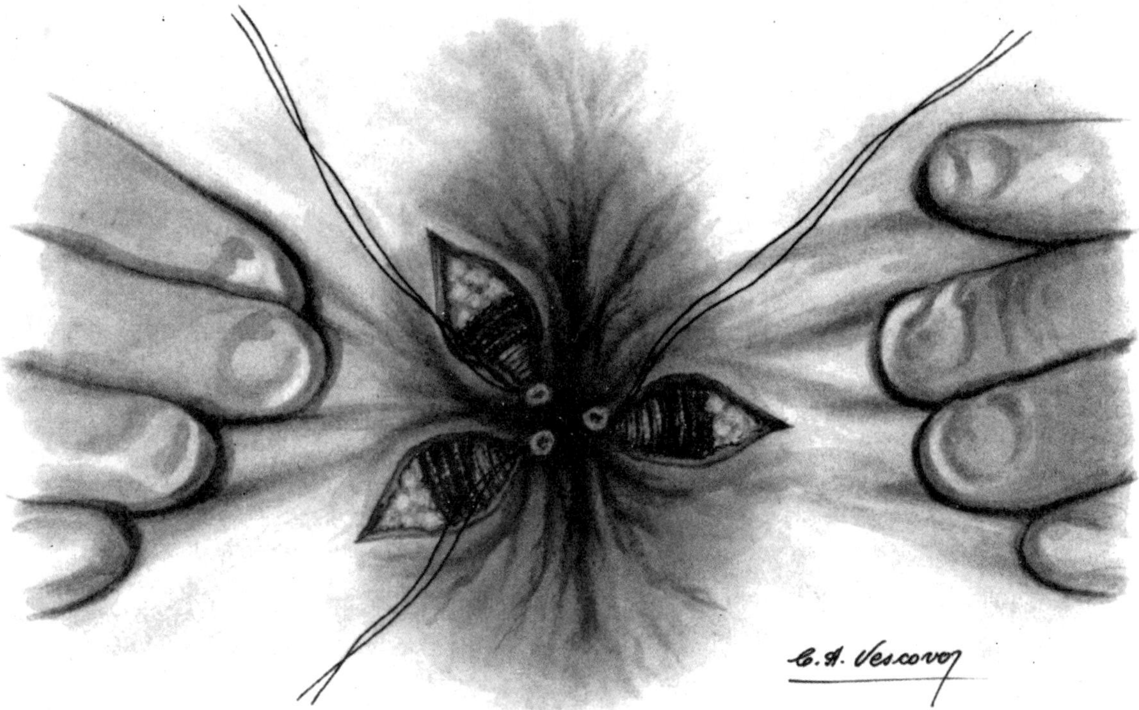

FIGURE 62.9

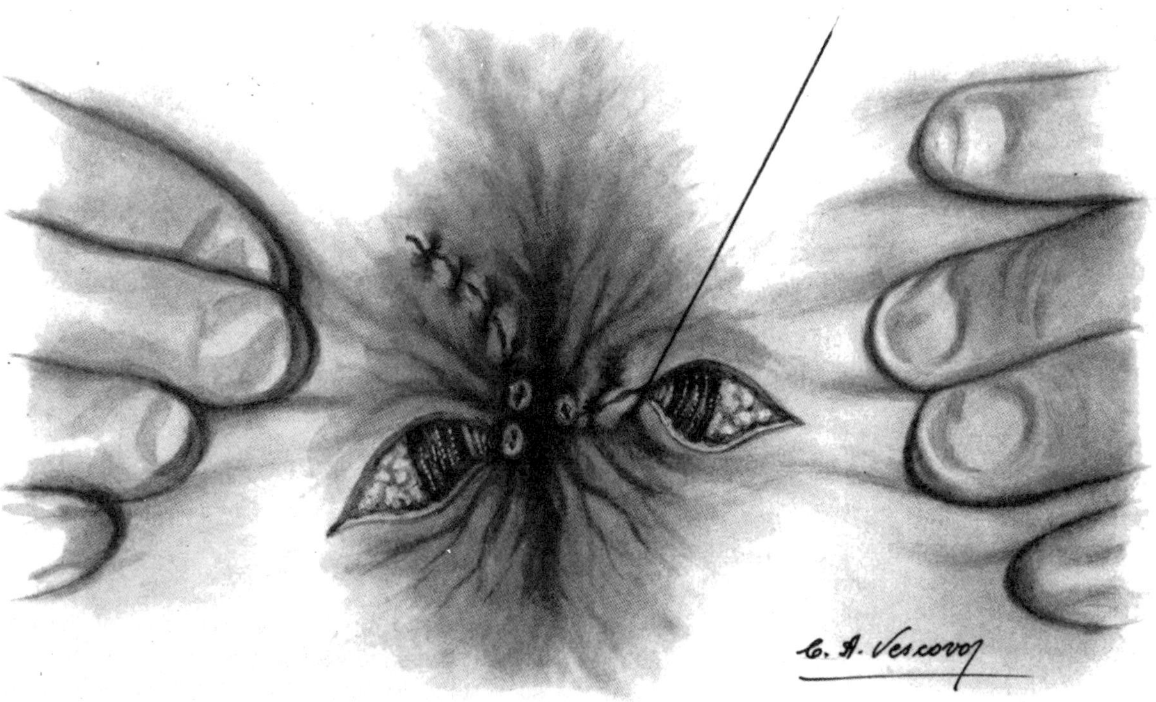

FIGURE 62.10

FIGURE 62.11 TREATMENT OF HEMORRHOID WITH ELASTIC BANDS (3, 5, 6, 18, 24)

This section shows the treatment of a first or second degree bleeding hemorrhoid using elastic bands. An anoscope has been introduced. A hemorrhoid ligator has been passed through the anoscope. The ligator has two drums or cylinders, an external and an internal one. Two elastic bands or rings have been placed in the internal drum. The dark colored elastic rings can be seen in drawing A, placed in the internal drum. An Allis clamp has been passed through the internal drum to grasp the selected hemorrhoidal group, about 10 mm above the pectinate line, to avoid pain. Traction is applied to the Allis clamp to introduce the hemorrhoidal group inside the drum. By manually adjusting the handles of the ligator a trigger effect is produced, leading to successive separation of the elastic bands, which are applied to the neck of the hemorrhoid, as seen in B. Compression by the elastic rings leads to necrosis and separation of the hemorrhoidal group.

Surgical Technique

FIGURE 62.12

Thrombosis of an external hemorrhoid. If the diagnosis is made within 24 to 48 hours and the patient has severe pain, surgical therapy is indicated. This consists of excision of the thrombus together with the skin and subcutaneous tissue, as shown by the broken line around the swelling.

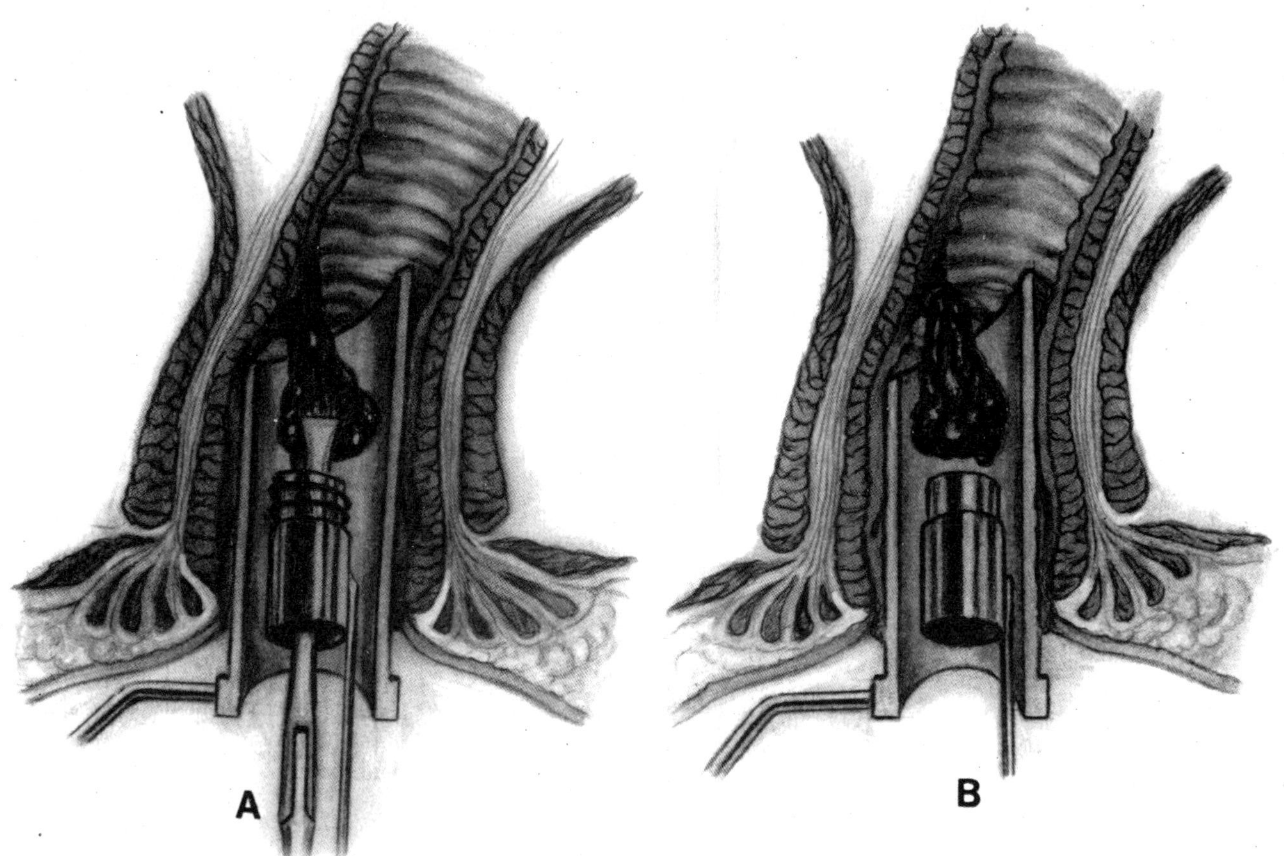

FIGURE 62.11 TREATMENT OF HEMORRHOID WITH ELASTIC BANDS (3, 5, 6, 18, 24)

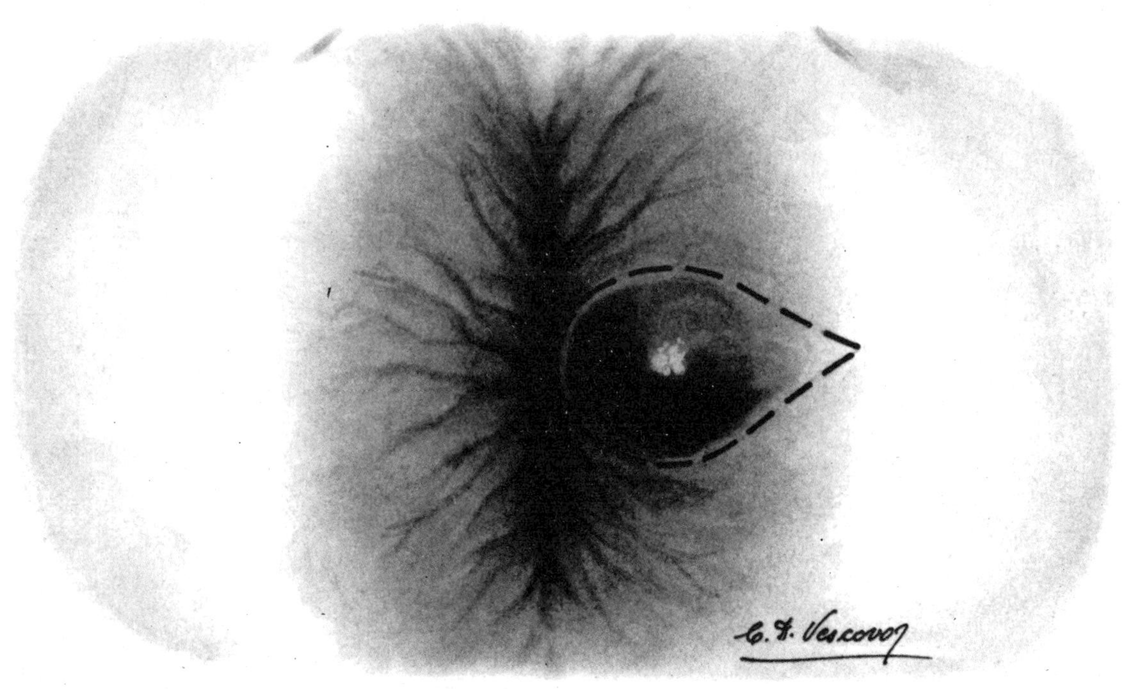

FIGURE 62.12

FIGURE 62.13
Using a scalpel, the skin and subcutaneous tissue around the swelling has been incised. The thrombus is removed en bloc together with the skin and subcutaneous tissue, using scissors.

Surgical Technique

FIGURE 62.14
Once the hemorrhoidal mass has been excised, hemostasis is completed with the electrocautery. The wound is left open.

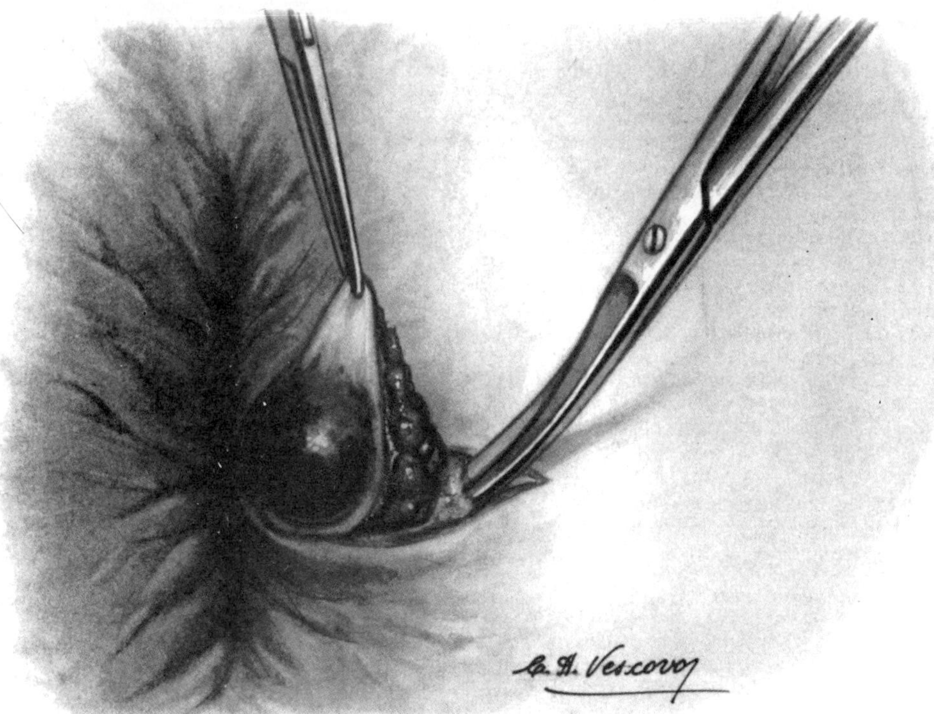

FIGURE 62.13

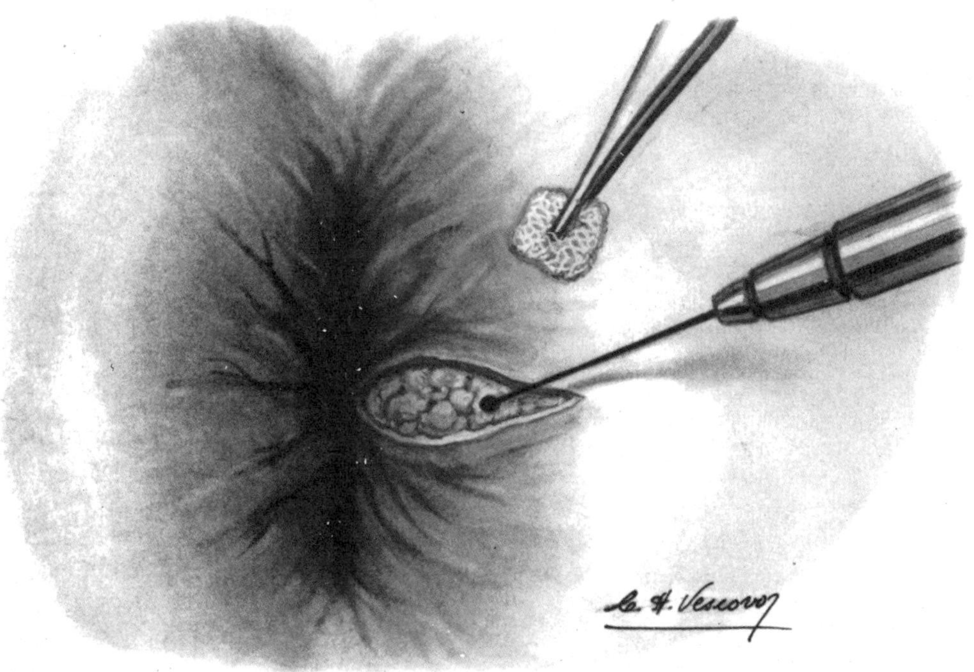

FIGURE 62.14

References

1. Alexander-Williams, J., Crapp, A.R. Conservative management of hemorrhoids. Injection, freezing and ligation. Clin. Gastroenterol. 4:595, 1975.
2. Allen-Mersh, T.G., Mann, C.V. Open haemorrhoidectomy (St. Mark's ligation/excision method). In Fielding, L.P., Goldberg, S.M. (Eds.) Surgery of the colon, rectum and anus. Ed. 5, p. 789. Butterworth-Heinemann, Oxford, 1993.
3. Barron, J. Office ligation of internal hemorrhoids. Am. J. Surg. 105:563, 1963.
4. Buls, J.G., Goldberg, S.M. Modern management of hemorrhoids. Surg. Clin. North Am. 58:409, 1978.
5. Chassin, J.L. Operative strategy in general surgery. Ed. 2, p. 733. Springer-Verlag, New York, 1994.
6. Corman, M.L. Colon and rectal surgery. Ed. 3, p. 54. Lippincott, Philadelphia, 1993.
7. Ferguson, J.A., Heaton, J.R. Closed hemorrhoidectomy. Dis. Colon Rectum 2:176, 1959.
8. Ferguson, J.A., Mazier, W.P., Granchrow, M.I., Friend, W.G. The closed technique of hemorrhoidectomy. Surgery 70:480, 1971.
9. Gabriel, W.B. The principles and practice of rectal surgery. Ed. 4. H.K. Lewis, London, 1948.
10. Goligher, J.C. Surgery of the anus, rectum and colon. Ed. 4, p. 93. Balliere Tindall, London, 1980.
11. Lau, W.Y., Chow, H.P., Poon, G.P., Wong, S.H. Rubber band ligation of three primary hemorrhoids in a single version. A safe and effective procedure. Dis. Colon Rectum 25:336, 1982.
12. Leicester, R.J., Nicolls, R.J., Mann, C.V. Infrared coagulation. Dis. Colon Rectum 24:602, 1981.
13. Mann, C.V. Open haemorrhoidectomy (St. Mark's ligation/excision method). In Todd, I.P. Fielding, L.P. (Eds.) Operative surgery. Ed. 4. vol. 3, p. 495. Mosby Butterworths, St. Louis, 1983.
14. Mazier, W.P. Hemorrhoidal disease. In Bauer J.J. (Ed.) Colorectal surgery illustrated. p. 309. Mosby–Year Book, St. Louis, 1983.
15. Milligan, E.T.C., Morgan, C.N. Surgical anatomy of the anal canal. Lancet 2:1150, 1934.
16. Milligan, E.T.C., Morgan, C.N., Jones, L.E., Oficer, R. Surgical anatomy of the anal canal and the operative treatment of haemorrhoids. Lancet 1:1119, 1937.
17. Milligan, E.T.C. Hemorrhoids. Br. Med. J. 2:412, 1939.
18. Nivatvongs, S., Goldberg, S.M. An improved technique of rubber band ligation of hemorrhoids. Am. J. Surg. 144:379, 1982.
19. Nivatvongs, S. Hemorrhoids. In Gordon, P.H., Nivatvongs, S. (Ed.) Principles and practice of surgery for the colon, rectum and anus. p. 179. Quality Medical Publishing, St. Louis, 1992.
20. Rudd, W.W.H. Ligation of hemorrhoids as an office procedure. Can. Med. Assoc. J. 108:56, 1979.
21. Russell, T.R., Donohue, J.H. Hemorrhoidal banding: A warning. Dis. Colon Rectum 28:291, 1985.
22. Smith, L.E. Hemorrhoids. In Fazio, V.W. Current therapy in colon and rectal surgery. p. 9. B.C. Decker, Toronto, 1990.
23. Steinberg, D.M., Liegois, H., Alexander-Williams, J. Long term review of the results of rubber band ligation of hemorrhoids. Br. J. Surg. 62:144, 1975.
24. Vernava, A.M. III, Madoff, R.D. Anorectal disease. In Bell, R.H., Rikkers, L.F. Mulholland, M.W. (Eds.) Digestive tract surgery. A text and atlas. p. 1421. Lippincott-Raven, Philadelphia, 1996.
25. Williams, N.S. Haemorrhoidal disease. In Keighley, M.R.B., Williams, N.S. (Eds.) Surgery of the anus, rectum and colon. Vol. 1, p. 295. W.B. Saunders, Philadelphia, 1993.

ANAL FISSURE

Anal fissure presents itself as a rupture of the squamous epithelium of the anal canal, extending from the anal margin to the dentate line. Anal fissure may be acute or chronic. The typical anal fissure commences acutely and is usually related with passage of a thick, hard fecal bolus. In some cases an acute anal fissure is related to the acute diarrheas.

Anal fissure produces intense pain beginning at defecation and lasting from a few minutes to several hours. The intense pain of the fissure is not related to the physical findings (30). Acute cases are usually cured by medical therapy. In case the pain does not disappear with medical therapy after 3 or 4 weeks, surgical treatment should be advised.

Acute anal fissure may become chronic, either because the treatment was not adequate or because the patient had excessive residual pressure due to an intense contraction of the internal anal sphincter (3). In the chronic stage the fissure looks like an elliptical ulcer with elevated borders and deeper than in the acute stage, where the pale transverse muscle fibers of the internal anal sphincter can be seen.

In men, anal fissures are located in the posterior anal commissure in 99% of cases, with only 1% in the anterior commissure. In women, 90% of cases are located posteriorly and 10% in the anterior anal commissure.

In addition to its preponderant posterior location, anal fissure is characterized by being strictly limited to the squamous mucosa of the canal (anoderm), between the anal margin and the pectinate line. Any fissure that extends beyond the endoderm or is not located posteriorly or anteriorly, having a lateral position, should be suspected of not being a primary fissure but due to some other underlying pathologic process such as Crohn's disease, ulcerative colitis, tuberculosis, syphilis, AIDS, and so on.

Chronic anal fissures frequently present a polypoid formation at the upper end, at the level of the pectinate line. This polypoid formation is firm, and is known as a hypertrophied papilla. It is formed by an infection of the underlying crypt that later invades the neighboring papilla, provoking an increase in its size and invasion by fibrous tissue, making it firmer in consistency. At the lower end of a chronic fissure, in the skin of the anal margin, a pathologic formation known as a sentinel pile is usually seen. It is due to a thickening of the skin of the anal margin caused by inflammation, stasis, and lymphedema, which is later invaded by fibrous tissue. This structure is not related to hemorrhoids. Because of its location in the lower angle of the fissure, it is known as a sentinel pile. If the fissure is chronic and, in addition to the ulceration, presents a hypertrophied papilla and a sentinel pile, it is said we are facing the fissure triad.

In 1951, Eisenhammer (7) proved that the muscle fibers in the bottom of the fissure did not belong to the external anal sphincter, as had been believed, but to the internal sphincter. These investigations were later confirmed by Morgan and Thompson, Goligher, and others (12, 21). Eisenhammer also demonstrated that it was not necessary to excise the fissure, that merely dividing the muscle fibers in the bottom of the fissure would lead to its healing with good results. Later, however, experience revealed that, even though this technique led to healing of the fissure, it frequently left some discomfort, which, even though not important, made the patient uncomfortable, since the anus became deformed, acquiring the shape of a key hole and allowing a fecal material and secretions to filter out through the groove left by division of the internal sphincter. This was accompanied by itching and soiling of underclothing (1, 3, 9, 15). In 1959, Eisenhammer (8) modified the technique. Instead of dividing the muscle fibers of the internal anal sphincter in the bottom of the fissure, he proposed transecting the internal sphincter laterally, without touching the fissure. Lateral section of the internal anal sphincter does not lead to the inconveniences previously mentioned. The Eisenhammer technique is now known as open lateral internal sphincterotomy.

In 1969, Notaras (22) proposed a modification of the Eisenhammer technique that consists of transecting the internal sphincter laterally by introducing a cataract knife as a stylet, which he called closed or subcutaneous lateral internal sphincterotomy (3, 12, 17).

Forced Dilation of the Anal Sphincter

In 1838, Récamier (27) of France proposed the use of forced dilation of the anal sphincter to treat chronic anal fissure. Though this procedure may offer good results as far as the pain is concerned (19), it has several inconveniences (6, 9, 18, 23, 24, 25)

1. Forced dilation is not effective in all cases.
2. Freedom from pain may not be long lasting.
3. Recurrence is frequent.
4. Injury to the sphincter may cause incontinence in 30% of patients.
5. It should not be done in patients over 55 years of age.
6. Forced dilation may affect the external sphincter, which is not related to the fissure.

At present this technique has been practically abandoned.

In the following, we will describe the closed or subcutaneous lateral internal sphincterotomy (Notaras) which is being performed more frequently. Later we will describe the open lateral internal sphincterotomy (Eisenhammer).

Surgical Technique

Anesthesia may be local, caudal, or general. The patient is placed in the lithotomy position.

Surgical Technique

FIGURE 62.15
Without any special preparation and the patient in the lithotomy position, a bivalved Eisenhammer speculum is introduced into the anus. Other bivalve speculums can be used such as the Parks, Goligher, or Ferguson, so that the valves are located to the right and to the left in order to inspect the fissure and look for some other condition. The drawing shows a typical chronic anal fissure situated between the pectinate line and the anal margin. The muscular fibers of the internal sphincter can be seen running transversely in the bottom of the fissure and whitish in color. A hypertrophied papilla can be seen at the superior end of the fissure and a sentinel pile can be seen in the lower end, both well developed.

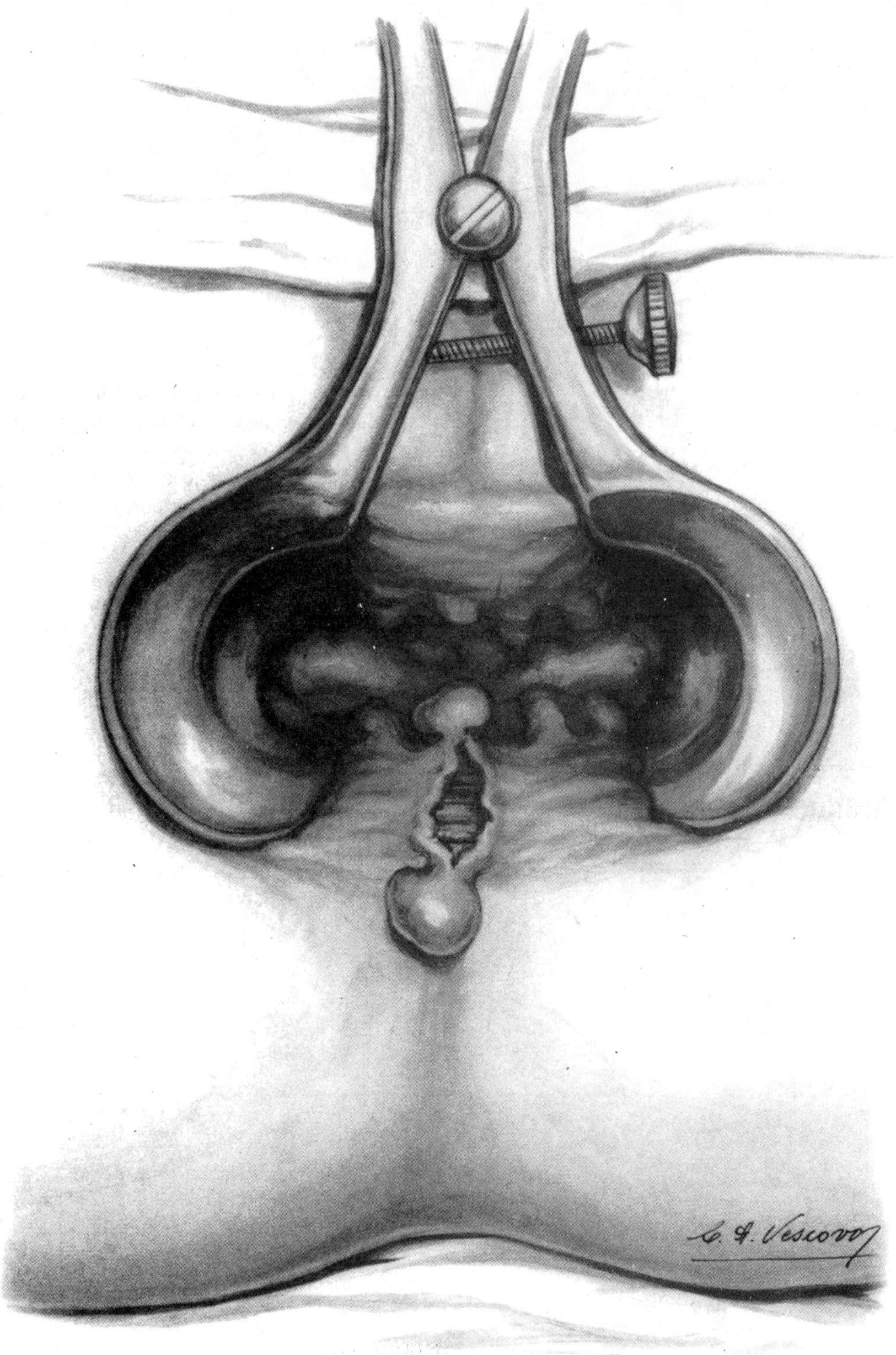

FIGURE 62.15

FIGURE 62.16
Once the lesion has been identified and evaluated, the retractor's position is changed so that one valve is applied to the anterior wall and the other to the posterior wall of the anal canal. The speculum is opened to a diameter of about 4 cm. This opening stretches the inferior border of the internal sphincter, making it palpable or, at times, visible. The intersphincteric sulcus separating the border of the internal sphincter from the subcutaneous portion of the external sphincter is found just outside the inferior border of the internal sphincter.

Surgical Technique

FIGURE 62.17
This section shows the internal anal sphincter with its inferior border and the external anal sphincter with its three portions, subcutaneous, superficial, and deep. The end of the clamp points out, as in the previous figure, the intersphincteric sulcus, through which a cataract knife will be introduced to transect the distal segment of the internal sphincter. The figure also shows the pectinate line, which is the limit of the sphincterotomy.

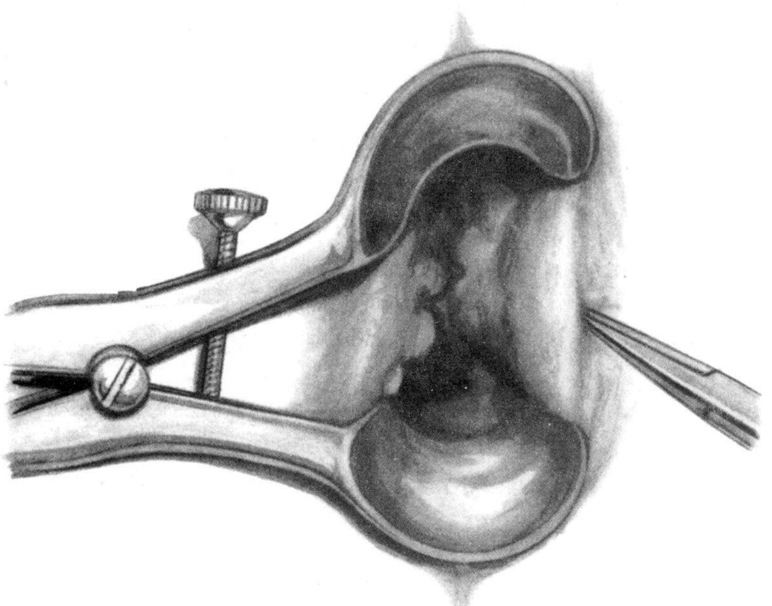

FIGURE 62.16

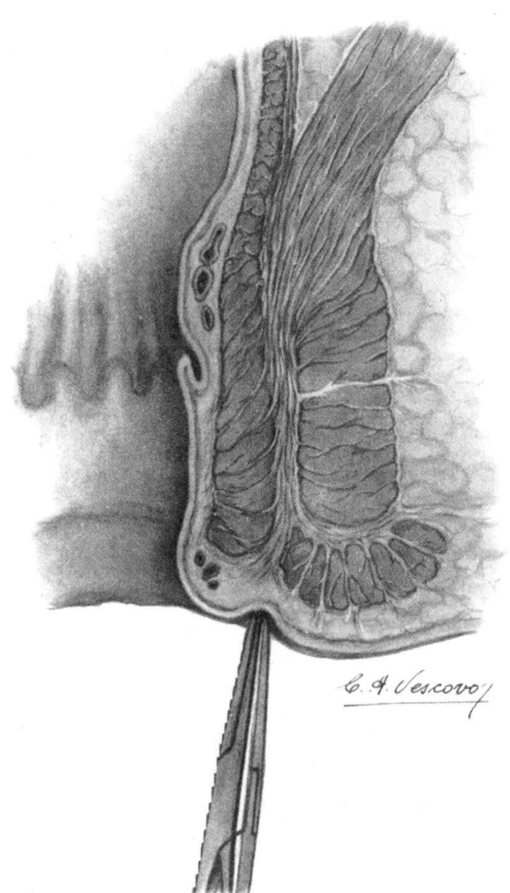

FIGURE 62.17

FIGURE 62.18
Drawing showing the moment the surgeon is about to introduce the scalpel into the intersphincteric sulcus. The usual site of insertion is at the 3 o'clock position with the patient in lithotomy. Some surgeons prefer to introduce the cataract knife into the right side, at the 9 o'clock position.

Surgical Technique

FIGURE 62.19
View of a section at the moment the surgeon has inserted the knife between the internal and the external anal sphincters, so that one of its sides faces toward the lumen of the anal canal. The end of the knife is inserted up to near the pectinate line. The surgeon uses the left index finger in the canal to feel the tissues transected by the knife.

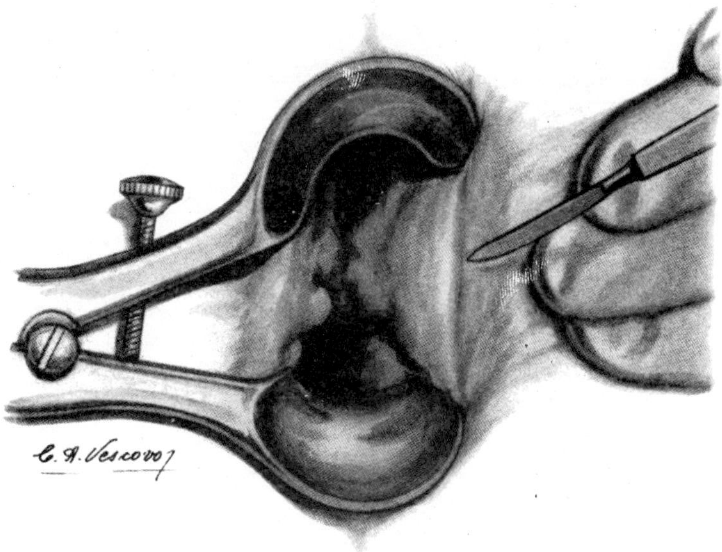

FIGURE 62.18

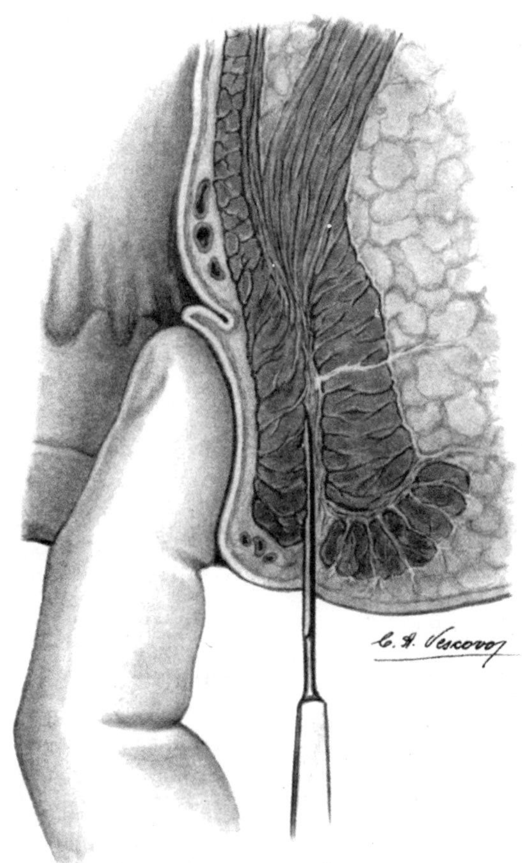

FIGURE 62.19

FIGURE 62.20

The knife has been inserted to the vicinity of the pectinate line. To transect the muscular fibers of the internal sphincter, the knife has to be rotated so that its cutting edge faces the lumen of the canal. The limit of transection of the sphincter is shown by a broken line. Once the transection is carried out, the surgeon's finger in the canal will feel emptiness and disappearance of the tension that was exerted by the inferior border of the internal sphincter. When the internal sphincter is sectioned, the surgeon's finger in the canal will feel the scalpel through the endoderm. Care should be taken to avoid injuring the endoderm, which may lead to postoperative fistula or abscess.

Surgical Technique

FIGURE 62.21

The scalpel has been removed. The surgeon's finger in the canal then completes the rupture of any muscle fibers that were not transected. Pressure with the finger facilitates hemostasis. In the original Notaras technique the scalpel is inserted between the endoderm and the sphincter. Upon reaching the pectinate line, it is rotated so that its edge faces outward to transect the internal sphincter. By this technique, there is danger of injuring the external sphincter.

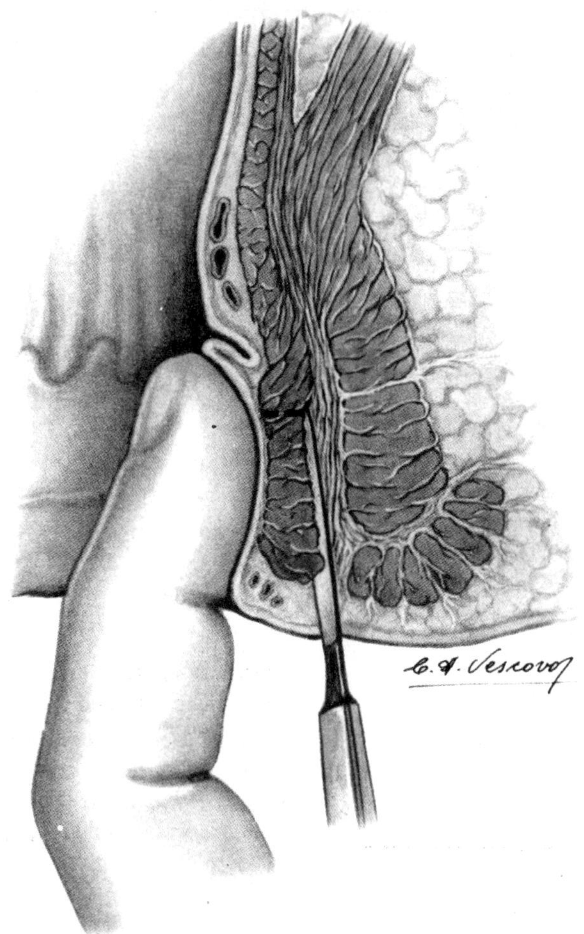

FIGURE 62.20

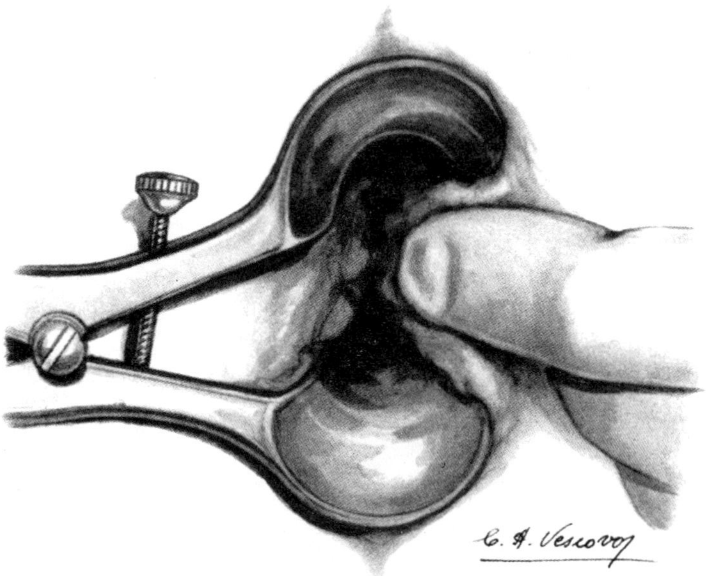

FIGURE 62.21

FIGURE 62.22
Schematic drawing of the previous figure to show how the pulp of the surgeon's left index finger compresses the area of transection of the internal anal sphincter. If bleeding is seen coming from the small wound of entrance of the scalpel, a rare occurrence, digital pressure is maintained for a few minutes to ensure hemostasis.

Surgical Technique

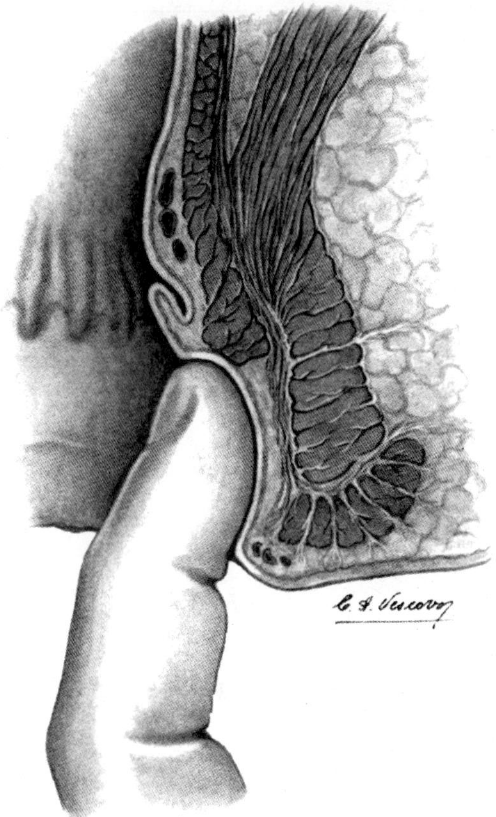

FIGURE 62.22

FIGURE 62.23
The patient is placed in the lithotomy position with an Eisenhammer speculum inserted so that one of its valves is applied toward the anterior wall and the other toward the posterior wall. A 3-cm-long radial incision is made at 9 o'clock including the distal part of the endoderm and the anal skin. The whitish fibers of the internal sphincter are easily identified.

Lateral Internal Sphincterotomy by the Open Technique

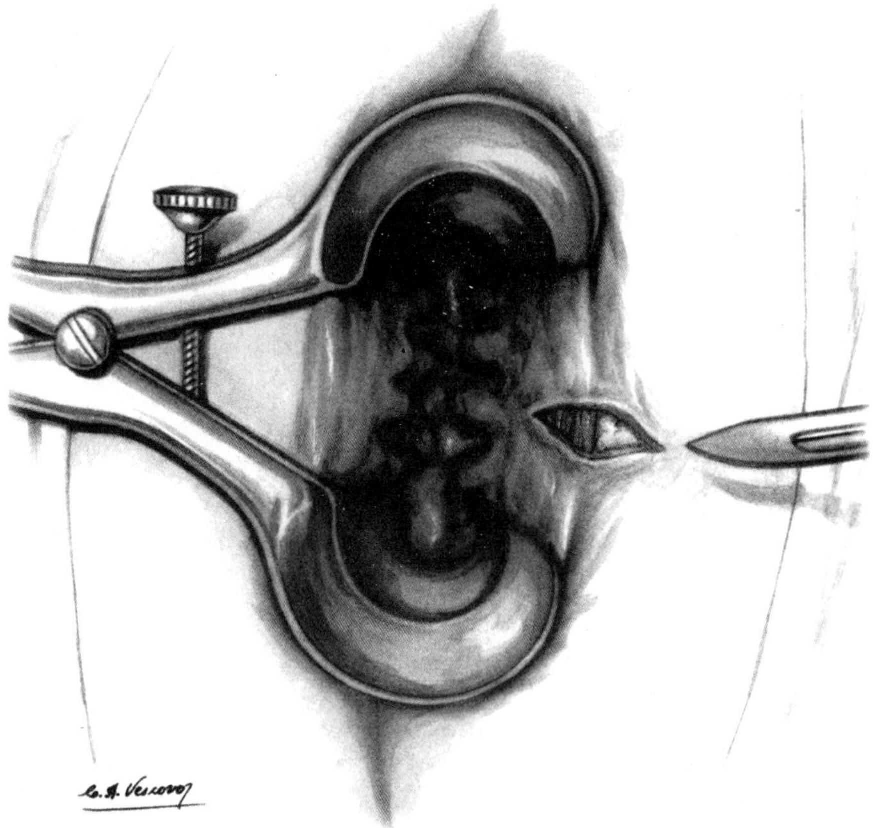

FIGURE 62.23

FIGURE 62.24
Using an Allis clamp, traction is applied to the inferior border of the internal sphincter. Between the endoderm and the internal anal sphincter a delicate scissors with blunt ends is introduced to separate these structures. Once these structures have been separated, the scissors are removed and then inserted between the internal and external sphincters. These two stages can be easier if a few cubic centimeters of saline solution are injected.

Lateral Internal Sphincterotomy by the Open Technique

FIGURE 62.25
Once the internal sphincter has been separated from neighboring tissues, its inferior border is grasped with Allis clamps and transected with straight scissors up to the pectinate line. The radial incision tends to close spontaneously and does not have to be sutured (insert).

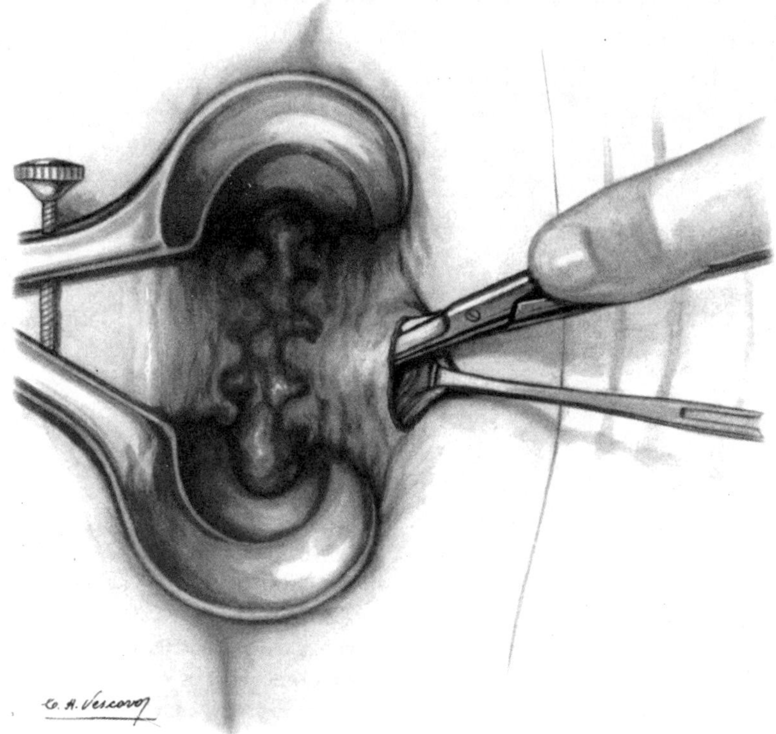

FIGURE 62.24

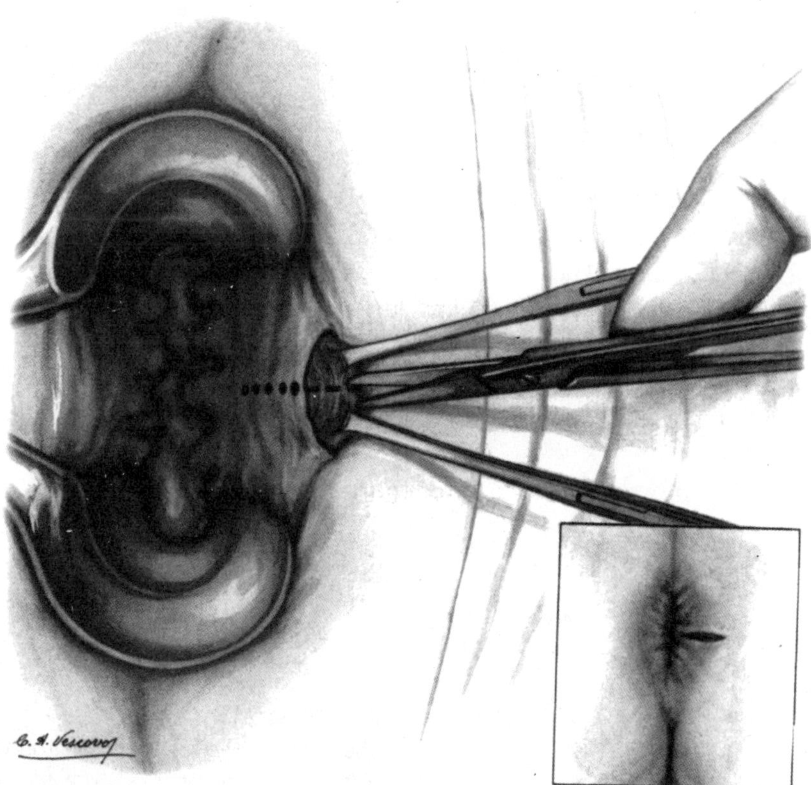

FIGURE 62.25

FIGURE 62.26 RESECTION OF THE SENTINEL PILE

If the sentinel pile is voluminous, it is advisable to resect it in the same procedure. This same attitude should be taken if there is a very hypertrophic papilla. If both are only moderately developed, they do not have to be removed. The sentinel pile is removed with scissors with no need to suture the defect. Hemostasis is by means of electrocautery. If the sentinel pile is very big, it can be removed, with a scalpel, in two halves.

Lateral Internal Sphincterotomy by the Open Technique

FIGURE 62.27

The sentinel pile has been split in two halves with a scalpel. Both halves are removed with scissors (see drawing). Hemostasis is by electrocautery.

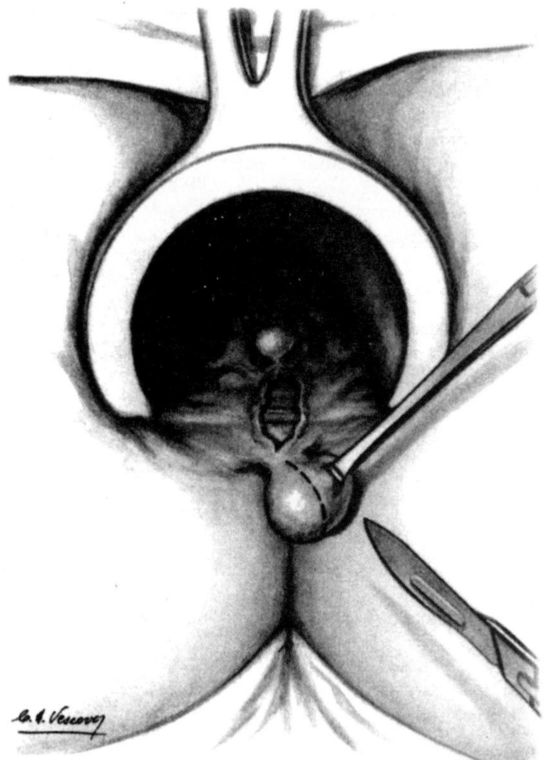

FIGURE 62.26 RESECTION OF THE SENTINEL PILE

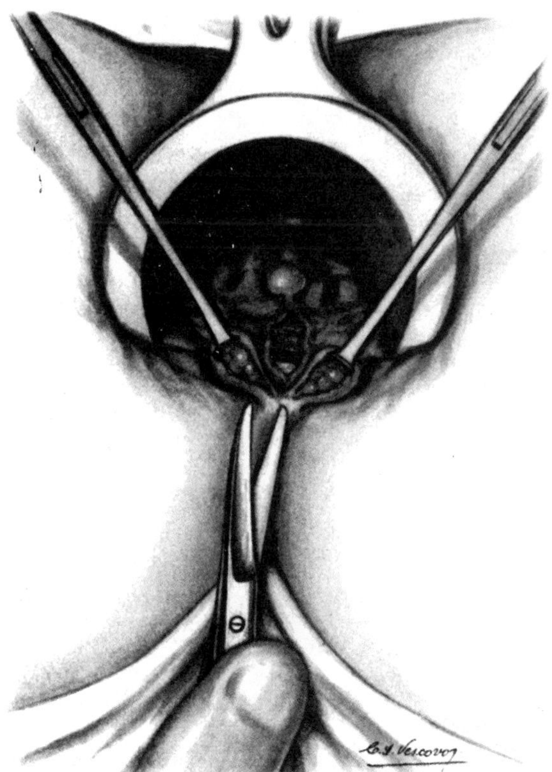

FIGURE 62.27

References

1. Abcarian, H. Surgical correction of chronic anal fissure: results of lateral and internal sphincterotomy versus fissurectomy–midline sphincterotomy. Dis. Colon Rectum 23:31, 1980.
2. Abcarian, H., Lakshaman, S., Read, D.R., Roccaforte, P. The role of internal sphincter in chronic anal fissures. Dis. Colon Rectum 25:525, 1982.
3. Arabi, J., Alexander-Williams, J., Keigley, M.R.B. Anal pressure in hemorrhoids and anal fissure. Am. J. Surg. 134:608, 1974.
4. Boulous, P.B., Araujo, J.G.C. Adequate internal sphincterotomy for chronic anal fissure: Subcutaneous or open technique? Br. J. Surg. 71:360, 1984.
5. Coller, J.A., Karulf, R.E. Anal fissure. In Fazio, V.W. (Ed.) Current therapy in colon and rectal surgery. p. 15. B.C. Decker, Philadelphia, 1990.
6. Corman, M.L. Colon and rectal surgery. Ed. 3, p. 116. Lippincott, Philadelphia, 1993.
7. Eisenhammer, S. The surgical correction of chronic internal anal sphincteric contracture. S. Afr. Med. J. 25:486, 1951.
8. Eisenhammer, S. The evaluation of internal anal sphincterotomy operation with special reference to anal fissure. Surg. Gynecol. Obstet. 109:583, 1959.
9. Etala, E. Tratamiento quirurgico de la fisura anal. Pren. Méd. Argent. 74:141, 1987.
10. Gabriel, W.B. Principles and practice of rectal surgery. Ed. 3, p. 129 H.K. Lewis, London, 1945.
11. Gliedman, M.L. Atlas of surgical techniques. p. 396. McGraw-Hill, New York, 1990.
12. Goligher, J.C. Surgery of the anus, rectum and colon. Ed. 4, p. 147. Macmillan, New York, 1980.
13. Goodsall, D.H., Miles, W.E. Diseases of the anus and rectum. Part I, p. 211. Longmans Green, London, 1900.
14. Gordon, P.H. Fissure-in-ano. In Gordon, P.H., Nivatvongs, S. (ed). Principles and practice of surgery for the colon, rectum and anus. p. 199. Quality Medical Publishing, St. Louis, 1992.
15. Gorfine, S.R. Anal fissures. In Bauer, J.J. (Ed.) Colorectal surgery illustrated. p. 347. Mosby–Year Book, St. Louis, 1993.
16. Hawley, P.R. The treatment of chronic fissure in ano. Br. J. Surg. 56:519, 1969.
17. Hoffman, D.C., Golisher, J.C. Lateral subcutaneous internal sphincterotomy in treatment of anal fissure. Br. Med. J. 3:673, 1970.
18. Keighley, M.R.B. Fissure in ano. In Keighley, M.R.B., Williams, N.S. (Eds.) Surgery of the anus, rectum and colon. Vol. 1, p. 364. W.B. Saunders, London, 1993.
19. Marby, M., Alexander-Williams, J., Buchmann, P., et al. A randomized controlled trial to compare anal dilatation with lateral subcutaneous sphincterotomy for anal fissure. Dis. Colon Rectum 22:308, 1979.
20. Milligan, E.T.C., Morgan, C.N. Surgical anatomy of the anal with special reference to ano-rectal fistulas. Lancet, 2:1213, 1934.
21. Morgan, C.N., Thompson, H.R. Surgical anatomy of the anal canal with special reference to the surgical importance of the internal sphincter and conjoint longitudinal muscles. Ann. R. Coll. Surg. Engl. 19:88, 1956.
22. Notaras, M.J. Lateral subcutaneous sphincterotomy for anal fissure. A new technique. Proc. R. Soc. Med. 62:713, 1969.
23. Notaras, M.J. The treatment of anal fissure by lateral subcutaneous internal sphincterotomy. A technique and results. Br. J. Surg. 58:96, 1971.
24. Notaras, M.J. Anal fissure. In Maingot, R. (Ed.) Abdominal operations. Ed. 7, vol. II, p. 2356. Appleton Century Crofts, New York, 1980.
25. Notaras, M.J. Lateral subcutaneous internal anal sphincterotomy for anal fissure. In Fielding, L.P., Goldberg, S.M. (Eds.) Surgery of the colon, rectum and anus. Ed. 5, p. 871. Butterworth-Heinemann, Oxford, 1993.
26. Oh, C. A modified technique for lateral internal sphincterotomy. Surg. Gynecol. Obst. 146:623, 1978.
27. Récamier, J.C.A. Extension, massage et percussion cadencé dans le traitement des contractures musculaires. Rev. Med. Franc. 1:74, 1838. (Translated into English in Dis. Colon Rectum, 23:362, 1980.)
28. Shrock, T.R. Benign and malignant diseases of the anorectum. In Fromm, D. (Ed.) Gastrointestinal surgery. Vol. 2, p. 606. Churchill Livingstone, New York, 1985.
29. Vagai, W., Mann, C. Closed lateral internal sphincterotomy without removal of sentinel pile for fissure in ano. Dis. Colon Rectum 3:91, 1981.
30. Vernava, A.M., Madoff, R.D. Anorectal disease. In Bell, R.H. Jr., Rikkers, L.F., Mulholland, M.W. (Eds.) Digestive tract surgery. p. 1421. Lippincott-Raven, Philadelphia, 1996.
31. Watts, J.M., Bennett, R.C., Goligher, J.C. Stretching of the anal sphincter in the treatment of fissure in ano. Br. Med. J. 2:342, 1965.
32. Welch, C.E., Ottinger, L.W., Welch, J.P. Manual of lower gastrointestinal surgery. p. 216. Springer-Verlag, New York, Heidelberg, Berlin, 1980.

ANORECTAL ABSCESSES AND FISTULAS

Anorectal Abscesses

Anorectal abscesses develop in the spaces around the anus and rectum. Abscesses and fistulas have similar origins. The abscess is considered to be the acute part of the septic process and the fistula the chronic part of the same process (7, 23, 25, 33).

The infection begins in the intersphincteric plane, in one of the anal glands. Some authors do not agree with that origin (13, 14). Anal glands are located in the submucosa, in the internal sphincter, and in the intermuscular space. There are eight or nine of these glands (13). Anal glands do not penetrate the smooth longitudinal fibers or the muscle fibers of the external anal sphincter. They lubricate the inside of the anal canal by depositing mucus in the crypts of Morgagni. From this intersphincteric focus infection spreads in several directions. Generally, the infection that starts as a small intersphincteric abscess spreads down to the perineum. Less frequently, the infection spreads upward, leading to the formation of a high intersphincteric or supralevator abscess. Lateral spread may occur through the external anal sphincter toward the ischiorectal fossa. The anal crypts are localized in the anterior or posterior wall of the anal canal, which means that most abscesses develop in the anterior or posterior wall of the anal canal.

Anorectal abscesses are classified according to their location, as

1. Perianal abscesses, located under the perianal skin.
2. Ischiorectal abscesses, located in the ischiorectal fossa.
3. Intersphincteric abscesses, located in the intersphincteric space.
4. Supralevator abscesses, located above the levator ani and below the pelvic peritoneum.

From these locations, the abscesses may spread in different directions.

Patients with superficial anorectal abscesses, either perineal or ischiorectal, usually complain of perineal pain, made worse on moving, by sitting, or during bowel movements. In contrast to the pain of anal fissure, the pain due to abscesses is continuous until the abscess is drained. Patients usually notice painful swellings in the anal or perianal region.

Deep abscesses such as the supralevators, which are infrequent, usually produce low abdominal pain without external swelling.

The presence of fever is related to the size of the abscess. Small abscesses are usually afebrile, while large abscesses usually develop fever, sometimes high.

Anorectal abscesses should be drained as soon as they are diagnosed. The surgeon should not wait for fluctuation because during that wait the abscess will contain pus, even without fluctuation. It should be kept in mind that drainage of an anorectal abscess may give rise to an anorectal fistula. Some authors (30) believe this occurs in 70% of abscesses, others less frequently (13, 14).

Perianal, ischiorectal, and intersphincteric abscesses are the most common. Supralevator abscesses are infrequent. The latter may have the same origin as other anorectal abscesses, or may be due to complications of conditions in some organs located in the lower abdomen such as colonic diverticula, Crohn's disease, gynecologic problems, and so on. The incidence of supralevator abscesses is not over 5% (13).

Perianal abscess is the most frequent anorectal abscess. Pus accumulates in the subcutaneous tissue of the anal margin. Perianal abscess may be localized in any perianal segment but is most frequent laterally, either right or left. Ischiorectal abscess is less frequent than perianal abscess but is usually larger, with 50 to 100 mL of pus.

Perianal and ischiorectal abscesses should be drained by an incision as close to the anus as possible so that, if a fistula develops, its tract will be as short as possible. Most surgeons remove a segment of skin to keep the incision from closing and the abscess from recurring. In order to effectively drain an abscess, a closed hemostatic clamp is introduced into the abscess and opened while still in the abscess to facilitate evaluation of the pus. The surgeon then inserts the right index finger inside the abscess to determine its extent, verify the presence of communication with other abscesses, and break any loculations. Ischiorectal abscesses are located farther away from the anal margin and are more prone to develop a fistula as a sequela.

Intersphincteric abscesses are drained by transecting the inferior portion of the internal sphincter using a technique similar to that used in treating chronic anal fissure.

To carry out drainage of supralevator abscesses, their origin must be determined before surgery, so that the surgical procedure to be performed can be selected. If the supralevator abscess has originated from an intersphincteric abscess that has spread upward, the abscess should be drained toward the rectal lumen. If the abscess arose from an ischiorectal abscess that spread upward, it should be drained through the ischiorectal fossa and not through the rectum, so as to avoid the formation of an extrasphincteric fistula. If the supralevator abscess developed as a complication of a colonic problem, from the broad ligament or from some other pelvic organ, it should be drained into the rectal lumen, through the ischiorectal fossa.

Anorectal Fistulas

Anorectal fistulas are made up of a tract communicating the skin with the inside of the anal canal. Generally, fistulas, like abscesses, are due to infection in an anal gland. The fistulous opening inside the anal canal is designated as the primary or internal orifice, while the opening in the perianal skin is known as the secondary or external orifice. Anorectal fistulas are classified according to their relation to the anal sphincters (17, 25).

1. *Intersphincteric Fistulas.* These are the most frequent fistulas, making up about 70% of anorectal fistulas. These fistulas originate in the anal canal, cross the intersphincteric plane, and exit in the perineal skin. Treatment of these fistulas is simple and results of surgery are excellent.
2. *Transphincteric Fistulas.* These fistulas make up about 25% of fistulas. After originating in the anal canal, they pass through both sphincters, through the ischiorectal fossa, to the perineal skin. Treatment of these fistulas is directly related to the extent to which they compromise the external anal sphincter. In cases with low fistulas that involve a small portion of the external sphincter, treatment consists of a fistulotomy, the same as in intersphincteric fistulas. In cases where the fistulous tract involves an important segment of the external anal sphincter, it will be necessary to place a seton around the upper portion of the external sphincter, to transect it 6 to 8 weeks later.
3. *Suprasphincteric Fistulas.* These constitute 5% of anorectal fistulas. These fistulas also originate in the pectinate line, spreading upward through the intersphincteric plane, over the puborectalis muscle, then descending through the ischiorectal fossa to the perineal skin. To treat these fistulas the internal anal sphincter should be transected and a seton placed in the external anal sphincter, to be transected in a second stage, 6 to 8 weeks later (35).
4. *Extrasphincteric Fistulas.* These fistulas represent about 1% of anorectal fistulas (35) and originate in the upper rectum, penetrating the levator ani muscle, remaining in a plane outside the sphincteric muscles,

and passing to the perineal skin through the ischiorectal fossa. These fistulas are due to pelvic infections caused by inflammatory conditions of the colon, Crohn's disease, and so on. In treating these fistulas it is necessary to treat the condition that caused them (35).

Goodsall's Rule

This rule states that if the cutaneous opening of an anorectal fistula is located anterior to an imaginary line running transversely through the middle of the anal orifice, the tract of the fistula will run radially toward the internal orifice. If the cutaneous opening of the fistula is posterior to the imaginary line, the fistula will generally run in a curvilinear course to meet the principal fistulous tract running posterior to the rectum.

Fistulotomy or Fistulectomy?

It is generally accepted that fistulotomy is the most adequate treatment for anorectal fistulas. No advantages have been shown if fistulectomy is performed. On the contrary, inconveniences have been observed due to resection of healthy tissue and injury to the external anal sphincter.

Surgical Technique

FIGURE 62.28 CORONAL SECTION OF THE ANORECTAL REGION

1, Anal margin; 2, pectinate line; 3, internal anal sphincter; 4, longitudinal fibers of the muscular layer of the rectum; 5, external anal sphincter with its 3 parts: deep, superficial, and subcutaneous; 6, anorectal ring made up of the internal fibers of the levator ani, the superior fibers of the external anal sphincter, and part of the internal sphincter.

Surgical Technique

FIGURE 62.29

Digital palpation of the anorectal ring. This ring is palpable in the posterior and lateral walls, not in the anterior wall.

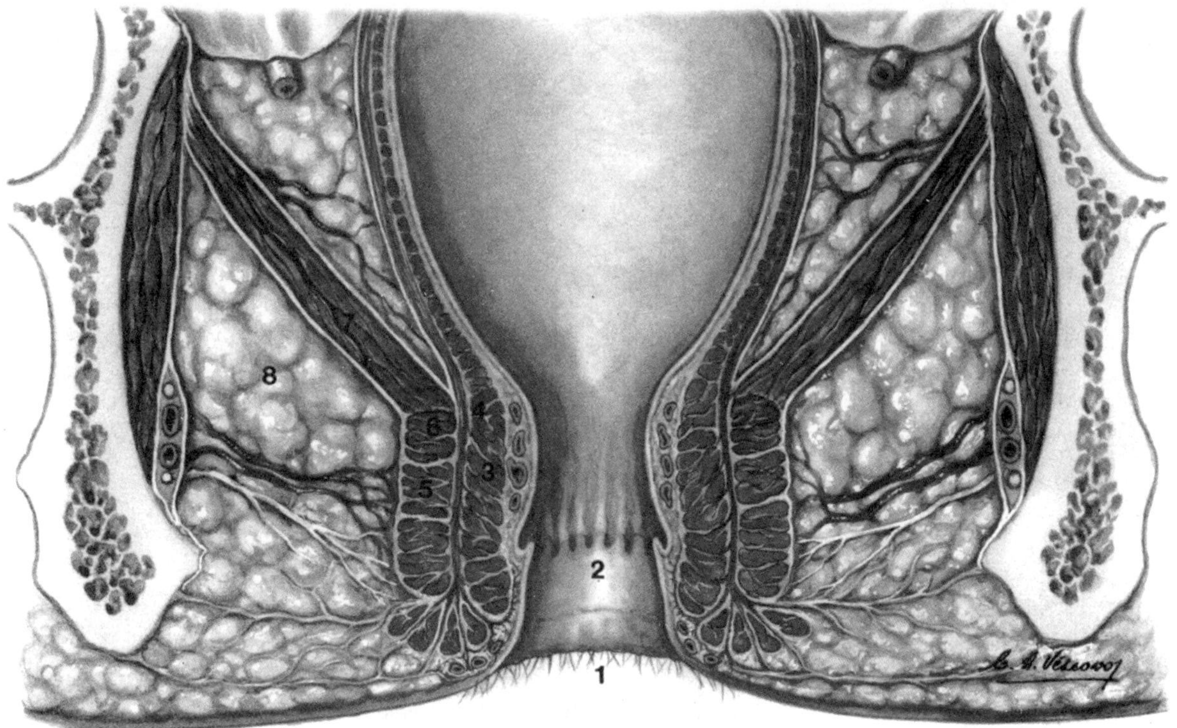

FIGURE 62.28 CORONAL SECTION OF THE ANORECTAL REGION

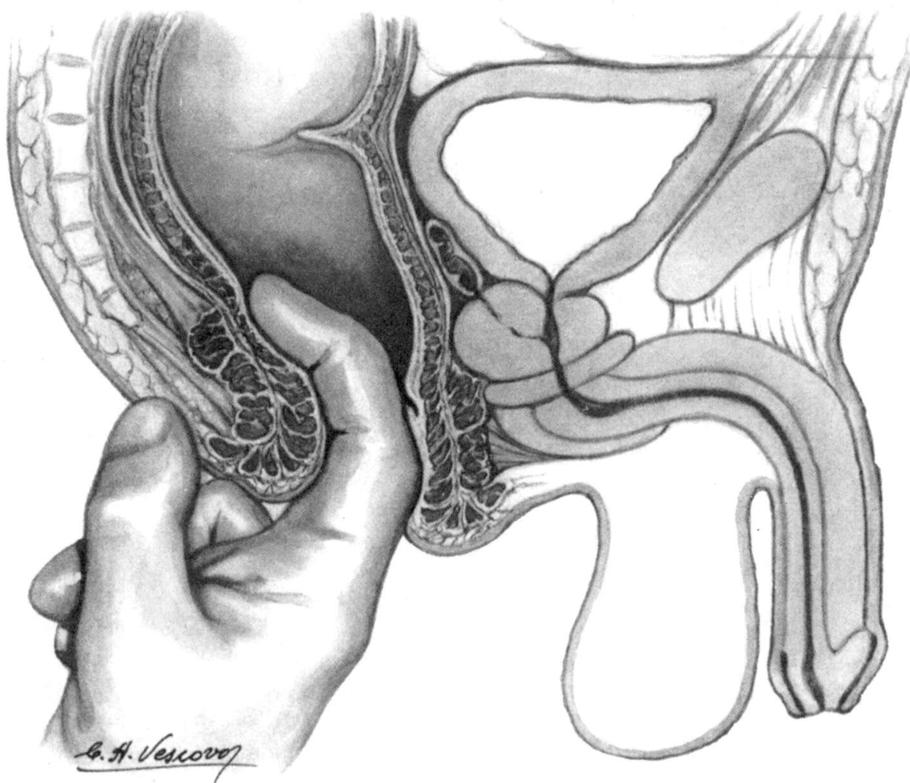

FIGURE 62.29

FIGURE 62.30
Anorectal abscesses: 1, perianal; 2, intersphincteric; 3, submucosal; 4, ischiorectal; 5, supralevator.

Surgical Technique

FIGURE 62.31
Opening of a large right ischiorectal abscess. The skin and subcutaneous tissue have been incised. A closed hemostatic clamp is introduced into the abscess and opened inside the abscess cavity to facilitate exit of the pus. The right index finger is then inserted to determine the size of the abscess and the presence of connections with other abscesses, and to break up any existing loculations.

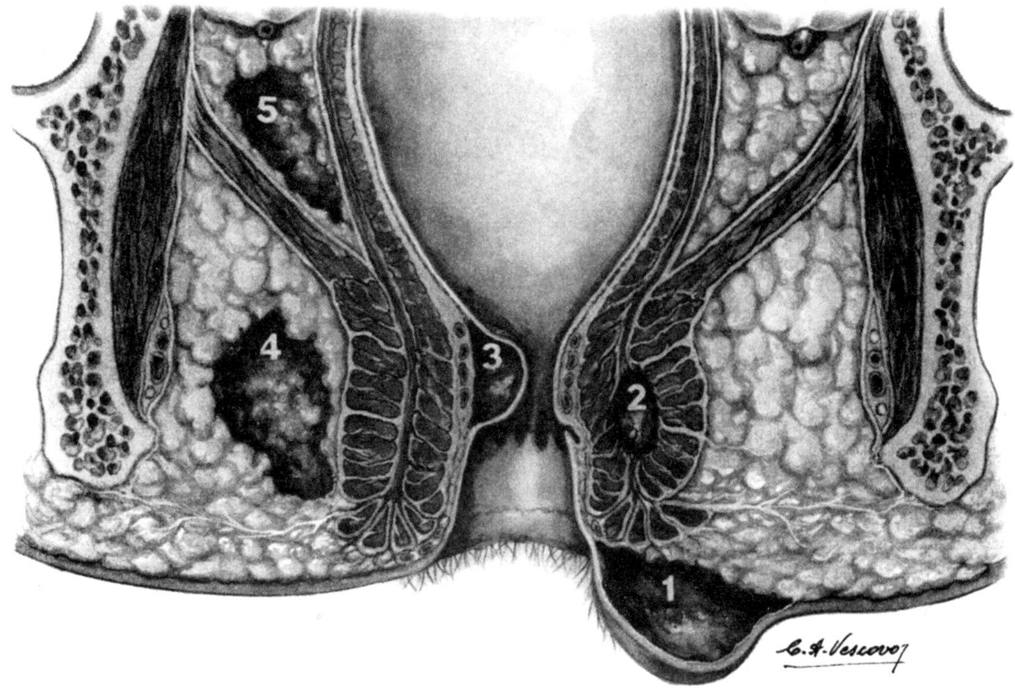

FIGURE 62.30

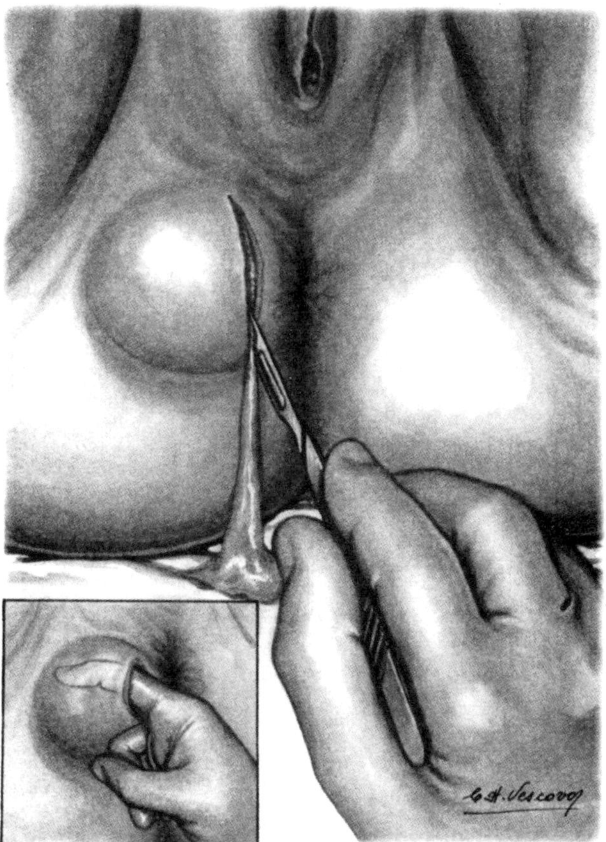

FIGURE 62.31

FIGURE 62.32
1, Intersphincteric fistula; 2, transphincteric fistula.

Surgical Technique

FIGURE 62.33
1, Suprasphincteric fistula; 2, extrasphincteric fistula in its course toward the perineal skin.

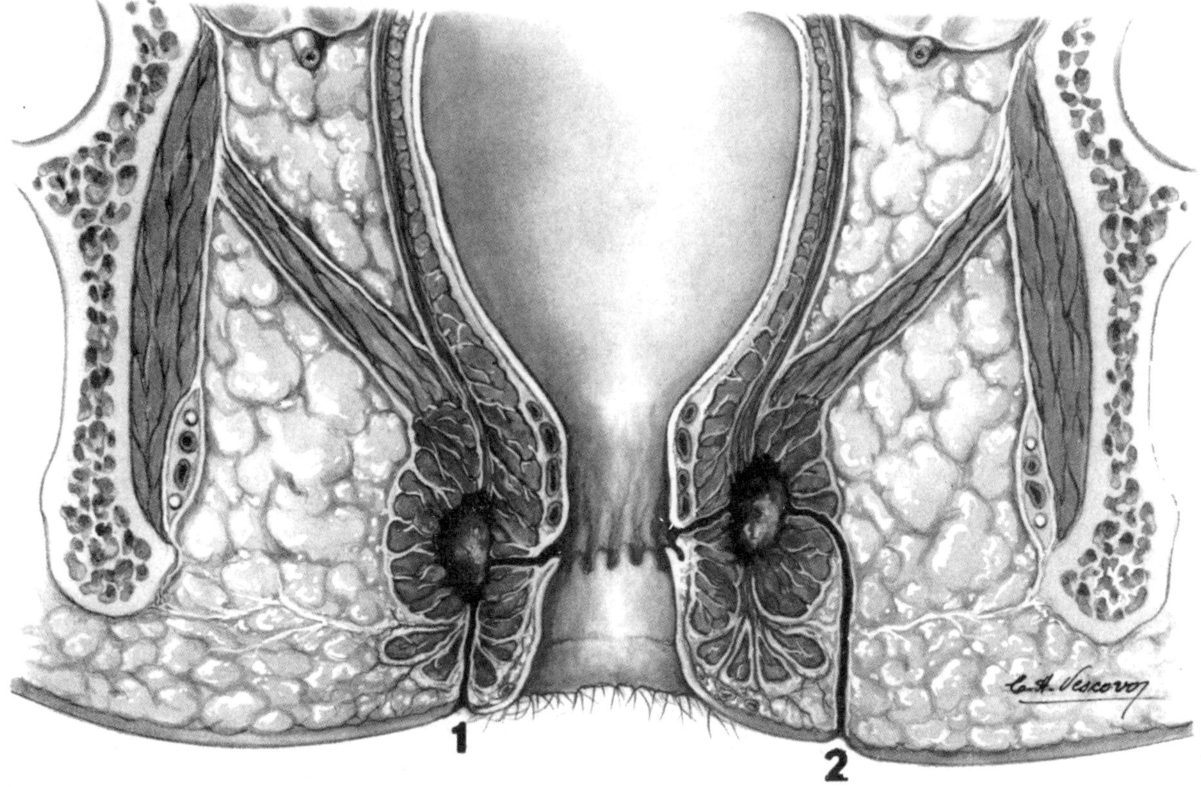

FIGURE 62.32

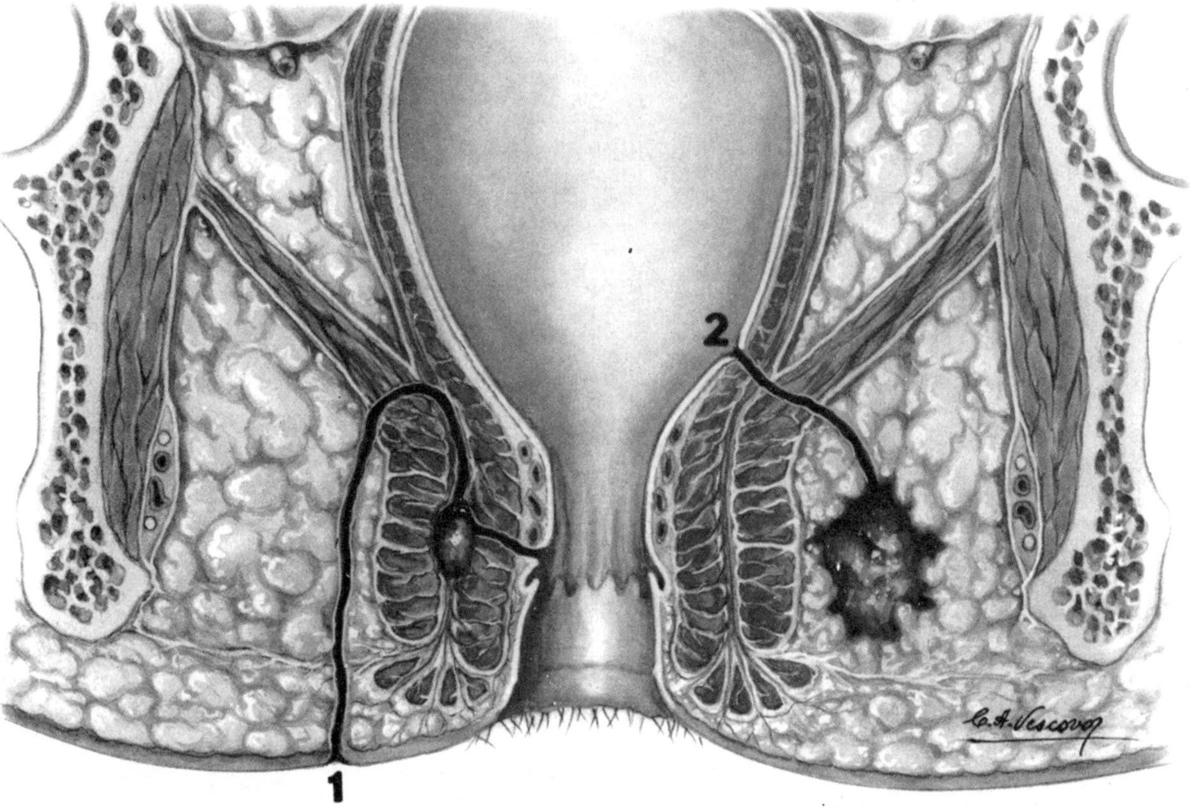

FIGURE 62.33

FIGURE 62.34
Low fistula.

Surgical Technique

FIGURE 62.35
High fistula.

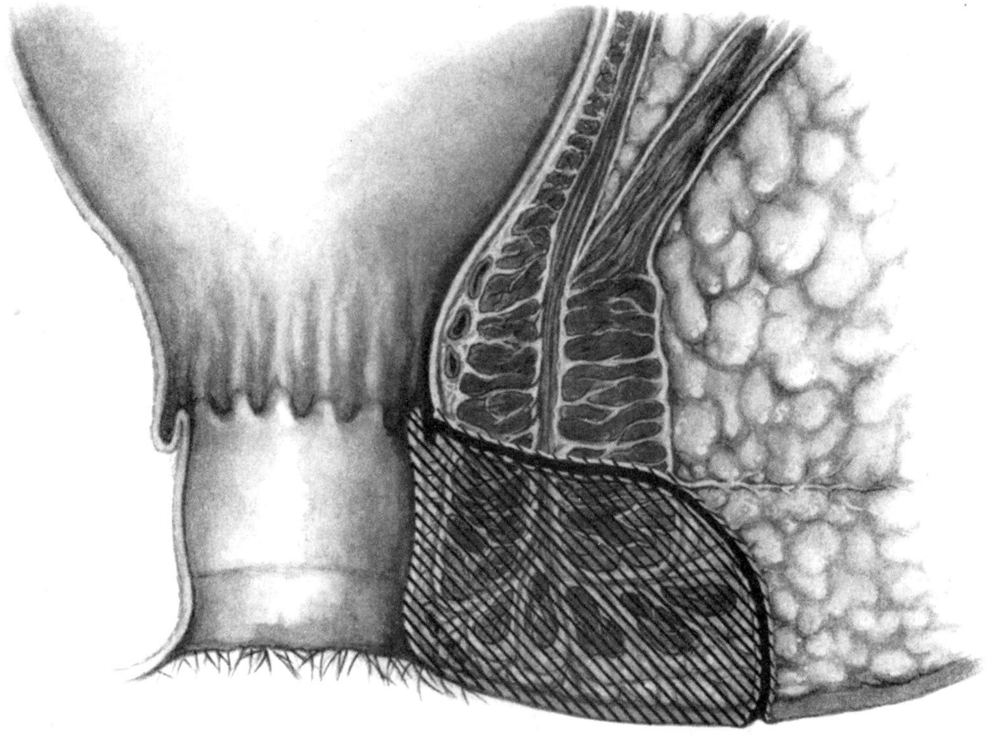

FIGURE 62.34

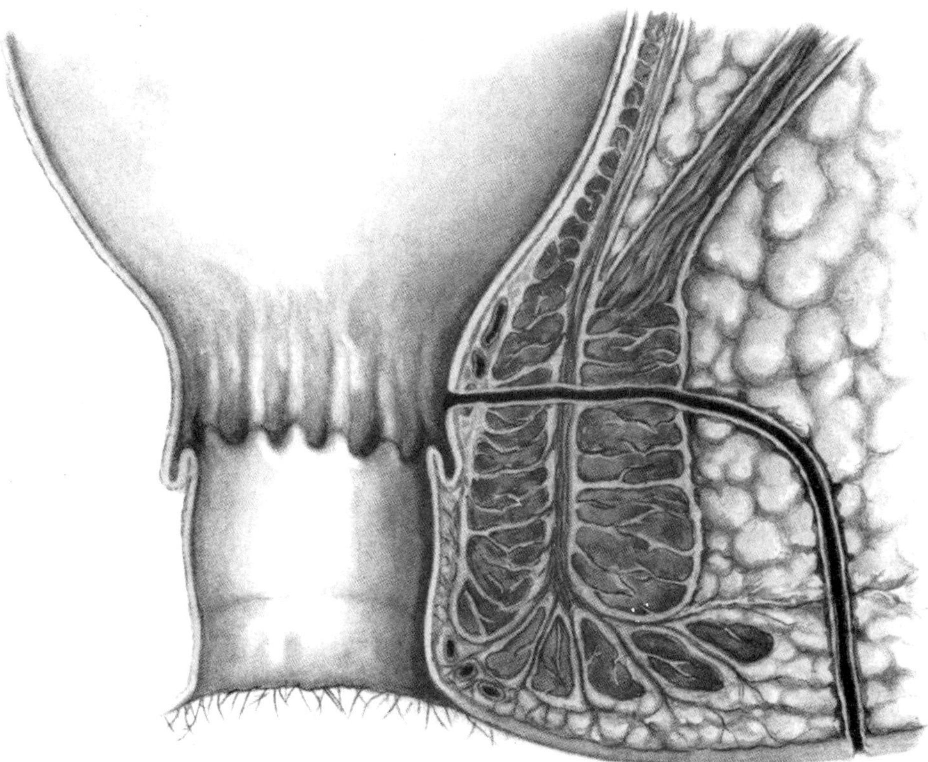

FIGURE 62.35

FIGURE 62.36
Surgery for a low fistula. The cutaneous or secondary orifice can be seen.

Surgical Technique

FIGURE 62.37
An explorer is being inserted through the external orifice.

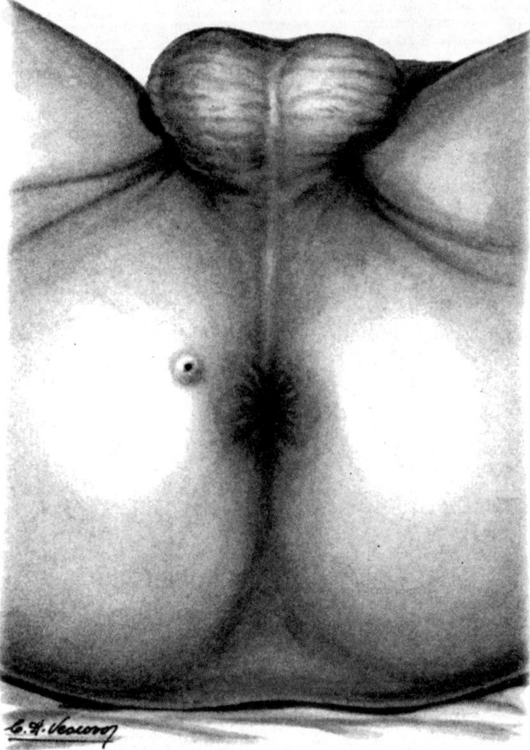

FIGURE 62.36

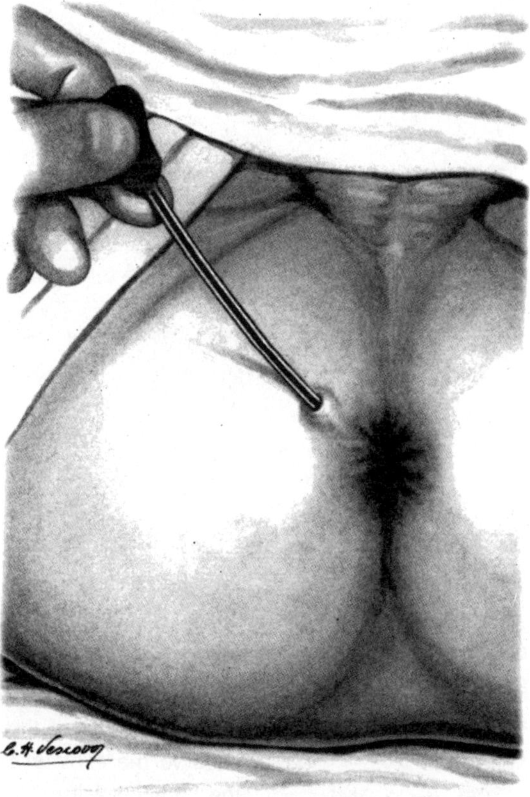

FIGURE 62.37

FIGURE 62.38
The surgeon holds the explorer with the left hand while, with the right index finger inserted in the anus, the primary orifice of the fistula is explored. If the internal orifice cannot be cannulated, attempts to identify it can be made by injecting hydrogen peroxide, milk, or saline solution, to observe if the fluid comes out of the internal orifice.

Surgical Technique

FIGURE 62.39
Coronal section of the anal region, in which it is possible to observe the explorer passing through the fistulous tract and the surgeon, with the help of the index finger in the rectum, tries to identify the internal orifice of the fistula.

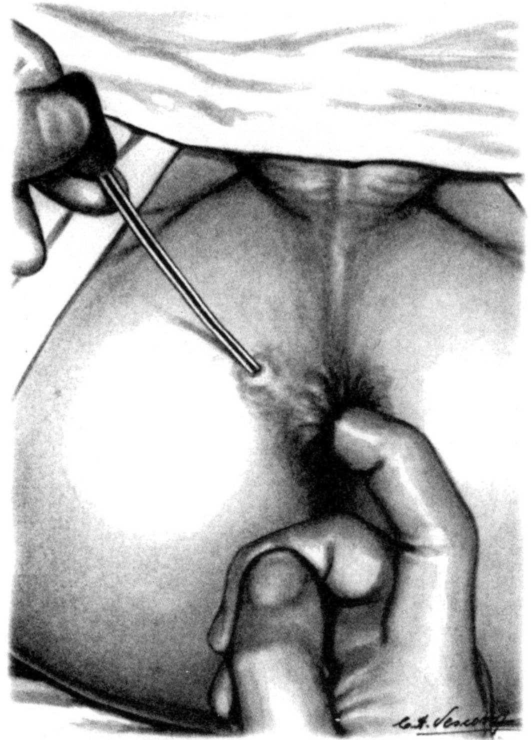

FIGURE 62.38

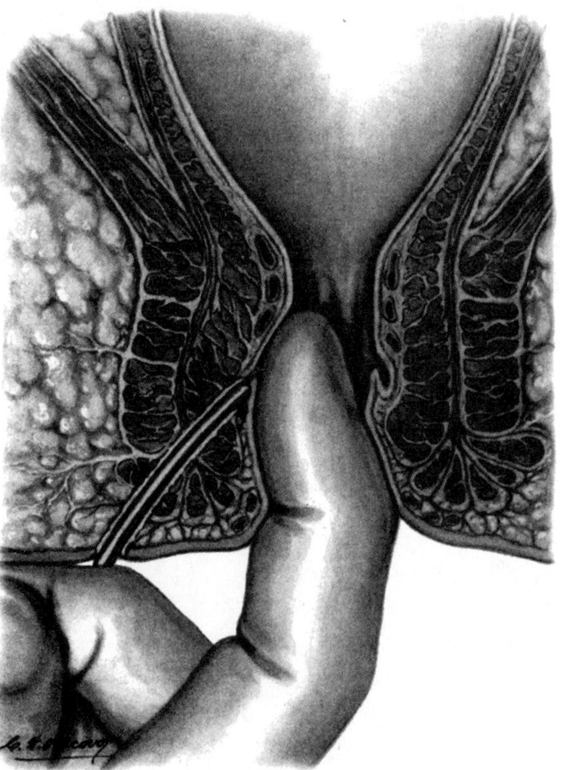

FIGURE 62.39

FIGURE 62.40
The explorer has been passed through the entire fistulous tract, as seen in the drawing, in order to carry out the fistulotomy.

Surgical Technique

FIGURE 62.41
The skin, the subcutaneous tissue, and the fistulous tract are being incised with a scalpel. Some surgeons do this with electrocautery.

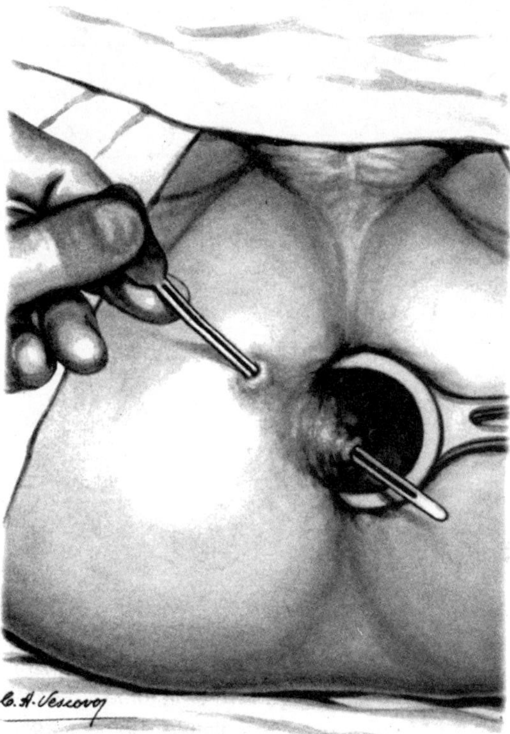

FIGURE 62.40

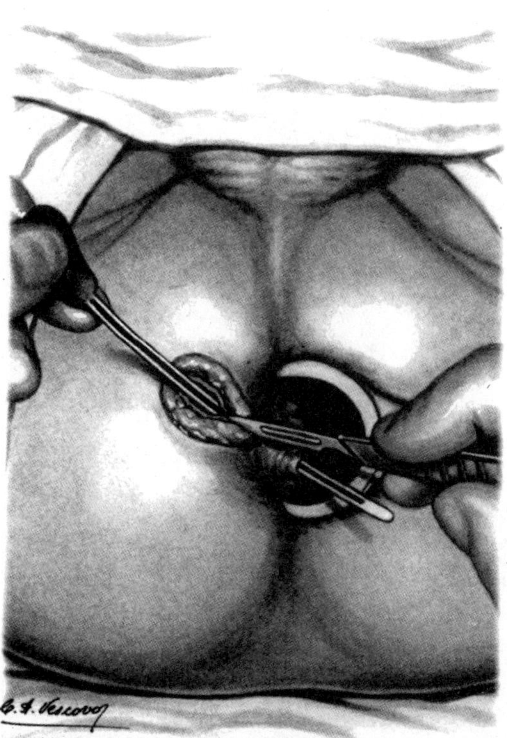

FIGURE 62.41

FIGURE 62.42
Once the fistulotomy is completed, a curette is passed over the fistulous tract to remove the granulation tissue of the fistula. Some surgeons complete the fistulotomy by suturing the wall on both sides of the fistula to the skin.

Surgical Technique

FIGURE 62.43
High anorectal fistula. An explorer has been passed through the tract of a high anal fistula.

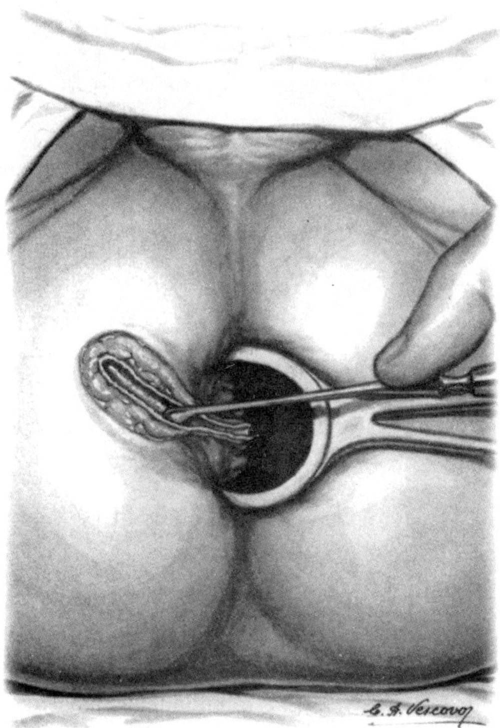

FIGURE 62.42

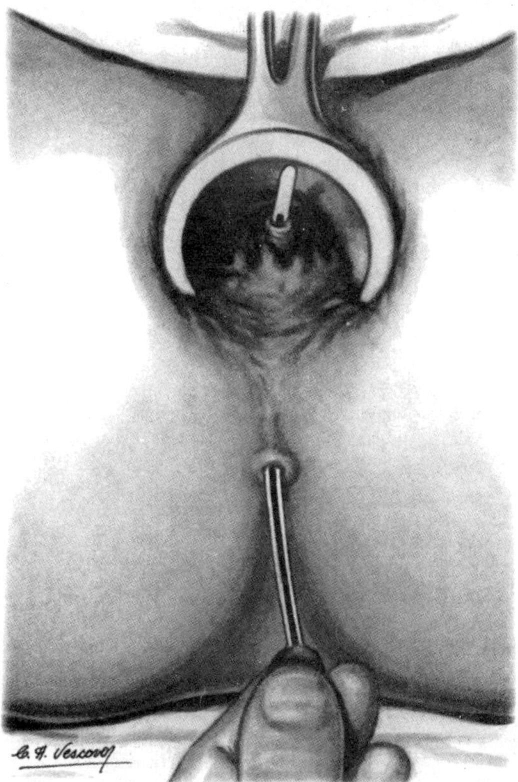

FIGURE 62.43

FIGURE 62.44
The low portion of the fistula and the inferior portion of the external anal sphincter are being incised. The upper segment of the sphincter will not be transected, and a heavy silk seton will be passed around it. Transection of this high segment of the sphincter will be done in 6 to 8 weeks.

Surgical Technique

FIGURE 62.45
A thick silk thread is being passed through the high portion of the external anal sphincter.

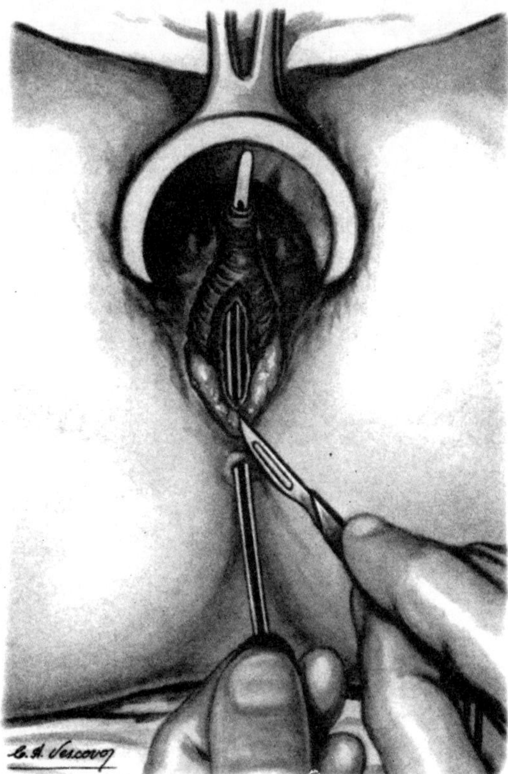

FIGURE 62.44

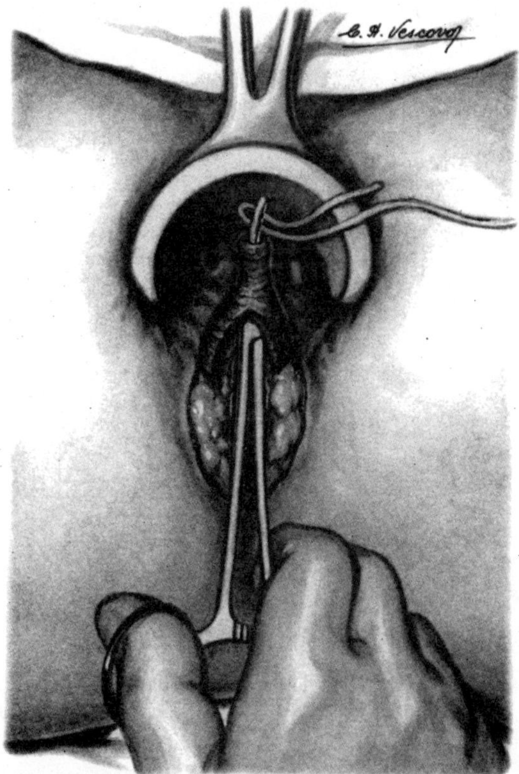

FIGURE 62.45

FIGURE 62.46
The silk suture has been loosely tied around the upper segment of the external anal sphincter. The drawing shows the fistulotomy of the low portion of the fistula.

Surgical Technique

FIGURE 62.47
Coronal section showing the ligature of the external anal sphincter with thick silk. Some surgeons use a rubber band that is periodically tightened around the upper segment of the sphincter.

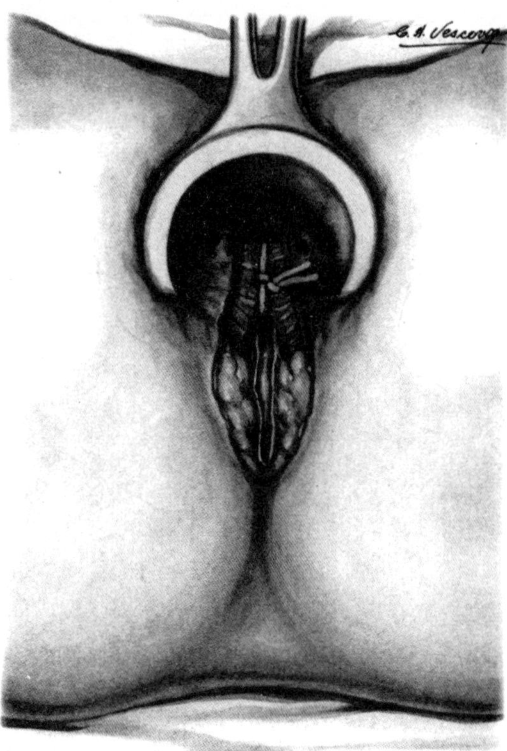

FIGURE 62.46

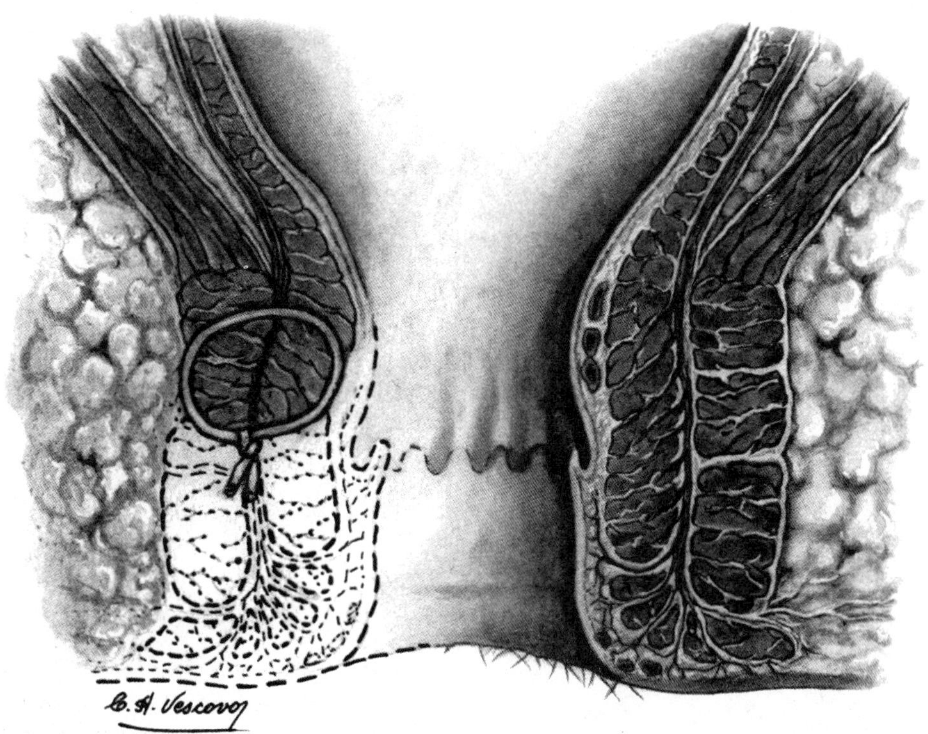

FIGURE 62.47

FIGURE 62.48
Six to eight weeks after ligating the upper segment of the external sphincter, it is transected. The previous ligation prevents the ends of the transected sphincter from retracting and separating because inflammatory tissue has developed fixing the muscle fibers.

Surgical Technique

FIGURE 62.49
The superior segment of the external sphincter has been transected. The sphincteric ends have not separated because they are fixed by local fibrosis.

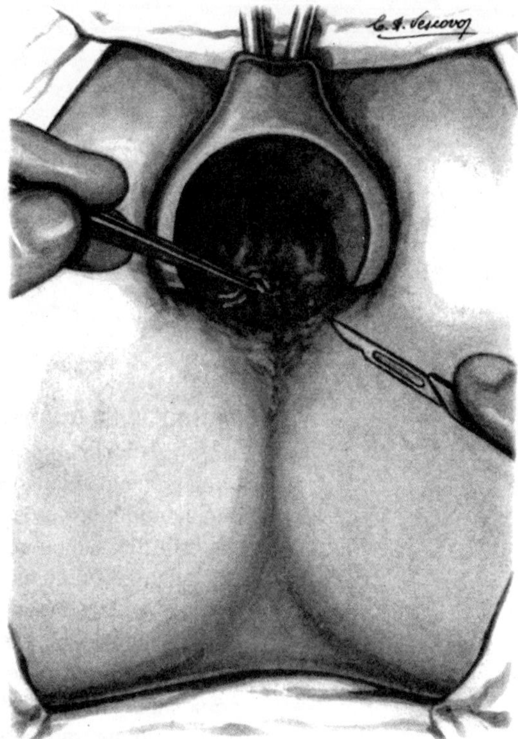

FIGURE 62.48

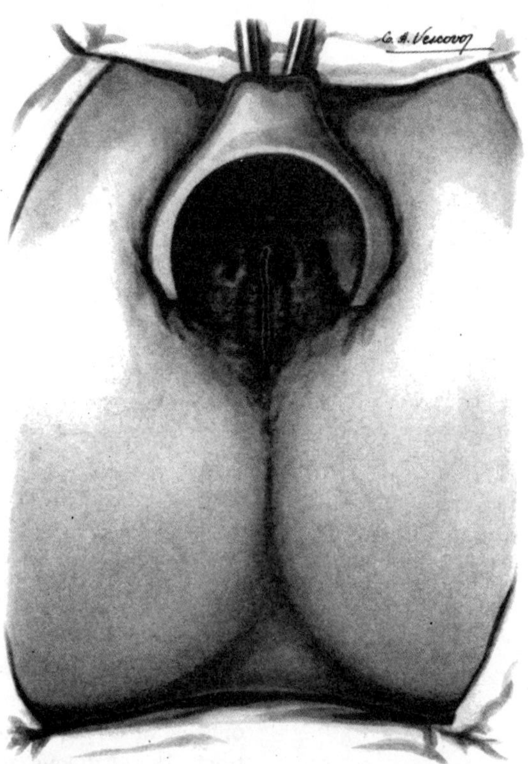

FIGURE 62.49

FIGURE 62.50 GOODSALL'S LAW
A transverse line passes through the middle of the anal orifice dividing the fistulous tracts into two groups: 1, fistulas with the cutaneous orifice posterior to the transverse line and 2, fistulas with the cutaneous orifice anterior to the transverse line. 1, Fistulas with a posterior orifice follow a curvilinear tract before communicating with the main fistulous tract, which opens into the anal canal in the posterior midline. This is why fistulas with a posterior orifice follow a horseshoe-shaped or a semi-horseshoe-shaped tract. 2, Fistulas with their cutaneous orifice anterior to the transverse line open directly into the anal canal, radially, without curves.

Surgical Technique

FIGURE 62.51 HORSESHOE FISTULA
As seen in the drawing, there are two posterior cutaneous orifices, which form a curvilinear tract joining the main fistulous tract. This fistulous tract runs straight and opens in the internal orifice in the pectinate line.

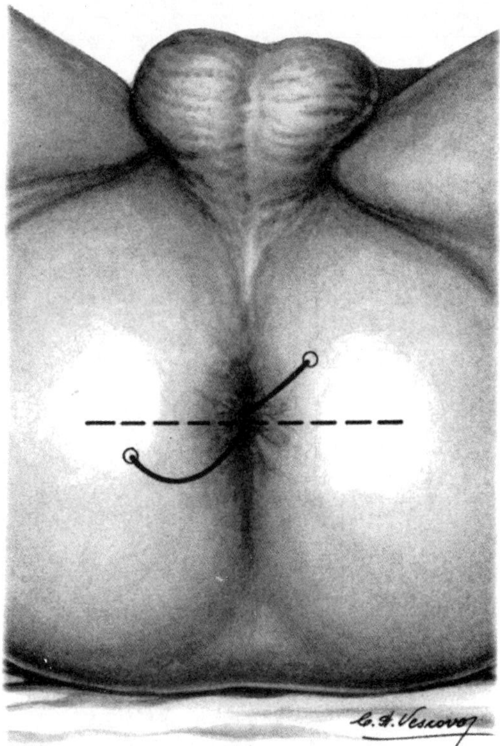

FIGURE 62.50 GOODSALL'S LAW

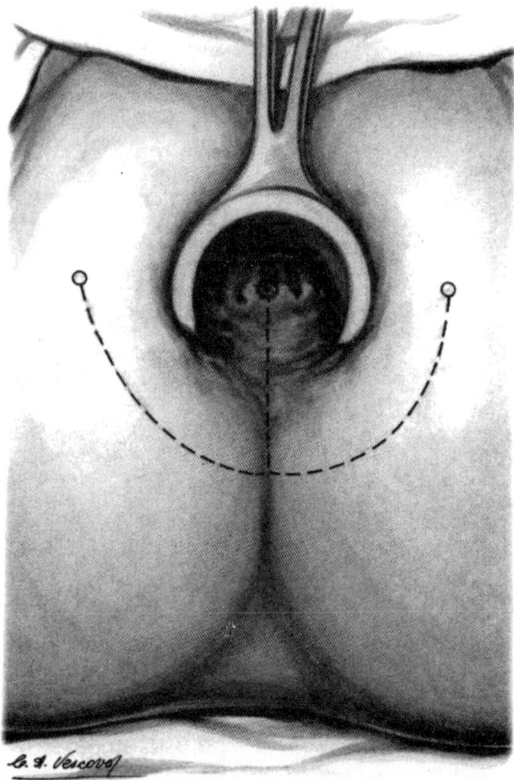

FIGURE 62.51 HORSESHOE FISTULA

FIGURE 62.52
The operation begins by performing the fistulotomy of the lateral curvilinear fistulous tracts.

Surgical Technique

FIGURE 62.53
Once the fistulotomy of the lateral fistulous tracts is completed, the principal fistulous tract is catheterized.

H

I

J

K

L

M

N

O

P

R

S

T